Textbook of Family Medicine

EIGHTH EDITION

Textbook of Family Medicine

EIGHTH EDITION

Edited by

Robert E. Rakel, MD

Professor
Department of Family and Community Medicine
Baylor College of Medicine
Houston, Texas

David P. Rakel, MD

Associate Professor
Department of Family Medicine
University of Wisconsin School of Medicine and Public Health
Madison, Wisconsin

ELSEVIER
SAUNDERS

1600 John F. Kennedy Blvd.
Ste 1800
Philadelphia, PA 19103-2899

TEXTBOOK OF FAMILY MEDICINE, EIGHTH EDITION   ISBN: 978-1-4377-1160-8

Copyright © 2011 by Saunders, an imprint of Elsevier Inc.
No part of this publication may be reproduced or transmitted in any form or by any means, electronic or mechanical, including photocopying, recording, or any information storage and retrieval system, without permission in writing from the publisher. Details on how to seek permission, further information about the Publisher's permissions policies, and our arrangements with organizations such as the Copyright Clearance Center and the Copyright Licensing Agency, can be found at our website: www.elsevier.com/permissions.

This book and the individual contributions contained in it are protected under copyright by the Publisher (other than as may be noted herein).

ISBN: 978-1-4377-1160-8

Notice
Knowledge and best practice in this field are constantly changing. As new research and experience broaden our understanding, changes in research methods, professional practices, or medical treatment may become necessary.

Practitioners and researchers must always rely on their own experience and knowledge in evaluating and using any information, methods, compounds, or experiments described herein. In using such information or methods they should be mindful of their own safety and the safety of others, including parties for whom they have a professional responsibility.

With respect to any drug or pharmaceutical products identified, readers are advised to check the most current information provided (i) on procedures featured or (ii) by the manufacturer of each product to be administered, to verify the recommended dose or formula, the method and duration of administration, and contraindications. It is the responsibility of practitioners, relying on their own experience and knowledge of their patients, to make diagnoses, to determine dosages and the best treatment for each individual patient, and to take all appropriate safety precautions. To the fullest extent of the law, neither the Publisher nor the authors, contributors, or editors, assume any liability for any injury and/or damage to persons or property as a matter of products liability, negligence or otherwise, or from any use or operation of any methods, products, instructions, or ideas contained in the material herein.

Previous editions copyrighted 2007, 2002, 1995, 1990, 1984, 1978, 1973 by Saunders.

Senior Acquisitions Editor: Kate Dimock
Senior Developmental Editor: Agnes Byrnes
Publishing Services Manager: Patricia Tannian
Senior Project Manager: John Casey
Designer: Lou Forgione

your source for books, journals and multimedia in the health sciences

www.elsevierhealth.com

Working together to grow
libraries in developing countries

www.elsevier.com | www.bookaid.org | www.sabre.org

ELSEVIER   BOOK AID International   Sabre Foundation

The Publisher's policy is to use paper manufactured from sustainable forests

Printed in China

Last digit is the print number: 9 8 7 6 5 4 3 2 1

Contributors

Syed M. Ahmed, MD
Professor, Department of Family and Community Medicine
Medical College of Wisconsin
Milwaukee, Wisconsin
Psychosocial Influences on Health

Irene Alexandraki, MD, MPH
Assistant Professor, Department of Medicine
University of Florida College of Medicine
Jacksonville, Florida
Endocrinology

Louis F. Amorosa, MD
Professor, Department of Medicine
University of Medicine and Dentistry of New Jersey
Robert Wood Johnson Medical School
New Brunswick, New Jersey
Diabetes Mellitus

Gregory J. Anderson, MD
Assistant Professor, Department of Family Medicine
Mayo Clinic College of Medicine
Rochester, Minnesota
Obesity

Roberto A. Andrade, MD
Assistant Professor, Department of Medicine–Infectious
   Diseases
Baylor College of Medicine
Houston, Texas
Care of the Adult HIV-Infected Patient

Bruce Bagley, MD
Medical Director for Quality Improvement
American Academy of Family Physicians
Leawood, Kansas
*Using Health Information Technology for Optimal
   Patient Care and Service*

Bruce Barrett, MD, PhD
Associate Professor, Department of Family Medicine
University of Wisconsin
Madison, Wisconsin
Herbs and Other Dietary Supplements

Richard Basilan, MD
Infectious Diseases Fellow
Department of Internal Medicine
University of Missouri
Columbia, Missouri
Infectious Diseases

J. Mark Beard, MD
Associate Professor, Department of Family Medicine
University of Washington
Seattle, Washington
Common Office Procedures

Wendy S. Biggs, MD
Associate Professor, Department of Family Medicine
Michigan State University
College of Human Medicine
Lansing, Michigan;
Associate Director
Midland Family Medicine Residency at MidMichigan
   Medical Center
Midland, Michigan
Medical Human Sexuality

Harold Bland, MD
Interim Chair, Department of Clinical Sciences
Professor and Education Director for Pediatrics
Florida State University College of Medicine
Tallahassee, Florida
Care of the Newborn

John F. Bober, MD
Associate Professor of Psychiatry
NEOUCOM, Akron Children's Hospital
Akron, Ohio
Behavioral Problems in Children and Adolescents

David A. Brechtelsbauer, MD, CMD
Associate Professor, Department of Family Medicine
Sanford School of Medicine of The University of South Dakota
Director of Geriatrics Training
Sioux Falls Family Medicine Residency
Sioux Falls, South Dakota
Delirium and Dementia

Jason N. Buchanan, MD
Assistant Professor, Department of Family
   and Community Medicine
Baylor College of Medicine
Houston, Texas
Gastroenterology

Jennifer J. Buescher, MD, MSPH
Associate Director
Clarkson Family Medicine Residency Program
Omaha, Nebraska
Care of the Newborn

Kara Cadwallader, MD
Clinical Associate Professor
Family Medicine Residency of Idaho
University of Washington
Department of Family Medicine
Seattle, Washington;
Medical Director, Planned Parenthood of the Great
  Northwest–Idaho
Boise, Idaho
Gynecology

William E. Carroll, MD
Adjunct Assistant Professor, Department of Neurology
The Ohio State University Medical Center
Medical Director, Neurology
Grant Medical Center
Columbus, Ohio
Neurology

Charles Carter, MD
Associate Professor, Department of Family Medicine
University of South Carolina School of Medicine
Residency Director
Palmetto Health Family Medicine Residency Program
Columbia, South Carolina
Urinary Tract Disorders

Douglas Comeau, DO
Assistant Professor, Department of Family Medicine
Faculty for the Primary Care Sports Medicine Fellowship
Boston University School of Medicine
Team Physician, Boston College
Boston, Massachusetts
Rheumatology and Musculoskeletal Problems

Renee Crichlow, MD
Assistant Professor
North Memorial Family Medicine Residency Program
University of Minnesota School of Medicine
Minneapolis, Minnesota
Preventive Health Care

Earl R. Crouch, Jr, MD
Chairman, Department of Ophthalmology
Eastern Virginia Medical School
Norfolk, Virginia
Ophthalmology

Eric R. Crouch, MD
Assistant Professor, Departments of Ophthalmology
  and Pediatrics
Eastern Virginia Medical School
Norfolk, Virginia
Ophthalmology

Alan K. David, MD
Professor and Chairman, Department of Family
  and Community Medicine
Associate Dean, Faculty Affairs
Medical College of Wisconsin
Milwaukee, Wisconsin
Hematology

Frank Verloin DeGruy III, MD, MSFM
Woodward-Chisholm Chair
Department of Family Medicine
University of Colorado School of Medicine
Aurora, Colorado
*Difficult Clinical Encounters: Patients with Personality Disorders
  and Somatoform Complaints*

Eric J. Dippel, MD
Midwest Cardiovascular Research Foundation
Davenport, Iowa
Cardiovascular Disease

Jonathan A. Drezner, MD
Associate Professor, Department of Family Medicine
University of Washington
Seattle, Washington
Sports Medicine

Denise M. Dupras, MD
Assistant Professor of Internal Medicine
Department of Internal Medicine
Mayo Clinic
Rochester, Minnesota
Clinical Problem Solving

Bernard Ewigman, MD, MSPH
Professor and Chair, Department of Family Medicine
University of Chicago
Chicago, Illinois
*Interpreting the Medical Literature: Applying Evidence-Based
  Medicine in Practice*

W. Gregory Feero, MD, PhD
Faculty, Maine-Dartmouth Family Medicine Residency
Augusta, Maine;
Special Advisor to the Director
National Human Genome Research Institute
National Institutes of Health
Bethesda, Maryland
Clinical Genetics (Genomics)

Robert E. Feinstein, MD
Professor, Department of Psychiatry
Senior Associate Dean of Education
University of Colorado, School of Medicine
Aurora, Colorado
Crisis Intervention, Trauma, and Intimate Partner Violence
*Difficult Clinical Encounters: Patients with Personality Disorders
  and Somatoform Complaints*

Blair Foreman, MD
Cardiovascular Medicine
Genesis Heart Institute
Davenport, Iowa
Cardiovascular Disease

Gregory M. Garrison, MD
Assistant Professor of Family Medicine
Department of Family Medicine
Mayo Clinic
Rochester, Minnesota
Clinical Problem Solving

Curtis Gingrich, MD
Clinical Assistant Professor, Department of Family Medicine
The Ohio State University College of Medicine
Executive Director of Medical Education
Grant Medical Center
Columbus, Ohio
Neurology

Andrea Gordon, MD
Assistant Professor, Department of Public Health
    and Family Medicine
Tufts University School of Medicine
Boston, Massachusetts;
Faculty Physician
Tufts University Family Medicine Residency Program
Malden, Massachusetts
Rheumatology and Musculoskeletal Problems

Thomas R. Grant, Jr., MD
Faculty, Department of Family and Community Medicine
Eastern Virginia Medical School
Norfolk, Virginia
Ophthalmology

Mary P. Guerrera, MD
Associate Professor and Director of Integrative Medicine
Department of Family Medicine
University of Connecticut School of Medicine
Farmington, Connecticut
*Complementary and Alternative Medicine: Integration
    into Primary Care*

Janelle Guirguis-Blake, MD
Clinical Associate Professor, Department of Family Medicine
University of Washington
...tle, Washington;
...Department of Family Medicine
...ly Medicine Residency Program
...ington
...lth Care

...rly G. Harmon, MD
...inical Professor
Departments of Family Medicine and Orthopaedics and Sports
    Medicine
University of Washington
Seattle, Washington
Sports Medicine

Kevin Heaton, DO
Resident, Department of Family Medicine
Boston Medical Center
Boston, Massachusetts
Rheumatology and Musculoskeletal Problems

Joel J. Heidelbaugh, MD
Clinical Associate Professor and Clerkship Director
Department of Family Medicine
University of Michigan
Ann Arbor, Michigan
Gastroenterology

Donald D. Hensrud, MD, MPH
Chair, Division of Preventive, Occupational, and Aerospace
    Medicine
Mayo Clinic
Associate Professor, Department of Preventive Medicine
    and Nutrition
College of Medicine
Rochester, Minnesota
Obesity

Vivian Hernandez-Trujillo, MD
Director, Division of Allergy and Immunology
Miami Children's Hospital
Miami, Florida
Allergy

Arthur H. Herold, MD
Associate Professor, Department of Family Medicine
College of Medicine
University of South Florida
Tampa, Florida
Interpreting Laboratory Tests

Paul J. Hershberger, PhD
Professor, Clinical Health Psychologist
Department of Family Medicine
Boonshoft School of Medicine
Wright State University
Dayton, Ohio
Psychosocial Influences on Health

Robert Holleman, MD
Assistant Professor of Pediatrics
University of South Carolina School of Medicine
Director, Division of Pediatric Nephrology
Residency Director, Palmetto Health Pediatric Residency
    Program
Columbia, South Carolina
Urinary Tract Disorders

Keith B. Holten, MD
Chief Medical Officer
Berger Health System
Circleville, Ohio
*Interpreting the Medical Literature: Applying Evidence-Based
    Medicine in Practice*

Jodi Summers Holtrop, PhD
Assistant Professor, Department of Family Medicine
College of Human Medicine
Michigan State University
East Lansing, Michigan
Nutrition and Family Medicine

Robert Holleman, MD
Assistant Professor, Department of Pediatrics
University of South Carolina School of Medicine
Director, Division of Pediatric Nephrology
Residency Director
Palmetto Health Pediatric Residency Program
Columbia, South Carolina
Urinary Tract Disorders

Keith B. Holten, MD
Director, University of Cincinnati–Affiliated Residency Program
Clinton Memorial Hospital
Wilmington, Ohio
Interpreting the Medical Literature: Applying Evidence-Based Medicine in Practice

Thomas Houston, MD
Clinical Professor, Department of Family Medicine and Public Health
The Ohio State University
Staff Physician, McConnell Heart Health Center
Columbus, Ohio
Nicotine Addiction

Mark R. Hutchinson, PhD
Professor and Director of Sports Medicine Services
Department of Orthopaedics
College of Medicine, University of Illinois at Chicago
Chicago, Illinois
Common Issues in Orthopedics

Wayne Jonas, MD
Professor, Department of Family Medicine
Georgetown University
Washington, DC;
Associate Professor, Department of Family Medicine
Uniformed Services
University of the Health Sciences
Bethesda, Maryland
The Primary Medical Home

Robert B. Kelly, MD, MS
Associate Professor, Department of Family Medicine
School of Medicine, Case Western Reserve University
Faculty, Family Medicine Residency Program
Fairview Hospital/Cleveland Clinic
Cleveland, Ohio
Patient Education

Sanford R. Kimmel, MD
Professor and Vice-Chair, Department of Family Medicine
University of Toledo College of Medicine
Toledo, Ohio
Growth and Development

Hoonmo Koo, MD, MPH
Assistant Professor, Department of Medicine–Infectious Diseases
Baylor College of Medicine
Houston, Texas
Infectious Diseases

Colin P. Kopes-Kerr, MD, JD, MPH
Director of Residency Education, Family Medicine Residency Program
Santa Rosa Family Medicine Residency Consortium
Physician, Department of Family Medicine
Kaiser Permanente Medical Center
Santa Rosa, California
Lifestyle Interventions and Behavior Change

Alicia Kowalhuk, DO
Assistant Professor, Department of Family and Community Medicine
Baylor College of Medicine
Medical Director, Insight Program
Harris County Hospital District
Medical Director, CARE Clinic
Santa Maria Hostel
Houston, Texas
Drug Abuse

Jennifer Krejci-Manwaring, MD
Assistant Professor, Division of Dermatology and Cutaneous Surgery
School of Medicine
University of Texas Health Science Center
San Antonio, Texas
Dermatology

Esther J. Lee, MD
Fellow in Endocrinology and Diabetes
University of Medicine and Dentistry of New Jersey
Robert Wood Johnson Medical School
New Brunswick, New Jersey
Diabetes Mellitus

Jeanne P. Lemkau, MD
Professor Emerita
Department of Family Medicine and Community Health
Boonshoft School of Medicine
Wright State University
Dayton, Ohio
Psychosocial Influences on Health

Phil Lieberman, MD
Clinical Professor, Departments of Medicine and Pediatrics
Division of Allergy and Immunology
University of Tennessee College of Medicine
Memphis, Tennessee
Allergy

Adriana C. Linares, MD, MPH, DrPH
Assistant Professor, Department of Family Medicine
Baylor College of Medicine
Houston, Texas
Contraception

David R. McBride, MD
Assistant Professor, Department of Family Medicine
Boston University School of Medicine
Director, Student Health Services
Boston University
Boston, Massachusetts
Infectious Diseases

David McCrary, MD
Infectious Disease Fellow, Department of Infectious Diseases
University of Missouri Health System
Columbia, Missouri
Infectious Diseases

Stephen P. Merry, MD
Assistant Professor of Family Medicine
Department of Family Medicine
Mayo Clinic
Rochester, Minnesota
Clinical Problem Solving

David Meyers, MD
Director, Center for Primary Care, Prevention,
    and Clinical Partnerships
Agency for Healthcare Research and Quality
Rockville, Maryland
Preventive Health Care

Gregg Mitchell, MD
Associate Professor, Department of Family Medicine
University of Tennessee
Jackson, Tennessee
Allergy

James L. Moeller, MD
Sports Medicine Associates, PLC
Auburn Hills, Michigan
Common Issues in Orthopedics

Arshag Mooradian, MD
Professor and Chair, Department of Medicine
University of Florida College of Medicine
Jacksonville, Florida
Endocrinology

Scott E. Moser, MD
Professor, Department of Family and Community Medicine
University of Kansas School of Medicine
Wichita, Kansas
Behavioral Problems in Children and Adolescents

Mary Barth Noel, MPH, PhD, RD
Professor and Senior Associate Chair
Department of Family Medicine, College of Human Medicine
Michigan State University
East Lansing, Michigan
Nutrition and Family Medicine

John G. O'Handley, MD
Clinical Associate Professor, Department of Family Medicine
The Ohio State University College of Medicine
Columbus, Ohio
Otolaryngology

John W. O'Kane, MD
Associate Professor, Department of Orthopaedics
    and Sports Medicine
University of Washington
Seattle, Washington
Sports Medicine

Justin Osborn, MD
Clinical Assistant Professor
Department of Family Medicine
University of Washington
Seattle, Washington
Common Office Procedures

Heather L. Paladine, MD
Assistant Clinical Professor of Medicine
Center for Family and Community Medicine
Columbia University Medical Center
New York, New York
Gynecology

Minal Patel, MD
Assistant Professor, Department of Family
    and Community Medicine
Baylor College of Medicine
Houston, Texas
Back: Cervical and Thoracolumbar Spine

Gabriella Pridjian, MD
Professor and Chair, Department of Obstetrics and Gynecology
Tulane University School of Medicine
New Orleans, Louisiana
Obstetrics

David P. Rakel, MD
Associate Professor, Department of Family Medicine
University of Wisconsin School of Medicine and Public Health
Madison, Wisconsin
The Primary Medical Home

Robert E. Rakel, MD
Professor, Department of Family and Community Medicine
Baylor College of Medicine
Houston, Texas
The Family Physician
Care of the Dying Patient
Establishing Rapport
Nicotine Addiction

Terry G. Rascoe, MD
Vice Chair, Department of Family and Community Medicine
Texas A&M University College of Medicine
Scott & White Memorial Hospital System
College Station, Texas
Interviewing Techniques

Karen Ratliff-Schaub, MD
Associate Professor, Department of Pediatrics
The Ohio State University College of Medicine
Medical Director, The Nisonger Center for Developmental
    Disabilities
The Ohio State University
Columbus, Ohio
Growth and Development

Brian C. Reed, MD
Assistant Professor and Vice Chair
Department of Family and Community Medicine
Baylor College of Medicine
Houston, Texas
Drug Abuse

Michael D. Reis, MD
Interim Chair, Department of Family
    and Community Medicine
Texas A&M University College of Medicine
Vice Chair, Department of Family Medicine
Scott & White Memorial Hospital System
College Station, Texas
Interviewing Techniques

J. Adam Rindfleisch, MD, MPhil
Assistant Professor, Department of Family Medicine
University of Wisconsin School of Medicine and Public Health
Madison, Wisconsin
Herbs and Other Dietary Supplements

R. Hal Ritter, Jr., PhD
Associate Professor, Department of Family
    and Community Medicine
Texas A&M University College of Medicine
Family Medicine Residency Behavioral Science Educator
Department of Family and Community Medicine
Scott & White Memorial Hospital System
College Station, Texas
Interviewing Techniques

William E. Roland, MD
Associate Professor of Clinical Medicine
Department of Internal Medicine
Division of Infectious Diseases
University of Missouri–Columbia School of Medicine
Associate Chief of Staff for Education
Harry S Truman Memorial Veterans Hospital
Columbia, Missouri
Infectious Diseases

Brian Rothberg, MD
Assistant Professor, Department of Psychiatry
University of Colorado Denver School of Medicine
Aurora, Colorado
Anxiety and Depression

George Rust, MD, MPH
Professor, Department of Family Medicine
Director, National Center for Primary Care
Morehouse School of Medicine
Atlanta, Georgia
Pulmonary Medicine

Zishan Samiuddin, MD
Assistant Professor, Department of Family
    and Community Medicine
Department of Psychiatry and Behavioral Sciences
Baylor College of Medicine
Houston, Texas
Care of the Adult HIV-Infected Patient

Gorge Samraj, MD
Associate Professor and Director
Family Medicine Obstetrics and Women's Health Program
University of Florida College of Medicine
Jacksonville, Florida
Endocrinology

Christopher D. Schneck, MD
Associate Professor, Department of Psychiatry
University of Colorado School of Medicine
Aurora, Colorado
Anxiety and Depression

Sarina B. Schrager, MD, MS
Associate Professor, Department of Family Medicine
University of Wisconsin
Madison, Wisconsin
Gynecology

Ann I. Schutt-Ainé, MD
Assistant Professor, Department of Obstetrics and Gynecology
Baylor College of Medicine
Houston, Texas
Contraception

Stacy Seikel, MD
Medical Director
The Center For Drug-Free Living
Clinical Assistant Professor
Department of Psychiatry and Addiction Medicine
University of Florida
Clinical Assistant Professor
Florida State University College of Medicine
Orlando, Florida
Alcohol Use Disorders

Ashish R. Shah, MD
Otolaryngology ENT
Ohio ENT
Columbus, Ohio
Otolaryngology

Krupa Shah, MD, MPH
Instructor in Medicine
Division of Geriatrics and Aging
University of Rochester School of Medicine
Rochester, New York
Back: Cervical and Thoracolumbar Spine

Nicolas W. Shammas, MS, MD
Adjunct Clinical Professor, Department of Internal Medicine
University of Iowa School of Medicine
Iowa City, Iowa;
Midwest Cardiovascular Research Foundation
Davenport, Iowa
Cardiovascular Disease

Kevin M. Sherin, MD, MPH, MBA
Director, Orange County Health Department
Clinical Professor of Family Medicine
Department of Family Medicine and Rural Health
Florida State University College of Medicine
Associate Professor, Department of Family Medicine
    and Department of Education
University of Florida
Orlando, Florida
Alcohol Use Disorders

Jeffrey A. Silverstein, MD
Orthopaedic Resident Physician
University of Illinois at Chicago
Chicago, Illinois
Common Issues in Orthopedics

Alan J. Smith, PhD, MEd
Assistant Dean and Director
Graduate Medical Education
Associate Professor of Family Medicine
University of Utah Health Sciences Center
Salt Lake City, Utah
Clinical Problem Solving

David A. Smith, MD
Professor, College of Family and Community Medicine
Texas A&M University College of Medicine
College Station, Texas
Delirium and Dementia

Douglas R. Smucker, MD
Associate Professor, Department of Family Medicine
University of Cincinnati College of Medicine
Cincinnati, Ohio
Interpreting the Medical Literature: Applying Evidence-Based Medicine in Practice

Abby Snavely, MD
Chief Resident, Department of Psychiatry
University of Colorado School of Medicine
Aurora, Colorado
Crisis Intervention, Trauma, and Intimate Partner Violence

James Stallworth, MD
Associate Professor, Department of Pediatrics
Director, Division of General Pediatrics
University of South Carolina School of Medicine
Columbia, South Carolina
Urinary Tract Disorders

Nancy G. Stevens, MD, MPH
Professor, Department of Family Medicine
Director, Family Medicine Residency Network
University of Washington
Seattle, Washington
Clinical Genetics (Genomics)

Melissa Stiles, MD
Professor, Department of Family Medicine
University of Wisconsin
Madison, Wisconsin
Care of the Elderly Patient

Elizabeth M. Strauch, MD
Vice President for Medical Affairs
Houston Hospice
Houston, Texas
Care of the Dying Patient

Jeff Susman, MD
Dean and Professor of Family Medicine
Northeast Ohio Universities College of Medicine
Rootstown, Ohio
Interpreting the Medical Literature: Applying Evidence-Based Medicine in Practice

David Swee, MD
Professor and Chair
Department of Family Medicine
University of Medicine and Dentistry of New Jersey
Robert Wood Johnson Medical School
New Brunswick, New Jersey
Diabetes Mellitus

Margaret Thompson, MD
Associate Professor, Department of Family Medicine
College of Human Medicine
Michigan State University
Grand Rapids, Michigan
Nutrition and Family Medicine

Evan J. Tobin, MD
Clinical Assistant Professor
Department of Otolaryngology–Head and Neck Surgery
The Ohio State University
Columbus, Ohio
Otolaryngology

Peter P. Toth, MD, PhD
Clinical Professor
Department of Family and Community Medicine
University of Illinois School of Medicine
Peoria, Illinois;
Director of Preventive Cardiology
Sterling Rock Falls Clinic
Sterling, Illinois
Cardiovascular Disease

Richard P. Usatine, MD
Professor, Department of Family and Community Medicine and Dermatology
School of Medicine, University of Texas Health Science Center
San Antonio, Texas
Dermatology

William C. Wadland, MD, MS
Professor and Chair, Department of Family Medicine
College of Human Medicine
Michigan State University
East Lansing, Michigan
Nutrition and Family Medicine

Steven Waldren, MD, MS
Director, American Academy of Family Physicians Center for Health Information Technology
Leawood, Kansas
Using Health Information Technology for Optimal Patient Care and Service

Kathleen Walsh, DO
Geriatric Medicine
The Monroe Clinic
Monroe, Wisconsin
Care of the Elderly Patient

Elizabeth A. Warner, MD
Associate Professor
Department of Internal Medicine
University of South Florida
Tampa, Florida
Interpreting Laboratory Tests

Gloria Westney, MD
Associate Professor, Department of Medicine
Morehouse School of Medicine
Atlanta, Georgia
Pulmonary Medicine

Russell D. White, MD
Professor of Medicine
Professor of Orthopedic Surgery
Director, Sports Medicine Fellowhip Program
Medical Director, Sports Medicine Center
Department of Community & Family Medicine
University of Missouri Kansas City School of Medicine
Head Team Physician, NCAA Division I Athletic Program
University of Missouri Kansas City
Kansas City, Missouri

Dave E. Williams, MD
Assistant Professor and Medical Director, Department
    of Family Medicine
Louisiana Health Sciences Center
School of Medicine
New Orleans, Louisiana
Obstetrics

George Wilson, MD
Professor and Chair, Department of Community Health
    and Family Medicine
University of Florida College of Medicine
Jacksonville, Florida
Endocrinology

Jane E. Wilson, MD, MPH
Potomac Physicians, P.A.
Baltimore, Maryland
Preventive Health Care

Tracy Wolff, MD, MPH
Medical Officer
U.S. Preventive Services Task Force Program
Center for Primary Care, Prevention, and Clinical Partnerships
Agency for Healthcare Research and Quality
Rockville, Maryland
Preventive Health Care

Philip Zazove, MD
Professor, Department of Family Medicine
University of Michigan Health System
Ann Arbor, Michigan
Clinical Genetics (Genomics)

Anthony Zeimet, DO
Assistant Professor of Clinical Medicine
Division of Infectious Diseases
University of Missouri–Columbia
Columbia, Missouri
Infectious Diseases

*To our wives, **Peggy** and **Denise***

To all primary care health professionals:
Our common goal is to achieve the very best outcome for our patients.

Preface

The *Textbook of Family Practice* was first published in 1973, just as the new specialty of Family Practice was being established. In 2005 the American Board of Family Practice changed its name to the American Board of Family Medicine, and this eighth edition reflects that name change.

For the first time this entire edition is available as an electronic version that can be accessed online. Additional material is available online, including 30 procedural videos from Elsevier's Procedures Consult.

In this edition, David Rakel, Associate Professor of Family Medicine at the University of Wisconsin, joins his father as co-editor.

This text is designed to be a resource for family physicians to help them remain current with recent advances in medicine. It will be especially valuable to the family physician preparing for certification or recertification by the American Board of Family Medicine.

Our goal is to serve as a resource for all health professionals responsible for providing primary care to patients, especially those professionals who may not have been adequately trained in the large variety of areas that make up comprehensive primary care.

Almost all authors are family physicians. For the clinical chapters we have continued the policy established in the first edition of having an authority in the field co-author the chapter with an experienced family physician to ensure that the information is current and relevant to the needs of the family physician.

The use of color in this edition enhances the rapid retrieval of essential information by highlighting Key Points and other essential information. Also included are more than 1000 tables and illustrations. The strength of recommendation taxonomy (SORT) in the Key Treatment boxes is used to indicate the strength of the evidence, focusing primarily on Grade A recommendations.

Although this text focuses on problems most frequently encountered by the family physician, significant attention is also paid to the diagnosis of potentially serious problems that would be dangerous if missed. Diagnosing a problem in its early, undifferentiated stage is much more difficult than after symptoms have progressed to the point that the diagnosis is evident. Early diagnosis and treatment decreases morbidity and is much more cost effective.

Our thanks to the staff at Elsevier and for their high standards and insistence on quality.

Robert E. Rakel, MD
David P. Rakel, MD

Contents

PART ONE

Principles of Family Medicine

The Family Physician

Robert E. Rakel

Key Points

- The rewards in family medicine come from knowing patients intimately over time and sharing their trust, respect, and friendship, as well as from the variety of problems encountered in practice that keep the family physician professionally stimulated and challenged.

- The American Board of Family Practice was established in 1969 and changed its name to the American Board of Family Medicine in 2004. It was the first specialty board to require recertification every 7 years to ensure ongoing competence of its diplomates.

- The American Academy of Family Physicians (AAFP) began as the American Academy of General Practice in 1947 and was renamed in 1971.

- Primary care is the provision of continuing, comprehensive care to a population undifferentiated by gender, disease, or organ system.

- The most challenging diagnoses are those for diseases or disorders in their early, undifferentiated stage, when there are often only subtle differences between serious disease and minor ailments.

- The family physician is the conductor, orchestrating the skills of a variety of health professionals that may be involved in the care of a seriously ill patient.

- The most cost-effective health care systems depend on a strong primary care base. The United States has the most expensive health care system in the world but ranks among the worst in overall quality of care because of its weak primary care base.

- The greater the number of primary care physicians in a country, the lower is the mortality rate and the lower the cost.

The family physician provides continuing, comprehensive care in a personalized manner to patients of all ages, regardless of the presence of disease or the nature of the presenting complaint. Family physicians accept responsibility for managing an individual's total health needs while maintaining an intimate, confidential relationship with the patient.

Family medicine emphasizes continuing responsibility for total health care—from the first contact and initial assessment through the ongoing care of chronic problems. Prevention and early recognition of disease are essential features of the discipline. Coordination and integration of all necessary health services (minimizing fragmentation) and the skills to manage most medical problems allow family physicians to provide cost-effective health care.

Family medicine is a specialty that shares many areas of content with other clinical disciplines, incorporating this shared knowledge and using it uniquely to deliver primary medical care. In addition to sharing content with other medical specialties, family medicine emphasizes knowledge from areas such as family dynamics, interpersonal relations, counseling, and psychotherapy. The specialty's foundation remains clinical, with the primary focus on the medical care of people who are ill.

The curriculum for training family physicians is designed to represent realistically the skills and body of knowledge that the physicians will require in practice. This curriculum is based on an analysis of the problems seen and the skills used by family physicians in their practice. The randomly educated primary physician has been replaced by one specifically prepared to address the types of problems likely to be encountered in practice. For this reason, the "model office" is an essential component of all family practice residency programs.

The Joy of Family Practice

If you cannot work with love but only with distaste, it is better that you should leave your work and sit at the gate of the temple and take alms from those who work with joy.

Kahlil Gibran (1883–1931)

The rewards in family medicine come largely from knowing patients intimately over time and sharing their trust, respect, and friendship. The thrill is the close bond (friendship) that develops with patients. This bond is strengthened with each physical or emotional crisis in a person's life, when he or she turns to the family physician for help. It is a pleasure going to the office every day and a privilege to work closely with people who value and respect our efforts.

The practice of family medicine involves the joy of greeting old friends in every examining room, and the variety of problems encountered keeps the physician professionally stimulated and perpetually challenged. In contrast, physicians practicing in narrow specialties often lose their enthusiasm for medicine after seeing the same problems every day. The variety in family practice sustains the excitement and precludes boredom. Our greatest days in practice are when we are fully focused on our patients, enjoying to the fullest the experience of working with others.

Patient Satisfaction

Attributes considered most important for patient satisfaction are listed in Table 1-1 (Stock Keister et al., 2004a). Overall, people want their primary care doctor to meet five basic criteria: "to be in their insurance plan, to be in a location that is convenient, to be able to schedule an appointment within a reasonable period of time, to have good communication skills, and to have a reasonable amount of experience in practice." They especially want "a physician who listens to them, who takes the time to explain things to them, and who is able to effectively integrate their care" (Stock Keister et al., 2004b, p. 2312).

Patient satisfaction correlates strongly with physician satisfaction, and physicians satisfied with their careers are more likely to provide better health care than dissatisfied physicians. If physicians do not enjoy their jobs, their patients are not likely to be happy with these physicians' job performance.

Physician Satisfaction

Physician satisfaction is associated with quality of care, particularly as measured by patient satisfaction. The strongest factors associated with physician satisfaction are not personal income, but rather the ability to provide high-quality care to patients. Physicians are most satisfied with their practice when they can have an ongoing relationship with their patients, the freedom to make clinical decisions without financial conflicts of interest, adequate time with patients, and sufficient communication with specialists (DeVoe et al., 2002). Landon and colleagues (2003) found that rather than declining income, the strongest predictor of decreasing satisfaction

Table 1-1 What Patients Want in a Physician

- Does not judge.
- Understands and supports me.
- Is always honest and direct.
- Acts as a partner in maintaining my health.
- Treats serious and nonserious conditions.
- Attends to my emotional as well as physical health.
- Truly listens to me.
- Encourages me to lead a healthier lifestyle.
- Tries to get to know me.
- Can help with any problem.
- Is someone I can stay with as I grow older.

Modified from Stock Keister MC, Green LA, Kahn NB, et al. What people want from their family physician. Am Fam Physician 2004;69:2310.

in practice is loss of clinical autonomy. This includes the inability to obtain services for their patients, control their time with patients, and the freedom to provide high-quality care.

In an analysis of 33 specialties, Leigh and associates (2002) found that physicians in high-income "procedural" specialties, such as obstetrics-gynecology, otolaryngology, ophthalmology, and orthopedics, were the most dissatisfied. Physicians in these specialties and those in internal medicine were more likely than family physicians to be dissatisfied with their careers. Among the specialty areas most satisfying was geriatrics. Because the population older than 65 years in the United States has doubled since 1960 and will double again by 2030, it is important that we have sufficient primary care physicians to care for them. The need for and the rewards of this type of practice must be communicated to students before they decide how to spend the rest of their professional lives. Overall, 70% of U.S. physicians are satisfied with their career, with 40% being very satisfied and only 20% dissatisfied (Leigh et al., 2002).

Development of the Specialty

As long ago as 1923, Francis Peabody commented that the swing of the pendulum toward specialization had reached its apex, and that modern medicine had fragmented the health care delivery system too greatly. He called for a rapid return of the generalist physician who would give comprehensive, personalized care.

Dr. Peabody's declaration proved to be premature; neither the medical establishment nor society was ready for such a proclamation. The trend toward specialization gained momentum through the 1950s, and fewer physicians entered general practice. In the early 1960s, leaders in the field of general practice began advocating a seemingly paradoxical solution to reverse the trend and correct the scarcity of general practitioners—the creation of still another specialty. These physicians envisioned a specialty that embodied the knowledge, skills, and ideals they knew as primary care. In 1966 the concept of a new specialty in primary care received official recognition in two separate reports published 1 month apart. The first was the report of the Citizens' Commission on Medical Education of the American Medical Association, also known as the Millis Commission Report.

The second report came from the Ad Hoc Committee on Education for Family Practice of the Council of Medical Education of the American Medical Association, also called the Willard Committee (1966). Three years later, in 1969, the American Board of Family Practice (ABFP) became the 20th medical specialty board. The name of the specialty board was changed in 2004 to the *American Board of Family Medicine* (ABFM).

Much of the impetus for the Millis and Willard reports came from the American Academy of General Practice, which was renamed the *American Academy of Family Physicians* (AAFP) in 1971. The name change reflected a desire to increase emphasis on family-oriented health care and to gain academic acceptance for the new specialty of family practice.

Specialty Certification

The ABFM has distinguished itself by being the first specialty board to require recertification, now called *maintenance of certification*, every 7 years, to ensure the ongoing competence of its members.

In the basic requirements for certification and recertification, the ABFM has included *continuing education* (CE), the foundation on which the American Academy of General Practice had been built when organized in 1947. A *diplomate* of the ABFM must complete 300 hours of acceptable CE activity every 6 years and one self-assessment module per year over the Internet to be eligible for recertification. Once eligible, a candidate's competence is examined by cognitive testing and a performance in practice evaluation. The ABFM's emphasis on quality of education, knowledge, and performance has facilitated the rapid increase in prestige for the family physician in the U.S. health care system.

The logic of the ABFM's emphasis on continuing education to maintain required knowledge and skills has been adopted by other specialties and state medical societies. All specialty boards are now committed to the concept of recertification to ensure that their diplomates remain current with advances in medicine.

The four components of "maintenance of certification" by the ABFM are professional standing, lifelong learning and self-assessment, cognitive expertise, and practice performance assessment. The ABFM also offers subspecialty certificates called *certificates of added qualifications* in five areas: adolescent medicine, geriatric medicine, hospice and palliative medicine, sleep medicine, and sports medicine. Combined residency programs are available at some institutions combining family medicine and emergency medicine or psychiatry. The combined residency makes candidates available for certification by both specialty boards with 1 year less of training than that required for two separate residencies, through appropriate overlap of training requirements.

Definitions

Family Medicine

Family medicine is the medical specialty that provides continuing and comprehensive health care for the individual and the family. It is the specialty in breadth that integrates the biologic, clinical, and behavioral sciences. The scope of family medicine encompasses all ages, both genders, each organ system, and every disease entity (AAFP, 2009).

In many countries, the term *general practice* is synonymous with *family medicine*. The Royal New Zealand College of General Practitioners emphasizes that a general practitioner provides care that is "anticipatory as well as responsive and is not limited by the age, sex, race, religion, or social circumstances of patients, nor by their physical or mental states." The general practitioner must be the patient's advocate; must be competent, caring, and compassionate; must be able to live with uncertainty; and must be willing to recognize limitations and refer when necessary (Richards, 1997).

Family Physician

The family physician is a physician who is educated and trained in the discipline of family medicine. Family physicians possess distinct attitudes, skills, and knowledge that qualify them to provide continuing and comprehensive medical care, health maintenance, and preventive services to each member of a family regardless of gender, age, or type of problem (i.e., biologic, behavioral, or social). These specialists, because of their background and interactions with the family, are best qualified to serve as each patient's advocate in all health-related matters, including the appropriate use of consultants, health services, and community resources (AAFP, 2009).

The World Organization of Family Doctors (World Organization of National Colleges, Academies and Academic Associations of General Practitioners/Family Physicians [WONCA]) defines the "family doctor" in part as the physician who is primarily responsible for providing comprehensive health care to every individual seeking medical care, arranging for other health personnel to provide services when necessary. The family physician functions as a generalist who accepts everyone seeking care, whereas other health providers limit access to their services on the basis of age, gender, or diagnosis (WONCA, 1991, p. 2).

Primary Care

Primary care is health care that is accessible, comprehensive, coordinated, and continuing. It is provided by physicians specifically trained for and skilled in comprehensive first-contact and continuing care for ill persons or those with an undiagnosed sign, symptom, or health concern (i.e., the "undifferentiated" patient) and is not limited by problem origin (i.e., biologic, behavioral, or social), organ system, or gender.

In addition to diagnosis and treatment of acute and chronic illnesses, primary care includes health promotion, disease prevention, health maintenance, counseling, and patient education in a variety of health care settings (e.g., office, inpatient, critical care, long-term care, home care). Primary care is performed and managed by a personal physician, using other health professionals for consultation or referral as appropriate.

Primary care is the backbone of the health care system and encompasses the following functions:

1. It is *first-contact care*, serving as a point of entry for the patient into the health care system.
2. It includes *continuity* by virtue of caring for patients in sickness and in health over some period.

3. It is *comprehensive care,* drawing from all the traditional major disciplines for its functional content.
4. It serves a *coordinative function* for all the health care needs of the patient.
5. It assumes *continuing responsibility* for individual patient follow-up and community health problems.
6. It is a highly personalized type of care.

In a 2008 report, Primary Health Care—Now More than Ever, the World Health Organization (WHO) emphasizes that primary care is the best way of coping with the illnesses of the 21st century, and that better use of existing preventive measures could reduce the global burden of disease by as much as 70%. Rather than drifting from one short-term priority to another, countries should make prevention equally important as cure and focus on the rise in chronic diseases that require long-term care and strong community support. Furthermore, at the 62nd World Health Assembly in 2009, WHO strongly reaffirmed the values and principles of primary health care as the basis for strengthening health care systems worldwide.

Primary Care Physician

A primary care physician is a generalist physician who provides definitive care to the undifferentiated patient at the point of first contact and takes continuing responsibility for providing the patient's care. Primary care physicians devote most of their practice to providing primary care services to a defined population of patients. The style of primary care practice is such that the personal primary care physician serves as the entry point for substantially all the patient's medical and health care needs. Primary care physicians are advocates for the patient in coordinating the use of the entire health care system to benefit the patient (AAFP, 2009).

Patients want a physician who is attentive to their needs and skilled at addressing them, and with whom they can establish a lifelong relationship. They want a physician who can guide them through the evolving, complex U.S. health care system.

The ABFM and the American Board of Internal Medicine have agreed on a definition of the generalist physician, and they believe that "providing optimal generalist care requires broad and comprehensive training that cannot be gained in brief and uncoordinated educational experiences" (Kimball and Young, 1994, p. 316).

The Council on Graduate Medical Education (COGME) and the Association of American Medical Colleges (AAMC) define generalist physicians as those who have completed 3-year training programs in family medicine, internal medicine, or pediatrics and who do not subspecialize. COGME emphasizes that this definition should be "based on an objective analysis of training requirements in disciplines that provide graduates with broad capabilities for primary care practice."

Unfortunately, the number of students entering primary care continues to decline. "In 2009, for the 12th straight year, the number of graduating U.S. medical students choosing primary care residencies reached dismally low levels" (Bodenheimer et al., 2009).

Physicians who provide primary care should be trained specifically to manage the problems encountered in a pri-

mary care practice. Rivo and associates (1994) identified the common conditions and diagnoses that generalist physicians should be competent to manage in a primary care practice and compared these with the training of the various "generalist" specialties. They recommended that the training of generalist physicians include at least 90% of the key diagnoses. By comparing the content of residency programs, they found that this goal was met by family practice (95%), internal medicine (91%), and pediatrics (91%), but that obstetrics-gynecology (47%) and emergency medicine (42%) fell far short of this goal.

Personalized Care

It is much more important to know what sort of patient has a disease than what sort of disease a patient has.

Sir William Osler (1904)

In the 12th century, Maimonides said, "May I never see in the patient anything but a fellow creature in pain. May I never consider him merely a vessel of disease" (Friedenwald, 1917). If an intimate relationship with patients remains the primary concern of physicians, high-quality medical care will persist, regardless of the way it is organized and financed. For this reason, family medicine emphasizes consideration of the individual patient in the full context of her or his life, rather than the episodic care of a presenting complaint.

Family physicians assess the illnesses and complaints presented to them, dealing personally with most and arranging special assistance for a few. The family physician serves as the patients' advocate, explaining the causes and implications of illness to patients and families, and serves as an advisor and confidant to the family. The family physician receives great intellectual satisfaction from this practice, but the greatest reward arises from the depth of human understanding and personal satisfaction inherent in family practice.

Patients have adjusted somewhat to a more impersonal form of health care delivery and frequently look to institutions rather than to individuals for their health care; however, their need for personalized concern and compassion remains. Tumulty (1970) found that patients believe a good physician is one who shows genuine interest in them; who thoroughly evaluates their problem; who demonstrates compassion, understanding, and warmth; and who provides clear insight into what is wrong and what must be done to correct it.

Ludmerer (1999a) focused on the problems facing medical education in this environment:

Some managed care organizations have even urged that physicians be taught to act in part as advocates of the insurance payer rather than the patients for whom they care (p. 881). . . . Medical educators would do well to ponder the potential long-term consequences of educating the nation's physicians in today's commercial atmosphere in which the good visit is a short visit, patients are "consumers," and institutional officials speak more often of the financial balance sheet than of service and the relief of patients' suffering (p. 882).

Cranshaw and colleagues (1995) discussed the ethics of the medical profession:

> *Our first obligation must be to serve the good of those persons who seek our help and trust us to provide it. Physicians, as physicians, are not, and must never be, commercial entrepreneurs, gate closers, or agents of fiscal policy that runs counter to our trust. Any defection from primacy of the patient's well-being places the patient at risk by treatment that may compromise quality of or access to medical care. . . . Only by caring and advocating for the patient can the integrity of our profession be affirmed (p. 1553).*

Caring

> *Caring without science is well-intentioned kindness, but not medicine. On the other hand, science without caring empties medicine of healing and negates the great potential of an ancient profession. The two complement and are essential to the art of doctoring.*
>
> (Lown, 1996, p. 223)

Family physicians do not just treat patients; they care for people. This caring function of family medicine emphasizes the personalized approach to understanding the patient as a person, respecting the person as an individual, and showing compassion for his or her discomfort. The best illustration of a caring and compassionate physician is "The Doctor" by Sir Luke Fildes (Figure 1-1). The painting shows a physician at the bedside of an ill child in the preantibiotic era. The physician in the painting is Dr. Murray, who cared for Sir Luke Fildes's son, who died Christmas morning 1877. The painting has become the symbol for medicine as a caring profession.

Compassion

> *The treatment of a disease may be entirely impersonal; the care of a patient must be completely personal.*
>
> Francis Peabody (1930)

Compassion means co-suffering and reflects the physician's willingness somehow to share the patient's anguish and understand what the sickness means to that person. Compassion is an attempt to feel along with the patient. Pellegrino (1979, p. 161) said, "We can never feel with another person when we pass judgment as a superior, only when we see our own frailties as well as his." A compassionate authority figure is effective only when others can receive the "orders" without being humiliated. The physician must not "put down" the patients, but must be ever ready, in Galileo's words, "to pronounce that wise, ingenuous, and modest statement—'I don't know.'" Compassion, practiced in these terms in each patient encounter, obtunds the inherent dehumanizing tendencies of the current highly institutionalized and technologically oriented patterns of patient care.

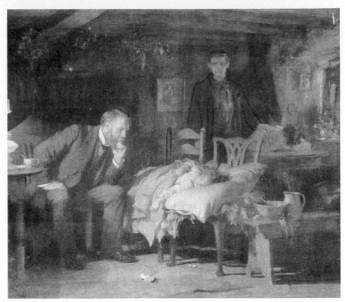

Figure 1-1 "The Doctor" by Sir Luke Fildes, 1891. © Tate, London, 2005.

The family physician's relationship with each patient should reflect compassion, understanding, and patience, combined with a high degree of intellectual honesty. The physician must be thorough in approaching problems but also possess a sense of humor. He or she must be capable of encouraging in each patient the optimism, courage, insight, and the self-discipline necessary for recovery.

Bulger (1998) addressed the threats to scientific compassionate care in the managed-care environment:

> *With health care time inordinately rationed today in the interest of economy, Americans could organize themselves right out of compassion. . . . It would be a tragedy, just when we have so many scientific therapies at hand, for scientists to negotiate away the element of compassion, leaving this crucial dimension of healing to nonscientific healers.*

Time for patient care is becoming increasingly threatened. Bulger (1998, p. 106) described a study involving a "good Samaritan" principle, showing that the decision of whether or not to stop and care for a person in distress is predominantly a function of having the time to do so. Even those with the best intentions require time to be of help to a suffering person.

Characteristics and Functions of the Family Physician

The ideal family physician is an explorer, driven by a persistent curiosity and the desire to know more (Table 1-2).

Continuing Responsibility

One of the essential functions of the family physician is the willingness to accept ongoing responsibility for managing a patient's medical care. After a patient or a family has been accepted into the physician's practice, the responsibility for

Table 1-2 Attributes of the Family Physician*

- A strong sense of responsibility for the total, ongoing care of the individual and the family during health, illness, and rehabilitation.
- Compassion and empathy, with a sincere interest in the patient and the family.
- A curious and constantly inquisitive attitude.
- Enthusiasm for the undifferentiated medical problem and its resolution.
- Interest in the broad spectrum of clinical medicine.
- The ability to deal comfortably with multiple problems occurring simultaneously in a patient.
- Desire for frequent and varied intellectual and technical challenges.
- The ability to support children during growth and development and in their adjustment to family and society.
- Assists patients in coping with everyday problems and in maintaining stability in the family and community.
- The capacity to act as coordinator of all health resources needed in the care of a patient.
- Enthusiasm for learning and for the satisfaction that comes from maintaining current medical knowledge through continuing medical education.
- The ability to maintain composure in times of stress and to respond quickly with logic, effectiveness, and compassion.
- A desire to identify problems at the earliest possible stage or to prevent disease entirely.
- A strong wish to maintain maximum patient satisfaction, recognizing the need for continuing patient rapport.
- The skills necessary to manage chronic illness and to ensure maximal rehabilitation after acute illness.
- Appreciation for the complex mix of physical, emotional, and social elements in personalized patient care.
- A feeling of personal satisfaction derived from intimate relationships with patients that naturally develop over long periods of continuous care, as opposed to the short-term pleasures gained from treating episodic illnesses.
- Skills for and a commitment to educating patients and families about disease processes and the principles of good health.
- A commitment to place the interests of the patient above those of self.

*These characteristics are desirable for all physicians, but are of greatest importance for the family physician.

care is total and continuing. The Millis Commission chose the term "primary physician" to emphasize the concept of primary responsibility for the patient's welfare; however, the term *primary care physician* is more popular and refers to any physician who provides first-contact care.

The family physician's commitment to patients does not cease at the end of illness but is a continuing responsibility, regardless of the patient's state of health or the disease process. There is no need to identify the beginning or end point of treatment, because care of a problem can be reopened at any time—even though a later visit may be primarily for another problem. This prevents the family physician from focusing too narrowly on one problem and helps maintain a perspective on the total patient in her or his environment. Peabody (1930) believed that much patient dissatisfaction resulted from the physician's neglecting to assume personal responsibility for supervision of the patient's care: "For some reason or other, no one physician has seen the case through from beginning to end, and the patient may be suffering from the very multitude of his counselors" (p. 8).

Continuity of care is a core attribute of family medicine, transcending multiple illness episodes, and it includes

responsibility for preventive care and care coordination. "This longitudinal relationship evolves into a strong bond between physician and patient characterized by trust, loyalty, and a sense of responsibility" (Saultz, 2003). Trust grows stronger as the physician-patient relationship continues and provides the patient a sense of confidence that care will always be in his or her best interest. It also facilitates improved quality of care the longer the relationship continues.

The greater the degree of continuing involvement with a patient, the more capable the physician is in detecting early signs and symptoms of organic disease and differentiating it from a functional problem. Patients with problems arising from emotional and social conflicts can be managed most effectively by a physician who has intimate knowledge of the individual and his or her family and community background. This knowledge comes only from insight gained by observing the patient's long-term patterns of behavior and responses to changing stressful situations. This longitudinal view is particularly useful in the care of children and allows the physician to be more effective in assisting children to reach their full potential. The closeness that develops between physicians and young patients increases a physician's ability to aid the patients with problems later in life, such as adjustment to puberty, problems with employment, or marriage and changing social pressures. As the family physician maintains this continuing involvement with successive generations within a family, the ability to manage intercurrent problems increases with knowledge of the total family background.

By virtue of this ongoing involvement and intimate association with the family, the family physician develops a perceptive awareness of a family's nature and style of operation. This ability to observe families over time allows valuable insight that improves the quality of medical care provided to an individual patient. A major challenge in family medicine is the need to be alert to the changing stresses, transitions, and expectations of family members over time, as well as the effect that these and other family interactions have on the health of individual patients.

Although the family is the family physician's primary concern, his or her skills are equally applicable to the individual living alone or to people in other varieties of family living. Individuals with alternative forms of family living interact with others who have a significant effect on their lives. The principles of group dynamics and interpersonal relationships that affect health are equally applicable to everyone.

The family physician must assess an individual's personality so that presenting symptoms can be appropriately evaluated and given the proper degree of attention and emphasis. A complaint of abdominal pain may be treated lightly in one patient who frequently presents with minor problems, but the same complaint would be investigated immediately and in depth in another patient who has a more stoic personality. The decision regarding which studies to perform and when is influenced by knowledge of the patient's lifestyle, personality, and previous response pattern. The greater the degree of knowledge and insight into the patient's background, as gained through years of ongoing contact, the more capable is the physician in making an appropriate early and rapid assessment of the presenting complaint. The less background information the physician has to rely on, the greater is the need to depend on costly laboratory studies, and the more likely is overreaction to the presenting symptom.

Families receiving continuing comprehensive care have a decreased incidence of hospitalization, fewer operations, and less physician visits for illnesses compared with those having no regular physician. This results from the physician's knowledge of the patients, seeing them earlier for acute problems and therefore preventing complications that would require hospitalization, being available by telephone or by e-mail, and seeing them more frequently in the office for health supervision. Care is also less expensive because there is less need to rely on radiographic and laboratory procedures and visits to emergency departments.

Continuity of care improves quality of care, especially for those with chronic conditions such as asthma and diabetes (Cabana and Jee, 2004). Because about 90% of diabetic patients in the United States receive care from a primary care physician, continuity of care can be especially important. Parchman and associates (2002) found that for adults with type 2 diabetes, continuing care from the same primary care provider was associated with lower Hb_{A1c} values, regardless of how long the patient had suffered from diabetes. Having a regular source of primary care helped these adults manage their diet and improve glucose control.

Collusion of Anonymity

The need for a primary physician who accepts continuing responsibility for patient care was emphasized by Michael Balint (1965) in his concept of *collusion of anonymity*. In this situation the patient is seen by a variety of physicians, not one of whom is willing to accept total management of the problem. Important decisions are made—some good, some poor—but without anyone feeling fully responsible for them.

Francis Peabody (1930) examined the futility of a patient's making the rounds from one specialist to another without finding relief because the patient:

> *. . . lacked the guidance of a sound general practitioner who understood his physical condition, his nervous temperament and knew the details of his daily life. And many a patient who on his own initiative has sought out specialists, has had minor defects accentuated so that they assume a needless importance, and has even undergone operations that might well have been avoided. Those who are particularly blessed with this world's goods, who want the best regardless of the cost and imagine that they are getting it because they can afford to consult as many renowned specialists as they wish, are often pathetically tragic figures as they veer from one course of treatment to another. Like ships that lack a guiding hand upon the helm, they swing from tack to tack with each new gust of wind but get no nearer to the Port of Health because there is no pilot to set the general direction of their course (pp. 21-22).*

Chronic Illness

The family physician must also be committed to managing the common chronic illnesses that have no known cure, but for which continuing management by a personal physician is all the more necessary to maintain an optimal state of health for the patient. It is a difficult and often trying job to manage these unresolvable and progressively crippling problems, control of which requires a remodeling of the lifestyle of the entire family.

About 45% of Americans have a chronic condition. The costs to individuals and to the health care system are enormous. In 2000, care of chronic illness consumed 75 cents of every health care dollar spent in the United States (Robert Wood Johnson Foundation Annual Report, 2002).

Comorbidity, the coincident occurrence of coexisting and apparently unrelated disorders, is increasing as the population ages. Those age 60 years or older have an average of 2.2 chronic conditions, and physicians in primary care provide most of this care (Bayliss et al., 2003).

Diabetes is one of the most rapidly increasing chronic conditions (Figure 1-2). Quality of life is enhanced when care of diabetic patients is provided in a primary care setting without compromising quality of care (Collins et al., 2009).

Quality of Care

Primary care provided by physicians specifically trained to care for the problems presenting to personal physicians, who know their patients over time, is of higher quality than care provided by other physicians. This has been confirmed by a variety of studies comparing the care given by physicians in different specialties. When hospitalized patients with pneumonia are cared for by family physicians or full-time specialist hospitalists, the quality of care is comparable, but the hospitalists incur higher hospital charges, longer lengths of stay, and use more resources (Smith et al., 2002).

In the United States, a 20% increase in the number of primary care physicians is associated with a 5% decrease in mortality (40 fewer deaths per 100,000 population), but the benefit is even greater if the primary care physician is a family physician. Adding one more family physician per 10,000 people is associated with 70 fewer deaths per 100,000 population, which is a 9% reduction in mortality. Specialists practicing outside their area have increased mortality rates for patients with acquired pneumonia, acute myocardial infarction, congestive heart failure, and upper gastrointestinal hemorrhage. Specialists are trained to look for zebras instead of horses, and specialty care usually means more tests, which lead to a cascade effect and a greater likelihood of adverse effects, including death. A study of the major determinants of health outcomes in all 50 U.S. states found that when the number of specialty physicians increases, outcomes are worse, whereas mortality rates are lower where there are more primary care physicians (Starfield et al., 2005).

McGann and Bowman (1990) compared the morbidity and mortality of patients hospitalized by family physicians and by internists. Even though the family physicians' patients were older and more severely ill, there was no significant difference in morbidity and mortality. The total charges for their hospital care also were lower.

A comparison of family physicians and obstetrician-gynecologists in the management of low-risk pregnancies showed no difference with respect to neonatal outcomes. However, women cared for by family physicians had fewer cesarean sections and episiotomies and were less likely to receive epidural anesthesia (Hueston et al., 1995).

Patients of subspecialists practicing outside their specialty have longer lengths of hospital stay and higher mortality

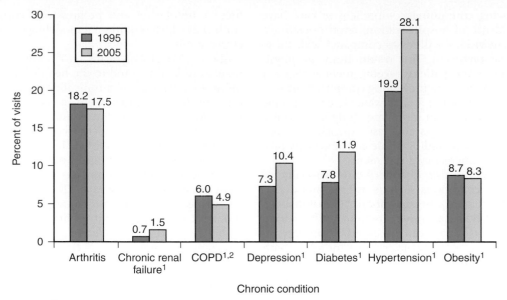

Figure 1-2 Percentage of office visits by adults 18 years and older with selected chronic conditions: United States, 1995 and 2005. *(From Cherry DK, Woodwell DA, Rechtsteiner EA. National Ambulatory Medical Care Survey: 2005 summary. Advance data from vital and health statistics. No 387. Hyattsville, Md, National Center for Health Statistics, 2007. www.cdc/gov/nchs/ahcd/oficevisitcharts/htm.)*

rates than patients of subspecialists practicing within their specialty or of general internists (Weingarten et al., 2002). The quality of the U.S. health care system is being eroded by physicians being extensively trained, at great expense, to practice in one area and, instead, practicing in another area, such as anesthesiologists practicing in emergency departments or surgeons practicing as generalists. Primary care, to be done well, requires extensive training specifically tailored to problems frequently seen in primary care.

As much-needed changes in the American medical system are implemented, it would be wise to keep some perspective on the situation regarding physician distribution. Beeson (1974) commented:

I have no doubt at all that a good family doctor can deal with the great majority of medical episodes quickly and competently. A specialist, on the other hand, feels that he must be thorough, not only because of his training but also because he has a reputation to protect. He, therefore, spends more time with each patient and orders more laboratory work. The result is a waste of doctors' time and patients' money. This not only inflates the national health bill, but also creates an illusion of doctor shortage when the only real need is to have the existing doctors doing the right things (p. 48).

Cost-Effective Care

The physician who is well acquainted with the patient provides more personal and humane medical care, and does so more economically, than the physician involved in only episodic care. The physician who knows his or her patients well can assess the nature of their problems more rapidly and accurately. Because of the intimate, ongoing relationship, the family physician is under less pressure to exclude diagnostic

possibilities using expensive laboratory and radiologic procedures than the physician unfamiliar with the patient.

The United States has the most expensive health care system in the world. In 1965 the cost of health care in the United States was just under 6% of the gross domestic product (GDP). It shot up to 16% of GDP in 2008 and continues to increase, with predictions it will reach 20% by 2015. Despite the most expensive health care, however, the United States ranks 29th in infant mortality, 48th in life expectancy, and 19th (of 19) in preventable deaths among industrialized nations.[*]

Although the rhetoric suggests it is worth this cost to have the best health care system in the world, the truth is that we are far from that goal. WHO ranks the quality of health care in the United States at 37th in the world, well behind Morocco and Colombia. (For the standing of all countries see www.photius.com/rankings/health ranks.html.) In a comparison of the quality of health care in 13 developed countries using 16 different health indicators, the United States ranked 12th, second from the bottom. Evidence indicates that quality of health care is associated with primary care performance. Of the seven countries at the top of the average health ranking, five have strong primary care infrastructures. As Starfield (2000) states, "The higher the primary care physician-to-population ratio, the better most health outcomes are" (p. 485).

Similarly, the greater the number of primary care physicians practicing in a country, the lower is the cost of health care. Figure 1-3 shows that in the United Kingdom, Canada, and the United States, the cost of health care is inversely proportional to the percentage of generalists practicing in that country. Great Britain has twice the percentage of family physicians but half the cost. Administrative overhead accounts

---

*www.aafp.org/online/news-now/professional-issues/20081223health-ceos.html. Accessed January 2010.

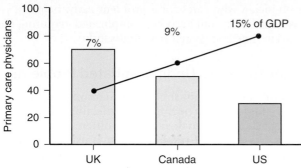

Figure 1-3 Inverse relationship between number of generalists and cost of health care in the United Kingdom, Canada, and the United States. *(From Organisation for Economic Cooperation and Development. OECD Health Data, June 2005. http://www.oecd.org/document/56/0,2340,en_2649_34631_12968734_1_1_1_1,00.html/ Accessed April 2006.)*

for a major part of the high overhead cost (31%) of U.S. health care (Woolhandler et al., 2003). For the same number of physicians, Canada has one "billing clerk" for every 17 in the United States (Lundberg, 2002).

Countries with strong primary care have lower overall health care costs, improved health outcomes, and healthier populations (Starfield, 2001; Phillips and Starfield, 2004). In comparing 11 features of primary care in 11 Western countries, the United States ranked lowest in terms of primary care ranking and highest in per-capita health care expenditures. The United States also performed poorly on public satisfaction, health indicators, and the use of medication (Starfield, 1994).

In the United States, the greater the number of primary care physicians, the lower is the mortality, and conversely, the higher the specialist/population ratio, the greater is the mortality. Adding one family physician per 10,000 people would result in 35 fewer deaths. Increasing the number of specialists, a process that continues in the United States, is associated with higher mortality and increasing cost. One third of the excessive cost is attributed to performance of unnecessary procedures (Starfield et al., 2005).

Uninsured Persons

The number of Americans without health insurance has been increasing by 1 million per year. In 2008 the number of uninsured persons was 46 million, or 16% of the U.S. population. The number of people who are *underinsured* (another 50 million) is growing even more rapidly. Contrary to widespread belief, the problem is not confined simply to unemployed or poor persons. More than one half of uninsured persons have annual incomes greater than $75,000, and 8 of 10 are in working families.

The United States is the only developed country that does not have universal health care coverage for all its citizens. According to Geyman, "Today's nonsystem is in chaos. A large part of health care has been taken over by for-profit corporations whose interests are motivated more by return on investment to shareholders than by quality of care for patients" (2002, p. 407).

The Institute of Medicine (IOM) report on the uninsured population, *Insuring America's Health: Principles and Recommendations*, called for "health care coverage by 2010 that is universal, continuous, affordable, sustainable, and enhancing of high-quality care that is effective, efficient, safe, timely, patient centered, and equitable. . . . While stopping short of advocating a specific approach, the IOM's Committee on the Consequences of Uninsurance acknowledges that the single payer model is the most effective in ensuring continuous universal coverage that would remain affordable for individuals and for society" (Geyman, 2004, p. 635).

Family physicians account for a larger proportion of office visits to U.S. physicians than any other specialty. However, Geyman (2004) observed problems:

The country's health care (non) system has undergone a major transformation to a market-based system largely dominated by corporate interests and a business ethic. The goal envisioned in the 1960s of rebuilding the U.S. health care system on a generalist base, with all Americans having ready access to comprehensive health care through a personal physician, has not been achieved. Overspecialization was a problem as long as 4000 years ago, when Herodotus in 2000 BC noted that "The art of medicine is thus divided: each physician applies himself to one disease only and not more."

Comprehensive Care

The term *comprehensive medical care* spans the entire spectrum of medicine. The effectiveness with which a physician delivers primary care depends on the degree of involvement attained during training and practice. The family physician must be trained comprehensively to acquire all the medical skills necessary to care for most problems. The greater the number of skills omitted from the family physician's training and practice, the more frequent is the need to refer minor problems to another physician. A truly comprehensive primary care physician adequately manages acute infections, biopsies skin and other lesions, repairs lacerations, treats musculoskeletal sprains and minor fractures, removes foreign bodies, treats vaginitis, provides obstetric care and care for the newborn infant, gives supportive psychotherapy, and supervises diagnostic procedures. The needs of a family physician's patient range from a routine physical examination, when the patient feels well and wants to identify potential risk factors, to a problem that calls for referral to one or more narrowly specialized physicians with highly developed technical skills. The family physician must be aware of the variety and complexity of skills and facilities available to help manage patients and must match these to the individual's specific needs, giving full consideration to the patient's personality and expectations.

Management of an illness involves much more than a diagnosis and an outline for treatment. It requires an awareness of all the factors that may aid or hinder an individual's recovery from illness. This approach requires consideration of religious beliefs; social, economic, or cultural problems; personal expectations; and heredity. The outstanding clinician recognizes the effects that spiritual, intellectual, emotional, social, and economic factors have on a patient's illness.

The family physician's ability to confront relatively large numbers of unselected patients with undifferentiated conditions and carry on a therapeutic relationship over time is a unique primary care skill. The skilled family physician has a higher level of tolerance for the uncertain than her or his consultant colleague.

Society benefits more from a surgeon who has a sufficient volume of surgery to maintain proficiency through frequent use of well-honed skills than from one who has a low volume of surgery and serves also as a primary care physician. The early identification of disease while it is in its undifferentiated stage requires specific training; it is not a skill that can be automatically assumed by someone whose training has been mostly in hospital intensive care units.

Interpersonal Skills

One of the foremost skills of the family physician is the ability to use effectively the knowledge of interpersonal relations in the management of patients. This powerful element of clinical medicine may be the specialty's most useful tool. Physicians too often are seen as lacking personal concern and as being unskilled in understanding personal anxiety and feelings. There is a need to nourish the seed of compassion and concern for sick people that motivates students as they enter medical school.

Family medicine emphasizes the integration of compassion, empathy, and personalized concern. Some of the earnest solicitude of the "old country doctor" and his or her untiring compassion for people must be incorporated as effective but impersonal modern medical procedures are applied. The patient should be viewed compassionately as a person in distress who needs to be treated with concern, dignity, and personal consideration. The patient has a right to be given some insight into his or her problems, a reasonable appraisal of the potential outcome, and a realistic picture of the emotional, financial, and occupational expenses involved in his or her care. The greatest deterrents to filing malpractice claims are patient satisfaction, good patient rapport, and active patient participation in the health care process.

To relate well to patients, a physician must develop compassion and courtesy, the ability to establish rapport and to communicate effectively, the ability to gather information rapidly and to organize it logically, the skills required to identify all significant patient problems and to manage these problems appropriately, the ability to listen, the skills necessary to motivate people, and the ability to observe and detect nonverbal clues (see Chapter 12).

Accessibility

The mere availability of the physician is therapeutic. The feeling of security that the patient gains just by knowing he or she can "touch" the physician, in person or by phone, is therapeutic and has a comforting and calming influence. Accessibility is an essential feature of primary care. Services must be available when needed and should be within geographic proximity. When primary care is not available, many individuals turn to hospital emergency departments. Emergency department care is fine for emergencies, but it is no substitute for the personalized, long-term, comprehensive care a family physician can provide.

Many practices are instituting open-access scheduling, in which patients can be seen the day they call. This tells the patient that they are the highest priority and that the problem will be handled immediately. It also is more efficient for

the physician who cares for a problem early, before it progresses in severity and becomes complicated, requiring more physician time and greater patient disability.

Diagnostic Skills: Undifferentiated Problems

The family physician must be an outstanding diagnostician. Skills in this area must be honed to perfection, because problems are usually seen in their early, undifferentiated state and without the degree of resolution that is usually present by the time patients are referred to consulting specialists. This is a unique feature of family medicine, because symptoms seen at this stage are often vague and nondescript, with signs being minimal or absent. Unlike the consulting specialist, the family physician does not evaluate the case after it has been preselected by another physician, and the diagnostic procedures used by the family physician must be selected from the entire spectrum of medicine.

At this stage of disease, there are often only subtle differences between the early symptoms of serious disease and those of self-limiting, minor ailments. To the inexperienced person, the clinical pictures may appear identical, but to the astute and experienced family physician, one symptom is more suspicious than another because of the greater probability that it signals a potentially serious illness. Diagnoses are frequently made on the basis of probability, and the likelihood that a specific disease is present frequently depends on the incidence of the disease relative to the symptom seen in the physician's community during a given time of year. Many patients will never be assigned a final, definitive diagnosis, because a presenting symptom or a complaint will resolve before a specific diagnosis can be made. Pragmatically, this is an efficient method that is less costly and achieves high patient satisfaction, even though it may be disquieting to the purist physician who believes a thorough workup and specific diagnosis always should be obtained. Similarly, family physicians are more likely to use a therapeutic trial to confirm the diagnosis.

The family physician is an expert in the rapid assessment of a problem presented for the first time. He or she evaluates its potential significance, often making a diagnosis by exclusion rather than by inclusion, after making certain the symptoms are not those of a serious problem. Once assured, some time is allowed to elapse. Time is used as an efficient diagnostic aid. Follow-up visits are scheduled at appropriate intervals to watch for subtle changes in the presenting symptoms. The physician usually identifies the symptom that has the greatest discriminatory value and watches it more closely than the others. The most significant clue to the true nature of the illness may depend on subtle changes in this key symptom. The family physician's effectiveness is often determined by his or her knack for perceiving the hidden or subtle dimensions of illness and following them closely.

The maxim that "an accurate history is the most important factor in arriving at an accurate diagnosis" is especially appropriate to family medicine, because symptoms may be the only obvious feature of an illness at the time it is presented to the family physician. Further inquiry into the nature of the symptoms, time of onset, extenuating factors, and other unique subjective features may provide the only diagnostic clues available at such an early stage.

The family physician must be a perceptive humanist, alert to early identification of new problems. Arriving at an early diagnosis may be of less importance than determining the real reason the patient came to the physician. The symptoms may be the result of a self-limiting or acute problem, but anxiety or fear may be the true precipitating factor. Although the symptom may be hoarseness that has resulted from postnasal drainage accompanying an upper respiratory tract infection, the patient may fear it is caused by a laryngeal carcinoma similar to that recently found in a friend. Clinical evaluation must rule out the possibility of laryngeal carcinoma, but the patient's fears and apprehension regarding this possibility must also be allayed.

Every physical problem has an emotional component, and although this factor is usually minimal, it can be significant. A patient's personality, fears, and anxieties play a role in every illness and are important factors in primary care.

The Family Physician as Coordinator

Francis Peabody (1930), Professor of Medicine at Harvard Medical School from 1921 to 1927, was ahead of his time. His comments remain appropriate today:

Never was the public in need of wise, broadly trained advisors so much as it needs them today to guide them through the complicated maze of modern medicine. The extraordinary development of medical science, with its consequent diversity of medical specialism and the increasing limitations in the extent of special fields—the very factors that are creating specialists—in themselves create a new demand, not for men who are experts along narrow lines, but for men who are in touch with many lines (p. 20).

The family physician, by virtue of her or his breadth of training in a wide variety of medical disciplines, has unique insights into the skills possessed by physicians in the more limited specialties. The family physician is best prepared to select specialists whose skills can be applied most appropriately to a given case, as well as to coordinate the activities of each, so that they are not counterproductive.

As medicine becomes more specialized and complex, the family physician's role as the integrator of health services becomes increasingly important. The family physician facilitates the patient's access to the whole health care system and interprets the activities of this system to the patient, explaining the nature of the illness, the implication of the treatment, and the effect of both on the patient's way of life. The following statement from the Millis Commission Report (Citizens' Commission, 1966) concerning expectations of the patient is especially appropriate:

The patient wants, and should have, someone of high competence and good judgment to take charge of the total situation, someone who can serve as coordinator of all the medical resources that can help solve his problem. He wants a company president who will make proper use of his skills and knowledge of more specialized members of the firm. He wants a quarterback who will diagnose the constantly changing situation, coordinate the whole team, and call on each member for the particular contributions that he is best able to make to the team effort (p. 39).

Such breadth of vision is important for a coordinating physician. She or he must have a realistic overview of the problem and an awareness of the many alternative routes to select the one that is most appropriate. As Pellegrino (1966) stated:

It should be clear, too, that no simple addition of specialties can equal the generalist function. To build a wall, one needs more than the aimless piling up of bricks, one needs an architect. Every operation which analyzes some part of the human mechanism requires it to be balanced by another which synthesizes and coordinates (p. 542).

The complexity of modern medicine frequently involves a variety of health professionals, each with highly developed skills in a particular area. In planning the patient's care, the family physician, having established rapport with a patient and family and having knowledge of the patient's background, personality, fears, and expectations, is best able to select and coordinate the activities of appropriate individuals from the large variety of medical disciplines. He or she can maintain effective communication among those involved, as well as function as the patient's advocate and interpret to the patient and family the many unfamiliar and complicated procedures being used. This prevents any one consulting physician, unfamiliar with the concepts or actions of all others involved, from ordering a test or medication that would conflict with other treatment. Dunphy (1964) described the value of the surgeon and the family physician working closely as a team:

It is impossible to provide high quality surgical care without that knowledge of the whole patient, which only a family physician can supply. When their mutual decisions . . . bring hope, comfort and ultimately, health to a gravely ill human being, the total experience is the essence and the joy of medicine (p. 12).

The ability to orchestrate the knowledge and skills of diverse professionals is a skill to be learned during training and cultivated in practice. It is not an automatic attribute of all physicians or merely the result of exposure to a large number of professionals. These coordinator skills extend beyond the traditional medical disciplines into the many community agencies and allied health professions as well. Because of his or her close involvement with the community, the family physician is ideally suited to be the integrator of the patient's care, coordinating the skills of consultants when appropriate and involving community nurses, social agencies, the clergy, or other family members when needed. Knowledge of community health resources and a personal involvement with the community can be used to maximum benefit for diagnostic and therapeutic purposes and to achieve the best possible level of rehabilitation.

Only 5% of visits to family physicians lead to a referral, and more than 50% are for consultation rather than direct intervention. Surgical specialists are sent the largest share of referrals at 45.4%, followed by medical specialists at 31% and obstetrician-gynecologists at 4.6%. Physicians consulted most frequently are orthopedic surgeons, followed by general surgeons, otolaryngologists, and gastroenterologists. Psychiatrists are consulted the least (Forrest et al., 2002; Starfield et al., 2002).

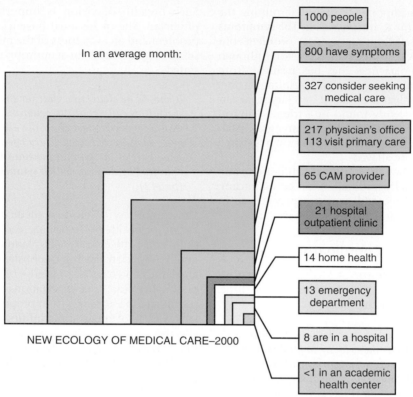

In an average month:

1000 people

800 have symptoms

327 consider seeking medical care

217 physician's office
113 visit primary care

65 CAM provider

21 hospital outpatient clinic

14 home health

13 emergency department

8 are in a hospital

<1 in an academic health center

NEW ECOLOGY OF MEDICAL CARE–2000

Figure 1-4 Number of persons experiencing an illness during an average month per 1000 people. *(From Green LA, Fryer GE Jr, Yawn BP, et al. The ecology of medical care revisited. N Engl J Med 2001;344:2021-2025.)*

The Family Physician in Practice

The advent of family medicine has led to a renaissance in medical education involving a reassessment of the traditional medical education environment in a teaching hospital. It is now considered more realistic to train a physician in a community atmosphere, providing exposure to the diseases and problems most closely approximating those she or he will encounter during practice. The ambulatory care skills and knowledge that most medical graduates will need cannot be taught totally within the tertiary medical center. The specialty of family practice emphasizes training in ambulatory care skills in an appropriately realistic environment, using patients representing a cross section of a community and incorporating those problems most frequently encountered by physicians practicing primary care.

The lack of relevance in the referral medical center also applies to the hospitalized patient. Figure 1-4 places the health problems of an average community in perspective. In any given month, 800 people experience at least one symptom. Most of these people are managed by self-treatment, but 217 consult a physician. Of these, eight are hospitalized, but only one goes to an academic medical center. Patients seen in the medical center (with most cases used for teaching) represent atypical samples of illness occurring within the community. Students exposed to patients in only this manner develop an unrealistic concept of the types of medical problems prevalent in society and particularly those composing primary care. It focuses their training on knowledge and skills of limited usefulness in later practice. Medical schools should accept the responsibility of providing health care for a defined population, and the dean's office should ensure that the curriculum is congruent with the health needs of that population.

Practice Content

Since 1975, the National Ambulatory Medical Care Survey conducted by the National Center for Health Statistics (NCHS) of the U.S. Department of Health and Human Services has annually reported the problems seen by office-based physicians (in all specialties) in the United States. More than 53% of all office visits in the United States were to primary care physicians (Figure 1-5). The 20 most common diagnoses seen by physicians in their office are shown in Table 1-3. Note that arthritis is fourth and diabetes mellitus sixth, reflecting the prominence of chronic diseases in practice. For those who think primary care is little more than caring for acute pharyngitis, note that it is 19th. When only chronic conditions are listed (Table 1-4), arthritis is second and diabetes fourth.

Primary care physicians manage an average of 1.65 problems per visit. Of visits to primary care physicians, 61% were for a medical examination, compared with 23% for surgical specialists. Although hypertension is the most common problem encountered in offices (see Table 1-3), primary care physicians checked the blood pressure at 60% of the visits, compared with only 20% of surgical specialists and 40% of visits to medical specialists (National Center for Health Statistics, 2002).

Available data concerning primary care indicate that more people use this type of medical service than any other and that, contrary to popular opinion, sophisticated medical technology is not normally either required or overused in basic primary care encounters. Most primary care visits arise

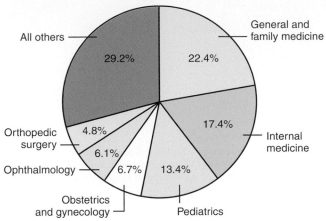

Figure 1-5 Percent distribution of office visits by physician specialty: United States, 2005. *(From Cherry DK, Woodwell DA, Rechtsteiner EA. National Ambulatory Medical Care Survey: 2005 Summary. Advance data from vital and health statistics. No 387. Hyattsville, Md, National Center for Health Statistics, 2007.* www.cdc.gov/nchs/ahcd/officevisitcharts.htm.)

Table 1-3 Rank Order of Office Visits by Diagnosis

1. Essential hypertension
2. Routine infant or child health check
3. Acute upper respiratory infections, excluding pharyngitis
4. Arthropathies and related disorders
5. Malignant neoplasms
6. Diabetes mellitus
7. Spinal disorders
8. Rheumatism, excluding back
9. General medical examination
10. Follow-up examination
11. Specific procedures and aftercare
12. Normal pregnancy
13. Gynecologic examination
14. Otitis media and eustachian tube disorders
15. Asthma
16. Disorder of lipoid metabolism
17. Chronic sinusitis
18. Heart disease, excluding ischemic
19. Acute pharyngitis
20. Allergic rhinitis

From Cherry DK, Woodwell DA, Rechtsteiner EA. 2005 Summary: National Ambulatory Medical Care Survey. National Center for Health Statistics, Advance Data Vital Health Statistics. No 387. Washington, DC, US Government Printing Office, 2007.

from patients requesting care for relatively uncomplicated problems, many of which are self-limiting but cause the patients concern or discomfort. Treatment is often symptomatic, consisting of pain relief or anxiety reduction rather than a "cure." The greatest cost-efficiency results when these patients' needs are satisfied while the self-limiting course of the disease is recognized, without incurring unnecessary costs for additional tests.

Patient-Centered Medical Home

The patient-centered medical home ((PCMH; see Chapter 2) has been proposed as an enhanced model of primary care by four medical organizations (family medicine, pediatrics,

Table 1-4 Rank Order of Chronic Conditions, All Ages

1. Hypertension
2. Arthritis
3. Hyperlipidemia
4. Diabetes
5. Depression
6. Obesity
7. Cancer
8. Asthma
9. Chronic obstructive pulmonary disease
10. Ischemic heart disease
11. Osteoporosis
12. Cerebrovascular disease
13. Congestive heart failure
14. Chronic renal failure

internal medicine, osteopathy) and is focused on reducing fragmentation of care and overcoming the reliance on specialty rather than primary care (Berenson et al., 2008; Rogers, 2008).

Primary care was encouraged to expand beyond its restrictive role as a provider of care to one that analyzes the needs of a community and focuses on those at risk of disease. This process was first described in the 1950s by Sydney Karf, who looked at the needs of his community in South Africa, whether or not they were his patients (Kark and Cassel, 1952). The process involves identifying the health problems of a community, such as diabetes or obesity, and developing a program to prevent the disease and care for people in the early stage, then evaluating the effectiveness of the program (Longlett et al., 2001).

Looking toward the Future

The pace of medical progress may result in tomorrow's innovations exceeding today's fantasies. Family medicine in the future will be different as a result of technology. Every patient and physician will be computer literate, with patients having access to the same sources of information as the physician. Patients are likely to have their own home page that contains their medical information and gives them access to whatever services they need (Scherger, 2005). Although the Internet is an excellent tool for consumers to access information about their health and for disseminating health care information, it will never be a substitute for a face-to-face discussion and physical examination. It cannot convey the worry in a voice or the subtle nonverbal clues to the real reason for the patient's distress. However, the Internet does allow the individual patient to be more active and involved in his or her own care.

The advent of the electronic medical record may be as significant as the discovery of penicillin (see Chapter 9). It will allow the family physician to incorporate the latest evidence-based recommendations into an individual's care, write electronic prescriptions, and be alerted to drug interactions while seeing a patient. Internet-based textbooks such as this one will provide immediate access to information during the patient visit.

References

The complete reference list is available online at www.expertconsult.com.

Web Resources

www.aafp.org

The American Academy of Family Physicians site with information for members, residents, students, and patients. Publishes the *American Family Physician, Family Practice Management Journal, Annals of Family Medicine,* and *AAFP News Now.* Sponsors the Family Medicine Interest Group (FMIG) for medical students at www.fmignet. aafp.org.

www.familydoctor.org

Consumer health information, including tips for healthy living, search by symptom, immunization schedules, and drug information.

www.theabfm.org

The American Board of Family Medicine, the second largest medical specialty in the United States. Site includes a link to *The Journal of the American Board of Family Medicine,* certification requirements, and reciprocity agreements with other countries.

www.photius.com/rankings/healthranks.html

The World Health Organization's ranking of the quality of health care in 190 countries. Also available are life expectancy, preventable deaths, and total health expenditure (as % of GDP).

www.globalfamilydoctor.com/

The World Organization of National Colleges, Academies and Academic Associations of General Practitioners/Family Physicians (WONCA). The World Organization of Family Doctors is made up of 120 organizations in 99 countries.

www.stfm.org

The Society of Teachers of Family Medicine, representing 5000 teachers, publishes *Family Medicine* and the *STFM Messenger.*

www.adfmmed.org

The Association of Departments of Family Medicine represents departments of family medicine in U.S. medical schools.

www.napcrg.org

The North American Primary Care Research Group (NAPCRG) is committed to fostering research in primary care.

CHAPTER 2

The Patient-Centered Medical Home

David P. Rakel and Wayne Jonas

The intuitive mind is a sacred gift, and the rational mind is a faithful servant. We have created a society in which we honor the servant and have forgotten the gift.

Albert Einstein

Key Points

- Continuous, health-oriented relationships are the foundation on which the medical home, or "health home," is built. This is the interpersonal environment.

- The patient-centered medical home brings together health professionals to work collectively toward the health needs of the community through the creation of health teams.

- A continuous self-reflective process is required for the physician leader to maintain joy in her or his work, which will translate into the quality of the health home.

- The health home can have the greatest impact on community health by working toward the incorporation of positive lifestyle behaviors. This is the behavioral environment.

- Patient empowerment is a way of interacting in which accurate information is provided in a manner that is understandable to the individual and that both respects and promotes the patient's ability to make decisions. A patient's decision making is the inner, personal environment, influenced by external issues such as culture, family, peer group, work, and payment for care.

- Creating an optimal healing environment (including inner, inter, behavioral, and external) within the medical home will encourage empowerment toward positive change.

History

The concept of the "medical home" was first described in *Standards of Child Care* by the American Academy of Pediatrics (AAP) Council on Pediatrics Practice in 1967. It defined "ideal care" for children with disabilities as a practice that provided care that was accessible, coordinated, family centered, and culturally effective.

The American Academy of Family Physicians (AAFP) used this concept to expand the characteristics based on discussions defining the future of family medicine. These characteristics described the "personal" medical home, which focused on bringing attention to the importance of continuous, relationship-centered, whole-system, comprehensive care for communities (Martin et al., 2004). In 2007 the AAP, AAFP, American College of Physicians (ACP), and American Osteopathic Association (AOA) collaborated to define further the foundational principles of the patient-centered medical home (PCMH; Table 2-1). The goal of the medical home is to emphasize the importance of primary care in improving quality of care, health outcomes, and patient experience, with improved cost-efficiency.

However, the ingredients of the medical home (or "health home") continue to be defined and modified based on the needs of the clinicians and communities who implement them. These ingredients and how they are delivered are key to the achievement of the lofty goals of the medical home and family medicine in general. This chapter discusses the most important ingredients for the medical home and the actions that the family physician must take to create one.

Healing, Curing, and the Goals of the Medical Home

Medicine in general and primary care in particular involve constant tension between diagnosis and elimination of the disease (cure) on one hand and alleviation of suffering in the context of disease and treatment (healing) on the other. In this context, *healing* means helping patients cope

Table 2-1 Principles of a Patient-Centered Medical Home

1. Access to care based on an ongoing relationship with a personal physician who is able to provide first-contact, continuous, and comprehensive care.
2. Care provided by a physician-led team of individuals within the practice who collectively take responsibility for the ongoing needs of patients.
3. Care based on a whole-person (holistic) orientation in which the practice team takes responsibility for either providing care that encompasses all patient needs or arranges for the care to be done by other qualified professionals.
4. Care coordinated and integrated across all elements of the complex health care system and the patient's community.
5. Care facilitated by the use of office practice systems (e.g., registries, information technology, health information exchange) to ensure that patients receive the indicated care when and where they need and want it in a culturally and linguistically appropriate manner.
6. Reimbursement structure that supports and encourages this model of care.

Modified from American College of Physicians. Joint principles of the patient-centered medical home, March 2007. http://www.acponline.org/advocacy/where_we_stand/medical_home/approve_jp.pdf.

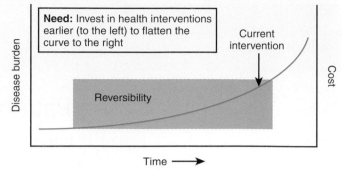

Figure 2-1 Profit in the current U.S. health care system is obtained focusing on the right of the curve. Investment toward the left of the curve will reduce disease burden and cost over time.

emotionally and practically with whatever condition they face, even when cure is not possible.

In *The Nature of Suffering and the Goals of Medicine*, Cassell (2004) elegantly describes this tension and the continual erosion of healing practices under the pressure to apply more specific, technologic cures. In *A Time to Heal*, Ludmerer (1999) documents how, despite decades of efforts in curriculum change, these core values of healing in medical education have failed to gain significant traction under the forces driving the payment for cure-seeking behaviors.

Thus, the physician seeking to create a medical home that balances cure and healing faces considerable challenges, especially in the delivery of healing. What are the essential components of such a health care home? How can they be delivered in the current medical context? What actions must the family physician take to create not only a practice that treats disease, but an optimal healing environment as well?

Balancing Treatment of Disease and Promotion of Health

Health is largely a result of positive lifestyle behaviors that are often challenging to change. Addressing issues such as smoking, obesity, substance abuse, and inactivity can reduce premature death by 40% (McGinnis et al., 2002; Schroeder, 2007). Positive lifestyle behaviors not only prevent premature death but also extend the average life expectancy by 14 years (Khaw et al., 2008). Currently, approximately 4 cents of every dollar spent for health care goes toward prevention and public health, with 96% spent on treating established disease (Lambrew, 2007). Two thirds of chronic disease is behavior related and could be mitigated by working interprofessionally to help guide patients toward healthy choices (McGinnis et al., 2002).

Behaviors that have the greatest impact on preventing chronic disease and its progression are (1) reducing exposure to toxic substances (tobacco, alcohol, drugs, pollution), (2) movement and exercise, (3) healthy diet, (4) psychosocial integration and stress management, and (5) early disease detection and intervention (Jonas, 2009; McGinnis, 2003). For these behaviors to have an impact, the health home will need to be financially supported and have the goal of health as its primary focus. This will require new forms of funding that go beyond the disease-focused throughput model of payment. A primary care clinic that only works from this model will encourage shorter office visits while promoting reliance on expensive technology that often suppresses symptoms without addressing its cause. The health home will push the curve in Figure 2-1 to the left and will involve professionals who specialize in health promotion (or creation) to flatten the curve and reduce the need for the "disease care" teams currently well established in the tertiary care setting.

Establishing an Optimal Healing Environment

An *optimal healing environment* (OHE) involves the delivery and context of medical treatment rather than the specific treatment itself. It focuses on creating healing in the process of disease treatment. This means optimizing the "meaning and context" effects of the care process rather than ignoring or dismissing them as "placebo" effects. An OHE involves attending to three primary domains of care delivery: (1) the "inner," personal environment of the team and patient; (2) the "inter," personal or relationship environment of care delivery; and (3) the "external" behavioral and physical environment of the medical home (Jonas et al., 2003).

Often, a "medicine" itself is given the most credit in medicine. A prescribed medication is valued for its "specific" medical influence, as deemed beneficial by randomized (placebo-)controlled trials (RCTs). This research focuses on the effects of the drug and attempts to control the context in order to reduce "nonspecific" (placebo) effects that may compromise the results. This helps physicians understand the specific effects of the drugs they prescribe, but it does not value those nonspecific effects that surround the prescribing of a medication. It is impossible, even undesirable, to remove all nonspecific effects from the patient encounter.

"Meaning" and "context" effects are rooted in relationship-centered care, including empathy, trust, empowerment, and hope. Research on one of the most frequently prescribed drugs in primary care, selective serotonin reuptake inhibitors (SSRIs), shows that these work only about 6% to 9% better than placebo (Kirsch et al., 2002; Turner et al., 2008). Both placebo and drug work well and are often almost 60%

Table 2-2 Optimal Healing Environments

Inner Environment to the Outer Environment						
Healing Intention	**Personal Wholeness**	**Healing Relationships**	**Healing Organizations**	**Healthy Lifestyles**	**Integrative Collaborative Medicine**	**Healing Spaces**
Expectation Hope Understanding Belief	Mind Body Spirit Family Community	Compassion Empathy Social support Communication	Leadership Mission Culture Teamwork	Diet Movement Relaxation Addictions	Person oriented Conventional Complementary Culturally appropriate	Nature Light Color Architecture
Enhance awareness expectancy.	Enhance personal integration.	Enhance caring communication.	Enhance delivery process.	Enhance healthy habits.	Enhance medical care.	Enhance healing structure.

Modified from Jonas WB, Chez RA. Toward optimal healing environments in health care. J Altern Complement Med 2004;10 Suppl 1:S1-S6.

effective. Therefore, if the drug only accounts for 9% of this effect, which factor accounts for the majority of the healing influence? Maybe researchers are not giving enough credit to the clinician and the nonspecific variables that surround the prescribing of the pill. Maybe it is simply the act of listening to people who are suffering and giving them a sense of understanding that there is something they can do to overcome the suffering. Maybe it is the interaction between two people before the medicine is prescribed that has the greatest healing effect. Psychiatrists gifted at developing a trusting relationship were found to have better effects with placebo in treating depression than their colleagues less talented at developing relationships who used active drug (McKay et al., 2006). Acupuncture delivered with a greater ritual produces better effects than the same points treated with less ritual (Kaptchuk et al., 2008; Kelley et al., 2009). Maybe it is the cost. Drugs that cost more (up to a certain point) work better in pain treatment than the same drugs that cost less (Waber et al., 2008).

Family physicians do not need to wait for further research to create an OHE for patient care. Physicians already know that the factors summarized in Table 2-2 will help encourage the healthy unfolding of complex systems. The most important part in influencing healing in others is focused on the left side of the table and starts with a self-reflective, internal process. Family physicians first need to understand the importance of continuously exploring their own health, so that they are prepared to do the same for their patients.

The Importance of Self-Care

To care deeply for others, we must know how to care for ourselves. As Cassell (2004) says, ". . . virtually all the doctor's healing power flows from the doctor's self-mastery." True primary care, therefore, also includes what we do for ourselves. Up to 60% of practicing physicians report symptoms of "burnout" (Shanafelt et al., 2003; Spickard et al., 2002). This is associated with emotional exhaustion, depersonalization (seeing patients as objects), reduced empathy, and the loss of meaning in work.

The characteristics lost in burnout are important ingredients in facilitating health and healing in others. If the health team physician leader is "burning out," the health home will not be healthy. When physicians practice healthy lifestyle behaviors, they are more likely to educate patients on the importance of these behaviors (Lewis et al., 1991) and to become more motivating to their patients toward positive change (Frank et al., 2000; Lobelo et al., 2009). Every family physician benefits from a self-reflective inquiry about personal balance toward health. This behavior will constantly be challenged and will require attention and "mastery."

Most primary care physicians are attracted into the field to make a difference in people's lives through continuous healing relationships. When the demands of the working environment tax the sense of control to maintain these relationships, stress and potential burnout can ensue. One remedy for this is to use the patient encounter to allow *meaning* to flow through the work. The healing-oriented primary care approach recognizes each patient as a unique individual with specific needs in the physical, emotional, and spiritual domains and sets aside both mental space and physical time to deal with those needs. To be aware of these personal needs is a mindful practice in which the physician is fully present in the moment with the patient, where each is able to reduce suffering in the other (Epstein, 1999). This "mindfulness" approach has been found to enhance well-being and physician attitudes in patient-centered care (Krasner et al., 2009). It requires that physicians create physical time in the health home to sit and listen to patient stories (Rakel, 2008).

Investing in Relationship

The medical home is just that, a "home" where someone feels welcome, known, and part of a community. The ongoing relationship with patients provides insight into the complexity of their health care needs and honors the interaction between multiple health perspectives. It allows the clinician to use evidence-based guidelines while realizing that variability is the norm. The best care for one individual may not be best for another. Patient-centered care recognizes that care should be focused on the needs of the individual patient, not simply on a disease state. Ideally, the goal should be "relationship centered," encouraging attention to the unique needs of the patient to be well. Thus, creating healing relationships is a core goal of an effective medical home (Chez and Jonas, 2005).

The evidence for the benefits of continuous, relationship-centered primary care is solid and growing. It has been found to improve quality of care (Starfield, 1991), reduce expenditures on diagnostic testing (Epstein et al., 2005), reduce hospital admissions (Gill and Mainous, 1998), and lower total health care costs (De Maeseneer et al., 2003). Having continuous, ongoing relationships with patients is often cited as the most rewarding aspect of being a family physician (Fairhurst and May, 2006). A systematic review of controlled trials on effective "team care," where relationship-centered factors are formalized in the care process, has demonstrated reduced mortality and morbidity, improved morale of health care workers, and reduced costs of health care (Safran et al., 2006).

One health care system that restructured its whole organization around establishing long-term, trusting, accountable relationships is the Southcentral Foundation Alaska Native Health Care model (Eby, 2007). This was the main request of the leaders of native Alaskans when they were asked what they wanted most in their public-owned health care system. Above all else, they valued the relationship with their physician, someone who "listens to them, takes time to explain things and who is able to coordinate effectively their overall care" (Gottlieb, 2007). The system made this its primary objective. After transforming their health model in 1999, urgent care and emergency department utilization decreased by 40%, specialist utilization by 50%, and hospitalization days by 30%. Customer satisfaction surveys showed that 91% rated their overall care as "favorable" (Gottlieb et al., 2008).

Empowerment

The greatest amount of suffering, disability, and cost occurs when the individual becomes more dependent on tertiary health care. The goal of the primary health team is to reduce this need. This requires that physicians empower individuals, families, and communities to understand what they can do to reduce the risk of disease and move the acuity curve in Figure 2-2 to the left. This will increase control of health by the individual, family, and community, with less dependence on the health care industry. To understand how best to work toward this goal, it is important to understand the process of empowerment.

Empowerment does not mean that patients do what is asked of them; this is *compliance*. Empowerment is the antithesis of compliance because noncompliance is two people working toward different goals. Empowerment is a way of interacting in which accurate information is provided in a manner understandable to the individual that both respects and promotes patients' ability to make decisions for themselves. A patient's decision making is the "inner," personal environment, influenced by external issues such as culture, family, peer group, work, and payment for care. Anderson and Funnell (2009) describe this well in their research on empowerment and diabetes care, reporting that 98% of diabetes care is "patient directed." When a patient is told to act a certain way, this is successful less than 5% of the time.

Empowerment is both a process and an outcome. The *process* requires that a health care partner recognizes individuals' unique needs and helps them think critically to make informed decisions on which they choose to act. This results in an *outcome* that individuals decide is best for them

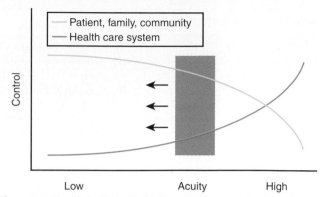

Figure 2-2 The Alaska Native Health Care model moved the slashed lines to the left, reducing dependence on the health care system and increasing control of the family. The goal is to flatten the curves to the right. The health care system should empower the family and community to maintain control of their health and make people less dependent on the "health rescue." *(Modified from Gottlieb K, Sylvester I, Eby D. Transforming your practice: what matters most. Fam Pract Manag 2008;15:32-38.)*

and their current situations. Health care practitioners cannot control their patients' decisions and thus cannot own the outcome. The clinician can recognize the psychosocial and emotional underpinnings that allow positive change to take place, then gradually and supportively work with the patient toward positive behaviors that the patient, family, and community can define with the guidance of their family physician. As the health guide of the community, the relationship-centered health home requires the development of health teams to facilitate this change.

Health Teams

Health-focused care requires that primary care physicians evolve beyond "physician-centered care" that is restricted by the dwindling access of the one-on-one physician visit. The family physician of the future can be a leader in the creation of a team of health professionals who provide multiple paths to access care (Figure 2-3) (Grumbach and Bodenheimer, 2004). This may involve group visits, phone contact, and information technology. The goal should be a proactive, collaborative team effort toward meeting patient goals, not just expecting adherence to treatment guidelines (Nutting et al., 2009).

In 2003 the Robert Wood Johnson Foundation supported research to bring behavior change initiatives into primary care to address inactivity, unhealthy eating, smoking, and risky drinking (Cifuentes et al., 2005). Lessons learned from 17 practice-based research networks showed that health behavior change resources are enthusiastically received by practices and patients (Cohen et al., 2005; Woolf et al., 2005), and that practices that use multifaceted team-based interventions are more effective in promoting healthy behaviors than those providing isolated therapy (Goldstein et al., 2004; Prada, 2006; Solberg et al., 2000; Woolf et al., 2005).

When working within teams, it is important to understand the difference among multidisciplinary, interdisciplinary, and transdisciplinary team models (Table 2-3). Traditional *multidisciplinary* teams are often focused on disease states and are limited to specific organ systems. In multidisciplinary teams, clinicians work in isolation, with limited

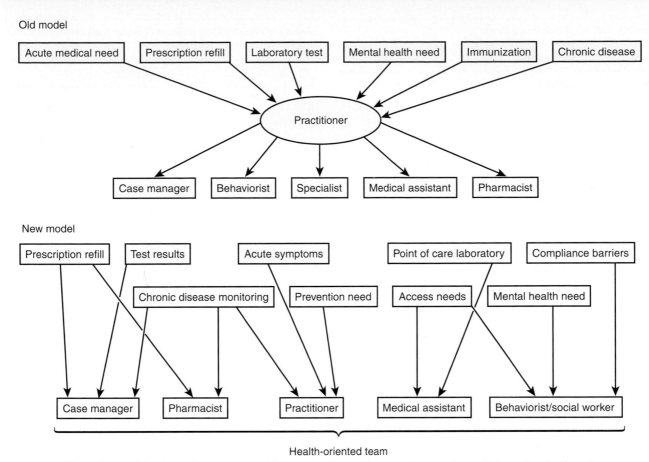

Figure 2-3 Traditional model versus new model of care showing multiple ways to access the health home (medical home).

communication and collaboration. These models tend to focus on body parts or systems in isolation, not recognizing their interdependency. Developing a common goal of health facilitation allows professionals to come together to develop *interdisciplinary* teams that encourage insight toward new ways of problem solving not previously in the group's collective consciousness. When this new insight develops, the interdisciplinary team becomes a *transdisciplinary* team as its members develop novel ways to create (or promote) health that transcend the "siloed" model of care (Choi and Pak, 2006; Soklaridis et al., 2007).

Who Should Compose the Health Team?

The family physician knows the population of the community served and their specific health care needs. This insight will define the professionals who will be of most benefit for health creation (promotion). For example, obesity is a significant health threat in many locales. A team of professionals working together toward sustained optimal weight for patients might include a registered dietician, an exercise physiologist, and a psychologist or mind-body practitioner, to understand the interplay between stress and eating. The process to develop a health-oriented team for musculoskeletal health (back pain) is summarized in Table 2-4.

The health team may look different from a disease team, but there will be obvious overlap. A health home may include a nutritionist who works with diabetic patients. This team member can also provide counseling for prediabetic persons and overweight youths, to prevent the expression of a disease that is often the result of lifestyle choices.

Health Team Models

There are many ways to develop health-oriented teams. The approach will depend on the needs of patients, the availability of team members, the size of the clinic, strategic planning, and the support of administration and clinic staff. Teams can be initiated in all sizes of clinics, from large, complex institutions to small, rural settings, and may take many forms. For example, a team may include only the family physician and two health coaches or medical assistants. This "teamlet" model extends the office visit to include communication before the visit, after the visit, and between visits (Bodenheimer and Laing, 2007). The teamlet uses these opportunities to address patient needs and develops appropriate strategies. The health team's common mission is working toward the greatest improvement in the patient's quality of life. If the group agrees to work toward uncovering root causes of symptoms, this common goal will progress to disease resolution.

The team does not need to share the same space as long as they maintain communication and build intermember relationships. This will help clinicians learn of each other's interests and talents in relation to common goals, fostering mutual understanding, trust, and respect. Without the team concept, there will simply be separate therapies and professionals working in isolation, causing fragmentation of care.

Table 2-3 Defining Disciplinary Teams

Term	Definition
Multidisciplinary team	**Additive.** "Comprised of more than two professionals from different health care disciplines who work with the same patient, set of patients, or clinical condition, but provide care independently of each other" (Interdisciplinary Team Building). For example, a patient may have visits with both a primary care practitioner (PCP) and physical therapist (PT). Although the PCP may view clinical notes or a report from the PT, the two disciplines usually do not interact.
Interdisciplinary team	**Interactive.** An ongoing and integrated care team of one patient, set of patients, or clinical condition. Team members develop collegial relationships with shared goals and joint decision making. They interact, supporting as well as questioning each other's opinions, and negotiate to develop health strategies based on the needs of the individual.
Transdisciplinary team	**Holistic.** Professionals learn from each other and in the process transcend traditional disciplinary boundaries, which may result in new knowledge. Often, the greater the difference between professions (epistemologic distance; e.g., engineering and humanities), the more likely insight will develop toward the creation of a new way to solve a problem.

Data from Choi BC, Pak AW. Multidisciplinarity, interdisciplinarity and transdisciplinarity in health research, services, education and policy. 1. Definitions, objectives, and evidence of effectiveness. 3. Discipline, inter-discipline distance, and selection of discipline. Clin Invest Med 2006;29:351-64; 2008;31:E41-E48.

Table 2-4 Health-Oriented Team Creation Worksheet (Example: Achieving Optimal Back Health)

Task	Action
Health need of my community	Achieving optimal back health
Identify professionals to address health need.	1. Manual practitioner 2. Physical therapist 3. Psychologist/"mindfulness" instructor 4. Health coach
Delineate the team-focused goal/mission.	To empower patients to learn how to achieve their ideal back function and health.
Name the health-oriented program.	"Back to Health" program
Create relationships between team members.	Team members to meet initially to develop program goal/mission and methods of interacting. Periodic meetings as needed for team building and interactions around patient issues.
Agree on team communication method.	Fax or e-mail will be sent to the team for referrals, findings, and discussion.
Follow up and promote sustainability.	Patient will meet periodically with health coach/nurse at the medical home to sustain lifestyle behaviors.

The most important ingredient in effective teams is trust—trust that each team member will play his or her particular part in care delivery and process improvement (Sargeant et al., 2008). Changing to an effective team approach takes humility and time and requires constant fine-tuning and quality improvement. However, the physician can begin in any domain that fits the readiness of the practice (see Table 2-4), and the effects will often spread to other domains. The following checklist provides some places to start in a practice assessment format.

The Health Home Checklist

- Create a "home" where those who enter feel known and welcome. Patients will remember how they *felt* in a health home longer than what they are told.
- Create a common mission supported by all health home members; for example, "To invest in a continuous healing relationship with the well-being of the community we serve."
- Provide multiple ways to access care from the most appropriate health professional (see Figure 2-3).
- Provide a variety of encounter visits that complement the one-on-one office visit. These may include group visits, e-mail, support groups, and health promotion or disease-focused programs.
- Create relationships through open communication with a team of health professionals who can positively influence lifestyle behaviors or address specific disease states.

- Provide a way for the consumers (patients) to have input into what health-related programs or services are implemented based on their perceived needs.
- Provide an opportunity to understand the most important areas that patients believe need to be addressed for their long-term health. (See the Health Agreement document online at www.expertconsult.com.)
- Learn to provide rapid and evidence-based information on lifestyle and complementary medicine in each team encounter.
- Review the space of the practice, and develop a plan to make it less stress inducing and more comfortable to the patient and team members.
- Make sure the health home that is created matches that which gives family physicians meaning and purpose in their work. This will translate across the medical home, encouraging team acceptance while reducing the risk of burnout.

Conclusion

Creating optimal healing environments with health-oriented teams honors the concepts of the medical home as primary care physicians transition to health as a critical focus (see Table 2-2). This is an exciting opportunity for professionals from varied disciplines to come together to work toward a common goal and honors specific expertise. The family physician's expertise in understanding the multiple, complex systems working toward the patient's unique goal of health leads the implementation of these model health homes.

The gift of primary care is the human connection that occurs within continuous healing relationships. Family physicians will succeed in providing efficient, cost-effective quality care if they invest in aspects of care that are the most valuable yet most difficult to measure. The most important area is the nonquantifiable process occurring between the practitioner and patient in which both are transformed (Scott et al., 2008).

EVIDENCE-BASED SUMMARY

- Positive lifestyle behaviors have the largest effect on reducing morbidity and mortality (Khaw et al., 2008; McGinnis et al., 2002; Schroeder, 2007) (SOR: A).
- Team-based interventions are more effective in promoting healthy behaviors than are those that provide isolated therapy (Woolf et al., 2005, Safran et al., 2006) (SOR: B).
- Relationship-centered care improves quality of care (Starfield, 1991) (SOR: B).
- Relationship-centered care reduces health care costs (De Maeseneer et al., 2003; Epstein et al., 2005) (SOR: B).

References

The complete reference list is available online at www.expertconsult.com.

Web Resources

www.pcpcc.net/content/emmi
Videos to educate staff and colleagues about the patient-centered medical home (PCMH).

www.transformed.com/resources/pcmh.cfm
Resources for transforming a medical practice to a medical home.

www.aafp.org/pcmh
Resources on PCMH from the TransforMED project and the AAFP.

www.transformed.com/mhiq/welcome.cfm
Module to calculate your medical home IQ. Gives a baseline practice assessment toward the creation of a medical home.

www.transformed.com/Delta-Exchange
A community of clinicians, tools, and resources to help clinics transform to a PCMH (requires a monthly fee).

www.cfah.org/pdfs/PACT_Guide_0109.pdf
Guide for creating a patient information guide about your medical home.

www.samueliinstitute.org/research/research-home/optimalhealing.html
A guide for creating an optimal healing environment in health care.

3 CHAPTER

Psychosocial Influences on Health

Syed M. Ahmed, Jeanne P. Lemkau, and Paul J. Hershberger

Chapter contents

Key Points

- Factors that influence health include age, gender, and sexual orientation.
- Religious, ethnic, and cultural groups affect individual functioning.
- Individuals are affected by family composition, structure, and functioning.
- The health of an individual is influenced by work and school status.
- Individuals are affected by their social support network and significant others.
- Financial resources, including health insurance status, affect health status.
- Personal and family history of major loss, trauma, or illness should be integrated into the assessment of a patient's health status.
- Psychological functioning, including personality, defensive style, and current mental status, warrant evaluation.
- Data about the patient's physical environment, including home, neighborhood, and environmental hazards, are essential.
- The physician should elicit an account of recent stressors and changes in the patient's life.
- Collaborative physician-patient relationships that emphasize physician listening form the context for sensitive psychosocial care.

- An overweight 11-year-old boy with abnormal lipids tells his family physician that his favorite activity is playing online video games.
- A middle-aged woman emphatically asserts that her blood pressure is elevated only when she has it taken in a medical setting.
- A single mother with a part-time job but no health insurance tells her doctor that she can only take medications that have a co-pay of a few dollars.

Psychosocial factors influence health. Assessing and treating patients in a manner that integrates psychosocial and biologic aspects of care are the essence of excellent family medicine and its greatest challenges. The following example is illustrative.

Mr. Ramirez is a 52-year-old man who lost his well-paying job as a software engineer several years ago. After 8 months of unemployment, he took a less satisfying job for less money. Mr. Ramirez has type 2I diabetes, diagnosed when he was 45 years old and well-controlled before he lost his job. He has taken diabetes education classes and can accurately describe what he must do to maintain good glucose control. Reluctantly, Mr. Ramirez acknowledges to his physician that he doesn't follow his diet as closely as he once did and more frequently eats fast food. He also misses the exercise facility at his former workplace and struggles with motivation to exercise. His marriage "isn't as good as it used to be," and he reports decreased interest in sex. When the physician asks him about feelings of depression, Mr. Ramirez says that he never thought he was a weak person, but he just doesn't enjoy things as he once did. His physician emphasizes the changes Mr. Ramirez has experienced in the past few years and the emotional toll of such stress. She briefly describes how stress and depression make diabetes more difficult to control, and how she and Mr. Ramirez can collaboratively work on strategies to improve his health and quality of life.

This case highlights the following three imperatives for providing care that is appropriately responsive to psychosocial issues:

1. The physician *sees the person first*, conceptualizing symptoms and behaviors in their social and psychological context and responding with sensitivity to the patient's experience and priorities.
2. The physician *understands the interactive nature of multiple biopsychosocial variables* and communicates this effectively to the patient.

3. The physician *fosters a supportive and empathic physician-patient relationship* to provide the foundation for gathering information and intervening effectively.

As the case illustrates, biomedical factors may be only a small part of what patients bring to their physicians. The *biomedical model,* based on the assumptions of mind-body dualism, biologic reductionism, and linear causality, has resulted in miraculous achievements of high-technology medicine, but primary care physicians who restrict their attention to purely medical considerations are of limited use to their patients. Nevertheless, the shift from a biomedical to a biopsychosocial paradigm has been a major challenge to modern medicine.

In 1977, psychiatrist George Engel proposed a *biopsychosocial model* that included social and psychological variables as crucial determinants of disease and illness. According to his new framework, the subsystems of the body interact to produce successively more complex biologic systems, which are simultaneously affected by social and psychological factors. The organism is thus conceptualized in terms of complex interacting systems of biologic, psychological, and social forces, and neither disease nor illness is seen as understandable only in terms of smaller and smaller biologic components. Engel (1980) believed that systemic interactions of biopsychosocial factors were relevant to all disease processes and to the individual's experience of illness. Accordingly, understanding a person's response to a disease requires consideration of such interacting factors as the social and cultural environment, the individual's psychological resources, and the biochemistry and genetics of the disorder in the population (Brody, 1999).

In the following section, we present a number of conceptual models and perspectives that emphasize different but overlapping psychosocial dimensions that influence health (Table 3-1). These models can aid practicing physicians in thinking about their patients in a psychosocial context and conceptualizing potentially helpful interventions. Subsequently, we elaborate on practical strategies for gathering and using psychosocial information in clinical practice and discuss a pragmatic approach to addressing psychosocial considerations in primary care. We conclude with brief discussions of evidence-based practice and how current challenges and trends in the health care system may affect the practice of family medicine.

Conceptual Models

The Biopsychosocial Model

As previously noted, the biopsychosocial model was proposed as a scientific paradigm by Engel (1977), who encouraged the clinician to observe biochemical and morphologic changes in relation to a patient's emotional patterns, life goals, attitudes toward illness, and social environment. Engel proposed that the brain and peripheral organs were linked in complex, mutually adjusting relationships, affected by changes in social as well as physical stimuli. Within this model, environmental and psychological stress is seen as potentially pathogenic for the individual. Emotions may serve as the organism's bridge between the meaning (or significance) of stressful events and the changes in physiologic function (Zegans, 1983). Engel urged physicians to evaluate the patient on biologic, psychological, and social factors in order to understand and manage clinical problems effectively (Wise, 1997). For example, a workplace accident could be seen as resulting from poorly designed equipment (social) and inattentiveness (psychological) brought about by low blood sugar (biologic). Similarly, the accident could result in damage to internal organs (biologic), distress (psychological), and lost income (social), any or all of which may become the focus of physician intervention.

Comprehensive evaluation of biopsychosocial dimensions would assess the following:

- *Biologic factors,* including genetics, medical history, and environmental factors that affect physiologic functioning (e.g., those causing cancer).
- *Psychological factors,* including affective, cognitive, and behavioral components, such as feelings, beliefs, expectations, personality, coping style, and health behaviors (e.g., exercise, diet, smoking), which are contributors to patients' experience of health and illness.
- *Social factors,* including access to health care, quality of available health care, social systems (e.g., family, school, work, church, government), social values, customs, and social support.

Further discussion of biologic influences on health is beyond the scope of this chapter. Psychological and social factors known to affect health are discussed next.

Psychological Factors

The numerous theories about personality in human history reflect a variety of cultural, religious, philosophic, and scientific perspectives. Two of these, "hardiness" and the five-factor model, are discussed here. We also review key features of the literature on the relationship between emotions and health.

Hardiness is one personality construct that has received considerable research support in explaining who does and who does not become sick under stress (Kobasa, 1979). Hardiness includes three characteristics (Table 3-2): (1) a strong sense of *personal control;* (2) *commitment,* a sense of purpose or involvement in events or activities; and (3) *challenge,* the ability to see change as an opportunity for growth. Kobasa and her colleagues (1982) demonstrated that people with high levels of the "three Cs" of control, commitment, and challenge tended to remain healthier than their less hardy

Table 3-1 Psychosocial Influences: Conceptual Models

Biopsychosocial model
Systems approach
Stress and coping model
Life span perspective
Ethnomedical cultural model

Table 3-2 The Three "C"s of Hardiness

Control: having a sense of personal control of the future.
Commitment: sense of commitment and purpose in life.
Challenge: seeing change as a challenge or opportunity.

Table 3-3 Five-Factor Model of Personality

1. Openness to experience: tendency to be curious and appreciative of a variety of experience.
2. Conscientiousness: proclivity to be self-disciplined, to plan, and to direct behavior toward achieving goals.
3. Extraversion: reference for being around other people, to be enthusiastic and socially energetic.
4. Agreeableness: inclination to be cooperative with others, strongly preferring harmony over disagreement.
5. Neuroticism: propensity to experience negative emotions on an ongoing and regular basis.

counterparts. Studies show that illness increased with stress and decreased with greater hardiness and exercise. A physician's knowledge of a patient's degree of hardiness may help in assessing the patient's response to stressors.

The most prominent approach to personality at present is the *five-factor model* (Goldberg, 1993). The five broad personality domains in this model, for which OCEAN can be an acronym, are *openness* to experience, *conscientiousness*, *extraversion*, *agreeableness*, and *neuroticism* (Table 3-3). Research on the relationship of these factors to health variables has generated several findings. *Conscientiousness* has been associated with longevity among healthy individuals and better functional status in those with physical illnesses or impairments, whereas *neuroticism* is consistently found to be negatively correlated with health (Goodwin and Friedman, 2006; Smith and Mackenzie, 2006). *Agreeableness, extraversion,* and *openness* to experience generally tend to have weaker associations with health and therefore are considered less relevant to understanding links between personality and health.

Because personality style is regarded as stable across the life span, physician focus on changing personality for health reasons is not a sensible pursuit. However, viewing personality from a broader perspective, with specific regard to how individuals experience and manage emotion, does offer the physician more latitude in intervention.

The experience of *chronic negative emotions* (depression, anxiety, and anger) tends to be associated with poorer health. There is an extensive research literature linking negative affectivity and pessimism to adverse health outcomes (Peterson et al., 1988; Salovey et al., 2000). Although the experience of negative emotions is a natural part of the human experience, effective management of such emotions through cognitive strategies, active coping, and social support can be learned, and medications can be a helpful adjunct when negative emotional states are prolonged or severe.

Likewise, a large body of research indicates that *positive* emotional states are associated with better health and longevity. Happiness, optimism, and positive attitudes toward aging have been associated with 7 more years of life (Danner et al., 2001; Levy et al., 2002). Almost three decades of research have shown that an optimistic outlook has a positive effect on coping and on mental and physical health outcomes (Peterson and Steen, 2002). Family physicians have long recognized the importance of mobilizing and maintaining patient hopefulness through encouraging words that foster positive expectations of medical treatment. Additionally, the demonstrated efficacy of placebos affirms the importance of this approach (Sobel, 1991).

Social Factors

A gradient between socioeconomic status (SES) and health is consistently found in epidemiologic studies (Marmot, 2004). Persons with less education and income tend to have poorer health than their better-educated and richer counterparts. Interestingly, subjective SES (i.e., individuals' perceptions of where they view themselves on the social ladder) has an even stronger relationship to health than objective SES (Singh-Manoux et al., 2005). Negative affect, stress, pessimism, and a decreased sense of control are among the factors thought to contribute to the relationship between lower subjective SES and poorer health (Operario et al., 2004).

In general, social support reduces stress and contributes to more positive health outcomes. *Social support* refers to the process by which a social network provides psychological and material resources to enhance an individual's ability to cope with stress (Cohen, 2004). Both quantity and quality of support are important, and sources of support include spouse, lover, friends, family, co-workers, and health care professionals. A person who has many friends but no confidant may have inadequate social support in a time of need. Some people report high levels of satisfaction with just a few close friends, whereas others require larger social networks.

There are several varieties of social support (Cohen, 2004). *Emotional support* involves the expression of caring, concern, and empathy toward the person and typically involves opportunities for the recipient to express emotions and vent. *Instrumental support* involves providing some type of direct assistance, which might include financial resources, transportation, or help with daily tasks. *Informational support* involves giving advice or providing relevant information to an individual.

Social support appears to undergird health by buffering the person against negative effects of stress, perhaps by affecting the cognitive appraisal of stress. When people encounter a strong stressor, such as a major financial crisis, individuals with high levels of social support may appraise the situation as less stressful than will those with low levels of support. Social support may further buffer the stress by modifying people's response to a stressor as they turn to friends for advice, reassurance, or material aid. Social integration, or participating in a broad range of social relationships, benefits health and well-being by enhancing self-esteem and fostering positive health behaviors in people who believe that others count on them. Social integration is beneficial, whether or not an individual is experiencing stress (Cohen, 2004).

Relationships also can involve significant negative social exchange and be harmful to health. For example, negative interactions in troubled marriages have adverse effects on cardiovascular, endocrine, and immune system function (Robles and Kiecolt-Glaser, 2003).

Misconceptions

Polan (1993) identified and addressed two common misconceptions about the biopsychosocial model. First, contrary to popular belief, the physician who is "humanistic" is not necessarily practicing biopsychosocial medicine. A physician can be ethical and caring but still neglect scientific knowledge from psychology, sociology, anthropology, and relevant data from the patient's life. For example, compassion by itself is of limited usefulness to a physician who needs an effective treatment plan for an asthmatic patient who smokes. Knowledge of the social environment and of the individual psychology of the patient is crucial.

The second common misconception is that people can be reduced to distinct biologic, psychological, and social categories, or that problems can then be expressed as a set of scientific principles from which diagnosis and treatment can be neatly derived. In fact, use of the biopsychosocial model *increases* rather than decreases the level of complexity required to understand patient status, introducing multiple avenues for intervention. Interpreting the biopsychosocial model as a new opportunity for reductionist thinking diminishes the power to inform more holistic treatment. Borrell-Carrio and colleagues (2004) proposed a biopsychosocially oriented clinical practice, based on self-awareness, active cultivation of trust, an emotional style characterized by empathic curiosity, self-calibration to reduce bias, cultivation of emotional sensitivity to assist with diagnosis and therapeutic relationships, use of informed intuition, and communication of clinical evidence to foster dialogue.

The Systems Approach

Humans are infinitely complex. Adequately conceptualizing a person in health or illness requires a systems approach that encompasses this complexity. The concept of *systems* was first developed by von Bertalanffy (1968) to refer to the dynamic interrelationships of various components. A systems approach rejects the notion of linear causality in favor of multidimensional and multidirectional models.

The systems approach has strongly influenced conceptualizations of family functioning. Smilkstein (1978) developed one of the first applications of "family systems" thinking for family medicine. Physician attention is important to the systemic interactions of family members and the impact of crisis, coping styles, and resources on family functioning. He incorporated these components into the "family APGAR"

(*a*daptation, *p*artnership, *g*rowth, *a*ffection, and *r*esolve), a simple instrument and mnemonic device for assessing the functioning of a family system in health and illness (not to be confused with the newborn Apgar score).

The Stress and Coping Model

General relationships among life stresses, coping resources, and health outcomes are presented schematically in Figure 3-1. This approach represents another example of the application of a systems model. As this model illustrates, health outcomes are impacted by how life stresses affect the individual. The effect of stress is moderated by the individual's appraisal and coping responses, personality, and the person's available social resources. Although the complex synergistic interactions that characterize these relationships are beyond the scope of this chapter, the major variables provide a basis for considering physician interventions.

Definitions of Stress

Stress has been variously defined as an environmental event, a response to an event or circumstances, and a process. One approach defines stress in terms of life events—as a stimulus—circumstances or events that require the person to adapt produce feelings of tension. These *stressors* may be major catastrophic events (e.g., natural disaster), major life events (e.g., death of a loved one), or recurrent daily hassles (e.g., need to manage a chronic medical condition).

Stress can also be seen as a response. For example, a person with a social phobia feels stressed in a social setting such as a party, experiencing a psychological state of nervousness with associated physical symptoms of dry mouth, palpitations, and sweating. This physiologic and psychological response to a stressor is often called *strain*.

A third approach emphasizes stress as a process in which "environmental demands tax or exceed the adaptive capacity of an organism, resulting in psychological and biologic

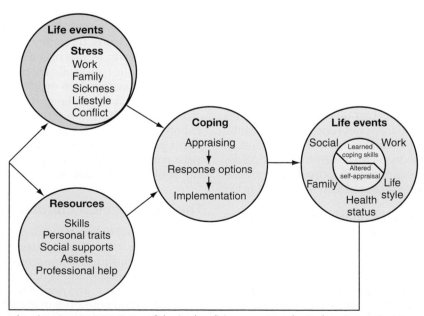

Figure 3-1 Stress, life events, and coping. *(From Tunks E, Bellissimo A. Behavioral medicine: concepts and procedures. Boston, Allyn & Bacon. Copyright © 1991 Person Education.)*

changes that may place persons at risk for disease" (Cohen et al., 1995). Within this approach, stress includes stressors and strains, along with the relationship between the person and the environment. The process involves transactions between the person and the environment, with each affecting and being affected by the other (Sarafino, 1990). "Adaptive capacity" is operationalized in terms of resilience and vulnerability; the physician considers aspects of a person's psychological makeup and social world that may render the patient more susceptible or more resilient (Steptoe, 1998).

Stress Appraisal and Coping

Every family physician sees patients under stress who present with a wide spectrum of stress-related symptoms and coping responses. How the individual interprets and copes with stress is as significant as the stressor itself. Cognitive appraisal of a stressor, rather than severity or duration alone, determines physiologic and behavioral responses (Epel et al., 1998).

Coping refers to how individuals manage the real or imagined discrepancy between environmental demands and their resources for addressing the stressful situation. According to Lazarus and Folkman (1984), adaptation to stress is mediated by appraisal (i.e., personal meaning of a stressor and one's sense of resources for dealing with it) and coping (i.e., thoughts and behaviors used to manage stress). With emotion-focused coping, a person directs energy to regulating internal feeling states, whereas with problem-focused coping, a person directs attention to reducing the stressor or expanding resources for dealing with it (Sarafino, 1990). The effect of stressful life events on health is determined by many factors related to coping, such as cognitive style, personality characteristics, and social and behavioral tendencies.

Personal Control

An individual's perception of the extent of his or her control in a stressful circumstance is a critical component of the appraisal process in coping. This includes control over the stressor or circumstances as well as control over one's responses, whether problem focused or emotion focused. How a person deals with the loss of control precipitated by stressful life events can affect health outcomes.

Personal control can be defined as the feeling that one can make decisions and take effective action to produce desirable outcomes and avoid undesirable ones (Rodin, 1986). Mobilizing a strong sense of personal control can significantly reduce the impact of stressors on the individual, particularly when the response is appropriate to the circumstance. Sarafino (1990) classified personal control into the following five types:

1. *Behavioral control* involves the ability to take concrete action to reduce the impact of a stressor; for example, using a special breathing technique to reduce pain.
2. *Cognitive control* involves the ability to use thought processes or strategies to modify the impact of a stressor. For example, focusing on a pleasant thought during suturing of a laceration may decrease the pain sensation.
3. *Decisional control* involves the opportunity to choose between alternative procedures or courses of action. For example, a victim of domestic violence may benefit from considering various options when and how she will leave her abuser.
4. *Informational control* involves the opportunity to obtain knowledge about a stressful event, what will happen, why, and what consequences are likely. For example, a patient may decrease anxiety regarding upcoming surgery when he learns more about managing discomfort from the procedure.
5. *Retrospective control* involves beliefs about causation of a stressful event after it has occurred. The attribution that the person makes about the adversity can affect future perspective and behavior. For example, attributing misfortune for factors that are temporary and specific leaves an individual feeling more optimistic than when misfortune is attributed to stable and global factors (Seligman, 1990).

Life stresses affect health outcomes. These effects are moderated not only by individual differences in genetics and pathophysiology, but also by psychosocial factors. Psychosocial influences include appraisal and coping, personality traits, cognitive styles, and resources (including social support).

The Life Span Perspective

The life span perspective emphasizes the importance of an individual's place on his or her personal developmental trajectory. Past development, current status, and anticipated developmental changes and challenges are taken into account. On the biologic level, changes in cellular functions occur from infancy through old age; decline in physical stamina is one manifestation of this dynamic change. On the psychological level, personality interacts with ongoing changes that occur across the life span (e.g., becoming a parent), and each developmental stage brings its own psychosocial challenges. Erikson's eight stages of development highlight the importance of trust issues in infancy, autonomy issues in early childhood, and issues of generativity and meaning in old age (Erickson, 1959). On the social level, family and peer relationships change throughout life, with significant implications for health, which may be either positive or negative. For example, the typical adolescent's shift toward greater reliance on peer relationships may lead to behaviors that endanger health, such as smoking or substance abuse. The death of a husband who has been physically abusive may lead to improved well-being for the surviving wife. The primary care physician needs to keep the life span model in mind and assist patients in addressing psychosocial factors that facilitate or block health and development.

The Ethnomedical Cultural Model

Every encounter between a patient and a physician is a cross-cultural transaction. Each person brings to the physician-patient relationship a unique mix of culturally embedded attitudes, knowledge, and beliefs. Ethnicity, gender, religion, language, education, and personal history shape expectations and behavior on both sides of the relationship. A physician's cultural proficiency is instrumental in establishing rapport and gathering information for accurate and comprehensive diagnosis and treatment (Carrillo et al., 1999). The patient's acculturation status and cultural background are important to understand, and physicians should become familiar with the dominant cultural groups they serve.

The ethnomedical cultural model emphasizes cultural concepts relevant to health and illness (Kleinman et al., 1978), including patient beliefs and expectations about the body, illness, and treatment. Berlin and Fowkes (1983) operationalize this model in clinical encounters with their LEARN acronym, exhorting physicians to do the following:

- Listen with empathy and understanding to a patient's perception of the problem by eliciting the patient's explanatory model for the illness.
- Explain your perceptions or explanatory model in language the patient can understand.
- Acknowledge the differences and similarities between your explanatory model and that of the patient, and discuss any significant discrepancies.
- Recommend treatment that you decide is optimal within your explanatory model.
- Negotiate treatment with the patient, seeking a compromise that is acceptable to the patient, is consistent with your ethical standards, and uses the patient's social network when necessary.

The ethnomedical cultural model highlights cross-cultural elements in all physician-patient interactions.

Integration of Psychosocial Issues in Clinical Practice

Wynne (2003) states, "In the 'real' world of health care, systems thinking is more needed than ever before, but its increased complexity challenges both clinicians and researchers to the depths of their resources." Knowledge, attitudes, beliefs, emotions, behaviors, relationships, and social environmental interact to affect the experience of illness or well-being. Accordingly, physicians' ability to promote health and relieve suffering depends on their ability to engage effectively in this complex web of interrelationships. This is a daunting task that depends on fostering a quality relationship over time, gathering sufficient biopsychosocial data about a particular patient, and integrating data with theoretic understanding to inform interventions.

The challenge for even the most astute physician is to assess and address psychosocially important issues within the limited time available for each patient. In a 10- to 15-minute period, a detailed evaluation of all relevant psychosocial factors is an impractical goal. Using a pragmatic approach that balances this goal with time constraints, a physician can maintain awareness of psychosocial cues and information in all patient encounters while restricting direct inquiry, depending on the specific situation. A physician may not need to elicit a detailed psychosocial assessment with every patient who presents with an upper respiratory infection, but knowing if the patient smokes would be useful, leading to further inquiry and potential smoking intervention.

Following pragmatic considerations, a physician should work collaboratively with patients to identify problems of highest priority and to address different issues in different encounters. For example, in the case of domestic violence, immediate needs for patient safety must be addressed. Addressing long-standing issues, such as dysfunctional means of coping with stress, must be a secondary concern in the face of the primary need to achieve safety. Similarly, every physician learns to place high priority on patient complaints of chest pain, adjusting questioning depending on the patient's age, gender, family history of coronary heart disease, and patient medical history. Nevertheless, the physician must look for psychosocial clues, evaluate stressors, and be aware of factors that suggest an anxiety or somatization disorder. These secondary factors can be addressed in more depth when the physician is assured that a cardiac crisis is not imminent.

Collection of Psychosocial Data

In family practice settings, the most common and natural approach to gathering psychosocial data is interviewing the patient over time. Freud suggested that the major achievements of healthy development were the abilities "to work and to love," and this is often a good place to start, even in the first contact with a physician. Where does this patient work, and how does he or she feel about the job, school, or household responsibilities? Who is "family" for this patient, and what is the nature of the support system? Detailed inquiries about work and love made in the context of the ongoing physician-patient relationship result in significant accretion of knowledge over time and make it easy to flag stressful changes in these important arenas.

Other important areas of inquiry include the patient's physical and social environment. Factors such as the quality of housing, neighborhood, food, and financial resources all affect patient safety, health care use, family stress, and physical health. Understanding the ethnic, religious, and political culture of a patient and family is important for guiding culturally appropriate care. Personal and family history, usually gathered gradually over time, can alert the physician to important family coping patterns, strengths, and liabilities. Of special importance is information on major personal family "dislocations," including losses, illness, and trauma. Knowledge of traumatic patient encounters with previous medical care may alert the physician to anticipate and manage potential crisis situations.

Information from patient dialogue can be supplemented by standard measures such as health questionnaires (e.g., SF 36), screening inventories (e.g., Beck Depression Inventory), and stress, coping, and social support tools. Other areas include interviews with family members, including structured assessments (e.g., family APGAR); review of existing records (e.g., school records); consultation with multidisciplinary colleagues (e.g., psychologist, occupational therapist); observation of the patient's environment through home visits; and consultation with cultural informants and translators when needed.

Interventions Using Psychosocial Data

A comprehensive review of interventions addressing psychosocial influences in health is beyond the scope of this chapter and would require discussions of clinical psychology, social work, nursing, occupational therapy, and public health. Even in optimal circumstances, competency can be achieved only within a limited range. Realistically, family physicians should achieve basic proficiency in selected interventional strategies and pursue additional training in areas of interest relevant to their specific practice needs. Here we discuss pragmatic interventions for practicing physicians based on the general model of stress, life events, coping, and health discussed earlier.

Because health outcomes are affected by stressful life events, coping (e.g., stress appraisal), and resources (e.g., personality, social support), addressing any dimension can have a positive effect on functioning. As stress increases relative to available support and coping capacities, disequilibrium results. Increases in stress or decreases in social support tend to destabilize functioning, and various factors can contribute to exacerbating or mitigating stress. For example, a new medical diagnosis is stressful, whereas a loving partnership is a source of support and will tend to ease stress. Some life events, such as the death of a supportive partner, affect several elements in the model, as the bereaved partner confronts a major loss (stress) without the person who had previously offered comfort in such times (decreased support). Accordingly, persons who are grieving are at higher risk for experiencing health problems (Rogers and Reich, 1988).

Interventions that should be part of the standard repertoire for family physicians are those that do no harm, usually help, and employ traditional skills. Specifically, physicians can work with patients directly to reduce stress, to enhance or mobilize social support resources, and to reinforce or model positive stress appraisal and coping. *Direct approaches* to stress reduction may include intervening in the patient's environment (e.g., arranging respite care for an older patient to relieve stress on his middle-aged daughter) and allaying a patient's unrealistic fears about an illness. *Social support* can be enhanced directly through the provision of more contact with the physician or indirectly through mobilizing the patient to increase contact with family or friends. Physicians can support *positive coping* through instilling hope, modeling optimism, and encouraging patients who adapt. Reminding patients of personal strengths previously used to confront crises is also helpful. The physician often can implement these strategies through the process of asking questions that allow the patient to respond in a broader perspective (e.g., "What do you remember doing to help you cope with the death of your good friend several years ago?"). Especially when behavior change is indicated, collaborating rather than giving advice is more likely to be effective. One collaborative approach that has demonstrated efficacy is motivational interviewing (Rollnick et al., 2008; Rubac et al., 2005).

In the provision of care within a biopsychosocial model, interdisciplinary teams, rather than solo practitioners, have the advantage, and physicians can have more positive impact on their patients' lives when they harness the wisdom of colleagues from other fields through referral or consultation. Depending on physician training, interest, and time, these basic categories of intervention can be supplemented by a wide range of psychosocial interventions, from family therapy to behavior modification.

Important Times for Psychosocial Interventions

Interventions that attend to psychosocial issues are especially important at specific times in the provision of family medical care. *Natural transitions in the family life cycle,* such as the birth of a child or the death of a spouse, call on the physician to provide empathic support, assess the patient's support system, normalize emotional reactions, and provide anticipatory guidance as patients confront changing family roles and functioning.

When adherence or lifestyle issues impinge on health, interventions that focus on biologic mechanisms alone are likely to be ineffective. The health effects of substance abuse, domestic violence, poverty, or inactivity are often best addressed through attention to social environment and psychological concerns.

A *dramatic change in patient symptoms* also indicates consideration of psychosocial factors. A psychosocial crisis can provoke an exacerbation of a chronic condition (e.g., rheumatoid arthritis), a new manifestation of illness (e.g., myocardial infarction), or emotional-psychiatric symptoms (e.g., anxiety, trouble sleeping) best treated through stress reduction and symptomatic care.

A *significant medical diagnosis* may precipitate emotional distress or psychosocial upheaval and requires physician attention to the context of the patient's life. Effective physician intervention may involve anticipating the nature of the potential family crisis, including family members in discussions with the patient, and addressing family needs for support. Timely provision of accurate information can enhance a patient's sense of control. Direct support by the physician during the initial adjustment phase can minimize more serious emotional disruption.

Patients living with chronic illness require sensitive psychosocial care. Managing a chronic health problem challenges a person's ability to adhere to a myriad of medical recommendations, making it more difficult to cope with other life stressors. Patients often deal with the predictable set of issues in highly idiosyncratic ways. Adequate attention to these issues can make medical management easier and more successful. These issues can often be effectively addressed within the physician-patient relationship and through judicious referral to support groups for chronically ill patients. Pollin (1995) identified eight emotionally charged issues that patients with chronic illnesses inevitably confront: control, self-image, dependency, stigma, abandonment, anger, isolation, and death. The professional stance useful in assisting the patient with each issue is important. In response to control issues, for example, professionals should help patients express their feelings of loss of control and to identify areas where they may feel powerless. Normalizing the patient's feelings and fears is the first step in helping address control issues. The goal of intervening in this issue is to reinforce the patient's confidence in being able to cope with the demands of the medical condition.

Evidence-Based Practice

Increasingly, high-quality data are available that support the therapeutic efficiency of a variety of general and specific behavioral interventions relevant to primary care practice (Trask et al., 2002). A systematic review by Di Blasi and colleagues (2002) on the consequences of nonspecific effects of the physician-patient relationship found that providing information and emotional support contributed to recovery or improvement from physical illness. Because coping with stress and managing chronic illness often involve behavior change, physicians may use "motivational interviewing" approaches to assist these patients (Rollnick et al., 2008).

Much research demonstrates the efficacy of psychosocial interventions in diseases historically viewed as purely medical, including cancer (Anderson et al., 2007; Edwards et al., 2008; Rehse and Pukrop, 2003; Spiegel et al, 1989) and diabetes (Bogner et al., 2007), as well as behavioral interventions such as exercise for cardiovascular disease (Taylor et al., 2004). Online resources are available to search for study results (see Web Resources at end of chapter).

Given the time constraints typically encountered by primary care physicians and the expertise required to use behavioral interventions effectively, the physician should be aware of behavioral health providers in the community in order to make effective and timely referrals. The evidence base for effective behavioral interventions in numerous psychiatric and psychosocial problems, as well as medical problems, continues to expand (e.g., mood and anxiety disorders, trauma victims). Highly effective treatments are underused when physicians underrefer to mental health professionals with specialized training and overrely on the use of psychotropic medicines alone. Unfortunately, even when guidelines are available that physicians could follow themselves, resistance to change impedes their implementation (Torrey et al., 2001).

EVIDENCE-BASED SUMMARY

- Providing information and emotional support contributes to the recovery and improvement from physical illness (SOR: A; Di Blasi et al., 2002).
- Negative emotions such as anger, anxiety, and depression are associated with poor health (SOR: B; Salovey et al., 2000).
- Positive emotions such as happiness, optimism, and a positive attitude have been shown to add 7 years to life (SOR: B; Danner et al., 2001; Levy et al., 2002).
- "Motivational interviewing" outperforms traditional advice-giving in addressing a broad range of behavioral problems (SOR: A; Rubac et al., 2000).
- Exercise-based rehabilitation for patients with cardiovascular disease is associated with reduced cardiovascular-related and all-caused mortality (SOR: A; Taylor et al., 2004).
- Treating depression in older patients with diabetes reduces mortality (SOR: A; Bogner et al., 2007).

The Patient-Centered Medical Home and Psychosocial Issues

The passage of federal health care reform in 2010 has made this issue even more controversial in the United States. Health care spending currently represents approximately 18% of the U.S. gross domestic product (GDP) and is projected to surpass 20% within a decade (Sisko et al., 2009). Concern about uninsured and underinsured persons remains, although new legislation to mandate insurance overage is scheduled to take effect in 2014.

Numerous perspectives exist on how the health care system needs to change, but a consensus is emerging that focuses on the importance of primary care and on managing chronic disease in the context of a high-quality physician-patient relationship (Bein, 2009). This consensus reflects the accumulating evidence that higher-quality health care at lower cost is achieved when primary care is emphasized (Starfield et al., 2005).

The concept of the patient-centered medical home (PCMH) embodies this emerging emphasis. As discussed in Chapter 2, the numerous components of a PCMH (or "health home") include the use of an electronic health record, better access and scheduling processes, use of evidence-based medicine, more point-of-care services (e.g., multidisciplinary teams, group visits), and an ongoing emphasis on quality improvement. Some argue that incremental change in this regard is insufficient, and that transformation of practices is necessary (Nutting et al., 2009). Such transformation would include a broad, population-based approach to preventive services and chronic care, beyond a "single patient at a time" approach. However, services are individualized to each patient based on the patient's goals and unique needs, which includes attention to the psychosocial factors that affect chronic disease prevention and management.

These trends represent an opportunity for family medicine to take a leadership role in health care reform, with an emphasis on psychosocial aspects. The PCMH philosophy is consistent with family medicine's long-standing emphasis on whole-person care in the context of a high-quality physician-patient relationship. Ideally, the family physician in a health home setting will address the psychosocial needs of patients in collaboration with ancillary providers, as needed.

Conclusion

To practice in a way that sensitively integrates psychosocial concerns, a physician needs to have a solid knowledge base in the social and behavioral sciences (Cuff and Vanselow, 2004). This general knowledge base complements specific knowledge of self, patients, practice, and community. Self-knowledge entails an honest assessment of the physician's knowledge base, skills, and attitudes relevant to comprehensive care. Acknowledging limitations in dealing with psychosocial issues in primary care is vital and can serve as an impetus to pursue further training and to develop appropriate collaborative relationships with other professionals. The responsible physician feigns neither knowledge nor empathy, but relies on an interdisciplinary network of professional and community resources to complement personal limitations.

Knowledge of each patient is also requisite to the provision of sensitive psychosocial care, with attention to life stresses, coping, personality, and social resources. As Osler (1904) emphasized, knowing what kind of person has a disease is as important as knowing the disease. Also, the physician needs to know the population, including demographic, socioeconomic, cultural, and epidemiologic dimensions. Addressing psychosocial issues in a practice that serves an ethnically diverse, indigent population presents different challenges than addressing the needs of an affluent population from a familiar ethnic and cultural background. Understanding the practice also entails knowing the health care economics and current systems of care, which inevitably introduce challenges to comprehensive care.

References

The complete reference list is available online at www.expertconsult.com.

Web Resources

www.cochranebehmed.org

Cochrane Behavioral Medicine Field. This evidence-based resource provides ready access to randomized controlled trials, meta-analyses, and systematic reviews of behavioral interventions for health problems.

www.motivationalinterview.org

This website offers extensive resources on the topic of motivational interviewing.

www.hbns.org

Health Behavior News Service. Disseminates the results of peer-reviewed research in the broad area of behavior and health.

www.aafp.org/pcmh

This resource of the American Academy of Family Physicians provides ready access to information about the patient-centered medical home movement.

www.cfah.org

Center for the Advancement of Health. Conducts research, communicates research findings, and advocates for policies that allow persons to benefit from health science research.

CHAPTER 4

Care of the Elderly Patient

Melissa Stiles and Kathleen Walsh

Family physicians are responsible for the care of increasing numbers of elderly patients and their unique and complex primary care needs. Older patients often have comorbidities, "polypharmacy," and psychological, social, and functional impairments. These can lead to variability in presentation of health problems and make diagnosis and treatment challenging for the family physician.

This chapter discusses common geriatric syndromes and outlines a process by which the family physician can effectively and efficiently care for the elderly patient. The main goal is to assist elderly persons to maintain function and quality of life with self-respect, preserving their lifestyle as much as possible. The chapter addresses functional assessment, falls, elder abuse, pressure ulcers, rational drug prescribing, and incontinence; geriatric conditions such as dementia, delirium, and depression are discussed in other chapters.

Geriatric Assessment

Key Points

- A comprehensive geriatric assessment includes a systematic approach assessing medical, functional, psychological, and social domains.

- A medication review is an essential component of a geriatric assessment.
- A multidisciplinary approach is used to identify intervention and management strategies.
- A questionnaire targeted to the geriatric assessment domains will expedite the patient visit.
- The goals of the geriatric assessment are to maintain function and preserve quality of life.

Longer life spans and aging "baby boomers" will double the population of Americans age 65 years and older over the next 25 years. The dramatic increase in life expectancy in the United States is the result of improved medical care and prevention efforts. In 2006, persons 65 years or older numbered 37.3 million and represented 12.4% of the U.S. population, about one in every eight Americans. The population 65 and over increased from 35 million in 2000 to about 40 million in 2010, a 15% increase, and then will increase to 55 million in 2020, a 36% increase for that decade. According to the Centers for Disease Control and Prevention (CDC, 2007), by 2030 there will be about 71.5 million older persons, more than twice their number in 2000 and about 20% of the U.S. population (Table 4-1).

There has been a significant shift in the leading causes of death for all groups from infectious disease and acute illnesses to chronic diseases and degenerative illnesses. Of the

Table 4-1 Population by Age and Gender: 2008*

Age	Both Genders		Male		Female	
	Number	%	Number	%	Number	%
All ages	299,106	100.0	146,855	100.0	152,250	100.0
Under 55 years	229,014	76.6	115,014	78.3	113,999	74.9
55 to 59 years	18,371	6.1	8929	6.1	9442	6.2
60 to 64 years	14,931	5.0	7150	4.9	7781	5.1
65 to 69 years	11,165	3.7	5238	3.6	5928	3.9
70 to 74 years	8423	2.8	3740	2.5	4683	3.1
75 to 79 years	7353	2.5	3200	2.2	4154	2.7
80 to 84 years	5559	1.9	2106	1.4	3453	2.3
85 years and over	4289	1.4	1479	1.0	2810	1.8

Data from U.S. Census Bureau, 2008 statistics. http://www.census.gov/population/www/socdemo/age/older_2008.html.
*Numbers in thousands; civilian noninstitutionalized population.

elderly population, approximately 8% experience severe cognitive impairment, 20% have chronic disabilities and vision problems, and 33% have restrictions in mobility and hearing loss (Freedman et al., 2002). There are also the predictable age-related structural and physiologic changes that occur with aging. External factors such as diet, occupation, social support, and access to health care can significantly influence the extent and speed of the physiologic decline (Arif et al., 2005; Sarma and Peddigrew, 2008; Tourlouki et al., 2009).

America's aging population is also marked by a more racially and ethnically diverse group of individuals. Simultaneously, the health status of racial and ethnic minorities lags far behind that of nonminority populations. The burden of many chronic diseases and conditions, such as hypertension, diabetes, and cancer, varies widely by race and ethnicity. Data from the 2004 National Health Interview Survey (NHIS) indicated that 39% of non-Hispanic white adults aged 65 years or older reported very good or excellent health, compared with 24% of non-Hispanic blacks and 29% of Hispanics.

There is a strong economic incentive for action. The cost of providing health care for an older American is three to five times greater than the cost for someone younger than 65. As a result, by 2030, the nation's health care spending is projected to increase by 25% because of these demographic shifts (CDC, 2006).

A comprehensive geriatric assessment is a systematic approach to the collection of patient data. The approach varies greatly, from single-physician evaluation with referral as needed, to full teams of professionals evaluating all patients. The geriatric assessment can assist in developing an individualized approach to each patient (Table 4-2). It is imperative to recognize the unique "blueprint" of what characterizes each elderly patient, including age, ethnicity, education, religious or spiritual beliefs, traditions, diet, interests/hobbies, daily routines, medical illness and disabilities, language barriers, functional status, marital status, sexual orientation,

Table 4-2 Goals of Geriatric Assessment

1. Focus on preventive medicine rather than acute medicine.
2. Focus on improving or maintaining functional ability and not necessarily on a "cure."
3. Provide a long-term solution for "difficult to manage" patients with multiple physicians, recurrent emergency department visits, and hospital admissions with poor follow-up.
4. Aid in the diagnosis of health-related problems.
5. Develop plans for treatment and follow-up care.
6. Establish plans for coordination of care.
7. Determine the need and site of long-term care as appropriate.
8. Determine optimal use of health care resources.
9. Prevent readmission into the hospital.

family and social support, occupation, life experiences, and socioeconomic position.

The geriatric assessment can be divided into four categories: medical, functional, psychological, and social. Within each of these categories are a number of approaches, including use of office-based instruments that can aid in collection of information and streamline the plan of care.

Medical Assessment

The medical assessment includes a review of the patient's medical record, medication history (past and present), and a nutritional evaluation. On average, elderly patients have four to six diagnosable disorders, which may require the use of several medications. One disorder can affect another, and in turn a collective deterioration of both can lead to overall poor outcomes. Review of the patient's medical record should focus on conditions that are more common in the elderly (geriatric syndromes) and in particular their risk factors.

Four shared risk factors—older age, baseline cognitive impairment, baseline functional impairment, and impaired mobility—have been identified within the five most common geriatric syndromes: pressure ulcers, incontinence, falls, functional decline, and delirium (Inouye et al., 2007). It is important that health care providers familiarize themselves with the common geriatric body area or system disorders that can directly influence these risk factors. Understanding the basic mechanisms involved in geriatric syndromes is essential to targeting therapeutic options.

During the medical assessment, the review of systems should be completed with special emphasis on sensory impairment, dentition, mood, memory, urinary symptoms, falls, nutrition, and pain. The U.S. Preventive Services Task Force (1996) recommends routine screening for visual and hearing impairment.

Hearing loss is the third most prevalent chronic condition in elderly people, after hypertension and arthritis, and its prevalence and severity increase with age. In persons age 65 to 75 years, the prevalence of hearing loss ranges from 20% to 40% (Cruikshanks et al., 1998; Rahko et al., 1985; Reuben et al., 1998), whereas in those over age 75, it ranges from 40% to 66% (Ciurlia-Guy et al., 1993; Parving et al., 1997).

Screening for hearing loss can be accomplished using two office-based methods: the audioscope (objective) and a validated short questionnaire (subjective). The audioscope is a handheld instrument that functions as an otoscope and audiometer and can be used to visualize the ear canal and eardrum and remove cerumen if necessary. The audioscope is easy to use, with 87% to 96% sensitivity and 70% to 90% specificity (Abyad, 1997; Mulrow, 1991). The Hearing Handicap Inventory for the Elderly–Short Version (HHIE-S) is a subjective, 10-item, 5-minute questionnaire with an overall accuracy of 75% in identifying hearing loss (Mulrow et al., 1990).

A formal audiologic evaluation should be offered to any patient who fails a hearing screening. The evaluation can assist in determining the need for further testing or management, including hearing aid, medical treatment, or surgical intervention.

Review of the patient's current medication list, including over-the-counter (OTC) medications, as well as any drug allergies or previous adverse drug reactions, is a necessary component of the geriatric assessment. *Adverse drug reactions* (ADRs; also adverse drug events) are a significant public health issue, especially in the elderly population (Thomsen et al., 2007). *Polypharmacy* is defined as taking more than four medications and is an independent risk factor for both delirium and falls (Inouye et al., 2000; Molyan and Binder, 2007).

Patients or family members should be asked to bring in all the patient's prescription medications and supplements at the initial visit and periodically thereafter. Clinicians can make sure patients have the prescribed drugs, but possession of these drugs does not guarantee adherence. Patients should be asked to demonstrate their ability to read labels (often printed in small type), open containers (especially the child-resistant type), and recognize their medications. Pillboxes may be helpful in organizing the patient's medications by the week or month.

Nutritional evaluation is an integral part of the geriatric assessment. The type, quantity, and frequency of food eaten should be determined. Malnutrition and undernutrition can lead to health problems that include delayed healing and longer hospital stays. A reliable marker of nutritional problems is weight loss, specifically, more than 5% in the past month and 10% or greater weight loss in the last 6 months (Huffman, 2002). Clinicians should ask about any special diets (e.g., low carbohydrate, vegetarian, low salt) or self-prescribed "fad" diets. A nutritional screen can aid in further assessment of the patient's nutritional health and help guide interventions (Figure 4-1). Additional questioning should include weight loss and change of fit in clothing; amount of money spent on food; and accessibility of grocers with a variety of fresh foods.

The ability to chew and swallow should also be evaluated. It may be impaired by xerostomia (dryness of mouth), which is common in elderly persons. Decreased taste or smell may reduce the pleasure of eating, so patients may eat less. Patients with decreased vision, arthritis, immobility, or tremors may have difficulty preparing meals and may injure or burn themselves when cooking. Patients worried about urinary incontinence may reduce their fluid intake and thus may eat less food.

Functional Assessment

A primary goal of the geriatric assessment is to identify interventions to help patients maintain function and stay at home in independent living situations. The functional assessment focuses on *activities of daily living* (ADLs) and risk screening for falls. The basic ADLs include eating, dressing, bathing, transferring, and toileting. The instrumental ADLs (IADLs) consist of shopping, managing money, driving, using the telephone, housekeeping, laundry, meal preparation, and managing medications (Katz, 1983). Home health and social services referral should be considered for patients who have difficulty with the ADLs. A simple method of screening patients for gait and mobility problems is to ask, "Have you fallen all the way to the ground in the past 12 months?" A positive screen should lead to a more thorough evaluation and consideration of a physical therapy referral (Ganz et al., 2007) (see Falls Assessment).

Psychological Assessment

The psychological assessment screens for cognitive impairment and depression, two conditions that significantly impact both the patient and the family. The most studied test to screen for cognition is the Mini-Mental State Examination, which is best for identifying patients with moderate or severe dementia. Depression can be readily screened with shorter versions of the original 30-item Yesavage Geriatric Depression Scale (GDS) (Yesavage et al., 1983). The five-item version of the GDS asks the following:

1. Are you basically satisfied with your life?
2. Do you often feel bored?
3. Do you often feel helpless?
4. Do you prefer to stay home rather than going out and doing new things?
5. Do you feel pretty worthless the way you are now?

A score of greater than two positive answers is positive (97% sensitivity, 85% specificity) (Rinalde et al., 2003). The Yale Depression Screen ("Do you often feel sad or depressed?") is a validated one-item GDS screening tool (Mahoney et al., 1994).

Social Assessment

It is important to assess the patient's living situation and social support when performing a geriatric assessment. The living situation should be evaluated for potential hazards,

Directions: Read the statements below. Circle the number in the YES column if it applies to you or the person you are completing the questionnaire for. Add the circled numbers for the total.

	YES
I have an illness or condition that made me change the kind and/or amount of food I eat.	2
I eat fewer than two meals per day.	3
I eat few fruits or vegetables or milk products.	2
I have three or more drinks of beer, liquor, or wine almost every day.	2
I have tooth or mouth problems that make it hard for me to eat.	2
I don't always have enough money to buy the food I need.	4
I eat alone most of the time.	1
I take three or more different prescribed or over-the-counter drugs a day.	1
Without wanting to, I have lost or gained 10 pounds in the last six months.	2
I am not always physically able to shop, cook, and/or feed myself.	2
TOTAL	

Total

0–2	Good! Recheck your nutritional score in six months.
3–5	You are at moderate nutritional risk. See what can be done to improve your eating habits and lifestyle. Your office on aging, senior nutrition program, senior citizens center or health department can help. Recheck your nutritional score in three months.
6 or more	You are at high nutritional risk. Bring this checklist next time you see your doctor, dietitian or other qualified health or service professional. Talk with them about any problems you may have. Ask for help to improve your nutritional health.

Figure 4-1 Nutrition questionnaires such as this (Determine Your Nutritional Health) can help in the assessment of the elderly patient's nutritional health. *(Courtesy Nutrition Screening Initiative, Washington, DC, 2007.)*

especially if the patient is identified as being at risk of falling. The social assessment also includes questions about financial stressors and caregiver concerns. Advance planning is a key component of the assessment and includes clarifying the patient's values and setting goals for care in case of future incapacity, including identifying the patient's "power of attorney" for health care.

Summary

A geriatric assessment can identify frequent problems, thus leading to earlier interventions for the common medical and social concerns of the elderly population. It is important to remember, however, that patients may underreport medical problems because they worry about losing their independence. Patients may also be reluctant to repeat their health concerns to their primary care physician because they fear being perceived as having an emotional or psychiatric illness. Often, older patients will rationalize their symptoms as being a "normal" component of aging.

The key to a successful geriatric assessment is to establish trust and effective communication between the patient and the physician. Allotting for adequate time during appointments and, if needed, scheduling frequent office visits are essential to the gathering of information. Inquiring about recent socioeconomic changes, functional losses, or life transitions is also important. The physician should obtain the patient's medical records before the first visit. A questionnaire targeted to the geriatric assessment domains should be completed by the patient, with family assistance if needed

(Figure 4-2). Language, education, social support, economic status, and cultural/ethnic factors play a vital role in the patient's health care outcome. A multidisciplinary approach is used to interventions and management. Preserving function and maintaining quality of life are the primary goals of the geriatric assessment (Miller et al., 2000).

Falls

Key Points

- Falls result in significant morbidity, mortality, and functional decline.
- Patients should be asked about history of falls and balance issues.
- Medication review is a key component of falls assessment.
- Multifactorial interventions can reduce the rate of falls.
- Exercise programs that focus on strength and balance training are most effective in preventing falls.

Epidemiology

Falls result in significant morbidity and mortality as well as an increased rate of nursing home placement. Each year, approximately 30% of persons over age 65 fall at least once, and the incidence increases with age. Up to 10% of falls result in serious injury. Falls are the leading cause of injury-related deaths in people over 65 years (CDC, 2005). In the United States, hip fractures currently account for more than 300,000

GERIATRIC HEALTH QUESTIONNAIRE

Date: _____ Birthdate: _____ Hosp #: _____

Name: _____ Address: _____

INSTRUCTIONS: PLEASE CIRCLE ANSWERS.

1. **General health:** In general, would you say your health is:
   Excellent / Very good / Good / Fair / Poor

   How much bodily pain have you had during the past 4 weeks?
   None / Very mild / Mild / Moderate / Severe / Very severe

2. **Activities of daily living:** Are you (I) independent (can do by myself); (A) require assistance (need help from another person); or (D) dependent (cannot do at all) with each of the following tasks?

Walking	I	A	D	Using telephone	I	A	D
Dressing	I	A	D	Shopping	I	A	D
Bathing	I	A	D	Preparing meals	I	A	D
Eating	I	A	D	Housework	I	A	D
Toileting	I	A	D	Taking medications	I	A	D
Driving	I	A	D	Managing finances	I	A	D

3. **Geriatric review of systems:**

   a. Do you have difficulty driving, watching TV, or reading because of poor eyesight? Yes / No

   b. Can you hear normal conversational voice? Yes / No

   Do you use hearing aids? Yes / No

   c. Do you have problems with your memory? Yes / No

   d. Do you often feel sad or depressed? Yes / No

   e. Have you unintentionally lost weight in the last 6 months? Yes / No

   f. Do you have trouble with control of your bladder? Yes / No

   Do you have trouble with control of your bowels? Yes / No

   g. How many falls have you had in the past year? _____

   h. Do you drink alcohol? Yes / No

   If yes, how many drinks per week? _____

4. Do you live with anyone? Yes / No

   If yes, who? Spouse / Child / Other / Relative / Friend

   Who would help you in an emergency? _____

   Who would help you with health care decisions if you were not able to communicate your wishes?

   _____

5. How many medicines do you take, including prescribed, over the counter, and vitamins? _____

   What is your system for taking your medications? Pill box / Family help / List or chart / None

6. Are you sexually active? Yes / No

7. Has anyone intentionally tried to harm you? Yes / No

8. Have you had a shot to prevent pneumonia? Yes / No

9. Please draw the face of a clock with all the numbers and the hands set to indicate 10 minutes after 11 o'clock.

Memory: 3 item recall after 1 minute   (pen, dog, watch)   # recalled _____

Patient signature _____ Date _____

Reviewing physician _____ Date _____

Figure 4-2 Geriatric health questionnaires assist in gathering pertinent information regarding the functioning of the elderly patient.

hospitalizations, with a 1-year mortality rate of up to 33% (Sattin, 1992; Tinetti et al., 1998). By 2050, it is estimated that the worldwide number of hip fractures will rise to 6.26 million. Direct medical costs related to falls in adults age 65 or older exceeded $19 billion in 2000 (Stevens et al., 2006).

Falls also cause functional limitations by both direct injury and indirect psychological consequences. Postfall anxiety leads to loss of self-confidence in ambulation and self-imposed limitations in activity. Postfall anxiety syndrome can also result in depression, social isolation, and increased risk of falls from deconditioning. Because the cause of falls is often multifactorial, the assessment and interventions target several areas (Nevitt et al., 1989).

Risk Factors

The multiple risk factors for falling can be categorized as intrinsic or extrinsic. *Intrinsic* risk factors include age-related physiologic changes and diseases that affect the risk of falling (Table 4-3). *Extrinsic* risk factors include medications and environmental obstacles. The risk of falling increases significantly in people with multiple risk factors. A prospective study found that 19% of older patients with one risk factor have a fall in a given year, compared with 60% of older patients with three risk factors (Tinetti et al., 1998).

Taking four or more prescription drugs is itself a risk factor for falling. Also, several medication classes have a higher potential to cause falls, including tricyclic antidepressants, neuroleptic agents, serotonin reuptake inhibitors, benzodiazepines, and class 1A antiarrhythmic medications. Narcotic analgesics, antihistamines, and anticonvulsants are also associated with increased risk for falls (Ensrud et al., 2002; Rubenstein and Josephson, 2002).

Physical restraints have been used in an attempt to reduce falling. Although the focus here is on community-dwelling elderly persons, it is worth noting that use of physical restraint in the nursing home and hospital setting does *not* reduce the risk of falling and is instead associated with an increased risk of injury (Neufeld et al., 1999). Since the 1980s, the use of physical restraints has been appropriately and dramatically reduced.

Screening

At present, no one screening test can be recommended to identify potential fallers (Gates et al., 2008). The two best predictors of falls are a history of falls and a reported abnormality in gait or balance (Ganz et al., 2007). "Have you had any falls in the past year?" is a simple screening question that can be answered by the patient or caregiver in a previsit questionnaire. For patients who have not fallen, the pretest probability of a fall in the upcoming year ranges from 19% to 36%. Also, asking the patient, "Have you noticed any problems with gait, balance, or mobility?" is another simple screening question. Answering "yes" to either screening question warrants further assessment (Tinetti, 2003).

Falls Assessment

Falls assessment should include a multifactorial evaluation beginning with the circumstances surrounding the fall(s), associated symptoms, risk factor assessment, and medication history (Table 4-4). The physician should ask about the environment (e.g., indoors or outdoors, dark or well lighted, time of day), environmental obstacles (e.g., throw rugs, door thresholds, stairs), and footwear worn at the time. The history should also include questions about prodromal symptoms (e.g., lightheadedness, dizziness), if there was a loss of consciousness or other symptoms of arrhythmias (i.e., palpitations). If available, obtain information from a witness. The evaluation should also include questions about risk factors, functional abilities and medication history (AGS et al., 2001).

Postural blood pressure and pulse are important assessments in the examination. Up to 30% of older persons have orthostatic hypotension, and although some may be asymptomatic, others become lightheaded and dizzy (Luukinen et al., 1999). The musculoskeletal examination should focus on range of motion in the legs, inflammatory or degenerative conditions of the leg joints, kyphosis, and abnormalities of the feet. The neurologic examination should include proprioception, coordination, muscle strength, and cognition. The cardiovascular examination should focus on detecting

Table 4-3 Intrinsic Risk Factors for Falls

Age-related changes in:
- Vision
- Hearing
- Proprioception
- Decreased blood pressure response to postural changes
- Delayed compensatory muscle response to postural changes

Age >80 years
Cognitive impairment
Depression
Functional impairment
History of falls
Visual impairment
Gait or balance impairment
Use of assistive device
Arthritis
Leg weakness

Table 4-4 Initial Evaluation of Falls

History
Circumstances of fall
Presence of risk factors
Medical conditions
Medication review
Functional abilities

Physical Examination
Postural blood pressure
Visual acuity
Cardiovascular examination: rhythm, murmurs
Neurologic examination: strength, proprioception, cognition
Musculoskeletal examination: range of motion (ROM), joint abnormalities
Gait and balance assessment

Diagnostic Studies
None required routinely.

potential causes of falls (e.g., arrhythmias, aortic stenosis). Visual acuity and hearing should be assessed. Disturbances in gait and balance can be identified through the patient or caregiver's direct report or a simple office-based assessment, such as the "get up and go" test (Podsiadlo and Richardson, 1991). This test may be scored, timed, or used as an overall assessment of the patient's gait, stability, balance, and strength. The patient is asked to stand from a seated position, walk about 10 feet (3 meters), turn around, walk back, and sit down again. If the patient needs to push off the chair or rock back-and-forth several times to arise, leg strength is diminished. The task should be completed within 10 seconds. Gait abnormalities, such as poor step height, decreased stride length, and shuffling, may be observed. A wide-based stance and slow, multiple-point turning may reveal poor balance.

Laboratory evaluation and imaging are based on the history and clinical findings. If an underlying metabolic abnormality is suspected (e.g., diabetes, anemia, dehydration), appropriate blood tests may assist in the diagnosis. If a patient is suspected of having syncope, cardiac rhythm monitoring (e.g., Holter or event monitor) is appropriate. An echocardiogram may be necessary for evaluation of a murmur. Neuroimaging with magnetic resonance imaging (MRI) or computed tomography (CT) is indicated for the evaluation of focal findings on neurologic examination.

Management

Evidence has demonstrated that a multifactorial approach and intervention strategy is needed to reduce the rate of falling in older patients (Figure 4-3). Because one of the most modifiable risk factors is medication use, medication review is a key component of management (Hanlon et al., 1997). The review should focus on decreasing the dose or discontinuing sedating medications. If orthostasis is present, adjustment of diuretics and antihypertensive medications should be considered. The role of vitamin D in fall prevention is questionable. Although, it probably does not decrease the risk of falls, except in patients with low levels of vitamin D, supplementation should be started in patients with osteopenia or osteoporosis (Gillespie et al., 2009).

Supervised exercise programs should be considered for patients at high risk for falls; exercise can reduce the physical risk factors (Rose, 2008). Specifically, programs that focus on two of three exercise components (strengthening, balance training, and aerobic/endurance training) for a minimum of 12 weeks have shown the most benefit (Costello and Edelstein, 2008). Finally, home hazard evaluation and intervention is an essential component in the assessment of falls in elderly

KEY TREATMENT

Risk factor assessment and multifactorial intervention reduces rate of falls (Gillespie et al., 2009) (SOR: A).
Exercise programs that target more than two components reduce rate of falls (Gillespie et al., 2009) (SOR: A).
Community-living elderly patients who have fallen or who have risk factors for falling should have their homes assessed for safety (Gillespie et al., 2001) (SOR: A).
All older individuals should be asked at least once yearly about falls (Tinetti, 2003, AGS et al., 2001) (SOR: C).

persons, particularly those with visual impairment and multiple risk factors (Gillespie et al., 2001; Stevens et al., 2001).

Elder Abuse

Key Points

- Elder abuse is underreported.
- Direct questioning for elder abuse is recommended.
- Physicians should recognize the physical and behavioral signs of abuse.
- A positive screen for elder abuse should be followed by a safety assessment.
- Physician reporting requirements regarding elder abuse vary by state.

Elder abuse is a significant public health issue that physicians need to identify and address in both outpatient and inpatient settings. The prevalence of elder abuse is difficult to determine because its definition varies across U.S. states and other countries and research is still limited in this area (Erlingsson, 2007). In a systematic review of international literature, estimates ranged from 3.2% to 27.5% based on population studies. More than 6% of the general population had reported abuse in the prior month (Cooper et al., 2008).

In the United States, the number of people age 65 and older who have been victims of elder abuse ranges between 1 and 2 million. In 2000, adult protective services (APS) departments received approximately 470,000 reports. Of the types of abuse, elder "self-neglect" is most often reported. A prospective, population-based cohort study found that elder self-neglect was associated with a 5.82 times increased risk for mortality in the year after a report of self-neglect (Dong et al., 2009). From incidence studies, it is estimated that for every case reported, about five go underreported (National Elder Abuse Incidence Study, 1998). Underreporting stems from both patient issues (familial secrecy, denial, fear, shame) and provider issues (lack of awareness) (Kahan and Paris, 2003). Primary care physicians have the opportunity to detect early signs of elder abuse in patients with whom they have well-established relationships (Stiles et al., 2002).

Definition

The National Center on Elder Abuse (2009) defines elder abuse as "a term referring to any knowing, intentional, or negligent act by a caregiver or any other person that causes harm or a serious risk of harm to a vulnerable adult." Although terms vary across states, elder abuse can be generally categorized into several types: physical abuse, emotional abuse, sexual abuse, exploitation, neglect, self-neglect, and abandonment (Table 4-5). Elder abuse is also classified by its setting. *Domestic* abuse occurs in the home of the victim. *Institutional* abuse occurs in a nursing home, hospital, assisted-living center, or group home.

Risk Factors

Awareness of risk factors for abuse can increase the chance of identification and early intervention. Although research is ongoing, several characteristics of both the victim and the

PREVENTION OF FALLS IN OLDER PERSONS LIVING IN THE COMMUNITY

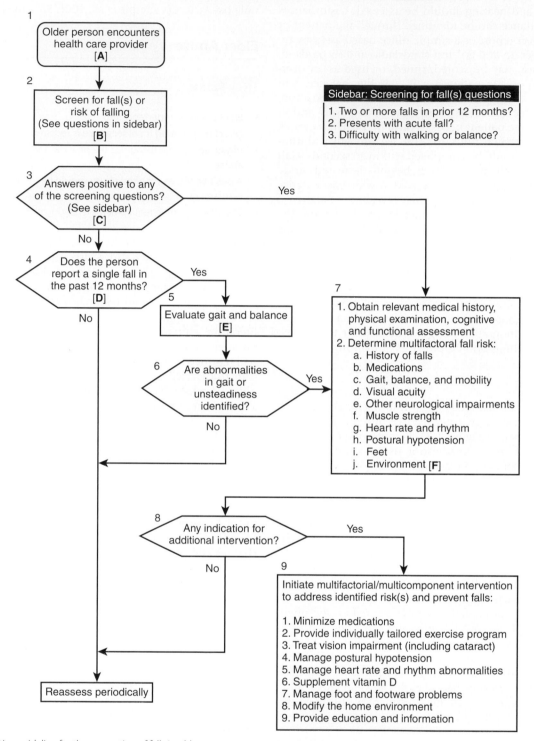

Figure 4-3 Practice guideline for the prevention of falls in older persons.
(From American Geriatrics Society (AGS), British Geriatrics Society, and American Academy of Orthopedic Surgeons Panel on Falls Prevention: Guideline for the prevention of falls in older persons. J Am Geriatr Soc 2001;49:664-672.)

abuser should trigger further screening questions. Risk factors associated with the *victim* include shared living situations, history of dementia, and social isolation. *Perpetrator* risk factors include a history of mental illness (specifically depression), alcohol abuse, and financial dependency (Lachs and Pillemer, 2004).

Screening

There is no consensus that asymptomatic patients should be screened for elder abuse. The American Medical Association (AMA, 1992) suggests that all outpatients be screened for family violence, but the U.S. Preventive Services Task

Table 4-5 Elder Abuse: Definitions

Physical abuse: Inflicting, or threatening to inflict, physical pain or injury on a vulnerable elderly person, or depriving the person of a basic need.
Emotional abuse: Inflicting mental pain, anguish, or distress on an elderly person through verbal or nonverbal acts.
Sexual abuse: Nonconsensual sexual contact of any kind.
Exploitation: Illegal taking, misuse, or concealment of funds, property, or assets of a vulnerable elder.
Neglect: Refusal or failure by those responsible to provide food, shelter, health care or protection for a vulnerable elder.
Abandonment: The desertion of a vulnerable elder by anyone who has assumed the responsibility for care or custody of that person.
Self-neglect: Characterized as the behavior of an elderly person that threatens his or her own health or safety.

Modified from National Center on Elder Abuse.
 http://www.ncea.aoa.gov/NCEAroot/Main_Site/Index.aspx. October 2009.

Table 4-6 Screening Questions for Elder Abuse

Are you afraid of anyone at home?
Are you alone a lot?
Has anyone at home ever hurt you?
Has anyone taken anything that was yours without asking?
Does anyone at home make you uncomfortable or afraid?
Has anyone ever forced you to sign a document that you did not understand?
Are you kept isolated from friends or relatives?

Table 4-7 Physical Signs of Elder Abuse

General
Weight loss
Dehydration
Poor hygiene
HEENT
Traumatic alopecia
Poor oral hygiene
Absent hearing aids, dentures, or eyeglasses
Subconjunctival or vitreous hemorrhage
Skin
Hematomas
Welts
Burns
Bruises
Bites
Pressure sores
Genitorectal
Inguinal rash
Fecal impaction
Musculoskeletal
Fractures
Contractures

HEENT, Head, ears, eyes, nose, throat.

Force (2009) concluded that there was insufficient evidence for or against screening for older adults or their caregivers for elder abuse. Patients should be screened if there is a suspicion of elder abuse. The questions should be open-ended, nonthreatening, and asked in a variety of ways to assess for the different forms of elder abuse (Table 4-6). A positive response should be followed by more direct questions as to the nature of the abuse. Direct questioning by physicians has been shown to increase reporting (Oswald et al., 2004).

Clinical Manifestations

Certain behavioral and physical signs should raise suspicion for elder abuse. Behavioral signs in the caregiver include answering for the patient, insisting on being present for the entire visit, failing to offer assistance, and displaying indifference or anger. Behavioral signs in the elderly patient include poor eye contact, hesitation to talk openly, or fearfulness toward the caregiver. Other indicators of possible abuse include confusion, paranoia, anxiety, anger, and low self-esteem. Physical signs that may signal neglect include poor hygiene, malnutrition, dehydration, pressure ulcers, and injuries (Table 4-7). Medication nonadherence may also be a warning sign for abuse.

Assessment

In suspected cases of abuse, the assessment includes a thorough history, physical examination, and functional, cognitive, and mental health assessments. The patient and the caregiver should be interviewed alone and separately (Abbey, 2009). Documentation begins with the description of the abusive or neglectful event, using the patient's words whenever possible. The duration, frequency, and severity of the abuse should be recorded. If injuries are present, a detailed description of the injuries and photographs, if available, should be documented. Assessment of functional dependence can be helpful in recommending resources, whereas evaluation of cognitive impairment is important in assessing both risk and capacity. The assessment should also include a mental health screening, with particular attention to depression, anxiety, insomnia, and alcohol abuse.

The elderly patient's caregiver should be assessed for caregiver stress and for risk factors for elder abuse, including alcohol abuse, depression, and financial dependency.

Management

Because the cause of elder abuse is often multifactorial, management involves a multidisciplinary approach with social workers and legal, financial, and APS representatives. The immediate management is determined by the safety and capacity assessments. Is the patient in any immediate danger? If so, acute hospitalization, safe home placement, and a protective court order may be indicated. If the patient lacks capacity, the physician should work with APS on options, including guardianship, financial management resources, and order of protection if indicated. In other cases, management should focus on utilizing community resources to maintain the patient in the least restrictive environment. The emphasis is to decrease social isolation and caregiver stress. Interventions can include respite care, home health or custodial services, counseling, and drug or alcohol rehabilitation.

Reporting Requirement

All 50 states have laws authorizing APS departments to intervene in cases of elder abuse. It is important for primary care physicians to know their state's requirements on mandatory reporting for elder abuse and which type of abuse (e.g., physical, emotional, sexual, financial) requires reporting. Higher rates of abuse have been documented in states that require public education regarding elder abuse and states that require mandatory reporting (Jogerst et al., 2003). Mandatory reporting laws in 42 states are controversial because they conflict with a competent elder's autonomy and with the physician-patient relationship. In such cases, physicians should explain their legal obligation to report and emphasize that the goal of reporting is to develop a care plan to assist the patient.

KEY TREATMENT

Direct questioning by physicians for elder abuse increases the rate of reporting (Oswald et al., 2004) (SOR: B).
Older individuals should be screened for elder abuse (AMA, 1992) (SOR: C).

Pressure Ulcers

Key Points

- Preventive measures can reduce the incidence of pressure ulcers in elderly patients.
- Classification is only one aspect of wound assessment.
- Assessment of pressure ulcers includes identification of risk factors.
- Pain assessment is an essential component of management.
- Risk factor modification is the key to management of pressure ulcers.

Pressure ulcers are a common and serious public health issue, especially in the elderly population. The reported incidence is as high as 22% in the nursing home population and range from 4.7% to 9% up to 32% in the hospitalized population (Allman, 1995, 1997; Coleman et al., 2002; Kaltenthaler et al., 2001). The treatment costs related to pressure ulcers exceed an estimated $5 billion annually in the United States (Xakellis et al., 1995). Prevention is paramount and can reduce the incidence of pressure ulcers by 50%. A thorough assessment of the wound and potential risk factors is the key to management.

Classification

Wound assessment begins with classification, as initially proposed in 1989 by the National Pressure Ulcer Advisory Panel (NPUAP) and then adopted for the Agency for Health Care Policy and Research (AHCPR) Pressure Ulcer Clinical

Practice Guidelines (1992 and 1994). The NPUAP revised the stage I classification in 1998 and added two stages in 2007: suspected deep tissue injury and unstageable. The six classifications are as follows:

Suspected deep tissue injury: Purple or maroon, localized area of discolored skin or blood-filled blister caused by damage to underlying soft tissue from pressure and shear. The area may be preceded by tissue that is painful, firm, mushy, boggy, and warmer or cooler compared with adjacent tissue.

Stage I: Intact skin with nonblanchable redness of a localized area, usually over a bony prominence. Darkly pigmented skin may not have visible blanching; its color may differ from the surrounding area. The area may be painful, firm, soft, and warmer or cooler compared with adjacent tissue. Stage I may be difficult to detect in individuals with dark skin tones.

Stage II: Partial-thickness skin loss involving the epidermis, the dermis, or both. The ulcer is superficial and presents clinically as an abrasion, blister, or shallow crater, without slough.

Stage III: Full-thickness skin loss involving damage or necrosis of subcutaneous tissue that may extend down to, but not through, underlying fascia. The ulcer presents clinically as a deep crater with or without undermining of adjacent tissue.

Stage IV: Full-thickness skin loss with extensive destruction, tissue necrosis, or damage to muscle, bone, or supporting structures (e.g., tendons, joint capsules). Slough or eschar may be present on some parts of the wound bed, often with undermining and tunneling.

Unstageable: Full-thickness tissue loss in which the base of the ulcer is covered with slough (yellow, tan, gray, green, or brown) and/or eschar in the wound bed.

A wound cannot be accurately staged if eschar or slough is present. The staging system is useful only for initial classification because wounds do not heal predictably (Ferrell, 1997). Thus, it is important to include other factors when describing the wound, to help assess treatment over time. These factors include size, type of exudate, and a description of the predominant tissue type. Size can be assessed by measuring the two largest diameters at right angles. The type and amount of exudate should be recorded. Exudate types include serous (clear or amber), sanguineous (bloody), or purulent (thick, yellow, and/or odiferous). The predominant tissue types are epithelial, granulation, necrotic, and eschar (AHCPR, 1992; Ferrell, 1997; Makelbust, 1997; NPUAP, 2007).

Risk Factors

An understanding of risk factors for pressure sore development is the key to prevention and management. Risk factors can be divided into extrinsic and intrinsic categories (Table 4-8).

Extrinsic Risk Factors

Extrinsic factors include direct pressure, shearing forces, friction, and moisture. Direct pressure results in hypoperfusion of the affected tissue, which can lead to hypoxia, acidosis, and if prolonged, tissue death and necrosis. Pressure sores most frequently occur over bony prominences below the

Table 4-8 Risk Factors for Pressure Sore Development

Extrinsic Factors
Pressure
Shear
Friction
Moisture

Intrinsic Factors
Age
Impaired mobility
Malnutrition
Sensory impairment

Table 4-9 Risk Factor Modification

Implement	Avoid
Support devices to reduce pressure	Donut-type devices
Frequent repositioning	Massage over bony prominences
Positioning devices such as pillows	Raising head of bed above 30 degrees
Lifting devices such as a trapeze	Dragging the patient during transfers

waist: the sacrum, greater trochanter, malleolus, heel, ischial tuberosity, and fibular head. Of note, heels are the second most common site for pressure ulcer development. As the prevalence of pressure ulcers at other sites has decreased or remained the same, prevalence of heel pressure ulcers has increased.

Shear forces result from traction on the skin, which causes a relative displacement of the underlying structures. This usually occurs when patients are positioned in bed more than 30 degrees, or seated, and then slide down. In these patients the underlying sacrum is at risk for pressure sore development. *Friction* between the skin and a stationary source such as bedclothes or sheets is another factor. Care must be taken to avoid friction, especially during transfers in and out of bed. Excessive *moisture* can lead to skin maceration and subsequent skin breakdown. Common causes include incontinence, diarrhea, and excessive perspiration (AHCPR, 1994; Patterson and Bennett, 1995).

Intrinsic Risk Factors

Intrinsic risk factors for pressure ulcer development include age, conditions that impair mobility, malnutrition, and sensory impairment. Skin changes associated with aging (e.g., epidermal thinning, diminished vascularity) increase the susceptibility of older persons to shearing forces, pressure, and friction. Immobility can cause infrequent position changes, thus exposing an older person to prolonged pressure. Malnutrition, specifically an inadequate intake of calories or protein, has been associated with the development of pressure sores (Thomas, 2001). AHCPR (1994) defines clinically significant malnutrition as a serum albumin level of less than 3.5 mg/dL, a total lymphocyte count of less than 1800 cells/mm^3, or body weight less than 80% of ideal weight. Supplementation of micronutrients involved in skin healing, such as ascorbic acid and zinc, has not been shown to prevent pressure sores or improve rates of healing. Sensory impairment, such as in diabetic neuropathy, can prevent an individual from responding appropriately to pressure-related discomfort (Patterson and Bennett, 1995; Reddy et al., 2006; Thomas, 1997, 2001).

Risk Factor Assessment Tools

The AHCPR's guidelines recommend that individuals with limited mobility be assessed on admission to hospitals, nursing homes, and home care programs for risk factors for pressure sore development. The most common assessment tool is the Braden scale (Pancorbo-Hidalgo et al., 2006). Risk factor identification and subsequent intervention are integral components of pressure sore prevention and management.

Management

The principles of pressure sore management include modification of risk factors, nutritional support, maintaining a wound environment optimal for healing, and pain control.

Risk Factor Modification

The primary goal is to reduce pressure, shear, and friction over high-risk bony prominences (Table 4-9). This can be accomplished by frequent turning and repositioning while in bed (every 2 hours), frequent repositioning while sitting (every hour), and use of a support device to lower surface pressure, such as foam, static air, alternating air, gel, or water mattress. Positioning devices such as pillows or foam wedges should be used to keep bony prominences (e.g., knees, ankles) from touching each other or high-risk areas from contacting the bed (e.g., heels). Donut-type devices should be avoided because the tissue within the ring can become necrotic from increased venous congestion.

Massage should be avoided over bony prominences because it can lead to deep tissue trauma. When positioning on the side, avoid pressure directly on the trochanter. To decrease the effect of shear forces, maintain the head of the bed at the lowest degree of elevation. To decrease the effect of friction lubricants, use protective films, dressings, or padding. Also, lifting devices such as a trapeze can be used to assist patients with limited mobility in transfers and repositioning (AHCPR, 1994; Bergstrom, 1997; Bluestein and Javaher, 2008; Reddy et al., 2006; Remsburg and Bennett, 1997).

Nutritional Support

Nutritional support emphasizing adequate protein and calorie intake is another key component of pressure sore management. Protein intake should be 1.0 to 1.5 g/kg/day. Caloric intake should be 30 to 35 kcal/kg/day. Some experts recommend supplementation with vitamin C and zinc, although evidence that either enhances wound healing is limited (AHCPR, 1994; Langer et al., 2003; Reddy et al., 2006; Thomas, 2001).

Debridement

Wound healing requires a moist environment, free of necrotic tissue and infection, which allow for granulation and reepithelialization. Debridement is often needed to remove necrotic tissue, slough, and eschar, which can be accomplished by sharp, mechanical, enzymatic, and/or autolytic techniques. The technique used depends on the patient's condition, location, clinical urgency and overall goals for patient care. Debridement is not recommended for heel ulcers that have stable, dry eschar without edema or signs of infection (AHCPR, 1994; NPUAP, 2007).

Sharp debridement is appropriate for removing areas of thick eschar and necrotic tissue in extensive ulcers. Care must be taken to control pain when using this technique. Also, surgical debridement may cause transient bacteremia, and prophylactic antibiotics may be needed for high-risk patients.

Mechanical debridement includes wet-to-dry dressings, hydrotherapy, wound irrigation, and dextranomers, which are small beads of highly hydrophilic dextran polymers (e.g., Debrisan). Wet-to-dry dressings may be painful when changed and need be discontinued when the wound bed is clean to avoid desiccation (Ovington, 2001). *Hydrotherapy* is appropriate for pressure sores with thick exudate or necrotic tissue. Care must be taken not to place the wound too close to the jets. Irrigation pressures need to be high enough to adequately cleanse the wound, but not too high to potentially cause tissue trauma. Safe and effective pressures are between 4-15 pounds per square inch (psi). Examples of safe irrigation devices include 35-mL syringe with 19-gauge needle or angiocatheter, water-jet device at the lowest setting, and saline squeeze bottle (250 mL) with irrigation cap.

Enzymatic debridement is accomplished by products that have proteolytic enzymes such as papain and urea (e.g., Accuzyme, Panafil) and collagenase. Typically used once daily, these products may damage healthy tissue and should not be used if infection is present. Thus, special care is needed in application, and use should be limited to short periods (<2 weeks).

Autolytic debridement involves the use of occlusive synthetic dressings that allow enzymes normally present within wounds to self-digest necrotic tissue. Occlusive dressings should not be used if the wound is infected or if there is a moderate amount of exudate (AHCPR, 1994; Cervo et al., 2000; Goode and Thomas, 1997).

Infection Control

In the majority of cases, infection can be prevented by adequate debridement and cleansing. Wounds should be cleansed daily and with dressing changes. Normal saline is the most appropriate solution for cleansing. Avoid skin cleansers or antiseptics that are cytotoxic, such as povidone-iodine, hydrogen peroxide, and acetic acid. Signs of a wound infection include delayed healing, increasing wound size, purulent exudate, pain, and foul odor. Initially, consider a trial of topical antibiotics, such as silver sulfadiazine cream (Silvadene), for 2 weeks. Superficial cultures of the wound are not helpful because they detect only the surface colonization. Ideally, bacterial tissue cultures should be performed to guide antibiotic coverage. Systemic antibiotics are reserved for patients with cellulitis, osteomyelitis, bacteremia, or sepsis (AHCPR, 1994).

Dressing Selection

Wound dressings provide a physiologically moist wound environment shown to enhance healing, reduce pain, debride necrotic tissue, and decrease infection rates in pressure sores. Dressing selection depends on the stage, amount of exudate, size, site, and condition of surrounding skin. No moist-dressing type has proved superior to the others (Bouza et al., 2005). The main categories of modern dressings are polyurethane films, hydrocolloids, amorphous hydrogels, hydrogel sheets, polyurethane foams, foamed gels, alginates, and hydrocolloid/alginate combinations (Table 4-10).

For deep, stage III and stage IV pressure sores, packing is often needed to eliminate dead space. This can be accomplished with saline-moistened gauze, calcium alginates, gels, and dextranomers. After packing, the wound is covered with an occlusive or semiocclusive dressing. If excessive exudate is present, the dressing must have absorptive properties to control exudate without drying the wound bed. Examples include saline-moistened gauze, alginates, and combination hydrocolloid/alginate dressings.

Pressure sores should be evaluated weekly by a health care professional. Reevaluation of the treatment plan should be considered if there are not signs of healing within 2 weeks of treatment (Ferrell, 1997; Goode and Thomas, 1997).

Pain Control

The overall management of a patient with a pressure sore includes pain assessment and control. Patients should be assessed for pain related to the pressure sore. Management includes the appropriate use of analgesics and eliminating or modifying the source of the pain. This can be accomplished by repositioning, using support surfaces, and using wound dressings shown to reduce pain. Pain should be anticipated before dressing changes and debridement. Appropriate analgesia should be provided as needed.

Adjunctive Therapy

Numerous modalities have been attempted to expedite the wound healing process, but their role remains unclear. Examples include electrical stimulation, hyperbaric oxygen, ultrasound, and hydrotherapy (Baba-Akbari et al., 2006; Kranke et al., 2004; Olyaee Manesh et al., 2006). Negative-pressure wound therapy has shown promise in the management of stage III and IV pressure ulcer (Banwell and Teot, 2003; Mendez-Eastman, 2004). Further research is needed to establish efficacy of adjunctive therapy for wound healing.

KEY TREATMENT

Assess all support surfaces and patient factors for increased pressure and modify appropriately (AHCPR, 1994, Reddy et al., 2006) (SOR: A).

Assess and manage the patient's nutritional status (AHCPR, 1994; Langer et al., 2003; Thomas, 2001) (SOR: B).

Assess all patients for pain related to the pressure ulcer treatment or its treatment (AHCPR, 1994; NPUAP, 2007) (SOR: C).

Table 4-10 Wound Dressing Properties

Wound Dressings	Absorbent Quality*	Debriding Action	Frequency of Dressing Change	Stage
Polyurethane films (e.g., Bioclusive, Opsite, 3M Tegaderm)	None	None	Every 7 days or less	I, II
Hydrogels (e.g., Dermagauze, Flexigel, 3M Tegagel)	Minimal to moderate	Autolysis	Every 7 days or less	II, III, IV
Hydrocolloids (e.g., Combiderm, Duoderm, 3M Tegaderm)	Minimal to large	Autolysis	Every 7 days or less	II, III, IV
Polyurethane foams (e.g., Allevyn, Curafoam, Optifoam)	Minimal to moderate	None	Every 7 days or less	II, III, IV
Alginates (e.g., Algicell, Kalginate, Sorbsan)	Minimal to large	Autolysis	Daily to every 3 days	II, III, IV

*None, minimal, moderate, or large.

Rational Drug Prescribing for Elderly Patients

Key Points

- Adverse drug events result in significant morbidity and a high rate of hospital admissions.
- Medications should be adjusted for the individual patient's renal function.
- Medication lists of elderly patients should be periodically reviewed, focusing on indications and side effects.
- One drug should not be used to treat the side effects of another medication.
- Pharmacists' recommendations should be incorporated in a rational drug-prescribing plan.

The primary care physician plays an important role in addressing an array of pharmaceutical issues and concerns for elderly patients, including polypharmacy, adverse drug reactions, adherence, and undertreatment of certain conditions.

Medication use is common in the elderly population and increases with age. A population-based survey showed that 44% of men and 57% of women over age 65 used five or more medications weekly (Kaufmann et al., 2002). Although persons over 65 represent only 13% of the general population, they account for more than 30% of U.S. drug expenditures, totaling over $73 billion in 2006 (MEPS, 2006). Polypharmacy is a major risk factor for *adverse drug events* (ADEs). Up to 10% of emergency department visits and 10% to 17% of hospital admissions are the result of ADEs (Hayes et al., 2007).

Pharmacokinetics and Pharmacodynamics

Knowledge of the physiologic changes that occur with aging is essential when prescribing medications to the elderly patient. Changes in pharmacokinetics and pharmacodynamics can result in increased or decreased amounts of medication and drug-drug interactions (Table 4-11).

Pharmacokinetics refers to the body's response to the drug and includes absorption, distribution, metabolism, and elimination (excretion). Age-related gastrointestinal and skin changes have minimal effect on drug *absorption*, except for drugs that require active gastrointestinal transport (vitamins,

Table 4-11 Pharmacokinetic Changes in Older Persons

Absorption generally does not change.
Longer half-life of lipophilic drugs.
Increased amount of water soluble and free (active) drug.
Decreased excretion.

minerals), which decreases with aging. The *volume of distribution* (Vd) is determined by degree of plasma protein binding and body composition. The changes in protein binding are not clinically significant, unless a condition (e.g., acute illness, malnutrition) is causing a marked decline in albumin. Water composition and lean body mass decrease with aging. Fat composition increases, resulting in a larger Vd of lipid-soluble drugs, such as benzodiazepines. Although liver function tests are unchanged, liver size and blood flow are somewhat reduced. The clinical significance is difficult to determine because there is such wide interindividual variation in hepatic metabolism. Drug *elimination* is mainly affected by a decrease in creatinine clearance. Also, decreased muscle mass causes a decrease in serum creatinine. Because serum creatinine may appear normal even when significant renal impairment exists, it is important to calculate clearance and adjust medication dosages accordingly (Cusak, 2004). The Cockcroft-Gault (1976) formula can be used to estimate creatinine (Cr) clearance:

$$\text{Cr clearance} = (140 - \text{Age[yr]}) \times$$
$$(\text{Actual body weight[kg]}) / (72 \times \text{Serum Cr[mg/dL]})$$

For women, multiply the result by 0.85. Of note, this formula is less accurate in extremely ill patients and those with moderate to severe renal insufficiency.

Pharmacodynamics refers to the end-organ response to a drug. Although not as well understood as pharmacokinetic changes, pharmacodynamic changes can lead to changes in receptor binding, a decrease in receptor number, and altered translation of response to a receptor. One clinical example involves beta-adrenergic blockers and beta-adrenergic agonists. With aging, there is a reduction in beta-adrenergic activity in the cardiovascular and respiratory systems that can result in less responsiveness to beta blockers and beta agonists (Cooney and Pascuzzi, 2009).

Common Prescribing Issues

Prescribing problems that can lead to ADEs include a failure to monitor medications appropriately, to prescribe clinically indicated medications, to educate patients, or to maintain continuity (Higashi et al., 2004). One well-researched problem is the use of inappropriate medications in elderly patients. In 1991, based on ADEs in the nursing home, an expert panel developed a list of drugs that should generally be avoided in the elderly population (Beers et al., 1991). These Beers Criteria were updated in 2002 to include ambulatory and nursing facility populations (Fick et al., 2003/04). Medications on the list are generally ineffective in elderly patients, have a higher risk for ADEs, or have safer alternatives (Table 4-12). The list also includes recommendations regarding medication dosages that generally should not be

Table 4-12 Drugs to Avoid or Limit in the General Elderly Population

Pharmacologic Agents	Comments
Drug Classes to Avoid	
Antihistamines	Nonsedating antihistamines (e.g., fexofenadine, loratadine) are considered safer.
Antispasmodics	May result in anticholinergic side effects, sedation, and generalized weakness.
Barbiturates	Highly addictive with many side effects; numerous other agents for sedation are preferred.
Gastrointestinal antispasmodic drugs (e.g., dicyclomine, hyoscyamine)	Highly anticholinergic
Long-acting benzodiazepines (e.g., chlordiazepoxide, diazepam)	Short-acting or medium-acting agents are preferred; start with smaller doses.
Muscle relaxants	May result in anticholinergic side effects, sedation, and generalized weakness.
Specific Drugs to Avoid	
Amitriptyline	Highly anticholinergic; use newer antidepressants or less anticholinergic tricyclics.
Chlorpropamide	Long half-life leads to increased risk of hypoglycemia; newer insulin secretagogues are preferred.
Dipyridamole	May cause dizziness and hypotension.
Disopyramide	Anticholinergic and negative inotropic properties.
Doxepin	Highly anticholinergic; use newer antidepressants or less anticholinergic tricyclics.
Indomethacin	Compared with other NSAIDs, risk of CNS, gastrointestinal, and renal side effects is greater.
Meperidine	Active metabolite normeperidine may accumulate and cause CNS stimulation and seizures.
Meprobamate	Highly addictive, may worsen depression; other anxiolytics preferred.
Methyldopa	Common side effects include depression, sedation, and edema; multiple antihypertensive options are available.
Pentazocine	Mixed narcotic agonist/antagonist with potent CNS effects.
Phenylbutazone	May cause severe bone marrow suppression; other NSAIDs are preferred.
Propoxyphene	Weak narcotic pain reliever (probably no better than acetaminophen alone) but has same side profile as other narcotics.
Reserpine	CNS side effects include sedation and depression; multiple antihypertensive options are available.
Ticlopidine	More toxic effects than aspirin or clopidogrel.
Trimethobenzamide	May cause extrapyramidal side effects; numerous alternative antiemetics are available.
Drugs to Limit	
Digoxin	Limit to 0.125 mg/day or less in most elderly patients.
Ferrous sulfate	Limit to 325 mg/day or less in most elderly patients.

CNS, Central nervous system; *NSAIDs*, nonsteroidal anti-inflammatory drugs.

Data from Beers MH: Explicit criteria for determining potentially inappropriate medication use by the elderly: an update. Arch Intern Med 157:1531-536, 1997; Fick DM, Cooper JW, Wade WE, et al: Updating the Beers criteria for potentially inappropriate medication use in older adults. Arch Intern Med 163:2716-2724, 2003.

exceeded and medications to avoid in certain comorbid conditions. It is important to note that this list is only a *guideline;* if a patient has been taking one of the medications without adverse effects, it may not need to be discontinued.

On the other end of the spectrum is failure to prescribe clinically appropriate medications. Common oversights include a failure to prescribe a beta blocker for a patient with congestive heart failure or with a history of a myocardial infarction, aspirin in a patient with known coronary heart disease, or ACE inhibitors for a patient with diabetes and proteinuria (Rosen et al., 2004; Sloane et al., 2004).

Principles of Prescribing

With patients seeing multiple providers across different clinical settings, it is essential that the medication list remain updated. In one prospective observational study, 74% of patients were taking at least one medication of which their primary physician was unaware (Bikowski et al., 2001).

At least once yearly, ask your older patients to bring in all their medications, including OTC medications. Use a checklist to review each medication (Table 4-13). With each medication, first and foremost, review the indication. Educating the patient about the indication can decrease ADEs and increase adherence (Garcia, 2006). Is the medication effective? Medications are often started for good clinical reasons but never revisited as to their efficacy. Are there side effects? Medications should be discontinued if there are intolerable side effects, and always consider an ADE as a cause of any new patient symptom. Avoid the "prescribing cascade," in which medications are started to treat an ADE. Does the medication require any laboratory monitoring? This may include direct drug levels (e.g., digoxin) or monitoring for side effects (e.g., electrolytes in patient taking hydrochlorothiazide).

Is the patient taking the medication? Medication nonadherence is a common and complex issue with both physician and patient factors. Depending on the definition, "nonadherence" ranges from 14% to 70% (DeSmet et al., 2007). Adherence is associated with the number of medications, cost, frequency of dosing, and patient's knowledge of the condition. It is important to obtain the patient's perspective and concerns about medications in a nonjudgmental manner (Erice Group, 2009). Methods to increase adherence have focused on educational interventions and external cognitive aids. For short-term therapies, written information, counseling about the medication's indication and potential side effects, and personal phone calls increased adherence. The same effect was not seen for patients taking long-term medications (Haynes et al., 2008; McDonald et al., 2002).

Finally, the checklist should include asking if the medication is still needed. Has the patient's condition changed to where you can stop unnecessary drugs, such as preventive medications in a hospice patient?

Continuity of pharmacists is as important as continuity of physicians in decreasing medication errors. Encourage patients to use one pharmacy, and inform the pharmacist of any medication changes. Seeking input from the pharmacist can reduce inappropriate prescribing (Garcia, 2006). With inpatient settings, pharmacists obtain more accurate medication histories from patients, reducing the rate and severity of ADEs (Carter et al., 2006; Reeder and Mutnick, 2008). Simplify the medication regimen by using once-daily dosing and generic drugs, if possible. Discontinue medications that have no indication or benefit (Carlson, 1996). When initiating medications, start one at a time at the lowest dose possible (Table 4-14).

The decision to prescribe a drug depends on many factors besides age, including the patient's functional status, comorbidities, other medications, and personal preferences and values. Physicians must be extremely vigilant in prescribing, especially for the frail elderly patient, carefully weighing the risks and benefits of any new medication. Periodic review of patients' medication list is essential to monitor for adverse effects, potentially inappropriate drugs, drug-drug interactions, and drug-disease interactions.

KEY TREATMENT

Current methods of improving medication adherence for chronic health problems are not predictably effective (Haynes et al., 2008; McDonald et al., 2002) (SOR: B).

Certain drugs should be avoided or limited in the elderly patient (Fick et al., 2003/04) (SOR: C).

Obtain local pharmacists' recommendations to reduce inappropriate prescribing and adverse drug events (Garcia, 2006) (SOR: B).

Reviewing a medication list regularly can reduce polypharmacy and inappropriate prescribing (SOR: B).

Urinary Incontinence

Key Points

- Incontinence is a common medical problem in the elderly population, affecting up to 30% of women and 15% of men.
- Older women are more likely to have urge and stress incontinence, and older men are more likely to experience overflow and urge incontinence.
- Acute episodes of incontinence are more likely the result of underlying medical conditions (e.g., infection, hyperglycemia) or new medications (e.g., diuretics).

Table 4-13 Medication Question Checklist

1. Is there a clear indication for this medication?
2. Is it working?
3. Are there side effects?
4. Is the patient taking the medication routinely?
5. Does the medication need lab monitoring?
6. Is it still needed?

Table 4-14 Principles of Rational Drug Prescribing for Elderly Patients

1. Periodically update and review the medication list.
2. Work with the community pharmacist.
3. Educate the patient about the medication.
4. Consider an adverse drug event (ADE) as a cause of any new patient symptom.
5. Simplify the medication regimen.
6. Start one medication at a time, at lowest possible dose.

- Specific health risks, including depression and falls, have been linked to urinary incontinence in the elderly patient.
- History, physical examination, urinalysis, and postvoid residual assessment are the key elements in categorization of incontinence.
- In the majority of patients, incontinence can be diagnosed and treated by the primary care provider.
- Treatment options for incontinence include behavior modification, pelvic floor exercises, pharmacologic agents, vaginal pessaries, periurethral bulking agents, and surgical procedures.
- Systemic hormone replacement therapy may exacerbate incontinence.

Urinary incontinence, defined as involuntary leakage of urine, affects 25% to 30% of all adults in their lifetime. The estimated prevalence of urinary incontinence in people over 65 years of age ranges from 35% in community-dwelling individuals to more than 60% for those who reside in long-term care facilities (Goode et al., 2008; Song and Bae, 2007; Tennstedt et al., 2008). Incontinence not only increases in prevalence with age, but also is considered part of a geriatric syndrome. Within the younger population a specific condition of the lower urinary tract or its neurologic control is often the cause of urinary incontinence. In older persons, however, incontinence is often secondary to physiologic age-related changes, comorbidities, medications, and functional impairments.

In 2000 the estimated total cost of urinary incontinence in the United States was $16.3 billion, with $12.4 billion spent on incontinence care for women alone. Routine incontinence care represented the largest expenditure (Hu et al., 2004). Women spend almost $750 annually out of pocket for incontinence management, have significantly decreased quality of life, and are willing to pay almost $1400 per year for a cure. The annual costs of incontinence care are greater than annual direct costs for breast, ovarian, cervical, and uterine cancer treatments combined (Subak et al., 2006, 2008; Wilson et al., 2001).

Urinary incontinence is associated with increased morbidity and mortality. Studies have demonstrated an association between urinary incontinence and worsening in overall function. Health-related quality-of-life measurements have been found to decline in individuals with urinary incontinence (DuBeau et al., 2009; Ko et al., 2005; Teunissen et al., 2006). This decline has been seen in those living independently, in assisted-living facilities, and in long-term care environments (DuBeau et al., 2006).

Specific health risks linked to urinary incontinence include depression, social isolation, urinary tract infections, pressure ulcers, falls and fractures, decreased sexual activity, sleep deprivation, and increased caregiver stress (Brown et al., 2000; Griebling, 2006; Ory et al., 1986; Spector, 1994). Urinary incontinence is also found to be a common reason for institutionalization of the elderly patient (Holroyd-Leduc et al., 2004).

Age-Related Changes in Urinary System

Specific age-related changes in the urinary system can directly influence urinary continence. The pelvic floor muscles can lose tone and predispose women to uterine, bladder, and rectal prolapse, causing secondary urge incontinence. Overall

Table 4-15 Medications Associated with Urinary Incontinence in Elderly Patients

Diuretics: polyuria, frequency, urgency
Angiotensin-converting enzyme (ACE) inhibitors: cough precipitating stress incontinence
Anticholinergics: urinary retention, overflow incontinence, stool impaction
Psychotropics: anticholinergic actions, sedation, immobility, delirium
Narcotic analgesics: urinary retention, fecal impaction, sedation, delirium
Alpha-adrenergic agonists: contraction of smooth muscle of urethra and prostatic capsule
Alpha-adrenergic blockers: urethral relaxation
Alcohol: polyuria, frequency, urgency, sedation, delirium, immobility
Caffeine: polyuria, bladder irritation

bladder capacity also tends to decrease, limiting total volume and therefore increasing urge to urinate. Prostatic hypertrophy predisposes older men to increases in postvoid residual volumes. Older incontinent persons may also experience increased involuntary bladder contractions, exacerbating the problem.

Presentation

Urinary incontinence presentations can be divided into acute ("transient") or chronic. Sudden onset of incontinence by potentially reversible and treatable conditions is referred to as *acute* urinary incontinence. Conditions contributing to acute incontinence include lower urinary tract conditions, stool impaction, delirium, fluid imbalance, impaired mobility, and medications (Table 4-15). These conditions not only precipitate acute urinary incontinence, but can also contribute to chronic incontinence.

Chronic incontinence can be divided into five types: urge, stress, overflow, functional, and mixed (Table 4-16).

Urge Incontinence

Urge incontinence is the most common type of incontinence identified in the older ambulatory patient. It is defined as an abrupt, urgent sensation to urinate and results in loss of urine, with both large and small amounts. Urinary frequency and nocturia are often associated with urge incontinence. *Detrusor overactivity* is also associated, caused by age-related smooth muscle changes, central inhibitory pathway lesions, history of pelvic irradiation, and bladder sensory or motor innervation deficits. Urge incontinence with an elevated postvoid residual volume can occur when detrusor overactivity and impaired detrusor contractility occur simultaneously. Urinary frequency and retention are common in these patients, particularly those receiving anticholinergic medications.

Stress Incontinence

Stress incontinence is the unintentional loss of urine. It is most often associated with weakening of the pelvic floor muscles and subsequent hypermobility of the bladder outlet and urethra. Stress incontinence occurs with physical movement or activity, such as coughing, sneezing, laughing, or heavy lifting. Stress incontinence is often seen in older women with previous vaginal deliveries or pelvic surgery. It

Table 4-16 Persistent Urinary Incontinence: Types, Causes, and Treatments

Types	Symptoms	Common Causes	Primary Treatment
Stress	Involuntary loss of urine with increases in intra-abdominal pressure (e.g., cough, laugh, exercise)	Urethral hypermobility Sphincteric dysfunction Radical prostatectomy	Scheduled voiding Pelvic muscle exercises Alpha-adrenergic agonist* Estrogen (topical)* Periurethral injection Surgical bladder neck suspension or sling
Urge	Leakage of urine because of inability to delay voiding after sensation of bladder fullness is perceived	Detrusor overactivity Neurologic disorders Spinal cord injury	Antimuscarinic drugs Topical estrogen (for severe vaginal atrophy or atrophic vaginitis) Bladder training (including pelvic muscle exercises)
Mixed	Combination of urge and stress symptoms	Combination of above causes	One or combination of above, targeting most bothersome symptom(s) first
Overflow	Leakage of urine resulting from mechanical forces on overdistended bladder, or from other effects of urinary retention on bladder and sphincter function	Detrusor failure Neurologic disorders Spinal cord injury Diabetes Anatomic obstruction	Bladder retraining Surgical removal of obstruction Intermittent catheterization Indwelling catheterization
Functional	Urinary accidents associated with inability to toilet, caused by impairment of cognitive or physical functioning, psychological unwillingness, or environmental barriers	Mobility impairment Cognitive impairment	Behavioral interventions with toileting assistance Environmental adaptations Undergarments and pads

*Controversial.

is also associated with lack of estrogen in the menopausal woman. Obesity can exacerbate the symptoms of stress incontinence.

Overflow Incontinence

Symptoms of overflow incontinence include weak urine stream, dribbling, urinary hesitancy, frequency, and nocturia. These symptoms may overlap with other types of incontinence, influencing the diagnosis. The etiology of overflow incontinence includes detrusor muscle weakness, bladder outlet obstruction, or both. Medications such as narcotics, anticholinergics, and alpha-adrenergic blockers can contribute to overflow incontinence.

Functional Incontinence

Functional incontinence refers to leakage of urine caused by factors not directly associated with the bladder. Cognitive impairment (e.g., dementia), mobility disorders (e.g., Parkinson's disease), and inaccessible bathrooms are the most common contributing factors in functional incontinence. Factors may be temporary, as in the patient with a lower extremity fracture who is not able to transfer independently on and off the toilet.

Mixed Incontinence

Mixed urinary incontinence is the combination of two types of incontinence simultaneously, typically stress and urge incontinence. Mixed incontinence is the most common type in women, and the causes of the two forms may or may not

be related. *Detrusor hyperactivity with impaired contractility* (DHIC) is a form of mixed incontinence specific to older adults. Symptoms include urinary frequency and urgency caused by uninhibited contractions of the detrusor smooth muscle. When patients try to void, the bladder does not contract sufficiently, and emptying is incomplete, leading to overflow incontinence.

Evaluation

The initial step in the clinical evaluation is the identification of patients with urinary incontinence. Many older patients do not complain about incontinence to their health care provider because they are embarrassed or believe their symptoms are just part of normal aging. Direct questioning during the review of systems can help identify urinary incontinence: Do you have trouble with your bladder? Do you lose urine when you do not want to? Do you find that you have to wear pads or adult diapers for protection? (Fantl et al., 1996; Kane et al., 2004).

A thorough history and physical examination are important in the clinical evaluation of older patients with urinary incontinence. The main objectives of the workup are to diagnose and treat reversible causes, establish the principal type of urinary incontinence to help guide treatment, identify patients who may need subspecialty referral, and improve overall quality of life for the patient. Once urinary incontinence has been identified, the evaluation should continue with a detailed incontinence history, including the type of leakage, frequency, duration, inciting factors, previous treatments, and overall treatment goals. The physical exam should include abdominal, genitopelvic, rectal, and neurologic evaluation. Health care providers need to be aware of the specific "red flags" to refer a patient for further urologic, gynecologic, or urodynamic evaluation (Table 4-17).

A urinalysis should be obtained in all patients to assess for urinary tract infections, hematuria, or other medical conditions that may be associated with urinary incontinence. Persistent hematuria should prompt additional evaluation, including upper urinary tract imaging and cystoscopy. A postvoid residual volume (with ultrasound or catheterization) helps to exclude overflow incontinence. In clinical practice, a postvoid volume of less than 50 mL is regarded as normal, and in general, residual volumes greater than 200 mL are considered abnormal (Fantl et al., 1996).

Voiding (bladder) diaries can provide valuable information for the clinician and patient. The diary includes documentation of each urination episode and any associated symptoms of incontinence for three 24-hour periods. If possible, the patient can also record the amount of fluid intake and output (Abrams and Klevmark, 1996). Several patterns of abnormality can emerge from the voiding diary. For example, frequent small volumes can occur in patients with overactive bladder syndrome, detrusor overactivity, and some painful bladder conditions (e.g., cancer). Frequent large-volume voids are associated with *polyuria*, as seen in patients with excessive fluid intake and conditions causing polyuria (e.g., diabetes, hypercalcemia). Obstructive sleep apnea, physiologic aging, congestive heart failure, and medications can all cause nocturnal polyuria (Bryan et al., 2004). A simple office tool that can help detect stress incontinence is the cough test. The patient is asked to produce a forceful cough with a comfortably full bladder to determine any urine leakage and potential stress incontinence.

Treatment

Several therapeutic options exist to help manage the different types of urinary incontinence. Many older adults prefer to start with conservative therapies such as behavioral modification techniques before considering medications or surgery. In many cases, several small behavioral changes together may lead to significant improvement in symptoms.

Behavioral Interventions

Particular beverages can aggravate the lower urinary tract symptoms in older adults. Alcohol, caffeine, and highly acidic citrus fruits and drinks are considered direct bladder-irritants and may worsen incontinence symptoms. Alcohol has diuretic properties, causing increased urinary frequency. Weight loss may be beneficial for some patients, in particular women with stress incontinence. *Nocturia* is a common complaint for many elderly patients with multifactorial causes (Sugaya et al., 2008). Minimizing late-afternoon and evening fluid intake may decrease nocturnal episodes for some patients. Reduced production of antidiuretic hormone has been seen in patients with obstructive sleep apnea. Treatment of the sleep apnea may help reduce nocturia symptoms (Kujuba and Aboseif, 2008).

In older patients with symptoms of urinary urgency, *timed voiding* is often suggested. Many patients experience symptoms only when the bladder is full, so voiding more frequently will reduce the amount of bladder distention and the sense of urinary urgency. Older patients with cognitive or mobility impairments will often need assisted-toileting programs. Providing physical assistance in going to the toilet on a regular basis can reduce incontinence episodes (van Houten et al., 2007). Some patients benefit from *bladder retraining*, in which they are taught to delay voiding at progressively longer intervals (Wallace et al., 2004). Bladder retraining can take months and has the most benefit for patients with urge incontinence and those with mixed incontinence when combined with pelvic floor exercises (Tuenissen et al., 2004). The patient is encouraged to focus on the sensations in the pelvis, complete pelvic floor contractions and wait until the urgency sensation subsides before proceeding to the toilet.

Pelvic floor muscle (Kegel) *exercises* remain one of the mainstays of behavioral therapy in the treatment of urinary incontinence. The exercises involve repetitive contractions and relaxations of the pelvic floor muscles. They have been found effective in stress, urge, and mixed incontinence (Hay-Smith and Dumoulin, 2006). A simply way to teach women to identify and isolate the pelvic floor muscles is by having the patient squeeze the examiner's finger during vaginal examination. Squeezing the examiner's finger by contracting the anal sphincter during a rectal exam can help both men and women isolate the pelvic floor muscles.

Pessaries in many different forms have been used for hundreds of years for the treatment of pelvic organ prolapse and urinary incontinence in women. The support offered by the pessary helps in correcting the angles and contacts between adjacent organs, thus minimizing bladder irritation and spontaneous contractions that lead to incontinence. Pessaries come in a variety of shapes and sizes and must be individually fitted for each patient by their health provider. Routine cleaning and care by either the patient or, in many cases, their provider is required. In many women, pessaries offer the advantage of avoiding surgery while providing functional support.

Many older adults with urinary incontinence use some type of pad or undergarment to help with their urinary incontinence. Although these products play an important role in the management of incontinence symptoms, patients should be encouraged to seek other types of treatment if appropriate. The cost of these products can be significant and is not covered by Medicare or most other insurance plans. However, it is important to realize that these absorbent products can help older adults maintain their functional independence and participate in their preferred activities.

Table 4-17 "Red Flag" Criteria for Referral of Older Patient with Incontinence to Subspecialist

Significant uterine, bladder, or rectal prolapse
Surgery or radiation involving lower urinary tract within past 6 months
Two or more symptomatic urinary infections in past 6 months
More than five red blood cells per high-power field (>5 RBCs/hpf) on repeated urinalysis in the absence of infection
Postvoid residual volume greater than 200 mL
Marked prostatic enlargement, prominent asymmetry, or induration of bladder lobes
Persistent symptoms after appropriate trials of behavioral or drug therapy

Pharmacologic Therapies

Various medications have been used to treat the different forms of urinary incontinence. However, most current medications are used for urge or mixed incontinence, because there is little evidence that adrenergic agonists help stress incontinence (Alhasso et al., 2005) (Table 4-18). The anticholinergic, antimuscarinic medications prescribed for urge incontinence work by blocking cholinergic receptors in the bladder, which in turn diminishes bladder contractility. This class of medications is effective but has adverse side effects (e.g., dry mouth, constipation) related to the cross-reactivity with muscarinic receptors in the salivary glands and colon (Alhasso et al., 2006). Additional side effects include dry eyes, blurry vision, and risk of urinary retention. Anticholin-

ergics in the elderly patient can also worsen cognitive function or cause drug-induced delirium, mimicking dementia. Newer medications that are theoretically more uroselective and preferentially bind to the muscarinic receptors in the bladder may be associated with fewer adverse side effects. Incontinence medications should not be prescribed to those patients with untreated closed-angle glaucoma and in memory-impaired patients already taking cholinesterase inhibitors, to prevent further deterioration of memory function. The anticholinergic agents and cholinesterase inhibitors work in direct opposition and, if taken together, can lead to rapid loss of cognitive function (Sink et al., 2008).

Alpha-adrenergic antagonists are helpful in treating urge incontinence in men with benign prostatic hypertrophy (BPH). Hypotension is a common side effect with traditional

Table 4-18 Drug Treatment for Urinary Incontinence

Generic Drugs (Trade Name)	Dosages	Mechanisms of Action	Type of Incontinence
Antimuscarinic			
Darifenacin (Enablex)	7.5-15 mg qd	Lessen involuntary bladder contractions and increase bladder capacity	Urge or mixed
Oxybutynin (Ditropan) (Ditropan XL) (Oxytrol transdermal)	2.5-5 mg tid 5-30 mg qd (extended release) 3.9-mg patch every 4 days	Lessen involuntary bladder contractions and increase bladder capacity	Urge or mixed
Solifenacin (Vesicare)	5-10 mg qd	Lessen involuntary bladder contractions and increase bladder capacity	Urge or mixed
Tolterodine (Detrol) (Detrol XL)	1-2 mg bid 2-4 mg qd (extended-release)	Lessen involuntary bladder contractions and increase bladder capacity	Urge or mixed
Trospium (Sanctura) (Santura XR)	20 mg bid 60 mg qd (extended release)	Lessen involuntary bladder contractions and increase bladder capacity	Urge or mixed
Estrogen			
Topical estrogen Topical cream	0.5-1.0 g qd for 2 weeks, then twice weekly	Strengthen periurethral tissues Increase periurethral blood flow	Urge, associated with severe vaginal atrophy or atrophic vaginitis Stress
Vaginal ring	One ring every 3 months		
Vaginal tablets	One 25-µg tablet qd for 2 weeks, then twice weekly		
Cholinergic Agonist			
Bethanechol (Urecholine)	10-30 mg tid	Stimulate bladder contraction	Overflow, with atonic bladder
Alpha-Adrenergic Antagonists			
Alfuzosin (UroXatral)	10 mg qd	Relax smooth muscle or urethra and prostate capsule	Urge, and symptoms associated with BPH
Tamsulosin (Flomax)	0.4 mg qd		
Terazosin (Hytrin)	1-10 mg qhs		

qd, Every day; *tid,* three times daily; *bid,* twice daily, *qhs,* every night at bedtime; *BPH,* benign prostatic hypertrophy.

alpha agents. The newer agents have less adverse side effects and should be used in older men who have low blood pressure or episodes of dizziness. The addition of an antimuscarinic drug can be considered in those men who are still symptomatic on alpha-antagonist therapy. For long-term treatment of overflow incontinence in men, 5α-reductase inhibitors alone or in combination have been shown to reduce the voiding symptoms from BPH as well as the incidence of urinary retention (McConnell et al., 2003).

The role of *estrogen* in the treatment of incontinence in the elderly patient remains uncertain. Topical estrogen is often prescribed for older women with urge incontinence related to atrophic vaginitis or severe vaginal atrophy. Conversely, combination estrogen/progestin oral hormone therapy has been associated with increased frequency of incontinence (Cody et al., 2009; Grady et al., 2001; Rossouw et al., 2002).

Surgical Treatment

The *sling procedure* is the primary form of open surgical treatment in women with stress incontinence. Several variations of the procedure exist with relation to the exact location of the sling and the nature of the graft material used to make the sling. The principal function of the sling is to increase the outlet resistance and thus prevent urine leakage during periods of increased intra-abdominal pressure. Initial success rates for the sling procedure range from 80% to 90% but decrease with time. Some women respond to other forms of therapy or elect to undergo another sling procedure (Anger et al., 2007).

Periurethral injection of bulking agents can be an effective treatment is some elderly women with stress incontinence. The procedure is minimally invasive and can be performed in the outpatient setting with rapid recovery and immediate results. To date, there is limited evidence that this can relieve stress incontinence in women (Keegan et al., 2007). One disadvantage is that treatment usually needs to be repeated with time. Injection therapy may be particularly useful in elderly women who are unable to undergo the more invasive sling procedure or who are symptomatic after a previous sling procedure. Older men with mild postprostatectomy stress incontinence may benefit from periurethral injection of bulking agents (Fantl et al., 1996).

KEY TREATMENT

Pelvic floor exercises help with all types of urinary incontinence in women (Hay-Smith and Dumoulin, 2006) (SOR: A).
Anticholinergic drugs are effective for overactive bladder syndrome, but are associated with common side effects (Alhasso et al., 2006) (SOR: A).
There is limited evidence that periurethral injection helps women with stress incontinence (Keegan et al., 2007) (SOR: A).

References

The complete reference list is available online at www.expertconsult.com.

Web Resources

www.ncbi.nlm.nih.gov/bookshelf/br.fcgi?book=hsahcpr&part=A5124
Agency for Health Care Policy and Research (AHCPR) Treatment of Pressure Ulcers Guideline.
www.npuap.org
National Pressure Ulcer Advisory Panel. Provides up-to-date information on the prevention and management of pressure ulcers.

www.aoa.gov
Administration on Aging. Offers comprehensive information about "seniors," including aging statistics and government programs.
www.ncea.aoa.gov/NCEAroot/Main_Site/Index.aspx
National Center on Elder Abuse. Provides information on the prevention, diagnosis, and management of elder abuse, including available resources for physicians, patients, and families.

Videos

www.fammed.wisc.edu/our-department/media/615/geriatric-assessment
Geriatric Assessment Podcast. An overview of geriatric assessment in the office setting.www.youtube.com/user/WIFamilyMedicine#p/u/4 3/xIMJ1aVvch8 Elder Abuse Podcast. An overview of the assessment and management of elder abuse.

CHAPTER **5**

Care of the Dying Patient

Robert E. Rakel and Elizabeth M. Strauch

Chapter contents

Medical education and our professional attitude regarding patient care are oriented primarily toward sustaining life and curing disease. This is reasonable, because not long ago the major causes of death were the infectious diseases, which usually attacked young people, who died before experiencing life. With the advent of antibiotics, it was possible to triumph over these diseases and prevent untimely death. Patients had a high probability of complete recovery. It is no surprise, therefore, that the medical profession emphasized preserving life at all costs and became preoccupied with the advancing technology that made such triumphs possible. Today, people no longer die of acute illness, but rather from chronic disease for which there is no cure. This calls for medicine to focus on improving the *quality* rather than the quantity of life and to recognize that the relief of suffering is superior to attempts to cure when there is limited likelihood of success. Patients with chronic diseases and those who are terminally ill will benefit most from supportive therapy.

In previous centuries, it was assumed that life should be lived so that one would be able to "die well," but contemporary American culture has refused to accept death as a normal occurrence. Children and young adults have been conditioned to consider death from the viewpoint of the observer or disinterested third party. An individual's attitude toward his or her own death depends largely on experiences in dealing with the deaths of relatives or friends. Rather than

a time of despair, sickness may be used as an opportunity for reflection. For some patients, it may be the first time they have faced their own mortality. Too often, however, this natural personal encounter has been depersonalized by removing the dying patient to an institutional setting.

Care of a terminally ill patient typically focuses on the disease, neglecting the patient as a whole person. The value of treatment must be interpreted on the basis of its net value to the individual. When additional treatments no longer provide benefits, the patient needs someone who provides personalized care with attention to the patient's emotional as well as physical comfort. The dying person often is isolated physically and emotionally from familiar surroundings and placed in a social setting that gives very low priority to an individual's personality, fears, and past experiences. Informed physicians, family, and friends can do much to help the terminal patient die with integrity and with dignity. However, if dying is really to be accepted as a normal component of the life cycle, reintegration of the dying patient into the routine course of living is necessary.

The concept of quality care does not always demand that death be regarded as an enemy to be fought with every weapon at a physician's disposal. An obsession with quantity of life can adversely affect its quality; at times, a graceful death with dignity is preferable to lingering torment (LORAN Commission, 1989, p. 27). Many people consider quality of life more important than quantity and want to leave while they still have something to say about it. Today, it is possible to keep people alive indefinitely, often without consideration for the quality of life.

The Physician's Attitude

Less than 10% of people die suddenly, whereas more than 90% experience a protracted life-threatening illness (Emanuel et al., 2003). Terminal illness is more taxing on the physician than sudden and unexpected death. Not surprisingly, an empathic family physician with a long patient relationship may be uncomfortable in dealing with the patient's impending death. Physicians are most uncomfortable when they feel helpless. Unfortunately, this leads to withdrawal from the patient who is terminally ill, because the physician inappropriately feels helpless and impotent, when in fact a great deal of comfort and help can be provided.

While expressing concern and compassion for a terminal patient, the family physician still must maintain composure and objectivity to remain effective. Osler (1904) referred to this as "calm equanimity" and added, "Our equanimity is chiefly exercised in enabling us to bear with composure the misfortunes of our neighbors" (p. 8). Medicine long has emphasized the need for physicians to remain objective and deal with problems factually; if a physician is unable to do so effectively, attempts to hide emotion may lead the physician to adopt a facade that appears unsympathetic and insensitive to the patient's needs. A son reported that "with the worsening of my father's condition, the physician stopped being friendly and warm; his visits became rare and brief; his manner became quite detached, almost angry" (Seravalli, 1988, p. 1729).

Physicians sometimes lose enthusiasm for care once an illness has been recognized as incurable. If this occurs, interaction with the patient diminishes at the very time emotional support is needed most. Time-motion studies indicate that nurses and other ward personnel also spend less time with the terminally ill patient when giving baths and providing routine care. Using videotape surveillance of terminally ill patients' rooms in a university hospital, Sulmasy and Rahn (2001) found that the average patient spent more than 10 hours alone while awake per day. Since abandonment is a major fear of terminally ill patients, we must remain aware of the need to reduce the time patients spend without human interaction by physicians, nurses, or family.

Compassion fatigue is a form of emotional exhaustion and diminished empathy more common in health professionals caring for dying patients. Symptoms parallel those of posttraumatic stress disorder (PTSD), that is, hyperarousal, in the form of disturbed sleep and irritability, avoidance of the patient, and intrusive thoughts or dreams relating to the provider's work with dying patients (Kearney et al., 2009).

During the terminal stages of a fatal illness, it is vital to the dying patient that the family physician maintain a warm and caring relationship and, through the strength of the doctor-patient bond, provide support for the patient.

The physician who is uncomfortable discussing impending death can discourage conversation in many subtle ways. Hospital rounds are made rapidly, perhaps in a superficial, lighthearted manner, never pausing long enough to give the patient an opportunity to express fears and concerns. Comments such as "everything will be all right" effectively close lines of communication with an intelligent patient who is fully aware of the seriousness of the situation. When the physician tells a patient, "Don't worry," the patient interprets this as, "Don't bother me." Patients are unlikely to initiate discussions regarding their fears of death or feelings of helplessness under such circumstances and will remain silent or will avoid these issues unless they think the physician is interested and will listen. The physician easily can squelch such conversation, but a slight indication of willingness to discuss the problems disturbing the patient often results in frank conversations, which relieve much of the patient's anxiety and reveal concerns that can be shared only with the physician.

The "Right Time" to Die

Simpson (1976) described the "how dare you die on me" syndrome, in which the patient has the "effrontery" to die before medical and nursing staff have used all the treatments in their repertoire. The patient is supposed to die "at the right time"—neither before all potential effective therapies have been tried nor too long after all palliative procedures have been utilized. Health professionals often need to feel that everything possible was done for the patient before death. These attitudes have developed because the health care process too often focuses more on professional expectations than patient needs.

We might consider what we have done to the patient who dies in the isolation of a laminar flow room, without having been able to touch another person's hand during his last few weeks of life. Such treatment is a *false-positive*, a treatment inappropriate to the real needs of the patient (Saunders, 1976).

However, it is impossible for physicians to provide adequate support during this difficult time unless they have come to grips with their own mortality. Studies by the Group for the Advancement of Psychiatry have revealed that physicians are afraid of death in greater proportion than patient controls (Aring, 1971). What better defense against death than to make one's full-time vocation fighting it?

Patients are often more willing to accept death than the physicians who treat them, and many fear that they will receive more aggressive treatment than they want. Based on interviews with seriously ill patients, 60% preferred that treatment focus on comfort, even if it meant shortening their lives. The other 40% wanted life-extending care. Of those preferring comfort care, only 41% reported that treatment matched their wishes (Teno et al., 2002). In another study, more than half of physicians interviewed admitted they had provided overly aggressive care to patients (Solomon et al., 1993).

Many if not most patients will choose toxic chemotherapy, even if there is only a slight chance of cure, or even if it would prolong their life by only a few months. The concern is that they may choose this route on the advice of their physician, even though they will be miserable for those remaining months. It is important to have a straightforward discussion with the patient about the quality and quantity of life with and without chemotherapy. More than 20% of Medicare patients with metastatic cancer had a new chemotherapy treatment regimen started in the 2 weeks before death (Earle et al., 2004).

Unfortunately, chemotherapy is better compensated than are discussions as to its need and potential side effects. It is no surprise that oncologists prefer third- or fourth-line chemotherapy to discussing hospice care. One patient received intrathecal chemotherapy 6 days before his death at a cost of $3400 (Harrington and Smith, 2008).

Communication

Key Points

- Abandonment is a major fear of dying patients, who spend an average of 10 awake hours alone per day.
- Listening and allowing patients to express their fears and concerns is of great therapeutic benefit.
- Touch and sitting with the patient convey support and compassion.
- Frequent assessment of the patient and family's desire for information must be accompanied by honest answers.
- Patients should be allowed as much control as possible to avoid fear of the unknown.
- When cure is not possible, much benefit can be derived from attention to daily symptom control.
- Avoid giving false hope, but remember that hope and humor can be therapeutic.

When to Tell the Patient

The issue today is not so much whether to tell patients they have a terminal illness, but rather how to share this information with them—because most patients know the nature of their disease process to some degree. Because they know their patients well, family physicians should be able to gauge patients' desire to be told and their capacity to withstand the shock of disclosure. When a terminal state of cancer is inevitable, most patients prefer to discuss such issues with their family physician rather than with their oncologist.

Patients who have end-of-life conversations with their family physician have lower health care costs during the final week of life. Better communication results in better quality of life and quality of death as well as lower cost (Zhang et al., 2009). End-of-life care is often fragmented among providers, leading to a lack of continuity of care and impeding the ability to provide high-quality, interdisciplinary care. Enhanced communication among patients, families, and providers is crucial to high-quality end-of-life care (National Institutes of Health, 2004).

A frank discussion of death or how long the patient is expected to live may not be necessary or even indicated. A good understanding between physician and patient may make open disclosure unnecessary. The physician's role may be primarily one of supporting patients during the progressive, terminal course of their illness. However, the physician who is uncomfortable with the subject of death should not use such a situation as an excuse to avoid discussing the issue. The family physician's primary responsibility is to take the time to evaluate the situation, make sure the patient's true desires have been assessed correctly, and provide whatever support is needed, based on the patient's concepts and needs rather than those of the physician (Table 5-1).

The physician who can deal with death honestly is able to focus more attention on the patient and can determine the patient's level of awareness by listening and observing nonverbal cues. Clues to the patient's wish to discuss the condition may simply be a deep sigh, a tear, or a shaky voice. The physician must be alert during busy hospital rounds for these or similar signs. The physician can pause to sit and encourage conversation if time permits, or return later when more time is available. Whenever possible, however, the response should be at that moment, because the patient is more likely to communicate freely in a spontaneous situation. Physicians who are uncomfortable in this situation may insulate themselves from the issue during hospital rounds by checking the bedside monitoring equipment, or otherwise directing attention away from the patient, effectively ignoring overt as well as subtle clues to the patient's needs.

Talking with patients about their death can be difficult, but end-of-life discussions with patients do not result in greater emotional or psychological stress. On the contrary, worse outcomes are found in those who do not have these conversations. Such discussions result in less aggressive medical care near death and earlier hospice referrals. Wright and colleagues (2008) showed that quality of life deteriorates with a greater number of aggressive end-of-life interventions and improves with longer hospice care. Patients who spend less than a week in hospice have the same quality of life as those who receive no hospice care.

When the patient is ready to discuss her or his impending death, physician and patient are probably past the most difficult stage, and the physician needs merely to listen, accept the patient's feelings, and respond to questions honestly. Most patients will raise questions that indicate how much they wish to know, provided the physician gives them the opportunity. The most supportive and facilitative act the physician can provide is to sit and ask the patient, "Do you have any questions?" When asked in a sincere manner, patients who are ready to talk about their death will take advantage of the opportunity, but they may be reluctant under other, more hurried circumstances.

Patients usually will indicate their desire to discuss their prognosis, as well as when they want to avoid the subject and focus on other topics. Even patients who fully accept their terminal process cannot remain constantly focused on that

Table 5-1 Useful Questions in Determining a Terminally Ill Patient's Needs and Wishes

• What do you fear most?
• What would you like to accomplish in the time left?
• Which is your highest priority?
• How can I help you achieve this?
• What has been most difficult about this illness for you?
• How is your family (wife, husband, daughter, etc.) dealing with your illness?
• Is religion important to you?

subject and must attend to more satisfying issues. Physicians should honor and respond to this need, just as they would respond to a desire to discuss pain or other problems.

What physicians say to dying patients is not nearly as important as their willingness to listen. One of the most comforting steps physicians can take in caring for the dying is to allow them to talk about their fears, frustrations, hopes, needs, and desires. *Talking about problems can be very therapeutic.* Patients who are permitted to examine and discuss their feelings about death and dying are grateful for the opportunity and usually become less anxious, experience less pain, and accept their situation more easily. If they are denied this opportunity, especially when the terminal process is obvious, they may be convinced that the time remaining is too terrible to be discussed, and their anxiety will be significantly increased. Often, terminally ill patients are more fearful of the manner in which death will occur (e.g., painful, alone and abandoned, weak and helpless) than they are of death itself.

Do all patients want to be told of their fatal illness, however? Surveys indicate that 80% to 90% of patients say they wish to be told, whereas many physicians prefer not to tell a patient that he or she is dying. Ward (1974) found that family physicians are more likely to discuss a fatal diagnosis with women than with men (22% vs. 7.5%) and more often with patients in the upper social class than the lower social class (24% vs. 5% for men; 30% vs. 26% for women). Many physicians who state that they theoretically believe in telling the patient of the terminal nature of the illness employ evasion in their actual practice as often as most other physicians. Because of this reluctance, which may be based on discomfort with the issue emanating from intensive conditioning to preserve health and maintain life, future medical students must be trained more adequately in assisting patients with the process of living just before death.

Most physicians will tell a patient that he or she has terminal cancer if the patient asks a direct question, but otherwise will evade the issue and discuss it openly only with the family. In many cases this is the most appropriate course of action; some patients clearly indicate that they cannot and do not wish to face the fact that they have an incurable disease. It is essential, however, that the physician evaluate the true nature of the patient's desire in the matter and neither avoid the issue when the patient wishes to discuss it nor force a discussion on an unwilling individual. "When the task of telling a patient about an onerous diagnosis is too easy, the doctor has become callous. When it is too difficult, he needs to examine his own guilt or anxiety" (Weisman and Brettell, 1978, p. 251).

Patients should be given adequate time to absorb the knowledge of the terminal nature of their illness and the opportunity to react appropriately before death intervenes. This is not possible if the physician procrastinates or rationalizes that it is better not to inform the patient. The process should not be allowed to advance to such a final a stage that inadequate time remains for individuals to react appropriately and put their affairs in order.

How to Tell the Patient

There is no need to answer questions the patient has not yet asked. One way to approach the subject is to ask patients what they think the problem is, or how sick they think they really are. The response may be straightforward ("I think I have cancer"), or the patient may indicate a wish to avoid the issue by saying, "I hope it's nothing serious." The patient's condition can be revealed gradually or in stages, such as telling the patient after surgery that there is a suspicion of cancer, but that further information will have to wait for the pathology report. The physician should observe the patient's response to this initial suspicion and, based on that reaction, choose a method for presenting subsequent information. Tumulty (1973) supported the concept of *gradualism* in informing a patient and the family of the terminal nature of the illness: "The total truth is revealed in small doses as the illness unfolds, affording the family the opportunity to get its feet under itself before another blow falls.... The patient and the family need to be eased into the truth... not slugged with it" (pp. 180-181).

Such a gradual disclosure is likely to lead to acceptance, whereas a harsh, sudden, or abrupt disclosure is likely to result in denial or severe depression. If the patient appears reluctant to accept the information, do not push the issue; merely make sure that openings for discussion are made available periodically and further information is provided when the patient is ready.

One statement is never appropriate: "There is nothing more that we can do." Such statements tell patients they are being abandoned and increase their feelings of isolation and vulnerability. There is *always* something the family physician can do to provide compassionate, comforting care to the patient and family, even if it is only sitting at the bedside so the patient does not feel abandoned. *Distress* can take many forms: physical, emotional, and spiritual, as well as anticipating symptoms that may arise, such as pain, constipation, anxiety, depression, and nausea. Family physicians also can help by stopping or avoiding treatments and diagnostic procedures that hold little promise of improving the patient's quality of life, such as taking vital signs or turning patients in bed when they are trying to sleep. If a test will not lead to a change in treatment, the test is not indicated.

Delivering "Bad News"

When giving "bad news" to a patient, do so privately and without interruption (see **eTable 5-1** online). Use language the patient can understand; allow the patient to be emotional; offer to help break the news to family and employer; and be sure that care providers know what the patient has been told (Field and Cassel, 1997).

Health care professionals caring for patients at the end of life should assess the patient's readiness to engage in the discussion and appreciate their level of understanding about the situation and how much they want to know. Once physicians know the patient's preferences, they can tailor the discussion appropriately, checking periodically for the patient's level of comprehension and desire for more. It is best to provide small amounts of information at a time, frequently assessing the patient's desire to continue. Also, besides comprehension, what are the patient's expectations?

When sharing information regarding a fatal diagnosis with a patient, eye contact, touch, and personal closeness are important. If possible, sit with the patient and hold her or his hand or touch the forearm. Such gestures convey a sense of support, closeness, and compassion, reinforcing verbal assurance that the patient will not be abandoned during the difficult time remaining. Be positive whenever possible (Table 5-2).

Table 5-2 Positive Language to Use with Dying Patients

• I will keep you as comfortable as possible.
• I will focus on maintaining your quality of life.
• I want to help you live meaningfully in the time you have left.
• I will do everything I can to help you maintain your independence.
• Maintaining your independence and dignity will be my top priority.
• I will do my best to fulfill your wish to remain at home.

Modified from Stone MJ. Goals of care at the end of life. Baylor University Med Center Proc 2001;14;134-137.

Sitting with the patient on the bed or at the bedside rather than standing puts the physician on the same level and conveys in a clear, nonverbal manner a willingness to talk and listen. In one study, physicians visited with hospitalized patients for exactly 3 minutes. Half the visits they sat down, and the other half they remained standing, a little removed from the bed. "Every one of the patients [with whom] the physician had sat down thought the physician had stayed at least 10 minutes. None of the ones [with whom] the physician remained standing estimated that it was as long" (Kübler-Ross, 1975, p. 20).

Prognosticating

One of the most difficult tasks in medicine is predicting how long someone with a terminal illness will live. People enjoy repeating stories of patients who survived long after the date their doctor predicted. In most cases, however, physicians tend to be overly optimistic, and short estimates are more accurate than longer ones (Evans and McCarthy, 1985).

Physicians overestimate survival more than 60% of the time and underestimate it only 17% of the time (Christakis and Lamont, 2000). In addition to physicians overestimating prognosis, many patients believe their treatment at the end of their life (e.g., radiation) is intended to be curative, when in reality it is palliative. The better that physicians know their patients, the more they overestimate survival, probably hoping the best for patients they know well. The longer the physician has been in practice, the more accurate the prognosis. Most patients want optimistic physicians, but at some point, this optimism may delay palliative treatment.

Attempts have been made to develop indexes (e.g., Karnofsky score) to assist the physician in making objective estimates that correlate with actual survival. However, no accurate method is currently available, largely because of the multiple variables that influence when a patient dies. A good policy is to provide a conservative estimate. It is better to have the patient and family proud that they "beat the odds" or exceeded the physician's prediction than to have the patient die earlier than anticipated.

Conspiracy of Silence

Honesty with the terminal patient will provide the greatest benefits. However, the physician frequently is torn between patient and family, with the patient saying, "Don't tell my wife because she can't handle it," while the wife is saying, "Don't tell my husband because he can't handle it." Although the wishes and desires of the family must be considered when deciding how to care for a dying patient, the physician's primary obligation is to the patient. The method of management must be based on the physician's knowledge of the patient and insight into the patient's desires, feelings, and approach to life. Despite all efforts at deception, the patient knows or will soon learn about his or her condition.

By cooperating with the family in a conspiracy of silence, information that really belongs to the patient is withheld. Only if the physician believes that the patient is not yet ready to cope with the information, or sincerely wishes not to be told, should the information be withheld; however, this is more often the exception than the rule. One patient said, "I knew it was cancer from the moment they started lying to me" (Lamerton, 1976, p. 28). Simpson (1976) described a 63-year-old woman whose family insisted she knew nothing of her inoperable gastric carcinoma. When visited by the physician, "She gave a dry chuckle: 'Only a little ulcer... and my relatives down from Wales to see me for the first time in 15 years, and the priest here at 6 in the morning?'" (p. 193). When such a charade continues, terminally ill patients become more and more isolated because they are unable to communicate their concerns and fears honestly and openly with those closest to them. The elaborate schemes some families and physicians develop to "protect" the patient lead to great tension within the family, as everyone attempts to perpetuate the lie while continuing to interact with the patient.

Similarly, failure to provide the information to the patient's family can lead to a decrease in the quality of their relationship in the time remaining, because the patient's tensions and fears are not understood by family members and friends. Dunphy (1976) described a patient with terminal cancer who asked that his wife not be told. He then quickly planned a world cruise, which they had wanted to take for some time. The wife, unaware of the reason for the hasty departure, was unhappy and complaining throughout the trip, while the husband saw himself as a silent martyr, trying to provide a final measure of happiness for his wife. Only after returning home and reminiscing on this miserable cruise did he tell his wife the truth and the reason for the precipitous departure. Had she been told earlier, their final days together could have been a pleasant and memorable experience. At a time when the terminally ill patient most needs closeness, a lie may serve to push them apart.

Denial

Most patients tend to deny the reality of their situation after being made aware of the terminal nature of their illness. Denial is one way of coping with or protecting oneself against overwhelming anxiety, which otherwise could be incapacitating. This reaction is more marked in the patient who is told abruptly without adequate preparation. Although denial is noted primarily when the patient first learns of impending death, it can appear in different degrees at different times. Even patients who have accepted the terminal nature of their illness will need to employ denial periodically to avoid feelings of hopelessness. The mental burden of impending death is too heavy to carry all the time, and periodic relief is necessary to carry on customary activities and enjoy the limited time left. As Aring (1971) noted, La Rochefoucauld said, "Neither the sun nor death can be looked at steadily."

Patients who avoid asking about their illness or prognosis when the physician offers every opportunity usually are experiencing denial. Excessive denial usually means that the patient subconsciously knows the truth but wants to avoid facing it consciously. Even when repeatedly given the accurate diagnosis, some patients deny ever having been told. This denial provides constant emotional protection until the patient is ready to face the truth.

"Watch with Me"

The greatest fear of the dying patient is that of suffering alone and being deserted. There is less fear of a painful death than of the loneliness and alienation that may accompany it. A patient particularly dreads being abandoned by the physician in the face of death and may need increasing levels of professional support as the illness progresses. This is particularly true if family and friends are not able to cope with the deteriorating condition and begin to avoid contact, thus contributing further to the patient's feelings of loneliness and abandonment. If the patient feels that no one is available to discuss the situation openly and honestly, despair is likely to ensue. The patient's fear of the unknown is easier to cope with if his or her apprehension can be shared with a caring physician who provides comfort, support, encouragement, and even a modicum of hope.

Each new problem of the dying patient should be viewed as a nuisance requiring relief or removal and approached with the vigor that one would devote to an acute, short-term illness. When a fresh complaint arises, the patient should be reexamined and attempts made to relieve the symptom so the patient will not feel unworthy of further attention. If everyday nuisances can be controlled or lessened, the patient will feel that there is sincere concern for making her or his remaining life pleasant. The physician should give attention to details such as improving the taste of food by fixing or replacing dentures or stimulating the patient's appetite; eliminating foul odors; and suggesting occupational therapy to avoid boredom.

The physician should take advantage of every opportunity to touch and examine the patient rather than standing apart. Gentle palpation of areas of pain or merely taking a pulse can convey a sense of concern and warmth and provide comfort for an apprehensive and lonely patient. The physician and other health professionals can provide much support merely through conversation. The tendency to withdraw and reduce conversation contributes to the patient's sense of loneliness. Silence is an enemy of dying patients and increases their separation from society. Conversation is a social bond that affirms life and reduces anxiety by providing a means of catharsis. Saunders (1976) summed up the needs of a dying patient with the words of one patient: "Watch with me," asking that he not be abandoned in his final days. The readiness to listen and personal, caring contact are comforts that cannot be matched by modern "wonder drugs" and procedures.

When dying patients notice that people are avoiding them, they may interpret it as rejection, because their condition has not improved, or as the loss of love from family and friends,

which is particularly traumatic because it tends to negate long-cherished relationships; the joys of a rewarding life can suddenly lose their value. The dying patient's contentment depends on maintaining warm relationships with loved ones as well as continuing other satisfying interpersonal relationships, including with the physician. If physicians and others withdraw from interaction with the terminally ill patient, much of the motivation for living disappears and is replaced by despair or terminal depression. The following plea to fellow health professionals is from a young student nurse who was terminally ill (Kübler-Ross, 1975):

> *I know you feel insecure, don't know what to say, don't know what to do. But please believe me, if you care, you can't go wrong. Just admit that you care…. All I want to know is that there will be someone to hold my hand when I need it. I am afraid. Death may get to be a routine to you, but it is new to me. You may not see me as unique!… If only we could be honest, both admit of our fears, touch one another. If you really care, would you lose so much of your valuable professionalism if you even cried with me? Just person to person? Then, it might not be so hard to die—in a hospital—with friends close by (p. 26).*

Patient Control

We need to provide options to patients so they can actively participate in their care and feel a sense of control.

Terminally ill patients have a need to believe that they are still in control of their affairs as much as possible, even though they have lost control of their bodies. They should be given the freedom to make choices and assume responsibility over as many aspects of their existence as possible. For many individuals, this is an essential part of living, and its loss may destroy their motivation to live. A terminally ill patient should be helped to focus on and cope with the realities of daily living, because these problems remain very real and can serve as a diversion from constant preoccupation with the prospect of death. When patients have understanding and insight into the treatment and feel they still have some control over the decision-making process regarding their lives, they are more likely to cooperate with prescribed treatment regimens.

It is often fear of the unknown that makes a patient suspicious and resistant to therapy. Patients also should be given the opportunity to settle their affairs. Studies have shown that 40% of terminally ill patients are most concerned about being a burden to their family and friends, and that 40% of the families of cancer patients become impoverished as a result of providing care for a family member (Emanuel et al., 2003). Concentration on financial business and putting the house in order is a pragmatic approach to active participation in the decision-making process. Some patients may have a burning desire to complete a cherished project, reconcile an estranged relationship, or visit particular places before they die. Positive motivation can be maintained by assisting them to focus on and deal with these issues.

A sense of control is more possible for the patient if pain is controlled and the patient is made comfortable. Sleep should not be forced with medication, because some patients resist going to sleep, fearing they may never awaken, while others frequently have terrifying dreams.

The Importance of Hope

Hope is one of the essential ingredients of human existence, without which life is dark and cold and frustrating. It maintains strength and gives substance to courage. In the presence of hope, suffering of all sorts still has some positive qualities. In its absence, suffering is a completely negative experience (Tumulty, 1973, p. 171).

Hope allows patients to face the shortness of their lives constructively. Twycross (1986) defined hope as having "an expectation greater than zero of achieving a desired goal." Hope can also be defined as the patient believing in what is still possible. Anything that contributes to a sense of meaning or purpose in life fosters hope. Thus, belief in God or a higher being provides hope and may give a sense of meaning to suffering for some patients.

The physician should not raise false hopes or be overaggressive in treating a terminal illness to help the patient maintain hope. Some patients find it best to plan for a little time and hope for more. A false sense of hope may deflect the patient and family from finding final meaning and value in their remaining lives together.

Even advanced cancer patients can maintain a positive outlook on life. The physician can help direct a patient toward an achievable goal, such as pain relief, support for the family from a hospice service, or making a trip to visit relatives.

Even laughter can contribute to hope. One patient said, "I may not have much control over the nearness of death, but I do have the power to joke about it." Also, recalling uplifting moments such as vacations or looking at old photograph albums can support hope. Memories of the past can serve to enrich the present (Herth, 1990).

Having one's individuality accepted, honored, and acknowledged fosters hope, whereas devaluation of personhood and a feeling of abandonment and isolation interfere with hope. Hope is also hindered by uncontrollable pain and discomfort. The continuation of pain after attempts to control it have failed contributes to the loss of hope (Herth, 1990).

Even when death is near, the patient can hope for a measure of happiness during the amount of time he or she has remaining. The physician can support the patient's hope for a good quality of life in the remaining time, for spiritual healing, and for a final phase of life that has integrity and dignity.

Hope is a potent force for patients to deal with their illness and to have a confiding relationship with a physician, spouse, or close friend, which can also help prevent depression. Every physician-patient encounter should leave the dying patient emotionally more able to deal with end-of-life issues. Always promote the patient's sense of hope (Ngo-Metzger et al., 2008).

Discussing Religious and Spiritual Issues

As patients approach the end of their life and grapple with their mortality, their spiritual and religious concerns may be awakened or intensified. Although some physicians may be uncomfortable discussing a patient's spiritual and religious concerns, they can listen respectfully without judgment or discussion of religious views. Patients who believe that the physician really understands their concerns no longer feel isolated or alone in their final days (Low et al., 2002).

One way to approach this issue is to ask the patient, "Is faith or religion important to you in this illness?" In a study of patients with advanced cancer, 88% reported that religion and spirituality were important factors in adjusting to their illness (Balboni et al., 2007). Although religious coping can offer patients a sense of meaning and comfort when facing a life-threatening illness, it is somewhat surprising that a high level of religiousness is associated with preference for aggressive end-of-life care such as mechanical ventilation. These patients may have a greater trust that God will heal them through the treatment even when near death (Phelps et al., 2009).

Prolonging Living or Prolonging Dying?

It has been a long time since pneumonia was accepted as "the old man's friend." As one organic system after another slowed to a halt, the aged person was released from nausea, pain, delirium, and the degradation of lingering deterioration by finally developing pneumonia and dying. The family doctor merely showed concern and support; before antibiotics, there was not much to do but stand by and "let nature take its course." With improved medical care, however, a dying process that might have taken only a few days in previous years now may drag out for months (Veatch, 1972). Modern technology allows improved medical care to be taken to unrealistic extremes; one person was kept alive in a vegetative state for over 37 years (LORAN Commission, 1989).

Protraction of the dying process is a modern epidemic. Some physicians seem to forget that their primary responsibility is to relieve suffering, not prolong it. Greater clinical skill often is required to provide daily supportive care than to cure acute illness. Tenderness and caring must be included in the protocols of terminally ill patients so that the ravaged patient is allowed to die peacefully, without tubing and respirators. Patients should be allowed "to experience those waning moments unencumbered by high-tech devices that serve only to impede their capacity for human interaction. Here it is the patient's comfort, not the caregiver's need 'to do something,' that should prevail" (LORAN Commission, 1989, p. 29).

In some situations, therapeutic restraint is necessary to permit a patient to die with dignity. When a cure is no longer possible, care should focus on the comfort of patient and family. At St. Christopher's Hospice in London, feeding is provided by human hands instead of nasogastric or intravenous tubes; "even if the patient does not get enough physical nourishment, he or she gets what is more important—the personal nourishment of someone who cares enough to sit by the bed several hours each day" (Nelson and Rohricht, 1984, p. 174).

Management of Symptoms

When fewer therapeutic options are available, the physician's involvement should increase. Even when no cure is possible, much can still be done to relieve pain and suffering.

Table 5-3 Common Symptoms in Seriously Ill Hospitalized Patients

Symptom	Percentage of Total Patients	
	At Any Time	**Severe and Frequent**
Pain	51%	23%
Dyspnea	49%	23%
Anxiety	47%	16%
Depression	45%	14%
Nausea	34%	6%

From Expert Consult—Cecil Medicine, after Desbiens NA, Mueller-Rizner N, Connors AF Jr, et al, for the SUPPORT Investigators. The symptom burden of seriously ill hospitalized patients. J Pain Symptom Manage 1999;17:248-255.

The family physician can help alleviate the fear, symptoms, and family stress that often make this a distressing time, keeping the patient as comfortable as possible and avoiding any impression of abandonment. A good death means being free of pain and unpleasant symptoms yet having the ability to make clear decisions and prepare for death.

Care of the dying patient can be one of the most rewarding aspects of the family physician's practice. Too often, however, the physician's discomfort with this stage of life contributes to the isolation and discouragement of the terminally ill patient. Unwarranted fears of respiratory depression, addiction, or tolerance prevent the prescribing of adequate amounts of analgesics. The resulting uncontrolled pain makes those final weeks a nightmare for all. Families may disintegrate as a result of the sleepless nights, fears, and guilt that come from trying to cope with uncontrolled symptoms.

Table 5-3 shows symptoms most often encountered in seriously ill hospitalized patients; some are predictable, and all are manageable to some extent. Rarely is a single symptom present, and most patients have two or more. Symptom severity can be decreased if anticipated and treated early. Eliciting and addressing the patient's concerns about anticipated suffering can often be as important as managing the symptoms. Good control of pain, nausea, and dyspnea can enable patients to die in the place of their choosing with comfort and dignity.

The keys to symptom control, as in all areas of medicine, are a careful history and physical examination to determine the various causes of discomfort, as well as a broad knowledge of the therapeutic agents available.

Pain Control

Key Points

- Analgesics should be given regularly and in adequate doses. When given for severe pain, analgesics do not cause addiction or respiratory depression.
- Oral morphine is the drug of choice for severe pain.
- NSAIDs are recommended for bone or joint pain; antidepressants or anticonvulsants for burning or shooting pain; anticholinergics for cramping abdominal pain or bladder spasms; and antihistamines for restlessness and generalized discomfort.
- Prevention and treatment of constipation is required for all patients receiving opioids.

Pain can be physical, psychological, emotional, or spiritual. It can also be a combination of chronic, somatic, visceral, and neuropathic pain. *Somatic* and *visceral* pain accounts for about two thirds of patients with pain and responds to conventional opioids. About 35% of patients have some degree of *neuropathic* pain, a shooting or stabbing, electric shock–like pain. *Chronic* pain is influenced by memories of past pain and the anticipation of future pain. The fear of worsening pain may distort the patient's perception of current discomfort. Frustration and anxiety may accentuate the pain. All these factors can lower the patient's pain threshold and greatly magnify even minor disturbances (Twycross, 1993).

Failure to treat the whole person often results in inadequate pain control for patients with terminal cancer. Fatigue, insomnia, anxiety, boredom, and anger all contribute to a lower threshold for pain. Rest, sleep, diversion, and companionship all help to increase the patient's tolerance for pain.

Analgesics should be given in adequate amounts to provide comfort. The approach of giving analgesic doses as needed should be abandoned in the treatment of dying patients, because it contributes to a lower pain threshold and a need for increasing doses to relieve the pain. When medication is given regularly in adequate doses, the anxiety and fear that accentuate pain are avoided, and lower doses of the drug are effective, because the patient no longer fears recurrent or "breakthrough" pain.

Nonpharmacologic Techniques

Nonpharmacologic pain management techniques include transcutaneous electrical nerve stimulation (TENS), exercise, heat, cold, acupuncture, cognitive therapies (relaxation, imagery, hypnosis, biofeedback), behavioral therapy, psychotherapy, music therapy, and massage. Cold works especially well for neuropathic pain; heat works well for muscle spasm.

Opioids

A symptom-oriented history and careful examination may reveal a number of different sources of pain. Oral candidiasis, decubitus ulcers, constipation, and infected wounds all have specific remedies. Most patients with pain from cancer (and many with pain from nonneoplastic illnesses) require an opioid analgesic. Opioids are often the safest analgesics available, usually causing only temporary sedation and increased need for laxatives. Opioid toxicity may manifest as myoclonus or nightmares; the patient may exhibit spontaneous jerking or pull the hand away when touched, which can be misinterpreted by others, making them reluctant to touch the patient. Morphine taken orally gives good relief for cancer pain but has some unwanted side effects, mainly constipation and nausea.

High doses of opioids may be necessary to obtain initial pain control in a patient with severe pain. Psychological dependence is rarely a problem in patients who receive appropriate opioid doses for chronic, severe cancer pain. When medication is given before the recurrence of pain, craving for medication does not occur. Physical dependence does occur with routine use, but withdrawal symptoms can be avoided by reducing a dose no more than a 20% in any 2-day period.

In the past, physicians feared scrutiny by the U.S. Drug Enforcement Administration (DEA) for using high doses of morphine to control pain. However, failure to use adequate doses of morphine may be a greater concern now because a physician was successfully sued for undertreatment of pain in a terminally ill patient. The proper combination of pain medications can relieve pain without clouding the mind or suppressing the spirit.

Concerns about addiction, respiratory depression, and tolerance usually are unwarranted in patients with severe pain (Twycross, 1993). If the dose is titrated carefully, the patient's pain (or dyspnea) usually can be controlled completely. Patients can still be alert and mentally clear even when they receive hundreds of milligrams of oral morphine every 4 hours (Bruera et al., 1990).

A number of effective oral opioid preparations are available (Tables 5-4 and 5-5). If hydrocodone, 5 to 10 mg every 4 hours, is not adequate, oxycodone, 5 to 10 mg every 4 hours, should be used. Oral morphine beginning with 15 to 20 mg every 4 hours is usually the next step, but hydromorphone is a good alternative. The morphine dose should be titrated upward until analgesia lasts the full 4 hours, even if large doses are required.

The particular drug used is less important than the method of administration. To *prevent* pain, and end the cycle of uncontrolled pain followed by oversedation, an oral narcotic should be administered on a regular schedule around the clock. "Booster" doses equal to about half the regular 4-hour dose can be used as needed for breakthrough pain.

Long-acting drugs such as methadone (half-life, 48-72 hours) can be prescribed every 6 to 8 hours but are often unsuitable for booster doses. They will accumulate over several days and are difficult to titrate, especially in patients who have fluctuating levels of pain or deteriorating renal or hepatic function. Methadone is a synthetic that has no cross-allergenicity with morphine and is less expensive than other sustained-release opioid products. It is available in oral and injectable forms and has been successfully used via other routes. It is metabolized in the liver and has no active metabolites, making it especially useful in patients with renal insufficiency (Toombs and Kral, 2005).

Slow-release morphine preparations such as MS Contin or Oramorph SR can provide excellent analgesia for 8 to 12 hours, and Kadian and Avinza will last 12 to 24 hours. The shorter-acting, slow-release tablets may be given rectally when the patient cannot swallow (Wilkinson et al., 1992). Small, soluble tablets or concentrated solutions of morphine or hydromorphone can be given sublingually when the patient is too weak to swallow and can be used for both 4-hour and booster doses.

Fentanyl, a synthetic opioid, is available for use as a transdermal patch (Duragesic), in 25-, 50-, 75-, and 100-µg/hr strengths, or a transmucosal lozenge on a stick (Actiq), in 200 to 1600-µg strengths. Because these products are expensive and deliver a wide variation of plasma levels (25-µg patch = 4 to 11 mg of oral morphine every 4 hours), they should be reserved for patients who cannot receive drugs by the oral or subcutaneous routes. However, the patches may

Table 5-4 Select Oral Opioids

Narcotic and Dose	Oral Morphine Equivalent (mg)
Codeine (30 mg) + acetaminophen (300 mg) (Tylenol No. 3)	1–2
Hydrocodone (5 mg) + homatropine (1.5 mg) (Hycodan)	1–2
Hydrocodone (5 mg) + acetaminophen (500 mg) (Vicodin)	1–2
Oxycodone (5 mg) + aspirin (325 mg) (Percodan)	8
Oxycodone (5 mg) + acetaminophen (325 mg) (Percocet)	8
Oxycodone (5 mg/5 mL) (Roxicodone)	8/5 mL
Hydromorphone (2 mg) (Dilaudid)	10
Fentanyl patches (50 µg/hr) (Duragesic)	15 q4h
Morphine	
Tablets (Lilly, Roxane, Purdue-Frederick)	10, 15, or 30
Syrup (Roxane, Purdue-Frederick)	10 or 20/5 mL
Solution (Roxane, Purdue-Frederick)	20/mL
Slow release (MS Contin [30 mg], Oramorph SR, Kadian)	10 q4h × 3

q4h, Every 4 hours.

not work in thin, malnourished elderly patients because they need a subcutaneous fat reservoir to work. There is no need to use injections when an adequate dose by mouth will work as well. Table 5-6 provides a checklist of items to remember when prescribing an opioid.

Two opioid agents that also are available orally are not recommended for cancer pain. Meperidine (Demerol) has a very low oral potency, a short duration of action, and a toxic metabolite that can cause tremors or even seizures (Kaiko et al., 1983). Pentazocine (Talwin, Talacen) is an agonist-antagonist agent that is no more potent than aspirin with codeine and has a high incidence of psychotomimetic effects (hallucinations, confusion) in cancer patients.

Co-Analgesics

Co-Analgesics are drugs that potentiate the analgesic effects of opioids for particular types of pain (Table 5-7)

Bone Pain

Nonsteroidal anti-inflammatory drugs (NSAIDs) are quite helpful in the alleviation of pain from lesions in bones or skeletal muscles. The nonacetylated salicylates (e.g., salsalate [Disalcid], choline magnesium trisalicylate [Trilisate]) are less toxic to the gastric mucosa and do not inhibit platelet function (Zucker and Rothwell, 1978) but are less potent analgesics. The newer nonsalicylate NSAIDs are more potent, more convenient, more expensive, and less toxic than aspirin.

Table 5-5 Dosing Data for Opioid Analgesics

Guidelines

1. Evaluate pain for all patients using a 0 to 10 scale:
   A. Mild pain: 1-3
   B. Moderate pain: 4-7
   C. Severe pain: 8-10
2. For chronic moderate or severe pain, do the following:
   A. Give baseline medication around the clock.
   B. Order 10% of the total daily dose for PRN administration given every 1 to 2 hours for the PO route or every 30 to 60 minutes for the SC or IV route.
   C. For continuous infusion, PRN administration can be the hourly rate every 15 minutes or 10% of the total daily dose every 30 to 60 minutes.
   D. Adjust the baseline upward daily in an amount roughly equivalent to the total amount used for PRN.
   E. Negotiate with the patient the target level of relief, usually achieving a level at least <4.
3. In general, the oral route is preferable, then transcutaneous, subcutaneous, and intravenous routes.
4. When converting from one opioid to another, some experts recommend reducing the equianalgesic dose by one third to one half and then titrating as in guideline 2.
5. Elderly patients or those with severe renal or liver disease should start on one half of the usual initial dose.
6. If parenteral medication is needed for mild to moderate pain, use one half of the usual starting dose of morphine or an equivalent.
7. Refer to the Physicians' Desk Reference for additional fentanyl guidelines.
8. Naloxone (Narcan) should be used only in emergencies: Dilute 0.4mg of naloxone with 9mL of normal saline; give 0.1mg (2.5mL) by slow IVP until effect; and monitor patient every 15 minutes. It may be necessary to repeat naloxone again in 30 to 60 minutes.
9. Short-acting preparations should be used in the initial period and postoperatively. Switch to long-acting preparations when the pain is chronic and after the total daily dose is determined.

Medication*	Equianalgesic Dose (for chronic dosing)		Usual Starting Doses† (for opioid-naive patients)		Comments	Pain	Half-life (hr)	Duration (hr)	Relative Generic Cost
	IM/IV (onset 15-30min)	PO (onset 30-60min)	Parenteral	PO					
Morphine	10mg	30mg	5-10mg IV/SC q3-4hr (2.5-5mg)‡	15-30mg q3-4hr (IR or oral solution (5-15mg)‡	Immediate-release tablets (10, 15, 30mg) Oral sol. (2mg/mL, 4mg/mL); conc. (20mg/mL), can give buccally Sustained-release tablets (15, 30, 60, 100, 200mg) q12hr Rectal suppositories (5, 10, 20, 30mg) Use cautiously in severe renal disease	Mod to sev	1.5-2	3-7	$ (IR) $ (liquid) $ (SR) $ (IV)
Oxycodone	Not available	20mg	Not available	10mg q4-6hr (5mg)‡	Immediate-release tablets (5mg) Immediate-release liquid (20mg/mL) Sustained-release (10, 20, 40, 80mg) q12hr Percocet (oxycodone/acetaminophen): 2.5/325, 5/325, 7.5/500, 10/650mg). Monitor total acetaminophen dose.	Mod to sev	No data	4-6	$ (comb w/APAP) $ (IR) $ (liquid) $$ (SR)

Drug					Comments	Pain severity	Half-life (hr)	Onset/Peak (hr)	Cost
Hydromorphone (Dilaudid)	1.5mg	7.5mg	1-2mg IV/SC q3-4hr(0.5-1mg)‡	4-8mg q3-4hr (2-4mg)‡	Immediate-release tablets (2, 4, 8mg); Immediate-release liquid (1mg/1mL); Sustained-release (12, 16, 24, 32mg); Acceptable with renal disease; high equi-analgesic potency	Mod to sev	2-3	4-5	$$ (IR) $$ (liquid) $$$$ (SR) $$ (IV)
Methadone	Oral/IV ratio of 2:1	**Oral 24-hr dose (mg) of morphine** / **Oral morph/meth ratio**: <30 → 2:1; 31-99 → 4:1; 100-299 → 8:1; 300-499 → 12:1; 500-999 → 15:1; >1000 → 20:1	Total: 5-10mg/24hr Can give by continuous infusion or intermittent dosing qid (half starting dose for elderly; limited availability)‡	5-10mg q12hr (2.5mg)‡	Tablets (5, 10, 40mg); Liquid (1, 2 10mg/mL); Generally given bid or tid. Long variable $T_{1/2}$; small dose change makes big difference in blood level. Always write or advise "hold for sedation." PRN is one sixth to one tenth of daily dose 2-3 times per day maximum. Acceptable in cases of renal disease. Request consult for high-dose conversion, IV conversion, or if prescriber is inexperienced.	Mod to sev	15-190 (huge variation)	6-12	$ (PO) $$$ (IV)
Fentanyl (Duragesic patch) (PO)	100µg (single dose) 200µg (cont infusion)	**Oral 24-hr MS dose (mg)** / **Initial patch**: 90 → 25µg/hr; 180 → 50µg/hr; 360 → 100µg/hr	50-100 µg IV q1-2hr (50mg)‡	25 µg/hr TD q72hr (not recommended for opioid naïve)‡	TD: see PDR for details of dose transition; 12-hr delayed onset and offset with patch. IV: very short acting; associated with chest wall rigidity. Include short-acting supplement for breakthrough pain. Oral: available but difficult to dose or control (request consult)	Mod to sev	3-4(IV) 12 (TD)	1-2 (IV) 48-72 (TD)	$$$ (TD) $ (IV) $$$
Meperidine (Demerol)	75-100mg	300mg	75mg IV/SC/IM q2-3hr (25-50mg)‡ Generally not recommended	Not recommended	Not recommended for standard analgesia; may be useful for shivering and procedural analgesia or sedation. Toxic metabolites accumulate with repeated doses and with renal or hepatic disease. Contraindicated with MAOIs	Mod to sev	3-4	2-4	$$(PO) $ (IV)

Table 5-5 Dosing Data for Opioid Analgesics —cont'd

Codeine (Tylenol No. 3) (Tylenol No. 4)	120mg (IM only)	200mg	30mg IM/SC q3-4hr (15mg)‡ IV contraindicated	30-60mg q3-4hr (15-30mg)‡	Codeine alone: schedule if prescription Tylenol No. 3 (30mg of codeine plus 300mg of acetaminophen) Tylenol No. 4 (60mg of codeine and 300mg of acetaminophen) Tylenol w/codeine sol. (12mg of codeine and 120mg of acetaminophen per 5mL) Monitor total acetaminophen dose	Mild to mod	3	4-6	$
Hydrocodone (Vicodin, Lortab)	Not available	30mg	Not available	5-10mg q4-6hr (5mg)‡	Vicodin (5mg of hydrocodone and 500mg of acetaminophen) Vicoprofin (7.5mg of hydrocodone and 200mg of ibuprofen) Lortab (hydrocodone/ acetaminophen: 2.5/500; 5/500; 7.5/500mg Norco (10mg of hydrocodone and 325mg of acetaminophen) Monitor total acetaminophen dose	Mild to mod	3.3-4.5	4-6	$$

*New York State currently requires triplicate reporting.
†Adult >50kg.
‡One-half dose for elderly patients or those with severe renal or liver disease.
IR, immediate release; IVP, intravenous push; MAOIs, monoamine oxidase inhibitors; meth, methadone; mod, moderate; morph, morphine; MS, morphine sulfate; PDR, *Physicians' Desk Reference*; sev, severe; sol, solution; SR, sustained release; TD, transdermal.
Adapted from Storey P: *Primer of Palliative Care*, 3rd ed. Glenview, IL, American Academy of Hospice and Palliative Medicine, 2004, p 11.

Table 5-6 Physician's Checklist when Prescribing Opioids

1. Has an appropriate starting dose been determined?
2. Is a co-analgesic needed?
3. Is an antiemetic needed?
4. Has a laxative been prescribed?
5. Is the drug regimen written out in sufficient detail?
6. Has the patient been warned about possible side effects that might occur initially?
7. Do the patient and family know what to do if the pain remains uncontrolled?
8. Have arrangements been made for follow-up after 1, 3, and 7 days— either by the physician or by a trained hospice nurse?
9. Does the patient know what to do if he or she needs help or advice before the next follow-up visit?
10. Is the patient confident that the pain will improve considerably, probably within a few days, certainly within 1 or 2 weeks?

Modified from Twycross RG. Symptoms Control in Far Advanced Cancer: Pain Relief, ed 2. London, Pitman, 1993.

Although no single agent has been shown to be consistently more efficacious, particular patients do seem to favor one drug over another. If swallowing large tablets becomes a problem, piroxicam (Feldene) capsules, naproxen (Naprosyn) suspension, or indomethacin (Indocin) rectal suppositories may be used. The cyclooxygenase-2 (COX-2) inhibitor celecoxib (Celebrex) offers comparable analgesia and less gastrointestinal toxicity but at a higher risk of stroke or heart attack (which may not be an issue in the final weeks of life) and a higher cost. Steroids may also be a helpful adjuvant for bone pain.

Neuropathic Pain

For the burning, stabbing, or shooting pain caused by nerve damage, an anticonvulsant such as gabapentin (Neurontin), 100 to 400 mg orally one to four times a day, or pregabalin (Lyrica) 50-100 mg orally three times a day, may be a useful addition (Rosenberg et al., 1997). Amitriptyline or nortriptyline, in doses smaller than those used to treat depression (10-50 mg at bedtime), are often effective, but newer agents such as venlafaxine (Effexor) or duloxetine (Cymbalta) may be effective for neuropathic pain and have fewer side effects. If swallowing problems arise, and a tricyclic drug is needed, doxepin (Sinequan) solution may be used. The addition of carbamazepine (200 mg three times daily) or valproate (Depakene, 250 mg three times daily) should be considered if the tricyclic agent alone is not adequate. Both doxepin and carbamazepine can be administered rectally in gelatin capsules (Storey and Trumble, 1992). A short course of steroids also has been helpful in treating difficult, opioid-resistant neuropathic pain.

Visceral Pain and Smooth Muscle Spasm

If smooth muscle spasms are not caused by a treatable condition, such as urinary tract infection from a nonessential Foley catheter, these are best treated with an anticholinergic agent such as dicyclomine (Bentyl) or oxybutynin (Ditropan). If only small doses are needed, Transderm Scop patches may be useful. For more severe cases, 0.6 to 1.6 mg of glycopyrrolate (Robinul) subcutaneously may be used (Storey et al., 1990). The physician must be alert for side effects such as dry mouth, constipation, and delirium.

Anxiety and Depression

If anxiety is severe enough to require drug therapy, a benzodiazepine such as lorazepam (Ativan), 0.5 to 1 mg two or three times a day, may be effective. Antidepressants such as nortriptyline (Pamelor), desipramine (Norpramin), and doxepin in low doses (25-75 mg at bedtime) have analgesic properties and can help with insomnia and agitation. Selective serotonin reuptake inhibitors (SSRIs) and serotonin-norepinephrine reuptake inhibitors (SNRIs) may also be effective. Mirtazapine may provide the advantage of improved sleep and appetite. Psychostimulants such as methylphenidate (Ritalin), 2.5 to 10 mg orally at 9 AM and 12 noon, take effect quickly and can relieve depression and pain in some terminally ill patients, especially when prognosis is limited (Block, 2000).

Grief and depression may appear similarly. The key to their differentiation is whether the patient is able to function. For example, a grieving patient will still function by taking the children to school or going to work and will temporarily improve on seeing the grandchildren, whereas depressed patients will not function appropriately.

In family members, *complicated grief*, also called "unresolved grief," is grief persisting more than 6 months and occurring at least 6 months after death. Normally, grief symptoms fade over time, but those of complicated grief linger or worsen, resulting in a chronic state of mourning. Although complicated grief can lead to depression, it may be distinct and associated with long-term functional impairment (Prigerson et al., 1995). Parents who have not successfully worked through their grief are at increased risk of mental and physical problems 4 to 9 years later (Lannen et al., 2008).

Dyspnea

As with pain, dyspnea can have many causes. When anemia, bronchospasm, and heart failure have been excluded or treated, the focus should be on symptom control. Oxygen has been shown to be helpful for controlling dyspnea in patients with hypoxia, but may be less convenient and more expensive than opioids. When the dose of opioid is titrated carefully to control the pain and is administered on a regular schedule, with additional doses available for breakthrough dyspnea, the patient can obtain excellent relief without significant respiratory depression (Bruera et al., 1990).

Evidence from 13 studies shows a valuable effect of morphine for dyspnea in advanced lung disease and terminal cancer. However, using nebulized versus oral opioids showed no additional benefit. Good-quality evidence shows that long-acting beta agonists are beneficial in the treatment of dyspnea in chronic obstructive pulmonary disease (Qaseem et al., 2008).

It may also be helpful to provide cool, moving air (open window, fan) and keep an unobstructed line of sight between

Table 5-7 Dosing Data for Co-Analgesics

Pain Source	Pain Character	Drug Class	Examples	Comments
Bones or soft tissue	Tenderness over bone or joint pain on movement	NSAIDs	Ibuprofen, 400mg q4hr	Inexpensive; large pills
			Sulindac (Clinoril), 200mg q12hr	Well tolerated; preferred in renal impairment
			Naproxen (Naprosyn susp, 125mg/5mL), 15mL q8hr	Liquid preparation
			Indomethacin (Indocin, 50-mg caps *or* susp), q8hr	Suppository; more gastritis?
			Piroxicam (Feldene, 20-mg caps), qd	Easiest to swallow; more gastritis?
			Choline magnesium trisalicylate (Trilisate susp, 500mg/5mL), 15mL q12hr	No platelet dysfunction; less problem with gastritis; less effective
			Celecoxib (Celebrex), 100mg q12hr	Less gastrointestinal toxicity; high cost
Nerve damage or dysesthesia	Burning or shooting pain radiating from plexus or spinal root	Tricyclic antidepressant	Amitriptyline (Elavil), 10-50mg hs	Best studied; sedating; start with low dose
			Doxepin (Sinequan), 10-50mg hs	10mg/mL susp available
			Trazodone (Desyrel), 25-150mg hs	Less anticholinergic effect; one third as potent as amitriptyline
		Anticonvulsant	Carbamazepine (Tegretol), 200mg q6-12hr	Absorbed from rectum, unlike phenytoin
			Valproic acid (Depakene), 250mg q8-12hr	Liquid available, can be absorbed rectally
			Gabapentin (Neurontin), 100-400mg qd to qid	Often effective but expensive
Smooth muscle spasms	Colic: cramping, abdominal pain bladder spasms	Anticholinergic	Scopolamine (Transderm-Scop), , 1-2 patches q3d	Transdermal patch
			Dicyclomine (Bentyl), 10mg q4-8hr	Capsules
			Oxybutynin (Ditropan), 5-10mg q8hr	Tablets
			Hyoscyamine (Levsin), 0.125mg q4-8hr	Sublingual available
Anxiety	Generalized restlessness and discomfort	Antihistamine	Hydroxyzine (Atarax or Vistaril), 10-30mg q4hr	Orally or by subcutaneous infusion

Caps, capsules; NSAID, nonsteroidal anti-inflammatory drug; susp, suspension.

the patient and the outside. Careful consideration should be given to the use of antibiotics for pneumonia in the terminally ill patient. Because dyspnea can be controlled well without antibiotics, the physician must decide whether the antibiotics will improve the quality of life or just prolong the dying.

Constipation

Constipation can be more easily prevented than treated. When mobility and oral intake decrease and opioid analgesics are required, virtually every patient will require regular doses of laxatives to avoid distressing constipation. The laxative should be given once or twice *every* day and the amount increased until an effective dose is found. Bulk laxatives are tolerated poorly and rarely are adequate for these patients. If docusate (Colace), 100 to 200 mg twice daily, is not effective, add senna (Senokot), 1 to 4 tablets twice daily. Sorbitol 70% or lactulose should be added in doses of 15 to 45 mL two or three times per day if the tablets are inadequate or cause excessive cramping. If a patient has gone several days without a bowel movement or is having small, frequent, liquid stools, an impaction may require manual removal. Bisacodyl (Dulcolax) 10-mg suppositories or sodium phosphate (Fleet) enemas may be needed occasionally until an effective oral regimen is found. Impaction may cause delirium, which can mimic pain. In these patients, the delirium may be improved with a simple enema.

Nausea and Vomiting

In patients with nausea and vomiting, the physician should first look for a reversible cause such as constipation or gastritis from NSAIDs. If increased intracranial pressure is the cause, the patient may require steroids. Overfeeding may be the problem if a nasogastric or gastrostomy tube is in place. Metoclopramide (Reglan) is the agent of choice when an enormous liver limits gastric emptying or slow motility is causing early satiety. Many patients whose nausea and vomiting have not responded to prochlorperazine (Compazine) or promethazine (Phenergan) will be relieved by haloperidol (Haldol), 0.5 to 2 mg orally or subcutaneously every 8 hours. Effective and expensive preparations (usually unnecessary for hospice patients) that are approved for the treatment of nausea associated with chemotherapy include ondansetron (Zofran), granisetron (Kytril), dolasetron (Anzemet), and palonosetron (Aloxi).

As with persistent pain, persistent nausea should be treated with regularly scheduled antiemetics. Combinations of antiemetics that have different modes of action may be needed. A combination of haloperidol with metoclopramide or dexamethasone may be effective. When oral antiemetics cannot be tolerated, rectal suppositories can be tried but rarely provide adequate control for persistent nausea and vomiting unless they are compounded from the potent agents just mentioned. Continuous subcutaneous infusions of metoclopramide, haloperidol, and the required opioid are more effective (Baines, 1988). Even vomiting associated with complete bowel obstruction can be controlled *without* a nasogastric tube or gastrostomy with a continuous subcutaneous infusion of narcotics, antiemetics, and anticholinergic agents (Baines et al., 1985). Octreotide (Sandostatin) has also been extremely effective.

Hiccup

Persistent hiccup can be caused by any lesion affecting the phrenic nerve and by gastric distention or systemic problems, such as uremia. Oral treatment may include baclofen (Lioresal), 10 mg every 8 hours; chlorpromazine (Thorazine), 25 to 50 mg every 4 to 6 hours; metoclopramide, 10 to 20 mg every 6 to 8 hours; or haloperidol, 1 to 2 mg every 4 to 6 hours.

Subcutaneous Route

When oral opioids or antiemetics cannot be tolerated because of nausea, vomiting, stupor, or extreme weakness, parenteral medications may be needed. Frequent intramuscular injections or frequent restarting of intravenous infusions can be painful and difficult to manage at home. In these cases medications can be administered subcutaneously, either by intermittent bolus or by continuous infusion. At least 50 mL of medication per day can be infused through a small-gauge butterfly needle under the skin of the upper chest, arms, abdomen, or thighs using a portable pump. Morphine and hydromorphone have been shown to be safe and effective when administered by this route (Bruera et al, 1988). Metoclopramide (60-90 mg/day), haloperidol (1-10 mg/day), and glycopyrrolate (0.4-2.0 mg/day) can also be administered subcutaneously.

Nutrition

Although uncontrolled pain is the principal complaint of many patients, the family's primary concern is often the patient not eating well. The causes of cancer cachexia are still poorly understood. Because patients seem to stop eating, lose weight, and eventually die, the natural assumption has been that even if physicians cannot effectively treat the cancer, they can at least treat malnutrition and thereby delay death.

The problem is that more harm than good can come from tube feedings or pushing multiple cans of supplement each day. The family may feel responsible if the patient loses weight and may feel guilty when the person dies. Unfortunately, the patient's final weeks become a struggle with the family over how much the person has eaten. One patient said, "Tell her to stop pushing that spoon into my face; I don't want any more!" This can be carried to extremes, such as inserting nasogastric tubes in patients who "do not cooperate." If they tug on the tube, their hands may be tied to the bed rails. A study of tube feedings in elderly patients revealed that, within 2 weeks, 67% of patients with nasogastric tubes had attempted self-extubation, and 43% had aspiration pneumonia. Gastric or jejunal tubes had a lower self-extubation rate (44%), but 56% of the patients had aspiration pneumonia, 31% had a leak or infection at the insertion site, and 50% had a clogged or kinked tube (Ciocon et al., 1988). Another comprehensive analysis found evidence of many risks and no benefits from tube feeding in patients with advanced dementia (Finucane et al., 1999). Large volumes of supplemental feeding can cause painful gastric distention, nausea, diarrhea, and copious pulmonary secretions.

There is no evidence that forced feeding of cancer or dementia patients prolongs life. Careful metabolic studies on force-fed cancer patients at the National Institutes of Health showed irreversibly increased metabolic rates from forced feeding. It was speculated that tumor growth was accelerated (Terepka and Waterhouse, 1956). Animal experiments have shown that growth rates of a variety of different cancers are nutrient dependent; the growth rate slows down with fasting or protein-free diets and speeds up with total parenteral nutrition (TPN) (Buzby et al., 1980; Stragand et al., 1979). In several trials, patients who received TPN plus chemotherapy were compared with those receiving chemotherapy alone. The TPN group died faster, especially patients with lung adenocarcinoma (Jordan et al., 1981), colorectal cancer (Nixon et al., 1981), and small-cell lung cancer (Shike et al., 1984). Pooling data on TPN and cancer through 1985, Klein and associates (1986) found that infections were more common in patients receiving TPN, and that these patients were less responsive to chemotherapy and had shortened survival. After reviewing all the clinical trials of parenteral nutrition in patients receiving cancer chemotherapy, the American College of Physicians (1989) concluded, "The evidence suggests that parenteral nutritional support was associated with net harm, and no conditions could be defined in which such treatment appeared to be of benefit. Thus, the routine use of parenteral nutrition for patients undergoing chemotherapy should be strongly discouraged."

What should be done to relieve the anorexia of advanced cancer? **eTable 5-2** lists a number of treatable causes of anorexia. Uncontrolled pain blunts any person's appetite and can be alleviated. Low-level nausea, oral candidiasis, and constipation can interfere with eating and can be treated effectively. Families can be taught to relieve xerostomia (dry mouth), using a small syringe filled with water or juice, and to prepare soft foods. Corticosteroids or megestrol have been beneficial to some but can cause side effects. The most important service the family physician can provide is to allay guilt. An appropriate statement would be: "I do *not* believe that how much time your husband has, or how comfortable he is, depends on how much he eats."

Where to Die

Death with dignity is easiest to accomplish when the patient dies amid the surroundings that gave meaning to his or her life and in the company of those whose companionship provided most of the rewards of living. Physicians too often deny this, however, in the medically conditioned struggle to prolong life. Medical technology has advanced to the point that too few patients are permitted to die at home, even though improved diagnostic techniques identify the irreversible nature of a terminal process at an earlier stage. A sorry commentary, reflecting the abuse of technology, is the case of a man who had built his house with his own hands and wanted to die there but was prevented from doing so while physicians exhausted their therapeutic armamentarium in an attempt to prolong his life a few days or weeks. The family physician must remain in charge as the patient's advocate when the consultants want to continue aggressive therapy, yet all the patient wants to do is go to sleep. The family physician must have the courage to discontinue aggressive therapy when the evidence points to its futility.

Charles Lindbergh is an excellent example of an individual who insisted on designing his final days in a manner that would preserve dignity and allow him to die as comfortably as possible. When dying of lymphoma, he refused to remain in a medical center on the East Coast and returned to his home in Hawaii, where he made final arrangements regarding his estate and discussed with friends and family the details of his memorial service and burial site. His death was as he preferred—quiet, dignified, private, and in the company of family and friends—a striking contrast to what it would have been had he not insisted on leaving the medical center.

Although 70% of Americans still die in institutions (39% in hospitals and 31% in nursing homes), polls show that 80% of them say they would rather die at home (Farber et al., 2002). Jacqueline Onassis is an example of a prominent person whose wish to die at home was respected. Similarly, Richard Nixon's wishes were respected when his physicians and family knew that he wanted no extraordinary means taken to keep him alive if he developed an illness that left him seriously debilitated, particularly intellectually.

Some patients do not want to be a burden to their families and pride themselves on being able to afford hospitalization or nursing home care. For some of these patients, the gradual withdrawal from family may be an emotional "letting go"

that is necessary for all concerned in their particular family and circumstances. In other cases, the spouse simply may not be equipped physically or psychologically to deal with the loved one dying in the house over time. The important aspect is a network of support for all concerned, with no arbitrary judgment about the best approach. The family physician will be sensitive to the style of living and the style of dying that seem most appropriate in a given case once the options have been explained to the patient and family.

Hospice Care

Key Points

- Hospice care is intended for patients with a prognosis of 6 months or less.
- Most patients are referred too late, with a reported median survival only 3 weeks.
- A primary goal of a hospice is to support the patient's wish to die at home.
- The hospice team gives around-the-clock support to the family, relieves them at times to prevent burnout, and provides follow-up bereavement care for up to 1 year.

"Hospice" originally meant a way station for pilgrims and travelers, where they could be replenished, refreshed, and cared for if needed. The Irish Sisters of Charity viewed death as one stage of a journey. They opened hospices for dying patients in Dublin in 1879 and in London in 1905. These were places where dying people could be cared for when such care could not be managed at home.

Cicely Saunders was trained as a nurse and social worker in London in the 1940s. She cared for a dying cancer patient who made a £500 donation to "be a window" in the special home for the dying they both knew was needed. Ms. Saunders went to medical school and then worked in St. Joseph's Hospice in London from 1958 to 1965. She discovered the effectiveness of interdisciplinary team support, scheduled doses of oral opioids, and other methods to relieve the symptoms and stresses of her patients and their families. She opened St. Christopher's Hospice in south London in 1967, and the modern hospice movement was born. In 2008 there were almost 5000 hospices in the United States alone.

The hospice concept can benefit patients and families wherever death takes place. A hospice program consists of palliative and supportive services that provide physical, psychological, social, and spiritual care for dying persons and their families. Services are provided by a medically supervised interdisciplinary team of professionals and volunteers and are available both in the home and in an inpatient setting. Home care is provided as necessary: on a part-time, intermittent, regularly scheduled, or around-the-clock on-call basis. The hospice concept is directed toward providing compassionate care for people facing a life-limiting illness or injury. Hospice and palliative care involve a team-oriented approach to expert medical care, pain management, and emotional and spiritual support expressly tailored to the patient's needs and wishes. Support is provided to the patient's loved ones as well. At the center of hospice and palliative care is the belief that each of us has the right to die pain-free and with dignity, and that our families will receive the necessary support to allow us to do so (www.nhpco.org, 2009).

The principal requirement for hospice admission is a life-limiting illness with a prognosis of 6 months or less, should the disease run its normal course, as certified by the patient's physician and the hospice physician. **eTable 5-3** lists the standards of a hospice program as developed by the National Hospice and Palliative Care Organization (NHPCO).

The interdisciplinary hospice team consists of a patient care coordinator, a nurse, a physician, a counselor, a volunteer coordinator, and spiritual support. Medical services are on call 24 hours a day, 7 days a week. Continuity of care by the same group of team members provides a familiarity that is comforting to the patient. Volunteers are an integral part of the program and provide many helpful services. Hospice services are covered by Medicare, Medicaid, and most insurance companies to some extent. Some hospices are able to provide charity care.

To qualify for hospice under the Medicare Hospice Benefit, a patient should have a life expectancy of less than 6 months. Again, however, referrals are usually made much too late. A study of five hospice programs in Chicago showed that the median survival after referral was only 24 days (Stone, 2001). In fact, 7% of patients referred to hospice die within hours of admission. This may be because survival estimates by physicians at admission are accurate only 20% of the time, 63% being optimistic and 17% pessimistic. The longer the physician had cared for the patient, the more optimistic the prediction. In 2009 the median length of stay in a hospice was only about 26 days, with one third enrolling in the last week of life and 10% on the last day of life (www.nhpco.org). Family physicians should discuss hospice care when there are still options, not at the end of life.

Support for the Family

Families and close friends of the dying patient also suffer and should be supported. A good policy is for the physician not only to be sensitive to the needs of family members before death, but to follow up with the family after the patient dies, either with a phone call, a letter, or a home visit.

Hospice care is not focused only on the patient; the unit of care is the patient and family. The physical, psychological, and interpersonal needs of both the patient and the family are addressed. After a patient's death, family members may experience increased morbidity and mortality, emphasizing the need for greater family support from the physician. Unfortunately, most physicians do not routinely contact the family after a patient's death, so this need often goes unrecognized.

The "widower effect" is the likelihood that the surviving spouse will die shortly after the death of the partner. However, spouses of partners who received hospice care lived longer than those whose spouse died without the benefit of hospice care, probably because hospice patients impose less stress on the family (Christakis and Iwashyna, 2003).

The hospice team provides follow-up bereavement care to the family up to 1 year after the patient's death. Family members who experience grief after the death of a loved one

are more vulnerable to physical and other emotional disturbances than at any other time in their lives. They need help dealing with the grief, guilt, and symptoms associated with this emotional turmoil. The bereavement services of a hospice team can minimize these problems and can help family members cope with the pain of memories that arise from time to time, especially at holidays, birthdays, and other stressful occasions.

A man dying of cancer did not tell family or friends in order to spare them. After his death, some admired his ability to suffer in silence, but many were angry and hurt, believing he did not think they were strong enough to suffer with him. The survivors not only were angry because he did not appear to need them, but also were hurt because he did not even say good-bye (New Age, 1989).

The most remarkable contribution of the hospice movement is not that it provides a special and compassionate setting in which terminally ill persons can die without heroic measures, but that the family becomes involved and comfortable in caring for the ill member. With the rapid increase of scientific and technologic competence in the field of medicine, families feel increasingly incompetent and impotent to deal with dying. The hospice movement has reversed this trend and helps family members work with community support services to provide home care for many of these patients. When symptoms cannot be controlled at home, the hospice inpatient unit can provide medical and nursing expertise in a homelike setting.

Selecting a Hospice

Most cities now have more than one hospice. Some organizations consist of volunteers with little or no medical expertise. Others have freestanding inpatient units and their own medical staffs. The questions in **eTable 5-4** will help in the selection of a hospice.

Some patients and their families resist entering hospice for fear that their care will be taken over by a stranger and their personal physician will no longer be involved. That fear should be addressed directly by the family physician (CA, 2009). Many hospices employ a physician board-certified in hospice and palliative medicine who can help with particularly difficult symptom problems. (See www.abhpm.org for a list of certified physicians in each area.)

Social support and resources in the community are discussed online at www.expertconsult.com.

Advance Directives

Key Points

- An advance directive is a legal document expressing a person's preferences regarding care in the event the person becomes unable to make decisions regarding care.
- The most important item is the appointment of a health care surrogate as the patient's proxy.
- Advance directives vary from simple to complex, but still cannot cover every possibility.
- A variety of state-specific advance care-planning documents are available on the Internet.

An advance directive is a legal document that allows competent adults to express their intentions regarding medical treatment in the event that they lose decision-making capacity because of a terminal illness. Types of advance directives are as follows:

Living will: A form regarding the limitation of life-sustaining medical treatment in the face of a life-threatening illness.

Health care surrogate: The appointment of a person to serve as the health care proxy (or medical power of attorney) to make medical decisions according to the incapacitated patient's preference.

Durable power of attorney: Designates a person to make health, financial, and legal decisions if the patient is unable to do so.

"Do not resuscitate" order: Determined by the physician and patient or the patient's health care surrogate or power of attorney.

If a person has only one action to take, it should be to appoint a health care surrogate as the person's proxy. Family physicians should encourage every patient to name a substitute decision maker, proxy, or surrogate who can represent the patient's wishes when needed. One problem is that often the surrogates named in the advance directive are not present to make decisions or are too emotionally overwrought to offer guidance.

Each state has its own laws governing advance directives, available at www.caringinfo.org. Other sites for useful advance directive information follow:
www.familycaregiversonline.com/legal-medical.html
www.uslivingwillregistry.com/forms.shtm

The Patient Self-Determination Act of 1991 requires hospitals and other health care institutions that receive Medicare or Medicaid funds to inform patients of their right to formulate an advance directive. The purpose is to encourage greater awareness and use of advance directives so that situations of ambiguity can be avoided (Field and Cassel, 1997). The act requires hospitals to provide written information to all patients concerning their rights under state law to refuse or accept treatment and to complete advance directives.

Almost 90% of Americans say that they would not want extraordinary steps taken to prolong their lives if they were dying, but only 20% have put that wish in writing in the form of a "living will." The version of the living will shown in Figure 5-1 has several advantages over others. It clarifies the person's preferences, and instead of locking elements arbitrarily in place, it leaves two witnesses as guardians of the individual's wishes and intentions, with discretion to use their judgment in the specific circumstances. This statement presumes goodwill on all sides and should be helpful to all concerned.

There is no one-size fits-all approach to advance care planning. Some people prefer a simple approach, and others choose a more comprehensive, step-by-step process. The simple approach prevents support measures from being undertaken that should never have been initiated. It is best to have a patient both complete a living will and designate a health care surrogate, to ensure that the person receives the desired medical care.

Although advance directives are not guarantees that the patient's wishes will be followed, without them, these wishes probably will not be followed. Since the case of Terri Schiavo, a 41-year-old woman whose feeding tube was removed in 2005 after a legal battle and political storm, patients are much more aware of the need to declare their feelings about life-sustaining treatment. The Schiavo case illustrates the importance of advance care planning to save both family and physicians considerable anguish.

Unfortunately, the legal restrictions arising out of the Schiavo case may be counterproductive. Courts in several states have now ruled that life-sustaining interventions must be continued in the absence of *clear and convincing evidence* that the patient would not want them. Despite efforts to make advance directives address a greater variety of terminal situations, it is almost impossible to state accurately the patient's wishes in every scenario. Advance directives are poorly equipped to cope with the complex clinical situations that often arise, emphasizing the need to appoint a health care surrogate.

In the past, end-of-life decisions were usually limited to deciding whether or not to use cardiopulmonary resuscitation (CPR). Now the range includes feeding tubes, hydration, hospitalization, antibiotic use, and terminal sedation. The more the family can focus on what the patient would want, instead of what makes the family members feel most comfortable, the better will be the final decision (Lang and Quill, 2004).

I wish to live a full and long life, but not at all costs. If my death is near and cannot be avoided, and if I have lost the ability to interact with others and have no reasonable chance of regaining this ability, or if my suffering is intense and irreversible, I do not want to have my life prolonged. I would then ask not to be subjected to surgery or resuscitation. Nor would I then wish to have life support from mechanical ventilators, intensive care services, or other life-prolonging procedures. I would wish, rather, to have care that gives comfort and support, that facilitates my interaction with others to the extent that this is possible, and that brings peace.

In order to carry out these instructions and to interpret them, I authorize _____ to accept, plan, and refuse treatment on my behalf in cooperation with attending physicians and health personnel. This person knows how I value the experience of living, and how I would weigh incompetence, suffering, and dying. Should it be impossible to reach this person, I authorize _____ to make such choices for me. I have discussed my desires concerning terminal care with them, and I trust their judgment on my behalf.

In addition, I have discussed with them the following specific instructions regarding my care:
[List instructions.]

Date _____ Signed _____

Witnessed by _____ and by _____

Figure 5-1 Example of a living will.

CPR can be lifesaving in some cases, but in most terminally ill patients, it is extremely unlikely to result in return of satisfactory cardiopulmonary function, survival to discharge from the hospital, or ability to live outside an institution. In a large multi-institutional study, physicians did no better than chance in identifying their seriously ill hospitalized patients' wishes to forgo CPR, and such wishes, even when known, rarely were respected when the physician believed that another course was more appropriate (Connors et al., 1995).

A relatively simple Advance Care Plan Document is available from Project GRACE (Guidelines for Resuscitation and Care at End-of-life) at www.projectgrace.org. A document that attempts to address a variety of clinical situations that may arise is the Medical Directive site at www.medicaldirective.org. This permits patients and physicians to download a scenario-based living will that includes six different scenarios to cover a variety of situations, plus a personal statement and a Health Care Proxy. See Web Resources for additional sites and more information.

Euthanasia and assisted suicide are discussed online at www.expertconsult.com.

EVIDENCE-BASED SUMMARY

- Regularly assess patients for pain, dyspnea, and depression at end of life (SOR: B; Qaseem et al., 2008).
- Use therapies of proven effectiveness to manage pain at end of life, including NSAIDs and opioids (SOR: A; McNicol et al., 2005; Nicholson, 2007; Qaseem et al., 2008; Quigley, 2007; Wiffen and McQuay, 2007).
- Use therapies of proven effectiveness to manage dyspnea at end of life, including opioids and oxygen (SOR: B; Qaseem et al., 2008; Cranston et al., 2008; Jennings et al., 2001).
- Use therapies of proven effectiveness to manage depression at end of life, including tricyclic antidepressants, SSRIs, or SNRIs (SOR: B; Qaseem et al., 2008).
- Ensure that advance care planning, including completion of advance directives, occurs for all patients with serious illness (SOR: C; Qaseem et al., 2008).
- Use anticonvulsant drugs as adjuvants in management of pain (SOR: B; Wiffen et al., 2005a, 2005b; 2005c).
- Use antidepressants as adjuvants in management of neuropathic pain (SOR: B; Saarto and Wiffen, 2007).
- Treat anxiety at end of life (SOR: C; Jackson and Lipman, 2004).
- Treat constipation at end of life with laxatives (SOR: B; Miles et al., 2006).
- Use therapies of proven effectiveness to manage nausea and vomiting at end of life (SOR: C; Perkins and Dorman, 2009).
- For patients receiving palliative radiotherapy, if pressure symptoms occur in the beginning of treatment, or if symptoms are expected during therapy, start steroid therapy (e.g., dexamethasone, 3-10 mg × 1-3 orally or parenterally) (SOR: A; Finnish Medical Society, 2003).
- Opioids are effective in the treatment of dyspnea (SOR: A; Finnish Medical Society, 2003).
- Opioids are effective in the treatment of dyspnea; starting dose with morphine solution is 12 to 20 mg; starting dose with long-acting morphine is 10 to 30 mg; and dose is increased by 20% to 30% (up to 50%) (SOR: A; Finnish Medical Society, 2003).

References

The complete reference list is available online at www.expertconsult.com.

Web Resources

www.aarp.org
American Association of Retired Persons. Consumer information regarding living wills, life after loss, and end-of-life issues.

www.aahpm.org
American Academy of Hospice and Palliative Medicine: A professional organization providing educational resources, jobmart, news and challenges in symptom management.

http://cancer.org
American Cancer Society (ACS). Includes complete listing of services offered.

www.americangeriatrics.org
American Geriatrics Society. Practice guidelines and educational materials to those caring for older adults.

www.ampainsoc.org
American Pain Society. Professional education regarding pain management and research.

www.asbh.org
American Society for Bioethics and Humanities. Educational materials for health care professionals engaged in academic bioethics and the health-related humanities.

http://cancer.net
American Society of Clinical Oncology. Patient information regarding symptom and disease management.

www.adec.org
Association of Death Education and Counseling. Educational resources on coping with loss, bereavement rituals, grief counseling and other end-of-life issues.

http://getpalliativecare.org
Center to Advance Palliative Care. Tells patients where to find palliative care.

www.abanet.org/aging
Commission on Law and Aging of the American Bar Association. Consumer information on elder abuse, guardianship law, Medicare advocacy, and cognitive impairment.

www.compassionandchoices.org
Compassion & Choices. Nonprofit organization to improve care and expand choice at the end of life, including links to Facing a Terminal Illness, Planning for the Future, and Help for a Loved One.

www.dyingwell.org

Dying Well. Dr. Ira Byock's website, includes resources on end-of-life care, grief and healing, and frequently asked questions about end-of-life experience and care.

www.hospicefoundation.org

Hospice Foundation of America. How to locate and choose a hospice, paying for hospice care, tools for caregivers, etc.

www.nahc.org

National Association for Home Care. Trade association representing interests and concerns of home care agencies and hospices, including regulatory, legislative, and educational resources.

www.cancer.gov

National Cancer Institute. Complete listing of cancer treatment and ongoing clinical trials for the public and health care professionals.

www.nfcacares.org

National Family Caregivers Association. Tips and tools for family caregivers and information on agencies that provide caregiver support.

www.nhpco.org

National Hospice and Palliative Care Organization, formerly National Hospice Organization. A professional organization that provides a large variety of educational programs and helps find a hospice or palliative care program.

www.caringinfo.org

National Hospice and Palliative Care Organization (NHPCO); layperson's guide to advance care planning. Supported by grant from the Robert Wood Johnson Foundation; provides free advance directives for each state and toll-free, multi-language Helpline..

www.nih.gov/nia

National Institute on Aging. Publications and clinical trials on aging and disease; an on-line searchable database of more than 300 organizations that provide help to the elderly patient.

www.projectgrace.org

Project GRACE. Guidelines for resuscitation and care at end-of-life. Includes an advance care plan document.

www.epec.net

The EPEC Project. Education of healthcare professionals on the essential clinical competencies in palliative care.

http://medicaldirective.org

The Medical Directive. Information on how to prepare a living will, with answers to common questions.

www.uslivingwillregistry.com

U.S. Living Will Registry. National registry that stores advance directives for access by medical professionals (membership required). Provides advance directive forms for all 50 states.

CHAPTER 6

Preventive Health Care

Janelle Guirguis-Blake, Tracy Wolff, Renee Crichlow,
Jane E. Wilson, and David Meyers

Chapter contents

Key Concepts in Evidence-Based Prevention

Key Points

- Because prevention involves intervention in a healthy, asymptomatic patient, clinicians should demand a high standard of evidence. Proposed prevention strategies must be proven to be effective in improving patient-oriented outcomes.
- The evidence-based recommendations of the U.S. Preventive Services Task Force are considered the "gold standard" for clinical preventive services, and the regularly updated recommendations can be accessed on their website or in *The Guide to Clinical Preventive Services.*
- Risk factor identification allows targeted, efficient, and cost-effective preventive service provision; patients who are more likely to develop a specific disease may preferentially benefit from preventive strategies, including screening, counseling, chemoprevention, and immunizations.
- To determine whether a screening test is a good assessment, test accuracy (i.e., sensitivity and specificity) and the prevalence of the disease in the population to be screened must be considered.
- Screening for colorectal cancer, breast cancer, and cervical cancer has proven to be effective in decreasing the morbidity and mortality rates of these cancers.
- Cardiovascular disease prevention requires treatment of modifiable risk factors, including hypertension, hyperlipidemia, and smoking, to prevent cardiovascular events and cardiovascular-related deaths.

- Smoking cessation counseling and medical treatment should be provided to all adults who smoke.
- Short, simple depression screening instruments accurately identify patients who can benefit from early identification and treatment.
- Using local health departments as a resource, a family physician's knowledge of his or her patient population is the best guide to developing a risk-based screening strategy for sexually transmitted infections (e.g., HIV, chlamydia, gonorrhea).
- Diabetes screening should be offered to adults with hypertension.
- All women age 65 years or older and women age 60 or older with risk factors should be routinely screened for osteoporosis.
- Intensive behavioral counseling about consuming a healthy diet should be offered to all adults with hyperlipidemia and other known risk factors for cardiovascular and diet-related chronic diseases.
- Prevention plays a critical role in caring for all age groups. Special concerns about children, pregnant women, and elderly persons include ethical issues, competing causes of mortality, and the role of shared decision making.
- Changing the health behaviors of Americans has the greatest potential impact of any approach for decreasing morbidity and mortality and for improving the quality of life across diverse populations.
- The health belief model, theory of reasoned action, transtheoretical model, and social cognitive theory involve behavioral change and can help family physicians counsel patients.
- Improving the quality, delivery, and effectiveness of prevention in the family physician's office practice requires changes in the office system.

Prevention and the Family Physician

Prevention is central to family medicine for several reasons. A key mission of family medicine is preserving health and maximizing function of patients throughout their lives. The most common causes of morbidity and mortality are preventable chronic diseases. Prevention is important across the life span and requires repeated and evolving messaging over time. Family physicians care for patients within a family and community context that is critical to linking preventive services in the clinic with community resources. Much of prevention involves supporting patients in making healthy lifestyle changes, and family medicine has a strong foundation of behavioral medicine.

Evidence-Based Prevention

Definitions

Prevention is often categorized as primary, secondary, and tertiary prevention. *Primary prevention* is defined as interventions that reduce the risk of disease occurrence in otherwise healthy individuals. Counseling patients to avoid smoking and prescribing fluoride to children to prevent cavities are examples of primary prevention. *Secondary prevention* includes screening to identify risk factors for disease or the early detection of a disease among asymptomatic and at-risk individuals. Evaluating and treating abnormal blood pressure in adults is an effective way to identify individuals at risk for heart disease and provides an opportunity to intervene before the disease occurs. Screening for colon cancer using colonoscopy to detect precancerous polyps and then removing the polyps is another example of secondary prevention. Individuals who receive primary or secondary prevention services have no obvious signs of illness; in clinical terms, they are asymptomatic.

In contrast, *tertiary prevention* services are provided to individuals who clearly have a disease, and the goal is to prevent them from developing further complications. For example, diabetes care, including regular retinal examinations, foot care, and management of blood sugar levels, is tertiary prevention because the care provided is focused on limiting the complications of a disease that has already been identified. Many believe tertiary prevention is outside the scope of traditional prevention and should be a part of disease management.

Because prevention involves an intervention in a patient who is asymptomatic, clinicians should demand a high standard of evidence that proposed prevention strategies, including screening, counseling, chemoprevention, and immunizations, have been proven to prevent disease. This is critical because all interventions, including preventive screenings and immunizations, have harms. Evidence-based prevention recognizes that doing something to healthy asymptomatic patients requires a good evidence base that the benefits of the intervention outweigh its harms. Benefits to patients should be improvements in patient-oriented outcomes—benefits that are meaningful to a patient's function and well-being—rather than in intermediate outcomes, such as improvements in laboratory test results.

Steps involved in systematically assessing the net benefit of a preventive service involve assessing the ability to detect a risk factor or early disease before it causes complications; understanding and quantifying the effectiveness of early identification to modify a risk factor or condition and early intervention (compared with waiting until the condition becomes clinically apparent); understanding and quantifying the harms that result from the preventive service, including those from additional confirmatory testing and treatment of the condition; and balancing the overall benefits and harms of this preventive service.

Preventive services also involve costs of time and money to the patient and the health care system. Even services such as counseling that, on face value, appear to require minimal cost, actually involve a considerable cost in time and personnel resources, especially for counseling services that require intensive and repeated multifaceted counseling sessions to be effective. The time and personnel costs of counseling interventions must be balanced against the cost savings resulting from prevention or delay of a costly chronic illness. A well-established set of criteria from the World Health Organization (WHO) can help in evaluating whether screening is appropriate for specific diseases (Table 6-1).

In general, evidence-based prevention involves evidence derived from populations, and what "works" for a population may or may not be appropriate for an individual patient. Often, the populations who choose to be a part of randomized, controlled trials and other clinical trials are carefully selected and monitored for adherence to treatments. At the same time, it is not feasible to do an N-of-1 trial for every patient who visits the clinic. When considering applying evidence-based prevention, like evidence-based medicine in general, it is important to ask if the evidence or guideline applies to the individual patient.

Preventive Services Task Force and Evidence-Based Prevention

The U.S. Preventive Services Task Force (USPSTF) is an independent panel of 16 private-sector experts in primary care, clinical prevention, and epidemiologic methodology

Table 6-1 World Health Organization Criteria for a Screening Test

1. The condition being screened for should be an important health problem.
2. The natural history of the condition should be well understood.
3. There should be a detectable early stage.
4. Treatment at an early stage should be of more benefit than at a later stage.
5. A suitable test should be devised for the early stage.
6. The test should be acceptable.
7. Intervals for repeating the test should be determined.
8. Adequate health service provision should be made for the extra clinical workload resulting from screening.
9. The physical and psychological risks should be less than the benefits.
10. The costs should be balanced against the benefits.

From Wilson JMG, Jungner G. Principles and Practice of Screening for Disease. Geneva, World Health Organization, 1968.

(Guirguis-Blake, 2007). The USPSTF addresses a broad array of prevention topics important to primary care practice, including cancer prevention. Their recommendations address primary and secondary preventive services performed in primary care settings or recognized in primary care settings and referred to specialists. The 16 experts come from the clinical fields of family medicine, general internal medicine, pediatrics, obstetrics and gynecology, preventive medicine, behavioral medicine, and nursing. The USPSTF releases recommendations on a variety of topics relevant to family medicine that address preventive services for children, adolescents, and adults, including pregnant women.

The purpose of the USPSTF is to provide evidence-based recommendations for the provision of preventive services to apparently healthy individuals in the primary care setting. Primary and secondary preventive services addressed by the USPSTF include screening, counseling, and preventive medications. The methodology of the USPSTF is rigorous and transparent and involves the following steps:

1. Creation of an analytic framework and key questions to determine the scope of the literature review.
2. Systematic review of all relevant literature answering the key questions.
3. Quality-rating bodies of literature supporting each key question.
4. Quantification of the magnitude of benefits and harms.
5. Balancing the net benefits and harms of a specific preventive service.

The recommendation is then linked to a letter grade that reflects the magnitude of net benefit (i.e., balance of benefits and harms) and the strength of the evidence supporting the provision of a specific preventive service (see Evidence-Based Summary).

Using screening for osteoporosis as an example, the task force created a set of key questions beginning with an overarching question: Does osteoporosis screening result in decreased mortality or disability from osteoporosis? Because no evidence directly answered this question, a chain of intermediate key questions was systematically searched. What is the accuracy of screening tests (e.g., dual-energy x-ray absorptiometry [DEXA] scans)? What is the effectiveness of treatment of these screen-detected cases in preventing osteoporosis-related fractures, fracture-specific mortality, or overall mortality? What harms are caused by screening for and treatment of osteoporosis (Figure 6-1)? For USPSTF to recommend screening, each link in the chain of evidence must be supported by evidence, and there must be fair- or good-quality evidence that the benefits outweigh the harms. Any break in the chain of evidence (e.g., single key question for which there is insufficient evidence) results in a conclusion of insufficient evidence for that preventive service.

Challenges in Evidence-Based Prevention

Evidence-based prevention faces three levels of challenges: determining which services are effective (i.e., state of the science); delivering the message to prioritize the effective services; and applying the evidence in clinical practice. Conducting systematic reviews of literature to determine which preventive services are effective is time and resource intensive. Such reviews favor a team approach rather than one clinician conducting these reviews alone. Prevention literature is limited in some areas, especially harms of preventive services, and because of these limitations, many guidelines use expert opinion as a type of evidence supporting recommendations.

Conflicting guidelines create confusing messages. For example, conflicting guidelines leave clinicians without clear direction about what to do in their practices. Clinicians may have difficulty determining the methodologies of each specific guideline (e.g., consensus opinion, evidence based, evidence informed) and deciding which guideline to use in their practices. Evidence-based guidelines with transparent methodology (e.g., USPSTF) are reproducible and more reliable for implementation. Prioritizing effective preventive services leads to decreased overuse of ineffective services and increased use of effective services.

Systems challenges, including a lack of linkages to community resources, delivery system support, and clinical information support (e.g., reminder systems, electronic health

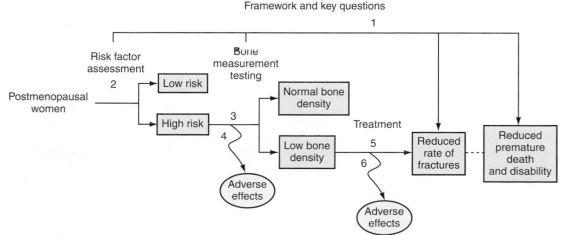

Figure 6-1 U.S. Preventive Services Task Force (USPSTF) framework for osteoporosis screening. Key questions addressed include the following: (1) Does screening using risk factor assessment or bone density testing reduce fractures? (2) Does risk factor assessment accurately identify women who may benefit from bone density testing? (3) Do bone density measurements accurately identify women who may benefit from treatment? (4) What are the harms of screening? (5) Does treatment reduce the risk of fractures in women identified by screening? (6) What are the harms of treatment?

records), make it difficult to apply evidence-based prevention in practice. A systematic approach to offering preventive services enables a busy clinician to prioritize the most effective services. A systematic team approach ensures that immunizations are administered on time, screening tests are done appropriately, and counseling services are offered to those who need them.

Statistical Concepts in Prevention

Expressing the Burden of Disease

Prevalence and Incidence

Several measures can quantify the burden of a disease in a particular community. *Prevalence* is the proportion of a defined group of people who have a condition or disease at a given point in time. Prevalence can be expressed in cases per 1000, 10,000, or 100,000 people or as a percentage. *Incidence* is the proportion of an initially disease-free group of people who develop the disease over a given period. Prevalence and incidence may describe the frequency and burden of disease in a population; however, incidence specifically communicates new cases of the disease over a specific period (e.g., new cases in a given year).

Tracking prevalence and incidence over time can help to determine health care strategies aimed at limiting the burden of a disease. For example, human immunodeficiency virus (HIV) prevalence has been rising over the past decade, partly because patients who previously would have died (from AIDS) within a few years of diagnosis now live longer. More effective treatment is prolonging life, and the rising prevalence is a sign of success of advances in therapy; health care strategies should continue to provide highly active antiretroviral therapy to treat HIV-infected patients. The incidence of HIV infection in particular communities is also increasing. This is a sign of increased transmission and means that more people are being infected; health care strategies should therefore focus on primary prevention of HIV infection.

Morbidity is the impact of the disease on health and functioning, and *mortality* is the degree to which a condition results in death. Some diseases may have a high prevalence but cause low morbidity, and other diseases may be rare but life-threatening conditions. Quantifying the burden of disease must take into account the number of people who are at risk for the disease and the consequences of the disease itself.

Expressing Screening Test Accuracy

When deciding whether an assessment is a "good screening test," the accuracy of the test and the prevalence of the disease in the population to be screened are important factors. The *accuracy* of a test is its ability to measure the actual value of the quantity being measured. Sensitivity and specificity are two measures used to express the accuracy of a screening or diagnostic test. *Sensitivity* is defined as the proportion of people with the target disorder who have a positive test result. *Specificity* is the proportion of people without the target disorder who have a negative test result. Sensitivity and specificity do not vary in relation to the prevalence of the condition being tested.

Positive and negative *predictive values* take into account the accuracy of the screening test and the prevalence of the disease, to express the likelihood that a test result is a true result rather than a false-positive or false-negative result. The *positive predictive value* is the proportion of people with a positive test result who have the target disorder. The *negative predictive value* is the proportion of people with a negative test result who are free of the target disorder. The positive predictive value is higher and the negative predictive value lower when a test is used in a population with a higher prevalence. Clinicians need to remember that in a population with a low prevalence of a specific disease, a positive test result is likely to be a false-positive result, even for a test with a high specificity.

Expressing the Yield of a Screening Test: Number Needed to Screen

"Number needed to screen" is a concept used to express the number of individuals who would need to be screened for a disease to prevent a single complication (morbidity or mortality) of that disease. The "number needed to treat" is a corollary concept that may be used for preventive medications (e.g., aspirin therapy). The number needed to treat is the number of individuals who would need to undergo the treatment or intervention to prevent a single case of disease (e.g., heart disease). This type of statistic may be useful for clinicians and patients when prioritizing different prevention or treatment options.

Risk Factors

A risk factor is a condition that is associated with an increased likelihood of a disease. For example, obesity is a risk factor for diabetes; obesity makes it more likely that a person will develop diabetes in his or her lifetime compared with someone who is not obese. Some risk factors are *causal;* the risk factor causes the disease. For example, smoking is a risk factor for and a proven cause of lung cancer; a smoker is many times more likely than a nonsmoker to develop lung cancer in his or her lifetime. Other risk factors are *associations;* people living at northern latitudes are more likely to have multiple sclerosis (i.e., there is no known causal relationship; it is simply an association). Risk factors for having a heart attack include gender, age, hypertension, smoking, and high cholesterol levels; other risk factors include sedentary lifestyle, obesity, and diabetes. Some risk factors are modifiable (i.e., can be changed), such as smoking, level of physical activity, and cholesterol levels, and others are nonmodifiable, such as age, gender, family history, and race. Some risk factors are *behavioral* risk factors, such as alcohol use, physical activity, and diet, and some type of change in behavior is required to modify these risk factors. Modifiable behavioral risk factors are significant contributors to most of the leading causes of death in the United States (Table 6-2). Preventive services strive to identify and change modifiable risk factors to prevent or delay disease.

When considering prevention programs, it is often cost-effective to target populations who have a higher risk of disease rather than to offer the service to the general population, in whom the risk factor or disease may be uncommon overall. For example, some sexually transmitted infections

Table 6-2 The 15 Leading Causes of Death—United States, 2006

1. Diseases of heart (heart disease)

2. Malignant neoplasms (cancer)

3. Cerebrovascular diseases (stroke)

4. Chronic lower respiratory diseases

5. Accidents (unintentional injuries)

6. Diabetes mellitus (diabetes)

7. Alzheimer's disease

8. Influenza and pneumonia

9. Nephritis, nephrotic syndrome and nephrosis (kidney disease)

10. Septicemia

11. Intentional self-harm (suicide)

12. Chronic liver disease and cirrhosis

13. Essential hypertension and hypertensive renal disease (hypertension)

14. Parkinson's disease

15. Assault (homicide)

Modified from Heron MP, Hoyert DL, Murphy SL, et al. Deaths: final data for 2006. National Vital Statistics Reports, vol 57, no 14. Hyattsville, Md, National Center for Health Statistics, 2009.

are rare in the general population but are more prevalent among certain groups of people. In some areas of the United States, gonorrhea has a prevalence of zero, whereas other areas have concentrated populations with gonorrhea. If community clinicians were asked to design a program to prevent gonorrhea, they might selectively screen those with risk factors or those living in communities with a documented high prevalence of gonorrhea. A key concept to consider is that even with a high sensitivity and specificity, screening for a risk factor or disease that is rare will result in a low positive predictive value. In other words, the yield of screening will be low, and false positives may outnumber true positives. It is therefore important to consider the burden of a risk factor or disease in a given population before deciding whether screening for that condition is worthwhile.

Preventive Services by Disease Category

Cancer

Almost one in every four deaths in the United States is caused by cancer, making it the second leading cause of death. It is estimated that approximately 1500 Americans die of cancer each day; a total of 562,340 cancer deaths were expected in 2009 (National Cancer Institute [SEER], 2009). The top causes of cancer-related deaths are presented in Table 6-3. Cancer has a significant impact on individuals, their families, and society as a whole. In 2001, there were an estimated 9.8 million people alive in United States who had received the diagnosis of cancer—some still had evidence of cancer, some were

in remission, and the remainder were cancer free. In 2009, an estimated 1,479,350 new cases of cancer were diagnosed. In the United States the lifetime risk of a cancer diagnosis is one in two for men and one in three for women (ACS, 2009). The National Institutes of Health (NIH) estimate that the direct and indirect overall cost of cancer in 2008 was $228 billion when total health expenditures and loss of productivity from morbidity and premature death were included.

Colorectal Cancer

Burden of Disease

Colorectal cancer is the fourth most common cancer in the United States and is the second leading cause of cancer deaths. In 2009, an estimated 49,920 people died of colorectal cancer, with the disease newly diagnosed in more than 146,000 patients. Incidence is low until age 45, after which the incidence increases with each year of life. A 50-year-old person has a 5% chance of having colon cancer and a 2.5% chance of dying of the disease (Pignone et al., 2002b). The colorectal cancer mortality rate rises 10 years after the incidence rises, and the stage at diagnosis influences prognosis. The estimated 5-year survival falls from 90% for Dukes stage A (localized) cancers to 8% in Dukes stage D cancers (presence of distant metastases). Risk factors for colorectal cancer include a first-degree relative with a history of colorectal cancer, a family history of hereditary nonpolyposis colorectal cancer or familial adenomatous polyposis, and patients with ulcerative colitis. However, most cases occur in persons of average risk.

Accuracy of Screening Tests

Sensitivity of screening with fecal occult blood testing (FOBT) varies with the frequency of testing and the method used. Sensitivity and specificity have been estimated at 40% and 96% to 98%, respectively. Hydration of the specimen increases sensitivity (60%) but reduces specificity (90%), producing more false-positive results (Pignone et al., 2002b).

Sigmoidoscopy visualizes only the lower half of the colon but has been estimated to identify 80% of all patients with significant findings in the colon because abnormal findings on sigmoidoscopy trigger examination of the entire colon (Pignone et al., 2002b). A colonoscopy has a sensitivity of 90% for large polyps and 75% for small polyps. Specificity for endoscopic screening is difficult to determine because many patients have polyps removed that would never have developed cancer. Newer stool study modalities with limited data include fecal DNA and fecal immunochemical tests.

Other screening tests for colorectal cancer include double-contrast barium enema, which has not reached the level of sensitivity of other modern screening procedures, and computed tomography (CT) colonography (i.e., virtual colonoscopy), which may have similar sensitivity as direct colonoscopy in finding colorectal cancer and large adenomas. Digital rectal examination (DRE) is not a recommended screening method for colorectal cancer because less than 10% of lesions are within the reach of an examiner's finger.

Effectiveness of Early Detection and Intervention

Screening for colorectal cancer reduces the incidence of and mortality from colorectal cancer by removing premalignant adenomatous polyps (USPSTF, 2008). Potential harms arise when false-positive screens lead to unnecessary invasive

Table 6-3 Age-Adjusted U.S. Death Rates and Trends for the Top 15 Cancer Sites[a]

Primary Site	Age-Adjusted Rate[b] 2002–2006	Trend (APC)[c] 1997–2006	Primary Site	Age-Adjusted Rate[b] 2002–2006	Trend (APC)[c] 1997–2006
Males, All Races			**Females, All Races**		
All sites	229.9	−1.7*	All sites	157.8	−1.1*
Lung and bronchus	70.5	−2.0*	Lung and bronchus	40.9	−0.1
Prostate	25.6	−4.0*	Breast	24.5	−1.9*
Colon and rectum	21.9	−2.8*	Colon and rectum	15.4	−2.7*
Pancreas	12.3	0.1	Pancreas	9.3	0.4*
Leukemia	9.8	−0.8*	Ovary	8.8	−0.3
Non-Hodgkin's lymphoma	9.0	−3.0*	Non-Hodgkin's lymphoma	5.7	−3.5*
Esophagus	7.8	0.4*	Leukemia	5.5	−1.2*
Urinary bladder	7.5	−0.2	Corpus and uterus, NOS	4.1	0.3*
Liver and IBD	7.5	2.1*	Brain and ONS	3.5	−1.4*
Kidney and renal pelvis	6.9	−0.6*	Liver and IBD	3.2	1.3*
Stomach	5.5	−3.7*	Myeloma	3.0	−1.5*
Brain and ONS	5.3	−1.1*	Stomach	2.8	−2.8*
Myeloma	4.5	−1.1*	Kidney and renal pelvis	2.7	−0.6*
Oral cavity and pharynx	3.9	−1.8*	Cervix uteri	2.5	−3.0*
Melanoma of the skin	3.9	0.2	Urinary bladder	2.2	−0.8*

Modified from Horner MJ, Ries LAG, Krapcho M, et al (eds). SEER Cancer Statistics Review, 1975–2006. National Cancer Institute. Bethesda, Md. http://seer.cancer.gov/csr/1975_2006/results_merged/topic_mor_trends.pdf.

IBD, Intrahepatic bile duct; ONS, other nervous system; NOS, not otherwise specified.

[a]Top 15 cancer sites selected based on 2002–2006 age-adjusted rates for the race/ethnic group.

[b]Mortality data used in calculating the rates are analyzed from U.S. mortality files provided by the National Center for Health Statistics, CDC. Rates are age-adjusted to the 2000 U.S. Std Population (19 age groups: Census P25-1130).

[c]The APC is the Annual Percent Change over the time interval. Mortality data used in calculating the trends are analyzed from US mortality files provided by the National Center for Health Statistics, CDC. Trends are based on rates age-adjusted to the 2000 U.S. Std Population (19 age groups: Census P25-1130).

*The APC is significantly different from zero ($p < .05$).

testing or false-negative results lead to false reassurance. Invasive screening procedures have risks such as bleeding and bowel perforation, which are even higher when therapeutic procedures (e.g., polypectomy) are performed (Pignone et al., 2002b).

Recommendation

The USPSTF strongly recommends screening for colorectal cancer in men and women 50 years to 75 years using FOBT, sigmoidoscopy, or colonoscopy. Screening may be initiated earlier for those with risk factors (e.g., 10 years before earliest diagnosis of family member). Screening methods include FOBT, flexible sigmoidoscopy, and colonoscopy (USPSTF,

2008). Unless individual risk factors indicate otherwise, there is insufficient evidence to continue screening after age 75. The American Academy of Family Physicians (AAFP), American College of Obstetrics and Gynecology (ACOG), and American College of Surgeons support similar recommendations (Pignone et al., 2002b).

The American Cancer Society (ACS) recommends screening average-risk adults beginning at age 50 with yearly FOBT or fecal immunochemical test annually, a flexible sigmoidoscope examination every 5 years, an FOBT plus flexible sigmoidoscopy every 5 years, a double-contrast barium enema every 5 years, a CT colonography every 5 years, or a colonoscopy every 10 years.

Cervical Cancer

Burden of Disease

The incidence of cervical cancer is decreasing but is still the 10th leading cause of cancer deaths. In the United States an estimated 11,000 new cases of cervical cancer were diagnosed in 2009, and 4070 of these patients will die from this preventable disease (ACS, 2009). Women who have never been screened represent a significant majority of those with diagnosed invasive cervical cancers and deaths caused by cervical cancer. The most important risk factor for this disease is infection with human papillomavirus (HPV). HPV is transmitted sexually, and 90% of squamous cell cervical cancers contain HPV DNA. Other risk factors for cervical cancer include early onset of intercourse, greater number of sexual partners, and cigarette smoking.

Accuracy of Screening Tests

The estimated sensitivity of a single conventional Papanicolaou (Pap) test ranges from 60% to 80% for high-grade lesions, and it is lower for low-grade lesions (Hartman et al., 2002). The available data on the accuracy of thin-layer cytology (e.g., ThinPrep, AutoCyte PREP), a newer screening test, indicate that it has a higher sensitivity but lower specificity compared with traditional Pap smears, but does result in fewer inadequate samples.

Effectiveness of Early Detection and Intervention

Early detection of cervical cancer is effective at decreasing morbidity and mortality because survival depends on the stage at diagnosis. More than 90% of women with local disease survive 5 years, but only 13% of women with distant disease at diagnosis survive 5 years (Hartman et al., 2002). Introduction of a screening program with Pap tests has consistently reduced morbidity and mortality across populations.

Increased detection of low-grade lesions and false positives are the primary potential sources of harm. Harms include increased evaluations, including repeated Pap tests and biopsies; psychological distress for the women with diagnosed low-grade lesions that may not be clinically important; and potential adverse effects from unnecessary treatment.

Two vaccines are designed to protect against the major strains of high-risk HPV. The quadrivalent HPV vaccine (types 6, 11, 16, 18) is currently approved by the U.S. Food and Drug Administration (FDA) for a three-injection series, which is maximally effective if given before the first sexual experience. Pap screening is still necessary even if the woman is fully vaccinated.

Recommendation

For cervical cancer in women who have been sexually active and have a cervix, USPSTF recommends screening within 3 years of onset of sexual activity or by age 21, whichever comes first, and screening at least every 3 years. They recommend against the use of routine Pap tests in low-risk women older than 65 years and in women who have had a hysterectomy for benign reasons (USPSTF, 2003). The AAFP (2008) endorses this recommendation. ACOG (2009) recommends starting at age 21 with screening every 2 years, then every 3 years for women over age 30 with three consecutive normal Pap smears. The ACS recommends initiating screening 3 years after a woman becomes sexually active or at age 21, with annual Pap tests (or biannual tests if using liquid-based preparation) until age 30 and then every 2 to 3 years thereafter (Hartman et al., 2002).

The USPSTF does not currently have recommendations regarding HPV vaccination. ACOG recommends HPV vaccination of females age 9 to 26 years against HPV. The ACS recommends beginning HPV vaccination series as early as 9 years at the discretion of the physician, with the understanding that it is still necessary to continue screening with the Pap test at the appropriate intervals even with the history of HPV vaccination.

The American Society for Colposcopy and Cervical Pathology suggests an option of using HPV screening as an adjunct to Pap smears in women age 30 and older. If HPV testing is negative, Pap smears can be spaced to every 3 years; however, if HPV screening is positive, Pap and HPV testing could be repeated in 1 year. ACOG endorses this option of using HPV testing as an adjunct in women 30 years and older.

Breast Cancer

Burden of Disease

Breast cancer is the second leading cause of cancer deaths in U.S. women; in 2008, an estimated 182,460 cases of invasive cancer and 67,770 cases of in situ breast cancer were diagnosed, with 40,480 breast cancer deaths (ACS, 2009). The risk for breast cancer increases with age: the 10-year risk for breast cancer is 1 in 69 for a woman at age 40 years, 1 in 42 at age 50, and 1 in 29 at age 60 (SEER, 2009). Several tools are available to predict risk of developing breast cancer for individual women (e.g., BRCAPRO, Gail, Claus, Tyrer-Cuzick). All these tools incorporate age and number of first-degree relatives with breast cancer into the calculations (Nelson et al., 2005). One example is found at www.cancer.gov/bcrisktool/.

Accuracy of Screening Tests

The prevalent methods of breast cancer screening are mammography, clinical breast examination (CBE), and self breast examination (SBE), or breast self-examination (BSE). The sensitivity of mammography ranges from 77% to 95% for cancers diagnosed over the following year, and specificity ranges from 94% to 97%. Sensitivity is lower in women younger than age 50 and in women taking hormone replacement because of increased breast tissue density. Specificity increases with shorter screening intervals and availability of prior mammograms. Adequate evidence suggests that teaching BSE does not reduce breast cancer mortality. The evidence for additional effects of CBE independent of mammography on breast cancer mortality is inadequate. The sensitivity of CBE ranges from 40% to 69% and specificity from 86% to 99% (Humphrey et al., 2002).

Effectiveness of Early Detection and Intervention

Trials evaluating the efficacy of mammography have limitations but have reported reductions in mortality of 15% to 32%, with a greater absolute risk reduction in older women. The number needed to invite for screening to extend one woman's life is 1904 for women age 40 to 49 years and 1339 for women age 50 to 59 years. Controversy still surrounds routine screening of average-risk women between ages 40 and 49; cancer-related mortality reduction has been observed in this age group, although false-positive results are a concern. BSE has not been shown to reduce breast cancer mortality or significantly alter the stage at diagnosis. CBE has not been evaluated independent of mammography; screening with CBE and mammography is comparable to using mammography alone (Humphrey et al., 2002; USPSTF, 2009).

Potential harms of breast cancer screening stem from false-positive results. Harms include unnecessary follow-up testing and invasive procedures, anxiety, and additional medical expense.

Recommendation

The USPSTF recommends the decision to start regular, biennial screening mammography before the age of 50 years should be an individual one and take patient context into account, including the patient's values regarding specific benefits and harms. USPSTF recommends biennial screening mammography for women aged 50 to 74 years. They recommend against teaching BSE (USPSTF, 2009). AAFP has endorsed USPSTF recommendations in the past. The American College of Physicians (ACP) recommends breast cancer risk assessment and individualized discussions of benefits and harms of mammography in women 40 to 49 years. ACS recommends annual mammography beginning at age 40, annual CBE after age 40, and insufficient evidence to recommend BSE. ACOG recommends mammography every 1 to 2 years for women age 40 to 49 years and annually after age 50 and CBE for all women, noting that BSE can be recommended.

The USPSTF recommends genetic counseling referral for women with a family history who may be at risk for BRCA mutation (USPSTF, 2005).

- Two first-degree relatives with breast cancer, one of whom received the diagnosis at age 50 or younger.
- A combination of three or more first- or second-degree relatives with breast cancer, regardless of age at diagnosis.
- A combination of both breast and ovarian cancer among first- and second-degree relatives.
- A first-degree relative with bilateral breast cancer.
- A combination of two or more first- or second-degree relatives with ovarian cancer, regardless of age at diagnosis.
- A first- or second-degree relative with both breast cancer and ovarian cancer at any age.
- A history of breast cancer in a male relative.

Lung Cancer

Burden of Disease

Lung cancer is the leading cause of all cancer deaths in the United States. ACS estimated 219,440 new cases and more than 159,390 deaths in 2009. Cigarette smoking is the main risk factor, with 87% of lung, bronchial, and tracheal cancers attributed to smoking (Humphrey et al., 2004). Other risk factors include family history and exposure to asbestos, radon, or passive smoke.

Accuracy of Screening Tests

Chest radiography with or without sputum cytology and low-dose computed tomography (LDCT) are being evaluated as methods of screening. LDCT sensitivity for detecting lung cancer is four times greater than the sensitivity of chest radiographs, but LDCT is associated with a greater number of false-positive results, more radiation exposure, and increased costs compared with chest radiography (Humphrey et al., 2004).

Effectiveness of Early Detection and Intervention

Chest radiography with or without sputum cytology and LDCT have not been shown to affect lung cancer mortality, even in high-risk populations. Both are associated with considerable harms because of the invasive procedures used to evaluate false-positive results (Humphrey et al., 2004).

Recommendation

The USPSTF (2004) found insufficient evidence to recommend for or against screening asymptomatic individuals for lung cancer. No other major organizations recommend any methods of screening for lung cancer (ACS, 2009).

Ovarian Cancer

Burden of Disease

Ovarian cancer is the fifth leading cause of cancer deaths in women, with an estimated 22,000 new cases and 14,600 deaths in 2009 (SEER, 2009). Most women have non-localized disease at diagnosis. Risk factors for developing ovarian cancer include having a first- or second-degree relative with ovarian cancer, being a carrier of the *BRCA1* or *BRCA2* gene mutations, and taking estrogens after menopause. Oral contraceptive use and parity have a protective effect, reducing the risk of disease (Nelson et al., 2004b).

Accuracy of Screening Tests

Determining the sensitivity and specificity of CA 125 blood level and transvaginal ultrasound as screening tests for ovarian cancer is difficult because thresholds for abnormal findings and lengths of follow-up differ among studies. Because the incidence of ovarian cancer in the general population is low, most women with positive screening test results do not have ovarian cancer.

Effectiveness of Early Detection and Intervention

No evidence indicates that any screening test reduces mortality from ovarian cancer. There is also insufficient evidence that any screening test that could detect early-stage cancer and lead to earlier diagnosis would reduce mortality. Screening for ovarian cancer is likely to result in a high false-positive rate, unnecessary surgery, and anxiety. Large, randomized controlled trials (RCTs) are underway to provide greater insight on methods of screening for ovarian cancer that may reduce morbidity and mortality.

Recommendation

The USPSTF (2004) recommends against routine screening for ovarian cancer. Routine screening is not recommended by any organization. ACS states that women with a strong family history may consider screening, and ACOG recommends that clinicians remain alert for early signs and symptoms of the disease (Nelson et al., 2004b).

Prostate Cancer

Burden of Disease

Prostate cancer is the second leading cause of cancer deaths in men. It was projected to result in 27,000 deaths and 192,280 new cases in 2009 (National Cancer Institute, SEER). Incidence increases with age, and more than 75% of cases are in men older than 65 years. Other risk factors include black race and having a first-degree relative with prostate cancer. Although a major cause of cancer death among men, many more men have a diagnosis of prostate cancer than die of it. Men in the United States have a 15% lifetime risk of diagnosis, but have only a 3% risk of dying of prostate cancer (Harris et al., 2001).

Accuracy of Screening Tests

The sensitivity and specificity of prostate-specific antigen (PSA) depend on the threshold set for a clinically significant abnormal value. Using the cutoff of 4.0 ng/mL has an estimated sensitivity of 63% to 83% and a specificity about 90% in the first screening. Sensitivity decreases with increasing age and the presence of benign prostatic hyperplasia. DRE evaluates only the posterior and lateral aspects of the prostate, has poor interoperator agreement, and detects less than 60% of prostate cancers (Harris et al., 2001). The combination of DRE with PSA increases the sensitivity but also increases the rate of false-positive results.

Effectiveness of Early Detection and Intervention

Screening with PSA and DRE can detect prostate cancer in its early stages, but it is not clear whether early detection improves health outcomes. Screening may result in several potential harms, including frequent false-positive results, biopsies, and anxiety. Treatment side effects may include erectile dysfunction, urinary incontinence, and bowel dysfunction. Treatment of all cases detected by screening is likely to result in many interventions for men who would never have experienced symptoms from their cancers (Harris et al., 2001).

Recommendation

The USPSTF concluded that the evidence is insufficient to recommend for or against routine screening for prostate cancer using PSA or DRE in men younger than age 75. ACS, AAFP, American Urological Association (AUA), and all other major organizations and societies concur with this recommendation of not recommending routine testing but consideration of shared decision making. USPSTF recommends against screening of men older than 75 (USPSTF, 2008).

Heart and Vascular Disease

Cardiovascular disease is a major public health burden and the leading cause of death in the United States; it is the underlying or contributing cause in approximately 60% of deaths (Wolff et al., 2009). Effective screening tests and early preventive interventions are available for early asymptomatic states and modifiable risk factors (Figure 6-2). An assessment of cardiovascular risk using validated prediction tools is an important first step in preventing cardiovascular events. The most studied tools are based on Framingham data and are available online* and can be incorporated into electronic medical record systems.

*http://hp2010.nhlbihin.net/atpiii/calculator.asp?usertype=prof.

Hypertension

Burden of Disease

Hypertension (HTN) is the most common cardiovascular disease and the most common reason patients visit family physicians (AAFP, 2002; AHA, 2005). Approximately 30% of adult Americans have hypertension; 7% of adults with HTN have never been told by their physician that they have high blood pressure (BP). Age is an important risk factor for hypertension: 7% of adults 18 to 39 years old have hypertension, versus 67% of adults age 60 and older (Ostchega et al., 2008).

The risk of death from coronary artery disease and stroke (cerebrovascular accident, CVA) is doubled with every 20–mm Hg systolic or 10–mm Hg diastolic increase in BP (Table 6-4). Elevated BP is also associated with heart failure and renal disease (JNC-7, 2004). Treatment and control of hypertension are less than ideal; 68% of hypertensive adults are treated with BP medications, and of those treated, 64% had their BP lowered to recommended levels (Ostchega et al., 2008).

Accuracy of Screening Tests

Office-based BP measurements are typically done with a sphygmomanometer. The accuracy depends on the examiner, patient factors, and the instrument used. Because of the resulting variability, two BP measurements at separate visits are necessary for diagnosis. Properly performed measurements are highly correlated with arterial BP and predict cardiac risk. Ambulatory monitoring may be more accurate and a better predictor of cardiac risk than office BP measurement, but it is subject to the same errors. A significant advantage of ambulatory monitoring is that it may identify patients with "white coat hypertension" (Sheridan et al., 2003).

Effectiveness of Early Detection and Intervention

No studies have examined the direct effect of screening on clinical outcomes; however, treating a patient for hypertension detected through screening appears to provide morbidity and mortality benefits. The benefits of screening and treatment depend on the degree of BP elevation and the presence of other cardiovascular risk factors, such as age, gender, lipid disorders, and diabetes. Potential harms from screening include labeling and exposure to the side effects of antihypertensive treatment.

Recommendation

The USPSTF (2007) recommends that clinicians screen all adults age18 and older for high blood pressure. AHA and AAFP make similar recommendations.

Hyperlipidemia

Burden of Disease

Of U.S. adults, 16% have a total cholesterol level greater than 240 mg/dL. Women have a higher prevalence of elevated total cholesterol than men (Schober et al., 2007). Low HDL is much more common in men than women (AHA, 2005). Total cholesterol levels higher than 200 mg/dL account for 27% of coronary heart disease (CHD) events in men and 34% in women. Elevated total cholesterol and low-density

---

Risk assessment tool for estimating 10-year risk of developing hard CHD
(myocardial infarction and coronary death)

The **risk assessment tool** below uses recent data from the Framingham Heart Study to estimate 10-year risk for "hard" coronary heart disease outcomes (myocardial infarction and coronary death). This tool is designed to estimate risk in adults aged 20 and older who do not have heart disease or diabetes. Use the calculator below to estimate 10-year risk.

Age:
☐ years

Gender:
☐ Female ☐ Male

Total cholesterol:
☐ mg/dL

HDL cholesterol:
☐ mg/dL

Smoker:
☐ No ☐ Yes

Systolic blood pressure:
☐ mm Hg

Currently on any medication to treat high blood pressure:
☐ No ☐ Yes

| Calculate 10-year risk |

Figure 6-2 Risk factors for cardiovascular disease. *(From the National Heat, Blood, and Lung Institute.http://hin.nhlbi.nih.gov/atpiii/calculator.asp?usertype=prof.)*

Table 6-4 Adult Blood Pressure Classification System (JNC-7)

Blood Pressure Class	Blood Pressure (mm Hg)		
	Systolic		Diastolic
Normal	<120	*and*	<80
Prehypertension	120-139	*or*	80-89
Stage 1 hypertension	140-159	*or*	90-99
Stage 2 hypertension	≥160	*or*	≥100

Modified from Chobanian AV, Bakris GL, Black HR, et al. The Seventh Report of the Joint National Committee on Prevention, Detection, Evaluation, and Treatment of High Blood Pressure: the JNC-7 Report. JAMA 2003;289:2560-2572.

lipoprotein (LDL) and low levels of high-density lipoprotein (HDL) increase the risk of CHD linearly (Pignone et al., 2001).

Accuracy of Screening Tests

Total cholesterol and HDL are the preferred screening tests and can be measured in fasting and nonfasting patients. Both values are reliable and do not vary substantially between fasting and nonfasting samples. In contrast, triglyceride levels vary 20% to 30% between fasting and nonfasting samples. Because LDL levels are calculated using the triglyceride value,

a fasting sample is needed to measure LDL accurately (Pignone et al., 2001).

Effectiveness of Early Detection and Intervention

Treating lipid abnormalities in persons with elevated cardiac risk reduces coronary events and mortality (Grundy et al., 2004). The benefits for persons with elevated lipid levels and low cardiac risk are less certain. Although typical initial interventions, lifestyle modifications such as diet and exercise appear to have minimal effect on abnormal lipid levels, and most adults will eventually require drug therapy. The harms of screening are not well defined, but a potential harm is drug treatment of persons who are unlikely to benefit because of low overall cardiac risk (USPSTF, 2008).

Recommendation

The USPSTF recommends screening all men older than 35 and men younger than 35 if they are at increased risk for CHD. Women older than 20 should be screened if they are at increased risk for CHD. The overall benefit of screening for lipid abnormalities for women not at increased risk and for younger men not at increased risk is small (USPSTF, 2008). AAFP agrees with the USPSTF recommendation. The third report of the National Heart, Lung, and Blood Institute's National Cholesterol Education Program's Expert Panel on the Detection, Evaluation, and Treatment of High Blood Cholesterol in Adults (Adult Treatment Panel III) recommended screening adults older than age 20 every 5 years (ATP III, 2002).

Abdominal Aortic Aneurysm

Burden of Disease

Approximately 9000 people die each year of abdominal aortic aneurysm (AAA), and most of them are men older than age 65. AAAs occur in 4% to 8% of older men and 0.5% to 1.5% of older women (Fleming et al., 2005). Major risk factors include age 65 or older, smoking (≥100 cigarettes in a lifetime), and male gender. Family history also increases risk in men and possibly in women (USPSTF, 2005). As many as one of every three untreated AAAs may rupture, and most of these individuals will die (Fleming et al., 2005).

Accuracy of Screening Tests

Ultrasound is a noninvasive test that accurately identifies AAA. It is 95% sensitive and 100% specific when appropriately performed. Physical examination is not an acceptable screening substitute (USPSTF, 2005). Patients without AAA on their initial ultrasound are unlikely to develop clinically important AAAs in their lifetimes (Fleming et al., 2005). Among men in the target age group (65-74 years), the number needed to screen to prevent one AAA-related death in 5 years is 500 smokers or 1783 nonsmokers (USPSTF, 2005).

Effectiveness of Early Detection and Intervention

Screening for AAA and surgical repair of large AAAs (≥5.5 cm) in men age 65 to 75 who have ever smoked leads to decreased AAA-specific mortality (USPSTF, 2005); whether screening affects all-cause mortality is uncertain. Although ultrasound can detect AAAs in women, women are unlikely to benefit from screening because they tend to develop AAAs at an older age. Screening studies have not shown a benefit for women (Fleming et al., 2005).

Screening can cause short-term anxiety. Surgical AAA repair carries a mortality risk of up to 5%. Perioperative cardiac and pulmonary complications are common, occurring in one third of patients (Fleming et al., 2005).

Recommendation

The USPSTF recommends screening for AAA in men between the ages of 65 and 75 years who have ever smoked, with no recommendation for or against screening men who never smoked, and recommending against routine screening in women (USPSTF, 2005). The Society for Vascular Surgery recommends screening all men age 60 to 85 years, women age 60 to 85 with risk factors for CHD, and men and women age 50 or older with a family history of AAA (Fleming et al., 2005).

Screening for AAA with ultrasound is part of a package of ultrasound screening offered by for-profit companies that is being marketed directly to patients. These packages usually include screening for carotid artery stenosis (CAS), AAA, and peripheral arterial disease (PAD). Patients may ask about these during visits to a family physician. Although there is evidence that screening for AAA in some populations is beneficial, evidence indicates that screening for CAS and PAD is harmful and thus not recommended (USPSTF, 2005, 2007).

Coronary Heart Disease and Cerebrovascular Disease

Burden of Disease

The epidemiology of cerebrovascular disease events is different for men and women. Men have a higher risk for coronary heart disease (CHD) and tend to have these events at a younger age than women. Women are more likely to die as a result of a myocardial infarction (MI); 38% of women die within 1 year of their first MI, versus 25% of men (Wolff et al., 2009).

Cerebrovascular disease is the third leading cause of death in the United States and approximately 500,000 people annually experience a first stroke (CVA). The mortality rate for cerebrovascular disease has declined by almost 70% since 1950, primarily because of reduced cigarette smoking and improved control of HTN. According to the Framingham data, the 10-year risk for initial ischemic stroke at age 55 years is 1.8% for women and 2.4% for men; at age 65 the risk increases to 3.9% for women and 5.8% for men (Wolff et al., 2009).

Accuracy of Screening Tests

Several screening mechanisms exist for CHD: electrocardiogram (ECG), exercise testing, and electron beam computed tomography (EBCT) for coronary calcium. The sensitivity of resting ECG abnormalities for CHD is low. The sensitivity of an exercise test ranges from 10% to 70% and the predictive value from 2.2% to 24%. False-positive results are more likely for young persons and women (Pignone et al., 2003). Evidence is limited on the use of nontraditional risk factors in CHD assessment, including ankle-brachial index (ABI), leukocyte count, fasting glucose level, periodontal disease, carotid intimal medial thickening, EBCT, homocysteine level, lipoprotein(a) level, and high-sensitivity C-reactive protein (hs-CRP) level. Screening for cerebrovascular disease with an ultrasound of the carotid artery to detect significant stenosis has a reported sensitivity of 86% to 90% and specificity of 87% to 94% (Wolff, 2007).

Effectiveness of Early Detection and Intervention

Although ECG and exercise stress tests can detect disease, the sensitivity and specificity of these tests limits their use in evaluating asymptomatic persons. False-positive results lead to invasive testing, and false-negative results lead to inappropriate reassurance. It is unclear that these assessments provide information beyond risk scoring, even for higher-risk persons. Although hs-CRP and ABI may reclassify some individuals into a higher or lower CHD risk category, evidence is lacking regarding the effect of screening or assessment with these or other modalities on outcomes (USPSTF, 2009).

Hormone replacement therapy does not prevent CHD in postmenopausal women (Anderson et al., 2004; Rossouw et al., 2002), and evidence does not support a benefit from vitamin supplements (Lee et al., 2005). There is good evidence that screening for CAS with an ultrasound leads to important harms, including strokes from confirmatory tests or surgery. For men at increased risk for CHD, aspirin prophylaxis decreases the rate of CHD events; and for women at increased risk of strokes, aspirin decreases the rate of strokes (Berger et al., 2006; USPSTF, 2009). The ideal dose is uncertain, but low doses (75 mg) are as effective as high doses

(325 mg). Smoking cessation, BP and lipid control, a healthy diet, and exercise have also been shown to be beneficial in preventing cerebrovascular disease events.

Recommendation

The USPSTF recommends against using ECG, exercise testing, or CT scanning to screen low-risk adults for CHD. Evidence is insufficient to recommend these techniques even for adults at increased risk (USPSTF, 2004). AAFP does not recommend routine ECG in asymptomatic children or adults as part of a periodic health examination (Pignone et al., 2003). USPSTF concluded that the evidence is insufficient for the use of nontraditional risk factors to screen asymptomatic men and women. They recommend against screening for asymptomatic CAS in the general adult population. USPSTF recommends the use of aspirin for men age 45 to 79 years and women age 55 to 79 when the potential benefit from a reduction in MIs or strokes, respectively, outweighs the potential harm from an increase in gastrointestinal hemorrhage (Table 6-5). It is important to discuss both the benefits and the harms with patients. Aspirin in younger men and women is not recommended because they are likely to experience more harm than benefit. There is no evidence to use aspirin for cardiovascular disease prevention in average-risk men and women 80 years or older (USPSTF, 2009).

Substance Abuse and Mental Health

Tobacco

Burden of Disease

Tobacco use, particularly cigarette smoking, is the leading cause of preventable death in the United States, and it results in approximately 443,000 premature deaths annually (CDC, 2008a). Among adults, approximately 41% of the smoking-attributable deaths are caused by cancer, 33% by cardiovascular disease, and 26% by respiratory disease (CDC, 2008a). Smoking during pregnancy results in almost 800 ($n = 776$) fetal deaths annually. An estimated 49,400 deaths annually from lung cancer and cardiovascular causes are attributable to second-hand smoke exposure (CDC, 2008a). Despite the known health effects, in 2007, an estimated 19.8% of U.S.

Table 6-5 10-Year Risk Levels* for Coronary Heart Disease (CHD, Men) and Stroke (Women)

Men		Women	
Age (years)	10-Year CHD Risk	Age (years)	10-Year Stroke Risk
45–59	>4%	55–59	>3%
60–69	>9%	60–69	>8%
70–79	>12%	70–79	>11%

*Level at which the number of cardiovascular disease events prevented is closely balanced to the number of serious bleeding events. Shared decision making is strongly encouraged with persons whose risk is close to (either above or below) these estimates of 10-year risk levels. As the potential cardiovascular disease reduction benefit increases above harms, the recommendation to take aspirin should become stronger.

adults continued to smoke (CDC, 2008b). The prevalence of smoking is higher among certain subgroups, including Native Americans and Native Alaskans, those with a lower level of education, adults age 25 to 44, and people living below the poverty level (CDC, 2008b).

Screening and Identification of Risk Group

Clinics that implement screening systems designed to identify and document a patient's tobacco use status increase the rate at which clinicians intervene with their patients who smoke. Including tobacco use as a "vital sign" increases the probability that tobacco use is routinely assessed and addressed. However, there is limited evidence that a screening system has a substantial impact on tobacco cessation rates (Fiore et al., 2008).

Effectiveness of Counseling Intervention

The optimal duration and frequency of tobacco counseling interventions is unknown, but good evidence indicates that even brief counseling interventions (<3 minutes) increase tobacco abstinence rates. Increasing the intensity of the counseling increases its efficacy (Fiore et al., 2008). The "5As" behavioral counseling framework provides a useful strategy for engaging patients in smoking cessation discussions (see later discussion).Providing problem-solving guidance and social support within and outside treatment is particularly important. Patients who are unwilling to try to quit should receive an intervention designed to motivate them to quit.

Several pharmacotherapies are safe and effective in helping adults to quit smoking. Nicotine replacement therapy—nicotine gum, transdermal patches, nicotine nasal spray, and nicotine inhalers—and sustained-release bupropion and varenicline are among the medications shown to be effective in increasing abstinence rates. There is limited evidence regarding the safety or efficacy of pharmacotherapy during pregnancy (Fiore et al., 2008).

Recommendation

The USPSTF recommends that clinicians screen all adults, including pregnant women, for tobacco use and provide tobacco cessation interventions for those who use tobacco products. The AAFP, American College of Preventive Medicine (ACPM), and the ACOG recommend a similar course of action. Brief smoking cessation interventions for adults and extended, tailored counseling for pregnant women are effective in increasing the proportion of smokers who successfully quit smoking and remain abstinent (USPSTF, 2009).

Alcohol

Burden of Disease

Alcohol abuse and *alcohol dependence* are associated with repeated negative physical, psychological, and social effects, and the effectiveness of interventions for alcohol dependence are well established. *Alcohol misuse*, such as "risky or hazardous" and "harmful" drinking, does not meet criteria for dependence but place individuals at risk for future problems. Across various primary care populations, the prevalence rates for risky drinking are 4% to 29%; for harmful drinking, 0.3% to 10%; and for alcohol dependence, 2% to 9%. Drinking alcohol influences tobacco use (and vice versa), and drinking onset during adolescence correlates with dependence as an adult and increases the risk of alcohol-related injuries. Alcohol misuse frequently coexists with depression or anxiety disorders (Whitlock et al., 2004).

Accuracy of Screening

Several effective screening instruments are available for use in the primary care setting. The Alcohol Use Disorders Identification Test (AUDIT) incorporates questions about consequences of drinking along with questions about quantity and frequency. Its specificity ranges from 78% to 96% and the sensitivity from 51% to 97%. The CAGE questionnaire (i.e., feeling the need to cut down, annoyed by criticism, guilty about drinking, and need for an eye-opener in the morning) is widely used in primary care. Specificity for CAGE ranges from 70% to 97% and sensitivity from 43% to 94%. The TWEAK and the T-ACE instruments are designed to screen pregnant women for alcohol misuse (Whitlock et al., 2004). The CRAFFT questionnaire has been validated for screening adolescents for substance abuse in primary care settings (Knight et al., 2003). Tools are available at http://www.niaaa.nih.gov/Publications/AlcoholResearch/. Biologic markers, such as carbohydrate-deficient transferring and serum γ-glutamyltransferase, are poor indicators of alcohol misuse.

Effectiveness of Counseling Intervention

Counseling interventions can be delivered wholly or partly in the primary care setting, and their effectiveness varies in terms of duration and frequency of the sessions. Effective interventions include feedback, advice, and goal setting, and most also include follow-up and further assistance. Depending on the intensity of the counseling, reduction in alcohol consumption ranges from three to nine drinks per week after 6 to 12 months of follow-up (Whitlock et al., 2004). The benefits of behavioral intervention for preventing or reducing alcohol misuse in adolescents are not known.

Recommendation

The USPSTF recommends screening and behavioral counseling interventions to reduce alcohol misuse by adults, including pregnant women, in primary care settings. They concluded that the evidence was insufficient to recommend for or against screening and behavioral counseling to prevent or reduce alcohol misuse by adolescents in primary care settings (USPSTF, 2004). The AMA, AAFP, and Canadian Task Force on Preventive Health Care (CTFPHC) also recommend screening adults for alcohol misuse and counseling for those who screen positive. ACOG recommends counseling all women about the harmful effects of drinking to the fetus and that abstinence is the best policy (Whitlock et al., 2004).

Screening adults for alcohol misuse in primary care settings can accurately identify patients at risk for increased morbidity and mortality, and brief behavioral counseling interventions with follow-up produce small to moderate reductions in alcohol consumption that are sustained for 6 to 12 months or longer (USPSTF, 2004).

Depression

Burden of Disease

Depressive disorders are common, chronic, and costly. Depression is the fourth leading contributor to the global burden of disease and a leading cause of disability. In the primary care setting, the point prevalence of major depression ranges from 5% to 9% for adults, and up to 50% of depressed patients are not recognized (Pignone et al., 2002a). The estimated prevalence of major depressive disorder is 2.0% in children younger than 13 years and 5.6% in adolescents age 13 to 18 (Williams et al., 2009). Risk factors for depression include female gender, family or personal history of depression, substance abuse, and chronic disease.

Accuracy of Screening

Several screening instruments are available and have a sensitivity of 80% to 90% and specificity of 70% to 85% (Pignone et al., 2002a). Instruments include the Beck Depression Inventory, the Zung Self-Assessment Depression Scale, and the General Health Questionnaire. Most instruments are easy to use and take less than 5 minutes to administer, although most depressed patients can be identified simply by asking about depressed mood and anhedonia (loss of pleasurable feelings). The Patient Health Questionnaire for Adolescents and the Beck Depression Inventory–Primary Care have demonstrated good sensitivity and specificity in primary care settings in adolescents (Williams et al., 2009). A review of these tools can be found in the article at http://www.aafp.org/afp/2002/0915/p1001.html.

Effectiveness of Early Detection and Intervention

There are effective treatments for patients with depressive illnesses detected through screening. Antidepressant medications include selective serotonin reuptake inhibitors (SSRIs) and tricyclic antidepressants (TCAs). Psychosocial and psychotherapeutic interventions are also effective treatments for major depression.

Clinicians who screen for depression should have systems in place to ensure that positive screening results are followed by accurate diagnosis, proper treatment, and adequate follow-up. All positive screening tests should be followed by full diagnostic interviews using standard diagnostic criteria to determine the presence or absence of major depression, dysthymia, or other psychological problems. The potential harms of screening include false-positive screening results, the inconvenience of further workup, and the potential adverse effects of labeling an individual "depressed."

Recommendation

The USPSTF (2002) recommends screening adults for depression in clinical settings that have systems in place to ensure accurate diagnosis, effective treatment, and follow-up. AAFP and CTFPHC endorse similar recommendations, and ACOG recommends that clinicians remain alert to symptoms of depression and ask questions about psychosocial stressors when taking a patient's history (Pignone et al., 2002a). USPSTF recommends screening adolescents (12-18 years of age) for major depressive disorder when systems are in place to ensure accurate diagnosis, psychotherapy, and follow-up. Routine screening has been recommended by Medicaid's EPSDT program and the American Academy of Pediatrics (AAP), and the American Medical Association (AMA) recommends screening for depression among adolescents who may be at increased risk for depression (USPSTF, 2009).

Screening for depression in adults and adolescents improves the accurate identification of depressed patients in primary care settings, and treatment of depressed patients identified in these settings decreases clinical morbidity. Screening should be offered to adults in clinical practices that have systems in place to ensure accurate diagnosis, effective treatment, and follow-up (USPSTF, 2002). Screening for major depressive disorder should be offered to adolescents when systems are in place to ensure accurate diagnosis, psychotherapy, and follow-up (USPFTF, 2009).

Infectious Diseases

Physicians need to consider which risk factors, both behavioral and demographic, place individual patients at increased risk of infection. Although the evidence base establishing risk factors for each sexually transmitted infection (STI) is based on the particulars of the individual studies examining each STI, clinicians may choose to consider high-risk sexual behaviors as having multiple current partners, having a new partner, using condoms inconsistently, having sex while under the influence of alcohol or drugs, and having sex in exchange for money or drugs. In addition to evaluation of a patient's modifiable behaviors, physicians should consider their patients' nonmodifiable demographics and social situation.

As noted earlier, all U.S. communities do not present the same infection risk. For example, both syphilis and gonorrhea have significantly higher prevalence rates in the South and many urban centers. Because of underlying social factors that increase STI risk, including poverty, discrimination, and social networks, black and Hispanic Americans have higher prevalence rates of most STIs. When considering screening for STIs, physicians should consult with local public health officials and use national, regional, and local epidemiologic data to tailor screening programs based on communities and populations they serve. In addition to behavioral risk factors, physicians should remember that for chlamydial infection and gonorrhea, all sexually active women age 24 years and younger are considered at increased risk (Meyers et al., 2008).

Chlamydial Infection

Burden of Disease

Chlamydia trachomatis infection is the most common sexually transmitted bacterial disease in the United States. In 2007, more than 1 million cases of chlamydial infection were reported to the Centers for Disease Control and Prevention (CDC), 370 cases per 100,000 population; an additional 2 million cases are thought to occur annually (Weinstock et al., 2004). Age is the strongest risk factor for infection in both men and women, with adolescent girls and women between ages 15 and 24 and men between 20 and 24 having the highest prevalence rates (CDC, 2009). It is important to note that higher rates of chlamydial infection and gonorrhea in younger women result not only from having more sex partners, but also from the relative immaturity of their immune systems and the presence of columnar epithelium on the adolescent cervix (Meyers et al., 2008). In addition to sexual activity and age, other risk factors for chlamydial infection include a recent history of STI, new or multiple sexual partners, inconsistent condom use, and exchanging sex

for money or drugs. Chlamydial infection is widely prevalent among all racial and ethnic groups in the United States, with higher prevalence rates among black and Hispanic populations. Increased prevalence rates are also found in incarcerated populations, military recruits, and patients presenting to public STI clinics (Meyers et al., 2007).

Although 75% of genital chlamydial infections in women are asymptomatic, *C. trachomatis* is a major cause of urethritis and cervicitis in women. Additionally, up to 40% of untreated cases of *C. trachomatis* may progress to pelvic inflammatory disease (PID). PID may result in ectopic pregnancy, infertility, and chronic pelvic pain. About 95% of men with *C. trachomatis* infection are asymptomatic. Genital infection in men occasionally results in acute urethritis or epididymitis and rarely in chronic complications such as prostatitis and reactive arthritis (Meyers et al., 2007).

Accuracy of Screening Tests

Nucleic acid amplification tests (NAATs), such as polymerase chain reaction (PCR) and transcription-mediated amplification (TMA), can identify chlamydial infection in asymptomatic women (nonpregnant and pregnant) and asymptomatic men. NAATs have high sensitivity (>80%) and specificity (>99%) and can be used with urine, vaginal, and cervical swabs (Meyers et al., 2007). It is important to remember that even with a test with high sensitivity, in a low-prevalence population, a positive screening result is more likely to be a false positive than an actual case. When screening a 20-year-old woman with no other risk factors other than her young age, given a prevalence rate of 1%, the positive predictive value for a positive chlamydial screen with an NAAT is only 47%. Point-of-care tests are becoming available that can be conducted in the office setting in about 30 minutes. Their sensitivity remains substantially lower than for laboratory-conducted NAATs, although their specificity is high (Mahilum-Tapay et al., 2007).

Effectiveness of Early Detection and Intervention

Screening and treatment for *Chlamydia* infection in high-risk, asymptomatic women has been demonstrated to reduce significantly their incidence of PID after 12 months of follow-up. There have been no published studies of the effectiveness of screening women not at increased risk. Although treatment of men eradicates infection, there is no evidence that screening men reduces transmission, acute infection, or sequelae in women. Potential harms of screening and treatment include the effects of false-positive test results, patient anxiety, unnecessary antibiotic use, and adverse drug reactions (Meyers et al., 2007).

Recommendation

The USPSTF recommends that clinicians routinely screen all sexually active women age 24 or younger (including pregnant women) and older asymptomatic women at increased risk for chlamydial infection. They recommend against routine screening in asymptomatic women age 25 and older (including pregnant women) who are not at increased risk. Although USPSTF found insufficient evidence to recommend for or against routine screening of men, they counsel clinicians and health care systems to focus on improving screening rates among women at increased risk, a group for whom the benefits of screening are certain (USPSTF, 2007).

The AAFP (2009) concurs with USPSTF. The CDC (2006) recommends annual screening for sexually active women 25 years old and younger and older women with new or multiple sexual partners.

Women with asymptomatic untreated chlamydial infection have high rates of morbidity from PID and its sequelae. Screening tests can accurately detect chlamydial infection in those at risk, and treatment is effective. All sexually active women age 24 and younger and all older women at increased risk for PID should be screened for chlamydial infection. The same risk factors and recommendation applies to pregnant women (USPSTF, 2007).

Gonorrheal Infection

Burden of Disease

In 2006, infection with *Neisseria gonorrhoeae* was the second most common reportable disease in the United States, with a reported rate just under 119 cases per 100,000 population. Unlike *Chlamydia* infection, which has seen increasing rates over the past decade, rates of *N. gonorrhoeae* infection have been stable since the mid-1990s. Infection rates are highest among girls and women between ages 15 and 24 years and men between 20 and 24 years. Although rates are increasing among white and Hispanic populations, the rate among blacks in 2006 (663 cases per 100,000) was almost 20 times higher than for whites. Other risk factors for infection include a history of previous gonorrhea or other STI, new or multiple sexual partners, inconsistent condom use, sex work, and drug use. The prevalence of gonorrhea varies widely among regions of the United States, with the South and Midwest having notably higher rates than the Northeast and West, and among communities (CDC, 2007).

In women, infection with *N. gonorrhoeae* is a major cause of cervicitis and PID. PID may cause ectopic pregnancy, infertility, and chronic pelvic pain. In men, gonorrhea can result in urethritis, epididymitis, and prostatitis. Gonorrheal infection is frequently asymptomatic in women. Infection in men can be asymptomatic as well, but less often than in women (Glass et al., 2005b).

Accuracy of Screening Tests

Culture isolates collected from endocervical swabs in women and urethral swabs in men remain an accurate screening test for genital gonorrheal infection. When transport conditions are suitable, the sensitivity is higher than 90%. Because culture remains the "gold standard," the specificity of culture is 100% when culture isolates are speciated. NAATs and nucleic acid hybridization tests have demonstrated sensitivity and specificity comparable to culture and compare better when transport conditions are not suitable for culture. Some newer tests can be used with urine and vaginal swabs, allowing screening without an invasive procedure (Glass et al., 2005b).

Effectiveness of Early Detection and Intervention

Screening can accurately detect gonorrheal infection, and antibiotic therapy can eliminate urogenital infections, prevent complications, and prevent further transmission. Potential harms of screening and treatment include false-positive test results, anxiety, and unnecessary antibiotic use (Glass et al., 2005b).

Recommendation

The USPSTF recommends that clinicians screen all sexually active women who are at increased risk for gonorrheal infection. Because of the lower burden of undiagnosed and untreated genital gonorrheal infection in men than women, USPSTF concluded that there was insufficient evidence to recommend for or against routine screening for gonorrhea in men at increased risk for infection. They recommend against routine screening for gonorrhea in men and women who are at low risk for infection (USPSTF, 2005).

Unlike chlamydial infection, which is relatively evenly distributed across the United States, gonorrheal infection demonstrates marked regional and local variation. USPSTF recommends that clinicians and health systems work with public health officials to understand the prevalence and distribution of gonorrhea in their communities and adjust their screening practices accordingly.

The AAFP and ACOG recommend screening sexually active women, including adolescents, at high risk for gonorrhea. The CDC recommends that clinicians screen all sexually active men who have sex with men for genital gonorrhea at least annually and for rectal and pharyngeal gonorrhea if they are at risk due to exposure. The Infectious Disease Society of America (IDSA) recommends that all HIV-positive individuals be screened for gonorrhea (Glass et al., 2005b).

Women with asymptomatic gonorrheal infection have high rates of morbidity from PID and its sequelae. Screening tests can accurately detect gonorrheal infection in those at risk, and treatment is effective. All high-risk, sexually active women (including pregnant women) should be screened for gonorrheal infection (USPSTF, 2005).

Human Immunodeficiency Virus Infection

Burden of Disease.

In 2007, about 37,000 people in the United States were diagnosed with acquired immunodeficiency syndrome (AIDS), raising the total to more than 1 million diagnosed cases since the recognition of AIDS in 1981. In 2006, more than 450,000 people in the United States were living with AIDS, and an additional 56,300 people were newly infected with HIV. From 2003 to 2007, the total number of new AIDS cases has remained relatively stable, but the proportion of HIV/AIDS cases has continued to increase steadily (CDC, 2009). With approximately 12,000 deaths in 2007, AIDS is not in the top 15 causes of death in the United States (Heron et al., 2009).

Those at increased risk for HIV infection include men who have had sex with men after 1975; men and women having unprotected sex with multiple partners; past or present injection drug users; men and women who exchange sex for money or drugs or have sex partners who do; individuals whose past or present sex partners were HIV infected, bisexual, or injection drug users; persons being treated for STIs; and persons with a history of blood transfusion between 1978 and 1985. Persons who request an HIV test despite reporting no individual risk factors may also be considered at increased risk, because this group is likely to include individuals not willing to disclose high-risk behaviors. A higher prevalence is seen in high-risk settings, such as STI clinics, correctional facilities, homeless shelters, tuberculosis clinics, clinics serving men who have sex with men, and adolescent health clinics with a high prevalence of STIs (Chou et al., 2005).

Accuracy of Screening Tests

Standard testing for HIV infection with the repeatedly reactive enzyme immunoassay, followed by confirmatory Western blot or immunofluorescent assay, has a sensitivity and specificity greater than 99%. False-positive test results are rare, even in low-risk settings. Compared with standard HIV testing, the reported sensitivities of rapid tests on blood specimens range from 96% to 100%, with specificities greater than 99.9%. Reported sensitivities and specificities of oral fluid HIV tests are also high (>99%) (Chou et al., 2005).

Effectiveness of Early Detection and Intervention

The wide adoption in the late 1990s of the use of highly active antiretroviral therapy (HAART) regimens with three or more agents has been associated with a marked decline in morbidity and mortality for HIV-infected patients in the United States. HAART regimens are consistently effective in reducing clinical progression and mortality in persons with CD4 cell counts less than 200 cells/mm^3. Appropriate prophylaxis and immunization against certain opportunistic infections have also been effective interventions in reducing morbidity (Chou et al., 2005).

Because false-positive test results are rare, harms associated with HIV screening are minimal. Potential harms of true-positive test results include increased anxiety, labeling, and deleterious effects on close relationships.

Although it is hoped that early diagnosis may lead to decreased transmission of HIV, evidence is lacking on the effect of increased screening leads on transmission (Chou et al., 2007). Additional evidence is also needed to clarify the balance of benefits and harms of early versus delayed treatment of asymptomatic patients with HIV infection.

Recommendation

The USPSTF strongly recommends that clinicians screen for HIV in all adolescents and adults at increased risk for HIV infection. They make no recommendation for or against routinely screening for HIV in adolescents and adults who are not at increased risk for HIV infection (USPSTF, 2005).

Counseling and HIV testing of high-risk individuals are recommended by the CDC and numerous professional organizations, including the AAFP, AMA, ACOG, ACP, and IDSA. The AAP considers all sexually active adolescents to be a high-risk group and recommends they be counseled and offered HIV testing. The CDC recommends that routine, voluntary testing be offered to all patients seen in health care facilities where the prevalence of HIV infection is 1% or greater and in settings serving client populations at increased behavioral or clinical HIV risk (Chou et al., 2005).

Standard and FDA–approved rapid screening tests accurately detect HIV infection, and interventions (e.g., HAART) reduce the risk of clinical progression and premature death. HIV screening should be offered to all adolescents and adults at high risk for HIV infection (USPSTF, 2005).

The following topics are discussed online at www.expertconsult.com:

- Syphilis infection
- Recommendations against routine screening for hepatitis B, C, and herpesvirus infections.

Metabolic, Nutritional, and Endocrine Conditions

Type 2 Diabetes Mellitus

Burden of Disease

The prevalence of type 2 diabetes in the United States is rising, particularly among adults with a body mass index (BMI) of 35 kg/m^2 or greater. From 1980 through 2006, the number of Americans with diabetes tripled, from 5.6 to 16.8 million (Norris et al., 2008). Patients with type 2 diabetes are at increased risk for microvascular and macrovascular disease. Microvascular disease leads to high rates of blindness, end-stage renal disease, and lower extremity amputations; macrovascular disease accounts for twofold to fourfold increased risk for heart disease and stroke in people with diabetes.

Accuracy of Screening Tests

Three tests have been used to screen for diabetes: fasting plasma glucose (FPG), 2-hour post-load plasma glucose (2-hour PG), and hemoglobin A$_{1c}$ (HbA$_{1c}$). Sensitivity and specificity are in the range of 75% to 80% for all three tests using these thresholds: FPG = 126 mg/dL, 2-hour PG = 200 mg/dL, and HbA$_{1c}$ = 6.4% (Harris et al., 2002). The American Diabetes Association (ADA) has recommended the FPG or 2-hour PG test for screening; the FPG is easier and faster to perform, more convenient, and acceptable to patients, and it is less expensive than other screening tests. The FPG is also more reproducible than the 2-hour PG test and has less intraindividual variation.

Effectiveness of Early Detection and Intervention

Early detection of diabetes has the potential to prevent complications of diabetes through early intensive control of cardiovascular disease risk factors and tight glycemic control. Aggressive blood pressure control in those identified with diabetes reduces the incidence of cardiovascular events and cardiovascular mortality. Patients with hyperlipidemia and diabetes who are treated with lipid-lowering agents have a similar reduction in the incidence of coronary heart disease (CHD) events as those without diabetes (RR reduction, 19%-42%) (USPSTF, 2008).

Intensive glycemic control in persons with clinically detected diabetes can reduce progression of microvascular disease. The benefits of tight glycemic control on microvascular clinical outcomes, such as severe visual impairment or end-stage renal disease, require long-term follow-up. There is inadequate evidence that early diabetes control as a result of screening provides an incremental benefit for microvascular clinical outcomes compared with initiating treatment after clinical diagnosis (USPSTF, 2008).

In patients who are screened and identified to have prediabetes, evidence indicates that lifestyle and pharmacotherapy can delay the progression of diabetes. However, there is little direct evidence that identifying persons with prediabetes will lead to long-term health benefits. Aggressive blood pressure control and lipid treatment therapy in patients with type 2 diabetes have been shown to reduce the incidence of CHD events in patients with diabetes (USPSTF, 2008). Potential harms of screening include psychological distress from a false-positive diagnosis and earlier exposure to potential adverse effects of treatment than if the diagnosis were made clinically.

Recommendation

The USPSTF (2008) recommends screening for type 2 diabetes in asymptomatic adults with sustained blood pressure (either treated or untreated) greater than 135/80 mm Hg. AAFP (2009) concurs with this recommendation. ACOG recommends FPG testing for women beginning at age 45 years, with an interval of 3 years. On the basis of expert opinion, ADA recommends screening every 3 years to detect prediabetes (IFG or IGT) or diabetes in persons age 45 and older, particularly in those with BMI of 25 kg/m² or greater. Screening is recommended in those overweight individuals younger than 45 years with one additional risk factor, including inactivity, family history of type 2 diabetes mellitus, membership in a high-risk ethnic group, gestational diabetes, hypertension, dyslipidemia, impaired glucose tolerance (IGT) or impaired fasting glucose (IFG), or a history of vascular disease (ADA, 2009).

Osteoporosis in Postmenopausal Women

Burden of Disease

One half of all postmenopausal women will have an osteoporosis-related fracture in their lifetime, including 25% who will develop a vertebral deformity and 15% who will suffer a hip fracture. *Osteoporosis* is defined as a bone mineral density (BMD) more than 2.5 standard deviations (SD) below the mean for a healthy woman, and *osteopenia* is a BMD between 1 and 2.5 SD below the mean. Among white women, it is estimated that 41% older than age 50 have osteopenia, and that 15% between ages 50 and 59 and 70% of those older than 80 have osteoporosis. Mexican American women experience similar rates. The rate among black women is approximately one-half the rate of the other groups. Including all races in the United States, an estimated 14 million women older than 50 years have osteopenia, and 5 million have osteoporosis (Nelson and Helfand, 2002).

Accuracy of Screening Tests

There are two major components of screening for osteoporosis: assessment of risk factors and BMD measurement. Older age, low body mass index (BMI), and not using estrogen replacement are associated with increased risk of osteoporosis and fracture. Other risk factors include white or Asian ancestry, positive family history, tobacco use, and low levels of weight-bearing physical activity (Melton et al., 1989). The WHO FRAX is a common assessment tool.[*] Other specific instruments, such as the Osteoporosis Risk Assessment Instrument (ORAI) and the Simple Calculated Osteoporosis Risk Estimation (SCORE) tool, use these risk factors to identify women at increased risk for fracture or low BMD. The ORAI has sensitivity of 94% and specificity of 41%, and the SCORE has sensitivity of 91% and specificity of 40% (Nelson and Helfand, 2002).

The BMD measured at the femoral neck by dual-energy x-ray absorptiometry (DEXA) is the most validated predictor of hip fractures. Several other methods for measuring BMD include single-photon absorptiometry, ultrasound, quantitative CT, single-energy x-ray absorptiometry, and peripheral quantitative CT. The results between tests are not highly correlated with one another, and the likelihood of a diagnosis of osteoporosis varies greatly depending on the site and type of test used, number of sites tested, brand of densitometer, and relevance of the reference range.

Effectiveness of Early Detection and Intervention

Treating osteoporosis with bisphosphonates reduces the risk of fracture (Nelson and Helfand, 2002). Estrogen, calcitonin, and selective estrogen receptor modulators have also been used to increase bone density and reduce fractures. The benefits of these treatments are greater for women at high risk for fracture than women at lower risk. Benefits of screening increase substantially with older age, particularly for women older than 65 and for women with important risk factors. In women age 60 to 64 who have risk factors, the benefits of screening are comparable to those of women age 65 to 69.

Several potential harms are associated with screening and treatment. An unwarranted diagnosis of osteoporosis may provoke anxiety. Potential harms may also arise from misinterpretation of BMD tests. Patients may have side effects from the medication; bisphosphonates often cause gastrointestinal side effects. The cost and inconvenience of undergoing multiple confirmatory tests must be considered.

Recommendation

The USPSTF (2011) recommends that women age 65 or older be routinely screened for osteoporosis, and that routine screening begin in younger women whose fracture risk equals that of a 65-year-old woman without risk factors. AAFP supports this position. The National Osteoporosis Foundation (NOF, 2008) recommends that adults over age 50 receive 1200 mg of calcium and 800 to 1000 IU of vitamin D₃ daily. NOF recommends BMD screening in women age 65 and older and men age 70 and older, as well as in postmenopausal women and men age 50 to 69 based on their risk factor profile. ACOG endorses the NOF guidance.

Obesity

Burden of Disease

Obesity is a substantial health problem in the United States, and the percentage of the population who is overweight or obese continues to rise. Defined as a BMI of 30 or higher, the prevalence of obesity in adults in the United States has increased from 13% to 27% over the past 40 years (McTigue et al., 2003). The prevalence of overweight rose from 31% to 34%. Obesity and overweight are associated with an increased risk of CHD, hypertension, stroke, type 2 diabetes, sleep apnea, musculoskeletal disorders, gallbladder disease, and several types of cancer. Obesity is associated with a decreased quality of life and social stigmatization.

Accuracy of Screening Tests

The BMI (weight [kg] ÷ height [m²]) is the most common test for obesity screening. It is easy to measure, highly reliable, and highly correlated with body fat and body fat mass. The waist-to-hip ratio is a good predictor of cardiovascular morbidity and mortality (McTigue et al., 2003). However, the BMI has been linked with the broadest range of health outcomes and is the most common indicator used in trials.

Effectiveness of Early Detection and Intervention

Counseling and behavioral interventions produce small to modest degrees of weight loss sustained over at least 1 year (McTigue et al., 2003). High-intensity or more

---

[*]www.shef.ac.uk/FRAX/tool.jsp?locationValue=1

frequent counseling promotes greater weight loss than low-intensity counseling. Moderate intentional weight loss (5%-10% of body weight) decreases the severity of the comorbidities associated with obesity and may reduce mortality. Pharmacotherapy also promotes modest weight loss (3-5 kg); discontinuing the medication may lead to rapid regain. Obesity surgery has been performed on patients with a BMI greater than 40 or with obesity-related comorbidities and has achieved dramatic weight loss.

Potential harms associated with screening and treatment include the stigma of being labeled "obese" and the detrimental health effects from cycles of weight loss followed by regain. Medications may cause adverse effects, and their long-term safety is not well known. A patient undergoing surgery may have complications, and 25% require reoperation within 5 years (McTigue et al., 2003).

Recommendation

The USPSTF (2003) recommends that clinicians screen all adult patients for obesity and offer intensive counseling and behavioral interventions to promote sustained weight loss for obese patients. AAFP (2008) concurs with this recommendation.

Healthy Diet Counseling

Burden of Disease

Consuming a healthy diet lowers the risks of morbidity and mortality from chronic disease. Four of the 10 leading causes of death—CHD, some types of cancer, stroke, and type 2 diabetes mellitus—are associated with unhealthy diets (Ammerman et al., 2002). Despite well-established benefits of consuming a healthy diet, more than 80% of Americans of all ages eat fewer than the recommended number of daily servings of fruit, vegetables, and grain products. Also, they consume more than the recommended number of calories from saturated fat and total fat (USDHHS, 2000).

Accuracy of Screening Tests

Several brief, validated dietary assessment instruments can identify dietary counseling needs, guide intervention, and monitor change among adult patients in primary care settings. (These can be found in the article at http://escholarship. org/uc/item/9s03p43r jgb.) Most of these instruments can be self-administered, are easily scored, have fewer than 40 items, and take 10 minutes or less to administer. Most assessments are subject to bias and may result in underreporting of calories.

Effectiveness of Early Detection and Intervention.

Medium- to high-intensity behavioral interventions produce consistent, sustained, and clinically important changes in dietary intake of saturated fat, total fat, fruits, vegetables, and fiber. The most effective interventions generally combine education, behaviorally oriented counseling, and patient reinforcement and follow-up (Ammerman et al., 2002). More intensive interventions and those of longer duration are associated with greater benefits and more sustained changes in diet. Self-reported dietary changes are often accompanied by improved lipids, BMI, and weight. Patients with hyperlipidemia and other risk factors for CHD and diet-related chronic disease benefit the most from dietary counseling, whereas patients at average risk for chronic disease generally achieve smaller changes in diet.

Recommendation

The USPSTF (2003) recommends intensive behavioral counseling for all adults with hyperlipidemia and other known risk factors for cardiovascular and diet-related chronic disease. Counseling may be done by the primary care provider or through referral to a specialist. The AAFP (2008) recommends intensive behavioral dietary counseling for adult patients with hyperlipidemia and other known risk factors for cardiovascular and diet-related chronic disease.

Physical Activity Counseling

Burden of Disease

Sedentary lifestyles are associated with increased risks of chronic diseases, including CHD, diabetes, obesity, and osteoporosis, and increased physical activity can reduce those risks (USDHHS, 2000). Despite the well-established benefits of exercise, only about 20% of adults achieved the recommended *Healthy People 2010* level of moderate exercise: 30 minutes of moderate physical activity on most days of the week; only 15% achieved a vigorous level of physical activity for 20 minutes on 3 days of the week (Eden et al., 2002).

Effectiveness of Counseling

Existing studies on physical activity counseling are inadequate to determine the overall efficacy, effectiveness, and feasibility of counseling in a primary care setting. Combining provider counseling with behavioral interventions such as patient goal setting, written exercise prescriptions, and individually tailored physical activity regimens may be the most effective way to change physical activity levels and warrants more research. Linking patients to community-based physical activity and fitness programs may enhance the effectiveness of primary care clinician counseling (Eden et al., 2002).

Recommendation

The USPSTF (2002) states that the evidence is insufficient to recommend for or against behavioral counseling in primary care settings to promote physical activity. Organizations that include the AAFP, U.S. Department of Health and Human Services *(Healthy People 2010)*, CDC, AAP, American Heart Association (AHA), and ACOG recommend that health care providers counsel all individuals about physical activity. These recommendations are based on the known health benefits of physical activity rather than on the effectiveness of counseling for promoting changes in physical activity (Eden et al., 2002).

Hormone therapy for the prevention of chronic conditions in postmenopausal women is discussed online at www.expertconsult.com.

Special Populations

Preventive Services for Children and Adolescents

Challenges in Evidence-Based Prevention

Prevention plays a critical role in all age groups. From a theoretic and practical perspective, however, greater emphasis should be placed on prevention in the earlier years because the potential benefit is greater. As people age, chronic diseases develop, and a greater proportion of health care becomes dedicated to disease management. Because prevention is most beneficial in the younger years, one would expect that the preventive services provided to children are supported by a strong evidence base. On the contrary, there is a relatively large evidence base for determining beneficial preventive services for adults, but aside from immunizations, the evidence base for childhood services is generally much more limited (Moyer and Butler, 2004).

Reasons for this lack of evidence base include length of follow-up required to realize reduction in disease outcomes, historical adoption and therefore standardization of many childhood preventive services, ethical considerations of not offering a potentially beneficial preventive service to children, methodologic challenges in determining developmentally appropriate outcomes in children, and the paradigm that knowledge alone represents a beneficial health outcome for families.

These evidence gaps in prevention highlight the challenge of child research rather than invalidate the importance of prevention in children. The message must be made clear to physicians, parents, and children—prevention is important at all ages. Several categories of preventive services are relevant to children: immunizations, counseling and anticipatory guidance, screening tests, and preventive medications. Chapters 22, 23, and 24 discuss care for children, including preventive services.

Immunizations

Immunizations, or vaccinations, usually are injections (oral in the case of the oral polio vaccine) that, when administered to an individual, elicit an immune response that protects the individual against the pathogen when future exposure occurs. Childhood is a particularly important time for immunizations because young children are still naïve to many viruses and bacteria, presenting an opportunity for primary prevention of disease.

The CDC National Immunization Program has an Advisory Committee on Immunization Practices (ACIP) that meets regularly and annually releases a Childhood and Adolescent Immunization Schedule (www.cdc.gov/vaccines/) (CDC, 2009). A catch-up schedule is available for children who have missed previous immunizations. The ACIP, AAP, and AAFP also release the annual Harmonized Childhood and Adolescent Immunization Schedule, which has been endorsed by the three organizations. Periodic preventive care visits by family physicians provide opportunities for administration of these immunizations.

Counseling and Anticipatory Guidance

Anticipatory guidance appropriately targeted to a child's developmental stage is a critical component of preventive care. Also, although good-quality evidence supporting the efficacy of most anticipatory guidance is limited, the standard of care is to provide such advice and counseling for parents (Moyer and Butler, 2004). Anticipatory guidance involves counseling caregivers to prepare for future normal child growth and development and to prepare caregivers for how these changes may need to be accommodated to promote development and to prevent injury or harm. Examples of anticipatory guidance include providing counseling to caregivers about various safety issues (e.g., use of infant and child car seats, bicycle helmets, water safety, poisoning prevention, childproofing the home), nutrition, appropriate dental care, and physical activity. Injury prevention is particularly important because unintentional injury is the leading cause of death for children and adolescents. In children 1 to 14 years old, the three leading causes of injury-related death are motor vehicle crashes, drowning, and fire.

Bright Futures (http://brightfutures.aap.org/web) is a well-known, frequently implemented example of a program that includes health supervision and anticipatory guidance dedicated to well-child care and prevention. The Bright Futures program was begun by the Maternal and Child Health Bureau (MCHB) of the federal government and is endorsed by the AAFP and AAP.

Preventive care of adolescents emphasizes anticipatory guidance and counseling. Important topics to discuss include sexual activity; alcohol, tobacco, and drug use; healthy eating and physical activity; injury prevention; and mental health. The evidence of the benefits of screening and counseling for these conditions in adolescence is not clear. The clinician must also ensure that immunizations are delivered to the adolescent according to the recommended schedule. Vaccination against hepatitis B should be administered if it was not given during infancy, and boosters for varicella; measles, mumps, rubella (MMR); tetanus, diphtheria, and pertussis are given as determined by the schedule. Adolescents, especially college students, are at increased risk for meningococcal meningitis. The risks of disease and the risks and benefits of immunization should be discussed with prospective college students.

Screening tests for infants and children are discussed online at www.expertconsult.com.

Preventive Medications

Preventive medications provide primary prevention of disease to average-risk or high-risk children. Preventive medications in childhood include fluoride for children with inadequately fluoridated drinking water and iron supplementation between ages 6 and 12 months for infants at high risk for iron deficiency anemia. Some preventive medications may be used in children with chronic diseases to prevent disease symptoms, progression, or complications; however, these medications may be considered disease management (i.e., tertiary prevention) rather than primary or secondary prevention.

Preventive Services for Pregnant Women

Preconception counseling and prenatal care largely focus on strategies to prevent or detect potential complications for the pregnant woman, fetus, and newborn. Routine preconception counseling may include risk assessment based on family history, counseling about use of folic acid for the prevention of neural tube defects, and counseling about the harms of smoking, alcohol use, and certain foods (e.g., fish with high levels of mercury) and drugs (prescription and illicit) on pregnancy outcomes.

Prenatal care includes screening tests, counseling, preventive medications, and immunizations. Screening laboratory tests include a complete blood cell count, blood type, Rh sensitivity, urinalysis for bacteriuria, screening for several STIs (e.g., syphilis, HIV, hepatitis B, gonorrhea [high risk], *Chlamydia* [high risk]), screening for neural tube defects, gestational diabetes mellitus, and group B streptococci (Kirkham et al., 2005).

Counseling is often anticipatory guidance for the upcoming stages of pregnancy, delivery, and the postpartum period. Counseling for breastfeeding is a key preventive component to prenatal care, as is the use of prenatal vitamins and influenza vaccine administration. Chapter 21 discusses care of the pregnant patient, including prenatal preventive services.

Preventive Services for Older Adults

An emphasis on a shared decision-making approach is especially important when considering preventive services for older adults. Family physicians and their older patients should consider issues that contribute to the complexity of prevention in older adults, including unique goals of prevention, life expectancy, comorbidities, potential for harm, and patient values and preferences (Harris et al., 2001).

The patient's values and preferences are always important, and shared decision making should occur *before* the preventive service is provided. Preventive aspirin therapy in elderly persons provides an illustrative example of the need for shared decision making. There are few studies on the use of aspirin for the prevention of cardiovascular disease in older adults. Older adults are at especially high risk of cardiovascular disease but also at high risk of gastrointestinal bleeding from aspirin. Some older men may decide that avoiding a myocardial infarction is of great value, and that having a gastrointestinal bleeding event is not a major problem, and they would probably decide to take aspirin (USPSTF, 2009).

Specific preventive services that are of special interest for older adults include immunizations. The CDC recommends the zoster vaccine for all adults over age 60, pneumococcal vaccine for adults over 65, and influenza vaccine annually for adults over 50 (ACIP, 2009). Other preventive interventions of special importance target common causes of disease and disability and include multifactorial interventions for older adults that improve physical function, maintain independent living, and reduce falls (AGS, 2001; Beswick et al., 2008; Gillespie et al., 2006).

Counseling

Although the leading causes of death in the United States remain heart disease, cancer, and cerebrovascular disease (stroke), in their landmark paper Actual Causes of Death in the United States, McGinnis and Foege (1993) concluded that 50% of U.S. mortality is caused by 10 lifestyle-related behaviors, including tobacco use, poor dietary habits, lack of physical activity, alcohol misuse, illicit drug use, and risky sexual practices. In a 2004 update, Mokdad and colleagues found that more than one third of U.S. mortality in 2000 was linked to four behaviors: tobacco use, alcohol consumption, poor diet, and physical inactivity. Changing the health behaviors of Americans has the greatest potential impact of any current approach for decreasing morbidity and mortality and for improving the quality of life across diverse populations (Whitlock et al., 2002).

A growing body of evidence demonstrates that brief interventions integrated into routine primary care can effectively address the most common and important health risk behaviors encountered in family medicine, including smoking cessation, healthy diet, regular physical activity, appropriate alcohol use, and responsible use of contraceptives. Simple, direct, and brief advice from the physician to change lifestyle habits has been shown to be effective in encouraging smoking cessation, reducing problem drinking, and modifying some cardiovascular risk factors associated with activity and diet (Whitlock et al., 2002). If 60% to 90% of practicing physicians regularly advised patients not to smoke, an additional 63,000 smokers would quit each year (Hollis, 2000). This approach works, and patients expect and want it. More than 95% of adults report that they expect their physicians to give them information about health behaviors and assistance in changing negative ones (Vogt et al., 1998). Not surprisingly, clinician advice has been associated with increased satisfaction with medical care.

Behavioral counseling interventions have expanded beyond the limits of one-on-one interactions between physicians and patients. Physicians' efforts are enhanced when the entire health care team takes appropriate and complementary roles in delivering interventions. For example, many components of successful interventions can take place outside the traditional physician-patient encounter. The patient can complete a health risk assessment while waiting to see the doctor; a trained staff member can do in-office counseling after the clinical encounter; a patient may be referred to a community-based program; and a follow-up visit or telephone call may be arranged. To emphasize the potential impact of a team approach, if a health care team member provides an additional 10 minutes of targeted assistance to one half of the patients who received brief advice on smoking cessation from the physician, the number of people expected to quit increases from 63,000 to 630,000 (Hollis, 2000). The use of additional resources, however, does not lessen the central importance of the clinician-patient relationship in promoting behavioral change. Effective clinician communication is essential in promoting behavior change.

Appreciating the impact of behavioral change interventions requires a broad population-based perspective. A family physician may become discouraged if only 5% to 14% of those receiving an intervention make clinically significant changes, such as quitting smoking. However, even modest effects result in tremendous benefits to the community when systematically applied to the large number of those in need. The potential for substantial public health benefit from office-based behavioral change interventions will be realized only when these interventions are applied broadly and regularly (see Chapter 7).

The "5As" Framework

In 2000, building on earlier work from the U.S. National Cancer Institute, the CTFPHC proposed a framework to guide physicians and health care systems in organizing their general approach to assisting patients with behavioral counseling interventions. In 2002, USPSTF adopted the

Table 6-6 The Five "A" Components of Behavior Counseling Interventions

Assess: Ask about or assess behavioral health risks and factors affecting choice of behavior change goals or methods.

Advise: Give clear, specific, and personalized behavior change advice, including information about personal health harms and benefits.

Agree: Collaboratively select appropriate treatment goals and methods based on the patient's interest in and willingness to change the behavior.

Assist: Using behavior change techniques, aid the patient in achieving agreed-on goals by acquiring the skills, confidence, and social or environmental supports for behavior change, supplemented with adjunctive medical treatments when appropriate (e.g., pharmacotherapy for tobacco dependence, contraceptive drugs or devices).

Arrange: Schedule follow-up contacts (in person or by telephone) to provide ongoing assistance or support and to adjust the treatment plan as needed, including referral to more intensive or specialized treatment. Intervention to help patients change unhealthy behaviors often requires repetition over time.

Modified from Whitlock EP, Orleans CT, Pender N, Allan J. Evaluating primary care behavioral counseling interventions: an evidence-based approach. Am J Prev Med 2002;22:267-284.

framework, known as the "5As," for evaluating the effectiveness of behavior counseling interventions (Table 6-6). The 5As framework is a powerful tool that can assist physicians in developing and evaluating their practice's behavior change interventions. USPSTF offers guidance on the evidence base for behavior change interventions for many specific behaviors.

Assessing Behavior

Systematic routine behavior risk factor assessment is the foundation for proactive behavioral counseling interventions and identifies all those in need of assistance. For example, having a system in place to identify and document tobacco use triples the odds of clinician intervention (Fiore et al., 2008). Assessment tools should be brief, easy to complete, and easily scored or interpreted. Assessment may range from a single focused question asked as part of taking the vital signs (e.g., Have you used tobacco products at all in the past 7 days?) to comprehensive tools known as health risk appraisals (HRAs). HRAs may be mailed or e-mailed to patients in advance of their appointments. Some are available for completion or scoring by computer; others are available on the Internet (e.g., HowsYourHealth.org, MyHealthyLiving.net).

Advising the Patient

Physicians are influential catalysts for patient behavior change. By providing explicit health behavior advice, physicians establish that lifestyle changes are an important part of health care and motivate patients to change. Advice is most powerful when personalized and linked to a patient's own concerns, experiences, or values. A warm, empathetic, and nonjudgmental style engenders cooperation and less resistance. By qualifying advice with remarks such as, "As your

physician, I feel I should tell you that . . . ," the physician conveys respect for and avoids undermining patient autonomy (Whitlock et al., 2002). Placing confidence in the patient's ability to change and acknowledging past successes build patient's self-efficacy. Advice messages should not be lectures and should be delivered in 30 to 60 seconds.

Agreeing with the Patient

Only when the patient and physician agree that change is desired should goals and options be explored. Assessing the patient's motivation to change may be useful at this point, because appropriate interventions for those who are ready to change and for those who are not are likely to differ. For people with multiple behavioral risks, agreement is needed about which behavior change to focus on first. Physicians should partner with patients in considering the potential interventions. When patients are actively involved in making health care decisions, their choices are based on realistic expectations and are aligned with their own values.

Additional Assistance

Additional assistance within or outside the patient visit is likely to produce better outcomes than advice-only treatment. Busy clinicians, however, often do not have time to provide more than brief counseling (1-3 minutes). Behavior change interventions should incorporate additional team members and linkage to community resources. Many health systems use dieticians, nurse care managers, social workers, and trained medical assistants to provide assistance to patients as part of behavior change interventions. Assistance may take the form of additional behavior-specific counseling, general patient motivation and activation, or referral to a community resource. In addition to traditional print materials, interactive computer and web-based programs that assist behavior change are becoming available.

Arranging Follow-up

Behavior change requires follow-up. The physician may simply inform the patient of plans to follow up at their next regularly scheduled visit, making a note in the chart. Usually, however, initial follow-up should be scheduled within a relatively short period. Depending on the change being undertaken, follow-up may consist of a phone call a few days after a scheduled quit date, an e-mail inquiring about progress, or an in-office visit. After the initial follow-up, future contacts may often be spaced at successively longer intervals.

Theories and Models of Behavior Change

Behavior change theories and models can help physicians conceptualize the complex context in which individual behavior change occurs and the variability among patients' acceptance of behavior counseling interventions (Table 6-7). Insights gained from applying the models may help clinicians clarify barriers and opportunities when working with a given individual and customize an intervention based on an individual's needs, such as determining which patients may respond best to a more intensive intervention.

Table 6-7 Theories and Models of Individual Behavior Change

Theory or Model	Focus	Key Concepts
Health belief model	Peoples' perceptions of the threat of a health problem and appraisal of the behavior recommended to prevent or manage the problem.	Perceived susceptibility Perceived severity Perceived benefits of action Perceived barriers to action Cues to action Self-efficacy
Theory of reasoned action, theory of planned behavior	People are rational beings whose intention to perform a behavior is strongly related to its actual performance through beliefs, attitudes, subjective norms, and perceived behavioral control.	Behavioral intention Subjective norms Attitudes Perceived behavioral control
Stages of change, transtheoretical model	Readiness to change or attempt to change a health behavior varies among individuals and within an individual over time. Relapse is a common occurrence and part of the normal process of change.	Precontemplation Contemplation Preparation Action Maintenance Relapse
Social cognitive theory, social learning theory	Behavior is explained by dynamic interaction among personal factors, environmental influences, and behavior.	Observational learning Reciprocal determinism Outcome expectancy Behavioral capacity Self-efficacy Reinforcement

Modified from Whitlock EP, Orleans CT, Pender N, Allan J. Evaluating primary care behavioral counseling interventions: an evidence-based approach. Am J Prev Med 2002;22:267-284.

Most behavior change theories focus on the diverse, interacting levels of influence on an individual's behavior. For example, the stages of change (transtheoretical) model emphasizes that change is an ongoing process with multiple stages that often include relapse and recycling into new efforts to change. The concept of self-efficacy stresses that individual behavioral change requires the belief that change is needed and possible. Many theories recognize the dynamic interaction between intrapersonal, interpersonal, and environmental issues, including factors such as age, race, ethnicity, and socioeconomic status.

Systems Change

Family Physicians within the Health Care System

Family physicians are responsible for providing care for acute illnesses and chronic conditions. They also provide preventive services, including screening, immunizations, and behavioral counseling. In the disease-based model of health care, preventive care is often viewed as a competing demand. Americans, however, made more than 480 million visits in 2002 to their primary care physicians. As a trusted and well-used source of information and care, the family physician has a tremendous opportunity to improve the health of individual patients and entire communities through the provision of preventive services.

The good news is that family physicians, despite limited face-to-face time with patients, already spend a significant amount of time promoting health behaviors. One large study found that physicians addressed health behaviors during one half of all visits, spending on average more than 10% of the visit promoting health (Stange et al., 2002).

Further improvements in the provision of preventive services require more than improving clinician knowledge and attitude. Improving the quality, delivery, and effectiveness of prevention in primary care office practice requires changes in the office system. The family physician and other primary care clinicians must be integrated into a larger health care delivery team.

Using the 5As Model in a System

Of the five steps in the 5As model (assess, advise, agree, assist, and arrange), the family physician is likely to be most effective when charged with focusing on the advise and agree steps. The staff member who triages the patient may be assigned the responsibility of administering a brief health risk assessment or reviewing a flow sheet of preventive services and noting on the chart if the patient is due for an immunization or screening test. During the visit, the prompted physician can advise the patient to be more physically active and explore the patient's motivation to change or recommend a flu shot or cholesterol test. Most importantly, other members of the health care team can assist patients in learning additional information, acquiring new skills, choosing between options, and creating a personalized action plan. Team members, including nurses, medical assistants, social workers, and care managers, can link patients to resources in the community to support health behavior change and arrange follow-up (see Chapter 2).

The Chronic Care Model

The chronic care model (CCM) has been proposed as a useful framework for considering the system changes necessary to construct a health care system that proactively promotes healthy behaviors and trains clinician and patients to work as partners in a collaborative care process (Glasgow et al., 2001) (Figure 6-3). The CCM identifies six essential elements of a health care system that together foster interactions between an informed, activated patient and a prepared, proactive health care team. The model defines six broad dimensions that must be considered when redesigning systems of care: organization of care, clinical information systems, delivery-system design, decision support, self-management support, and community resources (Wagner, 1998). As a model, the CCM does not provide a specific set of interventions; instead, it acts as a framework within

CHRONIC CARE MODEL

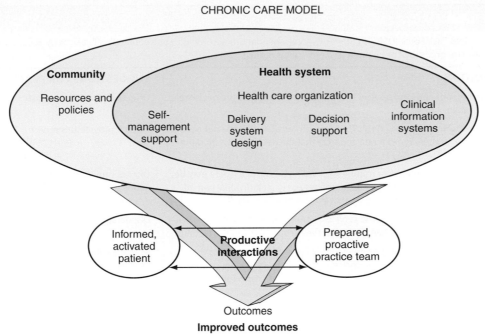

Figure 6-3 The chronic care model. *(Modified from Wagner EH. Chronic disease management: what will it take to improve chronic illness? Effect Clin Pract 1998;1:2-4.)*

which improvement strategies can be tailored to local conditions.

In an individual office, the application of the CCM toward improving the quality of preventive services may lead to any of the following:

- Developing a patient registry for child and adult immunizations (i.e., clinical information system).
- Implementing standing orders that all patients with diabetes receive a home glucose monitor and meet with a nurse educator (i.e., delivery system design).
- Referring all prenatal patients to a local La Leche League meeting (i.e., community resources).
- Designing a prompt to cue physicians to schedule a mammogram (i.e., decision support).
- Integrating achievement of prevention goals into physician performance bonuses (i.e., health system organization).
- Training physicians to use the techniques of motivational interviewing to set goals in collaboration with patients and identify personal barriers and supports after advising smokers to quit (i.e., self-management support).

Rethinking the Periodic Health Examination

Although the periodic health examination means many things to many people, most agree that it refers to a patient encounter focusing on health maintenance and disease prevention. Exactly which preventive services should be offered during such a periodic examination varies in practice; however, the services discussed in this chapter have been shown to improve patient-oriented health outcomes. Many of these services may be provided during regular office visits and in the context of a periodic health maintenance visit. Batteries

of tests (e.g., screening laboratory tests, ECGs) and general head-to-toe physical examinations often performed during preventive periodic health examinations (e.g., heart and lung auscultation, abdominal palpation) are not effective as general screening strategies in the general population. Instead, a customized preventive service package is most useful.

Conclusions

Preventive services should be tailored according to the individual patient's risk factors, preferences, and comorbid diseases. Although no "one size fits all" prevention plan can work for everyone, the following tenets remain true:

1. Prevention can lead to major health benefits, but all prevention attempts are not necessarily beneficial, and some services may be harmful.
2. Evidence for preventive service effectiveness can be used to prioritize preventive services for average-risk and high-risk patients in a family physician's practice.
3. Systems approaches using team models for provision of services, reminder systems, and electronic health records are critical to improving the use of evidence-based preventive services.
4. Counseling is a key component in prevention and requires health professionals trained in counseling modalities.

Providing evidence-based preventive services, including immunizations, screening tests, and behavior change interventions, is possible with planning, teamwork, and practice redesign.

EVIDENCE-BASED SUMMARY

The U.S. Preventive Services Task Force (USPSTF) grades its recommendations according to one of five classifications (A, B, C, D, I), reflecting the strength of evidence and magnitude of net benefit (benefits minus harms):

GRADE	DEFINITION	SUGGESTIONS FOR PRACTICE
A	USPSTF recommends the service. There is high certainty that the net benefit is substantial.	Offer or provide this service.
B	USPSTF recommends the service. There is high certainty that the net benefit is moderate, or there is moderate certainty that the net benefit is moderate to substantial.	Offer or provide this service.
C	USPSTF recommends against routinely providing the service. There may be considerations that support providing the service in an individual patient. There is at least moderate certainty that the net benefit is small.	Offer or provide this service only if other considerations support the offering or providing the service in an individual patient.
D	USPSTF recommends against the service. There is moderate or high certainty that the service has no net benefit or that the harms outweigh the benefits.	Discourage the use of this service.
I Statement	USPSTF concludes that the current evidence is insufficient to assess the balance of benefits and harms of the service. Evidence is lacking, of poor quality, or conflicting, and the balance of benefits and harms cannot be determined.	Read the clinical considerations section of USPSTF Recommendation Statement. If the service is offered, patients should understand the uncertainty about the balance of benefits and harms.

From U.S. Preventive Services Task Force Table of Recommended Preventive Services for 2001 to April 2009.

USPSTF CATEGORY A AND B RECOMMENDATIONS

SERVICE	POPULATION	COMMENTS
Screening for abdominal aortic aneurysm	Ever-smoking men ages 65-75 years: B	Never-smoking men ages 65-75: C Women: D
Screening for alcohol misuse	Adults: B	Adolescents: I
Aspirin for primary prevention of cardiovascular events	Men age 45-79 to prevent myocardial infarction (MI): A Women age 55-79 to prevent stroke: A	Men younger than 45 to prevent MI: D Women younger than 55 to prevent stroke: D Men and women 80+ to prevent cardiovascular disease: I
Screening for asymptomatic bacteriuria	Pregnant women: A	Nonpregnant women and men: D
Discussion of chemoprevention of breast cancer	Women at increased risk of breast cancer and decreased risk of adverse events: B	Women not at increased risk of breast cancer: D
Genetic risk assessment and BRCA mutation testing for breast and ovarian cancer susceptibility	Women whose family history is associated with increased risk for deleterious mutations in *BRCA1* or *BRCA2* genes: B	Women whose family history is not associated with increased risk for deleterious mutations in *BRCA1* or *BRCA2* gene: D
Screening for breast cancer with mammography	Women age 50+: B	Women 40-49: C Screening with clinical breast exam: I Breast self-exam: D
Counseling to promote breast-feeding	Interventions during pregnancy and after birth to promote and support breastfeeding: B	No subgroups
Screening for cervical cancer with Pap smear	Women younger than age 65 who are sexually active and have a cervix: A	Women over 65 who have had previous negative screens: D Women who have had total hysterectomy for benign disease: D Screening with new technologies: I Screening with HPV: I
Screening for *Chlamydia*	Sexually active nonpregnant women ≤24 and older nonpregnant women who are at increased risk: A	Pregnant women ≤24 and older pregnant women who are at increased risk: B Women ≥25 and older, whether or not they are pregnant, if they are not at increased risk: C Men: I
	Pregnant women <24 and older pregnant women who are at increased risk: B	Sexually active nonpregnant women <24 and older nonpregnant women who are at increased risk: A Women>25, whether or not they are pregnant, if they are not at increased risk: C

SERVICE	POPULATION	COMMENTS
Screening for colorectal cancer	Adults age 50-75: A	Adults 76-85: C Adults 85+: D Computed tomography colonography and fecal DNA testing as screening modalities for colorectal cancer: I
Screening for congenital hypothyroidism in newborns	Newborns: A	No subgroups
Prevention of dental caries	Preschool children, using oral fluoride supplementation in specific areas whose water is deficient in fluoride: B	Preschool children, using risk assessment: I
Screening for depression in adults	Adults within a system of care: B	No subgroups
Screening for depression in children and adolescents	Adolescents age 12-18: B	Children and adolescents age 7-11: I
Screening for type 2 diabetes	Adults with hypertension or dyslipidemia: B	Adults without hypertension or dyslipidemia: I
Intensive behavioral dietary counseling	Adults with hyperlipidemia or other risk factors for CVD: B	Routine behavioral counseling to promote a healthy diet: I
Folic acid supplementation	All women planning or capable of pregnancy: A	No subgroups
Screening for gonorrhea	Newborns: A Sexually active women, including those who are pregnant if they are at high risk: B	Men and women at low risk: D Men at high risk: I Pregnant women not at high risk: I
Screening for hepatitis: B	Pregnant women: A	General nonpregnant population: D
Screening for human immunodeficiency virus (HIV)	All adolescents and adults at increased risk: A All pregnant women: A	All adolescents and adults not at increased risk: C
Screening for hypertension	Adults ages 18+: A	No subgroups
Screening children and pregnant women for iron deficiency anemia	Asymptomatic pregnant women: B	Asymptomatic children age 6-12 months: I
Iron supplementation for children and pregnant women	Asymptomatic children age 6-12 months who are at increased risk: B	Asymptomatic children age 6-12 months who are at average risk: I Nonanemic pregnant women: I
Screening for lipid disorders in adults	Men 35+: A Women 45+: A Men 20-35: B Women 20-45: B	Men age 20-35 and women age 20-45 with no risk factors: C
Screening for newborn hearing	Hearing loss in newborns: B	No subgroups
Screening for obesity with intensive counseling and behavioral interventions	Adults: B Children >6 years old: B	Screening with low- to moderate-intensity counseling: I Counseling for overweight, not obese: I
Screening for osteoporosis	Women age 65+ and younger women with risk factors: B	Men: I
Screening for phenylketonuria in newborns	Newborns: A	No subgroups
Behavioral counseling to prevent sexually transmitted infections (STIs)	Sexually active adolescents and adults at increased risk for STIs: B	Non–sexually active adolescents and adults not at increased risk: I
Screening for sickle cell disease	Newborns: A	No subgroups
Screening for syphilis in pregnant women	All pregnant women and all persons at risk: A	All persons not at risk: D
Screen for tobacco use and provide tobacco cessation interventions	Adults: A Pregnant women: A	Screening for tobacco use or interventions to prevent or treat tobacco use among adolescents and children: I
Visual impairment to detect amblyopia, strabismus, visual field defect	Children younger than 5 years old: B	No subgroups

HPV, Human papillomavirus; *CVD*, Cardiovascular disease.

USPSTF CATEGORY D RECOMMENDATIONS: PREVENTIVE SERVICES NOT RECOMMENDED IN GENERAL POPULATION

SERVICE	POPULATION	COMMENTS
Screening for abdominal aortic aneurysm	Women: D	Ever-smoking men age 65-75: B Never-smoking men age 65-75: C
Aspirin for primary prevention of cardio-vascular events	Men younger than 45 to prevent myocardial infarction (MI): D Women younger than 55 to prevent stroke: D	Men age 45-79 to prevent MI: A Women age 55-79 to prevent stroke: A Men and women 80+ to prevent cardiovascular disease: I
Aspirin/NSAIDs to prevent colorectal cancer	Adults at average risk: D	No subgroups
Screening for bacterial vaginosis	Pregnant women at low risk for preterm delivery: D	Pregnant women at high risk for preterm delivery: I
Screening for asymptomatic bacteriuria	Men and nonpregnant women: D	Pregnant women: A
Beta-carotene supplements	Adults: D	Supplemental vitamins A, C, and E or folic acid or antioxidant combinations: I
Screening for bladder cancer	Adults: D	No subgroups
Screening for breast cancer	Women breast self-exam: D	No subgroups
BRCA mutation testing for breast and ovarian cancer susceptibility	Women whose family history is not associated with increased risk for deleterious mutations in *BRCA1* and *BRCA2*: D	Women whose family history is associated with increased risk for deleterious mutations in *BRCA1* and *BRCA2*: B
Carotid artery stenosis	Adults: D	No subgroups
Chemoprevention of breast cancer	Women not at increased risk of breast cancer: D	Women at increased risk of breast cancer and decreased risk of adverse events: B
Chemoprevention for hormone replacement therapy	Postmenopausal women: D Postmenopausal women who have had a hysterectomy: D	No subgroups
Screening for chronic obstructive pulmonary disease	Adults: D	No subgroups
Cervical cancer screening with Pap smear	Women over 65 who have had previous negative screens Women who have had total hysterectomy for benign disease: D	Women under 65 who are sexually active and have a cervix: A Screening with new technologies: I Screening with HPV: I
Screening for coronary heart disease (CHD)	Adults not at increased risk, using ECG, ETT, or EBCT: D	Adults at increased risk: I
Screening for colorectal cancer	Adults 85+: D	Adults 50-75: A Adults 76-85: C Computed tomography colonography and fecal DNA testing as screening modalities for colorectal cancer: I
Screening for genital herpes	Asymptomatic pregnant women: D Asymptomatic adolescents and adults: D	No subgroups
Screening for gonorrhea	Men and women at low risk: D	Sexually active women, including those who are pregnant if they are at high risk : B Newborns: A Men at high risk and pregnant women at low risk: I
Screening for hemochromatosis	Asymptomatic general population: D	No subgroups
Screening for hepatitis B infection	General population: D	Pregnant women: A
Screening for hepatitis C	Not at increased risk: D	Increased risk: I
Screening for idiopathic scoliosis	Adolescents: D	No subgroups
Screening for lead in childhood and pregnancy	Children age 1-5 years who are at average risk: D Pregnant women: D	Children age 1-5 years who are at increased risk: I
Screening for ovarian cancer	Women: D	No subgroups
Screening for peripheral arterial disease	General population: D	No subgroups

SERVICE	POPULATION	COMMENTS
Screening for prostate cancer	Men >75: D	Men <75: I
Postmenopausal hormone therapy for primary prevention of chronic problems	Postmenopausal women:Estrogen plus progestin or Estrogen alone: D	No subgroups
Screening for syphilis in pregnant women	All persons not at risk: D	All pregnant women and all persons at risk: A
Screening for testicular cancer	Men: D	No subgroups

Acknowledgments

The authors appreciate the invaluable work of the U.S. Preventive Services Task Force and the dedication of the members and staff that make this work possible.

References

The complete reference list is available online at www.expertconsult.com.

Web Resources

www.ahrq.gov/CLINIC/uspstfix.htm
Recommendations United States Preventive Services Task Force (USPSTF) prevention recommendations.

www.cdc.gov/vaccines
Center for Disease Control and Prevention (CDC) summary of vaccines, immunization schedules, and patient information.

www.thecommunityguide.org
The Community Task Force recommendations for evidence-based and community-based interventions for preventive health care.

http://hp2010.nhlbihin.net/atpiii/calculator.asp?usertype=prof
Ten-year cardiovascular risk calculator based on the Framingham data.

www.cancer.gov/bcrisktool/Default.aspx
Breast cancer risk calculator through the National Cancer Institute.

www.shef.ac.uk/FRAX/tool.jsp?locationValue=1FRAX: 10-year bone fracture risk calculator.

www.testandcalc.com/etc/tests/audit.asp
The Alcohol Use Disorders Identification Test (AUDIT).

www.howsyourhealth.org/
Survey of health habits that provides a summary letter that the user can print and bring to their physician appointment.

www.pubapps.vcu.edu/myhealthyliving/
Self-directed website to educate about the health benefits of nutrition, physical activity, avoiding tobacco, and limiting alcohol.

7 CHAPTER

Lifestyle Interventions and Behavior Change

Colin P. Kopes-Kerr

Key Points

- The two highest-yield strategies for prevention of chronic disease and death are (1) a routine annual cardiac risk assessment strategy for all adults, with intervention graded to level of risk, and (2) a strategy of primary prevention.

- The optimal strategy for the prevention of heart disease requires routine global cardiac risk assessment.

- A strategy of global cardiac risk assessment, with appropriate intervention graded to level of risk, closely approximates the effects of a primary prevention strategy.

In the hectic pace of modern family medicine, we may forget what first motivated us to become physicians. For many, it was an urge to do service, first by helping others live longer and healthier lives, then by comforting the sick and dying when we had nothing else to offer. This task often evolves into a tension between mastering the skills needed to treat illness and learning the strategies to prevent illness. Up to the present, the major emphasis in the training of primary care physicians has been on the treatment of disease.

This chapter approaches the problem of prevention from each of these perspectives: how to carry out effective prevention (1) from the traditional disease-oriented approach and (2) from a newer, general lifestyle approach. This discussion attempts to answer four practical and important questions for family physicians, as follows:

1. What is a healthy lifestyle?
2. What is the prevalence of a healthy lifestyle among patients?
3. What are the potential benefits for patients who have or who change to a healthy lifestyle?
4. What is the major obstacle to lifestyle changes in a family physician's office?

Prevention from the Disease-Oriented Perspective: A Focus on Heart Disease

To be effective, family physicians need to reduce mortality—from all causes, not just heart disease or stroke—for all their patients. Using the total number of deaths is the relevant measure of effectiveness for two reasons. First, it is simple, cleaner, and easier to measure; a person is either alive or dead. Second, the count is not affected by diagnostic error. The literature reviewed here focuses especially on *all-cause mortality* as a relevant measure of a healthy lifestyle.

In the United States the system for counting numbers of deaths is provided by the Centers for Disease Control and Prevention (CDC) through its Wisqars database. Simply type the search term leadcaus.html into Google, and the database will be the first link to appear. The variables for gender, age, ethnicity, and U.S. region can be changed to best fit where you are working.

The leading causes of death for all adults age 50 to 85 are listed in Table 7-1. A look at this list can provide a guide to action for your practice. If the number-one cause of death is heart disease, this may be the problem to address most vigorously, perhaps delaying other preventive activities until this is done. Alternatively, some might argue for a focus on cancer, because mortality from cancer is almost as high as from heart disease (and even higher in the age group 50-59), and cancer causes much more concern among patients.

However, good reasons exist not to focus on cancer. The first problem is that "cancer," when listed as the second leading cause of death in the United States, represents deaths from "all cancers." The disadvantage is that physicians have no good tools or tests that work against "all" cancers; the single exception is discussed later. Many mammograms are needed for breast cancer, many sigmoidoscopies or colonoscopies

Table 7-1 Ten Leading Causes of Death—United States, 2006*

Rank	Cause	Number
1	Heart disease	598,747
2	Cancer (all types)	520,129
3	Stroke	131,312
4	Chronic lung disease	121,824
5	Alzheimer's disease	72,388
6	Diabetes mellitus	67,295
7	Accidents	57,089
8	Pneumonia and flu	53,676
9	Chronic nephritis	42,123
10	Septicemia	31,594

Data from http://webapp.cdc.gov/sasweb/ncipc/leadcaus.html.

*All races, both genders; age groups: 50 to 85+.

for colon cancer, and many Pap smears for cervical cancer, to follow the conventional wisdom about how to reduce the effects of these cancers.

Such a strategy is only moderately effective. The risks of dying of breast cancer can be reduced by only 15% in the 3% of women who develop it in any decade after age 50 (Fletcher and Elmore, 2003). The risk of dying of colon cancer (incidence from 57 to about 320 for both genders ages 50-80 [Eddy, 1990]) can be reduced by only 16%. The single best strategy for reducing deaths from a cancer is cervical cancer screening; cervical cancer deaths can be reduced for the seven or eight invasive cervical cancers that occur annually per 10,000 population by 30% to 60% (Agency for Healthcare Research and Quality [AHRQ], U.S. Preventive Services Task Force [USPSTF], 2009).

Because these cancers are relatively rare, however, and because the tools are relatively inefficient, a cancer-focused approach to reducing overall mortality tends not to work. In fact, a 2002 review of cancer screening concluded that there is no evidence that cancer screening, as currently conducted, results in reductions of all-cause mortality (Black et al., 2002). Thus, even perfect compliance for all the traditionally recommended cancer programs may dramatically reduce a person's risk of dying of cancer, but it would not add a single day of life to this person's life span. Table 7-2 illustrates the failure of most cancer screening programs, even when they have a significant impact on the target cancer, to alter the ultimate bottom line: all-cause mortality.

Physicians are familiar with measuring the effectiveness of screening in terms of *relative risk* reductions. The most dramatic numbers relating to personal medical efficacy pertain to the interventions proven to work for established coronary artery disease (CAD), called *secondary prevention*. The most impressive numeric successes a good physician can achieve are the 20% to 40% reductions in heart disease events that result when persons with heart disease take statin medications regularly (4S Study, 1994; Heart Protection Study, 2002; Sheperd et al., 1994), or when patients who have had a heart attack use a beta-adrenergic blocker after their heart attack, which reduces the risk of recurrent myocardial infarction by 22% (Yusuf et al., 1988).

Secondary prevention is often preferable to physicians because benefits of *large effect size* can be seen after relatively short periods of intervention (only a few years). Physicians who focus on cancer prevention need to wait for 20 to 40 years to know how well the program worked. For example, Pap smears are recommended from age 21 to age 65 at about 3-year intervals; colon cancer screening is recommended annually from ages 50 to 75; and breast cancer screening typically from ages 40 to 85. The published data on efficacy refer to the entire lifetime of the screening program, so it takes a long time to see the benefit of what physicians do.

A short list of the most important interventions, those with large effect size in secondary prevention, are also summarized in Table 7-2. Physicians preferring the disease treatment model for medicine who want to believe their work is important and measurably effective should select at least one strategy from this table.

The prevention of heart disease, both primary and secondary, should be the first priority for primary care physicians. The critical question is how to do this. Most physicians focus on obvious risk factors, such as smoking, hypercholesterolemia, and diabetes. These same physicians are usually surprised to discover the evidence indicates that physicians who rely on a subjective "gestalt" for risk assessment usually make significant errors (Grover et al., 1994; Volpe et al., 2004). When physicians assess clinical coronary risk based on the major cardiac risk factors, they systematically tend to overtreat modest to severe elevations of a single risk factor, even when the global cardiac risk is quite low. Similarly, if they do only subjective risk factor assessment, physicians fail to offer treatment to many patients at high global cardiac risk merely because they lack any major risk factors or have only a mild abnormality of a few risks. A common example of misdirected treatment is prescribing a statin for a 40-year-old woman with a cholesterol level of 300 mg/dL but no other risk factors; according to the Framingham equation, she has a 10-year risk of a cardiac event of 2%, which is average for her age. To treat patients appropriately, the clinician must use one of the global risk calculators mentioned later.

Why focus on *global* cardiac risk? Leading national and specialty-based expert groups have endorsed this as the most important parameter for addressing cardiac health (Grundy et al., 1999). The Adult Treatment Panel Report (ATP II) of the National Cholesterol Education Program (NCEP), the Joint National Committee of the National High Blood Pressure Education Program, and the American Diabetes Association (ADA) all advocate "adjusting the intensity of risk factor management to the global risk of the patient." The NCEP Expert Panel on Detection, Evaluation, and Treatment of High Blood Cholesterol in Adults (ATP III, 2001) stated specifically, "A basic principle of prevention is that the intensity of risk-reduction therapy should be adjusted to a person's absolute risk. Hence, the first step in selection of LDL-lowering therapy is to assess a person's risk status. . . . In ATP III, a primary aim is to match intensity of LDL-lowering therapy with absolute risk." Hypertension experts John Laragh, Bruce Psaty, and Curt Furberg have directly

Table 7-2 Comparison of Disease-Specific Mortality and All-Cause Mortality Associated with Traditional Cancer and Cardiovascular Prevention Strategies

Intervention	Change in Disease-Specific Mortality*	Change in All-Cause Mortality†
Primary Prevention		
Pap smears	Cervical cancer: 20%-60% reduction after 17 or more Pap smears	0
Fecal occult blood testing (FOBT) Sigmoidoscopy Colonoscopy Digital rectal examination (DRE)	Colorectal cancer: 15% reduction after 20 or more FOBTs plus follow-up colonoscopy in patients with positive results	0
Mammography: 40-50 years Mammography: >50 years	Breast cancer: 16% reduction after 20 mammograms	0
Prostate-specific antigen (PSA) testing DRE	Prostate cancer: 0% reduction after 25 PSA tests	0
DRE, breast self-examination (BSE), physical examination	0% reduction after 40 years	0
Statins (AFCAPS/TexCAPS Study)‡	37% reduction in combined myocardial infarction, unstable angina, and stroke	0
Eight major lifestyle studies (see Tables 7-3 and 7-4): chronic disease and death	35%-83% reductions in coronary events 50%-71% reduction in stroke events 58%-93% reduction in onset of diabetes 36%-68% reduction in cancer deaths	40%-65%
Secondary Prevention		
4S Simvastatin Study§	34% reduction in major coronary events 42% reduction in coronary mortality in patients with heart disease	30%
West of Scotland Coronary Prevention Study (WOSCOPS)‖	Statins reduced coronary events by 31% and cardiovascular specific mortality by 32%.	0
The MRC/BHF Heart Protection Study¶	25% reduction in first-event rate for nonfatal myocardial infarction or coronary death, fatal or nonfatal stroke, and for coronary revascularization with 40-mg simvastatin in high-risk patients over 5 years in 20,536 U.K. adults age 40-80 years	12.9%
Beta blockers after myocardial infarction#	27% reduction of nonfatal infarction in 25 randomized trials (>23,000 patients)	22%

*All data from current U.S. Preventive Services Task Force (USPSTF) appraisal of the evidence and recommendations. http://www.ahrq.gov/clinic/uspstf08/colocancer/colors.htm#rationale; http://www.ahrq.gov/clinic/3rduspstf/cervcan/cervcanrr.htm; http://www.ahrq.gov/clinic/3rduspstf/breastcancer/brcanrr.htm; http://www.ahrq.gov/clinic/uspstf08/prostate/prostaters.htm.
†Black WC, Haggstrom DA, Welch HG. All-cause mortality in randomized trials of cancer screening. J Natl Cancer Inst 2002;94:167-173.
‡Downs JR et al., for AFCAPS/TexCAPS Research Group. Primary prevention of acute coronary events with lovastatin in men and women with average cholesterol levels: results of AFCAPS/TexCAPS. JAMA 1998;279:1615-1622.
§Scandinavian Simvastatin Survival Study Group. Randomised trial of cholesterol lowering in 4444 patients with coronary heart disease: the Scandinavian Simvastatin Survival Study (4S Study). Lancet 1994;344:1383-1389.
‖Shepherd J et al., for West of Scotland Coronary Prevention Study Group. Prevention of coronary heart disease with pravastatin in men with hypercholesterolemia. N Engl J Med 1994.
¶Heart Protection Study Collaborative Group. MRC/BHF Heart Protection Study of cholesterol lowering with simvastatin in 20,536 high-risk individuals: a randomised placebo-controlled trial. Lancet 2002;360:7-22
#Yusuf S, Wittes J, Friedman L. Overview of results of randomized clinical trials in heart disease. I. Treatments following myocardial infarction. JAMA 1988;260:2088-2093.

endorsed explicit global cardiac risk assessment as the new standard of care:

> Most current guidelines focus primarily on the management of individual cardiovascular risk factors, such as high blood pressure, hypercholesterolemia, or diabetes. A more appropriate clinical approach to reducing cardiovascular disease risk would be based on a comprehensive evaluation of risk profile, and accurate stratification of global (absolute) risk in individual patients. . . . The decision to treat a patient should be based on the level of global risk, rather than on the level of a single risk factor. . . . We proposed that global risk should be used as the main determination of whom to treat, how to treat, and how much to treat. . . . We propose to replace the single risk factor–based approach with the assessment of global

cardiovascular risk, both in the clinical management of individual patients and in guidelines. (Volpe et al., 2004)

Once the importance of carrying out some form of global cardiac risk assessment is accepted, a physician need only choose a method and use it consistently. A basic quality-of-care goal process standard would be to use the method of CAD risk assessment systematically for at least 85% of all adult patients over 85% of all years. There are many ways to carry out cardiac risk assessment—from the Framingham tables and equation (United States), by means of the NCEP ATP III risk calculator, to the Sheffield tables and the most recent technique, the QRISK calculator (United Kingdom) (Hippisley-Cox et al., 2008; Wallis et al., 1995). Many of these have been adapted for smart phones and personal digital assistants (PDAs) and are downloadable for free, so few major barriers to implementation exist, primarily time.

A time-efficient method that can be used in the office setting includes a preprinted list of the 10 major cardiac risk factors supported by the current literature. Consider making a list that can be incorporated into the patient's medical record, including the following:

- Age >55 (males); >65 (females)
- Male gender
- Family history of CAD
- Smoking
- Hypertension
- Diabetes
- Sedentary lifestyle
- Metabolic syndrome
- High cholesterol level
- Chronic renal insufficiency

Other considerations include major adverse life event and high perceived stress at work or home.

The purpose of this list is to classify all adults into one of three levels of risk: low, intermediate, or high. Where the dividing lines are drawn between categories is not as important as being *consistent*. In my practice, I consider up to three risk factors to be *low* risk, four to six factors to be *intermediate* risk, and more than six, *high* risk. This information (e.g., CAD Risk Score: "intermediate risk") should go directly into the problem list so that the physician can see it each visit. The intervention itself is relatively inexpensive, requiring only 1 to 2 minutes of physician (or better, medical assistant) time and involving simple laboratory tests—lipid panel and serum creatinine. I define the "metabolic syndrome" as a triglyceride level greater than 150 mg/dL and high-density lipoprotein (HDL) level less than 40 mg/dL for men (or <50 for women), according to the Reaven (2003) criteria. A serum creatinine is obtained to estimate glomerular filtration rate (GFR) and identify the presence of chronic renal insufficiency.

For patients at *low* global cardiac risk, nothing more is required than usual care, which should include conversations about diet, exercise, not smoking, and stress reduction. For persons at either intermediate or high risk, more is required. The physician should systematically apply the best evidence for reducing cardiac risk. This is now a sophisticated and effective set of measures.

For patients at *high* risk, it would be worth having a discussion about the formal "polypill" approach (Wald and Law, 2003). This strategy recommends daily intake of folic acid, a statin, aspirin (81 mg), along with half-doses of three different antihypertensives (hydrochlorothiazide, beta blocker, and ACE inhibitor). The proponents of this strategy claim that the polypill can reduce heart attacks and stroke (third leading cause of mortality) by more than 80% in both primary and secondary prevention. Although no reported randomized, controlled trials (RCTs) have yet proved this for primary prevention, one study showed major benefit in secondary prevention (Hippisley and Coupland, 2005), and more studies are under way.

All physicians should understand that the advances in conservative medical therapy for cardiovascular disease have kept pace and may well have outpaced the advances in the technology of heart disease (e.g., drug-eluted stents) with far fewer complications.

The power of global cardiac risk assessment lies in the synergies achieved with the simple medical interventions to address increased risk. Figure 7-1 illustrates how a single-intervention health promotion program using only "CAD Risk Assessment" and the appropriate conservative responses previously listed achieve multiple synergistic benefits across a large spectrum of diseases and the 10 leading causes of death.

The largest component of the previously described intervention program is basically the promotion of a healthy lifestyle. When applying the best evidence, it is impossible to prevent only heart disease. Appropriate interventions have a significant effect on almost all the 10 leading causes of death. Thus, even a single-minded focus on the prevention of just one disease (heart disease) inevitably leads to a broad focus on lifestyle behavioral changes.

Primary Prevention: A Focus on Lifestyle

Key Points

The five key elements of a healthy lifestyle are:

1. Not smoking.
2. Consuming 5 servings of fruits or vegetables each day.
3. Ten minutes of relaxation, silence, or meditation daily for stress reduction.
4. Maintaining BMI less than 30 kg/m^2 and working to bring it down toward 18.5 kg/m^2.
5. Exercising for at least 150 minutes a week (about 20 minutes daily), equivalent to at least brisk walking.

The five key elements may be simply communicated to patients by the numbers 0-5-10-30-150.

Only about 3% of the U.S. population has a healthy lifestyle as defined by criteria 1, 2, 4, and 5 above.

The potential benefits of a healthy lifestyle are:

- A 40% to 65% reduction in all-cause mortality.
- An 81% to 87% reduction in coronary heart disease events.
- A 67% reduction in all cardiovascular diseases.
- A 50% to 71% reduction in the risk of stroke.
- A 58% to 93% reduction in the risk of developing type 2 diabetes.
- A 36% to 60% reduction in cancer deaths.

A clinical practice may choose a broad, primary prevention approach rather than a single focus on prevention of coronary heart disease. Between 2000 and 2009, nine major

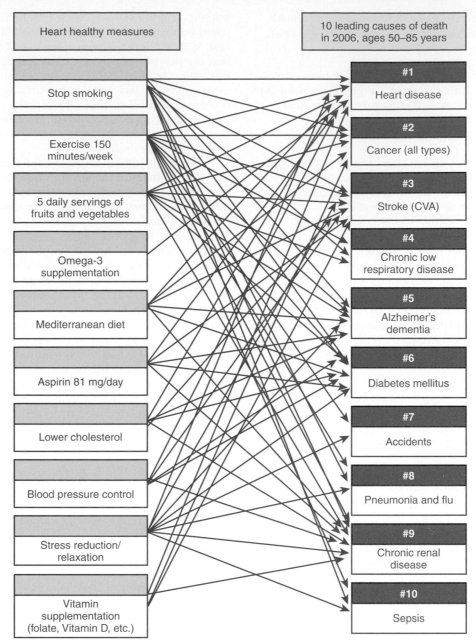

Figure 7-1 A single intervention with a simple, comprehensive medical approach to coronary risk has a significant impact on all 10 of the most common causes of death in the United States. A line is drawn from each of 10 potential cardiac risk interventions on the left side to all the causes of death that each intervention would also tend to reduce.

studies demonstrated that a healthy lifestyle is associated with large reductions in all-cause mortality and major reductions in multiple disease-specific outcomes. These studies succinctly define what should be understood by the term "healthy lifestyle." These primary prevention studies demonstrate that persons who have a number of healthy characteristics at the beginning of a period of observation enjoy remarkable benefits over periods ranging from 4 to 20 years.

The evidence chain begins with the Nurses' Health Study (Hu et al., 2001; Stampfer et al., 2000). In 84,129 participants followed up for 14 years, the effects of several lifestyle factors were analyzed, including not currently smoking, body mass index (BMI) less than 25 kg/m², alcohol consumption

at least 0.5 drinks per day, at least 0.5 hour daily of moderate to vigorous physical activity, and adhering to several dietary elements (increased intake of cereal fiber, marine omega-3 fatty acids, and folate; increased polyunsaturated/saturated fat ratio; and low *trans* fat intake and glycemic load). The group defined as "low risk" had all these characteristics. After 14 years, this low-risk group (3% of original study population) had an 83% reduction in coronary disease events. Another analysis of the same cohort showed that women at low risk also had a 91% reduction in the risk of developing diabetes.

In 2002 the Diabetes Prevention Program Research Group published the results of the only RCT among these lifestyle studies. This study focused solely on the outcome of type 2 diabetes among 3324 nondiabetic patients. The "standard" healthy lifestyle intervention consisted of written information provided at the beginning of the study and an annual 20- to 30- minute individual counseling session. The defined "standard" lifestyle goals included instructions to adhere to the U.S. Department of Agriculture (USDA) Food Guide Pyramid and the equivalent of an NCEP Step 1 diet; to reduce weight; and to increase physical activity. Subjects were randomized to standard lifestyle intervention plus metformin (875 mg twice daily), to standard lifestyle intervention plus placebo, or to "intensive" lifestyle intervention alone. The latter group was encouraged to achieve and maintain a weight reduction of at least 7% of initial body weight through a healthy low-calorie, low-fat diet and to engage in physical activity of moderate intensity, such as brisk walking, for at least 150 minutes per week. Subjects in this group also received a 16-lesson curriculum, taught by case managers on a one-to-one basis during the first 24 weeks after enrollment, with brief follow-up sessions monthly. After an average follow-up of only 2.8 years, the intensive lifestyle intervention was associated with a reduced incidence of diabetes (58% vs. 31% reduction with metformin, both compared to placebo). The intensive lifestyle intervention was significantly more effective than the standard lifestyle intervention plus metformin.

In the Healthy Aging: A Longitudinal Study in Europe (HALE Project), in 2539 participants age 70 to 95 at baseline, investigators found a 65% reduction in all-cause mortality and 67% to 77% reductions in disease-specific risks for coronary heart disease, any cardiovascular disease, and cancer in the group with four healthy lifestyle factors (never smoking, Mediterranean diet, 3-4 hours/week of moderate physical activity, and glass of wine or more daily) compared with the group with none of these healthy characteristics (Knoops et al., 2004).

The Women's Health Study analyzed smoking, alcohol use, exercise, BMI, and diet among 37,636 participants age 45 or older. After a mean of 10 years follow-up, there were risk reductions of 55% for total stroke and 71% for ischemic stroke; the risk-adjusted hazard ratio for participants who scored higher on an index of lifestyle factors than those who scored lower was 0.45 for total stroke and 0.29 for ischemic stroke (Kurth et al., 2006).

In the Health Professionals Follow-up Study, 42,847 men age 40 to 75 were followed over 16 years using similar healthy lifestyle criteria. "Low risk" was defined as the absence of smoking, BMI less than 25 kg/m^2, moderate to vigorous activity of at least 30 minutes a day, moderate alcohol consumption (5-30 g/day), and the top 40% of the distribution for healthy diet score. Compared with men with no healthy lifestyle factors, those with all five factors had an 87% reduction in the risk of developing coronary heart disease (Chiuve et al., 2006).

In the Atherosclerosis Risk in Communities Study (ARIC), the effects of four healthy lifestyle factors ($\geq$5 servings of fruits and vegetables per day, $\geq$2.5 hours of exercise per week, BMI of 18.5-30 kg/m^2, not smoking) were analyzed in 15,708 participants followed for only 4 years. Among subjects who had no healthy characteristics at baseline, those who changed their behavior and adopted a healthy lifestyle (all four habits) experienced a lower risk (40% reduction) of all-cause mortality and a 35% reduction in

cardiovascular disease (King et al., 2007). This study is particularly important because it indicates clearly that those with a relatively unhealthy lifestyle who change in midlife can still achieve dramatic reductions in health risks and longer life expectancy.

The European Prospective Investigation into Cancer and Nutrition (EPIC)–Norfolk study demonstrated significant reductions in all-cause mortality with increasing numbers of health factors in 20,244 participants followed for a mean of 11 years. The four factors analyzed were current nonsmoking status, engaging in regular physical activity, moderate alcohol use, and plasma vitamin C level greater than 0.88 ng/dL, as a surrogate for fruit and vegetable consumption. Individuals with all four factors had an advantage of approximately 14 years in chronologic age over those with only one of the four factors (Khaw et al., 2008).

Further follow-up analysis of the 43,685 individuals in the Health Professionals Follow-up Study and the 71,243 participants in the Nurses' Health Study showed that a healthy lifestyle was associated over time with a 69% reduction in the risk of developing an incident stroke among men and a 79% reduction of stroke risk among women (Chiuve et al., 2008).

The most recent major study in this line of evidence that changes in lifestyle behavior lead to remarkable changes in health outcomes is the "Healthy Living Is the Best Revenge" report. Ford and colleagues (2009) used data from 23,153 German participants age 35 to 65 from the European Prospective Investigation into Cancer and Nutrition (EPIC)–Potsdam study. They analyzed end points of type 2 diabetes mellitus, myocardial infarction, stroke, and cancer and the effect of four healthy lifestyle factors: never smoking, BMI less than 30 kg/m^2, 3.5 hours/week of physical activity or more, and adhering to healthy dietary principles (high intake of fruits, vegetables, and whole-grain bread; low meat consumption). Fewer than 4% of participants had zero healthy factors; most had one to three healthy factors, and 9% of the group had all four factors. During a follow-up of 7.8 years, after adjusting for age, gender, educational status, and occupational status, the hazard ratio for developing a chronic disease decreased progressively as the number of healthy factors increased. Participants with all four factors at baseline (vs. those with none) had a 78% lower risk of developing a chronic disease. The risk of developing diabetes was reduced by 93%, the risk of myocardial infarction by 81%, risk of stroke by 50%, and risk of cancer by 36%.

The results of these studies are summarized in Tables 7-3 and 7-4. Despite minor variations, there is now substantial consensus on what constitutes a "healthy lifestyle." Briefly stated, a healthy lifestyle consists of the following:

1. Not smoking
2. Five (5) servings of fruits and vegetables a day
3. Body mass index (BMI) less than 30 kg/m^2
4. About 150 minutes of exercise a week (~20 min/day)

Consider a fifth lifestyle factor: *stress reduction* or *relaxation.* The previous studies did not include this variable in their design most likely because of the difficulty in measuring effects. Nevertheless, substantial literature on this subject suggests (but does not prove) significant beneficial effects on blood pressure, smoking, alcohol abuse, cholesterol, psychosocial stress, atherosclerosis (measured by carotid artery

Table 7-3 Summary Data for the Eight Major Prospective Lifestyle Studies

Study	N	Ages	Follow-up (years)	Smoking	BMI (kg/m²)	Exercise (min/wk)	Diet	Other
Nurses' Health Study (2000)	84,129	30-55 in 1976	14	Not currently	<25	210	Top 40%*	Alcohol: ½ drink/day
Lifestyle or Metformin for Prevention of Diabetes (2002)	3234†	>25	2.8	Not specified	>24	150	NCEP Step 1 diet	—
Healthy Aging: A Longitudinal Study in Europe (HALE Project) (2004)	2339	70-95	10	Never, or quit >15 years	--—	200‡	Mediterranean Diet Score = 8§	Alcohol: >0 glass/day
Women's Health Study (2006)	37,636	>45	10	Never	<22, 22-24.9 25-29.9 30-34.9 > 35	Never/rare <1 time/wk 2-3 x/wk > 4 x/wk	Composite ‖	Alcohol: <1, 1-3, 4-10.5, >10.5
Health Professionals Follow-up (2006)	42,847	40-75 in 1986	16	Not currently	<25	210	Top 40% diet score¶	Alcohol: 5-30 g
Atherosclerosis Risk Factors in Communities (ARIC) (2007)	15,708	45-64	6	Not currently	18.5-30	>150	5 servings of fruits and vegetables daily	Alcohol: 1-14 units/wk
EPIC-Norfolk (2008)	20,244	45-79	11	Not currently	--—	210	Vitamin C level >50 mmol/L#	Alcohol: 1-14 units
EPIC-Potsdam (2009)	23,153	35-65	7.8	Never	<30	210	Composite**	—

*Diet criterion: highest 40% of the cohort for consumption of a diet high in cereal fiber, marine *n-3* fatty acids, and saturated fat, and low in *trans* fat and glycemic load.
†Subjects were selected based on criteria of age >25, BMI >24, and either fasting blood glucose or post–75-g glucose load; 2-hour postprandial glucose elevated but not diagnostic for diabetes.
‡Individuals with a score in the intermediate and the highest tertile on the Voorrips or Morris questionnaire were considered the low-risk group for physical activity.
§For the Mediterranean Diet Score, the subject must have had above-average consumption of the six positive variables: (1) polyunsaturated/saturated fatty acid ratio, (2) fruits, (3) vegetables, (4) legumes, (5) fish, and (6) grains. They also must have had below-average consumption of the two adverse factors: (7) red meat and (8) dairy products.
‖Considered six dietary factors: cereal fiber, folate, polyunsaturated/saturated fat ratio, omea-3 fatty acids, *trans* fats, and glycemic load, grouped into deciles and scored as 0 to 9.
¶Calculated a summary dietary score based on the Alternate Healthy Eating Index (AHEI).
#As a proxy for 5 servings of fruits and vegetables per day.
**A healthy diet was considered to consist of high intake of fruits and vegetables, whole-grain bread, and low consumption of meat.
NCEP, National Cholesterol Education Program; *EPIC,* European Prospective Investigation into Cancer and Nutrition.

intima-media thickness), angina, left ventricular hypertrophy, and overall mortality. A review of controlled trials using Transcendental Meditation (TM) techniques (many of which also compared TM to progressive muscle relaxation and other stress reduction techniques) found the following (Walton et al., 2004):

- Significant blood pressure reductions (11 mm Hg systolic and 6 mm Hg for diastolic) among elderly blacks (Alexander et al., 1996a; Schneider et al., 1995).
- A 13% reduction in cigarette use and smaller but significant reductions in drug and alcohol use (Alexander et al., 1994).
- Significant reductions in cholesterol after 11 months (Cooper and Aygen, 1979).
- A 30% reduction in psychosocial stress (Eppley et al., 1989).
- Implied reductions in atherosclerosis in patients with two or more risk factors for coronary heart disease of 33% after 1 year (Alexander et al., 1994, 1996a; Fields et al., 2002).

- Reduction in the likelihood of heart attack or stroke of 11% among elderly blacks (Alexander et al., 1994, 1996a).
- Greater exercise tolerance, maximal workload, delayed onset of ST-segment depression after 8 months (Zamarra et al., 1996).
- A highly significant reduction in all-cause mortality (Alexander et al., 1989, 1996b).

These studies are generally older, small in size, and of relatively poor methodologic quality (University of Alberta, 2007). However, these findings are supported by the INTER-HEART study, which identifies psychosocial stress as one of the nine leading risk factors for MI (Rosengren et al., 2004; Yusuf et al., 2004).

A relaxation or stress reduction variable is added to the basic lifestyle formula for two main reasons: (1) the mounting support from clinical research and (2) the epidemiologically well-established correlation of stress to overall morbidity and mortality (Figueredo, 2009). Also, a compelling commonsense belief among the general public holds that stress is bad for health and can be reduced by various behaviors.

Table 7-4 Outcomes of the Eight Major Prospective Lifestyle Studies

Study	Healthy Lifestyle at Baseline*	Major Findings
Nurses' Health Study (2000)	3%	83% reduction in coronary heart disease (CHD) events; follow-up study showed a 91% reduction in the risk of type 2 diabetes.
Lifestyle or Metformin for Prevention of Diabetes (2002)	—	58% reduction in diabetes compared to placebo; vs. 31% reduction with metformin and "standard" lifestyle intervention.
Healthy Aging: A Longitudinal Study in Europe (HALE Project) (2004)	—	65% reduction in all-cause mortality (all 4 points); 77% reduction in CHD; 67% reduction in all cardiovascular diseases; and 68% reduction in all cancers. The lack of any healthy lifestyle characteristics was associated with a population-attributable risk of 60% of all deaths, 64% of deaths from CHD, 61% from all cardiovascular diseases, and 60% from cancer.
Women's Health Study (2006)	4.7%	55% reduction of total stroke, 71% reduction ischemic stroke, and 27% increase in hemorrhagic stroke.
Health Professionals' Follow-up Study (2006)	—	87% reduction in men for CHD; 62% of coronary events might have been prevented with the five healthy lifestyle factors; in men taking medication for hypertension or hypercholesterolemia, 57% of all coronary events may have been prevented with a low-risk lifestyle. Compared with men who did not make lifestyle changes during follow-up, those who adopted two or more additional low-risk lifestyle factors had a 27% lower risk of CHD.
Atherosclerosis Risk Factors in Communities (ARIC) (2007)	8.5%	During 4 years of follow-up, total mortality and cardiovascular disease events were lower for new adopters (2.5% vs. 4.2%) and 11.7% vs. 16.5% compared to individuals who did not adopt a healthy lifestyle. New adopters had 40% lower all-cause mortality and 35% fewer cardiovascular events.
EPIC-Norfolk (2008)	—	Adjusted relative risks for all-cause mortality for men and women who had 3, 2, 1, and 0 risk factors compared to 4 healthy behaviors were 1.39, 1.95, 2.52, and 4.04, respectively. All 4 behaviors = 14 more years of life.
EPIC-Potsdam (2009)	9%	Subjects with all 4 factors at baseline had a 78% lower risk of developing a chronic disease: diabetes, 93% reduction; myocardial infarction, 81% reduction; stroke, 50% reduction; and cancer, 36% reduction.

*Prior data on the prevalence of healthy lifestyle characteristics among U.S. adults demonstrated that only 3% had all four healthy lifestyle factors: not smoking, 5 servings of fruits and vegetables a day, 150 minutes of exercise a week, and body mass index (BMI) of 18.5 to 25 kg/m². (Reeves MJ, Rafferty AP. Healthy lifestyle characteristics among adults in the United States, 2000. Arch Intern Med 2005;165:854-857.)

Currently, the data do not precisely define the minimum time needed in meditation or relaxation to achieve health benefits; many studies use 15 to 20 minutes daily (Lane et al., 2007). A reasonable conjecture of the "minimal effective dose," which follows the work of Depak Chopra (1993), is 10 minutes a day. Chopra believes that nothing more than 10 minutes of silence is required. Progressive increases in time will enhance the benefits, but a place to start is needed, as with the BMI criterion.

Thus, the revised list of essential components for a healthy lifestyle is as follows:

1. Not smoking
2. Five (5) servings of fruits and vegetables daily
3. Ten (10) minutes of relaxation or meditation exercise daily
4. BMI less than 30 kg/m²
5. Exercise for at least 150 minutes per week

This can be conveniently expressed by the simple numeric mnemonic 0-5-10-30-150, as follows:

0	Cigarettes a day
5	Servings of fruits and vegetables a day
10	Minutes of relaxation or meditation daily
30	BMI less than 30
150	Minutes of exercise a week

This is a concise notation for a prescription of 0 cigarettes a day, 5 servings of fruits and vegetables every day, 10 minutes of relaxation or meditation daily, a BMI less than 30, and 150 minutes of exercise each week. For a behavioral lifestyle intervention to be practical and acceptable to most physicians, it should be brief, easily memorable, and simple to communicate to patients.

The nine studies clearly indicate that certain lifestyle characteristics are associated with important reductions in both chronic disease and death. Also, only 3% to 9% of typical populations meet the varying requirements of a healthy lifestyle; the relevant number for the U.S. population from the national Behavioral Risk Factor Surveillance System is 3% (BRFSS, 2002). There is a huge population of people who do not have a healthy lifestyle and whom physicians can help by facilitating their transition to a healthier lifestyle.

Of the studies previously described, in many ways the ARIC Study and the Prospective Diabetes Group trial are arguably the most important. These studies show directly that subjects who previously had a suboptimal lifestyle up into middle age can experience proportional benefits in health outcomes by making changes in their behavior at that time. These studies do not, however, tell us that physicians can persuade patients to make corresponding changes in their behaviors.

After the Evidence: Motivational Interviewing

Key Points

The most promising technique of active listening to help patients change behavior is motivational interviewing.

The three essential tools of motivational interviewing are:

- A menu
- An importance "ruler"
- A confidence "ruler"

Resistance is to be expected and provides the physician with the best opportunity to assist patients to work on what they need to do for *themselves*.

The previous studies are adequate to meet information objectives, but this alone is insufficient. To help patients make changes in their lives—and each of these lifestyle habits represents major behavior change—it is necessary to help them discover their own motivations to make changes and to help build confidence in their ability to undertake the task. Providing information is a physician behavior that is usually well supported in traditional medical education and training. The pitfall, however, is that most primary care physicians were trained to use this information as the basis for giving *advice* to patients. Experience confirms that simply giving advice usually is ineffective, and to the contrary, the usually unwelcome advice often heightens resistance to new behaviors.

Physicians cannot provide the motivation for patients to undertake lifestyle change, so it is necessary to ask patients what they want to do. What are their reasons for continuing a lifestyle habit that they usually know is associated with some adverse effects on their health? All patients have such reasons, or the behavior would simply go away.

Unhealthy lifestyles are perpetuated when internally the "pros" in favor of a given behavior have reached a stalemate with the "cons," and a search for new behavior stops. The role of physicians is to help patients break the stalemate by creating opportunities for patients to reflect on their own behavior and values. A physician demonstrates respect for patients' autonomy and their right to make decisions for themselves when, after an examination of the pros and cons,

the physician accepts wherever patients are with change in their life and allows them to guide the clinician to the areas where they are most motivated to change. The greatest problem is that family physicians were never trained to do this; it does not just happen.

The way to make it happen is by listening. This is true regardless of which evidence physicians believe and what attitudes patients have. "Long before there was any scientific basis for health care, there were healers who had learned to listen carefully" (Rollnick et al., 2008, p. 65).

The most promising new technique of "active listening" for health care practitioners is *motivational interviewing* (MI). It is beyond the scope of this chapter to provide detailed instructions in the related skills, which must be experienced and practiced over at least a few months. This section discusses the underlying principles and simple ways to start implementing these skills in medical practice. The development of skills requires sufficient understanding of the basic theory of MI to try the related clinical style with patients. Patients will then provide enough direct and immediate feedback to help physicians quickly refine their skills. The relevant basics of theory and practice are readily accessible (Rollnick et al., 1999, 2008; see also Web Resources).

The clinical method of MI was first described in 1983 as an approach to problem drinking (Stockwell and Gregson, 1986). MI is a "skillful clinical style for eliciting from patients their own good motivations for making behavior changes in the interest of their health" (Rollnick et al., 2008, p. 6). MI is a collaborative partnership between patients and their physicians based on the assumption that motivation for behavioral change is "malleable" and is formed particularly in the context of relationships. In addition, MI requires of physicians a "certain detachment from outcomes—not an absence of caring, but rather an acceptance that people can and do make choices about the course of their lives" (Rollnick et al., 2008, p. 7).

Rollnick identifies four core guiding principles of MI, using the mnemonic RULE, as follows:

Resist the "righting reflex" (i.e., "Don't try to fix it, and don't give advice").

Understand the patient's motivations.

Listen; use empathic, active listening throughout the clinical interview.

Empower the patient.

The physician needs to support patients' beliefs that change is possible and will make a profound difference in their life.

The key change in physician behavior required is a transition from asking multiple, "get to the point," close-ended questions, often mistakenly assumed to be efficient, to a style that employs fewer and predominantly open-ended questions. This allows patients the time to tell their stories. The benefit for patients is the feeling of being heard. For physicians, the benefit can be greater patient satisfaction; patients often feel they had more time with the physician and received more attention, whether or not the visits are actually longer. The challenge is to allow the patient to be in control.

Another good example of a systematic approach to MI in the clinical setting is the Kaiser TPMG educational program. The Brief Negotiation Roadmap offers a practical six-step sequence for physicians in practice: (1) open the encounter; (2) negotiate the agenda; (3) assess readiness; (4) explore ambivalence; (5) tailor the transition; and (6) close the encounter. The Kaiser example offers a good illustration of the use of the three basic tools of MI: a "menu" for the agenda, a motivational "ruler," and a confidence "ruler."

The Process in Your Clinical Practice

The encounter for lifestyle change opens with the establishment of rapport and trust with your patient. You are assisting the patient to be in control of the encounter and trying to establish a partnership for what needs to be done, which only the patient can decide. Your role is to assess the patient's level of healthy lifestyle activity, educational needs, emotional state, and readiness to embark on change, and to reflect these back to the patient as they become clear.

A good way to open the discussion is to present a list of options (a "menu") that you and the patient might work on together for the encounter. Ask if this is acceptable. You can identify a patient's readiness for behavioral change simply by asking the patient about the positive aspects of the patient's current behavior and then listening. Follow this up with a similar question, What are the negative aspects of this behavior? To assess the current state of the tension between the positive and negative aspects, using a motivational "ruler," ask the patient how *important* it is to change the current behavior, on a scale of 1 to 10. If the patient rates the importance of change as only a 2 out of 10, you can ask, "Why isn't it a zero or a one?" If it is a 6, you can ask, "What would it take to make it a seven?" The goal of this interaction is simply to understand the patient's readiness for behavioral change and to facilitate the patient's recognition of his or her own ambivalence.

The uncovering of ambivalence is a useful step forward, not a failure on the physician's part. Ambivalence must exist, or the behavior would have changed already. Ambivalence is the reason for the encounter. The physician must try to understand what creates the tension that results in ambivalence. Ambivalence can be addressed; a clear "no" cannot. If the patient turns out not to be ready for change, the patient is probably right. Only the patient fully understands all the competing values in his or her life. Acknowledge that directly, asking such questions as, "Where does that leave you now?" or "What are you thinking/feeling at this point?"

If the patient is ready for change, you want to find out how much and how fast. Let the patient be in charge. A good question is, "How can I help?" If the patient does not have a specific task for you right now, you can always just offer information from a clinical perspective. Ask if this is acceptable. Try to reach mutual clarity about what to expect. "How confident are you that you can cut your smoking in half this week?" On a confidence scale (1-10), physicians are seeking a level of 7 out of 10, to indicate that the patient is really confident about making a change. If the answer is less than 7, you can gently suggest considering a lower goal. For example, "Well, if you only feel a confidence of 5 about cutting your smoking in half, how confident would you feel about reducing your smoking by two cigarettes a day this week?"

When you have a firm degree of confidence (≥7) about a mutually agreed goal, you are ready to close the encounter. Affirm the effort the patient is making to enhance the quality of his or her health. Affirm that you will be there for the patient at each turn on this path to lifestyle change.

Basic Steps toward Self-Motivation

1. Elicit agreement with the patient that it is acceptable to talk about behavior change for any issue.
2. Ask what the patient sees as positive aspects of his or her current behavior, then ask about the negative aspects.
3. Use the motivational RULE to assess how important it is now for the patient to make a change in the target behavior."
4. Ask how confident the patient is about making a change.
5. Resolve ambivalence. Revise the degree of anticipated change in the target behavior until the patient's confidence level is 7 or higher. If this is not possible, explicitly acknowledge that this may not be a good time to undertake change in this area.
6. Close the encounter with encouragement toward the patient's stated goal or an offer to be of assistance whenever the patient is ready.

Crux of the Lifestyle Dilemma: Do Physicians Believe in Primary Prevention?

Key Points

- Good, even great, evidence is not enough to lead to substantial lifestyle changes among patients.
- Traditional medical training has not prepared the majority of practice physicians in the science (evidence) of primary prevention or in the tools necessary to make it happen, such as motivational interviewing.
- Although many physicians say they believe in primary prevention, their behavior often belies this. Belief in the power and effectiveness of primary intervention strategies among primary care physicians cannot be assumed and must be explored individually with each physician.
- Physicians need to go through a series of steps, much as any patient who desires to change a behavior, to become proficient at primary prevention.
- The predicted results will reward the efforts for physicians who can take a day-by-day, long-term perspective on health.

Why not primary prevention now? Whether this means systematically performing CAD risk assessments on all adult patients, or whether the physician wants the broadest possible impact on multiple major chronic diseases through primary prevention, the rate-limiting step is the same: motivation. As with patients, too few physicians actively engage in either strategy. What would be required for lifestyle work to become a critical part of every patient encounter? Motivational interviewing theory suggests that the behavior is not important to physicians, or they lack skill in this technique.

The data cited have now been long available. Physicians do not lack an evidence base to justify such a behavior change; they lack the will. They should examine this phenomenon as a perfect problem to approach with MI skills.

The problem is usually couched in terms of patient compliance and patient resistance as the source of failure to adopt a healthy lifestyle. This may be true in part, but the physician also plays a role. The principles of MI, applied to patients, suggest that physicians need to understand patients' perspective better and, whatever their resistance, why they do want to take care of themselves (Rollinik et al., 2008; Ruback et al., 2005). One can never positively influence the behavior of another person without continuous, positive, empathic, nonjudgmental support.

Another barrier in providing primary prevention is that no one has directly observed a primary prevention "miracle." Although so important to the religious conversion experience, miracles just don't happen in primary prevention. Prevention of poor outcomes is not an observable event.

In usual practice, physicians derive the most satisfaction by testing or treating and seeing a prompt result. The relatively simple "instant gratification" of this approach is addictive. Give sublingual nifedipine, and the patient's blood pressure decreases; give insulin, and the sugar level is reduced. Tap on a reflex, and the tendon jumps; order a CT scan, and unseen abnormalities become apparent. Primary prevention offers no such satisfaction, even though it may be a favorite subject of interest, with a gratifying sense of sharing a deep belief.

Motivating physicians to move toward a primary prevention lifestyle and practice (these must go together) is similar to moving a smoker toward smoking cessation. All patients who are smokers should receive at every physician visit a straightforward, simple, clear, nonjudgmental message that giving up smoking is the single most important thing they could do for their health. This message should be accompanied by a simple question, "Would you like to talk about it?" Although average results from simple, brief counseling are 2.8% quit rates (Lancaster and Stead, 2004), because of the large patient populations, this rate is actually quite important. Physicians must be willing to accept intermediate behavioral outcomes in this range: 3% to 5% increases in smoking cessation (Butler et al., 1999), exercise (Hillsdon et al., 2007; Lawlor and Hanratty, 2001; Ogilvie et al., 2007; Peterson, 2007; Sherman et al., 2007), eating 5 servings of fruits and vegetables (Steptoe et al., 2003), other healthy nutrition practices (Hunt et al., 1995), reducing problem drinking (Fleming, 2005; Ockene et al., 1999), accident prevention (Miller and Galbraith, 1995), and general healthy lifestyle advice (Christian et al., 2008; Steptoe et al., 2001).

Each physician should reflect on the following questions:

1. "Do I believe that primary prevention can really work, and that it can substantially outperform other strategies to promote health?" As noted, belief is required. Exposure to high-quality primary prevention information can help, especially with urging from a colleague or mentor. We cannot assume that physicians believe; we have to ask. Belief is a journey, and the physician must explore personal history and professional socialization, first asking, "On a scale of 1 to 10, how great is my belief that primary prevention is the right thing to do and the key to the best results in medicine?"
2. "If I do believe in primary prevention, do I think it is *important*?" The physician must be convinced that this is a worthwhile focus. The physician's belief in the relative importance of preventive interventions is influenced by example, information, patient satisfaction, and organizational support. If primary prevention is *not* important, it does not deserve to be practiced. If the physician thinks it is even somewhat important, however, primary prevention warrants further consideration.
3. "If I believe in primary prevention, and I believe it is of paramount importance, am I convinced that I can do it?" Confidence is also relative and susceptible to both information and example. The physician needs to ask,

"On a scale of 1 to 10, how confident am I that I can integrate the behaviors necessary for primary prevention into my life and work flow?"

The evidentiary basis, practice, and strategies of motivational interviewing are new enough that many physicians are not even familiar with the term. Many of these physicians, however, intuitively respond to the process and may think,— "I've done that; I just didn't know what it was called." Usually, however, MI is only targeted at patients with high-risk medical conditions. As a strategy, it has succeeded dramatically for certain patients, but MI has not penetrated far into the U.S. health care environment since it was introduced to a wide audience in 1992. MI simply is not a formal part of most practices, mainly because the power of the intervention has been aimed at the wrong strata of system participants.

Insufficient data and insight surround the major question, "How do we nurture physicians in their career development to have firsthand knowledge of the power to change and evolve personally?" If the United States is to become a healthier country, current health care reform policies should address this question directly. Primary prevention can then become a natural, integral part of the health care process, an act as simple as breathing.

Summary

The answers to the four questions posed at the beginning of this chapter should now be fairly clear.

What is a healthy lifestyle?

A healthy lifestyle consists of five essential elements:

1. Not smoking (0 cigarettes)
2. Five (5) servings of fruits and vegetables daily
3. 10 minutes of relaxation, silence, or meditation daily for stress reduction
4. BMI less than 30 kg/m^2
5. 150 minutes of exercise over the course of each week.

This list may be communicated succinctly to patients by the simple numeric mnemonic 0-5-10-30-150.

What is the prevalence of a healthy lifestyle among patients?

For the general U.S. population, the prevalence of a healthy lifestyle defined by the four criteria above is 3%. This means that a large number of patients could benefit by being encouraged to adopt a healthy lifestyle.

What are the potential benefits for patients who have or who change to a healthy lifestyle?

The potential benefits of a healthy lifestyle are:

1. A 40% to 65% reduction in all-cause mortality.
2. An 81% to 87% reduction in coronary heart disease events.
3. A 67% reduction in all cardiovascular diseases.
4. A 50% to 71% reduction in stroke.
5. A 58% to 93% reduction in the risk of developing type 2 diabetes.
6. A 36% to 60% reduction in cancer deaths.

What is the major obstacle to lifestyle changes in a family physician's office?

The major obstacle to the behavioral changes required to live a healthy lifestyle is a lack of physician training and skills in motivational interviewing. This is the major challenge to the training of physicians for the 21st century. The effectiveness of improved training and greater organizational support in health care systems for healthy physician lifestyles, as well as enhanced listening and MI skills, should be a major focus of the primary care research agenda for the future.

EVIDENCE-BASED SUMMARY

- Individual global cardiac risk assessment performed regularly and followed by appropriate graded interventions is the most effective strategy for preventing heart disease (SOR: C).
- Living a healthy lifestyle or changing to one is potentially more effective than focused cardiac risk reduction, because it not only reduces adverse cardiac events and death to a similar degree, but also is associated with major reductions in chronic diseases (diabetes, stroke, all cardiovascular disease, and even cancer) as well as large proportional reductions in all-cause mortality (SOR: B).
- A healthy lifestyle consists of the following:
  Not smoking (SOR: A)
  5 servings of fruits or vegetables each day (SOR: B)
  10 minutes of relaxation, silence, or meditation each day (SOR: C)
  Maintaining a BMI less than 30 kg/m^2 (SOR: B)
- The most promising new technique of active listening to assist patients in making behavioral changes is motivational interviewing (SOR: C).

References

The complete reference list is available online at www.expertconsult.com.

Web Resources

http://webapp.cdc.gov/sasweb/ncipc/leadcaus.html
  Centers for Disease Control and Prevention (CDC) Wisqars database of U.S. deaths by cause, gender, age, ethnicity, and region.

U.S. Preventive Services Task Force (USPSTF, AHRQ) *reports on breast, cervical, colon, and prostate cancer:*

www.ahrq.gov/clinic/3rduspstf/breastcancer/brcanrr.htm

www.ahrq.gov/clinic/3rduspstf/cervcan/cervcanrr.htm

www.ahrq.gov/clinic/uspstf08/colocancer/colors.htm#rationale

www.ahrq.gov/clinic/uspstf08/prostate/prostaters.htm

Web-based cardiac global risk calculators:

http://hp2010.nhlbihin.net/atpiii/calculator.asp?usertype=prof
  Interactive Framingham Cardiac Risk Calculator.

www.qrisk.org United Kingdom Q-Risk Calculator.

www.health.gov/paguidelines/Report/Default.aspx
  U.S. Activity Guidelines for Adults (2008).

www.kphealtheducation.org/bnroadmap/index.html
  Brief Negotiation Roadmap: Behavioral Tools for Practitioners, Kaiser Health Foundation. A log-in (free) is required, but access is open to the public. This site includes interactive demonstrations, videos, and various tools for behavior change; a good place to start in learning the techniques of motivational interviewing.

www.signup4.net/Public/ap.aspx?EID=DONT10E
  A list of courses in motivational interviewing offered by Kaiser Regional Health Education; regularly updated.

www.motivationalinterview.org/
  Motivational interviewing resources for clinicians, researchers, and trainers.

www.Kopes-eticHealth.com
  The author's personal website featuring collected work on primary prevention, cardiac risk reduction, and other topics.

http://community.icontact.com/p/kopes-etichealth/newsletters/kopes-etichealth
  Archive of all the author's electronic newsletters for primary care physicians: *FP Revolution*. This electronic newsletter is published free twice monthly. You may sign up at www.Kopes-eticHealth.com.

8 CHAPTER

Interpreting the Medical Literature: Applying Evidence-Based Medicine in Practice

Jeff Susman, Bernard Ewigman, Keith B. Holten, and Douglas R. Smucker

Chapter contents

Key Points

- Interpreting the medical literature is a task any physician can do, particularly when using common, evidence-based summaries that are available at low or no cost.

- The studies should report statistically significant results that are applicable to the physician's population of patients and that should evaluate important patient-oriented outcomes, including potential harms.

- When potentially changing practice behavior, the physician should assess whether the evidence is from high-quality studies replicated over time.

- The medical literature is an evolving body of evidence, and each physician should develop a personal plan to keep up with important changes in medicine and strategies to answer more immediately important clinical questions at the point of care.

- Using summary measures, such as the number needed to treat or harm and attributable risk, can make decisions about patient care more collaborative and transparent

Building Clinical Evidence from Published Research

Evidence-based medicine (EBM)—asking clear, relevant clinical questions, finding appropriate studies, critically appraising the literature, and implementing changes in practice behavior—has become an essential part of medical care. Most busy physicians do not have the time or the background to answer critically the questions that arise in practice. Primary care physicians identify 2.4 clinical questions for every 10 encounters (Barrie and Ward, 1997), but they spend less than 15 minutes on average with each patient. Evidence about common primary care problems is accumulating at an overwhelming pace, and the broad scope of family medicine presents important challenges. Other barriers to the use of EBM include lack of evidence that is pertinent to an individual patient, quick access to information at the point of care, and potentially negative impacts on the art of medicine (McAllister et al., 1999). How can diligent physicians narrow the gap between their current behaviors and best practices?

In this chapter, hormone replacement therapy (HRT) for postmenopausal women is used as a case example to understand the evolution of medical practice and the changing landscape of evidence and to review concepts important to interpreting the medical literature. These concepts form the basis for practical EBM tools that family physicians can use to answer important clinical questions.

In Chapter 10, information from the Women's Health Initiative (WHI) about HRT is considered, and similar epidemiologic and statistical issues are covered. Chapter 10 emphasizes the importance of how risk data are framed or presented to the patient and the primacy of patient preference (i.e., ability to make informed decisions about therapy). Unfortunately, evidence concerning the ideal manner of presenting information to patients and clinicians and promoting informed decision-making is still scant. This chapter and Chapter 10 take a slightly different approach to similar clinical questions, and together, these two chapters provide the background for the motivated family physician

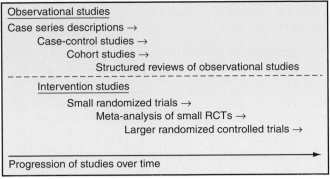

| Observational studies |
| Case series descriptions → |
| Case-control studies → |
| Cohort studies → |
| Structured reviews of observational studies |
| - |
| Intervention studies |
| Small randomized trials → |
| Meta-analysis of small RCTs → |
| Larger randomized controlled trials → |
| Progression of studies over time |

Figure 8-1 Common progression of research in building the strength of evidence; *RCTs*, randomized, controlled trials.

to better understand concepts of risk and probability and to foster enhanced physician-patient decision-making.

Evidence for interventions such as HRT usually begins with observational studies, including unblinded case series, case-control studies, and cohort studies, and it culminates in randomized, controlled trials (RCTs) (Figure 8-1). To better understand how we arrived at the current clinical understanding of HRT and its effects on heart disease, we review the progression of research studies and evidence over the past 30 years. A series of observational studies in the 1970s and 1980s led to regular prescribing of HRT to prevent a number of significant health conditions in postmenopausal women.

Case-Control Studies

Case-control studies are often the first step in a progression of building clinical evidence because they are relatively inexpensive and rapid studies to complete. Case-control studies always look backward in time (i.e., retrospective studies) to determine a statistical association between an *exposure* and an *outcome*. To complete a case-control study of the association of HRT and coronary heart disease (CHD), a researcher would identify a group of *cases* (i.e., women with CHD) and a group of *controls* (i.e., women without CHD) and look back in time to determine how many women in each group had taken HRT. The association between exposure (i.e., HRT) and outcome (i.e., CHD) in a case-control study is typically summarized by a statistical measure called an *odds ratio*. An odds ratio is an estimation of the true relative risk for the outcome in question. A common form of bias in a case-control study is *recall bias:* errors in accurately determining whether cases and controls had exposure to HRT in the past.

Cohort Studies

Cohort studies are often the next step in building the strength of evidence regarding an association between an exposure and an outcome. Cohort studies typically look forward in time (i.e., prospective studies) and are generally more expensive and take longer to complete than case-control studies. However, they provide a more accurate estimate of the relative risk for women who take HRT and those who do not. A cohort study is also an *observational study*—one that observes outcomes in groups but does not assign participants to a particular exposure or treatment. In a cohort study of HRT and CHD, a researcher would identify a group of women taking HRT and a similar group of women who

have chosen not to take HRT, and the researcher would then follow them over time and count the number of CHD events. Because outcome events may be uncommon in each group and may take many months to occur, cohort studies often require large numbers of participants and long follow-up periods to show significant differences between groups.

The primary statistical measure from a cohort study is *relative risk*. This is a ratio of the rate of CHD events among women who choose to take HRT divided by the rate among women who choose not to take HRT. A common form of bias in cohort studies related to prevention is the *healthy user bias*, when participants who choose one preventive measure (e.g., HRT) also tend to make healthier lifestyle decisions (e.g., diet, exercise) that may also prevent the measured outcome (i.e., CHD).

Beginning with case-control studies and then using larger cohort studies, observational research showed that HRT might reduce the incidence of CHD, fractures, and colorectal cancer. These observational studies also suggested that the same therapy might cause harm, with a slightly increased risk of breast cancer, stroke, and venous thromboembolism. On balance, however, even a small positive impact of HRT on preventing CHD was thought to far outweigh the potential adverse effects of HRT.

Structured Reviews and Meta-Analysis

After a number of studies are completed, whether cohort studies or initial small RCTs, these are often reviewed and summarized in publications called *structured reviews*. Occasionally, data from a series of studies are combined using a statistical technique called *meta-analysis*, which allows increased statistical power to determine the weight of evidence from a series of studies. The use of HRT was greatly increased during the 1990s based on a number of case-control and cohort studies and on three meta-analysis studies that further suggested that HRT was protective against CHD (Pettiti, 1998).

In 1991, an editorial in the *New England Journal of Medicine* concluded that "a consensus of epidemiologic reports has demonstrated that women who are given postmenopausal estrogen therapy have a reduction of about 40% to 50% in the risk of ischemic heart disease as compared with women who do not receive such therapy" (Goldman and Tosteson, 1991). HRT became a de facto standard for postmenopausal women through the 1990s.

The Power of Randomized, Controlled Trials

In RCTs, study participants are randomly allocated to two or more groups and then assigned to receive an intervention such as HRT or to receive no active treatment (i.e., placebo or to continue with their usual care). RCTs greatly add to the confidence of measured results because the structure of an RCT helps to eliminate many of the inherent biases that are in observational studies. For example, in cohort studies of HRT and CHD, it is hypothesized that women who choose to take HRT are generally healthier and have better healthy lifestyle practices than women who do not choose to take HRT. Because participants in an RCT are randomly assigned to treatment and control groups, they are less likely to have differences in other factors that might prevent or promote heart disease.

Table 8-1 Understanding Study Results

Typical summary rates from randomized, controlled trials:

$$\text{Incidence rate} = \frac{\text{Number of new cases of disease over a defined period}}{\text{Number of persons at risk during the period}}$$

$$\text{Relative risk (RR)} = \frac{\text{Incidence rate among the treated group}}{\text{Incidence rate among the placebo group}}$$

Summary measures that may be more meaningful for clinicians:

Attributable risk (AR), or risk difference =
  (Incidence rate among treated group) −
  (Incidence rate among placebo group)

Number needed to treat (NNT) or number needed to harm (NNH) =
    Reciprocal of AR, or 1 / AR

Table 8-2 Examples of Summary Rates from the Women's Health Initiative (WHI) Study

The following equations show how to take a summary rate commonly reported in published studies (i.e., relative risk) and calculate a summary measure (e.g., number needed to treat, number needed to harm) that may be more useful in describing the results to clinicians and patients. The example considers the average annual incidence rates and relative risk for coronary heart disease (CHD) events in the WHI study on the effects of hormone replacement therapy (HRT):

Average annual incidence among HRT − treated women
= 37 CHD events / year / 10,000 women

Average annual incidence among placebo − treated women
= 30 CHD events / year / 10,000 women

$$\text{Relative Risk of CHD} = \frac{37 \text{ CHD events / 10,000 women}}{30 \text{ CHD events / 10,000 women}} = 1.29 \text{ (adjusted)}$$

The relative risk describes a relative 29% increase in CHD events. It may be more useful to consider the absolute difference in incidence rates between the two groups to understand the magnitude of the potential risk for a given patient:

$$\text{Attributable risk (AR)} = \frac{37 \text{ CHD events}}{10,000 \text{ women}} - \frac{30 \text{ CHD events}}{10,000 \text{ women}}$$

$$= \frac{7 \text{ additional}}{10,000 \text{ women}} \text{CHD events}$$

The number needed to harm (NNH) can be calculated to describe, on average, how many women must be treated for 1 year to cause one additional CHD event attributable to HRT:

$$\text{NNH} = \frac{1}{7 \text{ CHD events / 1000 women}} = \frac{10,000}{7} = 1430$$

Data from Ebell MH, Messimer SR, Barry HC. Putting computer-based evidence in the hands of clinicians. JAMA 1999;28:1171-1172.

The decreased likelihood of a healthy user bias in an RCT may explain why HRT appeared to be protective in cohort studies but later proved to be harmful. Because RCTs have this inherent ability to remove many important potential forms of bias (but are not immune to biases themselves), a physician can have more confidence that they reflect the true association between the HRT treatment and CHD outcomes. Despite decades of work, dozens of observational studies, and structured reviews that strongly suggested a protective effect of HRT for CHD, a single, large RCT trumped them all and caused a sudden reversal in physicians' prescribing behavior.

The results of the WHI study, released in 2002, sent a shock wave through the medical community. For the first time, a large, randomized trial showed that HRT—given to otherwise fairly healthy postmenopausal women—caused a statistically significant increase in CHD events. Within days of the release of the WHI primary results, many women called their physicians to decide whether they should continue with HRT. Many physicians drastically changed their prescription of HRT based on the WHI; within 9 months, prescriptions of the most popular formulation of HRT decreased by as much as 61% (Majumdar et al., 2004). Perhaps more than any other single study in modern medical history, the WHI report dramatically changed a widespread, common medical practice.

Understanding the Statistical Significance of Study Results

Reports from RCTs such as the WHI study frequently include relative risk as a summary measure of differences between the treatment and placebo groups (Table 8-1). To arrive at the relative risk, the researcher first measures the incidence rate of an outcome in each of the two study groups (i.e., treatment and placebo). The incidence rate for each group is a ratio of the number of new outcome events, such as CHD events, divided by the number of patients at risk for the outcome in that group over a specific period. In multiyear studies, the average annual incidence rate is often reported as a summary measure. In a placebo-controlled RCT, the relative risk is then calculated as a ratio of the incidence rate for the treatment group divided by the incidence rate for the placebo group (Table 8-2).

How can a physician determine whether the reported relative risk from a study is significant enough to influence clinical decisions? Typically, the statistical significance of the summary measure is reported, which in this case is relative risk. Statistical significance is usually summarized in published studies by a p value for a given summary measure. The p value describes the statistical probability that the observed difference between the groups could have happened simply by chance alone. A p value of less than 0.05 is the arbitrary cutoff most often used for "statistical significance." A "$p < 0.05$" means that there is less than a 1 in 20 (5%) probability that a difference as large as that observed would have occurred by chance alone; a $p = 0.04$ means a 1 in 25 (4%) probability; a $p = 0.06$ means a 1 in 16 probability (6%).

Although frequently used, p values provide only limited information: the chance that any difference found is caused by chance, or random error. A p value alone gives no indication of the clinical significance of a finding and provides no information regarding the likelihood that a finding of "no difference" is caused by chance, or random error.

Confidence intervals are much more informative than p values. When relative risk is reported as the summary result of a study, the 95% confidence interval (CI) is often used to give an indication of the precision of the estimated relative risk. The 95% CI describes the range within which there is a 95% probability that the true relative risk (RR) is in that range. An RR of 1.0 indicates no difference. For example, if a study reported an RR of 2.5 with a 95% CI of 2.3 to 2.7, we could be reasonably certain (95% certain) that the true RR was no less than 2.3 and no greater than 2.7. Our conclusion would be that the estimated RR of 2.5 is fairly precise. However, if RR was reported as 2.5 with a 95% CI of 1.1 to 5.0, the true RR could be as low as 1.1 (almost no difference) or as high as 5.0 (a fivefold difference), an obviously imprecise estimate of the relative risk.

Confidence intervals also provide a better measure than *p* values of the precision for concluding that there is no difference in a relative risk. Any 95% CI that includes RR = 1.0 indicates that there may be "no difference." However, a RR of 1.1 with a 95% CI of 0.99 to 1.11 is almost certainly a finding of no difference (i.e., a narrow confidence interval), whereas an estimated RR = 1.4 with a 95% CI interval of 0.99 to 1.7 is much less precise (i.e., a wide confidence interval). Even though the 95% CI contains 1.0, there may still be a true difference, just not detected in this study.

Interpreting Study Results: Statistical and Clinical Significance

Although the WHI showed a statistically significant increase in the relative risk of CHD events among women who were randomly assigned to take HRT, it is important to consider the absolute difference in CHD events between the two groups to understand the strength of the association and to discuss the risk of HRT treatment with individual patients. Calculating *absolute risk* (in addition to relative risk) is a helpful way to understand the level of risk that HRT may add for a group of women who are at risk for CHD events (see Table 8-2).

In the WHI study, the relative risk of CHD for participants who took HRT was 1.29, with a 95% confidence interval that did not cross 1.0 (95% CI, 1.02 to 1.63). This figure (RR = 1.29) can generally be interpreted as HRT being associated with a 29% increase in CHD events. This summary measure was reported widely in medical journals and the mainstream press.

When reported in terms of relative risk, the weight of the association between HRT and CHD sounds ominous (i.e., a 29% increase). However, in terms of absolute risk attributable to HRT treatment, a less portentous picture emerges (see Table 8-2). In the WHI study, women taking HRT had an average rate of CHD events of 0.37% per year, an average of 37 events per 10,000 women each year, and those in the placebo group had an annual rate of 0.30%, or 30 events per 10,000 women each year. Although the adjusted RR of CHD is 1.29 (0.37 divided by 0.30), the *attributable risk* or risk difference between the two groups is 0.07% (0.37 minus 0.30). In other words, approximately seven additional cases of CHD occurred for 10,000 women using HRT during each year over the course of the study. The attributable risk of the treatment group can be summarized as the *number needed to harm* (NNH) or, if a study reports a beneficial effect, the *number needed to treat* (NNT). In this case the NNH was approximately 1430; on average, for every 1430 patients treated with HRT, one additional CHD event occurred (i.e., the inverse of the risk difference, 0.07, or 10,000 divided by 7) (see Table 8-2). The NNH or NNT is often a more understandable and

useful summary of study outcomes when physicians and patients weigh the risks and benefits of a particular therapy.

Other Keys to Interpreting Clinical Evidence

Pearls

- Use a personal digital assistant (PDA) or computer online, with bookmarks for helpful EBM sources, to apply evidence at the point of care.
- Although full access to the Cochrane Database can be expensive, helpful summaries are available for free.
- Attend an information mastery or EBM workshop to solidify your grasp of basic concepts and application of this information to daily practice.
- Becoming a reviewer of Clinical Inquiries, HelpDesk Answers, or PURLs can consolidate your skills in EBM.
- Make it a habit to spend 10 minutes each day reviewing important systematic reviews or evidence-based summaries of relevance to your practice.

One of the major tasks in interpreting whether the results of a study should change practice is to determine whether all relevant patient-oriented outcomes were considered. It is important to distinguish among physiologic outcomes (e.g., serum calcium), intermediate outcomes (e.g., bone density), and patient-oriented outcomes (e.g., fractures). Whenever possible, practice decisions should be based on outcomes patients would deem important. For example, in a trial of HRT for osteoporosis, a decrease in fracture incidence would be a more convincing outcome than a change in a physiologic parameter such as bone density. Likewise, all important harms (i.e., risks) and financial end points (i.e., costs and savings) should be reported. In a trial of a new antiresorptive agent, the rate of esophagitis, gastritis, and esophageal perforation may be important harms to elaborate, along with such measures as patient satisfaction, costs and savings of care, and global well-being.

When assessing the benefits and harms of such a new treatment, appropriate competing alternatives (including no treatment at all) should be compared. Typically, such a comparison may take the form of a "balance sheet," a table comparing each intervention in terms of benefits, harms, and economic end points. Many studies are randomized, placebo-controlled trials in which patients receive an active intervention or a placebo or sham intervention. Alternatively, a study may use an *active comparator*, an intervention already known to be effective. Each of these approaches has pros and cons, but the most important point to remember is that just because a study shows statistical significance in a single measure, it does not mean that appropriate patient-oriented outcomes were considered.

When a study shows no effect, the question of *power* is raised. Put in simple terms, power is the ability to detect the effect of an intervention; it depends on the number of patients in the study, the magnitude of effect of the intervention, and the variability of the effect from one subject to another. For some interventions, even a small effect may be important. For example, many nonpharmacologic treatments for hypertension (e.g., salt restriction) have relatively modest, but important effects. Clinicians should generally be skeptical of small studies that show negative results.

Examining the confidence intervals is the easiest way to assess whether the study sample was too small and therefore did not have the statistical power to detect a clinically important difference (as reflected by wide confidence intervals).

Even when a study is positive or shows statistically significant results, it is important to consider whether the findings are clinically significant and applicable to your practice. For example, if a study showed a drug reduces the risk of heart attack by one in a million patients, we would probably be skeptical about its utility. Likewise, the findings showing that daily borscht reduces fractures in a study done in Russian dockworkers may or may not be applicable in the United States. The acceptability of an intervention (e.g., electroconvulsive therapy for depression) may vary. Moreover, the ability to replicate the findings of a study done in a typical research setting is often reduced in real-world practice. An intervention for osteoporosis requiring daily injections may be demonstrated to be efficacious, but in the average practice setting, its effectiveness may be much more limited.

Clinicians frequently rely on the synthesis of many studies, rather than a single study, to change our practices. Such reviews can be *systematic,* in which rigorous attempts are made to uncover all studies, published and unpublished, in English and in other relevant languages, or they may be more limited reviews that consider only a portion of the published literature. Some use formal mathematical methods to combine the results of studies (i.e., meta-analysis), and others are *qualitative* and synthesize data according to an author's overall judgment. Common biases to consider related to published reviews include whether all sources of evidence were considered; how disparate results were combined; whether relevant patient-oriented outcomes were assessed; if there was adequate attention to the quality of the studies and their generalizability; and whether the authors analyzed why differences in outcomes may have occurred, based on such factors as study design, population, and intervention. Published reviews, including systematic reviews and clinical guidelines, have become increasingly important tools for the busy clinician.

Clinicians may hone critical appraisal skills through involvement with local journal clubs, working with the Family Physicians' Inquiries Network (www.fpin.org). Although it is important to understand basic concepts for interpreting medical literature, sifting through original research studies can be a tedious, impractical process for busy clinicians. Many practical EBM tools have emerged in recent years to help physicians quickly access comprehensive, expert reviews of published studies in the middle of a busy practice (Table 8-3). The ability to critique articles using a structured approach is facilitated by using widely available worksheets and tools (see Web Resources). Although many taxonomies exist for level of evidence, two of the most widely available are the Centre for Evidence-Based Medicine (CEBM) and the taxonomy used in this book. The Strength of Recommendation Taxonomy is specifically tailored to family medicine (Ebell et al., 2004).

Using Evidence at the Point of Care

Physicians have many sources of clinical information, from throwaway or non–peer-reviewed journals to evidence-based, searchable databases. Each of these has advantages, disadvantages, and different methods of access (Table 8-4).

Table 8-3 Distinguishing Characteristics of Evidence-Based Medicine

Characteristic	Description
Explicit methods	Databases are searched and search strategies described.
Focus on patient-oriented outcomes	Concentrates on clinical research that reports patient-oriented outcomes.
Systematic searches	The searches are systematic and thorough so that important evidence is not missed.
Standardized critical appraisal	Important sources of potential systematic and random error are assessed in each study.
Hierarchy of study design	More weight is given to stronger study designs.
Designation of levels of evidence	Each study is designated with respect to the strength of the study design and its quality of evidence.
Grading of accumulated recommendations	Each recommendation is graded according to the strength of the evidence from research studies that support the recommendation.
Verifiable findings	The explicitness of the methods of searching and critical appraisal allows others to verify or refute findings and recommendations.

One model to help busy physicians stay clinically current, called *information mastery,* has been advocated by Slawson and Shaughnessy (1999), Ebell and colleagues (1999), and Geyman (1999). In this model, physicians seek the answer to clinical questions through secondary sources of information that have been created by experts through a review of the medical literature. Secondary sources include the following (Table 8-5):

- Evidence-based summaries, such as Cochrane Collaboration reviews, Patient-Oriented Evidence that Matters (POEMs), Clinical Inquiries, and Priority Updates from the Research Literature (PURLs), as published in the *Journal of Family Practice.*
- Systematic reviews, including PubMed and Clinical Inquiries.
- Guidelines, written by professional societies and accessed through sites such as the National Guideline Clearinghouse (www.ngc.gov).
- Evidence-based databases, such as Essential Evidence Plus, DynaMed, and PEPID PCP.

The following example describes the type of relevant information that a busy clinician can access using two of these EBM resources.

Case Example

A 55-year-old woman sees you because she is experiencing severe vasomotor symptoms (i.e., hot flashes). These symptoms are keeping her awake at night. She had a total

Table 8-4 Examples of Reference Materials on Hormone Replacement Therapy for the Busy Physician

Type of Literature	Advantages	Disadvantages	Availability	Examples
Textbooks	Comprehensive review of topics	Long period from concept to printing; book/CD space requirements; cost; reading time	Print: hardcover and paperback	Berek Novak's *Gynecology* ($150)
Unsolicited medical journals	No cost	Some not peer reviewed; unpredictable topics; large volume of materials; may have industry sponsorship	Print; some articles online	*Female Patient* (complimentary)
Subscription peer-reviewed journals	Peer reviewed; pertinent	Cost and subscription management; stacks of journals; need to appraise critically	Print and online	*Obstetrics and Gynecology* ($368 annually for non-ACOG member)
Evidence-based searches	Peer reviewed; pertinent topics	Cost; CD management; summaries have learning curve	CD-ROM and online	Cochrane Reviews: abstracts (complimentary) and full reviews (subscription)
Searchable evidence databases	Searchable; rapid; focused search possible; point of care access	Learning curve for searches	PDA and online	Essential Evidence Plus ($79)

CD, Compact disk; *ACOG*, American College of Obstetricians and Gynecologists; *PDA*, personal digital assistant.

abdominal hysterectomy and oophorectomy 1 year ago because of uterine fibroids. She is concerned about the dangers of HRT. What is the current evidence to support HRT for this patient? How should you counsel this patient?

A PubMed search (http://www.ncbi.nlm.nih.gov/entrez/query/static/clinical.html) was performed using the "clinical queries" home page. Using the field *therapy* as the clinical study category and emphasis—*broad, sensitive search* were chosen. The search terms were *hormone replacement therapy* and *vasomotor symptoms*. An excellent, evidence-based summary from *Women's Health* (Pinkerton et al., 2009) reviews the use of estrogen and other hormonal replacement therapies, various antidepressants, clonidine, gabapentin, and dietary and herbal supplements. The search and review of this article took approximately 3 minutes.

Another PubMed reference found by doing a search (http://www.ncbi.nlm.nih.gov/sites/entrez) using the keywords *hormone replacement therapy* and the limit, *Meta-Analysis*, uncovered a recent Cochrane review. "Long-term hormone therapy for perimenopausal and postmenopausal women" summarizes the literature and discusses current recommendations on the use of HRT (Farquhar et al., 2009). This summary considered 19 trials of almost 42,000 women and concludes that in relatively healthy women, combined continuous hormone therapy (HT) significantly increased the risk of venous thromboembolism or coronary event (after 1 year's use), stroke (after 3 years), breast cancer, and gallbladder disease. Long-term estrogen-only HT significantly increased the risk of venous thromboembolism (after 1-2 years), stroke (3 years), and gallbladder disease (7 years) but did not significantly increase the risk of breast cancer. Furthermore, the authors conclude that "we need more evidence on the safety of HT for menopausal symptom control, though short-term use appears to be relatively safe for healthy

younger women." This evidence took another 3 minutes to review.

A search using the online version of UpToDate using the keywords *hormone replacement therapy* quickly led to a review, "Postmenopausal hormone therapy: benefits and risks." A detailed description of evidence and cross-links with specific topics was found, including patient education handouts. A link to a summary of treatment of women with menopausal symptoms (www.uptodate.com/online/content/topic.do?topicKey=r_endo_f/9609) concludes:

> *Most postmenopausal women, with the exception of women with breast cancer or known cardiovascular disease, who have symptoms of vaginal atrophy and/or vasomotor instability are good candidates for estrogen therapy (for the shortest duration possible depending upon symptoms). The recommendations outlined below are consistent with those of the North American Menopause Society.*

Likewise, using the Essential Evidence Plus search engine online uncovers 141 references when using the keywords *hormone replacement therapy*, including guidelines, evidence summaries, POEMs, and a patient education handout. A similar search at the FPIN website was also quite valuable. The decision of which platform and database to use is largely personal. Some of the distinctive characteristics of each resource are outlined in Table 8-5.

This case outlines how a physician with access to searchable databases can quickly review a wide array of clinical evidence and published guidelines. Such resources are based on systematic evaluations of evidence and can provide clinicians with practical guidance at the point of care. EBM, information mastery, and the application of knowledge at

Table 8-5 Examples of Evidence Sources

Information Source Access	Description	Cost
PubMed http://www.ncbi.nlm.nih.gov/pubmed/	Service of National Library of Medicine; 19 million citations back to the 1950s; includes links to many sites with full-text articles.	No charge
National Guideline Clearinghouse www.ngc.gov	Collection of guidelines, regularly updated; sponsored by Agency for Healthcare Research and Quality (AHRQ), U.S. Department of Health and Human Services.	No charge
U.S. Preventive Services Task Force (USPSTF) www.ahrq.gov/clinic/prevenix.htm	Federal prevention guidelines; public health focus; AHRQ is lead agency for project.	No charge
Bandolier www.medicine.ox.ac.uk/bandolier	British site; PubMed and Cochrane Library searched monthly for published systematic reviews and meta-analyses; excellent glossary, "What is series," covers common terms and acronyms.	No charge
Canadian Task Force on Preventive Health Care www.ctfphc.org	Canadian site; practical guide for health care providers, planners, and consumers for preventive health interventions.	No charge
Essential Evidence Plus www.essentialevidenceplus.com	Database of filtered, synopsized, evidence-based information; quarterly updates; searches a full spectrum of evidence-based resources, including POEMs and Cochrane abstracts, 325 diagnostic calculators and support tools, and summaries of evidence-based practice guidelines; POEMs are evidence-based summaries of single articles, not complete bodies of evidence; EBM presentation tools.	30 days free; $79/year
Cochrane Database www.cochrane.org/reviews/index.htm	An international, nonprofit, independent organization that produces and disseminates systematic reviews of health care interventions and promotes the search for evidence in the form of clinical trials and other studies of interventions.	$310/year; abstracts free; often available from institutions
TRIP (Turning Research into Practice) www.tripdatabase.com	British site; central search engine for high-quality medical literature from wide range of sources: evidence-based records, clinical guidelines, clinical questions and answers, electronic textbooks, and medical images; more than 13 million peer-reviewed journal articles	Free searches
ACP Journal Club www.acponline.org/journals/acpjc/jcmenu/htm	Tied to subscription to *Annals of Internal Medicine*; regular structured reviews of important articles and informed commentary; focused on internal medicine; sponsored by American College of Physicians.	$520/year
Family Physicians Inquiries Network (FPIN) www.fpin.org	Virtual learning community with growing point of care that answers clinical questions on basis of evidence-based content tools using structured, critical reviews of the literature; evidence graded and explicit; number of participants available (Clinical Inquiries and HelpDesk Answers); comprehensive point-of-care content (see PEPID below and PURLS); system identifies all new practice recommendations from newly emerging research findings.	Graduated trial available for handheld or online searching
DynaMed www.ebscohost.com/dynamed/	Point-of-care reference tool organized around over 3000 clinical topics; systematically reviews over 500 medical journals and provides useful summaries of the literature, in an increasingly evidence-based manner.	$395 for individual; discounts, trainee pricing available
UpToDate www.uptodate.com	Online, computer, and point of care accessible; comprehensive; qualitative reviews with many explicit descriptions of evidence, but recommendations not tied to a specific strength of recommendation taxonomy; expert opinion often mixed with more evidence-based recommendations.	$495; $195 for trainees
Physicians Electronic Portable Information Database (PEPID) PCP www.pepidonline.com	Online and handheld point of care accessible; integrated and hyperlinked; 2700 clinical topics, 6000-drug database, 1000 calculators and decision aids, all linked in a single application; includes all USPSTF recommendations; evidence based guidelines, all Clinical Inquiries, HelpDesk Answers, and Priority Updates from the Research Literature (PURLs) from FPIN.	$209.95

the point of care remain works in progress. By developing a basic understanding of these resources and tools, physicians' care for patients can be more effective, safe, and efficient.

Evidence Levels

A: Randomized, controlled trials (RCTs); meta-analyses; well-designed, systematic reviews
B: Case-control or cohort studies, retrospective studies, certain uncontrolled studies
C: Consensus statements, expert guidelines, usual practice, opinion

A glossary of EBM terms is provided in eAppendix 8-1 online at www.expertconsult.com.

Pitfalls

- Do not assume that statistical significance is the same as clinical significance.
- Do not rely on pharmaceutical representatives or experts who may be biased in their presentation of information.
- Consider the potential harms and economic effects of an intervention.
- Do not assume that results even from a well-done study are applicable to your population of patients.
- Do not fail to use the many comprehensive sources of evidence-based information.

References

The complete reference list is available online at www.expertconsult.com.

Web Resources

See also Table 8-5
fur2www.fpin.org
    Family Physicians' Inquiries Network.
www.ngc.gov
    National Guideline Clearinghouse.
www.mclibrary.duke.edu/subject/ebm?tab=appraising
www.cche.net/usersguides/main.asp
    Useful resources for critiquing articles using a structured approach.

www.cebm.net/index.aspx?o=1025
    Centre for Evidence-Based Medicine (CEBM) taxonomy for levels of evidence.
www.jfponline.com/Pages.asp?AID=1635
    The Strength of Recommendation Taxonomy, specifically tailored to family medicine.

9 CHAPTER

Using Health Information Technology for Optimal Patient Care and Service

Bruce Bagley and Steven Waldren

Chapter contents

Key Points

- Information technology must support the core office functions for finances, personnel, and clinical quality.
- Information management is essential for quality patient care and efficient practice operations.
- Well-organized clinical information at the point of care means better decisions for patients.
- Registries are required for a population approach to complete and timely care.
- Information technology must help the team with care management and care coordination tasks.
- Computers can enhance patient and care team relationships through communication, education, and self-management support.
- Quality measures and reporting capability must be embedded in the EHR.
- Decision support tools ensure patient safety and timely, evidence-based care.

We live in a world that is so rich with information that managing, filtering, and organizing the data has become our most important challenge as we strive to use information technology (IT) to help us deliver reliable, high-quality care to our patients.

In the past the goal for family physicians was to have the *electronic health record* (EHR) selected, implemented, and working efficiently. Unfortunately, many EHR systems focused primarily on recording the office visit and support for billing and coding decisions. Over time, systems evolved to provide better support for office workflow, electronic prescribing, and clinical information management. Real-time interoperability and widespread health data exchange

remain challenges for clinical practice and for the U.S. health care system.

Information technology and the installation of hardware and software in the practice should not be a goal in and of itself. Computers must be configured and connected to support the key management functions of the medical office for finances, personnel, and clinical quality. For this reason, we organize this chapter by considering each of the core functionalities required for efficient medical office functioning. We describe how health information technology should be used to greatest advantage and address the need for integration, connectivity, and data exchange.

Components of Patient Care

Care of the Individual

Individual patient care will continue to be at the heart of what we do as family physicians. Documenting, organizing and transmitting the record of patient care over time must be well done, efficient, and communicated clearly to others. Electronic health records should help physicians document an accurate and complete account of the patient's care, including history, physical findings, laboratory tests, imaging results, advice from other specialists, medications, preventive measures, and screening efforts. A problem and medication list helps to present this information in a tabular form for easy reference and summarizes most of the important information that should accompany the patient wherever he or she receives care. The personal health record should capture the majority of this information so that all providers have access, as needed.

Most EHR systems rely on templates to enter information in discrete, searchable fields. There is always tension between the need for providing sufficient detail (granular data) and the burden of entering too much detail without additional benefit to patients or physicians. At times, free text may be necessary to communicate precisely what is happening, such as a complex symptom history. Other information, such as routine physical findings, treatment plans, medications, and tests are more useful if entered in a tabular format (granular data) so that they can be identified and used to generate orders, check for allergies or interactions, feed decision support tools, and generate documents for transmission to others.

Personal health records for individuals are critical to ensure that important information about the patients' medical problems, current treatments, usual sources of care, and medications go with them whenever they need evaluation or treatment. Electronic health records should be able to interact with the personal health record to keep it accurate and up-to-date. In essence, the personal health record is a "snapshot" of the EHR at a point in time. It should be updated whenever there are any changes. The Continuity of Care Record (CCR) standard provides a format for the collection and transmission of this important data.

Care of a Population

In addition to caring for individuals, the office care team has the responsibility to monitor and manage their ability to care for the population they serve. This may apply to a particular condition (e.g., diabetes) or preventive services (e.g., immunizations, recommended screenings). Although the care each individual receives is important, the aggregate of the care that all patients with a particular condition receive is a better indication of the effectiveness of the overall approach to care.

Registries are used to track and organize information about all patients with a particular condition. For example, a registry for diabetes would include all patients in the practice who have been identified as diabetic. It should provide the office team with information about the patient's most recent visit (e.g., glycosylated hemoglobin and lipid levels, blood pressure results), eye exam date, and patient self-management goals. Many registries provide information for proactive contact with patients whose clinical parameters are missing or out of range. Registries provide the opportunity for patient care and contact between visits, in addition to highlighting needed services during the visit.

Ideally, EHRs should be able to integrate the registry function into the workflow and draw data from appropriate sources automatically. If this function is not integrated into the EHR, stand-alone and web-based products are available to help manage a population of patients.

Care Management Support

Patients often find themselves caught in a fragmented and disconnected health care system. Electronic systems can help track referrals to other specialists, laboratory test results, or imaging results to ensure that the recommended care has been accomplished. When patients are referred to other providers or to the hospital, they should be accompanied by the necessary clinical information so that the best decisions can be made, resulting in timely and efficient diagnostic testing or treatment.

Electronic health records should be able to produce a summary of important clinical information that is readable, transportable, and computable; the CCR standard provides a mechanism to do all three. The format allows data to be read by any browser software or to be converted to the readable formats of most EHRs.

Pharmacies now have the capability to capture and transmit data about prescription fills and renewal authorizations. If these data are made available to the physician, he or she can be on the alert for patients who have discontinued medications for a variety of reasons. Pharmacy benefits managers (PBMs) have data on formularies, drug prices, patient responsibility (co-payments), and coverage rules for each health plan contract. This information can be transferred to the EHR to aid in decision support for the physician as the prescription is generated.

Managing Patient Relationships

Electronic health records can store information about individual patient preferences, including primary language, end-of-life wishes, cultural beliefs or rituals, usual caregivers, nicknames, and extended family connections.

Secure e-mail can provide easy and efficient access to health care services and information for many patients. A *patient portal* allows patients to view sections of their EHR, request prescriptions or appointments, and report the results of home monitoring. Patient portals are also used to help direct patients to preferred Internet-based resources for education and support.

Patient self-management support shifts some of the responsibility for chronic illness care or lifestyle modification directly to the patient. Electronic systems can aid by sending automated reminders, education, and encouragement to patients between visits. Systems can track progress toward patient-oriented goals and report back to the office care team.

Social networking is now part of everyday life for a sizable portion of the U.S. population. Innovative uses of social networking can provide regular communication with patients, allowing for the development of support groups and enhancing interactions with patients between face-to-face visits. Just as the EHR must integrate into the physician workflow, the patient support strategies must integrate into their daily routines and tools.

Monitoring and Improving Quality and Performance

Measurement of clinical care has become increasingly important for documenting and improving the level of evidence-based care we provide. Performance measures should be built into the process of care to serve as reminders and permit the efficient capture of quality data for reporting. The National Quality Forum now endorses clinical performance measures for many of the common conditions that family physicians treat.

Comparative effectiveness research (CER) is used to determine if different treatments or procedures used in the care of the same condition have significantly different patient outcomes. If research shows that one treatment is clearly more efficacious than another, all physicians should be promoting that treatment for most patients. EHRs help researchers collect data at the point of care and provide a platform for public health surveillance.

Measurement is the key to any quality improvement effort, whether streamlining patient flow or improving health outcomes for diabetic patients. As a general rule, measures for clinical care require data that the physician would want to have available to make the best diagnostic and treatment recommendations for the patient. This information can be organized on a flow sheet or template in the EHR for the dual purpose of ease of access by the care team and ease of data collection for quality measures. *Quality measures* can be used for both internal quality improvement and external reporting. An increasing portion of physician compensation will be attached to performance measures over time, so the degree to which these measures can be integrated into the system of care will determine the quality of patient care and the level of practice revenue.

Decision Support

Family physicians must acknowledge that they cannot remember everything about every patient. Decision support tools integrated into the office workflow help determine the correct diagnosis, help avoid patient harm from medication interactions or allergies, and provide ready access to the latest treatment guidelines. Electronic prescription writers can be configured to help with dosing decisions related to age, weight, renal function, and concurrent medications. These tools can also provide information about cost, formulary compliance, and availability of generic substitutions.

Office Business and Management Functions

Key Points

- In addition to scheduling and billing functions, information technology must facilitate intraoffice communications and workflow.
- Automating repetitive tasks saves time, improves efficiency, and enhances other patient care.
- Systems should record and analyze a broad set of demographics to enhance the care of diverse populations.
- Electronic monitoring of information allows data-driven decision making about staffing and resource allocation.

Well-developed information systems have long been available for practice management functions such as billing, collections, scheduling, and general accounting. These functions can now be supplemented with information from the clinical record to improve quality, efficiency, and reliability. Intraoffice communication through e-mail and workflow support will help automate routine or repetitive tasks and eliminate wasted time looking for team members. Having all the necessary information enhances payment levels and reduces claim denials.

With patient populations becoming more diverse, family physicians need to expand the demographics they track. In addition to name, address, and payer information, physicians must now record data on primary language, family relationships, cultural preferences, and even genetic information that might affect treatment decisions or medication selection.

Computer systems should also provide the information needed to manage productivity and personnel. Family physicians should make decisions about staffing levels or adding clinicians based on reliable data. Calculations of patient panel size by clinician, productivity per full-time equivalent (FTE) provider, and supply/demand for appointments will support good business decisions.

Integrating and Connecting Systems and Functions

Key Points

- Information technology systems must be configured to integrate all the core office functions seamlessly.
- Easy access to the Internet and decision support tools enhances patient care.
- Interoperability or the efficient transfer of data among disparate computer systems is essential to achieve the full potential of health information technology.
- Continuing professional development and medical education must be integrated into patient care.

Workflow Management

In a typical day, the family physician's work involves face-to-face visits, outside inquiries from patients, ordering or checking of laboratory results, consultations with colleagues, prescription refills, and interactions with office staff. Managing all these tasks in an efficient manner allows the physician to spend more time with patients and still maintain a personal life.

Information technology can help organize and cue the work for easy access and disposition. Ideally, the system will have a "workflow screen" that shows all pending tasks in a well-organized way. The physician can then quickly choose to answer a message or check off lab reports while moving from one examination room to the next. Efficient intraoffice e-mail communication facilitates work distribution and completion by connecting the entire office staff in an asynchronous manner.

Organizing Information for Point-of-Care Decision Making

Most EHR systems can be configured to organize needed information for a particular patient or condition so that it is presented in a clear and concise way. Some templates actually integrate treatment goals or guidelines and provide highlights or reminders when the patient's parameters are out of range. For example, if you are seeing a diabetic patient whose BMI or blood pressure is high or whose LDL level is above the recommended target, you would get a prompt to modify the treatment plan. When help is needed about what test might substantiate a suspected diagnosis, the computer should be able to assist. Treatment plans and follow-up recommendations can be printed, transmitted, and tracked over time and provide reminders as needed for both patients and office staff.

Health Information Exchange

Having all the information about tests, medications, consultations, and hospitalizations is essential if we are to make the best decisions for our patients. To have timely transfer of data from one point of care to another, there must be real-time exchange of information that is managed securely. Many U.S. regions now have health information exchange projects, which should become more useful over time as more practices have fully capable EHR systems.

Professional Development

Family physicians must be committed to lifelong learning and professional development. Traditional classroom or lecture formats may not serve practicing physicians as well as online interactive learning environments. The ability to look up information quickly while the patient is present will be a necessary part of care in the future. Practice-based improvement and point-of-care learning are now required competencies for physicians of all specialties.

Conclusion

Information technology must support the core functions of medical care. Diagnostic and therapeutic decisions, patient self-management support, and follow-up are all aided by effective computer systems. Electronic health record use, electronic prescribing, and data availability at the point of care are fast becoming the "standard of care" that all family physicians must strive to achieve.

References

The complete reference list is available online at www.expertconsult.com.

Web Resources

http://healthit.ahrq.gov Agency for Healthcare Research and Quality (AHRQ) National Health-IT Resource Center. This AHRQ-funded site aggregates educational information on health information technology from many authoritative sources.

www.centerforhit.org American Academy of Family Physicians (AAFP) Center for Health-IT. AAFP's site devoted to health information technology has many resources to help physicians and practices through the EHR adoption life cycle.

www.ccrstandard.com Unofficial site for the American Society for Testing Materials (ASTM) Continuity of Care Record (CCR) standard.

www.ehealthinitiative.org/ehi-guides-e-prescribing.html eHealth Initiative e-Prescribers Guide. A definitive guide for physicians and other prescribers on electronic prescribing; discusses the values of e-prescribing as well as how to implement e-prescribing successfully.

www.aafp.org/online/en/home/publications/journals/fpm.html *Family Practice Management Journal.* The journal of the AAFP devoted to educating family physicians about the implementation and management of a successful practice, with a section devoted to computerization.

http://en.wikipedia.org/wiki/Patient_portal Wikipedia–Patient Portals.

10 CHAPTER

Clinical Problem Solving

Gregory M. Garrison, Denise M. Dupras, Stephen P. Merry, and Alan J. Smith

Key Points

- Taking care of patients requires clinical decision-making skills.
- Most physicians rely on "mindlines" formed by previous knowledge and experience.
- A lag exists between the publication of new evidence and its incorporation into clinical practice.
- Clinicians should use evidence-based medicine techniques to update their mindlines.

During a 15-minute follow-up visit for her diabetes, Mrs. Smith, a 78-year-old white patient who has a history of well-controlled type 2 diabetes mellitus, hypertension, asthma, and mild dependent edema, requests a refill of her hormone replacement therapy (HRT). Glancing at her chart, you note that she has been taking 0.625 mg daily of conjugated estrogen (Premarin) since a hysterectomy for excessive bleeding at age 53. She is also taking 1000 mg of metformin twice daily, 20 mg of lisinopril daily, 25 mg of hydrochlorothiazide daily, and fluticasone plus albuterol (Advair; 250/50 μg twice daily) and using an albuterol metered-dose inhaler as needed. Before reaching for your pen, you wonder if HRT is the right choice for Mrs. Smith.

Anyone engaged in primary care faces scenarios such as this on a daily basis. Such a seemingly simple request requires that clinicians rapidly assess the current medical evidence as it applies to the particular patient, communicate the risks and benefits using language the patient understands, and recommend a course of action based on the patient's preferences. This is a daunting task, but most clinicians do it without a second thought. By analyzing how clinical decisions are made, physicians can better understand how to integrate evidence-based medicine and patient preferences to improve the efficacy and efficiency of clinical practice.

Making Clinical Decisions

A typical family physician sees a patient every 15 minutes and addresses three separate problems during the visit (Beasley et al., 2004). Busy clinicians operating in such an environment must make snap decisions regarding patient care. Ethnographic studies of actual physician decision making in primary care offices indicate that physicians rely on "mindlines" to guide them (Gabbay and le May, 2004). Physicians develop these mindlines as a preconceived, conceptualized, and standardized approach to a particular clinical scenario. For example, for a child with fever and tonsillar exudates, one physician's mindline may be to treat with penicillin, and another physician's mindline may be to obtain a culture and treat if the results are positive for *Streptococcus*. The foundation of these mindlines is the tacit knowledge physicians acquire during their early training. For example, the best predictor of a clinician's knowledge about hypertension treatment is his or her year of graduation from medical school (Evans et al., 1984). Subsequently, these mindlines are continuously refined by patient care experiences, interactions with colleagues, discussions with trusted experts, and to a lesser extent, focused reading. Mindlines allow the clinician a mechanism to cope with the demands of a busy office practice. If not continuously updated and refined, however, such mindlines can quickly become stale and outdated.

A significant lag often occurs between the publication of landmark clinical studies that change medical practice and their general adoption by the medical community. Often, an opinion leader or trusted expert must adopt the new clinical practice first before others in the medical community feel comfortable changing their own practices (Slawson et al., 1994). This supports the concept that interactions with colleagues and discussions with trusted experts are the primary influence in shaping physician mindlines. The challenge is for the physician to use the tools of evidence-based medicine to shape her or his own mindlines and become an opinion leader.

To make sound clinical decisions, the clinician must first check his or her mindline. If there are knowledge gaps in the mindline, it can be updated by asking a focused clinical question and using the techniques of evidence-based medicine. Next, the clinician discusses potential risks and benefits of treatment options with patients, determining their preferences. By integrating the medical evidence with patients' preferences, a shared clinical decision is reached.

You recall learning in medical school that HRT reduced the risk of cardiovascular disease and osteoporosis. Because your patient, Mrs. Smith, is clearly at risk for both, you have always refilled her conjugated estrogen (Premarin) since first seeing her 25 years ago. When a bone density scan 4 years ago showed no evidence of osteopenia, you congratulated yourself for all those years of prescribing HRT. However, a colleague recently presented a paper at an educational conference and, based on the results of the Women's Health Initiative (WHI) study, recommended that all women be taken off estrogen replacement therapy. The estrogen was originally started because of concerns about osteoporosis, but now you wonder whether Mrs. Smith should continue it.

Focusing the Question

Key Points

- Identify the existence of a knowledge gap.
- Determine the information source most likely to answer the type of question.
- Develop a focused question consisting of four parts: patient's problem, intervention, comparison intervention, and outcome of interest.

Many studies have documented that important clinical questions arise during the day-to-day care of patients (Dee and Blazek, 1993). The number and types of questions depend on the clinical setting and the experience of the physician. The most common generic questions involve choosing which drugs to prescribe, determining the cause of a condition, and deciding what diagnostic study to order (Ely et al., 2000). Studies also show that answers are not sought for most questions that arise, but that physicians who seek answers are usually successful in finding them (Ely et al., 1999). Previous studies that documented little dependence on computerized resources for finding answers may reflect that the studies were conducted when computers were not extensively used in the course of routine patient care (Covell et al., 1985; Osheroff and Bankowitz, 1993).

After identifying a knowledge gap relevant to making a clinical decision, the next step is finding the information necessary to close the gap. To find the necessary information, an answerable question must be developed. There are two general types of clinical questions: background and foreground. *Background questions* are the "who, what, why, and how" questions usually answered in textbooks and asked by medical students; for example, What oral drugs are used in the treatment of diabetes? *Foreground questions* focus on the specifics surrounding care of a patient; for example, Which is more effective in reducing fasting blood sugar level in an obese patient with type 2 diabetes—metformin or glyburide? It is unlikely that a textbook could adequately answer this second question.

Being able to identify the type of question helps direct the physician to the best source of information for answers.

Most of the questions that arise out of patient care can be categorized as foreground questions, because they are specific to a particular patient's case. Although unlikely to be found in textbooks, the ability to answer these questions at the point of care is essential to providing the best care in a timely manner. A *focused clinical question* must be developed to find the information efficiently (Richardson et al., 1995). Unfortunately, this critical step is often overlooked, causing needless frustration when searching for answers among thousands of hits in a search engine. Sackett and colleagues (2000) propose that "educational prescriptions" be used to teach this important skill to physicians in training.

The four components of a focused clinical question are (1) the patient's problem, (2) the intervention, (3) the comparison intervention, and (4) the outcome of interest. *Patient-oriented outcomes* are always better than disease-oriented outcomes because they are *direct measures* rather than secondary markers. For example, a study documenting that a new drug reduces total cholesterol by 20% (secondary marker) is important, but not as persuasive as a study documenting a decrease in cardiovascular death (direct measure).

Whether Mrs. Smith should remain on estrogen therapy is a complex question. You know that the WHI study assessed multiple outcomes of importance for this patient population, including the impact of hormones on heart disease, fracture rates, venous thromboembolism, colon cancer, and breast cancer. The question of whether Mrs. Smith should keep taking estrogen cannot be answered without weighing the risks and benefits of the therapy and the importance of each of these outcomes to the patient. Mrs. Smith's primary concern is the prevention of osteoporosis because her mother had severe osteoporosis with multiple fractures during her life. This additional information helps to guide the development of a relevant, focused clinical question for Mrs. Smith: In postmenopausal women at risk for osteoporosis (i.e., the patient's problem), is continuation of estrogen replacement therapy (i.e., the intervention) better than changing to bisphosphonate therapy (i.e., the comparison intervention) for prevention of osteoporotic fractures (i.e., the outcome of interest)?

Finding the Evidence

Key Points

- Usefulness = (Relevance × Validity)/Work
- Conflicting evidence is often the result of "medical chatter."
- POEMs and guidelines require the least amount of work to find relevant and valid results.

Having identified a focused question, the astute clinician is ready to find the information needed to answer it. The usefulness of medical information can be modeled in the following equation (Slawson et al, 1994):

$$\text{Usefulness} = \frac{(\text{Relevance}) \times (\text{Validity})}{(\text{Work})}$$

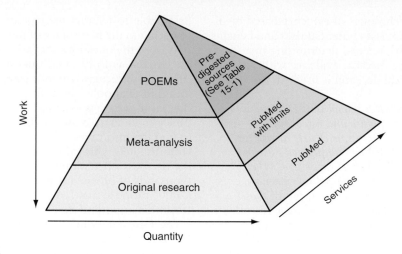

Figure 10-1 Evidence pyramid.

As the formula shows, busy clinicians should concentrate their efforts on easily obtained, valid evidence that is highly relevant (i.e., patient-oriented evidence). Such a strategy focuses attention on useful information and makes wise use of limited time and resources.

As shown in Figure 10-1, the work required to find useful medical information is inversely proportional to its quantity. At the bottom of the pyramid is original research. Although plentiful, much of it represents "medical chatter" among researchers (Slawson et al., 1994). Researchers are intimately familiar with published data in their narrow field of study and are able to place the article in its proper context. A busy clinician reading a single article in a relatively unfamiliar field is akin to overhearing a snippet of conversation at a dinner party. It may be dangerous to base decisions on such snippets without knowledge of the larger context. Checking the relevance and validity of such studies requires knowledge of statistical methods and study design. It is too time-consuming to be useful for answering clinical questions that arise during a patient visit.

At the next level of the pyramid are *systematic reviews* and *meta-analyses*. These types of studies focus on a single topic and attempt to draw conclusions from the volume of previously reported data. Although an improvement, the clinician still must explore the methodology used to select and analyze the data to ensure relevance to the clinical question. Often, these types of reviews focus on disease-oriented outcomes rather than patient-oriented outcomes, potentially making them less relevant. Disease-oriented outcomes, such as an increase in bone mineral density, may be a secondary marker for fracture risk, but they are inherently less relevant to the patient.

At the peak of the pyramid are *patient-oriented evidence that matters* (POEM) reviews (Table 10-1). Clinicians must decide if the POEM is relevant to their clinical question, but the amount of work required is greatly reduced. POEMs offer the most useful type of information for answering clinical questions that arise during patient visits. Unfortunately, a POEM does not exist for every clinical question. In these cases the clinician must step down the pyramid until relevant information is found.

The medical evidence often tells conflicting stories, as with HRT. This is particularly problematic at the original research or bottom level of the evidence pyramid. Differences in

Table 10-1 POEM* Sources

Source	Website
Free	
Bandolier	www.jr2.ox.ac.uk/bandolier
Cochrane Abstracts	www.cochrane.org/reviews/index.htm
National Guidelines Clearinghouse	www.guidelines.gov
Subscription	
American College of Physicians	www.acpjc.org
Clinical Evidence	www.clinicalevidence.org
Cochrane Reviews	www.cochrane.org/reviews/index/htm
Family Physicians Inquiries	www.fpin.org
Network InfoRetriever	www.infopoems.com
Journal of Family Practice	www.jfponline.com
Up To Date	www.uptodate.com

*Patient-oriented evidence that matters.

methodology, study populations, statistical power, and bias often explain the different conclusions and result in medical chatter. Putting such articles in their proper context is difficult at best for the practicing clinician. Moving up the evidence pyramid helps alleviate conflicting evidence, yielding results that are more reliable.

Often, minimal or no reliable medical evidence is available to answer a clinical question. In these cases, practicing clinicians must rely on their clinical experience and background medical knowledge—their mindlines.

Haynes (2001) defined another pyramid that is relevant to answering clinical questions. This is the pyramid of services for finding the best evidence. It is depicted as the third dimension of the evidence pyramid (Figure 10-1). At the bottom of the pyramid are tools to find the original studies.

The National Library of Medicine maintains a database of more than 15 million articles, called MEDLINE. Various engines are available to search MEDLINE and other databases for articles that may be used to answer clinical questions. For example, PubMed (www.pubmed.gov) provides tools to help clinicians search for meta-analyses and systematic reviews through the use of *limits* and *clinical queries* (Ebbert et al., 2003; Haynes and Wilczynski, 2005; Sood et al., 2004).

As in Mrs. Smith's case, there may not be a single study that addresses the specific question posed. In looking for the best evidence to inform clinical decision making, it is important to determine the standard of care for the patient's condition. Clinical guidelines, which are typically updated every 2 years, may be a useful resource. An excellent clearinghouse for clinical guidelines is sponsored by the Agency for Healthcare Research and Quality (AHRQ, www.guidelines.gov), although the listed guidelines are neither reviewed nor endorsed by AHRQ. Clinicians must critique the guidelines for validity and relevance in their own setting. This resource is higher up the services pyramid and reflects some interpretation and synthesis of original research and clinical practice.

You review the Institute for Clinical Systems Integration guideline for osteoporosis prevention and HRT at www.guidelines.gov, as well as the risk/benefit data from the www.WHI.org site (Figure 10-2). These guidelines tell you that HRT should not be used simply for prevention of osteoporosis in the absence of other significant menopausal symptoms. You reflect on your colleague's words: "Get everyone off that stuff!" It is time to have a discussion with Mrs. Smith regarding her estrogen therapy.

Incorporating Patient Preferences

Key Points

- There has been a cultural shift from paternalistic to shared decision making.
- The degree of shared decision making depends on risk, benefit, and a patient's preferences.
- Decision aids can help patients understand complex probabilities.

Until the 1980s, medical decision making was physician driven. Such decision making required and perhaps engendered patients' trust in their physicians. With such paternalistic care, patients effectively ceded decisional authority to their physician through implied consent. Physicians made the decisions, patients accepted them, and most patients preferred it that way. Many patients still prefer this type of interaction (Goldfarb, 2004). How many times do family physicians explain the risks and benefits of a procedure, only to have the patient respond, "So Doc, what would you do?"

In 1980 a small, influential group was formed: the Society for Medical Decision-Making. Over the years, the society's work has spawned two other movements: evidence-based medicine and shared decision making. *Evidence-based medicine* (EBM) seeks to provide physicians with the empirical data necessary to make wise clinical decisions through critical appraisal of the literature. *Shared decision making* occurs when physicians communicate the evidence to patients with sufficient clarity that they can become fully informed partners in their own health care decisions. Probabilistic evidence

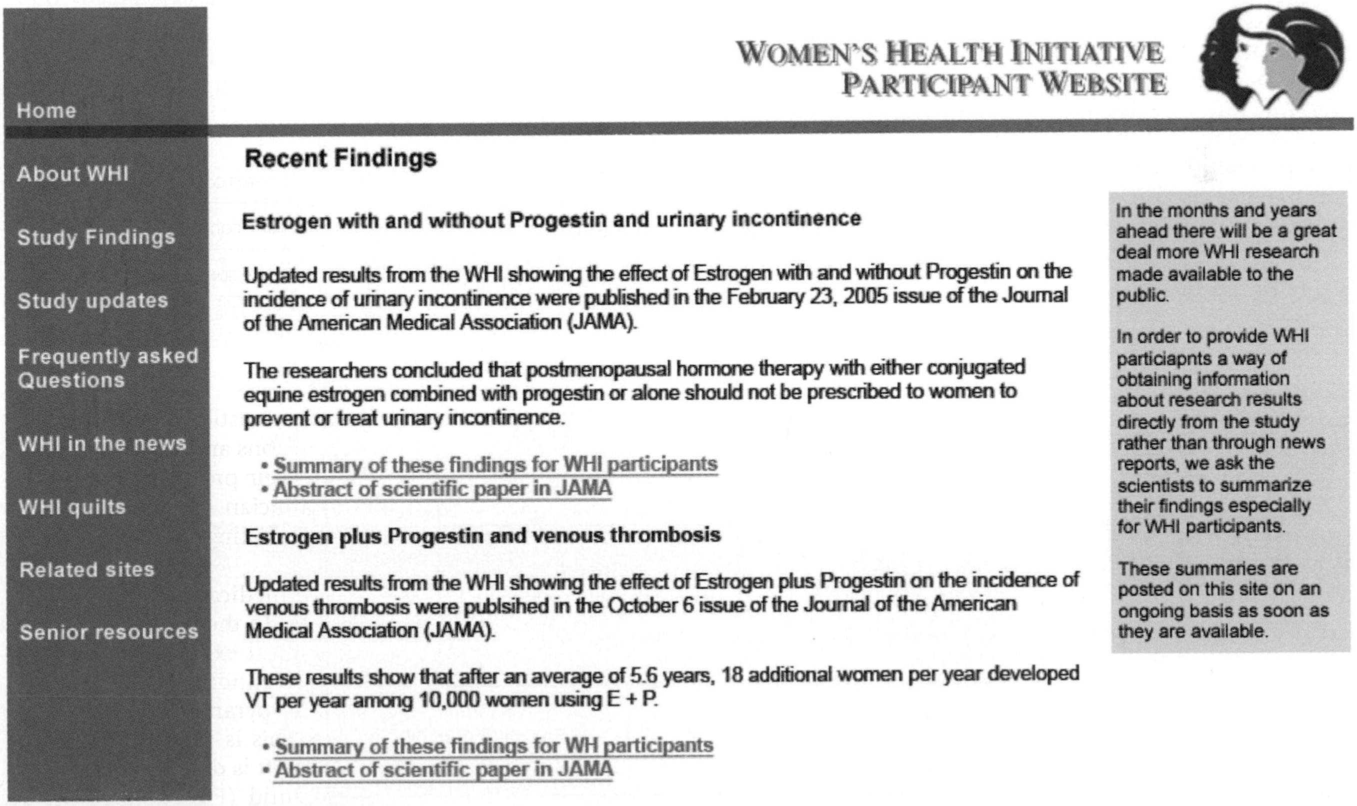

WOMEN'S HEALTH INITIATIVE PARTICIPANT WEBSITE

Home

About WHI

Study Findings

Study updates

Frequently asked Questions

WHI in the news

WHI quilts

Related sites

Senior resources

Recent Findings

Estrogen with and without Progestin and urinary incontinence

Updated results from the WHI showing the effect of Estrogen with and without Progestin on the incidence of urinary incontinence were published in the February 23, 2005 issue of the Journal of the American Medical Association (JAMA).

The researchers concluded that postmenopausal hormone therapy with either conjugated equine estrogen combined with progestin or alone should not be prescribed to women to prevent or treat urinary incontinence.

- Summary of these findings for WHI participants
- Abstract of scientific paper in JAMA

Estrogen plus Progestin and venous thrombosis

Updated results from the WHI showing the effect of Estrogen plus Progestin on the incidence of venous thrombosis were publsihed in the October 6 issue of the Journal of the American Medical Association (JAMA).

These results show that after an average of 5.6 years, 18 additional women per year developed VT per year among 10,000 women using E + P.

- Summary of these findings for WH participants
- Abstract of scientific paper in JAMA

In the months and years ahead there will be a great deal more WHI research made available to the public.

In order to provide WHI particiapnts a way of obtaining information about research results directly from the study rather than through news reports, we ask the scientists to summarize their findings especially for WHI participants.

These summaries are posted on this site on an ongoing basis as soon as they are available.

Figure 10-2 Women's Health Initiative (WHI) site.

alone should not guide decision making; patient preferences and values must be considered for a decision to be shared. As a result, shared decision making has been called an "ethical" process. The physician not only informs the patient before making the decision, but also seeks to empower the patient to become an active participant in decision making.

"Doctor," Mrs. Smith interjects as you finish clicking through the guideline pages. "I know you're concerned about me being on these hormones. But, I really am doing well, and I don't want to stop them unless I have to."

The cultural change toward active patient participation in medical decision making occurred rapidly. One survey of patients seeing their physician for chronic disease management between 1986 and 1990 found that 69% preferred "to leave decisions about my medical care up to my doctor." In contrast, a study only 10 years later found that 84% of women with node-negative breast cancer preferred a shared role in decision making regarding adjuvant chemotherapy. One week after using a decision aid to explore the risks and benefits, an additional 10% said they preferred a shared role in the decision (Arora and McHorney, 2000). This cultural shift toward greater patient involvement in clinical decision making may stem from the increased availability of medical knowledge in the public domain and an increasingly consumerist society (Guyatt et al., 2004).

Physician reactions to this cultural change range from self-interest in avoiding legal liability to selfless beneficence in seeking to include patient preferences (McGuire et al., 2005). Increased patient participation in medical decision making is associated with increased trust, higher patient satisfaction, and greater compliance with treatment, particularly lifestyle changes. In some cases, this leads to an improvement in disease outcomes (Epstein et al., 2004; O'Conner et al., 2003; Trachtenberg et al., 2005).

Shared decision making is substantially different from *informed consent*, a legal doctrine focused on disclosure of risk and benefit to the patient or the surrogate rather than on partnership in medical decision making. Shared decision making also differs from *medical consumerism*, in which patients obtain information from various media sources

before actively interviewing their physicians and making their own decisions about their health care. Shared decision making involves the creation of a physician-patient partnership, one of the six principal aims of health care in the 21st century, as identified by the Institute of Medicine's 2000 report (Sheridan et al., 2004).

A busy family medicine practice involves straightforward and complex medical decision making. The degree to which decision making is shared with the patient varies according to the risk of the intervention, certainty of the benefit, and the patient's desire for autonomy. Figure 10-3 illustrates how these three dimensions of risk, certainty of benefit, and patient preferences interact to determine whether shared decision making is necessary.

For decisions involving low risk and a single best course of action, shared decision making is unlikely to be helpful. Physicians are free to make the decision as long as they explain what needs to be done and why. The TV image of the wise family doctor making a diagnosis of strep throat and then sitting back in his chair to elicit patient involvement in the decision about whether to treat with penicillin is laughable to most patients, of little benefit, and a sure way to put the physician behind schedule.

Conversely, when multiple alternatives of almost equal benefit exist, the decision necessarily involves patient preferences. For example, in a young healthy patient with elevated lipid levels, the patient should share in the decision regarding initiation of a statin versus continued aggressive lifestyle changes. Such involvement is more likely to yield patient compliance with the mutually agreed course of action.

When the choice involves significant risk or moral beliefs and the certainty of benefit is low, the patient should be encouraged to make the decision, with the physician acting as an informant rather than a co-participant (Whitney et al., 2004). An excellent example occurs with first-trimester screening for Down syndrome and trisomy 18.

Physicians must be flexible, adjusting to the patient's desire for involvement in decision making. Some patients want collaborative decision making, whereas others feel more comfortable with traditional physician-directed decision making (McGuire et al., 2005). This is shown as the third dimension in Figure 10-3.

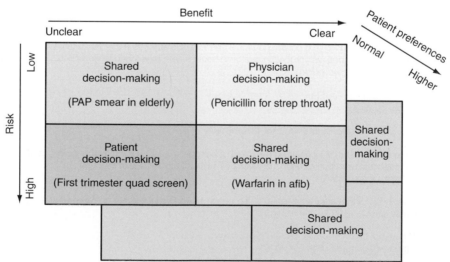

Figure 10-3 Shared decision-making model.

The desire to communicate data effectively to patients has resulted in development of many decision support tools, such as pamphlets, audio/videotapes (CDs), personalized counseling, smartphone apps, and interactive computer programs on the Internet. These tools inform patients about complex risk/benefit balances and help them determine their personal preferences and reach a decision by weighing the possible outcomes. An excellent example is the Atrial Fibrillation Treatment Decision-Making Aid offered by the University of Ottawa.* This tool informs patients about atrial fibrillation and strokes, estimates risks and benefits, and helps rank the patient's outcome preferences. Based on these data, a worksheet guides the physician and patient in a shared decision-making process (Ottawa Health Decision Centre, 2006, http://decisionaid.ohri.ca/).

Because working through such decision aids can be time-consuming and impede workflow in a busy clinic, they are often best assigned as homework, with a recheck visit at a later date to engage in shared decision making.

Mrs. Smith needs more patient-oriented evidence to help her share in the decision to continue or stop the HRT. Following the links on the Ottawa Health Decision Centre website, you bring up the decision aid, "Osteoporosis Decision Aid: Should I take hormone replacement therapy?" You print it, hand Mrs. Smith a pen, and head off to see your next patient while she ponders the information.

Decision making often is not as complex as Mrs. Smith's case, and no written decision aid may exist. A family physician may only have 2 or 3 minutes during a 15-minute patient encounter to explain the complex probabilities of risks and benefits for a particular intervention. Various statistical constructs have been proposed to communicate these probabilities to patients in an understandable manner.

The ideal format depends on the patient's condition and ability to understand probabilities. The relative risk ratio (RRR), absolute risk ratio (ARR), and *number needed to treat* (NNT) are reasonable constructs that can communicate the expected magnitude of benefit. Although the NNT has been proposed as an intuitive concept, a Danish trial showed that patients have difficulty understanding the magnitude of osteoporosis treatment benefit when presented in terms of NNT. Conversely, when explained as postponement of hip fracture, their treatment decisions reflected a better sense of the actual benefit (Christensen et al., 2003). Sheridan and colleagues (2003) similarly found that patients frequently misinterpreted the NNT but found the ARR and RRR more intuitive. The Evidence-Based Medicine Working Group has proposed more clearly communicating treatment benefit by using the construct of "likelihood of being helped versus harmed" (McAlister et al., 2000).

When you return to her examination room 15 minutes later, a satisfied Mrs. Smith declares, "I appreciate you giving me all the information, but what do you think I should do?" You review the decision aid with her, discussing the risk/benefit ratios; you note that she has identified the benefits of decreased fractures and

menopausal symptoms as more important than the risk of harm from blood clots, heart disease, stroke, or breast cancer. She states, "Doc, I know that my diabetes raises my risk of heart disease, but I just don't want to fall and break my hip and have to spend the rest of my life in a nursing home. Besides, I really enjoy not having the hot flashes."

You reflect for a moment on the Heart and Estrogen/ progestin Replacement Study (HERS) study results (Hulley et al., 1998) that showed a decrease in cardiovascular risk with HRT in years 3 to 5 of the study. You have heard some of the controversy surrounding the WHI results (2002) and the possibility that lower rates of cardiovascular disease might have been seen with longer exposures to estrogens if the trial had been continued.

You inform Mrs. Smith that you cannot really be sure, but because she has been receiving HRT so long, you do not believe her risk of heart attack is increased. You also make sure she understands the absolute risks of breast cancer and blood clots. She replies, "Well, Doc, I've been on estrogen for 25 years, and I never had a problem with my heart or my mammograms. I just don't want to wind up like my friends who've gone off estrogen and have hot flashes every night—you know what I mean?"

Clicking the pen, you say, "Well, Mrs. Smith, you seem to have a good understanding of your situation. Shall we continue that Premarin?"

Conclusion

Clinical decision making is the intersection of the science of evidence-based medicine and the art of shared decision making occurring within the bounds of the health care system (Figure 10-4). People yearn for a relationship with their physician, someone who listens to their needs and guides them through the medical system (Future of Family Medicine, 2004). Who is better equipped to perform outstanding clinical decision making and foster excellent physician-patient communication than the family physician? By forming close longitudinal relationships, family physicians have the opportunity to truly know their patients and to understand their values, their preferences, and their fears. When combined with evidence-based medical knowledge, it is no wonder patients trust and value their family physician.

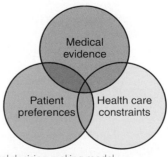

Figure 10-4 Clinical decision-making model.

References

The complete reference list is available online at www.expertconsult.com.

Web Resources

www.cochrane.org/reviews/index.htm
Cochrane Abstracts. Evidence-based systematic reviews of health care interventions.
Pros: Peer-reviewed evidence-based summaries.
Cons: Only abstracts available free, entire review is subscription service.

www.guidelines.gov
National Guidelines Clearinghouse. Evidence-based clinical practice guidelines.
Pros: Large library of clinical guidelines.
Cons: Evidence-based quality is not uniform and depends on guideline authors themselves; multiple guidelines for a single condition (e.g., hypertension yields 533 guidelines).

www.uptodate.com
Up To Date. Evidence-based peer-reviewed information resource; subscription based.

Pros: Comprehensive reviews on many topics with diagnostic and treatment information.
Cons: May not contain the latest evidence; may contain expert opinion.

www.fpin.org
Family Physicians Inquiries Network. Brief, structured evidence-based answers to clinical questions; subscription based.
Pros: Succinct reviews with evidence grading.
Cons: Although library is large, the questions answered may be extremely specific.

www.fpnotebook.com
Family Practice Notebook. Notes in outline form on a variety of topics.
Pros: Succinct information from a variety of sources.
Cons: No peer review; references may be sparse.

CHAPTER 11

Complementary and Alternative Medicine: Integration into Primary Care

Mary P. Guerrera

Key Points

- Terms and definitions that describe CAM are diverse and evolving.
- Integrative medicine combines CAM and conventional medicine.

The level of integration of conventional and CAM therapies is growing. That growth generates the need for tools or frameworks to make decisions about which therapies should be provided or recommended, about which CAM providers to whom conventional medical providers might refer patients, and the organizational structure to be used for the delivery of integrated care. The committee believes that the overarching rubric that should be used to guide the development of these tools should be the goal of providing comprehensive care that is safe and effective, that is collaborative and interdisciplinary, and that respects and joins interventions from all sources. (Institute of Medicine, 2005)

In these tumultuous times of health care reform, family physicians find themselves on a threshold: a place of great professional promise as well as uncertainty. Will they step through this historic doorway with newfound meaning and professional identity? Will they create new practice models, new ways of delivering care, and new methods of collaborating across the spectrum of healing practices and health professionals? Work is already underway with initiatives such as TransforMed and P4. In addition, the field of family medicine has taken the lead and is currently pioneering work bringing complementary and alternative medicine (CAM) and integrative medicine into residency training and clinical care (Benn et al., 2009).

How will these relatively new and evolving areas of health care optimize and revitalize the practice of family medicine? This chapter describes these new fields, assesses proposals by U.S. medical organizations, and addresses the challenges for practitioners applying current research techniques to these diverse and complex healing approaches and systems. Core principles and specific examples of CAM encountered by the practicing family physician are presented with relevant evidence and helpful tips.

Complementary and alternative medicine is based on multiple healing traditions practiced long before conventional Western medicine. Emerging from diverse cultural traditions worldwide, these approaches to health and healing offer the wisdom of their unique perspective on the human condition. Many traditional practices, including those of conventional medicine, share common roots and philosophies and uphold the sacred call to relieve the suffering of others. Family physicians should keep an open mind as they explore these dimensions of CAM.

What Is Complementary and Alternative Medicine?

Various definitions have been used to describe the array of approaches and philosophies commonly referred to as "CAM." As the field has evolved, so has the terminology. Unconventional, unproven, alternative, complementary, holistic, integrative, and integral are some of the most common examples of terms in current use.

Historically, medical pluralism has long existed in the United States (Kaptchuk and Eisenberg, 2001a). Over the past few decades, *alternative medicine* has become a more recognized entity within conventional medicine. Because of the public's growing use of CAM, the National Institutes of Health (NIH) created an Office of Alternative Medicine (OAM) in 1992, with the intention of bringing its scientific expertise "to more adequately explore unconventional medical practices" (NCCAM, 2000). Because of Americans' ongoing and increasing use of CAM, the OAM was expanded to the *National Center for Complementary and Alternative Medicine* (NCCAM) in 1998, guided by the following mission statement (2000): "We are dedicated to exploring complementary and alternative healing practices in the context of rigorous science, training researchers, and disseminating authoritative information to the public and professional communities." After a decade of work in the field, NCCAM has become a leading resource for helping the public and health professionals better understand this rapidly growing area of medicine. The center's name has led to the more widespread use and recognition of CAM as the defining term for this field. NCCAM's free website contains a wealth of information, including the following definitions (2000):

Complementary and alternative medicine is a group of diverse medical and health care systems, practices, and products that are not considered part of conventional medicine. Although some scientific evidence exists, the list of what is considered to be CAM changes continually as the therapies that are proved to be safe and effective become adopted into conventional health care and as new approaches to health care emerge.

Alternative medicine is used in place of conventional medicine. *Complementary medicine* is used together with conventional medicine.

Integrative medicine combines mainstream medical therapies and CAM therapies for which there is some high-quality scientific evidence of safety and effectiveness.

The NCCAM further classifies CAM into five categories, or domains (Figure 11-1). Examples of alternative or whole medical systems include homeopathy, naturopathy, and Ayurveda (**eAppendix 11-1** provides a glossary of CAM terms online at www.expertconsult.com). Although there are a variety of approaches to the complex taxonomy of CAM (Kaptchuk and Eisenberg, 2001b), the NIH system is most often used.

Another term, *holistic medicine*, also describes these practices and philosophy. The American Holistic Medical Association (AHMA), founded in 1978, is a membership organization for physicians and other health professionals seeking to practice a broader form of medicine than that currently taught in allopathic medical schools (Table 11-1). "Holistic medicine is the art and science of healing that addresses care of the

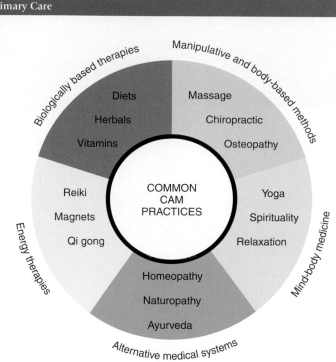

Figure 11-1 The National Center for Complementary and Alternative Medicine (NCCAM) groups complementary and alternative medicine (CAM) practices into five domains, recognizing that there can be some overlap among them. *Biologically based therapies* use substances found in nature, such as herbs, special diets, or vitamins (in doses outside those used in conventional medicine). *Energy therapies* involve the use of energy fields, such as magnetic fields or biofields (i.e., energy fields that some believe surround and penetrate the human body). *Manipulative and body-based methods* are based on manipulation or movement of one or more body parts. *Mind-body medicine* uses a variety of techniques designed to enhance the mind's ability to affect bodily function and symptoms. *Alternative or whole medical systems* are built on complete systems of theory and practice. Often, these systems have evolved apart from and earlier than the conventional medical approach used in the United States.

whole person—body, mind, and spirit. The practice of holistic medicine integrates conventional and complementary therapies to promote optimal health and to prevent and treat disease by addressing contributing factors" (AHMA, 2005).

In 1981, the nursing profession, guided by a group of nurses dedicated to bringing the concepts of holism to every arena of nursing practice, founded the American Holistic Nursing Association (AHNA). "Holistic nursing embraces all nursing that has as its goal enhancement of healing the whole person from birth to death. Holistic nursing recognizes that there are two views regarding holism: that holism involves identifying the interrelationships of the biopsychosociospiritual dimensions of the person, recognizing that the whole is greater than the sum of its parts, and that holism involves understanding the individual as a unitary whole in mutual process with the environment" (AHNA, 2005).

Integrative medicine, a term brought into popular use by Andrew Weil, MD, founder and director of the innovative University of Arizona Center for Integrative Medicine, describes how CAM and conventional medicine is practiced together (Rakel and Weil, 2003):

Integrative medicine is healing oriented and emphasizes the centrality of the doctor-patient relationship. It focuses on the least invasive, least toxic, and least costly methods to help facilitate health by integrating allopathic and complementary therapies. These are

Table 11-1 Important Events in Complementary and Integrative Medicine

Year	Event
1978	American Holistic Medical Association is founded.
1981	American Holistic Nurses Association is founded.
1992	U.S. Office of Alternative Medicine (OAM) is established.
1996	U.S. Food and Drug Administration (FDA) approves acupuncture needles for use by licensed practitioners.
1998	National Center for Complementary and Alternative Medicine (NCCAM) is established, replacing OAM..
1999	Consortium of Academic Health Centers for Integrative Medicine (CAHCIM) is formed in response to increasing public interest in complementary and alternative medicine (CAM) and grows to 46 members by 2010.
2000	American Board of Medical Acupuncture is established, with a certifying examination for physicians to demonstrate proficiency in the specialty of medical acupuncture.
2000	President Clinton appoints James S. Gordon, MD, to chair the first White House Commission on Complementary and Alternative Medicine Policy (WHCCAMP).
2002	WHCCAMP submits final report with administrative and legislative recommendations for maximizing the benefits of CAM for all Americans.
2005	Institute of Medicine (IOM) releases report on CAM in the United States. NCCAM releases 5-year strategic plan.
2006	CAHCIM sponsors the first North American Research Conference on Complementary and Integrative Medicine.
2009	IOM Summit on Integrative Medicine and the Health of the Public. CAHCIM sponsors a second research conference. NCCAM prepares its third strategic plan.

based on an understanding of the physical, emotional, psychologic, and spiritual aspects of the individual.

In general, the terms *holistic* and *integrative* seem to best convey the ideal blending of conventional and unconventional medicine "in that both imply a balanced, whole-person–centered approach and involve a synthesis of conventional medicine, CAM modalities, and other traditional medical systems, with the aim of prevention and healing as a basic foundation" (Lee et al., 2004).

The term *integral* has recently emerged in the literature. First noted several decades ago in the book *Mind, Body and Health: Toward an Integral Medicine* (Gordon et al., 1984), its original use may be traced to the work of Sri Aurobindo, an Indian mystic and political leader. The term has been popularized by contemporary philosopher and transpersonal psychologist Ken Wilber (2005), as applied in the context of his *integral theory*. Many thought leaders in the field of health and healing, including the Institute of Noetic Sciences (IONS), support these concepts and encourage further research into what may be considered the beginnings of a paradigm shift

in medicine (Schiltz, 2005). The following excerpt captures the essence of the deep change and transformation that integral medicine calls for (Wilber, 2005):

> *The crucial ingredient in any integral medical practice is not the integral medical bag itself—with all the conventional pills, and the orthodox surgery, and the subtle energy medicine, and the acupuncture needles—but the holder of that bag. Integrally informed health-care practitioners, the doctors, nurses, and therapists, have opened themselves to an entire spectrum of consciousness—matter to body to mind to soul to spirit—and who have thereby acknowledged what seems to be happening in any event. Body and mind and spirit are operating in self and culture and nature, and thus health and healing, sickness and wholeness, are all bound up in a multidimensional tapestry that cannot be cut into without loss.*

Family physicians know this to be true. They practice with the intention to care for the whole patient within the context of a continuous healing relationship while honoring the rich complexity and interplay of family, community, and environment. They acknowledge the personal and interpersonal effects of health and illness and are trained to consider the behavioral and social aspects of a person's life as well as the biomedical factors.

Now is the time not only to reclaim its roots, but also to move primary care into expanded dimensions and possibilities of health and healing. Family medicine is the ideal discipline to champion this movement and to actualize changes that will begin to heal the failing U.S. health care system. Whether it is called holistic, integrative, or integral, family physicians are collectively evolving toward a more compassionate and sustainable system of care that may ultimately be called *good medicine*.

Complementary and Alternative Medicine Use in the 1990s

Key Points

- Almost 40% of U.S. adults and 12% of children use CAM therapies.
- The number of adult Americans using CAM rose by 38% between 1990 and 1997 and has remained stable between 2002 and 2007.
- CAM is used more by women, by those with higher levels of education and income, and by those who were recently hospitalized.
- Most patients do not disclose CAM use to their physicians.
- Most patients use CAM *and* conventional care together.

The first major study of CAM use in the United States was conducted in 1990 by David Eisenberg and colleagues (1993), who published a landmark paper in the *New England Journal of Medicine*. Serving as a wake-up call to conventional medicine, the data from this national telephone survey of 1539 English-speaking adults estimated that one of three Americans (34%) had used a CAM therapy in the prior year. The study estimated that those using CAM had made 425 million visits to complementary medicine practitioners—more than all office visits to primary care physicians in that same time frame! The out-of-pocket costs for these CAM services were approximately $14 billion a year. The striking statistics alerted mainstream medicine and prompted further inquiry into the growing phenomenon of the public's use of CAM.

In 1997, Eisenberg and colleagues conducted a follow-up to the 1990 study, again using a national telephone survey of English-speaking adults (2055). The findings, published in the *Journal of the American Medical Association* in 1998, showed that the number of Americans using CAM rose by 38% (60 to 83 million) and that visits to CAM practitioners increased from an estimated 427 million to 629 million. Overall, 42% of Americans were estimated to be using at least one CAM therapy in the prior 12 months. With regard to costs, conservative estimates put expenditures for CAM professional services at $21.2 billion, with approximately $12.2 billion paid as out-of-pocket expenses (Eisenberg et al., 1998).

Most concerning was the finding that although CAM use had increased over the 7-year period, the number of patients informing their doctors of such use had not changed—approximately 60% to 70% of CAM users in 1990 and 1997 did not discuss their use of CAM with their physicians. Lack of communication was noted again in a 2006 NCCAM/American Association of Retired Persons (AARP) survey of adults 50 or older revealing only one-third of CAM users had talked to their physicians about their CAM use (AARP, 2007). Given this fact and the potential for untoward side effects, it is essential that physicians and all other health professionals ask patients about their use of CAM. In addition to NCCAM's "Time to Talk" campaign, several approaches have been suggested (Eisenberg, 1997); Table 11-2 lists an ABC format especially useful for the busy clinician (Sierpina, 2001).

Complementary and Alternative Medicine Use in the 21st Century

Data on the U.S. population's use of CAM was collected in 2002 and 2007. Considered the most comprehensive and reliable findings on American's use of CAM, these studies were conducted by the NCCAM and the National Center for Health Statistics (NCHS), part of the Centers for Disease Control and Prevention (CDC). For the first time, detailed questions regarding CAM were added into the 2002 edition of the NCHS National Health Interview Survey (NHIS), an annual study interviewing tens of thousands of Americans about their health- and illness-related experiences. The

2002 and 2007 studies were completed by ~30,000 families through adults 18 years or older who spoke English or Spanish. The study reflected CAM use during the 12 months before the survey. The 2007 survey included expanded questions on 36 types of CAM therapies commonly used in the United States—10 practitioner-based therapies, such as acupuncture, and 26 other, self-care therapies not requiring a practitioner. CAM therapies included in the surveys are listed in Table 11-3, and the terms are defined in eAppendix 11-1.

As shown in Figure 11-2, CAM use increased from 36% of U.S. adults in 2002 to 38% in 2007, or almost 4 of 10 adults (Barnes et al., 2004, 2008). For the first time, the 2007 survey collected data on CAM use in children (<18 years), showing 12% use, or 1 in 9 children. The top 10 CAM therapies for both adults and children are shown in Figure 11-3. Significant increases in adults' use of deep breathing, meditation, massage, and yoga occurred over the 5 years of the study. Another notable NCCAM/AARP study focused on CAM use in adults older than 50 years. Approximately two-thirds (63%) had used one or more CAM therapies (AARP, 2007). The most common reasons cited for not discussing CAM included: the physician never asked (42%), the patient did not know they should ask (30%), and there was not enough time during the office visit (19%). Of those using CAM, 66% did so to treat a specific condition and 65% for overall wellness. For details on CAM costs in the U.S., see **eFigures 11-1 to 11-3** online at www.expertconsult.com.

Table 11-2 Guidelines for Advising Patients Who Seek Alternative Therapies

Ask; don't tell.
Be willing to listen and learn.
Communicate and **c**ollaborate.
Diagnose.
Explain and **e**xplore options and preferences.

Table 11-3 Complementary and Alternative Medicine (CAM) Therapies Included in 2002 and 2007 National Health Interview Surveys

Acupuncture*	Natural nonvitamin and
Ayurveda*	nonmineral products (e.g., herbs,
Alternative practitioner*†	other products from plants,
Biofeedback*	enzymes)
Chelation therapy*	Naturopathy*
Chiropractic care*	Osteopathic manipulation*†
CAM†	Prayer for health reasons
Deep breathing exercises	Prayed for own health
Diet-based therapies	Others ever prayed for your health
Vegetarian diet	Participate in prayer group
Macrobiotic diet	Healing ritual for self
Atkins diet	Progressive relaxation
Pritikin diet	Qi gong
Ornish diet	Reiki*
Zone diet	Tai chi
Energy healing therapy*	Traditional healers*†
Folk medicine	Bontanica
Guided imagery	Curandero
Homeopathic treatment	Espiritista
Hypnosis	Hierbero
Massage*	Native American
Meditation	Shaman
Megavitamin therapy	Subador
Movement therapy†	Yoga
Alexander	
Feldenkreis	
Pilates	
Trager	

Definitions of these therapies are provided in the glossary of eAppendix 11-1.
*Indicates a practitioner-based therapy.
†Indicates addition to 2007 survey.

Who Is More Likely to Use CAM, and Why?

Consistent with data from the 2002 NHIS study, CAM use by adults in 2007 was more prevalent among women; adults age 30 to 69; those with higher education level, not poor, or living in the West; former smokers; and those hospitalized in the prior year (Barnes, 2008). CAM use was positively associated with number of health conditions and number of physician visits in the previous year. When concerned about cost or inability to pay for conventional care, adults were more likely to use CAM. For children, the 2007 data show no gender difference. For all therapies combined, CAM use was highest among adolescents age 12 to 17 years (16%) versus children age 5 to 11 years (11%) or preschool children age 0 to 4 years (8%). Children's use of CAM increased as their parents' education or income level increased, and when families were unable to afford conventional medical care. Children with a parent or other relative who used CAM were about five times as likely (23%) to use CAM as children whose parent did not (5%).

Figure 11-4 shows the disease or condition for which adults and children are most likely to seek CAM. The 2002 survey also addressed the important question: Why do people use CAM? Previous studies revealed general issues of the overuse of technology and a reductionist approach to care, managed-care time constraints limiting visits and eroding the physician-patient relationship, and the explosion of Internet-based information on CAM. Astin (1998) found that along with being more educated and reporting poor health status, most alternative medicine users were not dissatisfied with conventional medicine, but rather found these health care alternatives to be more congruent with their own values, beliefs, and philosophic orientations toward health and life. Only 4.4% reported relying primarily on CAM therapies for their health care. A subsequent study of patients using both CAM and conventional care also found that use of CAM did not primarily reflect dissatisfaction with conventional care (Eisenberg et al., 2001).

Reasons for CAM use reported in the 2002 NHIS study are shown in Figure 11-5, with slightly more than one half of all respondents believing CAM *combined with* conventional medicine would be helpful.

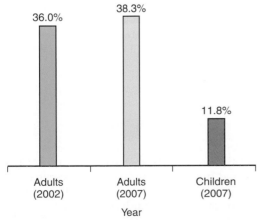

Figure 11-2 Complementary and alternative medicine (CAM) use by U.S. adults (2002, 2007) and Children (2007).
(From Barnes PM, Bloom B, Nahin R. Complementary and alternative medicine use among adults and children: United States, 2007. CDC National Health Statistics Report No 12. December 2008.)

Trends in CAM Use

The 2002 and 2007 NHIS data show that although the overall prevalence of CAM use by adults had remained relatively stable (36% and 38%, respectively), there have been significant increases in some therapies, including acupuncture, deep-breathing exercises, massage therapy, meditation, naturopathy, and yoga (see Figure 11-3). Several factors may account for this growth, including increasing state licensure of some of the practices and greater public awareness of their use through the press and Internet resources. Characteristics of adult and pediatric CAM users are similar in that education, poverty status, geographic region, number of health conditions, physician visits in the prior year, and delaying or not receiving conventional care because of cost are all associated with CAM use. Overall reasons for CAM use fall into two equal categories: (1) treating a variety of health problems, especially pain, and (2) promoting general health and wellness. Much of CAM use is "self-care" and is mostly used with conventional care.

Important U.S. Reports

Key Points

- The White House Commission on CAM created a blueprint for public policy and health care transformation in 2002.
- The Institute of Medicine's 2005 CAM report and 2009 summit called for expanding research, education, and clinical application.
- CAM challenges conventional research methods.
- CAM creates opportunities for innovative studies.
- The NIH National Center for Complementary and Alternative Medicine 2010 Strategic Plan will set an agenda for more CAM research.

Over the past two decades, several important reports have addressed CAM and integrative medicine in the United States. This section summarizes the major themes and recommendations.

White House Commission 2002 Report

The White House Commission on Complementary and Alternative Medicine Policy (WHCCAMP) 2002 report was the culmination of 18 months of in-depth work of a committee of 20 appointed commissioners. Their task was to provide the president, through the secretary of Health and Human Services, with a report containing legislative and administrative recommendations that would ensure a public policy that maximized the potential benefits of CAM to all. Specifically, the commission addressed the coordination of research to increase knowledge about CAM products; the education and training of health care practitioners in CAM; the provision of reliable and useful information about CAM practices and products to health care professionals; and guidance regarding appropriate access to and delivery of CAM. Table 11-4 lists the 10 guiding principles the commission endorsed for their process of making recommendations. The final report lists 29 recommendations and more than 100 action steps as a blueprint for shaping future CAM policy.

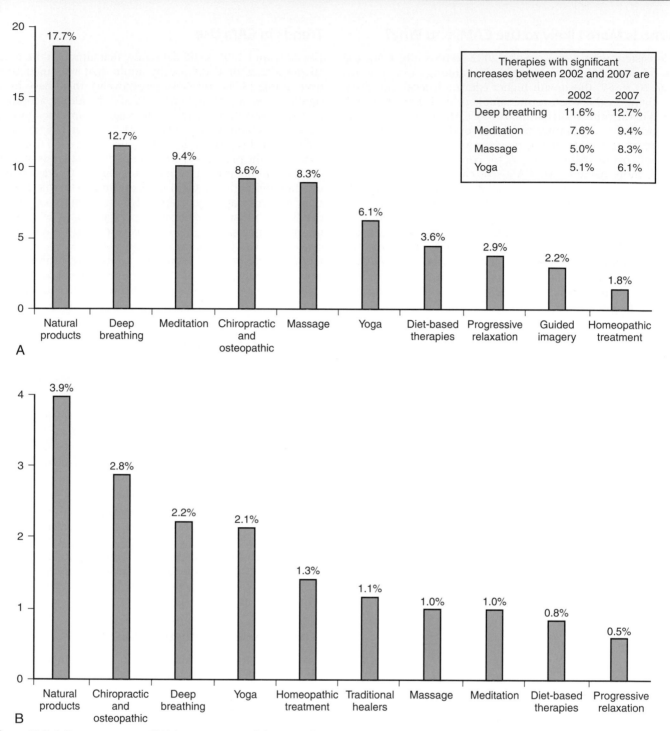

Figure 11-3 **A,** Ten most common CAM therapies among adults in 2007. **B,** Ten most common CAM therapies among children in 2007.
(From Barnes PM, Bloom B, Nahin R. Complementary and alternative medicine use among adults and children: United States, 2007. CDC National Health Statistics Report No 12. December 2008.)

Institute of Medicine 2005 Report and 2009 Summit

The Institute of Medicine (IOM) of the National Academy of Sciences acts as a private, nonprofit, society of scholars engaged in research dedicated to the promotion of science and technology for the public good. Because of the American public's increasing use of CAM and the many concerns regarding safety, efficacy, and information access, a report was commissioned and a committee charged to explore the emerging scientific, policy, and practice questions. The

300-page report released in 2005 gave specific recommendations in the domains of research, education, and clinical care; new and innovative approaches to research were considered essential. The IOM Committee Chair placed a "call to action" to researchers (Bondurant, 2005):

Ignoring CAM is not an option. The widespread use of CAM by patients is a mandate to the scientific community to improve our relatively weak scientific understanding of CAM practices. Moreover,

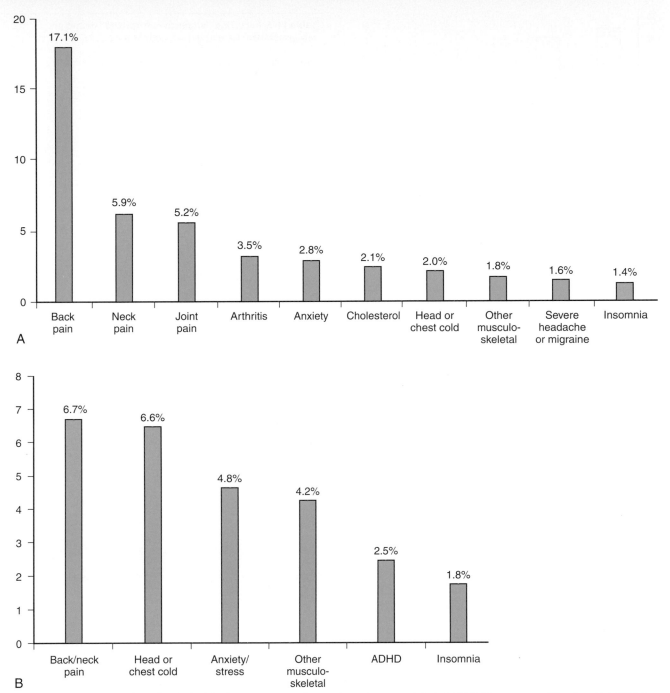

Figure 11-4 A, Disease or condition for which CAM therapies are most frequently used among adults in 2007. **B,** Disease or condition for which CAM therapies are most frequently used among children in 2007.

(From Barnes PM, Bloom B, Nahin R. Complementary and alternative medicine use among adults and children: United States, 2007. CDC National Health Statistics Report No 12. December 10, 2008.)

health professionals have a duty to their patients to bring these 2 worlds of contemporary medical practice together. The path to this outcome begins with adopting the same standards of evidence.

In 2009, IOM and the Bravewell Collaborative convened a 3-day summit, Integrative Medicine and the Health of the Public. More than 600 scientists, academic leaders, policy experts, health practitioners, advocates, and other participants from various disciplines examined the practice of integrative medicine, its scientific basis, and its potential for improving health. Note how the recurring themes and shared values listed in Table 11-5 resonate with the principles of family medicine and the foundations of the patient-centered medical home (PCMH). Family physician Victor Sierpina shared a vision for integrative medicine and the physician of the future (Table 11-6).

NCCAM Strategic Plan 2010

Now in its third cycle of 5-year strategic planning, NCCAM continues to explore CAM healing practices in the context of science, train CAM researchers, and disseminate authoritative information to public and professional communities.

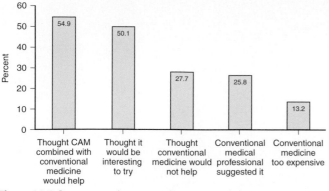

Figure 11-5 Reasons people use complementary and alternative medicine (CAM) therapies.
(From Barnes PM, Towell-Griner E, McFann K, Nahin RL: Complementary and alternative medicine use among adults: United States, 2002. CDC Advance Data Report No 343, 2004.)

Table 11-4 Guiding Principles: 2002 White House Commission on Complementary and Alternative Medicine Policy

1. A wholeness orientation in health care delivery
2. Evidence of safety and efficacy
3. The healing capacity of the person
4. Respect for individuality
5. The right to choose treatment
6. An emphasis on health promotion and self-care
7. Partnerships are essential for integrated health care
8. Education as a fundamental health care service
9. Dissemination of comprehensive and timely information
10. Integral public involvement

NCCAM's course for 2010–2014 is to create priority areas of CAM research to focus efforts that would best serve public need while meeting fiscal realities, as guided by four factors: (1) scientific promise, (2) extent and nature of practice and use, (3) amenability to rigorous scientific inquiry, and (4) potential to change health practices.

Nahin and Straus (2001) and Ahn and Kaptchuk (2005) discuss the unique challenges that CAM presents to conventional research approaches in evidence-based medicine (see Chapter 8). Many CAM study therapies are complex and heterogeneous compared with the more familiar single-drug trial of biomedicine. As such, innovative research strategies, such as those for sham acupuncture, will need to be continually developed. CAM may help the science of medicine to further evolve, as reflected on by Linde and Jonas (1999):

> *The continuing interface between orthodox and unorthodox medicine today provides the opportunity for new research strategies and methodologies to arise. By purposefully maintaining a creative tension between the established and frontier, we can advance scientific methods and more clearly define the boundaries and purpose of the scientific process for medicine.*

Table 11-5 Recurring Perspectives from IOM Summit on Integrative Medicine and the Health of the Public

Vision of optimal health: Alignment of individuals and their health care for optimal health and healing across a full life span.

Conceptually inclusive: Seamless engagement of the full range of established health factors—physical, psychological, social, preventive, and therapeutic.

Lifespan horizon: Integration across the life span to include personal, predictive, preventive, and participatory care.

Person-centered: Integration around, and within, each person.

Prevention-oriented: Prevention and disease minimization as the foundation of integrative health care.

Team-based: Care as a team activity, with the patient as a central team member.

Care integration: Seamless integration of the care processes, across caregivers and institutions.

Caring integration: Person- and relationship-centered care.

Science integration: Integration across approaches to care (e.g., conventional, traditional, alternative, complementary), as the evidence supports.

Policy opportunities: Emphasis on outcomes, elevation of patient insights, consideration of family and social factors, inclusion of team care and supportive follow-up, and contributions to the learning process.

From Institute of Medicine (IOM). Integrative Medicine and the Health of the Public: a summary of the February 2009 summit. Washington, DC, National Academies Press, 2009, p 5.

Table 11-6 How the Physician of the Future Will Function

The care process is…	The doctor's role will be…
Patient centered	A navigator
Team based	Part of a multidisciplinary team
High-touch, high-tech	Grounded in the community
Genomic and personalized Preventive Integrative	Support of social and environmental policies promoting health
And supports patients through…	**And will follow…**
Complementary and alternative practices	Evidence-based, outcome-focused practices
Belief that the body helps heal itself	Principles for creations of healing environments
	The lead of empowered patients

From Institute of Medicine (IOM). Integrative medicine and the health of the public: summary of the February 2009 summit. Washington, DC, The National Academics Press, 2009, p. 43.

Integrating Complementary and Alternative Medicine into Practice

Key Points

- Nutrition, mind-body medicine, and spirituality are core elements of integrative medicine practice.
- Strong evidence supports mind-body medicine for coronary artery disease, low back pain, and headache.
- Acupuncture is a safe and efficacious adjunctive treatment for several musculoskeletal conditions.
- Energy medicine researchers use current technologies to explore the frontiers of CAM.

Because the field of CAM and integrative medicine is so broad and includes so many different approaches and modalities, this section reviews core elements and then explores three common CAM modalities with evidence of efficacy: acupuncture, yoga, and homeopathy. Energy medicine, an important frontier of the CAM field, is also discussed.

Core Elements of Integrative Medicine

Nutrition, mind-body medicine, and spirituality are considered core elements of an integrative medicine approach and often are applied during patient consultation. These elements also tend to be cost-effective and patient empowering. Considered the foundation of good health and enhanced healing, nutritional principles are key elements in most treatment plans.

The adage "food is medicine" is becoming ever more important as the United States faces impending epidemics of diabetes and obesity. When the new food pyramid was released by the U.S. federal government (MyPyramid.gov), critics such as Walter Willett commented, "This is a huge lost opportunity to convey information about healthy food choices that could benefit Americans enormously.... The pyramid tells nothing of healthy food choices" (Mitka, 2005).

Other options are considered in the Healing Foods Pyramid (Figure 11-6). While developing the best nutrition advice for the diverse people seen at the University of Michigan's Integrative Medicine Clinic, family physician Monica Myklebust found various recommendations for the prevention and treatment of obesity, mood disorders, heart disease, diabetes, chronic pain, and inflammation. The result of her work is a user-friendly tool that brings all of these data together. Omega-3 fatty acids, antioxidants, medicinal seasonings, soy, chocolate, and tea are all considered. For example, green tea offers a variety of health benefits, with emerging evidence for prevention of cancer, stroke, and cardiovascular disease (Schneider and Segre, 2009). Health concerns regarding the sources of U.S. food and recommendations for organic and wild food are discussed. The Healing Foods Pyramid is available as a web-based interactive version (www.med.umich.edu/umim/clinical/pyramid). The top is left open to be filled in by what individuals feel may complete and customize their pyramid.

A particular aspect of nutrition that has received increasing attention for its value in lessening inflammation is that of fish oil (i.e., omega-6 and omega-3 fatty acids). Omega-3 fatty acids consist of eicosapentaenoic acid (EPA) and docosahexaenoic acid (DHA) and are mostly found in fatty fish, such as herring and salmon. Because inflammation plays a role in several common conditions, such as cardiovascular disease, asthma, arthritis, psoriasis, and inflammatory bowel disease, research has explored the role of omega-3 fatty acids in reducing symptoms and improving outcomes. Practical applications for recommending fish oil in the primary care setting included the following (Oh, 2005):

1. The American Heart Association recommends 1 gram (g) per day for all patients with documented coronary artery disease through diet or through supplementation.
2. For patients with mild or persistent hypertriglyceridemia, use of 2 to 4 g per day of fish oil may lower levels by 20% to 50% to reach ATP III goals.
3. For those with rheumatoid arthritis, doses of 2.6 to 6 g per day for at least 8 to 12 weeks are optimal and may reduce or eliminate nonsteroidal anti-inflammatory drug (NSAID) use.

Monitoring for clinical bleeding and for low-density lipoprotein (LDL) cholesterol and glycemic response should be considered for patients taking doses higher than 3 g/day, especially if they are diabetic. Unfortunately, because our waters are polluted with heavy metals, avoiding fish known to have high methyl mercury levels (especially by women who are pregnant and of childbearing age) is an important precaution when discussing fish oil use with patients (Williams, 2005). Along with fish oil consumption, other dietary modifications are also known to help lessen inflammation; Table 11-7 shows guidelines for prescribing an anti-inflammatory diet (Rakel, 2003; Rakel and Rindfleisch, 2006).

Mind-Body Medicine

The area of CAM with perhaps the most extensive research base is mind-body medicine, which encompasses a diverse array of practices that overlap many traditions and whole systems of care. Astin and colleagues (2003) concluded, "There is now considerable evidence that an array of mind-body therapies can be used as effective adjuncts to conventional medical treatment for a number of common clinical conditions." They found strong evidence to support mind-body approaches in the treatment of low back pain, coronary artery disease, headache, insomnia, preparing for surgical procedures, and in the management of disease-related symptoms of cancer, arthritis, and urinary incontinence.

Given the relative ease of learning and employing such techniques, NCCAM has made research into mind-body medicine a priority. Mind-body medicine approaches may enhance healing and optimize health. They may be recommended to most patients for health maintenance and disease management and could easily be incorporated into a PCMH through group visits or health coaches. In addition, a recent study of 70 primary care physicians who participated in an intensive mindfulness education program over 1 year showed dramatic improvements in mindfulness skills, burnout, mood disturbance, and empathy (Krasner et al., 2009). An accompanying editorial noted that the study "demonstrates that training physicians in the art of mindful practice has the potential to promote physician health *through* work." Also,

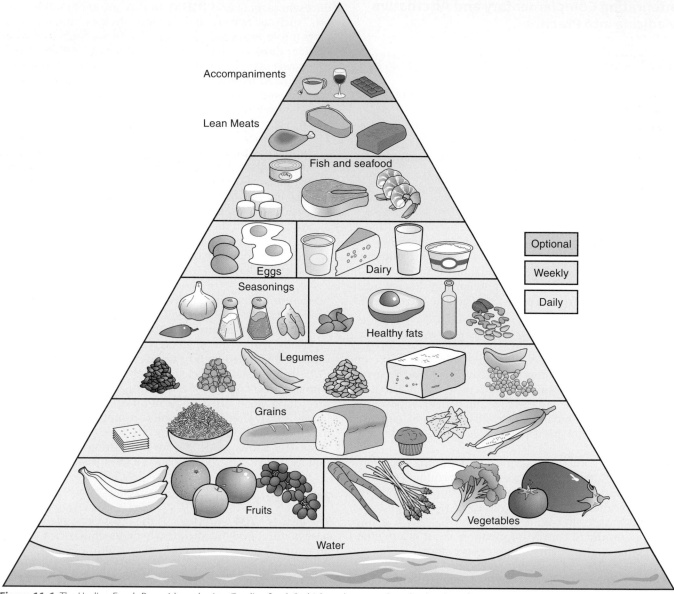

Accompaniments

Lean Meats

Fish and seafood

Optional

Weekly

Daily

Eggs

Dairy

Seasonings

Healthy fats

Legumes

Grains

Fruits

Vegetables

Water

Figure 11-6 The Healing Foods Pyramid emphasizes "healing foods," which are known to have healing benefits or essential nutrients; plant-based choices, which create the base and may be accented by animal foods; variety and balance of color, nutrients, and portions sizes; a healthful environment; and "mindful eating" to savor and focus on the food being eaten.

(Courtesy Monica Myklebust, MD, and Jenna Wunder, MPH, RD, University of Michigan Integrative Medicine Clinical Services, Regents of the University of Michigan. http://www.med.umich.edu/unim/clinical/pyramid/.)

recognizing and enhancing the meaning derived from the practice of medicine using these skills may "protect against burnout and promote patient-centered care for the benefit of both physicians and their patients" (Shanafelt, 2009).

Online **eAppendix 11-2** (www.expertconsult.com) highlights a well-known and well-studied mind-body technique called *mindfulness-based stress reduction* (MBSR) and includes a short audio sample of mindful breath work for the interested reader to try.

Spirituality

Another area thought to be integral to a whole-patient integrative medicine approach to care is spirituality. This broad and controversial subject is well reviewed (e.g., Sierpina and Sierpina, 2004); some key issues are considered here. Working definitions and terms from the Samueli Conference on Definitions and Standards in Healing Research (Dossey, 2003) include the following:

Spirituality encompasses the feelings, thoughts, experiences, and behaviors that arise from a search for that which is generally considered sacred or holy. Spirituality is usually considered to involve a sense of connection with an absolute, imminent, or transcendent spiritual force, however named, as well as the conviction that meaning, value, direction, and purpose are valid aspects of the universe.

Religion is the codified and ritualized beliefs and behaviors of those involved in spirituality, usually taking place within a community of like-minded individuals.

Table 11-7 Guidelines in Prescribing an Anti-Inflammatory Diet

1. Omega-3 and omega-6 fatty acids are essential polyunsaturated fatty acids (i.e., they cannot be made by the human body).
2. The ratio of omega-6 to omega-3 fatty acids in the average Western diet has steadily increased in the past 100 years. The standard American diet has a ratio of omega-6 to omega-3 of more than 20:1, but the ideal range is less than 4:1.
3. To follow an anti-inflammatory diet, take the following steps:
   a. Decrease red meat, poultry, and dairy intake.
   b. Increase the intake of omega-3 fatty acids, such as cold-water fish, flaxseed, walnuts, and green leafy vegetables.
   c. Even one meal of cold-water fish weekly reduces the risk of cardiac arrest. Consuming fish twice each week is ideal. If this is not possible, fish oil supplements can be taken at a dose of 500 to 2000 mg twice daily.
   d. An alternative is ground flax seeds or flaxseed oil. Flax should be freshly ground because it can spoil after exposure to light or heat. Supplementation can be provided with 500 to 2000 mg of flax oil twice daily.
   e. Reduce foods that contain omega-6 fatty acids, including the following:
      (1) Margarine.
      (2) Oils made from corn, cottonseed, grapeseed, peanut, safflower, sesame, soybean, or sunflower (avoid partially hydrogenated oils).
      (3) Foods with a long shelf life, such as crackers and chips.
   f. Cook with monounsaturated oils such as olive or canola oil.
4. Consider this dietary approach to treat the following:
   a. Heart disease or associated risk factors.
   b. Inflammatory rheumatic disorders.
   c. Autoimmune diseases.
   d. Chronic pain.
5. Low-carbohydrate, high-protein diets tend to have high omega-6 fat content and should be used with caution.
6. It may take up to 6 months to see the full clinical effects of an anti-inflammatory diet.

From Rakel D, Rindfleisch A: Integrative medicine. In Essential Family Medicine: Fundamentals and Case Studies. Philadelphia, Saunders, 2006.

Table 11-8 Spiritual Assessment Tools

FICA Mnemonic

F: Faith or belief—What is your faith or belief?

I: Importance and influence—Is it important in your life? How?

C: Community—Are you part of a religious community?

A: Awareness and addressing—What would you want me as your physician to be aware of?

How would you like me to address these issues in your care?

HOPE Mnemonic

H: Hope—What are your sources of hope, meaning, strength, peace, love, and connectedness?

O: Organized—Do you consider yourself part of an organized religion?

P: Personal spirituality and practices—What aspects of your spirituality or spiritual practices do you find most helpful?

E: Effects—How do your beliefs affect the kind of medical care you would like me to provide?

Three Questions

1. What helps you get through tough times?

2. Who do you turn to when you need support?

3. What meaning does this experience have for you?

Prayer is communication with an absolute, imminent, or transcendent spiritual force, however named. Such communication may take a variety of forms and may be theistic or nontheistic in nature, as in some forms of Buddhism. *Intercessory prayer* is an appeal to such a force to influence another person or thing. *Healing prayer* is an appeal to such a force for the healing and recovery of self or others. *Directed prayer* is offered with a specific outcome in mind. *Nondirected prayer* is offered with no specific outcome in mind, such as, "Thy will be done," or "May the best outcome prevail."

Given recent statistics on prayer from the 2002 National Health Interview Survey (NHIS) and Gallup Polls over the past six decades (showing that more than 90% of Americans believe in God or a universal spirit), it is not surprising that proponents and critics have agreed that taking a spiritual history is essential to a comprehensive and culturally sensitive medical consultation. Just as challenging as asking patients about substance abuse, domestic violence, and sexual practices, a spiritual history helps elucidate how spiritual beliefs or religious practices may impact health and health-related choices. Such discussions may be most relevant during times of a new diagnosis, loss of a loved

one, onset of depression, or terminal illness. Continuity of care and sensitivity to the biopsychosocial aspects of a patient's life foster the rapport to facilitate such discussion. Such inquiry may also help engage support systems or identify deep conflicts. Although not all physicians may be comfortable addressing spirituality with their patients, referrals to colleagues in pastoral care and chaplaincy are options to consider.

Interviewing seven physicians recognized as leaders in the field of healing research, Egnew (2005) found that "healing was defined in terms of developing a sense of personal wholeness that involves physical, mental, emotional, social and spiritual aspects of human experience." The central theme in the responses provided an operational definition of healing: "Healing is the personal experience of the transcendence of suffering."

Various models have been suggested as guides to taking the spiritual history (Table 11-8) (Anandarajah and Hight, 2001; Kinney, 1999; Puchalski and Romer, 2000).

Acupuncture, Yoga, and Homeopathic Remedies

Three areas of CAM are most likely to be encountered in the family physician's office: acupuncture, yoga, and homeopathic remedies (see Chapter 52 online for herbs and supplements). As shown in Table 11-9, these three areas are components of whole systems or *nonallopathic* medical systems of care: *acupuncture* within traditional Chinese medicine (TCM), *yoga* as a part of Ayurveda, and *homeopathic remedies* as the mainstay of homeopathy. Many

Table 11-9 Nonallopathic Medical Systems

Traditional Chinese Medicine

Philosophy: Qi and other substances flow through the body through various channels, or meridians. Yin and yang (i.e., passive and active) and the five elements (i.e., wood, fire, earth, metal, and water) have competing influences on various body parts. Excesses or deficiencies of these cause illness. Pain is blocked qi.

Diagnostics: A specific diagnosis is not needed. Information is gathered by the four kanbing: looking (i.e., observation of posture, coloring, gait, demeanor, appearance of the tongue); asking about the status of the 11 basic areas, including body temperature, sleep, fluid metabolism, pain, and digestion; listening to the body's sounds, including breathing, voice, and peristalsis; and palpation of the affected site and the pulse. The pulse is thought to have three parts that correlate with the status of different parts of the body.

Therapeutics: Acupuncture is the insertion of needles into various points along the qi meridians. Moxibustion is the burning of moxa (*Artemisia vulgaris*) on or near meridian points. Gua sha is pressing the skin with a hard, round-edged instrument to create petechiae. Cupping is the creation of a vacuum in a cup and applying the vacuum pressure to the skin. Tui na is manipulation or massage with specific hand movements. Plum blossom is a cluster of needles that is moved along a meridian. Herbal therapies typically are combinations of multiple herbs mixed specifically for the individual patient.

Ayurveda

Philosophy: The concept emerged in India 5000 years ago, and it incorporates five elements and three types of energy, or doshas. Vata is the dosha associated with movement, pitta governs metabolism, and kapha maintains structure. Diet, lifestyle, and relationships shape a person's energy and define health status. Ancient texts divide illnesses according to subspecialties, many of which are the same as for biomedicine.

Diagnostics: Factors that may have weakened the person's defenses are considered, such as genetics, trauma, diet, habits, seasonal affects, climate, age, balance of the doshas, emotions, metabolism, and acts of God. A full physical examination includes evaluation of pulses, speech and voice, eyes, tongue, and the appearance of the urine and feces.

Therapeutics: Approaches include prevention, detoxification, reestablishment of one's unique constitutional balance. Foods, emotions, and behaviors are used to adjust dosha levels. Panchakarma is used to remove aggravated doshas and toxins. Components of panchakarma include therapeutic vomiting, use of purgatives or laxatives, nasal administration of medications, blood purification (traditionally by blood-letting, now more often with teas), and therapeutic enemas.

Naturopathy

Philosophy: The body is able to heal itself by means of the healing power of nature. Healing occurs through a diet of natural, unrefined foods; adequate exercise; avoidance of environmental toxins; proper elimination of body wastes; and positive thoughts and emotions. Key principles in patient care include doing no harm, taking a preventive approach, and focusing on maintenance of health rather than just on the treatment of disease. The naturopath's goals are to educate, empower, and motivate.

Diagnostics: Methods may draw from any number of approaches, including laboratory testing not commonly performed in a biomedical setting.

Therapeutics: Approaches can include nutrition, botanicals, homeopathy, Chinese medicine, physical medicine (e.g., ultrasound, massage, manipulation), hydrotherapy (e.g., baths, steams, wraps, colonic irrigation), and various detoxification regimens.

Homeopathy

Philosophy: Homeopathy is based on the law of similars, which holds that medicines can produce the same symptoms in healthy people that they cure in those who are ill. Remedies are used in the smallest quantity possible, which can often mean they are diluted to the point that not even a molecule of the original therapeutic substance remains in solution.

Diagnostics: A detailed history is taken relating to the specific nature of symptoms. For example, otitis media is treated differently based on the mood of the child, which ear is sore, the nature of the fever, and the nature of the pain.

Therapeutics: A remedy that has elicited a similar set of symptoms in a healthy patient is given in minute quantity to the ill person. The degree to which a remedy is diluted is given as a Roman numeral. For example, a 6X solution has been diluted to one tenth of its strength six times (i.e., to 10^{-6} of the original strength), and a 200C solution has been diluted to 1/100 of its original strength 200 subsequent times (i.e., to 10^{-400} of its original strength).

From Rakel D, Rindfleisch A: Integrative medicine. In Essential Family Medicine: Fundamentals and Case Studies. Philadelphia, Saunders, 2006.

family physicians have pursued professional training in these fields and are now integrating new skills and perspectives into their practice. The Society of Teachers of Family Medicine (STFM) *Group on Hospital Medicine and Procedural Training* has proposed that acupuncture become an advanced procedure within the scope of family medicine training (Kelly, 2009).

Although challenging to research, trials have shown acupuncture efficacious as an adjunctive therapy in osteoarthritis of the knee (Berman et al., 2004) and as a complement to standard therapy for the debilitating effect of pelvic girdle pain during pregnancy (Elden et al., 2005). Cochrane reviews have shown that acupuncture benefits patients with chronic low back pain, neck pain, and headache (migraine

Table 11-10 Commonly Used Movement Therapies

Therapy*	Description	Research
Hatha yoga	Focuses on the use of postures (asanas) and breathing exercises (pranayama); traditionally used in India to purify the body and maximize the impact of meditation practice; many different schools; must be used with caution by those with glaucoma, retinal detachment, or at high risk for muscle strain or fracture.	Most trials are quite small. Positive benefits likely for musculoskeletal and other types of pain, lowering autonomic nervous system sympathetic tone; decreasing histamine effects of FEV_1 in asthmatic patients; reducing blood pressure; headaches, diabetes, osteoarthritis, rheumatoid arthritis; overall improvement in balance, endurance, and vitality.
Tai chi	Developed more than 5000 years ago; movement and breathing, often associated with specific flowing movement patterns, are used to affect the flow of energy, or qi.	Useful adjunctive therapy for arthritis and cardiovascular disease. Helpful for improving postural stability and decreasing fall risk in older adults.
Qigong (Qi gong)	Part of traditional Chinese medicine; also used to cultivate qi; includes breathing exercises, meditation, and physical movement; used in the martial arts and to generate energy to be used in healing.	Most studies conducted in China. Potentially useful for hypertension, decreasing overall stroke and mortality rates compared with controls, decreasing peripheral vascular resistance, increasing bone density; improvement of blood flow to brain (e.g., adjunctive treatment for memory loss, dizziness, insomnia, vertigo); improvement of cardiac output, ejection fraction, and valve function.
Feldenkrais	Developed by Moshe Feldenkrais in the 1950s; gentle movements and manipulation enlisted to retrain the body with new movement patterns.	Limited randomized trial–based research. Used to promote flexibility and posture, decrease back pain, and improve vocal cord function.

From Rakel D, Rindfleisch A. Integrative medicine. In Essential Family Medicine: Fundamentals and Case Studies. Philadelphia, Saunders, 2006.
*Other therapies include *Alexander technique*, which uses minimal effort to maximize efficiency of muscle use and alleviate problems associated with poor posture, and *Pilates*, which also uses exercises and other techniques used to strengthen postural muscles.
FEV_1, Forced expiratory volume in 1 second.

and tension) (Kelly, 2009). A meta-analysis evaluating 33 randomized, controlled trials (RCTs) of acupuncture for acute and chronic low back pain concluded that acupuncture effectively relieves chronic low back pain, although no evidence suggests that it is more effective than other active therapies (Manheimer et al., 2005).

Excellent reviews of acupuncture's theory, efficacy, and practice (Kaptchuk, 2002; Nielsen and Hammerschlag, 2004) cite the 1997 NIH Consensus Development Panel findings on acupuncture. After reviewing all available evidence from RCTs up to 1997, the panel concluded that clear evidence shows that acupuncture is efficacious for adult postoperative and chemotherapy nausea and vomiting and for postoperative dental pain. The panel also reported that acupuncture should be considered a useful adjunct for addiction, stroke rehabilitation, osteoarthritis, headache, low back pain, tennis elbow, menstrual cramps, carpal tunnel, and fibromyalgia (NIH, 1998).

Yoga, a widely popular and rapidly increasing CAM practice in the United States, has its roots in ancient India and is a Sanskrit word that means "yoke" or "union." The original goal of practicing these postures was to purify and prepare the body for higher states of consciousness. *Hatha yoga,* as described in Table 11-10 along with other types of movement therapies, has many different styles and is the most popular form taught and practiced in the United States today. Because most yoga instructors are not medical professionals, it is recommended to refer a patient to a teacher with several years' experience. A study

of the efficacy of yoga on pregnancy outcome (N =335) concluded that an integrated approach to yoga during pregnancy was safe and that it improved birth weight and decreased preterm labor and intrauterine growth retardation with no complications (Narendran et al., 2005). A recent study of 90 patients with chronic low back pain who participated in a 24-week trial of yoga twice a week showed those receiving the yoga intervention experienced decreased levels of pain, functional disability, and depression (Williams et al., 2009). The International Association of Yoga Therapists (IAYT) is a worldwide organization for yoga teachers, therapists, and researchers (www.iayt.org). The Yoga Alliance (www.yogaalliance.org), formed in 1999, sets minimum training standards for yoga teachers. Both organizations provide sound resources for professionals and the public.

Perhaps the most controversial of CAM therapies, *homeopathy* seems to defy biomedicine's attempts to decipher its mechanism of action. Particularly perplexing is the concept that the more dilute the remedy, the more potent is its effect. Founded by the German physician Samuel Hahnemann (1755–1843), homeopathy is still widely accepted and practiced in Europe and is now experiencing a renaissance in the United States. A brilliant linguist and scholar, Dr. Hahnemann developed the Principle of Similars, in which "like cures like" based on his medical translation work and personal experience of malaria symptoms after taking *Cinchona* bark, which was then the treatment for the disease. A critical overview of homeopathy by Jonas and colleagues (2003) reviewed the research regarding specific conditions and the placebo effect. After analyzing systematic reviews of clinical trials, the authors concluded, "Despite skepticism about the plausibility of homeopathy, some randomized, placebo-controlled trials and laboratory research report unexpected effects of homeopathic medicine. However, the evidence on the effectiveness of homeopathy for specific clinical conditions is scant, is of uneven quality, and is generally poorer quality than research done in allopathic medicine."

Known for his groundbreaking research showing homeopathic treatment of allergic rhinitis more effective than placebo (Taylor et al., 2000), David Reilly of Glasgow, Scotland, commented on the increasing scientific validation for homeopathy over the past decade. Noting that studies reviewed show positive evidence for overall effect and citing the growing prospective, observational research that indicates beneficial outcomes, Reilly (2005) points out that homeopathy can offer therapeutic options when conventional care has failed or reached a plateau, no conventional treatments exist, conventional treatments are contraindicated, side effects of conventional treatments are not tolerated, and patients are reluctant to accept conventional care. An important distinction clouds other areas of medical research: "The two dimensions of care need to be considered: the direct effects of the remedy and the therapeutic impact of the method of approach on the patient." Believing that the homeopathic approach is helping to reintroduce a holistic perspective in medical practice, Reilly concludes, "The evidence mosaic for homeopathy reinforces clinicians' and patients' experiential knowledge that this approach can make a valuable contribution to care, especially when applied with a whole person perspective and integrated with conventional knowledge."

Energy Medicine: Frontier Science of Complementary and Alternative Medicine

The practice of CAM presents many challenges to Western science. How does acupuncture work, and what is qi? How can dilute homeopathic remedies induce effects on biologic systems? What are the *chakras*, or energy centers, so integral to yoga and Ayurveda? These mysteries present us with opportunities for new discoveries and an expansion of our healing capacities (eAppendix 11-3). Many scientists are showing how research in biophysics and biomagnetism is helping to elucidate the subtle energies of

Table 11-11 Precautions in Complementary and Alternative Medicine

1. Primum non nocere (first, do no harm).

2. Patients may encounter complications if they abandon effective, conventional therapies in favor of complementary and alternative medicine (CAM).

3. Medicolegal issues and certification or qualification requirements of practitioners are important topics, not covered in this chapter.

biologic systems, including those of humans. Advanced technologies such as functional magnetic resonance imaging and infrared thermography are demonstrating amazing images that seem to correlate with empiric knowledge (eAppendix 11-4).

Open-minded scientists are helping to bridge the worlds of CAM and conventional medicine by linking research findings to those of clinical practice (Oschman, 2002). "Let us document each of these fascinating clues. We will connect the dots by describing an information system in the body that is the missing link for many phenomena that have seemed hopelessly inexplicable in the past. It is a system that is responsible for extraordinary feasts of perception, movement, and healing" (Oschman, 2003, p. xiv).

Conclusion

Complementary and alternative medicine is an evolving area of health care used by approximately 4 in 10 adults and 1 in 9 children in the United States. As a diverse system of varied approaches and philosophies of healing, CAM is usually incorporated into conventional health care as integrative medicine. CAM presents opportunities to expand the current research paradigm to meet the challenges of studying its multidimensional approach to health and healing. Prominent organizations such as the IOM have placed a call to action to the medical community to advance knowledge and clinical applications in this field. Family physicians, specialists in caring for the whole person though a continuous, healing relationship, are in the ideal discipline to advance the integration of safe and effective CAM into their repertoire to optimize the health of their patients (Table 11-11). Ultimately, complex terminology will subside as the essence of integrative medicine becomes good family medicine.

EVIDENCE-BASED SUMMARY

1. Fish oil supplementation can benefit heart health (Bucher et al., 2002; Wang et al., 2004), hypertriglyceridemia (Balk et al., 2004), and rheumatoid arthritis (Fortin et al., 1995; MacLean et al., 2004) (SOR: A).
2. Acupuncture should be considered as a treatment option for common painful conditions such as chronic low back pain (Furlan et al., 2005; Yuan et al., 2008), neck pain (Fu et al., 2009, Trinh et al., 2006) and headache (migraine, tension) (Linde et al., 2009a, 2009b) (SOR: A).
3. Green tea is associated with decreased risk of stroke and cardiovascular disease (Kuriyama et al., 2006) and may help prevent cancer of the breast (Sun et al., 2006a), gastrointestinal tract (Sun et al., 2006b), and prostate (Kurahashi et al., 2008) (SOR: B).
4. Yoga reduces functional disability, pain, and depression in people with chronic low back pain (Williams et al., 2009) (SOR: B).
5. Mindful communication may improve physician well-being and attitudes associated with patient-centered care (Kearney et al., 2009; Krasner et al., 2009) (SOR: C).

References

The complete reference list is available online at www.expertconsult.com.

Web Resources

www.nccam.nih.gov
> National Center for Complementary and Alternative Medicine, part of the National Institutes of Health (NIH). Offers excellent CAM resources for both patients and clinicians.

http://nccam.nih.gov/timetotalk/ "Time to Talk."
> NCCAM's educational campaign to encourage patients and clinicians to discuss their use of CAM. Download a toolkit for your office.

www.imconsortium.org
> Consortium of Academic Health Centers for Integrative Medicine. Includes 44 member institutions throughout North America who are advancing the field of integrative medicine in the domains of education, research, and clinical care.

www.integrativemedicine.arizona.edu
> Arizona Center for Integrative Medicine. Offers innovative education in integrative medicine.

12 CHAPTER

Establishing Rapport

Robert E. Rakel

Rapport comes from the French *en rapport*, which means "in harmony with." Rapport is most easily established during the patient's first visit, and achieving rapport enhances the likelihood that the patient will comply with the treatment plan. When rapport has been established, patients are more likely to forgive a less than perfect experience or an unexpected poor clinical outcome.

Even the most knowledgeable and skilled physician will have limited effectiveness if he or she is unable to develop rapport with patients. Unfortunately, rapport is one of those intangibles that is more than the sum of its parts. Rapport is not analyzed easily within any one body of knowledge. The basis of rapport, however, is the development of communication skills that instill in patients a sense of confidence and trust by conveying sincerity and an interest in their care and well-being. The patient's satisfaction and compliance with the physician's instructions (both measures of rapport) depend on the ability of the physician to communicate understanding, compassion, and genuine interest in the patient and to display a thorough approach to solving the patient's problems. Patient satisfaction also is related to the physician's efforts in educating patients about the disease process and motivating them to participate in their treatment.

Failure of communication between physician and patient also can affect the outcome of treatment, often as seriously as an error in treatment. More complaints against physicians result from a breakdown of the caring aspect of the doctor-patient relationship than from the technical quality of treatment.

Most complaints against physicians—and those that too frequently lead to legal action—are the result of a lack of communication between physician and patient. The potential for a serious problem always exists when a patient is inadequately informed regarding a diagnostic procedure, treatment, prognosis, or anticipated cost. The misunderstandings that result cause unnecessary expense and grief for both parties.

Similarly, the worries that result from distorted information can jeopardize the physician-patient relationship. When a patient is discussed on hospital rounds or with a colleague in the office, take care that the discussion is not within the patient's hearing distance or within that of other patients. Patients overhearing the conversation may believe the comments apply to them, or they may know the patient involved and relay the information in a distorted manner. Fragments of such conversations, overheard by the patient or others, are too easily taken out of context and can become the focus of fearful fantasies that only serve to increase uneasiness and apprehension.

Compassion, interest, and *thoroughness* are essential components of successful patient care. These features traditionally have been embodied in the term *bedside manner,* which also connotes qualities of concern, kindness, friendliness, wit, and cheerfulness, all of which result in an atmosphere of trust and confidence between physician and patient. The physician with the best bedside manner may be the one who makes no special effort to communicate these feelings but acts in a concerned, natural, and comfortable manner.

Oliver Wendell Holmes said that to be effective, the physician should "speak softly, be well-dressed, have quiet ways and have eyes that do not wander" (1883, p. 388). Lack of eye contact may be interpreted as a lack of concern. A good first impression is certainly a great help in establishing rapport. You do not get a second chance to create a first impression. The physician should approach the patient in an assured, confident (but not cocky or arrogant) manner and present a personal appearance that is acceptable to the patient. Empathetic frankness and honesty are important factors in instilling confidence and trust.

Personal appearance is a significant part of nonverbal communication. Patients consider house staff who wear white coats with conventional street clothes as more competent than those who wear scrub suits. If white coats are worn, the patient sees only the collar, tie, and shoes, and it is therefore important to keep these items neat.

Posture is also important in conveying an image of confidence and competence. Standing erect, moving briskly with head up and stomach in, is better than slouching. Energetic people seldom slump; they sit upright and appear alert. A listless or lethargic appearance can be interpreted as lack of concern.

Before entering the examining room or hospital room to see a patient, review the record briefly and become familiar with the patient's name and its proper pronunciation. If the pronunciation is unusual or difficult, place phonetic markings on the chart as a reminder for future use. Repeat the patient's name when first given it to confirm the pronunciation, and then use the name twice in the first minute to help it register. Review the medical record for particular aspects of the previous visit that should be remembered and commented on, such as the illness treated at that time, family conditions, or other problems. Patients will believe that the well-informed physician is truly interested in them. Additional courtesy, such as opening the door and assisting patients with their coats (especially elderly patients), shows a consideration that aids in establishing and maintaining rapport.

Respect

Patients should believe that their comments are being listened to, carefully considered, and taken seriously. They must believe that the physician values their comments and opinions before trusting him or her with information of a more personal nature. As long as the physician's attitude toward the patient embodies respect, concern, and kindness and a sincere effort is made to understand the patient's difficulties, the patient will overlook or forgive myriad other problems.

Oliver Wendell Holmes advised patients to "Choose a man who is personally agreeable, for a daily visit from an intelligent, amiable, pleasant, sympathetic person will cost you no more than one from a sloven or a boor, and his presence will do more for you than any prescription the other will order" (1883, p. 391).

A lack of confidence, rather than an excess of it, may lead physicians to appear aloof and unconcerned. Too often, physicians think that a godlike image of omnipotence is necessary for the maintenance of the patient's respect and confidence. It is usually a lack of self-confidence that causes physicians to retreat behind this protective image, which limits their ability to help. Secure physicians are freer to establish close personal relationships with patients without fearing their position will be threatened. A physician with a positive self-image is also willing to recognize and admit the limits of personal competence and feels comfortable seeking help from a colleague when such consultation is of value to the patient's care.

The bond of mutual respect is enhanced if the physician makes positive statements about other people. Patients find it difficult to respect a physician who is regularly detractive, making negative statements about other people or other physicians. Any comments that can be interpreted as "building yourself up by tearing someone else down" merely accomplish the reverse.

The effectiveness of physicians depends on the degree of their insight into the limitations of their personalities and the psychological defenses that distort their perceptions of patients. Physicians must recognize patients or situations that make them unreasonably angry or provoked (e.g., a whining, complaining individual who shows no interest in being rehabilitated, preferring a role of social dependency). The physician's emotions, if they go unrecognized, can serve as a barrier to the development of mutual respect. If the physician is aware of negative feelings toward a patient, an effort can be made to avoid showing signs of irritation or anger. It has been said that clenching of the physician's fist is a clinical sign of a hysterical patient. The physician should attempt to remain objective and analyze the situation for its diagnostic value.

Patients with trivial complaints or somatic manifestations of emotional disease sometimes are given less attention than those with clear-cut organic abnormalities. The frequency with which a physician complains about the triviality and inappropriateness of patients' problems has been found to be related to the volume of patients seen and the degree to which the physician feels overburdened. The more patients that physicians see and the more overloaded their practices, the more likely they are to describe patients' complaints as trivial, inappropriate, or bothersome. Physicians who have more time or take more time per patient, and who investigate the patient's complaints more thoroughly, frequently uncover significant factors and less often tend to view the complaints as trivial. Respect for patients involves taking their fears and apprehensions seriously and withholding value judgments. Patients who frequently seek help for nonspecific somatic and functional complaints may be depressed (Widmer et al., 1980).

Patient Satisfaction

A close relationship exists between rapport and patient satisfaction, and this chapter deals with the many facets of that relationship. It is important that the physician make an effort to understand what patients are "going through" (not only their pain and discomfort, but also the effect these have on their lives) and communicate this understanding to them.

Most studies indicate that patient satisfaction depends on information and the degree to which the patient understands the illness. Joos and associates (1993) found that patients whose desires for information and attention to emotional and family problems went unmet were significantly less satisfied with their physicians than those whose desires were met. Even patients with chronic diseases who had lived with the problem for years had questions they wanted answered. Their satisfaction was related more strongly to the desire for information and affective support than to whether the physician conducted examinations and tests. The greater the patients' satisfaction, the more likely they are to comply with treatment recommendations.

Although patient satisfaction is strongly associated with the length of the visit, it can be further enhanced by spending some time talking about nonmedical topics. Even brief chatting about the weather or something nonmedical can give the impression that more time was taken with the patient, thereby reducing the feeling of being rushed through the visit (Gross et al., 1998).

Patient Dissatisfaction

In a typical business, only 4% of customers voice their dissatisfaction. The other 96% say nothing, and 91% never return. This has led to many practices conducting regular patient satisfaction surveys so that problems can be identified.

Communication

The patient should be able to gain access to the clinician on the phone, by e-mail, or by an early appointment, without having to run an obstacle course created by an overly protective staff. Delay in returning a phone call may result in a patient remaining home all day waiting; if the call is not returned at all, the negative effect on rapport is great.

Unwillingness to make communication convenient for the patient usually results in a spiral of increasingly frequent attempts to reach the physician and mounting frustration for everyone. In contrast, physicians who give a high priority to communicating discover that most patients are considerate and even protective of the physician's time. At the beginning of a practice, patients do a certain amount of testing to determine a physician's accessibility; physicians who pass the test find that they are rarely inconvenienced by unnecessary calls or patient visits.

Verbal Communication

Much of the communication process in the clinical interview centers on verbal interchange. Symptoms, past medical history, family medical history, and psychosocial data are transmitted primarily by verbal means. The chief complaint is extremely important because it explains why patients believe they need the physician's help.

Patients who do not mention a concern and who withhold requests are less satisfied with their care and experience less improvement in their symptoms. Bell and colleagues (2001) found that 9% of patients had one or more unvoiced desires and were most hesitant to ask their physician for referrals and for physical therapy. These patients were also less likely to trust their physician. This is an important reason to be sensitive to subtle clues that the patient may be suppressing something important to them. What the patient does *not* say may be as important as what the patient says.

"Slips of the tongue" or major areas of omission (e.g., a married person who never mentions a spouse) may signify problem areas that, when explored, help establish the interviewer as a perceptive person who understands the underlying issues. The interviewer constantly must consider, "Why is the patient telling me that?" Even simple, casual remarks may be the patient's way of broaching issues of great concern; the man who says, "Oh, by the way, a friend of mine has been having some chest pain when he walks a lot. Do you think that sounds serious?" may actually be talking about his own concern that he is unable to face directly. A child may be brought to the office with a trivial problem so that the mother has a chance to discuss with the physician something that is troubling her; the child is a calling card, signaling the need to open the communication channel. The physician who is sensitive to these subtle clues and encourages the patient to discuss what is actually troublesome will find that the rapport established allows future interviews to be much more open and direct.

Hand-on-the-Doorknob Syndrome

The patient's parting phrase is sometimes a clue to the primary reason for the visit, or it may reflect another issue of great concern that is emotionally threatening and could not be voiced until adequate courage was summoned at the moment of departure. It sometimes surfaces as a last, desperate attempt to communicate because, with a hand on door, escape is readily accessible if the physician's reaction is unfavorable. Reasons for this hidden communication by the patient are important and must be recognized and addressed. Because of fear of rejection or humiliation, the patient may test the physician with minor complaints before mentioning the real reason for the visit (Quill, 1989). The physician must be alert to any unusual behavior during an interview (e.g., slips of the tongue, unexpected responses, overenthusiastic denials) and should search further for the underlying reason for the visit when a patient presents with a trivial complaint that appears inappropriate. It is a good practice to ask the patient routinely at the end of a visit, "Is there anything we have not covered, or anything else you would like to ask me?"

Patients with a fear of cancer, for example, often are unable to voice their concern to the physician. Instead, they present with somatic complaints or contrived reasons that necessitate a complete examination. They are hopeful that the examination will allay their fears without it being necessary to express them openly. A female patient presenting for a complete physical examination actually may be concerned over the possibility of a carcinoma of the breast, which her elder sister might have had at the same age or for which a friend recently had surgery. Such situations emphasize the need for a complete family history and a discussion of any patient concerns in an effort to allow these feelings to surface. Attention then should be paid to alleviating the anxiety. Apprehension regarding cancer is widespread, and the only cure for this fear often is a therapeutic conversation with the physician.

Physicians in private practice who have established rapport during an ongoing relationship with patients communicate more easily than do physicians seeing a patient for the first time in an emergency department (ED). Korsch and Negrete (1972) showed that ED physicians did more talking than the patients, although their perception was just the opposite. This was attributed to interaction with unfamiliar patients by house staff in a setting where the stress level is high and the orientation therapeutic. However, Arntson and Philipsborn (1982) found that physicians in private practice for 26 years who knew their patients and saw them in a low-stress situation for diagnosis or health maintenance also talked more than the patients (twice as long). One difference in the two settings was a strong, reciprocal affective relationship between physician and patient in the private office. If either made an affective statement, the other would respond similarly, whereas in the ED, patients expressed twice as many affective statements as did the physicians.

Vocabulary

The use of appropriate vocabulary assists in establishing rapport by ensuring easy and accurate communication. Phrasing questions in simple language appropriate to the patient's level of understanding and avoidance of medical jargon help establish a sense of working together. The patient's cultural background and educational level should be considered, and the physician should avoid using slang or a contrived accent, because the patient will detect the artificiality and consider this patronizing.

Patients prefer to be enlightened, and they demand maximum insight into their care. It is best to start all explanations at a basic level and proceed only as rapidly as the patient's understanding permits. An analysis of 1057 audiotaped patient interviews with 59 primary care physicians and 65 surgeons showed that in 9 of 10 cases, patients did not receive good explanations of proposed treatments or tests (Braddock et al., 1999).

Medical terminology should be avoided unless it is familiar to the patient. For example, some patients have interpreted "lumbar puncture" to mean "an operation to drain the lungs." No longer does the physician gain a therapeutic advantage by writing prescriptions in Latin or impressing the patient with medical terms.

Metaphors can be harmful and are often used without the physician being aware of the negative connotation, unknowingly raising the patient's anxiety level. Attempts to coerce a patient into having surgery with phrases such as "you are living on borrowed time" may cause anxiety and increase postoperative morbidity (Bedell et al., 2004).

Physicians should be sure of what patients mean to convey by their word selection and make certain they are operating at a common level of understanding. When the patient says he or she "drinks a little," inquire further to clarify "a little." If the patient "spits up blood," determine whether it is truly spitting or really vomiting. A major barrier to accurate interpersonal communication is the tendency of people to react to a statement from their own points of view, rather than attempting to interpret it from the speaker's vantage point. If a question exists regarding the clarity of the interpretation, it is best to repeat it to the speaker's satisfaction. Contract negotiators have found that when parties in a dispute realize that they are being understood and each party sees how the situation appears to the other, there is less need to exaggerate and act defensively. Korsch and Negrete (1972) found that some of the longest interviews between physician and patient were caused by failures in communication; they had to spend considerable time trying to "get on the same wavelength." An analysis of the conversations revealed that less than 5% of the physician's conversation was personal or friendly in nature, and that although most of the physicians believed that they had been friendly, fewer than half of patients had this impression.

Nonverbal Communication

Verbal communication occupies so much of daily social interaction that nonverbal communication often is ignored. However, much that is said is unspoken. Communications specialists have demonstrated convincingly that nonverbal messages play a major role in validating or contradicting verbal messages, with great influence as communication symbols in their own right.

Communication between two people is usually one-third nonverbal. What is said verbally often is emphasized nonverbally, and personal attitudes and emotions usually are communicated at the nonverbal level. Nonverbal communicative signals are under less censorship from conscious control than are verbal messages, so they are likely to be more genuine.

Charles Darwin held that there is a unique pattern of nonverbal actions for each emotion. In *Expressions of the Emotions in Man and Animals* (1872), Darwin suggested that emotional expressions are evolutionary remnants of previous adaptive behavior that persist even though currently useless. Snarling as a sign of aggression is one example. Although recent knowledge indicates that emotional expression is learned and genetically mediated, Darwin's idea of a unique pattern of actions has been shown for depression and anxiety and is likely in the future to be demonstrated for other emotional states.

Paralanguage

Paralanguage is the voice effect that accompanies or modifies talking and often communicates meaning. It includes velocity of speech (e.g., fast, slow, hesitant), tone and volume of voice, sighs and grunts, pauses, and inflections. Urgency, sincerity, confidence, hesitation, thoughtfulness, gaiety, sadness, and apprehension all are conveyed by qualities of voice. McCaskey (1979) believes that the literal interpretation (i.e., definition) of words accounts for only 10% of communication between two people, whereas facial expression and tone of voice account for up to 90% of the communication.

There is a real difference between verbal and vocal information. The *verbal message* refers to the words literally transmitted. The *vocal message* includes the emotional quality, the tone of voice, and the frequency and length of pauses—information that is lost when the words are written. Tone of voice, for example, can reverse the meaning of words. Sarcasm is a common example of a contradiction between vocal and verbal messages. Comparative studies have shown that when the vocal and verbal messages transmit contradictory information, the vocal is more accurate.

Physicians should be alert to subtle changes of tone, such as when patients ask whether everything will be all right. Are they asking for reassurance, showing fear, or doubting the diagnosis? Rather than concentrating exclusively on *what* patients are saying, the astute physician will concentrate on *how* they are saying it.

In a study of recordings of surgeons who had been sued and those who had not, the sued group could be identified by their tone of voice. They sounded dominant, whereas the nonsued group sounded less dominant and more concerned. "In the end it comes down to a matter of respect, and the simplest way that respect is communicated is through tone of voice" (Gladwell, 2005, p.43).

Touch

A close personal interest in the patient can be communicated by the appropriate use of touch. The most socially acceptable method in this country is a handshake, enabling the physician to establish early contact with the patient. The handshake, properly used, can convey to the patient sincerity and interest as well as security and poise. It is an inoffensive intrusion into the other person's area of privacy and can be extended under certain circumstances to include the application of the left hand to the lower or upper arm. This technique is often used by politicians to emphasize sincerity and concern (Figure 12-1). A variation of the politician's handshake is the "double-hander," which some equate to a miniature hug.

The handshake as a traditional greeting of friendship began by the raising of exposed hands by two approaching individuals to give evidence that they held no weapons. This proceeded to the grasping of hands or, in the Roman society, the forearms. In the United States, a firm handshake is most acceptable. Usually, the limp or "wet dishrag" handshake indicates lack of interest or insincerity, especially if it is rapidly withdrawn. A moist palm is a sign of nervousness or apprehension, and the "halfway there," fingers-only handshake indicates reluctance or indecision. However, the handshake continues to be modified culturally, and a person should be extremely wary of misinterpreting another person's handshake without understanding his or her cultural background.

In the past in China, the Confucian code of etiquette dictated that there should never be a touching of persons, and even today, Chinese officials may appear reluctant to grasp an extended hand; a Chinese man formerly shook his own hand (Butterfield, 1982). Some young people in the United States have modified the traditional palm-to-palm handshake to a grasping of the thumb and thenar eminence and continue to develop new variations reminiscent of the secret handshakes of fraternal groups.

Touching can be an effective method for communicating concern or compassion and can break down some of the defensive barriers to communication. Caution should be exercised, however, not to use it excessively or earlier than is socially permissible. If used without adequate preparation, touch can be interpreted as an invasion of privacy and a forward and inconsiderate act. During the physical examination, it is best to talk before touching by explaining to the patient what will be done next. Studies of primates have shown that touching gestures usually are considered nonaggressive and calming in nature. When used properly by the physician, touch can be facilitative and welcome.

The tremendous symbolic value of touch as a healing power was demonstrated during the Middle Ages, when people sought relief from scrofula (i.e., tuberculous lymphadenitis) through the king's touch, or royal touch, despite the notoriously low cure rates. This power has been transferred to physicians, and patients often feel better after a routine physical examination. Friedman (1979) stated that 85% of patients leaving a physician's office feel better even if they have not received medication or treatment, and 50% of patients in the waiting room feel better in anticipation of the help they will receive.

Touch, or "laying on of hands," may promote healing, especially if it is imbued by the patient with a special symbolic value. Franz Mesmer (1734–1815) was among the first to emphasize the medical importance of laying on of hands. Mesmer, however, believed that there was a magnetic power in his hands, which he called "animal magnetism" and which he applied to ailing individuals. His theory was unscientific, and although he became famous for successfully treating a number of hysterical patients, he finally was discredited by a committee that included Benjamin Franklin and Antoine Lavoisier. They found his treatments to be without magnetism and essentially useless. They did agree, however, that he had helped many people and had brought about many cures. They attributed these cures to unknown factors rather than to the animal magnetism he claimed. Mesmerism was the forerunner of hypnosis, initially called "artificial somnambulism," developed by Puysegur, a disciple of Mesmer.

The magic of touch can be good medicine, especially when combined with concern, support, and reassurance. *Stroking*, a special kind of touching, describes a physical or symbolic recognition of a person's finer attributes. A stroke may be a kind word, a warm gesture, or a simple touch of the hand. Infants deprived of touch and stroking suffer mental and physical deterioration. Adults also require stroking to maintain a healthy emotional state. Stroking occurs when an interchange between two people leaves one or both with a good or fulfilled feeling.

Lightly touching someone's elbow for less than 3 seconds can give you up to three times the chance of getting what you want (Pease and Pease, 2004). Elbow touching works better in places where touching is not the cultural norm, such as Great Britain and Germany.

Body Language

The astute physician will cultivate observational skills that enable the detection of hidden or subtle clues to diagnosis contained in the patient's nonverbal behavior. *Kinesics* is the study of nonverbal gestures, or body movements, and their meaning as a form of communication. However, specific gestures and their interpretation are of importance only when

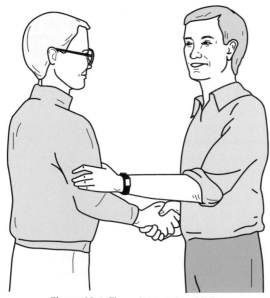

Figure 12-1 The politician's handshake.

judged in the context of the circumstances surrounding them. Body language alone does not reveal the entire behavioral image any more than verbal language does alone. Just as one word does not make a sentence or even have much meaning without the sentence, a single gesture has clinical relevance only as part of a sequence of actions. Although they have significance, individual signs are not reliable when they stand alone; they are meaningful only when considered in the context of a person's total behavioral pattern.

When there is *congruence* between the verbal and nonverbal message—when the gesture conveys the same message as the spoken word—communication and its meaning are probably in agreement. When a person indicates something different from the other, however, the *nonverbal* message usually is more accurate. Unless body language, tone of voice, and words spoken all match, look more closely for the reason.

Attempts by the patient to mask feelings can be detected readily by observing body behavior. True feelings are more likely to leak through conscious efforts to conceal feelings. Likewise, a physician's attempt at deception will be detected by patients and can destroy confidence and damage rapport. Positive verbal communication (e.g., "You're looking better today") accompanied by negative nonverbal cues will be interpreted by the patient as insincere. For example, a patient who is not told the true nature of a terminal illness usually knows it anyway and may distrust family, friends, and physician if they persist in the charade.

In a medical school commencement address, Alan Alda (star of TV's M*A*S*H) challenged new physicians to be able to read a patient's involuntary muscles as well as their radiographic studies. He asked, "Can you see the fear and uncertainty in my face? If I tell you where it hurts, can you hear in my voice where I ache? I show you my body, but I bring you my person. Will you tell me what you are doing and in words I can understand? Will you tell me when you don't know what to do?" (*Time*, May 28, 1979, p. 68). The physician will see the fear and uncertainty in the patient's face only if she or he is looking at the patient rather than the medical record. Alda's statement reflects the concern and compassion that patients desire. By using appropriate body language, the physician can convey this attention and concern in the most effective manner possible.

Body Position

The body position when sitting can show various degrees of tension or relaxation. The tense person sits erect with a fairly rigid posture. A person who is moderately relaxed has a forward lean of approximately 20 degrees and a side lean of up to 10 degrees. A very relaxed position (usually too relaxed for physicians interacting with patients) is a backward lean (i.e., recline) of 20 degrees and a sideways lean of more than 10 degrees.

Higher patient satisfaction is associated with a physician's forward body lean and rotation of the torso toward the patient. Larsen and Smith (1981, p. 487) found that "the patient also responds more favorably to the physician who relaxes his chin in his hands and gazes directly at the patient, rather than a physician who elevates his chin (unsupported) as if to imply a more superior status." Physicians whose communication styles have been considered patient oriented have been observed to change body position more frequently than physicians whose conversations were physician centered.

An attempt should be made, whenever possible, to sit rather than stand when interviewing a patient. Rapport is improved if the physician does not intimidate the patient by placing him or her in a submissive position. Patients feel more comfortable and less helpless speaking in a sitting position rather than prone. Sitting on the patient's bed is usually not recommended, but for some patients, it is an effective means of establishing closeness and conveying warmth in a relaxed yet attentive manner.

Mirroring

When good rapport exists between two people, each will mirror the other's movements. Some people unconsciously establish rapport with another by mirroring that person's movements or body posture (Key, 1980) (Figure 12-2). Disruptions in this mirroring may signal that one member disagrees with what the other has said or feels betrayed or insulted but cannot express this idea verbally. If the physician notices

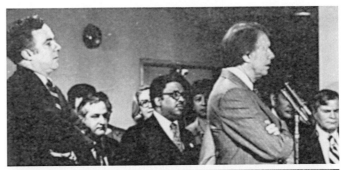
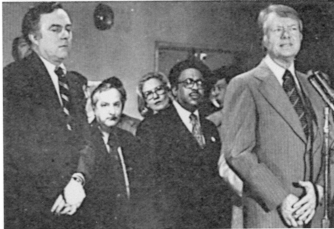
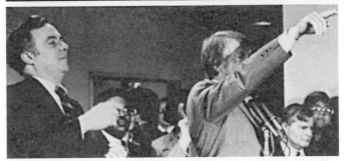

Figure 12-2 Joseph Califano *(left)*, Secretary of Health, Education and Welfare, mirrors his boss, President Jimmy Carter, through his posture and gestures. *(From Key MR [ed]: The Relationship of Verbal and Nonverbal Communication. New York, Mouton Publishers, 1980, p v.)*

this sudden disruption of mirroring activity by the patient, more attention should be focused on the comment that led to the change of position. Renegotiation or further explanation may be indicated. A powerful way to establish rapport is to match intentionally the body language of another.

Head Position

Typically, the head is held forward in anger and back in defiance, anxiety, or fear. It is down or bowed in sadness, submissiveness, shame, or guilt. The head tilted to one side indicates interest and attention (Scheflen, 1972) (Figure 12-3); under certain circumstances, this can be a flirtation. The erect head indicates self-confidence and maturity.

When listening to a patient, the physician should show interest and concern by an attentive position, which is best illustrated by sitting forward in the chair with an interested, attentive facial expression and the head slightly tilted. Darwin was one of the first to notice that animals assume a head tilt when listening intently.

Face

The human face can create more than 7000 expressions using 44 muscles (Cleese, 2001); some say 10,000 expressions are possible (Ekman, 2003).

Darwin (1872) proposed that cultures throughout the world express similar emotions or states of mind with remarkably uniform body movements. His information was gathered from missionary friends working with aborigines, persons under hypnosis, infants, and patients with mental disease. He also studied blind and deaf persons who, without benefit of learning from others, were observed to raise eyebrows when surprised and shrug their shoulders to indicate helplessness.

Darwin held that the facial expression of emotion, when undisguised, is independent of culture and is identical throughout the world. The facial expressions of joy, sadness, and anger are the same in the Australian aborigine, the American farmer, and the Norwegian fisherman (Ekman,

2006). Various cultures, however, do disguise the facial expression in different ways. In American culture, the mouth is used most often to disguise feelings. A person in a social gathering may be smiling, although inwardly sad or angry. The eyebrows, eyes, and forehead are least affected by these cultural disguises and are the most consistently dependable indicators of emotion. As Shakespeare wrote, "I saw his heart in his face" (*The Winter's Tale*, Act I, Scene II).

Ekman and Friesen (1975) found that the facial expressions of fear, disgust, happiness, and anger were the same in countries with widely disparate languages and cultures. They used composite facial photographs to show how each part of the face contributes to the expressions of emotion, especially surprise, fear, disgust, anger, happiness, and sadness. In American culture, when people want to disguise their true feelings and convey a more socially acceptable impression, they do so by smiling. This may be especially true in patients who are sad or depressed. Figure 12-4 is a composite showing sadness in the eyes, brow, and forehead being masked by a smile.

Smile

A genuine smile can be helpful in quickly establishing a friendly atmosphere and developing a warm, interpersonal relationship. A grin can be the physician's most effective weapon for breaking down resistance or apprehension in patients, especially children or young adults. A number of studies have shown that patients are more positively disposed to physicians who smile. The smile must be genuine, however; patients can easily spot a phony smile.

Smiles are controlled by the zygomatic major muscles that connect to the corners of the mouth and the orbicularis oculi muscles. The latter are not under conscious control and

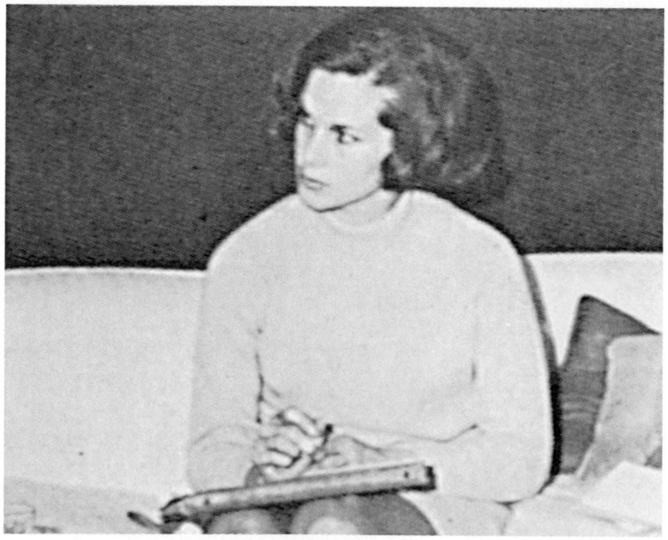

Figure 12-3 This woman signals attentiveness and seriousness by holding very still, cocking her head, and looking intently at the speaker.
(From Scheflen AE. Body Language and the Social Order—Communication as Behavioral Control. Englewood Cliffs, NJ, Prentice-Hall, 1972.)

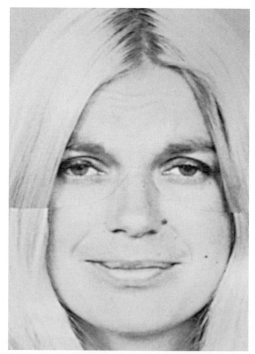

Figure 12-4 Masking sadness by smiling (see eyes and forehead).
(From Ekman P, Friesen WV. Unmasking the Face: a Guide to Recognizing Emotions from Facial Clues. Englewood Cliffs, NJ, Prentice-Hall, 1975.)

reveal a true smile that involves characteristic creases around the eyes. A genuine smile lights up the whole face; one that does not is more likely a deception (Ekman, 2005).

Micro-Expressions

Ekman and Friesen (1975) also described micro-expressions, a valuable indication of masking or deception. "Micro-expressions are caused by the face's all too rapid efficiency in registering inner feelings" (Morris, 1977, p. 110). Most facial expressions last more than 1 second, but micro-expressions last only about one fifth of a second (Ekman, 2003). This is approximately the time it takes to blink an eye, and micro-expressions easily can be missed if the physician is not carefully observing the patient. Micro-expressions tend to occur when emotion is concealed unwittingly by repression or deliberately by suppression. They can be seen if the patient begins to show a true facial expression, senses this, and immediately neutralizes or masks the expression. Some micro-expressions are complete enough to show the true emotion felt, but most often, they are squelched to such an extent that the physician has only a clue that the patient is concealing some emotion.

Most expressions last about 2 seconds (0.5-4 seconds). Surprise is the briefest expression (Ekman, 2003).

Eyes

The eyes are probably the principal organs of expression. They are so important to a person's appearance that when anonymity is desired, only the eyes need to be covered. The eyebrows have been shown to have 40 different positions of expression and the eyelids 23. Consider the magnitude of possible combinations when all facial elements are involved as indicators of expression. The message conveyed by each position can be further modified by the length of a glance and its intensity.

In most cultures, good rapport is enhanced when one's gaze meets the other's 60% to 70% of the time. When we talk, we maintain eye contact about 40% of the time and 80% when listening. Ninety percent of the gaze will be in a triangular area between the eyes and the mouth (Pease and Pease, 2004). On meeting, two people will scan each other's face for about 3 seconds, then briefly gaze downward. An upward eye break may be disconcerting or convey a lack of interest (Lewis, 1989). (See eFigure 12-1 online at www.expertconsult.com.)

The eyes can give more information for some emotions than others. Knapp (1978) found that the eyes were better than the brow, forehead, or lower face for the accurate portrayal of fear but were less accurate for anger and disgust. Even the lower eyelid alone can convey considerable information. In Figure 12-5, it is apparent that the person in B depicts more sadness than the one in A, but the pictures differ in only one respect: the lower eyelid.

It has long been known that *pupils* dilate when the person sees something pleasant and contract when something unpleasant is viewed. This involuntary signal can be a valuable indication of what is really going on. Asian jade dealers wore dark glasses so that no one could see their pupils dilate when they discovered an especially valuable piece of jade. Likewise, a magician doing card tricks can tell when a preselected card is seen by a subject because of the sudden pupil enlargement. In one experiment (Hess, 1975), the pupils of males dilated when the men were shown photographs of nude females and constricted for nude males. Homosexuals demonstrated the opposite. Dilated pupils also can indicate

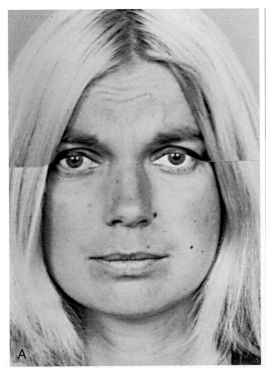 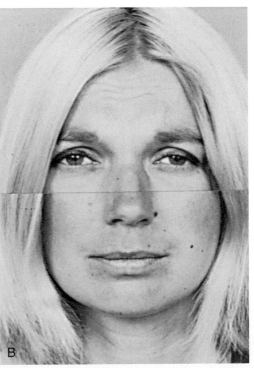

Figure 12-5 Sadness shown in the eyes and forehead (the mouth is neutral). The importance of the eyelids can be seen because the person on the right **(B)** is obviously sadder than the one on the left **(A)** but differs only in that a sad lower eyelid has been substituted for a neutral lower eyelid.
(From Ekman P, Friesen WV. Unmasking the Face: a Guide to Recognizing Emotions from Facial Clues. Englewood Cliffs, NJ, Prentice-Hall, 1975.)

that listeners are interested, whereas constricted pupils suggest that they do not like what is being said (or viewed).

Sincerity is expressed with the eyes. The best method for conveying sincerity is frequent eye contact, a technique most appropriately used when listening to the other person. One trait of good listeners is that they constantly look at the speaker. A listener who does not maintain eye contact but continues to look down or away from the speaker, may be shy, depressed, or indicating rejection of the speaker or the comments being made. One patient said, "I had one student doctor who looked at his toes instead of me. If he ever opens a practice, I don't believe I would trust him." Conversely, speakers frequently may break eye contact when talking and are permitted a distant stare when formulating ideas and selecting phrases. However, they still should try to make frequent, although less prolonged and intense, eye contact.

A special form of human-to-human awareness is conveyed by eye contact. Prolonged eye contact, or staring, can be offensive. Monkeys can be provoked to combat by a person staring at them because of the threat of aggression that this represents. Under other circumstances, however, staring can be flirtatious, emphasizing that the meaning of eye behavior depends on other factors in the situation.

The acceptability of eye contact varies significantly among different cultures. In the United States, focusing the eyes on the speaker indicates respect and attention, regardless of the age of the individuals involved. However, Mexican Americans tend not to maintain as much eye contact while listening as do other Americans and may look away from the speaker more often. This is not a sign of disrespect or inattention. In Latin American countries, a younger person may be thought disrespectful if his or her eyes meet those of the adult who is speaking. A physician could be considered seductive in that culture if he or she maintained steady eye contact while talking to a patient. In the United States, it is impolite to maintain eye contact with a stranger for more than 3 seconds, but Europeans believe that longer periods of eye contact are normal. The physician needs to consider the patient's cultural background when interpreting the meaning of eye contact behavior. Looking away from the speaker from time to time may be a sign of respect and sensitivity rather than the opposite. At the same time, the physician's failure to look a patient in the eye can be dehumanizing and can cause the patient to feel more like an object than a person. Patients are most comfortable when the physician looks at them approximately 50% of the time and are uncomfortable when eye contact is avoided.

The frequency of eye contact also can provide clues to whether the patient is anxious or depressed. The eyes of anxious patients blink frequently or dart back and forth. They look at the interviewer as frequently as low-anxiety patients but maintain eye contact for less time on each gaze. Similarly, the patient may interpret the physician's lack of eye contact as indicative of anxiety or discomfort, even rejection.

Frequent blinking of the eyes can be a sign of pressure or stress. In a political debate between Senator Bob Dole and President Bill Clinton in 1996, Dole blinked an average of 105 times per minute, showing more pressure than Clinton's 48 times per minute.

Depressed patients maintain eye contact only one-fourth as long as nondepressed patients. Downward contraction of the mouth and a downward angling of the head are also cues to depression. As with the anxious patient, there is no difference in frequency of eye contact in the depressed patient; the difference is only in the duration of contact.

Patients with abdominal pain caused by organic disease are more likely to keep their eyes open during palpation of the abdomen than those with nonspecific pain (Gray et al., 1988). The patient with genuine abdominal tenderness may apprehensively watch the physician's hand as it approaches the tender area.

Hands

The hands will be droopy and flaccid with sadness, fidgety or grasping in anxiety, and clenched in anger. When a speaker joins her or his hands, with fingers extended and fingertips touching, it is called *steepling* and indicates confidence and assurance in the comments being made (Figure 12-6).

Palms usually are held in the palm-in position. Turning the palms outward can be a subtle courting behavior (usually used by women), but it more likely indicates a warm and friendly greeting (Davis, 1975).

The hands of an anxious patient can be observed to shake when holding a pen, to twitch, or to be braced unnaturally. The white-knuckle pose of tightly locked fingers can be an effort to mask anxiety.

Hands can be a subtle indicator of the urge to interrupt. Be alert for this sign in a patient so that important information will not be suppressed, and the patient can be given every opportunity to supply valuable information. Indications of this urge to interrupt are a slight raising of the hand or perhaps the index finger only, pulling at the earlobe, or raising the index finger to the lips. The latter gesture also may indicate an attempt to suppress a comment and should alert the physician to inquire further and elicit the hidden information. A patient listening in "The Thinker" position, with the index finger across the lips or extended along the cheek, or one sitting with elbows on the table and hands clenched in front of the mouth, although listening intently, may not believe or understand the physician's words (Figure 12-7).

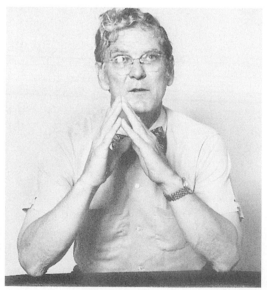

Figure 12-6 Steepling.

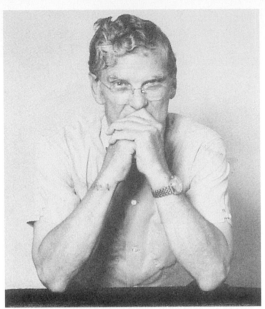

Figure 12-7 The defensive or "doubting Thomas" position.

The physician should take additional time to amplify the issue or explain the diagnosis or treatment regimen further.

Arms

Although folded arms are found in all cultures, this is considered a discovered action rather than an inborn trait because it is a natural position of comfort that is as easily discovered by the African tribesman as the New York banker. It is the subtle ways in which the arms are held that can give clues to underlying emotions. Crossed arms can be a defensive posture, indicating disagreement with another's view, or it can be a sign of insecurity. It can also be nothing more than a position of comfort and should, as with all other signs, be considered in the context of the individual's total behavior.

Notice the manner in which the arms are crossed. Are they relaxed in the normal position of comfort, or are they in a hugging posture, reflecting insecurity or sadness and indicating a need for reassurance? Anger can be seen in clenched fists that are held tightly against the body in a holding-back manner, preventing them from hitting (Figure 12-8). If the patient has assumed a position of resistance or defensiveness, sitting with arms and legs crossed and perhaps with body turned away, search for the reason for this defensiveness and try to eliminate it. Perhaps a recommendation that the patient stop smoking is threatening and difficult to accept. In that case, it is important to make an additional effort to explain the rationale for the recommendation; do not hurry over it with a brief comment or admonition.

Legs

Although crossing the legs is a common position of comfort, it can also indicate a shutting out of or protection against the outside world. If crossed legs in a patient confirm the total kinesic picture of resistance, including crossed arms and other signals discussed earlier (Figure 12-9), make every effort to identify the reason for the resistance and correct it before proceeding further. Likewise, locked ankles can indicate defensiveness. Diagnostic information obtained from a

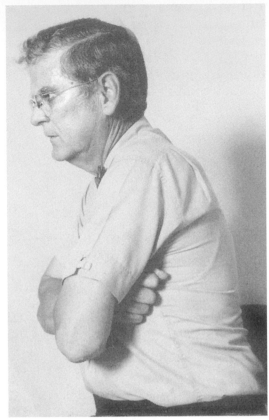

Figure 12-8 The resistant position, suggesting suppressed anger.

resistant patient is likely to be incomplete, and instructions are unlikely to be followed.

Notice the position of the feet and their movement. As with fidgety hand movements, anxiety is associated with the fidgety, constantly moving foot. An anxious or scared person may sit forward in the chair with feet placed in the ready-to-run position, with one foot in front of the other. The angry person is more likely to place the feet widely apart in a position of stability, whereas the feet of a sad person tend to move in a slow, circular pattern.

Gestures

The thumbs-up sign in the United States means "good going," but in some Islamic countries, it is the equivalent of an upraised middle finger. Similarly, the extended hand with palm forward means "stop" in the United States, but in West Africa, it is an insult greater than the upraised middle finger.

Joining the thumb and index finger in a circle to indicate "OK" is an insult in many Latin American countries and in France means zero or worthless. In Texas, raising the index and little finger with the middle two fingers folded down is the "Hook 'em Horns" gesture of the University of Texas Longhorns, but in parts of Africa this gesture is a curse and in Italy it means your spouse is unfaithful.

American television and the movies have dulled these differences worldwide, although some still exist. In the 1978 movie *Inglorious Bastards* (remade in 2009) the American posing as a German was detected because he displayed the number 2 using index and middle fingers, whereas Europeans would hold up the thumb and index finger with the thumb being number 1.

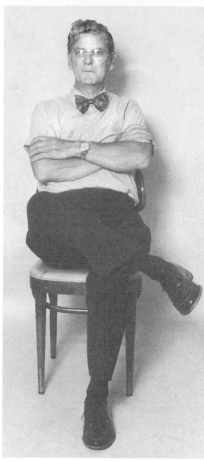

Figure 12-9 The defensive position.

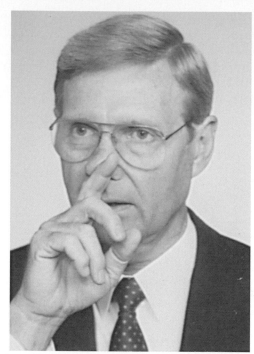

Figure 12-10 The nose rub, a variation of the respiratory avoidance response.

Preening

Preening gestures, such as the male pulling up socks, adjusting a tie, or combing hair and the female adjusting clothing or using a mirror to review makeup, may not necessarily be seductive in nature but can be an attempt to establish rapport and good interpersonal relations. If the preening is intended to be flirtatious, however, the woman may cross her legs, place a hand on her hip, caress her leg, or stroke the arm or thigh in some fashion. The flirtatious male typically uses gaze holding and head tilt to accentuate normal preening gestures or may stretch to make himself look larger. Both genders may use "accidental" touching as a flirting signal. When someone's attention is completely focused on the other, legs, knees, and feet are usually extended in the direction of the other. The physician should remain alert to the accentuation of normal preening gestures into courtship actions to identify the seductive patient and deal with the issue early, before unknowingly encouraging the patient to proceed further along this course.

Respiratory Avoidance Response

The respiratory avoidance response involves a frequent clearing of the throat when no phlegm or mucus is present. All animals exhibit a respiratory avoidance response as a means of clearing something unpleasant or undesirable from the respiratory tract. This action also can be a nonverbal indication of disgust or rejection. When physicians find themselves doing this, they should observe the accompanying circumstances and notice whether posterior pharyngeal mucus is truly present.

Nose Rub

Another component of the respiratory avoidance response is the nose rub (Figure 12-10). This involves a light or subtle rub of the nose with the index finger and signals rejection of a statement being made by the subject or by another individual. The nose rub to relieve an itch is usually vigorous and involves a repeated series of rubs, whereas that of the respiratory avoidance response is soft and consists of one or two light strokes, often involving nothing more than a light flick of the nose. Morris (1977, p. 111) described the nose flick as "a reflection of the fact that a split is being forced between inner thoughts and outward action." It can be associated with lying or with the struggle to appear calm while suppressing anger or discomfort. During Bill Clinton's testimony to the grand jury regarding his affair with Monica Lewinsky, he rarely touched his nose when telling the truth, but when he lied he gave a split-second frown, then touched his nose. During the testimony he touched it 26 times (Pease and Pease, 2004). Variations of the nose rub include pulling at the earlobe, scratching the side of the neck or rubbing one eye. Someone aware of the nose rub will often notice it in themselves and realize they are uncomfortable with what is being said by themselves or others. Watching for this during interviews on television may indicate the person being interviewed is uncomfortable with the question, or the person asking may realize it is a "testy" point.

This sign can be quite useful in patient interviewing. For example, the physician may ask a patient, "How are things at home?" The patient may answer, "Fine," but then clears his or her throat and lightly rubs the nose with the index finger. He or she is actually saying, "I don't like what you are asking me," or "I feel uncomfortable with my answer; things really aren't going very well at home." If there is a cause to pursue the issue further, a simple comment such as "Really?" or "You mean not even an occasional argument?" may lead to a flood of information masked by the previous response.

Verbal-Nonverbal Mismatch

Another indication that what a patient is saying may be in conflict with what is being felt is a verbal-nonverbal mismatch, such as when the patient answers "fine" to "how are things between you and your husband" while looking sad and avoiding eye contact (Quill, 1989). If the patient answered negatively to the question, "Have you ever had a venereal disease," and at the same time exhibited a nose rub, this topic should be followed up with a similar inquiry later, perhaps while doing the physical examination, when the patient may feel more comfortable after better rapport has been established.

Other clues that the patient may not be telling the truth or that there are repressed feelings are asymmetric facial expressions and a prolonged smile or expression of amazement. Almost all authentic facial expressions fade after 4 or 5 seconds (Ekman, 1985).

Neurolinguistic Programming

Neurolinguistic programming (NLP) involves the eye movements performed while thinking and depends on whether a person is thinking visually, aurally, or kinesthetically. A right-handed person who is visually oriented will look up and to his or her left when recalling something visually, but up and to the right if creating something visually or, in other words, making it up or lying. Similarly, a right-handed person will look sideways to his or her left when recalling sounds and sideways to the right when imagining sounds. A person who is looking up and to his or her right (i.e., your left) probably is imagining things he or she has never seen before. This technique is used by police investigators when interviewing suspects. A left-handed person will respond in opposite directions (Zellmann, 2004, Brooks, 1989) (Figure 12-11).

Detecting Lying

In addition to looking up and to the right to create an image or a fact, a person who is lying is also likely to do the following:

- Cover the mouth with hand.
- Rub or flick the nose.
- Scratch the neck.
- Pull at the ear, or rub behind the ear.
- Rub one eye.

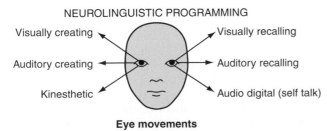

NEUROLINGUISTIC PROGRAMMING

Visually creating — Visually recalling

Auditory creating — Auditory recalling

Kinesthetic — Audio digital (self talk)

Eye movements

Figure 12-11 Neurolinguistic programming.

- Blink excessively (although absence of blinking is also possible).
- Have a micro-expression indicating something is different than what is said.
- Avoid making eye contact.
- Use arms and hands less.
- Be defensive rather than aggressive.
- Change manner or posture abruptly.

The liar will also rarely touch the other person or point a finger at them or others, and the story will not include negative details (Lieberman, 1998). The liar is not comfortable with silence and may speak more than normal to convince the other. Persons suspected of lying should be encouraged to talk because verbal and nonverbal clues will then be easier to detect (Vrij, 2005). Liars are also likely to slouch, unlike a confident person, who will sit upright. Remember that it takes a combination of verbal and nonverbal clues to detect lying, and no single action is likely to be dependable other than to raise doubt or suspicion.

Proxemics: Spatial Factors

Proxemics is the study of how people unconsciously structure the space around them. This structuring varies with every culture. North Americans, for example, maintain a protective "body bubble" of space about 2 feet in diameter around them when they interact with strangers or casual acquaintances. Violators of that space are considered intruders and cause the person to become defensive (Figure 12-12). In the Middle East, no such bubble exists, and it is proper to invade this area. In fact, not to do so may be interpreted as unfriendly and aloof. Arabs prefer to stand close enough to touch and smell the other person. Americans, however, if forced to stand close together, as on a crowded subway, will use their eyes (i.e., distant gaze) to maintain a more proper distance. An arm's length is a good measure of the appropriate personal distance for most people. A wife can stand inside her husband's bubble, but she will be unhappy if another woman invades this sphere of privacy, and vice versa.

Robert Frost said, "Good fences make good neighbors." In suburbs and small towns, people are more likely to talk to each other while in their backyards if a fence indicates the boundary than if there is a communal yard (McCaskey, 1979). Marking the boundary helps maintain territoriality and actually brings the neighbors closer together than when there is no fence.

Intimate space has been classified as that ranging from close physical contact to 18 inches, *personal space* from 18 inches to 4 feet, *social space* from 4 feet to 12 feet, and *public space* from 12 feet and beyond. Placing a desk between two people shifts personal space to social space. The office desk also can be a barrier to communication when it is placed between the physician and patient, thereby emphasizing the illusion of the physician's importance and power. There may be occasions when this is desired, but it usually is not necessary in a family physician's office. Office furniture should be arranged so that a minimum number of obstacles lie between physician and patient.

Automobiles magnify the size of one's personal space up to 10 times. Compare the relationship of two people having a conversation with that of "road rage" when one invades the other's space by cutting in front of them.

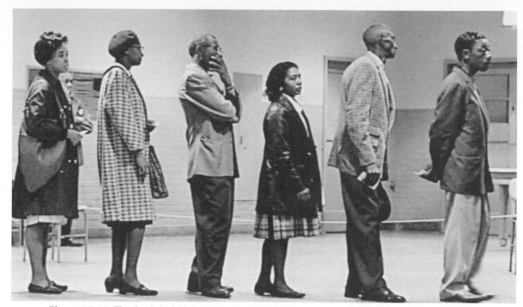

Figure 12-12 The "body bubble" surrounding strangers in a queue. *(Courtesy Magnum Photos, New York.)*

Hidden or Masked Communication and Patients' Expectations

Although the average person has a symptom about every 6 days, he or she visits a physician only once every 4 months. Some people visit a physician much more frequently than others for the same symptom. The group who visits more frequently tends to have a higher level of anxiety, fear, grief, or frustration. It is the physician's responsibility to search for, identify, and treat organic disease if it is present, but in about one half of cases, none will be found. It is equally important to identify the reason for these visits—the basis for the heightened concern or increased anxiety. A person may see a minor symptom as a potential catastrophe if she or he thinks it may be a sign of cancer similar to that causing a parent's death. Is the patient really there "just for a blood pressure check," or because of concern about the condition of his or her coronary arteries since a friend recently had an acute myocardial infarction? If the physician deals only with the symptoms, the real concerns may go undetected, and the result will be a dissatisfied and noncompliant patient.

Barsky (1981, p. 492) cautioned, "Patients who express dissatisfaction with their medical care should be questioned about this, as they may be dissatisfied because their real motivation in seeking care has not been illuminated." He also advised the physician to investigate the patient's current life stresses when visits are made if there is no change in clinical status.

Patients may come to a physician because of what they imagine is causing their symptoms rather than because of the symptoms themselves. Identifying what patients hope can be done for them—focusing on their expectations for the visit—often reveals hidden reasons for the visit. The physician should be sure to address the patient's expectations and make certain that the interpretation is correct. Rapport and satisfaction will be enhanced if the physician identifies and satisfies the patient's expectations for the visit. Dissatisfaction results when these expectations go unmet.

Listening Well

A good family physician must be a good listener. Of all the communication skills essential to rapport, the ability to listen well is probably the most important. All the information in the world about body language, vocal messages, and nonverbal cues is of limited value unless it helps the family physician be a better listener.

As Lown (1996) states, "In the brief time available to take a history, the aim is to obtain, in addition to essential facts, insight into the human being. This seems easy, but listening is the most complex and difficult of all the tools in a doctor's repertory. One must be an active listener to hear an unspoken problem" (p. 10). The appearance of readiness to listen is aided by bending forward and maintaining eye contact. The physician can discourage a patient from talking by looking away or writing in the medical record. Well-chosen questions can be rendered useless by inappropriate nonverbal behavior. Even great questions are of no value if you do not know how to listen.

For many people, the opposite of talking is not "listening" but rather "waiting to talk." It is impossible to listen attentively when you are planning what to say next. Besides, learning to listen is more difficult than learning to ask good questions (Dimitrius and Mazzarella, 1999).

The average listening efficiency of most people is only 25% because we do not concentrate on what is being said. Effective listening requires focus on what is being said and on voice tone, facial expression, and body movements. Hearing what someone says and truly listening to what they are saying is quite different (Zellmann, 2004).

Analyses of physician-patient interviews reveal that, on average, the physician rather than the patient does most of the talking, although when questioned, physicians usually imagine the reverse. In general, the less the physician says during an interview, the more the patient will say.

Boredom is one of the most difficult states to conceal. It is very difficult to appear attentive and interested if you are bored, and it takes considerable effort to appear interested (Dimitrius and Mazzarella, 1999).

Silence

Silence can be as effective a means of eliciting further information as direct questions. The timing is important, however, and silence should be used as a technique only when the physician is relatively certain that there is more information to follow the last statement. A shift of position or a nod and a smile, properly timed and coupled with silence, can be more effective than an encouraging comment. Nonverbal encouragement to continue is less distracting and may be more facilitative than the verbal form.

Attorneys use silence in the courtroom to get witnesses to say more than they had intended. They wait silently as if the witness has not given a complete answer, and usually they do receive additional information. Silence can be effective as long as the patient feels more inclined to fill the void than the physician. This is of value, however, only when there is more information to be obtained. It is said that Charles DeGaulle thought that silence was the ultimate power tool, and in his speeches, he gained control by looking at the audience, never breaking eye contact, and saying nothing.

Interruption

The patient may be following a line of thought and may be about to open up more but must stop and refocus if the physician captures the patient's attention with a question. The physician should interrupt a patient's statement only if it is necessary to change the conversation to a new topic, clarify an issue, elicit information not produced spontaneously, offer reassurance, or reduce patient anxiety.

Physicians usually use closed-ended questions to interrupt the patient and thereby inappropriately control the interview. Beckman and Frankel (1984) found that 69% of patients (52 of 74) had only 18 seconds to complete their initial complaint before being interrupted by their physician. This usually occurred after the patient stated only a single concern, and it effectively halted the further flow of information from the patient. This prematurely terminates opportunities for patients to present their primary concerns. Only one of the 52 patients subsequently returned to and completed the opening statement. In these recorded office interviews, only 23% of the patients were permitted to complete their list of problems uninterrupted; when they were,

the complete statements usually took less than 60 seconds, and none required more than 2.5 minutes.

Humor

The art of medicine consists of amusing the patient while nature cures the disease.

Voltaire

Humor can be helpful in establishing rapport and can strengthen the physician-patient relationship. It can be used to "break the ice" and is most useful if it communicates the feeling that "we are all in this together." Humor is an effective way for physicians to appear human while supporting and empathizing with their patients. Physicians who score high in empathy also tend to have a good sense of humor (Hampes, 2001). Empathic humor can promote a stronger physician-patient relationship and enhance the effectiveness of other, more traditional as well as nontraditional forms of therapy (Berger et al., 2004).

Care must be taken, however, because humor can be a two-edged sword that can cut either way if used inappropriately. The least risk is when the humor is self-deprecating or focused on neutral topics such as the weather or parking. It can even alienate the patient if they feel the joking around is inappropriate at the very time they want serious attention paid to their problem.

More research is needed on the value of humor in medicine so that we will know when and how to use it effectively. Norman Cousins, former editor of the *Saturday Review*, had ankylosing spondylitis. He received 3 hours of pain relief after watching comedy videotapes of "The Three Stooges" and "Abbott and Costello" but obtained only $\frac{1}{2}$ hour of pain relief from an oral analgesic. Some physicians write prescriptions for patients to laugh out loud three times each day. In India, Laughter Clubs convene at the beginning of each day to laugh out loud. Even a fake laugh makes one feel better throughout the day.

Physicians who express interest in patient opinions and who use humor more often are sued less often. Tasteful humor can reduce anxiety and create a bond of friendship, but humor used inappropriately can magnify the distance between patient and physician, especially if it belittles the patient.

Sections on Interviewing Effectively (including facilitating techniques) and Care with Caring can be found online at www.expertconsult.com.

References

The complete reference list is available online at www.expertconsult.com.

Web Resources

www.healthypeople.gov/document/html/volume1/healthcom.htm
   Federal government site on health communication strategies that is part of the Healthy People 2010 project.
www.changingminds.org
   Covers a variety of body language message clusters, including aggressive, attentive, deceptive, romantic, and submissive.
www.blifaloo.com/info/flirting-body-language.php
   Male and female flirting signals, eye contact, and mirroring. Also contains a link to "How to Detect Lies" plus tips on improving memory.

www.squidoo.com/bodylanguage
   "Body language it is important to know" with links to YouTube vignettes (e.g., dating tips, spotting a liar).
www.wikihow.com/Read-Body-Language
   Good overview of the major components of body language; includes a video demonstration.

13 CHAPTER

Patient Education

Robert B. Kelly

Chapter contents

Key Points

- Encouragement of healthy lifestyles by family physicians and acceptance of responsibility for health behaviors by patients are part of a new paradigm of the physician-patient relationship.
- Enhanced patient satisfaction and realistic expectations as a result of education can reduce risk of malpractice actions.
- Use a SOAPE note to document adding education to your plan.
- Match your message to each patient's stage of change.
- Use feedback, reinforcement, individualization, facilitation, and multiple channels when providing education.
- Learn brief techniques of motivational interviewing to be more successful in facilitating behavior change.

Family medicine has long embraced the concept of patient education as an integral part of patient care. It is an official policy of the American Academy of Family Physicians (AAFP) that "family physicians should take a leadership role in improving the health of the American public by providing accurate and meaningful patient education." The AAFP produces guidelines for residency curriculum in patient education; includes patient education materials in its journal, *American Family Physician;* and sponsors an award-winning resource (FamilyDoctor.org). The Joint Principles of the Patient-Centered Medical Home (2007) include patients' active participation in medical decision-making and the use of information technology to support patient education.

Patient education continues to evolve. Patients who are informed are more likely to be active participants in their care and adhere to treatment (Epstein et al., 2004). Although physicians have technical knowledge about medical conditions

and treatments, patients have more knowledge about their own experience, values, and cultural considerations. Effective patient-centered education requires physicians to individualize information according to each specific patient's needs, values, and culture, and consider these when working with patients to make treatment decisions (Falvo, 2004).

Rationale

Most people want to be better informed about every aspect of their health care. Apart from patients' expectations and satisfaction, there are a number of compelling reasons for physicians and other health providers to educate patients. The most important of these is better adherence to therapies (Gray et al., 2004; Rogers et al., 2005). Although the results of typical patient education efforts are modest (Haynes et al., 2002; Schroeder et al., 2004; van Eijken et al., 2003), education has the potential to improve health outcomes and reduce morbidity. Additional benefits to the physician include practice marketing through enhanced patient satisfaction (Aragon, 2003; Ganz, 2002) and prevention of malpractice actions (Eastaugh, 2004; Wissow, 2004).[11,12]

Existing data suggest that the most effective interventions available to clinicians for reducing the incidence and severity of the leading causes of disease and disability in the United States are those that address the personal health practices of patients (USPSTF, 1996). This implies movement of health care providers and patients toward a nontraditional relationship, in which encouragement of healthy lifestyles by providers and acceptance of responsibility for health behaviors by patients become the cornerstones of a new preventive care paradigm. Education of patients is critical to the implementation of this paradigm.

Opportunities

Education of the patient or the family can make a contribution to every medical interaction. Every recent medical school graduate is familiar with the SOAP note format (i.e., subjective data, objective data, assessment, and plan) for documenting a medical encounter. Adding education (E) to the plan by using a SOAPE note serves as a reminder to educate patients and to document the education.

All excellent family physicians are also excellent teachers of patients. Such physicians typically incorporate education continuously during the interaction with the patient, not as a separate step. When taking a history, the physician can assess attitudes, knowledge, and skills. When performing an examination, the physician can instruct about the purpose of the examination and the meaning of findings. When discussing a diagnosis, the physician can share its meaning and the process of decision making in approachable terminology. When suggesting therapy, the physician can assess understanding, willingness, and barriers to implementation.

Although patient education may largely occur in the context of individual provider-patient interactions, there are many additional opportunities to become involved in health education. Health education is a regular part of curricula in schools, may be found in workplace programs in many communities, and is routinely featured in the mass media. Family physicians who have become involved in health education can have greater impact from the ripple effects of networking in their community. Involvement can begin with small, manageable actions. Physicians can offer to come for question-and-answer sessions during health classes, offer to be a consultant to the school board regarding health curricula, or become a team physician for junior high or high school teams. Media involvement can come from volunteering to comment on current issues in health for local radio and television stations or from writing a regular health column for the local newspaper.

Within their own practice, many family physicians struggle to include all the education they want to provide. There are a variety of creative solutions to this problem. The physician can expand services to include group classes for common topics such as smoking cessation, perinatal care, and healthy diet. Group visits can be done for patients with chronic problems that need regular monitoring, such as diabetes and hypertension (Loney-Hutchinson et al., 2009). Also, patient education can be made the responsibility of the entire practice, involving office nurses, medical assistants, and receptionists as a team. Larger practices may have access to dieticians or pharmacists.

It is important not to overlook existing resources in the community that can be used to expand what is offered in the physician's office. These include national and local disease-specific support organizations such as the American Diabetes Association (ADA), American Heart Association (AHA), American Cancer Society (ACS), American Lung Association, Weight Watchers, and Alcoholics Anonymous (AA). Educational resources in the form of groups or short courses may also be sponsored by local libraries, YMCA chapters, churches, or other community organizations.

Principles of Patient Education

The system of patients accepting the advice of all-knowing physicians in an unquestioning and docile manner no longer applies. Instead, physicians should strive toward a doctor-patient partnership in which the patient sees the physician (and physicians see themselves) as a health consultant. In such a role, the question becomes how to educate most effectively. Research has consistently demonstrated that patient benefits are greatest when interventions follow sound educational principles, including the following (Simons-Morton et al., 1992):

Feedback means that the patient is informed about progress toward goals and objectives.

Reinforcement refers to encouragement or rewards for patient progress.

Individualization takes into account the needs, desires, and characteristics of the patient and demands that specific goals and objectives are negotiated for each patient.

Facilitation refers to materials, cues, and skill training that assist the patient in making changes.

Relevance to the learner means that the content is appropriate for an individual patient's circumstances.

Multiple channels imply combined learning strategies and a team approach to education.

These principles have been incorporated into the U.S. Preventive Services Task Force (USPSTF) recommendations for patient education and counseling shown in Table 13-1.

A Model of Health Behavior Change

Stages of Change

The purpose of patient education efforts often is to inform and to change behavior. Typically, the goal is to improve adherence to therapeutic regimens, encourage new lifestyles, or help the patient adopt other behaviors that prevent disease and disability. One of the most useful ways to understand the process of behavior change is the *transtheoretical model*, often called the "stages of change" model (Zimmerman et al., 2000). This model proposes stages called precontemplation, contemplation, preparation, action, and maintenance (Table 13-2). *Precontemplation, contemplation,* and *preparation* can be thought of as stages of motivation and readiness for change. In at-risk populations, typically 40% are precontemplators, 40% are contemplators, and 20% are in preparation (Prochaska and Velicer, 1997). Research has shown improvements in process and outcome measures when stage-matched interventions and recruitment methods are used (Prochaska et al., 2005). Although the model is described in a linear fashion, experience has demonstrated that patients naturally move back and forth among stages.

This model emphasizes the critical importance of the *stage of change*. Fortunately, it can usually be assessed with simple questions. Given typical constraints of time and resources in a primary care practice, most patient education efforts should focus on patients in the stage of *preparation*. Giving such patients the proper cue or knowledge to make a beneficial change is generally easy to provide. For simple

Table 13-1 USPSTF Recommendations for Patient Education and Counseling

Frame the teaching to match the patient's perceptions.
Fully inform patients of the purposes and expected effects of interventions and when to expect these effects.
Suggest small changes rather than large ones.
Be specific in recommending new behaviors.
Emphasize that it is easier to add new behaviors than eliminate established ones.
When feasible, link new behaviors to established ones.
Use the "power of the profession."
Obtain explicit commitments from the patient.
Use a combination of strategies.
Involve office staff.
Refer to community agencies, voluntary health organizations, reference material, and even other patients.
Monitor progress through follow-up contact.

From US Preventive Services Task Force: Guide to Clinical Preventive Services. Baltimore, Williams & Wilkins, 1996, p 953.

Table 13-2 Stages of Health Behavior Change

Precontemplation: Not intending to take action in the foreseeable future, usually measured as the next 6 months.
Contemplation: Intending to change in the next 6 months; aware of the pros and cons of changing, leading to procrastination.
Preparation: Intending to take action in the immediate future, usually measured as the next month; have a plan.
Action: Have made specific overt modifications to behavior within the last 6 months.
Maintenance: Working to prevent relapse, increasing confidence; typically lasts 6 months to 5 years.

From Prochaska JO, Velicer WF. The transtheoretical model of health behavior change. Am J Health Promot 1997;12:38-48.

behaviors (e.g., stretching before exercise), simple recommendations or an instructional pamphlet may be sufficient to accompany the physician's strong statement of support for the new behavior. For more complicated behaviors (e.g., dietary changes), one or more additional scheduled visits with the physician, a dietician, or other provider may be needed to set goals, convey knowledge or skills, and reinforce behavior change. A basic implementation of this thinking for health promotion has been called the "five As": *ask, advise, assess, assist,* and *arrange.* This approach has been promoted primarily for tobacco cessation (Kenford and Fiore, 2004).[19]

An important implication of the stages-of-change model is that encouraging action for patients in the precontemplation or contemplation stage is wasted energy. Instead, if the behavior is an important one, the goal should be to increase the patient's *readiness* for change. Research has shown that an increase in the "pros," or perceived benefits of change, is the most common finding when patients move from precontemplation to contemplation. Contemplators are usually weighing the perceived pros and cons of change in a manner that leaves them ambivalent about this decisional balance. Research indicates that movement from contemplation to action is most strongly associated with a decrease in the perceived cons of change. To reduce the cons for contemplators, the physician needs to identify these through open-ended questioning.

When and How to Intervene

When patients are unmotivated for change in the stage of precontemplation, the physician should decide whether to invest the time to intervene through assessment and attempted modification of beliefs, confidence, supports, or barriers. The decision often hinges on factors such as the level of risk for the patient, the time available at that visit, competing demands, and the physician's own experience and confidence level. At a minimum, an open-door policy should be adopted. The physician must convey the message that she or he is willing and ready to help the patient make changes when the patient becomes motivated to make them. Stage of change should be assessed on a regular basis as the patient is cared for over time.

If the physician takes up the challenge of the precontemplator, how can the pros and cons of change be assessed and addressed in the context of routine office visits? A useful approach for physicians is *motivational interviewing* (Miller and Rollnick, 2002). This approach is characterized by *collaboration* between physician and patient; by *evocation,* enhancing motivation by drawing on the patient's own perceptions, goals, and values; and by *autonomy,* in which the patient's right and capacity for self-direction are affirmed and informed choice is facilitated. Practical strategies for motivational interviewing can be integrated with a stages-of-change model of behavior change (Rollnick et al., 1999).

Because many patients are not motivated, and the health rewards of behavior change are often not immediate, physicians must also take steps to avoid "burnout." A long-term view is often helpful. The goal is to change readiness in increments over time and to be ready to detect a change in motivation that will allow meaningful change in behavior. It can also be the case that events will take place that cause a dramatic shift, usually caused by a change in perceived risk. These events are opportunities to explore health beliefs in the hope that they have changed. In the meantime, the best strategy is to be nonjudgmental, to feel rewarded for small changes that patients make, and to accept that some people will not change despite one's best efforts. If, for example, the annual smoking quit rate in a practice increases to 10% from a baseline of 5% of smokers per year, physicians should not despair about the other 90%, but instead congratulate themselves on doubling the rate of smoking cessation and leave the door open to the other 90%.

Planning for Patient Education in Your Practice

Key Points

- Employ all the people and places in your clinical setting—front and back office staff; waiting and examination room environments—to promote the most efficient and effective education for your patients.
- Familiarize yourself with resources in the community that can augment the education provided in your office.
- Consider how other family members will affect your patients' success in changing behaviors or learning how to self-monitor a chronic condition.
- Develop a simple system for you and your staff to store and retrieve printed patient education materials.
- Adjust your approach for patients with low health literacy.
- Explore Internet resources so that you can refer patients to reliable, high-quality sites.

Who Will Be Involved

Formal studies and anecdotal reports have consistently indicated that involvement of all of the office staff in patient education increases the total impact and saves the physician time. The physician always needs to be involved in defining the educational goals, delivering brief messages about the importance of goals, prescribing an educational process, and following up regularly to assess progress. Depending on the physician's interest and the nature of the problem, the education can be given by the physician or delegated to office nurses and other staff. Reception staff can suggest printed materials or other available modalities to patients while they wait or can be involved in giving patients printed materials prescribed by the physician. Group classes can be offered in the evening, organized around common topics within the practice. If these are run in conjunction with existing evening clinic hours, group classes can be a time-efficient method of delivering education to select patients. In larger practices, interested staff can form a patient education committee who uses a quality improvement process to foster patient education.

Available community resources should not be overlooked, including professionals such as dieticians and diabetes educators who may be hired on a full-time or part-time basis by a larger practice or who can split their time as a "circuit rider," spending a few hours each week at several practices. Many communities have existing programs for smoking cessation, weight loss, stress reduction, and exercise. Physicians can spend some of their time or their staff's time to become familiar with the programs, their costs, and schedules. In some cases, physicians' involvement as a medical consultant can lead to an improved program.

Remember that almost all patients have a family context. For example, whether a spouse smokes is an important factor in a smoking patient's efforts to quit. Similarly, if a patient needs to learn about dietary change to lower cholesterol and the spouse does all the food preparation for the household, the instruction will not be likely to affect the target behavior without involvement of that spouse.

Using Verbal Instruction

The most common form of patient education lies in talking to patients within the context of routine physician-patient contacts. This interaction serves as the foundation for further education that may be provided in the form of printed materials, video materials, classes, or other instructional modalities. Information must be given in a relevant way, embedded in expectations that are shared between provider and patient.

An atmosphere of acceptance, but not necessarily approval, is the first prerequisite to effective communication. This implies that the physician maintain a nonjudgmental stance when inquiring about the patient's experiences, beliefs, and behaviors. Physicians must demonstrate that they understand the patient's perspective, even if they do not agree with it. These crucial steps lead to a teaming with the patient toward achievement of common goals.

Medical jargon should be avoided. One approach to helping patients decode the jargon is to embed synonyms in the information provided; for example, "There is an atherosclerotic lesion *or blockage* in one of the coronary arteries, *the blood vessels that carry blood to the heart muscle itself.*"

Specificity and clarity are equally important principles. It is best *not* to use language such as, "Cut down on the fat you eat," "Exercise more," "Avoid heavy lifting," or even "Take your medicine three times each day." In the case of exercise, for example, the physician can indicate the type of exercise, how often to do it, how long to do it, how intensely to do it (e.g., by using a target pulse), and how to warm up and cool down before and after, as well as any warning symptoms. This level of specificity helps to ensure that a motivated patient will have the necessary information to change behavior effectively.

A final tip for effective verbal instruction is to keep checking the patient's understanding of the information. At a minimum, patients should be encouraged to ask questions and seek clarification. A better strategy is to ask patients to summarize their understanding of the information they have been given. Questions are most effectively stated in a way that accepts blame for any misunderstandings and is therefore not condescending: "Just so I can be sure that I've been clear about the information I've given you, would you repeat back to me in your own words what you are to do?" (Falvo, 2004).

Using Printed Materials

Printed materials are the next most frequently used patient education modality after verbal instruction. Unfortunately, these materials are often used alone, or without sufficient preceding verbal instruction, as a surrogate for provider-patient interaction. Printed materials can be classified into two types: prescriptive and nonprescriptive. Although there is some overlap between the two, *prescriptive* materials are usually given by the provider to the patient with a specific goal in mind. Their use is often triggered by the onset or recurrence of a medical problem. For example, if the patient has strained the lower back muscles, a brochure may be given that explains back mechanics, avoidance measures to prevent repeat injury, and a physical program to improve flexibility and strength during and after healing. This material can supplement the physician's instructions about the care of this injury.

In contrast, *nonprescriptive* materials are put out for patients to take freely or read as desired, usually in a waiting room or examination room area. These materials are more general and topic oriented, serving as "general health education" rather than patient education. Examples include a brochure that describes the four basic food groups and a pamphlet that describes common sexually transmitted diseases. Although serving more to *inform* than to change behavior, nonprescriptive materials may lead to patient questions and expand opportunities for patient education during the office visit.

Physicians are responsible for the accuracy of any materials they distribute. Hundreds of materials are available free of charge or at low cost. Sources of such materials are primarily pharmaceutical companies, national voluntary associations (e.g., ACS, AHA), and medical specialty societies such as the AAFP and American Academy of Pediatrics (AAP). Several issues are important to consider before using existing materials. First, is the content appropriate? Materials provided by pharmaceutical companies may advertise a product or present information in a biased way. Voluntary organizations' guidelines may not agree with the physician's judgments about proper screening and treatment. Second, is the material clearly presented, with a reading comprehension level appropriate for the patients served by the practice? A third type of concern is logistical. Will additional copies of the material continue to be available for replenishing supplies, or will the material go out of print? This is particularly a concern for pharmaceutical-funded campaigns. Is the format of the material suitable for storage and display in whatever system is used in the practice?

Writing Your Own

For a variety of reasons, a practice probably will want to develop some of its own printed materials. Besides the advantage of control over content and format, this also carries the responsibility for accuracy and development of a good product. Practices can begin with a planning process that identifies the most important needs, based on common educational issues and the quality and usefulness of existing materials for these issues. Because accuracy is critical, a recent literature search is done to broaden the knowledge base before starting to write. This is most important if a physician is writing about a topic for a nonprescriptive material to use in the waiting room. However, it remains a useful process for prescriptive materials, even if the goal is simply to put down in writing the physician's usual advice for a problem.

A common pitfall is to try to include too much information in the material. Restrict the content to three or four salient teaching points. Avoid jargon, extensive use of statistics, and fear messages. Be clear with advice and specific with instructions. Use short words and short sentences to improve readers' comprehension. Ideally, test material on colleagues and patients before final reproduction in quantity. Such a review process can be invaluable.

Simple line drawings with a few labels are usually more effective than complex illustrations, with the added benefit of better reproduction. Subheads help readers find information, and sparing use of bold and italic type help to emphasize terms when needed. Use the active tense, avoid negatives, and do not use absolutes such as *never*, *must*, and *always*. Expert writers recommend use of the first person in phrasing questions and the use of the second person in answering them: "How often and how long should *I* exercise?" "For best results, *you* should exercise for at least 30 minutes, at least 3 times each week." When laying out material, leave plenty of white space on the page, avoid long strings of capital letters, use a font with serifs, and use a 10- or 12-point type size.

Health Literacy

More than 90 million adults in the United States have poor literacy, leading to greater difficulty navigating the health care system and increased risk for poorer health outcomes (Andrus and Roth, 2002; Berkman et al., 2004). *Health literacy* refers to patients' ability to read and understand instructions, to give informed consent, and to comprehend, absorb, and retain information presented. Low–health literacy skills are not limited to patients with low intelligence, those with lower educational levels, or those of lower socioeconomic status.

Patients experience low literacy in a number of ways. Although some individuals may never have learned to read, others may be able to read the words but are unable to attach meaning to what is written. Difficulties may reflect differences in level of language use between the physician and patient or language barriers when the patient and physician are from different cultures. Regardless of the cause, if patients are unable to read or understand the material presented, they receive little benefit.

The best method of assessment of the degree of literacy involves observing, being alert to cues, and conducting sensitive and timely direct questioning. Several instruments have been developed to assess medical literacy (Davis et al., 1998). A good example is the *rapid estimate of adult literacy in medicine* (REALM), a word recognition test designed for patients in health care settings (Davis et al., 1993).

In some situations, visual presentation of concepts may help patients comprehend and remember information presented. In other cases, giving smaller amounts of information over several visits may be the most effective means to enhance patients' ability to absorb information. Written materials given to the patient should contain only essential information that is arranged in logical sequence and related to what the patient must know or do, rather than in-depth explanations.

When the literacy problem involves fluency or vocabulary, the physician should be especially cautious not to use jargon or assume that all "common" words or terms will be familiar to the patient. Using terms the patient knows and analogies of familiar themes may be helpful in assisting the patient to understand and remember concepts. When language is the specific problem, the physician may find it useful to use a third party fluent in both languages to assess the patient's understanding of the material presented.

Role of Computers

Most patients can access the Internet. Unfortunately, this easy access to information is a double-edged sword. Many sites provide opinion, hearsay, and outright falsehoods with the same authoritative style as peer-reviewed evidence from published medical research. Patients are poorly equipped to tell the difference.

As more and more of their patients go online, physicians should keep abreast of some of the more reliable web resources so that they can make useful recommendations to patients and respond to misinformation that patients may encounter. An extremely useful resource is familydoctor.org, produced by AAFP. Some group practices and even solo physicians have established their own websites that provide information to patients and links to other sites that may be useful.

Some computer-based electronic health record (EHR) systems have designed patient education as an integral part of the software. For example, the provider can be reminded to give recommended preventive health habit counseling based on the patient's age, gender, risk factors, and past documentation of counseling. Drawings, diagrams, pictures, graphic displays of growth parameters or laboratory data, and other visual aids can be called up on the computer screen to use in patient teaching in the examination room. A list of available educational materials can be automatically generated for the provider based on the reason for the visit, medications, orders, or diagnoses; the system can print these on demand and track which materials are given to the patient.

Other Materials and Modalities

It is helpful to supplement printed materials with models, anatomic charts, and other visual aids that can be used during the process of instruction. Such materials can be invaluable in trying to explain what a 3-ounce serving of meat looks like, or how a herniated lumbar disk presses on nerves in the back. Models and charts can be purchased from supply houses or sometimes are offered at no charge by pharmaceutical companies who market a related product.

Office Systems and Design

One of the ways to be most effective in patient education is to view the practice setting in its totality as an educational experience for patients. From this perspective, health providers can critically examine each physical area and each staff person for the potential to contribute to patient education. For example, in the waiting area, which typically has comfortable chairs and a magazine rack or television, physicians can add nonprescriptive educational brochures, decorate the walls with posters that reinforce simple educational messages, and even play educational programs or use computer-assisted instruction. Examination rooms can have posters and racks of printed materials, particularly materials that patients may hesitate to pick up while others are watching. Some practices use monthly or quarterly health themes and rotate posters and materials that relate to the theme.

Most practices need to establish some mechanism for storing, retrieving, indexing, and ordering printed materials. There is no single best way to do this. Physical systems range from racks to filing cabinets to shelves to computer-based programs that print materials on demand. Functionally, the important aspects of any system are that providers know what types of material are available, agree with their content, know how to find desired materials, periodically review existing materials for applicability and accuracy, and are able to order or produce more as stocks run low. It is often practical to delegate responsibility for many of these tasks to office personnel. Office staff may also be quite eager to participate in a patient education committee that identifies priority areas and reviews printed and other materials before they are added to the practice's resources.

References

The complete reference list is available online at www.expertconsult.com.

Web Resources

http://FamilyDoctor.org
www.MayoClinic.com
http://My.ClevelandClinic.org/health

http://PatientEducationCenter.org
www.RevolutionHealth.com
www.WebMD.com

14 CHAPTER

Interviewing Techniques

R. Hal Ritter, Jr., Michael D. Reis, and Terry G. Rascoe

Chapter contents

Key Points

- Listening is a key element for any successful interview.
- Building bridges of understanding helps to manage the various difficulties of the interview.
- Being sensitive to various forms of diversity, including disabilities, religious issues, and ethnicity, will enhance communication and participation by the patient.

The art of interviewing is a skill that is fully developed only through experience. Although various decision trees and protocols can be followed as the clinician seeks to confirm or rule out a preliminary hypothesis, the process of the interview often determines whether the therapeutic relationship is beneficial or deleterious to the outcome. Ritter and Wilson (2001) observed that listening is a key element in establishing the "three Rs" of interviewing: *rapport, respect,* and *relationship.* The quality of the relationship between the physician and patient is itself therapeutic, and the quality of this relationship will enhance or deter trust in the physician's care and the patient's adherence with the physician's recommendations.

Asay and Lambert (2009) discuss Michael Lambert's extensive, quantitative studies of contemporary psychotherapy, which validate that 30% of any therapeutic change is based on the quality of the relationship between the clinician and the client (LOE Grade A). This relationship is based on listening, mutual respect, empathy, and acceptance of the client.

Norfolk and associates (2007) note that the empathy necessary for rapport is based on trust and cooperation between physician and patient, and "rapport" is defined by the quality of the "doctor's understanding of the patient's perspective on his or her problem." Empathic skills "are *internal* diagnostic skills running parallel to those used to assess the patient's clinical presentation, and they allow the doctor to first identify significant clues to the patient's thoughts and feelings." These clues for understanding the patient's perspective may be verbal, nonverbal, or both (LOE Grade A).

In this regard, listening is a multisensory process. The physician listens to what is spoken, "listens" with the eyes for nonverbal behaviors, and "listens" with the fingers as examinations are completed. Rapport, respect, and relationship are enhanced by the physician taking the time to listen and understand the patient's concerns. This listening is often framed by a time constraint of 10 to 20 minutes in the examination room with the patient. It is not the actual amount of time the physician spends with the patient but the *perceived* quality of time that is critical to the patient's experience (Pollock and Grime, 2002). The physician conveys interest and concern for the patient by giving the *impression* of having time for the patient and being unhurried. Some patients feel disrespected by medical staffers who do not acknowledge the patient's own time commitments or personal beliefs and feelings (Lacy et al., 2004).

All interviews have content and a process. The *content* is the subject matter of the interview, or what is discussed. The *process* is rapport, or how the interview flows as the content is discussed. It is the nonverbal, emotional quality of the interaction. Rapport is a key to being a successful healer, especially in the current medical environment of technologic sophistication and managed-care limitations (see Chapter 12).

The Listening Environment

An important element in the listening environment is the physician's sense of attention with the patient, and whether the patient feels the physician is listening to his or her concerns (Table 14-1). If the physician is running behind schedule, has had several difficult encounters during the day, or is tired from lack of rest, the patient will often pick up on various subtleties in the physician's behavior that communicate a "lack of presence" to the patient (i.e., countertransference). Some patients may feel the need to help a hurried physician and may withhold important information (Pollock and Grime, 2002).

Health care providers generally seek to collect as much information as possible while avoiding unnecessary information gathering that uses up valuable time. However, the interpersonal dialogue during the interview is vitally important, and the additional information often provides essential clues for more effective differential diagnosis and therefore more comprehensive treatment planning and case management.

The following LISTEN paradigm is only a suggestion, and health care clinicians should modify it for their own practice situation and environment. The purpose of the paradigm is to provide a structural mnemonic that moves the conversation logically and holistically throughout the interview. As determined by the clinician, any particular part of the interview may be expanded as the situation warrants, and any part may be minimized. By covering each part at least minimally, the clinician can achieve a general overview of the functioning and strengths of the patient or client, as follows:

L: *Listening* is *active* and *empathic,* as the clinician maintains a friendly countenance and good eye contact, while responding in a *respectful* and *affirming* way to the person. Active listening includes verbal and nonverbal listening. It means to *look* and *listen,* to listen with the *eyes* and the *ears,* assessing the person's behavior and facial responses. It includes an assessment of dress, grooming, and observable hygiene, such as apparent body and clothing cleanliness, as well as dental health.

I: *Interpersonal* communication refers to the quality of the *interaction* between the clinician and the person

---

Table 14-1 Ritter LISTEN Paradigm for Interviewing and Assessment

L: Active listening, verbal and nonverbal, eyes and ears, respectful, affirming

I: Interpersonal interaction, mutuality, natural pacing, familial and social

S: Somatic, sensory, sense, sensitivity, body, behavior, healthy and unhealthy, reality, making sense, context

T: Thinking, cognition, intelligence, problem solving, daily living, self-care

E: Emotion, affect, expressiveness, congruence and consistency

N: Normal, now, present, resources, positive person strengths, cooperation in the healing process

Courtesy R. Hal Ritter, Jr, PhD, 2002, and Scott & White Memorial Hospital System.

---

throughout the interview. The clinician assesses the fluency and appropriateness of the person's speech and vocabulary. Does the conversation have a *natural flow* and *pacing?* Is it tense or strained? Does the person's hearing and understanding appear to be adequate for the conversation? Is the conversation characterized by a sense of *mutuality* and *care,* or is it more limited to just question and answer? The clinician inquires about the person's other interpersonal relationships, including *familial and social* (i.e., family and friends).

S: *Somatic, sensory, sense,* and *sensitivity* characteristics are highlighted. The clinician inquires about the person's *physical body* and *behavior* habits, *healthy and unhealthy,* such as exercise or substance abuse. What is the relevant medical history, including behavior? The interviewer assesses the person's *sensory experience* of the internal world, and his or her perception of the external world. Is the person in touch with internal and external *reality?* The clinician asks patients how they understand what is happening to them. How do they *make sense* of the experience of being interviewed or ill? What *meaning* does it have for them within their own personal history? The clinician is *sensitive* to the *contextual issues* such as family, gender, ethnicity, education, religion, and socioeconomic levels because they may influence the interviewing experience and the therapeutic process.

T: The clinician assesses the *thinking* or *cognitive abilities* of the person. Are reasoning and *problem* solving adequate for life decisions and for *daily living* and *self-care?* The clinician also assesses *intelligence* and evaluates whether there are deficits that may hinder adequate decision making.

E: *Emotion* is another area of focus. As the interview proceeds, the interviewer evaluates the *consistency* and *congruence* of the *affective* and *emotional* responses of the person during the conversation. How *expressive* is the person affectively? How well do the nonverbal behaviors match the emotional expressiveness in the person's voice throughout the conversation?

N: *Normal* and *now* are considered. The clinician assesses what the *normal resources* and *strengths* are for this person. How can these resources be used for collaboration in healing? The assessment is made in the *now,* in the *present:* How is this person *normal?* What *positive person strengths* do patients bring to the current situation for their potential *cooperation in the healing process?*

The Ritter LISTEN paradigm provides the clinician a moment-in-time assessment of this person, who is on a journey of growth and change. The conclusions are tentative because they do not indicate how the person will be in the future. Nevertheless, the LISTEN assessment provides information for holistic treatment planning and intervention (see Table 14-1).

The physical environment of the room should be welcoming and inviting, creating a sense of comfort to the patient. Sometimes, a nonmedical picture, such as a group picture of the staff or a family picture, can enhance the conversation.

In initiating the interview, the physician should sit down and strive to maintain good eye contact. By having comfortable chairs for the patient, the intention is conveyed that the physician desires for the patient to be comfortable during the visit. Taking notes on what the patient is saying is appropriate, but it should not interrupt the flow of the conversation or break a sense of continuity. By allowing patients to tell their story in the opening minutes of the interview, the physician gains a context for understanding how they view the problem being presented. Sometimes, the seemingly irrelevant information being presented by a patient becomes valuable contextual information for diagnosis, treatment, and compliance.

Maximizing the Time

When the physician invites the patient to move to the examination table, there is a cognitive shift for the patient that is explicit and implicit. Explicitly, it is a change of place that conveys that a shift is taking place in the process of the visit. Implicitly, it prepares the patient for the more physical aspects of the visit. It may even be appropriate for the physician to offer assistance to the patient during this transition.

As the physician examines the patient, each action is preceded by an explanation of what the patient can expect to happen next. These brief informative comments build respect and rapport because the patient is more at ease not having to guess what is going to happen. In this regard, each intervention is a request for informed consent. "I am now going to listen to your heart." The implied question is, "Is that all right?" Each statement carries this implied question, which is a way of being respectful and conveying the message that the patient is participating in the actual care being given and received. It is a collaborative and interactive conversation.

The Interview Process

As the physician talks with the patient, the natural flow of the conversation is itself a part of the diagnostic environment. How the patient interacts with the physician in the closeness and intimacy of the examination room is descriptive for how the patient relates with others outside the office context, whether at home or at work or at leisure and play.

During the interview, the physician's own feelings and intuitions can help the physician understand how the patient is dealing with the illness (Borrell-Carrió et al., 2004). Sometimes, in the scientific world of medicine, physicians may believe that keeping their own feelings out of the process is the best way to be objective and relevant. However, if the physician is mechanical and distant because of discomfort with personal sensitivity, the patient will quickly notice the distance.

Psychiatrist Harry Stack Sullivan (1954) observed that the work of the physician is to be a "participant-observer" in the process of the interview. The physician maintains a scientific observer perspective, while also being available and present to the patient as a fellow human in the journey of life. As the physician becomes more sensitive and aware of the interview process, there is the experience of "reciprocal emotion," the continuous reflecting of another's feelings. The openness of the interview is further enhanced by

the physician "mirroring" the body posture of the patient, such as crossing a leg, leaning forward, or leaning back (see Chapter 12).

Basic Communication

People often speak out of one particular language sensory system, and sometimes they express levels of understanding with a particular sensory language. In this regard, another form of mirroring is listening for which sensory system the patient is using and then joining that language system. Of particular importance are the visual, auditory, and kinesthetic language systems. For example, one person may say, "I *see* what you mean," and another may say, "I *hear* what you are saying," and another may say, "I am getting a *feeling* for what you mean."

When these sensory words are used, the physician can join that sensory system in the conversation: "Do you *see* what I am saying?" or "How do you *hear* what I am recommending?" or "How do you *feel* about my recommendations?" In each case, the physician is joining the patient's preferred way of expressing understanding.

The interviewing physician also learns to monitor personal feelings during the interview. Is there a hunch, an intuitive thought, or an uncomfortable feeling that is not logical, or even unrelated to the visit? It is important for the physician to pay attention to these internal messages so that important information is not missed. For example, a patient's seemingly harmless or even sarcastic remark about "most people in the medical field" may alert the physician to make an extra effort to build bridges of rapport, respect, and relationship with the patient, to increase the probability of compliance. A comment about car problems may mean follow-up appointments are at risk.

The conversational "give and take" during the interview provides the opportunity for the physician to learn about the context of the patient's life and relationships. More than just taking medical information, it is a *biopsychosocial* understanding of the patient (Brown, 2000; Engel, 1977, 1980). Coulehan and Block (2001) observe, "Good clinician communication *does* prevent malpractice suits. A patient who feels that the clinician listens to and understands him or her is not likely to sue that person, *even if there is a bad outcome*" [italics added].

Another element in the context of the relational environment is compassion, the "feeling with" the patient in the experience of illness and distress. As Rakel (2000) states:

> Good interpersonal skills enhanced by compassion enable the physician to dissect out the tangled mass of personal difficulties that so often form the core of functional disease or magnify the symptoms of an organic condition. We all know that a broken spirit underlies a great deal of the problems we encounter in practice.

The physician is the one who, by rapport, respect, and interpersonal relationship, humanizes for the patient the medical experience of laboratory and technology. The physician models for the patient a real person who is in a relationship with another real person.

The Participating Patient

Patients are more likely to accept recommendations from the physician if they feel they are a part of the process of treatment. Physicians often have different agendas than do patients for the clinic visit. The physician wants to find the problem, identify it, and bring hope and healing to the person. The patient wants to tell a story, to help better understand the illness, as well as find healing and recovery.

The patient can be encouraged to tell the story, even within the time constraints of the visit, with a statement such as, "We have about 15 minutes together today. How do you want to use this time? What do you want me to know?" In this way, the physician structures the time for the patient, and also gives the patient the freedom to express what he or she thinks is important. As the diagnosis and recommendations are made, the physician may ask the patient a question such as, "How do you want to participate in your treatment?" As Stone and colleagues (1998) observe, the physician is encouraging *adherence* rather than insisting on *compliance:* "Compliance implies an involuntary act of submission to authority, whereas adherence refers to a voluntary act of subscribing to a point of view."

Pearl
"Communicating your understanding of the patient's experience of the illness is one of the most therapeutic techniques we can use. 'The more I listen, the more my patients understand'" (Platt and Gordon, 2004).

Pitfall
Be careful not to lose the human being in the discussion of the disease entity. Avoid identifying the patient by the disease rather than by a personal description, such as the woman, man, boy, or girl who *has* the disease; the people are not the disease.

Pearl
The person is not the problem. The problem is the problem.

Difficult Patient Situations

Difficulties sometime arise during patients' visits that are not anticipated. For example, a patient may be feeling so poorly that without realizing it, cooperation is difficult. It is the physician's task to make the patient feel at ease and as comfortable as possible. In other cases the staff may not have fully prepared the patient for the physician. It is the physician's demeanor that sustains the interview with a sense of ease as the difficulty is addressed or the omitted information attained.

Sometimes, the patient is difficult from the very beginning because of the illness, personality, or the process of moving through the office system. Already under the stress of not feeling well, the negative attitude of the difficult patient is only exacerbated by the many small issues that may arise in the interview. Some patients are irritated about having to wait; having no clear diagnosis; or being denied their request for an antibiotic to treat a viral infection.

Psychiatrist Beryl Lawn (2004) says that the difficult patient is most often afraid; it is this deep fear that something is wrong that the patient cannot control. The personality of the difficult patient may lack the flexibility or resilience that is necessary for coping with other people and with day-to-day living. In the stress of the medical environment, difficult patients may become angry and try to take control of the process as a way of controlling their inner fears of inadequacy.

Sometimes, stepping back or to the side provides the upset patient with some personal space to regain composure. The physician then continues the interview, without trying to analyze or explain the difficult behavior. It is the work of reconnecting with the patient, of maintaining respect and working to establish rapport and relationship.

Another difficulty is the patient's ambivalence, such as hesitancy in making a medical decision or a lifestyle change decision. The physician may offer a respectful response such as, "I cannot decide for you. However, I do believe that it is an important decision, and I will respect whatever you decide." In this way, the physician assures the patient that medical treatment will be continued, regardless of how the ambivalence is managed. Some people are paralyzed by ambivalence, and they may remain at this point of indecision for some time. Some people do nothing until some externally imposed deadline, such as a job application drug screening, makes the decision for them (Ubel, 2002).

Whatever the difficulty, the physician maintains rapport, respect, and relationship with these difficult patients by listening for their concerns. By giving the impression of being unhurried and having time to listen, the physician maintains relationship and conveys to the patient that the physician-patient relationship will continue, undamaged by the present difficulty. In this way the relationship becomes a part of the healing process.

Barriers to Effective Communication

Time Demands

Time is one of the greatest challenges for the busy practitioner. Nothing disrupts effective communication more than patients' perception that the physician does not have time to address their problem.

Barriers

- Walk-in patients, who reduce physician time spent with prescheduled appointments.
- Insufficient length of time scheduled for complexity of the visit.
- Hidden agendas of the patient.
- Time for dictation and documentation.

Bridges

- Open-access scheduling. Predict urgent care needs, and create adequate same-day appointment times (Murray and Tantau, 2000).

- Improved triage on the phone. Have appointment staff ask patient if the scheduled amount of time will be sufficient to cover all the issues, or mark certain patients for an extended visit if they typically require extra time.
- Ask patients to bring a problem list with them, and ask them to show the list to the physician at the onset of the appointment. Items can be prioritized and time properly allotted for the visit. Schedule follow-up appointments for lower-priority items.
- Consider dictating or documenting while still in the room with the patient. This will lengthen the contact time with the patient and allow the patient to add any missing information to the record, as needed.

Interruptions

A continuous flow of information during the interview and examination is important for effective dialogue to occur. Interruptions in this process can distract the physician and inhibit open communication on the part of the patient.

Barriers

- Pagers going off
- Phone calls
- Knocks on the door

Bridges

- Consider having a triage nurse hold your pager while you are in the office. Pages can be answered promptly without interrupting the patient-physician communication. Urgent requests can be brought to your attention after the appointment has concluded, or the visit can be interrupted for emergencies. A bonus is that any additional information you may need, such as a chart or a laboratory report, can be brought to you at the time of the page information.
- Have a strict policy regarding phone interruptions. Most messages can be screened by staff, and if necessary, a brief message can be forwarded to you.
- Consider having several set times for answering messages. The staff can inform the caller of a time to avoid unnecessary callbacks.
- Knocks on the door disrupt the flow of the conversation, and they may alarm a patient if they occur during the more intimate parts of an examination. Limit door knocks to an absolute minimum.

Technology

New technologies, including electronic health records (EHRs) and handheld computers such as personal digital assistants (PDAs), have greatly improved data access. However, these same innovations may create barriers to meaningful interaction (Ventres et al., 2005).

Barriers

- Data (i.e., EHR) retrieval from a device requires loss of eye contact with the patient.
- Data entry into a device requires time and may be a distraction.

Bridges

- Always inform new patients what you are doing when viewing a computer screen. This assures the patient that you are actively retrieving information for the issues at hand.
- Try to maintain eye contact while viewing a paper chart or a computer device.
- Read back data, such as history, examination notes, and prescriptions, to the patient to summarize the visit and ensure accuracy.

Complementary and Alternative Medicine

The use of complementary and alternative medicine (CAM) therapies by patients has become commonplace. Discussions about the current or past use of CAM modalities is important for developing a clear understanding of the patient's beliefs and preferences and for avoiding potentially harmful interactions.

Barriers

- Negative or cynical attitude of the physician toward all CAM and toward patients who use CAM.
- Patient fears or indifference toward informing the physician about their use of CAM.
- Lack of a standardized history questionnaire that includes an inquiry about patient CAM practices.

Bridges

- Approach questions regarding CAM with an open and respectful tone, similar to taking a sexual history or inquiring about alcohol and tobacco use.
- Use a preprinted form or routinely ask patients to list all dietary supplements they take.

Religion and Spiritual Issues

There is currently more emphasis on being sensitive to the spiritual concerns of a patient (Levin et al., 1997; McCord et al., 2004). Some physicians believe that religion and spirituality discussions should be left to clergy and chaplains, who certainly should be included in patient care. However, Cumella (2002) suggests expanding Engel's biopsychosocial model to a biopsychosocial-spiritual model.

In the decade from 1994 to 2004, the percentage of U.S. medical schools offering curricula on spiritual history taking increased from 13% to 66% (Fortin and Barnett, 2004). In a 2004 survey, 43% of adults said they would welcome a discussion of spiritual matters with their physician during the taking of an initial medical history, and 77% said it is appropriate during a serious illness (McCord et al., 2004). However, only 10% report ever being asked by their physician about their faith and the possible impact their beliefs may have on their health care (Maugans and Wadland, 1991). Family physicians indicated that lack of time was the primary reason for omitting a spiritual history; 53% said a lack of training limited their ability to take a spiritual history, and 59% were concerned with projecting their own beliefs onto the patient (Ellis and Vinson, 1999).

However, taking a spiritual history can provide valuable information regarding a patient's perception of the disease and possible effects on treatment options and outcomes, as well as the availability of resources and social support for the patient. Some patients are not religious and have no interest in religion; some tend to become more religiously interested in times of crisis; and others are intensely religious. Some patients consider themselves to be spiritual, even though they do not identify with a particular religion or religious group.

Being religiously sensitive often includes being ethnically and culturally sensitive, and it is helpful for the physician to be comfortable with the level of religious concern that the patient may bring into the interview. For some patients and some physicians, all important decisions, including medical decisions, have some religious basis. When a physician is not sensitive to the patient's overall decision-making process, a patient who expresses appreciation at the end of the visit may then ignore all the physician's recommendations, because the patient feels the physician did not really understand what the illness means to the patient. In this regard, it is important for physicians to be aware of their own religious and spiritual heritage, whether it is absent, limited, or intense, because the values and beliefs and ethics of their religious heritage helped form their own decisions in patient care. Just as the patient's religion may influence medical decisions, so a physician's religious heritage may affect medical recommendations.

When taking a spiritual history, as with other elements of the review, it is often helpful to use open-ended questions that are nonjudgmental, such as the following:
Do you have a religious background?
Do you practice a particular faith?
Are you a spiritual person?

A "no" answer to these questions is probably a stop point for further questions. The physician may go on to another subject in the interview. However, if the answer is "yes," the physician may inquire about how the patient's religious heritage is a resource in a time of illness or may be relevant to medical decision making. If deemed appropriate, the physician may indicate her or his own religious heritage and then discuss how the patient and physician can relate to one another's religious backgrounds.

Some physicians may find the following brief interview assessment helpful (Pulchaski and Romer, 2000)—FICA:
Faith: Do you consider yourself to be a spiritual or religious person?
Importance: How important is your faith to you?
Community: Are you a part of a spiritual or religious community?
Address: How would you like me to address these issues in your health care?

Because religious faith and spirituality are an important part of some patients' lives and experiences, an awareness of this information further enhances the establishment of rapport, respect, and relationship, and it clarifies the physician's commitment to holistic treatment of the patient. It is what Odell (2003) calls "including versus imposing" the clinician's religious or spiritual views in the interviewing process.

Pearl

Any discussion of religion and spirituality should always seek to focus on the patient's beliefs, not on the physician's beliefs.

Cultural Competency

Cultural issues include disabilities and ethnicity. For example, there is a clear cultural divide in the deaf community between those who use sign language ("signers") and those who are referred to, often derisively, as "audists," or lip readers. The signers sometimes believe the audists have betrayed their disability by trying to "act as if it is not real." A signer is obviously deaf, but a lip reader is not. In addition to deaf patients, the following guidelines apply to patients with other physical and mental disabilities:

1. Be sensitive to patients with mental and physical disabilities.
2. Treat an adult as an adult. Do not patronize the patient.
3. Remember that a disability does not define intelligence.

One of the problems in being sensitive to cultural diversity is stereotyping similarities. Language, dress, or skin color may or may not be evidence of a particular ethnicity. Two people with the same skin color or the same language may be of totally different cultures. An American black, whose family has been in the United States for 200 years, has more in common with an American white than with a recent black immigrant from east Africa. A Hispanic person from Central America has an entirely different cultural experience than a Puerto Rican from New York City. A South Korean is very different from a Hmong from Laos, and a Japanese person and a Chinese person are not from the same culture or language.

The following recommendations address ethnicity in the primary care practice:

1. Provide pictures and magazines in the waiting room that reflect the cultural diversity of your patient population.
2. Provide written materials, such as home instructions and medication instructions, in the language of your patient population.
3. In all forms of diversity, avoid stereotyping similarities.
4. Pay attention to the languages that patients speak. If they speak only limited English, do not assume they understand what you are recommending medically. Ask questions. What is your country of origin? How long has your family been in the United States? What is your primary language?
5. Different cultures have different religious and cultural understandings of illness. How do you understand what the problem is that you are having?
6. Some cultural groups include other family members or healers in decision making. Being open and respectful, the patient is more likely to accept what the physician says. Ask questions to determine the situation. Are there others who will be included in the decision making for your medical care?
7. Be sensitive to the patient's language and to the patient's level of literacy when giving written instructions.
8. Thank the patient for coming and helping you understand their concerns.

Pearl

Avoid stereotypes and the myth of similarity.

Assessing for Unhealthy Alcohol Use

When physicians suspect that a patient has a problem with unhealthy alcohol use, they can ask a validated, single-question screening test (Smith et al., 2009): How many times in the past year have you had x or more drinks in 1 day? (for men, $x = 5$; for women, $x = 4$). Any response other than zero (0) is considered positive for unhealthy alcohol use. The question is 81.8% sensitive and 79.3% specific for disclosing unhealthy alcohol use. The single-question screen is recommended by the National Institute on Alcohol Abuse and Alcoholism (NIAAA) (LOE Grade A).

Interviewing Specific Groups

Because family medicine is a specialty of breadth as well as depth, the clinical interview can be challenging. Communicating effectively with patients and family members who have various communication abilities and various agendas is a challenging task that is never fully mastered. However, experience achieved through years of clinical practice does result in learned techniques that can help the clinical interview flow smoothly and create a pleasant experience for the patient and physician. The development of a healthy patient-physician relationship is itself therapeutic and is enhanced by the conduct of a productive clinical encounter. Successful approaches of practicing clinicians for communicating with typical patient types are listed in the Pearls.

General Interview Perspective: Be Careful

Be cautious when accepting the flattery of patients who are critical of the care they received from other physicians; these patients may have a long history of failed patient-physician relationships caused by unreasonable expectations.

Avoid being "inserted" into the middle of a family conflict by well-meaning family members. It is generally not helpful to agree to keep a secret ("Don't tell them I told you this, but..."). It is better to agree to discuss the subject and to insist on honesty with the patient ("Your daughter has shared with me that she is concerned about your drinking [or ability to live alone or angry outbursts]"). Playing along with the secret is usually unfair to patients and not in their best interest. Instead, it is often a perpetuation of the family's enabling behavior that has led to the perpetuation of the patient's problem, and at the least, it makes further communication with the patient and the formulation of plans difficult and uncomfortable.

Even though it may be tempting to appear an expert to the patient, a wise general policy is to avoid criticism of other health providers, whether verbally to the patient or in the medical record. When commenting on contentious issues and complex situations, appraisal from multiple perspectives is critical for understanding, and information should always be complete and in context. However, this broader perspective is almost never available at the patient interview.

Criticism of office staff behavior in the presence of the patient is inappropriate and may be damaging to the patient-physician relationship. Share constructive criticism only with staff members and only in private.

Age Considerations for the Interview

In the following age categories, various techniques are suggested for establishing and maintaining rapport, respect, and relationship between the physician and the patient. However, techniques are not magic bullets. They are baseline suggestions, tools for a lifetime of learning about the concerns and the medical needs of the people who come to the physician for care.

Infants and Babies

1. Babies' future behavior during physician appointments is in part determined by the cumulative experience of each office visit. Try to avoid unpleasant portions of examination when clinically acceptable.
2. Enter the examination room quietly, and keep movements slow and to a minimum.
3. Listen carefully to the caregiver. Parents tend to know when there is something wrong with their child. Pay attention to their concerns.
4. Babies are experts at body language; this is their primary form of communication.
5. Avoid invading the infant's space initially.
6. Smile at mom or dad and speak softly.
7. Sit down and try to get your face to the level of the baby's face while still maintaining appropriate distance.
8. Smile at the baby, and make eye contact.
9. Notice baby's body language. If appropriate, tickle or play with the baby.
10. Perform as much of the examination as possible with the baby in the caregiver's arms before moving to the examination table.
11. Minimize the need to restrain the baby during the examination; this should be the last resort.
12. Many smiles to the baby will help decrease fear and resistant behavior.

Toddlers and Children

1. If the child is playing with a toy or reading a book, pretend to be interested in the item. Do not take the item away from the child unless it is offered to you; promptly return it.
2. As you visit with the caregiver about the reason for the visit, observe the child for the current level of activity (e.g., sleepy, fussy, irritable, lethargic) and for developmental milestones. However, keep your attention on the caregiver while gathering history. Do not be distracted by a rambunctious child. If your eyes wander to the child, the parent may lose track of what he or she is thinking. The parent will focus attention on the child's behavior and may interpret your gaze as disapproval of the child's behavior. This subtle glance at the child is not a good way to maintain a positive relationship with the parent.
3. Ask the parent to hold the child in the lap to begin the examination; perform less invasive portions of examination

first to begin to build the child's trust, such as listening to the heart with the stethoscope, before touching the child with your hands.

4. If the child is very anxious about the examination, pretend to examine their stuffed animal, or examine their parent to demonstrate what you are doing, and then examine the child in the same fashion, such as looking in his ears.

5. Male clinicians particularly need to use a soft voice. Higher pitches tend to be less frightening. Play with the child during the examination; look for bunnies in the ears, or listen for breakfast in the tummy.

6. Save the most unpleasant portions of examination for last, such as a throat examination with a tongue depressor.

7. Offer the child a "peace offering" at the end of the visit, such as a sticker or other age-appropriate item.

8. End interview with positive gestures toward the child: wave bye-bye, "give me five," or other exit gestures.

Adolescents

When older adolescents are accompanied by parents, consider using the first few minutes of the interview to allow the parents the opportunity to verbalize their thoughts and concerns about the child. Then, politely, invite the parents to step outside the examination room while you complete the interview. You may want to bring the parents back into the room at the conclusion of the examination for any final discussions, while carefully keeping confidentiality issues in mind.

1. Greet the adolescent patient with a smile, good eye contact, and a firm handshake.

2. Depending on age and social skills, many adolescents are withdrawn and quiet. Frequently, if this behavior is ignored, and continued attempts are made to draw the patient into conversation, the behavior will improve.

3. For many adolescent interviews, the HEADSSS technique is a helpful way to structure the interview in a thorough and time-conserving manner (Lukefahr, 2005):
   Home: How is home life? Are both parents in the home? Siblings? Who else lives there? What is the atmosphere (e.g., friendly, supportive, conflicted, angry, critical)?
   Education or *employment:* How is school? Grades? Good student? Favorite and most difficult subjects? How get along with fellow students and teachers? Employment? After school? Odd jobs? Babysitting?
   Activities: School? Sports? Clubs? Community? Religious? Other?
   Drugs: Use any illegal substances? Legal? Tobacco? Alcohol? How often? Any use by family members in the home?
   Sexual status: Are you active sexually? Have you ever had any kind of sexual contact with another person, even once? Protection? Any worries about sexually transmitted diseases or pregnancy?
   Suicide: Have you ever considered hurting yourself or killing yourself? Ending your life? Any attempts? Previous family history of suicide? Hurting or killing someone else?
   Safety: Any violence or abuse in the home? Neighborhood?

4. Conclude the interview with the same good eye contact, a smile, and a firm handshake. Thank the patient for the conversation.

Pearl

The words and body language of the physician and staff should always reflect genuine concern and respect for the adolescent patient, regardless of the adolescent's appearance or behavior in the office.

Adult Patients

1. Briefly review the established patient's record before entering the room; it is important that the patient know you are at least somewhat familiar with his or her history.

2. Knock on the closed door of the examination room before opening; this demonstrates to the patient a respect for privacy, as well as your courtesy and concern.

3. Smile and maintain eye contact as you warmly shake the patient's hand and pleasantly greet him or her. Then, greet the others in the examination room in a similar fashion. Greeting the children demonstrates a family-centered approach to care.

4. Visit for a short time by exchanging pleasantries. Ask about the family, hobbies, and other activities.

5. Ask the patient, "How can I help you today?" or "What brings you here today?"

6. Allow the patient to speak freely for at least 2 minutes without interruption. (This is longer than it seems.)

7. Maintain eye contact, smile, and mirror the body position of the patient to communicate attentiveness and congruence.

8. Before concluding the interview and the examination, ask the patient if there is anything else he or she wants to discuss.

9. Conclude the interview with the same good eye contact, a smile, and a firm handshake.

Elderly Patients

1. Greet the patient with good eye contact, a smile, and a comfortable handshake.

2. Be aware that the elderly patient may be struggling in various degrees with issues regarding decreasing physical abilities, changing body image, cognition or mental function, loss of social friends and family to illness or death, and a deeper level of spirituality, especially regarding end of life.

3. Address patients using the surname and Mr., Mrs., or Ms.; do not call them by their first name unless they have previously made it clear that this is their preference. When in doubt, assume a more formal approach.

4. Visit for a short time by exchanging pleasantries. Ask about the patient's family, hobbies, and other activities.

5. Ask the patient, "How can I help you today?" or "What brings you here today?"

6. Allow the patient to speak freely for at least 2 minutes without interruption (this is longer than it seems).

7. Be aware of any visual or auditory acuity problems; adjust speech rate and tone accordingly.

8. If the topic is appropriate and time permits, consider discussing the patient's feelings regarding end-of-life issues. Offer help in developing a living will, and encourage patients to discuss their feelings with the closest family members.

9. Offer an elderly patient your hand as he or she moves to the examination table. Good practice is to have one hand on the patient's arm or hand and the other on the back. This is a caring gesture as the patient steps up and sits on the examination table, and it helps with positioning and balance.

10. Conclude the interview with the same good eye contact, a smile, and a comfortable handshake.

Specific Concerns

Demented Elderly Patients

1. Despite dementia, eye contact, a smile, and a comfortable handshake are still appropriate ways to greet the patient.

2. Next, greet the patient's caregiver-spouse, adult child, or nursing home staff member as you would a patient, and thank the person for being present.

3. If possible, arrange the examination room so the patient is nearest to you and the caregiver is seated farther away and out of the patient's peripheral visual field; this allows the caregiver to communicate by body language without the patient's awareness; the responses are necessary to determine the accuracy of the patient's responses to your questions.

4. If possible, address the patient rather that the caregiver, and ask the patient's permission before you begin talking with the caregiver about the patient. "Do you mind if I ask your daughter a few questions about how you're doing?"

5. Speak slowly and clearly and in short sentences.

6. Always remember to review the patient's current medications and to record each one accurately in the chart.

7. If patient is wheelchair bound, avoid moving the patient to the examination table; most examinations can be performed adequately without this difficult and time-consuming effort.

8. At the conclusion of the visit, remember to *ask the patient first* and then the caregiver if they have any questions.

9. Conclude the interview with the same good eye contact, a smile, and a comfortable handshake, *first with the patient* and then with the caregiver.

The Difficult Patient

1. Allow the difficult patient to vent his or her feelings.

2. Listen patiently and allow the patient to tell his or her story.

3. Avoid a judgmental attitude. View the patient's disruptive behaviors as an *opportunity* to learn more about his or her needs and concerns.

4. Maintain a calm and confident demeanor; control the expression of emotion to what is appropriate for a medical professional.

5. Ask family members or friends accompanying the patient for their perspectives.

6. Be patient during the interview; upset human behavior changes slowly.

7. Attempt to close the encounter with some type of agreed-on contract and plans for the next scheduled visit.

The Somatizing Patient

1. Patients who somatize experience emotional distress or difficult life situations as physical symptoms.

2. Up to 60% of somatizing patients have coexisting depression, and some studies have suggested an association between somatization disorder and a history of sexual or physical abuse (Kroenke et al., 1994).

3. Part of the pathophysiology of somatization is *the need to be sick*.

4. Realize that the patient is truly suffering, and acknowledge this through a concerned attitude.

5. The BATHE technique (background, affect, trouble, handling, empathy) is a helpful way to structure the clinical interview (Stuart and Lieberman, 2002).

6. Frequent, regularly scheduled visits allow patients to feel they are being followed closely and decrease the need for emergency department visits.

7. Patients' frequent requests for laboratory and x-ray studies are best addressed with compromise and assurance that the regular visits can ensure that any serious problem will be found early.

8. Patients' frequent telephone calls can be handled by discussing limits on the number and length of calls and by offering to increase (temporarily) the frequency of the office visits.

Giving Bad News

1. Breaking "bad news" is an unpleasant task that must be approached with the patient's best interest in mind.

2. Patients generally desire frank and empathetic disclosure of a terminal diagnosis or other bad news.

3. The **ABCDE** technique is used for sharing bad news (Rabow and McPhee, 1999):

   Advanced preparation. Be familiar with relevant clinical information, and be prepared to discuss basics of treatment and prognosis.

   Build a therapeutic environment and relationship. Have family support present; meet everyone. Warn that bad news is coming, and use appropriate touch.

   Communicate well. Learn what is already known. Share additional information frankly, using common language and compassion; allow for silence and tears. Ask the patient to restate what has been said. Allow time for questions.

   Deal with reactions. Assess and respond to emotional reactions. Be aware of body language. Be empathetic and supportive, and avoid criticizing other health professionals.

   Encourage and validate. Explore what the news means to the patient. Offer realistic hope. Inquire about patient's emotional and spiritual needs, and offer resources for assistance as indicated.

Conclusion

The art of interviewing is a skill that is learned, developed, and enhanced through clinical practice. It is an ongoing process that will change as the physician engages people of different ages from a variety of circumstances and with a variety of health concerns. Through each interview, listening is a key element for establishing and maintaining rapport, respect, and relationship with the patient. More than just a collection of techniques, listening is the ability to be fully present in the moment of the interview with the person who has come for help and care. It is the art of interviewing and building bridges of continuity to a long-term relationship of trust and care.

References

The complete reference list is available online at www.expertconsult.com.

15 CHAPTER

Interpreting Laboratory Tests

Elizabeth A. Warner and Arthur H. Herold

Chapter contents

The use of the clinical laboratory to evaluate patients for the presence or absence of disease transcends medical and surgical specialties. Physicians in all areas of medical practice are dependent on laboratory testing to arrive at a correct diagnosis. Because many factors increase the uncertainty associated with a test result, physicians need to understand the limitations of interpreting test results.

Clinical decision making using diagnostic laboratory testing is based on the assumption that a given test is accurate and precise. Diagnostic test *accuracy* is the ability of a test to distinguish patients with a disease from those who are disease free (Leeflang et al., 2008). Test accuracy is not necessarily fixed; accuracy may vary among patient populations and with different clinical conditions. *Precision* is a measure of the reproducibility of a test measurement when the same specimen is rechecked under the same circumstances. Sources of imprecision include biologic variability and analytic variability. *Biologic variability* is the variation in a test result in the same person at different times because of physiologic processes, constitutional factors, and extrinsic factors (McClatchey, 2002) (Table 15-1). *Analytic variation* refers to the variation in repeated tests on the same specimen and relates to analytic technique and

specimen processing. With current technology, biologic variation plays a larger role than analytic variation in most laboratory tests.

The Concept of "Normal"

The result of a laboratory test is compared with a reference standard, which traditionally has indicated values that are seen in healthy persons. Using the terms "normal results" or "normal range" implies that there is a clear distinction between healthy and diseased persons, when in reality there is considerable overlap.

The current standard of comparison for laboratory results is the *reference range*, which is frequently defined by results that are between chosen percentiles (typically the 2.5th to 97.5th percentiles) in a healthy reference population. Several problems are encountered when deriving a reference range. Often, the reference population is not representative of persons being tested. Differences in gender, age distribution, race, ethnicity, or the setting (hospitalized vs. ambulatory patients) between the reference population and the person receiving the test may be present. The person being tested

Table 15-1 Biologic Variables that Affect Test Results

Biologic Rhythms
Circadian
Ultradian
Infradian
Constitutional Factors
Age
Gender
Genotype
Extrinsic Factors
Posture
Exercise
Diet: caffeine
Drugs and pharmaceuticals: oral contraceptives
Alcohol use
Pregnancy
Intercurrent illness

From Holmes EA. The interpretation of laboratory tests. In McClatchey KD (ed). Clinical Laboratory Medicine, 2nd ed. Philadelphia, Lippincott–Williams & Wilkins, 2002, p 98.

Table 15-2 Probability that a Healthy Person Will Have an Abnormal Result with Multiple Tests

Number of Independent Tests	Probability of Abnormal Result (%)
1	5
2	10
5	23
10	40
20	64
50	92
90	99
Infinity	100

From Burke MD. Laboratory tests: basic concepts and realistic expectations. Postgrad Med 1978;63:55.

should be tested under similar physiologic conditions (e.g., fasting, sitting, resting) as the reference population. The size of the reference population may be too small to include a representative range of the population.

Two statistical methods, parametric and nonparametric, are generally used to define the reference intervals. The *parametric* method applies when the results of the sample population fits a normal gaussian distribution, with a bell-shaped curve around the mean. In this case, the 2.5th and 97.5th percentiles can be calculated using statistical formulas. When the reference values do not follow a normal distribution, *nonparametric* methods are used, arranging the results from the reference subjects in ascending order, and identifying values between the 2.5th and 97.5th percentiles as within the reference range.

Reference ranges for a particular test can be the manufacturer's suggested reference range or may be modified because of differences in the population using the laboratory. The Clinical Laboratory Improvement Act of 1998 (CLIA) has defined three requirements for reference values: the normal or reference ranges must be made available to the ordering physician; the normal or reference ranges must be included in the laboratory procedure manual; and the laboratory must establish specifications for performance characteristics, including the reference range, for each test before reporting patient results. Using the manufacturer's reference range is valid when the analytic processing of the test is the same as that done by the manufacturer and when the population being tested is similar to the reference population used to define the reference range. When selecting a reference range that includes 95%

of the test results, 5% of the population will fall outside the reference range for a single test. When more than one test is ordered, the probability increases that at least one result will be outside the reference range. Table 15-2 compares the number of independent tests ordered with the probability of an abnormal result being present in healthy persons.

Evaluating a Test's Performance Characteristics

Given that tests are not totally accurate or precise, one must have a way to quantify these shortcomings. A test's ability to discriminate diseased from nondiseased persons is defined by its sensitivity, specificity, and positive and negative predictive values. Table 15-3 shows how each is calculated. Sensitivity and specificity are inherent technical aspects of a test and are independent of the prevalence of disease in the population tested. However, given that diseases have a spectrum of manifestations, sensitivity and specificity are improved if the population is heavily weighted with patients who have advanced (vs. early) illness.

Sensitivity is defined as the percentage of persons with the disease who are correctly identified by the test. *Specificity* is the percentage of persons who are disease-free and correctly excluded by the test. The *positive predictive value* is defined as the percentage of persons with a positive test who actually have the disease, whereas the *negative predictive value* is the percentage of persons with a negative test who do not have the disease. Predictive value is influenced by the sensitivity and specificity of the test and the *prevalence* (the percentage of people in a population who at a given time have the disease).

Separating Diseased from Disease-Free Persons

Under ideal circumstances, sensitivity and specificity approach 100%. In reality, they are lower. The best currently available test to decide who is diseased or disease-free could be imperfect and have sensitivities and specificities in the 80% range. Moreover, discrepancies between a test's efficacy and its effectiveness are common. *Efficacy* is a test's performance under ideal conditions, whereas *effectiveness* is its performance under usual circumstances. Tests under development are evaluated under highly rigorous criteria, but in clinical practice, inadvertent error can be introduced into the technical performance or interpretation of the test results. Also, test values for the diseased and disease-free populations overlap.

A cutoff value may be chosen to separate "normal" from abnormal (Figure 15-1). This decision is arbitrary and involves selecting a balance between sensitivity and specificity. The receiver operating characteristic (ROC) curve is a graphic analysis used to identify a cutoff that minimizes false-positive and false-negative results (Figure 15-2). The sensitivity and specificity are calculated for a number of cutoff values, with the variables *1-Specificity* plotted on the *x* axis and *Sensitivity* plotted on the *y* axis. Each point on the curve represents a cutoff for the test. A perfect test would have a cutoff that allowed both 100% sensitivity and 100% specificity. This would be a point at the upper-left corner of the graph. The most efficient cutoff for a single test is the one that gives the most correct results, represented by the value that plots nearest to the upper-left corner of the graph.

The optimal cutoff depends on the purpose of the test and essentially is a risk/benefit analysis. In situations where disease detection is most important, the cutoff may be chosen that maximizes sensitivity at the expense of decreasing specificity. If disease exclusion is the goal, sensitivity and negative predictive value need to be maximized. It is important that negative results be *true* negatives as opposed to false negatives, so that a negative test has correctly excluded the individual as having disease. Similarly, if disease confirmation is the goal, specificity and positive predictive value are critical. It is important that positive results are *true* positives and not false positives, so that healthy persons are not misidentified, especially when treatments (e.g., surgery) have serious risks.

The predictive value of a test is directly related to the pretest probability of disease. When the prevalence of disease is high in the population, a positive test result is expected and a negative result is not expected, because the disease is common. Similarly, when the prevalence is low, a negative test result is anticipated because few people have the disease. These characteristics of predictive value become clinically useful when one compares the outcome of a positive or negative test result with the pretest probability of disease (Figure 15-3). Prevalence (pretest probability of disease) is plotted against predictive value for a positive and negative test. Note that a test result loses its ability to discriminate those who have disease from those who do not at the extremes of prevalence. If disease probability is low, a positive or negative result does not change the post-test probability much—it is still low. On the other hand, if disease probability is high, the post-test results, whether positive or negative, do not substantially alter an already high probability of disease being present. The predictive value has the greatest power to discriminate those with disease from those who are disease free in the mid-pretest probability range, near 50%. A positive test result suggests a higher post-test probability of disease than a negative result.

Table 15-3 Diagnostic Test Performance Characteristics

Finding	Disease Present	Disease Absent
Test positive	True positive (TP)	False positive (FP)
Test negative	False negative (FN)	True negative (TN)

Sensitivity = TP/(TP + FN); Specificity = TN/(TN + FP).
Positive predictive value = TP/(TP + FP); Negative predictive value = TN/(TN + FN).

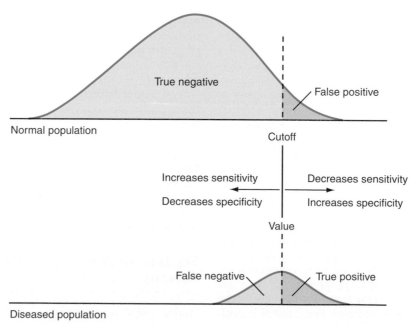

Figure 15-1 Effect of changing a test's cutoff value on disease classification.
(Modified from Cebul RD, Beck LH. Teaching Clinical Decision Making. Westport, Conn, Praeger, 1985, p 4.)

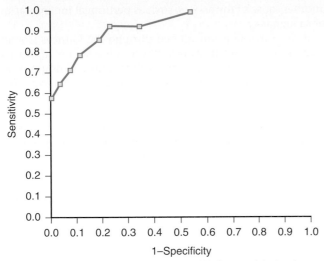

Figure 15-2 Receiver operating characteristic (ROC) curve showing the effect of changing the cutoff values for separating disease from no disease. *(From Tetrault GA. Laboratory statistics. In Henry JB (ed). Clinical Diagnosis and Management by Laboratory Methods, 20th ed. Philadelphia, Saunders, 2001.)*

Multiple Test Ordering

For many diseases, more than one test is available for diagnostic or screening purposes. The dilemma then becomes whether a positive result on several tests must be present before the diagnosis is confirmed, or whether a single positive test is sufficient to label the person as diseased. The various possibilities will have an impact on sensitivity and specificity if the tests are viewed separately. Consider the example in which two tests are available for the diagnosis of a disease. Three combinations can lead to an affirmative diagnosis:

1. If one of the two tests is positive, the diagnosis is made.
2. A positive result for both tests is required before the diagnosis is confirmed.
3. The second test is performed only if the first is positive, and the person is labeled as diseased only if the second is also positive.

The first combination will increase sensitivity and decrease specificity in comparison with each test alone, and the second combination will decrease sensitivity and increase specificity. These effects on sensitivity and specificity for multiple test ordering are similar to shifting the cutoff point for a single test.

The value of performing a second test only when the first is positive generally comes into play when the first test is significantly less expensive and easier to administer than the second but is less specific, although highly sensitive. The second test is highly sensitive and specific but more costly to perform on large populations, especially for screening purposes. An example is the enzyme-linked immunosorbent assay (ELISA) and Western blot test for human immunodeficiency virus (HIV) testing. The ELISA has a high sensitivity and is relatively inexpensive and easy to perform, but it is less specific. The Western blot test has high sensitivity and specificity, but it is more expensive and more difficult to perform. Using the ELISA first identifies almost everyone with the disease, whereas the Western blot excludes the fraction of persons incorrectly labeled as

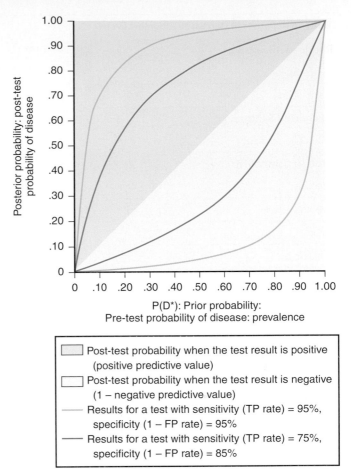

	Post-test probability when the test result is positive (positive predictive value)
	Post-test probability when the test result is negative (1 – negative predictive value)
	Results for a test with sensitivity (TP rate) = 95%, specificity (1 – FP rate) = 95%
	Results for a test with sensitivity (TP rate) = 75%, specificity (1 – FP rate) = 85%

Figure 15-3 The relationship between pretest and post-test probability of disease based on a positive or negative test result. *(From Sackett DL, Haynes RB, Guynett GH, et al. Clinical Epidemiology, 2nd ed. Boston, Little, Brown, 1991, p 92.)*

having disease (false positives) by the ELISA test. This testing sequence has improved sensitivity and specificity over each test alone and is more cost-effective than initially performing both tests.

Considerations for Ordering Tests

In addition to diagnostic accuracy, the other important consideration in test ordering is the ultimate effect on the patient. What actions will be taken, based on the test results? What are the expected benefits or harms that might occur, based on a positive or a negative result? Will ordering a particular test be more likely to help than harm the patient? Unfortunately, at present, randomized controlled trials (RCTs) that examine the outcomes of test-and-treatment strategies are not available for most clinical situations. Thoughtful systematic reviews of diagnostic test accuracy, linked with clinical evidence examining treatment options, may be the best available evidence to help guide decisions on diagnostic testing (Cornell et al., 2008).

The following section presents an overview of 40 commonly ordered tests. Each section discusses the physiologic significance of the test, a typical range of reference values, and a listing of some common disease states that might explain an abnormal result. The reference ranges for each

Table 15-4 Causes of Decreased Albumin Levels

Reduced Absorption
Malabsorption
Malnutrition
Decreased Synthesis
Chronic liver disease
Protein Catabolism
Infection
Hypothyroidism
Burns
Malignancy
Chronic inflammation
Increased Losses
Nephrotic syndrome
Cirrhosis
Protein-losing enteropathies
Hemorrhage
Dilutional
Syndrome of inappropriate antidiuretic hormone secretion (SIADH)
Intravenous hydration

test are intended as guides and may differ from the reference ranges used by different laboratories, depending on the reference population and the test methodology.

Albumin

Albumin is a transport protein that is produced mainly in the liver and maintains osmotic pressure. Albumin has a long half-life (20 days) and a small (~5%) daily turnover. In humans, albumin levels rise from birth up to age 1 year, thereafter remaining stable at approximately 3.5 to 5.5 grams per deciliter (g/dL) throughout adult life. Albumin levels are reduced with advancing liver disease, nephrotic syndrome, protein-losing enteropathy, malnutrition, and some inflammatory diseases (Table 15-4). Elevations of serum albumin are unusual except in dehydration.

In severe acute infection, reduced albumin production combined with increased catabolism causes a reduction in serum albumin levels beginning in 12 to 36 hours and reaching a maximum nadir in about 5 days. As a marker for malnutrition, however, albumin levels decline relatively late. Albumin levels are most helpful in the evaluation of edema, liver disease, and proteinuria.

The difference between the serum albumin level and the albumin in ascites fluid, the serum-ascites albumin gradient (SAAG), can help differentiate portal hypertension from other causes of ascites. SAAG greater than 1.1 g/dL is seen with portal hypertension; SAAG less than 1.1 g/dL suggests another cause of the ascites, such as peritoneal inflammation or malignancy.

Most of the albumin filtered through the kidneys is reabsorbed, so significant urinary albumin is a sign of abnormal renal function. Large amounts (>300 mg/dL) of albumin can be detected on standard urine dipsticks. *Microalbuminuria* is defined as a persistent increase of urinary albumin that is below the detectable range of the standard dipstick test. Microalbuminuria is a marker for early diabetic nephropathy and also predicts macrovascular disease. Urinary albumin can be assayed from a spot urine specimen, which is corrected by the urine creatinine, or a 24-hour urine collection. A 24-hour urinary albumin excretion in mg/day equates to the same numeric value for the spot urine albumin (mg)/creatinine (g) ratio. Therefore the reference ranges for each test are normal <30, microalbuminuria 30-300, and clinical albuminuria >300. Factors that may interfere with the test accuracy include strenuous or prolonged exercise, upright posture, hematuria, menses, genital or urinary infections, congestive heart failure, uncontrolled hypertension or uncontrolled hyperglycemia, and high protein or high salt intake.

Alkaline Phosphatase

Alkaline phosphatase (ALP) is found in a wide variety of tissues, including the liver, bone, intestine, and placenta. The reference value for ALP depends on age and gender, with higher levels in childhood, adolescence, and pregnancy. A typical reference range in an adult is 25 to 100 U/L. In adults, the source of an elevated ALP is the liver, bone, or medication (Table 15-5). Typically, hepatic elevations of ALP are suggestive of cholestatic liver disease or biliary tract dysfunction. Mild ALP elevations (one to two times above reference range) can occur with parenchymal liver disease, such as hepatitis or cirrhosis. Marked ALP elevations occur with infiltrative liver disease or biliary obstruction, intrahepatic or extrahepatic. A persistently elevated ALP level can be an early sign of primary biliary cirrhosis. In cholestatic liver disease, bilirubin and *gamma-glutamyltransferase* (GGT) levels are increased as well, with less prominent elevations in aminotransferase levels. To confirm a hepatic source of an elevated ALP level, one can simultaneously measure GGT, which is elevated in obstructive liver disease but not with bone disease. Imaging studies of the liver, by sonography or computed tomography (CT), can define an anatomic basis for obstruction in the setting of an elevated ALP level of hepatic origin.

Aminotransferases

Liver chemistry tests are widely used to assess hepatic function. Common markers of hepatocellular damage are the aminotransferases, *aspartate aminotransferase* (AST) and *alanine aminotransferase* (ALT). While AST is also found in other tissues, such as the heart, blood, and skeletal muscle, ALT is more specific for liver. The aminotransferases are released by hepatocytes with cell injury or death. The reference range is approximately 10 to 40 U/L for AST and 15 to 40 U/L for AST. The magnitude of the elevation of aminotransferases and the ratio of AST to ALT can help suggest the cause of liver disease. Mild elevation (<5 times the upper limit of normal) of the ALT or AST, with ALT > AST, is frequently found with chronic liver disease, including chronic viral hepatitis, fatty

Table 15-5 Causes of Increased Alkaline Phosphatase Levels

Bone Origin
Paget's disease
Osteomalacia
Rickets
Hyperparathyroidism
Metastatic disease
Liver Origin
Extrahepatic biliary obstruction
Pancreatic cancer
Biliary cancer
Common bile duct stone
Intrahepatic obstruction
Metastatic liver disease
Infiltrative diseases
Hepatitis
Primary biliary cirrhosis
Sclerosing cholangitis
Cirrhosis
Passive hepatic congestion
Other Causes
Drugs
Phenobarbital
Phenytoin
Chlorpropamide
Hyperthyroidism
Temporal arteritis

Table 15-6 Pattern of Liver Function Elevation

Test	Hepatocellular Disorders	Obstructive Disorders
Bilirubin	+	++
Aminotransferases	+++	+
Alkaline phosphatase	+	++
γ-Glutamyltransferase	+	++
Albumin	Decreased	Normal

liver, and medications. Probably the most common cause of persistently elevated unexplained aminotransferases is fatty infiltration of the liver. Less common causes of mildly elevated aminotransferases with ALT > AST include autoimmune hepatitis, hemochromatosis, alpha-1 antitrypsin disease, Wilson's disease, metastatic disease, and cholestatic liver disease. Mild aminotransferase elevations with AST > ALT are more suggestive of alcohol-related liver disease, but can also occur with cirrhosis and fatty liver. With alcoholic hepatitis, AST levels typically are approximately twice ALT levels, but the AST levels rarely are greater than 300 U/L. Marked elevations (greater than 15 times upper limit of normal) of AST and ALT suggest significant necrosis, such as seen in acute viral or drug-induced hepatitis, in ischemic hepatitis, or as can occur with acute biliary obstruction (Green and Flamm, 2002). However, the magnitude of elevation of the aminotransferases does not necessarily correlate with the severity of underlying liver disease or the prognosis. In fact, normal or minimally elevated aminotransferases may be seen in patients with end-stage liver disease. When AST is elevated without elevation of ALT, one should consider extrahepatic causes, particularly myocardial or skeletal muscle sources. When AST and ALT are elevated approximately the same, a hepatic origin is most likely. Table 15-6 compares the differences in liver function tests between hepatocellular and obstructive disorders.

Lactate dehydrogenase (LDH) is elevated in liver disease but is nonspecific; it is also found in skeletal muscle, cardiac muscle, blood, and some pulmonary disorders. Measurement of LDH rarely adds useful information to the evaluation of liver disease. GGT is a microsomal enzyme that is inducible by alcohol and certain drugs, including warfarin and some anticonvulsants. Although not specific for alcohol abuse, GGT is the most sensitive liver enzyme for alcohol abuse.

Amylase and Lipase

Pancreatic disease, particularly *acute pancreatitis,* is often associated with elevations in amylase and lipase. Table 15-7 lists common causes of elevated amylase and lipase. Lipase levels have greater sensitivity and specificity for pancreatic disease than amylase levels. Because there are many different assays for amylase and lipase, with different reference ranges, physicians should consult their laboratory's reference range to determine their upper limits of normal. Amylase and lipase values increase 3 to 6 hours after the onset of acute pancreatitis, both peaking at approximately 24 hours. Amylase levels fall to normal in 3 to 5 days; lipase levels return to normal in 8 to 14 days. Because of exocrine insufficiency caused by recurrent pancreatitis, amylase levels tend to be lower when alcohol is the cause of pancreatitis, as opposed to gallstone or drug-induced pancreatitis. Pancreatitis is likely when the amylase is elevated to three times the upper limit of normal. When lipase levels are more than five times normal, pancreatitis is virtually always present. A normal amylase value, however, does not exclude pancreatitis, especially when induced by hypertriglyceridemia.

Antinuclear Antibodies

Antinuclear antibodies (ANAs) are autoantibodies against parts of the cell's nucleus. Combined with clinical features, ANA testing can help diagnose certain collagen vascular

Table 15-7 Causes of Elevated Amylase and Lipase Levels

Amylase	Lipase
Pancreatic Diseases	
	Acute pancreatitis
	Chronic pancreatitis
Acute pancreatitis	
Chronic pancreatitis	
Pancreatic pseudocyst	
Pancreatic cancer	
Pancreatic trauma	
Nonpancreatic Diseases	
Salivary gland disorders	Acute cholecystitis
Intestinal perforation, ischemia, or obstruction	Intestinal infarction
Diabetic ketoacidosis	Perforated peptic ulcer
Perforated peptic ulcer	Renal failure
Ruptured ectopic pregnancy	
Renal failure	
Macroamylasemia	
Pregnancy	

Table 15-8 Conditions Associated with Positive Antinuclear Antibody (ANA) Test

ANA very useful for diagnosis
Systemic lupus erythematosus
Systemic sclerosis
ANA somewhat useful for diagnosis
Sjögren's syndrome
Polymyositis-dermatomyositis
ANA very useful for monitoring or prognosis
Drug-associated lupus
Mixed connective tissue disease
Autoimmune hepatitis
ANA not useful or has no proven value for diagnosis, monitoring, or prognosis
Rheumatoid arthritis
Multiple sclerosis
Thyroid disease
Infectious diseases
Idiopathic thrombocytopenia purpura
Fibromyalgia

From Solomon DH, Kavanaugh AJ, Schur PH, et al. Evidence-based guidelines for the use of immunologic tests: antinuclear antibody testing. Arthritis Rheum 2002;47:434-444.

disorders (Table 15-8). The likelihood that an ANA test will help with diagnosis depends on the pretest probability of disease. ANA tests are reported as negative (no staining) or positive at the highest cutoff of dilution of the serum that shows immunofluorescent nuclear staining. If positive, the description of the pattern is noted. When the ANA test is positive, testing for specific nuclear antigens should be guided by the clinical findings.

Although the ANA is 95% sensitive for *systemic lupus erythematosus* (SLE), it is not specific and is seen in other diseases. Higher titers are more specific for SLE but may be seen in the other autoimmune diseases. About 20% of normal people have an ANA titer of 1:40 or higher, and 5% have a titer of 1:160 or higher. Less than 5% of patients with definite SLE have a negative ANA titer. Because of the high prevalence of positive ANAs in normal people, physicians need to reserve the diagnosis of SLE for patients who have clinical findings compatible with SLE. ANA titers correlate poorly with relapses, remission, and severity of disease and are not helpful in monitoring the course or response to therapy. ANA testing should be ordered when a connective tissue disease is considered, but it is not generally helpful in the evaluation of nonspecific complaints, such as fatigue or back pain (Solomon et al., 2002).

For patients with a positive ANA titer, further testing for specific nuclear antibodies can be obtained, guided by the pattern of ANA staining and the clinical findings. The interpretation of testing for specific nuclear antigens can also be difficult; most of the "specific" antigens are not 100% specific for a particular disease and need to be interpreted in the clinical context. The anti-DNA test is highly specific for SLE, with about 95% specificity but only 50% to 60% sensitivity, and it can be used as a confirmatory test in patients with a positive ANA. Similarly, the anti-Sm (Smith) test is also highly specific for SLE, but with 30% sensitivity. Anti-SSA/Ro and anti-SSS/La are often used to diagnose Sjögren's syndrome but can also be found in SLE. Anti Scl-70 is found in scleroderma but is not a requirement for diagnosis.

Bilirubin

Bilirubin is produced by catabolism of hemoglobin in extrahepatic tissues. Hepatocytes conjugate the bilirubin, and it is then excreted into bile. Blood bilirubin levels are a function of production rate and biliary excretion. Total bilirubin is a combination of lipid-soluble *unconjugated* bilirubin and water-soluble *conjugated* bilirubin. Total bilirubin is less than 1.5 mg/dL and is normally primarily unconjugated bilirubin. The initial step in the evaluation of an elevated bilirubin level is to distinguish conjugated (direct) from unconjugated (indirect) hyperbilirubinemia.

Probably the most common cause of unconjugated hyperbilirubinemia is *Gilbert's syndrome,* a benign condition that affects up to 5% of the population. In Gilbert's syndrome, only the unconjugated bilirubin is elevated; the rest of the liver enzymes are normal. Other causes of unconjugated hyperbilirubinemia include hemolysis, ineffective erythropoiesis (as in megaloblastic anemias), or a recent hematoma. With normal hepatic function, hemolysis is not associated with bilirubin levels greater than 5 mg/dL. In an asymptomatic person with mildly elevated unconjugated hyperbilirubinemia (<4 mg/dL), a presumptive diagnosis of Gilbert's syndrome can be made if there are no medications that cause elevated bilirubin, there is no evidence of hemolysis, and the liver enzymes are normal (Green and Flamm, 2002).

Conjugated hyperbilirubinemia generally occurs with defects of hepatic excretion, including extrahepatic obstruction, intrahepatic cholestasis, cirrhosis, hepatitis, and toxins. Bilirubinuria is a fairly sensitive marker for biliary obstruction and may occasionally be found before jaundice is evident.

Blood Urea Nitrogen and Creatinine

Blood urea nitrogen (BUN) is a byproduct of protein metabolism and is produced by the liver. The reference range for BUN level is 7 to 18 mg/dL. A rise in BUN can be seen with worsening renal function. However, an elevated BUN level is not specific for intrinsic renal disease and can be seen with prerenal causes of azotemia such as hypovolemia and congestive heart failure, postrenal causes of obstructive nephropathy, and gastrointestinal bleeding. At low flow rates, the renal tubules will increase reabsorption of urea, thereby elevating BUN proportionately more than creatinine. BUN can also be reduced in severe liver disease, malnutrition, the syndrome of inappropriate antidiuretic hormone secretion (SIADH), or occasionally the third trimester of pregnancy.

Creatinine is a product of muscle metabolism, and production is related to muscle mass, age, gender, and race, and dietary meat intake. Creatinine is filtered by the glomerulus and secreted by the proximal tubule. Creatinine levels increase as renal function is reduced. At normal renal function, most of the urinary creatinine excretion is from glomerular filtration, with about 5% to 10% from tubular secretion. As the *glomerular filtration rate* (GFR) declines, a larger proportion of creatinine excretion comes from secretion; therefore, direct measurements of creatinine clearance overestimate GFR with progressive reductions in renal function. Some drugs, including cimetidine, trimethoprim, fenofibrate, salicylates, and pyrimethamine, can block the secretion of creatinine and falsely elevate creatinine levels, particularly in the setting of a low GFR. Although serum creatinine has long been used to estimate renal function, current guidelines from the National Kidney Foundation recommend using *estimated* GFR (eGFR) from serum creatinine to report kidney function. Many clinical laboratories now automatically report the eGFR using the Modification of Diet in Renal Disease (MDRD) equation. This equation uses age, serum creatinine, and gender to estimate the GFR, expressing GFR in mL/min/1.73 m^2. Limitations of the eGFR include lack of standardization of creatinine assays in different laboratories and underestimation of GFR in healthy persons. In addition, the equations were developed in persons with chronic kidney disease and may not accurately calculate GFR in elderly, nonwhite, or healthy persons (Stevens and Levey, 2005).

The BUN/creatinine ratio can help differentiate prerenal and postrenal causes of renal insufficiency from intrinsic renal disease. Ratios of 10:1 suggest intrinsic renal pathology; ratios greater than 20:1 suggest prerenal or postrenal causes.

Calcium

The total calcium level is a measurement of free (also called *ionized*) calcium, protein-bound calcium, and a chelated fraction. Approximately 50% of total calcium is ionized, 40% to 50% is bound to albumin, and 5% to 20% is bound to other ions. Only the free or ionized portion of calcium is physiologically active. Because of the binding of calcium with albumin, simultaneous measurements of calcium and albumin need to be performed to interpret calcium abnormalities. For every 1 g/dL that serum albumin is decreased below 4 g/dL, the estimated serum calcium is corrected by adding 0.8 mg/dL to the measured calcium level. An alternative is to measure ionized calcium levels in patients with abnormalities of serum albumin. The reference range for serum calcium is 8.5 to 10.5 mg/dL and for ionized calcium, 4.65 to 5.28 mg/dL. Serum calcium measurements are not precise enough to differentiate normal levels from mildly elevated calcium levels reliably; therefore a number of measurements are needed to confirm true mild hypercalcemia.

The etiology of *hypercalcemia* is either hyperparathyroidism or malignancy in more than 90% of hypercalcemic patients. In the ambulatory setting, most patients with hypercalcemia have hyperparathyroidism. Typically the hypercalcemia of hyperparathyroidism is modest, with calcium levels less than 11 mg/dL and minimal symptoms. Hospitalized patients are more likely to have malignancy as a cause of hypercalcemia. Calcium levels greater than 13 mg/dL are usually associated with malignancy. Intact *parathyroid hormone* (PTH, parathormone) levels can differentiate hyperparathyroidism from other causes of hypercalcemia. Nonhyperparathyroid causes of hypercalcemia will give low or "normal" intact PTH levels in a setting of hypercalcemia, whereas the PTH level will be increased in hyperparathyroidism. Occasionally, patients with a family history of hypercalcemia show a reduction in calcium excretion and have familial hypocalciuric hypercalcemia. Other causes of hypercalcemia are related to increased gastrointestinal (GI) absorption, increased bone resorption, and decreased renal excretion (Table 15-9).

Perhaps the most common cause of a low total calcium level is a *low albumin level*. When hypocalcemia is found, one should establish that the serum albumin is normal. If serum albumin is also reduced, one should perform the above correction to confirm true hypocalcemia. Another important cause of hypocalcemia is *hypomagnesemia*, which can lead to PTH resistance or reduced PTH secretion. Correction of the magnesium deficiency usually results in correction of the hypocalcemia. Other causes of hypocalcemia include chronic kidney disease, vitamin D deficiency, malabsorption, acute pancreatitis, transfusion with citrated blood, rhabdomyolysis, hypoparathyroidism, and pseudohypoparathyroidism, and occasionally bisphosphonate therapy.

Carcinoembryonic Antigen

Carcinoembryonic antigen (CEA), an oncofetal glycoprotein antigen, has been mainly used in the evaluation of patients with adenocarcinomas of the GI tract, especially colorectal cancer. CEA may be elevated in benign as well as malignant diseases (Table 15-10). CEA is not recommended as a screening test for occult cancer (including colorectal) because of its low sensitivity and specificity, but it may be used as supportive evidence in a patient undergoing diagnostic evaluation because of signs and symptoms of colon cancer. Its main value is in monitoring for persistent, metastatic or recurrent colon cancer after surgery. A preoperative elevation should return to normal in 6 to 12 weeks (CEA half-life, 2 weeks), if all disease has been resected. The liver metabolizes CEA, and therefore hepatic diseases can result in delayed clearance. Treatment (surgery, radiation, chemotherapy) may produce

Table 15-9 Causes of Calcium Abnormalities

Hypercalcemia
Hyperparathyroidism (primary and secondary)
Malignancies: breast, lung, prostate, renal, myeloma, T-cell leukemia, lymphoma
Drugs
Thiazide diuretics
Milk-alkali syndrome
Vitamin D intoxication
Granulomatous diseases
Sarcoidosis
Tuberculosis
Chronic renal failure
Immobilization
Hyperthyroidism

Hypocalcemia
Hypomagnesemia
Hypoparathyroidism
Malabsorption of calcium or vitamin D
Acute pancreatitis
Rhabdomyolysis
Hyperphosphatemia
Chronic renal failure
Transfusion of multiple units of citrated blood
Drugs
Loop diuretics
Phenytoin
Phenobarbital
Cisplatin
Gentamicin
Pentamidine
Ketoconazole
Calcitonin

Table 15-10 Conditions Associated with Elevated Carcinoembryonic Antigen (CEA) Level

Disease	Patients with Elevated CEA (%)
Carcinoma of entodermal origin (colon, stomach, pancreas, lung)	60-75
Colon cancer	
Overall	63
Dukes Stage A	20
Dukes Stage B	58
Dukes Stage C	68
Lung cancer	
Small cell carcinoma	About 33
Non–small cell carcinoma	About 67
Carcinoma of nonendodermal origin (e.g., head and neck, ovary, thyroid)	50
Breast cancer	
Metastatic disease	≥50
Localized disease	About 25
Acute nonmalignant inflammatory disease, especially gastrointestinal tract (e.g., ulcerative colitis, regional enteritis, diverticulitis, peptic ulcers, chronic pancreatitis)	Variable
Liver disease (alcoholic cirrhosis, chronic active hepatitis, obstructive jaundice)	Variable
Renal failure, fibrocystic breast disease, hypothyroidism	Variable
Healthy persons	
Nonsmokers	3
Smokers	19
Former smokers	7

transient artifactual elevations. CEA has a 97% sensitivity for detecting recurrence in the patient whose postoperative CEA value has returned to normal, and 66% sensitivity for recurrence in the patient with normal preoperative levels.

The adult reference range for CEA is 2.5 ng/mL or less for nonsmokers and 5.0 ng/mL or less for smokers. The degree of CEA elevation correlates with tumor bulk at diagnosis and therefore with prognosis. Values less than 5 ng/mL before therapy suggest localized disease and favorable prognosis, whereas levels greater than 10 ng/mL suggest extensive disease and a worse prognosis. About 30% of patients with metastatic colon cancer have normal CEA levels. Benign diseases do not usually produce CEA levels greater than 5 to 10 ng/mL. For an individual patient, repeat testing or longitudinal monitoring should be conducted at the same laboratory with the same methods because of variability among assays. A 20% to 25% increase in plasma concentration is considered a significant change. A rising CEA level may detect recurrent disease 2 to 6 months before it is clinically apparent.

Chloride

Chloride is the most abundant extracellular *anion*. Measurements of serum chloride are not useful for routine screening but may help in the evaluation of acid-base disturbances.

The reference range of chloride is 98 to 109 mmol/L. In volume expansion, serum chloride generally increases, and in volume depletion, serum chloride is reduced. *Hypochloremia* occurs with loss of chloride-containing body fluids, such as with prolonged vomiting, burns, diuretic use, and salt-wasting nephropathy. Hypochloremia is commonly seen with metabolic alkalosis. *Hyperchloremia* occurs with non–anion gap metabolic acidosis, usually related to diarrhea or renal tubular acidosis, and with administration of large amounts of sodium chloride.

Urine chloride levels are useful in the evaluation of metabolic alkalosis. Low urine chloride (<10 mmol/L) is present with chloride-responsive causes of alkalosis, such as vomiting with volume depletion. Elevated levels of urine chloride (>20 mmol/L) are present in conditions associated with mineralocorticoid excess, such as hyperaldosteronism and hypercortisolism.

Coagulation Studies

The most common coagulation studies, *prothrombin time* (PT) and *partial thromboplastin time* (PTT), are used to evaluate patients with clotting disorders or to monitor patients taking heparin or oral anticoagulants. It is helpful for the laboratory to know whether a patient is taking an anticoagulant at testing. Hospitalized patients with nonsurgical diagnoses, who do not have liver disease or a history of anticoagulant use, do not benefit from routine PT and PTT testing. These are poor screening tests for postoperative bleeding in patients without historical risk factors, physical findings, or a medication history that suggests an increased bleeding risk (Eckman et al., 2003). Preoperative PT and PTT should be reserved for patients with known or suspected coagulation disorders and those receiving anticoagulation therapy.

Prothrombin time, a simple and inexpensive test for evaluating the extrinsic coagulation pathway, is the time in seconds for citrated plasma to clot after the addition of calcium and thromboplastin. Test accuracy depends on proper collection and instrument technique. Common uses include monitoring anticoagulant therapy with warfarin, evaluating liver function (because the liver synthesizes most of the clotting factors), and screening for coagulation disorders of the extrinsic system. PT is prolonged by defects in factors I (fibrinogen), II (prothrombin), V, VII, and X. The normal range for PT is 11 to 13 seconds.

Previously, PT measurements exhibited variability across laboratories because of differences in thromboplastin sensitivity. To correct for the type of thromboplastin used, the World Health Organization (WHO) recommends using the *international normalized ratio* (INR) to report PT results for patients taking oral anticoagulants. Now widely accepted, the INR is calculated as follows:

$$INR = (Patient\ PT / Mean\ normal\ PT)^{ISI}$$

The ISI is the international sensitivity index of the thromboplastin used at the local laboratory. Provided by the test's manufacturer, ISI reflects the responsiveness of the thromboplastin used in the PT test. The reference range for the INR in the non-anticoagulated patient is 0.9 to 1.1. The PT is prolonged in persons with vitamin K deficiency, including those with fat malabsorption syndromes, recent broad-spectrum antibiotic use, and premature infants. In addition, the use of warfarin, many drugs and herbs, severe liver disease, alcoholism, deficiencies of clotting factors, and circulating anticoagulants can prolong the PT. The PT is not affected by platelet disorders or platelet count. The target INR varies with specific indications. In general, an INR goal of 2.5 (range, 2.0-3.0) is generally accepted for the treatment of venous thromboembolic disease and atrial fibrillation, and 3.0 (range, 2.5-3.5) for patients at risk for arterial thromboembolism, including those with mechanical heart valves.

The *activated* partial thromboplastin time (aPTT, or simply PTT) is a simple, inexpensive test for evaluating the intrinsic coagulation pathway, monitoring heparin therapy, screening for hemophilia A and B, and detecting clotting inhibitors. PTT is the time in seconds for citrated plasma to clot after a contact activator is added to plasma and incubated at 37° C for 5 minutes. Thromboplastin and calcium are added and the time to clot formation is recorded, which should be within 10 seconds of the control. PTT is abnormally prolonged in most patients with coagulation disorders (~90%) and is therefore the best screening test in persons suspected of having a clotting disorder. PTT screens for all coagulation factors that lead to thrombin formation except VII and XIII. These factors include factors I, II, V, VIII (antihemophiliac), IX (Christmas), X, and XII (Hageman). PTT is useful to evaluate patients with a known, suspected, or active bleeding disorder; consumptive coagulopathy (e.g., disseminated intravascular coagulation); disorder of fibrin clot formation; or fibrinogen deficiency. In addition, PTT is prolonged with deficiency of the Fletcher (prekallikrein) and Fitzgerald factors, warfarin or heparin therapy, lupus anticoagulant, and vitamin K deficiency. PTT is significantly shortened by hemolysis, is affected by high or low hematocrit, but is not affected by platelet dysfunction or count. A prolonged PT or PTT can be caused by either a factor inhibitor or a deficiency of a clotting factor. To differentiate the two, a mixing study can be performed. When the abnormality is corrected after mixing with normal blood, a factor deficiency is likely. Failure to correct after mixing suggests the presence of a factor inhibitor.

When monitoring heparin therapy, the most widely used target for anticoagulation is a PTT 1.5 to 2.5 times the upper limit of normal. Now, however, because of the great variation in thromboplastins used in different PTT assays, PTT results vary widely among laboratories. Therapeutic heparin levels, as measured by antifactor Xa units, are approximately 0.3 to 0.7 antifactor Xa IU/mL. With plasma concentrations of heparin at 0.3IU/mL, investigators have found that mean PTT values ranged from 48 to 108 seconds, depending on the laboratory methods used. The American College of Chest Physicians recommends against the use of a fixed PTT therapeutic range for the treatment of venous thrombosis; instead, they recommend that each laboratory determine the PTT range that corresponds to a therapeutic heparin level: 0.3 to 0.7 IU/mL by factor Xa dilution. Anti–factor Xa levels may also be used to monitor appropriate anticoagulation doses in patients with obesity or renal failure, because these groups are more likely to be over-anticoagulated using weight-based heparin dosing (Hirsch et al., 2008).

Cobalamin (Vitamin B$_{12}$) and Folic Acid Deficiency

A deficiency of vitamin B$_{12}$ or folic acid may be suspected when a macrocytic anemia (MCV >100 fL) is present. Vitamin B$_{12}$ and folate deficiency causes a megaloblastic anemia, which is one type of macrocytic anemia.

The hematologic picture is identical for both folate and vitamin B$_{12}$ deficiency. *Megaloblasts* are enlarged blastic cells (precursors to the erythroid and myeloid cell lines) found in the bone marrow and caused by aberrant DNA synthesis. The peripheral blood smear typically shows the presence of oval macrocytes, hypersegmented neutrophils (>5% neutrophils with 5 lobes or any neutrophil with 6 lobes). *Anisocytosis* (size variation) and *poikilocytosis* (shape variation) of the red blood cells (RBCs) are often present, so the RBC distribution width (RDW) is increased. The reticulocyte count is usually decreased. Thrombocytopenia is present in 12% and leukopenia in 9% of cases; occasionally, B$_{12}$ or folate deficiency will present with pancytopenia. Coexisting disease such as iron deficiency, inflammatory process, renal failure, or thalassemia trait also may normalize the mean corpuscular volume (MCV) value in the patient with vitamin B$_{12}$ or folate deficiency.

The clinician must distinguish folate from B$_{12}$ deficiency, because supplementing one will not correct the symptoms from deficiency of the other, i.e., folate replacement will not improve the neuropsychiatric abnormalities caused by vitamin B$_{12}$ deficiency. The neurologic signs and symptoms, such as paresthesias, memory loss, dementia, and weakness, may precede hematologic abnormalities. Vitamin B$_{12}$ and folate deficiency often coexist because some causes overlap (Table 15-11).

Because vitamin B$_{12}$ is a cofactor in the conversion of methylmalonic acid to succinyl coenzyme A (CoA) and homocysteine to methionine, deficiencies of vitamin B$_{12}$ will lead to increased levels of methylmalonic acid and homocysteine. Folate is required in the conversion of homocysteine to methionine, but not in the conversion of methylmalonic acid to succinyl CoA. Folate deficiency is associated with elevated homocysteine, but not methylmalonic acid. The reference range for vitamin B$_{12}$ is often listed as 200 to 900 pg/mL;

however, it is now recognized that a significant portion of patients with vitamin B$_{12}$ levels of 200 to 400 pg/mL have symptoms of vitamin B$_{12}$ deficiency.

Folate levels greater than 4 ng/mL are considered normal; levels of 2 to 4 ng/mL are indeterminate. A person in negative folate balance will become serum deficient before tissue folate stores decrease; therefore a low serum folate level indicates a negative folate balance, but not necessarily tissue folate deficiency. Intake of folate may normalize serum levels initially, so serum folate levels should be determined before a hospitalized or potentially deficient patient is fed, takes vitamins, or is given a transfusion. Measuring RBC folate levels is not recommended because it is difficult to interpret. Instead, testing for methylmalonic acid and homocysteine can help determine if patients with levels in the low-normal range actually have vitamin B$_{12}$ or folate deficiency. Folic acid is absorbed in the upper small bowel, whereas B$_{12}$ is absorbed mainly in the ileum with the help of intrinsic factor, which is secreted by the gastric parietal cells. Nutritional factors and malabsorption syndromes are principal reasons for deficiency of both vitamin B$_{12}$ and folic acid. Hemolysis will falsely elevate serum folic acid levels.

Complete Blood Count

The complete blood count (CBC) measures circulating blood cells, including RBCs, white blood cells (WBCs), and platelets (Table 15-12). Current technology uses electronic cell counters that can count and size the cells, providing an estimate of cell volume (MCV) and variation in cell size (RDW), and give a five-part WBC differential, including neutrophils, lymphocytes, monocytes, eosinophils, and basophils (Tefferi et al., 2005). Typically, peripheral blood smears are prepared for manual review only when requested or when automated hematology analyzers flag abnormal results. By analyzing large numbers of cells, current instruments can generate more accurate data than by manual review for most parameters. Indications for manual review of a blood smear include the evaluation of hemolysis, RBC inclusions, myelodysplasia, megaloblastic changes, thrombocytosis, throm-

---

Table 15-11 Cobalamin (Vitamin B$_{12}$) and Folate Deficiency

Most Common Cause	Vitamin B$_{12}$ Deficiency	Folate Deficiency
Inadequate intake	Strict vegetarian diet (rare) Alcoholism, elderly patients	Malnutrition Alcoholism
Increased need	Pregnancy, lactation	Pregnancy, lactation, infancy Neoplasia, hyperthyroidism, hemolysis
Defective absorption or storage	Decreased intrinsic factor (e.g., pernicious anemia, congenital deficiency of intrinsic factor, gastrectomy) Zollinger-Ellison syndrome Pancreatitis Ileal mucosal disease (e.g., sprue, regional enteritis, surgery, lymphoma) Tapeworm infestation, other parasites Bacterial overgrowth in blind-loop syndrome Drugs (e.g., colchicine, aspirin, metformin)	Malabsorption caused by: Drugs (e.g., anticonvulsants, antituberculosis agents, oral contraceptives, folate antagonist) Jejunal mucosal disease (e.g., amyloidosis, sprue, lymphoma, surgery) Liver disease (cirrhosis, hepatoma)

bocytopenia, leukocytosis, and immature or abnormal cells (Bain, 2005).

Red Blood Cells

A mild *anemia* is the most common abnormality found on a CBC. Factors that help determine whether further testing should be performed include the degree of anemia and the presence of other abnormalities in the CBC. The first step is to classify the anemia, based on MCV, as microcytic (<80 fL), normocytic (80-100 fL), or macrocytic (>100 fL). With a *microcytic* anemia, the most important test is the ferritin level, which is diagnostic of iron deficiency anemia when less than 12 ng/mL. With a *normocytic* anemia, potentially treatable causes should be excluded

(e.g., recent bleeding, hemolysis, renal insufficiency, vitamin deficiency). Other causes of a normocytic anemia (e.g., anemia of chronic disease, primary bone marrow disorder) may need a bone marrow biopsy for definitive diagnosis. For a *macrocytic* anemia, important determinations are the medication history, alcohol use, and vitamin B_{12} or folate deficiency.

Erythrocytosis refers to a hematocrit above the reference range. In *true* erythrocytosis, the total circulatory RBC mass is increased, whereas in *relative* erythrocytosis, the RBC mass is normal, but the plasma volume is decreased, so the hematocrit is elevated. With true erythrocytosis, elevated erythropoietin levels suggest a secondary cause and can help distinguish secondary erythrocytosis from polycythemia vera (Table 15-13).

Table 15-12 Complete Blood Count Components

Test	Description	95% Reference Range Conventional	Reference Range International
Hemoglobin (Hb)	Measure of oxygen-carrying capacity of blood expressed as grams per unit volume (usually deciliters; g/dL).	M: 13.5-17.5 g/dL F: 12.0-16.0 g/dL	135-175 g/L 120-160 g/L
Hematocrit (Hct)	Measure of solid elements of blood (mostly RBCs), as percentage of whole blood (remainder is plasma). Hct = MCV × RBC. Expressed in%, usually about three times Hb. Both Hct and Hb usually are low in anemia, but may not be apparent early in acute blood loss, because plasma volume needs about 12-24 hours to equilibrate.	M: 39%-49% F: 35%-45%	0.39-49, volume fraction 0.35-0.45, volume fraction
Red blood cell (RBC) mass	Erythrocyte count; true measure of cells/L.	M: 4.3-5.7 × 10^6 cells/μL F: 3.8-5.1 × 10^6 cells/μL	4.3-5.1 × 10^{12} 3.8-5.1 × 10^{12}
Red cell indices	MCH, MCHC, MCV. *Note:* In early anemia, MCV may change before Hb and Hct.		
Mean corpuscular hemoglobin (MCH)	Hb divided by RBC; represents the content (weight) of Hb in average RBC; not as useful as MCHC.	26-34 pg/cell	0.40-0.53 fmol/cell
Mean corpuscular hemoglobin concentration (MCHC)	Hb divided by Hct, concentration of Hb per unit volume of packed RBCs. Appearance of erythrocytes on peripheral smear is affected by Hb concentration in cell; low, hypochromic; normal, normochromic; high, hyperchromic.	31.37% Hb/cell or g Hb/dL RBCs	4.81-574 mmol Hb/L RBCs
Mean corpuscular volume (MCV)	Hct × 1000 divided by the RBC count; reflects RBC size; small, microcytic; normal, normocytic; large, macrocytic. *Note:* Presence of microcytosis and macrocytosis in same sample may result in normal MCV.	80-100 fL 1fL (femtoliter) = 10^{-15} L = 1 cubic micrometer (μm^3)	80-100 fL
Red cell distribution width (RDW)	Estimate of RBC size variability (anisocytosis); standard deviation (SD) of RBC size divided by MCV.	11.5-14.5	11.5-14.5
Reticulocyte count (%)	Expressed as percent of reticulocytes per 1000 RBCs counted.	0.5%-1.5%	0.005-0.015 (number fraction)
Reticulocyte count (absolute)	Reticulocyte (%) × RBC count; more meaningful expression of erythropoiesis.	50 × 10^3/μL	50 × 10^9/L
Platelet count		150-450 × 10^3/μL	150-450 × 10^9/L

Table 15-13 Classification of Erythrocytosis

Relative Erythrocytosis
Diminished plasma volume
Spurious polycythemia

Absolute Erythrocytosis
Genetic disorders
Familiar polycythemia
Primary marrow disorders
Polycythemia vera
Secondary conditions with appropriately increased erythropoietin
High altitude, pulmonary disease, congenital heart disease, sleep apnea syndrome, carboxyhemoglobin
High-affinity hemoglobin
Secondary conditions with inappropriately increased erythropoietin production
Erythropoietin producing tumors (renal carcinoma, cerebellar hemangioma, hepatoma)
Polycystic kidney disease

Modified from Cazzolo M. Serum erythropoietin concentration as a diagnostic tool for polycythemia vera. Haematologica 2004;89:1160.

White Blood Cells

The WBC count is often requested to support a diagnosis of infection or an inflammatory process. The WBC count is useful as a means of monitoring the course of a disease or response to treatment. The cell types that make up the WBC count include neutrophils (segmented and band forms), lymphocytes, monocytes, eosinophils, and basophils. *Bands* are immature neutrophils, and *segmented* forms are mature neutrophils. To diagnose neutropenia, the *absolute neutrophil count* (ANC) should be determined. The ANC is obtained from the cell counter or calculated by multiplying the total WBC count by the percentage of bands plus mature neutrophils (segmented forms):

$$\text{ANC} = \text{WBC count} \times (\%\ \text{Bands} + \%\ \text{Segmented forms})$$

When severe neutropenia, the ANC drops below 500 cells/mm³, and the patient is at risk for infections. Causes of neutropenia include drug reactions, bacterial and viral infections, hematopoietic diseases, cachexia, hypersplenism, and autoimmune diseases. Lymphocytopenia is present when the lymphocyte count is less than 1500 cells/mm³ in the adult or 3000 cells/mm³ in children. Causes of lymphocytopenia include immunosuppressant drugs, corticosteroid therapy, viral infections (including HIV), and genetic immunodeficiencies.

Leukocytosis, or an elevated WBC count, occurs when the total WBC count is greater than 10,000 cells/mm³. An elevated WBC count may be the result of a reactive process (leukemoid reaction) or leukemia. Leukemoid reactions can result from infections, toxic conditions, neoplasms, myeloproliferative diseases, and other hematologic disorders. The first step in the evaluation of leukocytosis is to determine what type of WBC is elevated. Leukocytosis may be caused by neutrophilia, eosinophilia, basophilia, monocytosis, or lymphocytosis (Table 15-14).

Platelets

Platelets, cellular fragments of the bone marrow precursor-cell megakaryocytes, are essential to clot formation and have a life span of about 10 days. Clinically, a disorder in platelets is usually suspected in a patient with excessive bleeding, typically from a mucocutaneous source or after trauma. Clinical evidence of bleeding does not occur until the platelet count drops below 50 to 70 × 10³/μL. Platelet counts of less than 10 to 20 × 10³/μL are associated with major spontaneous bleeding. *Thrombocytopenia* may be caused by disorders of production, distribution, or destruction (Table 15-15). In evaluating thrombocytopenia, first examine the peripheral smear for platelet clumping, or repeat the test using sodium citrate as the anticoagulant. *Thrombocytosis,* or an increased platelet count, may be caused by a reactive process or a myeloproliferative disorder. Reactive processes do not usually produce platelet counts greater than 1000 × 10³/μL. Common causes of thrombocytosis include iron deficiency, acute blood loss, inflammatory disorders, malignancies, splenectomy, and myeloproliferative disorders.

Carbon Dioxide or Bicarbonate

Acid-base disturbances are often recognized by abnormalities in the carbon dioxide (CO_2) content of blood, which is composed primarily of bicarbonate (HCO_3^-), with small amounts of carbonic acid and dissolved carbon dioxide. The reference range for CO_2 is 22 to 29 mmol/L. A reduced serum bicarbonate concentration frequently suggests *metabolic acidosis,* particularly when combined with a low pH. An elevated serum bicarbonate level frequently occurs with *metabolic alkalosis.* Bicarbonate is often used as a buffer for excess acid production, and levels are reduced in metabolic acidosis. In the evaluation of acidosis, calculation of the serum *anion gap* is helpful in determining the cause of the acidosis, as follows:

$$\text{Anion gap} = \text{Na} - (\text{Cl} + \text{CO}_2)$$

The normal range is 10 to 12 mmol/L. An increased anion gap generally indicates the presence of metabolic acidosis with elevation of unmeasured ions, such as lactic acid, phosphates, sulfates, and ketoacids. A normal anion gap acidosis is seen with bicarbonate losses and increased chloride resorption and most frequently occurs with chronic diarrhea, but also with certain types of renal tubular acidosis. Low anion gaps can occur with hypoalbuminuria, congestive heart failure, and occasionally, multiple myeloma.

An elevated serum bicarbonate level frequently occurs in the setting of metabolic alkalosis. Metabolic alkalosis can be generated by loss of acid, such as in vomiting, but normally the kidney corrects the abnormality promptly by excreting excess bicarbonate. To maintain a metabolic alkalosis, the kidney must not be able to excrete excess bicarbonate. This

Table 15-14 Common Causes of Leukocytosis or Leukopenia Stratified by White Blood Cell (WBC, Leukocyte)Type

Condition	Description
Leukocytosis	
Neutrophilia	Infections, leukemia, rheumatic and autoimmune disorders, neoplastic disorders, chemicals, trauma, endocrine and metabolic disorders, hematologic disorders, drugs
Eosinophilia	Infectious diseases, parasitic infections, allergic diseases, myeloproliferative and neoplastic diseases, cutaneous diseases, gastrointestinal diseases
Basophilia	Allergic reactions, chronic myeloid leukemia, myeloid metaplasia, polycythemia vera, ionizing radiation, hypothyroidism, chronic hemolytic anemia, splenectomy
Monocytosis	Infections, neoplastic disorders, gastrointestinal disorders, sarcoidosis, drug reactions, recovering from marrow suppression
Lymphocytosis	Viral infections, lymphocytic leukemia, other infectious diseases, neoplastic disorders
Leukopenia	
Neutropenia	Overwhelming bacterial infection, viral infection, drug reaction, ionizing radiation, hematopoietic diseases, hypersplenism, anaphylactic shock, cachexia, autoimmune disease
Eosinopenia	Acute stress (usually physical), acute inflammatory states, Cushing's syndrome, corticosteroids
Basopenia	Sustained treatment with glucocorticoids, acute infection or stress, hyperthyroidism
Monocytopenia	Onset of steroid therapy; hairy cell leukemia
Lymphocytopenia	Immunodeficiency disorders, adrenocortical hormone excess, chemotherapeutic drugs, irradiation, impaired drainage of intestinal lymphatics, advanced lymphomas and carcinomas

From Speicher CE. The Right Test, 3rd ed. Philadelphia, Saunders, 1998.

abnormality usually occurs in the setting of volume depletion, when sodium reabsorption is enhanced and the sodium must be accompanied by an anion to maintain electroneutrality. In the absence of available chloride in the urine, bicarbonate is reabsorbed with sodium, thereby maintaining the alkalosis. As mentioned earlier, urine chloride levels can assist in determining the cause of the metabolic alkalosis.

C-Reactive Protein

An acute-phase reactant glycoprotein, C-reactive protein (CRP) is associated with inflammation. CRP is one of the first proteins to become elevated after an inflammatory process has begun and disappears rapidly when inflammation subsides. In healthy persons, CRP levels are usually less than 0.8 mg/L and are often below the detection limit for standard assays. Serum levels may increase dramatically to exceed 100 mg/L in the presence of bacterial and viral infections, inflammation, severe trauma, surgery, neoplastic proliferation, tissue injury, or necrosis, and transplant rejection. Moderate elevations may be seen with myocardial infarction, autoimmune diseases, rheumatic fever, pregnancy, and postoperatively, as well as in obese persons and women taking estrogen replacement therapy or with an intrauterine device in place. CRP is not affected by age, race, or food intake and does not have significant circadian variation. Drugs that may reduce or suppress CRP levels by controlling inflammation include statins, fibrates, niacin, nonsteroidal anti-inflammatory drugs (NSAIDs), steroids, salicylates, angiotension-converting enzyme (ACE) inhibitors, and beta-adrenergic blockers. CRP has some advantages over erythrocyte sedimentation rate (ESR). The CRP rises before the ESR, returns to baseline sooner, and is less influenced by altered physiologic states.

The levels of CRP used to assess atherosclerotic risk are much lower than those associated with inflammation (Myers et al., 2004). More sensitive immunoassays were developed to measure levels lower than those detected in conventional assays. These *highly sensitive* CRP tests (hsCRP; Cardiac-CRP) can accurately measure to a lower limit of 0.3 mg/L. Many studies have found that hsCRP levels predict the long-term risk of myocardial infarction, ischemic stroke, peripheral vascular disease, and all-cause mortality in healthy subjects. The hsCRP also predicts outcomes in patients with stable coronary artery disease, acute coronary syndromes, and after percutaneous coronary intervention. In 2004 the American College of Cardiology and American Heart Association (AHA) recommended hsCRP testing to further evaluate patients judged to be at intermediate risk for the development of coronary heart disease (those with 10-year CHD risk of 10% to 20%). CRP levels are divided into tertiles: low risk (<1.0 mg/L), average risk (1.0-3.0 mg/L), and high risk (>3.0 mg/L). A CRP in the highest tertile is associated with a twofold risk of major coronary events compared with a CRP in the lowest tertile. Unexplained levels of hsCRP levels higher than 10 mg/L should be repeated and evaluated for noncardiovascular causes, such as infection or inflammation (Smith et al., 2004).

Erythrocyte Sedimentation Rate

The ESR is one of the oldest laboratory tests still in clinical use. The test measures the distance that erythrocytes (RBCs) fall in a column of anticoagulated blood in 1 hour. Plasma

Table 15-15 Causes of Thrombocytopenia

Decreased Production
Congenital disorders
Radiation or chemotherapy
Vitamin B_{12} or folate deficiency
Drugs
Systemic lupus erythematosus
Aplastic anemia
Acute leukemia
Lymphomas
Alcohol abuse
Viral infections (including HIV)
Increased Destruction
Immune thrombocytopenia
Drugs
Quinine
Quinidine
Heparin
Sulfa drugs
Valproic acid
Disseminated intravascular coagulation (DIC)
Hemolytic-uremic syndrome
Hemolysis, liver dysfunction, and low platelets (HELLP syndrome)
Sepsis
Cardiopulmonary bypass
Toxemia of pregnancy, eclampsia
Splenic Sequestration

Table 15-16 Factors Affecting the Erythrocyte Sedimentation Rate (ESR)

Increase	Decrease	No Effect
Anemia	Polycythemia	Body temperature
Macrocytosis	Microcytosis	Recent meal
Female gender	Spherocytosis	Aspirin
Advanced age	Extreme leukocytosis	NSAIDs
Second- and third-trimester pregnancy	Sickle cell disease	First-trimester pregnancy
Hypoalbuminemia	Excessive anticoagulant	
Tilted ESR tube	Short ESR tube	
High room temperature	Low room temperature Clotted blood sample	

NSAIDs, Nonsteroidal anti-inflammatory drugs.

proteins known as *acute-phase reactants* facilitate erythrocyte aggregation, which in turn affects the rate at which the solid component of blood will settle in a capillary tube. The plasma proteins most responsible for this aggregation (rouleaux formation), in decreasing order, are fibrinogen, beta (β-) globulins, alpha (α-) globulins, gamma (γ-) globulins, and albumin. Inflammatory, infectious, neoplastic, and collagen vascular diseases increase the ESR. The ESR is helpful in the diagnosis of *polymyalgia rheumatica* and *temporal arteritis;* otherwise, it is both nonsensitive and nonspecific. In studies of patients with biopsy-proven temporal arteritis, 90% of patients had an ESR greater than 30 mm/hr with mean ESR of 90 mm/hr. About 4% of patients with biopsy-proven temporal arteritis have a normal ESR (Smetana and Shmerling, 2002). When there is strong clinical evidence for temporal arteritis and a normal ESR, however, a temporal artery biopsy or a trial of corticosteroids should be considered. Although

used to follow the response to corticosteroid therapy in polymyalgia rheumatica and temporal arteritis, ESR should be used in conjunction with clinical findings. Typically, ESR drops within a few days of corticosteroid therapy, falling to a level that is higher than normal. In addition, relapse can occur without ESR elevation.

Table 15-16 lists physiologic, pathologic, and technical factors that alter ESR, which is higher in women than men and higher in older persons. To determine ESR for healthy adult men, age in years is divided by 2, and for women, age in years plus 10, divided by 2. Clinical considerations for using ESR have been defined (Brigden, 1998; Sox and Liang, 1986). It should not be used as a screening test for disease in asymptomatic persons. As a single test after a normal history and physical examination in asymptomatic persons, ESR contributes to disease detection of a serious illness in less than 6 of 10,000 persons. The underlying cause of an elevated ESR is usually apparent by the history and physical examination, especially for extreme elevations of about 100 mm/hr. Many cases of unexplained elevated ESR are transient and not associated with serious disease. If no obvious cause is seen for elevated ESR, repeating the test in several months is recommended, rather than searching for occult disease.

Fecal Occult Blood Test

The fecal occult blood test (FOBT) is used to detect blood loss in the stool that is not clinically apparent. Patients who report rectal bleeding or those with frank blood by rectal examination should undergo further diagnostic evaluation and do not need an FOBT. Although mainly used to screen for colorectal cancer, the FOBT is not specific for colorectal cancer. The two main FOBTs commercially available are the *guaiac-based tests*, which detect pseudoperoxidase in the heme portion of hemoglobin, and the more expensive *immunochemical tests*, which detect the globulin portion of human hemoglobin. Most RCTs using the FOBT as a screening test for colorectal cancer used guaiac testing. Newer methods using immunochemical testing are also used in clinical practice. Stool assays that identify colon neoplasia are still being developed and tested. Guaiac FOBT kits include Hemoccult and Hemoccult II SENSA; Hemoccult II has been widely used in clinical practice as well as RCTs.

The basis of the guaiac test is that the pseudoperoxidase of hemoglobin oxidizes guaiac to form a blue-colored quinone compound, after the addition of a hydrogen peroxide developer. The likelihood of a positive guaiac test is related to the amount of blood present in the stool. Normally, about 0.5 to 1.5 mL of blood is lost daily into the GI tract. The FOBT test requires approximately 2 mL/day of blood to be positive; to be consistently positive requires more. Several factors have an impact on FOBT performance characteristics. Bleeding from proximal gastrointestinal lesions, including the right colon, may allow for degradation of the heme, which will then not catalyze the guaiac reaction. The myoglobin or hemoglobin in red meat can give a false-positive reaction, although ingesting 8 oz of cooked red meat daily has only a 5% probability of giving a positive test result. Peroxidase-rich raw vegetables and fruits (turnips, parsnips, horseradish, artichokes, mushrooms, radishes, broccoli, cauliflower, beets, apples, oranges, bananas, melons, grapes, pears, plums, cantaloupe) may give a false-positive result if fecal specimens are tested immediately after collection. However, plant peroxidases are unstable with time; therefore, if a specimen is developed several days after collection, the likelihood of a false-positive test result because of plant peroxidases is reduced.

Gastric irritants such as aspirin, NSAIDs, and excessive alcohol consumption may also produce positive results. Oral iron supplements and acetaminophen do not affect the guaiac test. Ascorbic acid (vitamin C) in excess of 250 mg/day or multivitamins with vitamin C may cause a false-negative result because ascorbic acid is a reducing agent and interferes with the oxidation of guaiac. Other antioxidants should also be avoided. Antacids may also cause false-negative results.

The processes of collecting and processing FOBTs are important in the evaluation of the results. Delaying the processing of the slides allows for dehydration of the specimen, which allows degradation of peroxidase activity and will decrease the sensitivity of testing. The delay between preparation and laboratory testing should not exceed 6 days. The issue of rehydration of dried slides with water is controversial. Rehydration of slides increases sensitivity and decreases specificity (false-positive rate increases). Rehydration increases the positivity rate of Hemoccult II fourfold, from 2% to 3% to 8% to 16% (10% average), but this rate can be minimized if the patient adheres to a low-peroxidase diet. Proper patient instruction and preparation are essential during collection of specimens (Bresalier, 2002). Patients should not collect specimens until 3 days after menses have stopped or if obvious rectal bleeding or hematuria is noted. For 3 days before testing, patients should avoid ingesting red meat, vegetables with high amounts of peroxidase (broccoli, turnip, cantaloupe, cauliflower, radishes), aspirin, NSAIDs, and vitamin C. The detection of the blue color of a positive test may be affected by other factors, including a thick stool smear, exposure to high ambient temperatures, and black stools from iron ingestion.

As a screening test for colorectal cancer, FOBT has low sensitivity and specificity. Other GI lesions, including hemorrhoids, angiodysplasia, diverticular disease, and upper GI lesions, can lead to increased blood in the stool. Bleeding from colon cancers can be intermittent or undetectable, and other factors can give false-positive or false-negative readings. About 2% to 6% of asymptomatic adults have a positive FOBT test, 10% of whom have cancer and 20% to 30%, adenomas. The rest have upper GI sources of bleeding, nonneoplastic lower GI sources of bleeding (e.g., hemorrhoids), or no identified source of bleeding. The sensitivity of the FOBT in patients with colon cancer is approximately 30%.

With home-based testing, FOBT has best been studied using a regimen of three stools. Because only one specimen is obtained during a digital rectal examination (DRE), office collection is less sensitive than three at-home determinations. A study compared FOBT during DRE (without rehydration) in the office and home-based six-sample FOBT (with rehydration) to colonoscopy. The digital FOBT was positive in 6.4% of patients with adenomas with high-grade dysplasia and 9.5% of patients with cancer, whereas the home-based FOBTs were positive in 29.8% of patients with adenomas with high-grade dysplasia and in 42.9% of patients with cancer (Collins et al., 2005). A single digital FOBT has poor sensitivity and therefore cannot be recommended as the sole test for screening for colon cancer.

Because of the concerns about sensitivity and specificity with the FOBT, new tests have been developed. With a change in the developer fluid, the Hemoccult SENSA is more sensitive than Hemoccult or Hemoccult II but less specific. Newer fecal immunochemical tests (FITs; Hema Select, FlexSure, Insure) have been developed to increase the sensitivity and specificity over FOBT. These tests are based on an antigen-antibody reaction that is specific for human hemoglobin. They do not react with animal hemoglobin or peroxide-containing foods. Moreover, the FIT is not affected by ingestion of vitamin C, iron, or rehydration, and testing can be delayed for up to 30 days. Therefore, dietary restrictions and specimen handling are not critical issues. The FIT can detect stool hemoglobin at one-tenth the concentration of the FOBT. Some brands (e.g., Insure) detect the globulin portion of hemoglobin, which is degraded in the upper GI tract. Therefore, these tests are more specific for identifying bleeding from the colon.

Glucose

The reference range for a fasting plasma glucose level is between 70 and 99 mg/dL. *Hypoglycemia* is best documented by a plasma venous glucose level less than 50 mg/dL, although there is considerable variability in the level of hypoglycemia that causes symptoms. Asymptomatic hypoglycemia in a patient not taking insulin or oral hypoglycemic agents may be a laboratory artifact caused by ongoing metabolism of glucose in the specimen, especially if a delay has occurred in processing the specimen. The diagnosis of hypoglycemia is best made with typical symptoms associated with a laboratory confirmation of venous hypoglycemia, followed by relief of symptoms after ingesting glucose. The glucose tolerance test (GTT) can produce hypoglycemia in normal persons and should not be routinely ordered in the evaluation of hypoglycemia.

Hypoglycemia can be defined as iatrogenic, postprandial, or fasting. *Postprandial* hypoglycemia occurs after meals and is usually mild and self-limiting. *Alimentary* hypoglycemia occurs when patients have rapid gastric emptying. Insulin levels rise rapidly after a meal and fall more slowly than glucose levels, which results in hypoglycemia. *Fasting* hypoglycemia is seen much less often than reactive hypoglycemia and may be a harbinger of more severe disease, including insulin-producing pancreatic tumors and hepatic, adrenal, or renal insufficiency, or it may be the result of excess insulin or sulfonylurea administration. True fasting hypoglycemia needs to be confirmed by a prolonged fast, with simultaneous measurement of glucose and insulin. This technique can help determine whether the hypoglycemia is associated with excess insulin.

Diabetes mellitus is characterized by *hyperglycemia*. The American Diabetes Association has defined *normal* fasting plasma glucose as less than 100 mg/dL (5.6 mmol/L), *prediabetes* as 100 to 125 mg/dL (5.6-6.9 mmol/L), and diabetes mellitus as 126 mg/dL (7.0 mmol/L) or greater.

Glycosylated Hemoglobin (Hemoglobin A$_{1c}$)

The hemoglobin A$_{1c}$ (HbA$_{1c}$) fraction measures nonenzymatic glycosylation of hemoglobin, which is related to level of glucose concentration over the life span of the erythrocyte. The HbA$_{1c}$ fraction can be used to estimate glucose control in the previous 3 months. In persons with normal erythrocyte survival, the glucose levels in the last 30 days contribute to 50% of the HbA$_{1c}$, whereas the glucose levels in the preceding 90 to 120 days contribute only 10% to the HbA$_{1c}$ measurement. Although previously laboratories varied considerably in the reporting of HbA$_{1c}$ results, virtually all U.S. laboratories now have adopted the National Glycohemoglobin Standardization Program (NGSP) methods. Recent standards propose reporting HbA$_{1c}$ in the familiar percentage and in international units (mmol/mol), combined with the HbA$_{1c}$-derived average glucose (ADAG) (Saudek et al., 2008). Using NHANES III data that the population average for HbA$_{1c}$ was 5.17 with standard deviation (SD) of 0.45, the International Expert Committee (2009) selected an HbA$_{1c}$ of 6.5% (~3 SD above average) as the cutoff point to diagnose diabetes mellitus, with confirmation by a fasting glucose greater than 126 mg/dL or oral GTT greater than 200 mg/dL, or a repeat HbA$_{1c}$ greater than 6.5%. Goals for achieving optimal control of diabetes are controversial, but a reasonable goal in most persons is an HbA$_{1c}$ less than 7%. Conditions that shorten erythrocyte survival, such as hemolysis or recent bleeding, give a lower HbA$_{1c}$ level.

Helicobacter pylori

A spiral, urease-producing bacterium, *Helicobacter pylori* is associated with almost 90% of duodenal ulcers. Testing is indicated in patients with either active or previously documented peptic ulcer disease, in the evaluation of dyspepsia who have no "alarm features," and for patients with a history of gastric MALT (mucosa-associated lymphoid tissue) lymphoma (MALToma) (Chey and Wong, 2007). Several tests can be performed during endoscopy. Rapid urease testing of a biopsy specimen has sensitivity over 90% and specificity over 95%, with results available within 1 to 24 hours. The sensitivity of rapid urease tests is reduced by drugs that treat *H. pylori*, including bismuth, antibiotics, and proton pump inhibitors (PPIs). Histologic examination of gastric biopsies can also detect *H. pylori*. Culturing *H. pylori* has a lower yield, is more expensive, and is not widely done.

Serologic tests for immunoglobulin G (IgG) antibody to *H. pylori* are helpful in determining previous infection and have sensitivity of approximately 88% but specificity of only 70% to 80%. Even though titers may decline slowly after eradication of the organism with antibiotics, these tests have limited use in evaluation of the effectiveness of antibiotic therapy and cannot reliably distinguish current from past infection. The value of *H. pylori* antibody testing in the evaluation of uninvestigated dyspepsia depends on the prevalence of *H. pylori* infection. In areas of high prevalence (>20%), serologic testing may be cost-effective for a test-and-treat strategy. Antibody testing is inexpensive and has a very good negative predictive value.

Urease breath tests using carbon 13 (^{13}C)–urea or ^{14}C-urea can detect ongoing replication of *H. pylori*. These tests are most helpful in determining whether *H. pylori* has been successfully eradicated after a course of treatment, but they can also confirm active infection in the presence of positive serologic findings. After the ingestion of labeled urea, urease-producing *H. pylori* organisms break down the urea and produce labeled CO_2, which is absorbed into the circulation and exhaled, and can be measured by collecting an exhaled breath sample in a bag. False-negative breath tests may occur with the recent use of antibiotics, bismuth, or PPIs. Most studies find the sensitivity and specificity of the urease breath test to be greater than 95%.

Testing for *H. pylori* antigen in the stool by ELISA assays has been found to have sensitivity over 90% and specificity approaching 100%, thereby making it an accurate noninvasive method to diagnose active *H. pylori* infection in untreated patients. As in urease breath testing, recent antibiotics, PPIs, and bismuth can cause false-negative results. Stool tests can also be used to confirm eradication, but no sooner than 4 weeks after completion of therapy.

Hepatitis Serology

Hepatitis A virus (HAV), hepatitis B virus (HBV), and less often hepatitis C virus (HCV) are the usual causes of acute viral hepatitis. A person with symptoms of acute hepatitis should have these four hepatitis serologies performed: immunoglobulin M (IgM) anti-HAV, hepatitis B surface antigen (HBsAg), IgM anti-HBc, and anti-HCV. At present, stool and blood assays for HAV antigen are not available. The diagnosis of hepatitis A is made by the detection of IgM anti-HAV during acute illness. A positive anti-HAV with only IgG anti-HAV indicates previous infection.

In hepatitis B, HBsAg is the earliest serologic marker of infection and is present before elevation of the aminotransferases. If HBsAg is present for more than 6 months, the patient should be considered chronically infected (carrier). Antibodies to HBsAg (anti-HBs) indicate immunity to hepatitis B and appear several weeks to months after HBsAg disappears. The gap between the presence of HBsAg and anti-HBs is a window period; during this time antibody to hepatitis core antigen (anti-HBc) can be detected in the blood. Anti-HBc can be differentiated into an IgM anti-HBc, which indicates recent infection, and an IgG anti-HBc, which indicates previous infection. HBeAg, a subparticle of core antigen, is present only when HBsAg is present and is a marker for infectiousness. Anti-HBe appears after HBeAg disappears, indicates decreasing infectivity, a good prognosis, and remains detectable for years. HBV DNA testing can be used to follow titers in patients receiving antiviral therapy for chronic hepatitis B infection. *Hepatitis delta virus* (HDV) infection coexists with hepatitis B in about 4% of hepatitis B infections and carries an increased mortality rate. HDV depends on the presence of HBV for expression and replication and can cause acute or chronic infection. Previous vaccination for hepatitis B should produce a positive titer only for anti-HBs.

Hepatitis C occasionally presents as acute hepatitis, but more frequently is detected in the evaluation of patients with elevated aminotransferases or chronic liver disease. With chronic hepatitis, aminotransferases are often only mildly elevated and occasionally, normal. The diagnosis is made by detecting antibody to hepatitis C (anti-HCV). Anti-HCV does not differentiate acute from chronic infection and does not indicate immunity. In acute hepatitis C the antibody may not be detected initially, and the test may need to be repeated later to confirm infection. In a patient with abnormal liver enzymes and a risk factor for hepatitis C (e.g., injection drug use, hemophilia, history of blood transfusions before 1985), a positive anti-HCV is sufficient to make the diagnosis.

A quantitative HCV-RNA assay can be used for diagnosis of acute infection as early as 1 to 2 weeks after exposure, and before anti-HCV appears. Quantification of viral ribonucleic acid (RNA) by the reverse-transcriptase polymerase chain reaction (RT-PCR) also can confirm hepatitis C infection, as well as measure viral load. These tests are particularly useful in the absence of risk factors or abnormal liver enzymes, when antibody testing is indeterminate, or with immunodeficiency. In addition, quantification of viral RNA can assess response to treatment.

Human Immunodeficiency Virus

The diagnosis of HIV infection usually depends on the detection of antibodies to the virus. The recommended screening test for HIV infection is an initial enzyme immunoassay, the ELISA test, which can detect the presence of antibody to HIV 2 to 8 weeks after infection. HIV ELISA testing studies in blood donors have found specificities of 99.7% and 99.99% (Chou et al., 2005). An initially positive ELISA should be repeated, and repeatedly positive ELISAs need to be confirmed by a more specific test, most often the Western blot. A positive ELISA combined with a negative Western blot should be considered a false-positive HIV test and indicates that HIV infection is not present. A positive ELISA and an indeterminate Western blot result can be a marker for early HIV infection or advanced acquired immunodeficiency syndrome (AIDS), or it can be a false-positive test result. The predictive value of a positive HIV test depends on the prevalence in the population being tested.

Rapid HIV tests are currently available that check saliva, whole blood, and plasma. The whole-blood tests measure capillary blood with a finger stick and do not require centrifugation. These tests are interpreted visually, do not require instrumentation, and provide test results in minutes. Rapid tests may be preferred for testing in patients who are not likely to return for results of standard testing, for pregnant women at delivery with

no HIV testing during their pregnancy, and for testing during occupational exposure. Rapid tests for HIV have similar sensitivity and specificity to the standard ELISA tests. Clusters of false-positive oral rapid tests have been reported, emphasizing the need for confirmatory testing of positive rapid tests.

Tests to measure HIV directly include quantitative HIV RNA testing by PCR, which measures viral load or actual viral replication. Quantitative HIV RNA measurements are useful in evaluating indeterminate Western blot results and acute HIV infection, when the patient presents before seroconversion. Because neonates born to HIV-infected mothers often have maternal antibodies for months, early testing with HIV-1 DNA PCR can identify infants with HIV infection. In 2006 the U.S. Centers for Disease Control and Prevention (CDC) recommended routine, voluntary HIV screening for all patients age 13 to 64 in any health care setting.

Iron Studies

Iron deficiency is the most common type of anemia worldwide and therefore a significant cause of human morbidity. Other than menstrual blood losses, negligible iron is lost in a healthy person. Normally, regulation of iron absorption in the proximal small intestine controls iron balance. Iron deficiency results from increased need (growth of infancy or childhood, pregnancy), excessive loss (menstruation, hemorrhage, GI loss), inadequate intake (iron-deficient diet), or defective absorption (gastrectomy or sprue). In adult men or postmenopausal women with adequate iron stores, it takes 3 to 4 years for these stores to be depleted once negative iron balance starts.

During early *iron deficiency anemia*, the erythrocytes may be normochromic normocytic, and later the peripheral blood smear may show microcytosis, anisocytosis, poikilocytosis, and hypochromia. The reticulocyte count is low, and RDW is high (>16). Bone marrow stores of iron are decreased or absent. Serum iron has marked diurnal variation (higher in morning, lower later in day) and is increased transiently after meals. Because morning levels determine the reference range, iron levels should be performed on a fasting morning specimen. Obtaining a serum iron level without determining the level of transferrin (*total iron-binding capacity*, TIBC) is of limited value. Serum iron is decreased with inflammation, infection, and ascorbate deficiency and increased with iron ingestion, transfusions, liver disease, aplastic anemia, and ineffective erythropoiesis. TIBC is an approximation of transferrin and can be calculated when the transferrin is known, as follows:

$$TIBC(\ g/dL) = Transferrin(mg/dL) \times 1.25$$

The total iron-binding capacity or transferrin is not subject to diurnal fluctuation, but it is reduced in chronic inflammation and malnutrition. Iron deficiency is the only microcytic hypochromic anemia associated with absent iron stores (Brittenham, 2005). The serum ferritin is the best indirect marker for the assessment of iron stores. However, serum ferritin is an acute-phase reactant and can be elevated in some patients with liver disease, malignancy, or inflammatory or infectious diseases. Therefore, although a low ferritin (<12 µg/L) is highly specific for iron deficiency, elevated ferritin levels do not rule out iron deficiency. Hemolysis may cause falsely high levels of serum iron. Table 15-17 lists results of iron studies in common anemias.

Lipid Profile

Lipid levels are often obtained to evaluate cardiovascular risk. There are four major classes of lipoproteins: chylomicrons, very-low-density lipoprotein (VLDL) cholesterol (VLDL-C), low-density lipoprotein (LDL) cholesterol (LDL-C), and high-density lipoprotein (HDL) cholesterol (HDL-C). Approximately 60% to 70% of plasma cholesterol is carried as LDL-C. A direct association is seen between increased LDL-C and the risk of CHD. HDL-C functions in the reverse transport of cholesterol to the liver and carries apolipoprotein A-1. HDL-C accounts for about 20% to 30% of total cholesterol. HDL-C and CHD have a strong independent inverse relationship; for every 1-mg/dL decrease in HDL, the risk of coronary artery disease (CAD) increases 2% to 3%. The Adult Treatment Panel (ATP III) of the National Cholesterol Education Program (2001) has recommended lipid screening as a tool to promote cardiovascular disease risk reduction. The standard lipid profile, as recommended by the ATP III, consists of direct measurement of total cholesterol, HDL-C, and triglycerides, with a calculated LDL-C, obtained after a 9-hour fast. The basis for the LDL calculation is the recognition of the following:

$$Total\ cholesterol = HDL - C + LDL - C + VLDL - C + Chylomicrons$$

In the fasting state, chylomicrons approximate zero and drop out of the equation. The VLDL is estimated as the triglycerides (mg/dL)/5. The Friedewald formula for calculating LDL follows:

$$LDL = Total\ cholesterol - HDL - (Triglycerides/5)$$

The Friedewald formula for estimating LDL is not valid in the following three conditions: when there are chylomicrons present, when the triglycerides are over 400 mg/dL, and when there is dysbetalipoproteinemia (type III hyperlipidemia). Hypertriglyceridemia and dysbetalipoproteinemia lead to underestimations of the LDL. Using the Friedewald formula, some non-LDL lipoproteins—intermediate-density lipoprotein (IDL) and lipoprotein (a)—are included in the LDL calculation. Measurements of direct LDL, although more costly, give more accurate values than calculations using this formula in patients with hypertriglyceridemia. Recent analysis suggests that using nonfasting total cholesterol and HDL measurements give reliable assessment of CHD risk without the need to measure triglycerides (Di Angelantonio, 2009).

There are a number of sources of physiologic and analytic variation in lipid measurements. The physiologic variation is the amount that results can vary in one person, even under ideal testing circumstances, because of different physiologic states. The analytic variation is the variation in a measurement from the same sample using the same assay. Physiologic variations can result in lipid measurements 13% above or below a person's mean levels and are greater than analytic variations. The following conditions can affect the physiologic variation and should be considered when interpreting a lipid profile. Chylomicrons should be eliminated after a 12-hour fast; however, almost all the chylomicrons are removed after 9 hours. Failure to fast before the test elevates the triglycerides and leads to an underestimation of the LDL. The total cholesterol and HDL are not significantly different in the fasting or postprandial state. Testing should be done with standardization of body position. Lying down leads to dilution of the plasma, with an approximate 10% reduction in total cholesterol, LDL, and HDL and a 15% reduction in triglycerides. Most guidelines suggest performing the test 5 minutes after sitting. In addition, prolonged application of the tourniquet during venipuncture can cause elevation of the cholesterol; 2% to 5% increases in cholesterol have been noted after 2 minutes of tourniquet application. Dietary changes begin to become apparent in lipid measurements in approximately 1 to 2 weeks; therefore, patients should have a stable diet for 3 weeks before testing. Morning specimens are preferred because triglycerides have diurnal variation—lowest in the morning, highest in the afternoon. In addition, lipids are 8% higher in the winter than summer. Recent illness or surgery, including myocardial infarction, stroke, or cardiac catheterization, can lower lipid measurements for several weeks. For major illness or injury, it may be necessary to wait 2 to 3 months before measurement. Cholesterol levels decrease 24 hours after myocardial infarction and remain depressed for up to 12 weeks. The plasma cholesterol level is about 3% lower than the serum level. Lipid values may fluctuate by 3% to 9% with use of the same sample and assay. Table 15-18 lists drugs that can affect the lipid components. Major causes of secondary dyslipidemia include diabetes mellitus, hypothyroidism, nephrotic syndrome, and obstructive liver disease.

Table 15-17 Iron-Related Laboratory Measurements in Common Anemias

Type of Anemia	Serum Iron	Total Iron-Binding Capacity	Transferrin Saturation	Serum Ferritin	Serum Transferrin Receptor
Iron deficiency anemia	Low	High	Low	Low	High
Anemia of chronic disease	Low	Low	Low	High*	Low
Thalassemia	High	Low	High	High	High
Megaloblastic anemia	High	Low	High	High	High
Hemolytic anemia	High*	Low*	High*	High*	High

From Cook JD. The measurement of serum transferrin receptor. Am J Med Sci 1999;318:269-276.
*May fall within normal range.

Magnesium

Magnesium levels are not routinely included in standard chemistry panels, so abnormalities of magnesium frequently go unrecognized. The reference range of serum magnesium concentration is 1.7 to 2.2 mg/dL (1.5-1.7 mEq/L, or 0.75-0.95 mmol/L). The most common cause of *hypermagnesemia* is excess magnesium intake in a patient with chronic kidney disease (Table 15-19). Mild hypermagnesemia can also be seen in Addison's disease, hypothyroidism, and lithium intoxication. Symptoms of hypermagnesemia are seen with levels greater than 4 to 6 mg/dL.

Hypomagnesemia is more common than hypermagnesemia. The three mechanisms causing hypomagnesemia are reduced intestinal absorption from malnutrition or malabsorption, increased urinary losses, and intracellular shifts. Hypomagnesemia is typically associated with alcohol abuse, hypokalemia, hypocalcemia, chronic diarrhea, and ventricular arrhythmias. Symptoms occur with serum concentrations less than 1 mEq/L. Clinically, hypomagnesemia is associated with neuromuscular hyperirritability, including tremors, tetany, and rarely, seizures. In distinguishing renal wasting from extrarenal losses as the cause of hypomagnesemia, a 24-hour urine excretion of greater than 24 mg or a spot urine fractional excretion of magnesium greater than 2% suggests that the cause of hypomagnesemia is excessive renal losses. Drugs that cause hypomagnesemia include loop and thiazide diuretics (but not potassium-sparing diuretics), cisplatin, aminoglycosides, pentamidine, and cyclosporine.

Mononucleosis (Epstein-Barr Virus Infection)

Mononucleosis is a common viral infection, particularly in adolescents and young adults, and has an incubation period of 30 to 45 days and a prodrome of 7 to 14 days. Typically, mononucleosis is associated with an infection by the Epstein-Barr virus (EBV), which is a herpesvirus. Laboratory findings include leukocytosis, with more than half the leukocytes being lymphocytes. Approximately 10% to 15% of the mononuclear cells are atypical lymphocytes. Thrombocytopenia may develop with infectious mononucleosis. Almost 90% of patients with mononucleosis have abnormal liver enzymes. Mononucleosis is typically diagnosed by detecting a *heterophile antibody,* which is a nonspecific response to EBV infection. The heterophile antibody response is an IgM antibody that will agglutinate with the surface antigen of sheep and horse RBCs, but not with guinea pig kidney cells. Monospot tests are done with rapid slide agglutination procedures and horse RBCs to detect the heterophile antibody. Clinically, about 40% of patients have a positive heterophile antibody response at week 1, 60% at week 2, and 80% to 90% by week 3. The heterophile antibody usually persists for 3 to 6 months after an acute infection, less frequently up to 1 year. The heterophile antibody has an overall false-negative rate of 10% to 15%. However, in children under age 4 years, the heterophile antibody is falsely negative in 70% to 80% of cases. False-positive heterophile antibodies can occur with rubella, hepatitis, other viral infections, and lymphoma.

When the heterophile antibody is negative or the features of infectious mononucleosis are atypical, the disease can be confirmed with specific Epstein-Barr antibodies. Acute or recent infection is thought to be present if four serologic criteria are found: positive IgM to viral capsid antigen (VCA); high titers (>1:320) of IgG to VCA; positive early antigen antibody (anti-EA); and initial absence of antibody to Epstein-Barr nuclear antigens (EBNAs). The most useful EBV-specific antibody to diagnose acute mononucleosis is the IgM VCA, which appears soon after the onset of symptoms and has sensitivity of 91% to 98%

Table 15-18 Effects of Drugs on Lipid Values

Drug	Total Cholesterol	LDL Cholesterol	HDL Cholesterol	Triglycerides
Androgens	—	↑	↓	—
Antiepileptics	—	↑	↑	↑
Thiazide diuretics	↑/—	↑	—	↑
Beta blockers	—	—	↓	↑
Alpha blockers	↓/—	↓/—	↑	↓
Corticosteroids	↑	↑	↑	↑
Cyclosporine	↑	↑	—	—
C-19 Progestin	—	↑	↓	—
C-21 Progestin	—	—	↓	—
Oral estrogens	↓	↓	↑	↑
Phenothiazines	↑	—	↓	↑
Retinoids	↑	↑	↓	↑

Modified from Henkin Y, Como JA, Oberman A. Secondary dyslipidemia: inadvertent effects of drugs in clinical practice. JAMA 1992;267:961-968.
HDL, High-density lipoprotein; *LDL,* low-density lipoprotein.

Table 15-19 Causes of Magnesium Abnormalities

Hypermagnesemia
Overingestion (usually in setting of renal insufficiency)
Antacids
Cathartics
Laxatives
Renal insufficiency
Addison's disease
Hypothyroidism
Lithium intoxication

Hypomagnesemia
Gastrointestinal causes
Low-magnesium diet
Malabsorption
Diarrhea
Renal tubular disorders
Ketoacidosis
Alcohol abuse
Drugs
Diuretics
Digitalis
Cyclosporine
Cisplatin
Aminoglycosides
Carbenicillin
Amphotericin B

and specificity of 99%. Convalescent testing should document the appearance of IgG EBNA and disappearance of IgM VCA and anti-EA.

Syndromes mimicking infectious mononucleosis, but with negative heterophile antibodies, are considered *heterophile-negative* infectious mononucleosis. The most common syndromes are related to cytomegalovirus infection and toxoplasmosis. Occasionally, viral hepatitis, rubella, lymphoma, leukemia, and the drugs isoniazid and phenytoin can cause a mononucleosis-like syndrome. Because heterophile antibodies are not uniformly positive early in the disease, serial tests may often be needed weekly to confirm mononucleosis. Specific serologic tests for EBV are relatively expensive and take longer to obtain results, so they are generally reserved for unclear cases and are not necessary in most patients with infectious mononucleosis. In an adolescent or young adult with appropriate clinical symptoms, heterophile antibodies are 95% sensitive and specific.

Natriuretic Peptides (BNP and N-terminal pro-BNP)

Blood levels of natriuretic peptides are used in the evaluation of *heart failure*. Cardiac cells release natriuretic peptides, in response to stretch and wall tension. Ventricular myocytes release a pro–B-type natriuretic peptide (pro-BNP), which is cleaved into the active B-type natriuretic peptide (BNP) and the inactive N-terminal pro-BNP (NT–pro-BNP). Levels of both BNP and NT–pro-BNP increase with age and in renal insufficiency and are reduced in women and obese patients. Some medications, including spironolactone, ACE inhibitors, and angiotensin receptor blockers, lower BNP/NT–pro-BNP levels. Other conditions that increase natriuretic peptides include myocardial ischemia, atrial fibrillation, pulmonary embolus, pulmonary hypertension, chronic kidney disease, and sepsis.

The major established use of BNP testing is evaluating *acute dyspnea*, when the cause is uncertain, to differentiate whether the etiology is from heart failure versus another cause. A normal level in a patient with acute dyspnea has a high negative predictive value and suggests that heart failure is unlikely the etiology. Elevated levels of BNP and NT–pro-BNP also are predictive of death or increased cardiovascular events. The optimal cutoffs for BNP/NT–pro-BNP vary with age. BNP less than 100 pg/mL or NT–pro-BNP less than 400 pg/mL makes the diagnosis of heart failure unlikely. Levels of BNP greater than 400 pg/mL or NT–pro-BNP greater than 2000 suggest heart failure (Dickstein et al., 2008). Using BNP measures to guide therapy in patients with established heart failure did not improve overall survival, quality of life, or total hospitalization but did reduce hospitalizations for heart failure in patients less than 75 years old (Pfisterer et al., 2009).

Phosphorus

The usual serum phosphorus level is approximately 2.5 to 4.8 mg/dL in adults and 4.0 to 6.0 mg/dL in children. Disorders of phosphorus metabolism are caused by variations in dietary intake, phosphorus excretion, and transcellular shifts. Because postprandial phosphorylation of glucose can decrease serum phosphorus levels, fasting specimens are more accurate. *Hyperphosphatemia* most often occurs in the setting of reduced renal excretion from renal insufficiency. Other causes of hyperphosphatemia include excess phosphate ingestion, either orally or with phosphate-containing enemas, hypoparathyroidism, and spurious causes such as thrombocytosis. Less common causes include acromegaly, hyperthyroidism, acidosis, and massive cell lysis from hemolysis, rhabdomyolysis, and tumor lysis after chemotherapy.

Hypophosphatemia is defined as a serum phosphorus level below 2.5 mg/dL. Clinically significant hypophosphatemia occurs at levels less than 1.5 mg/dL. The three major mechanisms associated with hypophosphatemia are decreased intestinal absorption, increased phosphate loss from the kidney, and increased phosphorus shift into the bones. Decreased absorption occurs most often with antacid use. Persistent hypophosphatemia most frequently results from disorders causing increased phosphate loss in the kidney, including hyperparathyroidism, renal tubular disease, and chronic acidosis. Intracellular shifts into cells and bones, during acute respiratory alkalosis, hyperalimentation, intravenous carbohydrate administration, rapid tumor growth, or treatment of respiratory failure or diabetic ketoacidosis, can cause hypophosphatemia.

Potassium

Potassium is the most abundant *cation* in the body and has a much higher concentration in the intracellular space than in extracellular fluids. Normal potassium levels are maintained despite fluctuating potassium intake by adjustments in renal secretion of potassium. *Hyperkalemia* is defined as a serum potassium level greater than 5.1 mmol/L. Occasionally, hyperkalemia can be an artifact (pseudohyperkalemia) of phlebotomy, associated with thrombocytosis, leukocytosis, or hemolysis during phlebotomy. In a patient with hyperkalemia of no apparent cause, a plasma potassium level can eliminate these effects on the potassium measurement. Because the normal response to increased potassium intake is to increase excretion, hyperkalemia is not likely to be attributed to increased intake unless there is a deficiency in potassium excretion. Shifts of potassium from intracellular to extracellular fluids, such as with acute metabolic acidosis, crush injury, burns, insulin deficiency, beta-adrenergic blockade, and hemolysis, can be associated with a transient hyperkalemia. Persistent hyperkalemia is usually associated with decreased potassium excretion. Potassium excretion by the kidney is flow dependent; therefore, oliguria and anuria are important causes of hyperkalemia. Because aldosterone deficiency is an important cause of decreased potassium excretion, hyperkalemia is seen with hyporeninism, hypoaldosteronism, type 4 renal tubular acidosis, and drugs that inhibit aldosterone (Table 15-20).

Hypokalemia is associated with a serum potassium level of less than 3.5 mmol/L. Symptoms are nonspecific and include muscular weakness. Occasionally, hypokalemia is associated with sustained inadequate potassium intake, particularly in patients with alcohol abuse. Transient episodes of hypokalemia are associated with increased extracellular to intracellular potassium shifts and occur with catecholamine increase, hyperinsulinemia, and adrenergic drugs such as bronchodilators. More frequently, hypokalemia is a result of GI loss of potassium, such as with protracted vomiting, diarrhea, and laxative abuse. Other causes of hypokalemia include drugs, metabolic alkalosis, skin losses, and increased urinary losses. Hypomagnesemia is an important cause of refractory hypokalemia.

Pregnancy Tests

Current pregnancy tests use immunoassays with monoclonal antibodies to measure the beta subunit of human chorionic gonadotropin (hCG). Serum assays and sensitive urine assays can now detect pregnancy approximately 1 week after conception. Home pregnancy tests are generally sensitive enough to diagnose pregnancy accurately when done on the first day of the missed period. The most common reason for a false-negative pregnancy test is incorrect timing, such as performing the test too soon.

In the first 4 to 8 weeks of pregnancy, hCG levels double approximately every 2 days. Failure to double in 48 to 72 hours suggests an ectopic pregnancy or abnormal intrauterine pregnancy. For the first 2 weeks after conception, serum levels of hCG are higher than those in urine. However, beginning at approximately 3 weeks and for the remainder of the pregnancy, urine levels are higher than serum levels. Levels of hCG return to normal approximately 2 weeks after delivery. After an abortion, levels return to normal in approximately 3 to 8 weeks. Other conditions that can raise hCG levels include gestational trophoblastic neoplasms, such as hydatidiform mole and choriocarcinoma.

Prostate-Specific Antigen

Prostate-specific antigen (PSA) is a glycoprotein protease enzyme produced by the epithelial cells of the prostate. This protein circulates in the serum and can become elevated because of benign and malignant conditions of the prostate. From 50% to 90% of PSA is protein bound and the remainder is free. PSA is used as a tumor maker for the screening, diagnosis, and management of prostate cancer. PSA lacks specificity for cancer, however, because it can be elevated in benign conditions such as benign prostatic hypertrophy (BPH). Estimates suggest that a PSA higher than 4 ng/mL has sensitivity of 70% to 80% and specificity of 60% to 70% for prostate cancer. Factors other than prostate cancer can affect the PSA level (Table 15-21). Controversy surrounds the effect of the digital rectal examination (DRE) on PSA. Theoretically, digitally palpating the prostate gland should elevate the serum PSA. However, it appears that PSA elevations after DRE are probably not significant, so there is no recommendation to withhold PSA testing immediately after DRE.

Although elevations of the PSA are associated with increased risk of prostate cancer, the upper limit of normal of 4 ng/mL may be somewhat arbitrary. During an initial screening examination, prostate cancer was found in 27% of men with PSA levels of 4.1 to 9.9 ng/mL and 59% with PSA over 10 ng/mL (Hernandez and Thompson, 2004). However, prostate cancer is found in 23.9% of men with PSA of 2.1 to 3.0 ng/mL and 26.9% with PSA of 3.1 to 4.0 ng/mL (Thompson et al., 2004).

The positive predictive value (PPV) of the PSA is improved if used complementary to DRE (Table 15-22). The PPV is doubled if the patient also has an abnormal DRE. A normal PSA does not exclude cancer; 20% to 40% of men with organ-confined prostate cancer will have PSA within the reference range. One report of men with confirmed, untreated, clinically significant prostate cancer found these PSA values: less than 4 ng/mL (27%), 4 to 10 ng/mL (21%), 10 to 20 ng/mL (16%), and greater than 20 ng/mL (36%).

The use of PSA for screening for prostate cancer remains controversial. Although it is clear that PSA testing can lead to earlier detection of prostate cancer, it is not clear that early diagnosis and treatment offers significant reduction in prostate cancer mortality. Given that the lifetime risk of death from prostate cancer is only 3% in U.S. men, a large portion of men detected by screening may not have clinically significant disease.

In addition to screening, PSA is used to monitor the response to treatment for localized prostate cancer. After radical prostatectomy, PSA levels should become undetectable. Any detectable levels suggest residual or recurrent tumor and may occur months or years before it becomes clinically apparent. PSA levels fall after radiation therapy, although usually do not become

Table 15-20 Causes of Abnormal Potassium Levels

Hyperkalemia	Renal losses
Pseudohyperkalemia	Diuresis
Thrombocytosis	Renal tubular acidosis (proximal, distal)
Leukocytosis	Hypomagnesemia
Prolonged tourniquet use during venipuncture	Hyperaldosteronism
Hemolysis	Cushing's syndrome
Reduced excretion	**Nonrenal losses**
Oliguria	Diarrhea
Renal failure	Vomiting
Hyporeninemic hypoaldosteronism	Periodic paralysis
Adrenal insufficiency	Burns
Type IV renal tubular acidosis	**Cellular shifts**
Cellular shifts	Alkalosis
Acute acidosis	Beta-adrenergic therapy
Insulin deficiency	Catecholamine excess
Rhabdomyolysis	**Drugs**
Drugs	Thiazide diuretics
Beta blockers	Loop diuretics
ACE inhibitors	Epinephrine
Angiotensin receptor blockers	Albuterol
Spironolactone	Carbenicillin
Triamterene	Ticarcillin
Amiloride	Licorice
NSAIDs	Glucocorticoids
Heparin	Mineralocorticoids
Cyclosporine	
Pentamidine	
Hypokalemia	
Inadequate diet	
Malnutrition	
Alcoholism	

ACE, Angiotensin-converting enzyme; *NSAIDs,* nonsteroidal anti-inflammatory drugs.

undetectable. A PSA recurrence has been defined as three successive increases in the PSA level after radiation therapy.

Total Protein

Total protein includes albumin and globulin. The factors that affect the total protein level include changes in fluid status, the balance of protein synthesis and catabolism, and protein losses. While dehydration can cause a relative increase in serum protein concentration, volume expansion causes a relative decrease in protein concentration. Elevated protein levels in the absence of dehydration are usually related to increased globulin levels. As previously discussed, acute-phase reactants are proteins that are increased in inflammatory conditions and include C-reactive protein, haptoglobin, fibrinogen, ceruloplasmin, and α_1-antitrypsin.

Table 15-21 Noncancer Factors that May Influence Prostate-Specific Antigen

Factor	Change
Acute urinary retention	Increase
Androgens	Increase
Antiandrogens	Decrease
Bed rest	Decrease
Benign prostatic hypertrophy	Increase
Cirrhosis	Increase
Cystoscopy	Increase
Digital rectal examination	Not significant
Diurnal variation	No change
Ejaculation	Increase
Extensive exercise	Increase
Finasteride	Decrease
Physiologic variation	May fluctuate by 30%
Prostate needle biopsy	Increase
Prostatic massage	Increase
Prostatitis	Increase
Radial prostatectomy	Decrease
Radiation therapy	Increase initially then decrease
Transurethral resection of prostate	Increase
Transurethral ultrasound of prostate	No change
Urethral instrumentation	Increase

Table 15-22 Positive Predictive Value (PPV) of Total Prostate-Specific Antigen (PSA) for Prostate Cancer

Digital Rectal Examination	PSA Value		
	0.0-4.0 ng/mL	4.1-10 ng/mL	>10 ng/mL
Negative	9%	20%	31%
Positive	17%	45%	77%

Data from Oesterling JE. Prostate-specific antigen: a valuable clinical tool. Oncology 1991;5:112.

Serum protein *electrophoresis* separates proteins based on their mobility in an electric field and can provide a visual estimate of albumin and globin levels. The five bands on the electrophoresis column include albumin, α_1-globulin, α_2-globulin, β-globulin, and γ-globulin. The main component of the α_1 band is α_1-antitrypsin, which may increase with pregnancy, estrogen therapy, and inflammation. α_2-Globulin is composed of haptoglobin, ceruloplasmin, and α_2-macroglobulin. The main component of β-globulin is transferrin, which functions to transport iron. Transferrin levels are reduced in liver disease, nephrotic syndrome, protein-losing enteropathy, and starvation. Levels of transferrin are helpful in monitoring nutritional status in hospitalized patients. Elevations may be seen in iron deficiency anemia, pregnancy, and estrogen use. The β-lipoprotein band can be found in the α_2-globulin or β-globulin zone. The immunoglobulins are found primarily in the γ region. Diffuse elevations in the γ region can occur with chronic infections, liver disease, autoimmune disorders, and granulomatous diseases. A monoclonal spike in the γ region indicates proliferation of a single immunoglobulin, as seen in myeloma or a monoclonal gammopathy of uncertain significance. Immunoglobulin abnormalities noted on protein electrophoresis can be further characterized by *immunoelectrophoresis*.

Rheumatoid Factor and Anti–Cyclic Citrullinated Peptide Antibodies

The diagnosis of rheumatoid arthritis (RA) is usually made based on clinical findings, supported by laboratory testing. The mainstay of testing has been the IgM rheumatoid factor (RF), which is an autoantibody directed against the Fc portion of the IgG molecule. The sensitivity of RF is approximately 54% to 88% and the specificity 48% to 92%, depending on the method used (Lee and Schur, 2003). RF is not specific for RA and may be detected in the serum of persons with other rheumatoid conditions, chronic infections, or inflammatory conditions, as well as in healthy older adults.

Results are usually reported as a titer determined by using a tube dilution method. A significant titer is 1:80 or greater. In RA, titers are often 1:640 to 1:520 but can even be found up to 1:320,000. Very high titers more likely indicate severe disease or systemic involvement. Increasing serial titer elevations can be used to monitor RA disease progression, but not response to therapy. RF titers may decrease during remission, but only rarely do they become undetectable. The ESR is a better index of disease activity.

Anti–cyclic citrullinated peptide (anti-CCP) antibodies show promise in the diagnosis of RA. Citrulline is an amino acid produced by modification of arginine and is found in filaggrin, a component of keratin. Recently, sensitivity and specificity of anti-CCP antibodies was reported as 67% and 95%, respectively. The advantage of anti-CCP over RF is that it is much more specific for RA. Its optimal use is uncertain, but anti-CCP testing shows greatest benefit with false-positive RF, such as in hepatitis C with cryoglobulinemia. In patients with a moderate pretest probability of RA, positive anti-CCP significantly increases the likelihood of RA (Shmerling, 2009).

Sodium

Abnormal serum sodium levels are markers for impaired water balance. The reference range for serum sodium concentration is 135 to 145 mmol/L. In the evaluation of abnormal

Table 15-23 Classification of Hyponatremia

Clinical Findings	Causes
Volume depletion Tachycardia Hypotension Urine sodium <10 mEq/L Increased urine osmolarity *Volume overload* Edema Urine sodium <10 mEq/L Urine osmolarity high	Gastrointestinal losses: vomiting, diarrhea Renal losses: diuretics, chronic renal failure, salt-wasting nephropathies Skin losses: burns Third-space losses: pancreatitis Congestive heart failure, nephrotic syndrome, cirrhosis
Euvolemic	**SIADH**
No edema No evidence of dehydration Urine sodium >20mEq/L (unless Na-restricted diet) Urine osmolality > serum osmolality Normal thyroid and adrenal function	CNS disorders: infection, mass lesion, head trauma, acute intermittent porphyria Pulmonary: lung cancer, infection Drugs: chlorpropamide, opiates, nicotine, diuretics, phenothiazines, vincristine, carbamazepine, SSRIs
Psychogenic polydipsia	

CNS, Central nervous system; *SSRIs*, selective serotonin reuptake inhibitors.

Table 15-24 Classification of Hypernatremia

Total Body Sodium (Na)	Causes	Urine Measurements
Reduced total body sodium (both Na and water losses, but relatively more loss of water)	Gastrointestinal losses: diarrhea, lactulose Skin losses: excess sweating Renal losses: loop diuretics, osmotic diuretics	Urine Na <10 mEq/L Hypertonic urine Urine Na ≥20 mEq/L Hypotonic or isotonic urine
Normal total body Na (loss of water)	Renal losses: central or nephrogenic diabetes insipidus, lithium, demeclocycline, hypercalcemia, hypokalemia Nonrenal losses: insensible losses from skin or respiratory tract	Variable urine Na Variable urine tonicity Urine Na variable Hypertonic urine
Increased total body Na (addition of sodium)	Hypertonic intravenous fluids Hypertonic dialysate Saltwater drownings	Urine Na >20 mEq/L Hypertonic or isotonic urine

Modified from Schrier RW. Renal and Electrolyte Disorders, 4th ed. Boston, Little, Brown, 1992, p 43.

sodium levels, it is helpful to measure or calculate the plasma osmolarity, which typically has a range of 280 to 295 mOsm/kg H_2O.

$$Calculated\ osmolarity = (2 \times Na) + (BUN/2.8) + (Glucose/18)$$

In most cases, *hyponatremia* is associated with hypo-osmolality. Pseudohyponatremia can occur in the presence of other osmotically active substances, such as ethanol, methanol, mannitol, and glucose. Pseudohyponatremia is associated with an osmolar gap, which means the laboratory's measured osmolarity is greater than the calculated osmolarity by 10. In the setting of hyperglycemia, every 100-mg/dL rise in glucose lowers serum sodium by 1.6 mmol/L.

In hyponatremia associated with hypo-osmolarity, the determination of the patient's volume status is essential to determine the cause of hyponatremia (Verbalis, 2007).

Hyponatremia can occur in states of volume deficiency, euvolemic states, or hypervolemic conditions (Table 15-23). The clinical significance of hyponatremia depends on the severity and rate of development. In general, symptoms are seen when sodium levels are less than 120 mmol/L.

Hypovolemic hyponatremia is associated with low total-body sodium. The most common sources of sodium loss are the GI tract or kidney and, less often, third-space losses. With nonrenal losses, the kidney responds by reducing sodium and water excretion in the urine. In the absence of diuretic therapy, the urine sodium concentration is usually less than 30 mmol/L, and urine osmolarity is high. Hypovolemic hyponatremia responds readily to isotonic fluid replacement.

Hypervolemic hyponatremia can occur with advanced congestive heart failure, cirrhosis, nephrotic syndrome, and renal failure in the presence of total-body sodium overload and edema. In these disorders, effective renal blood flow is reduced, thus stimulating the release of antidiuretic hormone

Table 15-25 Causes of Hyperuricemia*

Overproduction
Myeloproliferative disorders
Polycythemia vera
Hemolytic anemia
Malignancies
Psoriasis
Toxemia of pregnancy
Ethanol

Decreased Excretion
Renal failure
Volume depletion
Hypothyroidism
Hyperparathyroidism
Diabetic ketoacidosis

Drugs
Thiazides
Furosemide
Aspirin (low dose)
Ethambutol
Pyrazinamide
Cyclosporine
Niacin
Vitamin B_{12} therapy

*Normal range: 3.5 to 5.1 mmol/L.

(ADH), which reduces renal excretion of water. Both sodium and water are increased, but water is increased proportionally more than sodium. In the absence of diuretic therapy, urine sodium is generally less than 30 mmol/L, and urine osmolarity is increased.

The most common cause of *euvolemic hyponatremia* is the syndrome of inappropriate ADH secretion (SIADH), which occurs when the stimulus for ADH secretion is not related to osmolarity or reduced renal blood flow. No edema is present, although mild volume expansion and a modest increase in weight are seen. Continued release of ADH occurs despite low plasma osmolarity. SIADH should be considered a cause of hyponatremia in the absence of evidence of volume loss, edema, and adrenal insufficiency or hypothyroidism. The major laboratory finding, in addition to hyponatremia, is urine that is not maximally dilute (i.e., urine osmolarity >100 mOsm/kg H_2O). The urine sodium level is greater than 30 mmol/L, assuming adequate sodium intake. Other clinical findings that suggest SIADH include a uric acid level less than 3 mEq/dL and BUN less than 10 mg/dL. Serum ADH levels are not helpful because most causes of hyponatremia are associated with elevated ADH levels. The major causes of SIADH are drugs and pulmonary and central nervous system diseases. SIADH can respond to fluid restriction or correction of the underlying disorder. Another cause of euvolemic hyponatremia is called *primary polydipsia*, which occurs in people who consume massive amounts of water and have very large volumes of urine. In general, plasma osmolarity is mildly decreased. These individuals have low urine sodium and dilute urine. The hyponatremia readily responds to a reduction in fluid intake.

Hypernatremia is a serious electrolyte abnormality, but it generally occurs in the setting of a significant underlying medical illness (Table 15-24). Determination of the patient's volume status is also critical in the evaluation of hypernatremia (Schrier, 1992). Hypernatremia can occur in the setting of reduced total-body sodium, normal total-body sodium, and increased total-body sodium. Hypernatremia is seen with reduced total-body sodium when sodium and water losses occur but more water than sodium is lost. For example, when a patient has significant diarrhea, hypernatremia can develop when the patient cannot ingest enough water to compensate for the loss. Clinical evidence of dehydration is noted, urine osmolarity is high, and the urine sodium level is low.

Water loss not connected with sodium loss is associated with hypernatremia and normal total-body sodium. Inadequate ADH secretion (central diabetes insipidus) or renal tubules unresponsive to ADH (nephrogenic diabetes insipidus) can lead to hypernatremia because of an inability to concentrate the urine. Uncommon disorders of the hypothalamus and pituitary can cause a high-set osmoreceptor in which osmotic, but not volume, regulation is impaired. The trigger for the release of ADH may be closer to 300 instead of the normal 285 mOsm/kg.

Less frequently, hypernatremia can occur in a setting of increased total-body sodium from an excessive exogenous sodium load. Hypertonic intravenous fluids, saltwater near-drowning, and hypertonic dialysis can cause hypernatremia.

Streptococcal Testing

"Pharyngitis" is a frequent office diagnosis, but the only common form of pharyngitis that requires antibiotic treatment is that caused by *group A beta-hemolytic streptococci* (GABHS). Approximately 15% to 30% of children and 5% to 10% of adults with sore throat have streptococcal pharyngitis. Suggestive clinical features include fever, no cough or rhinorrhea, tonsillar exudates or beefy-red pharynx, and tender anterior cervical lymphadenopathy.

For an acutely ill patient, the *rapid antigen detection test* (RADT) and traditional bacterial throat culture are available to identify GABHS. In the setting of pharyngitis and a typical syndrome, a positive culture or RADT is sufficient to begin treatment. The sensitivity of both is affected by throat swab technique. Using Dacron or rayon rather than cotton swabs will enhance the chances of detection. Testing should be done of both tonsils or tonsillar pillars and the posterior pharynx. Antigen or bacterial recovery from the throat is increased by rigorous swabbing. Avoid swabbing just the soft palate, tongue, buccal mucosa, or lips. The RADT has the advantage of giving immediate results, which allows for early antibiotic therapy and thus decreases the duration of illness, complications, and contagiousness. Current RADTs use immunoassay or nucleic acid testing to detect the group A streptococcal carbohydrate. This antigen disappears rapidly after antibiotic therapy, so a history of recent antibiotic use may give a false-negative result. The major limitation of rapid streptococcal tests is low sensitivity (75%-80% on average), but specificity is high (95%-98%). Therefore, a positive test can be accepted as evidence of disease and therapy begun without further testing. However, a negative result does not exclude the possibility of GABHS as the source of the pharyngitis. Children and adolescents with a negative RADT should have a throat culture for confirmation. Because of the low incidence of streptococcal pharyngitis and the extremely low risk of rheumatic fever in adults, the American Society of Infectious Diseases supports the use of RADT alone in adults, without confirmation by cultures (Bisno et al., 2002).

The throat culture is performed on sheep blood agar plate under aerobic conditions. If proper collection and plating technique are used, throat culture sensitivity is 95% to 96% and specificity 99.5%. With poor technique, sensitivity can be as low as 30%. To differentiate group A from other streptococci, a bacitracin disk is placed on this agar. Hemolysis is inhibited in over 95% of group A streptococci by bacitracin, whereas only 10% to 20% of groups C and G and a small percentage of group B are inhibited by bacitracin. Previous antibiotic use may diminish the colony count. If clinical conditions suggest the presence of other pharyngeal pathogens, such as *Candida albicans*, *Corynebacterium diphtheriae*, or *Neisseria gonorrhoeae*, the laboratory test should be altered because different collection and plating techniques are required. Throat culture results are generally reported 24 to 28 hours after plating. Antibiotic sensitivities are not routinely reported because GABHS is uniformly sensitive to penicillin.

Syphilis Testing

The sexually transmitted disease (STD) syphilis is usually diagnosed with serologic testing. Although darkfield microscopy can identify spirochetes in fluid obtained from lesions of primary syphilis, the test has many false-negative readings, and many physicians are not trained to perform these tests. PCR for *Treponema pallidum* DNA is now commercially available for diagnosing early syphilis, with early reports showing good sensitivity and specificity. The major serologic tests for syphilis are the nonspecific nontreponemal Venereal Disease Research Laboratories (VDRL) and rapid plasma reagin (RPR) tests, which measure antibody production to a cardiolipin-cholesterol-lecithin antigen, and the specific treponemal antibody tests, which measure antibodies against the spirochete *T. pallidum*. The usual screening for syphilis is a two-step process, beginning with the RPR or VDRL test, followed by treponemal antibody testing for confirmation.

The RPR or VDRL is reported as a titer of the highest dilution giving a positive test. The VDRL usually becomes positive approximately 1 to 4 weeks after the development of a chancre. The highest titers of nontreponemal tests are seen in secondary syphilis. The sensitivity of the RPR or VDRL is 78% to 86% in primary syphilis, 100% in secondary syphilis, and 95% to 98% in latent syphilis. Titers of VDRL or RPR parallel disease activity. After appropriate treatment of primary or secondary syphilis, titers decline and usually become negative within 1 year. A fourfold decline in titer 6 months after treatment suggests an adequate response to treatment of primary or secondary syphilis. A fourfold rise in titers after treatment suggests reinfection. Low titers may persist after treatment of late and latent syphilis. Approximately 20% of nontreponemal screening tests are false positive; false-positive tests usually have titers less than 1:8. Causes of false-positive nontreponemal tests include autoimmune disorders, HIV infection, infectious mononucleosis, endocarditis, and lymphoma.

The treponemal tests, such as the fluorescent treponemal antibody absorption (FTA-ABS) test or *T. pallidum* enzyme immunoassay (EIA), are used to confirm infection in a patient with a positive nontreponemal test. The FTA has a sensitivity of 84% in primary syphilis and almost 100% in other stages of syphilis. The specificity is 96%; approximately 1% of the population has a false-positive treponemal antibody, and it is not routinely used for screening. The treponemal tests are reported as positive or negative. Treponemal tests remain positive in 95% of patients, even after treatment, and are not used to monitor treatment response.

In neurosyphilis, cerebrospinal fluid (CSF) abnormalities include elevated protein, a lymphocytic pleocytosis, and a positive VDRL. The CSF VDRL is the preferred test because it is more specific than the CSF FTA. However, the sensitivity is low enough that a negative CSF VDRL does not rule out neurosyphilis. In congenital syphilis, the diagnosis can be difficult because both FTA and VDRL antibodies can be transferred passively to newborns, and their identification at birth in the baby does not necessarily indicate infection. Passively transmitted antibodies generally decline in the first 2 months of life. If titers rise after birth, congenital syphilis is likely. Testing using specific *T. pallidum* EIA IgM may allow earlier diagnosis of congenital syphilis.

Thyroid Testing

Currently available tests for assessing thyroid function measure functional activity of the thyroid, the hypothalamic-pituitary-thyroid axis, or thyroid hormone levels. The third-generation thyroid-stimulating hormone (TSH) test is the best method to confirm or exclude thyroid disease in an ambulatory population. TSH is produced by the pituitary and is inhibited by circulating thyroxine (T_4) and triiodothyronine (T_3). In general, a normal TSH level is approximately 0.5 to 5 mIU/L and excludes hyperthyroidism or primary hypothyroidism. Supersensitive tests measure TSH at levels at least as low as 0.01 mIU/L. TSH levels less than 0.1 mIU/L suggest hyperthyroidism. Levels of 0.1 to 0.5 mIU/L may represent subclinical hyperthyroidism or excess thyroid hormone administration. Levels of 6 to 10 mIU/L are often considered subclinical hypothyroidism, are usually associated with normal free T_4 levels, and are not usually associated with symptoms. In patients with subclinical hypothyroidism, the presence of thyroid antibodies suggests a risk of conversion to frank hypothyroidism of about 5% per year. Symptomatic hypothyroidism occurs with TSH levels greater than 10 mIU/L. The TSH test is also the best way to monitor the results of replacement or suppressive therapy. Although the TSH level is an excellent screen for thyroid function in ambulatory patients, it must be interpreted with caution in acutely ill patients. TSH levels should be used to diagnose thyroid disorders in acutely ill hospitalized patients only when less than 0.1 mIU/L or greater than 20 mIU/L.

Measurements of circulating thyroid hormone should be obtained to confirm abnormal TSH levels. Measurement of free T_4 levels measure the total amount of hormone in blood, free and protein bound. Total T_4 or T_3 levels can be misleading in the setting of protein-binding abnormalities, such as estrogen therapy and liver disease. An approximate reference range in the adult for free T_4 is 0.7 to 2.5 ng/dL and for free T_3 0.2 to 0.5 ng/dL. Free T_3 testing is usually not necessary. One exception is in early hyperthyroidism, when the TSH is suppressed, free T_4 is normal, and free T_3 is elevated.

Primary hypothyroidism accounts for more than 95% of cases of hypothyroidism and is associated with an elevated TSH and reduced free T_4. *Central hypothyroidism* (secondary or tertiary) is associated with low free T_4 and normal to low TSH. Primary hyperthyroidism is associated with a suppressed TSH and elevated free T_4. Subclinical hyperthyroidism is associated with a reduced TSH, but normal free T_4 and T_3 levels.

The radioactive iodine uptake scan measures 24-hour thyroid uptake of a labeled quantity of radioactive iodine. In normal persons, uptake is 8% to 30%. Lower limits of normal cannot be reliably differentiated from hypothyroidism in the radioactive iodine uptake scan. Its major value is to help identify causes of thyrotoxicosis associated with low levels of iodine uptake, such as thyroiditis and fictitious hyperthyroidism from overingestion of thyroid hormones. Other causes of reduced thyroid hormone uptake include recent iodine contrast administration and amiodarone.

Uric Acid

Uric acid is produced in the liver as a byproduct of purine metabolism. Measurement of uric acid is useful in the evaluation of *gout* and monitoring of certain types of chemotherapy. Uric acid levels are increased in situations with increased dietary purine intake, reduced excretion, or increased production. In addition, volume status affects uric acid secretion. With a decrease in extracellular volume, uric acid excretion declines, and serum uric acid levels increase. Conversely, volume expansion increases uric acid excretion and leads to *hypouricemia*. Several drugs inhibit the reabsorption of uric acid in the kidney and therefore lead to *uricosuria* (Table 15-25).

Progressively higher levels *of hyperuricemia* predict the likelihood of gout; however, most authorities believe that asymptomatic hyperuricemia should not be treated. At 37° C, saturation in plasma occurs when uric acid levels are greater than 6.8 mg/dL. Most patients with gout have uric acid levels greater than 7 mg/dL at some time, but they can have normal serum uric acid levels at the time of an acute gouty attack. Although a biologically significant uric acid level is greater than 6.8 mg/dL, the upper limits of "normal" based on population studies are 7.7 mg/dL for men and 6.8 mg/dL for women. The incidence of gout is approximately 5% per year in men with uric acid levels greater than 9 mg/dL, but only 0.5% per year with uric acid levels of 7.0 to 8.9 mg/dL.

A distinction between production of uric acid and reduced uric acid excretion as a cause of hyperuricemia may be helpful in evaluating patients with gout. This can be accomplished by measurement of 24-hour urinary uric acid and creatinine excretion. "Underexcretion" is identified when the *fractional excretion* (excretion of uric acid/excretion of creatinine) is less than 6%. When a person is consuming a regular diet, excretion of uric acid greater than 800 mg/day is considered *hyperuricosuria*. Follow-up testing for patients with hyperuricosuria can be repeated on a low-purine diet, with 24-hour excretion of uric acid greater than 600 mg indicating uric acid overproduction. Of patients with gout, an estimated 90% have reduced uric acid excretion, and less than 10% have overproduction of uric acid as the cause. Drugs that lower serum uric acid include losartan, amlodipine, fenofibrate, and atorvastatin.

Urine Drug Screens

The standard urine drug screen in a clinical setting is a panel of immunoassays designed to detect common drugs of abuse. The panel can include the five drugs required by federal workplace testing: amphetamines, cocaine, opiates, marijuana, and PCP. Other drugs that are prevalent in the community can be added to the panel, including benzodiazepines and barbiturates. Point-of-care testing kits can be ordered for office use that are individualized to the need of the practice. These point-of-care tests provide results in minutes and have generally good sensitivity. The manufacturers recommend follow-up testing with a different laboratory technique to confirm positive tests.

The guidelines that mandate testing procedures for federal workplace testing do not apply in clinical settings. For example, there are no required chain-of-custody policies to safeguard the processing of specimens in clinical settings. Clinical laboratories are not required to perform tests to ensure that the urine sample provided has not been diluted or adulterated. The cutoff points designated to define a positive and negative test are somewhat arbitrary, are chosen mainly to maximize sensitivity and specificity, and do not correlate with the degree of impairment or toxicity. Urine that contains a drug concentration below the cutoff will be reported as negative, even though the drug is present. With standard drug screens, the immunoassays can produce false-positive results. In workplace settings, positive screening tests are followed by more specific tests, such as gas chromatography/mass spectroscopy (GC/MS), and a specimen is not reported as positive unless the GC/MS is also positive. In clinical settings, confirmatory tests are not routinely available and are rarely ordered. Therefore, urine drug screens are designed to help the physician take care of the patient; they are not intended to be used for forensic or legal purposes.

Generally, drugs and their metabolites are detectable in urine tests for about 3 days after use. A notable exception is marijuana, which can be present in the urine for weeks after heavy use. Urine drug screens have significant limitations, which are not always recognized. For example, most immunoassays for "opiates" are designed to detect heroin and measure codeine, which is a byproduct of heroin and morphine metabolism. However, synthetic opioids such as fentanyl or methadone do not cross-react with codeine immunoassays and will produce a negative result. A negative urine drug screen for opiates might falsely lead the physician to believe that the person does not use any opioids. To help determine the sensitivity and the known false-positive results associated with a urine drug screen, the physician should review the package inserts (Warner and Sharma, 2009).

Vitamin D

Vitamin D is now recognized not only for its importance in preventing rickets, but also in preventing osteopenia, osteoporosis, muscle weakness, and falls. Testing levels of vitamin D can be considered in patients at increased risk of vitamin D deficiency, including elderly patients and those with osteoporosis, osteopenia, fat malabsorption, chronic kidney disease, and increased skin pigmentation. The term "vitamin D" includes vitamin D_2 and vitamin D_3. Vitamin D_2 (calciferol) is manufactured from the plant sterols in yeast, and vitamin D_3 (cholecalciferol) is manufactured from lanolin. Vitamin D is hydroxylated by the liver into 25-hydroxyvitamin D [25(OH)D], the major circulating form of vitamin D in the body. The kidney converts 25(OH)D into 1,25-dihydroxyvitamin D [1,25(OH)$_2$D], which is the active form of vitamin D.

The laboratory diagnosis of vitamin D deficiency relies on measuring the levels of 25(OH)D. Measuring 1,25(OH)$_2$D is not recommended in clinical practice because it is not a reliable indicator of vitamin D status. 1,25(OH)$_2$D has a half-life of only 4 hours, whereas 25(OH)D has a half-life of about 3 weeks. In addition, vitamin 1,25(OH)$_2$D levels can actually increase with vitamin D deficiency, because increasing PTH levels result in increasing levels of 1,25(OH)$_2$D.

The 25(OH)D is a measurement of vitamin D intake and that made in the body after sun exposure. Although some laboratories may report 25(OH)D_2 and 25(OH)D_3 levels, it is the total level that is used clinically to monitor vitamin D status. PTH rises when the 25(OH)D levels are less than 30 ng/mL. Although labs may list 20 to 100 ng/mL as the reference range for 25(OH)D, most experts define a preferred level of 25(OH)D as 30 to 60 ng/mL, with deficiency defined as less than 20 ng/mL and insufficiency as 20 to 20 ng/mL. Currently, a 25(OH)D greater than 30 ng/mL is considered the preferred level for both adults and children.

References

The complete reference list is available online at www.expertconsult.com.

Web Resources

www.nlm.nih.gov/medlineplus/laboratorytests.html
An overview for patients that explains basic laboratory principles, also gives links to other resources.

www.labtestsonline.org/understanding/analytes/microalbumin/test.html
Developed by American Association for Clinical Chemistry, site allows patients to search for explanation of specific tests.

www.ahrq.gov/CLINIC/uspstfix.htm
Homepage of the U.S. Preventive Services Task Force (USPSTF), which lists recommendations for screening tests.

PART TWO

Practice of Family Medicine

CHAPTER 16

Infectious Diseases

Anthony Zeimet, David R. McBride, Richard Basilan, William E. Roland, David McCrary, Hoonmo Koo

Chapter contents

BRONCHITIS

David R. McBride

Key Points

- Acute bronchitis is part of the continuum of "acute respiratory tract infection" most often caused by viruses.
- Antibiotics are not routinely recommended for the treatment of bronchitis.
- The cough of bronchitis may last up to 4 weeks.
- Beta-adrenergic agonists are not helpful unless patients have signs of bronchospasm associated with the infection.
- Acute exacerbations of chronic bronchitis with increased sputum production should be treated with antibiotics to decrease mortality.

Infections of the upper respiratory tract accounted for more than 36 million ambulatory medical visits in 2005, according to the National Ambulatory Medical Care Survey (Cherry et al., 2007). Although a large percentage of these infections are viral in origin, antibiotics are still prescribed for more than 50% of patients with *acute respiratory tract infection* (ARTI). *Acute bronchitis*, in the ARTI category, is defined as a respiratory infection in which cough is the predominant symptom and there is no evidence of pneumonia. Antibiotics are often prescribed despite limited evidence that they shorten the duration of acute bronchitis. With increasing incidence of antibiotic resistance, bronchitis allows physicians to practice "prescriptive restraint" and to provide supportive therapy. Consider using the phrase "chest cold" to help patients understand the viral and benign nature of this infection.

Chronic bronchitis is one of the manifestations of *chronic obstructive pulmonary disease* (COPD) and is defined clinically as cough and sputum production on most days for 3 months annually for 2 years. Chronic bronchitis is thought to be primarily inflammatory in origin, although infection may be associated with acute exacerbations; with increased sputum production and worsening dyspnea, antibiotics have proved effective in acute episodes. However, systemic corticosteroids are the mainstay of COPD exacerbation management.

The patient with acute bronchitis presents with cough, often productive. Patients may report clear or colored mucus in association with the presumed diagnosis of acute bronchitis. Despite what many patients believe, the color of sputum, even purulent sputum, is not predictive of bacterial infection. The cough of bronchitis can last up to 4 weeks, sometimes even longer. Typically, acute bronchitis is associated with other manifestations of infection, such as malaise and fever.

Respiratory viruses are thought to cause the majority of cases of acute bronchitis. Influenza A and B, parainfluenza, respiratory syncytial virus (RSV), coronavirus, adenovirus, and rhinovirus are common pathogens in the viral category. Clues to a specific virus may be found in the patient history; for example, RSV might be considered when there is household exposure to infected children. Influenza typically presents with sudden onset of symptoms, including fever, myalgias, cough, and sore throat.

Neuraminidase inhibitors are modestly effective in shortening the duration of influenza in ambulatory and healthy patients (by about 1 day), if initiated in the first 48 hours of illness. The resistance patterns of influenza A and B have shifted in the last several years and may vary based on yearly viral strains. Influenza B has remained, as of 2010, sensitive to zanamivir (Relenza) and oseltamivir (Tamiflu). Currently circulating strains of influenza A, both H1N1 and H3N2, and influenza B have generally remained sensitive to both oseltamivir and zanamivir (Fiore et al., 2011). Family physicians are advised to consider restraint in the prescribing of these agents, since resistance is of great concern. Yearly influenza immunization and cough etiquette and hygiene are likely the most useful techniques for influenza management.

Studies have identified other pathogens, such as *Mycoplasma pneumoniae* and *Chlamydophila pneumoniae*, in a small minority of cases of clinical acute upper respiratory illness with cough as the predominant symptom. No significant benefit has been found in treating these infections with antibiotics. An exception in the treatment of acute bronchitis-like illness with antibiotics is when confirmed or probable *Bordetella pertussis* is present. Early treatment with a macrolide antibiotic and patient isolation will likely decrease coughing paroxysms and limit spread of disease (Braman, 2006). Although common upper respiratory bacterial pathogens, such as *Moraxella (Branhamella) catarrhalis, Streptococcus pneumoniae,* and *Haemophilus influenzae,* may be isolated from patients with acute bronchitis, their relevance is questionable because these bacteria can be present in the respiratory tract of healthy individuals. Obtaining sputum for culture when bronchitis is the diagnosis generally is not useful.

Antibiotics may offer a modest benefit in the treatment of acute bronchitis, with many studies showing no statistical significance in the outcome of treated versus not-treated groups. Measures of function, such as duration of illness, loss of work, and limitation of activity, have not shown clinically significant improvement in those with acute bronchitis taking antibiotics. Coupled with cost and the potential for side effects, the use of antibiotics for acute bronchitis is not recommended. If a provider decides to use an antibiotic in a specific patient situation, narrow-spectrum respiratory agents are preferred, such as a first-generation macrolide or doxycycline.

Treating the symptom of cough in acute bronchitis is an important concern for patients. In adults with acute bronchitis with signs of airway obstruction, evidenced by wheezing on examination or decreased peak expiratory flow rate, beta-2 agonists may be helpful in alleviating cough. These agents are not helpful for children with acute cough or adults with cough and no evidence of airway obstruction. Side effects of tremor and an anxious feeling must be weighed against this benefit.

Patients often are primarily interested in alleviating symptoms caused by respiratory illness. Unfortunately, there is mixed evidence for the use of over-the-counter (OTC) and prescription cough medications. Dextromethorphan and codeine may be somewhat effective, although they have not been evaluated in randomized, double-blinded, placebo-controlled trials for acute bronchitis. Combination first-generation antihistamine-decongestant products may be effective for the cough associated with colds. Naproxen showed efficacy against cough in one upper respiratory model study (Sperber et al., 1992). Guaifenesin acts as an expectorant and may have some effect on cough by its mucus-thinning properties.

Chronic Bronchitis: Acute Exacerbation

Acute exacerbations of chronic bronchitis may be triggered by bacterial or viral infection or may be noninfectious. *H. influenzae* accounts for 50% of bacterial exacerbations with *S. pneumoniae* and *M. catarrhalis* causing an additional third (Moussaoui et al., 2008). For acute exacerbation of COPD associated with purulent sputum and increased shortness of breath, antibiotic therapy decreases mortality by 77% and treatment failure by 53% (Ram et al., 2009). This finding was true regardless of the antibiotic choice, although coverage for the organisms just noted seems rationale. Consideration of the frequency of beta-lactamase production within these organisms in a community is important. More recent meta-analysis shows that a shorter course, no longer than 5 days, is as effective as longer treatment with antibiotic (Moussaoui et al., 2008).

Other features of the management of acute exacerbation of chronic bronchitis include systemic corticosteroids, inhaled beta agonists and anticholinergics (e.g., ipratropium), and support for oxygenation status and ventilation. Patients with chronic bronchitis may have multiple hospital admissions and may remain colonized with both community-acquired and hospital-acquired organisms. It is advisable to reserve the use of antibiotics, unless absolutely necessary to prevent the development of resistant organisms.

KEY TREATMENT

Antibiotics for the treatment of bronchitis is not recommended because of the cost, potential for side effects, and lack of clinical benefit (Braman, 2006; Smith et al., 2009) (SOR: A).

In the treatment of *Bordetella pertussis,* early administration of a macrolide antibiotic and patient isolation will likely decrease coughing paroxysms and limit spread of disease (Braman, 2006) (SOR: A).

In adults with acute bronchitis with signs of airway obstruction, as evidenced by wheezing on examination or decreased peak expiratory flow rate, beta-2 agonists may be helpful in alleviating cough (Braman, 2006) (SOR: B).

For acute exacerbation of COPD associated with purulent sputum and increased shortness of breath, treatment with antibiotics decreases mortality by 77% and treatment failure by 53% (Ram et al., 2009) (SOR: A).

PNEUMONIA

Anthony Zeimet

Key Points

- Assessment tools for pneumonia severity (e.g., CURB-65) can help determine the treatment approach.
- The therapy of pneumonia is often empiric because the infecting organism is not readily isolated in more than 50% of cases.
- Chest radiography is one of the most useful diagnostic tools in pneumonia.

Community-acquired pneumonia (CAP) is defined as an acute infection of the pulmonary parenchyma and, along with influenza, is the seventh leading cause of death in the United States. Fever, cough, sputum production, pleuritic chest pain, and dyspnea are common symptoms of CAP. Nausea, vomiting, and diarrhea also may occur, and in elderly patients, CAP may present with mental status changes. Although its absence usually makes pneumonia less likely, fever can be absent in the elderly patient. Other physical examination findings include an elevated respiratory rate, conversational dyspnea, tachycardia, and rales. Egophony and dullness to percussion may be noted with focal consolidation. Typical laboratory findings include leukocytosis. The diagnosis of pneumonia is based on the presence of symptoms *and* the presence of an infiltrate on chest radiograph. If infiltrate is not present, consider obtaining a chest tomography scan (which has higher sensitivity) to rule in or rule out CAP. If negative, other diagnoses should be considered.

The most common microbiologic agent of pneumonia is often not isolated (Table 16-1). Furthermore, studies have shown that bacteriologic causes of pneumonia cannot be determined by radiographic appearance (i.e., "typical" vs. "atypical"). In the proper clinical setting, certain clinical microbes should be considered because they can affect treatment considerations and epidemiologic studies. These include *Legionella* spp., influenza A and B, and community-acquired methicillin-resistant *Staphylococcus aureus* (MRSA).

Certain diagnostic tests are performed based on clinical setting. Blood cultures are not routinely done in the outpatient setting but should always be done if the patient is being admitted to the hospital, ideally before antibiotics are given. The use of Gram stain and sputum culture remains controversial but can provide more evidence of a bacterial cause (e.g., many PMNs). If sputum cultures are being obtained, it is recommended that the physician have the patient expectorate directly into a specimen cup and have it sent immediately for processing. This can increase the yield of isolating *Streptococcus pneumoniae* among

Table 16-1 Most Common Etiologies of Community-Acquired Pneumonia

Patient Type	Etiology
Outpatient	*Streptococcus pneumoniae* *Mycoplasma pneumoniae* *Haemophilus influenzae* *Chlamydophila pneumoniae* Respiratory viruses*
Inpatient (non-ICU)	*S. pneumoniae* *M. pneumoniae* *C. pneumoniae* *H. influenzae* *Legionella* spp. Aspiration Respiratory viruses*
Inpatient (ICU)	*S. pneumoniae* *Staphylococcus aureus* *Legionella* spp. Gram-negative bacilli *H. influenzae*

Modified from Mandell LA, Wunderink RG, Anzueto A, et al. Infectious Diseases Society–American Thoracic Society Consensus Guidelines on Management of Community-Acquired Pneumonia in Adults. Clin Infect Dis 2007;44:S27-S72.
ICU, Intensive care unit.
*Influenza A and B, adenovirus, respiratory syncytial virus, and parainfluenza.

other respiratory pathogens. Other tests include urine antigen tests for *S. pneumoniae, Legionella pneumophila* serogroup 1, and nasal swab for influenza A and B. In young children, RSV, adenovirus, and parainfluenza in addition to influenza are common causes. Nasal swab for RSV and influenza can be rapidly done, but the other causes can be determined with viral cultures, serology, enzyme-linked immunosorbent assay (ELISA), and polymerase chain reaction (PCR), although results usually are received after resolution of the acute symptoms.

Perhaps the most important decision for clinicians is to determine the location of treatment. The American Thoracic Society (ATS) and the Infectious Diseases Society of America (IDSA) recommend use of the *pneumonia severity index* (PSI), which uses 20 variables to risk-stratify the patient into five mortality classes, or the *CURB-65*, which measures five clinical variables in this decision making. The CURB-65 may be the easiest and most convenient to use at the site of decision making. A score of 0 or 1 indicates treatment as an outpatient; a score of 2 requires hospital admission to the general medical ward; and a score of 3 or more indicates admission to an intensive care unit (ICU) (Box 16-1).

Treatment of CAP should be targeted toward the most likely etiology (Table 16-2). Outpatient therapy for patients who have no comorbidities and have not received antibiotics within the last 3 months includes doxycycline or a macrolide antibiotic. Use of a fluoroquinolone antibiotic (levofloxacin or moxifloxacin) should be reserved for patients with more complicated pneumonia and those requiring hospitalization. Patients who have comorbid conditions or recent antibiotic exposure, or who will be hospitalized, should receive a respiratory fluoroquinolone or combination therapy with a beta-lactam drug plus a macrolide, for 48 to 72 hours after fever abates (usually 5-7 days' total therapy). If an organism is isolated, therapy may be narrowed to cover the causative agent. The clinician should consider longer therapy and appropriate antibiotics to cover for infection by less common organisms such as *Staphylococcus aureus* or *Pseudomonas aeruginosa*. If the patient has no more than one abnormal value (temperature <37.8° C, heart rate <100, respiratory rate <24, SBP >90, O_2 saturation >90%, Po_2 >60 on room air) *and* the patient is able to maintain oral intake and has a normal mental status, the clinician can safely switch to oral therapy and discharge the patient from the hospital. Unless the etiology of the pneumonia is known, the physician should switch to oral antibiotics in the same class as the intravenous antibiotics used.

The U.S. Preventive Services Task Force (USPSTF) along with IDSA and ATS recommend annual influenza vaccinations to those over 50 years of age, those who are (or who reside with those who are) at high risk for influenza complications, and all health care workers. Furthermore, the pneumococcal vaccine should be given to all those over age 65. Smoking cessation is also important and should be discussed at each clinic visit.

KEY TREATMENT

Locally adapted guidelines should be implemented to improve the processing of care variables and relevant clinical outcomes in pneumonia (Mandell et al., 2007) (SOR: B).

Objective criteria or scores should always be supplemented with physician determination of subjective factors, including the patient's ability to take oral medication safely and reliably and the availability of outpatient support resources (Mandell et al., 2007) (SOR: B).

For patients with CURB-65 score of 2 or higher, more intensive treatment (i.e., hospitalization or, where appropriate and available, intensive in-home health care services) is usually warranted (Mandell et al., 2007) (SOR: C).

INFLUENZA

Anthony Zeimet

Key Points

- Concerns about development of resistant seasonal and H1N1 swine-derived influenza virus should be considered in the decision to administer antiviral medications to healthy patients with these infections.
- The abrupt onset of fever with chills, headache, malaise, myalgias, arthralgias, and rigors during "flu season" is sufficient to diagnose influenza.
- Prevention of influenza is generally with vaccination.

Influenza deserves special mention because it is an important cause of pneumonitis and can precede a bacterial pneumonia. Influenza viruses are medium-sized enveloped ribonucleic acid (RNA) viruses that consist of a lipid bilayer with matrix proteins with spiked surface projections of glycoproteins (hemagglutinins, neuraminidase) on the outer surface (Figure 16-1). Both influenza A and influenza B have eight segmented pieces of single-stranded RNA. The only difference between influenza A and influenza B is that B does not have an M2 ion channel. *Hemagglutinins,* three types of which typically infect humans (H1, H2, H3), bind to respiratory epithelial cells and allow fusion with the host cell. *Neuraminidase,* consisting of two types (N1, N2), allows release of virus from the infected cells.

A unique aspect of influenza is that antigenic variation occurs annually. Antigenic shift is caused by a genetic reassortment between animal and human influenza strains, producing a novel virus that generally causes the worldwide pandemics. Influenza viruses circulate mostly among humans, birds, and swine. Sometimes; a human strain and an animal strain can intermingle and create a new, unique virus. This is what happened during spring 2009, heralding the most recent pandemic and creating "Novel H1N1 Influenza" (swine influenza). Genotype analysis

---

Box 16-1 CURB-65 Criteria

Assign a value of 1 for each variable:
- Confusion: Is the patient disoriented to person, place, or time?
- BUN >20 mg/dl
- Respiratory rate > 30 breaths/min
- Blood pressure: systolic <90 or diastolic <60 mm Hg
- Age >65 years

Interpretation

- Score 0 or 1: outpatient treatment
- Score 2 : inpatient treatment on a general medical floor
- Score >3: inpatient treatment in an intensive care unit

BUN, Blood urea nitrogen.

Table 16-2 Guide to Empiric Choice of Antimicrobial Agent for Treating Patients with Community-Acquired Pneumonia (CAP)

Patient Characteristics	Preferred Treatment Options
Outpatient	
Previously Healthy	
No recent antibiotic therapy	Oral-based β-lactam, macrolide,* or doxycycline
Recent antibiotic therapy[†]	A respiratory fluoroquinolone‡ alone, an advanced macrolide* plus high-dose amoxicillin,§ or an advanced macrolide plus high-dose amoxicillin-clavulanate.¶
Comorbidities (COPD, diabetes, renal failure or congestive heart failure, or malignancy)	
No recent antibiotic therapy	An advanced macrolide* plus β-lactam or a respiratory fluoroquinolone
Recent antibiotic therapy	A respiratory fluoroquinolone‡ alone or an advanced macrolide plus a β-lactam**
Suspected aspiration with infection	Amoxicillin-clavulanate or clindamycin
Influenza with bacterial superinfection	Vancomycin, linezolid, or other coverage for MRSA or community-acquired MRSA
Inpatient	
Medical Ward	
No recent antibiotic therapy	A respiratory fluoroquinolone alone or an advanced macrolide plus a β-lactam††
Recent antibiotic therapy	An advanced macrolide plus a β-lactam, or a respiratory fluoroquinolone alone (regimen selected will depend on nature of recent antibiotic therapy)

Patient Characteristics	Preferred Treatment Options
Intensive Care Unit (ICU)	
Pseudomonas infection is not an issue	A β-lactam†† plus either an advanced macrolide or a respiratory fluoroquinolone
Pseudomonas infection is not an issue but patient has a β-lactam allergy	A respiratory fluoroquinolone, with or without clindamycin
Pseudomonas infection is an issue‡‡ (cystic fibrosis, impaired host defenses)	Either (1) an antipseudomonal β-lactam§§ plus ciprofloxacin, or (2) an antipseudomonal agent plus an aminoglycoside## plus a respiratory fluoroquinolone or a macrolide
Pseudomonas infection is an issue but the patient has a β-lactam allergy. Health care–associated exposure	Aztreonam plus aminoglycoside plus levofloxacin¶¶ or other respiratory quinolone Anti-*Pseudomonas* cephalosporin, carbapenem (not ertapenem) or β-lactam/β-lactamase inhibitor with anti-*Pseudomonas* activity plus vancomycin (for MRSA coverage) ± quinolone or aminoglycoside
Nursing Home	
Receiving treatment in nursing home	A respiratory fluoroquinolone alone or vancomycin (for *S. aureus* including MRSA) plus a β-lactam (cefepime or piperacillin/tazobactam if *Pseudomonas* is suspected; ceftriaxone if *Pseudomonas* is not suspected)
Hospitalized	Same as for medical ward and ICU

Data from Mandell LA, Wunderink RG, Anzueto A, et al. Infectious Diseases Society of America/American Thoracic Society consensus guidelines of community-acquired pneumonia in adults. Clin Infect Dis. 2007;44:S27-S72.

COPD, Chronic obstructive pulmonary disease; *MRSA,* methicillin-resistant *Staphylococcus aureus.*

*Azithromycin or clarithromycin.

[†]That is, the patient was given a course of antibiotic(s) for treatment of any infection within the past 3 months, excluding the current episode of infection. Such treatment is a risk factor for drug-resistant *Streptococcus pneumoniae* and possibly for infection with gram-negative bacilli. Depending on the class of antibiotics recently given, one or another of the suggested options may be selected. Recent use of a fluoroquinolone should dictate selection of a nonfluoroquinolone regimen, and vice versa.

‡Moxifloxacin, levofloxacin, or gemifloxacin.

§Dosage: 1 g orally (PO) three times daily (tid).

¶Dosage: 2 g PO twice daily (bid).

**High-dose amoxicillin (1 g tid), high-dose amoxicillin-clavulanate (2 g bid), cefpodoxime, cefprozil, or cefuroxime.

††Cefotaxime, ceftriaxone, ampicillin-sulbactam, or ertapenem.

‡‡The antipseudomonal agents chosen reflect this concern. Risk factors for *Pseudomonas* infection include severe structural lung disease (e.g., bronchiectasis) and recent antibiotic therapy, health care–associated exposures or stay in hospital (especially in the ICU). For patients with CAP in the ICU, coverage for *S. pneumoniae* and *Legionella* species must always be considered. Piperacillin-tazobactam, imipenem, meropenem, and cefepime are excellent β-lactams and are adequate for most *S. pneumoniae* and *H. influenzae* infections. They may be preferred when there is concern for relatively unusual CAP pathogens, such as *P. aeruginosa, Klebsiella* spp., and other gram-negative bacteria.

§§Piperacillin, piperacillin-tazobactam, imipenem, meropenem, or cefepime.

##Data suggest that older adults receiving aminoglycosides have worse outcomes.

¶¶Dosage for hospitalized patients, 750 mg/day.

of this strain determined that components came from an influenza virus circulating among swine herds in North America that combined with a virus circulating among ill swine in Eurasia, creating a new influenza strain capable of causing disease in humans. Because this virus had not previously infected humans, it had the potential to cause widespread morbidity and mortality worldwide. During pandemics, the U.S. Centers for Disease Control and Prevention (CDC) estimates an additional 10,000 to 40,000 deaths caused by influenza. Although higher than in non-pandemic years, mortality was significantly less than initially predicted in 2009.

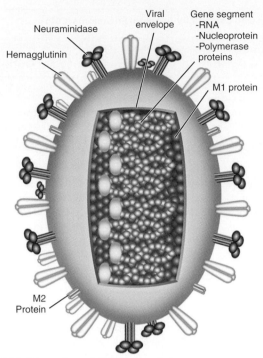

Figure 16-1 Schematic model of influenza A virus.
(From Treanor JJ: Influenza viruses, including avian influenza and swine influenza. In Mandell GL, Bennett JE, Dolin RD (eds). Mandell, Douglas, and Bennett's Principles and Practices of Infectious Diseases, 7th ed. Philadelphia, Churchill Livingstone, 2010, p 2266.)

The abrupt onset of fever, along with chills, headache, malaise, myalgias, arthralgias, and rigors during "flu season," is sufficient to diagnose influenza. As the fever resolves, a dry cough and nasal discharge predominate. A rapid nasal swab or viral cultures can be used to confirm the diagnosis of influenza but is rarely needed. In fact, the sensitivity of these rapid tests can range from 50% to 70%, so a negative test does not rule out influenza. The primary care physician needs to determine if the patient has influenza or the common cold, because symptoms of both illnesses generally overlap (Table 16-3).

Treatment of influenza is generally not necessary because it is usually a self-limiting condition. Treatment should be reserved for those with comorbidities who present within 48 hours of symptom onset. Neuraminidase inhibitors (zanamivir and oseltamivir) prevent the release of virus from the respiratory epithelium and are approved for both influenza A and influenza B. The M2 inhibitors (amantadine and rimantadine) are approved by the U.S. Food and Drug Administration (FDA) for the treatment of influenza A because these drugs block the M2 ion protein channel, preventing fusion of the virus to host cell membrane (influenza B has no M2 ion channel). The use of M2 inhibitors is limited because of increasing resistance among influenza A viruses, as well as causing central nervous system (CNS) problems that are usually exacerbated in elderly persons, who are more likely to seek treatment for influenza (Table 16-4).

The major complication of influenza is a secondary bacterial pneumonia or exacerbation of underlying COPD. Initial improvement in clinical symptoms followed by deterioration usually suggests a secondary bacterial pneumonia, which can usually be confirmed with a chest radiograph showing an infiltrate. Other, less common complications of influenza

Table 16-3 Common Cold versus Influenza Symptoms

Symptom	Common Cold	Influenza
Fever	Rare	Abrupt onset
Cough	Frequent, usually hacking	Frequent, usually severe
Sore throat	Frequent	Rare
Nasal congestion	Frequent	Rare
Sneezing	Frequent	Rare
Myalgia	Rare	Frequent
Headache	Rare	Frequent
Fatigue	Mild	Severe

include myositis, myocarditis, pericarditis, transverse myelitis, encephalitis, and Guillain-Barré syndrome.

Prevention of influenza is generally with vaccination. Box 16-2 outlines patients at risk for influenza complications who should be vaccinated yearly. Although anyone wanting an influenza vaccine should be vaccinated, during periods of vaccine shortage, high-risk groups have priority. A well-matched vaccine can prevent influenza among 70% to 90% of adults and decrease work absenteeism. Conversely, a poorly matched vaccine only prevents influenza in 50% of healthy adults. Proper hand hygiene and covering one's cough are two additional important components in preventing the spread of influenza virus.

KEY TREATMENT

Early treatment (within 48 hours of onset of symptoms) with oseltamivir or zanamivir is recommended for influenza A (Jefferson et al., 2006) (SOR: A).

Use of oseltamivir and zanamivir is not recommended for patients with uncomplicated influenza with symptoms for more than 48 hours (Kaiser and Hayden, 1999) (SOR: A).

Oseltamivir and zanamivir may be used to reduce viral shedding in hospitalized patients or to treat influenza pneumonia (Mandell et al., 2007) (SOR: C).

SYSTEMIC VIRAL INFECTIONS

Anthony Zeimet

Key Points

- Population-based vaccination programs have been highly effective in decreasing the incidence of many viral infections.
- Acyclovir can be used in adults and children with varicella to decrease symptoms if given in the first 48 hours after rash onset, but its benefit must be weighed against its cost and the possibility of development of viral resistance.
- Antiviral medications should be considered to decrease the incidence of postherpetic neuralgia, particularly in older patients.

Table 16-4 Treatment and Chemoprophylaxis Recommendations for Influenza

Agent/ Group	Treatment	Chemoprophylaxis
Neuraminidase Inhibitors		
Oseltamivir		
Adults	75-mg capsule twice daily (bid) for 5 days	75-mg capsule once daily (qd)
Children (age >12 mo)		
<15 kg	60 mg/day divided into 2 doses	30 mg qd
15-23 kg	90 mg/day in 2 doses	45 mg qd
24-40 kg	120 mg/day in 2 doses	60 mg qd
>40 kg	160 mg/day in 2 doses	75 mg qd
Zanamivir		
Adults	Two 5-mg inhalations (10 mg bid)	Two 5-mg inhalations (10 mg qd)
Children	Two 5-mg inhalations (10 mg bid)(age >7 yr)	Twp 5-mg inhalations (10 mg qd)(age >5 yr)
M2 Inhibitors (Adamantadines)[*]		
Rimantadine[†]		
Adults	200 mg/day as either a single daily dose or divided into 2 doses	200 mg/day as either a single daily dose or divided into 2 doses
Children		
1-9 yr	6.6 mg/kg/day (max, 150 mg/day) divided in 2 doses	5 mg/kg qd, not to exceed 150 mg
>10 yr	200 mg/day as either a single daily dose or divided into 2 doses	200 mg/day as either a single daily dose or divided into 2 doses
Amantadine		
Adults	200 mg/day as either a single daily dose or divided into 2 doses	200 mg/day as either a single daily dose or divided into 2 doses
Children		
1-9 yr	5-8 mg/kg/day divided into 2 doses or as a single daily dose (max, 150 mg/day)	5-8 mg/kg/day divided into 2 doses or as a single daily dose (max, 150 mg/day)
9-12 yr	200 mg/day divided into 2 doses	200 mg/day divided into 2 doses

Modified from Harper SA, Bradley JS, Englund JA, et al. Seasonal influenza in adults and children: diagnosis, treatment, chemoprophylaxis, and institutional outbreak management. Clinical Practice Guidelines of the Infectious Diseases Society of America. Clin Infect Dis 2009;48:1003-1032.
[*]The amantadines should be used only when influenza A (H1N1) infection or exposure is suspected. The amantadines should not be used for infection or exposure to influenza A (H2N3) or influenza B.
[†]Rimantadine has not been approved by the U.S. Food and Drug Administration for treatment of children, although published data exist on safety and efficacy in the pediatric population.

Box 16-2 Groups at risk for Influenza Complications[*]

Unvaccinated infants age 12 to 24 months

Persons with asthma or other chronic pulmonary disease, such as cystic fibrosis in children or chronic obstructive pulmonary disease in adults

Patients with hemodynamically significant cardiac disease

Patients with immunosuppressive disorders or receiving immunosuppressive therapy

Patient with human immunodeficiency virus (HIV) infection

Patients with sickle cell anemia and other hemoglobinopathies

Patients with disease requiring long-term aspirin therapy (e.g., rheumatoid arthritis, Kawasaki disease)

Patients with chronic renal obstruction

Patients with cancer

Patients with chronic metabolic disease, such as diabetes mellitus

Patient with neuromuscular disorders, seizure disorders, or cognitive dysfunction that may compromise the handling of respiratory secretions

Adults older than 66 years

Residents of any age of nursing homes or other long-term care facilities

Modified from Harper SA, Bradley JS, Englund JA, et al. Seasonal influenza in adults and children: diagnosis, treatment, chemoprophylaxis, and institutional outbreak management. Clinical Practice Guidelines of the Infectious Diseases Society of America. Clin Infect Dis 2009;48:1003-1032.
*Data suggest that the highest risk of both mortality and serious morbidity (e.g., hospitalization) occurs in severely immunocompromised patients (e.g., hematopoietic stem cell transplant patients) and very elderly (>85 years) residents of nursing homes; infants under age 24 months also have high hospitalization rates but lower case-fatality rates than the other two groups.

- Measles has had a resurgence in recent years and should be suspected when a patient presents with cough, coryza, conjunctivitis, and head-to-toe rash.
- Epstein-Barr virus and cytomegalovirus infections are generally not clinically distinguishable, and their treatment is primarily supportive.

Vaccinations have dramatically decreased the incidence of a number of historically common viral infections; smallpox has been eradicated through widespread vaccination. However, recent outbreaks of measles and mumps on college campuses underscore the need to remain vigilant in administering vaccines at the population level, even though no vaccine is available for many common viruses.

Varicella and Herpes Zoster

Varicella is one of the classic viral exanthems of childhood. Before routine vaccination, having chickenpox was one of childhood's "rites of passage." The virus, a herpesvirus (human herpesvirus 3), is effectively transmitted, causing outbreaks in schools and households.

Patients with primary varicella present with fever, headache, and sore throat. Generally within 1 to 2 days of onset of symptoms, a papulovesicular rash erupts diffusely. The classic description of the chickenpox lesion is "a dewdrop on a rose petal," suggesting a central vesicle on an erythematous base. Lesions continue to appear for 5 to 7 days. All lesions going from papule to vesicle to crusted lesion takes about

2 weeks. Patients are considered to be infectious, primarily through respiratory secretions, during the 2 days before symptoms appear and until all lesions are crusted.

Treatment of varicella is generally supportive. Control of spread may be a concern in group-living environments such as schools or residence halls. Isolation of the infected patient away from those susceptible to varicella infection is standard practice. Acyclovir can be started within the first 24 hours after rash eruption to achieve an attenuation of the infectious course. In children, this means a decrease in the duration of fever by about 1 day and a decrease in the number of lesions (Swingler, 2010). In adults, acyclovir decreases rash duration and the number of lesions, although the results are less significant than for children. Adult dosing of acyclovir for varicella is 800 mg five times daily. The marginal benefit must be weighed against the possible development of resistance at a population level and the cost of the medication. Complications of varicella can include secondary infection of skin lesions, pneumonitis, encephalitis, and dehydration from vomiting and diarrhea.

Varicella is prevented primarily through administration of vaccine. The vaccine is highly effective in children, with recommended dosing at 12 to 15 months with a second dose at 4 to 6 years. Varicella is now included in a measles-mumps-rubella (MMR) vaccine, which can be given between 12 months and 12 years of age. The varicella vaccine is a live, attenuated virus and should not be given to certain immunocompromised patients. The vaccine can also be administered to exposed immunocompetent contacts, although the benefit is clearer for children than adults. Severely immunocompromised patients exposed to varicella (particularly those with advanced HIV disease) may be given high-dose acyclovir to prevent development of disease.

Herpes zoster is a reactivation of the neurotropic varicella virus, typically in a dermatomal distribution. This is more common in elderly or immunocompromised patients but can occur in healthy people as well. Patients with zoster may note generalized malaise, hyperesthesia, numbness, tingling, and pain in the skin before development of a rash. The appearance of the rash is the same as for chickenpox, although most often isolated to a unilateral dermatome. The diagnosis of herpes zoster is clinical based on the history and the classic appearance of the rash. In immunocompromised patients, however, the rash may not be dermatomally isolated. When the diagnosis is unclear, viral culture can be obtained from the base of a lesion.

Antiviral medications are likely to decrease the incidence of *postherpetic neuralgia* and are recommended, particularly in elderly patients (Wareham, 2010). Valacyclovir (1 g three times daily) or famciclovir (500 mg every 8 hours) for 7 days is likely more effective than acyclovir in achieving this result. Either drug should be started as soon after the diagnosis as possible, preferably within 48 to 72 hours of rash onset. When patients have established postherpetic neuralgia, gabapentin and tricyclic antidepressants are helpful in alleviating the pain.

The rash of zoster is infectious to the touch. Patients should be advised to keep the rash covered until all the lesions have crusted. Zoster of the trigeminal nerve can extend to the eye and warrants immediate ophthalmologic intervention.

A vaccine to prevent herpes zoster in adults was released in 2006. The zoster vaccine differs from the varicella vaccine in that the amount of attenuated virus is 14 times higher in the zoster vaccine. The vaccine decreases the incidence of zoster by 50%. It is recommended for administration by the American Academy of Family Physicians (AAFP) to adults over age 60, regardless of prior varicella or zoster history. Although generally well tolerated, the vaccine is somewhat costly.

Measles

In 2008, more measles cases were reported than in any other year since 1997 (CDC, 2010). Measles is the "first disease" of childhood from the history of medicine. In adults, measles infection may be acquired in the face of waning immunity from remote immunization. A booster dose of MMR vaccine is recommended before college entry.

Clinically, measles presents with cough, coryza (nasal irritation and congestion), and conjunctivitis. Fever is common several days before the onset of the rash. The rash of measles typically spreads from head to toe and has an erythematous, papular appearance with a "sandpaper" feeling. Koplik's spots are erythematous papules with a bluish center on the oral mucosa and appear early in measles. Measles is highly contagious through droplets.

Lymphopenia and neutropenia are common laboratory findings with measles infection. Complications of measles include primary infections such as pneumonia, gastroenteritis, encephalitis, and the rare subacute sclerosing panencephalitis. Secondary infections such as otitis media, pneumonia, and adenitis may also occur.

Treatment is supportive, and the implications of measles infection are primarily in the public health realm. Patients with measles should be isolated for at least 4 days after the appearance of the rash. It is important to recognize that patients are contagious for 2 days before the development of symptoms. Careful verification of immunization status for close contacts is essential.

Epstein-Barr Virus and Cytomegalovirus

Clinical *infectious mononucleosis* is a common infection in adolescents and early adults. The clinical syndrome is most often caused by Epstein-Barr virus (EBV), although cytomegalovirus (CMV) may also be the source in this clinical syndrome, which includes fever, exudative tonsillitis, adenopathy (often including posterior cervical or occipital nodes), and fatigue. EBV is transmitted in oral secretions and may be transmitted sexually as well. B cells are infected with EBV either directly or after contact with epithelial cells, resulting in diffuse lymphoid enlargement.

The diagnosis of infectious mononucleosis is made by recognizing the clinical symptoms of fever, pharyngitis, and adenopathy along with the laboratory findings of greater than 50% lymphocytes with 10% or more atypical lymphocytes (Hoagland, 1952). Also, a positive serologic test for heterophile antibody assists the family physician in the diagnosis. To differentiate EBV from CMV mononucleosis, serology (IgG and IgM) may be obtained. Results of these tests are generally not available in time to have a significant benefit clinically.

Splenic enlargement as part of this lymphoid hypertrophy can lead to splenic rupture (0.1% risk) (Dommerby et al., 1986). Athletes with infectious mononucleosis must be managed carefully to avoid their participation in sports that could result in abdominal trauma. Other risks associated with infectious mononucleosis include upper airway obstruction, asymptomatic transaminase elevation, thrombocytopenia, and rash after the administration of ampicillin or amoxicillin. Routinely obtaining transaminase levels in patients without clinical hepatitis is of little value and can increase the overall cost of management.

Treatment of infectious mononucleosis is largely supportive. Patients should be instructed to treat fever with antipyretics, rest, and expect symptom duration of 2 to 4 weeks, although symptoms can last for several months. The use of steroids, such as prednisone, has shown limited benefit. Data suggest an initial benefit 12 hours after steroid administration, although this is lost within several days (Candy and Hotopf, 2006). Combination of steroid and an antiviral (valacyclovir) may have some positive effect on fatigue.

KEY TREATMENT

Acyclovir started within the first 24 hours after varicella rash eruption can attenuate the infectious course, decreasing duration of fever by 1 day and reducing the number of lesions (SOR: A).
Administration of varicella vaccine to a susceptible child within 3 days of exposure will likely modify or prevent disease (Macartney and McIntyre, 2008) (SOR: A).
Antiviral medications decrease the incidence of postherpetic neuralgia (Wareham, 2010) (SOR: B).

TUBERCULOSIS

David McCrary

Key Points

- The most common presentation of tuberculosis is pulmonary disease.
- Tuberculosis is diagnosed by acid-fast bacilli smears and cultures.
- Standard first-line agents to treat TB are isoniazid, rifampin, pyrazinamide, and ethambutol.
- High-risk patients with a positive purified protein derivative skin test or Quantiferon-TB Gold test should be treated for latent TB infection.
- The current recommendation for first-line treatment for latent TB is 9 months of oral isoniazid.

Tuberculosis skin testing should be interpreted without regard to bacille Calmette-Guérin (BCG) history, because BCG is administered in areas where TB is endemic and BCG does not provide complete protection from TB infection.

Tuberculosis (TB) is a disease that has plagued humans since antiquity, with evidence of spinal TB in neolithic and early Egyptian remains. At present, TB affects approximately one third of the world's population. TB is the world's second most common cause of death from infectious disease after human immunodeficiency virus or acquired immunodeficiency syndrome (HIV/AIDS). Tuberculosis is caused by *Mycobacterium tuberculosis*, an acid-fast bacillus. TB is acquired by inhalation of respiratory droplets. These respiratory droplets are spread by coughing. Brief contact carries little risk for acquiring TB, and infection generally does not occur in open air; open-air sanatoriums were the cornerstone of TB treatment before antimicrobial therapy.

Epidemiology

In the United States, TB incidence rates have been on the decline since 1992, coinciding with the control of HIV-induced AIDS by antiretroviral therapy. However, TB remains prevalent in certain high-risk groups (i.e. immigrants, IV drug use, homeless persons). Most cases of TB are in people age 15 to 49 years. TB in elderly persons is generally caused by a reactivation of latent infection acquired in the remote past, whereas TB in young children indicates ongoing active transmission in the community. Infection in children is more likely to progress to active TB and disseminated disease. Persons with HIV infection have a disproportionately higher risk for acquiring TB than the general population.

Presentation

Tuberculosis is most frequently manifested clinically as pulmonary disease, but it can involve any organ. Extrapulmonary TB accounts for about 20% of disease in HIV-seronegative persons but is more common in HIV-seropositive persons. Pulmonary TB typically manifest with fever, night sweats, chronic cough, sputum production, hemoptysis, anorexia, and weight loss. Chest radiographs in patients with pulmonary TB typically reveal upper-lobe cavitary lesions and can reveal infiltrates or nodular lesions, as well as lymphadenopathy (Figure 16-2). TB in the setting of advanced HIV co-infection does not generally manifest in the typical manner (Table 16-5).

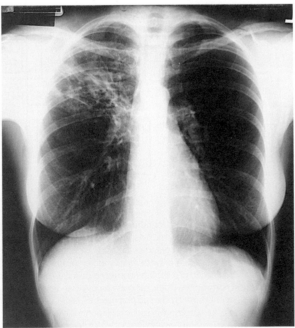

Figure 16-2 Chest radiograph showing right apical infiltrate typical of a patient with primary tuberculosis.
(From Fitzgerald D, Sterling T, Haas D. Mycobacterium tuberculosis. In Mandell GL, Bennett JE, Dolin R (eds). Mandell, Douglas, and Bennett's Principles and Practice of Infectious Diseases, 7th ed. Philadelphia, Churchill Livingstone, 2010, p 3141.)

Diagnosis

The diagnosis of pulmonary TB is made by the demonstration of acid-fast bacilli (AFB) in sputum and the growth of *M. tuberculosis* in culture. These patients typically have an abnormal chest radiograph, as previously described. *M. tuberculosis* is a slow-growing bacterium, and cultures can take up to 6 weeks to grow. A PCR assay developed for *M. tuberculosis* can be run on AFB smear–positive sputum to hasten the diagnosis of pulmonary TB. A positive PCR on AFB-positive sputum is diagnostic of pulmonary TB, but a negative test does not rule out the diagnosis.

Table 16-5 Clinical Manifestations of Active Tuberculosis in Early verus Late* Human Immunodeficiency Virus Infection

Sign	Early	Late
Tuberculin test	Usually positive	Usually negative
Adenopathy	Unusual	Common
Pulmonary distribution	Upper lobe	Lower and middle lobes
Cavitation	Often present	Typically absent
Extrapulmonary disease	10%-15% of cases	50% of cases

Modified from Murray JF. Cursed duet: HIV infection and tuberculosis. Respiration 1990;57:210-220.

*For practical purposes, "early" and "late" may be defined as CD4+ cell counts >300 cells/mm³ and <200 cells/mm³, respectively.

Treatment

Patients with AFB positive smears from sputum samples should be started on anti-TB therapy while awaiting results of PCR and cultures. The treatment of TB always uses multiple agents with anti-TB activity. Single agents should never be used. The standard first-line agents are isoniazid (INH), rifampin (RIF), pyrazinamide (PZA), and ethambutol (EMB) (Figure 16-3 and Table 16-6). If administered, INH should be given with pyridoxine (vitamin B_6; 25-50 mg orally daily) to prevent neuropathy. Treatment of active pulmonary TB is generally for 6 months regardless of HIV status, but treatment may need to be extended in certain situations.

Directly observed therapy (DOT) is the preferred mechanism of administration to ensure compliance. Many local county and state health departments have systems for DOT. Treatment of HIV-seropositive patients with TB who are receiving an antiretroviral (ARV) regimen that contains a protease inhibitor is complicated by the latter's interaction with rifamycins (particularly rifampin). Management of such patients should be coordinated with an infectious diseases specialist, who also should manage drug-resistant TB treatment.

Latent Tuberculosis Infection and Purified Protein Derivative

In the United States, latent tuberculosis infection (LTBI) is the most prevalent form of tuberculosis. LTBI is the term given to patients with a positive purified protein derivative (PPD) skin test without evidence of active TB. PPD has been used for more than 100 years and relies on delayed-type hypersensitivity (DTH) to *M. tuberculosis* cellular proteins.

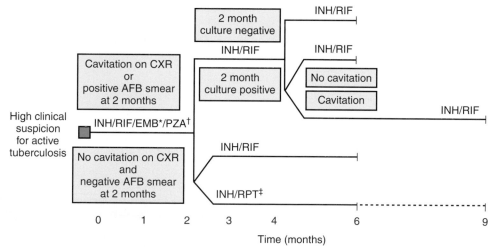

Figure 16-3 Treatment algorithm for tuberculosis. Patients in whom TB is proved or strongly suspected should have treatment initiated with isoniazid, rifampin, pyrazinamide, and ethambutol for the initial 2 months. A repeat smear and culture should be performed when 2 months of treatment has been completed. If cavities were seen on the initial chest radiograph or the acid-fast smear is positive at completion of 2 months of treatment, the continuation phase of treatment should consist of isoniazid and rifampin daily or twice weekly for 4 months to complete a total of 6 months of treatment. If cavitation was present on the initial chest radiograph and the culture at completion of 2 months' therapy is positive, the continuation phase should be lengthened to 7 months (total of 9 months of treatment). If the patient has HIV infection and the CD4+ cell count is less than 100/mm³, the continuation phase should consist of daily or three-times-weekly isoniazid and rifampin. In HIV-uninfected patients having no cavitation on chest radiograph and negative acid-fast smears at completion of 2 months of treatment, the continuation phase may consist of either once-weekly isoniazid and rifapentine, or daily or twice-weekly isoniazid and rifampin, to complete a total of 6 months *(bottom)*. Patients receiving isoniazid and rifapentine, and whose 2-month cultures are positive, should have treatment extended by an additional 3 months (total of 9 months).
*EMB may be discontinued when results of drug susceptibility testing indicate no drug resistance. †PZA may be discontinued after it has been taken for 2 months (56 doses).
‡RPT should not be used in HIV-infected patients with TB or in patients with extrapulmonary TB. Therapy should be extended to 9 months if 2-month culture is positive.
AFB, Acid-fast bacilli; *CXR,* chest radiograph (x-ray); *EMB,* ethambutol; *INH,* isoniazid; *PZA,* pyrazinamide; *RIF,* rifampin; *RPT,* rifapentine.
From Centers for Disease Control and Prevention (CDC). Treatment of tuberculosis. American Thoracic Society, CDC, and Infectious Diseases Society of America. MMWR 2003;52(RR-11):1-88.

Because PPD relies on DTH, any factor that reduces the DTH affects the host response to PPD. The most common clinical example is use of corticosteroids, which blunt the DTH response and can complicate PPD interpretation. Therefore, PPD testing should not be performed while a patient is taking corticosteroids. Also, TB testing should be targeted to those with higher risk of infection and should not routinely be done in those with low risk (ATS/CDC, 2000).

The PPD can also give false-positive results in patients with previous bacille Calmette-Guérin (BCG) vaccination or with infection by other mycobacterial infections. In the United States, this may cause difficulties in testing immigrants from countries who routinely use BCG vaccination programs. However, previous BCG vaccination should not change the interpretation of the PPD or willingness to treat such individuals accordingly.

Table 16-6 Recommended Treatment Regimens for Pulmonary Tuberculosis

Initial Phase				Continuation Phase			Rating* (Evidence)†	
Drugs	Interval and doses‡ (minimal duration)	Regimen	Drugs	Interval and doses‡ § (minimal duration)	Range of total doses (minimal duration)		HIV Positive	HIV Negative
Regimen 1								
INH RIF PZA EMB	7 days per week for 55 doses (8 wk) or 5 d/wk for 40 doses (8 wk)¶¶	1a	INH/RIF	7 d/wk for 126 doses (18 wk) or 5 d/wk for 90 doses (18 wk)¶	182-130(26 wk)		A (I)	A (II)
		1b	INH/RIF	Twice weekly for 36 doses(18 wk)	92-76(26 wk)		A (I)	A (II)¶
		1c**	INH/RPT	Once weekly for 18 doses(18 wk)	74-58(26 wk)		B (I)	E (I)
Regimen 2								
INH RIF PZA EMB	7 days per week for 14 doses (2 wk), then twice weekly for 12 doses (6 wk) or 5 d/wk for 10 doses (2 wk),¶ then twice weekly for 12 doses (6 wk)	2a	INH/RIF	Twice weekly for 36 doses (18 wk)	62-58(26 wk)		A (II)	B (II)¶
		2b**	INH/RPT	Once weekly for 18 doses(18 wk)	44-40(26 wk)		B (I)	E(I)
Regimen 3								
INH RIF PZA EMB	Three times weekly for 24 doses (8wk)	3	INH/RIF	Three times weekly for 54 doses (18wk)	78 (26 wk)		B (I)	B(II)
Regimen 4								
INH RIF EMB	7 days per week for 56 doses (8wk) or 5d/wk for 40 doses (8wk) ¶	4a	INH/RIF	7 days per week for 217 doses (31wk) or 5d/wk for 155 doses (31 wk)¶¶	273-195(39 wk)		C (I)	C (III)
		4b	INH/RIF	Twice weekly for 62 doses (31wk)	118-102(39 wk)		C (I)	C (III)

From American Thoracic Society, CDC, Infectious Diseases Society of America. Treatment of tuberculosis. MMWR 2003;52:1-77.

DOT, Directly observed therapy; *EMB*, ethambutol, *INH*, isoniazid; *PZA*, pyrazinamide; *RIF*, rifampin; *RPT*, rifapentine.

*Definitions of evidence ratings: *A*, preferred; *B*, acceptable alternative; *C*, offer when A and B cannot be given; *E*, should never be given.

†Definition of evidence ratings: *I*, randomized clinical trial; *II*, data from clinical trials that were not randomized or were conducted in other populations; *III*, expert opinion.

‡When DOT is used, drugs may be given 5 days per week and the necessary number of doses adjusted accordingly. Although there are no studies that compare five with seven daily doses, extensive experience indicates this would be an effective practice.

§Patients with cavitation on initial chest radiograph and positive cultures on completion of 2 months of therapy should receive a 7-month (31 weeks, either 217 doses [daily] or 62 doses [twice weekly]) continuation phase.

¶Five-days-a-week administration is always given by DOT. Rating for 5 day per week regimens is AIII.

¶¶Not recommended for HIV-infected patients with CD4+ cell counts <100 cells/μL.

**Options 1c and 2b should be used only in HIV-negative patients who have negative sputum smears at completion of 2 months of therapy and who do not have cavitation on initial chest radiograph. For patients started on this regimen and found to have a positive culture from the 2-month specimen, treatment should be extended an extra 3 months.

The DTH response can wane over time. To overcome this problem, nonreacting patients may undergo repeat PPD 1 week after their initial PPD. The diagnosis of LTBI is made by interpretation of a PPD and by ascertaining the patient's risk factors for progression to active TB if left untreated (Box 16-3). Interpretation of the PPD should be based on the area of induration and not the area of surrounding erythema. Persons whose PPDs have converted from negative to positive within 2 years are presumed to have been infected recently. The decision to use PPD means treating the patient for LTBI if the PPD test is positive.

Patients at increased risk for progression to active TB include those who have been recently infected (recent PPD converters); patients who are HIV seropositive; patients who have silicosis, diabetes, or chronic renal failure (including those receiving hemodialysis); solid-organ transplant recipients; patients with gastrectomy or jejunoileal bypass or head and neck cancer; injection drug users; patients with chest radiograph evidence of prior TB; and patients who weigh at least 5% less than ideal body weight. Patients taking chronic corticosteroid therapy and those who are to receive tumor necrosis factor alpha (TNF-α) blockers (e.g., infliximab) are also at risk. Patients taking corticosteroids also have higher risk of progression to active TB with larger doses and longer courses of corticosteroids.

Standard therapy for LTBI is INH, 300 mg orally daily for 9 months, regardless of HIV status. Again, INH should always be administered with pyridoxine to prevent neuropathy.

Interferon-γ Release Assays

To overcome the false-positive results and confusion of PPD testing in certain populations, newer interferon-gamma (IFN-γ) release assays such as the Quantiferon-TB Gold (QFT-G) test have been developed to detect latent *M. tuberculosis*.

QFT-G quantifies the release of IFN-γ from lymphocytes of the host's blood in response to three *M. tuberculosis* target antigens that are absent from BCG and most other nontuberculous *Mycobacterium* spp. The advantages of using QFT-G include one-time blood testing without the need for follow-up visit, no triggering of amnestic responses, and possibly more specific response to *M. tuberculosis*. However, QTF-G use in immunocompromised or anergic patients is limited, with indeterminate results. Some studies also show discordant results in individuals tested with both PPD and QTF-G. In general, QTF-G may be used in all circumstances in which the PPD is used. However, whether the QTF-G is truly more specific or sensitive than the PPD in latent or active TB is yet to be determined.

KEY TREATMENT

The treatment of choice for latent TB infection is daily isoniazid (INH) for 9 months (ATS/CDC, 2000) (SOR: A).
Short-course rifampin (Rifadin) plus INH (3 months) is equivalent to standard INH therapy and may increase compliance in patients with latent TB infection (Ena and Valls, 2005) (SOR: B).
Although uncommon in the United States, drug-resistant TB and multidrug-resistant TB underscore the need for combination drug therapy and directly observed therapy in patients with tuberculosis (CDC, 2007) (SOR: C).

SEXUALLY TRANSMITTED INFECTIONS

David R. McBride

Key Points

- The U.S. Preventive Services Task Force recommends "high-intensity" behavioral counseling to at-risk adults and adolescents to prevent sexually transmitted infections.
- Be specific in addressing patients' sexual practices so as to provide appropriate prevention advice.
- Regular screening for *Chlamydia* infection is recommended for all sexually active women under age 24, all pregnant women under 24, and at-risk pregnant and nonpregnant women over 24.
- The presence of STIs such as gonorrhea, *Chlamydia*, and herpes increases the likelihood of HIV transmission.
- Testing for HIV should be offered on an "opt out" basis in all health care settings.
- The majority of patients with herpes simplex virus infection will not show recognizable symptoms. Screening for HSV immunity is of questionable value.
- Urine is an acceptable specimen to test for gonorrhea and *Chlamydia* in both men and women.
- The human papillomavirus vaccine is effective in reducing incidence of HPV infection, and physicians should discuss the vaccine with young women and men and their families.
- Routine screening for the mere presence of HPV is not recommended outside the context of cervical cancer screening.

Box 16-3   Criteria for Tuberculin Positivity by Risk Group

Reaction ≥5mm of Induration

HIV-positive persons

Recent contacts of tuberculosis patients

Fibrotic changes on chest radiography consistent with prior tuberculosis

Patients with organ transplants and other immunosuppressed patients (receiving equivalent of ≥15 mg/day of prednisone for at least 1 month)

Reaction ≥10 mm of Induration

Recent immigrants (within 5 years) from high-prevalence countries

Injection drug users

Residents and employees of high-risk congregate settings (prisons and jails, nursing homes, hospitals and other health care facilities, residential facilities for patients with AIDS, and homeless shelters)

Children less than 4 years of age, or infants, children, and adolescents exposed to adults at high risk.

Reaction ≥15 mm of Induration

Person with no risk factors for tuberculosis

Modified from Centers for Disease Control and Prevention. Targeted tuberculin testing and treatment of latent tuberculosis infection. American Thoracic Society. MMWR 2000;49(RR-6):1-51.

The CDC estimates that 19 million new cases of *sexually transmitted infections* (STIs) occur each year. More than half are in young people age 15 to 24 years. The most important development in the primary prevention of STIs is immunization against human papillomavirus (HPV). The vaccine can prevent infection with certain strains of HPV that cause cervical cancer and genital warts. Trials are ongoing to determine the effectiveness of daily ARV therapy in preventing transmission of HIV. Vaccination investigation is ongoing for herpes simplex, *Chlamydia trachomatis,* and HIV. This breadth of research effort holds promise for the future in the prevention of STIs.

Prevention

The USPSTF recommends "high-intensity" behavioral counseling to at-risk adults and adolescents to prevent STIs. High-intensity counseling involves multiple sessions and often is delivered to groups of patients. Unfortunately, this type of intervention has limitations in its practicality for population-based delivery. No risk of harm was discovered in the delivery of counseling for STI prevention.

Vaccination is the most important form of primary prevention of common infectious diseases. Two vaccines are currently on the market for HPV prevention—one that protects against four viral subtypes (6,11,16,18) and is licensed for use in males and females 9 to 26 years of age, and the other against two subtypes (16,18), licensed for females 10 to 25 years of age. Hepatitis B is a sexually transmitted infection, and immunization is recommended for adolescents who have not been previously inoculated. This is a requirement in many states for school entry. Hepatitis A can be transmitted by oro-anal sexual contact, and vaccination should be offered to patients who are contemplating engaging in this sexual practice.

Recommendations surrounding the use of barrier methods for STI prevention should be tailored to the sex practices of the client. For example, a percentage of women use anal sex as a method of birth control but may not consider the need for condom use with this practice. The question, "Do you regularly use condoms?" has little relevance to infection control for many sexual practices. Evidence supports the advice to use barrier methods of latex or other approved material in a manner that prevents the exchange of blood and body fluids in decreasing STIs. Condoms confer a 30% risk reduction for herpes simplex and up to an 80% risk reduction for HIV, when used correctly (Weller and Davis-Beaty, 2002; Martin et al., 2009).

The secondary prevention of STIs is achieved through direct and nonjudgmental patient assessment and screening and avoiding assumptions about patient sexual practices. Screening is a tool to prevent the inadvertent spread of infection as well as the sequelae of undetected disease. Table 16-7 summarizes USPSTF and CDC recommendations for screening of STIs.

Genital Ulcers

Infectious genital ulcers are associated with herpes simplex virus (HSV), syphilis, chancroid, lymphogranuloma venereum, and granuloma inguinale. HSV is by far the most common, affecting 50 million people in the United States. HSV-1 and HSV-2 are chronic, neurotropic viral infections that enter through epithelium and come to rest in the dorsal root ganglia. Therefore, infection leads to lifetime presence of the virus, but the clinical manifestation of this condition

Table 16-7 Recommendations for the Screening of Sexually Transmitted Infections (STIs)

STI	Who to Screen?	Recommending Body
Chlamydia	All sexually active women under age 24. Women over 24 at increased risk. All pregnant women under 24 and those over 24 at increased risk. Insufficient evidence for or against screening men.	USPSTF
Gonorrhea	All sexually active women at increased risk. Insufficient evidence for screening women not at increased risk. Insufficient evidence for or against screening men at increased risk.	USPSTF
Syphilis	Strongly recommended for pregnant women and all patients at increased risk.	USPSTF
HIV	All individuals as a routine part of health care in all settings after informing the patient. Pregnant women as standard prenatal testing.	CDC
Herpes	Recommendation against screening for asymptomatic individuals.	USPSTF
Hepatitis B	Strongly recommended for pregnant women at their first prenatal visit.	USPSTF

Modified from US Preventive Services Task Force (USPSTF). Guide to Clinical Preventive Services, 2009. http://www.ahrq.gov/clinic/pocketgd09/pocketgd09.pdf; and Branson B et al. Revised recommendations for HIV testing of adults, adolescents and pregnant women in health-care settings. MMWR 2006;55(RR-14):1-17.

is variable. A small percentage of those with serologic evidence of HSV-2 (10%-25%) have had symptoms of clinical herpes infection. In addition, patients with HSV infection can shed the virus in the absence of symptoms, creating a prime opportunity for spread.

Herpes Simplex

Herpes simplex outbreak may be followed by a prodrome of malaise, fever, and regional lymphadenopathy before the appearance of grouped vesicles on an erythematous base. The vesicles are typically quickly broken and become ulcerated in appearance, with each vesicle usually less than several millimeters in size. True first-time infections tend to present more severely than secondary presentations of previously infected individuals, with a prodrome present in 80% of cases.

The lesions can be in any location around the genitals or rectum, on the proximal thighs and buttocks, inside the vagina, and in and around the mouth. The lesions are most often painful, particularly when on mucosal surfaces, or itchy. In women, herpes simplex can present with cervicitis-like symptoms with bleeding and discharge and cervical ulcerations on examination, or simply mucopurulent cervicitis. Herpetic lesions around the urethra tend to be extremely painful and can make urination difficult. Rectal HSV can be confused with irritation, perianal fissure, and even candidiasis because of its often beefy-red appearance and itching.

Vesicles typically appear 6 days after infection and can last up to 2 weeks in an initial infection. Subsequent outbreaks tend to have a shorter duration and to be less uncomfortable for patients. Confirmation of infection is helpful, but the diagnosis can be made primarily on the clinical appearance of the exanthema. Vigorous sample collection from an ulcer (which the patient may not appreciate) to be sent for PCR identification and typing is the most readily available method of laboratory diagnosis. Serum antibody testing is not useful in the initial HSV diagnosis because antibody levels will not be appreciable early in infection. The appearance of convalescent immunoglobulin G (IgG) and IgM levels several weeks after a suspected outbreak might help to support the diagnosis of HSV infection.

The value of screening for HSV immunity is debatable and should generally not be recommended for asymptomatic individuals. In addition, the USPSTF recommends against screening asymptomatic pregnant women for HSV to prevent transmission to the newborn. Given that many patients with HSV infection never manifest symptoms, the value of knowing that one is HSV seropositive is questionable. In addition, HSV-1 and HSV-2, although classically oral and genital, respectively, can "mix and match" based on sexual practices. It is often confusing for asymptomatic individuals to know that they have HSV antibody (Do I have cold sores? Do I have genital herpes? How should this change the way I live my life?). In monogamous couples with one partner known to be HSV positive and the other with unknown status, testing of the latter may indicate suppressive therapy in the seropositive partner if the other is found to be negative.

Regular barrier method use decreases transmission of herpes in both men and women, with patients using condoms 100% of the time having a 30% reduction in HSV acquisition from those who never use condoms (Martin et al., 2009). Serodiscordant couples may also decrease transmission through antiviral suppressive therapy to the HSV-positive partner (Table 16-8).

Syphilis

Syphilis is a spirochetal infection that has resurged since 2001, the nadir year since 1996. Syphilis infection rates are highest in men who have sex with men. Syphilis is much less common than the other STIs, with an infection rate of 5.6 per 100,000 population in the United States (vs. 496 per 100,000 for *Chlamydia*).

Syphilis presents in several stages. The *primary* phase of syphilis is a painless ulcer called a *chancre* (Figure 16-4). The chancre may be visible on the genitals, although it can also be inside the vagina, mouth, or rectum, making it difficult to find. This lesion will appear within 3 weeks of transmission and will last for several weeks untreated. The *secondary* phase of infection is disseminated and involves a diffuse macular rash, typically with palm and sole lesions, generalized lymphadenopathy,

fever, and condyloma latum (smooth, moist lesions on genitals without cauliflower appearance of condyloma acuminatum). *Tertiary* syphilis is often asymptomatic but affects the heart, eyes, and auditory system and can be associated with gumma formation. *Gummas* are soft, granulomatous growths in organs that can cause mechanical obstruction and weakening of blood vessel walls. Latent infection often involves the CNS.

Diagnosis of primary syphilis is challenging. The test of choice is darkfield microscopy, which is not readily available. Direct fluorescent (monoclonal) antibody (DFA) testing may be available. Antibody tests for syphilis, such as the rapid plasma reagin (RPR) and the less frequently used Venereal

Table 16-8 Treatment Guidelines for Herpes Simplex Infection

Drug	Initial Outbreak	Suppression	Recurrence
Acyclovir	400 mg tid for 7-10 days	400 mg bid	400 mg tid for 5 days 800 mg bid for 5 days 800 mg tid for 2 days
Valacyclovir	1.0 g bid for 7-10 days	500 mg once daily 1.0 g once daily	500 mg bid for 3 days 1.0 g once daily for 5 days
Famciclovir	250 mg tid for 7-10 days	250 mg bid	125 mg bid for 5 days 1.0 g bid for 1 day

Data from Centers for Disease Control and Prevention. Sexually transmitted disease treatment guidelines, 2010. MMWR 2010;59(No. RR-12).
tid, Three times daily; *bid*, twice daily.

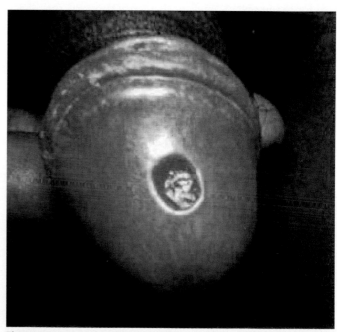

Figure 16-4 Primary chancre of syphilis.
(From http://www.stdptc.uc.edu/system/files/images/syphilisprimary%20chancre%20of%20 glans.thumbnail.jpg.)

Disease Research Laboratories (VDRL), are often not positive early in infection and thus cannot be used to rule out primary syphilis based on a single reading. Treponemal antigen testing (EIA) may be available in some laboratories. The fluorescent treponemal antibody absorption (FTA-ABS) test may also be negative in the early infection. Direct PCR for primary syphilis lesions has been tested but is not yet FDA approved. A physician may choose to treat presumptively if a painless chancre and risk factors are present and may then do a convalescent RPR test in 1 to 2 weeks to confirm the infection by the appearance of a positive reaction. One would expect a fourfold change in titer of either test to indicate the presence of disease.

Primary and secondary syphilis are treated with a single injection of penicillin G, 2.5 million units. Other regimens do not have proven effectiveness but can be used in the penicillin-allergic patient, including doxycycline, 100 mg twice daily for 14 days; ceftriaxone, 500 mg to 1 g intramuscularly (IM) daily for 8 to 10 days; or azithromycin, 2 g as a single oral dose, although resistance to azithromycin has been observed. Patients treated for primary syphilis should have periodic clinical follow-up and serologic testing to determine a fourfold decrease in RPR reactivity within 6 months.

Latent syphilis can be either *early*, meaning infection within the last year, or *late*, meaning infection beyond a year. Early latent syphilis is treated with a single injection of penicillin G, 2.4 million units. Syphilis of late latency or unknown duration is treated with three injections of penicillin G, 2.4 million units, in 3 consecutive weeks. For penicillin-allergic patients, doxycycline, 100 mg twice daily for 28 days, is required. Those with latent syphilis should have ophthalmic examination as well as evaluation for vascular gumma formation. Suspected neurologic involvement of latent syphilis must be evaluated with cerebrospinal fluid (CSF) examination and treatment with aqueous penicillin G, 3-4 million units intravenously (IV) every 4 hours for 10 to 14 days.

Partners of patients with newly diagnosed syphilis are at risk for infection. Partners within 90 days of a diagnosis of primary syphilis should be tested, but treated presumptively even if serologic testing is negative. For partners prior to 90 days before diagnosis, serology is generally reliable in detecting presence of infection and may guide treatment. Patients with secondary syphilis should inform partners within 6 months before diagnosis, or 12 months for those diagnosed with tertiary syphilis (Table 16-9).

Table 16-9 Diagnosis and Treatment of Syphilis

Stage	Clinical Manifestations	Diagnosis (Sensitivity)	Treatment
Primary syphilis	Chancre	Darkfield microscopy of skin lesion (80%) Nontreponemal tests (78%-86%) Treponemal-specific tests (76%-84%)	Penicillin G benzathine, 2.4 million units IM (single dose) Alternatives in nonpregnant patients with penicillin allergy: doxycycline (Vibramycin), 100 mg PO bid for 2 weeks; tetracycline, 500 mg PO four times daily for 2 weeks; ceftriaxone (Rocephin), 1 g IM or IV once daily for 8-10 days; *or* azithromycin (Zithromax), 2 g PO (single dose)
Secondary syphilis	Skin and mucous membranes: diffuse rash, condyloma latum, other lesions Renal system: glomerulonephritis, nephrotic syndrome Liver: hepatitis CNS: headache, meningismus, cranial neuropathy, iritis, uveitis Constitutional symptoms: fever, malaise, generalized lymphadenopathy, arthralgias, weight loss, others	Darkfield microscopy of skin lesion (80%) Nontreponemal tests (100%) Treponemal-specific tests (100%)	Same treatments as for primary syphilis
Latent syphilis	None	Nontreponemal tests (95%-100%) Treponemal-specific tests (97%-100%)	Early latent syphilis: same treatments as for primary and secondary syphilis Late latent syphilis: penicillin G benzathine, 2.4 million units IM once weekly for 3 weeks Alternatives in nonpregnant patients with penicillin allergy: doxycycline, 100 mg PO bid for 4 weeks, *or* tetracycline, 500 mg PO four times daily for 4 weeks
Tertiary (late) syphilis	Gummatous disease, cardiovascular disease	Nontreponemal tests (71%-73%) Treponemal-specific tests (94%-96%)	Same treatment as for late latent syphilis
Neurosyphilis	Seizures, ataxia, aphasia, paresis, hyperreflexia, personality changes, cognitive disturbance, visual changes, hearing loss, neuropathy, loss of bowel or bladder function, others	Cerebrospinal fluid examination	Aqueous crystalline penicillin G, 3-4 million units IV q4h for 10-14 days, *or* penicillin G procaine, 2.4 million units IM once daily, plus probenecid, 500 mg PO four times daily, both drugs given for 10-14 days

Data from Brown DL, Frank JE. Diagnosis and management of syphilis. Am Fam Physician , 2003;68:283-290.
IM, Intramuscularly; *IV*, intravenously, *PO*, orally; *q4h*, every 4 hours; *CNS*, central nervous system.

Chancroid

Chancroid may occur in regional outbreaks and presents with a painful genital ulcer and suppurative regional adenopathy. Herpes and syphilis should both be ruled out in the patient suspected of having chancroid infection. Chancroid is caused by *Haemophilus ducreyi* and there is currently no FDA approved test to directly detect this organism. Treatment with azithromycin (1 g as single dose), ceftriaxone (250 mg IM as a single dose), ciprofloxacin (500 mg twice daily for 3 days), or erythromycin (500 mg three times daily for 7 days) are all alternatives (Table 16-10). It may be necessary to perform incision and drainage on fluctuant inguinal nodes. Patients should be reexamined in 1 to 2 weeks to ensure healing of the primary ulcer(s) and resolution of the adenopathy. Partners who had contact with the infected patient starting 10 days before development of the patient's symptoms should be treated, regardless of the presence of symptoms.

Table 16-10 Treatment of Chancroid, Lymphogranuloma Venereum, and Granuloma Inguinale

Infection	Recommended Treatment	Alternate Treatment
Chancroid	Azithromycin, 1 g PO × 1 *or* Ceftriaxone, 250 mg IM single dose *or* Ciprofloxacin, 500 mg bid for 3 days *or* Erythromycin base, 500 mg tid for 7 days	—
Lymphogranuloma venereum	Doxycycline, 100 mg bid for 21 days	Erythromycin base, 500 mg PO four times daily for 21 days
Granuloma inguinale	Doxycycline, 100 mg bid for at least 3 weeks until all lesions have completely healed	Azithromycin, 1 g PO once weekly for 3 weeks until all lesions have completely healed *or* Ciprofloxacin, 750 mg PO four times daily for at least 3 weeks until all lesions have completely healed *or* Erythromycin base, 500 mg four times daily for at least 3 weeks until all lesions have completely healed *or* TMP/SMX, 1 DS bid for at least 3 weeks *or* until all lesions have completely healed

PO, Orally; *IM*, intramuscularly; *bid*, twice daily; *tid*, three times daily; *qid*, four times daily; *TMP-SMX*, trimethoprim-sulfamethoxazole; *DS*, double-strength tablet.

Lymphogranuloma Venereum and Granuloma Inguinale

Less common ulcerating STIs include lymphogranuloma venereum (LGV) and granuloma inguinale (Figure 16-5). LGV causes regional adenopathy and often an ulcer at the point of entry. Rectal LGV may cause a proctocolitis with anal pain, discharge, bleeding, and diarrhea. LGV is caused by *Chlamydia trachomatis* serotypes and can be detected by testing swabbed material from open lesions or aspirates from lymph nodes with culture, DFA, or nucleic acid detection. Treatment is noted above (Table 16-10). Granuloma inguinale, caused by *Klebsiella granulomatis*, is rare in the United States and causes progressive ulcerative disease of the genitals.

Urethritis and Cervicitis

A second STI category includes those causing the clinical presentation of vaginal discharge, pelvic pain, dyspareunia, and dysuria in women and penile discharge and dysuria in men, as well as possible rectal pain and discharge in men and women. Of this group, *Chlamydia trachomatis* is the most common, causing 1.2 million infections in the United States in 2008 (CDC, 2009). In fact, *Chlamydia* is the most frequently reported reportable infection.

Chlamydia trachomatis

The majority of women with *Chlamydia* infection are without symptoms. Many men are asymptomatic as well. Regular screening for *Chlamydia*, as recommended by the USPSTF, can significantly reduce the incidence of pelvic inflammatory disease (PID), one of the most serious sequelae of untreated infection. In women with untreated *Chlamydia* infection, in addition to PID, tubo-ovarian abscess, tubal scarring and ectopic pregnancy, and infertility can all result.

As previously mentioned, regular screening is currently recommended for all sexually active women under age 24, all pregnant women under 24, and at-risk pregnant and nonpregnant women over 24. *Chlamydia* testing can be performed on several liquid-based Papanicolaou (Pap) tests.

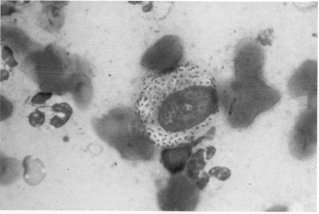

Figure 16-5 Biopsy of granuloma inguinale lesion revealing "Donovan bodies" consistent with *Klebsiella granulomatis*.
(From Mandell GL, Bennett JE, Dolin R (eds). Mandell, Douglas, and Bennett's Principles and Practices of Infectious Diseases, 7th ed. Philadelphia, Churchill Livingstone, 2010.)

Endocervical swabs for nucleic acid amplification are acceptable when a conventional Pap smear is being used. Given the recent liberalization of recommendations about Pap testing for women under 21 years of age, urine nucleic acid amplification is a readily available alternative for *Chlamydia* testing. This can easily be done at a contraceptive counseling clinic. Urine testing is also an acceptable method of testing for men, in addition to a urethral swab. Rectal *Chlamydia* infection can occur in individuals who practice receptive anal intercourse. An FDA-approved method of testing should be used for screening and diagnosis of this infection.

Asymptomatic *Chlamydia* infection is treated with either a single dose of azithromycin, 1 g orally, the drug of choice, or doxycycline, 100 mg twice daily, for 7 days (Table 16-11). *Patient-delivered partner therapy* (PDPT), the practice of dispensing treatment to diagnosed patients to treat their partner(s), has proved effective in reducing reinfection rates and further spread of infection. EPT is legally allowable in 21 states and potentially allowable in another 21.

Chlamydia infection may present symptomatically in men or women with symptoms of dysuria and with discharge and with pelvic pain and dyspareunia in women. The discharge of *C. trachomatis*, versus that of *Neisseria gonorrhoeae*, is said to be more mucoid than purulent, although this characteristic is not specific enough to provide diagnostic accuracy. Symptomatic *Chlamydia*, without evidence of PID, is treated the same as asymptomatic infection. Many practitioners will treat presumptively for *Chlamydia* and gonorrhea in patients who present with the symptoms previously mentioned while they wait for confirmatory testing.

Neisseria gonorrhoeae

Neisseria gonorrhoeae infection may be asymptomatic in both men and women. The current USPSTF recommendation is for screening women at risk. Men with penile gonorrhea typically present with purulent penile discharge and dysuria with *N. gonorrhoeae* infection. Mucopurulent discharge, dysuria, pelvic pain, and dyspareunia are typical symptoms in women. In patients who engage in anal intercourse, anal discharge, rectal pain, and bleeding can be presenting symptoms. Gonococcal pharyngitis is within the differential of exudative pharyngitis in sexually active patients. When symptomatic, throat pain, tonsillar exudates, and anterior cervical adenopathy may be present.

Testing for gonorrhea can be done using liquid-based Pap technologies, cervical or urethral swabs, or urine for nucleic acid amplification. In men with visible discharge, a Gram stain with white blood cells (WBCs) and gram-positive intracellular diplococci has a high degree of sensitivity. Culture testing may be preferred for suspected pharyngeal and rectal specimens pending FDA approval of other methods.

Again, physicians may opt to treat patients with mucopurulent cervicitis or urethritis presumptively for gonorrhea and *Chlamydia* while waiting for confirmatory testing. Fluoroquinolone therapy is no longer recommended because of widespread resistance (Table 16-11).

Because reinfection with gonorrhea is common for several months after treatment, it may be advisable to retest patients with confirmed gonorrhea in the 3 months after treatment. Similarly, STIs may be an indicator of risk behavior, and a complete risk history and testing for other STIs is advisable if not completed at the initial visit.

Nongonococcal Urethritis

In male patients with symptomatic urethritis, a causative agent may not be identified, a situation often referred to as nongonococcal urethritis (NGU). Technically, *Chlamydia* is included in this category. Organisms such as *Ureaplasma urealyticum* and *Mycoplasma genitalium* may be the cause and may be difficult to detect. Treatment for these infections is the same as for symptomatic *Chlamydia*, with azithromycin or doxycycline (Table 16-11). It is recommended that partners of patients with NGU should be evaluated and treated. In some cases, testing of partners may detect a specific organism as the cause of infection (e.g., *Chlamydia*).

Trichomonas vaginalis

Trichomonas vaginalis causes vaginitis in women, who may have a stereotypic frothy, green, and foul-smelling discharge. Many women are asymptomatic with trichomoniasis. In addition to causing asymptomatic infection in men, *T. vaginalis* may cause urethritis. This organism may be suspected in men when patients have repeated treatment failures and

Table 16-11 Treatment of Urethritis and Cervicitis

Infection	Recommended Treatment	Alternate Treatment
Chlamydia trachomatis	Azithromycin, 1 g PO × 1 *or* Doxycycline, 100 mg bid for 7 days	Erythromycin base, 500 mg PO four times daily for 7 days *or* Ofloxacin, 300 mg PO bid for 7 days *or* Levofloxacin, 500 mg PO once daily for 7 days
Neisseria gonorrhoeae: urethral, cervical, or rectal	Ceftriaxone, 125 mg IM × 1 Treat for *C. trachomatis* concurrently if this has not been ruled out.	Cefixime, 400 mg PO single dose
Neisseria gonorrhoeae: pharynx	Ceftriaxone, 125 mg IM × 1 *or* Treat for *C. trachomatis* concurrently if this has not been ruled out.	—
Nongonococcal urethritis	Azithromycin, 1 g PO single dose *or* Doxycycline, 100 mg PO bid for 7 days	Erythromycin base, 500 mg PO qid for 7 days *or* Ofloxacin, 300 mg PO bid for 7 days *or* Levofloxacin, 500 mg PO daily for 7 days
Trichomonas vaginalis	Metronidazole, 1 g PO × 1 *or* Tinidazole, 2 g PO × 1	—

Modified from Centers for Disease Control and Prevention. Sexually transmitted disease treatment guidelines, 2010. MMWR 2010;59(No. RR-12).

no other explanation for symptoms. Microscopic examination of vaginal discharge is 60% to 70% sensitive in women. A first voided urine specimen or urethral swab for microscopic exam may be helpful in identifying the protozoa. Culture for *Trichomonas*, which requires a special medium, may be necessary to identify this infection accurately in men. *Trichomonas* is effectively treated with a single 2-g dose of metronidazole (Table 16-11).

For non-STI causes of vaginal discharge, see the online discussion at www.expertconsult.com.

Pelvic Inflammatory Disease

Pelvic inflammatory disease can be caused by a number of organisms, including *Chlamydia*, and presents with pelvic pain and discharge. Findings that contribute to the diagnosis of PID include fever greater than 101° F, cervical or vaginal mucopurulent discharge, abundant WBCs on saline preparation of vaginal discharge, elevated erythrocyte sedimentation rate (ESR), elevated C-reactive protein (CRP), and evidence of *N. gonorrhoeae* or *C. trachomatis* infection. Hospitalization with parenteral antibiotics may be necessary in pregnant patients, patients in whom surgical emergency cannot be ruled out, those who do not respond to oral treatment, those who cannot tolerate oral treatment, and patients who have severe illness or tubo-ovarian abscess. When treating PID parenterally, improvement of symptoms for 24 hours may prompt a change to oral therapy (Table 16-12). Conversely, if oral therapy is not producing significant improvement within 2 to 3 days, admission for parenteral therapy may be necessary.

Human Papillomavirus

Patient awareness of human papillomavirus infection has greatly increased in recent years, in large part related to the patient-directed advertising of the HPV vaccine. HPV is likely the most common STI. Thirty types of HPV can infect the genital area, some causing genital warts, some causing malignancies of the genital organs, and most being asymptomatic. The gross categories most often used are "high risk" (most often types 16 and 18) and "low risk" (types 6 and 11) HPV infection, the former more often associated with genital cancer.

Prevention of HPV infection and cervical cancer was revolutionized with the release of the HPV vaccine, which is effective in reducing the incidence of HPV-associated disease. Currently, two vaccines are licensed in the United States. Gardasil (Merck), released in 2006, includes protection against viral types 6, 11, 16, and 18. It is approved for the prevention of vulvar and vaginal cancer and for the prevention of cervical cancer, cervical dysplasia, and genital warts in females age 9 to 26. The vaccine was recently approved for males of the same age range for the prevention of genital warts. More recently, Cervarix (GlaxoSmithKline) was approved for the prevention of cervical cancer and cervical dysplasia from HPV types 16 and 18 in women age 10 to 25. Ideally, the vaccine should be administered before initiation of sexual activity to prevent initial acquisition of these HPV types. Patients who are already sexually active may also receive the vaccine.

The transmission of HPV to men decreases with consistent condom use, from 53.9% in men who never use condoms to 37.9% in men who "always" use them. Unfortunately, HPV can infect skin that is not covered by the use of traditional barrier methods (Nielson et al., 2010). Male circumcision may decrease the transmission of HPV.

Patients have many questions about HPV, in particular about screening for asymptomatic infection. HPV infection occurs with high frequency in the sexually active population; up to 50% or more of sexually active individuals have HPV at some point in their life. In addition, HPV is effectively transmitted, even if contact does not involve genital-to-genital touching (i.e., manual stimulation can transmit the virus). Again, most HPV infections are without symptoms and resolve spontaneously through eradication by the intact immune system. For all these reasons, screening for the mere presence of HPV infection has minimal utility. There is no treatment for asymptomatic HPV infection.

The most common presentation of HPV infection is in the context of an abnormal Pap smear. HPV is directly linked to cervical dysplasia. For women over age 21 and under 35, HPV testing with high-risk viral detection is common. The presence of high-risk HPV informs further management of the Pap result. It is currently recommended that women over 35 be automatically tested for high-risk HPV infection at the Pap smear.

Patients may present with visible warts, or these may be detected at routine or STI screening. Genital warts are often cosmetically unacceptable to patients, even though they are infrequently functionally problematic. In some circumstances, wart burden can be high enough to cause physical discomfort or relative obstruction of the vagina or rectum.

Table 16-12 Treatment of Pelvic Inflammatory Disease (PID)

Route	Recommended Treatment	Alternate Treatment
Parenteral	Cefotetan, 2 g IV q12h *or* Cefoxitin 2 g IV q6h *plus* Doxycycline, 100 mg PO or IV q12h *or* Clindamycin, 900 mg IV q8h *plus* Gentamicin loading dose IV or IM (2 mg/kg) followed by maintenance dose (1.5 mg/kg) q8h; may use once-daily gentamicin dosing.	Ampicillin/sulbactam, 3 g IV q6h *plus* Doxycycline, 100 mg PO or IV q12h
Intramuscular	Ceftriaxone, 250 mg IM single dose, *plus* doxycycline, 100 mg bid for 14 days, with or without metronidazole, 500 mg bid for 14 days	Cefoxitin 2 g IM single dose plus probenecid 1 g orally concurrently administered plus doxycycline 100 mg bid for 14 days with or without metronidazole 500 mg bid for 14 days.

Data from Centers for Disease Control and Prevention. Sexually transmitted disease treatment guidelines, 2010. MMWR 2010;59(No. RR-12).
IV, Intravenously; *PO,* orally; *IM,* intramuscularly; *q6h, q8h, q12h,* every 6, 8, or 12 hours; *bid,* twice daily.

The treatment of warts is destructive and may serve to stimulate an immune response to the HPV-infected cells, which are typically "above" the surveillance mechanisms of the immune system in the epidermis. Office methods of treatment include cryotherapy and trichloroacetic acid or podophyllin resin application. Patients may apply podofilox 0.5% solution or gel or imiquimod 5% cream (Table 16-13). For more extensive cases of warts or intra-anal or intravaginal infections that are difficult to treat using the previous methods, surgical techniques may be necessary to achieve resolution. Untreated, warts may resolve spontaneously, remain the same, or worsen.

Ectoparasites

Patients with *pediculosis pubis,* or pubic lice, most often present with pruritus or with visible nits. Pubic lice are visible on inspection of the pubic area, as are nits, which are adherent to the hair shaft. Partners of patients with pubic lice should also be treated to prevent reinfection. Linens and clothing should be laundered or dry-cleaned or kept in a closed plastic container or bag for 72 hours.

Table 16-13 **Treatment of Genital Warts**

Provider applied
Cryotherapy
Trichloroacetic acid (TCA): small amount applied until wart whitens
Podophyllin resin, 10% to 25%
All these may be repeated every 1 to 2 weeks until warts are resolved.

Patient applied
Podofilox 0.5% solution or gel applied twice daily for 3 days, followed by 4 days of no therapy.
Imiquimod 5% cream applied once daily at bedtime three times a week for up to 16 weeks; washed off 6 to 10 hours after application.

Table 16-14 **Treatment for Ectoparasites**

Infestation	Recommended Treatment	Alternate Treatment
Pediculosis pubis	Permethrin 1% cream applied to affected area and washed off after 10 minutes *or* Pyrethrins with piperonyl butoxide applied to affected area and washed off after 10 minutes	Malathion 0.5% lotion applied for 8-12 hours and washed off *or* Ivermectin, 250 μg/kg orally once, repeated in 2 weeks
Scabies	Permethrin cream 5% applied to whole body, neck to soles of feet, and washed off in 8-14 hours, *or* Ivermectin, 200 μg/kg orally once, repeated in 2 weeks	Lindane 1% applied to whole body, neck to soles of feet, and washed off in 8 hours

Data from Workowshi KA, Berman SM. Sexually transmitted disease treatment guidelines. MMWR 2006;55(RR-11).

Scabies diagnosis can be challenging. Again, patients present with itching that can be anywhere on the body, although often in the genital area or on the buttocks when infection is sexual in origin. The pruritus associated with *Sarcoptes scabiei* is a result of sensitization to the mite droppings underneath the skin as the mite burrows. The classic "burrow" or linear papular eruption is not always present. Scraping of lesions with microscopic examination may be performed to identify the mite. As with pediculosis, close contacts should be treated. Linens and clothing should be laundered or dry-cleaned or isolated in plastic containers for 72 hours. The pruritus-associated with scabies can take several weeks to resolve after treatment. Patients living in group settings (dormitories or apartments) may reinfect one another as a result of inadequate primary treatment of all contacts (Table 16-14).

KEY TREATMENT

Regular barrier method use decreases transmission of herpes simplex virus in both men and women, with patients using condoms 100% of the time having a 30% reduction in HSV acquisition compared with those who never use condoms (Martin et al., 2009) (SOR: A).

For STIs other than syphilis, expedited partner therapy, the practice of administering medication to diagnosed patients to treat their partner(s), has proved effective in reducing reinfection rates and further spread of infection (CDC, 2006) (SOR: B).

Human papillomavirus vaccine is effective in reducing the incidence of HPV infection (Sundar et al., 2010) (SOR: A).

Imiquimod 1% or 5% increases wart clearance compared with placebo in people without HIV infection (Buck, 2010) (SOR: A).

Podofilox (Condylox) is more effective than placebo at clearing genital warts after 16 weeks (SOR: A).

The most common outpatient treatment for PID is ceftriaxone (250 mg IM) plus doxycycline (100 mg) twice daily for 14 days.

GENITOURINARY INFECTIONS

William E. Roland

Key Points

- Symptomatic urinary tract infections (UTIs) should be treated.
- Uncomplicated cystitis in women can be treated safely and effectively through telephone treatment protocols.
- Asymptomatic UTIs should be treated in pregnant women and in men about to undergo urologic surgery.
- Young children with UTIs might benefit from an etiologic workup (renal ultrasound, voiding cystourethrogram) if they are:
  - Boys of any age
  - Children of any age with a febrile UTI
  - Girls younger than 3 years with first UTI (difficulty verbalizing symptoms)
  - Children with recurrent UTI who have not been imaged previously
  - First UTI in children with a family history or with renal disease, abnormal voiding, poor growth, urinary tract abnormalities, or hypertension
- Acute prostatitis is usually caused by *Escherichia coli.*

Urinary tract infection (UTI) is defined as significant bacteriuria in the presence of symptoms. UTI accounts for a significant number of emergency department visits; an estimated 20% of women experience a UTI in their lifetime. The urinary tract is normally sterile. *Uncomplicated* UTI involves the urinary bladder in a host without underlying renal or neurologic disease. The bladder mucosa is invaded, most often by enteric coliform bacteria (e.g., *E. coli*) that ascend into the bladder via the urethra. Sexual intercourse can promote this migration, and cystitis is common in otherwise healthy young women. Frequent and complete voiding has been associated with a reduction in the incidence of UTI. *Complicated* UTI occurs in the setting of underlying structural, medical, or neurologic disease.

Signs and symptoms of a UTI include dysuria, frequency, urgency, nocturia, enuresis, incontinence, urethral pain, suprapubic pain, low back pain, and hematuria. Fever is unusual. Up to 30% of patients with symptoms of cystitis have a smoldering *pyelonephritis*, especially when symptoms have been present for more than 1 week. A patient with pyelonephritis usually appears ill, with fever, sweating, and prostration, along with costovertebral angle (flank) tenderness in most cases. The differential diagnosis of uncomplicated UTI includes use of diuretics or caffeine, interstitial cystitis, vaginitis, pregnancy, pelvic mass, PID, and benign prostatic hypertrophy (BPH).

If a UTI is suspected, the initial test of choice is urinalysis, although with classic signs and symptoms of infection in women, this test is not always necessary. Pyuria, as indicated by a positive result on the leukocyte esterase dip test, is found in the majority of patients with UTI. The presence of urinary nitrites is fairly specific for UTI. The combination of positive leukocyte esterase and nitrites improves sensitivity. On urine microscopy, levels of pyuria as low as two to five leukocytes per high-power field (2-5 WBCs/hpf) in a centrifuged specimen are significant in the female patient with appropriate symptoms, as is the presence of bacteriuria. Urine culture and sensitivity are not needed in simple UTIs. Cultures should be done in patients with recurrent UTIs, patients with pyelonephritis, and pregnant patients.

Antibiotic therapy can be given in a 3-day regimen for young, sexually active women. A 7- to 10-day course of antibiotics should be used in pregnant patients and patients with complicated UTIs. All the drugs listed in Table 16-15 can be used in a 3-day or 7- to 10-day course. Clinical practice guidelines that include telephone assessment and treatment have shown a decrease in unnecessary laboratory utilization while maintaining quality of care (Saint et al., 1999). Trimethoprim-sulfamethoxazole (TMP-SMX) has been a mainstay of UTI therapy, but in some localities, resistance of *E. coli* to TMP-SMX is 20% (Mehnert-Kay, 2005).

If a urine culture is done and the organism is resistant to the drug prescribed, a change in antibiotics is indicated only if the patient is still symptomatic. For symptomatic treatment, a bladder anesthetic can be used, such as phenazopyridine (Pyridium), 200 mg three times daily for 2 days. Patients should be warned that this produces an orange tinge in tears and urine. Patients should also be instructed to increase fluid intake.

Pyelonephritis is suggested by a failure of a short course of antibiotics. Signs and symptoms of pyelonephritis include shaking chills and fever higher than 38.5° C (101.3° F), flank pain, malaise, urinary frequency and burning, and costover-

Table 16-15 Treatment Regimens for Acute Uncomplicated Cystitis*

Otherwise Healthy Women†
3-Day Regimens
TMP-SMX, 160/800 mg q12h
Trimethoprim, 100 mg q12h
Fluoroquinolones‡
Ciprofloxacin, 100-250 mg q12h
Ciprofloxacin XR, 500 mg qd
Gatifloxacin, 200 mg qd
Levofloxacin, 250 mg qd
5-Day to 7-Day Regimens
Nitrofurantoin monohydrate/macrocrystals, 100 mg q12h
Nitrofurantoin macrocrystals, 50-100 mg qid
Amoxicillin, 250 mg q8h or 500 mg q12h
Cephalexin, 250 mg q6h, or other cephalosporin
Consider 7-day regimen.
Pregnant Women
Amoxicillin, 250 mg q8h or 500 mg q12h
Nitrofurantoin monohydrate/macrocrystals, 100 mg q12h
Nitrofurantoin macrocrystals, 50-100 mg qid
Cephalexin, 250 mg q6h, or other cephalosporin
TMP-SMX, 160/800 mg q12h
Other Patients
Male gender, diabetes, symptoms for 7 days, recent antimicrobial use, age > 65
TMP-SMX,§ 160/800 mg q12h
Fluoroquinolones, as per 3-day regimens
Cephalexin, 250 mg q6h, or other cephalosporin
Consider 7-day regimen.

From Hooton TM, Stamm WE. Diagnosis and treatment of uncomplicated urinary tract infection. Infect Dis North Am 1997;11:551.
TMP-SMX, Trimethoprim-sulfamethoxazole; *qd*, every day; *q12h*, every 12 hours; *q6h*, every 6 hours; *q8h*, every 8 hours; *qid*, four times daily.
*Treatments listed to be prescribed before etiologic agent is known (Gram stain may help); therapy can be modified when cause is identified.
†Characteristic pathogens are *Escherichia coli* (85%-90%) and *Staphylococcus saprophyticus* (5%-15%); other organisms account for less than 5% of cases and include *Proteus mirabilis, Klebsiella pneumoniae*, and *Enterococcus* spp.
‡Fluoroquinolones should not be used in pregnancy.
§Although classified as pregnancy category C, TMP-SMX is widely used; however, avoid its use in the first and second trimesters.

tebral angle tenderness. The infection can produce septic shock. A patient who is unable to tolerate oral intake should be hospitalized and given empiric IV antibiotics aimed at broad-spectrum gram-negative coverage, such as third-generation cephalosporins, fluoroquinolones, or aminoglycosides, while awaiting results of blood and urine cultures. A 14-day course of antibiotic therapy (IV or PO) is recommended.

Urinary Tract Infection in Pregnancy

Although the most common bacterial infection during pregnancy, the incidence of UTI in pregnancy is similar to that reported in sexually active nonpregnant women of childbearing age. Up to 40% of pregnant women with untreated bacteriuria in the first trimester develop acute pyelonephritis later in pregnancy. Premature births and perinatal mortality are increased in pregnancies complicated by UTI. Therefore, in pregnant women, asymptomatic bacteriuria alone should be actively sought and aggressively treated with at least one urinalysis, preferably toward the end of the first trimester.

Nitrofurantoin, ampicillin, and the cephalosporins have been used most extensively in pregnancy and are the regimens of choice for treating asymptomatic or minimally symptomatic UTI. TMP-SMX should be avoided in the first trimester because of possible teratogenic effects and should be avoided near term because of a possible role in the development of kernicterus. Fluoroquinolones are avoided because of possible adverse effects on fetal cartilage development. For pregnant women with overt pyelonephritis, admission to the hospital for parenteral therapy should be the standard of care; beta-lactam agents with or without aminoglycosides are the cornerstone of therapy. Prevention of UTI, including pyelonephritis, can be accomplished during pregnancy with nitrofurantoin or cephalexin taken prophylactically after coitus or at bedtime without relation to coitus. Such prophylaxis should be considered for patients who have had acute pyelonephritis during pregnancy, patients with bacteriuria during pregnancy who have had a recurrence after a course of treatment, and patients who had recurrent UTI before pregnancy that required prophylaxis.

Catheter-Associated Urinary Tract Infection

Catheter-associated UTIs are associated with increased mortality and costs. Risk factors for catheter-associated UTIs include the duration of catheterization, lack of systemic antibiotic therapy, female gender, age older than 50 years, and azotemia. To help prevent infection, urinary catheters should be avoided when possible and used only as long as needed. The catheter should be inserted with strict aseptic technique by trained persons, and a closed system should be used at all times. Treatment of catheter-associated UTI depends on the clinical circumstances. Symptomatic patients (e.g., those with fever, chills, dyspnea, and hypotension) require immediate antibiotic therapy along with removal and replacement of the urinary catheter if it has been in place for a week or longer. In an asymptomatic patient, therapy should be postponed until the catheter can be removed. Patients with long-term indwelling catheters seldom become symptomatic unless the catheter is obstructed or is eroding through the bladder mucosa. In patients who do become symptomatic, appropriate antibiotics should be administered and the catheter changed. Therapy for asymptomatic catheterized patients leads to the selection of increasingly antibiotic-resistant bacteria.

Recurrent Urinary Tract Infection

Recurrence of uncomplicated cystitis in reproductive-age women is common, and some form of preventive strategy is indicated if three or more symptomatic episodes occur in 1 year. However, risk factors specific to women with recurrent cystitis have received little study (Sen, 2008). Several antimicrobial strategies are available, but before initiating therapy, the patient should try such simple interventions as voiding immediately after sexual intercourse and using a contraceptive method other than a diaphragm and spermicide. Ingestion of cranberry juice has been shown to be effective in decreasing bacteriuria with pyuria, but not bacteriuria alone or symptomatic UTI, in an elderly population. Cranberry juice may be effective for preventing UTI in young, otherwise healthy women.

If simple nondrug measures are ineffective, continuous or postcoital—if the infections are temporally related to intercourse—low-dose antimicrobial prophylaxis with TMP-SMX, a fluoroquinolone, or nitrofurantoin should be considered. Typically, a prophylactic regimen is initially prescribed for 6 months and then discontinued. If the infections recur, the prophylactic program can be instituted for a longer period. An alternative approach to antimicrobial prophylaxis for women with less frequent recurrences (<4 a year) is to supply TMP-SMX or a fluoroquinolone and allow the patient to self-medicate with short-course therapy at the first symptoms of infection.

A minority of patients have *relapsing* UTI, as evidenced by finding the same bacterial strain within 2 weeks after completion of antimicrobial therapy. Two factors can contribute to the pathogenesis of relapsing infection in women: (1) deep tissue infection of the kidney that is suppressed but not eradicated by a 14-day course of antibiotics and (2) structural abnormality of the urinary tract, particularly calculi. Patients with true relapsing UTIs should undergo renal ultrasound, intravenous pyelogram (IVP), or voiding cystourethrogram, and longer-term therapy should be considered.

Urinary Tract Infections in Children

Urinary tract infection is one of the most common infections of childhood. Factors predisposing to UTI include taking broad-spectrum antibiotics (e.g., amoxicillin, cephalexin), which are likely to alter gastrointestinal and periurethral flora; incomplete bladder emptying or infrequent voiding; voiding dysfunction; and constipation. UTI in young children serves as a marker for abnormalities of the urinary tract. Imaging of the urinary tract is recommended in every febrile infant or young child with a first UTI to identify children with abnormalities that predispose to renal damage. Imaging should consist of urinary tract ultrasonography to detect dilation of the renal parenchyma. Voiding cystourethrography is often ordered but does not appear to improve clinical outcomes in uncomplicated UTIs (Alper and Curry, 2005).

Prostatitis

A common complication of UTI in men is prostatitis. Bacterial prostatitis is usually caused by the same gram-negative bacilli that cause UTI in female patients; 80% or more of such infections are caused by *Escherichia coli*. The pathogenesis of this condition is poorly understood. Antibacterial substances in prostatic secretions probably protect against such infections. A National Institutes of Health (NIH) expert consensus panel has recommended classifying prostatitis into three syndromes: acute bacterial prostatitis, chronic bacterial prostatitis, and *chronic pelvic pain syndrome* (CPPS). *Acute bacterial prostatitis* is a febrile illness characterized by chills, dysuria, urinary frequency and urgency, and pain in the perineum, back, or pelvis. The bladder outlet can be obstructed. On physical examination, the prostate is found to be enlarged, tender, and indurated. Pyuria is present, and urine cultures generally grow *E. coli* or another typical uropathogen.

Chronic bacterial prostatitis is a clinically more occult disease and may be manifested only as recurrent bacteriuria or variable low-grade fever with back or pelvic discomfort. Urinary symptoms usually relate to the reintroduction of infection into the bladder, with both pyuria and bacteriuria. A chronic prostatic focus is the most common cause of recurrent UTI in men. CPPS is the diagnosis for the large group of men who present with minimal signs on physical examination but have a variety of irritative or obstructive voiding symptoms; perineal, pelvic, or back pain; and sexual dysfunction. These men can be divided into those with and those without inflammation (defined as >10 WBCs/hpf in expressed prostatic secretions). The etiology and appropriate management in these patients, regardless of inflammatory status, is unknown.

KEY TREATMENT

Pregnant women should be screened for asymptomatic bacteriuria in the first trimester of pregnancy (Wadland and Plante, 1989) (SOR: A).

Pregnant women who have asymptomatic bacteriuria should be treated with antimicrobial therapy for 3 to 7 days (Nicolle et al., 2005) (SOR: B).

Pyuria accompanying asymptomatic bacteriuria should not be treated with antimicrobial therapy (Nicolle, 2003) (SOR: C1).

A 3-day course of TMP-SMX (Bactrim, Septra) is recommended as empiric therapy of uncomplicated UTIs in women, in regions where the rate of resistant *E. coli* is less than 20% (Warren et al., 1999) (SOR: C).

Fluoroquinolones are not recommended as first-line treatment of uncomplicated UTIs, to preserve their effectiveness for complicated UTIs (Warren et al., 1999) (SOR: C).

A randomized, placebo-controlled trial of 150 women over 12 months found that cranberry juice and cranberry extract tablets significantly decreased the number of patients having at least one symptomatic UTI per year (Stothers, 2002) (SOR: B).

TICK-BORNE INFECTIONS

William E. Roland

Key Points

- Laboratory findings in acute tick-borne infection often include a normal or low WBC count, thrombocytopenia, hyponatremia, and elevated liver enzymes.
- Doxycycline is the drug of choice for patients with RMSF.
- Appropriate antibiotic treatment should be initiated immediately with strong suspicion of ehrlichiosis.
- If left untreated, Lyme disease can progress to cognitive disorders, sleep disturbance, fatigue, and personality changes.

In the United States, more vector-borne diseases are transmitted by ticks than by any other agent. Tick-borne diseases can result from infection with pathogens that include bacteria, rickettsiae, viruses, and protozoa. Most tick-borne diseases are transmitted during the spring and summer months when ticks are active. A knowledge of which species of tick is endemic in an area can help narrow the diagnosis (Table 16-16).

Rocky Mountain Spotted Fever

Rocky Mountain spotted fever (RMSF) is the most severe and most often reported rickettsial illness in the United States. It is caused by *Rickettsia rickettsii*, a species of bacteria that is spread to humans by ixodid (hard) ticks (Figure 16-6).

Initial signs and symptoms include sudden onset of fever, headache, and muscle pain, followed by development of rash. The disease can be difficult to diagnose in the early stage. RMSF is most common among males and children. Risk factors are frequent exposure to dogs and living near wooded areas or areas with high grass. The presentation of RSMF is nonspecific, following an incubation of about 5 to 10 days after a tick bite. Initial symptoms can include fever, nausea, vomiting, severe headache, muscle pain, and lack of appetite. Later signs and symptoms include rash, abdominal pain, joint pain, and diarrhea. The rash first appears 2 to 5 days after the onset of fever. Most often it begins as small, flat, pink, nonitchy spots on the wrists, forearms, and ankles. The characteristic red spotted rash of RMSF is usually not seen until the sixth day or later after onset of symptoms. As many as 10% to 15% of patients never develop a rash (Figure 16-7). No widely available laboratory assay provides rapid confirmation of early RMSF, although commercial PCR testing is available. Therefore, treatment decisions should be based on epidemiologic and clinical clues. Treatment should never be delayed while waiting for confirmation by laboratory results. Routine clinical laboratory findings suggestive of RMSF include normal WBC count, thrombocytopenia, hyponatremia, and elevated liver enzyme levels. Serologic assays are the most often used methods for confirming cases of RMSF.

Doxycycline is the drug of choice for patients with RMSF. Therapy is continued for at least 3 days after fever subsides and until there is unequivocal evidence of clinical improvement, generally for a minimum total course of 5 to 10 days. Tetracyclines are usually not the preferred drug for use in pregnant women. Whereas chloramphenicol is typically the preferred treatment for RMSF during pregnancy, care must be used when administering chloramphenicol late during the third trimester of pregnancy because of risks associated with gray baby syndrome.

Ehrlichiosis

Three species of *Ehrlichia* in the United States are known to cause disease in humans. *Ehrlichia chaffeensis,* the cause of human monocytic ehrlichiosis, occurs primarily in southeastern and south-central regions and is primarily transmitted by the lone star tick, *Amblyomma americanum* (Figure 16-8). Human granulocytic ehrlichiosis is caused by *Anaplasma phagocytophila* or *Anaplasma equi* and is transmitted by *Ixodes* ticks. *Ehrlichia ewingii* is the most recently recognized human pathogen, with cases reported in immunocompromised patients in Missouri, Oklahoma, and Tennessee.

After an incubation period of about 5 to 10 days following the tick bite, initial symptoms generally include fever,

Table 16-16 Features of Common Tick-Borne Diseases in the United States*

Disease (Causative Agent)	Primary Vector(s)	Approx. Distribution	Incubation Period (Days)	Common Initial Signs and Symptoms	Common Laboratory Abnormalities	Rash	Fatality Rate (%)
Rocky Mountain Spotted fever (*Rickettsia rickettsii*)	American dog tick (*Dermacentor variabilis*), Rocky Mountain wood tick (*D. andersoni*); brown dog tick (*Rhipicephalus sanguineus*) in Arizona	Widespread in United States, especially in south Atlantic and south-central states	2 to 14	Fever, nausea, vomiting, myalgia, anorexia, headache	Thrombocytopenia, mild hyponatremia, mildly elevated hepatic transaminase levels	Maculopapular rash ; appears about 2 to 4 days after fever onset in 50% to 80% of adults and more than 90% of children; may involve palms and soles	5 to 10
Human monocytic ehrlichiosis (*Ehrlichia chaffeensis*)	Lone star tick (*Amblyomma americanum*)	Southern, south-central, mid-Atlantic, and northern states; isolated areas of New England	5 to 14	Fever, headache, malaise, myalgia	Leukopenia, thrombocytopenia, elevated serum transaminase levels	Rash appears in more than 30% of adults and in about 60% of children	2 to 3
Human granulocytic anaplasmosis (*Anaplasma phagocytophilum*)	Black-legged tick (*Ixodes scapularis* and *I. pacificus*) in United States	North central and Pacific states; New England	5 to 21	Fever, headache, malaise, nausea, vomiting	Leukopenia, thrombocytopenia, elevated serum transaminase levels	Rare	<1
Ehrlichia ewingii infection	Lone star tick	South Atlantic and south-central states; isolated areas of New England	5 to 14	Fever, headache, myalgia, nausea, vomiting	Leukopenia, thrombocytopenia, elevated serum transaminase levels	Rare	None documented

Modified from Chapman AS, Bakken JS, Folk SM, et al. Diagnosis and management of tick-borne rickettsial diseases: Rocky Mountain spotted fever, ehrlichioses, and anaplasmosis—United States. A practical guide for physicians and other health-care and public health professionals. MMWR 2006;55(RR-4):3.

*Treatment for these diseases is the same: adults should receive 100 mg of doxycycline (Vibramycin) orally or intravenously twice a day, and children who weigh less than 100 lb (45.4 kg) should receive 2.2 mg/kg of doxycycline orally or intravenously twice a day.

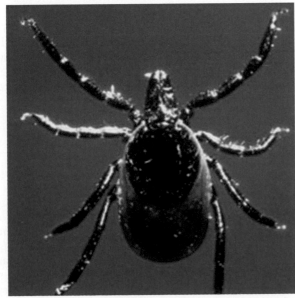

Figure 16-6 Ixodid tick

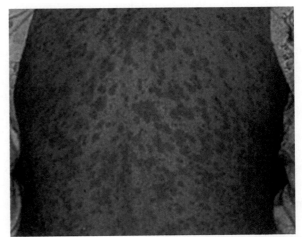

Figure 16-7 Image of a patient with Rocky Mountain spotted fever; note late rash on trunk.

(From Bratton R, Corey G. Tick-borne diseases. Am Fam Physician 2005;71:2323-2332.)

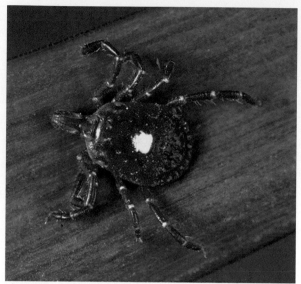

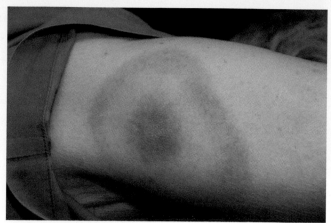

Figure 16-9 Target rash of erythema migrans in Lyme disease. *(From http://phil.cdc.gov/PHIL_Images/9875/9875_lores.jpg.)*

Figure 16-8 Lone star tick, *Amblyomma americanum.* *(From http://www.cdc.gov/ncidod/dvbid/stari/lone-star-tick-image.htm.)*

headache, malaise, and muscle aches. Other signs and symptoms can include nausea, vomiting, diarrhea, cough, joint pains, confusion, and occasionally rash. Laboratory findings indicating ehrlichiosis include leukopenia, thrombocytopenia, and elevated liver enzymes. Ehrlichiosis can be a severe illness, especially if untreated, and as many as half of all patients require hospitalization. Laboratory confirmation of ehrlichiosis requires serologic, molecular (PCR), or culture-based methods.

Appropriate antibiotic treatment should be initiated immediately when there is a strong suspicion of ehrlichiosis on the basis of clinical and epidemiologic findings. The treatment recommendations are the same as for Rocky Mountain spotted fever. Rifampin has been used successfully in a limited number of pregnant women with documented ehrlichiosis.

Babesiosis

Babesiosis is caused by hemoprotozoan parasites of the genus *Babesia*. The white-footed deer mouse is the main reservoir in the United States, and the vector is *Ixodes* ticks. Most infections are probably asymptomatic. Manifestations of disease include fever, chills, sweating, myalgias, fatigue, hepatosplenomegaly, and hemolytic anemia. Symptoms typically occur after an incubation period of 1 to 4 weeks and can last several weeks. The disease is more severe in immunosuppressed, splenectomized, or elderly patients. Diagnosis can be made by microscopic examination of thick and thin blood smears stained with Giemsa, looking for the parasite in red blood cells (RBCs). Options for treatment include clindamycin plus quinine or atovaquone plus azithromycin.

Lyme Disease

Lyme disease is caused by the spirochetal bacterium *Borrelia burgdorferi*. *Ixodes* ticks are responsible for transmitting Lyme disease bacteria to humans. In the United States, Lyme disease

is mostly localized to states in the northeastern, mid-Atlantic, and upper north-central regions, as well as northwestern California. Lyme disease most often manifests with a characteristic bull's-eye rash (erythema migrans) accompanied by nonspecific symptoms such as fever, malaise, fatigue, headache, muscle aches, and joint aches (Figure 16-9).

Lyme disease spirochetes disseminate from the site of the tick bite, causing multiple (secondary) erythema migrans lesions. Other manifestations of dissemination include lymphocytic meningitis, cranial neuropathy (especially facial nerve palsy), radiculoneuritis, migratory joint and muscle pains, myocarditis, and transient atrioventricular blocks of varying degree. If left untreated, the disease can progress to intermittent swelling and pain of one or a few joints (usually large weight-bearing joints such as the knee), cognitive disorders, sleep disturbance, fatigue, and personality changes. The diagnosis is based primarily on clinical findings, and it is often appropriate to treat patients with early disease solely on the basis of objective signs and a known exposure. Serologic testing may provide valuable supportive diagnostic information in patients with endemic exposure and objective clinical findings that suggest later-stage disseminated Lyme disease.

Treatment for 3 to 4 weeks with doxycycline or amoxicillin is generally effective in early disease. Cefuroxime axetil or erythromycin can be used for persons allergic to penicillin or who cannot take tetracyclines. Later disease, particularly with objective neurologic manifestations, can require treatment with intravenous ceftriaxone or penicillin for 4 weeks or more, depending on disease severity.

Tularemia

Tularemia is caused by *Francisella tularensis*, one of the most infectious pathogenic bacteria known. Most cases in the United States occur in south-central and western states. Humans can become infected through diverse environmental exposures, including bites by infected arthropods; handling infectious animal tissues or fluids; direct contact with or ingestion of contaminated food, water, or soil; and inhalation of infective aerosols. Inhaled *F. tularensis* causes pleuropneumonitis. Some exposures contaminate the eye, resulting in ocular tularemia; penetrate broken skin, result-

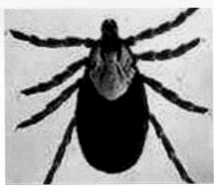

Figure 16-10 *Dermacentor andersoni* tick.
(From http://www.cdc.gov/ticks/images/rocky_mountain_wood_tick.jpg.)

ing in ulceroglandular or glandular disease; or cause oropharyngeal disease with cervical lymphadenitis. Untreated, bacilli inoculated into skin or mucous membranes multiply, spread to regional lymph nodes, multiply further, and then can disseminate to organs throughout the body.

The onset of tularemia is usually abrupt, with fever, headache, chills and rigors, generalized body aches, coryza, and sore throat. A dry or slightly productive cough and substernal pain or tightness often occur with or without objective signs of pneumonia. Nausea, vomiting, and diarrhea can occur. Sweats, fever, chills, progressive weakness, malaise, anorexia, and weight loss characterize continuing illness. Rapid diagnostic testing for tularemia is not widely available. Respiratory secretions and blood for culture should be collected in suspected patients and the laboratory alerted to the need for special diagnostic and safety procedures. Streptomycin (1 g IM bid for 10 days) is the drug of choice, and gentamicin is an acceptable alternative. Tetracyclines and chloramphenicol can also be used.

Colorado Tick Fever

Colorado tick fever is an acute viral infection transmitted by the bite of the *Dermacentor andersoni* tick (Figure 16-10). The disease is limited to the western United States and is most prevalent from March to September. Symptoms start about 3 to 6 days after the tick bite. Fever continues for 3 days, stops, and then recurs 1 to 3 days later for another few days. Other symptoms include excessive sweating, muscle aches, joint stiffness, headache, photophobia, nausea, vomiting, weakness, and an occasional faint rash. Routine blood tests might show a low WBC count, mildly elevated liver function, and mildly elevated creatine phosphokinase (CPK). Diagnosis is confirmed by testing blood for complement fixation immunofluorescent antibody staining to Colorado tick virus. Treatment is removal of the tick and treatment of symptoms.

Prevention of Tick-Borne Disease

Physicians should advise patients who walk or hike in tick-infested areas to tuck long pants into socks to protect the legs and wear shoes and long-sleeved shirts. Ticks show up on white or light colors better than dark colors, making them easier to remove from clothing. If attached, ticks should be removed immediately by using a tweezers, pulling carefully and steadily. Insect repellents such as DEET, alone or in combination with permethrin, may be helpful.

KEY TREATMENT

Appropriate antibiotic therapy should be initiated immediately when there is suspicion of Rocky Mountain spotted fever, ehrlichiosis, or relapsing fever rather than waiting for laboratory confirmation (Bratton and Corey, 2005; Spach et al., 1993) (SOR: C).

Treatment with doxycycline (Vibramycin) or tetracycline is recommended for RMSF, Lyme disease, ehrlichiosis, and relapsing fever (Bratton and Corey, 2005; Spach et al., 1993) (SOR: C).

Recommended actions to prevent tick-borne disease include avoidance of tick-infested areas; wearing long pants and tucking the pant legs into socks; applying diethyltoluamide (DEET) insect repellents; using bed nets when camping; and carefully inspecting oneself frequently while in an at-risk area (Bratton and Corey, 2005; Spach et al., 1993) (SOR: C).

Antibiotic prophylaxis is not routinely recommended for a tick bite to prevent Lyme disease, unless the risk of infection is high (Wormser et al., 2006) (SOR: B).

Recommended treatment for suspected tularemia is streptomycin or gentamicin given empirically before evidence of laboratory confirmation (Bratton and Corey, 2005; Spach et al., 1993) (SOR: C).

CELLULITIS

William E. Roland

Key Points

- Most cases of cellulitis are caused by staphylococci or streptococci, but other causes should be considered by clinical situation.
- Physicians must rule out more ominous causes of skin inflammation, such as necrotizing fasciitis and pyomyositis, when considering cellulitis.
- Edema-associated cellulitis is best treated by mobilizing edema fluid.

Cellulitis is an acute, spreading inflammation of the derma and subcutaneous issue. Patients complain of tenderness, warmth, swelling, and spreading erythema. In contrast to *erysipelas*, cellulitis usually lacks sharp demarcation at the border. Factors that predispose to cellulitis include trauma, an underlying skin lesion (furuncle, ulcer), or a complication arising from a wound, ulcer, or dermatosis. Occasionally, cellulitis results from a blood-borne infection that metastasizes to the skin.

Pain and erythema usually develop within several days and are often associated with malaise, fever, and chills. The area involved is often extensive, red, hot, and swollen. Patchy involvement with skip lesions can be seen. Regional lymphadenopathy is common, and bacteremia can occur. Several clinical entities resemble cellulitis, including pyoderma gangrenosum, gout, and insect bites. Necrotizing fasciitis and gas gangrene are surgical emergencies. Given that the predominant organism involved in most cases of cellulitis is a gram-positive coccus, clinical history and morphology on physical examination usually suffice in the diagnosis and treatment of cellulitis. A history of freshwater exposure may implicate *Aeromonas hydrophila* as the causative organism; saltwater exposure suggests *Vibrio* spp. Cellulitis in a patient with liver disease and shellfish ingestion moves *Vibrio vulnificus* to the top of the differential.

Patients with soft tissue infection should have blood drawn for laboratory testing if signs and symptoms of systemic toxicity are present (e.g., fever or hypothermia, tachycardia, hypotension). Laboratory testing should include blood culture and drug susceptibility tests; WBC count with differential; and measurement of creatinine, bicarbonate, CPK, and CRP levels. Hospitalization should be considered for patients with hypotension or an elevated creatinine level, low serum bicarbonate level, elevated CPK level (i.e., 2-3 times upper limit of normal), marked left shift, or CRP level greater than 13 mg/L (123.8 nmol/L). Gram stain with culture and culture of needle aspiration or punch biopsy specimens should be performed to determine a definitive etiology, and a surgical consult should be considered for inspection, exploration, and drainage. Findings that may signal potentially severe, deep, soft tissue infection and that may require emergent surgical evaluation include cutaneous hemorrhage, gas in the tissue, pain disproportionate to physical findings, rapid progression, skin anesthesia, skin sloughing, and violaceous bullae.

Radiologic studies may be helpful if abscess or osteomyelitis is a possibility. Ultrasonography is helpful in detecting a subcutaneous collection of fluid. Magnetic resonance imaging (MRI) is also useful in differentiating cellulitis from necrotizing fasciitis. The diagnosis of necrotizing cellulitis is by direct surgical examination or by frozen pathology sections.

Empiric antibiotics for immunocompetent patients with cellulitis should be targeted toward gram-positive cocci (Table 16-17). Broader coverage should be initiated for diabetic patients to include gram-positive aerobes, gram-negative aerobes, and anaerobes. Patients who present with severe infection or whose infection is progressing despite empiric antibiotic therapy should be treated more aggressively; the treatment strategy should be based on results of appropriate Gram stain, culture, and drug susceptibility analysis. In the case of *Staphylococcus aureus*, the physician should assume that the organism is resistant, and agents effective against MRSA, such as vancomycin, linezolid (Zyvox), or daptomycin (Cubicin), should be used.

The antibiotic may be switched from an intravenous drug to an oral drug when fever has subsided and the skin lesion begins to resolve, usually in 3 to 5 days. The total duration of therapy should be 7 to 14 days. Longer duration may be required if the response is slow or is associated with abscess, tissue necrosis, or underlying skin processes (infected ulcers or wounds). Treatment of cellulitis should include elevation and immobilization to decrease swelling. Patients with interdigital dermatophytic infections should be treated with a concomitant topical antifungal applied once or twice daily. Topical antifungals can also help reduce the risk of recurrence of the cellulitis. Support stockings, good skin hygiene, and prompt treatment of tinea pedis helps with prevention of cellulitis in patients with peripheral edema, who are predisposed to recurrence. In patients who continue to have frequent episodes of cellulitis or erysipelas, prophylactic treatment with penicillin V, 250 mg or 500 mg orally twice daily, or erythromycin, 250 mg once or twice daily (for penicillin-allergic patients), may be indicated.

KEY TREATMENT

Penicillin, given parenterally or orally depending on clinical severity, is the treatment of choice for erysipelas (Stevens et al., 2005) (SOR: A).

For cellulitis, a penicillinase-resistant semisynthetic penicillin (amoxicillin/clavulanate) or a first-generation cephalosporin should be selected, unless streptococci or staphylococci resistant to these agents are common in the community (Stevens et al., 2005) (SOR: A).

For suspected MRSA skin infections, oral treatment options include trimethoprim-sulfamethoxazole, clindamycin, and doxycycline (Stevens et al., 2005) (SOR: C).

FURUNCLES AND CARBUNCLES

David R. McBride

KEY POINTS

- The majority of furuncles and carbuncles are caused by *Staphylococcus* spp., increasingly, community-acquired methicillin-resistant *S. aureus*.
- Drainage of pus is of primary importance in treating skin and soft tissue infections.
- Culture of SSTIs is important in guiding antibiotic treatment when initial measures of drainage are not effective.
- For recurrent boils, consider referral to Infectious disease specialist, possibly to eradicate carriage state.

Furuncles, or boils, are infections of the skin and soft tissue usually associated with a hair follicle. *Carbuncles* are an extension of this skin and soft tissue infection continuum and involve more of the surrounding and subcutaneous tissue. The broad category *skin and soft tissue infections* (SSTIs) is used to describe this continuum that includes furuncles and carbuncles. SSTIs are common in both healthy and immunocompromised patients and likely initiate with some breach of the skin integrity, such as irritation of hair follicles from friction or microscopic trauma to the skin.

Up to 74% of furuncles and carbuncles are caused by community-acquired methicillin-resistant *Staphylococcus aureus* (CA-MRSA) (CDC, 2010). Other potential causative organisms include nonresistant *Staphylococcus* spp. and *Streptococcus* spp. It has become increasingly important to obtain culture of a lesion to direct antibiotic coverage given the increase in CA-MRSA.

There is no reliable historical or examination element that will distinguish a CA-MRSA from a methicillin-sensitive staphylococcal skin lesion. Stereotypically, patients report CA-MRSA lesions starting like a spider bite. Furuncles and carbuncles can occur anywhere on the body, although the axillae, groin, and buttocks are particularly common sites. In addition, practices that cause skin trauma (e.g., shaving, waxing) are often noted in patients with these SSTIs. Fever and malaise are uncommon with milder lesions but become more frequent with the increasing scope of localized infection.

Of primary importance in the management of carbuncles and furuncles is facilitation of drainage of any purulent material. With smaller lesions, this may be accomplished by heat application by the patient at home. As lesions increase in size and fluctuance, surgical drainage is essential to facilitate resolution of an SSTI. It is important to consider culture

Table 16-17 Antimicrobial Therapy for Impetigo and for Skin and Soft Tissue Infections (SSTIs)

| Antibiotic | Dosage | | Comments |
	Adults	Children*	
Impetigo†			
Dicloxacillin	250 mg qid PO	12 mg/kg/day in 4 divided doses PO	—
Cephalexin	250 mg qid PO	25 mg/kg/day in 4 divided doses PO	—
Erythromycin	250 mg qid PO‡	40 mg/kg/day in 4 divided doses PO	Some strains of *Staphylococcus aureus* and *Streptococcus pyogenes* may be resistant.
Clindamycin	300-400 mg tid PO	10-20 mg/kg/day in 3 divided doses PO	—
Amoxicillin/ clavulanate	975/125 mg bid PO	25 mg/kg/day of amoxicillin component in 2 divided doses PO	—
Mupirocin ointment	Apply to lesions tid.	Apply to lesions tid.	For patients with limited lesions
MSSA SSTIs			
Nafcillin or oxacillin	1-2 g q4h IV	100-150 mg/kg/day in 4 divided dose	Parenteral drug of choice; inactive against MRSA
Cefazolin	1 g q8h IV	50 mg/kg/day in 3 divided doses	For penicillin-allergic patients, except those with immediate hypersensitivity reactions
Clindamycin	600 mg/kg q8h IV or 300-450 mg tid PO	25-40 mg/kg/day in 3 divided doses IV or 10-20 mg/kg/day in 3 divided doses PO	Bacteriostatic; potential for cross-resistance and emergence of resistance in erythromycin-resistant strains; inducible resistance in MRSA
Dicloxacillin	500 mg qid PO	25 mg/kg/day in 4 divided doses PO	Oral agent of choice for methicillin-susceptible strains
Cephalexin	500 mg qid PO	25 mg/kg/day in 4 divided doses PO	For penicillin-allergic patients, except those with immediate hypersensitivity reactions
Doxycycline, minocycline	100 mg bid PO	Not recommended for children <8 yr	Bacteriostatic; limited clinical experience
TMP-SMZ	1 or 2 double-strength tablets bid PO	9-12 mg/kg (based on TMP component) in either 4 divided doses IV or 2 divided doses PO	Bacteriostatic; efficacy poorly documented
MRSA SSTIs			
Vancomycin	30 mg/kg/day in 2 divided doses IV	40 mg/kg/day in 4 divided doses IV	For penicillin-allergic patients; parenteral drug of choice for MRSA infections
Linezolid	600 mg q12h IV or 600 mg bid PO	10 mg/kg q12h IV or PO	Bacteriostatic; limited clinical experience; no cross-resistance with other antibiotic classes; expensive; may replace other second-line agents as preferred oral drug for MRSA infections
Clindamycin	600 mg/kg q8h IV or 300-450 mg tid PO	25-40 mg/kg/day in 2 divided doses IV or 10-20 mg/kg/day in 3 divided doses PO	Bacteriostatic; potential for cross-resistance and emergence of resistance in erythromycin-resistant strains; inducible resistance in MRSA
Daptomycin	4 mg/kg every 24 hours IV	Not applicable	Bactericidal; possible myopathy
Doxycycline, minocycline	100 mg bid PO	Not recommended for children <8 yr	Bacteriostatic; limited clinical experience
TMP-SMZ	1 or 2 double-strength tablets bid PO	9-12 mg/kg (based on TMP component) in either 4 divided doses IV or 2 divided doses PO	Bactericidal; limited efficacy data

Modified from Stevens D et al. Practice guidelines for the diagnosis and management of skin and soft-tissue infections. Clin Infect Dis 2005;41:1373-1406.

MSSA, Methicillin-susceptible *Staphylococcus aureus*; *MRSA*, methicillin-resistant *S. aureus*; *TMP-SMZ*, trimethoprim-sulfamethoxazole; *PO*, orally; *IV*, intravenously; *qid*, four times daily; *tid*, three times daily; *bid*, twice daily; *q4h*, every 4 hours; *q8h*, every 8 hours; *q12h*, every 12 hours.

*Doses listed not appropriate for neonates.

†Infection caused by *Staphylococcus* and *Streptococcus* spp. Duration of therapy is about 7 days, depending on clinical response.

‡Adult dosage of erythromycin ethylsuccinate is 400 mg qid PO.

of purulent material when performing incision and drainage in the event that the patient fails to improve and antibiotic coverage becomes necessary. Cure rates of lesions with drainage alone exceed 90%. Careful follow-up after drainage is essential to ensure clinical improvement; daily dressing changes in the office after surgical drainage is effective. The addition of postdrainage antibiotics has not shown much added benefit.

To prevent the spread of infection to others who come into contact with the patient recovering from an SSTI, an occlusive dressing to prevent leakage of lesion fluid and careful hygiene are indicated. There is no evidence that extensive cleaning of common spaces (e.g., locker rooms) prevents the spread of SSTI-causing bacteria more than routine cleaning measures. Towels and soiled clothing should be laundered in hot water, and any common equipment should be cleaned per manufacturer recommendations.

When lesions do not respond to heat, or when lesions are larger yet not amenable to drainage, antibiotics may be used. Reasonable first-line antibiotic coverage for nonfluctuant lesions may include dicloxacillin, first- or second-generation cephalosporins, macrolides, or clindamycin. In patients with suspected CA-MRSA, better choices include TMP-SMX, tetracycline, or clindamycin. It is important to note that up to 50% of CA-MRSA species will be resistant to clindamycin, particularly if the patient has been treated with other antibiotics in the previous weeks to months (Stevens et al., 2005). Oral administration of these antibiotics is acceptable in the nontoxic patient. Patient signs and symptoms that would warrant hospital admission include fever or hypothermia, tachycardia, or hypotension as signs of sepsis and lesions greater than 5 cm in size (Table 16-18).

For patients with recurrent SSTIs, evaluation for the presence of nasal carriage with a nasal culture is indicated. The value of eradication of bacterial carriage is unclear. Referral for infectious disease specialist evaluation may be indicated to guide decision making in the patient with recurrent furuncles and carbuncles.

KEY TREATMENT

Cure rates of fluctuant skin lesions with drainage alone is over 90%. Postdrainage antibiotics do not significantly improve outcomes (Stevens et al., 2005; Rajendran et al., 2007) (SOR: A). Trimethoprim-sulfamethoxazole (TMP-SMX), clindamycin, and tetracycline are first-choice antibiotics when CA-MRSA is suspected. Up to 50% of CA-MRSA species will be resistant to clindamycin, particularly in the patient previously treated with other antibiotics (Stevens et al., 2005) (SOR: C).

DIABETIC ULCERS

William E. Roland

Key Points

- The existence, severity, and extent of infection, as well as vascular status, neuropathy, and glycemic control, should be assessed in patients with a diabetic foot infection.

Table 16-18 Proposed Strategy for Management of Patients with Skin and Soft Tissue Infection (SSTI)

Class	Patient Criteria	Management	Antibiotic
1	Afebrile and healthy, other than cellulitis	Treat with common first-line antibiotics for SSTI if no drainable abscess. Surgical drainage with or without antibiotics.	Semisynthetic penicillin, Oral 1st/2nd-generation cephalosporin, macrolide, or clindamycin
2	Febrile and ill appearing, but no unstable comorbidities; lesion <5 cm	Surgical drainage of abscess if possible. Treat presumptively for MRSA and monitor closely for response. Inpatient management may be indicated.	Trimethoprim-sulfamethoxazole (TMP-SMX), tetracycline (TTC), or clindamycin
3	Toxic appearance or at least one unstable comorbidity or a limb-threatening infection	Hospital admission with broad-spectrum antibiotics with MRSA coverage; infectious disease (ID) consultation.	Broad-spectrum coverage, including vancomycin
4	Sepsis syndrome or life-threatening infection (necrotizing fasciitis)	Same as above, plus aggressive surgical debridement.	Same as above, with ID specialist guidance

Modified from McBride D. CA-MRSA lesions: what works, what doesn't. J Fam Pract 2008;57:588-592.

- Visible bone and palpable bone on probing suggest underlying osteomyelitis in patients with a diabetic foot infection.
- Before an infected wound of a diabetic foot infection is cultured, any overlying necrotic debris should be removed to eliminate surface contamination and to provide more accurate results.

Patients with diabetes are prone to skin ulcers caused by neuropathy, vascular insufficiency, and diminished neutrophil function. Minor wounds can be secondarily infected, leading to ulcer formation. These ulcers often have extensive undermining with necrotic tissues and are often close to the anus, thus promoting an environment suitable for multiple species of microorganisms, including anaerobes. Diabetic foot infections range in severity from superficial paronychia to deep infection involving bone. Non–limb-threatening infections involve superficial ulcers with minimal cellulitis (<2 cm from portal of entry), no signs of systemic toxicity, and no significant ischemia in the limb.

Common causes of infections are aerobic gram-positive bacteria, particularly *Staphylococcus aureus* and beta-hemolytic streptococci. Limb-threatening infections have extensive cellulitis, lymphangitis, ulcers extending to the subcutaneous tissues, and prominent ischemia. Infection in patients who have recently received antibiotics or who have deep, limb-threatening infection or chronic wounds are usually caused by a mixture of aerobic gram-positive, aerobic gram-negative (e.g., *Escherichia coli*, *Proteus* spp., *Klebsiella* spp.), and anaerobic organisms (e.g., *Bacteroides*, *Clostridium*, *Peptococcus*, and *Peptostreptococcus* spp.). Surgery is necessary to unroof encrusted areas, and the wounds need to be examined and probed to determine the extent of the infection and check for bone involvement (Dinh et al., 2008). Debridement or drainage should be promptly performed. Deep wound cultures should be obtained if possible. If deep culture is not feasible, Gram stain and culture from the curettage of the base of the ulcer or from purulent exudates may be needed to guide antibiotic therapy (Figure 16-11).

Plain radiography of the foot is indicated for detection of osteomyelitis, foreign bodies, and soft tissue gas. When plain radiography is negative but osteomyelitis is clinically suspected, radionuclide scan or MRI should be performed. MRI provides more accurate information regarding the extent of the infectious process. The presence of peripheral artery disease and neuropathy should be assessed.

The antibiotic regimen should be based on meaningful bacteriologic data. However, the initial regimen for a previously untreated patient with non–limb-threatening infection should focus on *S. aureus* and streptococci. Mild infections may be treated with dicloxacillin or cephalexin for 2 weeks. Amoxicillin/clavulanate may be used if polymicrobial infection is suspected. If MSRA is suspected, oral treatment options include TMP-SMX or doxycycline. For limb-threatening infections, broad-spectrum antibiotics are recommended for coverage of group B streptococci, other streptococci, Enterobacteriaceae, anaerobic gram-positive cocci, and *Bacteroides* spp. Treatment regimens include ampicillin-sulbactam or ertapenem (Invanz), clindamycin plus a third-generation cephalosporin, and clindamycin plus ciprofloxacin. Intravenous vancomycin should be added if MRSA infection is suspected. Ciprofloxacin as a single agent is not recommended.

In addition to antibiotic treatment, good glycemic control should be obtained and open wounds gently packed with sterile gauze moistened with ¼-strength povidone-iodine (Betadine) solution. Edema should be reduced by bed rest, elevation, and diuretic therapy as indicated. For prevention of diabetic foot ulcers, all patients with diabetes should have an annual foot examination that includes assessment for anatomic deformities, skin breaks, nail disorders, loss of protection sensation, diminished arterial supply, and inappropriate footwear.

KEY TREATMENT

Routine wound swabs and cultures of material from sinus tracts are unreliable and strongly discouraged in the management of diabetic foot infection (Pellizzer et al., 2001; Senneville et al., 2006) (SOR: B).

The empiric antibiotic regimen for diabetic foot infection should always include an agent active against *Staphylococcus aureus*, including MRSA if necessary, and streptococci (Abdulrazak et al., 2005; Lipsky et al., 2004). (SOR: A)

BITE INFECTIONS

David McCrary

Key Points

- The use of prophylactic antibiotics may be necessary in the initial management of bite wounds, particularly if the bite is on the hand or face or from a cat.
- First-generation cephalosporins (e.g., cephalexin) are not effective as monotherapy for bite wounds because of resistance issues.
- Avoid primary wound closure in the management of bite wounds.

It is estimated that bites account for 800,000 medical visits annually in the United States, making up 1% of emergency department visits. Bite wounds consist of lacerations, evulsions, punctures, and scratches. The microbiology of bite wounds is generally polymicrobial, with an array of potential bacteria from the environment, the victim's skin flora, and the biter's oral flora.

Animal Bites

Dog bites account for approximately 80% of all animal bites requiring medical attention, in which 85% are provoked attacks. Most dog bites occur on the distal extremities, but children tend to sustain facial bites. Patients who present for medical attention are often concerned about the care of disfiguring wounds or the need for appropriate vaccination (i.e., tetanus, rabies). However, up to 30% of medically treated wounds may become infected. These wounds are often contaminated with multiple strains of aerobic and anaerobic bacteria. Local signs of infection with erythema, edema, pain, and purulent drainage are common with animal bite wounds.

Although the most frequently isolated pathogen related to dog and cat bite wounds is *Pasteurella multocida*, the array of potential organisms is much greater. Anaerobes such as *Bacteroides tectum*, *Prevotella* spp., fusobacteria, and peptostreptococci can be isolated from animal bite wounds 75% of the time, mostly from wounds with abscess formation. *Capnocytophaga canimorsus* has also been associated with fatal infection from fulminant sepsis in asplenic patients. Wounds inflicted by cats are often scratches or tiny punctures located on the extremity and are likely to become infected and lead to abscess formation.

In the United States, venomous snakes bite approximately 8000 people yearly. Envenomation in such snakebites account for the majority of morbidity and mortality associated with such bites. However, infection of soft tissue structures may also occur as a result of oral flora from the snake, which tends to be fecal in nature because live prey usually defecate in the snake's mouth with their ingestion.

Human Bites

Human bites are not uncommon, especially in children. Human bites have a higher complication and infection rate than do animal bites. Human bite wounds most often affect the hand and fingers and in some cases may present as "love

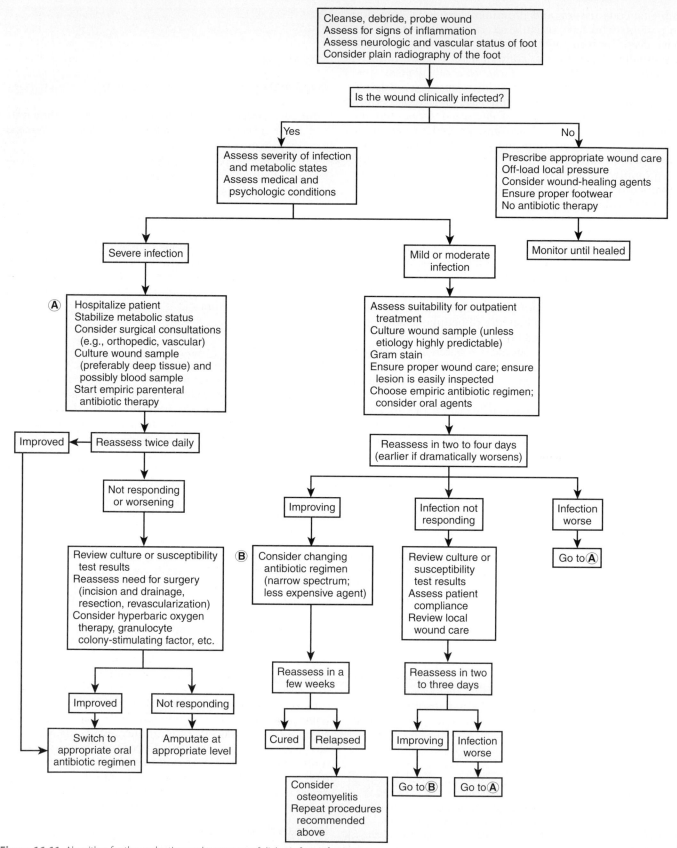

Figure 16-11 Algorithm for the evaluation and treatment of diabetic foot infection.
(Modified from Lipsky BA. Medical treatment of diabetic foot infections. Clin Infect Dis 2004;39(suppl 2):S110.

nips" to the breast and genital areas. Self-inflicted bites often include wounds of the lip and tissues surrounding the nail, such as paronychia. Also included in this are clenched-fist injuries or "fight bites," which result in small lacerations to the knuckles when striking a person in the mouth. Normal human oral flora, rather than skin flora, is the source of most bacteria isolated from human bite wound cultures (viridans streptococci, *Eikenella corrodens*).

Treatment

Management of bite wounds is the same as for any other wound: good wound care in the form of adequate irrigation and debridement of nonviable tissue as needed (Table 16-19). Bite wounds in general do not require primary closure, but after adequate irrigation and debridement, wounds may be approximated and closed by delayed primary or secondary intention. An exception to this rule may include bite wounds to the face. General wound management measures such as tetanus toxoid administration should also be employed. Bite wounds involving the hands should be evaluated by a hand surgeon, given the risk of adjacent tendon sheath, bone, or joint involvement and the dire consequences if such structures are involved.

The transmission of *rabies* through the bites of domestic pets in the United States and developed countries is rare. In fact, the dog strain of rabies is considered eliminated in the U.S. dog population, and cat bites are often managed through observation of the animal, without the immediate need for rabies *postexposure treatment* (PET). However, wild mammal exposure, especially bat, skunk, or raccoon, often warrants PET, which involves thorough cleaning of the bite wound, ideally with povidone-iodine solution, along with rabies immune globulin given at the wound site and rabies vaccine given on days 0, 3, 7, and 14.

Bite wounds should be considered contaminated wounds from presentation, given the oral microbial flora of humans and animals, and most patients should probably receive antibiotics early. Empiric antibiotics are used to eradicate oral flora inoculated from the mouth of the biter, whether human or animal, into the wound. All moderate to severe animal bite wounds, or wounds that have an associated crush injury or that are close to a bone or joint, should be considered contaminated with potential pathogens, and these patients should receive 3 to 5 days of "prophylactic" antimicrobial therapy. Gram stains with culture of bite wounds are specific but not sensitive indicators of bacterial growth. Nonetheless, Gram stain can be used to help guide initial empiric antibiotic therapy.

Amoxicillin–clavulanic acid (amoxicillin-clavulanate; Augmentin) or penicillin plus a penicillinase-resistant penicillin are normally first-line agents for empiric therapy directed at bite wounds. First-generation cephalosporins (e.g., cephalexin) are not effective as monotherapy because of resistance of some anaerobic bacteria and *E. corrodens*. A 5- to 10-day course of antibiotics is usually adequate for infections limited to the soft tissue, and a minimum of 3 weeks of therapy is required for infections involving joints or bones. Close follow-up is required in all bites to ensure adequate healing.

Of special consideration in human bite wounds is the potential for spread of viral pathogens, most notably *hepatitis*

B virus (HBV) and HIV, if the source person is positive. HBV exposure in this setting should be handled in the same manner as other exposures, with administration of HBIG and HBV vaccination. With regard to HIV, CDC guidelines for managing nonoccupational HIV exposure recommend handling each case individually in consultation with an infectious diseases specialist.

KEY TREATMENT

Use of antibiotic prophylactic after bites of the hand reduces the incidence of infection (Medeiros and Saconato, 2005) (SOR: B). Antibiotic prophylaxis after bites by humans reduces incidence of infection (SOR: C).

BONE AND JOINT INFECTIONS

Anthony Zeimet

Key Points

- The diagnosis of osteomyelitis is based on radiographic findings (plain radiograph or MRI) showing bony destruction along with histologic analysis and culture results.
- Chronic osteomyelitis is not an emergency, and antibiotics can be safely withheld until an etiologic diagnosis is established.
- Diabetic foot infections require a careful evaluation to assess perfusion and vascular supply, and corrective measures should be undertaken to reestablish adequate perfusion if necessary.
- In diabetic foot ulcers, if one can probe to bone, the patient most likely has osteomyelitis.
- Orthopedic hardware infections are best managed in conjunction with an infectious diseases specialist and orthopedic surgeon.

Osteomyelitis

Osteomyelitis is defined as progressive, inflammation leading to destruction of the bone, usually secondary to an infectious agent. Bacteria can enter bone through hematogenous seeding or a contiguous focus after trauma, implantation of a foreign device, or a local soft tissue infection. Acute osteomyelitis is defined as infection that evolves over a few weeks. Chronic osteomyelitis implies persistent infection of several weeks to months.

Hematogenous osteomyelitis occurs primarily in children within the metaphyses of long bones (tibia and femur) and vertebrae in adults. In addition to local signs of inflammation and infection, patients generally have various systemic signs, including fever, irritability, and lethargy. Physical findings include tenderness over involved area and decreased range of motion in adjacent joints. Chronic osteomyelitis usually occurs in adults, caused by an open injury to bone and surrounding soft tissue. Erythema, drainage around area, and bone pain are usually present on physical examination. Systemic symptoms occur less frequently.

The diagnosis of osteomyelitis is based on the clinical picture and supporting laboratory and radiologic findings. Leukocytosis and elevations in CRP and ESR may

Table 16-19 Management of Bite Wounds

History

Animal bite: Ascertain the type of animal, whether the bite was provoked or unprovoked, and the situation/environment in which the bite occurred. If the species can be rabid, locate the animal for 10 days' observation or sacrifice.
Patient: Obtain information on antimicrobial allergies, current medications, splenectomy, mastectomy, liver disease, and immunosuppression.

Physical Examination

Record a diagram of the wound with the location, type, and depth of injury; range of motion; possibility of joint penetration; presence of edema or crush injury; nerve and tendon function; signs of infection; and odor of exudate.

Culture

Infected wounds should be cultured and a Gram stain performed. Anaerobic cultures should be obtained in the presence of abscesses, sepsis, serious cellulitis, devitalized tissue, or foul odor of the exudate. Small tears and infected punctures should be cultured with a minitipped (nasopharyngeal) swab.

Irrigation

Copious amounts of normal saline should be used for irrigation. Puncture wounds should be irrigated with a "high-pressure jet" from a 20-mL syringe and an 18-gauge needle or catheter tip.

Debridement

Devitalized or necrotic tissue should be cautiously debrided. Debris and foreign bodies should be removed.

Radiographs

Radiographs should be obtained if fracture or bone penetration is possible to provide a baseline for future osteomyelitis.

Wound Closure

Wound closure may be necessary for selected, fresh, uninfected wounds, especially facial wounds, but primary wound closure is not usually indicated. Wound edges should be approximated with adhesive strips in selected cases.

Antimicrobial Therapy

Prophylaxis: Consider prophylaxis (1) for moderate to severe injury less than 8 hours old, especially if edema or crush injury is present; (2) if bone or joint penetration is possible; (3) for hand wounds; (4) for immunocompromised patients (including those with mastectomy, liver disease, or steroid therapy); (5) if the wound is adjacent to prosthetic joint; and (6) if the wound is in the genital area. Coverage should include *Pasteurella multocida, Staphylococcus aureus,* and anaerobes.
Treatment: Cover *P. multocida, S. aureus,* and anaerobes. Use oral medication if the patient is seen early after a bite and only mild to moderate signs of infection are present. The following can be considered for cat or dog bites in adults:
- *First choice:* Amoxicillin/clavulanic acid, 875/125 mg bid or 500/125 mg tid with food.
- *Penicillin allergy:* No alternative treatment for animal bites has been established for penicillin-allergic patients. The following regimens can be considered for adults:
  1. Clindamycin (300 mg PO qid) plus either levofloxacin (500 mg PO daily) or trimethoprim-sulfamethoxazole (2 double-strength tablets PO bid).
  2. Doxycycline, 100 mg PO bid.
  3. Moxifloxacin, 400 mg PO daily.
  4. In the highly penicillin-allergic pregnant patient, macrolides have been used, but the wounds must be watched carefully.

On emergency department discharge, a single starting dose of parenteral antibiotic, such as ertapenem (1 g), may be useful in selected cases. If hospitalization or closely monitored outpatient follow-up is required, intravenous agents should be used. Current choices include ampicillin/sulbactam and cefoxitin. The rising incidence of community-acquired *S. aureus* isolates that are methicillin resistant and therefore resistant to the drugs recommended here emphasizes the importance of susceptibility-testing any *S. aureus* isolates.

Hospitalization

Indications include fever, sepsis, spread of cellulitis, significant edema or crush injury, loss of function, a compromised host, and patient noncompliance.

Immunizations

Give tetanus booster (Td; tetanus and diphtheria toxoids for adults) if original three-dose series has been given but none in the past 5 years. Adults who have not received acellular pertussis vaccine (Tdap), should be given this instead of Td. Give a primary series and tetanus immune globulin if the patient was never immunized.
Rabies vaccine (on days 0, 3, 7, 14, and 28) with hyperimmune globulin may be required, depending on the type of animal, ability to observe the animal, and locality.

Elevation

Elevation may be required if any edema is present. Lack of elevation is a common cause of therapeutic failure.

Table 16-19 **Management of Bite Wounds—cont'd**

Immobilization
Immobilize the extremity, especially hands, with a splint.

Follow-up
Follow-up should occur at 24 hours and perhaps 48 hours for outpatients.

Reporting
Reporting the incident to a local health department may be required.

From Goldstein EJC. Bites. In Mandell GL, Bennett JE, Dolin RD (eds). Mandell, Douglas, and Bennett's Principles and Practice of Infectious Diseases, 7th ed. Philadelphia, Churchill Livingstone-- Elsevier, 2010.
PO, Orally; *bid*, twice daily; *tid*, three times daily; *qid*, four times daily.

be seen but can also be normal. Blood cultures may be positive in up to half of children with acute osteomyelitis. If plain radiographs show bone destruction and inflammation; the diagnosis of osteomyelitis is confirmed. Typical findings on plain-radiographs will include osteolysis, periosteal reaction, and sequestra (segments of necrotic bone separated from living bone by granulation tissue). Findings seen on plain radiographs usually denote a process that has been ongoing for at least 2 weeks. Bone scintigraphy (bone scan) is often performed on patients with suspected osteomyelitis; however, sensitivity is quite low, and a negative result can offer false reassurance to the physician, so its routine use is not recommended. If the plain-radiographs are negative but the suspicion for osteomyelitis is still high, an MRI scan should be considered.

Once the diagnosis of osteomyelitis has been made, the next step is to obtain an etiologic diagnosis. Histopathologic and microbiologic examination of bone is the "gold standard." Cultures of sinus tracts are not reliable for identifying the causative organism. Common causative bacteriologic organisms in neonates include *Staphylococcus aureus*, group B streptococci, and *Escherichia coli*. Later in life, *S. aureus* is most common, and in elderly persons, gram-negative organisms such as *Pseudomonas aeruginosa* and *Serratia* spp. have increased incidence.

Empiric antibiotics are rarely required for chronic disease but are often necessary for acute osteomyelitis. Ideally, surgical debridement of all necrotic tissue and inflammatory debris (pus) should be undertaken and multiple surgical cultures with bone histology samples obtained. Antimicrobial therapy will be dictated by test results. Generally, treatment is for 4 to 6 weeks. With the exception of the fluoroquinolone class of antibiotics, which achieve high serum levels with oral administration, bone antibiotic levels cannot exceed the minimum inhibitory concentration (MIC) for the infecting organism; therefore, antibiotics must be given intravenously. This underscores the importance in obtaining a bacterial diagnosis so that the appropriate antibiotic can be used for the duration of treatment. Acute osteomyelitis is usually readily curable; however, chronic osteomyelitis is generally more refractory to therapy and requires repeat debridement and antibiotic courses.

Diabetic Foot Osteomyelitis

Patients with uncontrolled diabetes are at increased risk for development of osteomyelitis, especially in the presence of neuropathy or venous or arterial insufficiency. *S. aureus* and beta-hemolytic streptococci are the predominant organisms, although other gram-positive or gram-negative aerobic or anaerobic bacteria may also be seen. Plain radiographs should be the initial test to evaluate for the presence of osteomyelitis, followed by MRI if negative. If there is a draining sinus, the "probe to bone" test should be performed with a sterile probe; if bone is palpated, the diagnosis of osteomyelitis is highly likely. Further evaluation of the diabetic patient should be to assess for vascular insufficiency with the use of ankle-brachial indices and transcutaneous oximetry. If significant compromise is found, arteriography followed by revascularization should be undertaken. Surgical debridement is again the cornerstone of treatment, along with antibiotics directed toward the causative microorganism.

Orthopedic Hardware Infections

Infections secondary to orthopedic hardware devices have become common problems with the increasing incidence of hip, knee, and shoulder replacement surgeries. Also, patients with traumatic injury resulting in a fracture often have hardware implanted to stabilize the bone. These patients present in one of the three following ways:

1. *Early:* Symptoms develop less than 3 months after surgery and have an acute presentation with pain, erythema, and warmth, usually caused by *S. aureus* and gram-negative bacilli.
2. *Delayed:* Symptoms develop 3 to 24 months after surgery, generally with subtle signs of infection, including implant loosening and persistent pain, and usually caused by less virulent organisms such as coagulase-negative staphylococci and *Propionibacterium acnes*.
3. *Late:* Symptoms develop 24 months after surgery and are usually caused by hematogenous seeding from skin, dental, respiratory, and urinary infections.

Treatment requires debridement of the surrounding tissue and hardware removal, although this cannot always be done in patients with bone instability. It is recommended that treatment of these infections be done in conjunction with an infectious diseases specialist working with the orthopedic surgeon.

Septic Arthritis

Septic arthritis is defined as infection within the joint space of two bones. The major causative organisms include *S. aureus* and in the sexually promiscuous individual, *Neisseria gonorrhoeae*. Intravenous drug users are likely to develop septic arthritis within unusual joints (e.g., sternoclavicular, sacroiliac). Rheumatoid arthritis, presence of joint prostheses, and steroid use are predisposing factors for development of septic arthritis.

Diagnosis is usually based on clinical presentation of a warm, swollen joint with limitation in range of motion. A joint aspiration should be completed and the synovial fluid sent for Gram stain with culture, WBC count with differential, and crystal analysis to rule out gout and pseudogout. Blood cultures should also be drawn before initiation of antibiotics.

Gonococcal arthritis usually presents as an acute arthritis involving one or more joints in a sexually active individual. Two thirds of patients have dermatitis with one or multiple, usually asymptomatic, lesions that progress from macular to papular and finally vesicular or pustular. Joint fluid, urethral, and rectal cultures should also be obtained. Treatment is generally with a third-generation cephalosporin intravenously until improvement, followed by oral therapy to complete a 1-week course of therapy.

Treatment of nongonococcal arthritis requires proper draining of the infected joint. This is often done surgically, although repeat needle drainage may also be successful if the joint is easily accessible. Treatment generally depends on the Gram stain and includes a third-generation cephalosporin, with the addition of vancomycin if gram-positive cocci in clusters are seen. Duration of therapy is 3 to 4 weeks.

KEY TREATMENT

Treatment of osteomyelitis requires surgical debridement followed by a 4- to 6-week course of intravenous antibiotic therapy (SOR: C). Septic arthritis is usually caused by a gonococcus in a sexually active adult, and use of a third-generation cephalosporin is the mainstay of therapy (Workowski and Berman, 2006) (SOR: A). Nongonococcal arthritis should be treated with surgical debridement or repeated needle aspirations, with a third-generation cephalosporin and vancomycin if gram-positive cocci are seen (Goldenberg, 1998) (SOR: B).

FEVER OF UNKNOWN ORIGIN

Anthony Zeimet

Key Points

- A comprehensive history and physical examination with laboratory and radiologic evaluation are important in the workup for fever of unknown origin (FUO).
- If routine information is unrevealing, more specific testing for FUO is undertaken based on the patient's age, travel history, and disease process to develop a differential diagnosis.

- The serum ferritin level (often elevated with malignancy) and naproxen test (reduces fever with malignancy) may be helpful in determining an underlying malignant process.
- Initiation of empiric antibiotics should be done only in specific FUO situations to prevent skewing culture results, thus maximizing isolation of the causative organism.

Patients who have a persistent fever despite workup are generally classified as having a "fever of unknown origin" (FUO). In 1961, Petersdorf and Beeson described 100 patients with persistent fever, otherwise known as fever of unknown origin. They introduced the standard, classic definition of FUO: fever higher than 38.3° C (101° F) on several occasions, persisting without diagnosis for at least 3 weeks, with 1 week of investigational study in the hospital setting. With advancing technology, this definition has been revised to allow for more than two outpatient visits, or 3 days if investigation is in the hospital setting. Most patients with FUO have chronic or subacute symptoms and can be safely evaluated in the outpatient setting, with a median time to diagnosis of 40 days.

The differential diagnosis of FUO is quite broad and extensive. Determining an etiologic diagnosis of an FUO depends on generating a differential diagnosis compatible with the patient's history and physical examination. The principal disease categories for FUO include infection (30% overall), neoplasms (18%), collagen vascular diseases (12%), and miscellaneous (14%) (Box 16-5). Because of this broad differential, a newer classification system divides FUO into four groups: classic, nosocomial, neutropenic, and HIV associated, which helps narrow the differential diagnosis. Furthermore, classic FUO can be broken down into three subgroups: infants and children, elderly, and travelers. Despite an extensive workup, the etiologic diagnosis usually remains elusive in 7% to 30% of patients (Box 16-4).

The diagnostic workup of FUO should begin with a thorough history and physical examination, including documentation of the fever. The patient may provide a diary noting the date and time of fever. Routine noninvasive investigations are recommended in all patients before diagnosing FUO (Box 16-6). Acute febrile illness is never called an FUO. The patient's medication profile is reviewed because numerous drugs can be the cause. If unrevealing, a workup is initiated based on the differential diagnosis for the patient's age, travel history, geographic location, and disease process. Dukes criteria for infective endocarditis have 99% specificity in patients with FUO. When the initial investigations are not helpful in identifying a cause, imaging should be considered, such as computed tomography (CT) scans of the chest, abdomen, and pelvis; CT may reveal an abscess or suggest an underlying malignancy. An elevated serum ferritin level can suggest a neoplasm or myeloproliferative disorder and, if normal, greatly decreases the chance that the patient has an underlying malignancy. Lower-extremity Doppler ultrasound should be considered in the sedentary or obese patient to rule out deep venous thrombosis. A temporal artery biopsy should be considered in the elderly patient to rule out temporal arteritis. Liver biopsy has a high diagnostic yield with minimal toxicity, whereas bone marrow cultures usually have a low yield and should be considered only in special situations.

Empiric therapy with antibiotics is rarely appropriate for the patient with FUO. A diagnosis is essential to guide

Box 16-4 Differential Diagnosis for Fever of Unknown Origin (FUO)

Classic

Infections: Abscesses, endocarditis, tuberculosis (TB), complicated urinary tract infection (UTI).

> *Geographic location:* Leishmaniasis (Spain), melioidosis (Southeast Asia, Australia), Kikuchi-Fujimoto disease (form of necrotizing lymphadenitis, Japan).

Connective tissue diseases: Juvenile rheumatoid arthritis (JRA, Still's disease), rheumatoid arthritis (RA), systemic lupus erythematosus (SLE), temporal arteritis, polymyalgia rheumatica (PMR).

Neoplasms: malignant neoplasm, lymphoma, leukemia.

Other: Familial Mediterranean fever in Ashkenazi Jews.

Infants and Children

Respiratory infections predominate if <12 years.

Kawasaki disease if <5 years.

JRA, (Still's disease) in the older child/young adult.

Elderly

Connective tissue diseases are more prominent.

Travelers

Infections: Malaria, hepatitis, pneumonia/bronchitis, UTI/pyelonephritis, dysentery, dengue fever, enteric fever, TB, rickettsial infection, acute human immunodeficiency virus (HIV) infection, amebic liver abscess.

Nosocomial

Postoperative urinary and respiratory tract instrumentation; use of intravascular devices; drug therapy; immobilization.

Septic thrombophlebitis, pulmonary embolus, *Clostridium difficile* colitis, drug fever.

Neutropenic

Fungal: 40% susceptible to empiric antifungals, 5% will be resistant to empiric therapy.

Bacterial: 10% not responding to empiric antimicrobial therapy and usually with cryptic focus.

Unusual pathogens: 5% will be toxoplasmosis (*Toxoplasma gondii*) reactivation, atypical mycobacterial, TB, fastidious pathogens (*Legionella, Mycoplasma, Chlamydophila*).

Viral: 5% of causes (HSV, CMV, EBV, HHV-6, VZV, RSV, influenza, parainfluenza).

Other: 10% will be transplant related (e.g., GVHD) following stem cell transplant, 25% will be undefined.

HIV Associated

Infections: *Mycobacterium avium* complex (MAC), *Pneumocystis carinii* pneumonia (PCP), cytomegalovirus (CMV), histoplasmosis, viral (HCV, HBV, adenovirus, HSV esophagitis, VZV encephalitis), TB, other fungi, cerebral toxoplasmosis, disseminated cryptosporidiosis.

Neoplasms: Lymphoma, Kaposi's sarcoma.

Other: Drug fever, Castleman's disease.

HSV, Herpes simplex virus; *EBV,* Epstein-Barr virus; *HHV,* human herpesvirus; *VZV,* varicella-zoster virus; *RSV,* respiratory syncytial virus; *GVHD,* graft-versus-host disease; *HCV,* hepatitis C virus; *HBV,* hepatitis B virus.

Box 16-5 Causes of Fever of Unknown Origin

Infections

Abscesses: Hepatic, subhepatic, gallbladder, subphrenic, splenic, periappendiceal, perinephric, pelvic, and other sites.

Granulomatous: Extrapulmonary and miliary tuberculosis, atypical mycobacterial infection, fungal infection.

Intravascular: Catheter-related endocarditis, meningococcemia, gonococcemia, *Listeria, Brucella,* rat-bite fever, relapsing fever.

Viral, rickettsial, and chlamydial: Infectious mononucleosis, cytomegalovirus, human immunodeficiency virus, hepatitis, Q fever, psittacosis.

Parasitic: Extraintestinal amebiasis, malaria, toxoplasmosis.

Noninfectious Inflammatory Disorders

Collagen vascular diseases: Rheumatic fever, systemic lupus erythematosus, rheumatoid arthritis (particularly Still's disease), vasculitis (all types).

Granulomatous: Sarcoidosis, granulomatous hepatitis, Crohn's disease.

Tissue injury: Pulmonary emboli, sickle cell disease, hemolytic anemia.

Neoplastic Diseases

Lymphoma/leukemia: Hodgkin's and non-Hodgkin's lymphoma, acute leukemia, myelodysplastic syndrome

Carcinoma: Kidney, pancreas, liver, gastrointestinal tract, lung, especially when metastatic

Atrial myxomas

Central nervous system tumors

Drugs

Sulfonamides

Penicillins

Thiouracils

Barbiturates

Quinidine

Laxatives (especially with phenolphthalein)

Factitious Illnesses

Injections of toxic material

Manipulation or exchange of thermometers

Other Causes

Familial Mediterranean fever

Fabry's disease

Cyclic neutropenia

From Dale DC. The febrile patient. In Goldman L, Ausiello D (eds). Cecil Textbook of Medicine, 22nd ed. Philadelphia, Saunders, 2004, p 1730.

treatment, and use of antibiotics may delay determining a causative infectious agent. The naproxen test (Naprosyn; 375 mg PO every 12 hours for 3 days) is helpful in determining if the fever is secondary to infection or malignancy. A dramatic decrease in the patient's temperature during the test generally indicates a malignant focus, whereas minimal or no response indicates an infectious etiology.

The prognosis of FUO depends on the etiologic category. Undiagnosed FUO has a very favorable outcome. Patients in whom diagnostic investigations fail to identify an etiology should be followed clinically with serial history reviews and physical examinations until the fever resolves or new diagnostic clues are found.

KEY TREATMENT

Diagnosis of FUO may be assisted by the Dukes criteria for endocar-ditis, CT scan of the abdomen, nuclear scanning with a technetium-based isotope, and liver biopsy (Mourad et al., 2003) (SOR: B).
Routine bone marrow cultures are not recommended in the FUO workup (Mourad et al., 2003) (SOR: B).
Empiric antibiotics should be initiated only in specific situations, to avoid skewing culture results and thus maximizing potential isola-tion of the causative organism (Mourad et al., 2003) (SOR: B).

COMPLICATED INTRA-ABDOMINAL INFECTIONS

Richard Basilan

Intra-abdominal infections may either be *uncomplicated* (limited to the gut lumen, such as gastroenteritis or colitis) or *complicated* (extending through to the peritoneum) (Sol-omkin et al., 2010). The clinical presentation of complicated intra-abdominal infections can range from mild symptoms such as nausea, mild abdominal pain, and cramping to life-threatening septic shock.

Clinical findings result from local or diffuse inflamma-tion with or without abscess formation. Fever and abdomi-nal pain are typically present, with additional symptoms depending on the organ involved. Elderly and immuno-compromised patients present with atypical, usually milder symptoms. Imaging studies form an important adjunct to diagnosis. Management involves empiric antibiotic coverage for bowel flora—mainly streptococci, enterococci, enteric gram-negative rods, and anaerobes—as well as controlling the source of infection, usually through surgery.

SPONTANEOUS BACTERIAL PERITONITIS

Richard Basilan

Key Points

- Spontaneous bacterial peritonitis usually occurs in the setting of ascites and chronic liver disease.
- Spontaneous bacterial peritonitis is a diagnosis of exclusion.
- Ascitic fluid culture yield improves with inoculation into blood culture bottles at bedside.

Spontaneous bacterial peritonitis (SBP) is a form of infec-tious peritonitis without a surgically correctable cause and is therefore a diagnosis of exclusion. The route of infection in SBP is usually not apparent and is often presumed to be hema-togenous, lymphogenous, by transmural migration through an intact gut wall from the intestinal lumen, or in women, from the vagina via the fallopian tubes (Levison and Bush, 2010). SBP occurs in the setting of ascites in most cases, and it is particularly common in patients with cirrhosis. In pediatric populations, those with postnecrotic cirrhosis or nephrotic syndrome are more often affected. In adults, almost 70% of patients who develop SBP have Child-Pugh class C liver dis-ease, and 10% to 30% of hospitalized patients with cirrho-sis and ascites have SBP (Mowat and Stanley, 2001). SBP is almost always caused by a single organism, typically enteric gram-negative rods, most often *E. coli*, followed by *Klebsiella pneumoniae*. Gram-positive cocci account for about 25% of

Box 16-6 Minimal Diagnostic Workup to Qualify as Fever of Unknown Origin

Comprehensive history
Physical examination
Complete blood cell count plus differential
Blood film reviewed by hematopathologist
Routine blood chemistry (including lactate dehydrogenase, bilirubin, and liver enzymes)
Urinalysis and microscopy
Blood (×3) and urine cultures
Antinuclear antibodies, rheumatoid factor
Human immunodeficiency virus antibody
Cytomegalovirus IgM antibodies; heterophil antibody test (if consis-tent with mononucleosis-like syndrome)
Q-fever serology (if exposure risk factors exist)
Chest radiography
Hepatitis serology (if abnormal liver enzyme test result)

From Mourad O, Palda V, Detsky A. A comprehensive evidence-based approach to fever of unknown origin. Arch Intern Med 2003;163:545-551.

episodes of SBP, and streptococci are isolated most often. SBP caused by anaerobes is rare. Growth of more than one organ-ism should raise the suspicion of secondary peritonitis.

Signs and symptoms of SBP are subtle and require a high index of suspicion. Fever greater than 100° F (38° C) is the most common presenting sign, occurring in 50% to 80% of cases. Abdominal pain, nausea, vomiting, and diarrhea are usually present. Peritoneal signs (abdominal tenderness or rebound tenderness) are common but may be absent in patients with ascites. In adults, mental status changes may also occur. SBP is often confused with acute appendicitis in children. In adults, SBP should be suspected in any patient with previously stable chronic liver disease who undergoes acute decompensation in clinical status.

Spontaneous bacterial peritonitis is diagnosed by analysis of ascitic fluid obtained by abdominal paracentesis. Infection has been typically defined as an ascitic fluid WBC count higher than 250 cells/mm³, which is considered diagnostic even when the culture of the ascitic fluid is negative. In cases where bloody fluid is obtained ("traumatic paracentesis"), the WBC count should be corrected by 1 WBC per 250 RBCs/mm³. The use of bedside dipstick for leukocyte esterase has a high false-nega-tive rate and is not recommended (Nguyen-Khac et al., 2008). Ascitic fluid culture yield can be increased by inoculating blood culture bottles with 10 mL of ascitic fluid at the bedside. Blood cultures should also be obtained as part of the workup.

After the diagnosis of peritonitis is established, second-ary peritonitis should be ruled out. CT of the abdomen with oral and intravenous contrast can help direct the surgeon to a particular source of infection, as opposed to doing a full exploratory laparotomy. A high ascitic fluid total protein (>1 g/dL) or amylase level is suggestive of secondary perito-nitis. The treatment of choice is generally a third-generation cephalosporin such as cefotaxime (2 g IV every 8-12 hours) or ceftriaxone (2 g IV once daily). Patients who have an ascitic fluid WBC count higher than 250 cells/mm³ should be given empiric intravenous antibiotics without delay. Oral amoxi-cillin–clavulanic acid can be used for mild, uncomplicated cases (Navasa et al., 1996). Duration of treatment varies from 5 to 14 days depending on clinical response. Patients usually respond to appropriate antibiotic therapy within 48 to 72 hours; otherwise, a repeat paracentesis should be performed. If the ascitic fluid WBC count does not decrease by more than 25%, alternative diagnoses should be considered. Prophylaxis with a fluoroquinolone or trimethoprim-sulfamethoxazole should be considered, particularly in high-risk patients (Garcia-Tsao and Lim, 2009).

KEY TREATMENT

Spontaneous bacterial peritonitis is treated with third-generation cephalosporins (cefotaxime or ceftriaxone), with ampicillin-sulbactam, fluoroquinolones, or carbapenems as alternative agents (Solomkin et al., 2010) (SOR: B).
Patients with diffuse peritonitis should undergo an emergency surgical procedure as soon as possible, even if ongoing measures to restore physiologic stability need to be continued during the procedure (Solomkin et al., 2010) (SOR: B).

Discussions of the following infections can be found online at www.expertconsult.com:

- Secondary bacterial peritonitis and intra-abdominal abscesses
- Cholecystitis
- Cholangitis
- Appendicitis
- Diverticulitis

CENTRAL NERVOUS SYSTEM INFECTIONS

Richard Basilan

Key Points

- Bacterial meningitis is life threatening and requires urgent medical attention and treatment.
- Viral encephalitis should be treated with acyclovir until herpes simplex virus is ruled out.
- Most brain abscesses are caused by streptococci and *Staphylococcus aureus*.
- The CNS infections most likely to be encountered in clinical practice include meningitis, encephalitis, and abscess.
- All CNS infections can be difficult to diagnose, and a high index of suspicion by the health care provider is sometimes indicated to ensure patient survival.
- MRI is the most sensitive neuroimaging test for encephalitis.
- Acyclovir should be started immediately and continued until HSV PCR testing is obtained.

Bacterial Meningitis

Meningitis can be acute, subacute, or chronic. In otherwise healthy children, the three most common organisms causing acute bacterial meningitis are *Streptococcus pneumoniae*, *Neisseria meningitidis*, and *Haemophilus influenzae* type b (Hib). Isolation of an organism other than these three organisms from the CSF of a child older than 2 months always requires an explanation or evaluation for unusual host susceptibility. Children with cochlear implants, asplenia, HIV infection, or CSF leak

from basilar skull or cribriform fracture are at greater risk for pneumococcal meningitis. Deficiencies in terminal components of complement lead to greater risk for meningococcal infection (Saez-Llorens and McCracken, 2008). In adults, the common etiologic agents of acute meningitis include *S. pneumoniae*, *N. meningitidis*, and *Listeria monocytogenes*.

Patients with acute meningitis most often present with fever, headache, meningismus, and altered mental status. Infants can present with nonspecific symptoms such as inconsolable crying, irritability, nausea, vomiting, and diarrhea. Lethargy, anorexia, and grunting respirations indicate a critically ill infant. Older children may complain of headache, vomiting, back pain, myalgia, and photophobia; may be confused or disoriented; and may verbalize specifically that the neck is stiff or sore. Seizures are noted in up to 20% to 30% of children before hospital admission or early in the course of the illness.

In contrast, patients with subacute or chronic meningitis may have the same symptoms with a much more gradual onset, lower fever, and associated lethargy and disability. *Mycobacterium tuberculosis*, *Treponema pallidum* (syphilis), *Borrelia burgdorferi* (Lyme disease), and fungi (e.g., *Cryptococcus neoformans*, *Coccidioides* spp.) are the most common agents (Tunkel et al., 2010).

Physical examination should look for papilledema, middle ear and sinus infections, petechiae (common with *N. meningitidis*), nuchal rigidity, and in infants, a bulging fontanel. Blood cultures should be taken. A lumbar puncture (LP) for CSF analysis should be done as soon as possible. A brain CT scan before LP is not necessary if the patient has no evidence of immunocompromise, CNS disease, new seizure, papilledema, altered consciousness, or focal neurologic deficit, and if a subarachnoid hemorrhage is not suspected. If neuroimaging is necessary, blood cultures should be taken and antibiotics given before the study; a delay in administration of antibiotics leads to a worse outcome. CSF should be sent for cell count, WBC differential, glucose, protein, and Gram stain with culture. Acid-fast bacilli stain and cryptococcal antigen may be obtained when indicated.

Empiric antibiotics for the initial treatment of bacterial meningitis are listed in Table 16-20, but these should be tailored to the isolated organisms whenever possible. Adjunctive dexamethasone is recommended for children and infants with Hib meningitis, but not if they have already received antibiotics. In adults, adjunctive dexamethasone is recommended for pneumococcal meningitis (Tunkel et al., 2004). Close contacts of patients with *N. meningitidis* should receive rifampin, 20 mg/kg (not to exceed 600 mg) twice daily for 2 days, or ciprofloxacin, 500 mg as a single dose, or ceftriaxone, 250 mg IM as a single dose. Unimmunized persons exposed to *H. influenzae* meningitis should receive rifampin (Turkel et al., 2010). Pregnant women should not receive rifampin or doxycycline.

A repeat LP should be done if no clinical response is seen after 48 hours of appropriate antibiotic therapy, particularly for patients with resistant pneumococcal disease and those who received dexamethasone. Neonates with gram-negative bacilli and patients with ventriculoperitoneal (VP) shunts require documentation of CSF sterility. The duration of antimicrobial therapy is 7 days for patients with *N. meningitidis* or Hib, 10 to 14 days for pneumococcal meningitis, and 14 to 21 days for *Streptococcus agalactiae*.

Table 16-20 Empiric Antibiotics for Initial Treatment of Bacterial Meningitis

Age/Risk Factors	Empiric Antibiotic Therapy
<1 month	Ampicillin + cefotaxime *or* amp + aminoglycoside
1 month to 2 years	Vancomycin + ceftriaxone *or* cefotaxime*
2 to 50 years	Vancomycin + ceftriaxone *or* cefotaxime*
>50 years	Ampicillin + vancomycin + ceftriaxone or cefotaxime*
Basilar skull fracture	Vancomycin + ceftriaxone *or* cefotaxime
Penetrating head trauma	Vancomycin + ceftazidime, cefepime, *or* meropenem†
Postneurosurgery status	Vancomycin + ceftazidime, cefepime, *or* meropenem
Cerebrospinal fluid (CSF) shunt	Vancomycin + ceftazidime, cefepime, *or* meropenem

Modified from Practice Guidelines for Bacterial Meningitis, CID 2004:39.
*Consider adding rifampin if dexamethasone is also given.
†Imipenem should be avoided because it increases the risk of seizures.

KEY TREATMENT

Adjunctive dexamethasone is recommended for children and infants with *H. influenzae* type b meningitis, but not if they have already received antibiotics (Tunkel et al., 2004) (SOR: A).
In adults, adjunctive dexamethasone is recommended for pneumococcal meningitis (Tunkel et al., 2004) (SOR: B).

Viral Meningitis Viral meningitis manifests similar to bacterial meningitis, although its course is rarely aggressive. The diagnostic process and examination are similar to those for bacterial meningitis. Viral meningitis is usually caused by enteroviruses, HSV, mumps virus, and HIV. Along with the signs of meningitis, signs that suggest a viral etiology include genital lesions (HSV-2), diarrhea, or a maculopapular rash (enteroviruses). Diagnosis is made by the history, examination, and CSF results. Early in the course, the CSF might show predominantly neutrophils that can resemble bacterial meningitis. Treatment is symptomatic. Suppressive therapy should be offered to patients with recurrent HSV meningitis.

Viral Encephalitis

Although encephalitis can also be caused by bacteria and fungi, the great majority of cases are caused by viruses. Herpes simplex accounts for 10% of cases. Patients present with fever, acute decreased level of consciousness, and occasionally, seizures and language, memory, or behavior disturbances. MRI is the most sensitive neuroimaging test for encephalitis and might show temporal lobe inflammation in early HSV encephalitis. CSF studies and electroencephalography (EEG) are also recommended for all patients with encephalitis. Herpes simplex PCR should be done, and acyclovir should be given immediately until HSV encephalitis

is ruled out. During late summer and early fall, doxycycline should be considered to cover for tick-borne illnesses, and testing should include the mosquito-borne encephalitides such as West Nile, St. Louis, Eastern equine, and Western equine. Treatment depends on the suspected etiologic agent but is generally supportive (Tunkel et al., 2008).

Brain Abscess

A brain abscess is a focal, intracerebral infection that develops into a collection of pus surrounded by a well-vascularized capsule. Although fungi and protozoa (particularly *Toxoplasma*) can also cause brain abscesses, bacterial causes are much more common. Streptococci are found in 70% of bacterial abscesses and are usually from oropharyngeal infection or infective endocarditis, whereas *Staphylococcus aureus* accounts for 10% to 20% of isolates and is more often found after trauma. Community-associated MRSA strains have been increasing. Enteric gram-negative bacilli (e.g., *E. coli; Proteus, Klebsiella,* and *Pseudomonas* spp.) are isolated in 23% to 33% of patients, often in patients with ear infection, septicemia, or immunocompromise and those who have had neurosurgical procedures.

Most clinical symptoms are caused by the size and location of the abscess rather than the systemic signs of an infection. Headache is the most common complaint and may be accompanied by fever, mental status changes, evidence of increased intracranial pressure (nausea, vomiting, papilledema), or focal neurologic deficits. Diagnosis is usually made by CT scan with IV contrast showing the characteristic hypodense center with a peripheral uniform ring enhancement, with or without a surrounding area of brain edema. MRI is becoming the preferred imaging modality because of increased sensitivity, particularly for detecting satellite lesions. Additional testing depends on risk factors and the likely underlying source of infection and may include blood cultures, chest imaging, testing for HIV and antibodies to *Toxoplasma,* and transesophageal echogram. Empiric therapy typically involves vancomycin, ceftriaxone, and metronidazole. Optimal management also includes surgical drainage for most abscesses, both to find an etiologic microorganism and to improve chances of cure (Turkel, 2010).

INFECTIOUS DIARRHEA

Hoonmo Koo

Key Point

- Most acute diarrheal illness is viral and can be managed symptomatically and with appropriate attention to hydration.
- Travelers' diarrhea is usually caused by diarrheogenic *Escherichia coli.*
- The infection in travelers' diarrhea is usually self-limited.
- Antibiotics may shorten the duration of diarrhea by 1 to 3 days.
- The most common cause of antibiotic-associated diarrhea is *Clostridium difficile.*
- Treatment of antibiotic-associated diarrhea involves discontinuing the offending agent, if possible.

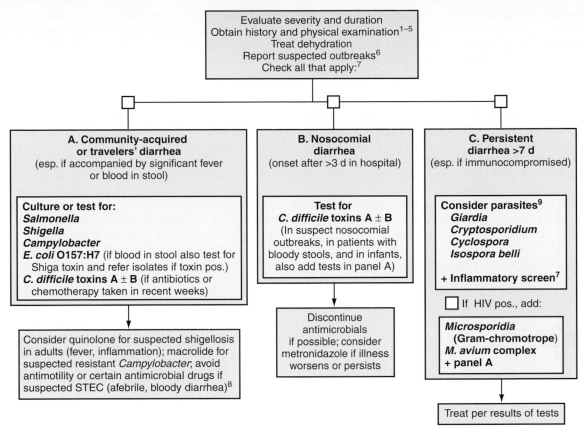

Figure 16-12 Recommendations for diagnosis and management of diarrheal illnesses. *HIV*, Human immunodeficiency virus; *Pos.*, positive. [1]Seafood or seacoast exposure should prompt culture for *Vibrio* spp. [2]Travelers' diarrhea that has not responded to empiric therapy with rifaximin, a quinolone, or azithromycin should be managed with the above approach. [3]Persistent abdominal pain and fever should prompt culture for *Yersinia enterocolitica* and cold enrichment. Right-side abdominal pain without high fever but with bloody or nonbloody diarrhea should prompt culture for Shiga toxin producing *E. coli* (STEC) O157. [4]Proctitis in symptomatic homosexual men can be diagnosed with sigmoidoscopy. Involvement in only the distal 15 cm suggests herpesvirus, gonococcal, chlamydial, or syphilitic infection; colitis extending more proximally suggests *Campylobacter*, *Shigella*, *Clostridium difficile*, or chlamydial (LGV serotype) infection, and noninflammatory diarrhea suggests giardiasis. [5]Postdiarrheal hemolytic uremic syndrome (HUS) should prompt testing of stools for STEC O157 and for Shiga toxin (send isolates to reference laboratory if toxin-positive but STEC-negative). [6]Outbreaks should prompt reporting to the health department. Consider saving culture plates and isolates and freeze whole stools or swabs at −70° C. [7]Fecal lactoferrin testing or microscopy for leukocytes can help document inflammation, which may be present in invasive colitis with *Salmonella*, *Shigella*, *Campylobacter*, or *C. difficile* colitis, and with inflammatory bowel disease. [8]Some experts recommend avoiding administration of antimicrobial agents to persons in the United States who have bloody diarrhea. [9]Commonly used tests for parasitic causes of diarrhea include fluorescence and EIA for *Giardia* and *Cryptosporidium*; acid-fast stains for *Cryptosporidium*, *Cyclospora*, *Isospora*, or *Mycobacterium* spp. (as well as culture for *Mycobacterium avium* complex); and special chromatrope or other stains for *Microsporidia*.
From Guerrant RL, Van Gilder T, Steiner TS, et al. Practice guidelines for the management of infectious diarrhea. Clin Infect Dis 2001;32:334.

Diarrhea is a common presenting complaint in the primary care physician's office. Not all causes of diarrhea are infectious, and not all infectious causes of diarrhea require specific antibiotic therapy. Diarrhea remains a major cause of morbidity and mortality, particularly for children in the developing world. Diarrhea is an alteration of normal bowel function, characterized by an increase in the water content, volume, or frequency of stools. *Acute* diarrhea is typically defined as present less than 14 days, and diarrhea is considered *chronic* when symptoms persist longer than 30 days (Figure 16-12).

Viral Gastroenteritis

Infectious diarrhea seen in the primary care physician's office is most frequently caused by viruses. A number of viral agents can cause diarrheal illness (Box 16-7). Rotaviruses are the principal enteric pathogens in children less than 5 years of age and the most important cause of hospitalization and infant mortality related to diarrheal illnesses. Noroviruses

---

Box 16-7 Viral Pathogens Causing Gastroenteritis

Established Pathogens

Adenoviruses (enteric types)

Astroviruses

Caliciviruses (Noroviruses)

Rotaviruses groups A, B, C

Cytomegalovirus

Likely and Emerging Pathogens

Coronaviruses

Enteroviruses

Picobirnaviruses, picotrirnaviruses

Pestiviruses

Toroviruses

From Guerrant RL, Bobak DA. Nausea, vomiting, and noninflammatory diarrhea. In Mandell GL, Bennett JE, Dolin R (eds). Principles and Practice of Infectious Diseases, 6th ed. Philadelphia, Churchill Livingstone, 2005, pp 1236-1249.

are the most common cause of food-borne disease worldwide.

Viral gastroenteritis is usually an acute self-limited illness, referred to as the "stomach flu." Enteric viruses are easily spread by fecal-oral transmission, through contamination of food and water, fomites, and person-to-person spread. Secondary attack rates can be high. Nausea and vomiting are the most prominent symptoms of viral gastroenteritis. Diarrhea, fever, headache, and constitutional symptoms may also be experienced. These viral infections can occur at any time during the year, but tend to occur more often in the winter. There is no specific therapy. Treatment is supportive, with particular emphasis on adequate replacement of fluids and electrolytes. If rehydration can be accomplished enterally, it is preferred.

Both the pentavalent bovine-human reassortment (RV5) and the oral, live-attenuated monovalent (RV1) rotavirus vaccines are effective for prevention of severe gastroenteritis. The RV5 vaccine series is recommended for children at ages 2, 4, and 6 months, whereas the RV1 vaccine should be administered to children 2 and 4 months of age.

Travelers' Diarrhea

Approximately 40% of travelers to developing regions of the world will develop diarrhea. Bacteria are responsible for approximately 80% of diarrhea acquired by travelers. Other important causes include viruses and parasites. The onset of the majority of cases of travelers' diarrhea is usually within 5 to 15 days after arrival. The presentation is typically a noninflammatory, nonbloody diarrhea associated with abdominal discomfort, fever, nausea, or vomiting. The duration is usually 1 to 5 days.

Enterotoxigenic *E. coli* is responsible for approximately 30% of travelers' diarrhea. Enteroaggregative *E. coli* is the second most common bacterial agent and causes 20% of cases. *Salmonella*, *Shigella*, and *Campylobacter* spp. are less often detected but are important causes of dysentery, particularly in Asia and Africa. *Dysentery* is severe inflammatory diarrhea manifested by fever and bloody stools. Most cases of travelers' diarrhea are self-limited, but chronic postinfectious irritable bowel syndrome may occur in up to 10% of those who experience diarrhea.

Prevention of travelers' diarrhea is an important component of pretravel counseling for high-risk countries. Food should be boiled, cooked, or peeled and water boiled to avoid consumption of fecal contamination. If a person develops travelers' diarrhea, a short course of antibiotics with rifaximin, ciprofloxacin, or azithromycin can shorten the duration of illness by 1 to 3 days. Antibiotic therapy is recommended for persons with bloody diarrhea or fever. Rifaximin, a nonabsorbed antibiotic, is not effective against invasive pathogens

and should not be administered for dysentery. Ciprofloxacin or azithromycin should be used for dysenteric symptoms based on local antimicrobial susceptibilities.

Antibiotic-Associated Diarrhea

Antibiotics are frequently prescribed in the primary care physician's office for a variety of infections. Unfortunately, antibiotics can alter the normal host microflora that can be protective against other infections. Antibiotic effects on the normal gastrointestinal tract microbiome can lead to antibiotic-associated diarrhea, which causes significant morbidity and mortality. Administration of antibiotics usually precedes symptoms of antibiotic-associated diarrhea by about 1 week but can be as distant as 2 or 3 months. Strong associations with clindamycin (Cleocin), cephalosporins, penicillins, and fluoroquinolones have been demonstrated, but any antibiotic can lead to antibiotic-associated diarrhea.

The most important cause of antibiotic-associated diarrhea is *Clostridium difficile*, an anaerobic, gram-positive, spore-forming rod. *C. difficile* is implicated as the cause in up to 25% of antibiotic-associated diarrhea cases, in 50% to 75% of antibiotic-associated colitis cases, and in more than 90% of antibiotic-associated pseudomembranous colitis cases. Risk factors for *C. difficile* diarrhea include antibiotics, health care exposure (recent stay in hospitals or long-term care facilities), older age (>60), and comorbid conditions.

The clinical presentation of *C. difficile* colitis is usually diarrhea, abdominal pain or cramping, and fever in a patient who recently received antibiotics. Leukocytosis is common and may be profound; levels can be consistent with leukemoid reaction. A rare but potentially fatal complication is toxic megacolon. *Toxic megacolon* manifests as acute colonic dilation to a diameter greater than 6 cm, associated with systemic toxicity and the absence of mechanical obstruction. With its high associated mortality, any patient who develops toxic megacolon requires immediate surgical evaluation for possible colectomy.

Diagnosis of *C. difficile* diarrhea is achieved by demonstration of *C. difficile* toxin A or B in the stool by enzyme immunoassay (EIA) or cell culture cytotoxicity assay in a symptomatic patient with a previous history of antibiotic use. Asymptomatic patients should not be tested. With the improved sensitivities of these diagnostic assays, one stool sample is usually sufficient to test for *C. difficile*, unless symptoms recur. Test of cure after therapy with repeat stool for *C. difficile* toxin is not recommended because stools may remain positive for *C. difficile* toxin despite clinical resolution. Endoscopy can demonstrate pseudomembranes in the colon. Pseudomembranes are diagnostic of *C. difficile* infection, but are often not present. Endoscopy may only reveal the presence of nonspecific colitis.

Clostridium difficile colitis is treated by discontinuing the offending agent(s) if possible and initiating antibiotic therapy (Box 16-8). Antimotility agents should be avoided. Oral metronidazole (Flagyl), 500 mg three times daily for 10 to 14 days, is recommended for mild-moderate *C. difficile* diarrhea. Severe diarrhea should be treated with oral vancomycin. Oral vancomycin is currently not recommended for all patients with *C. difficile* diarrhea because of concerns for the promotion of vancomycin-resistant enterococci (VRE) and its expense. About 10% to 20% of patients experience relapse

---

KEY TREATMENT

In travelers' diarrhea, in which enterotoxigenic *E. coli* or other bacterial pathogens are likely causes, prompt treatment with a fluoroquinolone, azithromycin, or rifaximin or, in children, azithromycin 10 mg/kg/day once daily can reduce the duration of an illness from 3 to 5 days to 1 to 2 days (DuPont, 2010) (SOR: A).

Box 16-8 Classification of *Clostridium difficile* Disease Severity and Treatment Recommendations

Severity Scoring

1 point

Requiring care in the ICU

T_{max} >38.3° C (100.9° F)

Albumin <2.5 mg/dL

WBC >15,000 cells/mm3

Age >60 years

2 points

Endoscopic or CT evidence of pseudomembranous colitis

Recommendations

For mild-moderate *C. difficile* diarrhea (≤1 point), treat with metronidazole (Flagyl) PO 500 mg tid.

For severe disease (≥2 points), use vancomycin 125 mg PO qid.

For patients who cannot receive oral medications, IV metronidazole 500 mg qid and vancomycin by nasogastric tube ± rectal enema should be administered.

ICU, Intensive care unit; *CT*, computed tomography; *PO*, by mouth; *IV*, intravenous; *qid*, four times daily; *tid*, three times daily; *WBCs*, white blood cells.

Modified from Zar FA, Bakkanagari FR, KMLST, et al. A comparison of vancomycin and metronidazole for the treatment of *Clostridium difficile*–associated diarrhea, stratified by disease severity. Clin Infect Dis 2007;45:302-307.

KEY TREATMENT

Treat mild-moderate *C. difficile* diarrhea with metronidazole (Zar et al., 2007) (SOR: B).

Vancomycin should be administered for severe *C. difficile* diarrhea (Zar et al., 2007) (SOR: B).

after therapy. For relapse, a repeat course of the original *C. difficile* treatment should be administered. Patients who have mild to moderate cases without volume depletion or systemic toxicity can be treated as outpatients.

Discussions of the following infections can be found online at www.expertconsult.com:

- Infectious viral hepatitis
- Endocarditis

References

The complete reference list is available online at www.expertconsult.com.

Web Resources

Standards, Practice Guidelines, and Statements Developed and/or Endorsed by Infectious Diseases Society of America. Systematically developed statements to assist practitioners and patients in making decisions about appropriate health care for specific clinical circumstances.

www.cdc.gov/std/
Up-to-date information on sexually transmitted diseases (STDs) and their treatment.

www.cdc.gov/tb/
Up-to-date information on tuberculosis and its treatment.

www.cdc.gov/ticks/-
Up-to-date information on tick-borne diseases and their treatment.

www.tripprep.com/scripts/main/default.asp
Information for travelers by destination and illness and an extensive listing of Travel Medicine providers throughout the world; requires free registration.

http://chestjournal.chestpubs.org/content/129/1_suppl
Evidence-based clinical practice guidelines from the American College of Chest Physicians.

www.mrw.interscience.wiley.com/cochrane/cochrane_clsysrev_subjects_fs.html
Comprehensive analyses of evidence related to bronchitis and many other conditions.

http://clinicalevidence.bmj.com/ceweb/index.jsp
Evidence-based reviews of the diagnosis and treatment of many common clinical problems.

www.mdcalc.com/curb-65-severity-score-community-acquired-pneumonia
CURB-65 score calculator to determine the severity of community-acquired pneumonia and need for hospitalization.

17 CHAPTER

Care of the Adult HIV-Infected Patient

Zishan Samiuddin and Roberto A. Andrade

Chapter contents

Key Points

- A behaviorally based, sexually transmitted infection, HIV affects multiple organ systems.
- No longer uniformly fatal, HIV disease is becoming a chronic condition that requires regular monitoring.
- Family physicians can expect to play a pivotal role in diagnosing HIV infection and monitoring age-related illnesses and medication side effects.

Know Syphilis in all its manifestations and relations, and all other things clinical will be added unto you.

WB Bean (1968)

Human immunodeficiency virus (HIV) infection may reasonably be called the "Syphilis" of the modern age. Both diseases are behaviorally based and sexually transmitted; both affect multiple organ systems; and both pose special clinical and public health challenges. This chapter discusses issues in the care of HIV-positive patients important to family medicine residents and physicians. Primary care physicians and trainees have treated HIV-positive patients since HIV was identified as the virus that causes acquired immunodeficiency syndrome (AIDS) and can expect to play a central role in coordinating the care of HIV-positive patients for the following reasons:

1. The Centers for Disease Control and Prevention (CDC) recommends universal voluntary testing of patients age 13 to 64 in all health care settings as of September 2006. This helps make HIV testing a routine part of medical care, decreases anxiety and stigma, encourages safer behaviors, and extends life. An additional benefit is reduced HIV transmission. Regular primary care physician visits present a unique opportunity for the patient to be tested and for the physician to assume responsibility for HIV testing.

2. As patients with HIV/AIDS age, they can expect to develop age-related illnesses that family medicine physicians are qualified and trained to monitor and treat.

3. Highly active antiretroviral therapy (HAART) prolongs lives but causes metabolic, cardiovascular, renal, hepatic, neuropsychiatric, and rheumatologic side effects that require monitoring and management.

4. HIV infection is transforming from a uniformly fatal illness to a chronic condition, with increasing numbers of people living with, and not dying from, HIV/AIDS. The care of patients living with HIV illness must now focus on common elements of chronic disease management.

Box 17-1 presents a timeline on HIV/AIDS and antiretroviral therapy.

Epidemiology

Key Points

- Of the 33 million persons living with HIV infection worldwide, 1 million live in the United States.
- Incidence of HIV infection in the United States has increased by 15%, whereas mortality has declined by 17% (2004–2007).
- Minorities and women are disproportionately affected by HIV infection.

About 33 million people worldwide are living with HIV/AIDS in 2007. Of these, 2.7 million have been newly infected, and 2 million people have died of HIV/AIDS. Developing

Box 17-1 Key Events in HIV/AIDS Crisis and Development of Therapy

1959	African man dies of a mysterious viral illness, now recognized as the ancestor of HIV.
1981	CDC reports "gay-related immune deficiency" (GRID) as the cause of outbreaks of deaths of gay men in California and New York.
	Cases soon appear among heterosexuals, intravenous drug users, and recipients of blood transfusions
1983	Montagnier and Gallo isolate retrovirus later named HIV.
	CDC warns about possible problems with the blood supply.
1985	HIV test is patented by Gallo's laboratory.
	Rock Hudson dies; Ryan White refused admission to school.
1987	Advent of zidovudine (AZT or ZDV) as first treatment for HIV infection.
1992	Combination therapy with zalcitabine (ddC) approved.
1993	Definition of AIDS revised by CDC.
	Concorde trials from Britain show that patients develop AIDS despite treatment with ZDV.
1996	Advent of protease inhibitors and "triple therapy" regimens.
	Viral reservoirs persist while viral loads remain undetectable.
1997	ACTG 076 shows AZT in pregnancy and during delivery reduces vertical transmission from 25% to 3%.
	CDC reports drop in annual AIDS deaths.
1998	First human trials of a vaccine begin.
	Generic HIV medications become available in Europe.
2001	First-entry inhibitor, enfuvirtide (Fuzeon), is developed.
2004	First generic antiretroviral approved by FDA.
	Combination drugs Truvada (emtricitabine and tenofovir) and Epzicom (abacavir and lamivudine) and new protease inhibitors Reyataz and Lexiva become available.
2005	As side effects of chronic HAART identified, experts recommend delay of HAART initiation.
2006	Current scientific opinion holds origin of HIV in the meat and bites of African monkeys.
2009	HIV genome is decoded.

countries account for more than 95% of these infections (UN AIDS, 2007). Since 1981, an estimated 1.7 million people have been infected; more than 1 million people in the United States are currently living with HIV/AIDS; and 565,927 have died of AIDS. The number of deaths has declined by 17% between 2003 and 2007. From 2004 to 2007, there has been an increase of 15% in the incidence of HIV/AIDS cases in the United States. This increase occurred mainly in persons age 40 to 44, who accounted for 15% of all HIV/AIDS cases, likely caused by both changes in reporting systems and increased HIV testing.

A disproportionate number of minorities and women are affected by HIV. Although the U.S. population is 13% black, blacks constituted 45% of newly diagnosed cases in 2006, with a rate of infection of 83.7 per 100,000. Of these, 60% are women. Blacks living with HIV/AIDS constitute about 60% of the adult HIV-positive population in 2007, with a rate of 76.7 per 100,000. Similarly, Hispanics, although constituting 12% of the population, reflect 17% of those persons newly infected with HIV in 2006 and 20% of those living with HIV/AIDS in 2007, with rates of 29.3 and 20 per 100,000, respectively. Year-end prevalence rates in 2007 were 185.1 per 100,000 population, with a range

between 2.2 in Samoa and 1750 per 100,000 in the District of Columbia.

Acquired immunodeficiency syndrome was diagnosed within 12 months of diagnosis of HIV infection for a larger percentage of Hispanics and male intravenous drug users (IVDUs) and men with high-risk heterosexual contact. Survival after AIDS diagnosis has increased in those who were diagnosed between 1998 and 2000, among men who have sex with men (MSM), and those who have acquired HIV perinatally. More whites survive 48 months after a diagnosis of AIDS than minorities. Survival has declined in IVDUs and with each year of age at diagnosis after age 35 (HIV/AIDS Surveillance Report, 2007).

Modes of Transmission and Relative Risk

Key Points

- Human immunodeficiency virus is transmitted through mucous membranes during anal, vaginal, and oral intercourse.
- Transmission of HIV also occurs through sharing injection equipment and needles. Vertical transmission occurs from mother to child.
- Blood, semen, vaginal fluid, breast milk, cerebrospinal fluid, amniotic fluid, and serosanguineous fluid can transmit HIV; saliva, tears, and sweat do not.
- The virus cannot survive outside the host, and 90% to 99% of infective HIV on dry surfaces is eliminated within hours. Insect bites and casual contact carry no risk.

As epidemic and scientific approaches to HIV infection evolved, the focus shifted from "risk groups" to "risky behaviors." This distinction is important, because risk *groups* can give a false sense of security by implying that certain groups of individuals are less vulnerable to infection. *Risky behaviors* is a more useful term, falling along a spectrum of "no risk" (e.g., complete sexual abstinence), "very low risk" (e.g., 100% use of latex condoms), to "very high risk" (e.g., unprotected receptive anal intercourse with ejaculation), with other behaviors in midspectrum. The physician serves as a source of accurate information to be provided in simple, nonjudgmental terms because ultimately the patient will decide the acceptable degree of risk.

The three main modes of transmission of HIV are as follows:
1. Through the mucous membranes during anal, vaginal, or oral sexual intercourse with an HIV-infected person. Average risk of transmission in heterosexual exposure is 1 in 1000 and increases with commercial sex workers to about 5 to 10 in 100. Co-infection with other sexually transmitted diseases (STDs), rough sex, and higher viral load increase risk, whereas condom use and male circumcision reduce risk. Uncircumcised men run risk similar to a woman, and circumcised men may transmit the virus to female partners four times as efficiently as uncircumcised men. Postmenopausal women are more susceptible because of thinning of the vaginal mucosa. Risk of infection per act has been suggested from cohort studies, so physicians should avoid discussing risks in numeric terms.

2. Through the veins while sharing needles or injection paraphernalia with an HIV-infected person.
3. Vertically from an HIV-infected mother to an infant during pregnancy, delivery, or through breastfeeding. High viral load, prolonged time after rupture of membranes, and chorioamnionitis increase risk of transmission, and peripartum prophylactic antiretroviral therapy decreases risk. Overall risk of transmission by breastfeeding is about 15% to 25% in 18- to 24-month-old infants.

Occupational exposure occurs by needle stick injuries (risk, 3:1000), infected blood or fluid splashing into the mouth or nose, or exposure to infected blood through a cut or an open wound. Mucous membrane exposure carries a risk of infection of about 9 in 10,000. Transmission of HIV through infected blood is extremely rare after routine screening of the blood supply was initiated in 1985. With risk of transmission as low as 2 per million, 16 annual infections are accounted for by infectious donations. Neither insect bites nor casual contact carry any risk.

Human immunodeficiency virus can be transmitted by blood, semen, vaginal fluid, breast milk, and serosanguineous body fluids. Contact with cerebrospinal fluid (CSF), amniotic fluid, and synovial fluid can be a risk factor for HIV transmission. Importantly, although HIV can be present in small quantities in saliva, sweat and tears, contact with these fluids does not transmit HIV. The virus cannot survive outside the host, and the amount of infective virus dried on surfaces is reduced by 90%-99% in a few hours.

Pathophysiology

Key Points

- Human immunodeficiency virus belongs to the viral group of Retroviridae, named for its capacity to synthesize DNA using RNA as a template. The subgroup is Lentivirinae, characterized by a long incubation period.
- HIV-1 is found globally, whereas HIV-2 is found mainly in western Africa, although cases of HIV-2 are being seen more frequently in the United States.
- HIV-1 is further subdivided into group M, O, and N, with group M (subdivided into 10 clades) causing most infections worldwide.
- Billions of virions are turned over daily in the virus, leading to frequent mutations and genetic variations.

Human immunodeficiency virus belongs to the group of viruses called *retroviruses,* so named because of their capacity to synthesize deoxyribonucleic acid (DNA) using ribonucleic acid (RNA) as a template, facilitated by the enzyme *reverse transcriptase.* Within the retrovirus class, HIV belongs to the lentivirus subgroup; lentiviruses are characterized by a long incubation period, allowing the infected person to spread the infection because they may remain unaware of their own HIV status (Chiu et al., 1985).

Of the two genetically distinct viral types of HIV, type 1 (HIV-1) is associated with global disease, whereas type 2

(HIV-2) is found mainly in western Africa, although cases of HIV-2 have started to appear in the United States. HIV-1 variants are further divided into group M (main), group O (outlier), and group N (non-M/non-O). As suggested by the name, group M causes most of the infections worldwide and is further subdivided into 10 subtypes, or *clades* (A-K). Clade C is the most common worldwide, and clade B is most frequently seen in North America and Europe. More than 20 sub-subtypes and *circulating recombinant forms* (CRFs) are seen in group M alone. *AE* is a recombinant subtype transmitted most effectively by heterosexual contact and most prevalent in Southeast Asia (Buonaguro et al., 2007). As billions of virions are turned over in the virus on a daily basis, mutations and genetic variations are quite common, a fact that becomes relevant when treatment is considered.

Life Cycle of HIV and Relevance to Treatment

Key Points

- Infection with HIV proceeds in a series of steps, the first step being virion binding to the host cell and releasing the viral RNA. Fusion inhibitors can interrupt this step.
- In step 2, HIV uses reverse transcriptase to convert viral RNA to DNA. RT inhibitors can prevent this step.
- The HIV DNA is then incorporated into the host genome to form the provirus, facilitated by integrase. The virus may remain latent until the CD4+ cell is immune activated, making viral proteins. Integrase Inhibitors interfere with this step.
- Transcription of DNA to RNA occurs in the nucleus. During translation, mRNA takes over the protein-making mechanism to form viral proteins as well as viral RNA. The products are then divided into functional units using viral protease. Protease inhibitors interrupt this step.
- The final step consists of assembly, budding, and pinching off of the viral proteins, RNA, and enzymes inside the host membrane to form the complete virion.

Human immunodeficiency virus gains access to CD4+ cells in stages (Berger et al., 1999; Smith and Daniel, 2006; Zheng et al., 2005). CD4+ cells are the main mediators of cellular immune response, helping T lymphocytes and B lymphocytes to perform their functions. The 800 to 1200 cells/mm^3 of blood in healthy people are usually decimated by HIV. Minor infections, such as herpes simplex virus, thrush, and vaginal candidiasis may occur as the CD4+ count falls below 500, when 50% of the immune reserve is depleted. With a worsening disease process and decreasing CD4+ count (<200), risk of life-threatening opportunistic infections and cancer increases. Research has focused on medications that can interrupt the life cycle and slow the infection of cells.

Step 1

The HIV adheres to and sequentially binds with the host CD4+ cell receptor and a co-receptor (CCR5 or CXCR4). Most wild-type viruses have the CCR5 co-receptor, but with prolonged infection, more and more CXCR4 appears.

Binding with the host CD4+ cell allows the virion to enter the cell and, aided by the co-receptor, to release the two copies of the viral RNA. Drugs called *fusion inhibitors* interrupt this step.

Step 2

Using the viral RNA as a template, HIV reverse transcriptase (RT) converts viral RNA to DNA in the cytoplasm. Smaller functional pieces of the HIV DNA split from the full copy of the DNA. *Reverse transcriptase inhibitors* (RTIs) are used to interrupt this step in the HIV life cycle. Nucleoside RTIs bind competitively and nonnucleoside RTIs (NNRTIs) bind noncompetitively with RT. NNRTIs are specific for HIV-1 and show no activity against HIV-2.

Step 3

The HIV DNA enters the cell nucleus and is incorporated into the host's DNA by the enzyme *integrase* to form the provirus. The virus may remain in a dormant state for many years if the cell is not activated. Once activated, the cell makes many thousands of virions, either for weeks or in a single burst that destroys the cell. *Integrase inhibitors* can prevent the incorporation of viral DNA into the host DNA.

Step 4

Activated CD4+ cells make more viral proteins by copying the DNA back to RNA. This step is called *transcription* and is controlled by both viral and host cell factors. This messenger RNA (mRNA) is transported back to the cytoplasm to be used as a template to make more viral proteins. This step is called *translation*. At this point the protein sequence of mRNA is changed back into the molecules that form envelope and core proteins. The enzyme that splices these large proteins into smaller functional proteins is called *protease*. This step can be prevented by *protease inhibitors* (PIs). HIV-2 carries many of the mutations that confer PI resistance, thus limiting PI activity.

Step 5

The core proteins, RNA, and enzymes just inside the cell membrane are combined with the viral envelope proteins within the host cell membrane. The virus then pinches off, and the process is repeated many times. The complete virus is thus a combination of viral as well as host cell components.

Classification and Staging of HIV/AIDS

Key Points

- The CDC classification uses CD4+ counts and specific HIV-related conditions to stage HIV illness. WHO guidelines use clinical observations.
- The CDC lists AIDS categories as A3, B3, C1, C2, and C3, with 23 AIDS-defining conditions. WHO includes primary HIV infection and four clinical stages.

The two classification systems currently in use to monitor the severity of HIV illness and assist with its management have been developed by the CDC (Table 17-1) and the World Health Organization (WHO) (Box 17-2). The CDC classification, last modified in 1993, uses CD4+ counts and specific HIV-related conditions, whereas the WHO classification, developed in 1990 and revised in 2007, is guided by clinical observations and can be used in settings where access to CD4+ tests is unavailable.

Category B: Symptomatic Conditions

These conditions must indicate defective cell-mediated immunity caused by HIV infection, or their clinical course and management must be complicated by HIV. Category B conditions include the following:

- Constitutional symptoms (fever >38.5° C or diarrhea) lasting more than 1 month
- Candidiasis: oropharyngeal or persistent or recurrent vulvovaginal
- Pelvic inflammatory disease
- Moderate or severe cervical dysplasia or carcinoma in situ
- Oral hairy leukoplakia
- Idiopathic thrombocytopenic purpura
- Peripheral neuropathy
- More than two episodes of multidermatomal herpes zoster
- Bacillary angiomatosis

Category C: AIDS-Defining Illnesses

Category C conditions include bacterial, viral, fungal infections, parasitic infestations, and some cancers.

Bacterial

- *Mycobacterium tuberculosis* infection at any site, pulmonary or extrapulmonary
- *Mycobacterium avium* complex disease; infection with *M. kansasii* or other species, disseminated or extrapulmonary
- *Mycobacterium,* any species disseminated or extrapulmonary
- Bacterial pneumonia, recurrent (>2 episodes in 12 months)
- Nontyphoid *Salmonella* septicemia, recurrent

Viral

- Cytomegalovirus disease (other than liver, spleen, or nodes) and retinitis with vision loss
- Herpes simplex virus (chronic ulcer persisting >1 month, bronchitis, pneumonitis, esophagitis)
- Progressive multifocal leukoencephalopathy

Fungal

- Candidiasis of the esophagus, bronchi, trachea, or lungs
- Coccidioidomycosis, disseminated or extrapulmonary
- Cryptococcosis, extrapulmonary
- Histoplasmosis, disseminated or extrapulmonary

Table 17-1 CDC Classification System of HIV/AIDS

CD4 Cell Count	Clinical Categories		
	A Asymptomatic Acute HIV or PGL	**B Symptomatic state Neither A nor C**	**C AIDS Indicator Conditions**
≥500 cells/mm³	A1	B1	C1
200-499 cells/mm³	A2	B2	C2
<200 cells/mm³	A3	B3	C3

Data from US Centers for Disease Control and Prevention. 1993 Revised classification system for HIV infection and expanded surveillance case definition for AIDS among adolescents and adults. MMWR 1992;41(RR-17):1-19.

- Isosporiasis, chronic intestinal (persisting for >1 month)
- Pneumonia, recurrent *(Pneumocystis jiroveci)*

Parasitic

- Cryptosporidiosis, chronic intestinal (persisting for >1 month)
- Toxoplasmosis of brain
- Isosporiasis, chronic intestinal (persisting for >1 month)

HIV-Related Conditions

- Encephalopathy, HIV related
- Wasting syndrome, HIV related (weight loss >10% body weight with either chronic diarrhea of >2 stools/day × 1 month or chronic weakness and documented fever >1 month)

Cancers

- Cervical cancer, invasive
- Kaposi's sarcoma
- Lymphoma (Burkitt's, immunoblastic, or primary lymphoma of brain)

Cancers and chronic renal failure associated with AIDS and lipodystrophy, insulin resistance, osteoporosis, and cardiovascular complications of HAART are being increasingly recognized and addressed.

Natural History and Clinical Course

Key Points

- About 20% of HIV-infected persons are unaware of their status because they look and feel healthy.
- Primary HIV infection manifests as a flulike syndrome 1 to 6 weeks after exposure.
- Symptoms include fever, pharyngitis, rash, myalgias, and meningismus; viral load is very high.
- The asymptomatic phase (8-12 weeks later) can persist for many years.
- The lower the viral set point, the better is the long-term prognosis.

More than one fifth of people infected with HIV are unaware of the infection because they look and feel healthy. Family physicians are likely to be the first health

---

Box 17-2 WHO Clinical Staging of HIV/AIDS

Primary HIV infection
Asymptomatic
Acute retroviral syndrome

Clinical Stage 1
Asymptomatic
Persistent generalized lymphadenopathy

Clinical Stage 3
Moderate unexplained weight loss (<10% body weight)
Recurrent respiratory infections (sinusitis, tonsillitis, otitis media, pharyngitis)
Herpes zoster
Angular cheilitis
Recurrent oral ulceration
Papular pruritic eruptions
Seborrheic dermatitis
Fungal nail infections

Clinical Stage 3
Severe, unexplained weight loss (>10% body weight)
Unexplained diarrhea longer than 1 month
Unexplained, persistent, constant or intermittent fever longer than 1 month (>37.6° C)
Persistent oral candidiasis
Oral hairy leukoplakia
Pulmonary tuberculosis
Severe presumed bacterial infections (pneumonia, empyema, pyomyositis, bone and joint infections, meningitis, bacteremia)
Acute necrotizing gingivitis, stomatitis, periodontitis
Unexplained anemia (hemoglobin <8 g/dL)
Neutropenia (<500 cells/mm³)
Chronic thrombocytopenia (<50,000 cells/mm³)

Clinical Stage 4
All the AIDS indicator conditions as defined by the CDC classification *and*
    Atypical disseminated leishmaniasis
    Symptomatic HIV-associated nephropathy
    Symptomatic HIV-associated cardiomyopathy
    Reactivation of American trypanosomiasis (meningoencephalitis or myocarditis)

Modified from World Health Organization. Case definitions of HIV for surveillance and revised clinical staging and immunological classification of HIV related disease in adults and children. Geneva, WHO, 2007. www.who.int/hiv/pub/guidelines/HIV.

professional contact for patients with primary HIV infection. Symptoms resemble a flu or mononucleosis syndrome. A high index of suspicion for HIV infection must be maintained in sexually active, injection drug–using patients or those with known HIV exposure. The incubation period from exposure to the development of the acute clinical illness, known as acute HIV syndrome, is usually 2 to 4 weeks (range, 1-6 weeks).

Common symptoms of primary infection, including fever, lymphadenopathy, pharyngitis, and a maculopapular rash, may occur in 50% to 70% of infected persons. Other symptoms include myalgias and arthralgias, headache, and diarrhea. HIV viral load reaches levels as high as several million RNA copies per milliliter during primary infection. During this period, HIV has seeded lymphoid tissues and various other body organs. Physical examination shows a rash that can involve the face, soles, palms, and trunk; malaise; fever of 40° C (104° F); lymphadenopathy; pharyngitis; oral, vaginal, or anal ulcers; and signs of meningismus. Oral or vaginal thrush may also occur. Cohort studies enrolling seroconverting patients have consistently shown that both the number and the duration of acute retroviral symptoms each independently increase the likelihood of later disease progression (Borrow et al., 1994; Douek, 2003; Koup et al., 1994; Zaunders et al., 2001, 2003). One study found a 78% likelihood of progression to AIDS within 3 years in patients with an acute viral syndrome lasting 14 days or more, whereas the chance of progression dropped to 10% in asymptomatic seroconverters (Lindback et al., 1994).

Patients enter an asymptomatic phase within 8 to 12 weeks after infection. This phase can persist for many years. At this stage, viral RNA is reduced (5000-15,000 copies/mL), even to an undetectable level. The balance between viremia and host response leads to the viral load being set at a relatively low, stable level called the *viral set point*. The lower the viral set point, the better is the long-term prognosis for the infected person (Mellors et al., 1996).

Depending on a variety of viral and host factors, viral replication overcomes immune response, and the viral load increases with an associated decrease in CD4+ lymphocytes (Figure 17-1). At counts less than 350 cells/mm³, thrush, herpes zoster, recurrent dermatoses, and other mucosal infections signify impaired immune function. Once the CD4+ count drops below 200 cells/mm³, the risk of developing life-threatening opportunistic infections increases greatly. This process can take years to develop, and long-term "non-progressors" have been identified. Proposed mechanisms causing CD4+ cell loss include direct infection by HIV, bone marrow toxicity leading to impaired lymphocytic regeneration, apoptosis from chronic immune activation, CTL activity against normal CD4+ cells, and ADCC killing of CD4+ cells carrying viral protein gp120 (Levy, 2006).

The final stage of HIV infection is the development of the CDC classification of AIDS. Median survival time after an AIDS-defining illness was about 12 months in the pre-HAART era (1981–1995), increasing to 60 months by 1995. An estimated 85% to 90% of patients will survive more than 6 years after a diagnosis of AIDS (CDC, 2006).

Diagnosis

Key Points

- Early HIV diagnosis increases access to care and decreases transmission.
- Approximately half of patients are diagnosed with AIDS within the first year of HIV diagnosis.
- Routine HIV testing using blood (or less often saliva or urine) helps reduce stigma and decrease anxiety.
- Infection is diagnosed by detection of HIV antigen in a two-step process, a preliminary EIA and a confirmatory Western blot.
- Rapid HIV testing removes the barrier of a return visit because results are available in 20 minutes.

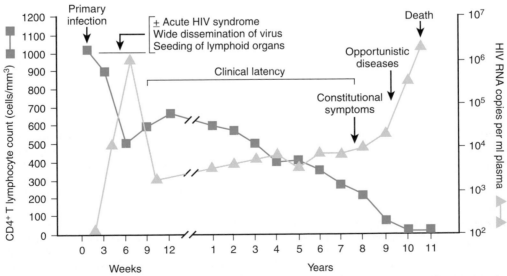

Figure 17-1 Typical course of HIV infection showing the relationship between the levels of HIV (viral load) and CD4+ T-cell counts over the average course of untreated HIV infection. NIAID publication showing clinical progression of HIV.
(Modified from Fauci AS et al. Immunopathogenic mechanisms of HIV infection. Ann Intern Med 1996;124:654-663.)

- The Oraquick and Multispot tests detect both HIV-1 and HIV-2; Reveal and Uni-Gold Recombigen tests detect HIV-1 only.
- As of September 2006, the CDC recommends voluntary testing in all health care settings after informing patients and allowing them to "opt out" if they choose.

Early diagnosis increases access to treatment and helps reduce HIV transmission, but it remains a challenge. Approximately half of HIV-positive patients are diagnosed with AIDS within the first year of HIV diagnosis (Klein et al., 2003; Samet et al., 2001). Many patients ignore the obvious link between sexual and drug use behavior. Taking a careful drug use and sexual history helps identify patients at high risk for HIV infection, and routine HIV testing helps remove the stigma of such identification (Box 17-3). Although blood tests are most common, tests using saliva or urine are also available.

Laboratory diagnosis of HIV that depends on the presence and detection of antibodies to HIV antigen is a two-step process. A specific test for the p24 antigen or HIV-1 RNA is also available but is not widely used. The highly sensitive enzyme immunoassay (EIA) constitutes the first step of the process; further testing is necessary only if the EIA is positive. If exposure occurred less than 3 months earlier and the test is negative, it is repeated in 3 months. EIA is repeated in duplicate if positive or indeterminate. A confirmatory Western blot test is done if the results of repeat testing are again positive or indeterminate. A positive Western blot is conclusive evidence for seropositivity. Indeterminate tests are repeated in a month. A Western blot discordant with EIA raises the possibility of HIV-2 infection.

The CDC estimates that 31% of people tested for HIV did not return for results in 2001 (CDC, 2003). Rapid HIV testing further removes the often-neglected barrier of repeat visits because results are available in about 20 minutes.

Box 17-3 Recommendations for HIV Screening

Patients in All Health Care Settings

Patients must be notified and then screened for HIV unless they decline (opt-out screening).

High-risk subpopulations should be screened for HIV at least annually.

Persons at high risk for HIV infection should have at least annual screening.

Using the general consent for medical care should be enough for HIV testing.

Prevention counseling should not be required with HIV diagnostic testing or screening.

Pregnant Women

All pregnant women must be routinely screened for HIV infection.

Patients must be notified and then screened for HIV unless they decline (opt-out screening).

Separate written consent for HIV testing should not be required if the patient has already signed a general consent for medical care.

Repeat screening in the third trimester is recommended in certain jurisdictions with elevated rates of HIV infection among pregnant women.

Modified from Centers for Disease Control and Prevention. Revised recommendations for HIV testing of adults, adolescents and pregnant women in healthcare settings. MMWR 2006;55(RR-14):1-17.

The U.S. Food and Drug Administration (FDA) has approved four rapid HIV screening tests: Oraquick (and Oraquick Advance), Reveal (and Reveal G2), Uni-Gold Recombigen HIV1/HIV2 Rapid Test, and Multispot HIV1/HIV2 Rapid Test. Oraquick and Multispot can detect both HIV-1 and HIV-2. If HIV antibodies are present, they bind to the HIV antigens affixed to the test strip membrane. This complex in turn binds to the colorimetric agent of the test kit and can be seen for a positive test. All these tests require confirmation if reactive. They are highly sensitive and specific, are interpreted visually, and require no instrumentation, making them highly convenient for office use. Oraquick and Uni-Gold are CLIA waived.

Approach to the Patient

Key Points

- Managing HIV/AIDS in the primary care setting helps decrease stigma and patient anxiety.
- Health promotion and disease prevention are becoming as important as managing chronic symptoms.
- A nonjudgmental attitude and strict confidentiality promote trust in the physician-patient relationship.
- Different aspects of the history and physical examination may need to be stressed with certain patients, including safer sex practices.
- HIV-specific history, physical examination, and laboratory tests must be obtained as indicated at each visit.

Family physicians are often the portal of entry into medical care, so they can be instrumental in assessing behaviors that put patients at risk for infection, diagnosing infection, and monitoring and treating the infected patient, even if the patient is referred to a specialist. Although controlling chronic symptoms and treating acute infectious episodes remain vital components of HIV care, health promotion and disease prevention are gaining equal prominence, now that novel and effective treatments are available, making the process of HIV care delivery analogous to that of such chronic illnesses as diabetes and hypertension. Also, managing HIV infection in the primary care setting serves to reduce social stigma and reduce patient anxiety.

The essential components of a successful long-term physician-patient relationship are trust that the physician will act in the patient's best interests, respect their wishes, be non-judgmental about their lifestyle and behaviors, and maintain the highest degree of confidentiality. The physician or other health care professional is responsible for providing a safe space for the patient to discuss sensitive information. Patients may avoid disclosing behaviors they think may be viewed disapprovingly by the professional. It is vitally important that patients are assured of confidentiality and questioned nonjudgmentally and respectfully. Culturally sensitive literature addressing the needs of local populations must be readily available, with pictures and posters showing familiar faces.

The first visit is crucial to establishing the tone of subsequent encounters. Aspects of the history that must be stressed may depend on time since diagnosis and the presence of symptoms. Recently diagnosed and asymptomatic patients need reassurance and accurate knowledge about the availability of current treatments. Life-threatening opportunistic infections

Table 17-2 HIV-Specific Patient History

Area of Questioning	Relevance
Date of diagnosis and mode of transmission Prior HIV-related illnesses and ART treatment history (reasons for discontinuation, side effects experienced) CD4+ counts and viral loads at diagnosis, nadir point, and most recently HIV-associated symptoms such as fever, night sweats, unintentional weight loss, generalized lymphadenopathy, diarrhea, and oral candidiasis History of travel to areas endemic for histoplasmosis, blastomycosis, and coccidioidomycosis	Assessing risk for other STDs, staging of illness, determination of HAART treatment options; assessing risk of immune suppression and disease progression Documentation and assessment of need for further testing and treatment
Detailed drug abuse history History of hepatitides and tuberculosis, including duration and adherence to chemoprophylaxis	Assessment of ability to adhere to treatment
Documentation of herbal and complementary medications	Determination of potential interactions with HAART
Number of pregnancies and HIV status during pregnancy	Determination of children at risk
Status of immunizations	Risk of infection in an immunocompromised patient
Psychiatric diagnoses	Ability to adhere to medication regimen
Living situation, employment, social support, pets. and daily diet	Ability to afford medications, risk of infections, nutritional status
Number of sexual partners and condom use, method of contraception, survival sex, persons to whom the patient has disclosed HIV status	Behaviors likely to increase reinfection and put partners at risk

ART, Antiretroviral therapy; *HAART*, highly active ART; *STDs*, sexually transmitted diseases.

(OIs) must be ruled out in symptomatic patients. A detailed treatment history, side effects experienced, and reasons for discontinuation of medications must be obtained from treatment-experienced patients. Screening for substance abuse and STDs must be addressed routinely. Behaviors that put others at risk for infection must be assessed (Table 17-2).

The physical examination must focus on organ systems most likely to be affected by HIV-related OIs and cancers. The examination may also reveal clues to potential complications and aid in staging the illness. Vital signs, including the presence of pain, are documented at every visit (Table 17-3).

Laboratory testing is important to monitor disease progress and the effects of HAART and to delineate treatment side effects, such as lipid, glucose, and renal abnormalities (Table 17-4).

Clinically stable patients need only be seen every 3 to 4 months. Recently diagnosed patients, those with acute illnesses, and those who are failing or have recently changed antiretroviral therapy may need to be seen more frequently. The 2009 guidelines allow follow-up visits to be extended to every 6 months, if the patient is virologically suppressed for more than 2 to 3 years (level 2).

Because 95% adherence maximizes the potential for long-term viral load suppression, adherence to therapy must be confirmed. Asking about doses missed in the prior 48 hours or 2 weeks may yield more accurate answers than inquiring in general about whether or not the patient is taking medications. Younger age, lack of social support, and chronic symptoms, including depression, are negative predictors of adherence. Race, ethnicity, gender, and inactive substance abuse do not predict adherence. Statistical risk factors for poor adherence should not lead to the decision to withhold treatment. Instead, the clinician must explore ways to counter the effects of these predictors.

Safer sex practices and specific instances of unprotected sex must be discussed. Interim problems and the status of previously discussed problems are also monitored.

Use of Antiretroviral Agents

Key Points

- Primary care physicians with appropriate experience and expertise can provide high-quality care to HIV-infected patients.
- U.S. DHHS guidelines are frequently updated and provide useful direction in treatment of HIV/AIDS patients.
- A few medication combinations should be avoided and certain drugs used with caution in special patient populations.
- Widespread use of HAART has decreased the prevalence of opportunistic infections in HIV/AIDS patients, but prophylaxis is generally advised for specific OIs.
- Once initiated, HAART must be continued indefinitely and lifelong.

The U.S. Department of Health and Human Services (DHHS) guidelines on the use of antiretroviral agents for HIV-infected adults (December 2009) provide guidance to HIV care practitioners on the optimal use of antiretroviral agents for the treatment of HIV infection in adults and adolescents in the United States. The recommendations are mostly based on studies in peer-reviewed journals (Guidelines Working Group, 2008).

Table 17-3 HIV-Specific Physical Examination

Component of Examination	Area of Relevance
Head, Eyes, Ears, Nose and Throat	
Oropharyngeal and gingival exam	Candidiasis and Kaposi's sarcoma
Funduscopy	Cytomegalovirus retinitis
Palpation of thyroid	Risk of anxiety or depression, which can interfere with adherence
Chest	
Auscultation for abnormal sounds or for absence of air movement	Pleural effusions, pneumonia, pneumothorax
Abdomen	
Hepatomegaly and splenomegaly	Evidence of hepatitis and cause of anemia
Anogenital exam and anal Pap test	Herpes simplex virus, human papillomavirus, or other STDs
Pelvic exam at first visit, in 6 months, and annually thereafter	Cancer, STDs, pelvic inflammatory disease
Baseline Neurologic Examination	
Dissociated sensory loss	Peripheral neuropathy
Fine motor skills	Dementia
Muscle strength	Myopathy, neuropathy
Psychiatric	
Mental status exam to rule out HIV-associated depression, anxiety, and psychosis	Impact on adherence to medications and appointments
Suicidal thoughts	Need for inpatient care
Behavioral changes	Intracranial pathology, side effects of medications, and laboratory abnormalities

STDs, Sexually transmitted diseases.

Despite the complexity of managing HIV-infected patients, an observational cohort study suggests that family physicians with appropriate experience and expertise in HIV care can provide high-quality care to patients with this complex chronic illness (Landon et al., 2005). Primary care providers without HIV experience, such as those who provide service in rural or underserved areas, should identify experts in the region who will provide consultation when needed. The following goals of therapy have broadened along with knowledge of HIV/AIDS and the epidemiology and long-term consequences of chronic infection:

1. To suppress HIV RNA (viral load) as low as possible (<48 copies/mL), for as long as possible.
2. To preserve or enhance immune function.
3. To delay clinical progression to AIDS.
4. To decrease risk of HIV transmission.
5. To decrease risk of nonopportunistic conditions.
6. To delay the selection of drug-resistant mutations by decreasing the rate of viral replication.

Achieving these goals has resulted in substantial reductions in HIV-related morbidity and mortality and has reduced vertical transmission (Mocroft et al., 1998; Mofenson et al., 1999; Palella et al., 1998, Vittinghoff et al., 1999).

The DHHS guidelines for initiating antiretroviral therapy (ART) include strength of evidence level for each recommendation (Table 17-5). There is strong evidence that patients with CD4+ count less than 200 cells/mm³ and those with a history of opportunistic illness will benefit the most from early ART. It is currently recommended that ART be initiated in patients with CD4+ count of 200 to 350 cells/mm³ (level 1) and 350 to 500 cells/mm³ (level 1/2) (Box 17-4).

Recent data from the ART Cohort Collaboration and North American AIDS Cohort Collaboration on Research and Design (NA ACCORD) suggest that deferring HAART at CD4+ count greater than 500 cells/mm³ was associated with increased risk of mortality. Following this research finding, current guidelines (level 2) recommend initiation of HAART at CD4+ counts of greater than 500. Half the panel members supported this course of action (1) because of the association between non–AIDS-defining illnesses, such as malignancies and liver and kidney disease, and (2) because currently available medications are much better tolerated for longer periods. Drawbacks to this recommendation are (1) the panel did not reach consensus; (2) the benefits of HAART initiation are still unclear; and (3) the results are from observational analyses.

Current antiretroviral medicines include nucleoside/nucleotide reverse-transcriptase inhibitors (NRTIs), nonnucleoside reverse-transcriptase inhibitors (NNRTIs), protease inhibitors (PIs), fusion inhibitors (FIs), CCR5 inhibitors, and integrase strand transfer inhibitors (INSTIs) (Table 17-6). All these groups except one is FDA approved and indicated in

Table 17-4 Routine Laboratory Testing for HIV-Infected Patients

Laboratory Investigation	Comments
Confirmation of HIV seropositivity	Baseline assessment
CD4+ cell count Quantitative HIV RNA	Test every 3 months and after 2 weeks of changes in treatment
Antiretroviral resistance testing	With virologic failure
Complete and differential blood count Chemistry panel with liver enzymes Urinalysis Lipid profile Glucose-6-phosphate dehydrogenase (G6PD) Hepatitis B surface antigen (HBsAg); surface and core antibody Hepatitis C antibody	Anemia with zidovudine Glucose and lipids with protease inhibitors (PIs) Nephrotoxicity with indinavir Baseline testing as clinically indicated
Electroencephalogram Chest radiograph	As clinically indicated
Serologic test for syphilis *Toxoplasma gondii* antibody	As often as clinically indicated
Pap smear: cervical and anal for women and anal for men	Annual test indicated

Table 17-5 Recommendations for Initiating Antiretroviral Therapy in Treatment-Naive Adults with Chronic HIV Infection

Measure	Antiretroviral Therapy Recommended (Rating)*
Patients with history of AIDS-defining illness	A
Patients with Asymptomatic HIV Disease:	
CD4+ cell count ≤200/µL	A
CD4+ cell count <350/µL but >200/µL	A
CD4+ cell count <500/µL but >350/µL	A/B
CD4+ cell count >500/µL	B
Other Patients (regardless of CD4+ T-cell count)	
Pregnant women	A
Patients with HIV-associated nephropathy	A
Patients co-infected with hepatitis B virus (HBV) when treatment is indicated	B

*Strength of recommendation: A, based on consistent and good-quality patient oriented evidence; B, based on inconsistent or limited-quality patient-oriented evidence; C, based on consensus, usual practice, opinion, and disease-oriented evidence.

antiretroviral-naive patients. FIs are only indicated in antiretro-viral-experienced patients. The latest guidelines provided significant changes from the previous version, especially on what combinations regimen to start in antiretroviral-naive subjects. Current standards of care in antiretroviral-naive patients recommend using three medications (three active agents), combining an NNRTI, a PI, or an INSTI with two NRTIs. This combination of "highly active antiretroviral therapy" has been labeled HAART.

Maraviroc was the only agent excluded by the 2009 guidelines as either a preferred or an alternative agent in antiretroviral-naive individuals. Maraviroc is a CCR5 inhibitor, comparable to efavirenz in terms of virologic response. Maraviroc blocks the CCR5 co-receptor but not the CXCR4 co-receptor. At this time, utility of maraviroc is limited because the Trofile test is required to screen for co-receptor use. Maraviroc will likely be recommended in future guidelines.

The number of preferred PIs was reduced to two: ritonavir-boosted darunavir and ritonavir-boosted atazanavir. Both of these are once-daily options, requiring only 1 capsule of 100 mg of ritonavir to enhance their pharmacokinetics. All other PIs were kept as alternative options for various reasons, including tolerability, toxicity, and efficacy. The dose of ritonavir used to boost PIs exerts negligible antiviral activity. However, it serves the important function of acting as a pharmacokinetic enhancer, increasing drug exposure and prolonging plasma half-life of the combined PI.

In terms of alternative options, it is important to keep in mind that most of these agents are occasionally preferred medications in different settings. A good example is the use of ritonavir-boosted lopinavir in pregnancy. In general, PIs remain valid options to initiate therapy. The PIs as a drug class have been associated with higher rates of adverse gastrointestinal events and potentially cardiovascular events, especially in populations with high cardiovascular risk.

Box 17-4 Antiretroviral Regimens for Treatment-Naive Patients

Preferred Regimens: Level 1

Ritonavir-boosted darunavir + tenofovir + emtricitabine

Ritonavir-boosted atazanavir + tenofovir + emtricitabine

Efavirenz + tenofovir + emtricitabine

Raltegravir + tenofovir + emtricitabine

Alternative Regimens: Level 2

Efavirenz + (abacavir *or* zidovudine)/lamivudine

Nevirapine + zidovudine/lamivudine

Atazanavir/ritonavir + (abacavir *or* zidovudine)/lamivudine

FPV/r* (once or twice daily) + *either* [(abacavir *or* zidovudine)lamivudine] *or* tenofovir/emtricitabine

LPV/r† (once or twice daily) + *either* [(abacavir *or* zidovudine)/lamivudine] *or* tenofovir/emtricitabine

Saquinavir/ritonavir + tenofovir/emtricitabine

*Fosamprenavir calcium and ritonavir.
†Lopinavir and ritonavir (Kaletra).

The preferred NNRTI continues to be efavirenz, with nevirapine (Viramune) remaining an alternative option. Efavirenz now comes coformulated with two other NRTIs, emtricitabine and tenofovir, in a single pill (Atripla) to be taken once daily as a complete antiretroviral regimen, which has increased prescriptions for Atripla. Atripla is not recommended for pregnant women because of potential CNS malformations; Physicians

Table 17-6 Antiretroviral Medicines

Generic (Brand)	Abbreviation
Nucleoside/Nucleotide Reverse-Transcriptase Inhibitors (NRTIs)	
Abacavir (Ziagen)	ABC
Emtricitabine (Emtriva)	FTC
Didanosine (Videx)	ddI
Lamivudine (Epivir)	3TC
Stavudine (Zerit)	d4T
Tenofovir (Viread)	TDF
Zalcitabine (Hivid)	ddC
Zidovudine (Retrovir)	ZDV
Abacavir and lamivudine (Epzicom)	ABC + 3TC
Emtricitabine and tenofovir (Truvada)	FTC + TDF
Lamivudine and zidovudine (Combivir)	3TC + ZDV
Nonnucleoside Reverse-Transcriptase Inhibitors (NNRTIs)	
Delavirdine mesylate (Rescriptor)	DLV
Efavirenz (EFV)	EFV
Etravirine (Intelence)	TMC-125

Generic (Brand)	Abbreviation
Nevirapine (Viramune)	NVP
Efavirenz, emtricitabine, and tenofovir (Atripla)	EFV + FTC + TDF
Protease Inhibitors (PIs)	
Atazanavir (Reyataz)	ATZ
Darunavir (Prezista)	TMC-114
Fosamprenavir calcium (Lexiva)	FPV
Indinavir sulfate (Crixivan)	IDV
Lopinavir and ritonavir (Kaletra)	LPV/r
Nelfinavir mesylate (Viracept)	NFV
Ritonavir (Norvir)	RTV
Saquinavir mesylate (Invirase)	SQV
Tipranavir (Aptivus)	TPV
Fusion Inhibitor	
Enfuvirtide (Fuzeon)	T-20
CCR5 Inhibitor	
Maraviroc (Selzentry)	
Integrase Strand Transfer Inhibitor	
Raltegravir (Isentress)	

Table 17-7 Antiretroviral Combinations to Avoid

Combination	Rationale for Avoidance
Atazanavir with proton pump inhibitors	Decrease in atazanavir absorption
Unboosted PIs with rifampin	Significant decrease in PI blood levels
Nevirapine in women with CD4+ >250 cells/mm³ or men with CD4+ >400 cells/mm³	Risk of serious and life-threatening hepatic events. Switching to nevirapine is possible once CD4+ count has increased beyond these levels with ART.
Efavirenz with itraconazole	Decrease in efavirenz blood levels
Abacavir in patients who are HLA 5701 positive	High potential for serious "abacavir hypersensitivity reaction"
Maraviroc in patients with dual/mixed or CXR4-utilizing virus	Because maraviroc is a CCR5 inhibitor, CXCR4-utilizing viruses respond inadequately or negligibly to treatment.

PIs, Protease inhibitors; *ART*, antiretroviral therapy.

must be cautious when prescribing efavirenz in fertile women because risk is highest during the first trimester. Nevirapine is not recommended in women with pretreatment CD4+ counts greater than 250 cells/mm³ or in men with CD4+ counts greater than 400 (level 2) because of a higher risk of serious hepatic events in these two groups (Table 17-7).

Both patient characteristics and physician preferences must necessarily be weighed when choosing between efavirenz and PIs. The preferred NRTI is emtricitabine coformulated with tenofovir, a one-pill-once-daily medication that has been compared with the other two coformulated NRTIs, lamivudine/zidovudine, and abacavir/lamivudine, because the former showed a better safety profile and virologic efficacy.

Once the antiretroviral regimen is selected, medication compliance becomes the most important factor in treatment success.

Table 17-8 Recommendations for Initiation and Discontinuation of Primary Prophylaxis of Most Common Opportunistic Infections (OIs)

OI	Initiation	Discontinuation	Drug of choice
PCP	CD4+ cell count <200 cells/mm^3	CD4+ cell count >200 cells/mm^3	TMP-SMX (Bactrim)
Toxoplasma gondii encephalitis	Seropositive for *T. gondii* and CD4+ cell count <100 cells/mm^3	CD4+ cell count >200 cells/mm^3	TMP-SMX (Bactrim) for PCP serves as primary prophylaxis. Suppressive regimen of choice for secondary prophylaxis is sulfadiazine plus pyrimethamine and leucovorin
MAC	CD4+ cell count <50 cells/mm^3	CD4+ cell count >100 cells/mm^3	Zithromycin, azithromycin
CMV retinitis	Primary prophylaxis is not routinely recommended; discontinuation of secondary prophylaxis can be considered in patients with a sustained response to HAART, defined as a CD4+ cell count greater than 100 to 150 cells/mm^3 for at least 6 months.		
Cryptococcus neoformans meningitis	Primary prophylaxis is not routinely recommended; discontinuation of secondary prophylaxis can be considered in patients with a sustained response to HAART, defined as a CD4+ cell count greater than 150 to 200 cells/mm^3 for at least 6 months.		

TMP-SMX, Trimethoprim-sulfamethoxazole; *PCP, Pneumocystis jiroveci (carinii)* pneumonia; *MAC, Mycobacterium avium* complex; *CMV*, cytomegalovirus.

An adequate response is expected between weeks 16 and 24 after initiation of ART. Other important factors for physicians treating HIV disease include close follow-up and monitoring of drug toxicities. Treatment success is defined as virologic suppression to undetectable HIV RNA (viral load) to the lowest detectable testing available (<48 copies/mL).

The wide use of HAART has helped decrease OI-related mortality in HIV-positive patients. OIs continue to cause morbidity and mortality for the following reasons:

1. Opportunistic infections are the main indicator of disease that drives many people who may be unaware of their HIV status to seek medical attention.
2. Highly active retroviral therapy may not be available to many patients for a variety of psychological and socioeconomic reasons.
3. Certain patients who are prescribed HAART may not experience virologic or immunologic response because of suboptimal adherence, pharmacokinetics, or unknown biologic issues.

Some OIs may cause a transient increase in viral load that may promote HIV disease progression and increase transmission. HAART becomes especially important to combat OIs for which specific treatments are unavailable.

Recommendations for the initiation and discontinuation of primary prophylactic medications are summarized in Table 17-8. Criteria to initiate or discontinue primary prophylaxis include the following:

1. Adequate CD4+ (immunologic) response.
2. The degree of virulence of the opportunistic agent. Thus the CD4+ cell count to minimize the risk of acquiring a specific illness will vary.

3. Other factors to consider in discontinuation of prophylaxis are the reduction of drug resistance, polypharmacy, drug to drug interactions, and cost.

Postexposure prophylaxis (PEP) of HIV infection in exposed individuals must be initiated within hours of exposure, if possible. The route of exposure may well be from mucous membranes, broken skin, or percutaneous route. The decision to initiate prophylaxis must be considered carefully because it is associated with potential morbidity and side effects. HIV testing must be performed at the time of exposure, at 6 and 12 weeks, and then 6 months later. Two-NRTI or three-drug (+ PI) regimens are recommended, depending on the severity of exposure.

Summary

Family physicians have treated HIV-positive patients ever since HIV was identified as the virus that causes AIDS in 1981 and continue to play a central role from the time of routine screening and diagnosis to the point where the disease stabilizes and becomes chronic. While consultation with a specialist may be needed for difficult-to-manage patients, family physicians can successfully care for HIV-positive patients. Acute retroviral infection may be difficult to differentiate from common community-acquired viruses. The approach to a patient must be respectful, nonjudgmental, and confidential. DHHS guidelines provide useful information about treatment of HIV with HAART. Treatment with HAART extends life and improves quality of life but is associated with significant morbidity and side effects.

KEY TREATMENT

Patients with a history of OI's and a CD4+ count less than 200 are likely to benefit most from HAART, but current recommendations suggest that HAART be initiated in those with count of 350 to 500 or even higher.

Current standards of care recommend using three medications (active agents), combining an NNRTI, a PI, or an INSTI with two NRTIs. Most antiretrovirals occasionally are preferred agents in different settings.

Darunavir or atazanavir boosted with ritonavir are the only two PIs preferred. The preferred NNRTI remains efavirenz.

Efavirenz now comes coformulated with emtricitabine (a preferred NRTI) and tenofovir in a once-daily pill (Atripla).

Adherence to the regimen becomes the most important factor once a regimen is selected.

Adequate response is expected at 16 to 24 months. Success is defined as suppression of viral load to 48 copies/mL.

Postexposure prophylaxis involves administration of two NRTIs with or without a PI.

References

The complete reference list is available online at www.expertconsult.com.

Web Resources

www.aidsetc.org
    A useful resource for clinical diagnosis and management.
www.aegis.org
    The largest HIV/AIDS website in the world; updated hourly.
www.aidsinfo.nih.gov
    Treatment guidelines, drug data, and information on clinical trials.

www.cdc.gov/hiv Free HIV/AIDS
    Publications and epidemiologic data.
www.thebody.com
    Excellent resource for patients.

CHAPTER 18

Pulmonary Medicine

George Rust and Gloria Westney

Chapter contents

Lung Disease in Primary Care

Breathing and heartbeat draw the line between life and death. Pulmonary disease, respiratory symptoms, and respiratory failure are common, high-impact conditions. For example, asthma is the most common chronic disease of childhood, respiratory failure causes many admissions to our nation's intensive care units (ICUs), and lung cancer is now the leading cause of cancer death for both men and women in America. Lung cancer accounts for 31% of cancer deaths in men and 25% of cancer deaths in women (American Cancer Society, 2002). In part because of the global spread of tobacco, the World Health Organization (WHO) estimates that chronic obstructive pulmonary disease will move from being the 12th leading cause of disease burden, as measured by lost disability-adjusted life-years (DALY), to being the fifth leading cause by 2020 (Murray and Lopez, 1996).

Roses are red, violets are blue;

Without your lungs, you would be too!

Smoking and Other Risk Factors for Lung Disease

The Centers for Disease Control and Prevention (CDC) describe smoking as the single most preventable cause of premature death in the United States, contributing to more than 400,000 deaths per year, or one in every five deaths. People who smoke suffer more than a 20-fold increase in risk of death from lung cancer and a 10-fold increase in risk of death resulting from bronchitis or emphysema (CDC, 1993). For women in the United States, there are more deaths caused by lung cancer than by breast cancer. Worldwide there were 5 million deaths attributable to smoking in 2000, almost 2 million of which were related to lung cancer and other lung diseases. WHO projects a doubling of smoking-related deaths by 2020 (Ezzati, 2003).

Smoking cessation is the most important factor in preventing lung and cardiovascular disease and all-cause mortality. Avoidance of secondary exposure to smoke, especially in the household, is also important in preventing childhood asthma and infections as well as adult cancers (DHHS, 2006).

Even simple physician advice to quit smoking provides a marginal benefit of 2.5% of patients quitting successfully (Lancaster and Stead, 2004). Interventions that combine counseling plus education or group strategies plus pharmacologic treatment with nicotine replacement or specific medications can achieve sustained quit rates of 25% to 30% (Hughes et al., 2004; Solomon et al., 2005; Stead and Lancaster, 2005). The Agency for Healthcare Research and Quality (AHRQ, 2008) has provided a comprehensive update to previous clinical guidelines for smoking cessation and treating tobacco dependence. Counseling is most effective when it includes both practical problem solving and social support. Pharmacologic treatment, such as nicotine replacement, bupropion, and varenicline, has proved effective but is most effective when combined with counseling or group programs. The Legacy Foundation reports that ex-smokers have an average of eight quit attempts before ultimately sustaining a tobacco-free lifestyle. Box 18-1 defines a strategy for helping patients to quit smoking by a simple mnemonic of "five As" (ask, advise, assess, assist, arrange).

Box 18-1 The Five As: Strategies to Help Patients Quit Smoking

Ask: Systematically identify all tobacco users at every visit.

Implement an office-wide system that ensures that, for *every* patient at *every* clinic visit, tobacco use status is queried and documented.

Advise: Strongly urge all tobacco users to quit.

In a clear, strong, and personalized manner, urge every tobacco user to quit.

Assess: Determine willingness to make a quit attempt.

Ask every tobacco user if he or she is willing to make a quit attempt at this time (e.g., within the next 30 days).

Assist: Aid the patient in quitting.

Help the patient with a quit plan; provide practical counseling; provide intra-treatment social support; help the patient obtain extra-treatment social support; recommend use of approved pharmacotherapy except in special circumstances; provide supplementary materials.

Arrange: Schedule follow-up contact.

Schedule follow-up contact, either in person or via telephone.

From Global Initiative for Chronic Obstructive Lung Disease: Executive Summary: Global Strategy for the Diagnosis, Management, and Prevention of COPD. Updated 2008. http://www.goldcopd.com/download.asp?intId=504.

Diagnostic Tools in Pulmonary Medicine

History and Physical Examination

Diagnosis starts with the patient history and physical examination. Pulmonary symptoms may be evaluated by traditional history-of-present-illness questions, such as character and quality of the symptoms, duration, onset, timing, exacerbating and alleviating factors, efforts at self-treatment, and the patient's own understanding of what is causing the symptoms. For example, the symptoms of asthma may be variously described by patients as shortness of breath, wheezing, whistling, "wheezling," chest tightness, tight breathing, or poor exercise tolerance. In addition, patients often self-medicate with over-the-counter (OTC) and prescription medications, as well as use herbal and nonmedicinal alternative therapies, which they typically do not report to their personal physician unless specifically asked (Braganza et al., 2003).

In addition to general history-taking, a detailed history of respiratory exposures and risk factors is essential. Smoking is perhaps the most important pulmonary risk factor. A detailed smoking history includes age of first smoking, quantity smoked, number of years as a smoker, other tobacco use, previous attempts to quit, and an assessment of the level of nicotine addiction. Family history can reveal relatives with immunoglobulin E (IgE)–mediated allergy or *atopy* (allergic rhinitis, asthma, eczema, nasal polyps, or aspirin hypersensitivity) or even more serious genetic risk factors, such as cystic fibrosis or α_1-antitrypsin deficiency. Perinatal history of premature birth, neonatal respiratory failure, and ventilator care can lead to bronchopulmonary dysplasia and chronic lung disease in children who survive neonatal intensive care.

Taking a good occupational history is also essential, asking the specific type of work the patient performs, as well as past jobs. In addition, the clinician should ask two key questions: "Have you ever been exposed to fumes, gases, or dusts?" and "Do your symptoms get better when you are away from work, during weekends and vacations?"

Physical examination begins with vital signs. For example, tachypnea out of proportion to fever may be the first presenting sign of childhood pneumonia. The degree of respiratory difficulty may also be observed in the form of obvious shortness of breath, the work of breathing, the use of accessory respiratory muscles, and the patient's need to take a breath in midsentence (described as *three-to-four-word dyspnea*). General examination can also reveal either peripheral or central cyanosis. Clubbing of the nails can indicate chronic lung disease. Morbid obesity may be associated with obstructive sleep apnea or right-sided heart failure *(cor pulmonale)*, or both.

Examination of the chest begins with inspection and progresses to percussion, palpation, and auscultation. Inspection can reveal chest deformities (pectus excavatum or flail chest) or spinal deformities (kyphosis or scoliosis) that interfere with breathing, or an enlarged anteroposterior (AP) diameter in adults with chronically hyperexpanded lungs. Adults with morbid obesity or prior chest trauma that restricts chest wall motion can have pulmonary function tests consistent with restrictive lung disease of extrapulmonary origin. Infants and children in respiratory distress can have retractions.

Palpation can identify thoracic wall abnormalities, mass lesions, or tenderness and show asymmetry of chest wall expansion. Percussion of lung fields should normally be resonant. Dullness to percussion can indicate fluid in the pleural space or consolidation of the lung itself, with fluid filling the normally air-filled alveolar spaces. Both these conditions also produce decreased breath sounds over the affected area. Hyperresonant lung fields on percussion can indicate the hyperexpansion of obstructive lung disease or even pneumothorax.

Auscultation should include listening over upper, middle, and lower lung fields of each lung posteriorly, as well as over the apices and mid–lung fields anteriorly. The right middle lobe of the lung and the lingula of the left lung can only be heard anteriorly. In addition to identifying areas of decreased breath sounds, the quality of lung sounds on auscultation can further differentiate underlying lung pathology. Normal (vesicular) lung sounds are continuous. Other continuous breath sounds include wheezing (sibilant or musical rhonchi) and bronchial (tubular) breath sounds ("Darth Vader" or snorkel breathing), which occur normally over the trachea or upper anterior chest wall. Discontinuous breath sounds include the sound of small alveolar sacs popping open in fluid-based lung consolidation, which are heard as adventitial lung sounds such as fine rales or crackles. This can occur in both bases, as in congestive heart failure, or in a more localized area, as in a lobar pneumonia. The sound has been described as similar to tufts of hair being rubbed together close to the ear.

Because decreased breath sounds and dullness to percussion can represent either fluid in the pleural space or consolidation of the lungs themselves, additional physical findings can help differentiate the two conditions. Vocal fremitus and tactile fremitus are increased in lung consolidation but decreased in pleural effusion. Localized egophony ("e-to-a" changes) indicates consolidation of that segment or lobe of the lung; it is not present in pleural effusion except in a small band just above the upper edge of the effusion.

Signs of bronchial inflammation, mucus, and obstruction in the bronchial tree include coarse crackles and wheezes (sonorous or musical rhonchi). Additionally, in normal vesicular breathing, the duration of the inspiratory phase is longer than the expiratory phase—typically 90% of the expired air is exhaled in the first second. Prolongation of the expiratory phase is an early sign of obstruction, even before wheezing develops. The diagnostic implications of these physical examination findings are summarized in Table 18-1.

Pulmonary Function Testing

Key Points

- Obstructive lung disease is diagnosed by demonstrating a ratio of forced expiratory volume at 1 second (FEV_1) to forced vital capacity (FVC) (or FEV_1/FEV_6 ratio) of less than 70%.
- Improvement in FEV_1 of at least 12% and at least 200 mL from prebronchodilator to postbronchodilator is considered evidence of reversibility of airway obstruction.
- Restrictive lung disease can be diagnosed using office spirometry if the FVC is reduced to less than 80% of predicted, in the presence of a normal FEV_1/FVC ratio (i.e., no obstruction).

Pulmonary function testing is essential for detecting lung disease and for differentiating obstructive from restrictive lung disease. Pulmonary function tests (PFTs) may be done in a hospital-based pulmonary function laboratory or, more often, in the outpatient setting using office spirometry. The simplest PFT is the *peak expiratory flow rate* (PEFR), measured by hand-held mechanical peak-flow meters given to patients for self-management and used in office settings and emergency departments (EDs) for quick assessment during acute exacerbations of asthma. PEFR is the maximum flow generated during expiration performed with maximal force ("Take a deep breath and blow out as hard and as fast as you can").

Previous office spirometry units were bulky and required frequent recalibration, but modern units are small, computerized, and often self-calibrating. Quality of testing is important. The patient should be seated comfortably and instructed appropriately. An adequate PFT must include three valid measures (quick start, good effort, maintenance of forced expiration for at least 6 seconds with no cough) and three relatively similar results (FVC varying by <200 mL).

Table 18-1 Physical Findings in Common Pulmonary Disorders

Disorder	Inspection	Palpation	Percussion	Auscultation
Bronchial asthma (acute attack)	Hyperinflation; use of accessory muscles	Impaired expansion; decreased fremitus	Hyperresonance; low diaphragm	Prolonged expiration; inspiratory and expiratory wheezes
Pneumothorax (complete)	Lag on affected side	Absent fremitus	Hyperresonant or tympanitic	Absent breath sounds
Pleural effusion (large)	Lag on affected side	Decreased fremitus; trachea and heart shifted away from affected side	Dullness or flatness	Absent breath sounds
Atelectasis (lobar obstruction)	Lag on affected side	Decreased fremitus; trachea and heart shifted toward affected side	Dullness or flatness	Absent breath sounds
Consolidation (pneumonia)	Possible lag or splinting on affected side	Increased fremitus	Dullness	Bronchial breath sounds; bronchophony; pectoriloquy; crackles

Modified from Hinshaw HC, Murray JF. Diseases of the Chest, 4th ed. Philadelphia, Saunders, 1980, p 23.

Results of office spirometry are presented both graphically and numerically, with actual values compared to values predicted by the patient's age, height, and gender. Figure 18-1 shows the points at which two critical values, *forced expiratory volume at 1 second* (FEV$_1$) and *forced vital capacity* (FVC), are measured on the time-volume curve. Figure 18-2 shows a typical flow-volume loop for patients that compares normal PFTs with obstructive lung disease and restrictive lung disease (Zoorob et al., 2002). Increasingly, the 6-second end point, or FEV$_6$, is being used as a reliable and reproducible surrogate measure that can replace FVC for patients unable to complete forced expiration beyond 6 seconds.

The key parameters of office spirometry are the FEV$_1$, the FVC, and the FEV$_1$/FVC ratio (percentage of exhaled volume blown out in first second of exhalation). The diagnosis of obstructive lung disease is made by demonstrating an FEV$_1$/FVC ratio (or FEV$_1$/FEV$_6$) of less than 70%. This means that the patient has exhaled less than 70% of FVC (full volume of air exhaled) in the first second of exhalation. Other tests of airway obstruction are the *mid-maximal expiratory flow rate* (MMEF, or FEF$_{25-75}$), which is the average expiratory flow over the middle half of expiration, that is, flow rate during the

time when 25% to 75% of the FVC is exhaled. This measure has been described as representing small airway obstruction, but it is less reproducible and has not been included in clinical guidelines for managing patients with obstructive lung disease. However, MMEF can be an early indicator of lung damage caused by smoking or occupational pneumoconioses. The FEF$_{25}$ and FEF$_{75}$ are moment-in-time measures of expiratory airflow and are therefore subject to significant patient-to-patient variability unrelated to clinical factors.

One other dimension of office spirometry in diagnosing and managing obstructive lung disease is to measure these parameters before and after a dose of inhaled beta-2 (β_2)–adrenergic agonist is given. Improvement in FEV$_1$ of at least 12% and at least 200 mL from prebronchodilator to postbronchodilator measurement is considered evidence of reversibility of airway obstruction. Complete reversibility helps establish the diagnosis of asthma, and it is also useful in guiding therapy by establishing the potential efficacy of medications. For example, some patients with chronic obstructive pulmonary disease (COPD) are more responsive to anticholinergic medications such as inhaled ipratropium, whereas others are more responsive to inhaled β_2-agonists such as albuterol.

For restrictive lung disease, the "gold-standard" test is the *total lung capacity* (TLC), which is a measure of maximal exhaled air (FVC) plus residual capacity (RC). However, this can only be tested in pulmonary function laboratories that can test the patient in a sealed chamber. For practical purposes in the primary care setting, restrictive lung disease can be diagnosed using office spirometry if the FVC is reduced to less than 80% of predicted in the presence of a normal FEV$_1$/FVC ratio (i.e., no obstruction). One other test that is available in pulmonary function labs but not in office spirometry is the *diffusion capacity* (DL$_{CO}$), which is a measure of the diffusion of carbon monoxide across the alveolar-capillary membrane. Clinical reductions in DL$_{CO}$ can occur with thickening of the alveolocapillary membrane, which can be a sign of interstitial fibrosis.

Chest Radiography and Other Diagnostic Imaging

Despite major advances in imaging technology, the chest x-ray film (CXR) is still an important diagnostic modality that can clearly reveal signs of pneumonia, COPD, heart

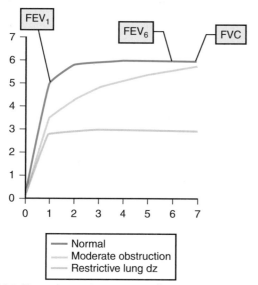

Figure 18-1 Time-volume spirometry curve showing measurement of FEV$_1$, FVC, and FEV$_6$ and curves for obstructive versus restrictive lung disease.

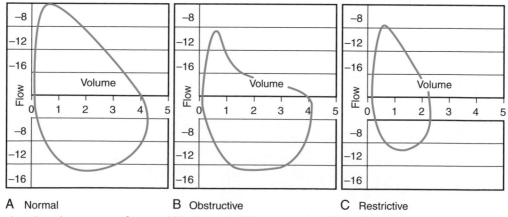

A Normal   B Obstructive   C Restrictive

Figure 18-2 Flow-volume loop showing curves for normal **(A)**, obstructive **(B)**, and restrictive **(C)** lung disease.

failure, tuberculosis, lung masses, and pleural effusion. Figure 18-3 shows a chest radiograph with right middle lobe pneumonia. Although the posteroanterior (PA) film shows some consolidation, it is attenuated by the overlying projection of a normal lower lobe. The lateral film, however, shows the classic wedge-shaped profile of a consolidated right middle lobe.

Chest radiography is also widely used in evaluating patients with suspected exposure to tuberculosis (TB), either because of symptoms, personal contact, or a positive intradermal purified protein derivative (PPD) test. Figure 18-4 shows the patchy infiltrates and hilar adenopathy typical of pulmonary TB, although TB can have a variety of presentations on chest x-ray films, including adenopathy, pleural scarring, infiltrates, cavitary lesions, and miliary TB.

Chest radiography can also be helpful in diagnosing nonpulmonary causes of shortness of breath, as in the case of congestive heart failure, with enlarged heart, bibasilar consolidation, small pleural effusions, and prominent pulmonary vasculature. In other conditions such as asthma, chest x-ray films can be quite normal despite significant respiratory compromise.

Increasingly, chest computed tomography (CT) scan plays an important role in diagnosing lung disease. High-resolution CT (HRCT) can identify pulmonary nodules and hilar lymph nodes at much smaller sizes than can chest radiography, and it is therefore important in diagnosing and staging lung cancers. CT can also detect lung abscess, vascular lesions, and pleural scarring or masses. Whereas early COPD or emphysematous changes can be difficult to detect with even HRCT, additional techniques such as minimum-intensity projection (MIP) can aggregate data from adjacent slices and, by subtracting vascular and other tissue densities not consistent with lung parenchyma and air, demonstrate small air pockets consistent with early emphysema.

Imaging modalities such as spiral CT have been demonstrated to be effective in detecting early lung cancer in patients with high-risk smoking histories, but as yet they have not demonstrated improvements in mortality that would justify this as a universal screening test for smokers in primary care practice. When small, noncalcified pulmonary nodules are detected by CT, the likelihood of malignancy is influenced by nodule size, density, number of nodules, and growth over time, combined with patient factors such as age, smoking history, gender, spirometry, occupational history, and endemic granulomatous disease (Libby et al., 2004).

Positron emission tomography scans using ^{18}F-fluorodeoxyglucose (FDG-PET) are becoming increasingly useful in evaluating lung cancers and lymphomas. The ability to define anatomy and metabolism, that is, glucose uptake within the

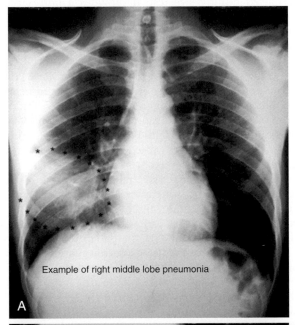

Example of right middle lobe pneumonia

A

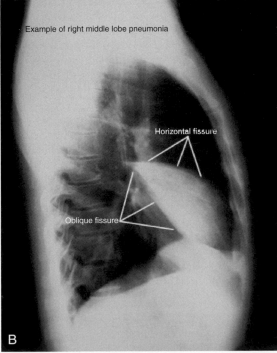

Example of right middle lobe pneumonia

Horizontal fissure

Oblique fissure

B

Figure 18-3 Posteroanterior (**A**) and lateral (**B**) chest radiographs showing right middle lobe pneumonia. *(From Department of Neurobiology and Developmental Sciences, University of Arkansas for Medical Sciences, Little Rock. http://anatomy.uams.edu/ anatomyhtml/xrays/xra_ atlas39.html and http://anatomy.uams.edu/anatomyhtml/xrays/ xra_atlas5.html.)*

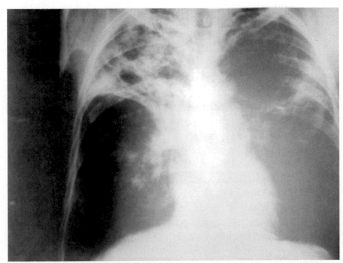

Figure 18-4 Chest radiograph showing tuberculosis, with upper lobe fibrotic patchy infiltrates and hilar adenopathy. *(From Centers for Disease Control and Prevention, Public Health Image Library, Image 2543. http://phil.cdc.gov/phil/home.asp.)*

tumor, makes the PET scan useful for staging, detecting node involvement, and defining resectability, tumor response to therapy, and tumor recurrence (Avril and Weber, 2005). Diagnosing solitary pulmonary nodules is a common challenge in primary care. A meta-analysis of studies comparing dynamic CT, magnetic resonance imaging (MRI), FDG-PET, and single-photon emission computed tomography (SPECT) scans based on positive and negative likelihood ratios for identifying malignant versus nonmalignant solitary nodules found that all four were similarly accurate (Cronin et al., 2008). Nuclear medicine studies such as gallium scans are also used extensively in evaluating pulmonary symptoms in patients with human immunodeficiency virus (HIV) infection or acquired immunodeficiency syndrome (AIDS) and are discussed in the section on HIV-related pulmonary infections in more detail.

Other imaging studies have more specific indications. One nuclear medicine study long used in primary care is the ventilation-perfusion (V/Q) scan. This is specifically performed to rule out pulmonary embolism, revealed by focal perfusion defects in adequately ventilated areas. This V/Q mismatch, in the absence of underlying lung pathology, is consistent with a high probability of pulmonary embolism. Unfortunately, patients can also demonstrate matching V/Q defects, which can occur when blood flow is shunted away from an under-ventilated area of the lung. Scans with no perfusion defect reflect a low probability for significant pulmonary embolism. Other tests are increasingly taking the place of the V/Q scan (see later discussion).

Bronchoscopy

Fiberoptic bronchoscopy allows direct visualization of the bronchial tree. It is useful for diagnosing conditions that require culture of a lower respiratory tract infection by bronchoalveolar lavage (BAL), or conditions such as bronchogenic carcinoma, that require tissue diagnosis by transbronchial biopsy. Sometimes these techniques are combined, as in the diagnosis of *Pneumocystis jiroveci (carinii)* pneumonia (PCP), for which the sensitivity of bronchoscopy with BAL is approximately 86% and with transbronchial biopsy is 87% (Broaddus et al., 1985). A comparative assessment of different bronchoscopic techniques in obtaining culture specimens in cases of ventilator-associated pneumonia found no significant difference between blind bronchial brushings and bronchoscope-assisted lavage, bronchoscope-directed brushings, or even blind endotracheal aspirates (Wood et al., 2003). Rates of complications (including hemoptysis and pneumothorax) with traditional bronchoscopy are in the range of 0.5% to 1.0% without biopsy and up to 6.8% with transbronchial biopsy (Pue and Pacht, 1995). In a pulmonary fellowship program, the rate of complications for all bronchoscopies performed (with and without biopsy) was 2.06% (Ouellette, 2006). Therapeutic interventions using bronchoscopy are also increasing, and lesions are treated through the bronchoscope with laser, cryotherapy, electrocautery, and stents (Rafanan and Mehta, 2000).

Newer diagnostic techniques include fluorescent bronchoscopy, which can be more sensitive for detecting early endobronchial tumors (Gilbert et al., 2004; Moghissi et al., 2008), and virtual bronchoscopy, which uses sophisticated software to reconstruct images from HRCT scan, to create three-dimensional imagery without invasive testing. This technique has been found useful in planning partial lung resection surgery, for example, but it cannot provide bronchoscopy's direct visualization of color, texture, or friability of the bronchial mucosa (Finklestein et al., 2004).

Measurement of Blood Gases

Measurement and monitoring of blood gases can be invasive or noninvasive. Transcutaneous pulse oximetry is the most widely used noninvasive test. It provides a fairly accurate measure of oxygen saturation (So_2) of hemoglobin at values ranging from 70% to 100% by measuring the difference between oxyhemoglobin and reduced hemoglobin in the absorption of light of specific wavelengths. So_2 of 98% corresponds to an arterial oxygen partial pressure (Pao_2) of 100 mm Hg, and 95% to a Pao_2 of 80 mm Hg, demonstrating the challenge of interpreting a test with a 95% confidence interval of ±5%. An oxygen saturation of less than 89% corresponds to a Pao_2 of less than 60 mm Hg. Decreased tissue perfusion or color changes caused by jaundice or intravascular dyes can degrade accuracy. Arterial oxygen levels can also be measured transcutaneously ($tcPo_2$) with a skin surface oxygen electrode, but its accuracy is also affected by tissue perfusion, skin temperature, and other factors.

Exhaled carbon dioxide can also be measured noninvasively, most often in the ICU for patients on mechanical ventilation or in operating rooms during general anesthesia. Capnography, colorimetric techniques, and CO_2 sensors can detect failure of mechanical ventilation or improper endotracheal tube placement, which generate hypercapnia secondary to hypoventilation.

The invasive technique most often used for measuring oxygen, CO_2, and acid-base blood chemistries is the arterial blood gas (ABG) measurement. Although it requires an arterial needle puncture and several milliliters of blood, it is highly accurate and reproducible. ABG measurement is indicated in any patient with acute respiratory distress or in managing the patient with respiratory failure. In addition to Pao_2 and arterial carbon dioxide partial pressure ($Paco_2$) measurements, ABG testing also provides a measure of pH, bicarbonate (HCO_3^-), and the anion gap, which can be used to detect respiratory (rather than metabolic) causes of acidosis and alkalosis. Patients with moderate to severe COPD can have chronic hypoxia plus chronic hypercapnia (decreased Pao_2 and increased $Paco_2$). They can also show signs of primary respiratory acidosis (reduced pH with elevated CO_2), and a compensatory metabolic alkalosis (partial normalization of the pH despite elevated $Paco_2$) mediated by renal HCO_3^- retention. Nomograms or software used in personal digital assistants (PDAs) allow simultaneous plotting of pH, CO_2, and HCO_3^- to facilitate interpretation of mixed respiratory and metabolic acid-base disturbances.

Common Pulmonary Symptoms

Shortness of Breath

A common presenting symptom in pulmonary disease is shortness of breath. The fundamental question in patients presenting with recent-onset or episodic shortness of breath is this: Is it a lung problem, a heart problem, or something else? The most common pulmonary causes of chronic or repeated episodes of shortness of breath include asthma, smoking-related COPD, chronic lung infections (TB and HIV-related infections), and occupational pneumoconiosis. Acute-onset shortness of breath can be caused by acute exacerbations of any of these chronic conditions, by acute infections such as pneumonia or acute bronchitis, or by spontaneous pneumothorax. Among otherwise healthy children, shortness of breath can be related to asthma, bronchiolitis, pneumonia, or upper-airway problems such as croup or epiglottitis. Chronic shortness of breath in children can be related to poorly controlled asthma, bronchopulmonary dysplasia from infancy, or chronic diseases (e.g., cystic fibrosis).

The cardiovascular system is the other organ system most often linked to shortness of breath. In adults, congestive heart failure (CHF) is a leading cause of recent-onset shortness of breath among middle-aged and older adults. In addition to shortness of breath, patients might report symptoms of wheezing from the pulmonary congestion, often referred to as *cardiac asthma*. Differentiating early CHF from pulmonary causes of dyspnea can be a challenge in middle-aged or older patients who smoke or have other chronic medical conditions. Other cardiac conditions associated with shortness of breath include pericarditis and cardiomyopathy, as well as congenital heart defects in infants presenting with respiratory distress. Vascular conditions include chronic pulmonary hypertension and pulmonary embolism in the setting of acute-onset shortness of breath.

Along with the history and physical examination, testing can help in ruling out pulmonary versus cardiac causes of dyspnea. Physicians often begin diagnostic testing with electrocardiogram (ECG) and even echocardiogram to rule out cardiac causes of shortness of breath, but simple history, auscultation of the heart and lungs, chest radiograph, and office spirometry can also assess for common pulmonary causes of shortness of breath. Improvement on weekends or non-workdays can suggest an occupational exposure, and a prolonged expiratory phase with expiratory wheezing suggests obstructive lung disease. Orthopnea and pedal edema suggest a cardiac cause. Bibasilar rales suggest fluid in the lower lung fields from CHF. ECG can approximate chamber enlargement and identify arrhythmias that might decrease ventricular filling time. Echocardiogram can measure ejection fraction and systolic or diastolic dysfunction indicating heart failure; local wall motion abnormalities suggesting ischemic disease; and valvular abnormalities. Levels of B-natriuretic protein (BNP) have a 90% sensitivity and 76% specificity for CHF; levels less than 100 pg/mL make CHF unlikely as the principal cause of shortness of breath or wheezing (Mueller et al., 2005). Chest radiograph can help rule out pulmonary or other thoracic mass lesions, lung infections, granulomatous or interstitial lung disease, pleural disease, pneumothorax, and cardiomegaly, supplemented with CT as needed. Although young patients with a normal physical examination have a low yield on chest radiography, up to 86% of patients older than 40 years with dyspnea have an abnormal chest x-ray film (Benacerraf et al., 1981). Spirometry showing an FEV_1/FVC ratio less than 70% is diagnostic of obstructive lung disease, and an FVC less than 80% of predicted value in the presence of a normal FEV_1/FVC ratio suggests restrictive lung disease.

Many patients present primarily with dyspnea on exertion. The 6-minute walking exercise test is a valid measure of exercise tolerance (compared with maximal exercise testing) in patients with COPD and other pulmonary conditions, as well as in various stages of CHF. It can be performed in primary care settings to assess functional disability and response to therapy (American Thoracic Society, 2002; Lipkin et al., 1986). In patients with pulmonary hypertension, the distance walked with encouragement in 6 minutes in a controlled environment is also a strong independent predictor of mortality (Miyamoto et al., 2000).

Formal cardiac ECG stress testing by exercise treadmill can quantify the level of exercise tolerance and diagnose cardiac ischemia or angina-equivalent conditions, in which a person has ischemia-induced shortness of breath but no chest pain. However, the test has a sensitivity of only 63% and specificity of 74% (86% specificity in the setting of three-vessel or left main coronary artery disease) (Gibbons et al., 1997). Other types of cardiac stress testing, such as exercise echocardiography or the nuclear medicine thallium treadmill test, can be more specific (see Chapter 27) (Mayo Clinic, 1996). The American College of Cardiology and American Society of Echocardiography published a recent consensus guideline on the appropriate use of stress echocardiography for specific clinical scenarios (Douglas et al., 2008). For patients unable to exercise, increased cardiac work may be induced pharmacologically, but dipyridamole and adenosine can each cause bronchospasm and should be avoided in patients with asthma or any other obstructive lung disease or undiagnosed pulmonary conditions (Tak and Gutierrez, 2004).

The presentation of patients with acute-onset shortness of breath requires more urgent evaluation. In addition to history and physical examination, a peak-flow test, chest x-ray film, ECG, complete blood count, and pulse oximetry or ABG testing may be done in short order. Further testing or treatment is guided by the differential diagnosis generated by this initial evaluation. Cardiac isoenzymes and troponin levels can help rule myocardial infarction in or out. If asthma is suspected, responsiveness to a trial of inhaled bronchodilator is both diagnostic and therapeutic. Antibiotics are initiated in cases of pneumonia or other pulmonary infection, and HIV testing can help in cases of suspected opportunistic infections (e.g., PCP).

Any suspicion of pulmonary embolism (PE) as a cause of acute shortness of breath requires specific diagnostic evaluation to allow quick intervention in this potentially life-threatening condition. Acute-onset shortness of breath coupled with pleuritic chest pain, hemoptysis, wedge-shaped pulmonary infarct lesions on chest radiograph, and an S1Q3 pattern and tachycardia on ECG can all point specifically to a diagnosis of PE, but most patients have a more nonspecific presentation. All patients with acute-onset shortness of breath with no apparent cause should be evaluated for PE. Physical examination for signs of deep venous thrombosis (DVT) (e.g., asymmetry in calf or thigh diameter, calf tenderness, Homans sign) are relatively insensitive and nonspecific, whereas other tests (e.g., D-dimer, CT angiography) can more accurately confirm the presence of significant underlying DVT. Clinical decision rules using objective scoring algorithms help establish pretest probability, which in turn enhances the predictive value of other tests for PE (Wells et al., 2000) (see later discussion).

Cough

Cough is also a common presenting symptom in primary care. Although cough can be part of a constellation of symptoms that leads to a specific diagnosis, it can also be the primary symptom in an undifferentiated patient. In these cases, the diagnosis must be obtained through a combination of careful history, physical examination, limited diagnostic testing, and often a trial of empiric therapy. Several elements of the history guide the initial differential diagnosis, especially a history of smoking, immunocompromise (HIV/AIDS or cancer chemotherapy), chronic pulmonary disease, medication use (ACE inhibitors), specific occupational exposures, or exposure to TB patients or TB-endemic areas.

Acute episodes of cough, defined as less than 3 weeks, are almost always caused by an acute infection (usually viral) or an acute exacerbation of chronic disease such as asthma or COPD, and the first rule should be to "do no harm" *(primum non nocere)* by treating conservatively and using time as a diagnostic test. Most episodes of acute cough caused by infection are viral in origin, mainly viral upper respiratory tract infections or acute bronchitis. Acute bacterial infections include sinusitis as well as bacterial overgrowth in exacerbations of chronic bronchitis or COPD. Fever, hemoptysis, or significant shortness of breath in association with cough indicates a chest radiograph or other immediate diagnostic evaluation. Frank hemoptysis can require urgent bronchoscopy for diagnosis and potentially for treatment (electrocoagulation of bleeding site). Without evidence of bacterial infection (clear evidence of sinusitis or pneumonia), previously healthy patients should generally be treated symptomatically without antibiotics, unless symptoms persist for more than 3 weeks.

Foreign body aspiration is a diagnostic consideration in children with either acute or chronic cough. Exacerbations of asthma, as well as infections by *Bordetella pertussis* (whooping cough) or *Bordetella parapertussis,* can lead to a persistent cough for as long as 3 to 8 weeks. Cough might indeed be the only symptom experienced by some patients with asthma (cough-variant asthma). In patients with underlying chronic bronchitis or COPD, antibiotics may be indicated during episodes of increased shortness of breath, wheezing, hypoxia, or limitations of activity if accompanied by a sudden change in sputum from thin and clear to thick or copious or yellow-green. Other subacute or chronic infections include bronchiectasis, which can manifest with a cough productive of mucopurulent, blood-tinged, or foul-smelling sputum. In children with chronic productive cough or recurrent pulmonary infections, cystic fibrosis must be considered. Survivors of premature birth with mechanical ventilation in neonatal intensive care may have chronic lung disease with acute exacerbations.

In adults, the most common causes of chronic cough in nonsmokers are postnasal drip, asthma, gastroesophageal reflux disease (GERD), and angiotensin-converting enzyme (ACE) inhibitors (Holmes and Fadden, 2004). Among smokers, chronic bronchitis, bronchiectasis, and bronchogenic carcinoma (lung cancer) must also be considered. Additional elements of the history can suggest other diagnoses. For example, occupational exposures can suggest specific diagnoses such as coal miner's lung or farmer's lung. Immigration from or travel to TB-endemic areas could suggest tuberculosis.

After the history and physical examination, a chest radiograph is the most valuable diagnostic test in evaluating the patient with chronic cough. Chest x-ray films can reveal infections (atypical pneumonia or TB), mass lesions (carcinoma), granulomatous disease (sarcoidosis), or evidence of occupational lung disease. Radiography can also reveal nonpulmonary causes of chronic cough, such as early CHF or pleural lesions. Office spirometry may also be performed to rule out obstructive lung disease.

In an otherwise healthy nonsmoker with chronic cough and a normal chest x-ray film, a trial of simple measures may be indicated. Persons being treated with an ACE inhibitor should be switched to alternative medication. Patients with occupational exposures should avoid the exposure or use protective equipment and should begin keeping a log to document the association of symptoms with days spent in workplace areas of exposure. Patients with signs of allergic rhinitis or postnasal drip may begin a simple trial of antihistamines. Patients with symptomatic GERD may begin taking a protein pump inhibitor (e.g., omeprazole) or H_2 antagonist. In some cases, chronic cough is the only symptom of GERD, and a successful trial of these agents is diagnostic.

Follow-up is essential, and the primary care practitioner must document instructions to patients that those who do not respond to empiric therapy in 2 to 3 weeks need further diagnostic evaluation. If asthma is suspected and initial office spirometry revealed normal pulmonary function, a simple approach is to ask the patient to keep a log of symptoms and peak flow meter readings, with peak flow tested within 30 minutes of rising each morning. In patients with an abnormal chest radiograph or in smokers with a normal radiograph and a chronic cough that does not respond to empiric therapy, a HRCT scan or even bronchoscopy may be indicated to rule out malignancy. Additional causes of chronic cough that might require further testing include sarcoidosis, TB, and other granulomatous or interstitial lung diseases, as well as pulmonary manifestations of autoimmune disease such as rheumatoid arthritis (RA) or systemic lupus erythematosus (SLE).

Patients with HIV/AIDS or other compromise of the immune system deserve specific evaluation (see Chapter 17). HIV testing may be indicated in patients with any risk factors, because pulmonary symptoms can be the first manifestation of symptomatic HIV disease. In patients known to be HIV positive, tests in addition to chest radiography and HRCT could include gallium scan, PET, bronchoscopy with BAL for stains and cultures, PPD, and sputum testing for PCP.

Obstructive Lung Disease

The most common chronic lung diseases that have a major global impact on disability and health care costs are three obstructive lung diseases: asthma, chronic obstructive pulmonary disease, and chronic bronchitis. Some patients have features of more than one of these conditions, such as the patient with asthma (acute episodes of reversible obstruction) who also has chronic bronchitis (cough productive of phlegm at least 3 months of the year for at least 2 years in a row), or the adult patient with asthma who is developing some level of irreversible decline in pulmonary function. COPD alone can ultimately result in pathologic signs of emphysema, a diagnosis previously made only with tissue pathology or large blebs on x-ray film but increasingly visible with various multislice HRCT techniques.

Asthma

Key Points

- Asthma is defined as an inflammatory, episodic, obstructive lung disease that is completely reversible.
- Self-management is focused on control of environmental triggers, regular peak-flow monitoring, and action plans, which can prevent or abort most flare-ups of asthma.
- All patients with persistent asthma (daytime symptoms more than twice a week or nocturnal symptoms more than twice a month) should be treated with daily long-term control medication, preferably an inhaled corticosteroid.
- Eliminating passive exposure to smokers is the most important intervention in eliminating environmental triggers.

Asthma is a chronic inflammatory airway disease characterized by recurring acute episodes of reversible airway obstruction, with return to normal lung function between episodes. Although bronchospasm is a component of the reversible airway obstruction, recent clinical guidelines have emphasized the inflammatory pathophysiology of asthma (National Heart, Lung and Blood Institute, 2007). Therefore the clinician must treat and prevent the inflammation that leads to mucosal edema, secretions, histologic remodeling of the airways, and bronchospasm of smooth muscle origin.

Epidemiology and Risk Factors

Asthma is the most common chronic disease of childhood and affects many adult patients as well. The prevalence of asthma is increasing rapidly worldwide. It now affects more than 300 million people and causes the loss of more than 15 million disability-adjusted life-years (DALY) each year (Global Initiative for Asthma, 2006). Asthma prevalence is increasing in many countries and is not decreasing globally, despite some indications of decreased emergency care utilization linked to improved care (Anandan et al., 2009). In the United States, National Health Interview Survey (NHIS) data (2002) suggest that 20 million Americans would report currently having asthma (72 per 1000 people). Asthma affects an estimated 6.1 million children nationally (83 per 1000). Across all age groups, asthma led to 1.9 million ED visits (National Hospital Ambulatory Medical Care Survey, 2002) and 4261 deaths in 2002, down from 4487 deaths in 2000 (National Vital Statistics System, 2002a). In 2003, asthma was the primary diagnosis for 469,738 hospitalizations in the United States, with an in-hospital mortality rate of 0.36% (Health Care Utilization Project, 2003). These hospitalizations alone generated charges of over $5.4 billion.

Asthma is also a high-disparity condition. Low-income, uninsured, and minority patients with asthma consistently receive worse care and have worse outcomes compared with asthma patients in the general population (Lang and Polansky, 1994). Hospitalization rates in the United States are 3.3 times higher for black than for white patients (National Vital Statistics System, 2002b). Publicly insured and uninsured patients are significantly more likely to be hospitalized and to seek ED care during acute exacerbations (Targonski et al., 1995).

The strongest risk factors for developing asthma are exposure to household smokers and a family history of asthma or atopy (asthma, atopic dermatitis, or allergic rhinitis). Family history of nasal polyps or aspirin hypersensitivity can also suggest risk for IgE-mediated atopic disease. Data are mixed on the impact of early childhood infections and bottle feeding versus breastfeeding on the development of asthma, although both are clearly associated with wheezing episodes in the first 3 years of life. Data showing a paradoxical protective effect of early childhood exposure to pets, farm animals, and bacterial antigens are still controversial (Adler et al., 2005; Platts-Mills et al., 2005; Remes et al., 2005; Waser et al., 2005).

Clinical Presentation and Diagnosis

A complete history in patients suspected of having asthma should include the frequency and severity of recent symptoms and should distinguish between daytime and nocturnal symptom frequency, a factor that is also important in staging asthma. A history of past or present smoking (tobacco or other drugs) is essential, as is an inquiry about current passive exposure to smokers in the household or occupational secondary exposure to tobacco smoke (e.g., bartenders, restaurant staff). The clinician should also inquire about activities, acute illnesses, or environmental exposures that trigger episodes, a family history of asthma or atopic disease, and a detailed occupational history. Some patients are also exposed to bronchial irritants through hobbies such as woodworking or oil painting.

Symptomatically, patients can present with complaints of chronic or acute episodic shortness of breath, wheezing, chest tightness, or a chronic cough (often at night). If they already have a diagnosis of asthma, they may report relief with rescue inhalers such as albuterol. Some patients, especially children, only have nocturnal cough, a syndrome known as *cough-variant asthma*, whereas others have symptoms precipitated mostly by exercise or by breathing in cold air.

On physical examination, the patient might have obvious difficulty breathing or audible wheezing during an acute episode. Patients with significant shortness of breath can have difficulty completing a full sentence without taking a breath, which could be described as "three-word dyspnea" (number of words the patient can say without taking a breath). Inspection can reveal nasal flaring, breathing through pursed lips, central or acral cyanosis, hyperexpansion of the chest, or use of accessory respiratory muscles. In more extreme cases, patients appear to have respiratory exhaustion, central or distal cyanosis, or even a blunting of mental status.

On auscultation, the earliest sign of airway obstruction is a prolonged expiratory phase (expiratory phase longer than inspiratory phase). A more obvious sign of asthma is expiratory wheezing. Wheezing can sometimes be brought out by forced expiration, performed by asking the patient to blow out forcefully while the examiner listens over the second intercostal space at the right costal margin. More severe cases of obstruction can result in both inspiratory and expiratory wheezing. In the most severe cases, wheezing might not be audible at all because airflow is minimal. In these cases, wheezing becomes much more prominent as airflow improves. Another sign of severity of an acute episode is *pulsus paradoxus*, defined as a decrease in systolic blood pressure of more than 20 mm Hg during inspiration.

A more objective measure of pulmonary function during an acute exacerbation of asthma is to measure the peak flow of air during forced expiration using a simple, low-cost peak-flow meter. Airflow is measured in liters per second. The best of three attempts is recorded as the peak-flow measurement. Results can be measured against nomograms based on the patient's age, gender, and height, but a better measurement is to compare the patient's peak flow during the acute episode against their baseline or best performance during a period of complete remission from asthma signs or symptoms.

When patients present with a history of asthma-like symptoms in the primary care setting, the diagnosis can be confirmed with office spirometry, a form of pulmonary function testing. The essential criterion for a diagnosis of airway obstruction is an FEV_1/FVC ratio of less than 70%. To diagnose asthma, the clinician must also demonstrate reversibility with inhaled bronchodilators, either through the patient's history or improvement in the forced expiratory volume of greater than 200 mL or 12%. Because asthma is defined as an obstructive lung disease that is completely reversible between episodes, testing in the office during asymptomatic periods might not demonstrate airway obstruction. In this case, it is helpful for the patient to use a peak-flow meter at home, testing three times each morning and recording the best value, as well as testing during symptom episodes. The record of these values can be reviewed with the family physician to aid in diagnosis, as well as for coaching the patient in self-management and prevention of future episodes.

Chest radiography is not always indicated if the patient has a classic history of episodic airway obstruction, especially if it is reversible with β-agonist rescue inhalers. In infants and children, however, the physician must distinguish upper-airway causes of obstruction from obstructive lung disease. Examples include croup or laryngotracheobronchitis, epiglottitis, and foreign bodies lodged in the upper airway. In infants and in older adults, the clinician must also exclude so-called cardiac asthma, which manifests as wheezing or other signs of airway obstruction related to pulmonary edema or CHF. In these patients, chest radiography is clearly indicated.

Patients older than 40 years who have new-onset asthma should have a complete workup to rule out other causes of airway obstruction. Many clinicians order a chest radiograph in all patients with new asthma, although there is a low rate of finding pathology in otherwise healthy older children and young adults. Chest x-ray films obtained during an acute episode of asthma can give false-positive findings of infiltrates or atelectasis.

Treatment

The National Asthma Education and Prevention Program (NAEPP) guidelines provide a comprehensive and evidence-based approach to the clinical care of asthma (National Heart Lung and Blood Institute, 1997; NAEPP Expert Panel Report 3, 2007). Unfortunately, there is a large gap between best-practice guideline-based care and usual care, as measured by compliance with these national guidelines (Thier et al., 2008) and by the clinical outcomes achievable when these guidelines are followed.

Acute Exacerbations

The mainstay of treatment for acute exacerbations of asthma is inhaled β-agonist medication such as albuterol. Although β-agonist medication is typically administered in the ED or physician's office with a nebulizer machine, a meta-analysis of controlled trials showed that a hand-held metered-dose inhaler (MDI) with a spacer device is at least as effective as a nebulizer in delivering albuterol and achieving a clinical response, as measured by pulmonary function and by clinical outcomes such as hospitalization (Castro-Rodriguez and Rodrigo, 2004). Adding ipratropium bromide to albuterol nebulizer treatments for patients with severe airflow obstruction in the acute ED setting produces additional bronchodilation, resulting in fewer hospital admissions (Plotnick and Ducharme, 2000; Rodrigo and Castro-Rodriguez, 2005).

Additional modalities of treatment include oxygen by nasal cannula or mask, and intravenous (IV) fluids for hydration. Short-term administration of systemic corticosteroids has also been demonstrated to be effective. Corticosteroids may be given intravenously (methylprednisolone), intramuscularly (dexamethasone or equivalent), or orally (prednisone or methylprednisolone). When given for 3 to 5 days as burst or pulse-dose therapy, steroids do not need to be tapered to prevent adrenal suppression. However, patients with chronic or severe exacerbations of asthma can require prolonged tapering to prevent rehospitalization for recurrence of airway obstruction.

Another treatment with evidence for efficacy in treating acute exacerbations of asthma is IV magnesium sulfate. A meta-analysis showed significant benefit in decreasing the rate of hospitalization of ED patients and in improving pulmonary function and clinical symptom scores (Cheuk et al., 2005). The most recent NAEPP Expert Panel Report (EPR-3, 2007) now recommends considering using IV magnesium sulfate or heliox-driven albuterol nebulizer treatments in patients who have failed to respond to 1 hour of conventional asthma therapy. Previous studies simply using heliox in place of oxygen did not prove beneficial (Rodrigo et al., 2003).

The benefit of other treatment options is less well documented. A meta-analysis showed that children treated with theophylline during hospitalizations for acute asthma exacerbations required more albuterol treatments and had longer hospital stays than children not treated with theophylline (Goodman et al., 1996).

Chronic Care and Disease Management

To achieve optimal outcomes, each patient should have a personal asthma care plan, which can be summarized in the mnemonic MAP (Box 18-2). The *management* plan refers to

---

Box 18-2 MAP for Asthma Care

Management Plan
- What do I do every day to control my asthma?

Action Plan
- What do I do when I have acute symptoms or my peak-flow meter values are dropping?

Prevention Plan
- What can I do to control asthma triggers and prevent acute flare-ups?

daily medications or activities such as measuring peak flow; an *action* plan is needed for specific steps to take in the event of increased symptoms or deteriorating peak-flow values; and a *prevention* plan focuses on understanding personal and environmental triggers, such as avoiding passive exposure to cigarette smoke and eliminating dust mite and cockroach antigens.

Appropriate chronic care requires appropriate staging of the clinical severity of asthma. Stage 1 is intermittent and stages 2, 3, and 4 all represent persistent (mild, moderate, and severe) disease. Criteria for classification of patients into stages 1 to 4 are shown in Figure 18-5 (NHLBI, 1997). This staging of asthma is done based on the level and frequency of symptoms or airflow obstruction before beginning treatment. The patient's step is determined by the *most severe* feature, and classification refers to symptoms *before* starting treatment. Pharmacologic treatment of asthma is linked to this classification, as shown in the treatment algorithm (Fig. 18-6).

A critical decision point is to decide if the patient has *persistent* disease as described by these criteria. Evidence suggests that primary care clinicians routinely underclassify the severity of asthma and thus undertreat with daily anti-inflammatory, long-term control medications. NAEPP guidelines suggest that only patients with truly intermittent disease—that is, patients with normal peak-flow readings, daytime symptoms no more than twice a week, and nighttime symptoms no more than twice a month—should be treated with intermittent medication alone. All other patients—those with mild, moderate, or severe persistent disease—should be treated with daily anti-inflammatory, long-term control medication such as an inhaled corticosteroid. One study has been cited as providing evidence allowing intermittent therapy of patients with mild to moderate persistent asthma, but the study results actually found that daily budesonide therapy produced greater improvements in prebronchodilator FEV_1, bronchial reactivity, sputum eosinophils, exhaled nitric oxide levels, scores for asthma control, and the number of symptom-free days, but not in postbronchodilator FEV_1 or in reported quality of life (Boushey et al., 2005).

A meta-analysis found that inhaled corticosteroids reduced asthma exacerbations by 55% compared with placebo or short-acting β-agonists, and long-acting β-agonists (LABAs) reduced flare-ups by only 26% (Sin et al., 2004). Similarly, a Cochrane Database review found that inhaled steroids at a dose equivalent to 400 μg/day of beclomethasone are more effective than leukotriene antagonists, and that inhaled corticosteroids should be considered first-line monotherapy for persistent asthma. Another Cochrane review found that patients with mild to moderate disease achieve similar levels of asthma control taking low doses (≤200 μg/day) as high doses (≥500 μg/day) of fluticasone, and that side effects are greater with higher doses. A dose equivalency chart for inhaled steroids is shown in Table 18-2. A new approach to monitoring therapy by measuring the fraction of exhaled nitric oxide (FE_{NO}) can allow better adjustment of inhaled-corticosteroid doses in the future (Smith et al., 2005). High-dose inhaled corticosteroids are useful primarily in weaning patients from oral steroids.

Other second-line long-term control agents include LABAs (salmeterol, formoterol), long-acting anticholinergics (tiotropium), leukotriene antagonists, inhaled mast cell stabilizers (cromolyn, nedocromil), and theophylline. Although each has demonstrated efficacy, none is as effective as inhaled corticosteroids. When low-dose inhaled corticosteroids are not providing complete remission, the clinician may add a second medication or increase the inhaled steroid dose to moderate levels. In a controlled trial of an inhaled LABA (formoterol) versus theophylline versus a leukotriene antagonist (zafirlukast) as second-line agents added to inhaled corticosteroid therapy, Yurdakul and colleagues (2002) found that the LABA was more effective in preventing exacerbations and had fewer side-effects than the other options. A Cochrane review of 12 controlled trials also found that LABAs were more effective than leukotriene antagonists as add-on therapy to inhaled steroids (Ram et al., 2005). Concern persists, however, that LABAs can increase mortality when used as monotherapy in the absence of inhaled corticosteroids (Abramson et al., 2003b). Randomized controlled trials now show that adding tiotropium bromide to low-dose inhaled corticosteroid (ICS) therapy is superior to doubling the dose of the ICS and equivalent to adding a LABA (Peters, 2010). The leukotriene synthesis inhibitor zileuton appears to improve pulmonary function and decrease need for β-agonist, but causes significant elevations of liver transaminases in 2% to 3% of patients (Nelson et al., 2007).

Immunotherapy also appears to be effective. A Cochrane review found that allergen immunotherapy reduces asthma symptoms and use of asthma medications at a level similar to that of inhaled corticosteroids (Abramson et al., 2003a). A newer third-line therapy is the once- or twice-monthly injection of monoclonal anti-IgE antibodies (omalizumab), an expensive therapy that is associated with a 98% to 99% reduction in free IgE and significantly fewer exacerbations of asthma, even allowing some patients to be weaned from inhaled corticosteroids (Walker et al., 2003).

KEY TREATMENT

Daily inhaled corticosteroids significantly reduce exacerbations and hospitalizations in patients with persistent asthma and are significantly more effective as first-line long-term control agents than any alternative agents (Sin et al., 2004) (SOR: A).

Long-acting β-agonists (LABAs) are more effective than leukotriene antagonists as add-on-therapy to inhaled steroids. Because most benefits of inhaled corticosteroid (ICS) are achieved at lower doses, adding a LABA to a low or medium dose of ICS is preferred over using a higher dose of ICS. LABAs should not be used as monotherapy because of higher risk of death (FDA black-box warning) (NAEPP EPR-3; Ram et al., 2005) (SOR: A).

Adding ipratropium bromide to albuterol nebulizer treatments for patients with severe airflow obstruction in the acute ED setting produces additional bronchodilation, resulting in fewer hospital admissions (Plotnick and Ducharme, 2000; Rodrigo and Castro-Rodriguez, 2005) (SOR: A).

Theophylline is an acceptable (but not preferred) alternative to LABA for second-line long-term control treatment in combination with inhaled corticosteroids, but theophylline or aminophylline should not be used in the acute treatment of ED or in-hospital patients (SOR: A).

Teaching patients to engage in effective self-management improves clinical outcomes (Gibson et al., 2002) (SOR: A).

Components of Severity		Classification of Asthma Severity (Youths ≥12 years of age and adults)			
			Persistent		
		Intermittent	Mild	Moderate	Severe
Impairment Normal FEV₁/FVC: 8–19 yr 85% 20–39 yr 80% 40–59 yr 75% 60–80 yr 70%	Symptoms	≤2 days/week	>2 days/week but not daily	Daily	Throughout the day
	Nighttime awakenings	≤2x/month	3–4x/month	>1x/week but not nightly	Often 7x/week
	Short-acting beta₂-agonist use for symptom control (not prevention of EIB)	≤2 days/week	>2 days/week but not >1x/day	Daily	Several times per day
	Interference with normal activity	None	Minor limitation	Some limitation	Extremely limited
	Lung function	• Normal FEV₁ between exacerbations • FEV₁ >80% predicted • FEV₁/FVC normal	• FEV₁ ≥80% predicted • FEV₁/FVC normal	• FEV₁ >60% but <80% predicted • FEV₁/FVC reduced 5%	• FEV₁ <60% predicted • FEV₁/FVC reduced >5%
Risk	Exacerbations requiring oral systemic corticosteroids	0–1/year (see note)	≥2/year (see note) ──────────────────────────────▶		
		◀── Consider severity and interval since last exacerbation. Frequency and severity may fluctuate over time for patients in any severity category. ──▶			
		Relative annual risk of exacerbations may be related to FEV₁			

Figure 18-5 Classification of asthma severity in adolescents 12 years or older and adults. *(From Guidelines for the Diagnosis and Management of Asthma; National Asthma Education and Prevention Program (NAEPP) Coordinating Committee, 2007.* http://www.nhlbi.nih.gov/guidelines/asthma/asthgdln.htm.

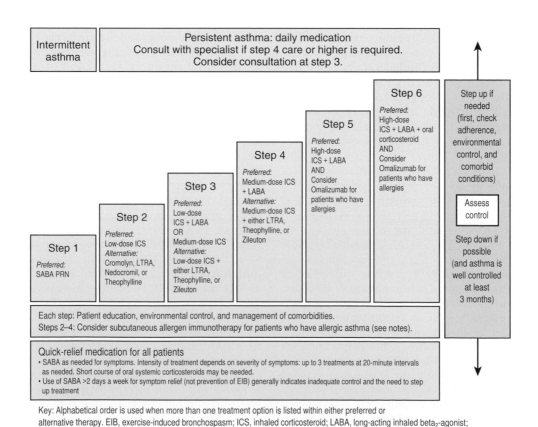

Figure 18-6 Stepwise approach for managing asthma in adolescents (≥12 years) and adults. *(From Guidelines for the Diagnosis and Management of Asthma; National Asthma Education and Prevention Program (NAEPP) Coordinating Committee, 2007. http://www.nhlbi.nih.gov/guidelines/asthma/asthgdln.htm.)*

Table 18-2 Estimated Comparative Daily Doses for Inhaled Corticosteroids for Adolescents (Age ≥12 Years) and Adults

Drug	Amount	Daily Dose (µg)		
		Low	Medium	High
Beclomethasone HFA	40 or 80 µg/puff	80-240	>240-480	>480
Budesonide DPI	90, 80, or 200 µg/inhalation	180-600	>600-1200	>1200
Flunisolide	250 µg/puff	500-1000	>1000-2000	>2000
Flunisolide HFA	80 µg/puff	320	>320-640	>640
Fluticasone				
HFA/MDI	44, 110, or 220 µg/puff	88-264	>264-440	>440
DPI	50, 100, or 250 µg/inhalation	100-300	>300-500	>500
Mometasone DPI	200 µg/inhalation	200	400	>400
Triamcinolone acetonide	75 µg/puff	300-750	>750-1500	>1500

From National Heart, Lung and Blood Institute, NHI, Expert Panel 3 (EPR3). Guidelines for the Diagnosis and Management of Asthma. National Asthma Education and Prevention Program (NAEPP) Coordinating Committee, 2007. http://www.nhlbi.nih.gov/guidelines/asthma/asthgdln.htm.
HFA, Hydrofluoroalkane; *DPI*, dry powder inhaler; *MDI*; metered-dose inhaler.

Prevention

Even though dust mites are usually mentioned as a controllable environmental trigger, a Cochrane review of 49 controlled trials found no evidence that either physical or chemical methods aimed at reducing exposure to house dust mite allergens had any benefit (Gotzsche et al., 2004). On the other hand, a controlled trial of an intervention to reduce cockroach and dust mite allergens *and* passive exposure to tobacco smoke among urban children with atopic asthma was effective in reducing both allergens in the home and asthma symptom-days (Morgan et al., 2004). Teaching patients to self-monitor and self-manage their asthma using an action plan and ongoing review with their physician is effective in reducing exacerbations and symptoms (Gibson et al., 2002). As with most pulmonary diseases, the most effective preventive strategy is to eliminate smoking as a risk factor from the patient, the household, and the workplace.

Chronic Obstructive Pulmonary Disease and Chronic Bronchitis

Key Points

- Because of the global spread of tobacco addiction, chronic obstructive pulmonary disease (COPD) will become the world's third leading cause of death by 2020.
- Quitting smoking reduces progressive loss of pulmonary function in patients with COPD, even in long-time smokers.
- The 6-minute walk test correlates strongly with quality of life and functional limitations in patients with COPD and other chronic lung diseases.
- Nocturnal home oxygen therapy improves symptoms and survival in patients with hypoxia at rest. Pulmonary rehabilitation improves symptoms but not survival.

- Inhaled corticosteroids, long-acting β2-agonists, and long-acting anticholinergics (tiotropium) each decrease exacerbation rates by 20% to 25% in patients with moderate to severe COPD, although patients may differ in their response to each therapy.

Consensus statements from the Global Initiative for Chronic Obstructive Lung Disease (GOLD standards, 2005) define chronic obstructive pulmonary disease as a postbronchodilator FVC of less than 80% of predicted in a patient with evidence of airway obstruction (FEV_1/FVC ratio <70%) that is not completely reversible. Although some patients with asthma, especially those who smoke, can progress to varying degrees of irreversibility consistent with COPD, the underlying pathophysiology and inflammatory mechanisms in asthma are distinct from those found in patients with COPD.

Epidemiology and Risk Factors

In large part because of the global spread of tobacco addiction, WHO estimates that COPD will move from the 12th to fifth leading cause of disability by 2020 (Murray and Lopez, 1996), also becoming the world's third leading cause of death.

Smoking is the most important risk factor for COPD and causes ongoing damage in COPD patients, as measured by an accelerated decline in FEV_1 compared with nonsmokers or ex-smokers. Among COPD patients who have quit smoking, exposure to secondhand smoke can also be a trigger factor for acute exacerbations. Variation in environmental air quality (ozone and small particulates) is also a factor associated with acute exacerbations of COPD. In many countries, air pollution can be a major source of smoking-equivalent damage to the respiratory tract in impoverished settings where daily cooking over indoor fires or charcoal is common. Other trigger factors for acute exacerbations include acute upper respiratory infections, sinusitis, exposure to dust or pet dander, and intercurrent illness. However, once patients reach a more severe stage of illness in which pulmonary reserves are minimal, almost any small change (e.g., fatigue, stress, change in weather) can trigger an exacerbation.

The other major risk factor for development of COPD is the inherited disorder α_1-antitrypsin deficiency. The recognition of this disease and its cellular mechanisms of injury to the lung have led to a specific understanding of protease and antiprotease imbalance as one mechanism of disease progression of emphysematous COPD. Any patient who develops COPD without a significant smoking history, any patient with a strong family history of COPD, and any patient developing clinically significant COPD before age 45 should be screened for α_1-antitrypsin deficiency. A detailed discussion of genetic counseling of patients with α_1-antitrypsin deficiency or carrier state can be found in the American Thoracic Society and European Respiratory Society (2003) consensus standards.

Clinical Presentation

Chronic obstructive pulmonary disease includes the two overlapping clinical conditions of chronic *bronchitis* and *emphysema*, which can coexist in the same patient. A practical clinical approach is to diagnose COPD by documenting obstruction that is not completely reversible on clinical examination and pulmonary function testing, then assessing whether the patient also has a component of chronic bronchitis, that is, cough productive of phlegm at least 3 months of each year for at least 2 years. Some patients meet this criterion for chronic bronchitis before developing clinical or spirometric evidence of obstructive lung disease. The international GOLD guidelines no longer categorize this as stage 0 COPD, because of insufficient evidence that patients will inevitably progress to obstructive lung disease.

Often, patients who smoke have had a chronic smoker's cough for years and present for medical treatment only when symptoms such as shortness of breath on exertion or at rest begin to appear. The hallmark symptom of symptomatic COPD is progressive and persistent shortness of breath. Because of the built-in reserve of the pulmonary system, such functional disability often is not noticed until there is a substantial decline in pulmonary function and substantial damage to lung parenchyma. Still, the U.S. Preventive Services Task Force (USPSTF) recommends not screening routinely with spirometry for obstructive lung disease or declining lung function.

Comorbidities are often present, and they must be comanaged with COPD if patients are to have optimal clinical outcomes and quality of life. For example, CHF can eventually occur after years of elevated right-sided pulmonary pressure (right-sided failure leading ultimately to biventricular failure), or patients might simply experience smoking-related myocardial infarctions and coronary ischemia in parallel with their COPD. Symptomatic COPD has a powerful adverse effect on quality of life, and a substantial percentage of patients with COPD develop comorbid depression. Chronic hypoxia and air hunger can also generate significant anxiety.

Diagnosis and Staging

By the time many patients present for treatment, the diagnosis of COPD is apparent. In addition to symptoms of dyspnea, chronic productive cough, and functional limitations, patients can show physical findings of lung hyperexpansion

(increased lung span on percussion, increased thoracic AP diameter, and use of accessory muscles of respiration). Extrathoracic signs include peripheral or central cyanosis, nail clubbing, and signs of increased central venous pressure or even right-sided heart failure. Box 18-3 presents the differential diagnosis and distinguishing features of COPD suggested by the GOLD guidelines. Any patient who develops

---

Box 18-3 Differential Diagnosis of COPD* (GOLD Guidelines)

COPD

Onset in midlife

Symptoms slowly progressive

Long smoking history

Dyspnea during exercise

Largely irreversible airflow limitation

Asthma

Onset early in life (often childhood)

Symptoms vary from day to day

Symptoms at night and early morning

Allergy, rhinitis, and/or eczema are also present

Family history of asthma

Largely reversible airflow limitation

Congestive Heart Failure (CHF)

Fine basilar crackles on auscultation

Chest radiograph shows dilated heart, pulmonary edema

Pulmonary function tests indicate volume restriction, not airflow limitation

Bronchiectasis

Large volumes of purulent sputum

Often associated with bacterial infection

Coarse crackles/clubbing on auscultation

Chest radiograph or CT shows bronchial dilation or bronchial wall thickening

Tuberculosis (TB)

Onset all ages

Chest radiograph shows lung infiltrate

Microbiologic confirmation

High local prevalence of tuberculosis

Obliterative Bronchiolitis

Onset in younger age, nonsmokers

May have history of rheumatoid arthritis or fume exposure

CT on expiration shows hypodense areas

Diffuse Panbronchiolitis

Most patients are male and nonsmokers.

Almost all have chronic sinusitis.

Chest radiography and HRCT show diffuse small centrilobular nodular opacities and hyperinflation

From Global Initiative for Chronic Obstructive Lung Disease: Executive Summary: Global Strategy for the Diagnosis, Management, and Prevention of COPD, Updated 2008, p 39. http://www.goldcopd.com/Guidelineitem.asp?l1=2&l2=1&intId=996.
*These features tend to be characteristic of the respective diseases but do not occur in every case. For example, a person who has never smoked may develop COPD, especially in the developing world where other risk factors may be more important than cigarette smoking, and asthma may develop in adult and even elderly patients.
COPD, Chronic obstructive pulmonary disease; *CT,* computed tomography; *HRCT,* high-resolution computed tomography.

COPD without a significant smoking history, or any patient developing COPD before age 45, should be screened for α_1-antitrypsin deficiency. HRCT can help identify granulomatous or interstitial lung diseases or provide evidence of bronchiectasis.

Spirometry is the key to making a formal diagnosis, as well as for staging the severity of illness. COPD may be diagnosed when obstructive lung disease is not fully reversible, defined as a postbronchodilator FVC of less than 80% of predicted in a patient with evidence of airway obstruction (FEV_1/FVC ratio <70%). A pattern of restrictive lung disease (FVC <80% of predicted in presence of normal FEV_1/FVC ratio) would suggest alternative diagnoses, such as pulmonary fibrosis, sarcoidosis, autoimmune conditions, or primary CHF.

Although there are several classification systems for severity of COPD, the American Thoracic Society (ATS) guidelines and the international GOLD standards are similar (Fig. 18-7). They are based on spirometric criteria—the presence of obstruction and the level of impairment in FEV_1—and correlate strongly with quality of life and functional limitations. The 6-minute walk test is another way to stage COPD by its impact on daily activities. A distance of less than 149 meters walked in 6 minutes of encouraged walking indicates more severe functional limitation, and a distance farther than 350 m indicates minimal limitation (Celli et al., 2004).

Treatment

Acute Exacerbations

The course of COPD is characterized by patients' daily coping with chronic obstruction, punctuated by episodic exacerbations that can be life threatening and only partially responsive to treatment. Initial evaluation includes the patient's assessment of the severity of symptoms, plus physical examination, chest radiograph, and ABG tests. Predicting which patients can be safely discharged from the ED versus those who need to be hospitalized requires evaluation of both clinical and psychosocial indicators (Smith et al., 2000).

Chest radiography can reveal underlying causes of an acute exacerbation, such as pneumonia or CHF. ABGs are useful in assessing initial hypoxia and hypercapnia, but also in monitoring the patient's response to judicious use of supplemental oxygen administered by nasal cannula or mask. Although relief of hypoxia reduces symptoms and improves cardiac function, it can also decrease the respiratory drive in a patient with chronic hypercapnia and partially compensated respiratory acidosis. For this reason, ABGs should be repeated within 30 minutes after starting oxygen, and ongoing hypoxia may be monitored with pulse oximetry (although oximetry becomes less accurate at So_2 levels <70%).

An immediate response is expected from inhaled β_2-agonist therapy in asthma, but the response to bronchodilators in acute exacerbations of COPD can be modest. Some patients are more responsive to anticholinergic bronchodilators such as ipratropium, and others respond to β_2-agonist agents, so these therapies are often combined in the acute setting. At home, patients can increase the dose or frequency of current medications or add a short-term agent to their chronic therapy (e.g., adding albuterol doses to LABA, or adding ipratropium to chronic tiotropium therapy). Spacer devices or mechanical nebulizer delivery systems may be used. Treatment of acute exacerbations of COPD with systemic corticosteroids (administered orally or parenterally) can reduce treatment failures by more than 50% and improve short-term dyspnea and PFTs, but there is some increase in adverse effects (Wood-Baker et al., 2005). Continuing these systemic steroids beyond 2 weeks has not been shown to have significant benefit.

Other acute treatments for COPD exacerbations include methylxanthines such as theophylline and aminophylline, which have a positive effect on the central drive to breathe, on diaphragmatic contractility, and on some mechanisms of bronchial inflammation. However, they probably do not significantly affect cyclic adenosine monophosphate (cAMP)–mediated bronchodilation. Antibiotics are indicated if there are signs of pneumonia, sepsis, or other bacterial infection. Recent changes in sputum production (copious, thick,

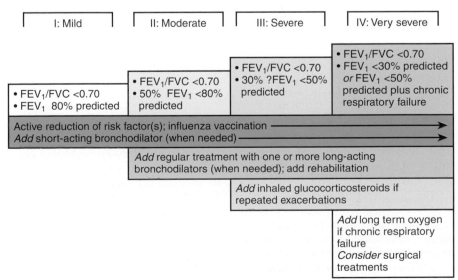

Figure 18-7 Classification and therapy at each stage of chronic obstructive pulmonary disease (COPD). Postbronchodilator FEV_1 is recommended for the diagnosis and assessment of severity of COPD. *(From Global Initiative for Chronic Obstructive Lung Disease: Global Strategy for the Diagnosis, Management and Prevention of COPD. Updated 2008. http://www.goldcopd.com/download.asp?intId=504.)*

multicolored, or blood tinged) just before the exacerbation can indicate bacterial overgrowth of chronically inflamed bronchial mucosa, another indication for antibiotics. Because of chronic bacterial colonization, second- and third-generation antibiotics may provide greater benefit.

Indications for hospitalization include severity of underlying illness, significant worsening during this exacerbation, failure of home or outpatient treatment efforts, significant comorbidities (CHF, arrhythmias, or electrolyte imbalance), and underlying pneumonia or other acute causes. Indications for admission to the ICU, or perhaps even intubation and mechanical ventilation, include severe dyspnea unresponsive to initial therapy, change in mental status (e.g., confusion, lethargy), or severe or worsening hypoxia (Pao_2 <40 mm Hg), hypercapnia ($Paco_2$ >60 mm Hg), or respiratory acidosis (pH <7.25). In a meta-analysis of treatment strategies for the patient hospitalized with an exacerbation of COPD, Quon and colleagues (2008) found that systemic corticosteroids decreased treatment failures by 46% and hospital stay by 1.4 days, although risk of hyperglycemia increased almost sixfold. Antibiotics also decreased treatment failures by 46% and in-hospital mortality by 78%. Noninvasive positive-pressure ventilation (NPPV) reduced the risk of intubation by 65%, in-hospital mortality by 55%, and hospital stay by 1.9 days. Noninvasive intermittent positive-pressure ventilation (NIPPV) is an option for treating moderate to severe respiratory failure in patients who have normal mental status, are stable hemodynamically, and do not have high risk for aspiration. About 80% of patients improve symptomatically within 4 hours of initiating NIPPV (Putinati et al., 2000; Wijkstra, 2003). On the other hand, chronic nocturnal use of NIPPV has yet to show significant benefit (Wijkstra et al., 2003).

Perhaps just as important as managing the pulmonary disease is to make sure other conditions do not complicate the exacerbation. Unless there are specific contraindications, a patient hospitalized for COPD exacerbation should be started on subcutaneous heparin to prevent DVT. Cardiac monitoring is often indicated in the ED and beyond to assess and treat related arrhythmias or cardiac ischemia. Electrolyte abnormalities are quite common, especially in the setting of rapidly changing $Paco_2$ and acid-base balance. The incidence of pneumonia in ICU patients ranges from 7% to 40%, and the mortality rate from ventilator-associated pneumonia can be as high as 50%. Prophylactic antibiotics can reduce the incidence of respiratory infections in ICU patients by up to 50%, but antibiotics do not reduce mortality (Liberati et al., 2004).

Chronic Care and Disease Management

Each patient with COPD also needs an ongoing care plan, which includes the MAP elements described for asthma patients (daily management plan, action plan for acute exacerbations, and prevention plan). The treatment of acute exacerbations is described earlier, but each patient should have an individual action plan for increasing symptoms, to prevent hospitalization. Such action plans might include symptoms or signs that would trigger a call to the physician, as well as use of short-acting β_2-agonists (albuterol, terbutaline), short-acting anticholinergic (ipratropium), or oral steroids. Use of short-course antibiotics triggered by changes in phlegm (increased sputum or change in sputum from clear to yellow-green) is common but untested by controlled trials.

A meta-analysis of controlled trials assessed the impact of various modalities of treatment for COPD (Sin et al., 2003). Outcome measures included hospitalizations, exacerbation rates, and health-related quality of life. Inhaled corticosteroids, long-acting β_2-agonists (salmeterol, formoterol), and the long-acting anticholinergic tiotropium each decreased exacerbation rates by 20% to 25% in patients with moderate to severe COPD. The greatest effect was in patients with FEV_1 of 1 to 2 L. Combining inhaled corticosteroids with a long-acting β_2-agonist provided modest additional benefit (30% reduction in exacerbations). Tiotropium may be added to inhaled corticosteroids and LABAs as triple therapy. Oral theophylline also appears to have some beneficial effects not only as a bronchodilator but also in increasing diaphragmatic muscle contractility and the central drive to breathe. As a result, there are improvements in FEV_1, Pao_2, and $Paco_2$, although these must be weighed against potentially significant side effects of theophylline, such as nausea, tremors, and palpitations.

Nonpharmacologic therapies have shown mixed results. Home oxygen therapy decreases dyspnea and increases survival significantly in those with hypoxia at rest (Pao_2 <60 mm Hg), but not in those with only exertional or nocturnal hypoxia (Crockett et al., 2000). NPPV has not been shown to improve COPD outcomes except in severely hypercapnic patients ($Paco_2$ >55 mm Hg, or 50-54 mm Hg in presence of nocturnal oxygen desaturation or multiple hospitalizations in past year). Pulmonary rehabilitation focuses on improving strength, cardiopulmonary fitness, and exercise tolerance, and nutrition improves health status, as measured by the St. George's Respiratory Questionnaire (SGRQ) and Chronic Respiratory Questionnaire (CRQ), but does not appear to decrease hospitalization or mortality rates (Lacasse et al., 2001). Pulmonary rehabilitation appears to be beneficial in COPD and other chronic pulmonary diseases and is recommended by Joint ACCP/AACVPR Evidence-Based Clinical Practice Guidelines (Ries, 2007).

One disease management program using self-management and telephone follow-up showed a 36% reduction in hospitalizations and a 45% reduction in mortality in COPD patients (Bourbeau et al., 2003), but other trials of disease management programs have not shown such benefit. Despite evidence of significant nutritional deficits in patients with moderate to severe COPD, neither nutritional supplements to increase antioxidants (vitamin E or beta-carotene) nor nutritional supports to increase caloric intake have been demonstrated to improve outcomes or functional status in patients with COPD.

Surgical therapy using lung volume reduction surgery can improve quality of life and exercise tolerance in selected patients with FEV_1 less than 30% to 40% of predicted values (Fishman et al., 2003; Geddes et al., 2000; Goldstein et al., 2003). However, surgery does not improve 5-year mortality and can actually worsen short-term mortality (National Emphysema Treatment Trial Research Group, 2001).

Treatment guidelines for each stage of COPD are summarized in Figure 18-7.

Prevention

Smoking cessation is the most important factor in preventing COPD, as well as the cornerstone of COPD treatment to prevent exacerbations and progressive loss of pulmonary function (Man et al., 2003). The decline in pulmonary function as measured by FEV_1 can be halved (from 60 to 30 mL/year) if COPD patients quit smoking (Anthonisen et al., 1994). Avoidance of secondary exposure to smoke, especially in the household, is also important. Physician advice to quit smoking alone has some impact, and combined interventions (counseling plus education or group strategies plus pharmacologic treatment with nicotine, bupropion) can achieve at least 25% long-term quit rates even in COPD patients. Use of spirometry for screening and early diagnosis of COPD to enhance smoking cessation interventions among smokers has not been shown to increase smoking cessation rates or other clinical outcomes.

Influenza vaccine should be administered every year; it can reduce hospitalizations and deaths from pneumonia, cardiovascular disease, and all causes by 30% to 40% (Govaert et al, 1994; Nichol et al, 2003). Pneumococcal vaccine is also indicated in all patients with COPD, and patients should be revaccinated after 10 years if the first pneumococcal vaccine was administered before age 65 years. Vaccination rates are increasing nationwide, but they are still significantly lower among the uninsured and among racial and ethnic minority populations (CDC, 2003b). Family physicians can improve vaccination rates in their own practice by establishing standing orders for influenza and pneumococcal vaccination (CDC, 2003c; 2009).

One critical role for the family physician in the chronic management of COPD is to facilitate open discussions with the patient and family members about end-of-life issues such as therapy during acute exacerbations. Although this has become routine in the management of cancer patients, the 5 year survival of patients with severe stages of COPD (as well as heart failure and other chronic organ failure) is often worse than that of many cancers. Many patients have a strong desire to avoid mechanical ventilation, only to end up intubated, unconscious, and having difficulty being weaned from the ventilator. Often, family members are asked to assist in end-of-life decision making when complications occur during a protracted downturn in the course of COPD, even though they have not previously discussed such issues with the patient. Facilitating such family discussions, providing templates for living wills and health care power of attorney forms, and referring for legal or psychological or pastoral counseling can dramatically ease a family's confusion and pain during these episodes and ultimately in dealing with the patient's death.

Acute Respiratory Failure

Acute respiratory failure can be the result of acute pulmonary infections, exacerbations of chronic pulmonary disease, or other conditions, such as pulmonary embolism, tension pneumothorax, or sepsis.

Clinical Presentation and Diagnosis

The clinical presentation of acute respiratory failure is usually obvious, although some patients slip into respiratory failure while being treated for initially less serious respiratory distress such as pneumonia or acute exacerbations of CHF, asthma, or COPD. Acute respiratory failure can have either or both of two components: inadequate oxygenation (hypoxia) and

---

KEY TREATMENT

Smoking cessation is the best intervention to slow the long-term rate of decline in FEV_1 (Anthonisen et al., 1994) (SOR: A).

Among patients with COPD, inhaled corticosteroid use for at least 24 weeks is associated with a significantly increased risk of serious pneumonia but not death, especially among those using the highest dose of ICS and those with the lowest baseline FEV_1 (Drummond, 2008; Singh, 2009) (SOR: A).

Patients with COPD receiving LABAs showed significant benefits in airflow limitation measures, health-related quality of life, and use of rescue medication, but the anticholinergic drug tiotropium decreased the incidence of severe COPD exacerbations even more than LABAs (Rodrigo, 2008) (SOR: A).

Tiotropium reduces the rate of decline of FEV_1 in patients with GOLD stage II COPD (Decramer, 2009). Unfortunately, inhaled anticholinergics may also be associated with a significantly increased risk of cardiovascular death, myocardial infarction, or stroke in COPD patients (Singh et al., 2008) (SOR: A).

All patients should be counseled on smoking cessation; combining effective behavioral therapies (behavioral group therapy, social support) with pharmacologic therapy (nicotine replacement therapy, antidepressants) (Hughes et al., 2004; Lancaster and Stead, 2004; Stead and Lancaster, 2005) (SOR: A).

Pulmonary rehabilitation, including patient education and cardiopulmonary exercise training, significantly improves clinical outcomes and health-related quality of life (Lacasse et al., 2001) (SOR: A).

Home oxygen therapy helps patients with resting Pao_2 less than 60 mm Hg but not patients with normal oxygen levels or with hypoxemia only on exertion (Crockett et al., 2000) (SOR: A).

---

inadequate ventilation (resulting in hypercarbia and respiratory acidosis). Although patients might initially present with severe shortness of breath, the hypoxia and increased $Paco_2$ can ultimately lead to suppression of respiratory centers in the brain, as well as lethargy, stupor, or coma.

An especially serious form of respiratory failure that can occur is acute respiratory distress syndrome (ARDS), which can occur in patients with severe trauma, especially those who have received massive blood transfusions, overwhelming pneumonia, septic shock, and the acute chest syndrome associated with sickle cell disease.

Indications for intubation and mechanical ventilation include hypoxia and hypoventilation unresponsive to pharmacologic intervention and supplemental oxygen delivery by mask or cannula. Patients unable to protect their own airway because of central nervous system (CNS) depression or inadequate gag reflex might also need intubation. The detailed management of mechanical ventilation is beyond the scope of this chapter, but ventilation can be thought of in terms of ventilator settings that increase or decrease *ventilation* (ventilator mode, respiratory rate, and tidal volume) and ventilator settings that improve *oxygenation*: forced inspiratory oxygen concentration (Fio_2) and continuous positive airway pressure (CPAP) or positive end-expiratory pressure (PEEP).

Weaning patients from the ventilator, especially those with chronic lung disease, can be challenging. Reintubation carries risks of trauma and of ventilator-associated pneumonia. Protocols based on objective criteria (vs. individual clinical judgment) significantly reduce time, costs, and complications related to weaning patients from mechanical ventilation.

Other Chronic Bronchial Diseases

Bronchiectasis

Bronchiectasis is both a chronic airway infection and a disease of chronic lung inflammation. Bronchiectasis might be more common outside the United States (Tsang and Tipoe, 2004). Clinical course can be progressive or indolent. Cough is the predominant symptom, and some patients have significant hemoptysis or shortness of breath, or both. Malodorous (fetid) breath is a characteristic symptom. Bronchiectasis not associated with a genetic disorder is designated non–cystic fibrosis bronchiectasis.

Antibiotics are given over the long term, using antipseudomonal antibiotics either orally or as aminoglycosides nebulized for inhalation. Macrolide antibiotics such as azithromycin appear to have antibiotic and anti-inflammatory effects in treating bronchiectasis. A Cochrane review found a small but significant benefit for prolonged antibiotic therapy in the treatment of patients with purulent bronchiectasis (Evans et al., 2003). Sputum cultures should be monitored for the presence of fungal (aspergillus) and mycobacterial organisms as well, because they can complicate the polymicrobial mix of organisms in these patients (Morrissey and Evans, 2003). Bronchodilators, oxygen, and even noninvasive pulmonary ventilation may be tried when bronchial obstruction becomes a major component of pulmonary impairment. Surgical resection of affected lung segments can be helpful in patients with localized disease (Greenstone, 2002).

Cystic Fibrosis

Cystic fibrosis (CF) is a genetic disease attributed to autosomal recessive defects on a single gene of chromosome 7. It affects membrane functions in mucus-secreting glands (e.g., sweat glands), the pancreas, and gastrointestinal and respiratory tracts. Diagnosis of CF is suspected in the presence of pancreatitis and chronic or recurrent lung infections in infants or children. Definitive diagnosis may be made with a sweat chloride test. Treatment of CF has improved significantly over the past decades. Patients now routinely live into adulthood, and now more adults are living with CF than children. Family physicians and internists (in partnership with subspecialists) are increasingly involved in the care of patients with this complex condition.

Specific treatment modalities for CF include physical therapy, nutrition therapy, mucolytics, antibiotics, and increasingly, anti-inflammatory therapies. Self-administered airway clearance techniques appear to be as effective as chest physiotherapy (Main et al., 2005). Antibiotics must be broad-spectrum and antipseudomonal agents and often are given in combination during exacerbations or acute infections. In recent years, inhaled tobramycin has become effective antibiotic therapy in bronchiectasis and CF. Aminoglycosides also appear to suppress the expression of the CF transmembrane conductance regulator. Anti-inflammatory therapy includes oral corticosteroids and ibuprofen; azithromycin has both antibiotic and anti-inflammatory properties. Inhaled corticosteroids, methotrexate, and protease replacement do not appear to be effective (Prescott and Johnson, 2005). Viral vectors or other methods may soon allow delivery of gene therapy directly to the respiratory tract to achieve cure or long-term relapse in CF patients.

Acute Infectious Diseases

Bronchiolitis in Children

Bronchiolitis is a viral infection associated with bronchial obstruction. It occurs most often in the fall and winter. About half of all children experience bronchiolitis during the first 2 years of life, with a median age of 6 months. *Respiratory syncytial virus* (RSV) is the most common causative organism, but other viruses (adenovirus, influenza, parainfluenza, and rhinovirus) can also cause bronchiolitis.

Clinical Presentation

Typically, an infant or toddler presents with routine signs and symptoms of upper respiratory infection, such as cough, sneezing, rhinitis, and low-grade fever. Dyspnea and irritability and perhaps audible wheezing soon follow. Tachypnea and nasal flaring are typical, along with signs of airway obstruction, such as a hyperexpanded chest and wheezing on auscultation, with a prolonged expiratory phase. Chest radiograph can show air trapping, peribronchial thickening, atelectasis, and patchy infiltrates. Premature infants and children with chronic disease are at special risk for respiratory failure or complications such as bacterial pneumonia, and up to 5% of patients require hospitalization for severe respiratory distress.

Treatment

Infants with mild bronchiolitis may be managed at home using fluids, antipyretics, and β_2-agonists if needed. Indications for hospitalization of children with bronchiolitis include age younger than 6 months, hypoxemia (Pao_2 <60 mm Hg or So_2 <92%), rapid deterioration, apnea, or poor oral intake.

Hospitalized infants should receive fluids (orally or intravenously) and supplemental humidified oxygen. Aerosolized bronchodilators, including aerosolized epinephrine, decrease airway obstruction. Aerosolized ribavirin may be used in infants or children with underlying risk factors, but a meta-analysis of eight randomized, controlled trials (RCTs) found no benefit for antiviral agents in general use. A systematic review of glucocorticoid treatment found no benefit in any subgroup of patients with bronchiolitis (Patel et al., 2004), and glucocorticoids do not appear to prevent post-bronchiolitic wheezing (Blom et al., 2007). Epinephrine treatment is better than placebo and might have a slight advantage over salbutamol in treating bronchiolitis in outpatient settings, but benefit has not been proved in hospitalized patients (Hartling et al., 2004). A Cochrane review concluded that nebulized hypertonic (3%) saline may significantly reduce the length of hospital stay and improve other clinical indicators in infants with acute viral bronchiolitis (Zhang et al., 2008).

Some patients ultimately have asthma, with the first episode diagnosed as bronchiolitis, but RSV has not been shown to be a causative agent of chronic asthma. A systematic review found treatment with RSV immune globulin to be effective in preventing hospitalizations and admission to the ICU but not in lowering mortality (Wang and Tang, 1999). Children with severe apnea or respiratory failure might require intubation and mechanical ventilation. Antibiotics are only indicated if secondary bacterial infection occurs.

Prevention

Smokers in the household predispose infants to bronchiolitis, and families should be counseled to make all homes with infants or children smoke free. In a small group of infants with underlying lung disease, heart disease, or low birth weight, monthly RSV hyperimmune gamma globulin has been proved to offer some protection from severe disease. Although influenza is a relatively infrequent cause of bronchiolitis, expanded recommendations for influenza vaccination include all children aged 6 to 23 months as well as all close contacts of children from birth through 23 months of age.

Acute Bronchitis

A frequently diagnosed infection in children and adults, acute bronchitis is typically a viral respiratory infection with lower tract symptoms, such as cough, phlegm, hoarseness, or wheezing. This syndrome should be distinguished from acute exacerbations in patients with chronic bronchitis, who are more vulnerable, who might be colonized with different bacterial flora in the respiratory tract, and who might require more aggressive treatment. In acute bronchitis in otherwise healthy patients, viral causes predominate. RSV and rhinovirus are common causative organisms even during influenza season.

Treatment of acute bronchitis in otherwise healthy patients should be primarily supportive because the condition is largely self-limited. Patients with underlying pulmonary disease, or even smokers, may have a higher rate of pulmonary complications (e.g., secondary pneumonia) or exacerbation of COPD. Options for symptomatic treatment include air humidifiers, cough suppressants, and antipyretic analgesics. Although β-agonists are sometimes prescribed, there is no evidence for a treatment benefit in the absence of measurable airway obstruction.

Antibiotic use is controversial. Because the most frequent cause is viral, bronchitis has often been overtreated with antibiotics, which would be a preventable source of antibiotic resistance. However, in patients with a productive cough persisting beyond 10 to 14 days, treatment with antibiotics may be indicated to treat bacterial co-infection, especially in smokers or in patients with underlying pulmonary disease. In a study of community-acquired acute bronchitis in France, polymerase chain reaction (PCR) testing revealed that 4.1% of patients were infected with *Chlamydia pneumoniae* and 2.3% with *Mycoplasma pneumoniae* (Gaillat et al., 2005).

A systematic review of RCTs comparing antibiotic therapy with placebo in the treatment of acute bronchitis or acute productive cough without underlying cause found a significant benefit for the antibiotic therapy, as measured by days of illness, persistent cough, and abnormal lung findings on examination (Smucny et al., 2004). An increase in adverse effects in the antibiotic-treated group compared with the placebo group outweighed many of these benefits, however, and caution in using antibiotics unnecessarily to prevent the spread of antibiotic-resistant bacteria is still valid at the population level. The specific choice of antibiotic seems to have little impact, despite known patterns of bacterial resistance in most communities. A systematic review of controlled trials that compared azithromycin to amoxicillin or amoxicillin–clavulanic acid in patients with clinical evidence of acute bronchitis, pneumonia, and acute exacerbation of chronic bronchitis found no significant advantage for using the macrolide antibiotic (Panpanich et al., 2004).

Pneumonia

Key Points

- Pneumonia causes over a million hospitalizations per year in the United States.
- Influenza vaccine should be administered every year to patients older than 50 years and to those with chronic lung disease, diabetes, immune dysfunction, or other chronic organ failure.
- Patients should be revaccinated with pneumococcal vaccine after 10 years if the first vaccine was administered before age 65 years.
- Although atypical pathogens commonly cause community-acquired pneumonia, controlled trials show that beta-lactam antibiotics are as effective as macrolides and quinolones in most cases.

Pneumonia is an infection of the lungs that leads to consolidation of the usually air-filled alveoli. It occurs in all age groups and can be caused by various agents, including viruses, bacteria, mycobacteria, mycoplasma, and fungi. Systemic viral infections such as influenza A or B in adults and measles or varicella in children can also lead to bacterial pneumonia.

Epidemiology and Risk Factors

As shown in Table 18-3, pneumonia is the principal diagnosis for more than 1 million hospitalizations per year in the United States, with aggregate charges for these hospitalizations of almost $23.5 billion per year (Health Care Utilization Project, 2002). In-hospital death occurs in 5.6% of these hospitalizations, and more than 10% of cases are in patients over age 85.

Clinical Presentation

Patients with pneumonia can present with cough, fever, dyspnea, or malaise. Cough can be productive or nonproductive, and blood tinged or with frank blood. The clinical presentation of pneumonia in otherwise healthy patients often follows one of two patterns that can indicate the cause. A rapid onset of cough and shortness of breath with a high fever can indicate classic bacterial lobar pneumonia such as that produced by a pneumococcus. Physical findings once consolidation occurs include decreased breath sounds, dullness to percussion, and egophony on the affected side. The white blood cell (WBC) count is often elevated (>15,000), with a predominance of neutrophils. A smoldering onset with low-grade fever and fewer constitutional symptoms can indicate an atypical pneumonia, which can be caused by organisms such as respiratory viruses or by *Mycoplasma*, *Chlamydia*, or *Legionella* species.

Patients with new-onset pneumonia can be categorized by whether they are living at home in a community setting or living in a nursing home or other institutional setting. Patients who have had prolonged hospitalizations or who

Table 18-3 Outcomes for Hospital Patients with Pneumonia*

Age Group (yr)	Total Discharges	Length of Stay (mean days)	Aggregate Charges ($)	In-Hospital Deaths
All discharges	1,171,546 (100%)	5.4	29,864.341,883	41,273 (3.52%)
<1	33,756 (2.88%)	3.5	491,074,183	—
1-17	109,351 (9.33%)	3.3	1,665,455,923	213 (0.19%)
18-44	108,599 (9.27%)	4.9	2,835,259,274	997 (0.92%)
45-64	261,175 (22.29%)	5.5	7,328,896,664	5626 (2.15%)
65-84	465,118 (39.70%)	5.9	12,728,150,823	20,142 (4.33%)
85+	192,791 (16.46%)	5.9	4,797,255,969	14,271 (7.40%)

*Except pneumonia caused by tuberculosis or sexually transmitted diseases.
Data from Healthcare Cost and Utilization Project (HCUP). Weighted U.S. estimates from HCUP Nationwide Inpatient Sample, 2007. Agency for Healthcare Research and Quality, Rockville, Md. http://hcupnet.ahrq.gov/.

live in nursing homes may be colonized with gram-negative organisms (e.g., *Serratia, Pseudomonas*), anaerobes, or multidrug-resistant bacteria.

Patients with pneumonia can be further categorized by whether they are immunocompetent or immunocompromised. Patients with immunodeficiencies (including HIV/AIDS) can present with opportunistic organisms including *Pneumocystis jiroveci (carinii)*, cryptococci, *Coccidioides immitis*, atypical mycobacteria, and fungi. Alcoholism can predispose patients to lung infections with *Haemophilus influenzae* or to aspirated anaerobic organisms such as *Peptostreptococcus* or *Bacteroides*.

In children, signs of pneumonia can include malaise, cough, chest pain, tachypnea, and intercostal retractions. Children with viral pneumonias have a less toxic appearance, with low-grade fever, wheezing, and cough. Children with bacterial pneumonia appear more acutely ill, with a high-grade fever, chills, cough, and dyspnea. The earliest diagnostic clue in children may be tachypnea disproportionate to degree of fever.

In infants, potential causes of pneumonia are tied to specific periods in the first few months of life. Pneumonia in the newborn is often linked to bacteria that colonize the mother's vaginal flora. Group B streptococcal infections can occur within the first 48 hours of life or appear at 7 to 10 days after birth. Other neonatal infections include gram-negative organisms such as *Escherichia coli*. Although *Chlamydia* infections of the eye can appear in newborns at 1 to 2 weeks of age, chlamydial pneumonia is typically diagnosed in infants age 6 to 8 weeks. Other causes of pneumonia in infants age 1 to 3 months include *Ureaplasma urealyticum* and cytomegalovirus (CMV).

Viral pneumonias are most common in preschool and older children. Viral upper respiratory infections or bronchiolitis can also predispose to a bacterial pneumonia. Bacterial pathogens are responsible for only 10% to 30% of all cases of infectious pediatric pneumonia. *Streptococcus pneumoniae* has been the most common bacterial cause of childhood pneumonia, but it is declining in the face of universal pneumococcal vaccination. *H. influenzae* type B pneumonia is associated with bacteremia and other deep tissue infections (e.g., meningitis, arthritis, cellulitis) but also has declined significantly with universal immunization. *Staphylococcus aureus* causes an aggressive pneumonia that can be complicated by acute respiratory failure, pneumatoceles, or empyema. Staphylococcal pneumonia typically occurs after a staphylococcal skin infection or a systemic viral illness such as varicella (chickenpox) or measles.

Diagnosis

Cases of pneumonia are often diagnosed presumptively based on the clinical presentation and perhaps a radiograph. Chest x-ray findings in viral pneumonias include patchy or streaky, often bilateral, interstitial patterns and hyperinflation of the lungs. Bacterial pneumonias show classic lobar consolidation and alveolar infiltrates, although x-ray findings typically lag behind the clinical course by 1 to 2 days and can be completely normal on day 1. Parapneumonic pleural effusions can also occur.

Sputum Gram stain and culture may be performed but have a low yield. Some bacterial agents such as *Legionella* may be identified by antigen detection from blood samples. *Mycoplasma pneumoniae* may be diagnosed with a positive cold agglutinin test of peripheral blood. Sputum smears and cultures for acid-fast bacilli (AFB) are appropriate when there has been possible contact with tuberculosis patients, in TB-endemic areas, or when clinical findings suggest TB. Invasive procedures (e.g., BAL, lung aspiration, bronchoscopy) are reserved for special circumstances, such as diagnosing pneumonia in the immunocompromised host or in ventilator-associated pneumonias.

Treatment

Although treatment of community-acquired pneumonia (CAP) is common in primary care, there are many controversies. Clearly, many patients may be managed on an outpatient basis (Segreti et al., 2005). Use of a formal instrument such as the pneumonia severity index (PSI) or CURB-65 (see Box 16-1) can more accurately identify patients eligible for outpatient treatment (IDSA/ATS, 2007). The choice of oral antibiotic in the outpatient setting must cover common causes of bacterial pneumonia. Many treatment guidelines suggest using antibiotics that cover atypical organisms such as *Mycoplasma* and *Legionella*, but there is insufficient evidence to support any specific antibiotic strategy in the outpatient treatment of CAP (Bjerre et al., 2004). Treatment should be continued for a minimum of five days, and at least 48-72 hours beyond the patient's last signs of fever or clinical instability.

In cases of pneumococcal pneumonia with bacteremia, there is limited evidence to suggest that dual therapy with a beta-lactam antibiotic and an antibiotic with coverage of atypical organisms results in lower case-fatality rates than using a β-lactam alone. A meta-analysis of studies comparing the effectiveness of a β-lactam antibiotic with antibiotics active against atypical pathogens in nonsevere CAP found no advantage for the antibiotics that were active against atypical pathogens (Shefet et al., 2005). This was true even on subgroup analysis for patients infected with *M. pneumoniae* and *C. pneumoniae*, but there was a significantly lower treatment failure rate in the small number of patients with *Legionella* infections (relative risk [RR], 0.40) treated with a macrolide antibiotic (Mills et al., 2005). Patients with significant comorbidities or chronic organ failure and those at risk for drug-resistant *S. pneumoniae* should be treated with a respiratory fluoroquinolone or combination of β-lactam and macrolide antibiotic (IDSA/ATS, 2007).

Indications for hospitalization of any patient include failure to respond or tolerate oral antibiotics, moderate to severe respiratory distress, significant deficit in oxygenation (alveolar-arterial [A-a] O_2 gradient), more than one area of lobar consolidation, empyema, immunosuppression, abscess formation, pneumatocele, underlying cardiopulmonary disease, and high-risk PSI score. Two additional factors are the patient's age (e.g., infants <2 months, elderly patients) and comorbidities (underlying pulmonary or cardiovascular disease).

Even in the hospital, not all patients must be treated with intravenous antibiotics (Marras et al., 2004). The patient might require hospitalization for dehydration or oxygen therapy, but in select cases, oral antibiotics may be equally effective, cost less, and require fewer days in the hospital than IV antibiotic therapy. Other patients may start receiving IV antibiotics in the hospital, but an algorithm that provides for an early switch to oral antibiotics and early discharge can reduce hospital stay.

Treatment of neonatal pneumonia should target group B streptococci and gram-negative organisms such as *E. coli*. Older children with suspected bacterial pneumonia should be treated with antibiotics that provide appropriate coverage for *H. influenzae* and *S. pneumoniae*. Pneumonia in children older than 5 years should also include macrolide coverage for *M. pneumoniae*. When symptoms recur or persist for longer than 1 month, further evaluation for an underlying condition should be undertaken (TB skin test, serum immunoglobulin, bronchoscopy, barium swallow, sweat chloride test).

Prevention

Approximately half of all cases of adult pneumonia can be prevented by annual administration of influenza vaccine, plus a one-time pneumococcal vaccine when indicated (Vu et al., 2002). Vaccination with inactivated influenza vaccine is appropriate for all age groups, but the live, attenuated influenza vaccine is approved for use only in healthy patients age 5 to 49 years. The CDC recommends that influenza vaccine be given to all children from 6 months to 18 years of age, all adults over age 50, and other persons at higher risk for complications of influenza (Box 18-4).

Health care workers are an important source of transmission of influenza from infected patients to other medically vulnerable patients. Therefore, they also should be immunized, preferably with inactivated vaccine if they have close contact with severely immunocompromised persons. Health care workers or family members vaccinated with live, attenuated influenza vaccine should avoid contact with severely immunosuppressed patients for at least 7 days after vaccination.

Two types of vaccine are available for immunizing against invasive pneumococcal disease. For children younger than 2 years, universal vaccination with heptavalent (7 serotypes) pneumococcal vaccine is recommended. For other indications and age groups, pneumococcal polysaccharide vaccines currently cover 23 serotypes of the disease. ACIP recommends the pneumococcal polysaccharide vaccine for all patients older than 2 years with pulmonary, cardiac, immune, or other medical risk factors, immunocompromised persons, and those older than 65 years. Specifically, the indications for pneumococcal polysaccharide vaccine are as follows:

- Adults 65 years or older
- Immunocompetent adults or children 2 years or older who are at increased risk for illness and death associated with pneumococcal disease because of chronic illness
- Adults or children 2 years or older with functional or anatomic asplenia
- Adults or children 2 years or older living in environments in which the risk for disease is high
- Immunocompromised adults or children 2 years or older who are at high risk for infection

A systematic review suggests that pneumococcal vaccination does not significantly reduce all-cause mortality or overall rates of pneumonia, but it is specifically effective in preventing invasive pneumococcal disease (Dear et al., 2003).

Box 18-4. Groups Who Should Receive Seasonal Influenza Vaccine[*]

All children age 6 months to 18 years

All persons age 50 years or older

Women who will be pregnant during the influenza season

Persons who have chronic pulmonary (including asthma), cardiovascular (except hypertension), renal, hepatic, cognitive, neurologic/neuromuscular, hematologic, or metabolic disorders (including diabetes mellitus)

Persons who have immunosuppression (including medication induced or HIV)

Residents of nursing homes and other long-term care facilities

Health care personnel

Household contacts and caregivers of children younger than 5 years and adults 50 years or older, with particular emphasis on vaccinating contacts of children less than 6 months

Household contacts and caregivers of persons with medical conditions that put them at higher risk for severe complications from influenza

*Centers for Disease Control and Prevention (CDC) recommendations, for all persons without contraindications in the groups listed.

Older patients should be revaccinated with pneumococcal polysaccharide vaccine after 10 years if the first pneumococcal vaccine was administered before age 65. Elderly persons with unknown vaccination status should be administered 1 dose of vaccine. Children older than 2 years at highest risk for serious pneumococcal infection and likely to have a rapid decline in pneumococcal antibody levels (asplenia, renal failure, HIV, cancer chemotherapy) should also be revaccinated after 3 to 5 years.

KEY TREATMENT

Treating uncomplicated community-acquired pneumonia with a macrolide or respiratory quinolone has no proven treatment advantage over cephalosporin or aminopenicillin therapy (Mills et al., 2005; Shefet et al., 2005), unless patients have significant comorbidities or other risk factors (IDSA/ATS, 2007) (SOR: A).

Oral antibiotic therapy for uncomplicated CAP is safe and effective in outpatient or inpatient settings in patients younger than 65 years with no preexisting lung disease or other chronic disease with stable vital signs and no evidence of hypoxia or sepsis ((Bjerre et al., 2004; Marras et al., 2004) (SOR: A).

Influenza vaccination and pneumococcal vaccine are demonstrably effective among elderly patients and those with chronic disease (Vu et al., 2002) (SOR: A).

Chronic Infectious Diseases

Tuberculosis

Key Points

- Eighty percent of TB cases come from 22 high-burden nations, and one third of cases occur in India alone.
- Sputum cultures can confirm the diagnosis of TB, but they also are important for identifying patterns of drug resistance.
- Polymerase chain reaction techniques looking for genetic polymorphisms can provide more rapid diagnosis of drug-resistant TB.
- Latent infection (positive skin test in asymptomatic patient with normal chest radiograph) is treated with 6 to 9 months of isoniazid or 4 months of rifampin.
- Treatment of active pulmonary TB requires a multidrug regimen for 6 to 12 months; cultures should be negative in 80% of patients within 2 months.

Tuberculosis is caused by infection with *Mycobacterium tuberculosis*, transmitted by airborne exposure from close contact with infected patients. Pulmonary infection is the most common form, although extrapulmonary TB from hematogenous spread (meningitis, peritonitis, renal or adrenal TB, spinal TB [Pott's disease], others) can occur in young children, elderly people, persons in high-endemic areas, and patients with impaired immunity or malnutrition.

Epidemiology and Risk Factors

In many parts of the world, TB is one of the most common causes of fatal respiratory infection; 80% of cases come from 22 high-burden nations, and one-third occur in India alone.

WHO (2005) estimated 8.8 million new TB cases worldwide in 2003, including 674,000 HIV-infected patients, with 1.7 million deaths attributed to TB. TB cases are falling or stable in most regions but increasing in Africa. In North America, TB rates rose during the 1980s, but since 1992, TB rates have been in decline.

Children, elderly people, and immunocompromised patients are especially vulnerable. In the United States, 22% of TB cases occur in older adults, with the highest rates in elderly residents of long-term care facilities (Thrupp et al., 2004). The most important risk factor for developing TB is having household or other close contact with a patient who has active TB.

Clinical Presentation

Tuberculosis can be a life-threatening infection. For pulmonary TB, symptoms include cough, fever, dyspnea, night sweats, and weight loss or failure to gain weight. The few physical findings other than weight loss can include wheezes, rales, or signs of consolidation in the affected lung field. Hematogenous spread can lead to signs of extrapulmonary infection. Patients with an initial diagnosis of CAP might instead have TB. Patients with CAP who have symptoms suggesting TB or who do not respond to antibiotic treatment, who have upper lobe infiltrates or cavitary lesions, who come from endemic areas, or who have persistent cough or hemoptysis should be evaluated for TB (Kunimoto and Long, 2005).

For patients with symptoms or with a positive PPD, chest radiograph and sputum cultures for AFB are required. Typical chest x-ray findings include hilar or mediastinal lymphadenopathy, patchy infiltrates, apical scarring, and pleural effusions, but a cavitary lesion or miliary pattern (typical millet-seed granulomas scattered diffusely throughout lung fields) more specifically suggests TB.

Diagnosis

Skin testing is still the best method of testing for latent infection by prior exposure to *M. tuberculosis.* Intradermal testing with 5 tuberculin units (0.1 mL) of PPD is more accurate than multiprong tine testing. Interpretation depends on the patient's risk of disease. Patients with a history of direct exposure to active cases of TB, or with impaired immunity such as HIV, should be considered to have a positive test if the area of induration is greater than 5 mm at 48 to 72 hours. Most other patients should be considered positive with induration greater than 10 mm. Very-low-risk patients (age >5 years, no history of exposure, normal immune system, low rates of TB in population) may be considered positive only with induration greater than 15 mm. These criteria are summarized in Box 18-5 (CDC, 2000). Persons vaccinated with bacille Calmette-Guérin (BCG) vaccine may still be accurately tested with PPD skin testing. For high-risk populations, a percentage tuberculin response higher than 15 on the QuantiFERON-TB test (QFT) performed on venous whole blood is moderately correlated with a positive skin test. Neither PPD nor QFT is recommended as routine screening in low-risk populations (CDC, 2003a).

Clinical diagnosis in endemic areas is often based on history of exposure, clinical signs, AFB smears, and chest x-ray findings. Sputum cultures can confirm the diagnosis and also

Box 18-5 Criteria for Tuberculin Positivity by Risk Group

Reaction ≥2 mm of Induration

HIV-positive patients

Recent contacts of TB patients

Fibrotic changes on chest radiograph consistent with prior TB

Patients with organ transplants and other immunocompromised patients (receiving equivalent of ≥15 mg/day of prednisone for ≥1 month)*

Reaction ≥10 mm of Induration

Recent immigrants (i.e., within last 5 yr) from high-prevalence countries

Injection drug users

Residents and employees[†] of high-risk congregate settings

    Prisons and jails

    Nursing homes and other long-term care facilities for elderly persons

    Hospitals and other health care facilities

    Residential facilities for AIDS patients

    Homeless shelters

Mycobacteriology laboratory personnel

Persons with high-risk conditions

    Silicosis

    Diabetes mellitus

    Chronic renal failure

    Some hematologic disorders (e.g., leukemias, lymphomas)

    Other specific malignancies (e.g., head/neck or lung carcinoma)

Weight loss ≥10% of ideal body weight

Gastrectomy

Jejunoileal bypass

Children <4 yr of age, or infants, children, and adolescents exposed to high-risk adults

Reaction ≥15 mm of Induration

Persons with no risk factors for TB

*Risk of TB in patients treated with corticosteroids increases with higher dose and longer duration.

†For persons who are otherwise at low risk and are tested at the start of employment, a reaction of ≥15 mm induration is considered positive.

---

are important for identifying patterns of drug resistance. In infants and young children, sputum AFB smears and cultures plus gastric aspirates each morning for 3 days yields the diagnosis only 50% of the time. Other cases may need to be treated presumptively, based on exposure, symptoms, and chest radiograph. In culture-negative cases of TB, it is essential to find the index case and to obtain sputum cultures and drug sensitivities from that patient to guide therapy for patients with negative cultures but active disease.

Laboratory diagnosis of TB historically has relied on the use of sputum smears for AFB and culturing of the *M. tuberculosis* organism. Culture results can require 2 to 8 weeks, but more rapid methods can detect early growth within 5 to 14 days (Katoch, 2004; Schluger, 2003). Gene amplification using PCR techniques can be performed on sputum samples for rapid results, as well as on cerebrospinal fluid (CSF), gastric or pleural aspirates, and urine. PCR is highly sensitive (95%-98%) for diagnosing TB from sputum in smear-positive and culture-positive cases, but it has lower sensitivity (57%-78%) for smear-negative and culture-positive cases (Rattan, 2000). PCR may also be used on organisms obtained from early growth on positive cultures to detect drug resistance more rapidly, taking advantage of the genetic polymorphisms in the *M. tuberculosis* organism, which are almost always associated with drug resistance. Although positive results are highly specific, failure to detect mutations does not entirely rule out drug resistance (Hazbon, 2004; Nachamkin et al., 1997).

Treatment

A positive PPD skin test in an asymptomatic patient with a normal chest x-ray film and negative HIV test represents latent infection with no active disease. A 6- to 9-month course of isoniazid is effective in treating this latent infection and in preventing the development of active TB. Isoniazid therapy is associated with clinical hepatitis in approximately 0.6% of treated patients (Smieja et al., 1999). An effective alternative is rifampin for 4 months. The short course of two drugs, rifampin and pyrazinamide for 2 months, is no longer recommended because of evidence of increased liver toxicity with this combination (CDC, 2001). Treatment of positive PPD latent infection is indicated even in patients with prior history of BCG vaccination and is also effective in patients co-infected with HIV (Wilkinson et al., 1998).

Treatment of active pulmonary TB requires a multidrug regimen for 6 to 12 months. For uncomplicated pulmonary TB, a short-course protocol of four drugs (isoniazid, rifampin, pyrazinamide, ethambutol) for the first 2 months and two drugs (isoniazid, rifampin) for the next 4 months is effective. Treatment with intermittent therapy 2 days per week has been less effective than daily therapy in RCTs (Mwandumba and Squire, 2001). Repeat cultures should be obtained after 2 months of treatment, when 80% of patients have negative cultures. Cavitary lesions, or persistent positive cultures after 2 months of therapy, are indications for an extended 9-month course of treatment. New drugs entering the pipeline of clinical trials include long-acting rifamycins and fluoroquinolones.

Directly observed therapy (DOT) is indicated for patients with specific risk factors for treatment failure caused by noncompliance, but RCTs in a variety of settings have not clearly demonstrated benefit over traditional public health strategies (Volmink and Garner, 2003). Enhanced DOT appears to be more effective. Box 18-6 lists strategies of social supports, barrier reduction, compliance monitoring, and incentives that can be blended in a broad-based strategy to ensure treatment compliance and cure (ATS, CDC, IDSA, 2003). WHO reports an 82% success rate for TB treatment worldwide, although the prevalence of multidrug-resistant TB is increasing.

Treatment of patients who have positive PPD and x-ray evidence of TB but negative sputum smears depends on the level of clinical suspicion for active TB. When suspicion is high, multidrug therapy should be initiated pending culture results. If cultures come back negative but the patient shows clinical or radiographic signs of improvement after 2 months of treatment, the patient is assumed to have culture-negative TB, and treatment should be completed using isoniazid and rifampin. If culture remains negative and there is no sign of clinical or radiographic improvement, treatment may be

Box 18-6 Broad-Based Strategy to Ensure Tuberculosis Treatment Adherence and Cure

Enablers

Interventions to assist the patient in completing therapy.

Transportation vouchers

Child care

Convenient clinic hours and locations

Clinic personnel who speak the languages of the populations served

Reminder systems and follow-up of missed appointments

Social service assistance (referrals for substance abuse treatment and counseling, housing, and other services)

Outreach workers (bilingual/bicultural as needed; can provide many services related to maintaining patient adherence, including provision of DOT, follow-up on missed appointments, monthly monitoring, transportation, sputum collection, social service assistance, and educational reinforcement)

Integration of care for tuberculosis with care for other conditions

Incentives

Interventions to motivate the patient, tailored to individual patient wishes and needs and thus meaningful to the patient

Food stamps or snacks and meals

Restaurant coupons

Assistance in finding or provision of housing

Clothing or other personal products

Books

Stipends

Patient contract

DOT, Directly observed therapy.

From American Thoracic Society, Centers for Disease Control and Prevention, Infectious Diseases Society of America. Treatment of tuberculosis. Am J Respir Crit Care Med 2003;167:603-662, and MMWR 52(RR-11):1-77. http://www.cdc.gov/mmwr/preview/mmwrhtml/rr5211a1.htm.

KEY TREATMENT

A 9-month course of isoniazid or a 4-month course of rifampin is effective in preventing developmetnt of active TB in asymptomatic patients with a positive PPD test and negative chest x-ray film (i.e., latent infection), even in patients with HIV co-infection (Smieja et al., 1999; Wilkinson et al., 1998) (SOR: A).

Treatment with intermittent therapy 2 days per week has been less effective than daily therapy in RCTs (Mwandumba and Squire, 2001) (SOR: A).

BCG vaccine effectively reduces infection rates by about 50% in highly endemic populations (Colditz et al., 1995) (SOR: B).

AIDS-Related Infections

Key Points

- Specific opportunistic infections are associated with HIV, and bacterial community-acquired pneumonias are also common.
- More than half of HIV-infected patients with CD4+ counts less than 200 cells/μL experience an AIDS-related opportunistic infection within the next 2 years.
- Tuberculosis is common in HIV patients. TB worsens the clinical course of HIV infection, and HIV infection complicates TB management.
- High-resolution CT scan is the best imaging study for diagnosing HIV-related pulmonary infections.
- Inactivated influenza and pneumococcal vaccines are recommended for HIV-infected patients who are still able to mount a significant immune response.

HIV/AIDS by definition compromises our host defense capacity for fighting otherwise-benign infections. Some of the most common opportunistic infections in patients with HIV/AIDS affect the lungs as their target organ.

Epidemiology and Risk Factors

Table 18-4 shows the relationship between opportunistic infections (OIs) and specific levels of immunocompromise as measured by CD4+ lymphocyte counts; 200 cells/μL is a critical threshold for prophylactic treatment (Clumeck and Wit, 2003). More than half of HIV patients with CD4+ counts below this level experience an AIDS-related OI in 2 years.

Human cases of *Pneumocystis carinii* pneumonia (PCP) are now understood to be caused by *Pneumocystis jiroveci.* Most healthy children have been infected asymptomatically with *P. jiroveci* by age 4 years (Pifer et al., 1978), allowing cases in HIV patients to occur either by reactivation or by new exposure. Without antiretroviral therapy or PCP prophylaxis, more than 70% of HIV-infected patients could be expected to experience PCP, with 20% to 40% mortality (Phair et al., 1990).

Clinical Presentation

A wide range of clinical presentations can occur with OIs in HIV/AIDS. PCP can manifest with cough, tachypnea, and fever. Chest films may be relatively normal early in the course of disease but eventually may show diffuse, bilateral, symmetric interstitial infiltrates in a butterfly pattern. Hypoxia,

discontinued after 2 months. For patients at low suspicion of TB, no treatment is indicated pending culture results. If cultures remain negative and the patient is asymptomatic with no progression on chest x-ray film, a standard course of treatment for latent TB (isoniazid for 9 months or rifampin for 4 months) is indicated (Fig. 18-8).

Prevention

The most important elements of prevention are screening for exposure, detection and follow-up of active cases, and prophylaxis of infected but clinically asymptomatic patients. PPD testing and treatment of latent infection is a more effective strategy than BCG vaccination in patient populations with relatively low incidence of pulmonary TB, but in highly endemic areas, infant BCG vaccination strategies can reduce childhood TB infection rates by as much as 50% (Colditz et al., 1995). Patients with a positive PPD but no symptoms and a negative chest film should be treated with isoniazid daily for 9 months or rifampin for 4 months. Maintaining an effective public health infrastructure, including TB surveillance, screening, and contact tracing, is essential. Sputum culture and sensitivity testing is an increasingly relevant component of an effective public health strategy to identify and contain the spread of multidrug-resistant TB.

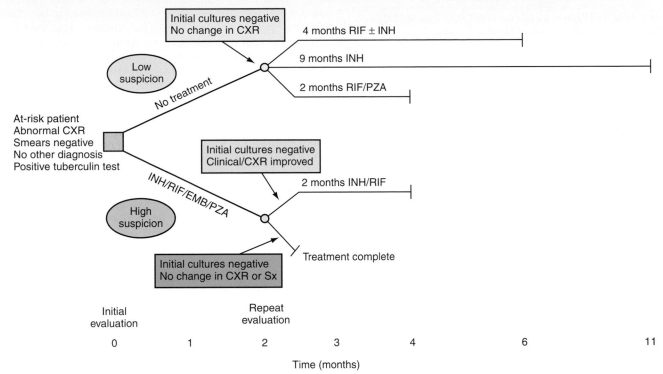

Figure 18-8 Treatment algorithm for inactive tuberculosis (TB) and for active, culture-negative pulmonary TB. *(American Thoracic Society, Centers for Disease Control and Prevention, and Infectious Diseases Society of America: Treatment of tuberculosis. Am J Respir Crit Care Med 2003;167:603-662, and MMWR 52(RR-11):1-77. http://www.cdc.gov/mmwr/preview/mmwrhtml/rr5211a1.htm.)*

Pao_2 less than 70 mm Hg, and an increased A-a O_2 gradient are typical. Pneumothorax occurring in a patient infected with HIV suggests PCP, which typically produces pneumatoceles as lung tissue is destroyed.

Clinicians should also have a high index of suspicion for pulmonary TB in HIV-infected patients. Presentation of pulmonary TB is fairly typical (upper lobe patchy infiltrates with or without cavitation) in patients with CD4µL, whereas patients with more severe immune suppression often have atypical lung presentations (lobar infiltrates or miliary pattern) or extrapulmonary forms of TB. In severely immunocompromised patients, sputum AFB cultures can be positive even in the presence of normal chest radiograph.

The attention to OIs should not diminish clinical suspicion for bacterial pneumonia as a cause of significant morbidity and mortality in HIV-infected patients. *S. pneumoniae, H. influenzae, Pseudomonas aeruginosa,* and *S. aureus* are the most frequently isolated organisms (Rimland et al., 2002). Patients present with typical symptoms such as fever, tachypnea, cough, and constitutional symptoms and a pattern of lobar pneumonia or other infiltrates on chest x-ray film.

Diagnosis

Diagnosis of PCP may be obtained from laboratory testing, histopathology, and imaging studies. Histochemical stains and direct immunofluorescent studies can confirm the organism's presence in induced sputum, but sensitivities are much greater (90%-99%) when specimens are obtained from BAL or transbronchial biopsy (Cruciani et al., 2002). Open lung biopsy is the "gold standard" and may be safer than bronchoscopic techniques for patients with bleeding disorders.

Nuclear medicine and CT studies are also used extensively in evaluating pulmonary symptoms in patients with HIV/AIDS. For example, HRCT scan can show a patchy, ground-glass appearance or characteristic pneumatoceles in PCP. Gallium-67 scintigraphy is also useful. In a study of 57 immunocompromised patients with pulmonary infections, the first-choice diagnosis suggested by CT was accurate in most fungal infections (95.0%) and PCP (87.5%), but was less accurate for bacterial (73.7%) and viral (75.0%) infections, and missed both cases of mycobacterial infection (Demirkazik et al., 2008). A gallium scan showing diffuse increased uptake in the lungs of an HIV-infected patient can also suggest PCP. Sensitivity is high (>90%), but specificity can be as low as 51%. Features of an abnormal gallium scan that increase specificity and positive predictive value include increased uptake in the lungs in the presence of a normal chest film, intensity of uptake in the lung (greater than liver uptake), and a diffuse heterogeneous pattern. In a comparative study of gallium scanning versus HRCT in HIV/AIDS patients with pulmonary symptoms but normal or near-normal chest radiographs, HRCT resulted in both higher positive predictive values (86%) and negative predictive values (88%) than gallium scintigraphy (62% and 73%) (Kirshenbaum et al., 1998).

Sequential thallium and gallium scanning may be performed when Kaposi's sarcoma is suspected. The combination of a positive thallium and negative gallium scan is highly specific for Kaposi's sarcoma, but sensitivity is decreased by the presence of opportunistic infections, which can make the gallium scan positive as well. Other nuclear imaging studies include cell-surface peptide receptor-binding molecules radiolabeled with indium or technetium (van de Wiele et al., 2002).

Table 18-4 Risk Factors Associated with Development of Major Opportunistic Infections in HIV-Infected Patients

Infection	CD4+ Count Risk Threshold (cells/mm³)	Other Risk Factors
Pneumocystis jiroveci (carinii) pneumonia (PCP)	≤200	Prior PCP Present CD4+ cells <14% Fever of unexplained etiology Presence of oral candidiasis
Mycobacterium tuberculosis	Any	Tuberculin skin test (PPD) positive Exposure to infectious contact
Mycobacterium avium complex	≤50	Prior respiratory or gastrointestinal colonization Prior opportunistic disease High viral load (>105 copies/mL)
Cytomegalovirus (CMV) disease	≤50	Seropositive (IgG antibodies to CMV) CMV viremia Prior opportunistic disease High viral load (>105 copies/mL)
Cryptococcal meningitis	≤50-100	Environmental exposure
Toxoplasmosis	≤100-200	Seropositive (IgG antibody to *T. gondii*)
Candida esophagitis	≤100	Prior *Candida* colonization High viral load (>105 copies/mL)
Cryptosporidiosis	≤100	Environmental exposure (contaminated water, soil, animal exposure)
Histoplasmosis	≤100	Exposure (endemic areas: Midwest, Southwest U.S.)
Coccidioidomycosis	≤100	Exposure (endemic areas: Southwest U.S., Mexico)

Prevention and Treatment

The treatment of HIV is covered in Chapter 17. However, there are specific opportunities for preventing pulmonary OIs in HIV-infected patients. Antiretroviral therapy (ART) has transformed HIV/AIDS into a chronic disease in which CD4+ counts can often be maintained above levels at which OIs are likely. For preventing pulmonary complications, prophylaxis regimens that were effective in decreasing OI rates in the pre-ART era still play a role in the care of patients with more advanced disease. ART has resulted in dramatic decreases in HIV-related mortality and OIs, but specific challenges are raised by the cost and complexity of the drug regimens as well as drug-drug interactions, particularly when mixing prophylactic antibiotics or antituberculous agents with protease inhibitors.

When an OI leads to the initial diagnosis of HIV/AIDS, treatment with ART and agents effective against the OI may be begun simultaneously. Fever and worsening of clinical symptoms several weeks after ART initiation may be related to recovery of the patient's immune function, described as an "immune reconstitution or reactivation syndrome," and must be differentiated from treatment failure or progression of disease by measuring serial CD4+ counts and RNA viral loads.

Trimethoprim-sulfamethoxazole (TMP-SMX) prophylaxis has been demonstrated to prevent episodes of *P. jiroveci* pneumonia and to enhance survival in patients with low CD4μL (D'Egidio et al., 2007). Oral dapsone or inhaled pentamidine are alternatives for patients unable to tolerate TMP-SMX. It is also used to treat PCP infections, although side-effects of TMP-SMX are significantly higher in HIV/AIDS patients. Corticosteroids are added for patients with significant respiratory distress or hypoxemia.

Tuberculosis worsens the clinical course of HIV infection, and HIV infection complicates the management of TB (Sharma et al., 2005). All HIV-infected patients should undergo PPD testing for latent infection with *M. tuberculosis*. A PPD reaction greater than 5 mm is considered positive in an HIV-infected patient. If chest x-ray film is negative and there are no other signs of active pulmonary or extrapulmonary TB, an appropriate treatment regimen for latent TB should be initiated. Treatment of latent TB reduces significantly the risk of developing active TB in HIV patients with a positive skin test (Volmink and Woldehanna, 2004). Regimens are similar to those used in HIV-negative patients, but if isoniazid is chosen, the duration of treatment is 9 months rather than 6 months. Standard treatment regimens for active TB appear to be effective in HIV patients as well, but trials will determine the optimum duration, regimen, and dosing frequency in patients with TB and more severe HIV-related immunocompromise. Treatment with rifampin should be avoided or undertaken with great caution in patients receiving protease inhibitors or nonnucleoside reverse-transcriptase inhibitors (NNRTIs). Dosage of rifabutin should be decreased with these agents. Detailed guidelines for the combined treatment of TB and HIV are available and frequently updated (CDC, 2007).

Mycobacterium avium complex (MAC) infections can be prevented with clarithromycin or rifabutin prophylaxis, although there is increasing resistance to clarithromycin. Disseminated MAC infection often manifests with signs in multiple organ systems. Localized pneumonia can occur in patients with more intact immune function receiving ART.

Although other prophylactic regimens are available to prevent systemic viral or fungal infections, a survival benefit has not been demonstrated. Inactivated influenza and 23-valent pneumococcal vaccines are recommended for HIV patients who are still able to mount a significant immune response and should be initiated early in the disease, with annual influenza vaccine each year thereafter. Live vaccines should not be used.

KEY TREATMENT

Treatment of latent tuberculosis (positive skin test) reduces risk of progression to active TB in HIV/AIDS patients (Volmink and Woldehanna, 2004) (SOR: A).

Influenza vaccine is indicated for HIV-AIDS patients (SOR: A).

Treatment of asymptomatic HIV-infected patients with trimethoprim-sulfamethoxazole significantly reduces pulmonary infections with *Pneumocystis* pneumonia (Grimwade et al., 2003) (SOR: A).

Fungal Infections of the Lung

Endemic mycoses (histoplasmosis, coccidioidomycosis, and paracoccidioidomycosis) can cause primary pulmonary infections in exposed patients as well as reactivation syndromes in patients with HIV or other causes of immune suppression. The incidence of these infections has decreased with the widespread use of ART for HIV infection. Fungal infections related to *Aspergillus* spp. are more widespread geographically, but the incidence of aspergillosis has also decreased with increasing ART use.

Epidemiology and Risk Factors

Histoplasmosis *(Histoplasma capsulatum)* is most common in basins of the Ohio and Mississippi rivers. Blastomycosis *(Blastomyces dermatitidis)* is found in this same area of the United States as well as in portions of Canada. Coccidioidomycosis *(Coccidioides immitis)* is prevalent in desert areas of the southwestern United States, and paracoccidioidomycosis *(Paracoccidioides brasiliensis)* is the most common endemic mycosis in Central and South America. Airborne exposure to local soil is a risk factor. In South Asia and Southeast Asia (especially India, China, Thailand, and Vietnam), *Penicilliosis marneffei* is another significant endemic mycosis affecting HIV/AIDS patients (Randhawa, 2000).

Aspergillosis occurs most often in the context of immune suppression, especially in HIV-infected patients with CD4+ lymphocyte counts less than 50 cells/μL. Leukopenia, systemic corticosteroids, bone marrow transplantation, and broad-spectrum antibiotic therapy also increase risk for aspergillosis.

Clinical Presentation

Presentation of any of the endemic mycoses depends on the patient's underlying immune status, as well as on the degree of exposure. For example, in patients with significant immune suppression (CD4+ lymphocyte counts <150/μL), histoplasmosis can manifest with signs and symptoms of disseminated multiorgan infection, whereas patients with more intact immune symptoms can have more localized pulmonary symptoms and signs. Blastomycosis is often a self-limited infection, but it can lead to chronic pneumonia or skin, musculoskeletal, or CNS involvement (Pappas, 2004). Cough, dyspnea, and fever, with or without weight loss or night sweats, are the most common symptoms (Baumgardner et al., 2004). Coccidioidomycosis similarly can manifest as a self-limited pulmonary infection. In the case of intense exposure or in immunosuppressed patients, it can manifest as a severe fulminant pulmonary infection with ARDS or as a disseminated infection (peritonitis, lymphadenopathy, skin nodules, meningitis, musculoskeletal or liver involvement).

Respiratory disease caused by *Aspergillus* can take the form of pseudomembranous tracheitis or invasive pneumonia. Pseudomembranous tracheitis can lead to airway obstruction. Both respiratory syndromes are associated with cough, fever, dyspnea, and hemoptysis, and pneumonia also produces hypoxia. Chest x-ray films can show diffuse interstitial infiltrates or even signs of pulmonary infarction caused by fungal invasion of vascular tissue.

Diagnosis

In disseminated histoplasmosis, *Histoplasma* antigen is detectable in blood or urine with 85% to 95% sensitivity. For isolated pulmonary histoplasmosis, BAL or transbronchial biopsy may be required. *Coccidioides* organisms may be cultured or seen on histopathologic tissue stains or detected by serologic tests of blood or CSF. *Aspergillus* spp. may be cultured from sputum samples, which is sufficient for diagnosis in the presence of a typical clinical syndrome and no alternative diagnosis. More definitive diagnosis may be made by BAL (50% sensitivity) or open-lung biopsy.

Treatment

Acute, uncomplicated pulmonary histoplasmosis may be treated with watchful waiting in patients with normal immune systems (Wheat et al., 2004). Severe disseminated histoplasmosis or severe diffuse pulmonary histoplasmosis is treated with the liposomal form of amphotericin B for 3 to 10 days, followed by 12 weeks of oral itraconazole therapy, and then lifelong itraconazole prophylaxis. New antifungal agents such as voriconazole, caspofungin, and micafungin are potential alternatives (Herbrecht et al., 2005; Ruhnke, 2004). Detailed treatment guidelines for the management of histoplasmosis and blastomycosis infections are available from IDSA (Chapman et al., 2008; Wheat et al., 2007).

For coccidioidomycosis and blastomycosis, amphotericin B is usually chosen for initial therapy. Less serious infections might respond to fluconazole or itraconazole, and some treatment success has been demonstrated with voriconazole (Bakleh et al., 2005). Meningitis is treated with fluconazole or intrathecal amphotericin B. The CDC recommends treatment with voriconazole for invasive aspergillosis.

Prevention

The most important means of preventing fungal pulmonary infections is the ART of HIV/AIDS. HIV patients treated for histoplasmosis or coccidioidomycosis require chronic suppressive therapy with itraconazole or alternative antifungal therapy for life. TMP-SMX prophylaxis for PCP might also be protective against paracoccidioidomycosis. Education and protective gear (protective masks) during digging, excavation, and construction projects or cave exploration in endemic areas can help prevent acute pulmonary infections caused by high-level environmental exposures.

Vascular Disease

Pulmonary Embolism

Key Points

- Clinical decision rules using objective scoring algorithms help establish pretest probability and enhance the predictive value of other tests for pulmonary embolism (PE).
- A negative *quantitative* D-dimer test by ELISA less than 500 μg/L can effectively rule out PE in patients with low or intermediate pretest probability of disease.

- High-resolution CT scan with contrast can be performed on the lungs and the deep veins of the legs at the same time in a PE protocol.
- Hemodynamically stable patients with submassive PE may be treated with dose-adjusted intravenous or fixed-dose subcutaneous heparin.
- Hemodynamically unstable patients with massive PE may be treated with thrombolytics or embolectomy.
- Prophylactic therapy is not effective if initiated after a clot has begun to form, so venous thromboembolism prophylaxis with subcutaneous heparin should be part of standard hospital admitting orders unless specifically contraindicated.

In the 19th century, Rudolf Virchow defined the pathologic process of pulmonary embolism, in which blood clots, usually from deep vein thromboses (DVTs) in one or both legs, break off and are trapped in the pulmonary arterial system, leading to pulmonary infarct, decreased oxygenation of venous blood returning from the periphery, and elevated right-sided pressures in the heart (Dalen, 2002). Two thirds of emboli reach both lungs and lodge in large or intermediate pulmonary arteries, most often in the lower lobes.

Epidemiology and Risk Factors

In 2003 there were 98,921 hospitalizations in the United States during which pulmonary embolism was diagnosed, generating charges of nearly $2 billion. In-hospital mortality was 3% (Health Care Utilization Project,, 2003). The importance of rapid diagnosis and treatment was underscored by Dalen and Alpert in 1975, who estimated that only 6% of PE deaths at that point in medical history occurred in patients diagnosed and treated for PE (Dalen, 2002).

The most important cause of pulmonary embolism is DVT, and both conditions are included under the broader term *venous thromboembolism* (VTE). Virchow's triad of risk included hypercoagulability, stasis, and vascular injury. Patients can develop DVT after surgery (especially hip or pelvic surgery), major trauma, prolonged hospitalization or bed confinement, or even prolonged sitting in a confined space (air travel, bus or car trips, medical school lectures). Patients at highest risk are those with a past history of DVT. Additional risk factors include smoking, cancer, obesity, pregnancy, heart disease, stroke, burns, and medications (e.g., estrogen therapy). Patients with inherited risk include those with antithrombin III deficiency, hyperhomocysteinemia, protein C or protein S deficiency, and factor V Leiden mutation, as well as those with acquired hypercoagulable states such as the antiphospholipid syndrome.

Clinical Presentation

Any suspicion of PE as a cause of acute shortness of breath requires specific diagnostic evaluation and quick intervention in this potentially life-threatening condition. Acute-onset shortness of breath coupled with pleuritic chest pain, hemoptysis, wedge-shaped pulmonary infarct lesions on chest radiograph, and S1Q3 pattern with tachycardia on ECG can all point specifically to a diagnosis of PE, but most patients have a nonspecific presentation. Collateral circulation from bronchial arteries makes pulmonary infarction relatively uncommon. Massive PE can lead to acute right ventricular failure and cardiovascular collapse. Pa_{O_2} greater than 80 mm Hg in room air and a normal A-a O_2 gradient make the diagnosis less likely but do not completely exclude PE. All patients with acute-onset shortness of breath with no apparent cause should be evaluated for PE.

Diagnosis

Diagnosing PE includes an evaluation for DVT. Physical examination for signs of DVT (asymmetry in calf or thigh diameter, calf tenderness, Homans sign) are relatively insensitive and nonspecific, and other tests (venous Doppler ultrasonography or spiral CT with contrast) can more accurately confirm the presence of significant underlying DVT.

Once suspected, PE must be confirmed or ruled out with a high degree of certainty. Failure to treat could be life threatening, but treatment carries significant risks as well. Clinical decision rules using objective scoring algorithms help establish pretest probability (high, intermediate, or low), which in turn enhances predictive value of other tests for PE (Ebell, 2004). One common decision tool uses only history and physical examination variables (Wells et al., 2001), and another scoring system adds variables from chest x-ray and arterial blood gas measurements (Wicki et al., 2001).

Several qualitative, semiquantitative, and quantitative laboratory methods are available for measuring D-dimer. Any negative D-dimer test can help exclude the diagnosis of PE in patients with low pretest probability of disease, but for patients with moderate pretest probability, only quantitative D-dimer test by enzyme-linked immunosorbent assay (ELISA) less than 500 µg/L can effectively rule out PE. Spiral CT with contrast and magnetic resonance angiography (MRA), two alternative imaging studies widely replacing V/Q scan, are more accessible and accurate in patients with underlying heart or lung disease, and perhaps more accurate for centrally located than peripheral emboli. Spiral CT also offers the advantage of potentially diagnosing other conditions, and when ordered in a PE protocol, may be combined with CT of the lower extremities to evaluate possible DVTs. Table 18-5 summarizes the results of strategies for excluding the diagnosis of PE (using criteria of post-test probability <5%) or for confirming the diagnosis (post-test probability >85%) (Roy et al., 2005).

Treatment

The options for treatment of PE include anticoagulation, thrombolysis, and (rarely) surgery. With controlled trials ongoing, no clear recommendation yet exists for thrombolysis in all cases of PE. One trial of alteplase plus heparin showed significantly decreased mortality in patients with submassive PE, compared with patients treated only with heparin (Konstantinides et al., 2002). However, a meta-analysis of all RCTs comparing thrombolytic therapy with heparin in patients with PE showed a survival benefit only in studies that included hemodynamically unstable patients (patients with massive PE). In trials that excluded these patients, there was no benefit found for thrombolysis (mortality slightly worse for thrombolytic therapy) (Wan et al., 2004). Treatment of DVT with thrombolytics has also been studied, and although venous blood flow may be improved and post-DVT syndrome decreased, there is a significant risk of hemorrhagic complications such as stroke.

Table 18-5 Diagnostic Tests to Exclude or Confirm Diagnosis of Pulmonary Embolism (PE)

Pretest Probability Based on Objective Clinical Decision Rules	Exclude Diagnosis (PE <5%)	Confirm Diagnosis (PE >85%)
Low clinical probability (10%)	Negative D-dimer (quantitative or semiquantitative) Negative spiral CT scan Negative MRA Low-probability V/Q scan	Positive pulmonary angiogram (no other test is adequate to confirm positive diagnosis of PE in a patient with low prior probability)
Moderate clinical probability (35%)	Quantitative D-dimer<500µg/L (by ELISA method) Normal or near-normal lung scan Negative spiral CT scan *in combination with* negative venous Doppler ultrasound of leg veins	Positive spiral CT scan High-probability V/Q scan Positive MRA Positive venous Doppler ultrasound of leg veins
High clinical probability (70%)	Negative pulmonary angiogram (no other test is adequate to exclude or rule out diagnosis of PE in a patient with a high prior probability)	Positive spiral CT scan High-probability V/Q scan Positive MRA Positive echocardiogram ultrasound

CT, Computed tomography; *ELISA,* enzyme-linked immunosorbent assay; *MRA,* magnetic resonance angiography; *V/Q,* ventilation/perfusion ratio.

In massive PE with cardiovascular collapse, thrombolysis is often used, but emergency pulmonary embolectomy is an option in settings where cardiothoracic surgery can be mobilized rapidly. Dauphine and Omari (2005) reported on 11 patients with massive PE treated with emergency embolectomy. Of the seven patients who did not have preoperative cardiac arrest, all survived to hospital discharge. One of the four patients who experienced cardiac arrest preoperatively also survived to discharge.

For patients who are hemodynamically stable and have less than massive pulmonary emboli, the initial treatment choice is dose-adjusted, intravenous unfractionated heparin or fixed-dose, subcutaneous low-molecular-weight (LMW) heparin. A meta-analysis comparing these two therapies in venous thromboembolism treatment found odds ratios favoring LMW heparin in both the rate of recurrence and the rate of bleeding complications, but these differences were not statistically significant (Erkens and Prins, 2010). LMW heparin by fixed-dose subcutaneous injection is at least as safe and effective as traditional dose-adjusted, unfractionated heparin therapy. Anticoagulation with warfarin is indicated for at least 3 to 6 months after an initial PE episode, and lifetime therapy may be warranted for patients with hypercoagulability or recurrent episodes. Patients with recurrent episodes unresponsive to anticoagulation might benefit from surgical placement of an inferior vena cava filter.

Prevention

Primary prevention of PE begins with prevention of DVT. Trauma, hip or pelvic surgery, general surgery, and hospitalization or prolonged bed rest put patients at significant short-term risk. Many cases of VTE can be prevented in these patients if prophylaxis is initiated promptly. Prophylactic therapy is not effective if it is initiated after a clot has begun to form, so it is crucial to include VTE prophylaxis (subcutaneous heparin as well as mechanical interventions) on admitting orders for most patients admitted to a hospital for surgery or for serious medical conditions. Clinicians currently underutilize prophylactic therapies recommended in various clinical guidelines. They should order heparin prophylaxis on admission automatically unless there is a specific contraindication or the patient is clearly not at risk, rather than ordering prophylaxis only when risk factors are obvious (Tooher et al., 2005). Once DVT begins in the legs, prompt diagnosis and therapy can provide effective secondary prevention of the more life-threatening PE.

KEY TREATMENT

Deep vein thrombosis prophylaxis begun routinely on hospital admission, unless specifically contraindicated, can prevent many in-hospital PE episodes (Tooher et al., 2005) (SOR: A).
An algorithm using clinical indicators, quantitative D-dimer test, and various imaging studies (spiral CT with contrast, MRA, venous Doppler ultrasound) can effectively rule in (>85% probability) or rule out (<5% probability) PE (Roy et al., 2005) (SOR: A).

Pulmonary Hypertension

Pulmonary hypertension is diagnosed when pulmonary artery pressures exceed normal levels, and symptoms ensue. The condition may be either primary or secondary to other causes, which can be pulmonary, cardiac, or systemic in origin.

Epidemiology and Risk Factors

Secondary causes of pulmonary hypertension include chronic lung disease (COPD and chronic bronchitis), cardiac disease (congenital defects, mitral stenosis, left atrial myxoma), autoimmune or inflammatory conditions such as scleroderma and SLE (Paolini et al., 2004), and granulomatous disease such as sarcoidosis. Certain drugs (fenfluramine) can also cause the condition, as can chronic liver disease with portal hypertension. Some patients experience pulmonary hypertension as a complication of arterial clotting or chronic damage from single or multiple episodes of PE.

Primary pulmonary hypertension is diagnosed when there is no obvious cause of the condition, and there is a familial form of the disease as well. Persistent pulmonary hypertension of the newborn occurs in 1.9 neonates per 1000 live births and results from shunting through a patent foramen ovale and ductus arteriosus, with or without pulmonary hypoplasia (Greenough and Khetriwal, 2005).

Clinical Presentation

Symptoms include easy fatigability, exertional dyspnea, chest pain, dizziness or lightheadedness, and syncope. Underlying pulmonary or cardiac disease can mask the diagnosis in early stages. Pulmonary hypertension is often diagnosed late with signs of right-sided heart failure. Patients with COPD, pulmonary fibrosis, sarcoidosis, or recurrent PE who have evidence of right-sided heart failure (cor pulmonale) should be evaluated for pulmonary hypertension as well.

Diagnosis

In the primary care office, patients can have signs of right-sided chamber enlargement on ECG. Echocardiogram may also suggest increased right-sided pressures and decreased cardiac index and can be performed both at rest and during exercise. It may also reveal cardiac causes of secondary pulmonary hypertension (Bossone et al., 2005). Definitive diagnosis is made by recording of a pulmonary artery pressure greater than 25 mm Hg on catheterization.

Treatment

Nonspecific treatments of pulmonary hypertension include loop diuretics, digoxin, and anticoagulant therapy with warfarin when indicated. Traditional therapies include dihydropyridine calcium channel blockers such as nifedipine or amlodipine, which can modestly decrease pulmonary arterial pressures in vasoresponsive patients but can also cause sudden death in nonvasoresponsive patients (Humbert, 2004; Malik et al. 1997).

Other therapies include prostacyclins such as epoprostenol and treprostinil; both are pulmonary and systemic vasodilators, but must be given by continuous intravenous infusion through an indwelling catheter or by subcutaneous injection (treprostinil) (Paramothayan et al., 2005). Iloprost is an inhaled form of prostacyclin apparently with fewer side effects that can improve exercise capacity and symptom scores, but it requires frequent dosing (Baker and Hockman, 2005). Side effects and economic costs are significant obstacles to the use of all these agents. Bosentan is a nonselective endothelin receptor antagonist, and sitaxsentan is a selective endothelin receptor antagonist. Both improve functional status and physiologic measures in pulmonary hypertension (Liu and Cheng, 2005).

Sildenafil, which inhibits phosphodiesterase type 5 in the pulmonary vasculature, has also been approved for this indication based on results of a controlled trial that showed it improved 6-minute walk distance, New York Hearth Association (NYHA) functional class, pulmonary artery pressure, cardiac index, and oxygenation. Sildenafil (2005) is also less expensive than the prostacyclins and endothelin receptor antagonists. Dipyridamole also has some phosphodiesterase type 5 activity.

Inhaled nitric oxide is a selective pulmonary vasodilator that is often used to treat persistent pulmonary hypertension of the newborn. In adults with pulmonary hypertension, a 2-year trial of inhaled nitric oxide therapy combined with dipyridamole demonstrated improvements in exercise capacity, symptoms, and hemodynamic measures (Perez-Penate et al., 2005). A European consensus panel has released guidelines for the use of nitric oxide in this condition (Germann et al., 2005).

Surgical therapies may be general (lung transplant) or specific, as in the repair of congenital shunting lesions, mitral stenosis, or atrial defects. Pulmonary thromboendarterectomy is effective in some patients with pulmonary hypertension associated with saddle pulmonary embolus (Olsson et al., 2005).

Other Pulmonary Diseases of the Pulmonary Vasculature

Wegener's granulomatosis is a vasculitis (inflammatory condition) of the vascular bed that can manifest either with shortness of breath or hemoptysis or with progressive pulmonary fibrosis caused by repeated small hemorrhages at the alveolar level. It is now categorized as a systemic antineutrophil cytoplasmic antibody (ANCA)–associated small-vessel vasculitis, and it usually combines pulmonary features with glomerulonephritis. Tissue biopsy of either the lung or the kidney may be diagnostic. Clinical manifestations result from the combination of vasculitis, glomerulonephritis, and necrotizing granulomas of the respiratory tract. CT may be more sensitive than MRI for diagnosis of pulmonary lesions.

Diffuse alveolar hemorrhage may result from autoimmune collagen vascular disease or vasculitis, Goodpasture's syndrome, and other vasculitides. *Goodpasture's syndrome* results from the formation of anti–glomerular basement membrane antibodies, which can also attack the lung capillary membranes. Primary pulmonary vasculitides affect mostly small vessels, but systemic conditions can affect vessels of all sizes. *Churg-Strauss syndrome* is a small-vessel vasculitis that often manifests first as asthma. Most patients also have maxillary sinusitis, allergic rhinitis, or nasal polyposis. Gastrointestinal, neurologic, and cardiac involvement often follows. The condition responds well to systemic steroids, but patients can require long-term low-dose prednisone as maintenance therapy (Guillevin et al., 2004).

Pulmonary Complications of Sickle Cell Disease

Patients with sickle cell disease have complications that can manifest with pulmonary signs and symptoms. For example, patients with sickle cell disease are especially vulnerable to capsular bacteria such as *Streptococcus pneumoniae* (pneumococcus) and *Haemophilus influenzae,* and they can present with acute lobar pneumonia, sepsis, or even pneumonia-related ARDS. Pneumococcal and Hib vaccines, in combination with penicillin prophylaxis, have significantly reduced (but not eliminated) rates of serious infections with these organisms (Hord et al., 2002).

Acute chest syndrome is an acute complication of sickle cell disease. One third of patients with this syndrome have an identified infectious cause. Less than one in 10 has a documented fat embolism. Postulated mechanisms in most patients with no identified cause include hypoxia-induced pulmonary vasoconstriction, with microclot formation and decreased levels of nitric oxide and other chemical mediators of vasodilation, inflammatory response, and cellular protection (Stuart and Setty, 2001). Hydroxyurea therapy promotes production of hemoglobin F (HbF) and appears to decrease the likelihood or severity of acute chest syndrome. Nitric oxide therapy might be of use acutely in acute chest syndrome or chronically in the treatment of pulmonary hypertension, but there is inadequate evidence from controlled trials.

Among adults with sickle cell disease, pulmonary hypertension is a significant cause of morbidity and appears to be a significant predictor of mortality, even with relatively modest elevations of pulmonary artery pressure. The pulmonary hypertension can be caused by widespread thrombosis of small arteries, although the cause is uncertain in many cases (Adedeji et al., 2001). Pulmonary hypertension complicates other chronic hemolytic anemias as well (Machado and Gladwin, 2005).

Malignant Disease

Lung Cancer

Key Points

- Lung cancer is the leading cause of cancer deaths in U.S. men and women.
- Smoking is the most serious and prevalent risk factor for lung cancer.
- Any pulmonary symptoms persisting beyond 3 weeks are indications for diagnostic evaluation. Smokers and patients older than 40 years should receive a more aggressive workup.
- High-resolution CT is more sensitive than chest radiography for diagnosing lung cancer. CT also provides anatomic detail for staging and operability.
- Patients with stage I, non–small cell carcinoma have 50% 5-year survival with appropriate surgical resection.
- The family physician plays a central role in facilitating family conversations about diagnostic and treatment options, advance directives, palliative care, and other end-of-life decisions.

Epidemiology and Risk Factors

Although not the most common cancer, lung cancer is the leading cause of cancer deaths in men and women in the United States. Lung cancer surpassed breast cancer as a cause of death among women in the 1990s because of increased smoking among women and better detection and treatment of breast cancer with decreased mortality. Smoking is clearly the most serious and prevalent risk factor for the development of lung cancer. According to the CDC, from 2000 to 2004, smoking resulted in an estimated annual average of 269,655 deaths among males and 173,940 deaths among females in the United States. The top three smoking-attributable causes were lung cancer, ischemic heart disease, and COPD (CDC, 2008).

Clinical Presentation

Smokers are at significant risk for lung cancer, but other patients can develop lung cancers as well, especially if they have significant secondary exposure to tobacco smoke or other carcinogens. History of asbestos exposure is a specific risk factor for the development of mesothelioma. Patients can present with respiratory symptoms such as a cough, hemoptysis, or shortness of breath, or they can present with constitutional symptoms such as fatigue and unexplained weight loss. In some cases a chest radiograph done for other reasons reveals a pulmonary nodule or mass lesion. In patients with metastatic pulmonary lesions, the symptoms of the primary cancer may be predominant or occult.

Diagnosis

Any pulmonary symptoms persisting beyond 3 weeks are an indication for a more extensive evaluation, and smokers and patients older than 40 years should receive a more aggressive workup. Diagnostic evaluation can begin with chest x-ray film, but a negative film does not rule out lung cancer or provide tissue diagnosis or staging. HRCT scanning is a more sensitive test for identifying lung cancers even at asymptomatic stages. HRCT can also provide some anatomic detail for staging and determining operability of the cancer. Tissue diagnosis is essential not only for confirming the presence of malignancy but also for determining the histopathology. Fiberoptic bronchoscopy with biopsy brushings and washings is highly accurate for diagnosing centrally located bronchogenic carcinoma in the proximal bronchial tree. Transbronchial biopsy can reach deeper tissues for diagnosis of metastatic pulmonary nodules or even lymph node biopsy. Peripheral pulmonary lesions or pleural lesions can be reached by CT-guided needle biopsy or by surgical open-lung biopsy.

The combination of tissue biopsy and imaging studies yields both the histopathologic type and the stage of cancer. The non–small cell lung cancers may be further classified into various histopathologic cell types, such as adenocarcinoma and squamous cell carcinoma. Staging of non–small cell cancers is summarized in Table 18-6 (American Cancer Society, 2005).

Treatment

General treatment principles and guidelines provide a framework for the primary care practitioner. Histopathology and stage at diagnosis drive treatment options. For example, surgical resection is not generally effective in treating small cell carcinomas of the lung, which may respond better to chemotherapy. On the other hand, a stage I, non–small cell carcinoma might have as much as a 50% 5-year survival rate with appropriate surgical resection. The European Respiratory Society and European Society of Thoracic Surgeons have published extensive clinical guidelines for evaluating any lung cancer patient's fitness for combined surgery and chemoradiotherapy (Brunelli, 2009).

Treatment options in addition to surgery include radiation therapy and chemotherapy. Response to any therapy differs by cell type (e.g., squamous cell vs. adenocarcinoma), stage of disease, and whether the tumor is primary or secondary. Metastatic pulmonary nodules from estrogen receptor–positive breast cancer may be treated quite differently from primary adenocarcinoma of the lung, although both generally receive some form of chemotherapy. The primary care practitioner must maintain a close working

Table 18-6 Staging and 5-Year Survival Related to Lung Cancers

Clinical Stage	Defining Characteristics	Average 5-Year Survival
Non–Small Cell Cancers		
I	Carcinoma confined to lung tissue; no spread to other organs or adjacent structures, and no lymph node involvement. Substages A and B refer to size of tumor.	51%
II	Carcinoma confined to lung tissue; no spread to other organs or adjacent structures, but positive lymph node involvement. Substages A and B refer to size of tumor.	26% 8% } 17%
III	Carcinoma with spread to adjacent structures, such as chest wall, diaphragm, mediastinum, or contralateral lung. Stage IIIA may still be operable; IIIB is inoperable.	
Stage IV	Metastatic to distant organs or tissue beyond the thoracic cavity	2%
Small Cell Cancers		
Limited	Limited to one lung or one side of the chest with no distant spread	10%-20%
Extensive	Spread beyond one lung to distant organs	1%-2%

From Lung and bronchus cancer: survival rates by race, sex, diagnosis-year, stage and age. SEER Statistics in Review, 1975–2003. National Cancer Institute. http://seer.cancer.gov/csr/1975_2003/results_merged/sect_15_lung_bronchus.pdf.

relationship with medical and surgical oncologists to help guide patients and families through various treatment options.

One specific role for the family physician is to help the patient and family address psychosocial needs in a proactive manner. The family physician may facilitate the first conversation between the patient and the patient's family in which the word "cancer" is mentioned or an ongoing conversation in which issues of death and dying can be addressed. The family physician must find the balance in encouraging the family to maintain hope but also in helping the family to develop contingency plans for potential crises, such as respiratory arrest or loss of function that leave the patient unable to live independently at home. Health care power of attorney and advance-directive documents are a much-needed complement to living wills, which cover only a narrow set of circumstances at the end of life. The family physician can help ensure that pain and other forms of discomfort are managed appropriately and can work closely with patient, family, oncologist, nurses, hospice, and the patient's faith community to manage proactively the balance between preserving life and preventing suffering, especially in a patient with a terminal illness.

Prevention

Smoking causes lung cancer (Khuder, 2001). Never smoking is the most important preventive measure available, but smoking cessation reduces the risk of all the major histologic types of lung cancer (Khuder and Mutgi, 2001). Beta-carotene and vitamin E do not prevent lung cancer, and in therapeutic doses beta-carotene might be associated with a slight increase in cancer (Albanes et al., 1995).

Regular chest x-ray screening with or without sputum cytology does not improve mortality rates (Manser et al., 2003). Studies suggest that routine screening of smokers with spiral CT every 6 months does increase detection of early stage cancer and might improve mortality by increasing the percentage of non–small cell cancers that are operable (Gohagan et al., 2005). Patients with stage I, non–small cell lung cancers may have a 5-year survival rate of 50%, but only 15% of lung cancers are found at this stage without routine screening.

Another aspect of preventing lung cancer deaths is the rates at which patients of different racial and ethnic groups receive potentially curative surgery in stage I disease. African American patients, for example, have significantly lower rates of surgery and significantly higher mortality rates. Causes of these racial disparities include patient factors (locus of control, acceptability of surgery, health beliefs about risks of opening such cancers to air during surgery), provider factors (biased treatment recommendations or assumptions about what patients might want), systemic or institutional factors (lack of insurance, poverty), and perhaps most importantly, the patient-physician dyad (issues of respect, trust, and effective communication influence the outcome of negotiating the treatment plan).

KEY TREATMENT

Smoking causes lung cancer. Never smoking is the most important preventive measure available, but smoking cessation also reduces the risk of all the major histologic types of lung cancer (Khuder, 2001) (SOR: A).

Routine screening of smokers with chest radiograph or sputum cytology does not improve survival. Use of frequent spiral CT suggests increased detection of early-stage cancer and improved mortality in non–small cell cancers (Manser et al., 2003; Gohagan et al., 2005) (SOR: A)

Beta-carotene and vitamin E do not prevent lung cancer and in therapeutic doses might be associated with a slight increase in cancer (Albanes et al., 1995) (SOR: B)

Occupational Lung Disease

Key Points

- At least 10% of asthma cases in adults can be attributed to occupational causes.
- The two key questions are, "Have you ever been exposed to fumes, gases, or dusts?" and "Do your symptoms get better when you are away from work, such as during weekends and vacations?"

- Asbestosis passed coal miner's lung as the leading cause of death from occupational pneumoconiosis in the United States.
- Because most occupational masks or respirators are imperfect and workers often remove them, preventive strategies should focus on worksite air-quality improvement.

Neoplasms of the lung are most frequently either primary lung carcinomas or metastatic lesions that arise in other organs. Lung carcinomas may be further divided into small cell and non–small cell cancers. Overall, survival for patients with lung carcinoma is only 15%, in part because lung cancers are often diagnosed at inoperable stages. Respiratory exposures cause a significant percentage of occupational illness and disability. Although a causative relationship cannot always be proved, a presumptive diagnosis may be made in the presence of typical signs and symptoms, confirmed by spirometry, chest radiography, or other diagnostic tests, in the presence of a work-related exposure known to cause pulmonary disease.

Taking a good occupational history is essential. In the occupational history, ask the specific type of work the patient performs and other jobs the patient has performed in the past. Two key questions are, "Have you ever been exposed to fumes, gases, or dusts?" and "Do your symptoms get better when you are away from work, such as during weekends and vacations?" Clinically, occupational lung diseases can be divided into five major groups (National Institute for Occupational Health and Safety [NIOSH], 1999): work-related asthma, pneumoconiosis, hypersensitivity pneumonitis, acute irritant or inhalant toxicity, and work-related cancers.

Work-Related Asthma

At least 10% of asthma cases in adults can be attributed to occupational exposures, so an occupational history should be obtained in every patient with asthma. Diagnostic criteria are the same as for other causes of asthma or airway obstruction, including spirometry (FEV_1/FVC ratio <0.7) and evidence of reversibility.

Chemical and natural agents can cause asthma or aggravate preexisting asthma. These include chemicals used in cleaning or manufacturing processes. Occupational exposures causing work-related asthma include dust exposures (e.g., cotton dust, wood sawdust, cement powder, bakery flour), organic exposures (e.g., molds and fungi in agricultural grains), chemical exposures (e.g., solvents, plastics, epoxies, ammonia, chlorine, petroleum vapors), and fumes from welding or other industrial sources (van Kampen et al., 2000), as shown in Figure 18-9 (NIOSH, 2004a). Peak-flow meter readings measured at the same time each day on workdays, weekends, and vacation days can help establish the occupational cause of disability for insurance purposes.

Occupational Pneumoconioses

The occupational pneumoconioses are diffuse parenchymal lung diseases caused by airborne exposure to inorganic materials such as asbestos, silica, and coal dust. In 1998 and 1999, asbestosis passed coal workers' pneumoconiosis (coal miner's lung) as the leading cause of death from occupational pneumoconiosis in the United States. Men accounted for 98% of these deaths. The rise in deaths caused by asbestosis is illustrated in Figure 18-10 (NIOSH, 2004b). Other occupational lung diseases are linked to heavy metal dust or fumes in specific syndromes such as berylliosis (beryllium) and stannosis (tin). Byssinosis, or brown-lung disease, occurs most often among workers in yarn, thread, and fabric mills from exposure to cotton dust.

Patients with occupational pneumoconioses may first develop symptoms of cough and dyspnea, with signs of small-airway disease or overt airway obstruction on pulmonary function testing. As the disease progresses, patients may also develop spirometric evidence of restrictive lung disease as well as chest x-ray changes. Removing the patient from the exposure or workplace is the most important step for preventing progression of disease. These pneumoconioses respond poorly to corticosteroids. Smoking significantly worsens the progression of occupational pneumoconiosis (Wang and Christiani, 2000).

Hypersensitivity Pneumonitis

Exposure to organic materials such as fungi, plant proteins, animal danders, or other organic dust can cause a similar type of diffuse parenchymal lung disease known as hypersensitivity pneumonitis. Examples include farmers'

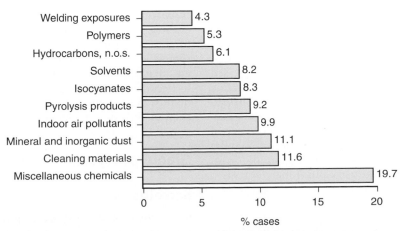

Figure 18-9 Causes of work-related asthma, 1993–1999. *(From National Institute for Occupational Safety and Health. Distribution of agent categories most often associated with work-related asthma cases for all four SENSOR reporting States [California, Massachusetts, Michigan, New Jersey], 1993–1999. Worker Health Chartbook, 2004. http://www2a.cdc.gov/niosh-Chartbook/imagedetail.asp?imgid=206.)*

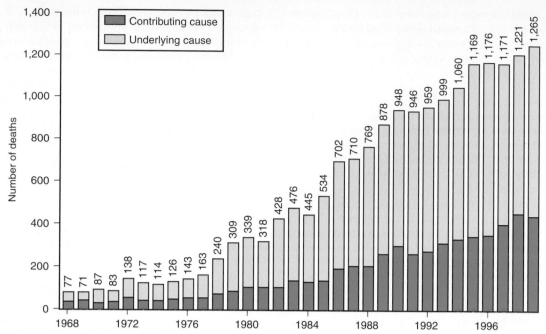

Figure 18-10 Asbestos as a contributing or underlying cause of death in the United States, 1968–1999. *(From National Institute for Occupational Safety and Health: Number of deaths of U.S. residents aged 15 or older with asbestosis recorded as an underlying or contributing cause on the death certificate, 1968–1999. Worker Health Chartbook, 2004. http://www2a.cdc.gov/NIOSH-Chartbook/imagedetail.asp?imgid=217.)*

lung, mushroom workers' lung, and bird fanciers' disease. Although fewer than 100 deaths per year in the United States are directly attributed to hypersensitivity pneumonitis, the number of cases and resulting short-term or long-term disability are potentially much higher.

Acute Irritant or Inhalant Toxicity

A number of acute pulmonary exposures each year are related to inhaled exposures to irritant chemicals. For example, when certain household chemicals such as bleach and ammonia are mixed, chlorine gas can be produced. Chlorine and chlorinated chemicals cause direct injury to tissues throughout the respiratory tract, including the bronchial mucosa. Injury can fill the alveolar sacs with fluid in a noncardiac form of pulmonary edema, or "chemical pneumonitis."

The large surface area of the alveolar sacs in close approximation to the pulmonary capillary system also provides a portal of entry to systemic toxicity from certain inhaled agents. For example, organophosphate and carbamate chemicals, whether used as nerve gas or as agricultural pesticides, can be absorbed readily throughout the respiratory tract. More than 5000 persons died within a week after inhaling methyl isocyanate gas released from a factory in Bhopal, India, in 1984. Pulmonary toxicity can also occur as a consequence of systemic exposures. For example, patients exposed to the toxic pesticide paraquat through skin absorption or by ingestion through the gastrointestinal tract often die from pulmonary hemorrhage or progressive pulmonary fibrosis.

Work-Related Cancers

The most obvious form of cancer associated with occupational inhalation exposures is mesothelioma, which is most often linked to asbestos exposure. Asbestos-related malignant mesothelioma accounted for an estimated 21,500 deaths in the United States from 1985 to 2009 (Lilienfeld et al., 1988). Persons with an occupational history of welding, pipefitting, shipbuilding, or other exposure to asbestos are at risk.

Lung cancers have also been associated with various occupational exposures, including welding or smelting fumes, coal dust, silica dust, and organic solvents. A more common exposure that has more recently been recognized as occupational is secondary exposure to tobacco smoke. Bartenders, restaurant staff, and others who work in smoke-filled environments are at significant risk for tobacco-related disease, including lung cancers, even if they have never personally smoked.

Prevention

Smoking significantly worsens the progression of occupational pneumoconioses such as black lung disease (coal miner's lung) and silicosis. Because most occupational masks or respirators are imperfect even when worn (and workers often remove masks intermittently for comfort), preventive strategies that rely on daily consistent use of respirators or masks in occupational settings are less effective than worksite air-quality improvement (e.g., increased ventilation, air filters, decreased dust or toxin production) in preventing occupational lung disease.

Granulomatous Diseases

Sarcoidosis

Sarcoidosis is defined as a multisystem granulomatous inflammatory disease of unknown etiology. It is the most common granulomatous disease of the lungs not attributed to a known infectious cause such as tuberculosis.

Risk Factors

Sarcoidosis can be found worldwide, but regional and racial/ethnic variations in epidemiology and clinical manifestations are intriguing. For example, it affects persons of Scandinavian origin and African Americans at much higher rates than other populations, with an incidence of 35.5 per 100,000 in African Americans and a slight female predominance. Several occupational and environmental exposures have been studied as possible risk factors for sarcoidosis, but none has been conclusively identified. Genetic susceptibility has also been difficult to define. The HLA class II antigens have been most often associated with susceptibility and prognosis in sarcoidosis, although not in all subpopulations (ATS/ERS/WASOG, 1999). The Sarcoidosis Genetic Analysis study (SAGA) suggested specific genetic loci related to sarcoidosis susceptibility in African Americans (Gray-McGuire et al., 2006); other studies show promise of characterizing susceptibility loci in a broader range of racial/ethnic groups (Iannuzzi, 2007).

Clinical Presentation

Sarcoidosis typically presents in early adulthood, between ages 20 and 40. Although the disease is systemic, a spectrum of clinical manifestations may suggest the prognosis. The onset of fever, arthralgias, bilateral hilar adenopathy on chest radiograph, and a raised, reddish skin lesion along the anterior tibial surfaces (erythema nodosum) characterize *Löfgren's syndrome,* an acute, self-limiting form of sarcoidosis that often undergoes spontaneous remission and has a favorable prognosis. The insidious onset of dyspnea, dry cough, hilar adenopathy and infiltrates on chest film, new skin lesions of the trunk and extremities, and complaints of recent vision changes characterize a chronic progressive form of sarcoidosis marked by multiple flares of disease requiring repeated treatment throughout the patient's lifetime.

Symptoms that bring patients to medical attention most often emanate from the lungs, skin, or the eyes (uveitis and lacrimal gland enlargement). Diagnosis of sarcoidosis may be delayed if symptoms are attributed to more common lung diseases such as asthma or chronic bronchitis (Judson et al., 2003). Pulmonary symptoms may result from bronchial obstruction, either external compression caused by adenopathy or granulomas within the airways. Progressive disease may cause damage to the lung parenchyma, with a restrictive pattern of pulmonary function and decreased diffusion capacity, consistent with progressive interstitial lung damage. Clinical features associated with a worse outcome include the presence of lupus pernio, chronic uveitis, hypercalcemia or nephrocalcinosis, nasal mucosal involvement and bone cysts. Neurosarcoidosis and cardiac involvement can be especially challenging to diagnose.

Diagnosis

The diagnosis of sarcoidosis is one of exclusion. The disease is established when clinical and radiographic findings are supported by a tissue biopsy specimen showing *noncaseating granuloma* (NCG), although NCG inflammation may be seen in biopsies from fungal infection, foreign body inclusions, and other noninfectious granulomatous diseases such as Langerhans cell histiocytosis (also referred to as eosinophilic granulomatosis or pulmonary histiocytosis X) and Wegener's granulomatosis. Tissue biopsy can usually be obtained from the lung, a palpable lymph node, a skin lesion, or the eye (conjunctiva or lacrimal gland). Percutaneous fine-needle aspiration specimen is less frequently obtained from the liver or from retroperitoneal or abdominal nodes by CT guidance. Biopsy from a CNS or cardiac location requires specialty consultation.

Along with clinical symptoms and biopsy, chest x-ray findings are added to support the diagnosis of sarcoidosis. The Scadding staging system classifies chest radiographs into stage 0 (normal), stage 1 (bilateral hilar adenopathy), stage 2 (adenopathy and infiltrates), stage 3 (infiltrates alone), and stage 4 (fibrosis and retractions). A chest film showing bilateral hilar adenopathy in HIV-negative patients with negative skin test and cultures for TB is suggestive, but lymphoma and other causes must be ruled out. HRCT can confirm the size and location of adenopathy as well as granulomas and early pulmonary fibrosis.

Transbronchial biopsy can document pathology and endobronchial involvement of the respiratory mucosa. Fine-needle aspiration of endobronchial lymph nodes is being used increasingly. Endobronchial ultrasound to localize more peripheral adenopathy enhances accuracy. Analysis of BAL fluid showing a C4/C8 lymphocyte ratio greater than 3.5 has high specificity for sarcoidosis. Open-lung biopsy is usually not needed but can be diagnostic. Several biomarkers and cytokine profiles that may be helpful in the diagnosis and disease activity in sarcoidosis are under investigation (Bargagli et al., 2008). The serum angiotensin-converting enzyme (ACE) level has historically been used and is often elevated in initial cases, but it is not fully reliable as the disease progresses. A sarcoidosis assessment instrument has been developed to help clinicians better characterize organ involvement in patients with sarcoidosis (Judson et al., 1999).

Treatment

Some sarcoidosis patients may require no treatment, or only intermittent nonsteroidal anti-inflammatory drugs (NSAIDs) for joint and constitutional symptoms. Topical corticosteroids may be effective for anterior uveitis and some skin lesions. Inhaled corticosteroids and bronchodilators are often used when cough is a prominent symptom in patients with pulmonary involvement, but response has been equivocal. Systemic therapy is needed for the majority of patients. Systemic corticosteroids are first-line therapy and, for patients with pulmonary involvement, improve symptoms, pulmonary function, and chest x-ray signs of disease.

Second-line therapies include cytotoxic agents and other immunomodulating agents (Baughman et al., 2008). Methotrexate and hydroxychloroquine can be used as steroid-sparing agents. In patients with cardiac or neural sarcoidosis, treatment regimens that include cytotoxic therapy (e.g., cyclophosphamide) are needed. Other treatment strategies include agents that inhibit tumor necrosis factor alpha (infliximab, adalimumab, etanercept) (Nunes et al., 2005). Comorbid illnesses and multiorgan involvement are common in sarcoidosis (Cox et al., 2004; Westney et al., 2007), so health-related quality-of-life instruments should be used to monitor global response to therapy (DeVries and Drent, 2007), and multidisciplinary team-based care is recommended.

Interstitial Lung Diseases

Interstitial lung diseases (ILDs) represent a broad range of acute and chronic lung disorders. The pathology may display varying degrees of pulmonary inflammation and fibrosis, leading ultimately to end-stage lung disease. ILDs are classified under the larger designation of *diffuse parenchymal lung disease*, which includes disorders from known causes (occupational and environmental exposures, as well as progressive infections), and unknown causes (sarcoidosis, lymphangioleiomyomatosis, pulmonary histiocytosis X, eosinophilic pneumonia, idiopathic interstitial lung diseases). The idiopathic ILDs have been subclassified by the American Thoracic Society and European Respiratory Society (2002) into the following clinicopathologic entities, in order of relative frequency: idiopathic pulmonary fibrosis (IPF), nonspecific interstitial pneumonia (NSIP), cryptogenic organizing pneumonia (COP), acute interstitial pneumonia (AIP), respiratory bronchiolitis-associated interstitial lung disease (RB-ILD), desquamative interstitial pneumonia (DIP), and lymphoid interstitial pneumonia (LIP).

Epidemiology and Risk Factors

Occupational risk factors and specific occupational lung diseases are reviewed in previous sections. Various medications, chemotherapeutic agents, and radiation therapy can all cause diffuse parenchymal lung disease and may result in end-stage lung disease with pulmonary fibrosis. Other causes include autoimmune connective tissue disorders (SLE, RA), granulomatous diseases (sarcoidosis, pulmonary Langerhans cell histiocytosis, eosinophilic granuloma), and metabolic diseases (Gaucher's, Niemann-Pick), congenital neoplasia (tuberous sclerosis, neurofibromatosis) malignancy (lymphangitic carcinomatosis, bronchoalveolar carcinoma, pulmonary lymphoma), and certain drugs (bleomycin, nitrofurantoin, amiodarone). Among the interstitial lung diseases, idiopathic pulmonary fibrosis occurs more often in patients over age 60 and in men more than women. Cigarette smoking, chronic aspiration, various environmental exposures (metal and wood dust), and numerous viruses (Epstein-Barr, influenza, CMV) have been implicated as potential risk factors. The remaining ILDs rarely occur and are designated as separate disease entities based on specific clinicopathologic differences (Lynch et al., 2005).

Clinical Presentation

The hallmark symptoms of ILDs are the insidious onset of progressive shortness of breath and exertional dyspnea with paroxysmal dry cough. A careful history may elicit symptoms of an earlier viral prodrome in patients that may also include cough with varying sputum production and systemic symptoms such as fever or weight loss. On physical examination, most patients can have the typical dry, end-inspiratory ("Velcro") crackles most appreciable in the lung bases. The finding of cyanosis and accentuated second heart sound, right ventricular heave, and lower-extremity edema suggest late phases of the disease caused by chronic hypoxemia and pulmonary fibrosis.

Diagnosis

The usual diagnostic approach for all ILDs is a thorough history and physical examination along with chest radiographic and pulmonary function studies. The chest film typically shows bilateral, often asymmetric reticular opacities in the peripheral and basal lung areas. A normal-appearing radiograph may rarely be encountered but does not exclude microscopic presence of an ILD. Often, x-ray abnormalities can be seen years before the development of symptoms, so past films should be reviewed. HRCT features of idiopathic pulmonary fibrosis may be distinct and include bibasilar subpleural honeycombing, traction bronchiectasis (as illustrated in Fig. 18-11), thick intralobular septa, and minimal ground-glass opacities. If the HRCT pattern shows a predominance of ground-glass opacification, especially located away from the subpleural areas, diagnoses such as nonspecific interstitial pneumonia, bronchiolitis obliterans organizing pneumonia (BOOP), or hypersensitivity pneumonitis should be considered. In some cases, fibrotic scarring and nodules create a mass lesion that must be distinguished from carcinoma or other neoplasm.

The typical PFT pattern is that of a restrictive ventilatory defect with decreased lung flow and volume, increased FEV_1/FVC ratio, and decreased DL_{CO}. Biopsy may be necessary to exclude malignancy or to rule in specific conditions such as sarcoidosis. Documenting pulmonary function, exercise capacity (6-minute walk test), and relationship of the ILD to any occupational or environmental exposure are all essential for helping patients receive appropriate worker's compensation or disability support when needed.

Treatment

Smoking cessation is essential, and pulmonary rehabilitation may improve quality of life and functional capacity for patients with any ILD. Pharmacologic options include single-agent or combination corticosteroid therapy and immunomodulating or antifibrotic agents (azathioprine, cyclophosphamide, colchicine, D-penicillamine). Overall, these therapies have shown marginal to no benefit in cases

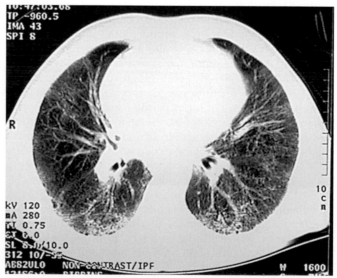

Figure 18-11 Computed tomographic scan of a patient with idiopathic pulmonary fibrosis.

of idiopathic pulmonary fibrosis, whereas patients with other ILDs may have a better response (Davies et al., 2003). A meta-analysis of 390 patients with pulmonary fibrosis did find that interferon gamma-1b therapy significantly reduced mortality (Bajwa et al., 2005). Causes of death identified for pulmonary fibrosis in one study included respiratory failure (39%), cardiovascular disease (27%), lung cancer (10%), pulmonary infection or emboli (6%) (Panos, 1990).

Unilateral lung transplantation may enhance survival and functioning in patients with advanced interstitial fibrosis with chronic respiratory failure, whereas pulmonary fibrosis with pulmonary hypertension may require bilateral lung transplantation (Alalawi et al., 2005). One-year survival after lung transplantation is 75%, with 44% of patients surviving 5 years or longer (Trulock, 2001).

Lung Manifestations of Autoimmune Connective Tissue Disorders and Other Systemic Diseases

Many connective tissue diseases can have an impact on the lungs and pleura or on pulmonary function. Rheumatoid arthritis, for example, can cause interstitial lung disease because of a fibronodular inflammatory response or even larger rheumatoid nodules. Inflammation can also lead to pleural effusion or scarring, and pleural biopsy can reveal rheumatic nodules. Patients with RA can also develop one of several varieties of inflammatory interstitial pneumonia.

Systemic lupus erythematosus can affect the lungs. The inflammatory response of SLE is more vasculitic in nature, which can manifest as pulmonary hemorrhage, thromboembolic disease, or an inflammatory pleuritis with effusion.

Other autoimmune diseases with pulmonary manifestations include mixed connective tissue disease (MCTD), Sjögren's syndrome, and progressive systemic sclerosis (scleroderma). Progressive systemic sclerosis can manifest with thickening and tightening of the skin of distal extremities, sclerodactyly, Raynaud's phenomenon, and multiorgan involvement of lungs, skin, kidney, heart, and gastrointestinal tract. Sixty percent of patients have shortness of breath; others have cough, pleuritic chest pain, or hemoptysis. Lung CT scan in progressive systemic sclerosis and other autoimmune conditions can show pleural scarring and ILD, especially a ground-glass fibronodular pattern and honeycombing.

Diseases of the Pleura and Extrapulmonary Space

Key Points

- In international settings, the most common cause of pleural disease is tuberculosis.
- More than 200 mL of pleural fluid may be detected by physical examination or by blunting of the costophrenic angles on upright chest x-ray film. Decubitus positioning of the patient can reveal as little as 10 mL of fluid on the dependent side.
- Thoracentesis may be done blindly if pleural fluid layers out to at least 1 cm on decubitus radiograph. Otherwise, ultrasound guided thoracentesis may be indicated.

- An exudate is diagnosed in pleural fluid by finding a pleural/serum protein ratio greater than 0.5 and a pleural/serum LDH level greater than 0.6 (or pleural LDH >200 IU/dL) or pleural protein greater than 3 g/dL.
- Purulent fluid in the pleural space is indicated by a high neutrophil count and pH less than 7.2, which can require a chest tube along with antibiotics.
- Rapid drainage of more than 1 L of fluid from large pleural effusions (or air from pneumothorax) can result in reexpansion pulmonary edema.

The lungs are lined by visceral pleura, and the inside of the thoracic cavity is lined by parietal pleura. Normally, these two are closely adjacent, with only enough fluid for lubrication in the space between them.

Epidemiology and Presentation

Outside the United States, the most common cause of pleural disease is tuberculosis. In the United States, TB is still significant, but other disorders, such as pneumonia, HIV-related infections, connective tissue disease (especially lupus), and malignancies (mesothelioma, peripheral lung cancer) must also be considered. Pleural effusions can be caused by systemic sources of transudate (CHF, hepatic failure with ascites, autoimmune disease) or by local inflammatory processes (parapneumonic effusion, pancreatitis, neoplasia).

Four major categories of pathology arise from the pleura or pleural space: pleural fluid (transudate, exudate, hemorrhage, or chylous effusion), pneumothorax, pleural scarring, and pleural mass.

Diagnosis

Pleuritic disease is suggested by thoracic pain on inspiration. More than 200 to 300 mL of fluid in the pleural space may also be detected by physical examination. Decreased breath sounds with dullness to percussion could suggest pleural fluid or lung consolidation, but pleural effusion may be distinguished by the presence of decreased tactile and vocal fremitus. Often, there is a small (1-2 cm) zone at the top edge of the pleural effusion where traditional signs of consolidation may be heard, including egophony. A pleural rub may be heard in areas of inflammation but disappears when significant fluid cushions the movement of visceral pleura against parietal pleura. For pneumothorax, significant air must be present in the pleural space to detect hyperresonance, although breath sounds are often decreased on the affected side. In the 1% to 2% of cases producing *tension pneumothorax*, in which air is able to enter the space but not equilibrate with either extrathoracic or bronchial air pressures, the clinician may detect tracheal shift, cardiac shift, or decreased heart sounds.

Chest radiography reveals blunting of the costophrenic angles and visible fluid when about 200 mL of fluid has accumulated in the pleural space. Decubitus positioning of the patient can reveal as little as 10 mL of fluid on the dependent side on chest films. Thoracentesis may be done blindly if the fluid layers out to at least 1-cm thickness on decubitus radiograph. Otherwise, ultrasound-guided thoracentesis may be indicated.

Pneumothorax is also visible on chest x-ray film, especially when it exceeds 10% or more than 100 mL of air is present in the pleural space. On radiographs, 2.5 cm of air space between the thoracic wall and the lung is equivalent to a 30% pneumothorax. This is best visualized on upright PA and lateral films or occasionally on the nondependent side when patients are in the decubitus position. Other imaging studies (CT, MRI) can give more anatomic detail in patients with mass lesions or scarring. These studies are also somewhat more sensitive than radiography in detecting small amounts of air in pneumothorax.

Diagnostic thoracentesis can help determine the type of fluid and potential causes. *Transudates* are serous fluids often associated with inflammatory conditions. Transudative fluid is thin and mildly yellow or straw colored, through which one can read newsprint. More specific laboratory criteria for differentiating exudate from transudate include a pleural/serum protein ratio greater than 0.5, pleural/serum lactate dehydrogenase (LDH) level greater than 0.6 (or measured pleural LDH >200 IU/dL), and pleural protein greater than 3 g/dL.

Exudates indicate the presence of white blood cells and often a response to infection such as pleural abscess or TB. Parapneumonic effusions may be inflammatory transudates initially or may progress to exudative fluid as WBCs and even the infectious organism itself spread to the pleural space. Infectious exudates are suggested by pH higher than 7.2, which can be an indication for chest tube drainage. More specifically, TB may be suggested by an exudative pleural effusion with elevated WBC count, more lymphocytes than granulocytes, and pleural glucose/serum glucose ratio less than 0.5. Hemorrhage into the pleural space is indicated by the gross or microscopic presence of red blood cells, although poor technique can result in a bloody tap that is not diagnostic. For mass lesions or scarring, pleural biopsy may be obtained (revealing granulomas or malignancy) either percutaneously with needle or surgically in an open biopsy.

Treatment

Treatment most importantly targets the underlying condition. For example, the inflammatory pleural effusions of SLE may be treated with systemic corticosteroids or other anti-inflammatory agents. Antibiotics treat pneumonia and parapneumonic effusions, although purulent fluid or abscess in the pleural space can require chest tube drainage in addition to antibiotics.

Other indications for chest tube placement include pneumothorax compromising ventilation, exceeding 25%, or recurring after initial needle thoracostomy. Trauma with hemorrhage into the pleural space can also require a chest tube, or even open-chest surgery to identify and treat the source of bleeding. Some pleural effusions may be treated with therapeutic pleural tap rather than chest tube. In these cases, up to 1 L of fluid may be drained through a pleural needle and catheter. For these therapeutic taps, attaching the thoracostomy needle to a tube and vacuum bottle may be more efficient and cause less risk of bleeding or pleural injury from movement of the needle during the procedure than the traditional technique of using a large syringe and stopcock to remove 30 to 50 mL at a time. Rapid drainage of large pleural effusions or pneumothorax can result in reexpansion pulmonary edema.

Patients with recurrent pneumothorax may require surgery to repair a specific defect. Patients with malignant pleural effusion that has recurred after complete reexpansion may benefit from pleural sclerosis, instilling agents such as bleomycin or tetracycline. Pleural stripping is rarely used because of the high rate of complications.

Disorders of Breathing

Sleep apnea may be obstructive or central in origin, or a combination of both. The effects of recurrent apnea extend well beyond simple fatigue or sleep deprivation, causing significant cardiovascular and neurologic disease. Patients with *obstructive* sleep apnea are often but not always obese. They experience episodes of intermittent apnea, often associated with snoring, especially during deeper stages of sleep. In addition to obesity, adenoidal or tonsillar enlargement, macroglossia, and laxity of the soft palate and pharyngeal tissue can contribute to sleep apnea. Stroke, brain tumors, trauma, cerebral edema, and other CNS disorders can affect breathing at the *central* level as well. Brainstem infarctions can lead to respiratory arrest and death. *Cheynes-Stokes respirations* describe an undulating pattern of breathing of increased depth and frequency alternating with waves of shallow, slower breathing and even apnea.

Many patients with obstructive sleep apnea have elements of central apnea as well. For example, alcohol and sedatives can exacerbate the respiratory depression and contribute to pharyngeal muscle laxity. In addition, patients with chronic obstructive sleep apnea can develop chronic CO_2 retention that further depresses respiration. Patients with the classic "pickwickian syndrome" (obesity and hypoventilation syndrome) have a constellation of signs, including morbid obesity, obstructive apnea, polycythemia, pulmonary hypertension, and right-sided heart failure. Patients can present with symptoms of daytime drowsiness, sleepiness, or feeling inadequately rested. Family members often bring the problem to the attention of the patient or the family physician, having observed loud snoring and interruptions in breathing during sleep. Sometimes a motor vehicle crash resulting from somnolence while driving brings the condition to light. Depression can also develop.

In addition to symptoms related to loss of sleep or upper airway obstruction, sleep apnea can contribute to other major causes of morbidity and mortality. Bradyarrhythmias are common, and hypoxia can lead to ventricular arrhythmias or even myocardial ischemia or stroke. When episodic hypoventilation becomes frequent or chronic, with resultant hypoxia and hypercapnia, a metabolic response may counteract the respiratory acidosis associated with hypoventilation; the kidneys retain bicarbonate to foster a compensatory metabolic alkalosis. Systemic and pulmonary hypertension may be intermediate outcomes that lead to more serious cardiac complications.

Formal diagnosis of sleep apnea can be made in a sleep laboratory using multichannel recording (polysomnography) of EEG, ECG, airflow, upper airway muscle tone, and oximetry. Home oximetry alone might not be adequately sensitive. The most essential treatment is significant weight reduction to decrease obesity. Other behavioral treatments include avoiding supine sleep and avoiding alcohol or sedatives. Nasal CPAP is effective for patients who tolerate it. Various oral or dental devices are also available, but data on effectiveness are limited. Surgical procedures attempt to reduce airway obstruction at the palate or tonsillopharyngeal or adenoidal

levels. The American Academy of Sleep Medicine (AASM) has published clinical guidelines with evidence-based recommendations and algorithms for the evaluation, diagnosis, treatment and follow-up of patients with sleep disorders (Epstein et al., 2009).

References

The complete reference list is available online at www.expertconsult.com.

Web Resources

www.guidelines.gov Provides clinical guidelines for pulmonary function testing and treatment.

www.thoracic.org/sections/publications/statements/index.html American Thoracic Society; general pulmonary guidelines.

www.nhlbi.nih.gov/guidelines/asthma/or www.nhlbi.nih.gov/about/naepp/ Clinical guidelines for asthma.

www.goldcopd.com Global Initiative for Chronic Obstructive Lung Disease (COPD); Global Strategy for the Diagnosis, Management, and Prevention of COPD (GOLD guidelines).

www.thoracic.org/sections/publications/statements/resources/idsaats-cap.pdf Information on community-acquired pneumonia.

www.cdc.gov/flu/professionals/and www.cdc.gov/vaccines/vpd-vac/pneumo Centers for Disease Control and Prevention; pneumococcal and influenza vaccines.

www.thoracic.org/sections/publications/statements/pages/mtpi/rr5211.html American Thoracic Society; tuberculosis information.

www.cdcnpin.org/scripts/tb/cdc.asp CDC tuberculosis information.

http://meded.ucsd.edu/clinicalmed/lung.htm; www.med.ucla.edu/wilkes Physical examination and lung auscultation.

www.aafp.org/afp/2004/0301/p1107.html Interpretation of spirometry.

www.nlhep.org/resources-medical.html#spirometry National Lung Health Education Program; spirometry information.

http://phil.cdc.gov/phil/quicksearch.asp Pulmonary imaging (e.g., chest radiograph, CT)

www.uams.edu/radiology/education/teaching_cases/default.asp University of Arkansas Medical Sciences, Department of Radiology Teaching Cases.

http://medinfo.ufl.edu/year1/rad6190/topics/lect4.shtml University of Florida Anatomy by Diagnostic Imaging course.

www.lungusa.org/ American Lung Association; community and patient resources.

www.nlm.nih.gov/medlineplus National Institutes of Health MedlinePlus online service.

Otorhinolaryngology

John G. O'Handley, Evan J. Tobin, and Ashish R. Shah

Emergencies

Key Points

- Drooling, posturing, and air hunger are classic signs of epiglottitis.
- A lateral neck radiograph showing a thumbprint sign can be diagnostic of epiglottitis.
- Although most peritonsillar abscesses should be drained, smaller and early abscesses may respond to medical therapy.
- Acute onset of wheezing in a child with no history of asthma should alert the clinician to a possible airway foreign body.
- A high index of suspicion is required for the timely diagnosis of retropharyngeal abscess.
- Adolescent boys with recurrent epistaxis may have a juvenile nasopharyngeal angiofibroma.

Epiglottitis

Epiglottitis (or "supraglottitis") is a condition that requires prompt attention by the physician. Epiglottitis results from bacterial (and rarely viral) infection of the supraglottic structures, that is, the epiglottis and arytenoid cartilages. A high level of suspicion is necessary to make a diagnosis and avoid significant morbidity. Rapid decompensation and complete loss of the airway are the sequelae of most concern. The physician should always be suspicious when a patient presents with fever, sore throat, and difficulty swallowing, and when the severity of oropharyngeal physical findings is not in proportion to the symptoms. Croup, tonsillitis, peritonsillar abscess, and other neck infection may be incorrectly diagnosed in these patients. Epiglottitis occurs mainly in children age 2 to 7 years, although infants, older children, and adults can be affected. Mortality rates of 6% to 7% have been reported in adults.

Signs and symptoms of epiglottitis include rapidly developing sore throat, high fever, restlessness, and lethargy. A "supraglottic," muffled voice is common. Many patients have difficulty with their saliva and drool. Classically, these patients are in a sitting position leaning forward, because this position tends to alleviate obstructive symptoms from the supraglottic swelling. They may show signs of "air hunger" or may have stridor.

Differential diagnosis includes tonsillitis, peritonsillar abscess, retropharyngeal abscess, airway foreign body, and

Table 19-1 Distinguishing Features of Epiglottitis and Croup

Feature	Epiglottitis	Croup
Cause	Bacterial	Viral
Age	1 year to adult	1 to 5 years
Location of obstruction	Supraglottic	Subglottic
Onset	Sudden (hours)	Gradual (days)
Fever	High	Low grade
Dysphagia	Marked	None
Drooling	Present	Minimal
Posture	Sitting	Recumbent
Toxemia	Mild to severe	Mild
Cough	Usually none	Barking, brassy, spontaneous
Voice	Clear to muffled	Hoarse
Respiratory rate	Normal to rapid	Rapid
Larynx palpation	Tender	Not tender
Clinical course	Shorter	Longer

From Berry FA, Yemen TA. Pediatric airway in health and disease. Pediatr Clin North Am 1994;41:153.

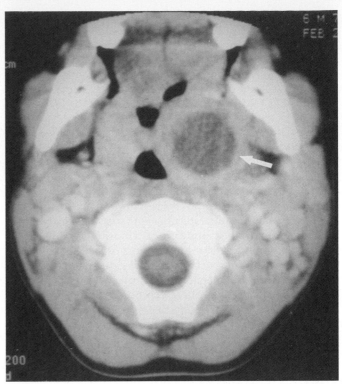

Figure 19-1 Large left peritonsillar abscess *(arrow)* that required surgical drainage.

croup. Physical examination with laryngoscopy is extremely useful in differentiating these diagnoses. Endoscopy should not be performed if there is concern of impending airway obstruction. Endoscopy will typically show erythema and edema of the epiglottis and arytenoid cartilages. Other findings include laryngeal tenderness on neck palpation, although palpation should be avoided when the diagnosis is being considered.

Any time the diagnosis of epiglottitis is in question, otorhinolaryngologic (ear-nose-throat, ENT) and infectious disease consultations are warranted. Placement of a tongue depressor has been known to precipitate acute airway obstruction and should be avoided entirely if epiglottitis is strongly suspected. Differentiation from croup can be difficult because there is considerable overlap of symptoms (Table 19-1) (Berry and Yemen, 1994). A lateral extended neck radiograph can help in the diagnosis. X-ray evidence includes the classic "thumbprint" sign. If epiglottitis is suspected or lateral neck radiography is confirmatory, the patient should be taken to the operating room (OR) for orotracheal intubation in the presence of an anesthesiologist and an otorhinolaryngologist. In any case of airway obstruction, cricothyrotomy or tracheotomy can be lifesaving, because orotracheal intubation can be difficult and sometimes impossible. Some patients, usually adults, may be treated expectantly with intravenous (IV) medications and intensive care unit (ICU) observation as long as personnel are available for control of the airway if necessary. If airway stability is questionable, observation is not recommended.

After control of the airway is achieved, cultures of the epiglottis should be obtained and directed antibiotics instituted. *Haemophilus influenzae* type b (Hib) is common and can be beta-lactamase producing. Other, less common organisms include beta-hemolytic streptococci, *Streptococcus pneumoniae*, and *Staphylococcus aureus*. Antibiotics should be administered parenterally; effective antibiotics include cefotaxime, ceftriaxone, ampicillin plus sulbactam, or ampicillin plus chloramphenicol. Steroids can be useful for edema and inflammation, but their effectiveness has not been proved in controlled studies..

The incidence of epiglottitis in children is decreasing since the introduction of the Hib vaccine in the late 1980s. However, the incidence has remained stable or slightly increased in adults.

Peritonsillar Abscess

A peritonsillar abscess is the accumulation of pus in the peritonsillar space that surrounds the tonsil. The same organisms responsible for common tonsillar infections— *Streptococcus* and *Staphylococcus* species and anaerobes—are also found in peritonsillar abscesses.

The typical signs and symptoms of peritonsillar abscess include fever, sore throat for 3 to 5 days, dysphagia, odynophagia, and a muffled, "hot potato" voice. Trismus is extremely common. Examination confirms asymmetric tonsils and peritonsillar edema and erythema. The soft palate and uvula are swollen and displaced away from the side of the abscess. It is often difficult to distinguish between abscess and peritonsillar cellulitis. If possible, it is helpful to palpate because fluctuance indicates a loculation of pus. Diagnosis is often made by clinical impression, but computed tomography (CT) can be confirmatory and useful when the diagnosis is uncertain (Fig. 19-1).

If untreated, a peritonsillar abscess may spontaneously drain, progress to involve the deep neck, or even lead to airway obstruction. The most important part of the treatment is drainage of the abscess cavity by needle aspiration, incision and drainage, or tonsillectomy. Cultures of the aspirate can be obtained, and broad-spectrum antibiotics should be started. Appropriate antibiotics include ampicillin-sulbactam (Unasyn) or clindamycin (Cleocin). Many patients present with dehydration, and parenteral fluids should be given if necessary. Analgesics should be prescribed as needed. One or two doses of IV corticosteroids may be given to decrease inflammation and pain.

Children presenting with peritonsillar abscess should be admitted to the hospital. Treatment with IV hydration and parenteral antibiotics is appropriate initially. Patients with peritonsillar cellulitis/phlegmon or early abscess often demonstrate a rapid response to treatment, whereas those with a well-formed peritonsillar abscess do not improve. Drainage is necessary in nonresponders. Abscesses in cooperative adults can be drained under local anesthesia in the emergency department (ED) or office and treated in an outpatient setting. Children usually require general anesthesia for drainage, and a tonsillectomy may also be performed. An elective tonsillectomy is often recommended for any patient with a peritonsillar abscess to prevent recurrence, especially with a history of recurrent tonsillitis, although few, if any, controlled studies support this recommendation.

Sudden Sensorineural Hearing Loss

Although most types of hearing loss are nonurgent problems, sudden sensorineural hearing loss (SSNHL) deserves special note because it is considered "otologic emergency." Any patient complaining of sudden hearing loss requires prompt evaluation. An obvious cause such as cerumen impaction or middle ear fluid can be treated appropriately and routinely. If a cause is not identified, sudden sensorineural hearing loss should be suspected and prompt ENT referral arranged. SSNHL is thought to be secondary to vascular, thromboembolic, viral, or autoimmune causes. It may also be the result of ototoxicity. Without treatment, hearing returns in one third of patients, partial hearing returns in one third, and there is no improvement in the remaining third. Early intervention with oral corticosteroids (and possibly antivirals, directed at the herpesvirus [Awad et al., 2008]) appears to improve outcomes, although few controlled studies have been done. The Cochrane Collaboration believes that there is a lack of good-quality evidence to support the use of steroids and that more research is needed (Wei et al., 2006). Finally, for patients who do not respond to systemic steroids, controlled studies do support the use intratympanic infusion of corticosteroids, demonstrating improved outcomes (Xenellis et al., 2006). Intratympanic steroids are also appealing for patients with contraindications to oral steroids (e.g., "brittle diabetics")

Foreign Bodies

Swallowing or aspiration of objects is most common in children but also occurs in the adult population. These objects can become lodged anywhere in the upper aerodigestive tract.

Esophagus

The most common location for esophageal foreign bodies is at the level of the cricopharyngeal muscle. Other regions include the anatomic narrowings of the esophagus, such as

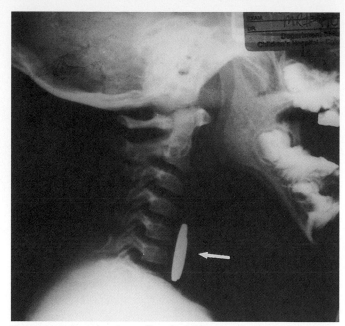

Figure 19-2 Lateral neck x-ray film of a child presenting with gagging and drooling, showing two coins *(arrow)* in the esophagus near the cricopharyngeal junction.

the gastroesophageal junction, and the area of indentation of the esophagus by the left main stem bronchus and the arch of the aorta. Coins are by far the most common objects found in the esophagus in children. Chicken or fish bones are more common in adults.

The diagnosis of an esophageal foreign body is primarily based on the medical history and physical examination, with the aid of radiologic studies. Parents might witness ingestion of the foreign body and subsequent coughing, gagging, refusal to eat, or drooling. Often, however, the incident goes unwitnessed, and reliance on other diagnostic techniques is necessary.

Plain radiographs (including lateral films) are often diagnostic in pediatric patients because most esophageal foreign objects are radiopaque (Fig. 19-2). Other radiologic findings that can suggest a foreign body include increased soft tissue density in the prevertebral space, mediastinal widening, air-fluid levels in the esophagus, and paraesophageal air. Disk batteries *require a high index of suspicion* because they can cause significant tissue injury and lead to esophageal perforation *if they are not removed emergently*. They have a classic appearance when viewed laterally, approximating a dime resting on a nickel (similar to the appearance of Fig. 19-2).

If there is sufficient evidence of an esophageal foreign body, ENT consultation is indicated for rigid esophagoscopy and removal. When radiolucent objects have been ingested, contrast esophagography might be indicated, although esophagograms can give a false-negative result and can also complicate visualization during rigid esophagoscopy.

Airway

As with esophageal foreign bodies, airway foreign bodies are much more common in infants and young children. Many deaths from foreign-body aspiration occur in the home before medical intervention can be administered. The most

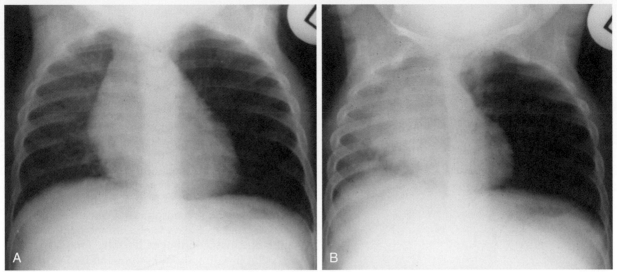

Figure 19-3 Inspiratory **(A)** and expiratory **(B)** radiographs of 8-year-old boy with left airway foreign body (peanut). No foreign object is visible on plain films, but the expiratory film shows overinflation of the left lung with mediastinal shift to the contralateral side.

frequently aspirated foreign bodies are foods, with nuts leading the list. Foreign bodies aspirated into the airway are usually found lodged in the bronchial tree but can also be found in the larynx or trachea. If the event is witnessed and results in complete airway obstruction, a Heimlich maneuver should be administered; however, the event is often not witnessed. Symptoms can include hoarseness, persistent cough, wheezing, or stridor if the foreign body is lodged in the trachea or larynx. Because the potential for morbidity and mortality is substantial, this condition requires urgent diagnosis and timely intervention to prevent catastrophe.

Any time a small child presents with wheezing or noisy breathing without a previous history of reactive airway disease, an airway foreign body should be included in the differential diagnosis. Typically, patients and parents recount a transient episode of coughing during eating that then subsided; the patient might even be symptom free for a time, then later have symptoms such as coughing or wheezing.

The most important diagnostic step for identifying a foreign body is a high index of suspicion. Careful auscultation of the lung fields is essential because subtle asymmetric differences may be found. Because most airway foreign bodies are radiolucent, chest radiographs can be normal, but abnormalities such as hyperinflation, atelectasis, or pneumonia can be present (Fig. 19-3). If plain radiographs are equivocal or normal and the patient is in stable condition, airway fluoroscopy can be helpful.

Consultation with a physician experienced in foreign body removal is required. Definitive treatment of airway foreign bodies is direct laryngoscopy and rigid bronchoscopy to identify and remove the object.

Epistaxis

Although epistaxis is usually nothing more than a minor annoyance, some episodes are severe enough to require urgent medical attention and intervention. In rare cases, epistaxis can also be a life-threatening emergency.

Predisposing factors for epistaxis include trauma (facial trauma or self-inflicted digital trauma), dry weather,

hypertension, bleeding dyscrasias (factor deficiencies, hereditary hemorrhagic telangiectasia, lymphoproliferative disorders), anticoagulation therapy (acetylsalicylic acid, heparin, warfarin), and intranasal tumors. Special consideration should be given to adolescent boys with recurrent epistaxis and nasal obstruction, because these symptoms might be the result of a juvenile nasopharyngeal angiofibroma. These are benign but locally aggressive tumors. All these potential risk factors should be considered because they must be addressed to treat the patient appropriately.

Epistaxis is classified according to its location. Bleeding from the anterior nasal cavity is most common and usually originates from a rich plexus of vessels at the anterior septum called *Kiesselbach's plexus* (Fig. 19-4). Bleeding from this location, although troublesome, is less likely to be severe and is usually easier to control than posterior epistaxis. Posterior epistaxis originates from the posterior two thirds of the nasal cavity and can be quite severe and much more difficult to control.

Initial management of epistaxis includes assessment and stabilization of vital signs. Rarely, severe bleeding can lead to airway compromise or hemodynamic compromise, or both, especially in patients with underlying cardiopulmonary dysfunction. The airway should be assessed and stabilized, urgently if necessary. Hypertension, if severe, should be controlled, with care taken to avoid subsequent *hypotension*. Hematologic studies, including complete blood count (CBC), prothrombin time, and partial thromboplastin time, should be ordered. Intravenous access should be established, allowing administration of fluids as well as IV medications, if necessary during treatment.

Treatment

Effective treatment requires adequate visualization and patient cooperation. The level of intervention by the primary care physician depends on level of experience, comfort level, and availability of appropriate supplies and equipment. ENT consultation should be considered when any of these prerequisites cannot be met. The patient should be reassured and

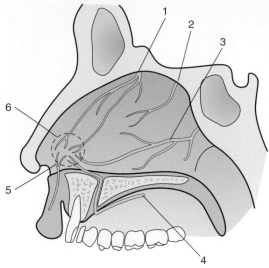

Figure 19-4 Kiesselbach's plexus. *1* and *2,* Anterior and posterior ethmoid arteries; *3,* septal branch of the sphenopalatine; *4,* greater palatine; *5,* branch from superior labial; *6,* Kiesselbach's plexus. *(From Colman BH, Hall IS (eds): Hall and Colman's Diseases of the Ear, Nose and Throat, 15th ed. Philadelphia, Churchill Livingstone, 2000, p 82.)*

given an explanation of the planned treatment. This results in better cooperation and decreases patient anxiety, improving treatment success. A bright headlight, nasal speculum, large nasal (Frazier tip) suction, and bayonet forceps are required. If the patient is monitored and stable, a small dose of IV narcotics titrated for analgesia and anxiolytic effect may be given. Extreme caution should be taken not to oversedate the patient. Also, instrumentation of the nose can lead to a significant vasovagal response that may be accentuated in a hypovolemic patient given narcotics. It is advised to err on the side of caution with regard to narcotic medication both during and after treatment.

All clots should be suctioned. They can be quite tenacious and require forceps for removal. The nasal cavity should next be topically anesthetized and decongested (a mixture of 4% lidocaine and phenylephrine works well). If a bleeding site is easily identified, it may be cauterized with a silver nitrate stick.

Anterior Packing

If suction, decongestion, and cautery do not stop the bleeding and the site is still thought to be anterior, an anterior nasal pack should be placed. This can be done with 0.5-inch petroleum gauze coated in antibiotic ointment. Alternatively, a variety of preformed packs are available. Merocel nasal packs or prepackaged inflatable packs are usually readily available and quite effective. Remembering that the nasal cavity extends *posteriorly* from the nostril and not *superiorly* facilitates placement. The pack should be coated in antibiotic ointment before placement.

Placement of the pack can be quite uncomfortable for the patient. Discomfort can be minimized by ensuring optimal decongestion and topical anesthesia of the nasal cavity. If using a Merocel pack, it is sometimes helpful to hydrate and expand the pack *before* placing it. This can be done with sterile saline or phenylephrine. Although the pack appears quite large after it is expanded, it decompresses readily and slides in easily once it is covered in antibiotic ointment. The

entire length of the pack needs to be grasped with the bayonet forceps if this technique is employed. Preexpansion of the pack also minimizes further abrasions and bleeding that can occur with placement of the firm pack. This technique is especially advantageous if a septal deviation or spur exists on the bleeding side. Regardless of what type of pack is used, care must be taken not to distort or overstretch the nasal ala (nostril) once the pack is in place. This causes significant discomfort and can result in necrosis of the nostril.

After the pack is in place, the patient should be observed for further bleeding. If the patient remains stable, has no significant comorbid conditions, and has only a unilateral anterior pack, the patient may be discharged with mild narcotic pain medications and antibiotics for prophylaxis against toxic shock syndrome and sinusitis. The pack should be removed 2 to 5 days later, with instructions to use nasal saline and nasal ointment liberally for the next 2 weeks. Recurrent bleeding should prompt an ENT consultation.

Posterior Packing

If the bleeding is not controlled with an anterior pack, the origin of the bleeding may be posterior, requiring an *anterior-posterior pack.* An anterior-posterior pack is inserted similar to a nasogastric tube, then inflated with the *minimum amount* of saline to stop the bleeding. The recommended maximum amount of inflation should not be surpassed.

If a preformed anterior-posterior pack is not available or not effective, a traditional anterior-posterior pack may be placed. The posterior pack is necessary essentially to seal off the posterior nasal cavity and provide a buttress to prevent the anterior pack from slipping posteriorly. A Foley catheter and balloon is slid into the nasal cavity and serves as the posterior pack and buttress. Once the Foley catheter is in place, it is inflated with 5 to 10 mL of saline (or air) and pulled snugly to seal the posterior nasal choana. A large anterior pack is then placed, which should quickly control the bleeding.

Placement of a posterior pack requires experience, and even if it is successfully done, ENT consultation is indicated to assist with further bleeding, pack removal, and to monitor for pack complications. Anterior-posterior packs are associated with significant patient discomfort and potential complications during and after insertion. Local complications, including necrosis of the alae, septum, and palate, can occur, and close observation is required to prevent them. Hypoxemia can also result. Supplemental oxygen and monitoring of oxygen saturation is indicated. Patients with preexisting cardiopulmonary disease require closer observation, often in the ICU. The patient might require judicious doses of narcotics for pain and antibiotics for infection prophylaxis.

Other Techniques

Rarely, epistaxis cannot be controlled with packing, requiring further intervention. This can include intraoperative endoscopic cautery, endoscopic or open arterial ligation, or angiography with selective embolization of the offending vessel. There are advantages and disadvantages to each of these techniques. In general, the surgical techniques are usually favored over embolization if there are no significant contraindications to surgery. All the surgical techniques have very high success rates. Embolization is also effective when performed by an experienced invasive radiologist, but it does carry the relatively low risk of inadvertent embolization of the internal carotid artery system and subsequent ischemic cerebral injury, which can be devastating.

Head and Neck Trauma and Respiratory Embarrassment

Key Points

- The ABCs of trauma include *a*irway, *b*reathing, *c*irculation, and *c*ervical spine clearance.
- Laryngeal and pharyngoesophageal injuries must be suspected in blunt or penetrating neck injuries.
- Intravenous access should be established and volume replacement initiated quickly.
- Isolated facial injuries can result in significant bleeding and can be associated with orbital or central nervous system injury.
- Overlooked facial fractures can result in long-term functional and cosmetic defects.

The ABCs of trauma should be remembered when treating a patient with cervicofacial trauma. This includes evaluation and treatment of *a*irway, *b*reathing, *c*irculation, and *c*ervical spine. The most pressing issue after significant face, head, or neck trauma is the potential for respiratory compromise, secondary to several causes. Altered mental status can lead to aspiration of blood or secretions with or without central hypoventilation. Comminuted facial fractures (midface or mandibular) can distort the oral and pharyngeal airway sufficiently to cause obstruction. An undetected expanding pharyngeal or neck hematoma can cause airway obstruction by extrinsic compression of the trachea or pharynx. Blunt or penetrating neck injuries can cause laryngeal fracture, bleeding, or hematoma, leading to critical airway obstruction.

Potential airway obstruction must be addressed quickly because complete obstruction can progress rapidly. The diagnosis is clinical because hypoxemia and carbon dioxide retention are late signs. Extensive facial edema or ecchymosis should arouse concern for facial fracture. A muffled voice can be the result of expanding hematoma. Laryngeal or tracheal injury should be suspected if the patient has a change in the voice, hemoptysis, subcutaneous emphysema, or stridor.

Stabilization of a compromised airway should be accomplished as soon as possible. Endotracheal intubation may be attempted, with plans for emergent cricothyrotomy as necessary. If time permits, the on-call anesthesiologist, trauma surgeon, or otorhinolaryngologist should be consulted to assist in airway management. Blind intubation (especially nasotracheal) or insertion of a laryngeal mask airway (LMA) is not recommended because this further compromises the already tenuous airway if intubation is unsuccessful. Although tracheotomy is the preferred procedure when endotracheal intubation is impossible or contraindicated, cricothyrotomy is also acceptable and can be lifesaving.

There is potential for significant blood loss after severe head and neck trauma. Intravenous access should be established and volume replacement initiated quickly. Bleeding from facial wounds can be controlled with direct pressure and suture ligation of arterial bleeding. Management of epistaxis is discussed earlier. Bleeding from the neck, or evidence

of expanding hematoma, implies a major vessel injury and requires immediate operative exploration by a trauma surgeon, vascular surgeon, or otorhinolaryngologist.

Unrecognized pharyngeal and esophageal injury can result in life-threatening infection. These injuries might not be obvious on initial evaluation and require a very high index of suspicion. Contrast studies and endoscopy are usually required to confirm the diagnosis. Treatment can include repair of the injury or external drainage to allow healing.

Isolated facial injuries are rarely life threatening but still can result in significant bleeding and, rarely, airway compromise and permanent disability. Significant facial trauma should be evaluated in the ED. The potential for intracranial and cervical spine injuries should be considered when major facial injuries are present. Trauma of the periorbital region requires ophthalmologic evaluation. All lacerations should be inspected, cleaned, and sutured. Antibiotics should be used if contamination is likely.

Deeper injuries can result in facial nerve transection. If facial nerve weakness is detected, plastic surgery or ENT consultation is necessary for expedient nerve exploration and repair. The parotid salivary duct can also be injured and requires repair over a stent. Facial fractures should be evaluated with CT (both axial and coronal images). Possible mandibular fractures should be evaluated with plain x-ray films, including panographic (Panorex) films. Overlooked and untreated facial fractures can result in significant long-term functional and cosmetic deficits. Oral surgery consultation is sometimes required, especially with injury to the teeth or altered dental occlusion.

The Ear

Key Points

- In smokers with otalgia, the clinician should suspect laryngopharyngeal carcinoma.
- A white mass behind the tympanic membrane might be a cholesteatoma.
- Pneumatic otoscopy is most useful in confirming middle ear fluid.
- Tympanometry and acoustic reflex testing are complementary to audiometry in determining the location of hearing loss.
- A neoplastic process should be considered when a presumed infection does not respond to usual medical treatment.

Physical Examination

See the discussion online at www.expertconsult.com.

Otalgia

While the vast majority of patients with otalgia have an otologic cause, the clinician must recognize that otalgia may be *referred*. Sensory innervation of the ear includes cranial nerves V, VII, IX, and X, and therefore disorders of structures with similar innervation can cause otalgia. It is imperative that the physician not simply attribute otalgia to an ear infection unless the physical examination supports this diagnosis. Otalgia can result from dysfunction of the nose, sinuses, oral cavity, pharynx, larynx, dentition, temporomandibular joints, and salivary glands. These structures must be thoroughly assessed, especially if the examination of the ear appears normal. This is especially true in smokers, whose initial symptom of laryngopharyngeal carcinoma may be otalgia. Otolaryngologic referral for laryngoscopy may be indicated with suspected referred otalgia. (See **eBox 19-1** and **eBox 19-2** online at www.expertconsult.com for differential diagnosis of otalgia.)

Tumors of the Ear

Tumors of the ear are rare. Classification is based on their location (external ear, middle ear, inner ear). A tumor of the external or middle ear is often easily diagnosed by visualizing a lesion on otoscopy. In some cases, symptoms may mimic infection (pain, otorrhea). Tumors of the inner ear can manifest with symptoms of hearing loss, tinnitus, disequilibrium, or facial weakness. (**eBox 19-3** online lists tumors of the ear by location.)

Vertigo

Key Points

- The most common cause of persistent vertigo is a peripheral vestibular disorder (38% to 56%).
- Central vestibular causes of vertigo represent less than 10% of all causes.
- Head movement always worsens the feeling of true vertigo.
- Benign paroxysmal positional vertigo is the most common cause of peripheral vestibular vertigo and is twice as common in women as men.
- Pneumatic otoscopy can cause nystagmus and vertigo in the presence of a perilymph fistula.
- Tinnitus is primarily caused by sensorineural hearing loss but occasionally can be the symptom of a vascular abnormality, hypermetabolic state, medication, or intracranial mass.

The sense of balance or equilibrium occurs when there is normal and harmonious function of several systems and organs in the body. These include the musculoskeletal system, the cardiovascular system, the central nervous system, the eyes, and the ears. Abnormal function of any of these can result in the sensation of dizziness or disequilibrium. The term *vertigo* is reserved to describe a perceived sensation of motion, usually spinning, of the person relative to the environment, or vice versa. Causes of disequilibrium can be categorized into one of three groups: *peripheral* (inner ear or labyrinthine), *central nervous system* (CNS), or *systemic* (e.g., cardiovascular, metabolic). Although not pathognomonic of a labyrinthine disorder, true vertigo most often indicates aberrant function of the inner ear.

Because patients use "dizzy" to describe many sensations, the actual sensation is best clarified by a detailed history (Box 19-1). The major studies on the causes of persistent dizziness, from Drachman and Hart (1972) to Davis (1994), all describe four diagnostic categories: lightheadedness, presyncope, disequilibrium, and vertigo. The investigators all conclude that the most common cause of persistent dizziness is a peripheral vestibular disorder (38%-56% of cases) followed closely by a psychogenic disorder (6%-33%). In about 25% of patients, the complaint is the result of the combined

Box 19-1 History for "Dizziness"
Description of the sensation (including associated symptoms)
Onset (acute, gradual)
Duration (date sensation was first noted, length of time it lasts)
Intensity (how troubling is it?)
Exacerbations (activities, positions, circumstances that worsen the situation)
Remissions (activities, positions, circumstances that make sensation better)
Medications (prescription, herbal, over the counter)
Other medical problems (e.g., diabetes, hypertension, heart disease)
Psychosocial (any stressors?)

effects of multiple sensory deficits, medications, or orthostasis, leading to complaints of presyncope, lightheadedness, or disequilibrium. Finally, central vestibular etiologies are unusual and represent less than 10% of all causes.

A thorough medical history allows the physician to distinguish between true vertigo (a sensation of spinning) and other sensations, such as presyncope, lightheadedness, and unsteadiness. The physical examination and laboratory evaluation are guided by the accuracy of the history. A sensation of vertigo originates from within the vestibular system but can be either *peripheral* (vestibular nerve and inner ear) or *central* (cerebellum, brainstem, thalamus, and cortex).

Questions regarding hearing and neurologic deficits can help elicit which part of the vestibular system is involved (Wiet et al., 1999) (see **eTable 19-1** online). Peripheral vertigo tends to be episodic, whereas central vertigo is constant. Neurologic symptoms or loss of consciousness do not occur with peripheral vertigo but are possible with central vertigo. Nystagmus, which is labeled by the direction of the fast component, can be present in both types of vertigo and can be horizontal or rotary; vertical nystagmus occurs only in central vertigo.

The physical examination should include assessment of orthostatic blood pressure changes, a complete ocular examination, tuning fork tests (Weber's and Rinne's), pneumatic otoscopy (elicits vertigo in patients with perilymphatic fistula), balance tests (Romberg's), gait (including tandem walking), and cranial nerve evaluation. The Dix-Hallpike maneuver (see **eFig. 19-3** online) is especially helpful in diagnosing benign paroxysmal positional vertigo (BPPV). Head movement always worsens the feeling of true vertigo. If it does not, the dizziness can be attributed to a cause other than vestibular dysfunction.

Laboratory testing can include an audiogram if no specific cause of vertigo can be found after the medical history and physical examination. Electronystagmography (ENG) is an objective study of the vestibular system and can help localize a vestibular lesion. Electrodes placed about the eye sense the movements of nystagmus as either spontaneous or initiated by maneuvers such as caloric testing, positioning, optokinetics, and pendulum tracing. A brain MRI scan is indicated in patients with unilateral otologic symptoms and in those unresponsive to treatment. Blood tests, when necessary, can include CBC, rapid plasma reagin (RPR), vitamin B_{12} level, folate level, drug screens, and heavy metal testing when indicated.

Meniere's Disease

Meniere's disease is characterized by episodic severe vertigo lasting hours, with associated symptoms of unilateral roaring tinnitus, fluctuating low-frequency hearing loss, and aural fullness. Typical onset is in the fifth decade of life. The cause is uncertain but is speculated to result from allergic, infectious, or autoimmune injury. The histopathologic finding includes *endolymphatic hydrops*, which is thought to be caused by either overproduction or underresorption of endolymph in the inner ear.

Meniere's disease is a clinical diagnosis mostly based on history. Testing may be obtained to support the diagnosis and rule out other disorders. Audiometry often demonstrates a low-frequency sensorineural hearing loss. An FTA-ABS test may be obtained to rule out syphilis. ENG may demonstrate a unilateral peripheral vestibular weakness on caloric testing. When the diagnosis is uncertain, a brain MRI with contrast is obtained to evaluate for a retrocochlear lesion. The differential diagnosis of Meniere's disease includes acute labyrinthitis, neurosyphilis, labyrinthine fistula, autoimmune inner ear disease, vestibular neuronitis, and migraine-associated vertigo.

Although Meniere's disease has a highly variable clinical course, most patients have long symptom-free periods between clusters of episodes. The majority of patients have an excellent prognosis, with symptoms burning out over several years. However, some patients have a disabling course with frequent and severe attacks. On average, a moderate sensorineural hearing loss is the end result. The disease may become bilateral in about 45% of cases (wide variability exists).

Treatment of an acute episode involves vestibular suppressants and antiemetics. As with any vestibular disorder, vestibular suppressants should be limited for use during acute symptoms because of their addictive potential and impairment of central compensation. Maintenance therapy includes reduction of sodium intake to less than 1500 mg/day and a diuretic such as hydrochlorothiazide-triamterene (Dyazide). Patients are also instructed to minimize caffeine, alcohol, nicotine, and chocolate. Allergy treatment may be helpful in some patients. Most patients have adequate control of symptoms with this regimen.

Patients who fail conservative measures may be candidates for procedures and surgical treatment. Gentamicin, a vestibulotoxic aminoglycoside antibiotic, may be injected transtympanically into the middle ear to permeate into the inner ear. Control of vertigo may result in 90%, but with a risk of hearing loss. Endolymphatic sac decompression or shunting through a mastoidectomy appears to benefit most patients with minimal risk to hearing. Although a generally accepted procedure, adequate studies are lacking on its effectiveness. More invasive interventions, including vestibular nerve section and labyrinthectomy, are reserved for patients with severe disease who do not respond to other measures (Sajjadi and Paparella, 2008).

KEY TREATMENT

Treatment of acute episodes of Meniere's disease involves vestibular suppressants and antiemetics (SOR: A).
Maintenance therapy includes reduction of sodium intake and use of a diuretic (SOR: A) (Thirlwall and Kundu, 2006).

Vestibular Neuronitis

Acute vertigo associated with nausea and vomiting (but without neurologic or audiologic symptoms) that originates in the vestibular nerve is known as *vestibular neuronitis*. Vestibular neuronitis can occur spontaneously or can follow viral illness. Nystagmus is horizontal, with the fast component beating away from the affected side. The symptoms peak within 24 hours and usually last 3 to 4 days. Autopsy studies have shown cell degeneration of one or more vestibular nerve trunks, a finding similar to that seen in Bell's palsy, which affects the facial nerve. A short course (3-5 days) of vestibular suppressants (e.g., meclizine [Antivert], diazepam [Valium]) and antiemetics such as promethazine (Phenergan) can provide symptomatic relief in the acute setting.

Distinguishing between vestibular neuronitis and bacterial labyrinthitis or labyrinthic ischemia is important. The diagnosis of *bacterial labyrinthitis is* based on hearing loss and otitis media or meningitis, and *labyrinthic ischemia* can be distinguished by hearing loss plus associated neurologic symptoms with a history of vascular disease.

Benign Paroxysmal Positional Vertigo

The most common cause of peripheral vestibular vertigo in adults is benign paroxysmal positional vertigo. BPPV occurs in all age groups but more often between ages 50 and 70. The incidence of BPPV is 11 to 64 per 100,000 persons per year and is twice as common in women as men (Froehling et al., 1991). It is caused when otoconia particles from the utricle or saccule lodge in the posterior semicircular canal and is also referred to as *canalithiasis*. This causes the canal to be a gravity-sensing organ, and head movement results in displacement of the otoconia and a sensation of vertigo.

The Dix-Hallpike maneuver reproduces this vertigo in the patient, resulting in nystagmus (see **eFig. 19-3**). Characteristics of the nystagmus of BPPV include fatigability, a latency period of 1 to 5 seconds before nystagmus begins after the head is moved, short duration of nystagmus from 5 to 30 seconds, and reversal of the nystagmus components when the patient is returned to the sitting position. If these characteristics are not present and treatment is not successful, BPPV cannot be diagnosed. In such a case, a CNS lesion is possible. BPPV can be the residual effect of Meniere's disease, ear surgery, vestibular neuronitis, or ischemia of the inner ear. Head trauma, even when it is minor, can lead to BPPV. However, one third of cases are idiopathic.

Treatment of BPPV consists of performing repositioning maneuvers with the goal of returning the otoconia to the utricle or saccule (Yacovino, 2009). In addition, the patient may attempt to reposition the otoconia at home by sitting upright on the bed and rapidly lying supine with the affected ear facing downward. After 1 minute, the head should be repositioned with the opposite ear facing downward, and the patient should wait another minute. The patient should then return slowly to the upright seated position and repeat this exercise four more times. The entire process is completed twice daily until the symptoms have abated.

An expert panel convened by the American Academy of Otolaryngology–Head and Neck Surgery Foundation recommended against "routinely treating BPPV with vestibular suppressant medication such as antihistamines or benzodiazepines" (Bhattacharyya et al., 2008). Because of the variability of symptoms, the clinician must judge each case independently. Resolution occurs in a few weeks or months, and the condition is benign, although it can recur.

KEY TREATMENT

Unless the diagnosis of BPPV is uncertain, radiographic imaging and vestibular testing are not recommended (SOR: B).
Patients with BPPV should be treated with an otoconia-repositioning maneuver (SOR: B) (Bhattacharyya et al., 2008).
Residual dizziness after successful repositioning procedures abates within 3 months without further treatment (SOR: B) (Seok, 2008).

Perilymph Fistula

Rapid changes in air pressure (barotrauma), otologic surgery, violent nose blowing or sneezing, head trauma, or chronic ear disease may cause leakage of perilymph fluid from the inner ear into the middle ear and result in episodes of vertigo. Associated signs and symptoms are variable but can include a sudden pop in the ear followed by hearing loss, vertigo, and sometimes tinnitus. Diagnosis can be determined by a fistula test, in which negative and positive pressures are applied to the tympanic membrane using pneumatic otoscopy, causing nystagmus and vertigo.

Labyrinthitis

As with vestibular neuronitis, labyrinthitis causes sudden and severe vertigo. In contrast to vestibular neuronitis, the patient also has tinnitus and hearing loss. The hearing loss is sensorineural, is often severe, and can be permanent. Labyrinthitis is caused by inflammation within the inner ear. The cause is most often a viral infection but can be bacterial. Bacterial labyrinthitis usually results from extension of a bacterial otitis media into the inner ear. A noninfectious *serous* labyrinthitis can also occur after an episode of acute otitis media. Other, less common causes include treponemal infections (syphilis) and rickettsial infection (Lyme disease).

Symptomatic treatment of labyrinthitis is similar to that for vestibular neuronitis. Antibiotics are recommended if a bacterial cause is suspected. As with acute otitis media, bacterial labyrinthitis can, in rare cases, lead to meningitis. Few other conditions cause the constellation of hearing loss, tinnitus, and vertigo, but cerebrovascular ischemia, meningitis, brain abscess, and encephalitis should all be considered. Although the vertigo should resolve over days to weeks, hearing loss and tinnitus can persist.

Drugs known to be ototoxic can cause acute onset of hearing loss and disequilibrium, although this is not true labyrinthitis. These drugs include salicylates, aminoglycosides, loop diuretics, and various chemotherapeutic agents. This cause should be considered in patients who complain of hearing loss or dizziness while taking these medications.

Tinnitus

Tinnitus is a term used to describe an internal noise perceived by the patient. It is usually, but not always, indicative of an otologic problem. Tinnitus is most often subjective, that is, heard only by the patient. However, it can be objective and

---

Box 19-2 Causes of Tinnitus

Subjective

Otologic: Presbycusis, noise-induced hearing loss, Meniere's disease, otosclerosis
Metabolic: Hyperthyroidism, hypothyroidism, hyperlipidemia, vitamin deficiency
Neurologic: Basilar skull fracture, whiplash injury, multiple sclerosis, meningitic effects
Pharmacologic: Aspirin, nonsteroidal anti-inflammatory drugs, aminoglycosides, tricyclic antidepressants, loop diuretics, heavy metals, oral contraceptives, caffeine, cocaine, marijuana
Dental: Temporomandibular joint syndrome
Psychologic: Depression, anxiety

Objective

Vascular abnormalities: Arteriovenous malformation, glomus tumors, stenotic carotid artery, vascular loops, persistent stapedial artery, dehiscent jugular bulb, hypertension
Tympanic muscle disorders: Palatomyoclonus, idiopathic stapedial muscle spasm
Patulous eustachian tube
Central nervous system anomalies: Congenital stenosis of the sylvian aqueduct, type 1 Arnold-Chiari malformation

From Lucente FE, Har-El G: Essentials of Otolaryngology. Philadelphia, Lippincott–Williams & Wilkins, 1999, p 110.

---

heard by the patient and the examiner. In most cases, tinnitus is secondary to bilateral sensorineural hearing loss and requires no further evaluation. In rare cases, tinnitus can be a symptom of a vascular abnormality (aneurysm or arteriovenous malformation), hypermetabolic state, or intracranial mass that, if not evaluated, could result in delayed treatment. Middle ear and rarely external ear pathology can also cause tinnitus, as can numerous medications (Box 19-2). The patient's medications should be reviewed.

Evaluation of tinnitus begins with a complete medical history, including duration of symptoms, possible inciting event (e.g., acoustic trauma), and accompanying symptoms (e.g., vertigo, hearing loss, headache, vision changes). Specific questions regarding the tinnitus are critical: Is it unilateral or bilateral? What is the quality of the tinnitus (pitch, volume)? Does it sound like a heartbeat or rushing blood? Does it change? A complete ENT evaluation should be performed, and audiometry is mandatory.

In general, if the tinnitus is bilateral, not particularly intrusive, not pulsatile, and associated with symmetric hearing loss, it is likely secondary to the hearing loss itself. The hearing loss requires further evaluation with magnetic resonance imaging (MRI) with contrast if it is asymmetric.

In cases of *pulsatile* tinnitus with normal otoscopy, magnetic resonance angiography (MRA) is performed to evaluate for vascular abnormalities. If otoscopy identifies a retrotympanic mass, a temporal bone CT is obtained to evaluate for a vascular mass or abnormality. Blood tests can be performed to rule out anemia or hyperthyroidism, which can result in a hypermetabolic state and cause tinnitus secondary to increased blood flow near the cochlea. Auscultation of the neck, periauricular area, and chest may identify a bruit or murmur, indicating a need for a carotid duplex ultrasound study or echocardiogram, respectively. Most cases of arterial pulsatile tinnitus are secondary to atherosclerotic carotid artery disease. Venous pulsatile tinnitus often improves with digital pressure over the internal jugular vein. Etiologies include idiopathic venous hum, a high-riding jugular bulb, or benign intracranial hypertension.

Effective treatment of tinnitus is difficult and usually requires various approaches. Finding and eliminating potential causes (especially pharmaceutical) is imperative. Patients should be counseled to avoid caffeine and nicotine. No single medicine has been proved effective in treating tinnitus. Antidepressants have shown promise, especially if depression coexists. Intravenous lidocaine eliminates tinnitus in some patients but is not practical and has obvious potential side effects. Various homeopathic treatments and nutritional supplements are effective in some cases, but most have not been evaluated in controlled studies. Hearing aids are beneficial in *masking* the tinnitus if hearing loss exists. Tinnitus maskers can be purchased that essentially drown out the tinnitus with various distracting noises. Biofeedback and a technique called *tinnitus retraining therapy* are helpful for some patients. These techniques can be learned through various publications or at a tinnitus treatment center. All patients with obtrusive tinnitus are encouraged to join the American Tinnitus Association, the largest tinnitus support group and an excellent source of reliable information.

Disorders of the External Ear

Otitis Externa

The most common cause of pain in the external ear is acute otitis externa. It affects 3% to 10% of the patient population. The pain is caused by inflammation and edema of the ear canal skin, which is normally adherent to the bone and cartilage of the auditory canal. The inflammatory reaction can be caused by bacteria, fungi, or contact dermatitis (see **eTable 19-2** online).

Cerumen protects the canal by forming an acidic coat that helps prevent infection. Factors that predispose to otitis externa include absence of cerumen, often from excessive cleaning by the patient; water, which macerates the skin of the auditory canal and raises the pH; and trauma to the skin of the auditory canal from foreign bodies or use of cotton swabs.

When a bacterial organism is suspected, treatment consists of cleaning the ear canal of any debris or drainage and then instilling antibiotic drops with or without steroids. Because the most common bacterial organisms in this infection are *Pseudomonas aeruginosa* and *Staphylococcus aureus*, drops containing ciprofloxacin or neomycin/polymyxin B are effective against these pathogens, combined with a steroid to decrease inflammation, pain, and pruritus (Ciprodex, Cortisporin, Coly-Mycin, Pediotic). A recent study found Ciprodex to be more effective against *P. aeruginosa* than neomycin/polymyxin B/hydrocortisone (Dohar et al., 2009).

The clinician must use judgment in assessing the severity of the infection and treat accordingly. If the infection spreads beyond the auditory canal, oral antimicrobials are indicated. If clinical improvement is not apparent after 48 hours, the patient needs to be reexamined for additional treatment or referral to an otorhinolaryngologist.

Fungal infections compose less than 10% of external otitis cases. The most common fungi are *Aspergillus niger* and *Candida* species and are more prevalent in tropical climates. Itching is a more common complaint than pain in fungal ear infections. Thorough cleaning of the ear canal is the primary duty of the physician in this infection. Drops that are effective include 2% acetic acid with or without a steroid. Clotrimazole drops or powder can also be used to treat fungal infections of the canal (van Bolen et al., 2003).

Approximately 90% of necrotizing (malignant) otitis externa is seen in immunocompromised patients such as diabetic patients, patients with acquired immunodeficiency syndrome (AIDS), and those receiving chemotherapy. Systemic antibiotics are mandatory in these cases. Antipseudomonal antimicrobials should be administered intravenously in the hospital setting, and surgical debridement is often necessary. Complications from necrotizing otitis externa include facial nerve palsy, mastoiditis, meningitis, and even death (Quick, 1999).

Other conditions that affect the external auditory canal include impacted cerumen, seborrheic dermatitis, psoriasis, contact dermatitis, and staphylococcal furunculosis. Symptoms and signs include pruritus, edema, scaling, crusting, oozing, and fissuring of the external auditory canal. Treatment of the underlying disease is the primary goal. Corticosteroid preparations are indicated for seborrheic dermatitis, psoriasis, and contact dermatitis. Oral antibiotics and sometimes incision and drainage are required for staphylococcal furunculosis.

KEY TREATMENT

Ciprofloxacin/dexamethasone 0.1% (Ciprodex Otic) applied ototopically in patients with acute otitis externa is more effective against *Pseudomonas aeruginosa* (most common isolate) than neomycin/polymyxin B/hydrocortisone (Cortisporin Otic) (SOR: A) (Dohar et al., 2009).

Using drops that have a steroid plus an antibiotic or acetic acid improves the cure rate compared to an antibiotic or acetic acid alone (SOR: A) (van Bolen et al., 2003).

Auricular Hematoma

Blunt auricular trauma, most commonly in wrestlers and boxers, may shear the perichondrium from the underlying cartilage, leading to a hematoma. The presence of a fluctuant swelling with loss of normal auricular landmarks helps to distinguish a hematoma from ecchymosis. If left untreated, an auricular hematoma may cause fibrosis and neocartilage formation, leading to a deformity of the auricle termed *cauliflower ear*. Therefore, treatment in a timely manner is recommended.

Although a Cochrane review could not define the best treatment for an acute auricular hematoma, a frequently successful treatment involves incision and drainage with dental rolls sutured to the anterior and posterior auricle (Fig. 19-5). Needle aspiration alone will often lead to recurrences. The bolster is usually left in place for 4 to 7 days, with the patient permitted to return to wrestling or boxing with headgear. Prophylactic antistaphylococcal antibiotics are given. For a long-standing hematoma or a cauliflower ear, debridement of fibrosis and cartilage is necessary (Jones and Mahendran, 2008).

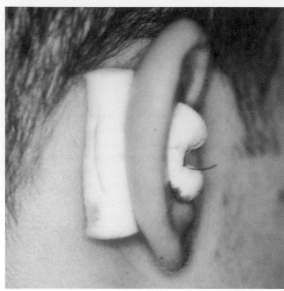

Figure 19-5 Photograph of 16-year-old boy who sustained auricular hematoma in wrestling match. He underwent incision and drainage with placement of dental rolls.

KEY TREATMENT

Successful treatment of auricular hematoma is incision and drainage with dental rolls sutured to the anterior and posterior auricle (SOR: B) (Jones and Mahendran, 2008).

External Auditory Canal Foreign Bodies

A common problem seen in family physicians' offices is a patient with an external auditory canal foreign body. A wide variety of objects can be found. In one study of 191 patients with aural foreign bodies, 27 different objects were discovered (Ansley and Cunningham, 1998). The most common were beads, plastic toys, pebbles, insects (especially cockroaches), popcorn kernels, earrings, paper, peas, cotton, pencil erasers, and seeds. When a patient presents with a chronic dry cough that has not responded to the usual measures, the physician should look for an aural foreign body (causing irritation of the ninth cranial nerve).

Removal of an external auditory canal foreign body is simplified if the object is in the lateral one third of the external auditory canal. Objects within the medial two-thirds pose a greater challenge. A variety of instruments can be used, depending on the object, including cerumen loops, alligator forceps, and otologic-tip suctions. Irrigation with body-temperature sterile water often dislodges the object. Hygroscopic objects such as vegetables, beans, and other food matter can swell and make the object even more impacted and should not be irrigated. Disk batteries should be removed immediately because of the possibility of liquefaction necrosis of the external auditory canal. Aural irrigation is contraindicated because wetting of the battery leads to leakage of electrolyte solution.

Smooth, round objects pose a difficult problem because, in trying to remove them, they are often pushed farther into the canal. Aural irrigation or even cyanoacrylate glue on the tip of a straightened paper clip is effective in removing objects that are difficult to retrieve. Methods to remove cockroaches or other insects include microscope immersion oil, mineral oil, or lidocaine. The effect of mineral oil or microscope immersion oil is to drown the insect, whereas lidocaine tends to make cockroaches crawl rapidly out of the canal (Bressler and Shelton, 1993). Otomicroscopy is often required for safe removal.

Depending on their age, fewer than 35% of patients should require anesthesia. The younger the patient, the more likely anesthesia will be required. Objects with sharp edges are best removed with an operating microscope with the patient under general anesthesia. Complications of foreign body removal include canal wall trauma and tympanic membrane perforation. Immobilization of the patient is the key to successful removal of aural foreign bodies, and at least two assistants are necessary.

Cerumen

Glandular secretions from the outer one third of the external auditory canal and desquamated epithelium combine to form cerumen. Cerumen is necessary to provide a hydrophobic and acidic environment to protect the underlying external ear canal epithelium and prevent infection. The external auditory canal is self-cleaning, with cerumen slowly pushed laterally to the external meatus.

Cerumen impaction is the symptomatic accumulation of cerumen in the external canal or an accumulation that prevents a needed assessment of the ear. Complete occlusion is not necessary. Symptoms may include hearing loss, tinnitus, pruritus, fullness, otalgia, cough, odor, and dizziness. Impaction often results from instrumentation with cotton-tipped applicators, which should be discouraged. Elderly patients with changes to external canal epithelium, patients with external canal abnormalities (e.g., osteomas, exostoses, stenosis), and users of hearing aids and earplugs are also at risk for impaction. Excessive cerumen production as a primary problem is relatively rare.

In most people, cleaning the external meatus with a finger in a washcloth while bathing is sufficient to maintain the ear canals. Treatment of cerumen impaction by the clinician may involve ceruminolytic agents, irrigation, or manual removal. Ceruminolytic agents include water-based, oil-based, and non-water-, non-oil-based solutions. A Cochrane review found that any type of ear drop (including water and saline) is more effective than no treatment, but study quality was lacking. Office irrigations may be performed using a large syringe with a large angiocatheter tip. The type of irrigant solution used is probably not critical, although a tepid or warm temperature is important to prevent the patient from becoming vertiginous from a labyrinthine caloric response. Instilling a ceruminolytic 15 minutes before irrigation may improve the success rate. Irrigations should not be performed in those with tympanic membrane perforations or previous ear surgery. Of note, irrigation with tap water has been implicated as a causative factor in malignant otitis externa. Therefore, instilling an acidifying ear drop after irrigation in diabetic patients is recommended. Manual removal requires knowledge of ear anatomy and special care to avoid trauma. A handheld otoscope with a curette and other instruments may be used. Otolaryngologists will often use binocular microscopy to aid with visualization. Those patients inquiring about ear candling should be informed that it has not been shown to be effective and presents a risk of thermal injury to the ear (Burton and Doree, 2008).

Frostbite

The ears, nose, and cheeks, in that order, are most at risk for frostbite. Exposure to subfreezing temperature is the main risk factor, but wind chill also greatly affects heat loss from the skin by convection. Protective clothing greatly diminishes the risk.

There are three grades: grade I frostbite, in which the skin is erythematous and edematous; grade II frostbite, in which the skin blisters and forms bullae; and grade III frostbite, which results in local necrosis of the dermis over 1 to 2 weeks. To assess the severity of frostbite, the physician must examine the tissue from several hours up to 2 days after the typical skin blanching occurs.

Treatment consists of quickly warming the ear with gauze soaked in saline at 38° to 40° C (100.4°-104.0° F). Any blisters that form should be allowed to reabsorb spontaneously. Topical antibiotic ointment can be applied, and viability of the tissue should be assessed periodically.

Lacerations

When there is trauma to the ear requiring suture closure, careful realignment is mandatory to maintain the auricular contour. The extent of the injury should be evaluated thoroughly with the tissue anesthetized with 1% lidocaine (without epinephrine). This allows a careful evaluation of the wound as well as a meticulous suture closure. Lacerations involving only the skin can be closed with everting nonabsorbable sutures. An earlobe that is torn from earring trauma can be closed in layers using absorbable chromic gut suture to close the dermis and nonabsorbable 5-0 or 6-0 suture to close the skin. Lacerations that involve cartilage, perichondrium, and skin must also be closed in layers but might best be referred to a specialist in otorhinolaryngology or to a plastic surgeon.

Disorders of the Middle Ear

Key Points

- Tympanic blistering (bullous myringitis) is simply a variant of acute otitis media (AOM) and should be treated as such.
- The most common infection in children seen in a physician's office is AOM.
- Three criteria are necessary for the diagnosis of AOM: acute onset, middle ear effusion, and signs or symptoms of middle ear inflammation.
- Severe AOM is defined as moderate to severe otalgia and fever greater than 39° C (102.2° F).
- When the diagnosis of AOM is uncertain (<2 criteria), observation is allowed in nonsevere illness.
- Amoxicillin is the drug of choice in treating AOM (80-90 mg/kg/day in 2 divided doses).
- Influenza vaccine decreases the number of cases of AOM in children 6 to 24 months of age.
- Surgical treatment is necessary for all middle ear and mastoid cholesteatomas.

- Antihistamines, decongestants, antibiotics, and corticosteroids are not recommended for routine use in otitis media with effusion.
- All traumatic perforations of the tympanic membrane require audiologic evaluation to rule out sensorineural hearing loss.
- Sudden sensorineural hearing loss is an otologic emergency.
- Facial weakness in the setting of AOM can require myringotomy with or without tube insertion in addition to broad-spectrum antibiotics.

Bullous Myringitis

Bullous myringitis refers to painful inflammatory bullae on the tympanic membrane. The blebs appear hemorrhagic. It was formerly thought that bullous myringitis was caused by *Mycoplasma pneumoniae* infection. Roberts (1980), however, summarized six studies involving 858 patients with bullous myringitis, and *M. pneumoniae* was isolated from only one. The cause is usually viral but can be bacterial in some cases. Studies have confirmed that bacterial cultures from bullous fluid are similar to cultures from middle ear fluid taken from patients with acute otitis media. The main isolates are *Streptococcus pneumoniae*, *Haemophilus influenzae*, and beta-hemolytic streptococci. The tympanic blistering is probably a nonspecific reaction and simply a variant of acute otitis media that should be treated as such.

It is important to distinguish bullous myringitis from acute otitis externa, which requires topical treatment, and from herpes zoster oticus, which can lead to cranial neuropathy and requires antiviral treatment. Neither of these conditions is usually limited to only tympanic membrane involvement.

KEY TREATMENT

No evidence supports the role of *Mycoplasma pneumoniae* as the causative agent in bullous or hemorrhagic myringitis (SOR: A) (Kotikoskie et al., 2004).

Bullous myringitis should be treated with antimicrobials used to treat acute otitis media (SOR: A).

Otitis Media

Acute Otitis Media

The most common infection for which children are seen in a physician's office is acute otitis media (AOM). The annual cost of AOM in the United States is an estimated $5 billion (Bondy et al., 2000). By age 7 years, 93% of children have had at least one episode of AOM, and 75% have had recurrent infections. AOM can occur at any age, but the highest incidence is between 6 and 24 months in the United States.

The primary cause of bacterial colonization of the middle ear is eustachian tube dysfunction. Abnormal tubal compliance in addition to delayed innervation of the tensor veli palatini muscle leads to collapse of the eustachian tube. Aerobic and anaerobic organisms, as well as viruses, can contribute to middle ear infection (Heikkinen et al., 1999). The three most common bacteria involved in AOM are *S. pneumoniae* (25%-40% of cases), *H. influenzae* (10%-30%), and *Moraxella catarrhalis* (2%-15%) (Klein, 2004). Risk factors most often associated with AOM are child care outside the home and parental smoking. Box 19-3 lists the common risk factors for AOM. A viral upper respiratory infection usually precedes an episode of AOM.

Three criteria are necessary to confirm the diagnosis of AOM: acute onset, presence of middle ear effusion, and signs or symptoms of middle ear inflammation (American Academy of Pediatrics [AAP], 2004; Level of evidence [Grade] B). Middle ear effusion can be diagnosed by direct visualization of air-fluid levels behind the tympanic membrane, a bulging drum, lack of movement on pneumatic otoscopy, or a flat tympanogram readout that indicates no tympanic membrane movement and therefore the presence of middle ear effusion. Redness of the tympanic membrane, pain, and fever are the most common signs and symptoms of middle ear inflammation (see **eBox 19-4** online). Erythema of the tympanic membrane without middle ear effusion is myringitis or tympanitis and is a separate diagnosis from AOM. Ear pain in the presence of a normal-appearing, flaccid tympanic membrane indicates causes other than AOM (Box 19-4).

The standard of care for the treatment of AOM in children older than 2 years is not to treat with antibiotics at the first visit, but to treat the pain and either observe the patient or prescribe an antimicrobial agent depending on certain criteria. The decision either to begin antibiotics or to observe the patient without them is based on the certainty of diagnosis, severity of symptoms, and age of the patient (AAP, 2004). (Table 19-2).

When all three criteria for the diagnosis of AOM are met (acute onset, middle ear effusion, and inflammation), the diagnosis is certain, and antibiotic therapy is indicated for any child 2 years old or younger (AAP, 2004; Grade A). For children older than 2 years, observation is an option if the illness is not severe and the parents can be relied on to report the patient's status and can obtain medication if necessary. Severe illness is defined as moderate to severe otalgia and fever higher than 39° C. (102.2° F.) When two or fewer diagnostic criteria are present, diagnosis is considered uncertain, and observation is allowed for children 6 months and older with nonsevere illness.

Box 19-3 Common Risk Factors for Acute Otitis Media (AOM)

Male gender

Bottle-feeding, especially in the supine position

Exposure to upper respiratory tract infections (e.g., daycare setting, winter season)

Genetic factors

Ethnic factors (e.g., Inuit or Native American)

Parental smoking

Allergy

Craniofacial abnormalities (e.g., cleft palate)

Previous episode of AOM, particularly during the preceding 3 months)

Use of a pacifier

From O'Handley JG. Controversies in the management of otitis media. Prim Care Rep 1999;5:43.

Box 19-4 Causes of Otalgia Other than Acute Otitis Media

Abscessed teeth

Cervical arthritis

Dental malocclusion

Nasopharyngeal carcinoma

Sinus infection

Sore throat

Temporomandibular joint disorders

Table 19-2 Treatment of Acute Otitis Media

Features	Treatment
Low-Risk Patients	
Older than 6 years, no antimicrobial therapy within past 3 months, no otorrhea, not in daycare, and temperature <38° C (<100.5° F)	Amoxicillin: 40-50 mg/kg/day in divided doses for 5 days
High-Risk Patients	
Younger than 2 years, in daycare, treated with antimicrobials within past 3 months, otorrhea, or temperature >38° C (>100.5° F)	Amoxicillin: 80-90 mg/kg/day in divided doses for 10 days
Treatment Failure	
Signs and symptoms persisting after 3 days	Amoxicillin–clavulanic acid (Augmentin): 80-90 mg/kg/day for 10 days Cefuroxime axetil (Ceftin): 20-30 mg/kg/day bid for 10 days Ceftriaxone (Rocephin): 50 mg/kg intramuscularly for 1 dose
Penicillin-Allergic Patient	
Any	Cefuroxime axetil: <2 years, 125 mg bid; ≥2 years, 250 mg bid TMP-SMX (Bactrim, Septra): 8 mg/kg TMP, 40 mg/kg SMX, per 24 hours in 2 doses Cefprozil (Cefzil): 30 mg/kg/day in 2 doses Cefaclor (Ceclor): 40 mg/kg/day in 3 doses Cefixime (Suprax): 8 mg/kg/day as a single dose

TMP-SMX, Trimethoprim-sulfamethoxazole; *bid*, twice daily.

Resistance of *Streptococcus pneumoniae* to penicillin is an increasing problem and ranges from 15% to 50% depending on the area. The mechanism of resistance is based on an alteration of penicillin-binding proteins rather than the production of beta-lactamase, as occurs with *H. influenzae* and *M. catarrhalis*. Resistance rates are higher in children than in adults, especially if the children are in daycare or have received antimicrobial therapy in the previous 3 months (Dowell and Schwartz, 1997).

The dose to treat AOM is 80 to 90 mg/kg/day in two divided doses (AAP, 2004). This allows the drug to overcome resistance in the causative organism (Dowell et al., 1999). For patients with a penicillin allergy, alternative medications include cefdinir, cefpodoxime, or cefuroxime. A meta-analysis found that first-generation cephalosporins have cross-allergy with penicillin, although the cross-allergy with second- and third-generation cephalosporins is negligible (Pichichero and Casey, 2007). Macrolides are not recommended for AOM in children because *H. influenzae* is the dominant organism causing AOM in this age group. Middle ear fluid becomes sterile 3 to 6 days after starting treatment (Carlin et al., 1991), so duration of therapy for uncomplicated AOM is 5 to 7 days, except for the child with an episode of AOM in the past 30 days, for whom a 10-day course of therapy is recommended (Pichichero and Brixner, 2006).

If the initial antibiotic fails to resolve symptoms in 72 hours (pain, fever, redness and bulging of the tympanic membrane, otorrhea), high-dose amoxicillin–clavulanic acid is recommended. Alternatives in penicillin-allergic patients include the antibiotics cited earlier. Patients who do not respond to amoxicillin–clavulanic acid therapy should be treated with intramuscular ceftriaxone for 3 days. This antibiotic in a single dose can also be used initially if the child is vomiting or unable to keep down oral medication. Doses of antimicrobials are given in Table 19-2.

Influenza vaccine has been shown to decrease the number of cases of AOM in immunized patients compared to controls and is recommended for all children age 6 to 24 months.

KEY TREATMENT

Antibiotics are most beneficial in children younger than 2 years with bilateral acute otitis media (AOM) and/or otorrhea (SOR: A). For most other children with mild disease, close observation and follow-up is an option (SOR: A) (Vouloumanou et al., 2009).
Administration of the seven-valent pneumococcal vaccine (PCV7) in infancy reduces the risk for AOM by 6% to 7%. Administering PCV7 to older children with a history of AOM appears to have no benefit in preventing further episodes (SOR: A) (Jansen et al., 2009).
Second- and third-generation cephalosporins may be used to treat AOM in penicillin-allergic patients (SOR: A) (Pichichero and Casey, 2007).
Uncomplicated AOM may be treated for 5 to 7 days (Pichichero and Brixner, 2006).
SOR: A

Otitis Media with Effusion

Otitis media with effusion (OME) is defined as persistent middle ear fluid without pain, fever, or redness of the tympanic membrane. It is often the result of AOM but can occur de novo. About 90% of children have OME before they reach school age. About 80% to 90% of cases resolve within 3 months and 95% within 1 year. Table 19-3 provides the Agency for Health Care Policy and Research (AHCPR) guidelines for treatment of OME.

Tympanometry can be used to judge the presence of middle ear fluid. It is important to document the affected ear, the duration of the effusion, and the presence and severity of symptoms associated with OME. The latter include a feeling of fullness in the ear, popping, mild pain, hearing loss, balance problems, and delayed language development.

If OME persists for 3 months, a comprehensive hearing evaluation should be performed. A 40-decibel (dB) loss (or worse) in hearing bilaterally mandates referral for evaluation for polyethylene (PE) tube placement. Management of hearing loss between 6 and 39 dB depends on parent or caregiver preferences and can include strategies to improve the listening and learning environment or referral for tube placement. If the hearing loss is 5 dB or less, repeat testing in 3 months may be performed if the middle ear effusion continues at that time. Follow-up testing is recommended every 3 to 6 months until the effusion resolves, unless significant hearing loss occurs or there is evidence for structural abnormalities of the eardrum or middle ear. In these patients, PE tube placement is the preferred course.

When referring to a surgeon, the primary care physician must provide an adequate history of the duration of the middle ear effusion, developmental state of the child, and pertinent information such as a history of AOM. Physician and parental expectations for the referral should be clarified. Ultimately, the decision for PE tube placement should be based on a consensus among all parties involved. The possibility of repeat surgery after tube extrusion is 20% to 50%, and with reoperation, adenoidectomy is recommended in children with normal palates because it reduces the need for future surgery by 50%.

KEY TREATMENT

Otitis media with effusion is best diagnosed with pneumatic otoscopy.
In children with craniofacial abnormalities, visual impairment, autism, speech delay, or hearing impairment, appropriate management of OME is critical (AAFP et al., 2004).
Antihistamines and decongestants have not been shown to be effective and are not recommended for treatment of OME.
Antibiotics and corticosteroids are also not recommended for routine management of OME because they do not provide long-term efficacy. SOR: A; B

Recurrent Otitis Media

Three episodes of AOM within 6 months with complete resolution between episodes or four episodes in 12 months defines recurrent otitis media. Although the evidence is conflicting, a double blind, placebo-controlled study comparing once or twice daily amoxicillin prophylaxis with placebo showed no benefit to using antibiotics. The authors recommended discouraging amoxicillin prophylaxis in children with recurrent otitis media not only because it is ineffective but also to prevent the acquisition of resistant pneumococci (Roark and Berman, 1997).

Tympanostomy tubes may be considered and may be beneficial in cases of recurrent AOM requiring multiple rounds of antibiotics within 6 to 12 months, especially if the episodes are severe.

Table 19-3 AHCPR Guidelines for Treatment of OME

Duration of OME	Treatment
6 weeks	Observation or antimicrobial therapy Hearing evaluation optional
3 months	Referral for hearing evaluation; with 20-dB hearing loss, patient should receive antimicrobial therapy or PE tube
4 to 6 months	Referral for PE tube if there is hearing loss

AHCPR, Agency for Health Care Policy and Research; *OME*, otitis media with effusion; *PE*, polyethylene.

Box 19-5 Complications of Otitis Media

Acute mastoiditis
Brain abscess
Epidural abscess
Facial nerve paralysis
Labyrinthitis
Meningitis
Sigmoid sinus thrombophlebitis
Subdural abscess
Subperiosteal abscess
Cholesteatoma

Chronic Suppurative Otitis Media

Chronic suppurative otitis media (CSOM) is the presence of persistent purulent otorrhea through a perforated tympanic membrane or tympanostomy tube. A persistent tympanic membrane perforation may result from acute otitis media, chronic eustachian tube dysfunction, or trauma. A cholesteatoma or rarely a tumor may also result in CSOM. Otorrhea may also be from chronic otitis externa, which may be difficult to distinguish from CSOM until treatment is initiated. Causes of otorrhea from the middle ear may not always be from middle ear bacterial infection (see **eTable 19-3**).

Associated symptoms often include hearing loss and tinnitus. Increasing pain, vertigo, or facial palsy imply a possible impending complication of CSOM (discussed later) and requires urgent otolaryngologist consultation. Binocular otomicroscopy allows better visualization and suctioning of purulent material compared to routine otoscopy. Imaging is reserved for medical treatment failures or if a complication is suspected. CT is helpful to evaluate for bony erosion. MRI is indicated with suspicion of CNS involvement.

Initial management should include culture and sensitivity of the discharge to allow appropriate antibiotic selection. If chronic otitis externa is suspected, the specimen should also be sent for fungal culture. Empiric antimicrobials should be started with coverage against the usual pathogens, which include *S. pneumoniae, H. influenzae, S. aureus, Pseudomonas* spp., and anaerobes. A Cochrane review demonstrated that ototopicals are superior to oral antibiotics. Quinolone ototopicals are safe for use in the middle ear. Topical aminoglycosides carry a risk of ototoxicity, but in some cases their use outweighs the risk. Systemic antibiotics may be required in severe cases or when copious drainage impairs administration of ototopicals. Aural toilet with an acetic acid solution (1 part distilled water, 1 part white vinegar) may be helpful to clear debris and provide antisepsis (Macfadyen et al., 2006a, 2006b).

If otorrhea resolves but a tympanic membrane perforation persists, the patient may be offered a tympanoplasty (tympanic membrane repair) to reduce the risk of recurrence and improve hearing. If medical therapy fails to control inflammation, a tympanomastoidectomy may be indicated to eradicate infection, aerate the middle ear and mastoid, and repair the tympanic membrane. *Chronic tympanostomy tube otorrhea* is treated the same as typical CSOM. In recalcitrant cases, however, tube removal or replacement may be indicated.

Also, adenoidectomy may be considered because chronic adenoiditis may act as a nidus for infection.

Complications

Although rare since the advent of antibiotics, complications of otitis media must be recognized early to avoid significant potential morbidity and mortality (Box 19-5). Chronic or recurrent otitis media can result in scarring of the tympanic membrane *(myringosclerosis or tympanosclerosis)*, which alone is usually of no consequence. If scarring involves the ossicles, however, hearing loss can result. Tympanic membrane retraction or perforation can also occur.

Intratemporal Complications

Extension of the infection into the mastoid air cells can lead to *acute mastoiditis*. The signs and symptoms of acute mastoiditis are fever and postauricular tenderness, erythema, and edema. It is important to recognize that acute mastoiditis is a clinical and not a radiologic diagnosis. Therefore, inflammatory changes on a temporal bone CT must be correlated with examination findings to be called acute mastoiditis. Furthermore, acute mastoiditis must be distinguished from an auricular cellulitis secondary to acute otitis externa. *Facial paralysis* may result from AOM or CSOM because of inflammation along the facial nerve as it courses through the middle ear space. Treatment of acute mastoiditis and facial nerve paralysis includes IV antibiotics, insertion of a tympanostomy tube for drainage, and sometimes emergent mastoidectomy. Infection within the middle ear space can extend into the inner ear, leading to labyrinthitis. Symptoms may include vertigo, tinnitus, and sensorineural hearing loss. Expeditious initiation of broad-spectrum antibiotics and in some cases insertion of a tympanostomy tube may be necessary. *Petrositis* is a rare complication involving inflammation of the petrous apex mastoid air cells. *Gradenigo's syndrome*, which includes retro-orbital pain, otorrhea, and cranial nerve VI palsy, may result. Treatment includes IV antibiotics and surgical drainage.

Intracranial Complications

The most serious complications of otitis media involve CNS extension of the infection and include sigmoid sinus thrombosis, meningitis, and brain abscess. Warning signs of an impending CNS complication include increasing pain, headache, spiking fever, or altered mental status. Evaluation may include MRI and lumbar puncture. Suspicion of CNS complication often requires urgent neurosurgical, ENT, and infectious diseases consultations. High-dose IV antibiotics and sometimes urgent surgery (mastoidectomy or craniotomy) are required to prevent significant morbidity or mortality. Otitic meningitis is a major cause of morbidity in the pediatric population. Fortunately, vaccines against *H. influenzae* type B and *Pneumococcus* spp. (Prevnar) have decreased these occurrences.

A "cholesteatoma" is a destructive epithelial cyst in the middle ear that may extend to the mastoid air cells. The term is a misnomer because of the lack of cholesterol and presence of only squamous epithelium and keratin debris. The external ear canal and outer layer of the tympanic membrane are lined with squamous epithelium. Keratin debris is continuously sloughed as new epithelial cells mature. In a normal ear the debris slowly migrates to the external meatus, where it is washed away. In contrast to the external ear, the middle ear space is lined with respiratory epithelium, which produces no keratin debris. Cholesteatomas form when squamous epithelium is abnormally located within the middle ear space, allowing the keratin debris to accumulate.

Cholesteatomas often result in CSOM with findings of purulent otorrhea, polyps, and granulation. However, some cholesteatomas are dry, with the finding of a white mass visible behind the tympanic membrane or a white mass or crusting on the tympanic membrane itself. A cholesteatoma must be differentiated from *myringosclerosis*, which is usually flat, white scarring on the tympanic membrane. Enzymatic properties, inflammation, and pressure may lead to bone erosion and hearing loss. If left untreated, serious problems may result, including facial nerve paralysis, labyrinthine fistula, and intracranial complications (see Complications of otitis media).

Congenital cholesteatomas occur without a history of tympanic membrane perforation or retraction and are postulated to result from congenital rests of epithelium in the middle ear space. These may occur in children with no significant history of otitis media and are usually diagnosed as an incidental white mass behind the tympanic membrane.

Primary acquired cholesteatomas result from prolonged eustachian tube dysfunction. Negative middle ear pressure results in a *retraction pocket* of the tympanic membrane, usually at the region of the pars flaccida. Squamous epithelium may become trapped and accumulate in the retraction pocket, resulting in a cholesteatoma. Any retraction pocket of the tympanic membrane requires further evaluation to prevent progression to cholesteatoma.

Secondary acquired cholesteatomas occur as a result of a tympanic membrane perforation. In some cases, a perforation of the tympanic membrane may allow the outer squamous epithelium to migrate into the middle ear space, leading to cholesteatoma formation.

Although aggressive medical treatment may reduce inflammation, surgical treatment is necessary for almost all cholesteatomas. In less advanced cholesteatomas, the external auditory canal is spared in surgery, a "canal wall up" tympanomastoidectomy. Close follow-up is required because of the risk of recurrence from microscopic disease or persistent eustachian tube dysfunction. In more advanced disease, the posterior canal is removed, termed a "canal wall down" tympanomastoidectomy (modified radical and radical mastoidectomy). The canal wall–down procedures are more likely to result in a conductive hearing loss, but the mastoid cavity becomes accessible through a larger external canal, thereby exteriorizing the cholesteatoma. Typically, semiannual mastoid bowl debridement is necessary to remove squamous and ceruminous debris to prevent inflammation.

Traumatic Tympanic Membrane Perforations

Traumatic perforation of the tympanic membrane may result from barotrauma (water skiing/diving injuries, blast injuries, blows to side of head), ear canal instrumentation (cotton-tipped applicators, bobby pins, paper clips, cerumen curettes), or otitis media (see earlier discussion). The patient usually complains of acute pain that subsides quickly, associated with bloody otorrhea. Severe vertigo can occur but is transient in most cases. Persistent vertigo suggests inner ear involvement (perilymphatic fistula). Hearing loss and tinnitus are also common.

Findings may include fresh blood in the canal and around the perforation. Any medial canal clots or debris should not be removed or irrigated except under microscopy. Secondary bacterial infection may require treatment with ototopical antibiotics. Topical fluoroquinolones are safe for use in the middle ear. Audiologic evaluation is necessary to rule out sensorineural hearing loss. If a tuning fork examination indicates sensorineural hearing loss or is unreliable, the patient should be referred for complete audiologic and ENT evaluation.

In uncomplicated cases the perforation is expected to heal spontaneously over days to weeks. The patient should be instructed to keep the ear dry during this time. If the perforation has not healed after several weeks, a tympanoplasty to close the perforation and, if necessary, repair ossicles is indicated. Repair of the perforation may improve hearing, reduce infection, and prevent cholesteatoma formation.

Barotrauma and Barotitis

Changes in altitude while flying (or scuba diving) can lead to rapid changes in middle ear pressure, leading to accumulation of serous middle ear fluid or blood. Symptoms may include aural fullness, otalgia, and conductive hearing loss. In most cases the fluid is resorbed, although this may take several weeks. *Autoinflation* maneuvers (popping the ears) may hasten recovery. Oral and topical decongestants, nasal steroid sprays, or a short course of corticosteroids may be helpful. Antibiotics are indicated only if there are signs of infection. If fluid persists or is troublesome to the patient, a myringotomy allows the fluid to be drained. Tympanostomy tube insertion may be indicated for persistent middle ear fluid.

Rarely, a rapid change in middle ear pressure can lead to the creation of a *perilymphatic fistula* between the inner and middle ear. The patient complains of severe vertigo and hearing loss (sensorineural) (see Vertigo). Urgent ENT consultation is indicated.

Hearing Loss

Hearing loss results from an interruption in the transmission of sound or subsequent nerve impulses in one or more areas of the ear. Recognition and treatment of hearing loss are imperative; unrecognized or untreated hearing loss may result in severe psychosocial ramifications in both adults and children. In the elderly population, hearing loss may lead to social withdrawal and depression. In the pediatric population, hearing loss may cause speech or cognitive delays. Hearing loss also has significant safety implications when it interferes with awareness of warning sounds (e.g., car horns, sirens, fire alarms). The four types of hearing loss follow:

1. *Conductive hearing loss* (CHL) occurs when there is a failure of normal propagation of acoustic energy through the conducting portions of the ear, which include the external auditory canal and the middle ear.
2. *Sensorineural hearing loss* (SNHL) occurs from dysfunction of the inner ear, which may be caused by a failure of the generation of nerve signals in the cochlea by the cochlear hair cells or propagation of electrical signals along the cochlear division of the eighth cranial nerve.
3. *Mixed hearing loss* (MHL) occurs when hearing loss results from both CHL and SNHL.
4. *Central hearing loss* can result from ischemic or traumatic brain injuries.

Hearing loss may be subclassified according to whether it is *acquired* or *congenital*. Hearing loss is further classified based on its *severity* (mild, moderate, severe, profound), *sidedness* (right, left, bilateral), *stability* (stable, progressive, fluctuating), and *cause*.

Evaluation includes noting the onset and duration of the hearing loss, any inciting events, the subjective severity of the hearing loss, and any psychosocial impact. Associated ear symptoms, medical history, and a history of ototoxic medication exposure are also important. Although history and examination provide clues to the etiology of the hearing loss, comprehensive audiometric evaluation is essential to making a diagnosis. Box 19-6 lists the most common types of CHL and SNHL.

Otosclerosis

Otosclerosis is caused by sclerotic fixation of the stapes and is the most common cause of CHL in the adult population with no previous history of trauma or infection. It is autosomal dominant in inheritance and more common in women than in men. Otosclerosis is usually bilateral and progressive. Treatment options include no treatment, amplification (hearing aid), fluoride treatment (stabilizes but does not improve hearing), and surgery (stapedectomy). Stapedectomy involves removing and replacing the stapes with a tiny prosthesis. This procedure has a success rate of greater than 95%. Risks of surgery, although rare, include worsened hearing, tympanic membrane perforation, changes in taste, and disequilibrium.

Sudden Sensorineural Hearing Loss

See Emergencies.

Presbycusis

Presbycusis is an all-inclusive term to describe the process of hearing loss related to aging. An estimated 30% to 35% of adults age 65 to 75 and 40% to 50% of adults older than 75 have hearing loss. Symptoms of presbycusis include gradu-

---

Box 19-6 Common Types of Conductive and Sensorineural Hearing Loss

Conductive Hearing Loss

Cholesteatoma
Cerumen impaction
Foreign body in ear canal
Ossicular problems
Otitis media with effusion
Otosclerosis
Retracted tympanic membrane (eustachian tube dysfunction)
Tumor of the ear canal or middle ear
Tympanic membrane perforation
Tympanosclerosis

Sensorineural Hearing Loss

Acoustic neuroma
Diabetes
Hereditary (congenital) loss
Idiopathic loss
Meniere's disease
Multiple sclerosis
Noise-induced loss
Ototoxicity
Perilymphatic fistula
Presbycusis
Syphilis

---

ally decreasing hearing acuity, especially for higher-pitch tones (women's and children's voices) and in certain situations (with background noise). Tinnitus is common.

The cause of presbycusis is likely multifactorial, but ultimately the loss of cochlear *hair cell* function is thought to be the cause in most cases. Hair cell damage or loss can result from chronic noise exposure, genetic predisposition, and ototoxic medications. The hearing loss may also be caused by neurovascular injury from chronic conditions such as hypertension or diabetes, which can affect the cochlea or cochlear nerve. Hormonal conditions such as hypothyroidism should be considered, as should unusual conditions such as tertiary syphilis. Central auditory problems might be the cause, from dementia, cerebrovascular disease, or cerebrovascular accident (CVA, stroke).

Although the term "presbycusis" implies sensorineural loss, conductive hearing loss should also be considered, including cerumen impaction, chronic OME, and otosclerosis (see Box 19-6).

Acoustic Neuroma

An acoustic neuroma (or more precisely, *vestibular schwannoma*) is a benign tumor that arises from the Schwann cells of cranial nerve VIII. Acoustic neuromas account for about 10% of all intracranial tumors. They are most commonly diagnosed in middle age. They are slightly more common in women than men. They are usually sporadic but may be associated with neurofibromatosis 1 or 2 (NF-1, NF-2). Most patients with NF-2 will develop bilateral acoustic neuromas. Acoustic neuromas in NF-1 are much less common.

The primary symptoms of vestibular schwannoma are asymmetric hearing loss (sensorineural) and tinnitus. The hearing loss is usually gradual in onset and progressive but can occur suddenly. Disequilibrium is not usually the chief complaint on presentation, but patients often admit to mild unsteadiness. Larger tumors can cause dysesthesia around the ear or facial weakness, or both. If the neuroma is diagnosed late, patients can manifest cerebellar symptoms and symptoms of mass effect and obstructing hydrocephalus.

After a complete neuro-otologic examination and audiologic evaluation, an MRI scan of the brain with fine cuts through the internal auditory canal with gadolinium contrast is necessary for diagnosis.

Treatment options include observation, surgery, or stereotactic radiotherapy. Most vestibular schwannomas require treatment to prevent cerebral complications from future growth. If the patient is aged or infirm, watchful waiting may be considered. Very small tumors may be observed because the rate of growth is often slow. Surgical treatment involves either a translabyrinthine resection if hearing is poor or a craniotomy for hearing preservation. Stereotactic radiotherapy has the obvious advantage of avoiding major surgery. Success is similar to surgery for smaller tumors. Shortcomings of this treatment include delayed facial paresis, tumor recurrence (which requires routine monitoring), and the potential for radiation-induced malignancies in the future.

Hearing Loss from Acoustic Energy

Excessive noise exposure is an important and usually preventable cause of hearing loss. Hearing loss can result from chronic or acute noise exposure, usually causing injury at the level of the cochlear hair cells. However, acute acoustic trauma can also cause injury to the tympanic membrane and middle ear structures.

Chronic noise exposure may be recreational or vocational. The Occupational Safety and Health Administration (OSHA) has established guidelines for safe limits for acute and chronic noise exposure to prevent occupational noise-induced hearing loss. Exposure to noise of 90 dB or less is permissible for up to 8 hours per day. As the noise intensity increases, the permissible duration of exposure decreases. OSHA outlines procedures for hearing protection and monitoring. These standards also can help provide guidelines to minimize excessive recreational noise exposure. Recreational activities known to cause excessive noise include hunting or target shooting with firearms, use of power tools or power lawn equipment, attendance at sporting venues, motor racing events, action movies, or concerts and listening to loud music on headphones. Hearing protection or avoidance is recommended for such activities.

Acute exposure to excessively loud noise can cause conductive or sensorineural hearing loss. CHL can result from a blast-type injury that leads to tympanic membrane perforation or ossicle injury. The conductive component of the hearing loss is usually reparable, but severe acoustic trauma can also cause sensorineural loss. SNHL from acute acoustic trauma is usually the result of temporary hair cell dysfunction or permanent injury, leading to transient or permanent *threshold shifts,* respectively. A concussive or blast injury (e.g., slap, airbag deployment to ear) can result in the formation of a labyrinthine fistula from the inner ear into the middle ear, which causes severe vertigo and SNHL. Most fistulas close spontaneously with bed rest, but some require middle ear exploration and repair. However, the sensorineural hearing loss is usually permanent.

Hearing Loss in the Pediatric Population

Congenital hearing loss is often hereditary but may be secondary to an intrauterine insult or infection. Of the hereditary variety, the majority are autosomal recessive and nonsyndromic. Risk factors for congenital hearing loss include family history of hearing loss, facial abnormalities, ICU admission, history of meningitis, syndromes known to be associated with hearing loss, low Apgar scores at birth, medications known to cause hearing loss (e.g., aminoglycosides), elevated bilirubin, some prenatal maternal infections, or suspicion of hearing loss.

Universal newborn hearing screening using otoacoustic emissions and auditory brainstem response allows early identification of impaired children. Intervention by age 6 months appears to improve language development. A temporal bone CT is often obtained to evaluate for inner ear malformations that would predispose the patient to further hearing loss with even mild head trauma. A genetics evaluation and counseling may be indicated. Mutations of the Connexin-26 gene, an autosomal recessive disorder, accounts for a significant percentage of nonsyndromic hereditary hearing loss. Hearing loss may coexist with other conditions (e.g., renal, ophthalmologic, thyroid, infectious, cardiac), so other testing may be indicated based on clinical suspicion.

In children with a significant hearing loss, hearing aids are recommended. A cochlear implant may be indicated for those with hearing so poor to be considered unaidable. A cochlear implant is a surgically implanted device that receives sound, converts it to electrical signals, and directly stimulates the cochlea. Results are excellent in properly selected patients.

An important and often unrecognized cause of hearing loss in children is chronic OME. Children with either unilateral or bilateral middle ear effusions refractory to medical treatment for more than 3 months should have audiometric testing. Myringotomy with tube insertion is indicated if bilateral CHL is found and should be considered in some cases of unilateral loss as well.

Treatment of Hearing Loss

Individual treatments for specific causes of hearing loss vary greatly. This section gives a brief overview of options available to improve hearing in patients with the most common causes of hearing loss.

Surgery is often performed for CHL. Myringotomy with or without tube insertion corrects hearing loss in cases of OME. The procedure is performed under brief general anesthesia in children or under local anesthesia for most adults. A tympanoplasty is performed for tympanic membrane perforations and to reconstruct ossicles with a prosthesis. A stapedectomy with placement of a prosthesis is often a successful option in patients with otosclerosis.

Cochlear implantation is indicated for profound SNHL in patients who do not benefit from conventional hearing aids. The procedure is indicated for adults and children as young as 12 months old.

Table 19-4 Causes of Facial Paralysis in Order of Occurrence

Cause	Percentage	Characteristics
Idiopathic (Bell's palsy)	60-85	Acute onset; viral prodrome (60% of cases)
Trauma	20-50	Acute-onset paralysis or paresis of previously functioning nerve
Herpes zoster	10-15	Ramsay Hunt syndrome with cranial nerve VII involvement, vestibular(vertigo), cochlear (hearing loss)
Tumor	10-15	Slow progression to complete paralysis
Birth	10-15	Part of congenital syndrome or birth trauma at delivery
Infection	4	Mastoiditis, otitis media, direct cranial nerve VII infection, Lyme disease
Brain lesion (central nervous system)	<10	Supranuclear or in brainstem

From Brody R, Har-El G. From Lucent FE, Har-El G. Essentials of Otolaryngology. Philadelphia, Lippincott Williams & Wilkins, 1999, p 131.

A variety of styles of hearing aids are used to rehabilitate hearing loss in patients with SNHL and CHL. The simplest (and least expensive) are larger, behind-the-ear aids with analog amplification of sound. The most complex (and most expensive) are completely-in-the-canal aids with programmable digital amplification. Several other types of aids fall between these two extremes. A certified audiologist, under the supervision of an otorhinolaryngologist, assists the patient with proper selection of an appropriate hearing aid.

Facial Nerve Paralysis

Facial paralysis occurs for various reasons. Possible causes are listed in Table 19-4. The eponym "Bell's palsy" is reserved for cases of idiopathic facial paralysis. It has been shown, however, that many if not most cases of idiopathic facial paralysis are actually caused by reactivation of latent herpesvirus living in the facial nerve or geniculate ganglion.

Although the most common cause of facial paralysis is indeed Bell's palsy, it is incumbent to rule out *other* potentially serious causes of facial paralysis before making this *diagnosis of exclusion*. Initially, a complete history and physical examination are required, including otologic and neurologic evaluation. The patient should be questioned regarding history of recurrent cold sores, which suggest herpetic involvement. Recent travel (especially camping) should be noted because Lyme disease is an often-overlooked cause of facial paralysis. Involvement of facial nerves is a concern in patients with a history of chronic otitis media or cholesteatoma. Other symptoms should be noted. Otalgia is common with Bell's palsy and does not always imply that the ear is involved. Of course, questions regarding risk factors for cerebrovascular disease or previous CVA should be obtained.

Evaluation of facial nerve function requires careful attention and comparison between the two sides of the face. The patient should be evaluated at rest and with voluntary movement. The patient should be asked to wrinkle the nose, raise the eyebrows, squeeze the eyes shut, and purse the lips to assess all branches of the facial nerve. The facial skin should be assessed, because a rash can indicate *herpes zoster oticus* (Ramsay Hunt syndrome). The eyes should be inspected to rule out exposure keratitis from lack of eye closure and dryness. If keratitis is suspected, ophthalmologic consultation should be obtained to prevent loss of vision. A complete neurologic examination must be done. If other neurologic deficits are found, neurology consultation is indicated. Lesions in the auditory canal should raise suspicion of herpes zoster oticus or malignancy of the external auditory canal with facial nerve involvement. Otitis externa and facial weakness can represent malignant otitis externa, especially if the patient is diabetic or immunocompromised. Signs of otitis media imply involvement of the facial nerve as it courses through the middle ear. The parotid gland and rest of the neck should be checked to rule out a parotid salivary gland mass that involves the facial nerve. Any of these associated ear findings should prompt ENT consultation because early intervention can improve outcome. Audiometry is recommended in the evaluation of facial paralysis because of the proximity of cranial nerves VII and VIII in the temporal bone.

In cases in which no identifiable cause is found, the diagnosis of Bell's palsy is made (though this diagnosis is not certain until a facial or acoustic neuroma has been ruled out either with return of facial function or with MRI scan). In the past, Bell's palsy was treated expectantly because the cause was not clear, making treatment difficult. Evidence now indicates that most Bell's palsy cases are secondary to a reactivation of the herpes simplex virus in the geniculate ganglion, causing neural edema and neurapraxia. On the basis of this research, treatment with antivirals and steroids are thought to improve outcomes. If no contraindications to steroids exist, prednisone (1 mg/kg, up to 60 mg, for approximately 7 days with a 7-day taper) is reasonable. In addition to steroids, an oral antiviral with activity against the herpesvirus is given (200 mg acyclovir [Zovirax] five times daily or valacyclovir [Valtrex] 500 mg twice daily for 7-10 days). Of the utmost importance is protection of the eye. Moisturizing eyedrops and nightly lubrication should be prescribed. Any signs of irritation should prompt an ophthalmology evaluation.

If the facial weakness is secondary to Ramsay Hunt syndrome, treatment is similar to that of Bell's palsy, but the clinical course and expected outcomes differ. This syndrome is caused by herpes zoster (rather than herpes simplex) involvement of the facial (geniculate), vestibulocochlear, and/or trigeminal ganglia. The infection causes pain and eventually vesicular eruptions around the auricle and external ear canal. Vesicles may appear only in the pharynx or hard palate in some cases. Facial weakness and at times dense paralysis are common. Hearing loss, tinnitus, and persistent vertigo also occur in 20% to 30% of patients (Adour, 1994). As with Bell's palsy, prompt initiation of oral steroids and acyclovir should begin when the diagnosis is suspected. This therapy can lessen vertigo and improve recovery of facial nerve function, although outcomes are not as favorable as for Bell's palsy. Some patients struggle with persistent facial weakness, pain, and hearing loss (Robillard et al., 1988).

In cases of facial paralysis associated with otitis externa or otitis media, treatment differs. If malignant otitis externa is suspected, the patient requires hospital admission, control of diabetes, and infectious diseases and ENT consultation. IV antibiotics and sometimes surgical debridement are required. CNS complications are possible.

Facial weakness in the setting of AOM requires treatment with a broad-spectrum antibiotic covering the usual pathogens of otitis media. In addition, a myringotomy with or without tube insertion is thought to hasten resolution and improve outcomes by allowing decompression of the infection. This also allows a culture to be done and antibiotic sensitivities determined. If facial weakness occurs in the setting of chronic otitis media or known cholesteatoma, topical and systemic antistaphylococcal and antipseudomonal antibiotics should be started and an urgent ENT consultation obtained in hopes of preventing permanent facial paralysis and further complications.

Expected outcome for true Bell's palsy is full return of function in 80% of patients. The remaining 20% have variable recovery. If recovery is incomplete, MRI is indicated to rule out neoplastic process (most likely a facial neuroma) that could mimic Bell's palsy. Patients with diabetes mellitus have a higher incidence of Bell's palsy and often have a poorer outcome. Permanent facial weakness is also more common after herpes zoster oticus. Outcomes of facial paralysis secondary to the other causes discussed are variable and depend on the severity of the pathology, the patient's general state of health, and the response to treatment.

In patients who have poor return of facial function, rehabilitation is necessary. The most important goal is protection of the eye, followed by improved cosmesis. Ophthalmologic and ENT involvement is continued (Almeida et al., 2009).

The Nose and Paranasal Sinuses

Key Points

- A CT scan of the sinuses is not necessary to diagnose uncomplicated acute sinusitis. CT should be considered when the diagnosis is uncertain, treatment has failed, or a complication or neoplasia is suspected. MRI is useful in evaluation of sinus tumors.
- Adenoid hypertrophy is a common cause of nasal symptoms in children, but in an adult can indicate a lymphoproliferative disorder or HIV infection.
- A nasal foreign body should be suspected in a child who presents with recent unilateral nasal obstruction, rhinorrhea, and odor.
- Nasal polyps can be seen with asthma, cystic fibrosis, and rarely neoplasia.
- After allergen avoidance and antihistamines, topical corticosteroids are the mainstay of treatment for seasonal allergic rhinitis.
- Leukotriene receptor antagonists can reduce the symptoms of allergic rhinitis.
- Treatment to restore mucociliary function in sinusitis is as important as antimicrobial therapy.

- Unlike adults, children with sinusitis rarely complain of facial pain.
- Prompt diagnosis and treatment of a nasoseptal hematoma can prevent subsequent cartilage destruction.

History

Signs and symptoms of most nasal and sinus disorders include nasal congestion, rhinorrhea, bleeding, facial pressure, halitosis or pain, headache, cough, otalgia, facial or periorbital swelling, altered (diminished, absent, or distorted) sense of smell, or postnasal drainage. Initial evaluation of the patient with nasal complaints begins with a complete history, with specific questions directed at the timing and chronicity of the symptoms and modifying factors. The patient should be questioned specifically about previous nasal trauma.

Patients should be asked about prescription and over-the-counter nasal, sinus, and allergy medications. Many patients try OTC remedies before seeking medical advice. Excessive use of decongestant nasal sprays can exacerbate and even cause nasal obstruction secondary to *rhinitis medicamentosa* and rebound nasal congestion. The patient should also be questioned about previous nasal surgery. Rarely, the patient admits to unorthodox self-treatment that may be significant (e.g., peroxide irrigation, overzealous nasal cleaning). This can explain continued symptoms and may indicate an underlying problem. The underlying problem may be true nasal pathology or rarely may be obsessive-compulsive disorder manifesting as repeated nasal cleaning.

Information about past medical history and social history is also necessary. Knowledge of the patient's work environment may be relevant. Exposure to chemicals or fumes can cause nasal symptoms. Woodworkers are known to have a higher incidence of sinonasal carcinoma. A history of environmental allergies or immune dysfunction is relevant. Many medical conditions (e.g., asthma, autoimmune disorders) are associated with sinonasal dysfunction. Other conditions (e.g., hypertension) will limit the use of decongestants. History of migraine is noteworthy because migraine headaches can be confused with sinus pain. Some prescriptions can exacerbate or even cause nasal dysfunction, especially medications (antihistamines, diuretics, antidepressants) that can lead to excessive nasal dryness (sicca). Drug allergies should be noted. Previous nasal surgery, if done, may not have been successful or even led to increased problems. Cigarette smoking and excessive use of alcohol and caffeine have negative effects on mucociliary function that can lead to congestion. A history of nasal or facial trauma is important. Previous or current use of intranasal cocaine can lead to significant pathology and symptomatology.

Physical Examination

See the discussion online at www.expertconsult.com.

Radiography

Plain radiographs do not approach the sensitivity and specificity of CT but are useful in some cases. Plain films are often ordered in cases of facial trauma, especially isolated nasal trauma. The films can be complementary to the physical examination.

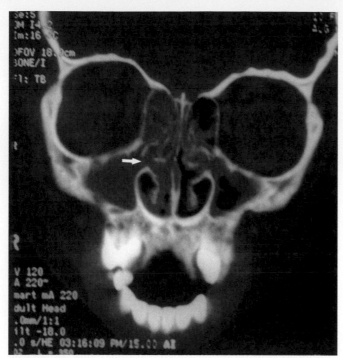

Figure 19-6 Coronal computed tomography scan showing complete opacification of the right maxillary and ethmoid sinuses with partial opacification of the left maxillary and ethmoid sinuses. Arrow indicates ostiomeatal complex.

Plain radiographs of the sinuses are still useful in certain circumstances. Plain sinus radiographs are reasonably accurate in assessing the maxillary and frontal sinuses in cases of *acute* sinusitis. Complete opacification or an air-fluid level in one of these sinuses usually indicates acute sinusitis. However, the relatively low sensitivity and specificity of plain films, especially in evaluating the ethmoid sinuses, have limited their usefulness.

Computed tomography has become an invaluable diagnostic tool for evaluating chronic nasal and sinus problems and has essentially supplanted the use of plain sinus films. CT of the sinuses allows unparalleled imaging of the complicated anatomy of the nose and paranasal sinuses. It has also increased understanding of the pathophysiology of sinusitis. CT scanning can show areas of mild mucosal thickening in the sinuses (indicating chronic sinusitis), complete opacification (seen in acute sinusitis, polyps, or sinus tumors), bone erosion, or abscess formation in adjacent critical structures such as the orbit or brain (Fig. 19-6). CT can show whether the *ostiomeatal complex* (the "bottleneck" of normal sinus drainage) is patent or obstructed and shows the myriad nasal and sinus normal variants, some of which predispose to sinonasal pathology.

Computed tomography of the sinuses should be ordered when the diagnosis of chronic sinusitis is suspected, medical treatment of sinusitis has failed and surgery is being contemplated, a complication of sinusitis is suspected, or a nasal or sinus mass is suspected. CT is not required as a confirmatory test in the treatment of uncomplicated acute sinusitis except in certain circumstances. The scan is helpful, however, in cases of *recurrent acute sinusitis* or when the diagnosis is not certain. Obtaining a scan during a patient's presumed

infection allows the diagnosis to be confirmed or ruled out. Although some abnormalities require further treatment occasionally, the scan identifies abnormalities or variations of normal anatomy that require no intervention. Mucus retention cysts, for example, are seen in up to 20% of the population. Unless they are large or infection is suspected (the patient complains of pain in the vicinity of the cyst), no treatment is required.

Magnetic resonance imaging is not particularly helpful in evaluating sinusitis and has two main limitations in evaluating inflammatory sinus conditions. First, MRI often tends to be too sensitive, showing mucosal thickening that is clinically insignificant. Second, MRI fails to show bony anatomy, which is critical in diagnosis and surgical planning in chronic sinusitis. MRI is useful in evaluating suspected sinonasal tumors and fungal infections of the sinuses. The limitations of MRI and its relatively high cost compared with CT do not justify its routine use in evaluating chronic sinusitis. When incidental sinusitis is noted on an MR image and the degree of sinusitis is severe, is asymmetric, or the patient is symptomatic, treatment (and sometimes ENT referral) is indicated.

Clinical Problems

Complaints related to the nose and sinuses are among the most common seen in a family medicine practice. Acute rhinitis (the common cold), allergic rhinitis, and sinusitis compose the vast majority of these complaints and, taken together, result in an enormous socioeconomic impact in terms of missed workdays and schooldays and pharmaceutical costs. Nasal complaints are usually related to nasal congestion, rhinorrhea, bleeding, facial pressure or pain, headache, cough, otalgia, facial or periorbital swelling, altered (diminished, absent, or distorted) sense of smell, or postnasal drainage.

Epistaxis

See also earlier Emergencies section. (p. 300). Epistaxis can be caused by trauma, dry weather, hypertension, bleeding dyscrasias, anticoagulation therapy, and intranasal tumors. Adolescent boys with recurrent epistaxis and nasal obstruction might have juvenile nasopharyngeal angiofibroma. Epistaxis typically responds to conservative treatment, including nasal hydration with saline mist, nasal ointment, environmental humidification, avoidance of digital trauma, and control of hypertension if present. If bleeding continues to be a problem, the patient should be referred to an ENT consultant for a complete evaluation of the nasal cavities and possible cautery. Screening blood studies for coagulopathy may be necessary.

Nasal Obstruction

The sensation of unilateral or bilateral nasal obstruction is relatively common and can range from mildly annoying to extremely frustrating to the patient. Nasal obstruction may be associated with other symptoms such as rhinorrhea, lost or altered sense of smell, or facial discomfort. Nasal obstruction may result from pathology of the nasal cavity or nasopharynx. (**eTable 19-4** online summarizes the most common causes, associated signs and symptoms, and treatment for nasal obstruction).

Physical Examination

See the discussion online at www.expertconsult.com.

Treatment

Successful treatment of nasal obstruction depends on making a correct diagnosis. Once the diagnosis has been established, a treatment plan should be developed. If the nasal obstruction is secondary to one of the various types of rhinitis, it is treated medically. This includes nasal steroids, antihistamines, leukotriene inhibitors, mucolytics, oral decongestants, topical decongestants, and nasal saline. These medications may be used alone or in various combinations. The choice of medications is determined by the severity of symptoms and the patient's medical history, response to treatment, and wishes. Oral steroids can be used in select severe cases but are associated with potential significant side effects. Nasal decongestant sprays are very effective for treating severe nasal congestion but should be used sparingly and never for longer than 3 days, to prevent rebound nasal obstruction (rhinitis medicamentosa). Allergy testing is done when allergies are suspected and the standard regimen is largely ineffective. Antibiotics are administered if a bacterial infection is suspected (acute rhinosinusitis).

Adenoid Hypertrophy

Adenoid hypertrophy is common in children. If identified in an adult, adenoid hypertrophy could indicate a lymphoproliferative disorder or HIV infection. The patient may present with nasal symptoms or symptoms of eustachian tube dysfunction. In the pediatric population, adenoid hypertrophy causes chronic or recurrent nasal obstruction, rhinorrhea, snoring, cough, or otitis media. The diagnosis is usually clinical but can be confirmed with lateral neck radiograph. If symptoms are severe or persistent, adenoidectomy is indicated; improvement is usually dramatic.

Foreign Body

A nasal foreign body should be suspected in a child with or without a history of previous nasal problems who presents with recent unilateral nasal obstruction, rhinorrhea, and odor. The nasal foreign body might not be visible secondary to the presence of mucosal edema, mucus, or pus.

If the foreign body is identified, removal may be attempted in a cooperative child. If removal is not possible or the diagnosis is uncertain, ENT consultation should be obtained. The ENT evaluation may be done in the office setting or in the operating room, depending again on patient cooperation and degree of suspicion. The nasal cavity is suctioned, decongested, and anesthetized with topical lidocaine. Endoscopy may be done. If the foreign body is seen, removal is undertaken.

If old enough, asking the child to blow the nose after decongestion might remove the foreign body or at least move it anteriorly. Removal can be difficult, and experience helps. Problems that can hinder removal include bleeding that obscures visibility. The foreign body can also be inadvertently pushed posteriorly. Softer foreign bodies, such as food matter and tissue paper, can disintegrate, requiring piecemeal removal.

A headlight and bivalve nasal speculum are recommended. Suction should be available. A small alligator or bayonet forceps is sometimes used, but may simply push the foreign body posteriorly. In many cases a useful instrument is a small, ball-tipped, right-angle probe, actually an otologic surgical instrument called an "attic hook." This can be gently passed posterior to the foreign body, turned 90 degrees, and then used to pull the foreign body anteriorly and out of the nose.

Once the foreign body is removed, the nasal cavity should be reinspected for retained, more distal foreign bodies. The other nasal cavity and ears should also be inspected because the child might be a "repeat offender." Antibiotics are recommended if there is evidence of obvious infection or complete removal is not certain and reexamination is planned.

Nasal Vestibulitis

A low-grade infection of the anterior nasal vestibule will cause chronic irritation, crusting, and sometimes bleeding. The examination typically shows mild erythema, cracking, and yellow crusting just inside the nostril, but it may be fairly normal. The etiology is usually *Staphylococcus aureus* but may be fungal. Herpetic infections are typically more severe and not as protracted. Treatment is with OTC topical antibiotic ointment (without neomycin because of patient sensitivity) and avoidance of irritating the area. If symptoms continue, methicillin-resistant *S. aureus* (MRSA) infection is possible and should respond to mupirocin ointment. Continued symptoms require ENT consultation.

Choanal Atresia

Choanal atresia is a common cause of nasal obstruction in children but can also be seen in adults. If bilateral, it manifests shortly after birth as an airway emergency, because neonates are "obligate nasal breathers" and cannot tolerate nasal obstruction. Typically they will oxygenate well while crying but will become cyanotic when crying stops and they cannot feed. This condition requires urgent ENT consultation. The airway is stabilized and the atresia repaired shortly thereafter. If unilateral, the atresia can go undiagnosed until later in childhood or even adulthood. The patient will report a lifelong history of nasal obstruction and rhinorrhea. Diagnosis is made with endoscopy and CT. Treatment is surgical.

Nasal Polyps

Nasal polyps are the result of nasal mucosal inflammation and edema. On examination, nasal polyps are usually silver-gray in color and may be translucent. If there is associated infection, polyps can appear erythematous or may be obscured by mucus. Polyps cause significant and sometimes complete nasal obstruction but are painless and insensate. Nasal polyps predispose the patient to sinusitis and often cause anosmia.

The exact cause of nasal polyps is unclear. Polyps are often associated with reactive airway disease and less often with environmental allergies. In children the presence of polyps should prompt testing for cystic fibrosis. Sinonasal tumor or fungal involvement should be considered, especially if the polyps are unilateral. If polyps are identified, further evaluation includes allergy and asthma testing and CT scan.

Medical treatment is initially offered but is often inadequate. Initial treatment includes topical steroids, allergy treatment, and treatment of sinusitis. In many patients, endoscopic sinus surgery is an important adjunct to medical treatment and results in significant improvement in symptoms. Unfortunately, polyps often recur after surgery, requiring repeated removal.

Deviated Septum

Most patients have some degree of asymptomatic septal deviation, but in some patients it is severe enough to cause symptoms of obstruction. Septal deviation is usually the result of previous nasal trauma. The trauma might have seemed relatively minor at the time or might have resulted in a nasal fracture. Some deviated septums are congenital. Physical examination may clearly demonstrate the septum obstructing the nasal airway if anterior. If more posterior, nasal endoscopy or CT may be necessary to make the diagnosis. Any patient complaining of persistent nasal obstruction deserves further evaluation, especially if the cause is not immediately evident. Symptomatic septal deviation is readily treatable with outpatient surgery.

Septoplasty is done through an intranasal incision, allowing deviated portions of cartilage and bone to be replaced to the midline or removed, resulting in a symmetrically patent nasal airway. Septoplasty is often combined with a turbinate reduction procedure. The procedures are usually well tolerated. Postoperative pain, formerly a greater problem, usually resulted from the need for nasal packing and removal. Newer devices such as soft-silicone (Silastic) splints now cause much less postoperative discomfort than traditional packing.

In pediatric patients, septoplasty is not usually recommended because of concern about disrupting nasal and facial growth, although this risk appears to be low. For this reason, "limited" septoplasty may be considered in select patients.

Hypertrophied Turbinates

Inferior turbinate hypertrophy is relatively common in adults and children. This usually occurs with chronic inflammation, usually resulting from allergy or rhinosinusitis. Turbinate hypertrophy usually responds to medical treatment addressing the primary problem. If the turbinates remain significantly hypertrophied despite medical treatment, turbinate reduction is offered, using cautery, radiofrequency treatment, fracture, excision, laser treatment, or cryotherapy. Submucosal resection of a portion of the conchal bone and stromal tissue seems to provide the greatest success.

Rhinitis

Allergic Rhinitis

Seasonal allergic rhinitis affects 10% to 30% of adults and up to 40% of children in the United States. Although half the patients with allergic rhinitis have symptoms for only 4 months per year, 20% experience symptoms more than 9 months per year. Direct medical costs of treating this condition plus indirect costs of lost productivity and absences from work or school are estimated at up to $2.4 billion per year in the United States. Unfortunately, seasonal allergic rhinitis is not self-limiting and often coexists with more serious conditions such as asthma, sleep apnea, nasal polyps, sinusitis, and OME.

Understanding the immunologic mechanisms of seasonal allergic rhinitis directs the physician to the appropriate therapy. Allergens such as pollens are deposited on the nasal mucosa and processed by macrophages. The allergens are then brought to T lymphocytes and B cells, the latter producing immunoglobulin E (IgE), which in turn attaches to receptors on mast cells and basophils, causing the release of histamine and other inflammatory substances. The action of these substances on the nasal mucosal cells and nerve endings produces the localized symptoms of nasal discharge, nasal congestion, sneezing, and itching. This is considered the early or immediate phase of the allergic reaction. The delayed-phase response can occur 6 to 8 hours after the initial exposure, even when there are no allergens present. A continued influx of immune cells into the nasal mucosa causes a recurrence of symptoms.

The annual cycle of allergens causing allergic rhinitis begins in the early spring with the flowering of deciduous trees, followed by the release of pollen from grasses during the summer months and from weeds during the late summer months and early fall. Mold spores can be present throughout the year but increase during the warm months.

The diagnosis of seasonal allergic rhinitis is made primarily by history. Differentiation from the common cold is through examination of the nasal mucosa. A pale-pink to blue, boggy nasal mucosa usually indicates allergic rhinitis, whereas a red mucosa is more likely the result of a viral infection or nonallergic vasomotor rhinitis. A horizontal nasal crease on the nose of children and allergic "shiners" are other physical signs to look for in making the diagnosis. Seeing eosinophils under the microscope from a nasal smear using a Wright's stain also points to a diagnosis of allergic rhinitis. Skin testing for specific allergens may be done when the symptoms warrant. The term *perennial rhinitis* simply indicates that the symptoms are present throughout the year and are often caused by allergens (dog or cat dander, mold, dust mites).

The treatment is the same for perennial rhinitis and for seasonal allergic rhinitis. The link among seasonal allergic rhinitis, asthma, and sinusitis is based on the one-airway theory. Because the mucosa in each of those areas consists of basement membrane, a capillary system, mucous glands, goblet cells, and nervous innervation, each area reacts similarly to allergens and responds to like treatments.

After allergen avoidance, antihistamines are most often used to treat seasonal allergic rhinitis. They can also be beneficial for asthma, although they have not been traditionally used as part of asthma treatment. The second generation of nonsedating antihistamines has shown clear benefits in treating seasonal allergic rhinitis and asthma (Grant et al., 1995). (**eTable 19-5** online shows the onset of action, sedating properties, cardiac side effects, and dosage regimens of first- and second-generation antihistamines.) Cetirizine (Zyrtec) and loratadine (Claritin) can be taken with food, whereas fexofenadine (Allegra) is less well absorbed when taken with food. A topical antihistamine, azelastine (Astelin) has shown efficacy in treating allergic rhinitis.

Adding a decongestant such as pseudoephedrine or phenylephrine can help relieve nasal congestion through its vasoconstrictor properties. The patient should be cautioned about

Table 19-5 Doses for Nasal Corticosteroids

Nasal Spray	Age: Dosage
Mometasone furoate (Nasonex)	2-12 yr: 2 sprays each nostril qd (200 µg/day)
Fluticasone propionate (Flonase)	4-16 yr: 1-2 sprays each nostril qd (100-200 µg/day) ≥15 yr: 2 sprays each nostril qd (200 µg/day)
Budesonide (Rhinocort, Pulmicort)	≥6 yr: 2 sprays each nostril bid or 4 sprays each nostril qd (256 µg/day)
Beclomethasone diproprionate (Beconase, Vancenase, Beconase AQ)	6-12 yr: 1 spray each nostril bid (168 µg/day) ≥12 yr: 1 or 2 sprays each nostril bid (168 or 336 µg/day)
Flunisolide	6-14 yr: 1 spray each nostril tid or 2 sprays each nostril bid (1500-2000 µg/day) ≥14 yr: 2 sprays each nostril bid or tid (200-300 µg/day)
Triamcinolone acetonide (Nasacort AQ)	2-5 yr: 1 spray each nostril daily 6-12 yr: 2 sprays each nostril qd (200 µg/day) ≥12 yr: 2 sprays each nostril qd or bid (220-440 µg/day)

qd, Daily; *bid,* twice daily; *tid,* three times daily.

side effects such as nervousness, irritability, and insomnia when taking decongestants. Decongestants should be used carefully in patients with hypertension and with symptoms of prostatic hypertrophy.

Topical corticosteroids are effective in reducing the inflammation of the late-phase reaction (Weiner et al., 1998). The onset of action is within 24 to 72 hours, with full effects within 1 to 2 weeks. The initial dose may be two to three times daily for the nasal corticosteroids, followed by a reduction in the dose for maintenance (Jacobsen, 2001). The main side effects of corticosteroid nasal sprays are epistaxis (5% of patients) and nasal dryness (10%). These can be managed by using saline nose drops or a small amount of petroleum jelly before insufflation of the corticosteroid. No sign of nasal mucosal atrophy has been seen after as long as 1 year of therapy.

There is no evidence that nasal corticosteroids suppress adrenal function, but because of the concern about the effect of topical corticosteroids on the hypothalamic-pituitary-adrenal axis, several newer nasal corticosteroids have been developed to be less well absorbed. Mometasone (Nasonex) and fluticasone (Flonase) are less than 2% bioavailable, whereas budesonide (Rhinocort) and beclomethasone (Beconase, Vancenase) are 11% and 17% bioavailable, respectively. Age-appropriate dosages for the nasal corticosteroids are shown in Table 19-5.

Leukotriene receptor antagonists have been shown to inhibit the early phase of antigen response and to attenuate the late-phase inflammatory response. Several randomized, placebo-controlled trials have proved that antileukotrienes can reduce the symptoms of allergic rhinitis and improve the quality of life (Meltzer, 2002). In addition, they reduce nasal congestion and improve the sense of smell. Zafirlukast (Accolate) and montelukast (Singulair) are effective when patients either refuse or fail antihistamines and nasal sprays and can be used in combination with antihistamines. Zafirlukast can cause liver enzyme abnormalities and should not be prescribed for children younger than 12 years. Montelukast has no serious side effects and can be prescribed for children as young as 6 years.

Patients who respond poorly to pharmacotherapy, who develop adverse side effects, or who simply wish to use an alternative to pharmacotherapy may consider immunotherapy. They must realize the commitment to this therapy is 3 to 5 years, and that local reactions are seen in 15% of patients and systemic reactions in 0.5%. A cost comparison between immunotherapy and medication done under the auspices of the American Academy of Allergy, Asthma, and Immunology demonstrated a significant reduction in cost of single-injection immunotherapy over medication in allergic rhinitis (Huggins and Looney, 2004).

The family physician is crucial to the diagnosis and treatment and can educate patients about the importance of allergen avoidance, adherence to the treatment regimen, and potential side effects of the medications.

KEY TREATMENT

As immunotherapy for allergic rhinitis, montelukast shows efficacy similar to loratadine but less than intranasal fluticasone.
Montelukast used concomitantly with loratadine or cetirizine shows increased benefit compared with either drug alone (Nayak and Langdon, 2007).
Intranasal steroids continue to be the mainstay of treatment for allergic rhinitis. For steroid-intolerant patients, however, montelukast with loratadine or cetirizine can produce comparable results.
Intranasal antihistamine therapy is effective for both allergic rhinitis and vasomotor rhinitis (Kaliner, 2007).
SOR: A

Vasomotor Rhinitis and Idiopathic Rhinitis

The term "vasomotor rhinitis" is a misnomer because there is no inflammation. The primary symptoms are a feeling of nasal congestion and rhinorrhea. Box 19-7 lists some of the conditions that are included in the category of vasomotor rhinitis. Allergy skin tests in patients with vasomotor rhinorrhea are negative, with less than 25% eosinophils present on a nasal swab. These patients do not fully respond to topical or systemic corticosteroids. The condition suggests hyperactivity of parasympathetic tone, blockage of sympathetic tone with vasodilation of submucosal venous sinusoids, and excessive seromucous secretions from the mucous glands. A good analogy to vasomotor rhinorrhea is functional bowel disease. Treatment is with systemic decongestants and antihistamines or topical anticholinergic agents such as ipratropium bromide (Atrovent 0.06% nasal spray). Because of the persistence of symptoms, patients should be warned about excessive use of OTC nasal sprays, which can lead to rhinitis medicamentosa.

Rhinitis Medicamentosa

The prolonged use of topical decongestants for the nose can itself induce nasal stuffiness. The condition is caused by *rebound swelling* after dissipation of the decongestive effect

Box 19-7 Conditions Included under Vasomotor Rhinitis

Drug-induced rhinitis (reserpine, nonselective β-blockers, antidepressants, oral contraceptives)

Irritant rhinitis (smoke, gases)

Temperature- and humidity-induced rhinitis

Emotion- and stress-induced rhinitis

Hormonal rhinitis (pregnancy, premenstrual, hypothyroidism)

Idiopathic rhinitis

Modified from Mikaelian AJ. Vasomotor rhinitis. Ear Nose Throat J 1999;68:207.

of the nasal spray. Increasing the dose of the spray is the patient's response to the rebound swelling, and the vicious cycle is difficult to break without education and medical help.

To treat rhinitis medicamentosa, the patient must stop using the topical decongestant to allow recovery of the damaged nasal mucosa. To relieve the subsequent rebound mucosal swelling, topical and oral corticosteroids are recommended. The length of time needed to successfully treat rhinitis medicamentosa varies depending on the duration the patient has used nasal decongestants. It takes at least 2 weeks to reverse the edema and histamine sensitivity. Other forms of treatment include systemic antihistamines or decongestants, corticosteroid injection into the inferior turbinate, and nocturnal sedation. Surgery is helpful if nasal septal deviation is present. Graf and colleagues (1995) achieved a 100% success rate at the end of 6 weeks of nasal corticosteroid therapy and avoidance of nasal decongestants. It takes time and patience to educate the patient about rhinitis medicamentosa, and both are essential for the treatment to be successful.

Atrophic Rhinitis

Elderly patients are more prone to develop atrophic rhinitis, which leads to nasal congestion, crusting, and foul odor. Treatment consists of saline nose sprays and topical antibiotics. Atrophic rhinitis can also result from previous nasal surgery, use of cocaine, and autoimmune or systemic inflammatory disorders (e.g., lupus, Wegener's granulomatosis). If the cause is unclear, further workup is indicated.

Sinusitis

Symptoms of rhinitis and sinusitis are often very similar and even difficult to differentiate in many cases. Sinusitis implies inflammation of the mucosa of one or more of the paranasal sinuses. This usually coexists with rhinitis and is actually more accurately referred to as *rhinosinusitis*. Studies have shown that CT scans of patients with uncomplicated viral upper respiratory infections (URIs) have mucosal thickening and opacification of the sinuses. For this reason, most URIs are technically considered *viral rhinosinusitis*. In most cases, these changes resolve with time and symptomatic treatment. The terms *rhinosinusitis* or *sinusitis* are typically used when a bacterial infection of the sinuses is suspected. About 5% of viral URIs will progress to bacterial rhinosinusitis. An estimated 20 million cases of bacterial sinusitis occur in the United States annually, accounting for 9% and 21% of all pediatric and adult antibiotic annual prescriptions, respectively (Sinus Partnership, 2004).

Inflammatory conditions of the paranasal sinuses cause significant socioeconomic impact annually, secondary to considerable medical expense and missed workdays. Chronic sinusitis can be quite debilitating. Studies have shown that quality-of-life scores of patients with chronic sinusitis are often similar to those of other, more severe conditions (CHF, COPD). Chronic sinusitis can also exacerbate coexisting medical conditions, most notably reactive airway disease.

Sinusitis represents one of the most common disorders requiring antibiotic treatment in adults. The challenge to the clinician in evaluating the patient with possible sinusitis is to differentiate viral URI, allergic rhinitis, and even a migraine headache, which do not require antibiotics, from bacterial sinusitis, which does respond to antibiotic treatment. There still seems to be a public perception that antibiotics hasten recovery from the common cold. Some physicians prescribe antibiotics in these situations, not wanting to disappoint the patient and seeing no significant risk. In fact, evidence suggests that there is a greater likelihood of *harming rather than benefiting* the patient with inappropriate use of antibiotics (Scott and Orzano, 2001). The emergence of bacteria highly resistant to broad-spectrum antibiotics has forced the medical community to modify its behavior regarding the treatment of URIs. Antibiotics should not be prescribed unless a bacterial infection is certain or at least probable. The patient should be educated about the rationale for this and usually responds favorably.

The underlying cause of most cases of sinusitis is mucociliary dysfunction and sinus obstruction. The maxillary sinuses, anterior ethmoid sinuses, and frontal sinuses all drain through small ostia that converge into a small channel called the *ostiomeatal unit*, which then empties into the middle meatus, beneath the middle turbinate . Obstruction at the ostiomeatal unit leads to obstruction of these sinuses and secondary infection. The posterior ethmoid sinuses and sphenoid sinuses are usually affected later. Sinusitis most often follows a viral URI or an episode of allergic rhinitis. Mucosal edema, impaired local immunity, and ciliary dysfunction lead to impaired sinus drainage and mucus stasis, followed by bacterial infection. Less frequently, sinusitis can result from direct bacterial contamination from an infected tooth or trauma.

Sinusitis is classified into *acute* (symptoms up to 3 weeks), *subacute* (symptoms from 3 to 6 weeks), and *chronic* (symptoms longer than 6 weeks) cases. Cases of acute sinusitis that clear completely only to develop again quickly are referred to as *recurrent acute sinusitis*. Although the types of sinusitis share many characteristics, there are several critical differences in pathogenesis and treatment.

The most important risk factor for the development of sinusitis is rhinitis (e.g., viral, allergic). Other risk factors include anatomic abnormalities (abnormality within the sinuses, septal deviation, choanal atresia, foreign body, adenoid hypertrophy), nasal polyps (which can also occur secondary to chronic sinusitis), conditions of local or systemic immunodeficiency, cystic fibrosis, primary ciliary dysfunction (Kartagener's syndrome), secondary ciliary dysfunction (cigarette smoking, nasal decongestant abuse, cocaine abuse), gastroesophageal reflux disease (GERD), systemic inflammatory conditions (sarcoidosis, Wegener's granulomatosis), dental disease, and nasal or sinus tumors. Any of these conditions can mimic or cause rhinosinusitis. Further workup or referral is indicated if a patient continues to struggle with nasal or sinus symptoms despite medical therapy.

The diagnosis of sinusitis is initially clinical. Imaging and cultures are not initially indicated (Reider, 2003). In 1996 the Task Force on Rhinosinusitis sponsored by the American Academy of Otolaryngology–Head and Neck Surgery developed diagnostic criteria for sinusitis. The signs and symptoms of sinusitis are divided into major and minor. *Major* signs and symptoms include facial pain and pressure, nasal congestion and obstruction, nasal discharge, discolored posterior discharge, anosmia or hyposmia, fever (acute only), and purulence on intranasal examination. *Minor* signs and symptoms include headache, otalgia or ear pressure, halitosis, dental pain, cough, fever (nonacute), and in children, fatigue and irritability. The diagnosis of sinusitis is *probable* if the patient has two or more major factors *or* one major and two or more minor factors. A *suggestive* history is indicated by the presence of one major factor or two minor factors.

Microbiology of sinusitis varies according to its chronicity. Acute sinusitis is most often *initially* viral. If symptoms persist, the likelihood of bacterial infection increases. Bacteria most often involved in acute sinusitis are *Pneumococcus* spp., *Haemophilus influenzae*, and *Moraxella catarrhalis*, with beta-lactamase production common in all these. Chronic sinusitis is caused by the same bacteria as in acute sinusitis, but anaerobic bacteria, *Pseudomonas* spp., and staphylococci become involved more often. The incidence of antibiotic-resistant bacteria, including MRSA and multidrug-resistant *Pneumococcus*, seems to be increasing. Polymicrobial infections are not uncommon.

Sinusitis can also be caused by fungi. *Invasive* fungal sinusitis (caused most often by *Aspergillus* or *Mucor* spp.) can be seen in patients with impaired immune function and poorly controlled diabetes. It is life threatening even with aggressive medical and surgical treatment. Much more common is a more indolent fungally mediated sinusitis. *Allergic fungal sinusitis* is seen in patients with normal immune function. This is often seen in association with nasal polyps and is thought to be the result of an aberrant immune response to the fungus rather than a true infection. Patients do not always have type I hypersensitivity to fungi. Secondary bacterial infection is often associated with this problem.

Rarer causes of sinusitis are secondary to mycobacterial or parasitic infection.

Complications of Sinusitis

Most cases of sinusitis would resolve with or without medical treatment. Sinusitis is usually treated, however, to avoid potential complications and hasten recovery. The proximity of the paranasal sinuses to the orbits and brain potentially allows infection to spread to these locations. Orbital and CNS involvement of sinusitis can lead to loss of vision and can be life threatening and therefore requires early recognition and treatment. Table 19-6 lists the potential complications of sinusitis and treatment recommendations. A high degree of clinical suspicion is required in cases of possible complicated sinusitis, especially in young children. Patients with a recent URI who present with periorbital erythema, vision change, increasing or severe headache, high fever, or altered mental status require *urgent evaluation* and treatment. Ophthalmologic, infectious diseases, and ENT consultations are obtained in cases of orbital complication. Periorbital and

Table 19-6 Complications of Sinusitis

Complication	Physical Findings	Treatment
Periorbital cellulitis	Periorbital erythema, edema	Antibiotics: PO or IV
Orbital cellulitis	Erythema, edema, proptosis ± vision loss	IV antibiotics, close observation
Orbital abscess	Erythema, edema, proptosis ± vision loss	IV antibiotics + drainage, FESS
Cavernous sinus thrombosis	Erythema, edema, proptosis + vision loss	IV antibiotics + FESS
Meningitis	Headache, altered mental status, nuchal rigidity, fever	IV antibiotics ± FESS
Intracranial abscess	Headache, altered mental status, high fever	IV antibiotics + drainage, FESS
Mucocele or pyocele	Facial swelling ± fever ± pain	Drainage

FESS, Functional endoscopic sinus surgery.

orbital cellulitis usually can be managed with intravenous antibiotics. The more severe orbital complications, however, usually require drainage procedures in combination with IV antibiotics. Surgical drainage also allows cultures to be obtained. Recovery from orbital complications is usually complete with prompt and aggressive treatment. Permanent vision impairment can occur even after appropriate treatment.

The CNS complications require neurosurgical, ENT, and infectious diseases consultation. High-dose IV antibiotics are administered. Surgical drainage of the sinuses is sometimes recommended to treat the nidus of the infection and identify the exact pathogen. Recovery from CNS complications is more variable and depends on the patient's age and medical history, severity of the infection, and response to treatment.

Although not always complicated infections, sphenoid and frontal sinusitis deserve special mention. In some cases, drainage of the frontal sinuses is compromised. Chronic and recurrent frontal sinusitis can lead to both intracranial and ophthalmologic complications if untreated. Large *mucoceles* or *mucopyeloceles* can also form within the frontal sinus, causing disfigurement and diplopia. These conditions usually require surgical drainage. Similarly, sphenoid sinusitis can rarely be aggressive. The carotid artery and optic nerves traverse the lateral walls of the sphenoid sinuses. The sphenoid sinus occupies a space inferior and anterior to the cranial vault. Acute or long-standing sphenoid sinusitis can progress to CNS or eye complications, or both. If frontal or sphenoid sinus involvement is noted on CT scan, ENT evaluation is usually indicated.

Medical Treatment of Acute Sinusitis

Treatment of acute sinusitis is almost always medical. Medical treatment of sinusitis, in general, is intended to restore normal mucociliary function, eradicate infection, and improve patient symptoms. Treatment to restore mucociliary function is critical and is as important as antibiotic treatment.

Improved mucociliary function allows the patient's local immunity to function better and often leads to resolution of the infection.

The patient's medical history, including allergies, must be considered. Patients with poorly controlled hypertension or coronary artery disease may not tolerate decongestants. In acute cases of sinusitis, mucociliary function can be improved by a combination of medications, including oral or topical decongestants (topically for less than 3 days), mucolytics (guaifenesin), and nasal toilet (saline mist or irrigations). Nasal saline irrigations are available over the counter or can be homemade. Both 0.9% isotonic saline and hypertonic saline irrigations are extremely beneficial. Nasal steroids are *not indicated* for acute sinusitis but may decrease symptoms and hasten recovery in some patients. Antihistamines are usually not helpful, unless there is a strong allergic component, and can actually be counterproductive by increasing mucus viscosity and mucosal dryness. Oral steroids are usually not indicated in acute sinusitis, but they may be helpful in select patients.

This leaves the practitioner with the responsibility of using good clinical judgment to appropriately prescribe antibiotics to treat acute sinusitis. Antibiotics are empirically chosen based on the expected pathogens and local antibiotic-resistance patterns. The high incidence of beta-lactamase–producing strains of *H. influenzae* and *M. catarrhalis* and the penicillin-resistant pneumococci must be considered. More prudent use of antibiotics seems to have resulted in a plateau of the emergence of antibiotic resistance of these pathogens. MRSA seems to be more common, however, especially in chronic sinusitis.

According to Cochrane Collaboration recommendations for treatment of acute sinusitis, antibiotics provide a minor improvement in simple, acute (uncomplicated) sinus infections. However, 8 of 10 patients improve without antibiotics within 2 weeks. The small benefit gained may be overridden by the negative effects of antibiotics, both on the patient and on the population in general. For acute sinusitis confirmed by radiology or nasal endoscopy, current evidence is limited but supports the use of *intranasal steroids for acute sinusitis* as a monotherapy or as an adjuvant therapy to antibiotics. Clinicians should weigh the modest but clinically important benefits against possible minor adverse events when prescribing therapy.

Many antibiotics are indicated for the treatment of acute bacterial rhinosinusitis. In addition, there are antibiotics that do not have Food and Drug Administration (FDA) approval for treatment of sinusitis but are still appropriately used.

The Sinus and Allergy Health Partnership (2004) made the following comprehensive recommendations regarding the treatment of acute rhinosinusitis:

1. A bacterial infection should be suspected if symptoms of a viral URI do not improve after 10 days, or if symptoms worsen after 5 to 7 days.
2. Antibiotic resistance is common. Specifically, intermediate resistance of *Streptococcus pneumoniae* to penicillin (PCN) is 15%, and complete resistance is estimated at 25%. Resistance of *S. pneumoniae* and *Haemophilus influenzae* to trimethoprim-sulfamethoxazole (TMP-SMX) is common, as is resistance of *S. pneumoniae* macrolides. Beta-lactamase production of *H. influenzae* and *Moraxella catarrhalis* is 30% and 100%, respectively.
3. Selection of an antibiotic should be based on severity of symptoms, whether the patient has received an antibiotic in the last 4 to 6 weeks, and the response to current antibiotic therapy after 72 hours. Mild symptoms include rhinorrhea and fatigue. Moderate symptoms include congestion, low-grade fever, and facial pain.
4. The widespread use of fluoroquinolones for mild sinusitis may promote resistance to this class of antibiotics.
5. Antibiotic choices for adults with mild disease and no recent antibiotics include amoxicillin (1.75-4 g/day, with or without clavulanate), cefpodoxime proxetil, cefuroxime axetil, or cefdinir. TMP-SMX, doxycycline, azithromycin, erythromycin, and clarithromycin may be considered in PCN-allergic patients, but the failure rate may be as high as 20% to 25%. Failure of therapy should prompt reevaluation of the patient or a switch in therapy.
6. Antibiotic choices for adults with moderate disease or with mild disease who have received recent antibiotics include amoxicillin-clavulanate (4 g/day) or a respiratory fluoroquinolone (levofloxacin or moxifloxacin). Ceftriaxone (1-2 g parenterally for 5 days) or combination therapy for gram-positive and gram-negative bacteria may also be considered. Failure of therapy should prompt reevaluation of the patient, CT scan, endoscopy with culture, or a switch in therapy.
7. Antibiotic choices for children with mild disease and no recent antibiotics include amoxicillin (90 mg/kg/day, with or without clavulanate), cefpodoxime proxetil, cefuroxime axetil, or cefdinir. TMP-SMX, doxycycline, azithromycin, erythromycin, and clarithromycin may be considered in PCN-allergic patients (especially immediate type I hypersensitivity), but the failure rate may be as high as 20 to 25%. If the patient has a true type I hypersensitivity to beta-lactams, desensitization, sinus culture, CT scan, or other intervention may be necessary. Less severe reaction may allow use of another beta-lactam antibiotic. Failure of therapy should prompt reevaluation of the patient or a switch in therapy.
8. Antibiotic choices for children with moderate disease or with mild disease who recently received antibiotics include amoxicillin-clavulanate (90 mg/kg/day). Cefpodoxime proxetil, cefuroxime axetil, or cefdinir may be used if there is a nonsevere PCN allergy (rash). Cefdinir is preferred because of high patient acceptance. Ceftriaxone (50 mg/kg/day parenterally for 5 days) or combination therapy for gram-positive and gram-negative bacteria may also be considered. Failure of therapy should prompt reevaluation of the patient, CT scan, endoscopy with culture, or a switch in therapy.

As recurrence or severity of the infection increases, broader-spectrum antibiotics are indicated. Macrolides, fluoroquinolones, augmented penicillins, and cephalosporins are useful in these cases. Culture-directed antibiotic treatment may be indicated in more refractory cases. Obtaining a culture usually requires an ENT referral, because simply swabbing the nasal cavity is not reliable. Cultures can be obtained from an endoscopically guided middle meatus swab. Maxillary sinus aspiration can also be done but is more invasive and not much more accurate than a middle meatal culture. Adjunctive treatment to help improve mucociliary function becomes more important as recurrence increases.

KEY TREATMENT

The American Academy of Otolaryngology–Head and Neck Surgery produced a consensus statement of Clinical Practice Guidelines for Treatment of Presumed Sinusitis (Rosenfeld et al., 2007). The following summary guidelines are for acute viral sinusitis (VRS), presumed acute bacterial rhinosinusitis (ABRS), and chronic rhinosinusitis (CRS). The key symptoms of sinusitis were rhinorrhea, nasal obstruction, and facial pressure or pain.

STRONGLY RECOMMENDED TREATMENT

The quality of data supporting the benefits of treatment outweighing the potential harm is strong (Grade A, B):
1. Clinicians should attempt to differentiate between viral and bacterial sinusitis.
2. The level of pain should be assessed when treating ABRS.

RECOMMENDED TREATMENT

The benefits of treatment outweigh the risks, but the data are not as strong (Grade B, C):
1. Imaging studies are not recommended for cases of uncomplicated VRS.
2. If a decision is made to treat ARS, amoxicillin should be used as first-line therapy if no PCN allergy.
3. If the patient worsens or fails to improve in 7 days, antibiotics should be started or changed.
4. The clinician should attempt to differentiate CRS from recurrent ARS.
5. The clinician should assess the patient with CRS or recurrent ARS for conditions or anatomic abnormalities that would predispose the patient to these conditions.
6. The clinician should obtain a CT scan when evaluating a patient with recurrent ARS or CRS.
7. The patient should be educated on control measures for ARS and CRS.

OPTION

There is only weak evidence that the benefit of treatment outweighs the risk (Grade D):
1. Symptom relief should be offered when treating VRS.
2. Symptom relief should be offered when treating ARS.
3. Observation without use of antibiotics may be done in cases of uncomplicated ARS with temperature less than 101° F (T <38.3° C).
4. Diagnostic nasal endoscopy should be employed in the evaluation of recurrent ARS or CRS.
5. Testing should be done for allergy and immune system dysfunction in patients with recurrent ARS or CRS.

SOR: B

Medical Treatment of Chronic Sinusitis

Medical treatment of chronic sinusitis is based on the same principles as for acute sinusitis: improvement of mucociliary function and eradication of bacteria. If chronic sinusitis is suspected, CT scan of the paranasal sinus should be ordered to confirm the diagnosis before further treatment is initiated; treatment of chronic sinusitis requires more aggressive therapy, with potential side effects. This contrasts with acute sinusitis, for which CT is not necessary before treatment. In addition to confirming the diagnosis and severity of the infections, CT can identify abnormalities that can predict a poorer response to medical treatment. This includes a posterior septal deviation, polyps, allergic fungal sinusitis, and various sinus abnormalities. The scan may also arouse suspicion of sinonasal mass or tumor, which would require earlier ENT evaluation. For all these reasons, referral to an ENT should also be considered as risk of recurrence or chronicity increases.

Medical treatment of chronic sinusitis requires more diligence than for acute sinusitis. Mucociliary improvement is accomplished with the same medications as for acute sinusitis. It is noteworthy that there are *no* medications with indications for treatment of chronic sinusitis (and relatively few for acute sinusitis). Topical and systemic steroids can be used to improve drainage in cases of chronic sinusitis by decreasing mucosal inflammation, edema, and mucus production. Most topical nasal steroids must be used daily for several weeks to have significant benefit. Although oral steroids significantly improve symptoms, the effects may be short-lived, and the potential side effects must be considered. Patients with known allergies should be aggressively treated. It should be remembered, however, that antihistamines cause mucosal drying and mucus stasis. These may need to be stopped in patients with acute exacerbation of chronic sinusitis. Saline irrigations are extremely helpful. Allergy and asthma medications such as leukotriene inhibitors and IgE antagonists can also benefit coexisting sinusitis.

The efficacy of antibiotics in treating chronic sinusitis has not been validated in controlled studies in adults. Two consensus statements do report that antibiotic treatment is likely beneficial in adults but *not in children* (Duiker, 2004; Grade B). Because of the apparent benefit, antibiotics are typically used to treat chronic sinusitis in adults. An antibiotic with activity against staphylococci, as well as the more typical pathogens (with predicted antibiotic resistance), must be chosen. In cases of nasal polyps, an antibiotic with antipseudomonal activity may be necessary. Although no antibiotics have FDA indications for "chronic sinusitis," appropriate choices include macrolides, broader-spectrum cephalosporins, fluoroquinolones, and augmented penicillin. "Older" antibiotics, such as TMP-SMX, clindamycin, doxycycline, and linezolid, may be quite useful in documented staphylococcal infections. Also, the addition of rifampin may be useful in treating documented staphylococcal infections.

Once chronic rhinosinusitis is suspected, ENT consultation is indicated to assist in medical management and to offer surgical options if indicated. Also, simply obtaining a middle meatal culture is extremely helpful in choosing an appropriate antibiotic. Treating chronic sinusitis requires a longer course of antibiotic treatment, often 3 to 8 weeks.

According to Cochrane Collaboration recommendations for medical treatment of chronic sinusitis, *nasal saline irrigations* for the symptoms of chronic rhinosinusitis are well tolerated. Although minor side effects are common, the beneficial effect of saline appears to outweigh these drawbacks for the majority of patients. The use of topical saline could be included as a treatment adjunct for the symptoms of chronic rhinosinusitis.

Failure of Medical Treatment of Sinusitis

When medical treatment of recurrent acute sinusitis or chronic sinusitis is not successful, further evaluation and treatment are indicated. An ENT consultation should be obtained for patients unresponsive to medical treatment of chronic sinusitis. The risk factors listed previously should be considered and modified if possible. Allergy testing should be arranged. Immunologic testing may be indicated. Pulmonary evaluation may be helpful if the patient has poorly controlled reactive airway disease.

If CT has not been done, a scan of the sinuses should be ordered to evaluate the anatomy of the sinuses. If CT has already been done, and symptoms have changed or significant time has elapsed since the first scan, a repeat scan may be helpful. Before repeating the scan, ENT consultation should be considered because the consultant might have a preference for type of scan ordered. A standard sinus CT scan often contains only coronal views; more detailed scans may be necessary for surgical planning.

The CT scan will show any evidence of chronic mucosal edema of the sinuses or even complete opacification. Partial or complete bilateral sinus opacification is typically seen in cases of long-standing chronic sinusitis or polyposis. Unilateral opacification or bony erosion is more worrisome for neoplastic disease or fungal sinusitis. The size of the turbinates and position of the nasal septum can also be assessed. In cases of medical failure or intolerance to continued aggressive medical treatment, surgery should be considered. *Endoscopic sinus surgery* (ESS), or *functional* ESS (FESS), has become the mainstay of surgical intervention for chronic sinusitis. Although earlier external surgical techniques are still occasionally indicated, FESS has the advantage of leaving no external scars and specifically addresses the critical area within the sinuses: the ostiomeatal unit. The procedure is typically done under general anesthesia but can be done under local anesthesia. Success rates of greater than 90% are expected and have been reported in many studies. Some patients experience relapse of their condition, especially if they had nasal polyps. Revision surgery is offered in these cases and is usually quite successful.

Successful sinus surgery often results in fewer and less severe infections and improved response to future medical treatment. The procedure is often done with septoplasty and turbinate surgery and is well tolerated. Advancements in minimally invasive surgical techniques have allowed preservation of more normal tissue and less surgical morbidity. Nasal packing is often not necessary. When used, resorbable packs are typically applied, obviating the need and discomfort of pack removal. Potential complications of ESS include bleeding, scarring leading to further sinus blockage, loss of smell, and rare orbital and CNS injury. For this reason, surgery is undertaken only after appropriate medical treatment and careful patient consideration.

According to Cochrane Collaboration recommendations for chronic rhinosinusitis, FESS as currently practiced is a safe procedure. The limited evidence suggests that FESS has not been demonstrated to confer additional benefit to that obtained by medical treatment (with or without sinus irrigation) in chronic rhinosinusitis. More randomized, controlled trials (RCTs) comparing FESS with medical and other treatments are required, with long-term follow up.

Advances in medical and surgical treatment deserve mention. Newer allergy and asthma medications (leukotriene inhibitors and IgE antagonists) show promise in the future treatment of chronic sinusitis. New antibiotics continue to be released to treat antibiotic-resistant bacteria. Compounding pharmacies have made available topical antibiotic and antifungal formulations that are quite effective in some patients. Topical treatment is appealing because it delivers extremely high concentrations of antibiotic to the target area,

minimizing systemic side effects and, theoretically, development of resistance. Topical treatment seems more effective in patients with sinus surgery that created open sinuses, allowing antibiotic delivery. Research into the genetics of sinusitis continues and should lead to further advances in treatment.

Surgical advances include improved power surgical debriders that spare normal mucosa, have more efficient surgery, and reduce blood loss. Packing materials have improved and often are resorbable. Image-guided surgery has become more commonplace. Balloon techniques allow dilation of the sinus ostia without tissue removal. Although not a substitute for an experienced surgeon, these advances often allow more focused and safer surgery.

Pediatric Sinusitis

Although the sinuses are not completely developed until adolescence, children can still develop sinusitis, usually involving the ethmoid and maxillary sinuses. Young children can have 5 to 10 episodes of acute rhinitis (viral URI) in a year. The usual symptoms of a URI lasting longer than 2 weeks can indicate development of bacterial sinusitis. Other symptoms indicating sinusitis in children include nighttime cough and foul breath. Children rarely complain of facial pain, which is common in adults.

Diagnoses other than sinusitis should also be considered in children with prolonged URI-type symptoms. Previously undiagnosed choanal atresia or stenosis can be present. Unilateral or bilateral nasal foreign bodies can also cause these symptoms. Environmental allergies should be considered, as should immunodeficiency, GERD, and cystic fibrosis. Many children with asthma also have coexisting sinusitis, which can complicate asthma management. Recurrent sinusitis can cause or worsen asthma exacerbations.

Chronic adenoid hypertrophy or chronic adenoiditis can mimic sinusitis in children. Adenoid hypertrophy can also *cause* sinusitis secondary to nasal obstruction, mucus stasis, and subsequent infection. This can occur with or without the presence of tonsil hypertrophy. Adenoid hypertrophy can lead to facial changes caused by chronic mouth breathing. Children with long-standing nasal obstruction tend to have an elongated, narrow face with open-mouth breathing, the "adenoid facies." Differentiating chronic adenoiditis from sinusitis can be difficult because the symptoms may be identical and the disorders often coexist.

According to Cochrane Collaboration recommendations, limited evidence suggests that *intranasal corticosteroids* may significantly improve nasal obstruction symptoms in children with moderate to severe adenoidal hypertrophy. This improvement may be associated with a reduction of adenoid size. The long-term effect of intranasal corticosteroids in these patients remains to be defined.

Medical treatment of pediatric acute sinusitis is similar to that for adults: decongestants, nasal saline irrigations or mist, and antibiotics (Duiker, 2004). The pathogens are similar to those of adults: pneumococci, *H. influenzae,* and *M. catarrhalis*. Coexisting problems (e.g., allergies) should be controlled. Diligence on the part of the parents is required because children might not tolerate nasal saline sprays willingly. If compliance is ensured, medical treatment should result in improvement in the vast majority of patients.

Children who fail medical therapy should be referred to an otorhinolaryngologist. Often, adenoidectomy is recommended. In properly selected patients, this procedure has a high success rate in greatly improving symptoms. For children unresponsive to medical treatment and adenoidectomy, a CT scan should be obtained. If significant sinusitis exists, the child likely has chronic sinusitis. Medical treatment should be reattempted because it might be more effective once the obstructing adenoids have been removed. If not previously done, the child should be screened for allergies, immune deficiency, and cystic fibrosis.

The efficacy of antibiotics in the treatment of pediatric chronic sinusitis has not been validated. Unlike adults with chronic sinusitis who likely benefit from longer courses of antibiotics, evidence-based research indicates that this is not the case for children (Duiker, 2004).

If symptoms persist, ESS is considered. The surgery targets the ostiomeatal unit in hope of improving sinus drainage and aeration. A ciliary biopsy may also be done to evaluate for ciliary dyskinesia. Cultures should also be obtained to tailor postoperative antibiotics. In properly selected patients, sinus surgery has an extremely high success rate. Although rare, significant risks, including bleeding and orbital and intracranial injury, must be considered. Surgery may be especially beneficial in children with coexisting pulmonary disease (asthma or cystic fibrosis).

Sinonasal Tumors

Intranasal and sinus tumors often manifest with symptoms identical to those of more benign sinonasal conditions. Nasal obstruction, facial pressure or pain, and bloody rhinorrhea are common symptoms of a neoplastic process within the nasal cavity or sinuses. Because these symptoms are also common with sinusitis, a high index of suspicion is required, and diagnosis is often delayed.

Tumors of the external nose are usually related to prolonged exposure to the sun. Basal cell and squamous cell carcinoma are most common (see Chapter 33). Intranasal tumors can be benign or malignant. The most common growth within the nasal cavity is the *benign squamous papilloma,* caused by the human papillomavirus (HPV). This typically appears as an exophytic lesion within the nose, often at a junction between squamous and respiratory epithelium, and causes irritation and bleeding. Treatment consists of simple excision, and recurrence is uncommon. Malignant degeneration is extremely unlikely.

A much more aggressive papillary lesion is an *inverted papilloma.* These tumors often manifest as unilateral polyps and can cause symptoms of nasal obstruction, bleeding, and sinusitis. These lesions require excision because they can be locally destructive, and malignant degeneration can occur. Endoscopic excision is usually possible, although external approaches are sometimes required.

The *juvenile nasopharyngeal angiofibroma* is a tumor that occurs exclusively in adolescent boys. The tumor is located within the nasopharynx but typically causes nasal symptoms. Patients present with nasal obstruction and recurrent epistaxis. Because nosebleeds and nasal obstruction are both common problems, a high index of suspicion is required to make a timely diagnosis. These tumors can be extremely aggressive, and surgical excision is required. Recurrences are possible, and radiation therapy is recommended for some patients.

Malignant tumors of the nose and sinuses include squamous cell carcinoma, adenocarcinoma, adenoid cystic carcinoma, hemangiopericytoma, osteosarcoma, and malignant melanoma. Again, early symptoms are similar to those of sinusitis, which often results in delayed diagnosis. The prognosis ranges from extremely good to extremely poor, depending on tumor type and stage. Orbital and intracranial extension often occurs. Both regional and distant metastases result in poorer prognosis. Aggressive treatment is required and involves combined treatment with surgery and radiation, sometimes with chemotherapy.

Nasal Polyps

Nasal polyps result from inflammation, with resultant exuberant swelling of the respiratory epithelium of the nasal and sinus mucosa. Typically, polyps cause symptoms of nasal obstruction and anosmia and can lead to sinusitis. Once formed, polyps have a grayish, translucent appearance. Nasal polyps are typically bilateral and are painless and insensate if touched. Typical nasal polyps are benign. Suspicion of neoplasia or fungal infection should be higher in cases of unilateral polyps. Their exact cause is not completely understood. Nasal polyps are often seen in atopic patients. Some patients are found to have nasal polyps, aspirin sensitivity, and asthma—the "asthma triad." Nasal polyps often coexist with chronic sinusitis. If seen in pediatric patients, nasal polyps should raise suspicion of cystic fibrosis.

Treatment of polyps consists of the usual medical treatment of sinusitis and allergies if present. *Oral steroids for nasal polyps* may reduce the need for surgery, but there are concerns about possible side effects with long-term oral steroid use. The side effects of short courses of oral steroids are less clearly defined. Duiker (2004) found only one trial that met inclusion criteria, involving 80 participants, about 75% of whom were randomized to receive oral prednisone. Quality-of-life and nasal symptom scores improved with a significant reduction in polyp size after 2 weeks of treatment versus no steroid treatment. However, the trial was small and of low methodologic quality. Oral steroids often result in temporary shrinkage of the polyps. Regrowth typically occurs shortly after the steroids are stopped. Topical nasal steroids are also sometimes effective in shrinking polyps or stabilizing their growth. Newer, more potent leukotriene inhibitors have shown promise in slowing or even reversing polyp growth in some patients, although these medications are not indicated for this use. If the polyps cause significant symptoms of nasal obstruction or sinusitis, ESS should be considered to remove the polyps and eradicate any chronic infection within the sinuses. Surgery also allows a biopsy to be done.

Although polyps often recur after ESS, the patient's subjective improvement is marked, and recurrence is often slow. In addition, the response to medical treatment is often greatly improved once the polyps have been removed. Revision surgery (and sometimes multiple surgeries over years) may be necessary.

Nasal Trauma

Traumatic injuries to the nose are extremely common and usually of little long-term significance. In some patients, however, trauma can result in significant cosmetic and functional problems. In severe cases, nasal trauma can result in severe bleeding and cerebrospinal fluid (CSF) leakage and can even be life threatening.

Evaluation of a patient who has sustained nasal trauma requires a thorough history. The mechanism of injury must be understood. If the injury was recent, the patient must be examined for signs of cervical, mandibular, maxillary, orbital, or intracranial injury. Bleeding can be quite severe after isolated nasal trauma but usually stops spontaneously or with only digital pressure.

Initial evaluation includes assessment of the gross appearance of the face, with special attention to the possibility of other facial fractures (orbital, zygomatic, mandibular). Obvious deformity of the nose should be noted, although marked edema obscures this in some cases. Radiographs may be ordered, but their utility is variable because nondisplaced fractures usually require no treatment, and displaced nasal fractures are usually obvious on examination.

Intranasal examination is done to rule out the presence of a septal hematoma or CSF leakage. A septal hematoma results when bleeding occurs between the septal perichondrium and the underlying cartilage. The hematoma can be unilateral or bilateral. It results in a widened septum with nasal obstruction. Successful treatment requires prompt diagnosis followed by incision and drainage and packing to prevent reaccumulation. If untreated, and especially if bilateral, the hematoma leads to ischemic necrosis of the cartilage or can result in abscess formation. This can ultimately result in loss of enough septal cartilage to cause external nasal collapse, called saddle nose deformity. Because it is extremely difficult to repair, avoiding saddle nose deformity is paramount.

Severe bleeding after nasal trauma can result from a vascular injury of the ethmoidal, the sphenopalatine, or rarely the carotid arteries. ENT consultation should be obtained if severe bleeding persists. *CSF leakage* is diagnosed when clear drainage is seen dripping from one or both sides of the nose. Leakage can increase in a more dependent position. Nasal CSF leakage requires urgent ENT and neurosurgical consultation. It often resolves spontaneously but can lead to life-threatening problems such as pneumocephalus (air within the cranial vault), meningitis, and brain abscess.

Isolated nasal deformity after nasal trauma results from displacement of the nasal bones, the external nasal cartilages, or the septum. The nasal bones can often be repositioned with excellent results by performing a *closed reduction*. This is done under local or general anesthesia, usually after the initial edema has subsided and before the bones have set (7-10 days after injury). Sometimes an *open reduction*, which involves refracturing the nasal bones, is required. If the septum is greatly deviated, it can be repaired at the same time. If significant nasal deformity persists, a formal *rhinoplasty*, which more precisely addresses all aspects of the external nose, can be done later. In children with nasal fractures, closed reduction is usually recommended sooner than for adults because their fractures heal more quickly. Repair should be done within 7 days of the injury, if possible. Open reduction is generally not recommended in children because of concern for affecting future nasal growth. If necessary, rhinoplasty is delayed until nasal growth is complete, which is shortly after puberty.

KEY TREATMENT

Radiographic imaging is not recommended in patients who meet the clinical criteria for acute bacterial rhinosinusitis.
Diagnosis of ABRS can be made if signs or symptoms are present 10 days beyond the initial onset of upper respiratory symptoms, or if there is a worsening within 10 days after an initial improvement ("double sickening") (Rosenfeld et al., 2007).
Amoxicillin is the first line of treatment for most adults with ABRS (SOR: B).

Oral Cavity and Pharynx

Key Points

- The Infectious Diseases Society of America now recommends the rapid antigen test alone to confirm the presence of group A beta-hemolytic streptococcal (GABHS) pharyngitis in adults.
- Cephalosporins appear to be superior to penicillin in bacterial eradication and clinical cure in GABHS pharyngitis.
- Motor disorders of the esophagus are more likely to cause difficulty swallowing liquids, whereas mechanical obstruction produces dysphagia with both solids and liquids.
- From 23% to 60% of patients presenting with a globus sensation have gastroesophageal reflux disease.
- Snoring is the most common symptom of obstructive sleep apnea and is more common in men than women.

Physical Examination and Radiography

See the discussion online at www.expertconsult.com.

Acute Pharyngitis and Tonsillitis

Viral agents cause the majority of sore throats. Even when exudates are present, less than 15% of children and 10% of adults have documented group A beta-hemolytic streptococci (GABHS) as the cause. In children younger than 3 years, the predominance of a viral cause is even higher than in school-age children.

Pharyngitis caused by GABHS (*Streptococcus pyogenes*) has its peak incidence in late winter and early spring. The incubation phase is 2 to 5 days and leads to sudden onset of sore throat, painful swallowing, fever, and chills. Less frequent symptoms include headache, abdominal pain, and nausea. On physical examination, a purulent white exudate is often seen on the tonsils, and the anterior cervical nodes are tender and enlarged. There is sometimes a scarlet fever rash (a diffuse, erythematous, macular, rough rash that tends to coalesce) and soft palate petechiae. Scarlet fever is the result of exotoxin-producing strains of GABHS. Pastia's lines are caused by prominence of the rash in the flexor creases of the antecubital space or axilla. A strawberry tongue is another sign of GABHS.

A throat culture is the "gold standard" for diagnosing GABHS infection. A 5% sheep blood agar plate is used to plate the throat swab and can be read in 24 hours (sensitivity 96%). Serologic tests (antistreptolysin O [ASO] titer) are accurate but not practical to use in diagnosing an acute infection because of the time involved in obtaining results.

Rapid antigen detection tests or optical immunoassays (OIAs) are the most popular tests for detection of GABHS. Although most manufacturers claim 95% to 97% true negatives (specificity), clinical trials suggest a lower figure of 90%. True positives (sensitivity) are claimed to be 90% to 95%, but again, clinical trials show closer to 60% to 80% sensitivity.

Scoring systems based on features of sore throat have been developed. The Centor criteria for screening consist of tonsillar exudates, tender anterior cervical lymphadenopathy, absence of cough, and history of fever (Centor et al., 1981). These findings in patients with sore throat can help determine the likelihood of GABHS. When three or four Centor criteria are met, the physician may use a rapid antigen detection test. However, Centor found that only 56% of adults with all four criteria had a positive throat culture, and only 30% to 34% of adults with three criteria had a positive culture. Therefore, 60% of adults with three or four Centor criteria are probably culture negative (Bisno, 2003). The negative predictive value of two or fewer Centor criteria is very high, and testing or treatment would not be indicated. The Infectious Disease Society of America (IDSA) now recommends the use of the rapid antigen test alone to confirm the presence of GABHS in adults (Bisno et al., 2002).

A study comparing five management strategies (no treatment or testing, empiric treatment with penicillin, throat culture, OIA with culture if results negative, OIA alone) found empiric therapy the least cost-effective and culture the most cost-effective strategy when GABHS prevalence was 10%. OIA alone was as effective as OIA followed by throat culture when OIA was negative (Neuner et al., 2003). Once a test result is positive, treatment with penicillin or a cephalosporin is recommended because there has been no incidence of in vitro resistance to these drugs.

Treatment for GABHS is penicillin VK, 250 mg two or three times daily in children and 500 mg three or four times daily in adolescents and adults for 10 days. Intramuscular penicillin G benzathine, 600,000 U for a child weighing less than 60 lb (27 kg) or 1.2 million U for patients weighing more than 60 lb, can be used if compliance is a problem or if the child cannot swallow or is vomiting. Mixing the benzathine penicillin with 300,000 U procaine penicillin alleviates some of the discomfort. Penicillin-allergic patients can use erythromycin, 40 mg/kg in two or four divided doses daily for 10 days. In recurrent disease, cephalexin, 12.5 mg/kg or 250 mg three or four times daily for 10 days, can be prescribed. Alternative antibiotics include cefpodoxime (Vantin), cefprozil (Cefzil), cefuroxime axetil (Ceftin), cefixime (Suprax), cefaclor (Ceclor), ceftibuten (Cedax), loracarbef (Lorabid), azithromycin (Zithromax), clarithromycin (Biaxin), and amoxicillin–clavulanic acid (Augmentin). Cephalosporins appear to be superior to penicillin in terms of bacterial eradication and clinical cure (Pichichero and Brixner, 2006).

After treatment, 15% of throat cultures remain positive for GABHS. This is considered a carrier state. One effective way to eliminate the carrier state is to use clindamycin (Cleocin), 20 mg/kg/day in three divided doses (maximum, 450 mg/day) for 10 days (Tanz et al., 1998). Contagiousness to others is inversely proportional to the length of time that GABHS is carried. Culturing contacts is indicated only when the contact is symptomatic. Pets have been considered a reservoir for GABHS, but some evidence casts doubt on this supposition (Wilson et al., 1995).

Although antimicrobial treatment is believed to decrease the suppurative (peritonsillar abscess) and immunologic (acute rheumatic fever, acute glomerulonephritis) sequelae of GABHS infection, much is not known. Acute rheumatic fever had become rare until 1986, when its incidence increased; any explanation is mere speculation. There is good evidence that antimicrobial treatment shortens the symptomatic period of GABHS and plays a part in preventing acute rheumatic fever. However, acute rheumatic fever can still occur in the presence of appropriately diagnosed and treated cases of GABHS pharyngitis and even in the absence of a symptomatic infection.

Only specific serotypes of GABHS (12, 49, 55, 57, Red Lake strain) cause acute glomerulonephritis (AGN) because of an antigen-antibody deposition on the kidney glomerular membrane. When a patient does have GABHS infection caused by one of these strains, only 15% develop AGN. Edema, hypertension, and rusty urine are the hallmarks of AGN and occur 10 days after the infection. Prompt treatment of GABHS pharyngitis with penicillin does not appear to prevent AGN. Treatment is symptomatic to control the blood pressure and edema.

The indications for tonsillectomy after GABHS infections are six episodes within 1 year or three to four episodes within each of 2 years (Pichichero, 2004). The severity of the infections and the total number of missed workdays or schooldays should also be taken into account when considering tonsillectomy.

Viral causes of pharyngitis include rhinovirus (20% of all pharyngitis) and coronavirus, adenovirus, and parainfluenza virus (5% of all pharyngitis) (Middleton, 1996). Coxsackievirus A can cause 1-mm to 2-mm red-ringed vesicles on the tonsils, uvula, and soft palate and is known as herpangina. Coxsackievirus A16 is the major cause of hand, foot, and mouth disease, a 1-week illness with 4-mm to 8-mm ulcers on the tongue and buccal mucosa and vesicles on the palms and soles. Incubation time for this illness is 4 to 6 days.

A type of pharyngitis similar to coxsackievirus A16 pharyngitis is caused by herpes simplex virus (HSV). Painful, shallow, red-bordered ulcers develop on the soft palate, gums, lips, or buccal mucosa and cause fever, pain, and lymphadenopathy. Acyclovir (Zovirax), 200 mg five times daily for 5 days; famciclovir (Famvir), 125 mg twice daily for 5 days, or valacyclovir (Valtrex), 500 mg twice daily for 5 days, can be used in severe cases of herpes stomatitis and lessen the duration of symptoms and viral shedding.

Epstein-Barr virus (EBV) as a cause of pharyngitis can mimic GABHS infection. It can also occur concurrently with GABHS infection. Studies have shown the two infections occurring together in 2% to 33% of cases. Prodromal symptoms to severe sore throat include malaise, anorexia, chills, and headache. Fatigue, lymphadenopathy, and hepatosplenomegaly can follow in 5 to 14 days. Pharyngitis with tonsillar hypertrophy and a membranous white tonsillar exudate lasts 5 to 10 days. Lymphadenopathy and hepatosplenomegaly can persist 3 to 6 weeks. Contact sports should be avoided for 6 weeks because of the possibility of splenic rupture. Complications that occur in less than 2% of patients with EBV infection include thrombocytopenia, hemolytic anemia, Guillain-Barré syndrome, Bell's palsy, transverse myelitis, and aseptic meningitis. Hepatitis can be seen in 20% to 50% of patients with EBV infection.

Diagnosis is made on clinical grounds supported by positive antibody tests. A CBC shows atypical lymphocytes, and

Box 19-8 Bacterial Causes of Pharyngitis Other than GABHS*

Group C β-hemolytic streptococci
Group G β-hemolytic streptococci
Anaerobes (*Peptostreptococcus, Fusobacterium,* and *Bacteroides* spp.)
Arcanobacterium haemolyticum
Chlamydia pneumoniae
Corynebacterium diphtheriae
Corynebacterium haemolyticum
Mycoplasma pneumoniae
Neisseria gonorrhoeae
Francisella tularensis (tularemia)
Yersinia enterocolitica
Haemophilus influenzae (epiglottitis)

*Group A β-hemolytic streptococci.

a monospot test is positive in 95% of cases of infectious mononucleosis (Middleton, 1996). Steroids (and rarely urgent tonsillectomy) are indicated when the tonsillar hypertrophy causes pharyngeal obstruction or when other life-threatening complications occur. Amoxicillin should be avoided because it often causes a rash in patients with infectious mononucleosis.

When the symptoms point to infectious mononucleosis but the monospot test or EBV titer result is negative, the patient may be infected with cytomegalovirus (CMV). The illness lasts 2 to 6 weeks and is characterized in older patients by higher fever and greater malaise but milder pharyngitis than with infectious mononucleosis. A CMV-specific immunoglobulin M (IgM) antibody test is the best means of diagnosing this infection. In immunocompromised patients, ganciclovir (Cytovene) or foscarnet (Foscavir) can control the infection. Bacterial causes of pharyngitis other than GABHS are shown in Box 19-8.

KEY TREATMENT

Although current treatment guidelines recommend oral penicillin V or intramuscular penicillin G benzathine as drugs of choice for GABHS, strong evidence supports cephalosporins as a first choice for this infection (SOR: A) (Casey and Pichichero, 2007).
In countries with low rates of rheumatic fever, 3 to 6 days of oral cephalosporins to treat GABHS has comparable efficacy to the usual 10-day oral penicillin regimen (SOR: A) (Altamimi et al., 2009).
Once-daily amoxicillin (750 mg to 1 g) for 10 days is as good as twice-daily or three-times-daily dosing (SOR: A)(Lennon et al., 2008).

Abnormalities of the Oral Region (eTable 19-6)

Swallowing Disorders

Patients who experience difficulty swallowing solids or liquids have *dysphagia*. About 7% of Americans experience dysphagia in their lifetime, and 30% to 40% of nursing home residents have swallowing disorders. Motor disorders of the esophagus are more likely to cause difficulty in swallowing liquid, whereas mechanical obstruction causes dysphagia with both solids and liquids.

Pharyngeal muscle weakness or CNS disease can lead to difficulty beginning the act of swallowing. The proximal one third of the esophagus is composed of striated or voluntary muscles, the middle one third is a combination of striated and smooth muscles, and the distal one third is entirely smooth muscle tissue. The two sphincters involved in swallowing are the upper and lower esophageal sphincters (UES and LES).

Food sticking in the throat is known as *oropharyngeal dysphagia,* and 80% of the cases are the result of neuromuscular disease (see **eBox 19-5** online for causes) (Trate et al., 1996). Inability to move solids from the esophagus to the stomach is referred to as *esophageal dysphagia,* which is more common than oropharyngeal dysphagia (see **eBox 19-6** online for causes). The history is extremely important in determining the cause of the dysphagia. If dysphagia is associated with chest pain, especially difficulty swallowing cold liquids, diffuse esophageal spasm is the most likely diagnosis.

A constant sensation of a lump in the throat is known as *globus hystericus* and is not necessarily associated with the act of swallowing. This diagnosis can be made only by ruling out anatomic or motor abnormalities of the pharynx, larynx, or esophagus. From 23% to 60% of patients presenting with a globus sensation have GERD as the origin (Ahuja et al., 1999). **eBox 19-7** online lists head and neck symptoms related to GERD versus gastroesophageal symptoms.

If the food bolus sticks in the distal esophagus, a stricture, malignancy, or ring is most likely the cause. Achalasia or degeneration of the nerve cell bodies of the myenteric plexus leads to esophageal dilation and food retention associated with increased tone of the LES.

Motor disorders of the esophagus cause progression of dysphagia over months to years. A carcinoma should be suspected when there is a rapid progression of dysphagia for solids in an older person with anorexia and weight loss; a history of smoking and alcohol use makes this diagnosis more likely. Medication-induced esophagitis is characterized by acute retrosternal pain exacerbated by swallowing. The most common medications associated with this syndrome are the tetracyclines (doxycycline, minocycline), potassium chloride pills, iron preparations, quinidine and its derivatives, aspirin, and nonsteroidal anti-inflammatory drugs (NSAIDs).

Another mechanical reason for dysphagia is an *esophageal web,* a thin diaphragm most often in the proximal esophagus. When associated with iron deficiency anemia, the condition is known as *Plummer-Vinson syndrome. Pulsion diverticula* are usually seen at the level of the cricopharyngeal muscle and occur predominantly in men older than 50 years. Regurgitation of food and liquid immediately after swallowing is the hallmark of this condition, with large diverticula that can cause almost complete obstruction. A *Zenker's diverticulum* originates from the posterior aspect of the esophagus and is bounded superiorly by the cricopharyngeal muscle and inferiorly by the inferior pharyngeal muscle. Treatment is usually surgical.

Dysphagia in the pediatric population is often secondary to tonsillar hypertrophy or esophageal foreign body. Diagnostic studies include a barium esophagram with views of the pharynx, esophagus, and stomach. To detect rings and early strictures, a barium-coated tablet or marshmallow can reveal the site of narrowing. When there is radiographic evidence of a lesion, esophagogastroscopy is indicated.

If no abnormality is found, esophageal manometry should be performed. The goal of esophageal manometry is to assess the characteristics of esophageal contractions and to define the LES and the UES and their response to swallowing. Only about 50% of patients show a definitive abnormality with this test. Provocative testing with manometry involves infusion of edrophonium, esophageal balloon dilation, or acid perfusion into the esophagus. Recording esophageal pH in an ambulatory setting can indicate if acid reflux episodes are present at the same time as the patient's symptoms.

The management of swallowing difficulties is directed toward the specific cause involved. eTable 19-7 lists the treatments for the various causes of dysphagia.

Snoring and Obstructive Sleep Apnea

Snoring is extremely prevalent but is also the most common symptom of obstructive sleep apnea. OSA occurs when the upper airway collapses during sleep, leading to obstruction, hypoventilation, and hypoxemia. OSA has been associated with development or exacerbation of hypertension, coronary artery disease, pulmonary hypertension, poor concentration, impotence, obesity, depression, and increased risk of motor vehicle crashes. It is a potentially serious medical condition that can be overlooked if not specifically sought.

Men have OSA more than women, and children can also be affected. Adults with OSA are often overweight or stocky. They are told that they snore loudly, and episodes of respiratory obstruction or gasping might be witnessed by a family member. Symptoms of OSA include loud snoring, daytime fatigue, morning headache (secondary to hypoxemia), restless sleeping habits, and frequent catnaps (often unintentionally, sometimes while driving).

Physical examination should be performed with attention to the patient's body habitus. The oral cavity should be inspected for tonsillar hypertrophy and evidence of excess soft palate tissue. The size and position of the tongue should be noted. The nose should be inspected for nasal obstruction. The size and position of the mandible and its relationship to the neck should be evaluated.

Strong suspicion of sleep apnea should be confirmed with an overnight sleep study or polysomnogram. The sleep study measures intensity of snoring, presence of apnea or hypopnea (partial apnea), oxygen saturation, sleep efficiency, and cardiac rhythm. The data are compiled and analyzed by a sleep specialist. A numeric value of the total number of apneas and hypopneas is derived, called the apnea-hypopnea index or *respiratory distress index* (RDI). An RDI of less than 5 is considered normal. An RDI greater than 5 with or without oxygen desaturation indicates sleep apnea. Some patients are found to have normal RDI values but have snoring with disrupted sleep. This condition has been described as "upper airway resistance syndrome." Treatment is similar to that for OSA.

Treatment for OSA is either nonsurgical or surgical. Nonsurgical methods are always attempted first and include weight loss and assisted nighttime ventilation by continuous positive airway pressure. CPAP essentially splints the collapsed airway open with positive pressure, given as the patient initiates inhalation. It is generally well tolerated, safe, and extremely effective in compliant patients. Unfortunately, some patients either do not tolerate CPAP or choose not to use it. Surgery is a potential option in these patients.

Numerous surgical procedures exist for the treatment of OSA. The gold standard is tracheotomy, which bypasses the upper airway obstruction and is almost always successful in eliminating sleep apnea. Obviously, most patients do not

see this as an appealing solution. For patients with severe OSA and morbid obesity, however, a tracheotomy can give extremely satisfying results. More popular procedures have been devised to try to eliminate (rather than bypass) the upper airway anatomic obstruction. Uvulopalatopharyngoplasty is used most often and entails removal of redundant oropharyngeal tissue, including the tonsils, the uvula, and a strip of soft palate. Its success depends on the severity of the OSA and the patient's anatomy. Other procedures use laser or radiofrequency tissue ablation to eliminate excess pharyngeal tissue. If nasal obstruction exists, it is corrected. In severe cases, procedures directed at the tongue base and facial skeleton have been effective in properly selected patients.

The Larynx

Key Points

- Most cases of acute stridor are secondary to inflammatory disorders such as croup, epiglottitis, and tracheitis.
- Neoplasia must be considered in adults with voice or swallowing complaints.
- Visualization of the laryngopharynx is required to evaluate any patient with persistent or severe stridor or with voice or throat symptoms.
- Parainfluenza virus is the most common cause of croup.
- Laryngomalacia is the most common cause of chronic stridor in neonates.
- Vocal cord nodules are always bilateral; polyps and cysts are usually unilateral.
- It is essential to elicit smoking and alcohol histories in patients with voice complaints because of the association with cancer.
- Although often idiopathic or iatrogenic, vocal cord paralysis requires thorough investigation.
- Vocal cord dysfunction is often misdiagnosed as asthma.

Initial Evaluation

Hoarseness, stridor, foreign body (globus) sensation, and dysphagia are all symptoms of laryngeal or hypopharyngeal pathology. When a patient presents with any of these persistent symptoms, a complete past medical and social history is essential. In addition, if hoarseness has persisted, laryngoscopy is indicated. Laryngoscopy can be performed indirectly using a mirror. If the hypopharynx and larynx are not adequately visualized with the mirror because of an excessive gag reflex, direct flexible fiberoptic laryngoscopy can be performed. A topical vasoconstrictor (e.g., 0.5% ephedrine) with a topical anesthetic (e.g., topical lidocaine) can be applied in the nose to improve patient comfort; however, this is not always necessary. The flexible fiberoptic nasopharyngoscope is then passed through the pharynx to visualize the larynx.

Radiography

Indications for imaging the larynx include evaluation of laryngeal tumors and traumatic laryngeal injuries. CT or MRI is performed to evaluate depth of invasion with tumors. CT is the preferred method for imaging malignant and nonmalignant disease, although MRI has certain indications. Traumatic injuries are best evaluated by CT scan. The modalities to assess stridor are directed by the history and physical examination. Available imaging techniques include chest radiography (PA and lateral films), neck radiography (PA and lateral films), and fluoroscopy. Contrast esophagography may be necessary to evaluate for vascular anomalies that can cause airway and esophageal compression or to rule out tracheoesophageal fistulas.

Special Studies

Airway fluoroscopy is useful for evaluating pediatric stridor. Fluoroscopy provides a dynamic picture of the entire airway from the nasopharynx to the carina. This facilitates the identification of obstructive lesions or foreign bodies during both phases of respiration.

A more specialized examination called video laryngeal stroboscopy (VLS) is performed by a speech/language pathologist. This technique allows highly detailed views of the larynx and also allows evaluation of the gross movement of the vocal cords and their vibratory motion. VLS is an excellent modality to photo-document lesions of the laryngopharynx. VLS is also helpful to voice therapists in identifying and following patients with voice disorders, including hoarseness and paradoxical vocal cord dysfunction (see later discussion).

Finally, direct laryngoscopy using a rigid laryngoscope can be performed, usually in the OR. Indications include the need for further evaluation and biopsy of pathology of the larynx.

Laryngitis

Laryngitis is the most common cause of acute hoarseness. It is secondary to diffuse swelling of the larynx. Viral infections are the most common cause and are often associated with other upper respiratory tract symptoms. Treatment is conservative, and recommendations include relative voice rest and avoidance of inhalational substances such as cigarette smoke or other irritating substances. Humidification may be helpful. Symptoms from viral laryngitis usually improve within days; if hoarseness persists longer than the typical several days, the physician should consider other causes, such as bacterial infection with respiratory organisms (e.g., *M. catarrhalis*, *H. influenzae*). For this reason, a course of antibiotics directed at these pathogens may be helpful, especially if symptoms persist even after conservative treatment.

Other uncommon infectious causes of laryngitis include tuberculosis and syphilis. Fungal infections can also localize to the larynx. Of these, *Candida albicans* is the most common and is found in immunocompromised patients, patients using inhaled steroids, and those using long-term, broad-spectrum antibiotics. Characteristic findings on examination include a diffuse reddened mucosa covered by white patches. Topical treatment includes nystatin, miconazole, or clotrimazole; systemic therapy includes fluconazole or ketoconazole.

Stridor

Stridor is noisy breathing. Stridor is a symptom, not a definitive diagnosis. It results from turbulent airflow and results from some degree of airway obstruction, usually at the level of the laryngopharynx or trachea. Stridor can affect both adults and children, but children present special diagnostic and therapeutic challenges because the antecedent history may be limited, physical examination is more challenging, and their small airways are more susceptible to critical obstruction. Because of the small airway diameter in infants and children, even small and subtle abnormalities can cause stridor and obstruct the airway.

It is helpful to localize stridor in the respiratory cycle. In general, *inspiratory* stridor typically is caused by an obstruction at or above the level of the true vocal cords, whereas *expiratory* stridor is usually localized to the more distal tracheobronchial tree. Biphasic stridor is usually caused by an obstruction at the true vocal cords, typically at the immediate subglottic level.

The medical history provides valuable information in the evaluation of stridor. In the pediatric population, a history should include questions about cyanosis, feeding difficulty, failure to gain weight, and retractions. Time of onset of stridor, birth history, prematurity, and need for immediate intubation at birth may help to identify the cause of stridor. A past medical history of smoking or ethanol abuse in an adult patient should raise the suspicion of a neoplastic process. Factors that tend to exacerbate the stridor are noted. These include change of intensity of stridor when in different positions, when crying, and when feeding. Previous intubation or laryngotracheal trauma can lead to acquired subglottic or tracheal stenosis. The presence of fever and a history of acute onset may be significant for an infectious process, including epiglottitis, croup, or tracheitis. New-onset stridor or increased stridor may portend impending airway distress, which would require more immediate workup, close monitoring, and possibly the need to stabilize the airway.

The severity of the obstruction and the need for intervention are sometimes difficult to determine. A child with a partially obstructed airway can have stridor but may not appear to be in respiratory distress. Intervention might or might not be needed. Examination should include documentation of stridor in the phase of respiration and whether suprasternal or intercostal retractions are present. The patency of the nose, oral cavity, and oropharynx should be noted. Large tonsils and adenoids can contribute to obstruction of the airway. The neck should be palpated for any masses that can cause extrinsic compression. Significant obstruction can cause signs of tachycardia, tachypnea, confusion, restlessness, or obtundation. Visualization of the larynx is paramount. Flexible fiberoptic laryngoscopy is the most useful modality in the workup of stridor. This usually requires an ENT consultation. It is easily performed in infants and adults.

There are many causes of stridor in the adult and pediatric population. The differential diagnosis includes lesions affecting various parts of the airway (see **eBox 19-8** online). Pediatric patients are more likely to have congenital causes of stridor, whereas any age group may have stridor secondary to trauma; inflammation; neoplasia, polyps, or papillomas; and foreign bodies. Common congenital anomalies include laryngomalacia, true vocal cord paralysis, subglottic stenosis, laryngeal webs and clefts, subglottic hemangiomas, anomalous great vessels, and complete tracheal rings. Most cases of acute stridor are caused by inflammatory disorders, including croup, epiglottitis, and tracheitis. Chronic causes of stridor are more likely to be congenital, neoplastic, or from airway stenosis.

The most common cause of acute stridor in the pediatric population is *croup* (laryngotracheobronchitis). The parainfluenza virus is the most common cause and affects primarily the subglottic area but can also affect other portions of the laryngotracheal complex. Stridor can be inspiratory or biphasic and is often associated with a barking cough. Radiographs usually show the typical subglottic narrowing caused by edema. The typical age group is 6 months to 2 years, but the condition can be seen in children up to 5 years. The infection and inflammation are usually self-limiting, and conservative management is recommended. Evidence supports the routine use of corticosteroids in most children with croup (Husby et al., 1993). Intervention at an earlier phase of the illness reduces the severity of symptoms and the rates of return to a health care practitioner for additional medical attention, ED visits, and hospital admissions. Many children respond to a single, oral dose of dexamethasone. For those who do not tolerate the oral preparation, nebulized budesonide or intramuscular dexamethasone are reasonable alternatives.

According to Cochrane Collaboration recommendations regarding glucocorticoids for croup, dexamethasone and budesonide are effective in relieving the symptoms of croup as early as 6 hours after treatment. Fewer return visits and (re)admissions are required, and hospital stay is shortened. Dexamethasone is also effective in patients with mild croup (SOR: A).

Severe cases of croup can manifest with significant respiratory distress or even obstruction. Therapy in these patients requires hospitalization (ICU in some cases); treatment includes corticosteroids, supplemental oxygen, fluids, humidification, nebulized racemic epinephrine aerosols, heliox, and occasionally intubation. Complications from croup include airway obstruction, pneumonia, pulmonary edema, and cardiac failure.

Laryngomalacia is the most common cause of chronic stridor in neonates and is characterized by high-pitched inspiratory stridor that can be intensified with agitation, feeding, and placement in the supine position. The disorder is caused by immaturity of the laryngeal cartilages and is typically seen on examination as an omega-shaped epiglottis and floppy aryepiglottic folds that partially obstruct the laryngeal inlet on inspiration. The key to the diagnosis lies in the history and typical findings on flexible fiberoptic laryngoscopy. Airway fluoroscopy provides a dynamic evaluation of the laryngotracheal complex and often shows a component of tracheomalacia as well (laryngotracheomalacia). Treatment is rarely needed, because the problem is self-limiting and resolves by 18 months of age. Gastroesophageal reflux is extremely common, because the increased pressure gradient needed for adequate ventilation causes an increase in acid reflux into the esophagus. This exacerbates the condition by causing a component of reflux laryngitis. Rarely, failure to thrive because of feeding problems, cor pulmonale, or persistent desaturations while asleep can indicate the need for surgical intervention to improve the airway. Even if uncomplicated laryngomalacia is suspected, ENT evaluation is still recommended to confirm the diagnosis.

True *vocal cord paralysis* is another common cause of congenital stridor and usually occurs at birth to 2 months of age. In newborns, the cause is usually injury to the vagus nerve sustained at birth, or it can be secondary to CNS abnormalities. Unilateral paralysis is fortunately more common than bilateral paralysis, which causes airway obstruction. The diagnosis is confirmed by flexible fiberoptic laryngoscopy. Workup also includes barium swallow, neck and chest radiography, and cardiology consultation to rule out a cardiothoracic cause of vagal paralysis. Treatment is rarely necessary because most patients improve or compensate adequately with the opposite vocal cord. Bilateral vocal cord paralysis manifests with a high-pitched stridor. MRI of the brain should be included in the workup to rule out hydrocephalus and Arnold-Chiari malformation. Emergent airway intervention by intubation or tracheotomy might be necessary.

Adults may also be affected by vocal cord paralysis, either unilateral or bilateral. Possible etiologies include neoplastic processes, traumatic injuries to the recurrent laryngeal nerve, or idiopathic causes. If the cause is known (e.g., occurring after cervical surgery resulting in recurrent laryngeal nerve injury), further workup may not be recommended. If the cause is not clear, imaging of the brain, neck, and chest is ordered to rule out a compressive lesion affecting the recurrent laryngeal nerve.

Recurrent respiratory papillomatosis occurs in all ages but is more common in children. It is the most common benign tumor of the airway and is usually found on the true vocal cords and supraglottic and subglottic areas. The causative agent is human papillomavirus. Symptoms usually begin with hoarseness or aphonia and progress to stridor and dyspnea at a later stage of disease. Treatment is by endoscopic removal using the carbon dioxide laser or pulsed dye laser (PDL), and recurrence is common. It can progress to complete airway obstruction and eventually death. Repeated procedures are required. Interferon has been used for severe cases. The antiviral drug cidofovir has demonstrated efficacy against recurrent respiratory papillomatosis and is considered a promising new adjuvant treatment for this disease. The HPV vaccination program in the female adolescent population may lead to a decreased incidence of pediatric laryngeal papillomas by reducing the vertical transmission of the virus from mother to baby.

Subglottic tracheal stenosis is caused by cicatricial scarring of the subglottic trachea and can be congenital or acquired. This area is often affected because the cricoid cartilage is the only complete ring in the trachea and is the narrowest segment in the airway. Acquired subglottic stenosis is most frequently a result of long-term intubation, with traumatic injury to the subglottic segment causing pressure necrosis and subsequent scarring. It may be idiopathic. Subglottic stenosis can occur in adults or children. Patients with severely stenotic segments causing significant respiratory symptoms usually require surgical intervention that includes splitting the subglottis with short-term stents, use of cartilage grafts, or placement of long-term stents.

Although many of the etiologies previously listed may also cause stridor in the adult population, most often an adult who presents with stridor will have this symptom secondary to subglottic tracheal stenosis, inflammation or edema of the larynx, neoplasia, or vocal cord paralysis. The workup is tailored to the history and endoscopic findings. In general, treatment of stridor depends on the etiology. The critical issue is stabilizing the airway in hopes of preventing catastrophe. Some conditions may respond to medical treatment, but any patient with stridor should be treated as having an impending airway obstruction until proved otherwise. ICU observation may be required, with personnel available to stabilize the airway by intubation or tracheotomy. ENT consultation is recommended for further evaluation and more definitive treatment.

Laryngeal Trauma

Injury to the airway is an important cause of death in patients with head and neck trauma. Laryngeal trauma must be recognized early to avoid catastrophic sequelae. Securing the airway is the most important initial step in the management of these injuries to preserve life. The most preventable factor in morbidity and mortality is likely a delay in diagnosis. Less severe laryngeal injuries may initially go undiagnosed, whereas major injuries can lead to early mortality.

Blunt trauma is a common cause of death in motor vehicle crashes. The mechanism of blunt laryngeal trauma is typically caused by a hyperextension of the neck (i.e., against the dashboard) with compression and fixation of the larynx against the cervical spine, which leads to fracture or comminution of cartilage with associated soft tissue injury. Laryngotracheal disruption can occur from "clothesline" injury, which can occur with motorcycle and snowmobile accidents.

Penetrating trauma is becoming more common with an increase in civilian violence. Knife and gunshot wounds are the most common cause of death in homicide cases. Other traumatized structures in the neck can include the great vessels, the esophagus, and the cervical spine.

Signs of laryngotracheal trauma include tenderness over the larynx, anterior neck contusion, subcutaneous emphysema, palpable fractures or crepitus, loss of thyroid prominence, tracheal deviation, and hemoptysis. Symptoms include hoarseness, shortness of breath, inability to tolerate the supine position, and dysphagia.

Examination should include flexible fiberoptic laryngoscopy in every patient, if possible, to evaluate the anatomy and function of the larynx. Diagnostic imaging includes cervical spine films, chest films, and CT scan. Unless physical examination and flexible fiberoptic laryngoscopy are normal, CT should be done in most cases. The decision to take a patient to the OR is based on history, physical examination, flexible fiberoptic laryngoscopy, and CT scanning.

As with any trauma patient, management of the airway is of primary importance. Some controversy still exists on the optimal management of the airway. Most authors recommend awake/local tracheotomy as the safest and least traumatic method of securing the airway in an adult patient with laryngeal trauma. Some reports recount the disastrous outcome of a lost airway after attempted oral or nasal intubation in patients with laryngeal trauma. However, many still advocate intubation as the initial method of securing the airway. Emergency cricothyroidotomy can be performed if time does not permit a formal tracheotomy.

Hoarseness

All patients who present with hoarseness should be questioned about the history, the duration, and the progression of symptoms. Hoarseness may be categorized as chronic or acute. Acute hoarseness is rarely secondary to a malignant process. Acute hoarseness usually results from vocal abuse, laryngitis, or smoking. Malignancy should be considered in patients with chronic hoarseness, but the differential also includes GERD, polyps, nodules, neurologic disorders, papillomas, and functional voice disorders (see **eTable 19-8** online).

Other symptoms can coexist with hoarseness. Cough can be secondary to irritation of the vocal cords from acute or chronic inflammation but can also indicate cancer of the larynx or lung. Dysphagia or odynophagia can be present from disorders of the pharynx and esophagus. Hemoptysis with hoarseness should be considered secondary to a malignancy until proved otherwise. A history of smoking and vocal abuse is an important consideration. Clear visualization of the larynx by indirect or direct laryngoscopy is absolutely necessary for all patients who present with hoarseness that does not resolve on its own or with medical therapy. This can require referral to an otorhinolaryngologist unless the family physician has training and experience in the procedures.

An unusual cause of voice problems is *spasmodic dysphonia* (or laryngeal dystonia). The exact etiology is unknown but is thought to be a CNS condition classified under "focal dystonias." It typically causes a harsh staccato voice but may cause breathiness. Spasmodic dystonia responds poorly to voice therapy but has been shown to respond very well to botulinum toxin injections into the larynx, done endoscopically or externally. The treatment weakens the muscles and lessens the symptoms for several months. Repeat injections are usually done, and response to treatment can decrease over time.

Vocal Cord Paralysis

Vocal cord paralysis can manifest itself as hoarseness. However, many patients are able to maintain a relatively normal voice because of compensation from the opposite vocal cord. Patients can present with shortness of breath while conversing, cough when swallowing, aspiration, or recurrent pneumonia. They may complain of the inability to hold a breath while exerting against a closed glottis (Valsalva maneuver). Visualization of the larynx by indirect or flexible fiberoptic nasolaryngoscopy usually reveals an immobile, sluggish vocal cord in a paramedian position.

Paralysis can result from peripheral (recurrent laryngeal or vagus) nerve involvement or a CNS disorder (e.g., CVA). Approximately 90% of vocal cord paralyses result from dysfunction of the peripheral nerve. Most causes of paralysis are found after a careful history and physical examination (see **eBox 19-9** online). Because of the course of the recurrent laryngeal nerve around the arch of the aorta on the left and around the subclavian artery on the right, a chest x-ray film is initially necessary to rule out compression from an intrathoracic process invading or compressing the nerve. CT or MRI may be useful for imaging the brain or the course of the recurrent laryngeal nerves. VLS is very useful and often yields further diagnostic and prognostic information.

Surgical trauma remains the most common cause of unilateral vocal cord paralysis. This is common after thyroidectomy, carotid artery surgery, or transcervical spine procedures. Neoplastic processes, including thyroid, lung, and esophageal cancers, must always be ruled out as a cause of either compression or invasion. Skull base tumors and mediastinal lesions are less common causes of paralysis. Careful palpation of the neck to rule out masses and evaluation of other cranial nerves help identify these problems.

KEY TREATMENT

The American Academy of Otolaryngology–Head and Neck Surgery produced a consensus statement of Clinical Practice Guidelines for Hoarseness (Dysphonia).

STRONGLY RECOMMENDED TREATMENT

The quality of data supporting the benefits of treatment outweighing the potential harm is strong (Grade A, B):
1. Clinicians should not routinely prescribe oral antibiotics to treat hoarseness.
2. Voice therapy should be employed for patients with hoarseness that affects voice-related quality of life.

RECOMMENDED TREATMENT

The benefits of treatment outweigh the risks, but the data are not as strong (Grade B, C):
1. Hoarseness should be diagnosed in a patient with an altered quality of voice.
2. Patients with hoarseness should be assessed with history or physical exam with attention to previous factors or treatments that may have affected the recurrent laryngeal nerve or larynx. This may include neck or chest surgery or radiation therapy, endotracheal intubation, tobacco use, or occupational vocal overuse.
3. The clinician may perform laryngoscopy (or refer) if hoarseness persists after 3 months, or sooner if suspicion of serious illness is high.
4. CT or MRI should not be performed until the larynx has been visualized (these tests may not be necessary).
5. Antireflux medications should not be prescribed in the absence of other signs or symptoms of reflux.
6. Clinicians should not routinely prescribe oral corticosteroids to treat hoarseness.
7. Laryngoscopy should be performed before recommending voice therapy.
8. Clinicians should advocate for surgery as an option in cases of suspected malignancy, soft tissue lesion, or glottic insufficiency.
9. Patients should be referred for possible treatment with botulinum toxin in cases of spasmodic dysphonia.

OPTION

There is only weak evidence that the benefit of treatment outweighs the risk (Grade D):
1. The clinician may perform laryngoscopy (or refer) at any time after diagnosis of hoarseness.
2. Antireflux medications may be prescribed in patients with hoarseness if there are signs of chronic laryngitis with laryngoscopy.
3. Patients with hoarseness should be educated on control and prevention methods.

SOR: A; B.

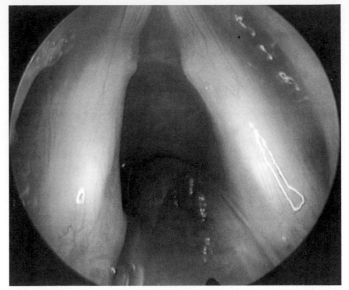

Figure 19-7 Intraoperative photograph of true vocal cords with nodules in 25-year-old teacher.

Bilateral vocal cord paralysis typically manifests with significant respiratory distress caused by obstruction of the glottis from bilateral medialization of vocal cords. Many of these patients need emergent establishment of the airway by intubation or tracheotomy. Causes of bilateral vocal cord paralysis include thyroid or cervical spine surgery or CNS disorders. Hydrocephalus or an Arnold-Chiari malformation can cause bilateral paralysis via brainstem herniation with stretching of the vagus nerves. Treatment in these circumstances is aimed at stabilizing the airway and treating the underlying problem, with the paralyzed cord usually returning to normal function after a few months.

There are numerous surgical techniques to improve vocalization. Endoscopic injection of autologous, allogenic, or alloplastic substances can provide temporary and even permanent improvement by medializing the weak vocal cord so that the mobile vocal cord can make contact. Open surgical approaches can also be performed for permanent unilateral paralysis, with excellent results. Medialization of the vocal cord with the use of alloplastic materials is now common. Surgical options to correct permanent bilateral vocal cord paralysis include removal of a portion of the arytenoids or vocal cords to open the airway; permanent tracheotomy is a last resort.

Vocal Cord Nodules

Vocal cord nodules result from long-term vocal overuse or abuse. Nodules are typically seen as symmetric raised areas at the anterior aspect of each vocal cord. These occur more often in women, boys, lecturers, coaches, and professional singers. The most common symptom is hoarseness and a persistent raspy voice. Smoking, allergies, and GERD tend to aggravate the condition and can prevent healing.

Nodules are always bilateral and classically occur at the junction of the anterior one third and posterior two thirds of the vocal cords (Fig. 19-7). Nodules must be distinguished from polyps, which are smooth and often unilateral, and granulomas, which tend to be located more posteriorly on the vocal cord. Treatment is initially conservative. The patient is referred for voice therapy, which consists of counseling, vocal reeducation, relative voice rest, and psychotherapeutic rehabilitation. Most patients respond after several sessions of voice therapy, but satisfactory improvement can take up to 12 to 18 months. Measures to control acid reflux and avoidance of irritating substances such as cigarette smoke are also routinely recommended. Surgery is reserved for rare patients who do not respond to voice therapy and consists of endoscopic removal. Postoperative voice therapy and acid reflux control are always indicated after surgical removal of nodules.

Reflux Laryngitis

Reflux laryngitis, also known as *laryngopharyngeal reflux* (LPR), is a relatively common condition. Many patients do not have the classic symptoms of GERD, including heartburn, and the correct diagnosis is often initially overlooked. Constant throat clearing may be the only presenting symptom. Other manifestations include a feeling of a lump in the throat with a choking sensation *(globus pharyngeus)*, odynophagia, dysphagia, chronic cough, and hoarseness. The patient may also complain of postnasal drainage. Spicy foods, fats, caffeine, chocolate, beer, milk, and orange juice are known to exacerbate the condition by lowering LES pressure. Several medications increase reflux of acid into the esophagus, such as beta blockers, calcium channel blockers, diazepam, and progesterone. Obesity and sleep apnea also predispose the patient to GERD and reflux laryngitis.

A careful history and examination allow the diagnosis to be made. Findings on indirect or flexible fiberoptic laryngoscopy are nonspecific and include edema, erythema, and redundancy of the mucosa around the arytenoids and postcricoid area. Occasionally, small granulomas are present posteriorly near the vocal processes of the arytenoids. Studies that help confirm the diagnosis of GERD include barium swallow, pH probe, esophageal manometry, and esophagoscopy. Gastroenterology consultation may be necessary.

Often the diagnosis of reflux laryngitis cannot be confirmed or excluded with a trial of empiric therapy. The treatment for reflux laryngitis consists of diet and lifestyle modifications and acid-reducing medications. Diet modification includes avoidance of foods and substances known to increase acid reflux. Lifestyle modifications include avoidance of eating near bedtime, elevation of the head of the bed 6 to 10 inches (15-25 cm), weight loss, and avoidance of tight-fitting clothing. Medical therapy usually begins with a trial of H_2 blockers or preferably daily dosing of proton pump inhibitors (PPIs). Refractory or severe cases usually respond well to twice-daily PPI therapy. Although most patients respond to treatment, resolution of symptoms can take several months after initiating proper treatment. It is critical that visualization of the larynx be obtained early if the patient's symptoms persist, to rule out more serious pathology such as neoplasia.

Cancer of the Larynx

Squamous cell carcinoma is by far the most common malignancy of the larynx. Laryngeal cancer accounts for 1% to 4% of all malignancies detected every year. Peak age group is between 60 and 65 years old, and it is more prevalent in men than in women (8:1), although the incidence in women is rising. Malignancies of the larynx are most common in smokers and alcohol abusers. When both these factors are present, the risk of developing cancer becomes 50% greater than the additive risk of each. Only 2% to 5% of laryngeal cancer patients have no history of smoking. Thus, it is extremely important to elicit smoking and alcohol histories in patients with head and neck complaints.

Hoarseness can be a very early symptom, making most cancers of the larynx curable because they are detected early. For this reason, hoarseness should never be simply attributed to "laryngitis" without proper evaluation. Other symptoms, including sore throat and referred otalgia, can exist without hoarseness. These patients are often treated incorrectly with antibiotics for an extended period and referral is delayed, thereby increasing morbidity and mortality.

Detection of cancer requires visualization of the larynx. Indirect or direct laryngoscopy usually shows a discrete, well-circumscribed exophytic lesion in the endolarynx, most frequently on one of the true vocal cords. A critical concern is potential airway obstruction in bulky tumors; emergent airway intervention is fairly common. The neck should be palpated to evaluate for cervical lymphadenopathy. Metastasis to the lungs or brain is also possible.

Several modalities of treatment exist for laryngeal cancer. Carcinoma in situ and leukoplakia can be treated with laser vaporization. Invasive carcinoma is usually treated with radiation or surgery or both, depending on the stage of disease. Numerous partial-laryngectomy surgical techniques are available that have high cure rates and preserve the voice. Total laryngectomy with a permanent tracheostomy is reserved for late-stage and recurrent tumors. Speech restoration is still possible after total laryngectomy. In some institutions, cancers of the larynx are treated initially with radiation, with significant rates of cure and voice preservation. Radiation therapy and chemoradiation can also be used to preserve the larynx, avoiding total laryngectomy. Studies to determine the ideal chemo/radiation treatment are ongoing. Patients unresponsive to radiation or chemotherapy are treated surgically, usually with total laryngectomy. Neck dissection is required in patients with cervical metastases.

The Neck

Physical Examination

See the discussion online at www.expertconsult.com.

Neck Masses

Proper evaluation of a neck mass includes obtaining a complete history and performing a thorough examination of the neck and all mucosal surfaces. Imaging options include CT with contrast, MRI with contrast, and ultrasound, which may assist in the diagnosis and help define the extent of a lesion. Classification includes congenital, inflammatory, and neoplastic disorders. In general, pediatric neck masses are usually inflammatory, followed by congenital lesions. Neoplasia occurs less often in pediatric patients. In adults, neoplasia is by far the most common entity, with inflammatory causes less common and congenital masses rare.

Congenital Neck Masses

Congenital neck masses are common in children but can occur in any age group. These are the most common cause of noninflammatory neck masses in the pediatric population. Classifying these into midline or lateral location helps in the workup because congenital neck masses occur in consistent anatomic sites (see **eBox 19-10** online).

Midline Neck Masses

Thyroglossal duct cysts are the most common anterior midline neck masses in children. They are remnants of the descending tract of the thyroid gland from the foramen cecum at the base of the tongue to its normal position in the lower neck.

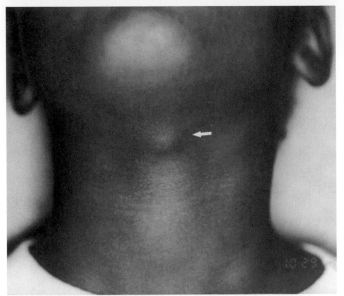

Figure 19-8 Photograph of 9-year-old child with midline neck mass *(arrow)* near the hyoid bone. Swallowing produced movement in the mass. Surgical excision with pathologic evaluation demonstrated a thyroglossal duct cyst.

Cysts or fistulas can occur anywhere along this tract and can intermittently become infected. Physical examination usually reveals a 2-cm to 4-cm mass in the anterior neck that moves with swallowing and elevates with tongue protrusion (Fig. 19-8). Treatment is surgical excision of the cyst and the tract, including the midhyoid bone, to the base of the tongue (Sistrunk procedure). There have been reports of neoplastic transformation of these cysts. Recurrence is possible.

Dermoid cysts typically develop along midline embryonic fusion planes and are composed of ectodermal and mesodermal embryonic remnants. Their usual location in the neck is in the submental area. They are also found frequently along the dorsum of the nose. Dermoid cysts tend not to move with swallowing or elevate with tongue protrusion, unlike thyroglossal duct cysts. Treatment is surgical excision.

Ranulas are cystic lesions that are usually present in the floor of the mouth. They can become "plunging" and extend through muscle planes into the upper midneck area. Plunging ranulas are thought to occur from mucus extravasation from a blocked salivary duct. Physical examination of a plunging ranula reveals a cystic mass in the submental area with or without a cystic mass in the floor of the mouth.

Lateral Neck Masses

Branchial cleft cysts are common congenital abnormalities found in the lateral neck area and are caused by failure of obliteration of the embryonic branchial clefts during development. Abnormalities can also manifest as sinus tracts or fistulas in the skin. These can become intermittently infected, especially after URIs.

Second branchial cleft abnormalities are by far the most common. These usually manifest as masses anterior to the sternocleidomastoid muscle with or without a fistulous opening. The sinus tract passes between the external and internal carotid arteries and ends in the tonsillar fossa. Treatment is complete surgical excision of the cyst and sinus tract after control of infection with appropriate antibiotics. First branchial cleft cysts are less common and manifest as a duplication abnormality of the external auditory canal (type I) or as an infected mass near the angle of the mandible with a sinus tract passing superiorly through the parotid salivary gland (type II).

Lymphangiomas (cystic hygromas) are congenital lymphatic masses often found in the neck. They usually manifest during the first year of life and often enlarge after a URI. They can also increase in size after hemorrhage into the cystic cavities. Lymphangiomas form from a failure of complete development and subsequent obstruction of the lymphatic system. They are most frequently found as an asymptomatic mass in the posterior triangle of the neck but can also be found anteriorly, causing airway or swallowing problems. Physical examination reveals a nontender, fluctuant, soft, spongy mass without discrete margins. Surgery is the mainstay treatment for lymphangiomas, although other modalities of interest include intralesional injection sclerotherapy and systemic interferon.

Hemangiomas are the most common congenital malformations. Most are cutaneous, but they can also be found in deep tissues. The most common deep location in the head and neck is the masseter muscle. Hemangiomas are characterized by appearance at or after birth, followed by a rapid proliferative phase at 6 to 18 months of age. The lesion then reaches a plateau phase, followed by a slow, involutional phase over 6 to 8 years. Even large, uncomplicated lesions left untreated usually undergo almost complete resolution. Conservative management is almost always recommended.

Certain locations, including the nasal tip, lips, and eyelids, can cause severe functional or cosmetic deformities, and referral for removal may be appropriate. Massive lesions can cause high-output heart failure or a consumptive coagulopathy (Kasabach-Merritt syndrome), whereas others can become ulcerated, infected, or hemorrhagic. Other forms of treatment for complicated lesions include interferon alfa-2b and corticosteroids. Cutaneous lesions may be treated with laser therapy.

Neoplastic Neck Masses

Benign lesions in the head and neck include *lipomas* and *fibromas* and require no treatment unless they cause significant functional or cosmetic deformity. Sebaceous cysts and epidermal inclusion cysts are also common and usually need to be excised because of the high incidence of recurrent infection.

All neck masses in adults should be presumed to be malignant until proved otherwise. The most common malignant neck mass in adults is metastatic *squamous cell carcinoma.* Primary tumors are usually found in the upper aerodigestive tract or skin. Smoking and alcohol abuse are etiologic factors. Careful examination of all mucosal surfaces of the head and neck is crucial to identify the primary tumor site. Endoscopy with biopsies is the first step in the diagnosis; surgical treatment of the primary site involves neck dissection, radiation, or both.

Lymphomas are one of the most common malignancies of the neck in children but can occur at any age. Patients can present with lymphadenopathy associated with constitutional symptoms (night sweats, fever, weight loss), hilar adenopathy, or hepatosplenomegaly. Diagnosis is confirmed by excisional biopsy. Most head and neck lymphomas are treated with a combination of radiation and chemotherapy.

Rhabdomyosarcoma is a common childhood neoplasm with peak incidence at age 5 years. Early symptoms include a painless, enlarging mass or symptoms related to obstruction by tumor. Approximately 35% of rhabdomyosarcomas manifest in the head, neck, and orbit. Embryonal rhabdomyosarcoma and botryoid sarcoma (a variety of embryonal rhabdomyosarcoma) are most common in the head and neck, accounting for 75% of cases. Other forms include alveolar and pleomorphic. Diagnosis is made by excisional biopsy, and treatment is multimodal, including surgery, radiation, and chemotherapy.

Carotid body tumors are paragangliomas that arise from the adventitia of the common carotid bifurcation. They are thought to arise from derivatives of neural crest cells and are members of the diffuse neuroendocrine system. They can be associated with other tumors of similar origin, including medullary thyroid carcinoma, parathyroid adenoma, and pheochromocytoma, in up to 7% of cases. Familial incidence is 8% to 10%, and inheritance is autosomal dominant. A high incidence of bilateral carotid body tumors occurs in familial paraganglioma syndromes, and 1% to 3% of these tumors actively secrete substances such as catecholamines or serotonin. Symptoms of catecholamine secretion include headache, perspiration, palpitations, pallor, and nausea. Screening for blood and urinary catecholamines should be performed to rule out a secreting tumor or pheochromocytoma. Symptoms of serotonin secretion are carcinoid syndrome, including diarrhea, flushing, severe headaches, and hypertension.

Other tumors of the head and neck arise from neurogenic tissue. These include schwannomas, neurofibromas, neurofibrosarcomas, and neuroblastomas. These tumors can manifest with associated cranial nerve deficits. Treatment is surgical excision.

Inflammatory Neck Masses

Reactive lymph nodes from a viral infection should be treated expectantly, whereas bacterial infections such as streptococcal tonsillitis or pharyngitis should be treated with appropriate antibiotics. In some cases, inflamed lymph nodes can suppurate and become abscessed, requiring incision and drainage. Masses thought to be reactive lymph nodes not responding to conservative management (antibiotics) often need referral for further evaluation to obtain a definitive diagnosis.

Cervical lymphadenitis can be caused by atypical mycobacteria, which may appear as a subcutaneous abscess with erythematous overlying skin (Fig. 19-9). Treatment includes excisional biopsy and appropriate antibiotics according to culture sensitivities. Incisional drainage is contraindicated and can cause chronic fistulization.

Cat-scratch disease is another pediatric infection that can manifest with lymphadenopathy. Most patients recount exposure to a cat, and many have a cutaneous lesion representing an inoculation site. The diagnosis is made by serologic testing for *Bartonella henselae*. The disease is self-limited.

Tuberculous cervical lymphadenitis (scrofula), caused by *Mycobacterium tuberculosis*, can manifest with bilateral lower lymph node enlargement. It is usually associated with pul-

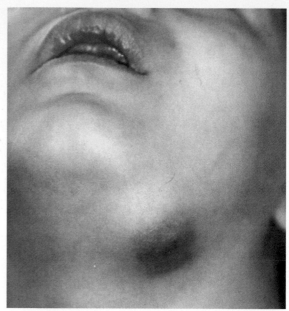

Figure 19-9 Photograph showing cervical adenitis with overlying skin erythema in a young child. Cultures revealed atypical mycobacteria.

monary involvement, and treatment is with a multidrug regimen. Nodes not responding to treatment should be excised.

Patients infected with *human immunodeficiency virus* (HIV) can present with asymptomatic lymph node enlargement. Persistent lymphadenopathy in AIDS patients is common, and most are followed if the nodes remain stable. Because of the higher incidence of non-Hodgkin's lymphoma and Kaposi's sarcoma in these patients, any suspicious neck masses with other constitutional symptoms should be referred for biopsy and tissue diagnosis. Fine-needle aspiration biopsy is appropriate, with indeterminate cytology requiring open excisional biopsy. Other possible causes of neck lymphadenopathy in immunocompromised patients include histoplasmosis, tuberculosis, atypical mycobacterial infections, and toxoplasmosis.

Sarcoidosis is a granulomatous disease that causes cervical lymphadenopathy and may be the presenting sign in 10% to 15% of cases. This disorder typically affects the African American population. Other findings include fever, sinusitis, parotid swelling, and hilar adenopathy on chest x-ray films. Diagnosis is classically made by tissue biopsy showing noncaseating granulomas. High angiotensin-converting enzyme level is common but not diagnostic. Other studies include cytoplasmic antineutrophil cytoplasmic antibody (c-ANCA) to rule out other granulomatous diseases, purified protein derivative and acid-fast bacillus stains to rule out tuberculosis, and Venereal Disease Research Laboratory (VRDL) and RPR tests to exclude syphilis.

Disorders of the Salivary Glands

The salivary glands consist of the paired parotid, submandibular, and sublingual glands and the minor salivary glands. Disorders of the salivary glands can be categorized into inflammatory, metabolic, and neoplastic problems (see **eBox 19-11** online). The history and physical examination facilitate differentiation among these categories.

Inflammatory Disorders

Acute sialoadenitis is a common cause of painful enlargement of the parotid and submandibular glands. The organism is usually *S. aureus,* but it can also be caused by *S. pneumoniae* and other bacteria. The infection is secondary to salivary stasis caused by decreased production (dehydration, poor oral hygiene) or intrinsic or extrinsic obstruction (stones, strictures, masses). Patients present with exquisite tenderness over the gland, fever, and sometimes skin erythema. Purulence can be expressed from the duct with manual massage of the gland. Treatment includes antistaphylococcal antibiotics, adequate hydration, massage of the gland, sialagogues, and warm compresses. Abscess can occur and requires incision and drainage.

Mumps is a relatively common cause of painful unilateral or bilateral parotid gland enlargement in children. It is caused by a paramyxovirus, and diagnosis is confirmed by elevation of antibodies to the S and V virus antigens or by isolation of the virus in the urine. The incubation period is 2 to 3 weeks, and infection lasts 7 to 10 days. Treatment is conservative, with close follow-up to observe for possible complications such as pancreatitis, meningitis, orchitis, and hearing loss.

Sialolithiasis is a cause of intermittent salivary gland enlargement and is usually associated with eating. Most calculi occur in the submandibular duct, and most are radiopaque. Calculi arising in the parotid duct are less common and tend to be radiolucent. Symptoms include recurrent, unilateral, tender salivary enlargement that subsides within 24 to 48 hours. Physical examination usually reveals a palpable stone in the duct of the gland. Sialography is successfully diagnostic if a calculus is not palpable. CT scan and ultrasound are also effective in identifying calculi. Treatment depends on the location of the obstruction. Calculi near the terminal orifice are easily removed transorally. Symptomatic calculi located near the hilum of the gland usually require excision of the gland.

Patients with HIV infection can present with enlargement of salivary glands. Glands can become infiltrated with benign lymphoid tissue or *lymphoepithelial cysts.* The cystic lesions often occur in the tail of the parotid gland, and aspiration can provide temporary relief of symptoms. These patients are treated conservatively because cysts tend to recur after excision or aspiration procedures. Differential diagnosis of salivary gland enlargement in HIV-infected patients includes non-Hodgkin's lymphoma and Kaposi's sarcoma. Fine-needle aspiration or excisional biopsy of suspicious masses is performed for diagnosis of malignancy.

Included in the differential diagnosis of inflammatory lesions of the major salivary glands are tuberculosis, cat-scratch disease, CMV infection, and first branchial arch cysts and sinuses.

Autoimmune Disorders

Sjögren's syndrome is characterized by xerostomia (dry mouth) with or without parotid gland enlargement. Chronic inflammatory cells and lymphocytes infiltrate the glands, leading to fibrosis and atrophy of the parenchyma. Xerophthalmia suggests involvement of the lacrimal gland and causes a gritty or painful sensation of the eye. Primary Sjögren's syndrome involves the exocrine glands, only without association with other connective tissue disorders. Secondary Sjögren's syndrome is often associated with rheumatoid arthritis and other autoimmune disorders.

The SS-A and SS-B autoantibodies are positive in most cases of primary Sjögren's syndrome. Other useful laboratory tests include rheumatoid factor, antinuclear antibody, thyroid globulin antibody, and thyroid antimicrosomal antibody titers. Lip biopsy can confirm the diagnosis of Sjögren's syndrome, and referral to an immunologist is appropriate. Treatment includes proper oral hygiene, mouth rinses, and medications that stimulate salivary flow. Steroids are useful for severe cases.

Other causes of xerostomia include surgery and irradiation of the head and neck. Several common classes of medications can cause mouth dryness as a side effect. These include antihistamines, analgesics, anticonvulsants, antidepressants, and antihypertensives. Systemic disorders that can be associated with xerostomia include dehydration, diabetes, anemia, and overall debilitation.

Neoplastic Disorders

Most salivary gland neoplasms arise in the parotid gland, and most are benign. Approximately 80% of parotid gland tumors are benign, with *pleomorphic adenoma* (mixed tumor) being the most common in adults. *Hemangiomas* are the most common benign tumor in children, but malignancy in children is more likely than in adults when a solid mass is found in the salivary gland. Other benign tumors include Warthin's tumors (papillary cystadenoma lymphomatosum) and oncocytomas. The most common malignancy in adults and children is *mucoepidermoid carcinoma.* Other malignancies include adenoid cystic carcinoma, malignant mixed tumor, and squamous cell carcinoma. Treatment of salivary gland neoplasms is surgical excision.

Thyroid Masses

Careful examination for thyroid abnormalities should be performed on each patient in routine office visits. *Thyroid nodules* occur in about 5% to 10% of the population; of these, approximately 10% are malignant. Differential diagnosis of thyroid masses is presented in Box 19-9. Risk factors for malignancy include exposure to radiation and family history of medullary carcinoma. Factors that increase the possibility of carcinoma include hoarseness; age younger than 20 years or older than 45 years; male gender; presence of a firm hard nodule; and vocal cord paralysis.

The most common disorder in patients who present with a thyroid nodule is *nontoxic multinodular goiter.* The presence of multiple nodules is helpful in diagnosis, but only one dominant nodule may be apparent on physical examination. Nontoxic multinodular goiter may be endemic in iodine-deficient areas or sporadic. Nodularity is thought to be secondary to repeated episodes of deficiency of thyroid hormone, causing increased levels of thyroid-stimulating hormone (TSH), which results in hyperplasia of the gland. Symptomatic compression on the trachea or esophagus can occur. Surgery is reserved for functional problems caused by compression or to rule out malignancy. Chest radiography and CT are helpful in evaluating substernal extension of goiter.

Graves' disease is an autoimmune disease that causes diffuse thyroid enlargement, hyperthyroidism, infiltrative ophthalmopathy, and myxedema. It is the most common cause

341

Box 19-9 Thyroid Masses

Degenerative
Graves' disease
Nontoxic multinodular goiter

Thyroiditis
Acute thyroiditis
Chronic lymphocytic throiditis (Hashimoto's)
Fibrous thyroiditis (Riedel's)
Subacute thyroiditis (granulomatous, lymphocytic)

Neoplastic
Benign
Follicular adenoma

Malignant
Anaplastic carcinoma
Follicular carcinoma
Lymphoma
Medullary carcinoma
Papillary carcinoma

of hyperthyroidism and is more common in women age 20 to 50. Treatment modalities include antithyroid medications, radioactive iodine ablation, or surgical excision when medical treatment fails.

Thyroiditis can cause nodular enlargement of the thyroid gland. Subacute thyroiditis may be a cause of intermittent hyperthyroidism from the release of stored thyroid hormone. Chronic lymphocytic (Hashimoto's) thyroiditis can cause diffuse nodular enlargement of the thyroid. Measurement of antithyroid microsomal antibodies is helpful but not specific for this disorder. Fibrous (Riedel's) thyroiditis is a rare cause of thyroid enlargement, and distinction from neoplasia can be difficult.

Neoplasms of the thyroid are classified as malignant or benign tumors. Follicular adenoma is the most common benign tumor. Malignancies include papillary (65%), follicular (20%), medullary (5%), and anaplastic (10%) carcinomas.

Medullary carcinoma is associated with an elevated calcitonin level, with pheochromocytoma and parathyroid hyperplasia in multiple endocrine neoplasia (MEN) IIA, and with pheochromocytoma, mucosal neuromas, ganglioneuromatosis, and marfanoid body habitus in MEN IIB. Measurement of urinary catecholamines, vanillylmandelic acid, and metanephrine levels is necessary to aid in the diagnosis of pheochromocytoma, which must be treated before surgery for medullary thyroid carcinoma. Hypercalcemia is diagnosed by measuring serum calcium levels.

Initial evaluation of a suspected or palpable nodule includes a thyroid ultrasound and TSH level. If the TSH level is low, a radioiodine scan is obtained. If the nodule corresponds to an area of increased uptake, a biopsy is not necessary because almost all "hot" nodules are benign. Ultrasound will define the number and size of nodules and identify characteristics suggesting malignancy.

Fine-needle aspiration biopsy (FNAB) is indicated for nodules larger than 1 cm or with suspicious ultrasound or examination features. Ultrasound guidance may be used to improve the diagnostic yield for difficult-to-palpate nodules (see **eFig. 19-9**). FNAB is highly accurate. Results are reported as benign, indeterminate, malignant, or nondiagnostic. Benign nodules should be followed with serial examination and ultrasound. Repeat FNAB is indicated with a significant size change. An indeterminate diagnosis may represent a follicular lesion. Follicular neoplasms are not distinguishable as benign or malignant because fine-needle aspiration fails to identify the critical factor of vascular or capsular invasion. Therefore, a thyroid lobectomy may be necessary for diagnosis. Alternatively, a radioiodine scan may be obtained and surgery performed if the nodule is "cold." Nondiagnostic aspirates should undergo repeat FNAB. A malignant diagnosis often requires a total thyroidectomy with central compartment lymphadenectomy. Postoperative radioactive iodine is often given. Risks of thyroid surgery include recurrent laryngeal injury and hypoparathyroidism.

Prognosis for papillary thyroid carcinoma is excellent, especially in younger patients. Prognosis is good for medullary and follicular carcinoma and universally poor for anaplastic carcinoma (Cooper et al., 2006).

References

The complete reference list is available online at www.expertconsult.com.

Web Resources

www.entnet.org
The American Academy of Otolaryngology–Head and Neck Surgery
Contains resources for physicians seeking information on ENT topics, as well as a section on patient education.

www.UTMB.edu/oto/
Dr. Quinn's Online Textbook of Otolaryngology, The Texas Nasal and Sinus Center, The Centers for Cancers of the Head and Neck, The Center for Audiology and Speech Pathology
Contains up to date information on all aspects of otolaryngology.

www.nidcd.nih.gov
The National Institute on Deafness and other Communication Disorders

Contains information about hearing, balance, smell, taste, voice, speech, and language

www.medlineplus.com
A service from the National Library of Medicine. Contains the most accurate database of the scientific medical literature plus a guide to over 9,000 prescription and OTC medications.

www.cochrane.org
The Cochrane Collaboration. Contains reviews of the latest literature in the field of otolaryngology.

CHAPTER 20

Allergy

Vivian Hernandez-Trujillo, Gregg Mitchell, and Phil Lieberman

Key Points

- Symptoms of allergic rhinitis include allergic shiners, allergic salute, pale nasal mucosa, loss of taste or smell, nasal speech, eustachian tube dysfunction, and disrupted sleep.
- Ophthalmologist referral should be provided to prevent cornea complications.
- Treatment of acute rhinitis includes environmental control, medications, and immunotherapy.
- Use environmental controls such as air conditioning with change of filters, HEPA filters, and masks with microfoam filters for dust allergy.
- Wash linens in hot water, using impermeable encasings for pillows and mattresses.
- Avoid fans and cool-mist vaporizers, and remove carpets.
- Oral second-generation antihistamines provide less sedation than previous drugs.
- Medications include intranasal steroids, topical antihistamines, leukotriene modifiers, and decongestants.
- Immunotherapy is directed at specific allergens with possible resolution of allergy.

The allergic patient differs from nonallergic patients in several ways (Box 20-1). The cause is unknown, but these abnormalities clearly are associated with abnormal cytokine production (Table 20-1). The result of these abnormalities is that allergic persons suffer from diseases such as allergic rhinitis and allergic asthma.

It must always be remembered, however, that these diseases are defined by their *phenotype*, and for each allergic disease, there is an almost identical phenotypic expression unrelated to allergy, including allergic and nonallergic (intrinsic) asthma, allergic and nonallergic rhinitis, and IgE-mediated and non–IgE-mediated anaphylactic events. Thus, when approaching the patient, the physician must always consider the mechanism of production of the symptoms because subtle differences may exist in treatment between allergic and nonallergic forms of disease, often with significant differences in prognosis.

The most important aspect of establishing the diagnosis of each of these illnesses is the history. The distinction between the allergic and nonallergic forms can only be conclusively determined by allergy testing. The most sensitive and least expensive (per test) means of assessing the presence of allergy is the allergy skin test. In vitro testing is often helpful, however, as a screening procedure.

The other important phenomenon to recognize is that the major allergic diseases (allergic rhinitis, allergic asthma, and anaphylaxis) are all increasing in incidence. The cause is unknown, but several hypotheses have been proposed. The *hygiene hypothesis* postulates that the rise in allergic disease is related to infection control in infants and children (e.g., through vaccination) and improved public health (e.g., through hygienic measures). Another hypothesis is that the allergic response is the same response used to defend against parasites. With a reduction in parasitic disease in more technically developed countries, a population has arisen that is free from exposure to parasites but still maintains a vigorous antiparasitic immune response that is aberrantly directed against the normally harmless organic substances such as pollen, animal dander, and food. Regardless of the mechanism, the burden of allergic disease in developed countries has increased rapidly since the 1970s.

Box 20-1 Abnormalities Described in Allergic Patients

Predisposition to manufacture large amounts of IgE directed against formerly harmless substances (e.g., pollen and food)

Abnormalities in the autonomic nervous system

  Hyporesponsive beta-adrenergic system

  Hyperresponsive alpha-adrenergic system

  Hyperactive cholinergic responses in the airways

  Hyperreleasability of mast cells and basophils

Table 20-1 Cytokine Production Abnormalities and Effects in Allergic Patients

Cytokine	Effects
Increased production of IL-4	Enhanced IgE production
Increased production of IL-13	Enhanced IgE production
Increased production of IL-5	Enhanced eosinophil activity and prolongation of the life of eosinophils
Increased production of IL-9	Bronchial hyperreactivity

Ig, Immunoglobulin; *IL,* interleukin.

Allergic Rhinitis

Allergic rhinitis is a symptom complex caused by airborne antigens. It occurs as *seasonal rhinitis* (hay fever) when pollens are in high concentration in the air. When it is intermittent or continuous without seasonal variation, it is termed *perennial allergic rhinitis.* Often occurring in families with an allergic history, perennial allergic rhinitis and mixed perennial and seasonal rhinitis were found to be twice as common as seasonal allergic rhinitis (Skoner, 2001).

Manifestations

In seasonal allergic rhinitis, exposure is followed by complaints of paroxysmal sneezing, a watery nasal discharge with congestion, and nasal pruritus. Conjunctival and pharyngeal itching often occurs. Less specific symptoms are postnasal drainage or fullness or aching in the frontal areas.

The patient might exhibit an *allergic salute,* an upward thrust of the palm against the nares to relieve itching and open the nasal airways and a gaping expression from mouth breathing. *Allergic shiners* or Dennie's lines are wrinkles beneath the lower eyelid. Speech can have a nasal quality. In children, nasal irritation can result in nose picking and recurrent epistaxis. Sleep disruption is often associated with nasal obstruction and mouth breathing. Patients might have sleep apnea–like symptoms, including restless sleep, snoring, or nighttime coughing, associated with postnasal mucus drainage and mild hoarseness. The nasal mucosa is typically moist, with enlarged, pale turbinates and serous discharge. Because the sense of smell is impaired, appetite may be decreased. Maxillomandibular alignment problems (overbite or underbite) result from chronic symptoms.

In perennial allergic rhinitis, nasal congestion, itching, obstruction, and frequent sniffing may be associated with a loss of sense of taste or smell, with decreased hearing and a popping sensation in the ears. A lower sneezing threshold often occurs with altered autonomic reflexes in perennial allergic rhinitis. Paroxysms of sneezing and rhinorrhea can result from changes in ambient temperature, head movement, odors from perfume, tobacco smoke, irritants, alcohol, and exposure to small quantities of antigen. Exercise reverses nasal congestion temporarily, from minutes to hours.

The turbinates are usually swollen and edematous and may be mistaken for nasal polyps, which are pearl-gray gelatinous masses and unusual in uncomplicated allergic rhinitis. Below the turbinates, the floor of the nostril is often prominent as a result of mucosal edema. One third to one half of children with allergic rhinitis have eustachian tube obstruction and resultant serous otitis. Otoscopy reveals a retracted or bulging tympanic membrane, impaired mobility, or a fluid level. In patients with intact tympanic membranes, tympanometry to measure middle ear pressures provides an indirect measure of eustachian tube function (Lazo-Saenz et al., 2005). The edematous nasal mucosa can obstruct the ostia, resulting in congestion or sinusitis with pressure symptoms or headache that is particularly notable with bending forward. Up to one third of patients have a lower respiratory tract component, including exercise-induced and mild persistent asthma.

Diagnosis

A seasonal history or an association with an inhaled allergen is helpful. It is often difficult to associate specific allergens with perennial rhinitis, although late-evening or early-morning symptoms may be seen with dust allergy. Occasionally, improvement of symptoms with a change in environment, such as a vacation, indicates the presence of environmental allergens. A nasal smear, stained with Hansel's stain to identify eosinophils, can support a diagnosis of nasal allergy, but it is not itself diagnostic. An elevated peripheral eosinophil count may be helpful; however, marked allergic symptoms can occur in the absence of blood eosinophilia.

Treatment

Nonspecific Measures

Removing known allergens is of prime importance because it can eliminate symptoms. When exposure is unavoidable, environmental control should reduce symptoms and prevent exacerbations. The patient or the family must assume responsibility for environmental control, so an understanding of allergens is helpful. Commonly inhaled allergens include pollens, which can produce symptoms of seasonal allergic rhinitis, conjunctivitis, and asthma. Allergenic pollens come from trees, grasses, and weeds. Pollens from flowering plants are insect-borne and are not important allergens. Pollen prevalence is usually determined by gravity slides, which sample pollen fallout without regard to wind direction, speed, and turbulence, so that daily reports of pollen prevalence often do not reflect the true concentration in the air or individual exposure.

Inhaled fungal allergens in fungus-sensitive subjects can produce seasonal symptoms during situations that promote fungal growth, such as humid and rainy weather and exposure to hay, mulch, commercial peat moss, and compost. Indoors, areas of spore formation can be identified at sites of water condensation such as shower curtains, window moldings, and damp basements. In addition, cool-mist vaporizers can serve as sources of fungal contamination.

A prime role for the patient and family is controlling house dust. House dust is a heterogeneous mixture of bacteria, fibrous matter of plant and animal origin, human epidermis, food remnants, fungi, insect debris, and animal dander and contains one major source of antigen: the dust mite. Mites are ubiquitous in households and are most prevalent in bedding, mattresses, carpeting, and upholstered furniture, particularly where warmth and humidity are high. Air conditioners and dehumidifiers are useful for these patients. High-efficiency particulate air (HEPA) filters are effective in removing dust and animal dander. Fans should not be used so that these lightweight particles can settle. Minimizing clutter and removing carpets are also effective measures. Linens should be washed in hot water (130° F, 55° C). Impermeable cases can be used for pillows and mattresses. The use of a mask over the nose and mouth with replaceable microfoam filters significantly reduces the effects of temporary exposure to inhaled allergens such as dust or pollens.

Animal allergens are derived from dried saliva on shed cat fur, rodent urine, and epidermal material from farm animals. The allergic respiratory reactions produced by animal allergens are species specific. Finished furs and wools are not allergenic. Feathers are often nonallergenic when fresh, and they produce allergic symptoms only after degradation. A careful history to identify environmental allergens is important for advising avoidance and treatment.

Control of Symptoms

Antihistamines are effective for symptomatic control of allergic rhinitis, whether it is seasonal or perennial (Bousquet et al., 2008; Wallace et al., 2008; SOR: A). For optimal results, antihistamines should be used before exposure to the known allergen. Complete control might not be achieved when patients use antihistamines only sporadically. During the implicated season, around-the-clock administration provides maximal symptomatic relief. Because compliance is always an issue, the new second-generation antihistamines offer a convenient dosing regimen (Table 20-2). These groups of drugs, with specific binding properties, allow little to no penetration into the central nervous system (CNS), thus greatly reducing their side effects, primarily sedation. The second-generation antihistamines also have anti-inflammatory effects.

Fexofenadine (Allegra), an analog of terfenadine, is safe and effective. Through its effects on T cells, fexofenadine can decrease airway inflammation. Loratadine (Claritin) is available as a once-daily (qd) product. It provides safe and effective control of most symptoms of allergic rhinitis if taken regularly. Desloratadine (Clarinex), also a once-daily medication, is a metabolite of loratadine. In murine models, desloratadine inhibits bronchial hyperresponsiveness and airway inflammation. Cetirizine (Zyrtec), a metabolite of hydroxyzine, is available in once-daily dosing. Cetirizine has anti-inflammatory properties and may be effective in patients with allergic rhinitis and reactive airway disease. Cetirizine's chemical properties, however, allow greater CNS penetration, and sedation is its chief side effect (16% vs. 4% for fexofenadine and loratadine). Levocetirizine (Xyzal), also

Table 20-2 Second-Generation Oral Antihistamines for Treatment of Allergic Rhinitis

Drug (Brand)t	Formulation	Dosing Frequency	Age of Patient
Cetirizine*(Zyrtec)	5 mg/5 mL syrup 5-mg, 10-mg chewable tablet 10-mg tablet	Once daily (qd) qd qd	6 months
Desloratadine (Clarinex)	2.5 mg/5 mL syrup 5-mg tablet	qd qd	6 months
Fexofenadine (Allegra)	30-mg, 60-mg tablets 180-mg tablet	Twice daily qd	6 years
Levocetirizine (Xyzal)	2.5 mg/5mL syrup 5-mg tablet	qd qd	6 months
Loratadine* (Claritin)	5 mg/5 mL syrup 10-mg reditablet	qd qd	2 years

*Available as over-the-counter (OTC) generic drug.

a once-daily medication, is a metabolite of cetirizine. Less sedation is associated with it than cetirizine.

Herbal medications have been used with effectiveness in treating perennial and seasonal allergic rhinitis. Butterbur (32 mg daily) was effective in treating seasonal allergic rhinitis when compared to cetirizine (10 mg daily) in 125 patients. After 2 weeks, patients treated with butterbur had improved vitality, general health, and physical activity as well as less sedation (Schapowal, 2002; SOR: A).

Second-generation antihistamines are available in combination with alpha-adrenergic decongestants and might be more effective in this form than antihistamines alone. Alpha-adrenergic drugs are also effective applied topically. Topical vasoconstrictors (sprays and drops) are best restricted to temporary use, such as when taking an airplane trip or during a severe flare-up of symptoms. Unfortunately, the side effect profile increases in these combinations. Intranasal antihistamines have the most rapid onset of action and are as effective as oral second-generation antihistamines in the treatment of seasonal allergic rhinitis (SOR: A). Azelastine (Astelin), available in a nasal spray formulation, decreases nasal airway resistance and is an effective treatment for rhinitis. Olopatadine (Patanase) is another topical antihistamine with effectiveness against symptoms of rhinitis. Leukotriene receptor antagonists, such as montelukast (Singulair), are also effective for the treatment of perennial and seasonal allergic rhinitis (Wallace et al., 2008).

Topical intranasal glucocorticoids—beclomethasone, fluticasone, mometasone, triamcinolone, flunisolide, ciclesonide, and budesonide—are the most effective medication in the treatment of allergic rhinitis (Wallace et al., 2008; SOR: A). Their effectiveness is directly related to proper and daily use, posing problems with patient compliance. Side effects are related primarily to nasal dryness and epistaxis. Using saline as a moisturizer can relieve these side effects. The therapeutic effects are generally not immediate, and some patients must take these medications for 1 to 3 weeks before they achieve maximum benefit.

When symptoms are severe and not responsive to trials of topical therapy, oral glucocorticoid therapy can be used as a last resort and only for limited duration. The rationale for glucocorticoid therapy for allergic rhinitis is that the condition, although mediated by immunoglobulin E (IgE), has a dual component: the immediate phase of edema and hypersecretion and a late inflammatory phase (Ciprandi et al., 2005). This dual reaction occurs in asthma as well.

Specific Immunotherapy

When skin tests identify sensitivity to an unavoidable inhalant allergen, immunotherapy may be indicated for treating allergic rhinitis. Its efficacy has been shown to be 80% for controlling pollen symptoms and 60% for controlling mold and house dust symptoms. Immunotherapy is therefore more effective in seasonal allergic rhinitis than perennial allergic rhinitis. When considering immunotherapy, the ease of control of other therapies should be weighed against the frequency and severity of symptoms as well as the possibility of complete resolution of allergy with immunotherapy.

KEY TREATMENT

Oral antihistamines, including fexofenadine, cetirizine, loratadine, levocetirizine, and desloratadine, improve symptoms (e.g., runny nose, nasal pruritus, sneezing and quality of life in patients with seasonal allergic rhinitis compared with placebo (SOR: A).
Herbal medications have been used with effectiveness in treating perennial and seasonal allergic rhinitis (SOR: A).
Inhaled corticosteroids were more effective than oral antihistamines in treating most nasal symptoms of seasonal allergic rhinitis, including nasal congestion, runny nose, pruritus, and sneezing (SOR: A).
Immunotherapy is effective against allergic rhinitis and can prevent the development of asthma in children (SOR: A).

Nasal Polyps

Key Points

- Nasal polyps may be associated with aspirin sensitivity.
- Nasal polyps can aggravate sinus disease.
- Topical glucocorticoids are important in long-term treatment.
- Polyps can recur after polypectomy.

Perennial allergic rhinitis may be associated with nasal polyps, but usually only when it is complicated by sinus infection. In adults, polyps may be associated with sensitivity to aspirin manifested by aggravation of rhinitis, asthma, and even shock.

Nasal polyps often develop in the absence of or only coincidentally with allergy. Polyps arise from diseased ethmoid and maxillary sinuses and are easily visible in the nasal cavity. Nasal polyps can cause obstruction and aggravate the preexisting sinus disease. The size of nasal polyps may be reduced by brief treatment with systemic glucocorticoids and by daily use of topical glucocorticoids for longer periods.

If sinus infection or the underlying allergic factors are not appropriately controlled, polypectomy may be necessary. Unfortunately, polyps tend to recur without sinus surgery.

Nonallergic Rhinitis

Key Points

- Symptoms of nonallergic rhinitis include chronic nasal obstruction and eosinophils on nasal smear, in the absence of allergy.
- Topical glucocorticoid steroid therapy is useful in treatment of NARES.
- Aggravating factors include physical changes or irritants for vasomotor rhinitis.
- Ipratropium bromide is best for controlling symptoms of vasomotor rhinitis.

Some patients with perennial rhinitis are not atopic by history or skin testing. Chronic nasal obstruction is the predominant symptom, and the condition may be associated with sinus disease and nasal polyps. Although there is no evidence of allergy by skin testing, numerous eosinophils are present, and the diagnosis is readily made by examining the nasal secretions for eosinophils and eosinophilic cationic protein (Kramer et al., 2004). The condition is also called *nonallergic rhinitis with eosinophilia* (NARES). A substantial number of patients have chronic rhinitis with rhinorrhea, postnasal drainage, and chronic or intermittent nasal obstruction. Symptoms are aggravated by many physical or irritant factors, such as cold air, odors, and smoke. Skin tests are negative, and no eosinophils are present in the tissue or secretions.

Topical glucocorticoid therapy is much more effective than antihistamines or decongestants for NARES. As with asthmatic patients, patients with associated sinus disease and nasal polyps are at risk for adverse reactions to aspirin and nonsteroidal anti-inflammatory drugs (NSAIDs). Patients with NARES are also at risk for obstructive sleep apnea (Wallace et al., 2008). Ipratropium bromide (0.03%) spray solution, fluticasone, and azelastine nasal sprays have all been shown to be effective treatment. Some patients benefit from antihistamine-decongestant combinations. The regular use of buffered saline lavage can also provide satisfactory symptomatic relief.

Allergy in the Eye

Key Points

- Symptoms of eye allergy include pruritus, erythema, and lacrimation.
- Treatment includes oral antihistamines plus topical medications such as mast cell stabilizers or H_1 blockers.

Conjunctivitis is the usual ocular reaction to airborne allergens. As in other forms of allergic inflammation, the mast cell plays a key role. Itching is the first symptom and may be associated with lacrimation. Dilation of the conjunctival blood vessels produces a "red" eye. Transudation of fluid through vessel walls results in edema of the conjunctiva, and exuded cells with increased glandular mucus secretions result in ocular discharge. In most atopic patients, conjunctivitis and allergic rhinitis occur together, but some patients are bothered only by eye symptoms. In contrast to other forms of conjunctivitis, the secretions contain eosinophils.

Vernal conjunctivitis is so called because of its occurrence in spring and summer. It is characterized by a bilateral recurrent inflammation of the conjunctiva. Vernal conjunctivitis typically occurs between ages 5 and 20 years. It often spontaneously resolves in 10 years. More than 50% of children with vernal conjunctivitis also have an atopic disorder such as allergic rhinitis, eczema, or asthma. Signs and symptoms include acute itching, tearing, photophobia, and excess mucus production. The patient often has a sense of a foreign body in the eye.

The topical conjunctival appearance establishes the diagnosis, which is confirmed by cytologic smears showing numerous eosinophils. In the tarsal (palpebral) form, there are flat-top cobblestone papillae; in the limbal form, there may be gelatinous hypertrophy and limbal papillary hypertrophy often associated with white dots (Trantas' dots). Although vernal conjunctivitis is usually self-limiting, corneal complications can occur, and ophthalmology consultation should be obtained. Although conjunctivitis is typically seasonal and common in atopic patients, no allergens have been identified as causal or aggravating factors.

The usual therapy for allergic conjunctivitis is an oral antihistamine with a topical medication (Table 20-3). Cromolyn (Opticrom) and lodoxamide 0.1% (Alomide) are mast cell stabilizers. Topical H_1 histamine blockers are also effective for treating allergic conjunctivitis. Ophthalmic histamine blocker solutions include emedastine (Emadine) and levocabastine (Livostin). Azelastine (Optivar), epinastine (Elestat), ketotifen (Zaditor, Claritin Eye, Zyrtec Itchy Eye) and olopatadine (Patanol, Pataday) are dual-acting drugs, preventing mast cell release and exerting antihistamine activity as well. Ketorolac (Acular) is a NSAID. Regular daily use is necessary to obtain maximum positive results with all topical agents. In severe cases and in vernal conjunctivitis, a soluble steroid such as fluorometholone ophthalmic solution (0.1%) is effective. The dose should be titrated to the minimum required to control symptoms. Use should be intermittent because glucocorticoids can lead to the development of cataracts, potentiate a secondary bacterial infection or a herpes simplex keratitis, and increase intraocular pressure. Steroid eyedrops should always be used under supervision by an ophthalmologist.

Asthma

The definition of asthma has undergone many changes over the years, but three elements are key to the diagnosis: reversible airway obstruction, airway inflammation, and increased airway responsiveness to a variety of stimuli. Physicians must remember that not all wheezing is asthma, and not all asthma has wheezing. Asthma is a chronic inflammatory disorder of the airways in which many different cells play a role. In patients with asthma, this inflammation causes breathlessness, chest tightness, recurrent episodes of wheezing, and cough, particularly at night. These symptoms are usually associated with variable airflow limitation that is partly reversible with treatment or sometimes spontaneously. This inflammation causes an associated increase in airway

responsiveness to a variety of stimuli (Busse et al., 2007). Data from the Centers for Disease Control and Prevention (CDC) have shown an increase in the prevalence of asthma in the United States from 1980 to 2001. However, there has been no increase in mortality and hospitalization rates since 1997 (cdc.gov/asthma; see also Chapter 20).

Diagnosis

Because of the lack of any specific symptom or sign to define asthma by history or physical examination, some patients are mistakenly thought to have asthma. Numerous other diseases must be considered in the differential diagnosis of asthma (Box 20-2). Although parental history of asthma is present in half of children with asthma, the positive predictive value of this history ranges from 11% to 37% (Burke et al., 2003). The diagnosis of asthma should occur in three stages. First, suggestive symptoms referable to the chest with precipitating factors should raise the possibility of asthma. Second, further testing should be performed to confirm the diagnosis. Third, the patient should have symptomatic improvement with the appropriate asthma therapy (see Classification). When all the stages have been performed and meet the criteria, the diagnosis of asthma can be made.

Table 20-3 Ophthalmic Solutions Useful in the Treatment of Allergic Conjunctivitis

Drug (Brand)	Formulation	Dosage
Mast Cell Stabilizers		
Cromolyn (Opticrom)	4%	1-2 gtt OU every 4-6 hr daily
Lodoxamide (Alomide)	0.1%	1 gtt OU qid
H₁ Histamine Blockers		
Emedastine (Emadine)	0.05%	1 gtt OU qid
Levocabastine (Livostin)	0.5 mg/mL	1 gtt OU bid
Combination Stabilizers/Blockers		
Ketotifen (Zaditor)	0.025%	1 gtt OU bid 8-12 hr apart
(Zyrtec Itchy Eye)	0.025%	1 gtt OU bid 8-12 hr apart
(Claritin Eye)	0.025%	1 gtt OU bid 8-12 hr apart
Epinastine (Elestat)	0.05%	1 gtt OU bid
Olopatadine (Patanol)	0.1%	1 gtt OU bid 6-8 hr apart
(Pataday)	0.2%	1 gtt OU qd
Azelastine (Optivar)	0.05%	1 gtt OU bid
Nonsteroidal Anti-Inflammatory Drugs		
Ketorolac (Acular)	0.5%	1 gtt OU qid

OU, Each eye; *gtt*, drops; *qid*, four times daily; *bid*, twice daily; *qd*, once daily.

Box 20-2 Differential Diagnosis of Asthma

Infants and Children

Allergic rhinosinusitis
Cystic fibrosis
Foreign body
Gastroesophageal reflux disease
Heart disease
Paradoxical vocal cord motion
Tumor
Viral bronchiolitis

Adults

ACE inhibitor–induced cough
Chronic obstructive pulmonary disease
Congestive heart failure
Eosinophilic pulmonary infiltration
Gastroesophageal reflux disease
Mechanical obstruction of the airway
Paradoxical vocal cord motion
Pulmonary embolism

ACE, Angiotensin-converting enzyme.

Box 20-3 Factors that Can Precipitate Asthma

Environmental allergens such as pollen, molds, house dust mites, cockroach excreta, and animal danders
Environmental changes or climate change
Exercise
Exposure to irritants (e.g., tobacco smoke), strong odors, and air pollutants
Exposure to medication: salicylates, NSAIDs, β-blockers
Exposure to occupational chemicals or allergens
Exposure to some food additives
Gastroesophageal reflux disease
Menses
Pregnancy
Sinusitis
Strong emotional feelings
Viral respiratory infections

NSAIDs, Nonsteroidal anti-inflammatory drugs.

Table 20-4 Severity of Any Spirometric Abnormality Based on FEV1*

Degree of Severity	FEV_1 (% Predicted)
Mild	>70%
Moderate	60-69%
Moderately severe	50-59%
Severe	35-49%
Very severe	<35%

From Brusaco V, Crapo R, Viegi G: Interpretative Strategies for lung function tests. Eur Respir J 2005;26:948-968. American Thoracic Society. Available at www.thoracic.org/sections/publications/statements/pages/pfet/pft5.html.
*Forced expiratory volume in 1 second.

Precipitating Factors

All patients suspected of having asthma should be questioned about early warning signs and precipitating factors. Early warning signs of an attack include symptoms such as cough, scratchy throat, and nasal stuffiness, especially if an attack follows an upper respiratory tract infection. Many other precipitating factors can provoke asthma symptoms or an acute attack (Box 20-3). Identification of these precipitating factors can help patients manage their asthma by learning their early warning signs and avoiding any exposure that triggers an exacerbation. These symptoms and identification of triggers are the first stages of diagnosis of asthma.

Confirmatory Testing

Pulmonary function testing is the "gold standard" for the diagnosis and management of asthma and is the second stage in the diagnosis of asthma. The only exclusion for obtaining pulmonary function tests should be the lack of an ability to perform the testing, most often determined by the patient's age (usually <4 years).

Spirometry is the most useful test in diagnosis of asthma. Spirometry includes measurements forced expiratory volume of air in 1 second (FEV_1) and forced vital capacity (FVC), the amount of air one can expel during forced expiration. FEV_1 is the most important value for the assessment of airflow obstruction. It declines in direct and linear proportion of worsening airway obstruction and increases with successful treatment of airway obstruction. Degrees of airway obstruction are defined according to the percentage of predicted FEV_1 achieved by the patient (Table 20-4) (American Thoracic Society [ATS], 2005).

Administration of a bronchodilator such as albuterol is indicated when performing spirometry. Improvement of FEV_1 by 12% or 200 mL after administering a bronchodilator suggests significant reversibility of the airway obstruction. Another useful value is the FEV_1/FVC ratio. A reduced ratio below the

5th percentile of the predicted value suggests obstructive airway disease. A reduced FVC with a normal or increased FEV_1/FVC ratio (>5% of predicted value) suggests a restrictive pattern of lung disease (ATS, 2005). Additional testing by bronchoprovocation may be considered if one suspects a patient has asthma but spirometry testing is normal. The only absolute contraindications to methacholine bronchoprovocation testing are severely reduced airflow (FEV_1 <50%), acute coronary syndrome or stroke in the past 3 months, uncontrolled hypertension, or known aortic aneurysm.

Peak-Flow Monitoring

The home use of peak-flow meters is helpful in the self-management of asthma but not in the diagnosis. The National Asthma Education and Prevention Program (2007) recommends daily monitoring for patients with moderate to severe persistent asthma. There is no evidence that peak-flow monitoring improves patient outcomes over self-monitoring of symptoms. However, if a practitioner provides a peak-flow meter, the patient should be properly instructed in its use (Busse et al., 2007). The patient should establish a baseline peak flow in the absence of asthma symptoms. Three zones on the meter are then set—green, yellow, and red. The green

Components of severity		Classifying Asthma Severity and Initiating Therapy in Children								
		Intermittent		Persistent						
				Mild		Moderate		Severe		
		Ages 0–4	Ages 5–11	Ages 0–4	Ages 5–11	Ages 0–4	Ages 5–11	Ages 0–4	Ages 5–11	
Impairment	Symptoms	≤2 days/week		>2 days/week but not daily		Daily		Throughout the day		
	Nighttime awakenings	0	≤2x/ month	1–2x/ month	3–4x/ month	3–4x/ month	>1x/week but not nightly	>1x/ week	Often 7x/week	
	Short-acting beta$_2$-agonist use for symptom control	≤2 days/week		>2 days/week but not daily		Daily		Several times per day		
	Interference with normal activity	None		Minor limitation		Some limitation		Extremely limited		
	Lung function • FEV$_1$ (predicted) or peak flow (personal best) • FEV$_1$/FVC	N/A	Normal FEV$_1$ between exacerbations >80% >85%	N/A	>80% >80%	N/A	60–80% 75–80%	N/A	<60% <75%	
Risk	Exacerbations requiring oral systemic corticosteroids (consider severity and interval since last exacerbation)	0–1/year (see notes)		≥2 exacerbations in 6 months requiring oral systemic corticosteroids, or ≥4 wheezing episodes/1 year lasting >1 day AND risk factors for persistent asthma	≥2x/year (see notes) Relative annual risk may be related to FEV$_1$	→			→	

Recommended step for initiating therapy (See "Stepwise Approach for Managing Asthma" for treatment steps.) The stepwise approach is meant to assist, not replace, the clinical decisionmaking required to meet individual patient needs.	Step 1 (for both age groups)	Step 2 (for both age groups)	Step 3 and consider short course of oral systemic cortico- steroids	Step 3: medium-dose ICS option and consider short course of oral systemic cortico- steroids	Step 3 and consider short course of oral systemic cortico- steroids	Step 3: medium-dose ICS option OR step 4 and consider short course of oral systemic cortico- steroids
	In 2–6 weeks, depending on severity, evaluate level of asthma control that is achieved. • Children 0–4 years old: If no clear benefit is observed in 4–6 weeks, stop treatment and consider alternative diagnoses or adjusting therapy. • Children 5–11 years old: Adjust therapy accordingly.					

Figure 20-1 Classifying asthma severity and initiating therapy in children. *(From Busse WW, Boushey HA, Camargo CA, et al. Guidelines for the Diagnosis and Management of Asthma. National Asthma Education and Prevention Program, Expert Panel Report 3. NIH Pub No 08-5846, October 2007.)*

zone is 80% to 100% of the patient's "personal best" and reassures the patient to continue the current regimen. The yellow zone is 50% to 80% of personal best and should signal the patient to change the measurement plan according to the clinician. The red zone is less than 50% of the personal best and should signal the patient to seek medical attention. The use of the peak-flow meter can help give some patients objective findings of the severity of their asthma.

Treatment

Classification

Asthma is classified into four categories based on subjective symptoms of frequency and severity and objective measurements of pulmonary function (Figs. 20-1 and 20-2).

Classification is initially based on the highest step at which any feature occurs, realizing that clinical features for individual patients can overlap. An individual patient's classification can and should change over time so the patient can move to a lower classification with adequate therapy.

The goal of asthma therapy is to maintain control of asthma with the least amount of medication and the least risk for adverse side effects. Obtaining control of asthma can be difficult to define for the patient and the clinician. Several keys to the definition of controlled asthma are prevention of troublesome symptoms (cough or wheezing), maintenance of normal pulmonary function, maintenance of normal activity levels, prevention of recurrent exacerbations, and meeting patients' and families' expectations of asthma care.

Components of severity		Classification of Asthma Severity ≥12 years of age			
			Persistent		
		Intermittent	Mild	Moderate	Severe
Impairment **Normal FEV₁/FVC:** 8–19 yr 85% 20–39 yr 80% 40–59 yr 75% 60–80 yr 70%	Symptoms	≤2 days/week	>2 days/week but not daily	Daily	Throughout the day
	Nighttime awakenings	≤2x/month	3–4x/month	>1x/week but not nightly	Often 7x/week
	Short-acting beta₂-agonist use for symptom control (not prevention of EIB)	≤2 days/week	>2 days/week but not daily, and not more than 1x on any day	Daily	Several times per day
	Interference with normal activity	None	Minor limitation	Some limitation	Extremely limited
	Lung function	• Normal FEV₁ between exacerbations • FEV1 >80% predicted • FEV₁/FVC normal	• FEV₁ >80% predicted • FEV₁/FVC normal	• FEV₁ >60% but <80% predicted • FEV₁/FVC reduced 5%	• FEV₁ <60% predicted • FEV₁/FVC reduced 5%
Risk	Exacerbations requiring oral systemic corticosteroids	0–1/year (see note)	≥2/year (see note) ⟶		
		← Consider severity and interval since last exacerbation. ⟶ Frequency and severity may fluctuate over time for patients in any severity category.			
		Relative annual risk of exacerbations may be related to FEV₁.			

Recommended step for initiating therapy (See "Stepwise Approach for Managing Asthma" for treatment steps.)		Step 1	Step 2	Step 3 and consider short course of oral systemic corticosteroids	Step 4 or 5
		In 2–6 weeks, evaluate level of asthma control that is achieved and adjust therapy accordingly.			

Figure 20-2 Classification of asthma severity. *(From Busse WW, Boushey HA, Camargo CA, et al. Guidelines for the Diagnosis and Management of Asthma. National Asthma Education and Prevention Program, Expert Panel Report 3. NIH Pub No 08-5846, October 2007.)*

Classification of asthma is the last stage in the diagnosis of asthma. Patients with asthma should respond to traditional treatment based on the stage of asthma. The National Heart, Lung and Blood Institute (NHLBI) provides the current clinical guidelines (Figs. 20-3 and 20-4) (Busse et al., 2007). The physician should keep the following points in mind when using the NHLBI guidelines:

1. The stepwise approach is intended to assist, not replace, the clinical decision making required to meet individual patient needs.
2. Classify severity; assign the patient to the most severe step in which any feature occurs.
3. Gain control as quickly as possible (a course of short systemic corticosteroids may be required); then step down to the least medication necessary to maintain control.
4. Minimize the use of short-acting inhaled β₂-agonists. Overreliance (e.g., use of short-acting inhaled β₂-agonist every day, increasing use or lack of expected effect, or use of approximately one canister a month even if not using it every day) indicates inadequate control of asthma and the need to initiate or intensify long-term-control therapy.
5. Provide parent education on asthma management and controlling environmental factors that make asthma worse at all points of care (e.g., allergens, irritants).
6. Consultation with an asthma specialist is recommended for patients with moderate or severe persistent asthma. Consider consultation for patients with mild persistent asthma.

Intermittent Asthma: Step 1

For intermittent asthma, short-acting inhaled β₂-agonists taken as needed are usually sufficient therapy so long as they are used less than twice a week (SOR: A). If therapy is repeated more often than every 6 weeks, a step-up in long-term care is recommended. Patients with intermittent asthma have symptoms of asthma less than twice per week, two or fewer nocturnal awakenings per month, and peak-flow measurements that are normal (peak expiratory flow rate [PEFR] >80% of predicted normal) (Busse et al., 2007).

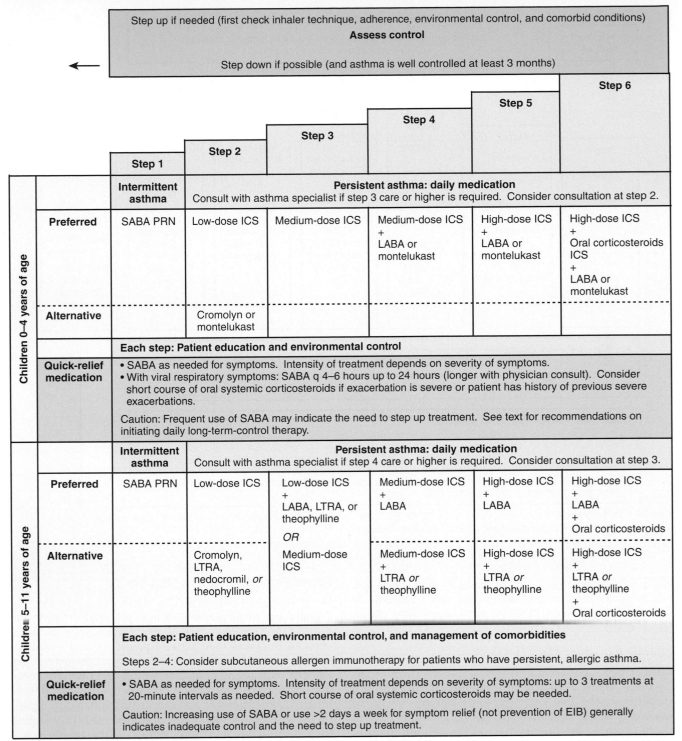

Figure 20-3 Step therapy for children with asthma. *(From Busse WW, Boushey HA, Camargo CA, et al. Guidelines for the Diagnosis and Management of Asthma. National Asthma Education and Prevention Program, Expert Panel Report 3. NIH Pub No 08-5846, October 2007.)*

Mild Persistent Asthma: Step 2

Patients with mild persistent asthma should receive daily treatment with inhaled corticosteroids (SOR: A). Leukotriene modifiers (cromolyn and nedocromil) may be considered as alternative, not preferred, controller medications for those with persistent asthma. Inhaled corticosteroids are now the preferred controller medication based on their greater efficacy. Long-term use of inhaled corticosteroids within labeled doses is safe for children in terms of growth, bone mineral density, and adrenal function. The most important factor in monitoring symptom control is the use of short-acting β_2-agonists, which should be less than twice per week. Mild persistent asthma is defined when a patient has asthmatic symptoms requiring relief

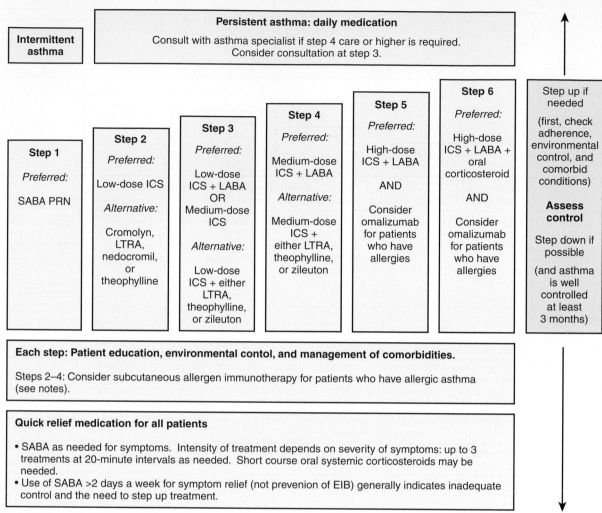

Figure 20-4 Step therapy for adults with asthma. *(From Busse WW, Boushey HA, Camargo CA, et al. Guidelines for the Diagnosis and Management of Asthma. National Asthma Education and Prevention Program, Expert Panel Report 3. NIH Pub No 08-5846, October 2007.)*

with an inhaled bronchodilator more than twice per week, nocturnal awakenings more than twice a month, or observed fluctuation in PEFR of more than 20% (Busse et al., 2007).

Moderate Persistent Asthma: Step 3

Moderate persistent asthma is defined as daily symptoms of asthma, daily need for bronchodilator medications, asthmatic attacks that interfere with activity, nocturnal awakenings more than once per week, or PEFR 60% to 80% of normal. Any one of these criteria should prompt the consideration of escalating asthma therapy. However, physicians should first review the patient's inhaler technique and adherence to therapy and determine if environmental factors are worsening the condition. Consultation with an asthma specialist may be considered to help with therapeutic options. Currently the preferred treatment option is addition of a long-acting inhaler β$_2$-agonist at a low to medium dose of inhaled corticosteroid (SOR: A). Other options include increasing the dose of inhaled corticosteroids with or without adding a long-acting β$_2$-agonist or adding a leukotriene modifier (SOR: B) (Busse et al., 2007).

Severe Persistent Asthma: Step 4 or 5

Severe persistent asthma is defined as waking from sleep 4 to 7 nights per week; frequent asthma exacerbation even from minor exposures to viruses, allergens, exercise, or air pollutants; an FEV$_1$ less than 60% of predicted; and inability to achieve normal lung function despite appropriate treatment. Patients with severe persistent asthma usually have continuous symptoms that should be treated with high doses of inhaled corticosteroids and long-acting inhaled β$_2$-agonists (SOR: B). If the asthma is not controlled, oral corticosteroids to gain and maintain control is the next therapeutic option. Current evidence suggests using omalizumab to avoid using systemic corticosteroid therapy in those patients with allergies (SOR: A). For patients who require long-term systemic corticosteroids, clinicians should use the lowest possible dose to control symptoms and monitor patients closely for adverse side effects (Busse et al., 2007).

Management of Asthma in Children

More than half of children with asthma develop symptoms before their fifth birthday. However, diagnosis can be difficult because there are no reliable tests for children at this age, and diagnosis must rely solely on clinical presentation. Among children younger than 5 years, the most common cause of asthma symptoms is a viral upper respiratory tract infection. Based on expert opinion, daily long-term control therapy should be initiated in young children who consistently require symptomatic treatment more than twice per week and those who experience severe exacerbations that occur less than 6 weeks apart. Therapy is recommended for children who had more than four episodes of wheezing in the past year that lasted more than 1 day and affected sleep and who have a positive asthma predictive index. A positive asthma predictive index is either one of two major risk factors (parental history of asthma or physician diagnosis of atopic dermatitis) or two of three minor risk factors (wheezing apart from colds, peripheral blood eosinophilia higher than 4%, or evidence of sensitization of foods) (Busse et al., 2007). Therapy may be given by metered-dose inhalers with a spacer; evidence suggests they are as good as or better than nebulizers for children with asthma (SOR: A) (Hsu et al., 2004).

Management of Asthma Exacerbation

Asthma exacerbations consist of episodes of progressively worsening shortness of breath, cough, wheezing, or chest tightness. These exacerbations are characterized by decreases in FVC and PEV_1 that can be measured by peak-flow meters. Peak-flow monitoring can help grade the severity of an exacerbation. Early treatment is the best strategy for effective treatment of asthma exacerbations. Patients should receive a written action plan to guide self-management of exacerbation, especially patients with persistent asthma or any history of a severe exacerbation. Patients should be able to recognize the early indicators of an exacerbation, such as a decline in PEFR. There should be prompt communication between the clinician and patient during any abrupt worsening of asthma, as well as availability of a short course of systemic corticosteroids even before this communication takes place. The goals of treating an exacerbation are correction of any significant hypoxemia, rapid reversal of airflow obstruction, and reduction of the likelihood of recurrence of severe airflow obstruction by intensifying therapy.

The NHLBI expert panel recommends increasing the frequency of inhaled β_2-agonists and initiating or increasing oral corticosteroid treatment. The panel does not recommend drinking large volumes of liquids or breathing warm, moist air. They also discourage the use of over-the-counter (OTC) products such as antihistamines, cold remedies, or bronchodilators. For patients who present to emergency departments (EDs), the clinician should obtain a brief targeted history as well as objective data such as peak-flow measurement and pulse oximetry. Clinicians should be aware of risk factors for asthma-related deaths: previous intubation or intensive care unit (ICU) admission for asthma, two or more hospitalizations, or more than three ED visits in the past year, use of more than two canisters of short-acting β_2-agonist per month, low socioeconomic status, illicit drug use, major psychosocial problems, and comorbidities such as cardiovascular or chronic lung disease. Chest radiographs should be obtained only in patients suspected of having a more complicated process such as pneumothorax, pneumonia, or congestive heart failure. Treatment of exacerbations in the ED should

include nebulizer therapy with short-acting β_2-agonists and nebulized anticholinergics such as ipratropium bromide (SOR: A) (Busse et al., 2007). However the NHLBI does not recommend continued use of nebulized anticholinergics during hospitalization. In general, patients should be discharged if their FEV_1 or PEFR has returned to greater than 70% of their predicted personal best and they are in no respiratory distress.

Exercise-Induced Bronchospasm

Exercise-induced bronchospasm is a bronchospastic event that usually occurs during or minutes after vigorous activity. The peak of the bronchospasm occurs 5 to 10 minutes after stopping the activity and usually resolves by 30 minutes. The goal of management is to allow patients to participate in any activity they choose without being hindered by asthma symptoms.

Beta-2 agonists used shortly before exercise help prevent exercise-induced bronchospasm in more than 80% of patients. Cromolyn or nedocromil taken shortly before exercise are acceptable options but should be considered alternatives. If symptoms are not controlled with these options, long-term controller medications such as an inhaled corticosteroid or leukotriene modifier may be considered. A warm-up period before exercise can benefit patients who can tolerate continuous exercise with minimal symptoms (Busse et al., 2007).

> **KEY TREATMENT**
>
> Pulmonary function testing is the "gold standard" for the diagnosis and management of asthma and should be performed in all patients over 4 years of age (SOR: C).
> Minimize the use of short-acting inhaled β_2-agonists for asthma patients (SOR: C).
> Short-acting inhaled β_2-agonists should be used less than twice a week for asthma, or step therapy should be increased (SOR: C).
> Inhaled corticosteroids are the preferred therapy for all patients with persistent asthma (SOR: A).
> Asthma exacerbations should be treated with oral corticosteroids (SOR: A).
> Nebulized ipratropium can be used for asthma exacerbation in the ED setting but should not be used in the inpatient setting (SOR: A).

Paradoxical Vocal Cord Motion

Paradoxical vocal cord motion is defined by an inappropriate adduction of the true vocal cords on inspiration and adduction on expiration. The functional airway obstruction results in marked inspiratory stridor and wheezing, and the symptoms are similar to asthma. Often misdiagnosed as refractory asthma, paradoxical vocal cord motion appears to be psychogenic and occurs most often in young women with a history of prior psychiatric illnesses (e.g., depression, personality disorder, posttraumatic stress disorder, sexual abuse, generalized anxiety). Diagnosis is made by direct laryngoscopy with visualization of the cords throughout the respiratory cycle. Treatment is difficult because there are no published studies on the efficacy of psychodynamic therapy or pharmacologic treatment.

Anaphylaxis

Anaphylaxis has been traditionally defined as an acute, systemic, immediate hypersensitivity reaction produced by IgE-mediated degranulation of mast cells and basophils (Lieberman, 1998). The term *anaphylactoid* has referred to a clinically similar event not mediated by IgE-induced mast cell and basophil degranulation. An alternative classification by the World Allergy Organization (Johansson et al., 2004) eliminates anaphylactoid and refers to all events as *anaphylactic*, subdividing them into immunologic and nonimmunologic episodes. Immunologic episodes are then further subdivided into those caused by IgE-mediated mast cell and basophil degranulation and those resulting from other immunologic processes. An example of a non-IgE immunologically mediated event is a transfusion reaction. An example of a nonimmunologic event is a reaction to the administration of radiocontrast that can directly degranulate mast cells and basophils without intervening IgE.

Manifestations

Almost all patients with anaphylaxis express cutaneous symptoms, the most common of which are urticaria and angioedema. However, anaphylactic events can occur without any cutaneous manifestation. The most common cause is probably the rapid onset of hypotension and shock, which diverts blood flow from the skin. Anaphylaxis can clearly be the cause of syncope without any other manifestation and therefore must be considered as a cause of any syncopal episode. Table 20-5 lists signs and symptoms of anaphylaxis and their frequency (Lieberman et al., 2005).

Criteria have been established for the diagnosis of anaphylaxis (Box 20-4) (Sampson et al., 2006). Anaphylaxis usually requires at least two-system involvement; in most cases the skin is involved, and respiratory, vascular, or gastrointestinal symptoms accompany skin involvement. Single-system involvement (usually the skin) may be sufficient when this symptom appears after exposure to a known allergen (e.g., person known to be allergic to shellfish who develops urticaria within 30 minutes of shellfish ingestion); the diagnosis of anaphylaxis can be made without two-system involvement. This concept is important because rapid administration of epinephrine in such a patient might prevent further manifestations.

The differential diagnosis and most common causes of anaphylaxis are shown in Boxes 20-5 and 20-6. The most frequent cause of anaphylaxis is foods, and the next most common is drugs. The most common food to cause anaphylaxis in adults is shellfish. In children, peanuts are the most common offenders. As many as 50% of cases of anaphylaxis occur without a known cause despite intense investigative efforts (Webb et al., 2004). Laboratory testing can be useful to establish a diagnosis of anaphylaxis and to rule out other causes of symptoms caused by conditions that mimic anaphylaxis (Table 20-6). The most common test to confirm a diagnosis of anaphylaxis is serum tryptase, with high specificity but low sensitivity. Plasma histamine and 24-hour urinary histamine metabolites can also be measured.

Table 20-5 Signs and Symptoms of Anaphylaxis and Frequency of Occurrence

Signs and Symptoms	Percent
Cutaneous	**90**
Urticaria and angioedema	85-90
Flushing	45-55
Pruritus without rash	2-5
Respiratory	**40-60**
Dyspnea, wheeze	45-50
Upper airway angioedema	50-60
Rhinitis	15-20
Abdominal	
Nausea, vomiting, diarrhea, cramping abdominal pain	25-30
Miscellaneous	
Dizziness, syncope, hypotension	30-35
Headache	5-8
Substernal pain	4-6
Seizure	1-2

Box 20-4 Diagnosis of Anaphylaxis

Acute onset of an illness (minutes to hours) with involvement of skin and mucosal tissue (e.g., hives, generalized itch and flush, swollen lips, tongue, and uvula)

and

Airway compromise (e.g., dyspnea, wheeze or bronchospasm, stridor, reduced lung functions)

or

Reduced blood pressure or associated symptoms (e.g., hypotonia, syncope)

Two or more of the following after exposure to known allergen for that patient (minutes to hours):

   History of severe allergic reaction

   Skin or mucosal tissue involvement (e.g., hives, generalized itch or flush, swollen lips, tongue, uvula)

   Airway compromise (e.g., dyspnea, wheeze/bronchospasm, stridor, reduced lung function)

   Reduced blood pressure or associated symptoms (e.g., hypotonia, syncope)

   In suspected food allergy: gastrointestinal symptoms (e.g., cramping abdominal pain, vomiting)

   Hypotension after exposure to known allergen for that patient (minutes to hours)

   Infants and children: low systolic blood pressure (age specific)

   Adults: systolic blood pressure less than 100 mm Hg

Caution: These criteria describe classic cases of anaphylaxis. Other presentations can also indicate anaphylaxis. Physicians must remember the potential for false-positive symptoms or signs resulting from panic, vasovagal episodes, and other causes.

Box 20-5 Differential Diagnosis of Anaphylaxis

Anaphylaxis

Vasodepressor and vasovagal reactions

Other forms of shock

    Hemorrhagic

    Hypoglycemic

    Cardiogenic

    Endotoxic

Flushing syndromes

Carcinoid

Red man syndrome caused by vancomycin

Postmenopausal

Alcohol induced

Vasointestinal peptide and other vasoactive peptide–secreting gastrointestinal tumors

Nonorganic diseases such as panic attacks

Box 20-6 Most Common Causes of Anaphylaxis

Foods

Shellfish

Peanuts

Tree nuts

Fish

Drugs

Antibiotics (especially beta-lactams)

Nonsteroidal anti-inflammatory drugs

Physical Causes

Exercise

Cold

Heat

Sunlight

Idiopathic

Treatment

Special equipment is necessary to deal with anaphylactic events that occur in the office (Box 20-7). An algorithm for the management of the acute episode is shown in Figure 20-5.

On suspicion that an anaphylactic event has occurred, therapy should be initiated immediately (Box 20-8). The airway, circulation, and level of consciousness should immediately be assessed. Oxygen should be started and the patient placed in the recumbent position with feet elevated. The recumbent position is important because death has been associated with the upright position. The upright position allows decreased venous return to the heart, resulting in pulseless ventricular contractions and arrhythmias.

Simultaneous with assessment, epinephrine should be administered. Intramuscular (IM) injection in the lateral thigh gives a more rapid peak level than subcutaneous or deltoid IM injection; therefore the lateral thigh is the preferred site of injection. For adults, the dose is 0.2 to 0.5 mL of a 1:1000 aqueous epinephrine preparation. For children, the

Table 20-6 Tests Used to Confirm a Diagnosis of Anaphylaxis

Test	Comment
Tests Used to Rule in Anaphylaxis	
Serum tryptase	Peaks at 60 to 90 minutes after onset of symptoms. May be elevated up to 6 hours. Ideal time to obtain blood is 1 to 2 hours after symptoms begin.
Plasma histamine	Begins to rise 5 to 10 minutes after onset of symptoms. Remains elevated only up to 60 minutes.
24-hour urinary	May be assayed in urine for up to 24 hours after initiation of histamine metabolite symptoms.
Tests Used to Rule out Other Conditions	
Serum serotonin	Rules out carcinoid.
Urinary 5-hidroxyendolicetic acid	Rules out carcinoid.
Serum vasointestinal hormonal polypeptide panel*	Rules out vasoactive polypeptide–secreting gastrointestinal tumor or medullary carcinoma of thyroid.
Plasma-free metanephrine and urinary vanillylmandelic acid	Rules out paradoxical response to pheochromocytoma.

*For example, pancreastatin, pancreatic hormone, vasointestinal polypeptide, and substance P.

dose is 0.01 mg/kg to a maximum of 0.3 mg. A more precise dosage regimen has been recommended by the Resuscitation Council of the United Kingdom (Box 20-9). If symptoms do not improve, this dose can be readministered at 5-minute intervals (or more frequently if the physician deems necessary). After several injections, if there is no response, an intravenous (IV) infusion of epinephrine may be considered. An infusion can be prepared by adding 1 mg (1 mL of 1:1000 dilution of epinephrine) to 250 mL of D5W, yielding a concentration of 4.0 µg/mL. This solution is infused at a rate of 1 to 4 µg/min (15-60 drops/min with microdrop apparatus), increasing to a maximum of 10.0 µg/min for adults and adolescents. For children, the dose is 0.01 mg/kg (0.1 mL/kg of 1:10,000 solution up to 10 µg/min); maximum recommended dose is 0.3 mg.

Epinephrine is mandated and the drug of choice for anaphylaxis. Other drugs include H_1 and H_2 antagonists; a combination of both is more effective than an H_1 antagonist alone for vascular manifestations. Diphenhydramine, 25 to 50 mg for adults and 1 mg/kg for children, can be given by slow IV infusion. Ranitidine can be administered in a dose of 1 mg/kg in adults and 12.5 to 50 mg in children, infused over 10 to 15 minutes. No controlled studies have demonstrated efficacy of corticosteroids, but they should help in prolonged reactions. Although there is no established dose, the suggested dose equivalent is 1 to 2 mg/kg of methylprednisolone every 6 hours.

For persistent hypotension, fluids or other vasopressors (or both) should be administered. For adults with persistent hypotension, 1 to 2 L of normal saline can be administered

Box 20-7 Equipment and Medication for Therapy of Anaphylaxis in the Office

Primary

Epinephrine solution (aqueous) 1:1000 (1-mL ampules and multidose vials)

Epinephrine solution (aqueous) 1:10,000 (commercially available preloaded in a syringe)

Tourniquet

1-mL and 5-mL disposable syringes

Oxygen tank and mask or nasal prongs

Diphenhydramine injectable

Ranitidine or cimetidine injectable

Injectable corticosteroids

Ambubag, oral airway, laryngoscope, endotracheal tube, no. 12 needle

Intravenous setup with large-bore catheter

IV fluids: 2000 mL of crystalloid solution, 1000 mL of hydroxyethyl starch

Aerosol beta-II bronchodilator and compressor nebulizer

Glucagon

Electrocardiogram

Normal saline: 10-mL vial for epinephrine dilution

Supporting

Dopamine

Suction apparatus

Sodium bicarbonate

Aminophylline

Atropine

IV setup with needles, tape, and tubing

Nonlatex gloves

Optional

Defibrillator

Calcium gluconate

Neuroleptic agents for seizures

Lidocaine

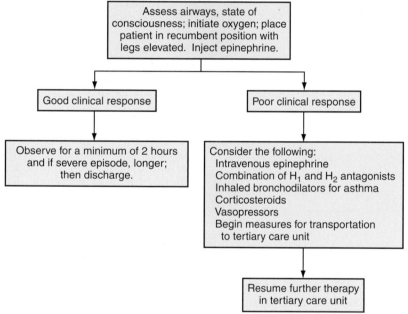

Figure 20-5 Algorithm for managing an episode of anaphylaxis.

at rates of 5 to 10 mg/kg in the first 5 minutes. After resolution of symptoms, patients should be observed because biphasic reactions can occur in up to 23% of cases (Scranton et al., 2009). The observation period should range from 6 to 24 hours, depending on the severity of the reaction (Tole and Lieberman, 2007).

Patients who have experienced episodes of anaphylaxis and who are at further risk of future events (e.g., insect sting hypersensitivity, food allergy) should have a prescription for an epinephrine autoinjector and should be instructed in its use. In addition, such patients should not take, if at all possible, drugs that might increase the severity of any future event or interfere with the use of epinephrine to treat such an event (Table 20-7).

KEY TREATMENT

Epinephrine should be the first medication used in the treatment of anaphylaxis (SOR: A).

Patients should be placed in supine position and oxygen administered, if needed (SOR: A).

Treatment with IV fluids, antihistamines (both H_1 and H_2), and corticosteroids should be considered after epinephrine administration (SOR: A).

Glucagon or atropine should be considered in anaphylaxis recalcitrant to treatment (SOR: A).

Box 20-8 Therapy for Anaphylaxis

Immediate Action

Assessment
Check airway and secure if needed.
Rapid assessment of level of consciousness
Vital signs

Treatment

Epinephrine
Supine position, legs elevated
Oxygen
Tourniquet proximal to injection site

Dependent on Evaluation

Start peripheral intravenous fluids.
H_1 and H_2 antagonist
Vasopressors
Corticosteroids
Aminophylline
Glucagon
Atropine
Electrocardiographic monitoring
Transfer to hospital

Hospital Management

Medical antishock trousers (MAST)
Continued therapy with above agents and management of complications

Box 20-9 Dosing Recommendations for Intramuscular Epinephrine in Anaphylaxis

Adults

0.5 mg (0.5 mL of 1:1000 concentration)

Children

Age ≥12 years

0.5 mg (0.5 mL of 1:1000 concentration)
or
0.3 mg (0.3 mL of 1:1000 concentration) if child is small or prepubertal

6-12 years

0.3 mg (0.3 mL using a 1:1000 concentration)

6 months to 6 years

0.15 mg (0.15 mL of 1:1000 concentration)

Age <6 months

0.15 mg (0.15 mL of 1:000 concentration)

Modified from the Working Group of Resuscitation Council of the United Kingdom, 2008.

Table 20-7 Drugs that Can Worsen or Complicate Therapy in Anaphylaxis

Drug Class	Effect
Beta blockers	Can worsen hypotension or wheeze and simultaneously decrease the β-adrenergic response to epinephrine as well as accentuate its α-adrenergic response.
ACE inhibitors	ACE metabolizes kinins that are activated during anaphylactic events; therefore an ACE inhibitor can worsen episodes.
ACE blockers	Although there is no clear-cut admonition regarding ACE blockers, theoretically they can have an effect similar to an ACE inhibitor.
Monoamine oxidase inhibitors	Interfere with catabolism of epinephrine and thus complicate calculation of correct dose of these drug inhibitors.
Tricyclic antidepressants	Prevent catecholamine reuptake and therefore can accentuate effect of a dose of epinephrine, thus complicating calculation of a proper dose.

ACE, Angiotensin-converting enzyme.

References

The complete reference list is available online at www.expertconsult.com.

Best Evidence Sources

Agency for Healthcare Research and Quality
Clinical Evidence Concise
Family Physicians Inquiries Network Clinical Inquiries

Journal of Family Practice Applied Evidence
National Guideline Clearinghouse
TRIP (Turning Research into Practice) Database

Web Resources

www.acaai.org
  American College of Allergy, Asthma and Immunology for information on the diagnosis and treatment of allergic diseases.
www.cdc.gov/nchs/fastats/asthma.htm
www.cdc.gov/ASTHMA/healthcare.html
  Center for Disease Control and Prevention Statistics.

www.nhlbi.nih.gov/guidelines/asthma/asthgdln.pdf
  National Heart, Lung and Blood Institute and National Asthma Education and Prevention Panel: Expert Panel Report 3: Guidelines for the Diagnosis and Management of Asthma, 2007.
www.thoracic.org/sections/publications/statements/pages/pfet/pft5.html
  American Thoracic Society information for interpretative strategies for lung function tests.

CHAPTER 21

Obstetrics

Dave E. Williams and Gabriella Pridjian

Key Points

- The United States ranks 30th in infant mortality.
- The causes of infant mortality are preterm birth, birth defects, sudden infant death syndrome, respiratory distress syndrome, and maternal pregnancy complications.

The American Academy of Family Physicians (AAFP) describes the specialty of family practice as the enhanced expression of general medical practice that is uniquely defined within the context of the family. Providing care across the continuum of the family life cycle, the family physician provides care to the pregnant woman as part of the full expression of the field. The family physician incorporates a comprehensive approach to maternity care that includes the assessment and management of psychosocial and biomedical risk factors. The family physician provides care to patients with low-risk pregnancies and equips them to birth their children without unnecessary interventions.

The family physician brings a unique approach to the management of the pregnant woman, who is often a healthy individual undergoing a natural process. This approach is patient centered, prevention oriented, educational, and noninterventional. Nationwide, approximately 29.6% of all family physicians provide routine obstetric services as part of their hospital care (AAFP, 1998). This number has been steadily declining, with regional variations reflecting the needs of the population and local attitudes. The majority of family physicians do not desire to practice obstetrics because of lifestyle issues, increasing costs of malpractice insurance, and difficulty obtaining hospital privileges. However, the family physician may be asked to counsel or care for the pregnant woman, even if not part of daily practice. It becomes incumbent on the individual practitioner to have a fundamental knowledge and appreciation of the field of obstetrics, including the obstetric emergency. Given that the family physician may be the sole provider of obstetric services, particularly in rural or underserved areas, the need to maintain the knowledge and skills to treat the problems and emergencies unique to obstetrics becomes increasingly important. The Advanced Life Support in Obstetrics (ALSO) course developed in 1990 effectively incorporates the techniques of other established life support courses as it applies to obstetric care.

For the successful practice of obstetrics, it is imperative for the family physician to practice in concert with an obstetric specialist. A collaborative relationship among obstetricians, family physicians, and in some cases, nurse midwives is essential for provision of consistent, high-quality care to pregnant women. Access to reliable consultation and suitable referral facilities for the complicated patient will optimize patient care and outcomes.

The integration of prenatal care into the clinical practice of the family physician not only reflects the full scope of the field but also provides a continuous infusion of pediatric patients into the practice. It serves as a model for the training of medical students and residents interested in the practice of obstetric care in the context of family practice.

This chapter provides an overview of the field of obstetrics that includes prenatal, intrapartum, and postpartum care of the pregnant woman. An evidence-based approach to areas of controversy and empiric practice is used while addressing the unique needs of family physicians, emphasizing their contribution and role in the research and development of the obstetrics literature.

Woman and Child Health

The health of a nation is often reflected in the health of its mothers and newborns. The World Health Organization (WHO) often uses a nation's maternity and neonatal morbidity and mortality statistics as a proxy for the health status of its population. It is an important summary reflecting social, political, health care delivery, and medical outcomes in a geographic area. The United States, despite its economic wealth and medical resources, consistently ranks poorly in such measures as maternal and infant mortality rates. In 2005 in the United States, 28,384 infants died before reaching their first birthdays, an infant mortality rate (IMR) of 6.9 per 1000 live births. Despite a more than 9% reduction in IMR between 1995 and 2005, the United States ranks 30th, after such select countries as Japan, the Scandinavian countries, and Canada (Box 21-1). In 2005, the U.S. IMR was more than three times as high as that in Singapore (2.1 per 1000 live births), the country with the lowest reported IMR. This number reflects in part the continuing disparities in health access and delivery for U.S. citizens (National Center for Health Statistics [NCHS], 2009).

Box 21-1 International Infant Mortality Rate (IMR)*

1. Singapore (2.1)
2. Hong Kong (2.4)
3. Sweden (2.4)
4. Japan (2.8)
5. Finland (3.0)
6. Norway (3.1)
7. Czech Republic (3.4)
8. Portugal (3.5)
9. France (3.6)
10. Belgium (3.7)
11. Greece (3.8)
12. Germany (3.9)
13. Ireland (4.0)
14. Spain (4.1)
15. Austria (4.2)
16. Switzerland (4.2)
17. Denmark (4.4)
18. Israel (4.6)
19. Italy (4.7)
20. Netherlands (4.9)
21. Australia (5.0)
22. England, Wales (5.0)
23. New Zealand (5.1)
24. Scotland (5.2)
25. Canada (5.4)
26. Cuba (6.2)
27. Hungary (6.2)
28. Northern Ireland (6.3)
29. Poland (6.4)
30. United States (6.9)
31. Slovakia (7.2)
32. Chile (7.9)
33. Puerto Rico (9.3)
34. Costa Rica (9.8)
35. Russian Federation (11.0)
36. Romania (15.0)

From National Center for Health Statistics. http://www.cdc.gov/nchs/hus.htm.
*Under 1 year of age; rankings are from lowest to highest IMR (per 1000 live births). Countries with the same IMR receive the same rank. Some of the variation in IMRs is caused by differences among countries in distinguishing between fetal and infant deaths.
Note: U.S. data used in this table is final mortality data. After 1994, Peristats uses period-linked birth/infant death data to calculate IMRs. Rates in table may vary slightly from other rates on PeriStats: www.marchofdimes.com/peristats.

The causes of infant mortality are multiple, with birth defects being the leading cause, with a 2005 rate of 134.6 per 100,000 live births. Preterm birth (birth at <37 completed weeks of gestation) or low birth weight (LBW) is the second leading cause of infant mortality in the United States. Preterm birth rates differ by race; during 2003–2005 (average), IMR (per 1000 live births) in the United States was highest for black infants (13.3), followed by Native Americans (8.4), whites (5.7), and Asians (4.8) (NCHS, 2010). This persistent disparity contributes to the relative high IMR in the United States compared with similarly developed countries. Other causes of infant mortality include sudden infant death syndrome, respiratory distress syndrome, and maternal pregnancy complications. These five causes accounted for more than half of all infant deaths in 2005 (Fig. 21-1). Despite gains, the rate of preterm birth, birth defects, and LBW remain relatively constant. This indicates a need for further health initiatives to address the health needs of the pregnant woman and the unborn.

Preconception Counseling

Key Points

- Preconception care is an integral part of prenatal care and permits health promotion and early identification of risk factors that can then be treated before pregnancy
- Folic acid supplementation should be started before conception, if possible, or immediately on diagnosis of pregnancy.

Ideally, women should plan pregnancy and discuss this plan with their physicians. Often, however, this option is not considered. It becomes the task of the physician to anticipate the potential and discuss preparation for pregnancy just as for methods of birth control. Primary care physicians are in

the best position to anticipate the need for this counseling, being most aware of ongoing medical problems and social concerns of the women in their care. Indeed, the practice of preconception care has been formally recommended since at least 1989 (Caring for Our Future, 1989). However, we believe that preconception care, in particular education, should begin at the time a woman reaches reproductive age, not only when she announces the desire to become pregnant.

The preconception period is an ideal time for education and counseling regarding cessation of cigarette, alcohol, or drug use. Often, the incentive of a healthier pregnancy is sufficient impetus for change in behavior. Although many women are able to cease cigarette, alcohol, or drug use during the pregnancy, the majority will resume use after delivery or breastfeeding. This is an opportune time for the family physician to reinforce further health-conscious behavior.

The preconception use of folic acid supplementation was formally recommended by the U.S. Centers for Disease Control and Prevention (CDC) in 1991 and others (American Academy of Pediatrics, Committee on Genetics, 1999). Evidence supports a reduction in neural tube defects by 50% when folic acid stores are replenished before pregnancy (Milunsky et al., 1989). It is now recommended that all reproductive-age women take 0.4 mg of folic acid daily (CDC, 1992). This is easily accomplished by prescribing prenatal vitamins before pregnancy as well as throughout gestation. Alternately, over-the-counter (OTC) vitamins can also be used because many now contain this higher amount of folic acid. For couples with one or more children with a neural tube defect or a family history, there should be a referral for specific counseling. From 2 to 4 mg of folic acid daily is recommended for these women at least 1 month before pregnancy and during the first 3 months of pregnancy.

Many genetic disorders are now amenable to prenatal diagnosis through direct analysis of the underlying mutations, analysis of their protein products, or abnormal metabolites. Genetic counseling should include a systematic assessment of family history of both parents. This can be through a targeted questionnaire or formal genetic counseling by a genetic counselor or geneticist (Box 21-2). The family physician should be aware of the ethnic makeup of the practice and especially familiar with disorders in these groups (Table 21-1). When targeted screening reveals an area of potential concern, formal genetic counseling should be obtained. With advances in discovery of the genetic basis for many diseases, the list of disorders amenable to prenatal diagnosis grows daily.

> **KEY TREATMENT**
>
> Folic acid supplementation is 0.4 mg for women without risk factors and up to 4 mg for those with risk factors (SOR: A).

Nutrition

There is sufficient data to confirm that poor nutrition during the prenatal period is associated with adverse pregnancy outcome, specifically *intrauterine growth restriction* (IUGR) and preterm delivery. Specific nutritional guidelines have been developed based on a woman's prepregnancy weight or, more specifically, her body mass index (BMI) (Table 21-2).

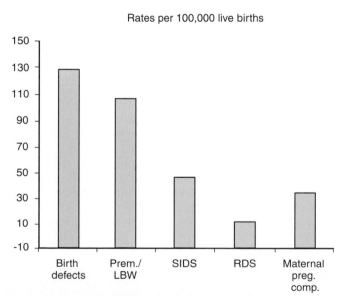

Rates per 100,000 live births

Figure 21-1 Infant deaths by cause of death, United States, 2005. Rates per 100,000 live births. *SIDS,* Sudden infant death syndrome; *RDS,* respiratory distress syndrome; *Maternal Preg. Comp,* material complications of pregnancy. *(Modified from National Center for Health Statistics. Period-linked birth/infant death data.* www.marchofdimes.com/peristats. *Accessed March 2010.)*

Box 21-2 Genetic Screening/Teratology Counseling

1. Will you be 35 at the time of your baby's birth?
2. What medications, prescribed, herbal, or over the counter, have you taken since your last menstrual period?
3. How much alcohol, cigarettes, or street drugs have you used since your last menstrual period?
4. Have you had miscarriages or stillborns? How many?
5. Do you have any metabolic disorders (such as diabetes or phenylketonuria)?
6. Have you been ill or had any infections since your last menstrual period?
7. What are the ethnic backgrounds of you and the baby's father? Are you related in any way?
8. Do you, the baby's father, or anyone in either of your families have:
   a. Neural tube defects (meningomyelocele, spina bifida, or anencephaly)?
   b. Congenital heart defects?
   c. Down syndrome?
   d. Tay-Sachs disease (Jewish, Cajun, French Canadian)?
   e. Sickle cell disease or trait (African American)?
   f. Thalassemia (Italian, Mediterranean, Asian or African American)? (MCV <80?)
   g. Muscular dystrophy?
   h. Cystic fibrosis?
   i. Huntington's chorea?
   j. Fragile X, mental retardation, or autism?
   k. Other chromosomal or inherited disorders or birth defects?

Table 21-1 Genetic Screening/Teratology Counseling

Ethnic Group	Higher Risk	Carrier Frequency
Caucasian	Cystic fibrosis	1 in 25
African American	Sickle cell disease Beta thalassemia	1 in 12
Southeast Asian	Alpha thalassemia	1 in 20
Mediterranean (Italian, Greek)	Beta thalassemia	1 in 25
Ashkenazi Jewish	Tay-Sachs disease Gaucher's disease type 1 Canavan's disease Cystic fibrosis	1 in 30 1 in 12 1 in 40 1 in 25

Table 21-2 Recommended Total Weight Gain for Pregnant Women

Phenotype	BMI	Weight Gain	
		lb	kg
Underweight	<18.5	28-40	13.7-18.2
Normal weight	18.5-24.9	25-35	11.4-15.9
Overweight	25-29.9	15-25	6.8-11.4
Obese (all classes)	≥30	11-20	5-9.1

Modified from Institute of Medicine, National Academies of Science. Weight gain during pregnancy: reexamining the guidelines, 2009.
BMI, Body mass index.

Caloric intake of an extra 300 kcal daily is sufficient for adequate maternal weight gain and fetal growth.

The practice of prenatal supplementation of vitamins and minerals is widespread, although many nutritionists believe it is unnecessary. Only the following two supplements are recommended in an adequately nourished female with a singleton pregnancy:

1. Iron, 30 mg/day, in the second and third trimester to meet the fetal demands for erythropoiesis.
2. Folic acid, 400 µg/day, in the preconception period and during the first trimester for prevention of birth defects.

However, because many U.S. women do not consume adequate vitamins and minerals (Block and Adams, 1993), and specific assessment of nutritional intake is often difficult, supplements are now widely used. Recommended daily allowances for pregnant women have been established and continue to be reevaluated (Table 21-3). Care must be taken to avoid toxicity of the fat-soluble vitamins, in particular vitamin A (retinol), where "more" is not necessarily better. Daily doses of retinol greater than 10,000 IU, approximately 3000 retinol equivalents (RE), have been associated with birth defects (Rothman et al., 1995). Women who do not consume sufficient milk products may benefit from calcium supplementation. This can easily be accomplished by prescribing an antacid that is made of calcium carbonate, most easily taken in chewable form. This will not only replenish calcium stores but also treat reflux esophagitis, which often occurs in the latter half of pregnancy.

Recent data suggest that supplementation with omega-3 fatty acids, specifically docosahexaenoic acid (DHA) plus eicosapentaenoic acid (EPA), may be beneficial (Dunstan et al., 2008). Both DHA and EPA may be beneficial for fetal brain development and are found in large amounts in wild fish. However, increased fish intake in pregnancy **is** not recommended because of the risk of increased mercury ingestion. Therefore, supplementation would be required. Large, well-controlled studies are needed before recommendation in pregnancy, but supplementation may be considered on an individual basis. The U.S. Food and Drug Administration (FDA, 2004) has formally warned women of childbearing age, pregnant and lactating women, and young children to avoid eating swordfish, shark, king mackerel, and tilefish and to consume no more than one 6-ounce can of albacore tuna per week. In all pregnant women, nutritional risk factors should be addressed, including low starting BMI, prior LBW infants, adolescence, religious and cultural dietary restrictions, medical illnesses requiring dietary manipulation, substance abuse, and eating disorders (Kolasa and Weismiller, 1995). Certain woman may benefit from formal dietary counseling from a dietician/nutritionist.

KEY TREATMENT

Iron (30 mg/day) is recommended in the second and third trimesters (SOR: A).
Folic acid (400 µg/day) is recommended in the preconception period and first trimester (SOR: A).

Table 21-3 Recommended Dietary Allowances for Women

	Nonpregnant (15-50 yr)	Pregnant (Singleton)	Lactating (first 6 mo)
Energy, kcal	1900-2200	+300	+500
Protein, g	44-50	60	65
Vitamin A, µg RE	800	800	1300
Vitamin D, µg*	5-10	10	10
Vitamin E, mg TE	8	10	12
Vitamin K, µg	55-65	65	65
Vitamin C, mg	60	70	95
Thiamin, mg	1.1	1.5	1.6
Riboflavin, mg	1.3	1.6	1.8
Niacin, mg NE	15	17	20
Vitamin B$_6$, mg	1.5-1.6	2.2	2.1
Folate, µg	400	400	400
Vitamin B$_{12}$, µg	2.0	2.2	2.6
Calcium, mg	800-1200	1200	1200
Phosphorus, mg	800-1200	1200	1200
Magnesium, mg	280	300	355
Iron, mg	15	30	15
Zinc, mg	12	15	19
Iodine, µg	150	175	200
Selenium, µg	50-55	65	75

Data from Report of the Subcommittee on the Tenth Edition of the RDAs, Recommended Dietary Allowances, National Academy of Sciences, with modifications from ACOG Committee Opinion #196, 1998; and CDC. Use of folic acid for the prevention of spina bifida and other neural tube defects, MMWR 1991;40:513-516.
*As cholecalciferol.
RE, Retinal equivalents; *TE*, alpha-tocopherol equivalents; *NE*, niacin equivalents.

Medical Risk Assessment

The preconception period is the ideal time to assess and counsel the prospective pregnant woman regarding medical disorders or risks she may encounter during the pregnancy. Of medical problems that have substantial impact on the fetus, hypertensive disorders and diabetes are among the most common.

Hypertension may have many effects on the pregnancy depending on the degree of abnormality. Fetal effects range from none to increased miscarriage, IUGR, abruptio placentae, and fetal death. Underlying blood pressure disorders should be treated appropriately before pregnancy. Some hypertensive, reproductive-age women are treated with angiotensin-converting enzyme (ACE) inhibitors. This class of therapeutics can cause significant risk to the developing fetus. These medications should be stopped and alternate medications started if needed. Women with preexisting hypertension should be referred for concurrent care with a physician experienced in managing hypertension in pregnancy.

Diabetes can also have many effects on the developing fetus. The preconception control of the maternal metabolism, reflected as normal blood glucose values before and after meals and normal hemoglobin A$_{1c}$, has been shown to decrease the incidence of diabetes-associated embryopathy to almost that of a nondiabetic pregnant woman (Mills et al., 1988). Women with preexisting diabetes should be referred for specialized care if pregnancy is contemplated.

Less attention is directed to emotional and psychiatric disorders. Pregnancy may be a stressor that precipitates an acute event or worsens ongoing anxiety or depression. This is more likely in the postpartum period.

KEY TREATMENT

Preconception care is an integral part of prenatal care and permits health promotion and early identification of risk factors that can then be treated before pregnancy, such as diabetes or hypertension (SOR: A).

Women with preexisting diabetes should be referred for specialized care if pregnancy is contemplated (SOR: C).

Routine Prenatal Care

In most Western countries, women attend between 7 and 11 prenatal visits, although recent data suggest that a reduced number of antenatal visits could be introduced into clinical practice without adverse effect to the mother and child (Carroli et al., 2001). Obstetric care provided by obstetricians, family physicians, and midwives has been found to be equally effective; however, patients were slightly more satisfied by the care provided by midwives and family physicians (Villar et al., 2004). Prenatal care services typically include screening and treatment for medical conditions and identification and interventions for behavioral risk factors associated with poor birth outcomes (e.g., smoking, poor nutrition).

One of the most important goals of prenatal care is recognizing which women have high-risk pregnancies and triaging these women to appropriate care (Kontopoulos and Vintzileos, 2004). It is important to identify the women at risk for adverse outcomes and refer them to appropriate specialty care. Adequate prenatal care has been shown to increase the chances that a woman has a healthy pregnancy and baby.

First Prenatal Visit

The first prenatal visit is one of the most important, particularly if the woman has not had preconception care (Box 21-3). The first prenatal visit should occur shortly after

Box 21-3 Expert Panel Recommendations for First Prenatal Visit

Risk Assessment for All

Medical History

Medical/surgical update
Nutrition update
Current pregnancy to date*

Psychosocial History

Smoking
Alcohol
Drugs
Social support
Extremes of physical work, exercise, and other activity
Stress

Physical Examination

Blood pressure*
Weight
Breast examination*
Pelvic examination for uterine size, dating, abnormalities*

Laboratory Tests

Recommended for all:
Hemoglobin/hematocrit
Urine culture
Recommended for some:
Rh screen
Syphilis test
Blood glucose level
Gonococcal culture

Health Promotion Activities and Information for All

Avoidance of teratogens
Safer sex*
Physical and emotional changes in pregnancy*
Sexuality*
Self-help strategies for discomforts (for some)
Fetal growth and development
Classes on nutrition, physical changes, exercise, psychological adaptation
Nutritional counseling (some or all)
Preparation for screening and diagnostic tests
Content and timing of visits*
Need to report danger signs*

*Accepted by panel but not specifically reviewed.
From Rosen M, Merkatz I, Hill J. Caring for our future: a report by the expert panel on the content of prenatal care. Obstet Gynecol 1991;77:785.

Box 21-4 Recommendations for Exercise in Pregnancy

1. Established exercise routines can be continued with mild to moderate intensity.
2. High-intensity or high-impact routines should be avoided or reduced.
3. The supine position should be avoided in the second and third trimesters.
4. Hyperthermia should be avoided.
5. Weight-bearing exercise should minimize strain because joints are more lax.
6. Routines should be designed to minimize risk of maternal trauma (falling).
7. Adequate nutritional intake to compensate for pregnancy should be assured.
8. Resumption of prepregnancy routines in the postpartum period should be gradual.

Modified from ACOG Technical Bulletin No. 189, 1994.

pregnancy. Preparation for the birthing process is a key theme around which to discuss care issues and choices such as breastfeeding. Structured educational programs to promote breastfeeding have unclear effectiveness. Pregnant women should be counseled about the risks of possible teratogens, including smoking, alcohol, and drug use, including exposure to medications, prescriptions, OTC drugs, and herbal remedies. Good handwashing is always encouraged because this is one of the best ways to avoid community-acquired infectious diseases. Appropriate immunizations such as influenza and novel influenza A (H1N1) virus should be offered. Common exposures such as workplace conditions and use of hot tubs and saunas should be explored. Exercise should also be encouraged if there is no obstetric contraindication (Box 21-4). Intercourse during pregnancy should be actively addressed because some women are reluctant to discuss this topic even with their physician. Sexual activity can generally continue during pregnancy except for few situations, such as placenta previa and preterm labor. Counseling regarding sexually transmitted diseases (STDs) and their avoidance should occur. Nutrition should be individualized, with an estimate of desirable weight gain given to the pregnant woman.

The estimated date of delivery (EDD) should be calculated by accurate determination of the last menstrual period (LMP). The first day of the LMP is a good clinical sign from which to calculate EDD, remembering that it must be adjusted for cycles shorter or longer than 28 days. The EDD can be calculated by Nagle's rule, that is, subtracting 3 months and adding 7 days to the first day of the LMP. EDD should then be extended by the number of days longer than a 28-day cycle or shortened by the number of days shorter. This approach should be considered if there is uncertainty about the LMP.

The physical examination during the first prenatal visit should include careful assessment of uterine size. If there is a discrepancy between menstrual age and uterine size, ultrasound should be considered early in the pregnancy to resolve the issue of dating. Recent evidence suggests that early sonography provides more accurate dating, which is important for timing screening tests and interventions and for optimal management of complications such as

the woman discovers she might be pregnant and should be viewed as a continuation of preconception counseling. Home pregnancy test kits have a sensitivity and specificity of at least 95%; many can detect pregnancy by the fifth menstrual week. The most important aspects of the first prenatal visit include education, risk assessment, appropriate laboratory testing, and establishment of gestational age.

Education is an important component of prenatal care, particularly for women who are pregnant for the first time. Frequency of prenatal visits should be explained, with information about the physiologic changes that occur during post-term pregnancies (Neilson, 2004). Late ultrasound, after 24 weeks, is not as sensitive for confirming gestational age. Additionally, any irregular bleeding or abdominal pain should prompt the practitioner to obtain sonographic confirmation of viability of the pregnancy as well as its normal intrauterine location.

A history and directed physical examination should be performed to detect conditions associated with increased maternal and perinatal morbidity and mortality. The first prenatal examination provides an opportunity for cervical cancer screening with a Papanicolaou (Pap) test in women who have not been screened recently. However, Pap tests performed in pregnant women may be less reliable. Risk factors should then identify other testing that might be done at this time, including blood glucose, sickle cell screening, Tay-Sachs screening, and surveillance for other infectious diseases.

Routine fetal heart auscultation, urinalysis, and assessment of maternal weight, blood pressure, and fundal height generally are recommended, although the supportive evidence varies (Kirkham et al., 2005). Women should be offered ABO and Rh blood typing and screening for anemia during the first prenatal visit. Genetic counseling and testing should be offered to couples with a family history of genetic disorders, a previously affected fetus or child, or a history of recurrent miscarriage. All women should be offered prenatal serum marker screening for neural tube defects and aneuploidy. Women at increased risk for aneuploidy should be offered amniocentesis or chorionic villus sampling (CVS). Counseling about the limitations and risks of these tests, as well as their psychologic implications, is necessary. Folic acid supplementation beginning in the preconception period and early pregnancy reduces the incidence of neural tube defects. Laboratory testing during the first prenatal visit consists of assessment of hemoglobin and hematocrit to identify anemia; blood D(Rh) type; serologic tests for syphilis, and rubella immunity; hepatitis B, and urinalysis. Testing for human immunodeficiency virus (HIV) infection should be offered and highly recommended because perinatal transmission can be decreased with appropriate medical intervention. During the pelvic examination, a Pap smear (if not done in past 6 months) as well as cultures for *Neisseria gonorrhoeae* and *Chlamydia* should be taken.

Follow-up Prenatal Visits

According to the report of the Expert Panel on Prenatal Care (Rosen et al., 1991), low-risk primigravid women should have at least 10 prenatal visits; low-risk multiparous women should have at least eight visits. Again, however, data suggest that antenatal visits could be reduced without adverse effect to the mother and child (Carroli et al., 2001). Women with psychosocial issues or pregnancy complications should be seen more frequently. In the first two trimesters, prenatal visits may be 5 to 6 weeks apart if no problems have been ascertained. Frequency of visits should increase after 30 weeks, with weekly visits after 37 weeks. Specific recommendations are noted in Table 21-4. Routine visits for low-risk women should be scheduled at times that recommended laboratory testing could be accomplished. Prenatal screening for chromosomal abnormalities is available in the first trimester between 10 weeks, 2 days and 13 weeks, 6 days. Structural defects of the fetus (in particular neural

Table 21-4 Expert Panel Recommendations for Visits throughout Pregnancy

Activity	Week/Trimester
Check for any exposure to infection.[*]	
Physical Examination	
Blood pressure	24[†]
Weight	Each visit
Fundal height/growth	16[†]
Fetal lie/presentation/engagement/heart rate[*]	24[†]
Cervical examination	41[*]
Laboratory Tests	
Hemoglobin/hematocrit	24-28
Rh sensitivity[‡]	26-28
Diabetic screen	26-28
Repeat syphilis[‡]	Third trimester
Repeat gonococcal and HIV[‡]	36
Serum alpha fetoprotein	14-16
Ultrasound[*]	When indicated
Health Promotion Activities	
Teratogen avoidance	Each visit
Safer sex[*]	Each visit
Maternal seatbelt use	Each trimester
Smoking cessation[‡]	Each trimester
Work/nutrition counseling[‡]	Each visit
Signs of preterm labor	Second/third trimester
Physical/emotional changes[*]	First/third trimester
Sexuality counseling[*]	First half of pregnancy
Fetal growth/development	Each visit
Self-help for discomforts[‡]	Each visit
General health habits	Each visit
Breastfeeding	26[†]
Infant car seat safety	Each visit
Childbirth/parenting classes	32
Family roles adjustment	38
Information about laboratory tests[*]	Before testing
Birth plan[*]	Third trimester
Labor (when to call/where to go)[*]	Third trimester

From Rosen M, Merkatz I, Hill J. Caring for our future: a report by the expert panel on the content of prenatal care. Obstet Gynecol 1991;77:785.
[*]Accepted by panel but not specifically reviewed.
[†]That week and each week thereafter.
[‡]For some.
HIV, Human immunodeficiency virus.

tube defects) and karyotypic abnormalities in the form of alpha-fetoprotein based tests (Quad screen, see below) can be obtained at 16 to 18 weeks. Screening for gestational diabetes is recommended at 26 to 28 weeks of gestation, as well as screening for anemia with a hemoglobin or hematocrit. Antibody screening, $Rh_0(D)$ immune globulin (RhoGAM) prophylaxis for D-negative mothers, and repeat testing for infectious diseases for at-risk mothers are recommended at this time.

At 36 weeks' gestation, rectocervical cultures for group B streptococci (GBS) should be obtained. If cultures are positive, antibiotic prophylaxis during labor is given. For women without a penicillin allergy, penicillin (5 million units, then 2.5 million units IV every 4 hours) is administered during labor. If there is a penicillin allergy, sensitivities to clindamycin and erythromycin should be obtained and one of these agents used. If the organism is resistant to these antibiotics, women with a serious penicillin allergy should receive vancomycin; women with a minimal reaction from penicillin (e.g., rash) should receive a first-generation cephalosporin intravenously during labor (ACOG, 2002a, Schrag et al., 2002). Women with GBS bacteruria or a prior child affected with GBS sepsis should be treated during labor without screening cultures.

The clinical components of routine prenatal visits are controversial. Most guidelines recommend routine assessment with fundal height and maternal weight and blood pressure measurements, fetal heart auscultation, urine testing for protein and glucose, and questions about fetal movement. The assessment of uterine growth and size should be performed at every prenatal visit. Documentation of fetal heart tones is also recommended with each prenatal visit. Before 12 weeks' gestation, the size of the uterus is estimated by bimanual pelvic examination. The ability to assess the presence of fetal heart tones using Doppler ultrasound before 12 weeks is variable. After 12 weeks and before

20 weeks, adequate uterine growth is assessed by location of the uterine fundus in the lower abdomen (Fig. 21-2). Fetal heart tones should be reliably heard during this period. At 20 weeks of gestation, most women have a palpable fundus at the umbilicus. After 20 weeks, fundal height is measured using the distance from top of the symphysis pubis to top of the fundus. The number of completed weeks of gestation should equal this measurement in centimeters (±2 cm). This measurement should be performed as accurately as possible. The most common reasons for inconsistency between menstrual age and fundal height is an inaccurate menstrual-age assignment and inaccurate measurements caused by maternal obesity. Larger-than-expected fundal height may also be caused by multiple gestation, uterine fibroids, polyhydramnios, or a large-for-gestational-age (LGA) fetus. Smaller-than-expected fundal height should warrant an exploration for etiologies such as oligohydramnios, IUGR, and fetal demise.

By 30 weeks' gestation, the fetus is large enough that it can be palpated through the maternal abdomen. Position of the fetus should be documented at this and subsequent visits. This is easily done in most women by Leopold's maneuvers (Fig. 21-3). The first maneuver involves palpation of the uterine fundus to identify the fetal part that is there. The palpating hands then glide downward laterally to perform the second maneuver, location of the fetal back. In the third maneuver the hands are cupped around the presenting part

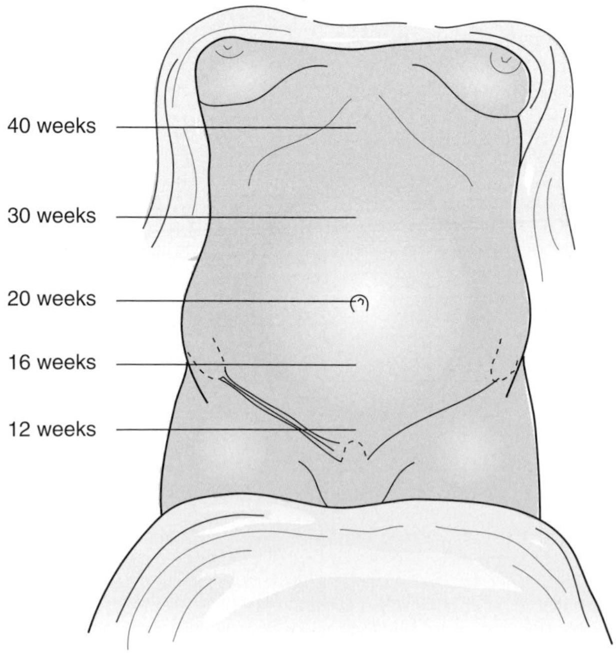

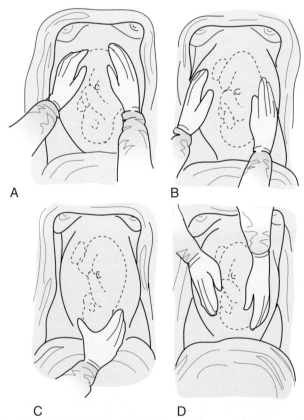

A B

C D

Figure 21-3 Leopold's maneuvers for determination of fetal position. **A,** First maneuver: palpation of the uterine fundus to identify the fetal part. **B,** Second maneuver: location of the fetal back. **C,** Third maneuver: cupped hands to determine the presenting part and station. **D,** Fourth maneuver: palpation of the cephalic prominence to determine the degree of flexion.

40 weeks

30 weeks

20 weeks

16 weeks

12 weeks

Figure 21-2 Fundal growth at various weeks of gestation.

at the level of the symphysis pubis to determine the presenting part as well as its degree of descent into the pelvis. If the presenting part is cephalic, the fourth maneuver will determine its degree of flexion. The examiner now turns 180 degrees to face the mother's legs, and the cephalic prominence is palpated. Another aid in ascertaining the position of the fetal back is the location of the fetal heart tones by Doppler sonography or auscultation. These sounds are best heard through the fetal back; in the left lower uterus in left occiput anterior, transverse, and posterior positions of the fetal head; and the right lower uterus in right occiput positions. The evidence supporting the previous practices is variable but continues as the standard of care (Kirkham et al., 2005).

By the end of gestation, the practitioner as well as the woman should know the presentation of the fetus. This avoids emergent management when she presents in labor with a nonvertex presentation. Internal digital cervical examination can also verify presentation of the fetus and may be done when needed. Unless indicated, however, routine cervical examination to determine cervical readiness for labor need not be done until 41 weeks' gestation.

Prenatal Genetic Diagnostic Testing

If specific risk factors for fetal abnormalities are identified in the mother, appropriate counseling and specific diagnostic testing should be offered. The most common reason to offer prenatal genetic diagnosis is advanced maternal age; a somewhat linear increase in nondisjunction in meiosis increases the risk of a conception with aneuploidy (abnormal chromosome number). This is one reason why older women have a higher rate of spontaneous first-trimester miscarriage. It is also why older women are more likely to give birth to a child with a chromosomal abnormality, most often Down syndrome (trisomy 21).

Women of advanced maternal age are those 35 or older at the anticipated birth of their baby. This group of women should be given specific counseling and offered diagnostic testing in the form of amniocentesis or CVS to ascertain the well-being of their fetus.

Amniocentesis

Genetic amniocentesis is typically performed at 14 to 20 weeks of gestation but can also be done any time after 20 menstrual weeks. After ultrasound examination of the fetus and placenta, an area of skin overlying a pocket of amniotic fluid is cleaned with iodine solution. With ultrasound guidance throughout the procedure, a 22-gauge spinal needle is used to remove 20 mL of amniotic fluid. Special care is taken to avoid the fetus, umbilical cord, and the large placental vessels. In experienced hands, the pregnancy loss rate attributed to the procedure is about 1 in 300. The entire testing time for a chromosomal analysis is about 10 to 12 days. Alternately, the supernatant may be assayed for metabolites to diagnose other disorders that run in the family if identified on counseling. Earlier amniocentesis (at 11 to 13 weeks) has been successfully performed but is not recommended any longer because of the recent initial reports regarding a slightly higher rate of clubfoot in these newborns.

EVIDENCE-BASED SUMMARY

- Early amniocentesis performed before 14 completed weeks of gestation is not considered a safe alternative to second-trimester amniocentesis or chorionic villus sampling (CVS) (SOR: A).
- CVS should *not* be performed before 10 completed weeks of gestation (SOR: B).
- CVS should always be performed under direct ultrasound control (SOR: B).
- Third-trimester amniocentesis does not appear to be associated with significant risk of complications leading to emergency delivery (SOR: B).

Chorionic Villus Sampling

In CVS, another technique for obtaining fetal tissue for genetic evaluation, the chorionic villi, or placental cells, are aspirated. With ultrasound guidance, CVS can be performed at 10 to 13 menstrual weeks transabdominally with a spinal needle or transvaginally with a catheter designed and approved for this purpose. Chromosomal analysis of the villous cells can be completed in 7 days. Thus the advantage to CVS is the early gestational time of the procedure and availability of the results. The procedure-related fetal loss rate is approximately 1 in 125 tests (Jackson et al., 1992).

Maternal Biochemical Screening

Low-risk women can be offered screening for genetic abnormalities of the fetus by biochemical testing in the first or second trimester and ultrasound nuchal translucency screening (first trimester) and targeted ultrasound evaluation of fetal anatomy, best done at 18 to 20 weeks' gestation. The general consensus is that women of any age should have access to any screening or diagnostic testing (as previously described) if they choose to accept the underlying risks.

Biochemical testing is the measurement of certain chemicals in the mother's blood found to be predictive of fetal abnormality. The quadruple screen is a maternal blood test in which one maternal sample drawn at 15 to 20 weeks (but most sensitive at 16 to 18 weeks) is assayed for alpha fetoprotein, estriols, and beta subunit of human chorionic gonadotropin (hCG). Normal ranges vary for each gestational week. Maternal serum alpha-fetoprotein (MSAFP) elevations can result from open neural tube defects such as spina bifida or anencephaly, when the protein leaks from the fetal tissue into the amniotic fluid through the amniochorion and into the maternal system. A lower-than-expected MSAFP suggests Down syndrome. The addition of β subunit of hCG and estriols has improved sensitivity for the detection of chromosomal abnormalities (Table 21-5). This test should be offered to any pregnant women with appropriate counseling regarding sensitivity and specificity. Women with abnormal tests should be referred for targeted ultrasound and possibly amniocentesis.

First-trimester ultrasound and biochemical screening are now available for clinical use, specifically the "First Trimester Screen" performed between 10 weeks, 2 days and 13 weeks, 6 days of gestation. Testing involves an ultrasound measurement of the nuchal translucency (lymphatic fluid at fetal neck) (Fig. 21-4) and laboratory measurement of pregnancy-associated plasma protein A (PAPP-A) and β subunit

Table 21-5 Second-Trimester Quadruple-Screen Results

Biochemical Results

	α-Fetoprotein	Estriols	β-HCG	Inhibin A
Down syndrome	Decreased	Decreased	Increased	Increased
Trisomy 18	Decreased	Decreased	Decreased	No change to decreased
Open neural tube defect*	Increased	**	**	**

Capabilities Statistics

	Detection Sensitivity	False-Positive Rate	Positive Predictive Value
Down syndrome	77%-79%	3%-5%	3.7%
Trisomy 18	60%	2%-4%	2.2%
Open neural tube defect*	90%	4.0%	2.5%

*Most sensitive at 16 to 18 weeks of gestation.
**Not used for neural tube defect screening.
HCG, Human chorionic gonadotropin.

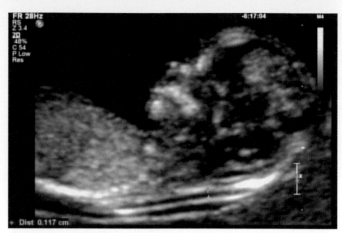

Figure 21-4 Transabdominal ultrasound assessment of nuchal translucency (NT). The measurement in this figure is normal. An increased measure (>3 mm) is associated with an increased risk of chromosomal abnormalities, complex congenital heart disease, and other genetic syndromes.

of hCG. The First Trimester Screen has about 85% sensitivity for Down syndrome detection at 4% false-positive rate. Several tests are also available that combine a first-trimester screen with a second-trimester screen for even higher sensitivity. Physicians should become familiar with the sensitivity, specificity, and availability of the test most suitable for their practices.

EVIDENCE-BASED SUMMARY

- First-trimester screening using both nuchal translucency measurement and biochemical markers is an effective screening test for Down syndrome in the general population (SOR: A).
- Women found to have increased risk of aneuploidy with first-trimester screening should be offered genetic counseling and the option of chorionic villus sampling or second-trimester amniocentesis (SOR: A).

Drug and Chemical Exposures in Pregnancy

Pregnant women frequently ask about the effect of drug and other chemical exposures on the unborn infant, whether environmental, OTC, or prescription. Many of these are everyday exposures at the workplace, in the community, or as a result of medical treatment and management.

The consequences can range from the most innocuous to actually jeopardizing the pregnancy. The physician should be prepared to answer these pregnancy-related questions and advise their patients appropriately.

The consequences of a chemical exposure may be related to the nature of the agent and the timing, dose, and duration of the exposure. The effect can range from minor morphologic abnormalities and growth deficiency to severe malformation and loss of the pregnancy. Thalidomide has obvious effects on the fetus, causing a third of fetuses to have limb reduction defects. Furthermore, the effect of a drug may be subtle or delayed (Welch et al., 1993). Diethylstilbestrol (DES) is associated with the development of uterine structural abnormalities and clear cell carcinoma of the vagina in daughters whose mothers took this medication.

Much of the knowledge about chemical exposures and effects on reproduction and fetal development comes from research on experimental animals. This poses great uncertainty given genetic variability and species-specific responses. Given these limitations, the health care provider must carefully weigh the evidence before using a drug. To help the practitioner classify a drug for use, the U.S. Food and Drug Administration (FDA, 1980) developed a risk factors index. The abbreviated definitions of these categories are as follows:

Category A: Controlled studies in women fail to demonstrate a risk to the fetus.

Category B: Animal reproduction studies have not demonstrated a fetal risk, but there are no controlled studies in pregnant women; or animal reproduction studies have shown adverse effect that was not confirmed in controlled human studies.

Category C: Studies in animals have revealed adverse effects on the fetus, and there are no controlled studies in women. Drugs should be given only if the potential benefit justifies the potential risk to the fetus.

Category D: There is positive evidence of human fetal risk, but the benefits from use in pregnant women may be acceptable.

Category X: Studies in animals or humans have demonstrated fetal abnormalities, or there is evidence of fetal risk based on human experience. The drug is contraindicated in women who are or who may become pregnant.

Table 21-6 Drugs and Exposures in Pregnancy

Agent	Recommendation	Comments
Antihistamines	Acceptable	Most are category B.
Decongestants	Acceptable	Pseudoephedrine preferred.
Cough medication with guaifenesin	Acceptable	—
Acetaminophen	Acceptable	Preferred analgesic and antipyretic.
Aspirin	Avoid	Increases risk of bleeding; no benefit in preeclampsia; may be prescribed in low doses for specific conditions.
NSAIDs	Avoid	Premature closure of ductus arteriosus.
Cephalosporins	Acceptable	—
Sulfonamides	Avoid in third trimester.	Kernicterus in newborn.
Tetracyclines	Avoid	Discoloration of teeth.
ACE inhibitors	Avoid	Stillborn, renal abnormalities, renal failure in newborn.
Immunizations	Avoid live, attenuated viruses.	Measles, mumps, rubella.
Allergy shots	Acceptable	Alteration in maintenance dose may be necessary.

Modified from Hueston WJ, Eolers GM, King DE, McGlaughlin VG. Common questions patients ask during pregnancy. Am Fam Physician 1995;51:1465-1470.
ACE, Angiotensin-converting enzyme; *NSAIDs,* nonsteroidal anti-inflammatory drugs.

This classification is an oversimplification, and the individual practitioner will need to weigh the available data in the management of the pregnant woman. Few absolutes are possible in the field of human teratology; however, current recommendations for common drug categories in pregnancy are summarized in Table 21-6. It is important to emphasize that it is difficult to demonstrate an actual cause-effect relationship between a specific drug and an adverse pregnancy outcome. At no time, however, should a drug be considered safe because no data exist.

Infections in Pregnancy

Although a woman is subject to many of the same infections during pregnancy as when not pregnant, specific infectious diseases have implications on fetal development and complications of pregnancy, such as premature labor and premature rupture of membranes. Certain infections in pregnancy can be teratogenic to the fetus, particularly if infections occur in the first trimester. These agents have been given the acronym of TORCH for toxoplasmosis, other (e.g., syphilis), rubella, cytomegalovirus, and herpesvirus. Although not teratogenic, HIV may be transmitted to the fetus and may be lethal in the child.

Toxoplasmosis

The causative agent of toxoplasmosis is *Toxoplasma gondii,* a parasite that usually infects rodents. Based on serologic studies, approximately one third of reproductive-age women have had toxoplasmosis. In the United States, maternal infection is thought to occur in about 0.5%. Congenital toxoplasmosis can only occur when active infection occurs during pregnancy. Recognizable damage to newborns is estimated to occur in about 1 in 10,000 births; incidence of infected but asymptomatic newborns is unknown. Maternal infections that occur in the first trimester are more likely to cause abortion and significant fetal damage. Infections later in pregnancy tend to be asymptomatic at birth.

A pregnant woman can contract toxoplasmosis by eating raw meat containing the cysts of the organism or by fecal-oral transmission of the oocytes from an infected cat. Cats that are fed cooked or canned food are most often not infectious. Those that obtain rodents from the wild are more at risk. Pregnant women should avoid changing cat litter and handling cats, particularly those cats allowed to roam outdoors. Maternal toxoplasmosis may be asymptomatic or may present as a mononucleosis-like syndrome. Congenital disease ranges from overwhelming, including seizures, microcephaly or hydrocephaly, chorioretinitis, hepatosplenomegaly, jaundice, microphthalmia, and cataracts, to less symptomatic, which usually involves chorioretinitis. Prenatal ultrasound or postnatal brain scan can also show intracranial calcifications. The placenta should be examined pathologically for cysts of *T. gondii* (Beasley and Egerman, 1998).

The diagnosis of toxoplasmosis is serologic, looking for immunoglobulin G (IgG) and IgM by enzyme-linked immunosorbent assay (ELISA). Some assays have a high level of false-positive results. Laboratories well versed in performing these serologic tests should be used. Pyrimethamine and sulfadiazine can treat women who acquire the infection prenatally. Effectiveness of treatment protocols for prevention of congenital infection appears variable (Wallon et al., 1999). Screening of all pregnant women is not recommended at this time.

Syphilis

Syphilis is a treatable infection caused by *Treponema pallidum,* a motile spirochete. In the pregnant woman, infection is most often sexually transmitted. The infection is described in four stages: primary, secondary, latent, and tertiary or late. It is rare to see pregnant women in tertiary or late syphilis (Sheffield and Wendel, 1999).

Pregnancy has little effect on the course of syphilis, but syphilis has a substantial effect on pregnancy and the fetus. Stages with spirochetemia are the most deleterious for the fetus. This is most often seen in late primary syphilis and in secondary syphilis. An increase in miscarriage, hydrops fetalis, stillborn, and preterm delivery of an infected fetus can be seen. Penicillin is the only antibiotic currently recommended for syphilis treatment in pregnancy because of its safety, efficacy, and transplacental passage to treat the fetus (CDC, 1999). Penicillin-allergic women should undergo desensitization first. Whenever treatment adequacy is questioned in pregnancy, repeat therapy should occur because congenital syphilis is a preventable disorder. All women with syphilis should be carefully evaluated for other STDs, in particular HIV, as the treatment and surveillance is different in co-infection and the possibility of neurosyphilis must be carefully evaluated.

Rubella

Congenital rubella was first recognized in 1941, when after a rubella epidemic, a large number of children born to infected mothers were noted to have cataracts. Immunization against the rubella virus in the United States, Canada, and many European countries has decreased maternal rubella and thus congenital rubella. In the United States, only a few cases of congenital rubella are reported per year. Attention is now directed at its eradication in developing countries (Banatvala, 1998).

Although maternal infection can be subclinical, it usually presents 14 to 21 days after exposure with a maculopapular rash that begins on the face and spreads to the neck, trunk, arms, and legs. It is associated with lymphadenopathy, malaise, arthralgias, and petechiae. There is no therapy other than supportive. Pregnant women found not to have immunity to rubella should be instructed to avoid individuals who have viral illnesses. Suspected infection should be documented by specific rubella IgG and IgM measurement or by viral culture of the mother.

Maternal rubella acquired in the first trimester of pregnancy has a high risk of conferring damage to the developing fetus, and documented cases should be counseled and pregnancy interruption offered. In congenital rubella syndrome, many abnormalities can be found, such as cataracts, chorioretinitis, microphthalmia, congenital heart disease, myocarditis, microcephaly, deafness, mental retardation, and bone lesions, as well as signs of systemic infection (pneumonitis, hepatosplenomegaly, hepatitis, thrombocytopenia) (Stamos and Rowley, 1994).

Cytomegalovirus

Two percent of pregnant women will develop primary cytomegalovirus (CMV) infection, obtained by direct contact or respiratory aerosol from an infected individual. They will most often be asymptomatic or have mild generalized symptoms such as fatigue, malaise, fever, lymphadenopathy, and pharyngitis. Approximately 50% of fetuses whose mothers seroconvert during pregnancy will develop CMV infection, but only 10 to 15% of these will have damage from the infection. Hearing loss is the most common manifestation.

Fetal infection and damage are more likely in the first and second trimesters. Although hearing loss is the most common presentation, congenital CMV can also present with microcephaly or hydrocephalus, microphthalmia, mental retardation, and brain calcifications. Overwhelming fetal infection at birth, known as cytomegalic inclusion disease, is uncommon, is most often caused by maternal primary infection late in gestation, and is often fatal.

Recurrent CMV infection in pregnancy can also cause infection of the fetus, but rarely fetal damage (Stagno, 1982).

Thus, documented immunity to CMV with serologic studies performed before a pregnancy can be reassuring to women at risk of exposure, such as child care providers or health care workers. General screening for CMV in pregnancy is not recommended at present. Suspected CMV infection should be documented by serology or cultures of the cervix, amniotic fluid, or maternal urine.

Herpesvirus

Herpes simplex virus type 2 (HSV-2) is the causative agent in most cases of genital herpes, with a few cases caused by HSV-1, which most often causes oropharyngeal herpes. Primary infection is most deleterious for both mother and fetus and can present as fever, malaise, inguinal lymphadenopathy, and urinary retention. At 2 to 10 days after exposure, vesicles containing numerous viral particles painfully erupt on the cervix, vagina, perineum, or rectum; ulcerate; and remain open 1 to 3 weeks. Herpetic lesions in recurrent disease last a shorter period and are most often not associated with systemic symptoms.

The fetus is most susceptible to herpesvirus infection and damage during viremia, which most often occurs in primary herpes. At that time, herpes-specific maternal IgG is not adequate for transplacental passage and protection of the fetus from serious disease. The fetus may also acquire a herpetic infection from delivery through an infected vaginal canal. If this occurs during a primary episode, the risk of congenital infection is about 50%; if during a recurrent infection, the risk is much less than 8%. Congenital herpes may be localized to skin, eyes, and oral cavity and may involve the central nervous system (CNS). Congenital infection may be disseminated and is often fatal or entirely asymptomatic (Riley, 1998).

Various surveillance protocols have been attempted to decrease perinatal transmission at delivery. At present, at labor and delivery, a careful evaluation of the genital tract for ulcers is performed. If any active lesions are found, the baby is delivered by cesarean section (Roberts et al., 1995). Prenatal use of acyclovir is controversial, but it has been used with informed consent in pregnant women with systemic disease or frequent episodes of recurrent disease.

Human Immunodeficiency Virus

Human immunodeficiency virus is a retrovirus transmitted through infected secretions, most often sexually. The most serious consequence of HIV infection in pregnancy is transmission to the fetus resulting in the birth of an HIV–congenitally infected newborn. Maternal HIV is not teratogenic or associated with increased fetal loss (except end-stage disease). The goal in pregnancy is identification of HIV disease and prevention of perinatal transmission. At-risk women include hemophiliacs, intravenous drug users, prostitutes, and female partners of infected men. Although most often seen in urban areas, HIV infection in women is rising throughout the United States.

Screening for HIV is recommended and should be offered to all pregnant women. At-risk women should be screened more than once during the pregnancy. Testing for IgG antibody with ELISA is the basis of screening for an HIV infection. Western blot or another, more specific test confirms all positive tests. If a pregnant woman is found to have HIV infection, specific counseling should be given, often best done in a center familiar with its treatment and management. Interruption of pregnancy should be offered. In ongoing pregnancies, specific therapy should be instituted to prevent perinatal transmission.

Zidovudine administration in HIV-infected pregnant women from 14 to 34 weeks' gestation decreased perinatal HIV transmission from 25.5% to 8.3% (Connor et al., 1994). The regimen included antepartum zidovudine (100 mg orally five times daily), intrapartum zidovudine (2 mg/kg body weight intravenously over 1 hour, then 1 mg/kg/hr until delivery). Zidovudine is given to the newborn (2 mg/kg orally every 6 hours for 6 weeks). This therapeutic regimen is currently used in pregnancy. However, combination therapy, including reverse-transcriptase inhibitors, is recommended by some experts (Rose, 1998).

Pregnant women on zidovudine therapy must be followed for bone marrow suppression and liver toxicity on a monthly basis. Although long-term studies are not available, the drug appears safe for the fetus. The quantity of viral load (HIV-1 RNA) in the mother appears to be a significant risk factor to fetal infection (Mofenson et al., 1999). Mode of delivery is controversial, with many experts recommending cesarean section to those women with high viral load. During vaginal delivery, artificial rupture of membranes and placement of a scalp electrode onto the fetal head are contraindicated. Amniocentesis and breastfeeding are also contraindicated in HIV-infected women.

EVIDENCE-BASED SUMMARY

- Pregnant women should be offered screening for HIV infection early in pregnancy because appropriate antenatal interventions can reduce maternal-to-child transmission (SOR: A).
- Women diagnosed as HIV positive during pregnancy should be informed that interventions such as antiretroviral therapy, cesarean section, and avoidance of breastfeeding can reduce the risk of mother-to child HIV transmission (SOR: A).
- Amniocentesis and breastfeeding are contraindicated in HIV-infected pregnant patients (SOR: A).

Influenza and Novel Influenza A (H1N1) Virus

The influenza virus poses a particular threat to the pregnant patient. The majority of pregnant women with novel influenza A (H1N1) or the regular seasonal influenza virus infection will present with typical acute upper respiratory, influenza-like illness (e.g., cough, sore throat, rhinorrhea) and fever. Other symptoms can include body aches, headache, fatigue, vomiting, and diarrhea. Most pregnant women have an uncomplicated disease course. However, pregnant women appear to be at higher risk for severe complications from influenza infection, and for some, illness might progress rapidly and may be complicated by secondary bacterial infections, including pneumonia and evidence of fetal distress. Case reports of adverse pregnancy outcomes and maternal deaths have been associated with severe illness and death. Ideally, pregnant women who have suspected novel influenza A (H1N1) virus infection should be tested for influenza, although commercially available rapid-testing kits have limited sensitivity.

Treatment should not be delayed pending results of testing or withheld in the absence of testing. Antiviral treatment is most effective when started as early as possible after the onset of symptoms (i.e. within first 2 days). The highest priority is to treat pregnant women with influenza-like symptoms as soon as possible. The currently novel influenza A (H1N1) virus is sensitive to the neuraminidase inhibitor antiviral medications zanamivir (Relenza) and oseltamivir (Tamiflu). Pregnancy should not be considered a contraindication to oseltamivir or zanamivir use. Because pregnant women may be at higher risk, the benefits of treatment or chemoprophylaxis with oseltamivir or zanamivir outweigh the theoretic risks of antiviral use. The Advisory Committee on Immunization Practices recommends that 2009/10 H1N1 monovalent flu and the seasonal flu vaccine be given to all pregnant women at any time during pregnancy. The American College of Obstetricians and Gynecologists (ACOG) and AAFP also recommend routine vaccination of all pregnant women. The nasal spray vaccine is not approved for use by pregnant women. Pregnant women should not receive nasal spray vaccine for either seasonal flu or 2009/10 H1N1 flu.

KEY TREATMENT

Pregnant women with confirmed, probable, or suspected novel influenza A (H1N1) infection should receive antiviral therapy with oseltamivir (Tamiflu) (CDC, 2009) (SOR: C).

Immunizations in Pregnancy

Immunizations that are not live, attenuated viruses are not contraindicated in pregnancy. Measles, mumps, and rubella (MMR) are the most common vaccines with live, attenuated viruses and should be avoided during pregnancy, although retrospective assessment of risks to the fetus has not documented a significant risk. Vaccines made of viral coat and not the complete virus are safe to administer in pregnancy; for example, influenza vaccinations are recommended. However, the pregnant woman should receive the injected vaccine and not the nasal spray, which is the live, attenuated virus.

Medical Disorders in Pregnancy

Many medical disorders can be seen in the pregnant woman; few are incompatible with pregnancy. In the management and care of the pregnant woman with a medical illness, it is important to understand the normal physiology of pregnancy and the effect of the disorder on the pregnancy, and vice versa. Common medical problems in pregnancy include anemia, asthma, hypertension, diabetes, and pyelonephritis. Women with moderate to severe preexisting medical illness should be referred for evaluation to a physician experienced in managing the disorder in pregnancy.

Anemia

Iron deficiency anemia during pregnancy has been associated with an increased risk of LBW, preterm delivery, and perinatal mortality. Normal physiologic changes in intravascular volume cause a physiologic anemia of pregnancy.

However, a severe anemia with maternal hemoglobin (Hgb, Hb) levels less than 6 g/dL has been associated with abnormal fetal oxygenation, resulting in nonreassuring fetal heart rate pattern, reduced amniotic fluid volume, fetal cerebral vasodilatation, and fetal death. In normal singleton pregnancy, blood volume increases approximately 36%, plasma volume 47%, and red blood cell (RBC) mass 17%, causing a relative hemodilution throughout pregnancy, but most pronounced after 28 weeks' gestation. Thus, Hb, hematocrit (Hct), and RBC count will be lower than normal, but RBC indices, specifically the mean corpuscular volume (MCV), mean corpuscular hemoglobin (MCH), and mean corpuscular hemoglobin concentration (MCHC), remain normal. Iron, iron-binding capacity, and ferritin remain unchanged. Hb less than 15 mg/dL and Hct less than 33% is generally considered nonphysiologic anemia in pregnancy.

The most common nonphysiologic anemia encountered in pregnancy is iron deficiency. *Iron deficiency anemia* is suspected when the RBC indices are low and there are microcytic, hypochromic RBCs on the peripheral blood smear. This anemia is confirmed by a low serum iron concentration, high total iron binding capacity, and low ferritin. Risk factors for iron deficiency anemia in otherwise healthy women include poor nutrition, menstrual loss, and short interconceptual period. Reproductive-age women have low-normal to abnormal iron stores for this reason. Iron requirements in pregnancy put an increased demand on maternal iron stores because iron is actively transported across the placenta to the fetus regardless of maternal stores. Iron supplementation decreases the prevalence of maternal anemia at delivery, and without iron supplementation in pregnancy, many women will become iron deficient. The recommendation is 30 mg of elemental iron in the form of simple salts such as ferrous sulfate, gluconate, or fumarate. Iron deficiency anemia should be treated with 60 to 120 mg of elemental iron in two or three divided doses daily, which can cause gastric irritation and constipation. More frequent administration has not been shown to improve absorption. Because iron demands in pregnancy are highest after 20 weeks' gestation, depending on the degree of anemia, full-dose iron therapy can be delayed until that time, when pregnancy-associated nausea and vomiting should have subsided. Dietary modifications or stool softeners may be required when pregnant women take large doses of iron.

The failure to respond to appropriate iron therapy should prompt further investigation and may suggest an incorrect diagnosis, coexisting disease, malabsorption (sometimes caused by enteric-coated tablets or concomitant antacids), patient noncompliance, or ongoing blood loss. Hypochromic, microcytic RBCs with an MCV of less than 80 suggest thalassemia. Hemoglobin electrophoresis should also be performed when evaluating hypochromic, microcytic anemia. Iron deficiency anemia and beta-thalassemia can coexist. Megaloblastic anemia from folic acid deficiency is unlikely in the pregnant woman because many reproductive-age women take at least 400 µg of folic acid daily. Any other anemia may occur in pregnancy. Its diagnosis and therapy should be prompt to ensure a healthy outcome for the fetus. Hereditary anemias have the additional implication of possible inheritance by the fetus that should be addressed with the pregnant woman.

EVIDENCE-BASED SUMMARY

- Iron supplementation decreases the prevalence of maternal anemia at delivery (SOR: A).
- Iron deficiency anemia during pregnancy has been associated with an increased risk of low birth weight, preterm delivery, and perinatal mortality (SOR: B).
- Severe anemia with maternal hemoglobin levels less than 6 g/dL has been associated with abnormal fetal oxygenation; thus maternal transfusion should be considered for fetal indications (SOR: B).

Data from ACOG, 2008a.

Asthma

Asthma is caused by reversible airway obstruction from bronchial smooth muscle contraction, excessive secretions, and edema in response to various stimuli, most often infectious or allergic. Airway obstruction is most severe in expiration, making breathing difficult and fatiguing. Asthma is a chronic illness with acute exacerbations.

Approximately 4% of pregnant women will have asthma with severity varying from mild to life threatening. One third of pregnant asthmatic patients will experience exacerbations of their disease (Stenius-Aarnaila et al., 1988). Women with severe asthma are more likely to have disease exacerbation while pregnant. Additionally, moderate to severe asthma can have a significant effect on pregnancy, including an increase in preterm labor, LBW, perinatal mortality, and preeclampsia.

In normal pregnancy, progesterone causes an increase in tidal volume and thus minute ventilation, to make more oxygen available for the fetus (Table 21-7). These changes result in a mild respiratory alkalosis that should be taken into account when interpreting blood gas values (Table 21-8).

Table 21-7 Pulmonary Function Changes in Pregnancy

Parameter	Nonpregnant Value	Pregnant Value
Tidal volume (V_T) (amount of air moved in one respiratory cycle)	450 mL	600 mL
Respiratory rate (breaths/min)	16-18	Same
Minute ventilation (volume of air moved/min)	7.2 L	9.6 L
Forced expiratory volume in 1 second (FEV_1)	80%-85% of VC	Same
Peak expiratory flow rate (PEFR)	380-550 L/min	Same
Forced vital capacity (FVC) (largest amount of air that can by exhaled after maximum filling of lungs)	3.5 L	Same
Residual volume (RV) (amount of air left in lungs after maximum expiration)	1000 mL	800 mL

Modified from Cugell DW, Frank NR, Gaensler EA, Badger TL. Pulmonary function in pregnancy. I. Serial observations in normal women. Am Rev Tuberc 1953;67:568.

Evaluation and management of acute asthma should include objective assessment of maternal lung function and fetal well-being; avoidance or control of environmental precipitating factors; pharmacologic therapy; and patient education (Clark, 1993). The best respiratory parameter to measure for assessment of the degree of obstruction in asthmatic patients is FEV_1 (see Table 21-7). This requires formal pulmonary function testing, so it is not a practical tool for monitoring. However, this value can be estimated by measuring the peak expiratory flow rate (PEFR) using an inexpensive portable peak-flow meter. Women with moderate to severe asthma should monitor their PEFR several times daily while pregnant. Normal PEFR for pregnant as well as nonpregnant women is 380 to 550 L/min. PEFR can be used to diagnose an exacerbation early, as well as for evaluation of therapy.

Pharmacologic therapy in the pregnant asthmatic patient is similar to that in the nonpregnant woman. The main goal of therapy is to maintain adequate oxygenation for the mother and fetus. The arterial oxygen partial pressure (PaO_2) should be kept above 60 mm Hg and oxygen saturation (SO_2) at least 95%. In acute exacerbations during pregnancy, the clinician should have a lower threshold for hospital admission and intubation. Women in the late second trimester and the third trimester should also have fetal monitoring.

Ultrasonography to detect IUGR of the fetus in the moderate to severe asthmatic patient is warranted. If IUGR is diagnosed, antenatal testing should be performed. During labor and delivery, the F-series prostaglandins, in particular prostaglandin $F_{2\alpha}$ (Hemabate), should be avoided because it stimulates bronchial smooth muscle to constrict. Instead, prostaglandin E_2 (Prostin E_2), which causes bronchodilation, should be used.

Chronic Hypertension

Historically, there have been many classifications of hypertension in pregnancy with no apparent consensus. In this chapter we use the now-accepted classification as developed by the National Institutes of Health (Report of the National High Blood Pressure Education Program Working Group on High Blood Pressure in Pregnancy). Hypertension during pregnancy is categorized as (1) preeclampsia/eclampsia, (2) gestational hypertension, (3) chronic hypertension, or (4) preeclampsia superimposed on chronic hypertension (Box 21-5). These categories identify different disorders that at times overlap but with different epidemiologic characteristics, pathophysiology, and risks for mother and baby. Pregnancy-induced hypertensive disorder is an older, less specific term no longer in general use.

Preexisting hypertension often complicates pregnancy. A diagnosis of chronic hypertension is made when hypertension precedes pregnancy or is diagnosed before 20 weeks of gestation. In normal pregnancy, arterial blood pressure (BP) and peripheral vascular resistance (PVR) fall shortly after implantation of the conception. Normal first-trimester and early second-trimester BP ranges from 92 to 114 mm Hg systolic, 46 to 66 diastolic sitting, and 103 to 123 systolic, 47 to 67 diastolic supine. At 28 to 30 weeks' gestation, BP in normal pregnant women increases to near prepregnancy range. It is generally accepted that BP greater than 130/80 mm Hg at any time during pregnancy is abnormal.

Fetal effects of chronic or essential hypertension depend on severity of hypertension and range from none to IUGR, fetal distress, abruptio placentae, prematurity, and fetal death (Haddad and Sibai, 1999). Women with preexisting hypertension have approximately a 20% chance of developing superimposed preeclampsia. The maternal and fetal morbidity and mortality are higher in chronic hypertension with superimposed preeclampsia than in each disorder alone.

Most women with chronic hypertension will present at their first prenatal visit with the diagnosis. As many as one third of pregnant women with essential hypertension will become normotensive in the first half of pregnancy. Often, their antihypertensive medications can be discontinued and only restarted when elevations recur, typically after 28 weeks. Controversy exists as to whether medical treatment of essential hypertension in pregnancy improves fetal outcome or decreases the risk of superimposed preeclampsia. However, maternal complications can occur when diastolic BP is persistently elevated. Thus, it is generally accepted that therapy to decrease maternal BP be instituted or modified to keep maternal diastolic BP lower than 100 to 105 mm Hg. A profound drop in maternal BP over a short period should be avoided to prevent decreased cardiac output to the placenta and fetus.

Alpha-methyldopa (Aldomet), a central-acting, alpha-adrenergic, false neurotransmitter, is the drug of choice for treatment of chronic hypertension in pregnancy. The initial starting dose is 250 mg every 8 hours. This dose can be increased to 2 g/day if needed. If adequate control cannot be obtained, a second drug, most often nifedipine or hydralazine, can be added. Also, with its safety confirmed in pregnancy, labetalol is gaining popularity for use as first-line single-agent therapy. ACE inhibitors and diuretics for BP control are contraindicated in pregnancy (Witlin and Sibai, 1998).

Obstetric management includes baseline laboratory studies early in pregnancy that will later help in diagnosis of superimposed preeclampsia. Specifically, in addition to routine prenatal testing, this includes renal function studies, liver enzymes, platelets, uric acid, and 24-hour urine test for protein and creatinine clearance. If chronic hypertension is a new diagnosis, pheochromocytoma should be ruled out by catecholamine levels in serum or 24-hour urine (Keely, 1998). Early ultrasonography to confirm dating and intermittently to evaluate

Table 21-8 Normal Arterial Blood Gas Values in Pregnancy

	pH	PCO_2 (mm Hg)	PO_2 (mm Hg)
Normal	7.40	35-40	75-100
Pregnancy	7.45	27-32	90-108

Box 21-5 Classification of Hypertensive Disorders in Pregnancy

Chronic hypertension
Preeclampsia/eclampsia
Preeclampsia superimposed on chronic hypertension
Gestational hypertension
1. Transient hypertension of pregnancy if preeclampsia is not present at delivery and blood pressure returns to normal by 12 weeks postpartum.
2. Chronic hypertension if the elevation persists.

fetal growth will aid in the diagnosis of IUGR. Women with moderate to severe hypertension benefit from more frequent prenatal visits as well as home BP monitoring. Antenatal testing should be performed at least for women with superimposed preeclampsia or IUGR. Preterm delivery may occur.

KEY TREATMENT

Alpha-methyldopa (Aldomet), a central-acting alpha-adrenergic, false neurotransmitter, is the drug of choice for treatment of chronic hypertension in pregnancy (SOR: C).

Gestational Diabetes

Gestational diabetes, or diabetes diagnosed in pregnancy, affects 3% to 5% of pregnant women. Pregnancy is a state of increasing insulin resistance predominantly caused by placentally produced hormones, in particular human placental lactogen, which increases with placental mass and gestational age. Although most women can compensate, a small subset of pregnant women cannot. Early impairment of glucose metabolism may have no maternal signs or symptoms, but can have fetal effects that include macrosomia, fetal distress, and fetal demise.

Screening for gestational diabetes by a glucose challenge is recommended at 26 to 28 weeks of gestation. There is little evidence supporting earlier screening. The U.S. Preventive Services Task Force (USPSTF), however, concludes that the current evidence is insufficient to assess the balance of benefits and harms of screening for gestational diabetes mellitus (GDM), either before or after 24 weeks' gestation and recommends that clinicians should discuss screening for GDM with their patients and make case-by-case decisions. Discussions should include information about the uncertainty of benefits and harms as well as the frequency of positive screening test results. Women who are obese, older than 25, have a family history of type 2 diabetes or gestational diabetes, or are members of certain ethnic groups, such as Hispanics, native Americans, Asians, and African Americans, are at increased risk for gestational diabetes.

The initial screening test is performed in a nonfasting state. The pregnant woman is asked to drink a mixture containing 50 g of glucose; 1 hour later a plasma glucose level is performed. If the result is 140 mg/dL or greater, the more definitive 100-g 3-hour glucose challenge is performed. The pregnant woman should have at least 3 days of adequate carbohydrate intake, fast the night before the test, and receive 100 g of glucose. Venous blood glucose is determined fasting and at 1, 2, and 3 hours after the glucose challenge. Two abnormal values make the diagnosis of gestational diabetes (Table 21-9). Different studies have various thresholds for making the diagnosis, and clinicians should review their institutional norms (Carpenter and Coustan, 1982) (Table 21-10). Women at high risk for gestational diabetes, such as those with glucosuria, prior gestational diabetes, obesity, or strong family history, should be screened earlier in pregnancy. If negative, testing should be repeated in the latter half. The evidence supporting this practice is variable.

Initial therapies of gestational diabetes are diet and, if not contraindicated in the pregnancy, exercise in the form of walking, as well as support from diabetes educators and nutritionists and increased surveillance in prenatal care. The daily recommendation is 30 to 35 kcal/kg lean body weight. If fasting blood sugar cannot be maintained below 105 and

Table 21-9 Screening for Gestational Diabetes[*]

Test	Abnormal Glucose Level (mg/dL)
50-g glucose, 1-hour challenge	≥140
100-g glucose, 3-hour challenge[*]:	
Fasting	≥105
1 hour	≥190
2 hour	≥165
3 hour	≥145

From National Diabetes Data Group, 1979.
[*]Two abnormal values needed for diagnosis of gestational diabetes.

Table 21-10 Diagnosis of Gestational Diabetes Mellitus

OGTT	NDDG[*]	Carpenter[†]
Fasting	105	95
1 hour	190	180
2 hour	165	155
3 hour	145	140

[*]National Diabetes Data Group, 1979.
[†]Carpenter MW, Coustan DR. Criteria for screening tests for gestational diabetes. Am J Obstet Gynecol 1982;144:768-773.
OGTT, Oral glucose tolerance test.

2-hour postprandial blood sugars below 120 mg/dL, insulin therapy is begun. Hemoglobin A_{1c} can be performed every 4 to 6 weeks but will not be elevated unless there is fasting hyperglycemia. At least weekly evaluation of blood sugar is recommended because insulin resistance increases with advancing gestation. Ultrasonography to assess fetal size should be performed every 4 to 6 weeks. Women requiring insulin should have antenatal testing in the third trimester. Good blood sugar control is also important to decrease the incidence of metabolic newborn complications such as hypoglycemia, hypocalcemia, polycythemia, and hyperbilirubinemia.

The family physician should remember that women who have had gestational diabetes have a 30% to 60% chance of developing type 2 diabetes mellitus in their lifetime (O'Sullivan, 1979). Postpartum and yearly glucose tolerance testing is recommended in these women. Weight loss and exercise have been shown to decrease their risk.

EVIDENCE-BASED SUMMARY

- The current evidence is insufficient to assess the balance of benefits and harms of screening for gestational diabetes mellitus (GDM), either before or after 24 weeks gestation.
- Screen for GDM using risk factor analysis and, if appropriate, use of an oral glucose tolerance test (OGTT) (SOR: C).

Data from American Diabetes Association (ADA), 2008; and U.S. Preventive Services Task Force (USPSTF), 2008.

Pyelonephritis

Asymptomatic bacteriuria can be found in 3% to 5% of pregnant women and up to 10% of those with sickle cell trait. Asymptomatic bacteriuria is most often caused by *Escherichia coli*. Antibiotic therapy is similar to that in the nonpregnant state. Cephalosporins, ampicillin, and nitrofurantoin (Macrodantin) are frequently used medications that are safe in pregnancy. It appears best to treat asymptomatic bacteriuria in pregnancy for 5 to 7 days. Untreated, 30% of women with asymptomatic bacteriuria will progress to pyelonephritis. Hormonal and anatomic changes of pregnancy causing hydronephrosis and hydroureter are responsible for the higher incidence of pyelonephritis in the pregnant woman. A urinary pathogen count of at least 100,000 colonies/mL is considered significant, although pyelonephritis also occurs at counts as low as 20,000 to 50,000 (Cunningham and Lucas, 1994). Periodic cultures for screening should be performed in women with sickle cell trait, recurrent urinary tract infection, recurrent asymptomatic bacteriuria, or urine dipstick suggesting bacterial growth, such as positive nitrite.

Pyelonephritis in pregnancy requires hospitalization because of frequently associated dehydration, nausea, vomiting, and premature labor, as well as the uncommon but serious risk of endotoxic shock and endotoxin damage of alveolocapillary membranes leading to pulmonary edema and a clinical picture of adult respiratory distress syndrome (Gurman et al., 1990). Pregnant women with pyelonephritis require hospitalization for aggressive hydration and parenteral antibiotics. Antibiotic treatment is similar to those of other-adult regimens. Intravenous antibiotic therapy with a cephalosporin or an extended-spectrum penicillin until symptoms improve and the fever has completely resolved is usually sufficient for initial therapy. Because 25% of patients with mild acute pyelonephritis who are pregnant have a recurrence, these patients should have monthly urine cultures or antimicrobial suppression with oral nitrofurantoin (Macrodantin), 100 mg daily, until 4 to 6 weeks postpartum. Fluoroquinolones should be avoided because of concerns about their teratogenic effects on the fetus. Oral antibiotics are then prescribed for 7 to 10 additional days. For seriously ill women, the addition of an aminoglycoside at the onset of therapy may be warranted until sensitivities of the offending organism are available. Renal function as well as peak and trough aminoglycoside levels should be followed.

Complications of Early Pregnancy

Ectopic Pregnancy

An ectopic pregnancy occurs when the fertilized ovum implants on any tissue other than the endometrial lining of the uterus. Overall, 95% of all ectopic pregnancies are tubal, 1.5% abdominal, 0.5% ovarian, and 0.03% cervical (Breen, 1970). A *heterotopic pregnancy* is a coexisting intrauterine and extrauterine pregnancy. Historically, there is an increasing incidence reported in the literature to a current rate of about 1 in 4000 pregnancies. This increased rate is thought to be associated with the use of ovarian stimulation and with assisted reproductive technologies. Ectopic pregnancies are responsible for more than 10% of all maternal deaths in the United States (Koonin et al., 1997).

The rate of ectopic pregnancy in women with known history of pelvic inflammatory disease (PID) is 6 to 10 times higher than in women with no prior history. PID usually results from invasion by either gonorrhea or chlamydia from the cervix into the uterus and tubes. The infection in these tissues causes an intense inflammatory reaction. Bacteria, white blood cells, and other fluids fill the tubes as the body combats the infection. During the healing process, however, the delicate tubal mucosa is permanently scarred. The fimbriated end of the fallopian tube as well as the lumen may become partially or completely blocked with scar tissue. If PID is treated very early and aggressively with intravenous (IV) antibiotics, the tubal damage might be minimized and fertility preserved. Other conditions associated with ectopic pregnancies include progestin-bearing intrauterine devices (IUDs), previous tubal surgery, and tubal ligation.

Diagnosis

A common clinical presentation of a woman with an ectopic pregnancy is the classic triad of amenorrhea, abdominal pain, and irregular vaginal bleeding. All women with these symptoms should be evaluated for possible ectopic gestation.

Serum quantitative hCG is often used to help identify those women with ectopic pregnancies. An isolated hCG level is not of much use unless it is above the threshold where one should visualize an intrauterine pregnancy with ultrasound. This threshold may vary depending upon type of hCG assay used and sonographic technique (Peisner and Timor-Tritsch, 1990). Two hCG levels drawn 48 hours apart are more informative. The general rule is a doubling of values in 48 hours. However, one must be careful to give pregnancies with a slow hCG rise every chance possible because they may turn out to be normal. A plateauing of hCG is consistent with an ectopic gestation or abnormal intrauterine pregnancy; ultrasound can be used to differentiate the two.

Serum progesterone levels are of some value in making the diagnosis of ectopic pregnancy (Stovall et al., 1989). A progesterone level less than 15 ng/mL is seen in 81% of ectopic, 93% of abnormal intrauterine, and 11% of normal intrauterine pregnancies. Less than 2% of ectopic pregnancies and less than about 4% of abnormal intrauterine pregnancies will have a progesterone level of 25 ng/mL or greater. Therefore a single progesterone value less than 15 ng/mL is probably an abnormal pregnancy and should prompt further evaluation. A single value greater than 25 ng/mL probably indicates a normal pregnancy.

Ultrasound

Key Point

- Routine screening ultrasound in low-risk pregnancies is not associated with a decrease in perinatal mortality, birth weight, or preterm birth.

With high-resolution vaginal sonography, a normal singleton pregnancy can be seen by $5\frac{1}{2}$ to 6 weeks of pregnancy ($1\frac{1}{2}$ to 2 weeks after the missed period). By this time, the quantitative hCG level has reached the *discriminatory zone*, or the level above which a gestational sac is always visualized. The discriminatory zone may vary from institution to institution because of differences in equipment and assays, but ranges from 800 to 1000 IU/L (Second International Standard), or 1000 to 2000 IU/L (First International Reference Preparation) (Nyberg et al., 1985; Peisner and Timor-Tritsch, 1990).

As many as 20% to 30% of ectopic gestations have no detectable sonographic abnormality. The typical ultrasound findings for ectopic pregnancy are a unilateral mass, fluid in the cul de sac, and no evidence of intrauterine pregnancy. Conclusive diagnosis of an ectopic gestation by sonography can only be made if a fetus or fetal cardiac motion is seen outside the uterus. With vaginal ultrasound, this only occurs in about 20% of ectopic pregnancies.

Management

Treatment for ectopic pregnancy can be medical or surgical. Methotrexate, a folate antagonist, is often used in the medical management of ectopic gestation. It inhibits the rapidly growing trophoblast cells of the early placenta. Several treatment protocols are accepted (Buster and Pisarska, 1999). Most side effects seen with low-dose methotrexate therapy are mild and transient. Resolution of the ectopic state has been reported in about 70% to 95% of cases treated, depending somewhat on selection criteria.

The surgical approaches for ectopic pregnancy include laparoscopy for both confirmation and treatment and occasionally, laparotomy. The procedure of choice is salpingostomy, reserving salpingectomy for women not wanting future fertility.

Spontaneous Abortion

First-trimester miscarriage is a common event. All women with clinically recognized pregnancies have approximately a 15% chance of spontaneous pregnancy loss in the first 3 months of pregnancy (Evans and Beischer, 1970). The risk is lower for younger women and higher for older mothers. Because women can present with symptoms of spontaneous miscarriage even before they are aware of pregnancy, all family physicians should be well versed in its assessment and management.

There are many causes of spontaneous pregnancy loss in the first trimester; sporadic chromosomal aneuploidy accounts for about 60%. The remaining 40% have various etiologies, including chronic maternal illness (e.g., diabetes, connective tissue disorder), uterine structural malformations, certain infections, inadequate progesterone production, and possibly other, less-well-understood causes such as immunologic "rejection" and environmental factors.

Diagnosis

First-trimester miscarriage can be further defined according to stage of pregnancy loss and associated symptoms.

Threatened abortion is diagnosed when the pregnant woman presents with vaginal bleeding, lower back discomfort, or midline pelvic cramping. On examination, the cervical os is closed, and the pregnancy is viable (by Doppler ultrasound). About 25% of women will have some degree of bleeding in the first trimester, about half of whom will miscarry. The remaining women may have a slightly higher risk

of perinatal complications, such as preterm labor and IUGR. The risk of congenital malformations is not increased.

Inevitable abortion occurs when there is profuse bleeding requiring surgical intervention or overt rupture of membranes. Although the cervical os may be initially closed and tissue has not passed, the miscarriage is inevitable.

Incomplete abortion is diagnosed when products of conception have passed the level of the cervical os. There is often heavy vaginal bleeding, midline cramping, and an open cervical os.

Complete abortion occurs when all the gestational products have passed. This is ascertained by examination of the passed products of conception, pelvic ultrasonography to ascertain emptiness of the uterus, and at times retrospectively with falling quantitative hCG levels.

"Missed abortion" is a poor term still in use to describe retention of a nonviable pregnancy for longer than 4 weeks. Ultrasound scans of these women provide a more specific and usually earlier diagnosis, such as empty sac or an embryonic gestation, or fetal demise.

Septic abortion is diagnosed when there is infection of the uterus and products of conception. This occurs most often with incomplete abortions. Fever, uterine tenderness, foul discharge, and leukocytosis should aid the practitioner in making this diagnosis.

Recurrent spontaneous abortion is reserved for those women who have had three or more first-trimester losses. This diagnosis should prompt further evaluation for etiology.

Management

The goal of management of early miscarriage is assurance of complete emptying of the uterus in the least traumatic manner, avoidance of excessive blood loss, prevention of infection, and administration of adequate emotional support. Women with threatened abortions are reassured somewhat that the loss is neither imminent nor inevitable. Bed rest is encouraged, but no evidence supports its value in prevention of miscarriage.

When there is profuse bleeding or sepsis, women with inevitable, incomplete, or septic abortions require prompt surgical treatment in the form of dilation and curettage (D&C), or in some, curettage alone. IV antibiotics should be used when appropriate. Rarely, blood transfusion is required. Certain women may benefit from oral antibiotics and methylergonovine (Methergine) on discharge.

When the diagnosis is missed abortion or incomplete abortion without hemorrhage or infection, the choice is surgical intervention versus natural spontaneous completion of the miscarriage. In well-selected women, no convincing evidence suggests one method is preferable. Many practitioners give these patients the option of D&C or spontaneous resolution. D&C has risks of anesthesia, cervical trauma, uterine scarring, and perforation; spontaneous resolution has risks of infection and hemorrhage. If products of conception for karyotype analysis are required for the evaluation of recurrent losses, surgical approach is more successful in producing uncontaminated tissue for culture.

Those women who are Rh(D)-negative and less than 13 weeks' gestation should receive 50 µg of D immune globulin intramuscularly when the abortion is diagnosed, to prevent sensitization. If beyond 13 weeks, 300 µg is used.

This treatment can be omitted if the father is known to be D-negative as well. Iron therapy should be given to women when heavy bleeding occurs or is anticipated.

Molar Pregnancy

A molar pregnancy, or *hydatidiform mole,* is uncommon. A *gestational trophoblastic disease* (GTD), it occurs predominantly in older women. In the United States, molar pregnancy occurs in about 1 in 1800 pregnancies (Grimes, 1984). Molar pregnancy can be classified as complete or incomplete, which are two distinct entities etiologically and pathologically. A *complete* or hydatidiform mole has no fetal components, consists entirely of hydropic placental villi, is frequently associated with medical complications, and has a 15% to 20% risk of GTD (Jones, 1987). In an *incomplete* mole, a fetus, usually abnormal, is often present. The placenta may be hydropic or small, and there is a 5% to 10% risk of GTD.

A hydatidiform mole is most often diagnosed in the first trimester because of symptoms of excessive nausea and vomiting, vaginal bleeding, uterine size larger than expected, and sonographic findings of no fetus but a large placenta with numerous small cysts. These findings should prompt quantitative hCG evaluation, which is often elevated. Evacuation of the uterus with careful attention to levels of hCG postevacuation is important to detect GTD, usually invasive mole, occasionally choriocarcinoma. Pregnancy is avoided for 1 year after a complete mole.

An incomplete mole is most often diagnosed in the second trimester and occasionally the third trimester. There may be an abnormal placenta, fetal growth and structural abnormalities, or signs and symptoms of preeclampsia.

Complications of Late Pregnancy

Preterm Labor

Preterm labor is defined as uterine contractions occurring before 37 weeks of gestation that cause cervical change. Cervical change can be diagnosed if an initial examination reveals a cervix that is at least 2 cm dilated or 80% effaced, or if interval cervical examinations document progression of effacement or dilation. Preterm contractions without cervical advancement can also occur; these do not require intervention. The distinction may be difficult, in particular at the onset of contractions.

Certain women are at higher risk of developing preterm labor (Box 21-6). These women should be assessed more frequently in the prenatal period and instructed on signs and symptoms of premature labor. While many tests to identify women at risk of preterm labor have been proposed and evaluated, only ultrasound for cervical length and fetal fibronectin have been shown to be effective (ACOG, 2001; Iams et al., 1996). A short cervix by transvaginal ultrasound and positive cervicovaginal fetal fibronectin test is predictive of an increased risk of preterm delivery in the index pregnancy.

Assessment of patients thought to be in premature labor involves monitoring for premature contractions as well as fetal heart rate while they are in the right or left lateral recumbent position. Complete history and physical exam should be performed to find any treatable causes

Box 21-6 Risk Factors for Preterm Labor
Low socioeconomic status
Uterine anomalies
African American ethnic group
Uterine leiomyoma
Poor nutritional state
Bacterial vaginosis
Low maternal weight (less than 50 Kg)
Multiple gestation
Poor pregnancy weight gain
Bacteriuria or urinary tract infection
Prior preterm labor
Placenta previa or abruptio
Cocaine use
Polyhydramnios
Nicotine use
Poor prenatal care

of premature labor as well any contraindications to tocolytic therapy. Urinalysis, as well as culture, is obtained and antibiotic therapy instituted if the urinalysis is suspicious. If there is a possibility of rupture of membranes, a sterile speculum examination of the cervix should be performed and vaginal fluid for nitrazine and ferning obtained. Cultures for GBS, *Chlamydia,* and possibly herpesvirus and *Neisseria gonorrhoeae* are often performed in this setting. If there is no historical or physical evidence of rupture of membranes, digital examination of the cervix with careful assessment of consistency as well as dilation and effacement is performed. Chorioamnionitis should be ruled out by assessing degree of uterine tenderness, leukocytosis, maternal fever, and fetal well-being.

In a woman at 22 to 35 weeks' gestation, before digital examination, assessment of the presence of fetal fibronectin can be determined. *Fetal fibronectin* is released from the interface of the chorion and decidua in women likely to deliver preterm. Fetal fibronectin can be determined in 1 hour by most hospital laboratories and is used predominantly for its high negative predictive value. Thus, if a fetal fibronectin is negative, the woman will likely not deliver for at least 7 to 10 days; if positive, closer surveillance or treatment is warranted.

Management

Hydration appears to decrease the frequency of preterm contractions, but it does not decrease the rate of preterm birth. Intermittent digital cervical examinations should be performed either to confirm the diagnosis of preterm labor or to monitor progression. The frequency of these examinations has not been established and should be based on the clinical situation. However, a digital examination should always be performed at discharge to assess any cervical change.

If preterm delivery is a possibility, antibiotic prophylaxis for group B streptococci should be administered (ACOG, 2002a). Betamethasone is also recommended, 12 mg intramuscularly every 24 hours for two doses to accelerate fetal lung maturity in patients between 24 and 34 weeks of gestation (Liggins and Howie, 1972).

If a diagnosis of preterm labor is made and contractions do not subside with bed rest and hydration, pharmacologic therapy is considered. Contraindications to stopping labor include chorioamnionitis, abruptio placentae, heavy vaginal bleeding, severe or chronic hypertension, and fetal demise. Although many tocolytic drugs are available, terbutaline and magnesium sulfate are used often.

Terbutaline at 0.25 mg can be administered subcutaneously every 20 to 30 minutes for three doses. If this is successful, oral therapy can be instituted at doses of 2.5 to 5.0 mg every 2 to 6 hours. Doses should be individualized, allowing maximal efficacy and low side effects. Through beta-1 receptors, beta agonists increase heart rate and thus stroke volume, increase fat breakdown, drive intravascular potassium into cells, and decrease gastrointestinal motility. Through beta-2 receptors, bronchial and uterine smooth muscle relaxation and glycogenolysis occurs. Certain maternal cardiac disorders are a contraindication to this therapy. Women taking beta-adrenergic agonists experience tachycardia, jitteriness, and occasionally nausea and vomiting. Maternal heart rate of 120 beats/min or greater is a contraindication for further dosing, and the interval or quantity may need modification. Fetal heart rate elevations can also be seen.

Intravenous magnesium sulfate therapy can also be used for preterm labor. There is no clear-cut greater efficacy of one tocolytic versus another. Magnesium sulfate relaxes uterine smooth muscle by competitive inhibition of the action of calcium. The dose should be adjusted so that contractions are decreased or abolished but maternal toxicity is not reached. This can be done by frequent examination of deep tendon reflexes, which should be present but depressed. Complete loss of deep tendon reflexes can herald further toxicity, and dosing should be decreased. Plasma magnesium levels can also be performed and should be kept between 5 and 8 mg/dL. Because it is excreted predominantly by the kidney, the plasma magnesium level is influenced by urine output as well as infusion rate. Calcium gluconate should be readily available in case of magnesium toxicity. Women receiving IV magnesium experience warmth, flushing, and poor muscle tone; some develop diplopia, nausea, and vomiting. The majority of these side effects occur with the loading dose. Magnesium sulfate therapy is typically used for 24 hours, then discontinued. Long-term tocolytic therapy has not been shown to be efficacious.

Intrauterine Growth Restriction

Fetuses with IUGR are those that fall below the 10th percentile for weight for a given gestational age. IUGR occurs when a fetus does not meet its growth potential (Vandenbosche and Kirchner, 1998). Some below-10th-percentile fetuses are not growth-restricted but constitutionally small, have reached their growth potential, and are healthy. Often, it is difficult to differentiate the two states.

Although mild growth abnormalities are generally tolerated well by the fetus, more severe growth abnormalities can be associated with poor outcome, including fetal distress, fetal demise, and postnatal developmental abnormalities (Botero and Lifshitz, 1999). The growth-restricted fetus should be identified so that appropriate management can be instituted to ensure the best outcome. Factors that influence fetal growth can be divided into the following three categories:

1. Maternal factors affecting nutrient availability to the fetus, such as poor nutrition and cigarette smoking (Chomitz et al., 1995),
2. Maternal factors influencing placental growth and function, such as maternal hypertension, diabetes with vascular involvement, and connective tissue disorders.
3. Fetal factors interfering with adequate utilization of nutrients despite their availability, such as fetal infection or genetic disorder.

Growth restriction has also been described as asymmetric and symmetric. *Asymmetric* or "head-sparing" IUGR occurs because of fetal autoregulation of blood flow. The initial response to lack of adequate delivery of oxygen and nutrients to the fetus results in shunting of blood flow to important organs such as the brain and adrenal glands. Muscle and other viscera such as kidneys are somewhat underperfused, resulting in smaller body than head, smaller muscle mass, and oligohydramnios due to underperfusion of the fetal kidneys and decreased fetal urine output. If inadequate delivery of oxygen and nutrients is early, persistent, or profound, all organs and tissues of the body will be affected and *symmetric* IUGR ensues. IUGR from fetal infection or genetic disorder is often symmetric as well because all the tissues of the body are often affected.

Diagnosis

The physician can suspect IUGR based on lack of appropriate growth of the uterine fundus. Poor fundal growth with or without risk factors for IUGR should prompt ultrasound evaluation. Women at risk for IUGR should have early sonography to confirm their estimated day of delivery to aid in diagnosis. For example, a woman at 30 weeks' gestation has her first ultrasound for possible IUGR. The fetus is found to be 27 weeks by all parameters measured. It would be

---

EVIDENCE-BASED SUMMARY

- There are no clear "first-line" tocolytic drugs to manage preterm labor; clinical circumstances and physician preferences should dictate treatment (SOR: A).
- Antibiotics do not appear to prolong gestation and should be reserved for group B streptococcal prophylaxis in patients in whom delivery is imminent (SOR: A).
- Neither maintenance treatment with tocolytic drugs nor repeated acute tocolysis improves perinatal outcome; neither should be undertaken as a general practice (SOR: A).
- Tocolytic drugs may prolong pregnancy for 2 to 7 days, which may allow for administration of steroids to improve fetal lung maturity and consideration of maternal transport to a tertiary care facility (SOR: A).
- Cervical ultrasound examination and fetal fibronectin testing have good negative predictive value; thus, either approach or both combined may be helpful in determining which patients do not need tocolysis (SOR: B).
- Amniocentesis may be used in women in preterm labor to assess fetal lung maturity and intra-amniotic infection (SOR: B).
- Bed rest, hydration, and pelvic rest do not appear to improve the rate of preterm birth and should not be routinely recommended (SOR: B).

Data from ACOG, 2003.

difficult to decide if the fetus is symmetrically growth-restricted or just due 3 weeks later. Overall, ultrasound for diagnosis of IUGR is 80% to 90% sensitive, depending on the measurements used. The abdominal circumference, a soft tissue measurement, is the first routinely measured parameter to fall behind normal growth in IUGR. Estimation of fetal weight, calculated using the abdominal circumference, can be plotted on fetal growth curves to evaluate its percentile for a specific gestational age.

Management

The only treatment modality thought to be of benefit for IUGR is bed rest in a lateral recumbent position. This position prevents vena caval compression by the gravid uterus and allows maximal venous return to the heart, maximizing cardiac output and uteroplacental perfusion. Certain fetuses with growth restriction caused by significant maternal illness may benefit from improvement of the maternal condition. Antenatal testing is recommended for IUGR fetuses. If antenatal testing is abnormal or persistent oligohydramnios is present, delivery may be warranted before term. Otherwise, these fetuses are delivered at 38 to 40 weeks, depending on the degree of growth restriction.

Preeclampsia

Preeclampsia is one of the most common causes of perinatal morbidity and mortality. The etiology for preeclampsia remains unknown. However, placental dysfunction may initiate systemic vasospasm, ischemia, and thrombosis that eventually damages maternal organs and causes placental infarction, IUGR, and death. Preeclampsia complicates 5% to 10% of all pregnancies. It occurs at both extremes of reproductive age but is greatest in women younger than 20. Risk factors for preeclampsia include extremes of maternal age, nulliparity, African American race, multiple gestation, molar pregnancy, preexisting medical conditions (hypertension, diabetes, renal disease, connective tissue disorders, vascular disease), and prior or family history of preeclampsia or eclampsia.

The disorder is typically suspected in the presence of hypertension and proteinuria in the pregnant woman without history of preexisting chronic hypertension. Edema is no longer considered a reliable clinical sign and is often seen after the 20th week of gestation without signs of a hypertensive disorder. Historically, mild preeclampsia was diagnosed with a systolic BP rise of 30 mm Hg or diastolic BP rise of 15 mm Hg. Consensus statements now describe mild preeclampsia as an absolute reading of 140/90 mm Hg or greater in a pregnant woman with proteinuria greater than 0.3 g in a 24-hour urine collection. Again, nondependent edema is no longer considered a diagnostic criterion. Severe preeclampsia consists of a systolic BP greater than 160 mm Hg or diastolic BP greater than 110 mm Hg, complicated by significant proteinuria (>5.0 g/day) and evidence of end-organ damage. Signs and symptoms indicating severe preeclampsia include headache, visual disturbances, confusion, right upper quadrant (RUQ) or epigastric pain, impaired liver function, proteinuria, oliguria (<500 mL/24 hr), pulmonary edema, microangiopathic hemolytic anemia, thrombocytopenia, oligohydramnios, and IUGR.

Pregnant women with hypertension documented before pregnancy may develop preeclampsia. Chronic hypertension with superimposed preeclampsia is responsible for 15% to 30% of hypertensive disease in pregnancy. Treatment for mild preeclampsia involves bed rest and surveillance to assess development of complications. Delivery is carefully delayed until fetal maturity, development of severe preeclampsia, or other complications occur. In most cases, treatment of severe preeclampsia is delivery.

During labor and delivery, women with preeclampsia should receive IV magnesium sulfate for seizure prophylaxis, with a loading dose of 4 g infused over 15 to 20 minutes, then continuous infusion at 2 g/hr, similar to the preterm-labor magnesium therapy protocol (Box 21-7). Blood pressure should be carefully evaluated and treated with IV hydralazine if levels are persistently above 110 mm Hg diastolic. Severe preeclamptic women should generally deliver within 24 hours. Postpartum therapy with magnesium sulfate is recommended for 12 to 24 hours depending on degree of severity.

HELLP Syndrome

If unrecognized, preeclampsia can progress to a syndrome of hemolysis, elevated liver enzymes, and low platelets (HELLP syndrome). This is another complication in seemingly stable patients. The HELLP syndrome is noted in 5% to 10% of patients with preeclamptic symptoms. Such patients often present with RUQ and epigastric pain and a peripheral blood smear consistent with a microangiopathic hemolytic anemia. There may be decrements in the platelet count and increments in the transaminase (AST, ALT) and lactic acid dehydrogenase (LDH) enzymes. This is a life-threatening emergency that requires prompt delivery of the baby.

Eclampsia

Another serious complication of preeclampsia is development of seizures or coma. This is known as eclampsia. Eclampsia occurs in approximately 0.2% of pregnancies and

---

Box 21-7 Magnesium Sulfate Protocol for Preterm Labor

1. Continuous electronic fetal and contraction monitoring.
2. Patient in lateral recumbent position.
3. Nothing by mouth initially; then clear liquids if muscle tone adequate to prevent aspiration.
4. Intravenous fluids begun with lactated Ringer's 5% dextrose solution.
5. Four grams (range, 2-6) of $MgSO_4 \cdot 7H_2O$ in 500 mL of 5% dextrose administered over 15 minutes as loading dose.
6. Continuous infusion of 1 to 3 g/hr of $MgSO_4 \cdot 7H_2O$ after initial load.
7. Calcium gluconate readily available.
8. Accurate intake and output.
9. Frequent assessment of deep tendon reflexes.
10. Frequent examination of lungs for early signs of pulmonary edema.
11. Plasma magnesium levels monitored as clinically indicated.
12. Continue protocol for 24 hours. Change to oral beta-adrenergic agent if needed.

terminates 1 in 1000 pregnancies. The seizures and mental status changes of eclampsia are thought to result from hypertensive encephalopathy. Perinatal mortality is 2.0% to 8.6% (Sibai et al., 1981). Maternal mortality is less than 2%, with intracranial hemorrhage the major cause.

Gestational Hypertension

Gestational hypertension is defined as systolic BP of 140 mm Hg or greater and/or a diastolic BP of 90 mm Hg or greater, in the absence of proteinuria, in a previously normotensive pregnant woman at or after 20 weeks of gestation. Gestational hypertension is considered severe with sustained elevations in systolic BP of 160 and/or diastolic of 110 mm Hg or greater. Women with BP greater than 140/90 mm Hg without proteinuria or end-organ damage may ultimately develop preeclampsia. These initially normotensive women usually become hypertensive late in pregnancy, during labor, or within 24 hours postpartum and note a return to normal BP within 10 days postpartum. If preeclampsia does not develop, the diagnosis of gestational hypertension is made. The diagnosis of gestational hypertension is a temporary one and should be used during pregnancy only in women who do not meet criteria for preeclampsia or chronic hypertension.

Abruptio Placentae

Abruptio placentae (placental abruption) refers to separation of a normally located placenta before birth of the fetus. This event occurs in 1 in 129 births. Severe abruption results in a fetal mortality of 0.2%. Bleeding into the decidua basalis leads to separation of the placenta. Hematoma formation further separates the placenta from the uterine wall and compresses these structures, compromising the blood supply to the fetus leading to increased intrauterine pressure, uterine tenderness, frequent uterine contractions, fetal distress, and demise. The severity of fetal distress correlates with the degree of placental separation.

When the abruption is extensive, retroplacental blood may penetrate the thickness of the uterine wall into the peritoneal cavity because of increased intrauterine pressure. This phenomenon is called "couvelaire uterus." The myometrium becomes weakened and rarely may rupture, leading immediately to a life-threatening obstetric emergency. In near-complete or complete abruption, fetal death is inevitable unless immediate delivery by cesarean section is performed. Abruptio placentae received renewed awareness with the causal relationship to cocaine (Kline, 1997).

Abruptio placentae is a clinical diagnosis. Painful vaginal bleeding in the third trimester is the hallmark. Because ultrasound for this disorder has a high false-negative rate, this complication is diagnosed primarily on the findings of vaginal bleeding, abdominal pain, uterine tenderness, uterine contractions, and fetal distress. In one prospective study, almost 80% of patients with abruptio placentae presented with vaginal bleeding, 66% with uterine or back pain, and 60% with fetal distress (Hurd et al., 1983). Other evidence of abruptio placentae can include idiopathic preterm labor, uterine hypertonicity, and fetal demise. The monitoring of uterine contractions may reveal a high baseline pressure with concurrent contractions often 1 to 2 minutes apart.

Etiology

From 40% to 50% of women with abruptio placentae have underlying hypertension. Maternal trauma is the cause in 1.5% to 9.4%. The remainder can be associated with excessive alcohol consumption, cocaine use, sudden decompression of the uterus (as in delivery of first twin), retroplacental bleeding from needle puncture after amniocentesis, and possibly tobacco use. In a small group, no underlying association is found; abnormalities of uterine blood vessels and decidua likely exist in this idiopathic group.

Management

The management of abruptio placentae is primarily supportive and entails both aggressive hydration and monitoring of maternal and fetal well-being, with the expeditious delivery of the fetus if indicated (Turner, 1994). Maternal and fetal death may result from hemorrhage and coagulopathy. Coagulation studies should be performed to look for disseminated intravascular coagulation (DIC). Packed RBCs should be typed and held. If the fetus appears viable but compromised, urgent cesarean delivery should be considered. Recommended laboratory testing includes complete blood count with platelets, prothrombin and partial thromboplastin time, fibrinogen, fibrin degradation products, D-dimer, blood type, and Kleihauer-Betke acid elution. D(Rh)-negative mothers benefit from administration of D immune globulin (Pearlman et al., 1990).

Placenta Previa

Placenta previa is a life-threatening condition that presents in three forms (Fig. 21-5). When the cervical os is completely covered with placenta, it is classified as a *complete* or *total* placenta previa. *Partial* placenta previa occurs when the placenta covers a portion of the cervical os. A *marginal* placenta previa is one that extends just to the edge of the cervix. Placental implantation in the lower uterine segment is termed *low-lying placenta*. The incidence of placenta previa is about 1 in 200 to 250 pregnancies and is associated with potentially serious consequences from hemorrhage, separation of the placenta, or emergency cesarean delivery (Iyasu et al., 1993).

Placenta previa is usually diagnosed when the patient complains of painless vaginal bleeding in the third trimester. A smaller number of patients present with excessive bleeding in labor. Usually the initial bleeding is not profuse enough to be fatal and spontaneously ceases, only to recur later. The average first bleed occurs at 27 to 32 weeks of gestation. Women with a centrally implanted placenta previa tend to have earlier episodes of bleeding, which are more severe. Another suspicious aspect of the history includes an abnormal lie, in particular transverse or breech presentation.

Risk Factors

There are a few predisposing factors for placenta previa. They include advanced maternal age, increased parity, uterine abnormalities, multiple gestation, tobacco abuse, prior placenta previa, and previous uterine surgery.

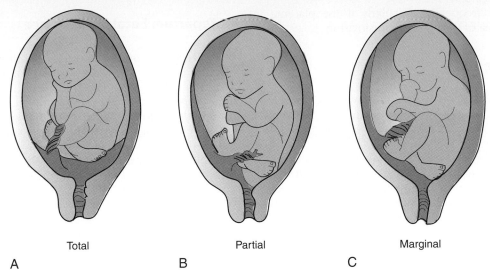

Total   Partial   Marginal

A   B   C

Figure 21-5 Various types of placenta previa. **A,** Cervical os is completely covered by the placenta. **B,** Cervical os is partially covered by the placenta. **C,** Placenta extends to the edge of the cervical os.

Ultrasound

Transabdominal ultrasound is a simple, precise, and safe method to visualize the placenta. It has an accuracy of 93% to 98% (Bowie et al., 1978). False-positive results can result from focal uterine contractions or bladder distention. The accurate assessment of placental position can also be difficult with a placenta implanted on the posterior uterine wall. In the patient whose placental edge is not well visualized and is not actively bleeding, the transvaginal approach may be used. The bladder should be empty, and initially the vaginal transducer should be inserted into the vagina to visualize the cervix. Once the closed cervix is visualized, deeper insertion of the probe will aid in visualization of the placenta. The use of the vaginal approach is safe and accurate in diagnosis of a placenta previa.

During routine second-trimester sonography, placenta previa is frequently diagnosed. Typically at 16 weeks' gestation, the placenta occupies 25% to 50% of the uterine surface area. As the third trimester approaches, growth of the lower uterine segment outflanks growth of the placenta, allowing apparent "migration" of the placenta (placental migration) away from the cervical os. For this reason, although 5% of pregnancies are diagnosed with complete previa by second-trimester ultrasound, 90% of these resolve by term (Rizos et al., 1979). When second-trimester sonography suggests a placenta previa, transvaginal ultrasound can be helpful in making a more accurate diagnosis before term.

Vasa Previa

Vasa previa is a rarely reported condition in which fetal blood vessels unsupported by the umbilical cord or placental tissue traverses the fetal membranes below the presenting part, covering the cervical os. It almost always coexists with a velamentous insertion of the umbilical cord. Vasa previa leads to fetal exsanguination from tearing of the large-caliber fetal vessels when the membranes rupture spontaneously or

artificially. This event has an associated fetal mortality of 33% to 100% (Bright and Becker, 1991).

When pulsatile vessels are palpated preceding the fetal vertex during digital examination, vasa previa should be considered along with cord presentation. Vasa previa must be included in the differential diagnosis of all cases of third-trimester bleeding. The blood that is lost can be tested for the presence of fetal hemoglobin, but often there is insufficient time to accomplish this. Vasa previa is often a retrospective diagnosis made after emergent cesarean delivery for fetal distress. Fetal mortality and morbidity from vasa previa may be reduced if there is a high index of suspicion, reliable method of diagnosis, and prompt surgical intervention (Messer et al., 1987).

Placenta Accreta, Increta, and Percreta

These three conditions are forms of abnormal placental attachment in which the trophoblasts invade beyond the normal location into the uterine muscle to varying degrees. Abnormal blood supply to the inner lining of the uterus and prior trauma to both the endometrium and myometrium (the muscle layer) appear to alter lower uterine physiology and influence placental implantation. The most common risk factor is a previous cesarean delivery or prior uterine surgery.

The risk of maternal death is 3%. In cases of bladder involvement with a placenta percreta, the risk of maternal death increases to 20%. The leading immediate causes of death are uterine bleeding and DIC. Placenta accreta, increta, or percreta is often the etiology of retained placenta (Breen et al., 1997). During manual extraction, the placenta fragments without complete separation, resulting in uncontrolled hemorrhage.

The major factor affecting outcome is the degree of placental invasion. A minimally invasive placenta (accreta) can often be removed manually or by curettage. Invasion deeper in the myometrium (increta) or through the myometrium (percreta) more often requires hysterectomy. The increased rate of cesarean deliveries is making abnormalities of placental attachment more frequent, particularly if the placenta is attached in the area of the prior uterine incision.

Multiple Gestation

At least 1 in 80 births is a twin gestation. With assisted reproductive technologies, this rate has now increased to almost 1 in 50 to 60. Approximately two thirds to three quarters of twins are dizygotic.

Twin gestation presents unique challenges. Monozygotic twins have twice the anomaly rate of dizygotic twins or singletons. Women with a twin gestation are more likely to miscarry early in gestation and more likely to deliver prematurely. Half of mothers of twins experience premature labor. Bed rest is often recommended after 5 months of gestation to aid in preterm-labor prevention. Education regarding associated signs and symptoms is important in this group. The average gestational age of delivery for a twin gestation is 36 menstrual weeks.

Women with a twin gestation are also at higher risk for chronic hypertension, pyelonephritis, gestational diabetes, and placenta previa. They should take supplemental iron, particularly in the latter trimesters, even if they are not iron deficient. Growth discordance can also occur, from twin-twin transfusion syndrome or more often simply from different placental implantation and different accessibility to nutrients. Serial ultrasound studies for growth approximately every 6 weeks is recommended. Twin fetuses with growth discordance should have antenatal testing.

The majority of twins will present both head first, cephalic-cephalic (Fig. 21-6, *A*), or first one cephalic, second one breech (cephalic-breech, 21-6, *B*). Any other combination can be seen, although cephalic-transverse (21-6, *C*), and breech-cephalic are the most likely in this remaining group. Once well into the third trimester, the first presenting fetus most often stays in its position; the second fetus often changes position, occasionally even during early labor. Twins who are cephalic-cephalic can be delivered vaginally. Those who are cephalic-breech and cephalic-transverse can also be attempted vaginally by skilled operators in carefully chosen women. When the first fetus is presenting other than cephalic, delivery is often best accomplished by cesarean section. Breastfeeding has been successful in many women with twins and should be encouraged.

Antepartum Fetal Surveillance

The three most common methods used to evaluate fetal well-being in utero are the nonstress test, contraction stress test, and biophysical profile (Babbitt, 1996). Vibroacoustic stimulation and fetal movement counts are also useful adjunctive tools in the evaluation of fetal well-being.

The indications for antepartum fetal surveillance are multiple and reflect conditions that are associated with increased fetal morbidity and mortality (Smith-Levitin et al., 1997). Conditions that lead to fetal hypoxia, uteroplacental insufficiency, and death are all indications for increased fetal surveillance. There are no absolute protocols for increased fetal surveillance, but there are certain accepted practices for given maternal-fetal risks. For example, weekly antenatal testing beginning the 32nd week of gestation is often performed in women with low to moderate risk (e.g., gestational diabetes, chronic hypertension, mild preeclampsia). For women with higher risk of abnormal outcome, earlier and more frequent antenatal testing is indicated, requiring an individualized approach.

Nonstress Test

Most often the nonstress test (NST) is used as the primary tool in antepartum fetal surveillance. It has been used to document second-trimester and third-trimester fetal well-being for the past 40 years. It serves as a surrogate measure of the developing fetal autonomic nervous system and the adequacy of the uteroplacental function (Myrick and Harper, 1996).

The NST is more specific than sensitive and thus a better indicator of fetal health than fetal illness. The test itself is read as reactive or nonreactive and may be repeated at intervals as a screen for high-risk maternal conditions. A reactive or reassuring NST is defined as one with at least two accelerations above baseline fetal heart rate of 15 beats/min for 15 seconds, in a 20-minute period. If a reactive pattern is not present at the end of the first 20 minutes, attempts may be made to arouse the fetus. Fetal rest periods, reportedly 30 to 40 minutes in duration, must be excluded for the fetus to demonstrate a reactive NST. Because fetuses can have normal sleep cycles lasting up to 40 minutes, NST might require over an hour to complete

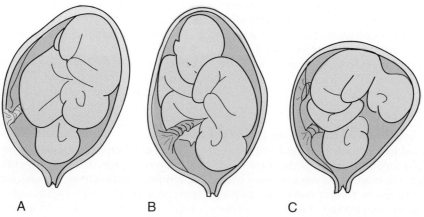

A   **B**   **C**

Figure 21-6 Three common twin presentations: **A,** cephalic-cephalic; **B,** cephalic-breech; **C,** cephalic-transverse.

if it is initially nonreactive. It is important to differentiate whether a nonreactive tracing truly represents a compromised fetus versus a temporary behavioral state (Knuppel et al., 1982).

The absence of fetal accelerations with the exclusion of a fetal sleep state denotes a nonreactive test. There are no contraindications to the NST as a primary screening tool, and it is easily reproducible, relatively inexpensive, and acceptable to most patients. Maternal narcotics, extreme prematurity, and fetal cardiac or CNS anomalies may also be responsible for a nonreactive NST. A nonreactive NST does not indicate fetal jeopardy but should be viewed as an indication for further evaluation. This evaluation may take the form of a biophysical profile or contraction stress test.

Biophysical Profile

The biophysical profile (BPP) is an ultrasound assessment of fetal well-being. It was originally designed to mimic the Apgar score for postnatal assessment. The BPP is technically more difficult to perform and interpret but provides a greater degree of certainty of fetal well-being. During a 30-minute examination, certain behavioral patterns associated with a healthy fetus are documented. The test is scored with five components, each worth 2 points (Table 21-11). Indicators such as amniotic fluid volume, fetal breathing, fetal heart rate, movement, and tone are evaluated. A score of 8 or 10 is reassuring; a score of 6 is suspicious and indicates a need for further evaluation; and a score of 4 or less is ominous, indicating the need for immediate intervention. A low score may also reflect the fetus's behavioral state during the test, such as normal sleep or sedation from maternal use of narcotics or CNS depressants. However, a decreasing score has been well correlated with poor outcome and with increasing degrees of fetal acidemia.

Modified Biophysical Profile

The modified BPP consists of the NST and the amniotic fluid index. It has proved to be an excellent means of fetal surveillance and identifies a group of patients at increased risk for poor perinatal outcome and small-for-gestational-age (SGA) infants. It has proved to be as effective as a full BPP in assessing fetal well-being.

Contraction Stress Test

With the increasing popularity of the NST, the contraction stress test (CST), also known as the *oxytocin challenge test* (OCT), is most often used as a supplementary tool in fetal surveillance. The CST is more cumbersome to perform, is difficult to interpret, and has several contraindications. This test is used to assess the reserve of the marginally compromised fetus when subjected to the stress of several uterine contractions (Collea and Holls, 1982; Lagrew, 1995). The goal of CST/OCT is to achieve three contractions in a 10-minute period through oxytocin infusion or nipple stimulation and look for late decelerations.

The CST is considered to be negative if no late decelerations are noted. A negative (normal) CST is a good indication of adequate fetal well-being as judged by fetal distress in labor, Apgar scores, and absence of meconium. The CST

Table 21-11 Components of the Biophysical Profile*

Parameter	Normal (score = 2)	Abnormal (score = 0)
Nonstress test	Two or more accelerations of at least 15 beats/min above baseline for at least 15 seconds.	Less than two accelerations of sufficient height and duration.
Amniotic fluid volume	At least one amniotic fluid pocket is 2 × 2 cm or greater in perpendicular plane.	No 2 × 2–cm pockets, *or* AFI less than 5.0.
Fetal breathing movements	Sustained fetal breathing for at least 30 seconds.	Less than 30 seconds of fetal breathing
Fetal body movements	At least three limb or gross body movements.	Less than three limb or body movements.
Fetal tone	Extremities in flexion at rest and at least one episode of extension of extremity or spine with return to flexion.	Extension at rest or no return to flexion after movement.

Modified from Norman LA, Karp LE. Biophysical profile for antepartum fetal assessment. Am J Fam Physician 1986;34:83-89.

*Scoring of latter four components is done sonographically in 30-minute observation period. Total score of 8 to 10 is reassuring; score of 6 is suspicious; and score of 4 or less is ominous.

AFI, Amniotic fluid index (sum of largest vertical pocket in each of four quadrants of uterus).

is considered positive if late decelerations accompany 50% or more of contractions. A positive CST is predictive of fetal compromise and distress in labor in up to 80% of cases and in specific clinical situations indicates need for delivery of the fetus. The presence of fewer decelerations indicates a suspicious study. The latter two conditions mandate need for further evaluation. Contraindications to a CST include risk of preterm labor, placenta previa, classic uterine scar or full thickness scar from previous uterine surgery, incompetent cervix, and multiple gestation (Babbitt, 1996).

Vibroacoustic Stimulation

Vibroacoustic stimulation is an artificial burst of noise produced by a handheld battery-powered artificial larynx (Birnholz and Benacerraf, 1983). This device is portable and easy to apply to the maternal abdomen and provides a stimulation that combines both sound and vibration. The goal is to alter the fetal behavioral state, waken a sleeping fetus, and provoke accelerations in the heart rate. Use of this device is associated with a significant increase in the number of reactive NSTs and a significant decrease in overall testing time. The use of vibroacoustic stimulation in achieving fetal heart rate accelerations has been found to be equally predictive of a favorable fetal outcome as spontaneously generated fetal heart rate accelerations (Smith et al., 1986).

Normal Labor and Delivery

Labor, whether preterm or term, is defined as the presence of sufficient uterine contractions in frequency, intensity, and duration to bring about effacement and dilation of the cervix. Control of normal labor is complex and, despite advances in medical science, poorly understood. Evidence supports prostaglandin (PG) involvement, in particular PGE_2 and $PGF_{2\alpha}$, as well as other mediators (Ulmsten, 1997).

Before the onset of labor, the fetal head may descend into the pelvis, and the height of the fundus will diminish. This lightening may occur acutely and may be very obvious to the pregnant woman, or it may occur over several weeks. An increase in pelvic pressure is experienced at this time. *False labor,* or irregular, short contractions that occur often before true labor, may in fact aid in cervical effacement and shortening of the cervical canal that begins as funneling at the internal cervical os. With impending true labor, cervical effacement and early dilation may allow the passage of a blood-tinged mucous termed "bloody show." Most women go into true labor within 3 days of a bloody show. Bleeding described as "heavy as the beginning of a menstrual period" may be pathologic, and the pregnant woman should be evaluated for placenta previa, abruptio placentae, or other causes of vaginal bleeding.

Contractions of active labor most often occur every 2 to 3 minutes, last about 1 minute, and have a mean of 40 mm Hg in intensity. However, some women successfully deliver babies with less frequent and intense uterine contractions. Frequent contractions of 1 to 2 minutes apart may be a sign of the increased intrauterine pressure associated with abruptio placentae. Adequate relaxation between contractions is imperative to allow oxygenated blood to enter the intravillous spaces and transfer to the fetal compartment. During the course of labor, uterine contractions cause cervical effacement and then dilation to a full 10 cm to allow passage of the fetal head, the largest diameter of the fetus to pass through the birth canal.

Progress of Labor

The degree and rate of cervical dilation measures the progress of labor. Labor can be divided into stages that are somewhat predictable in the nulliparous and multiparous woman (Table 21-12 and Fig. 21-7). The first stage of the labor course can be subdivided into the latent phase and the active phase.

First Stage of Labor

Latent Phase

The latent phase of the first stage of labor is variable in length, but usually less than 20 hours for a nullipara and 14 hours for a multipara. Little cervical dilation is seen, but cervical preparation for labor occurs with changes in consistency caused by changes in collagen and connective tissue. An increase in effacement as well as the anterior positioning of the cervix is also noted. Conduction anesthesia given in this phase may prolong or arrest progress. In normal pregnant women, latent-phase labor is best experienced at home. Clear liquids instead of heavy meals are encouraged during this time.

Table 21-12 Stages of Labor

Stage	Onset	Completion
First (latent and active phases)	Active labor	Complete dilation
Second	Complete dilation	Delivery of baby
Third	Delivery of baby	Delivery of placenta
Fourth*	Delivery of placenta	Contracted uterus

*Not always considered a stage.

Instructions for coming to the hospital include vaginal bleeding like a period, rupture of membranes, painful contractions at least 3 to 4 minutes apart, and decreased fetal movement. A subset of women may have a prolonged latent phase that can be treated with morphine in a hospital setting. Often this treatment accelerates transition to the active phase.

Active Phase

The active phase of the first stage of labor is the segment of rapid dilation, the progress of which is not affected by sedation or conduction anesthesia. This phase usually occurs at about 4 to 5 cm of cervical dilation. In general, nulliparous women dilate at least 1.2 cm per hour and multiparous 1.5 cm/hr (Friedman, 1978). Progress of the active phase depends on strength and frequency of uterine contractions, size, position, and attitude of the fetal head, as well as size and shape of the bony pelvis. Because of the different diameters of the pelvic inlet, midplane, and outlet, the fetal head must turn at different times of descent to negotiate the bony structure. Flexion of the fetal head during this process is crucial because this diminishes its anteroposterior (AP) diameter and permits easier descent. The cardinal movements of the fetal head during labor include engagement, descent, flexion, internal rotation, extension, external rotation, and expulsion.

Either continuous electronic fetal monitoring (EFM) or intermittent auscultation can be used to monitor the fetus in the active phase of labor (ACOG, 1995a). Instead of continuous EFM in this phase, in low-risk mothers with normal labor, the fetal heart may be auscultated after a contraction and recorded every 30 minutes; the frequency should be increased to every 15 minutes in higher-risk labors. Fetal heart rate decelerations should prompt even more frequent auscultation or continuous EFM. Auscultation rather than continuous EFM will allow mobility during labor, which may improve maternal comfort. IV fluids in the normal gravida can be reserved for women with long labor who become dehydrated despite oral liquids, those who require conduction anesthesia or large doses of pain medication, and those in whom complications develop or are suspected.

Second Stage of Labor

The second stage of labor involves maternal expulsive forces during uterine contractions to aid in the descent and ultimate delivery of the fetus. Instead of continuous monitoring, the fetal heart should be auscultated and recorded every 15 minutes in normal, low-risk pregnancies, and every

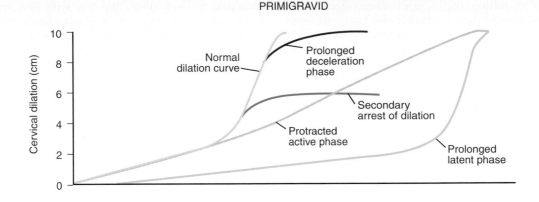

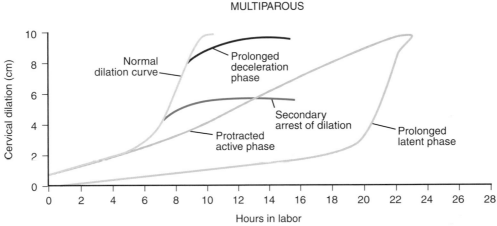

Figure 21-7 Composite curves of normal and abnormal labor progress. *(From Scherger J, Levitt C, Acheson L: Teaching family-centered perinatal care in family medicine. Part 2. Fam Med 1992;24:369.)*

10 minutes in higher-risk pregnancies. The second stage of labor averages 20 minutes for the multipara and 50 minutes for the nullipara. Although pushing for longer than 2 hours without an epidural or 3 hours with an epidural in a nullipara should alert the practitioner to possible cephalopelvic disproportion, pushing can continue longer in cases of adequate fetal heart rate and continued progress in descent.

Third Stage of Labor

The third stage of labor begins with the delivery of the baby. Appropriate equipment for resuscitation should be available. Maternal pushing with contractions will cause the fetal head to bulge the perineal tissues with increasing pressure to distend the opening of the vaginal canal and allow the fetal head to deliver. It is only when the head is stretching these tissues should the decision for episiotomy be made. The fetal head delivers with extension, after which the practitioner suctions the fetal mouth, pharynx, and nose. If meconium is present, wall suction to a DeLee trap is used for suctioning, and the fetus is not stimulated to breathe before a laryngoscope is used to assess the presence of meconium below the cords. After delivery of the fetal head and suctioning is complete, the neck of the fetus is explored for nuchal cords, which are preferably reduced if possible. If too tight to reduce, the cord must be clamped, then cut. The anterior shoulder of

the fetus is then delivered with gentle downward traction, but predominantly with maternal expulsive forces to avoid excessive pulling on the fetal neck, which can be associated with brachial plexus injury. Hyperflexion of the legs at the hip joint will allow the anterior shoulder to deliver more easily. After delivery of the anterior shoulder, the posterior shoulder is delivered usually quite easily with gentle upward traction. Excessive maternal efforts at this point can cause perineal lacerations. Thus the mother is instructed to push hard for the delivery of the anterior shoulder and gently for the posterior shoulder. Once the shoulders are delivered the remainder of the body escapes easily. The baby can then be placed on the mother's abdomen where warm towels await. The timing of clamping of the cord is controversial. As long as the baby is kept on the maternal abdomen, excessive blood shifts through an unclamped cord will usually not occur. The cord can then be clamped. Cord blood is obtained, as well as cord pH if desired.

The placenta should then be allowed to separate spontaneously. During this time, inspection of the vaginal canal and cervix for tears can be started, but adequate inspection for lacerations should be done after delivery of the placenta. Signs of placental separation include lengthening of the cord, gush of blood, and change in contour of the uterine fundus. Separation of the placenta from the maternal decidua is most likely from shearing forces as the now-smaller uterus contracts. After separation, uterine contractions decrease the size of the implantation site to arrest bleeding from this area. Maternal expulsive forces may be required to deliver the placenta along with gentle traction on the cord. Uterine massage and immediate breastfeeding will aid in maintaining a contractile state of the uterus and decrease uterine atony. In some cases, oxytocin may be required to maintain uterine contractility. After separation of the placenta, the episiotomy (if cut) and any lacerations should be repaired.

Fourth Stage of Labor

Some consider the first hour after delivery of the placenta the fourth stage of labor. Risk of uterine atony is highest during this period. The patient should be watched carefully for excessive vaginal bleeding, an enlarging boggy fundus, and hypotension. Massage of the uterine fundus most often is sufficient to return it to a contracted state and stop bleeding. Oxytocin may be added to the IV fluids in doses of 20 or 40 units/L of fluid and the IV rate increased, or if no IV fluid is needed, 20 units of oxytocin can be given intramuscularly (IM). Alternately, methylergonovine (Methergine), 0.2 mg, can be given IM every 20 minutes if the mother is not hypertensive. Finally, if no resolution to bleeding, 250 µg of prostaglandin $F_{2\alpha}$ (Hemabate) can be given IM every 15 to 20 minutes as needed for up to 3 doses.

Induction of Labor

Physicians have turned to induction of labor as a means of preventing complications from conditions such as prolonged rupture of membranes, fetal demise in utero or severe preeclampsia, or a post-term pregnancy. For example, post-term delivery beyond 42 weeks' gestation poses risks to both mothers and babies, including increased perinatal death, increased cesarean deliveries, perineal injuries from macrosomia, and labor dystocias. The onset of labor can be stimulated in different ways. Less interventional approaches, such as stripping of the amniotic membranes, may be effective but not predictable and thus may not be sufficient in women who need prompt delivery. Stripping of the membranes requires the cervix to be dilated sufficiently to introduce the examining finger. Potential risks include rupture of membranes, infection, and bleeding. However, this technique appears safe, in particular for those gravidas approaching postdates (El-Torkey and Grant, 1992).

In most cases the pharmacologic induction of pregnancy should be reserved for a medical or obstetric indication, such as hypertension, diabetes, premature rupture of membranes, postdates, fetal demise, and IUGR. Logistic and psychosocial factors, such as distance from the hospital and rapid labors, are also indications. Absolute contraindications for induction of labor are similar to those for spontaneous labor and vaginal delivery. In pregnancy, at term before induction of labor, fetal maturity should be confirmed. Gestational age of at least 39 weeks should be confirmed by early positive pregnancy test, early ultrasound, or early fetal heart tone auscultation. In some cases, fetal lung maturity studies from amniotic fluid may be required.

Success of induction is mainly a factor of parity and cervical readiness at the time of induction. A scoring system developed by Bishop in 1964 to assess the cervix has become popular (Table 21-13). A Bishop's score of 9 or greater is favorable for induction. Women with low scores benefit from cervical ripening with prostaglandins before induction.

Prostaglandin E_2 is now approved by the FDA for cervical ripening. Dinoprostone (Prepidil) is 0.5 mg of modified PGE_2 in 2.5 mL of gel that is placed intracervically and repeated once in 6 to 12 hours if the Bishop's score does not change appreciably. Intracervical dinoprostone may or may not cause uterine contractions. Its effect on cervical consistency appears unrelated to the number of contractions. Alternately, dinoprostone may be given intravaginally (Cervidil) as a slow-release, 12-hour vaginal insert that may be removed if uterine hyperstimulation occurs. Previous cesarean section is not a contraindication for use. If spontaneous labor does not ensue, an oxytocin infusion may then be used.

Misoprostol (Cytotec), a synthetic PGE_1 FDA approved for prevention of gastric ulcers, has been used off-label for cervical ripening and labor induction. Several protocols have been developed. It is a potent uterotonic agent that may be associated with increased incidence of uterine rupture. Misoprostol is best not used in women with prior cesarean section or uterine surgery.

EVIDENCE-BASED SUMMARY

- Patients should be counseled that walking during labor does not enhance or improve progress in labor and that it is not harmful (SOR: A).
- Continuous support during labor from caregivers should be encouraged because it is beneficial for women and their newborns (SOR: A).
- Active management of labor may shorten labor in nulliparous women, although it has not consistently been shown to reduce the rate of cesarean delivery (SOR: B).
- Amniotomy may be used to enhance progress in active labor but may increase the risk of maternal fever (SOR: B).
- Intrauterine pressure catheters may be helpful in the management of dystocia in select patients, such as obese women (SOR: C).
- Women with twin gestations may undergo augmentation of labor (SOR: C).

KEY TREATMENT

Prostaglandin E (PGE) analogs are effective for cervical ripening and inducing labor (SOR: A).

Low-dose or high-dose oxytocin regimens are appropriate for women in whom induction of labor is indicated (SOR: A)

Before 28 weeks' gestation, vaginal misoprostol appears to be the most efficient method of labor induction regardless of Bishop's score, although high-dose oxytocin infusion is also acceptable (SOR: A).

Approximately 25 µg of misoprostol should be considered as the initial dose for cervical ripening and labor induction; frequency of administration should be no more than every 3 to 6 hours (SOR: A).

Intravaginal PGE_2 for induction of labor in women with premature rupture of membranes appears to be safe and effective (SOR: A).

The use of misoprostol in women with prior cesarean delivery or major uterine surgery has been associated with an increase in uterine rupture and therefore should be avoided in the third trimester (SOR: A).

Misoprostol (50 µg every 6 hours) to induce labor may be appropriate in some situations, although higher doses are associated with an increased risk of complications, including uterine tachysystole with fetal heart rate decelerations (SOR: B).

Data from ACOG, 2009.

Table 21-13 Bishop's Pelvic Scoring for Elective Induction of Labor

Score	Dilation	Effacement	Station	Position	Consistency
0	Closed	0-30%	−3		
1	1-2 cm	40%-50%	−2	Posterior	Firm
2	3-4 cm	60%-70%	−1, 0	Midposition	Moderately firm
3	5+ cm	80+%	+1, +2	Anterior	Soft

The Bishop's score generally follows this scale:

Modifiers

A point is added to the score for each of the following:
Preeclampsia
Each prior vaginal delivery
A point is subtracted from the score for:
Postdates pregnancy
Nulliparity
Premature or prolonged rupture of membranes
Interpretation

Indications for Cervical Ripening with Prostaglandins

1. Bishop's score <5
2. Membranes intact
3. No regular contractions

Indications for Labor Induction with Pitocin

1. Bishop's score ≥5
2. Rupture of membranes

Cesarean Rates	First-Time Mothers	Women with Past Vaginal Deliveries
Scores of 0 to 3	45%	7.7%
Scores of 4 to 6	10%	3.9%
Scores of 7 to 10	1.4%	0.9%

Points for each parameter are added. A score of 9 or greater is favorable for induction.

Modified from Bishop EH. Pelvic scoring for elective induction. Obstet Gynecol 1964;24:266.

Oxytocin has been available for labor induction for 40 years. Administered appropriately, it is as safe as spontaneous labor. Many protocols are available for IV oxytocin infusion for induction of labor, from low-dose constant infusion (Mercer et al., 1990) to higher-dose incremental infusion (Muller et al., 1992; Satin et al., 1994). Steady-state levels after IV infusion occur about 40 minutes after the start of infusion. Starting doses range from 0.5 to 2 mU/min with incremental increases of 1 to 2 mU/min every 30 to 60 minutes (ACOG, 1995b). The goal is to achieve two to four uterine contractions in 10 minutes. All protocols share certain precautions. Continuous fetal heart rate and uterine contraction monitoring is mandatory. Hyperstimulation can occur even after a stable infusion rate has been established. Often, contraction intensity and frequency will increase spontaneously after the pregnant woman reaches the active phase or if the amniotic membranes rupture, necessitating a decrease in the oxytocin infusion rate. Hyperstimulation associated with fetal heart rate decelerations requires discontinuing or lowering of the infusion until recovery. Prolonged use of high doses of oxytocin can cause water intoxication because of its biochemical similarity to antidiuretic hormone.

Amniotomy alone or in conjunction with oxytocin has been shown to decrease the length of labor. In some cases, amniotomy alone can stimulate normal labor, omitting the need for oxytocin. Risks of early amniotomy is cord prolapse and chorioamnionitis. In clinical practice, the decision between induction and expectant management should include favorability of the cervix, maternal parity, and complicating medical or obstetric issues, as well as patient or physician convenience and preferences.

Abnormalities of Labor and Delivery

Dysfunctional Labor

A dysfunctional pattern of labor is defined as a deviation from the norm for the different phases of labor described earlier (see Fig. 21-7). In the latent phase of the first stage of labor, a prolonged or protracted course can be seen. In the active phase of the first stage of labor, both a protracted course and an arrested course can be seen (O'Brien and Cephalo, 1991). The disorders for each of these phases are examined separately.

Prolonged Latent Phase

The latent phase of the first stage of labor is variable in length, but usually less than 20 hours for a nullipara and 14 hours for a multipara. It is defined by the onset of regular contractions and is terminated by the onset of the active phase. The rate of dilation is usually 0.6 cm/hr or less. This phase is considered prolonged if it falls outside these parameters. The possible etiologies include an unripe cervix, false labor, sedation, and uterine inertia. The management of this condition is primarily conservative unless there is an expeditious need to deliver the fetus. This includes rest, observation, and possibly oxytocin augmentation. Maternal rest can be induced by a therapeutic dose of morphine, to provide a respite from the stresses of early labor and to promote sleep. The vast majority of these patients will declare themselves and either progress into labor or cease contractions, and then the diagnosis of false labor can be made. Amniotomy should be avoided in this phase because it increases the risk for chorioamnionitis. A prolonged latent phase in itself is not an indication for cesarean section.

Protracted Active Phase

The active phase of labor is defined as dilation of the cervix occurring at a rate of at least 1.2 cm/hr for nulliparous women and 1.5 cm/hr for multiparous women. A slower rate of dilation is known as protracted active phase or *primary dysfunctional labor*. The etiologies of a protracted active phase include fetal malposition (e.g., occiput posterior), relative cephalopelvic disproportion (CPD), inadequate uterine contractions, and anesthesia. Historically, debate has surrounded its management. The current trend is active management with oxytocin to optimize uterine contractions. A protracted active phase is a frequent predecessor of secondary arrest of cervical dilation and is associated with an increased risk of operative delivery.

Secondary Arrest of Cervical Dilation

The cessation of cervical dilation for 2 hours with a history of previously normal dilation is termed *secondary arrest*. The management of this condition varies considerably; however, an initial assessment and examination of the patient (including vaginal) are probably warranted, to document cervical dilation, fetal station, presentation, and position. Placement of an intrauterine monitor should be considered to assess the adequacy of uterine contractions. Alternative measures include ambulation, amniotomy, and oxytocin augmentation if the uterine contractions are judged inadequate. There is a high association with CPD, and a significant number of these patients will need operative delivery.

Abnormalities of the Second Stage of Labor

The second stage of labor is defined as the interval between the complete dilation of the cervix to the delivery of the infant. As with previous stages of labor, abnormalities in

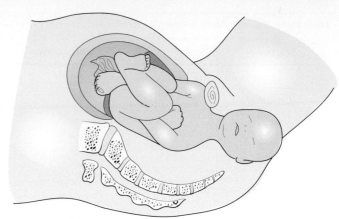

Figure 21-8 Shoulder dystocia. Impaction of the anterior shoulder against the pubic symphysis.

this stage include a protracted rate or a complete "arrest of descent," or the more common term *failure of descent*, used to describe an unchanged station. The evaluation of descent disorders should include maternal and fetal well-being, adequacy of contractions, obstructive etiologies (e.g., distended bladder), and cephalopelvic relationships. Other mitigating factors include maternal exhaustion, ineffective pushing, conduction anesthesia, and perineal resistance. There is also a high incidence of CPD with this condition and an increased risk of operative deliveries.

A *protracted descent* is more difficult to gauge but is defined by a rate of less than 1 cm/hr in nullipara women and less than 2 cm/hr in multiparous women. This diagnosis should prompt an evaluation for such causes as CPD, macrosomia, and inadequate pushing.

Shoulder Dystocia

Shoulder dystocia is defined as the impaction of the anterior shoulder against the pubic symphysis after the delivery of the head and occurs when the breadth of the shoulder is greater than the biparietal diameter of the head (Fig. 21-8). It is a life-threatening event associated with significant morbidity and mortality that needs to be recognized early and managed promptly. The overall incidence of shoulder dystocia is 0.3% to 1% but increases to 5% to 7% for newborns with macrosomia (birth weight >4500 g). Although a number of factors are associated with its occurrence, their predictive values are low, making it incumbent on the practitioner to be ever vigilant.

Several maternal and fetal complications are associated with shoulder dystocia (Carlan, 1991). Maternal complications are usually a consequence of soft tissue damage. The attempt to deliver the baby can result in an extension of an episiotomy to a fourth-degree laceration, with disruption of the anal sphincter and rectal mucosa. Other complications include hemorrhage secondary to uterine atony, vaginal lacerations, and rarely uterine rupture.

Fetal complications tend to be more profound. Brachial plexus injury can occur. Most resolve within 6 months with adequate physical therapy. However, the injury may persist as a source of lingering disability. Erb's palsy is the most common brachial plexus injury and involves the fifth and sixth cervical roots. Klumpke's palsy involves injury to the

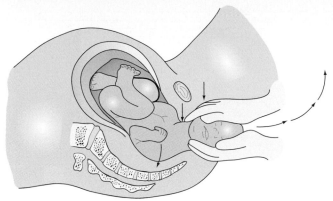

Figure 21-9 Shoulder dystocia. Release of the anterior shoulder from behind the pubic symphysis.

Box 21-8 Indications for Electronic Fetal Monitoring

Maternal

Hypertension

Insulin-dependent diabetes

Asthma

Other maternal diseases

Advanced maternal age

Epidural analgesia

Absence of prenatal care

Multiple gestations

Fetal

Premature rupture of membranes

Abnormal presentation

Prematurity

Postdates pregnancy

Oxytocin use

Intrauterine growth restriction

Meconium

eighth cervical root and the first thoracic fibers. Clavicular fracture may occur spontaneously or intentionally and may rarely result in damage to the underlying tissue. Prolonged fetal hypoxia secondary to a delay in the delivery can result in severe neurologic damage and even death.

Conditions that predispose to development of shoulder dystocia are related to either a macrosomic fetus or a contracted pelvis. Importantly, however, approximately one half of all shoulder dystocias occur with normal-weight fetuses and are unanticipated. Predisposing conditions include prepregnancy weight of greater than 180 pounds, excessive maternal weight gain, a history of diabetes or abnormal glucose tolerance, advanced maternal age, or a post-term pregnancy.

The key to management of this condition is anticipation and preparation. Warning signs include a prolonged second stage of labor or use of a vacuum or forceps. Once a shoulder dystocia becomes apparent, a number of maneuvers can be used to disimpact the shoulder (Fig. 21-9). The McRoberts maneuver is a time-honored and proven technique that is ideal in initial management (Gherman et al., 1997). It involves the flexion of the maternal thighs onto the abdomen, which increases the inlet diameter, straightens the lumbosacral lordosis, and removes the sacral prominence as a possible obstruction to delivery. This procedure is often done with suprapubic pressure to dislodge the offending shoulder from behind the maternal pubic symphysis. In contrast to suprapubic pressure, fundal pressure, which often serves to exacerbate the condition, should not be exerted. Other measures include the Woods' screw maneuver, an attempt to apply pressure to the back of the posterior shoulder to rotate the fetus, free the anterior shoulder, and attempt delivery obliquely. Alternately, delivery of the posterior arm can be attempted. Finally, as a measure of last resort, the Zavanelli maneuver, the cephalic replacement of the fetus followed by cesarean delivery, can be attempted.

Electronic Fetal Monitoring

Electronic fetal monitoring, developed at Yale University in the 1960s, was introduced into clinical practice in the early 1970s as an indirect measure of fetal oxygenation. EFM allowed the early detection of abnormal fetal heart rate patterns potentially associated with hypoxia and metabolic acidosis. Use of EFM has quickly become the standard of care for the management of high-risk pregnancies and a standard practice for low-risk pregnancies. In 2002 the National Center for Health Statistics estimated that approximately 85% of women in labor had EFM (NCHS, 2003). When used, EFM is predictive of a good outcome but not accurate or predictive of a bad outcome. In other words the false-positive rate of EFM is high for predicting adverse fetal outcomes. Recognizing the limitations of this technology, ACOG (2005) concurred that EFM appears to have no inherent benefit over auscultation properly performed in low-risk women. Furthermore, USPSTF (1996) could not recommend its routine use for the management of low-risk deliveries.

The use of EFM is associated with an increase in the rate of surgical interventions (vacuum, forceps, cesarean delivery), increased cost, and possibly increased legal risk; however, it is not associated with a decrease in the incidence of cerebral palsy. If the monitoring is done internally, there is increased risk of uterine perforation and scalp abscess in the neonate.

The multiple reasons for EFM may be subdivided into maternal and fetal indications (Box 21-8). EFM is indicated mainly for the monitoring of high-risk patients in labor, as well as for abnormalities in structured intermittent auscultation and when inadequate staffing is available to maintain the protocol for intermittent auscultation.

Interpretation of Fetal Heart Rate Recordings

A systematic approach in evaluation of the fetal heart rate (FHR) recordings is recommended to optimize interpretation. Studies have demonstrated poor reliability and consistency among various expert interpreters, even in controlled settings. The initial recommendations in 1997 by a National Institute of Child Health and Human Development (NICHHD) work group have been revised and updated by a 2008 work group cosponsored by the Society for Maternal-Fetal Medicine, in part to simplify and standardize FHR

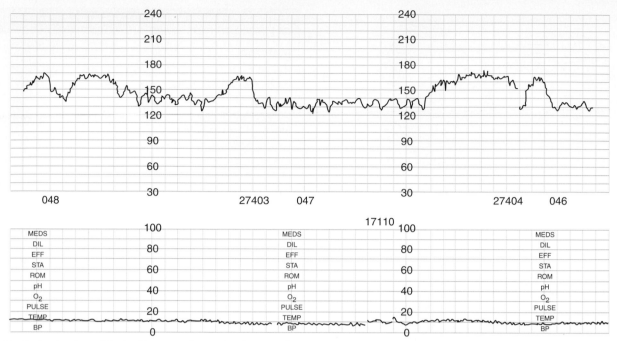

Figure 21-10 Accelerations of the fetal heart rate above a baseline rate of 130 to 140 beats per minute. Good variability is present.

interpretation. Five features of the FHR that need to be assessed: baseline, variability, accelerations, decelerations and its sub-classifications, and corresponding contractions. As of 2008, FHR recordings can be considered as belonging to one of three categories: normal (NICHHD Category I), indeterminate (Category II), and abnormal (Category III). *Normal* tracings are associated with a normal pH and fetal well-being, and current management should continue. *Indeterminate* tracings and *abnormal* tracings suggest the need for further evaluation and possible intervention. This evaluation may include vaginal examination, checking maternal vital signs, giving oxygen, changing maternal position, administering fluids, scalp stimulation, and determination of scalp pH measurement. An NICHHD Category II tracing will represent a significant fraction of those encountered in clinical care and will include all tracings that do not belong in categories I and II. An abnormal (NICHHD III) tracing usually indicates the need for the previous measures and consideration of expedited delivery.

Baseline Fetal Heart Rate

Normal baseline FHR ranges from 110 to 160 beats/min. A baseline change is interpreted as one that persists for 10 minutes or more and occurs between or in the absence of contractions. An FHR of less than 110 beats/min is considered *bradycardia*. FHR is a function of the autonomic nervous system. The vagus nerve provides an inhibitory affect, whereas the sympathetic nervous system provides an excitatory influence. As the gestation advances, the vagal system gains dominance, resulting in a gradual decrease in the baseline. Stressful events such as hypoxia, uterine contractions, and head compression evoke a baroreceptor reflex, with resulting peripheral vasoconstriction and hypertension causing bradycardia. Stimulation of peripheral nerve receptors can cause acceleration of FHR (Fig. 21-10). An FHR baseline greater than 160 beats/min is defined as *tachycardia*. This is

seen with certain maternal and fetal conditions, such as chorioamnionitis, maternal fever, and fetal tachyarrhythmias.

Variability of Fetal Heart Rate

The baseline FHR fluctuates constantly under normal conditions, described as its *variability*. This variability is often a good indicator of a healthy nervous system. Variability is the oscillation of the FHR around the baseline with amplitude of 6 to 25 beats/min. Variability reflects vagal efferent impulses only. Uncomplicated loss of variability is often caused by fetal quiescence (sleep state), CNS depressants (e.g., diazepam, morphine, magnesium sulfate), or parasympatholytic agents (e.g., atropine). The uncomplicated loss of variability is associated with no risk or minimal risk of acidosis and low Apgar scores. The presence of decreased variability in combination with late or severe variable deceleration is an ominous finding. Clinically variability is one of the most important indicators of fetal well-being, and the majority of babies with good variability do well regardless of the presence of decelerations.

Recent guidelines do not recommend the use of or differentiation between short-term and long-term variability in the assessment of fetal well-being (NICHHD, 2008). In the assessment of variability, the following categories are now recommended, reflecting the amplitude of the FHR tracing around the baseline (Fig. 21-11):

Absent: Amplitude range is undetectable.
Minimal: Amplitude range is detectable, but 5 beats/min or less.
Moderate: Amplitude is 6 to 25 beats/min.
Marked: Amplitude range is greater than 25 beats/min.

Bradycardia

Bradycardia is defined as FHR less than 110 beats/min for at least 10 minutes. *Mild* bradycardia ranges between 100 and 110 beats/min. Mild bradycardia with normal variability is

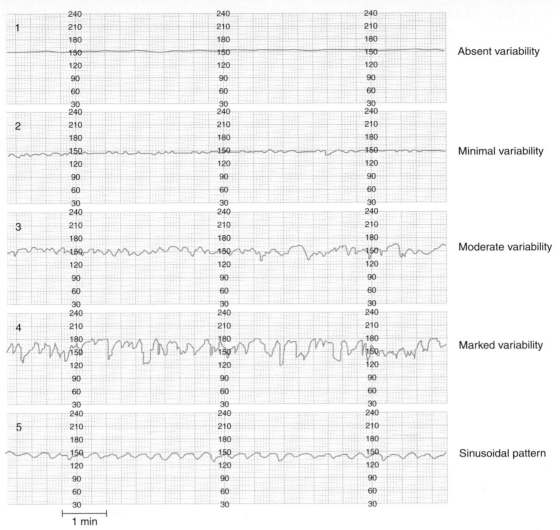

Figure 21-11 Variability in fetal heart rate (FHR). Definitions from National Institute of Child Health and Human Development. *(Redrawn from Cunningham FG, Leveno KL, Bloom SL, et al. Williams Obstetrics, 2nd ed. New York, McGraw-Hill, 2005.* http://www.accessmedicine.com.

not associated with fetal acidosis and is considered reassuring. *Moderate* bradycardia of 80 to 100 beats/min is considered a nonreassuring pattern. Bradycardia less than 80 beats/min is considered ominous and is often a terminal event (Fig. 21-12). There are numerous etiologies for fetal bradycardia (Box 21-9).

Tachycardia

Fetal tachycardia is defined as a baseline FHR of greater than 160 beats/min for at least 10 minutes. *Mild* tachycardia is a FHR of 160 to 180 beats/min; in *severe* tachycardia the FHR is greater than 180 beats/min. Fetal tachycardia greater than 200 beats/min is usually caused by fetal tachyarrhythmia or rarely a congenital anomaly and seldom results from fetal hypoxia. There are numerous etiologies of fetal tachycardia (Box 21-10).

Accelerations

Accelerations are transitory increases in FHR associated with fetal movement, scalp or acoustic stimulation, and uterine contractions. Accelerations are considered reassuring and are associated with fetal well-being. Accelerations form the basis of a reactive NST, defined as the presence of two or more accelerations of 15 beats/min above baseline for at least 15 seconds (see Fig. 21-10).

Early Decelerations

Early decelerations are caused by a vagal response to fetal head compression resulting in a slowing of FHR. These decelerations have a smooth, uniform shape that is a mirror image of the corresponding contraction. They begin with the onset of a contraction, nadir at the peak of the contraction, and promptly return to baseline. Early decelerations are considered reassuring and are associated with a good outcome.

Variable Decelerations

Variable decelerations are characterized by an acute fall in FHR with a rapid down slope and a variable recovery. These have variable shapes, at times described as being "v," "u," or "w" (Fig. 21-13). They also have a variable relationship with contractions. Variable decelerations may be classified according to their depth and duration as *mild* when the

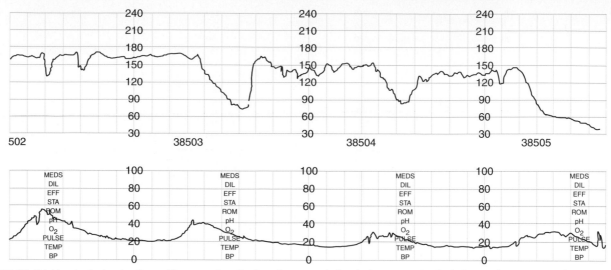

Figure 21-12 Fetal heart rate decelerations with contractions. Bradycardia occurred after the last contraction (only the initial segment is visible).

Box 21-9 Etiology of Fetal Bradycardia
Prolonged cord compression/cord prolapse
Hypothermia
Tetanic uterine contractions
Paracervical block
Epidural and spinal analgesia
Maternal seizure
Rapid descent
Vigorous vaginal examinations
Congenital heart disease
Fetal heart block
Severe hypoxia

Box 21-10 Etiology of Fetal Tachycardia
Chorioamnionitis
Hyperthyroidism
Parasympatholytic drugs (atropine, atarax)
Sympathomimetic drugs (terbutaline)
Fetal tachyarrhythmia
Maternal anxiety
Maternal fever
Fetal infection
Prematurity
Fetal hypoxia
Idiopathic

depth is greater than 80 beats/min and duration less than 30 seconds. Variable decelerations are considered *moderate* when the depth is 70 to 80 beats/min and duration is 30 to 60 seconds. Variable decelerations are *severe* when the depth is less than 70 beats/min and duration longer than 60 seconds.

Variable decelerations are the most commonly encountered pattern, occurring in 50% to 80% of all deliveries. They are almost always caused by umbilical cord compression. Variable decelerations are noted to be common with nuchal cord, short or prolapsed cord, or when the membranes have been ruptured. Segments of FHR accelerations just before and after the variable deceleration (shoulders) indicates a healthy response.

Late Decelerations

Late decelerations are consistent with NICHHD Category III, abnormal FHR tracing, and are associated with uteroplacental insufficiency. These are provoked by uterine contractions and are associated with decrease in uterine blood flow or placental dysfunction. A late deceleration is a symmetric, gradual fall in FHR beginning at or after the contraction peak, with a slow return to baseline only after the contraction has passed (Fig. 21-14). Postdate gestation, preeclampsia, chronic hypertension, and diabetes mellitus are among the many causes of placental dysfunction. The management

of late decelerations include turning the patient on her side to physiologically increase cardiac output and uterine blood flow, administering IV fluids to correct hypotension, discontinuing oxytocin infusion, and administering oxygen.

Sinusoidal Patterns

Sinusoidal patterns are rare but particularly ominous, belong to the NICHHD Category III, and are associated with a high rate of fetal morbidity and mortality. Sinusoidal patterns are characterized by a smooth, undulating, sine-wave pattern of 2 to 5 cycles/min and amplitude of 5 to 15 beats/min, with a notable absence of variability (Fig. 21-15). They occur with fetal anemia or severe hypoxia and need to be differentiated from a "pseudosinusoidal" pattern, which is a benign, uniform variability pattern with the preservation of beat-to-beat variability. Sinusoidal patterns are often ominous but are occasionally seen after the administration of narcotics to the mother.

Contractions

Contractions are classified as *normal* (no more than five contractions in a 10-minute period) or *tachysystole* (more than five contractions in a 10-minute period, averaged over a 30-minute window). The term "hyperstimulation" is no

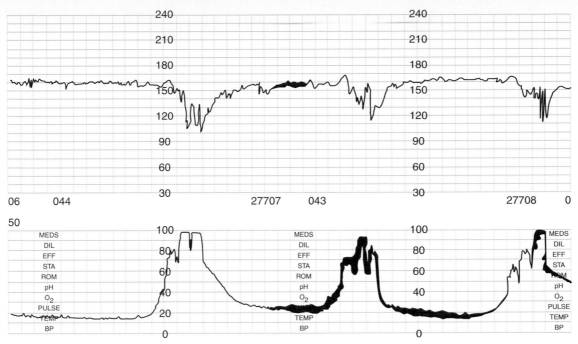

Figure 21-13 Variable decelerations of fetal heart rate.

longer accepted and should be discontinued. Tachysystole is qualified by the presence or absence of decelerations, and it applies to both spontaneous and stimulated labor.

EVIDENCE-BASED SUMMARY

- The false-positive rate of electronic fetal monitoring (EFM) for predicting adverse outcomes is high (SOR: A).
- The use of EFM is associated with an increase in the rate of surgical interventions (SOR: A).
- Compared with structured intermittent auscultation, continuous EFM shows no difference in overall neonatal mortality (SOR: A).
- Continuous EFM reduces neonatal seizure rates (SOR: A).
- Fetal pulse oximetry has not shown a reduction in cesarean delivery rates (SOR: A).
- The use of EFM does not result in a reduction of cerebral palsy rates (SOR: A).
- The labor of women with high-risk conditions should be monitored continuously (SOR: B).
- Reinterpretation of the fetal heart rate tracing, especially knowing the neonatal outcome, is not reliable (SOR: B).
- The use of fetal pulse oximetry in clinical practice cannot be supported at this time (SOR: B).

Data from ACOG, 2005, 2009b; Alfirevic et al., 2006; East et al., 2007; and Macones et al., 2008.

Vaginal Birth after Cesarean

A trial of vaginal birth after a previous cesarean delivery (VBAC) is an accepted method of delivery for most women with a prior low-transverse cesarean delivery. Factors that increase morbidity in VBAC should be understood so that practical decisions can be made regarding the best route of delivery for each patient. ACOG (2004) suggests the following criteria for selection of appropriate candidates: one previous cesarean delivery, adequate pelvis, no uterine scars, and immediate availability of both a physician to perform an emergency cesarean delivery and facilities and anesthesia to support an immediate cesarean delivery. Use of prostaglandin cervical ripening is discouraged in these women because of the small increased risk of uterine rupture associated with these medications when used with a scarred uterus.

The AAFP (2005) reviewed a trial of labor after cesarean (TOLAC) and compared TOLAC with elective repeat cesarean section (ERCS) and formulated the following recommendations:

Most women with one previous cesarean delivery with a low-transverse incision are candidates for VBAC and should be counseled about VBAC and offered a trial of labor; epidural anesthesia may be used for VBAC (SOR: A).

Women with a vertical incision within the lower uterine segment that does not extend into the fundus are candidates for VBAC (limited or inconsistent scientific evidence, SOR: B).

The use of prostaglandins for cervical ripening or induction of labor in most women with a previous cesarean delivery should be discouraged. Because uterine rupture may be catastrophic, VBAC should be attempted in institutions equipped to respond to emergencies with physicians immediately available to provide emergency care. After thorough counseling that weighs the individual benefits and risks of VBAC, the ultimate decision to attempt this procedure or undergo a repeat cesarean delivery should be made by the patient and her physician. This discussion should be documented in the medical record. VBAC is contraindicated in women with a previous classic uterine incision or extensive transfundal uterine surgery (primarily consensus and expert opinion, SOR: C).

After careful patient selection, preparation, and management, 7 or 8 of 10 women with uterine scars deliver vaginally. The strongest predictor of the safety of VBAC is the

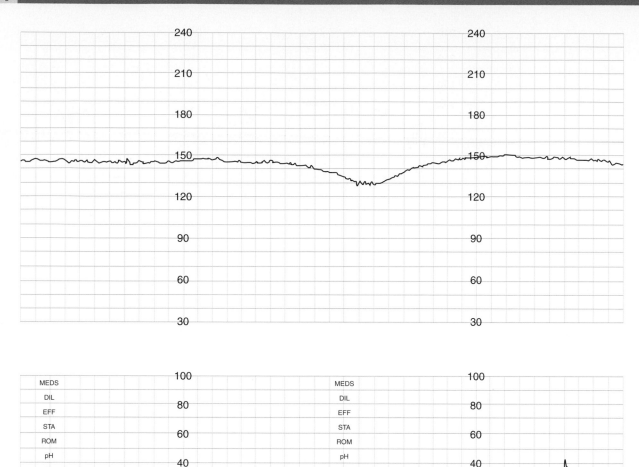

Figure 21-14 Late deceleration of fetal heart rate.

location of the previous uterine scar. Safety of TOLAC in women with history of one cervical low-transverse cesarean has been documented. Rupture of these incisions is low,

---

EVIDENCE-BASED SUMMARY

- Most women with one previous cesarean delivery with a low-transverse incision are candidates for vaginal birth after cesarean (VBAC) and should be counseled about VBAC and offered a trial of labor (SOR: A).
- Epidural anesthesia may be used for VBAC (SOR: A).
- Women with a vertical incision within the lower uterine segment that does not extend into the fundus are candidates for VBAC (SOR: B).
- The use of prostaglandins for cervical ripening or induction of labor in most women with a previous cesarean delivery should be discouraged (SOR: B).
- After thorough counseling about benefits and risks of VBAC, the decision to attempt this procedure or undergo a repeat cesarean delivery should be made by the patient and her physician (SOR: C).
- VBAC is contraindicated in women with a previous classic uterine incision or extensive transfundal uterine surgery (SOR: C).

Data from Wall et al., 2005.

0.5% (Pridjian, 1992). Information is insufficient to determine whether TOLAC is safe for VBAC candidates with two or more prior low-transverse cesarean sections, previous low-vertical incision, multiple gestation, breech presentation, or suspected macrosomia.

Oxytocin use and epidural anesthesia are not contraindicated in women attempting VBAC, although they should be used cautiously in this setting. An internal uterine pressure monitor is recommended when labor is enhanced or induced medically. The most common signs and symptoms of uterine rupture are fetal decelerations and distress, heavy vaginal bleeding, decreasing station or complete loss of the presenting part, loss of contraction intensity as documented by internal pressure monitor, uterine or pelvic pain in between contractions, and bloody urine.

Women who are most likely to have a successful VBAC are less than 40 years old, have had one prior cesarean delivery, undergo spontaneous labor, have a baby no greater than 4000 g, and had a prior cesarean section that was not for failure to progress or CPD in the active phase of labor. Based on the available data, the overall outcomes from TOLAC and ERCS are so similar that the two birthing methods appear medically equivalent. As a consequence, women's preferences for the method of delivery must be explored

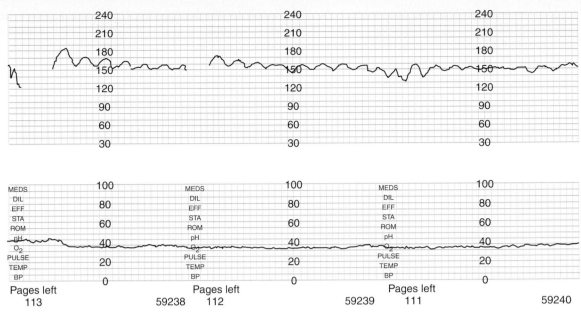

Figure 21-15 Sinusoidal fetal heart rate pattern.

and respected throughout pregnancy and during the delivery process. Women should be encouraged to undergo a TOLAC, but they should also have the opportunity to weigh the potential harms and benefits of TOLAC versus ERCS. A decision to have a cesarean delivery should be supported.

Intrapartum Procedures

Obstetric Anesthesia

At present, many pregnant women are choosing to receive analgesia to relieve the pain of childbirth through several methods. More than 50% of women in labor are reported to choose intrapartum epidural analgesia at many U.S. institutions. This probably reflects changing societal expectations and increasing participation in the birth process on the part of both anesthesiologists and certified registered nurse anesthetists.

Pain during the first stage of labor is attributable to uterine contractions and cervical dilation. Afferent impulses from the cervix and uterus are transmitted to the spinal cord via the tenth thoracic to first lumbar (T10-L1) segments. Pain is conducted along the paracervical and inferior hypogastric plexus. During the second stage, pain also occurs from distention and stretching of pelvic structures and the perineum. Second-stage pain is principally somatic in nature and is transmitted through the spinal second to fourth sacral (S2-S4) segments.

Therapeutic modalities to manage the pain of childbirth include systemic narcotics, local anesthesia, and psychological methods (Howell, 2000). Systemic narcotics used to manage pain during labor include meperidine (Demerol, 25 mg IM or IV) and nalbuphine (Nubain, 10 mg IV). Narcotics should be avoided at or near delivery because they can cause nausea, vomiting, decreased gastric motility, and respiratory depression and can interfere with the mother's ability to concentrate and cooperate. Fetal effects include respiratory and CNS depression and temperature instability. Naloxone (0.01 mg/kg) can be administered to depressed newborn as an IV bolus for counteracting the effect of narcotics.

A pudendal block provides analgesia to the vaginal introitus and perineum. Usually done in the second stage of labor, 5 mL of 1% lidocaine is injected into the pudendal canal, the location of the pudendal nerves and vessels. Care is taken to aspirate for blood before instilling the anesthetic solution. It takes approximately 10 minutes for anesthesia to establish. Infection at the injection site, intravascular injection, and maternal overdose are the major potential complications.

Neuraxial or epidural analgesia is popular among both physicians and patients (Vincent and Chestnut, 1998). The anesthesiologist's goal for epidural analgesia during the first stage of labor is to provide segmental sensory anesthesia of the T10 to L1 dermatomes. The dose of anesthetic necessary to achieve effective labor analgesia will depend on the intensity and location of the patient's pain. These in turn depend on the amount and rate of cervical dilation; the strength, frequency and duration of uterine contractions; and the position of the fetal head at the time epidural analgesia is placed. Typically, bupivacaine (Marcaine) or ropivacaine (Naropin), with or without a small dose of a lipid-soluble opioid such as fentanyl (Sublimaze) or sufentanil (Sufenta), establishes effective analgesia with minimal motor block. Maintenance of epidural analgesia may be achieved with intermittent bolus injections, continuous infusion, or patient-controlled dosing frequency.

Although epidural analgesia provides superior pain relief during labor, much controversy surrounds its drawbacks. These include the increased duration of labor, increased need for oxytocin augmentation, and increased rate of cesarean section for failure to progress. The most common complications, however, are maternal hypotension and headache from inadvertent puncture of the dura.

Contraindications to epidural analgesia include patient refusal, active maternal hemorrhage, maternal septicemia or untreated febrile illness, infection at or near needle insertion site, and maternal coagulopathy.

Psychological methods of pain relief include Lamaze, natural-childbirth methods, acupuncture, biofeedback, and

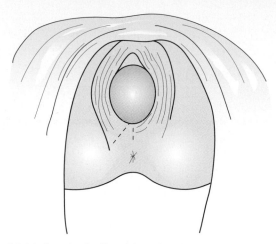

Figure 21-16 Crowning fetal head distending the perineal tissues. Broken lines depict the location of the incision for a midline (median) or mediolateral episiotomy.

Box 21-11 Categories of Perineal and Vaginal Lacerations

First degree: Confined to the superficial skin or mucosa; repair usually not required unless extensive or bleeding.

Second degree: Involves the mucosa and deeper tissues of the vagina and perineum.

Third degree: Involves the anal sphincter.

Fourth degree: Involves the rectal mucosa and usually transects the anal sphincter.

---

self-hypnosis. These techniques are useful in decreasing maternal anxiety and may reduce the amount of analgesia needed.

Episiotomy

An episiotomy is a surgical incision in the perineum to enlarge the introitus at delivery. Episiotomy is one of the most common medical procedures performed in the United States. There are two types of episiotomies (Fig. 21-16). The midline or *median* episiotomy is the most common in the United States. It involves an incision from the posterior aspect of the vagina downward, directly toward the anus, approximately half the length of the perineum. The *mediolateral* episiotomy is a diagonal incision toward either side of the midline, done to prevent tearing into the rectum. The mediolateral incision may serve to decrease the incidence of third- and fourth-degree extensions but is more difficult to repair and is associated with more blood loss, pain, slow healing, and dyspareunia. It is performed when the fetal head is crowning 3 to 4 cm. An average incision extends 5 to 6 cm into the vagina. Lacerations and extensions of episiotomies are described according to the extent of tissue involvement (Box 21-11).

Historically, episiotomies were performed for a number of indications. These include the substitution of an anticipated ragged spontaneous laceration for a more controlled straight surgical incision, reduction in the second stage of a labor, and reduction in subsequent pelvic relaxation and trauma to pelvic musculature.

The literature since 1980 does not substantiate the alleged benefits of episiotomy (Argentine Episiotomy Trial Collaborative Group, 1993), as supported by more recent review by the Agency for Healthcare Research and Quality (Viswanathan et al., 2005). The reputed long-term and short-term benefits have not been substantiated. Episiotomy is used in approximately one third of vaginal deliveries to hasten birth and prevent tearing of the perineum during delivery, but in fact it fails to accomplish any of the other maternal or fetal benefits traditionally ascribed to it (Klein et al., 1994). Episiotomies fail to prevent perineal damage, pelvic floor relaxation, reduction of the second stage of labor, and protection of the newborn from either intracranial hemorrhage or intrapartum asphyxia. Also, episiotomy does not protect women against urinary or fecal incontinence, pelvic organ prolapse, or difficulties in sexual function in the first 3 months to 5 years after delivery. Furthermore, in primigravid women, episiotomy appears to be causally associated with third-degree and fourth-degree lacerations.

In summary, episiotomy is an unproven, controversial surgical procedure best restricted to specific fetal and maternal indications. Most data do not support its routine application, making its use a decision best left to the individual physician and patient (Sleep et al., 1984).

The repair of an episiotomy should be approached with standard surgical principles. After appropriate positioning of the patient and with adequate lighting, the practitioner should determine the extent of the wound. Efforts should be made to assess the adequacy of the anesthesia. Sites of uncontrolled bleeding should be identified and hemostasis ensured. In the repair the practitioner should aim to use the least amount of suture material possible and achieve wound approximation without dead space. Several techniques of repair are accepted. Typically, an anchoring, hemostatic stitch of an absorbable or delayed-absorbable material such as 2-0 chromic catgut or polyglycolic acid is placed at the apex of the vaginal incision, and the vaginal mucosa is approximated in a continuous interlocking fashion to the hymenal ring (Fig. 21-17, *A*). Polyglycolic acid sutures may be superior to chromium catgut for episiotomy suturing. Compared with surgical repair using catgut or chromic suture, repair using 3-0 polyglactin 910 (Vicryl) suture results in decreased wound dehiscence and less postpartum perineal pain. This suture can then be tied or brought through to repair the deep layer of the perineum (Fig. 21-17, *B*). The deep perineal tissues are then approximated with interrupted or continuous stitches in the muscle and fascia. Finally the skin is approximated with a subcuticular stitch, knotted and buried inside the vagina above the hymenal ring (Fig. 21-17, *C*).

Diagnostic Ultrasound

Sonographic examination with the appropriate indication is an appropriate skill that enhances the diagnostic and therapeutic capabilities of family physicians who practice obstetrics. Even physicians who do not deliver babies are faced with clinical questions for which diagnostic ultrasound is indicated. Studies do not support the routine use of sonography in low-risk prenatal care; however, societal expectations and the relative ease of access to this technology have made it an established aspect of obstetric care. The Radius study group evaluated the use of screening ultrasounds in 15,151 low-risk pregnancies and found no difference in perinatal mortality, birth weight, or preterm birth. The study did not evaluate its use in high-risk pregnancy (Ewigman et al., 1993).

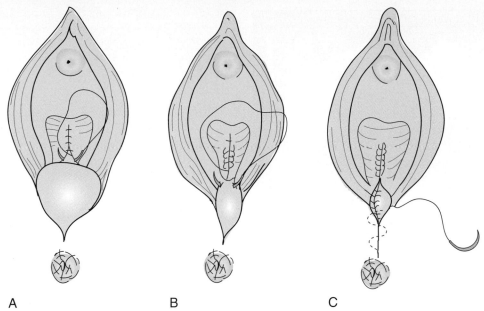

Figure 21-17 Episiotomy repair. **A,** Placement of the vaginal portion of the sutures. **B,** Deep perineal repair. **C,** Superficial perineal repair.

Box 21-12 Indications for Obstetric Ultrasound

1. Determination of gestational age
2. Diagnosis
   - Suspected miscarriage or fetal demise
   - Vaginal bleeding
   - Pelvic pain
   - Suspected multiple gestation
   - Suspected hydatidiform mole
   - Suspected ectopic pregnancy
   - Size-date discrepancy
   - Uterine or pelvic mass or abnormality
   - Congenital anomalies
   - Fetal presentation
3. Antenatal monitoring
   a. Biophysical profile (BPP)
   b. Intrauterine growth retardation (IUGR)
   c. Fetal macrosomia
4. Adjunct to obstetric procedures
   - Chorionic villus sampling
   - Amniocentesis
   - Cephalic version
5. ACOG* recommends ultrasound at 18 weeks for all patients.
   - Confirm dates and fetal survey.

From http://www.fpnotebook.com/OB/Rad/ObstrcUltrsnd.htm.
*American College of Gynecologists and Obstetricians.

The obstetric ultrasound has numerous indications and benefits in prenatal care (Box 21-12). Benefits include estimation of fetal age through biometry (accurate to within 1 week under 20 weeks, ±2 weeks at 20-28 weeks, and ±4 weeks after 28 weeks). In the hands of an experienced sonographer, the gestational sac size or the crown-rump length has proved a reliable measure of gestational age (Fig 21-18). Again, early ultrasound may provide more accurate dating, which is important for timing screening tests and interventions and for optimal management of complications such as post-term pregnancies (Neilson, 2004). Prenatal diagnosis and evaluation of fetal anomalies, growth anomalies (e.g., size vs. date discrepancies), fetal assessment (e.g., BPP, confirmation of fetal demise), maternal factors (e.g., diagnosis of ectopic pregnancy), and uterine anomalies are other indications and benefits.

The overutilization or recreational use of ultrasound technology may pose a medical-legal risk, particularly in the hands of an inexperienced provider.

Operative Vaginal Deliveries

Indications for operative vaginal delivery in a low-risk mother are nonreassuring FHR, maternal exhaustion, and prolonged second stage, which is generally 3 hours for a nulliparous woman and 2 hours for a parous woman.

Essential for safe operative vaginal delivery is optimal readiness. The laboring woman should understand the reasons why operative delivery has been chosen, with documentation in the chart. She should then be placed in a position in which her legs are maximally open, preferably in stirrups, with the perineum at the edge of the bed. Usual washing and draping is performed. The bladder is emptied. Adequate anesthesia makes placement of instruments easier and improves maternal cooperation. Pudendal block is often adequate for procedures when the fetal head is at the outlet. However, conduction anesthesia is often used. The cervix should be completely dilated and the membranes ruptured. Station, position, and attitude of the fetal head should be known. The fetal head should be engaged. Palpation, maternal sensation, or contraction monitoring can help identify the timing of contractions. Facilities for cesarean section should be available. Decision to use forceps or vacuum is based on operator skill, availability of instruments, and fetal-maternal considerations, including pelvic shape and size, fetal head position, and availability of anesthesia.

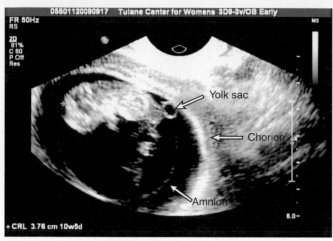

Figure 21-18 The crown-rump length (CRL) is denoted by crosses. Care should be taken to view the entire fetus in the midsagittal plane so as not to undermeasure. Conversely, the yolk sac is not a part of the CRL, so its inclusion will falsely increase the measurement.

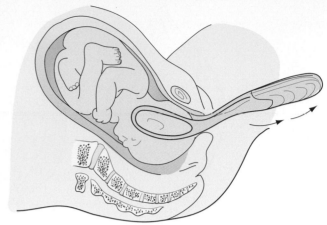

Figure 21-19 Outlet forceps delivery. The direction of traction is first downward so that the fetal head negotiates the pubic symphysis and then upward to deliver in extension.

Forceps Delivery

Currently, forceps deliveries are divided into outlet, low, mid, and high forceps, determined by the station of the fetal head. In an *outlet* forceps delivery the fetal head has reached the pelvic floor and is seen at the introitus without separating the labia. The fetal head may be right, left, or straight occiput anterior or posterior, and delivery is accomplished without rotation of greater than 45 degrees. A *low* forceps delivery is one in which the fetal head is at least +2 cm (on a 0 to +5 cm scale of station), but not on the pelvic floor. Rotation may be greater than or less than 45 degrees. A *mid* forceps delivery occurs when the head is engaged, but less than +2 cm station. A *high* forceps delivery, when the fetal head is unengaged, is no longer performed in modern obstetrics.

The choice of forceps to use is based on the operator's training and the type of forceps delivery. Typically, Simpson (or Simpson-DeLee) or Elliot forceps are used for low and outlet deliveries. After requirements for operative vaginal deliveries are met, the operator faces the maternal perineum with forceps held in the position desired. The left blade is generally placed first. The operator's right hand is fitted between the fetal head and the left vaginal side wall, and the left blade is placed by holding the handle at 12 o'clock and rotating counterclockwise as the blade slips between the fetal head and the operator's right hand. After adequate placement, the majority of the blade is no longer visible. In a similar fashion, the operator's left hand then aids in placement of the right blade. When properly placed, the handles should come together easily. Appropriate placement is then ascertained. The sagittal suture should be equidistant from both blades and perpendicular to the shanks, with the posterior fontanelle exactly between the two blades. The posterior fontanelle should be palpable about 1 fingerbreadth above the interdigitated shanks. Failure to apply the forceps symmetrically will increase risk of injury and failure of the technique.

Holding the handles together with moderate pressure, the operator rotates the fetal head if needed so that the occiput is directly anterior or posterior (sagittal suture is perpendicular to the floor). This rotation should be done during uterine muscle relaxation, just before a contraction. A mild degree of flexion of the fetal head during rotation will make rotation easier. With a contraction and additional expulsive forces from the mother, the operator applies traction. Traction direction should be guided by the maternal pelvis. Initial traction is downward (toward the floor) until the fetal head clears the symphysis pubis. Then, traction is directed more upward as the fetal head delivers with extension (Fig. 21-19). Although in some cases early episiotomy is beneficial to forceps delivery, most often episiotomy should be cut if needed when the fetal head is bulging the perineal tissues. In many cases, removal of the forceps at this time will preclude need for episiotomy. Removal of the forceps before delivery of the head should be in the opposite direction and order of placement. Maternal expulsive forces during a contraction can then often deliver the remainder of the fetal head. The vagina and cervix should be carefully inspected for lacerations.

Vacuum Extraction

Vacuum extractors currently in widespread use in the United States are those with a soft cup made of silicone or plastic. They are smaller and more flexible than the classic Malstrom metal cup. Vacuum can be easily applied. Although these cups tend to dislodge somewhat more frequently than the Malstrom metal cup, less scalp trauma is noted with their use. Often, vacuum delivery can be performed with little to no anesthesia. However, requirements of operative vaginal delivery still apply. For the best results, the vacuum cup should be placed over the sagittal suture about 3 cm from the posterior fontanelle. This can be difficult in fetal heads descending with asynclitism (lateral deflection). After placement of the cup, an examining finger is used to ascertain that no cervical, vaginal, or perineal tissue is trapped in the cup. With a contraction, after adequate vacuum is generated, downward and then upward traction should be applied to the fetal head (Fig. 21-20). The fetal head should be allowed to rotate if needed during descent. Forceful rotation of the fetal head using the suction cup is generally not recommended because of the increased risk of scalp injury. Removal of the cup is easily accomplished once suction is

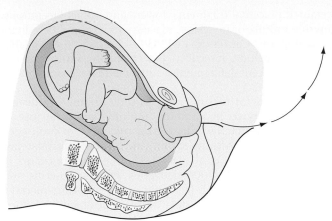

Figure 21-20 Vacuum extraction with J-shaped direction of traction, similar to forceps delivery.

discontinued. The cervix and vagina should be examined carefully for lacerations.

The Puerperium

The postpartum period, or puerperium, is the time during which the mother's altered anatomy, physiology, and biochemistry returns to the nonpregnant state. This process has its onset at the third stage of labor and is completed 6 weeks after delivery. These changes are normal and should not be confused with a pathologic condition. The woman undergoes physiologic and emotional changes that need to be monitored by her primary care physician.

Within the first 24 hours, the mother's pulse rate drops and her temperature may be slightly elevated. Generally, the white blood cell count increases during labor, with a marked leukocytosis (to 20,000/μL) occurring in the first 24 hours postpartum. The vaginal discharge is grossly bloody (lochia rubra) for the first 3 or 4 days. During the next few to 10 days, the lochia becomes more serous and pinkish brown and decreases in amount (lochia serosa). Finally, 7 to 10 days postpartum, the lochia becomes pale yellow–white and decreases even more in volume. Urine output temporarily increases and might contain protein and sugar, reflecting a maternal diuresis. This loss of fluid with the accompanying decrease in intravascular volume artificially elevates the hematocrit for a few days. The uterus involutes progressively; after 5 to 7 days, it should be firm and nontender, extending midway between the symphysis and umbilicus. By 2 weeks the uterus should no longer be palpable abdominally. Contractions of the involuting uterus are often painful and can require analgesics. Care should be exercised in choice of analgesia so as not to interfere with the maternal-infant bond or breastfeeding.

The mother is observed for 1 hour after completing the third stage of labor and given periodic uterine massage to make sure that the uterus contracts and remains contracted, preventing excess bleeding. If desired, breastfeeding can be initiated at this stage to promote uterine contraction, minimize bleeding, and promote involution of the uterus. If the uterus does not remain contracted with massage alone, oxytocin can be administered, either 10 units IM or dilute oxytocin with IV drip (10 or 30 U/1000 mL of IV fluid) at 125 to 200 mL/hr for 1 to 2 hours. Recent trends in the active management of labor encourage the administration of oxytocin before delivery of the placenta. This has been found to promote the delivery of the placenta and decrease incidence of uterine atony and postpartum hemorrhage (Prendiville et al., 2000). If general anesthesia was used for operative delivery, the mother is monitored (preferably in a recovery room or a labor, delivery, recovery, and postpartum room); oxygen and blood are tested for compatibility, and IV fluids must be readily available after delivery.

After the first 24 hours, postpartum recovery is rapid. A regular diet after a normal vaginal delivery can be offered as soon as the patient requests food. Full ambulation is encouraged as soon as possible. Showers can be encouraged, but vaginal douching is prohibited during the early postpartum period. Discomfort from an episiotomy can be relieved with hot sitz baths several times a day and analgesia. Drugs may be offered for pain as necessary but should be limited in breastfeeding mothers, because most drugs are secreted in breast milk. Meperidine (Demerol) is not the preferred analgesic for use in breastfeeding women because of the long half-life of its metabolite in infants. Repeated exposure to analgesics, especially meperidine, can result in drug accumulation and toxic effects in young or compromised infants because of their underdeveloped hepatic conjugation.

Bladder care is important. Urine retention, bladder overdistention, and catheterization should be avoided if possible. Rapid diuresis can occur, especially when oxytocin is discontinued. The woman must be encouraged to void and must be monitored to prevent asymptomatic bladder overfilling. The woman should be encouraged to defecate before leaving the hospital, although with early discharge, women often leave before a bowel movement has occurred. Laxatives may be needed for constipation. If a bowel movement has not occurred within 3 days, a mild cathartic may be given. Hemorrhoids can be minimized by maintaining an appropriate diet and good bowel function and can be treated with warm sitz baths. Regional anesthesia (spinal or epidural) delays ambulation and can delay spontaneous urination. Catheterization is recommended if significant urine output is not achieved by 12 hours and a distended bladder is apparent.

A complete blood count should be performed before discharge to verify that the woman is not significantly anemic. Women who have been determined to be seronegative should be immunized against rubella on the day of discharge. If the woman has Rh-negative blood, is not sensitized, and has an infant with Rh-positive blood, she should be given Rh_0D immune globulin 300 μg within 72 hours of delivery to prevent sensitization.

Rh(D) blood typing and antibody testing are strongly recommended for all pregnant women during their first visit for pregnancy-related care. The USPSTF found good evidence that Rh(D) blood typing, anti-Rh(D) antibody testing, and intervention with Rh(D) immunoglobulin are appropriate, prevent maternal sensitization, and improve outcomes for newborns. The benefits substantially outweigh any potential harm (USPSTF, 1989).

The breasts might become painfully engorged during early lactation, when the amount of milk is beginning to increase. If the mother is not going to breastfeed, lactation can be suppressed by firmly supporting the breasts, because gravity stimulates the let-down reflex and encourages milk flow. Many mothers find that tight binding of the breasts and restriction of oral fluid intake followed by firm support are effective, with symptoms lasting only 3 to 5 days.

The postpartum period can be complicated by the "baby blues," a common self-limited mood disorder. This is characterized by mild depressive symptoms, tearfulness (often for no discernible reason), anxiety, irritability, mood lability, increased sensitivity, and fatigue. The "blues" typically peak 4 to 5 days after delivery, can last hours to days, and usually resolve by the tenth postnatal day.

The "blues" is distinct from postpartum major depression, which occurs in approximately 10% of childbearing women (O'Hara et al., 1990). It can begin from 24 hours to several months after delivery. Its onset can be abrupt and symptoms severe, and it can be associated with lack of interest in the infant, suicidal or homicidal thoughts, hallucinations, or psychotic behavior. True psychosis probably reflects the exacerbation of preexisting mental illness in response to the physical and the psychological stress of pregnancy and delivery. Psychotherapy or pharmacotherapy is indicated, alone or in combination. Selective serotonin reuptake inhibitors may be associated with congenital heart anomalies and should be used with caution in pregnancy. All women should be routinely assessed during the antenatal period for a history of depression.

Prevention of pregnancy for several months to allow complete recovery is in the woman's best interest. *Rubella immunization mandates a delay of 3 months before a woman becomes pregnant.* Therefore, although intercourse may be resumed as soon as desired and comfortable, contraception is required because pregnancy is possible. Oral contraceptives may be started at discharge. A low-dose estrogen or progesterone-only preparation is desirable. A diaphragm should be fitted only after complete involution of the uterus, at 6 to 8 weeks; meanwhile, foams, jellies, and condoms may be used. In mothers who are not breastfeeding, earliest ovulation usually occurs about 4 weeks postpartum, 2 weeks before the first menses. However, conception has been reported as early as 2 weeks postpartum, so ovulation can occur earlier. Breastfeeding mothers tend to ovulate, then menstruate, usually at 10 to 12 weeks postpartum. The duration of anovulation is influenced by the frequency of breastfeeding, the duration of feedings, and the proportions of supplemental feeding.

Postpartum Hemorrhage

Traditionally, postpartum hemorrhage (PPH) was defined as blood loss greater than 500 mL in a vaginal delivery and greater than 1000 mL in a cesarean delivery. However, studies have revealed that an uncomplicated delivery often results in blood loss of more than 500 mL without any compromise of the mother's condition (Pritchard et al., 1962). Clinically, these findings led some authors to adopt a broader definition for PPH. Any bleeding that results in signs and symptoms of hemodynamic instability, or bleeding that could result in hemodynamic instability if untreated, is considered PPH. The loss of these amounts within 24 hours of delivery is termed *early* or *primary* PPH, and such losses are termed *late* or *secondary* PPH if they occur 24 hours after delivery or later. This section focuses primarily on early PPH.

The most common causes of PPH are uterine atony and lacerations of the vagina and cervix. Other causes include retained placental fragments, lower genital tract lacerations, uterine rupture or inversion, placenta accreta, and hereditary coagulopathy. Causes of late PPH (24 hours to 6 weeks after delivery) include infection, placental site subinvolution, retained placental fragments, and hereditary coagulopathy (ACOG, 1998a).

Risk factors for uterine atony include uterine overdistention secondary to hydramnios, multiple gestation, use of oxytocin, fetal macrosomia, high parity, rapid or prolonged labor, intra-amniotic infection, and use of uterine-relaxing agents (Combs et al., 1991). Uterine rupture occurs in approximately 1 in 2000 deliveries. Previous uterine surgery is a significant risk factor for uterine rupture, placenta accreta, and PPH. Other risk factors include obstructed labor, multiple gestations, abnormal fetal lie, and high parity.

Risk factors for hemorrhage at the time of cesarean delivery include preeclampsia, disorders of active labor, a history of previous hemorrhage, obesity, use of general anesthesia, and intra-amniotic infection.

Adequate intravascular access should be obtained in women who have significant risk factors for PPH. Active management of the third stage of labor has been shown to decrease the incidence of PPH. Early administration of oxytocin, early cord cutting and clamping, and controlled cord traction have been shown to decrease PPH by two-thirds (Soriano et al., 1996).

In the event of hemorrhage, supplemental oxygen should be administered to enhance cellular oxygen delivery. Heart rate and blood pressure should be monitored closely. Initial laboratory evaluation includes a complete blood count with platelet concentration. Blood type and crossmatch should be performed if not previously obtained. Fibrinogen, fibrin split products, prothrombin time, and partial thromboplastin time should be measured (ACOG, 1998a).

Excessive vaginal bleeding after placental delivery should prompt vigorous fundal massage while the patient is rapidly given 10 to 30 units of oxytocin in 1 L of IV fluid. If the fundus does not become firm, uterine atony is the presumed (and most common) diagnosis. Uterine atony should be initially managed by bimanual uterine massage and compression in addition to the oxytocin. If IV or IM oxytocin proves ineffective, other uterotonic agents, such as methylergonovine and prostaglandin derivatives (15-methyl $PGF_{2\alpha}$), may be used as second-line treatment (ACOG, 1998a). Methylergonovine may be administered in a dose of 0.2 mg IM every 2 to 4 hours. Methylergonovine can cause cramping, headache, and dizziness. This agent is contraindicated in hypertensive disease states because it induces vasoconstriction, which can lead to severe hypertension.

15-Methyl prostaglandin $F_{2\alpha}$ (Hemabate), may be given in a dose of 0.25 mg IM every 15 to 90 minutes (no more than eight doses). $PGF_{2\alpha}$ may also be given by intramyometrial injection at cesarean delivery or transabdominally after vaginal delivery. Prostaglandin E_2 can cause vasodilation and exacerbation of hypotension; therefore, 15-methyl $PGF_{2\alpha}$ is preferred. Because oxygen desaturation has been reported with use of $PGF_{2\alpha}$, patients should be monitored by pulse oximetry.

Continuing hemorrhage in a patient with a firm uterine fundus can indicate a hidden vaginal or cervical laceration. This type of injury is usually easy to identify and repair with adequate lighting, exposure, and assistance. If no laceration is present and the fundus is firm, the uterus requires gentle but thorough manual exploration for retained placenta, which should be removed. Uterine rupture is occasionally evident and requires immediate surgery.

An occult uterine inversion might also be discovered on vaginal examination, or it can manifest frankly. Uterine inversion is somewhat more common in primiparas and has no clear association with the mismanagement of labor. Because uterine inversion can quickly lead to shock, the physician should order brisk IV hydration and grasp the uterus in the palm, with the thumb anterior. The uterus is then firmly pushed back up into the abdominal cavity and held in place for several minutes (Brar et al., 1989). Magnesium sulfate, 0.25 mg IV, has been reported to assist in the repositioning of the uterus (Catanzarite et al., 1986).

If uterine and vaginal exploration is nondiagnostic, if uterine inversion is excluded, and if the fundus is firm, rarer causes of hemorrhage should be considered. Puerperal *hematomas* typically cause a vulvar or vaginal mass, and an occult retroperitoneal hematoma can manifest with severe abdominal pain and shock after delivery. The diagnosis is confirmed on laparotomy. Visible hematomas less than 4 cm and not expanding may be managed with ice packs and observation. Larger or expanding hematomas must be incised, irrigated, and packed, and any obvious bleeding vessels must be ligated. If venipuncture sites are oozing, coagulopathy should be considered.

Surgical intervention is undertaken for direct indications, such as uterine curettage for suspected retained placental tissue or for hemostasis if medical therapy fails. The most common indications for emergency hysterectomy include uterine atony, placenta accreta, uterine rupture, and the extension of a low-transverse uterine incision.

KEY TREATMENT

Uterotonic agents should be the first-line treatment for postpartum hemorrhage caused by uterine atony (SOR: C).

Management of PPH may vary greatly among patients, depending on etiology and available treatment options, and often a multidisciplinary approach is required (SOR: C).

When uterotonics fail following vaginal delivery, exploratory laparotomy is the next step (SOR: C).

In the presence of conditions known to be associated with placenta accreta, the obstetric care provider must have a high clinical suspicion and take appropriate precautions (SOR: C).

Data from ACOG, 2006.

References

The complete reference list is available online at www.expertconsult.com.

Web Resources

www.guidelines.gov
U.S. federal health guidelines; contains links to a variety of medical care and evidence-based guidelines for many clinical problems, in addition to obstetrics.

www.ahrq.gov/
Agency for Healthcare Research and Quality; contains clinical information, research findings, survey data, and funding opportunities.

www.uptodate.com
Subscription program offering clinical information focused on primary care but also including a variety of other clinical specialties.

www.marchofdimes.com/peristats/
Excellent source of free access to national, state, and city maternal and infant health data; includes graphs, quick facts, maps, and state summaries.

www.aafp.org
American Academy of Family Physicians; includes continuing medical education (CME) opportunities, clinical information, and links to the *American Family Physician, Family Practice Management,* and the *Annals of Family Medicine.*

Care of the Newborn

Jennifer J. Buescher and Harold Bland

Chapter contents

Whether present at the delivery or taking care of a new infant in the newborn nursery, the family physician plays an important part in newborn care during the early days of life. At the moment of birth, the newborn infant undergoes many changes and is vulnerable in the new environment. This chapter discusses these physiologic changes as well as the basics of neonatal resuscitation. The initial examination, common benign findings in the newborn period, developmental dysplasia of the hip, and audiology screening are described. Signs and symptoms of concern and common problems in the newborn period, including group B streptococcal infection and hyperbilirubinemia, are discussed, as well as infant safety, parent education, hospital follow-up, and care after discharge from the neonatal intensive care unit.

Preconception and Intrapartum Health

Key Points

- Oral folic acid supplementation before conception prevents neural tube defects.
- All pregnant women should be offered prenatal screening for trisomy 21 (Down syndrome) and neural tube defects.

- Pregnant women should be counseled against using tobacco, alcohol, or illicit drugs.
- Routine prenatal screening for group B streptococcal colonization significantly reduces early-onset neonatal GBS infection.
- Preexisting maternal illness (e.g., diabetes, hypo- and hyperthyroidism, hypertension) should be monitored closely during pregnancy.

A healthy newborn baby begins with a healthy pregnant mother. Family physicians are in the unique position of caring for women as they plan their families, during pregnancy, during childbirth, and after their infant is born. Preconception and intrapartum health care increase the likelihood of delivering a happy and healthy newborn.

Preconception Counseling

Preconception counseling regarding genetic diseases such as cystic fibrosis and Huntington's disease, as well as the dangers of tobacco, alcohol, and substance abuse, should be addressed with women of childbearing age. All women considering pregnancy should be encouraged to take in 400 μg (0.4 mg) of folic acid per day. Oral folic acid supplementation before conception can significantly decrease the risk of neural tube defects

(Czeizel and Dudas, 1992; MRC Vitamin Study Research Group, 1991). Women who have had a previous pregnancy affected by a neural tube defect should take 4000 µg (4.0 mg) of folic acid daily beginning 1 month before pregnancy (Centers for Disease Control and Prevention [CDC], 1992).

During pregnancy, maternal illness can adversely affect the fetus and lead to adverse neonatal outcomes. Maternal hypertension, preeclampsia, alcohol and tobacco use, illicit drug use, and autoimmune diseases can cause *intrauterine growth restriction* (IUGR) and preterm birth. Children born to women with diabetes mellitus or gestational diabetes are at risk for shoulder dystocia, operative delivery, hypoglycemia, and birth trauma (American College of Obstetricians and Gynecologists [ACOG], 2005). Maternal hyperglycemia at delivery also puts the infant at risk for hypoglycemia. Poorly controlled maternal hypothyroidism and hyperthyroidism are associated with low birth weight (LBW) and preterm delivery (ACOG, 2005). Fetal alcohol syndrome is directly caused by maternal alcohol use and abuse, and other illicit drug use is associated with preterm birth, congenital abnormalities, neurobehavioral abnormalities, and neonatal drug withdrawal syndromes (ACOG, 2005). Box 22-1 lists the more common human teratogens seen in the United States.

Intrapartum care should include regular fundal height measurements to monitor the growth of the fetus. Routine screening obstetric ultrasound is not recommended because of insufficient evidence of benefit or harm (ACOG, 2005). However, ultrasound is a useful and safe diagnostic test for investigating concerns about fetal growth, estimating gestational age, observing fetal anomalies, and studying other intrapartum conditions.

All pregnant women should be offered prenatal screening for trisomy 21 (Down syndrome) and neural tube defects. For most women, maternal serum quadruple analyte screen (quad screen) is the most appropriate screening test. The quad screen measures serum levels of alpha fetoprotein (AFP), human chorionic gonadotropin (hCG), unconjugated estriol, and inhibin-A. Inhibin-A was added to the prior triple screen to improve the detection of trisomy 21. For women younger than 35, the triple screen detects approximately 75% of trisomy 21, 90% of anencephaly, and 80% of spina bifida if measured between 16 and 18 weeks' gestation (Benn et al., 2003; Graves et al., 2002). Using the quad screen, approximately 85% of trisomy 21 cases can be detected. The quad screen also has a false-positive rate for trisomy 21 of 8.2% after correction of major gestational errors, so a positive quad screen indicates a 1.9% risk for true trisomy 21 (Benn et al., 2003).

Routine prenatal screening for group B streptococci (GBS) significantly reduces early-onset neonatal GBS infection (Schrag et al., 2002b). Women who test positive for GBS or who have had a previous child with invasive GBS disease should receive intrapartum antibiotics for at least 4 hours before delivery (Schrag et al., 2002a). Management of the infant born to a mother colonized with GBS is discussed later.

KEY TREATMENT

Oral folic acid supplementation before conception prevents neural tube defects (Czeizel and Dudas, 1992; MRC Vitamin Study Research Group, 1991) (SOR: A).

Routine prenatal screening for colonization by group B *Streptococcus* species significantly reduces early-onset neonatal GBS infection in neonates (Schrag et al., 2002b) (SOR: A).

Box 22-1 Selected Teratogenic Agents in Humans

Drugs and Environmental chemicals

Androgenic hormones
Angiotensin-converting enzyme (ACE) inhibitors
Angiotensin receptor blockers (sartans)
Antiepileptics
    Carbamazepine*
    Diphenylhydantoin
    Trimethadione
    Valproic acid
    Phenobarbital*
Antineoplastics
Cigarette smoking
Cocaine
Coumarin anticoagulants (warfarin)
Diethylstilbestrol
Etretinate
Fluconazole, high dose
Iodides and goiter
Lithium*
Mercury, organic
Methimazole
Methylene blue via intra-amniotic injection
Misoprostol
Penicillamine
1,3-*cis*-Retinoic acid (isotretinoin)
Tetracyclines
Thalidomide
Toluene abuse

Infections

Cytomegalovirus
Herpes simplex virus types 1 and 2
Parvovirus B19 (erythema infectiosum)
Rubella virus
Syphilis
Toxoplasmosis
Varicella virus

Maternal factors

Alcoholism
Type 1 diabetes mellitus
Folic acid deficiency
Phenylketonuria
Sjögren's syndrome

Modified from Shepard T. Catalog of Teratogenic Agents. 11th ed. Baltimore, Johns Hopkins University Press, 2004.

*Denotes agents that produce less than 10 defects in 1000 exposures.

Transition from Fetus to Newborn

Key Points

- A separate provider trained in neonatal care and resuscitation should be present and responsible only for the infant during every delivery.

- The ABC principles of neonatal resuscitation are airway, breathing, and circulation.
- The Apgar score should not be used as a substitution for assessing the ABCs in neonatal resuscitation.
- Resuscitation efforts should not be delayed or interrupted to assign an Apgar score.
- Routine endotracheal intubation and tracheal suction do not prevent meconium aspiration syndrome and may harm the vigorous infant.

During the first hours after delivery, the newborn must adapt to extrauterine life. This adaptation includes a highly coordinated series of physiologic changes during which the infant is particularly vulnerable. Health care providers trained to assess and manage newborns should be available during the delivery and immediate neonatal transition period for all infants.

Circulatory Changes

In utero, a series of central shunts moves oxygenated blood coming from the placenta through the umbilical vein to supply the brain and other organs. Most oxygenated blood bypasses the liver via the ductus venosus and enters the left side of the heart (bypassing the lungs) through the foramen ovale. The poorly oxygenated blood returning from the lungs bypasses the heart through the ductus arteriosus and returns to the placenta to obtain oxygen from the maternal circulation (Moore and Persaud, 1993).

On delivery, the fetal circulation must adapt to self-oxygenation, and the central shunting must cease. When the umbilical cord is clamped and cut, absent blood flow within the umbilical vein leads to the closure of the ductus venosus. The umbilical vessels functionally close by 2 to 3 days of life.

With the initial newborn breath, the aeration of the lungs drives fluid within the air space of the lungs into the pulmonary interstitium. An increase in the partial pressure of oxygen (P_{O_2}) within the pulmonary vasculature causes vasodilation and a progressive decrease in pulmonary vascular resistance. Increasing P_{O_2}, along with circulating prostaglandins, stimulates the constriction and closure of the ductus arteriosus. Pulmonary blood now flows preferentially to the heart, rather than directly into the aorta through the ductus arteriosus (Moore and Persaud, 1993; Thureen et al., 2005).

In the normal infant the ductus arteriosus might remain partially open during the first several hours of life and cause a soft systolic murmur. It can take the normal infant a few hours to clear the lungs of excess fluid, causing fine crackles to be heard on lung examination and a transient elevation of the respiratory rate. As pulmonary vascular resistance falls, systemic vascular resistance increases. When left atrial and ventricular pressures increase above right atrial pressures, the foramen ovale closes. Poorly oxygenated blood from the superior and inferior vena cava can now flow into the pulmonary arteries (Moore and Persaud, 1993). The foramen ovale typically becomes fully sealed within the first month of life.

Neonatal Resuscitation

The successful transition to extrauterine life depends heavily on the ability of the neonatal pulmonary system to adapt quickly and provide oxygen to the infant. Any illness or injury

---

Box 22-2 Neonatal Resuscitation Supplies and Equipment for Delivery of a Term Infant

Suction equipment

Bulb syringe
Mechanical suction and tubing
Suction catheters
8-F feeding tube and 20-mL syringe
Meconium aspirator

Bag and mask equipment

Neonatal resuscitation bag with a pressure-release valve or pressure manometer
Face masks, newborn and premature sizes
Oxygen source with flow meter and tubing

Medications and supplies to be immediately available if necessary

Epinephrine 1:10,000
Isotonic crystalloid for volume expansion
Sodium bicarbonate 4.2%
Naloxone hydrochloride (0.4 mg/mL)
Dextrose 10%
Normal saline for flushes
Umbilical vessel catheterization supplies
Syringes and needles

Miscellaneous

Gloves and appropriate personal protection
Radiant warmer or other heat source
Firm, padded resuscitation surface
Clock
Warmed linens and dry blankets
Stethoscope
Oropharyngeal airways

Intubation equipment

Laryngoscope with straight blades, no. 1
Extra bulbs and batteries for laryngoscope
Endotracheal (ET) tubes, sizes 2.5, 3.0, 3.5, and 4.0 mm
Materials to secure ET tube in place

Modified from Kattwinkel J (ed): Textbook of Neonatal Resuscitation, 5th ed. Elk Grove Village, Ill, American Academy of Pediatrics and American Heart Association, 2006.

---

that interferes with oxygenation puts the infant at great risk and should be identified and treated promptly. It is important that with every delivery, at least one person trained in neonatal care and resuscitation be assigned to care specifically for the infant. Caregivers should have immediate access to the necessary equipment for a complete resuscitation. If there is concern that the newborn will be at high risk for complications (e.g., thick meconium, fetal heart rate decelerations, known fetal anomalies), appropriate equipment should be set up and ready to use immediately (Box 22-2).

The American Academy of Pediatrics and American Heart Association developed specific protocols for neonatal resuscitation (AAP and AHA, 2006). An adapted resuscitation algorithm is given in Figure 22-1. This chapter does not cover the protocol in sufficient detail to produce competency in neonatal resuscitation and should not be used as a substitute

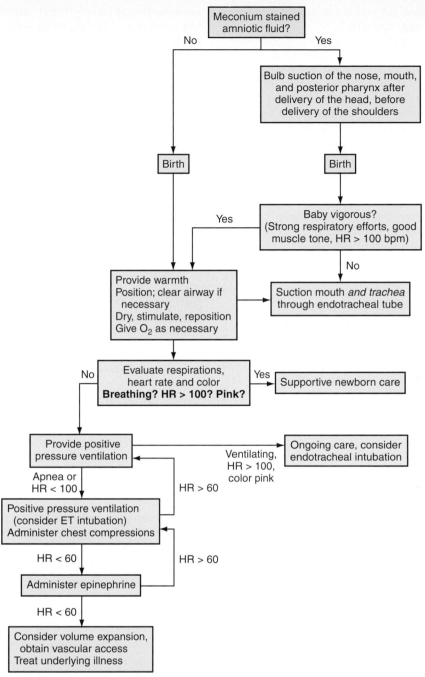

Figure 22-1 Algorithm for neonatal resuscitation. *ET,* Endotracheal; *HR,* heart rate.
(Modified from John Kattwinkel J (ed). Textbook of Neonatal Resuscitation. 5th ed. American Academy of Pediatrics and American Heart Association, Elk Grove Village, Ill, 2006.)

for participation in the AAP/AHA Neonatal Resuscitation Program (NRP). The ABCs of neonatal resuscitation are the same as adult resuscitation: clear and position the *airway,* make sure the infant is *breathing* (whether spontaneously or with support), and ensure *circulation* of oxygenated blood.

Initial stabilization procedures after every delivery should include warming and drying the infant, removing wet towels quickly, and providing tactile stimulation to encourage vigorous breathing and good muscle tone. After necessary resuscitation is completed, all neonates should receive chemoprophylaxis for ophthalmia neonatorum with 1% tetracycline ophthalmic ointment, 0.5% erythromycin ophthalmic ointment, or 1% silver nitrate aqueous solution. All three

medications have similar efficacy; however, silver nitrate is preferred in areas with appreciable incidence of penicillinase-producing *Neisseria gonorrhoeae.* Silver nitrate is more likely than tetracycline or erythromycin to cause a transient chemical conjunctivitis in the first 1 or 2 days of life (AAP, 2003a).

Infants should also receive 1.0 mg of vitamin K intramuscularly early after delivery to prevent vitamin K–deficiency bleeding (VKDB, previously hemorrhagic disease of the newborn) (AAP, 2003b; Puckett and Offringa, 2000). Concerns about a correlation between intramuscular (IM) vitamin K and childhood leukemia have not been validated, and there is insufficient data to show that oral vitamin K prevents late-onset VKDB; therefore, IM vitamin K should be administered to all newborns (AAP, 2003b).

The Apgar Score

The Apgar score is widely used as a part of the early assessment of the newborn (Table 22-1). A score of 0, 1, or 2 is assigned to each of the five physical signs at 1 and 5 minutes after birth. The Apgar score should not be used as a substitute for assessing the ABCs in neonatal resuscitation, and resuscitation efforts should not be delayed or interrupted to assign an Apgar score. However, the Apgar score does allow a quick and consistent way for different providers to describe an infant's condition. A score of 7 to 10 is considered normal. If the 5-minute Apgar score is abnormal, less than 7, appropriate resuscitation measures should be continued and Apgar scores assigned every 5 minutes until the infant is stabilized.

Although the Apgar score provides a systematic way for different providers to describe an infant's condition in the first minutes of life, it correlates poorly with future neurologic outcomes (AAP and ACOG, 1996). A poor Apgar score alone cannot be used to diagnose asphyxia in the newborn or predict the development of cerebral palsy. However, the Apgar score is correlated with early infant death. In a large population study of term infants, an abnormal 5-minute Apgar score correlated with a significantly increased risk of death in the first 28 days of life. Even in infants with the lowest scores, however, death within 28 days is uncommon, occurring in 244 of 1000 infants with 5-minute Apgar scores of 0 to 3 (Casey et al., 2001).

Resuscitation of the Infant Born through Meconium-Stained Amniotic Fluid

Meconium staining of the amniotic fluid is a common complication during delivery of term infants, and approximately 5% to 12% of these infants develop *meconium aspiration syndrome* (MAS) (Wiswell et al., 2000). Risk factors for meconium staining of the amniotic fluid include maternal hypertension, maternal diabetes, maternal chronic respiratory or cardiovascular disease, maternal heavy smoking, preeclampsia or eclampsia, oligohydramnios, IUGR, poor biophysical profile, and abnormal fetal heart rate patterns (Gelfand et al., 2004). MAS is a life-threatening disease for otherwise healthy term newborns, and appropriate resuscitation of the infant at risk for MAS is important (see later discussion). All infants at risk for MAS and showing respiratory distress or bradycardia after delivery should undergo standard neonatal resuscitation procedures. In the depressed infant, tracheal suctioning to remove visible meconium can decrease the incidence and the severity of MAS (AAP and AHA, 2006). However, when the infant is *vigorous* at birth—defined as heart rate greater than 100, spontaneous respiration, and spontaneous movements or extremity flexion—routine endotracheal intubation and tracheal suction does not prevent MAS (Wiswell et al., 2000).

KEY TREATMENT

In the vigorous infant, routine endotracheal intubation and tracheal suction do not prevent meconium aspiration syndrome and can harm the infant (Wiswell et al., 2000) (SOR: A).

Initial Newborn Evaluation

Key Points

- A comprehensive physical examination of the newborn should be completed and discussed with the parents within the first 12 to 18 hours of life.
- The newborn examination should include observation of the infant at rest, including resting muscle tone, skin color, and respiratory effort.
- Periodic breathing is a normal breathing pattern in the newborn.
- A normal infant may need several hours to clear the lungs of excess fluid, and fine pulmonary crackles can be a normal physical finding.
- A soft systolic murmur can be a normal physical finding in the first hours of life, as the ductus arteriosus remains partially open.
- Asymmetric limb movements and reflexes should prompt further evaluation.
- All newborns should be screened for hearing loss before discharge.

Once the infant has been stabilized immediately after delivery, maternal and infant bonding should be encouraged. Initiating breastfeeding within the first 60 minutes after birth can increase the chances of successful breastfeeding (Sinusas and Gagliardi, 2001).

Within the first 12 to 18 hours of life, a comprehensive physical examination should be completed and discussed with the parents. During the examination, the infant should be kept in a comfortable environment. Keeping the infant quiet and calm is important for adequate examination in the newborn period. The examination should begin with observation of activity, skin color, muscle tone, and respiratory effort while the infant is quiet. Listening to the heart and lungs should be completed next, disturbing the infant as little

---

Table 22-1 Apgar Score

Sign	Score*		
	0	**1**	**2**
Heart rate	Absent	<100 beats/min	≥100 beats/min
Respirations	Absent	Irregular and slow	Strong breaths, crying
Muscle tone	Limp	Some flexion	Good flexion, active motion
Reflex irritability to tactile stimulation	No response	Grimace	Cough, sneeze, cry,
Color	Blue or pale	Blue extremities, pink body	Completely pink

*Apgar scoring should be completed at 1 and 5 minutes. The normal Apgar score at 5 minutes is 7 or higher. If the 5-minute Apgar is less than 7, continue resuscitative efforts and assign additional scores every 5 minutes for up to 20 minutes after birth.
Modified from Kattwinkel J (ed). Textbook of Neonatal Resuscitation. 5th ed. Elk Grove Village, Ill, American Academy of Pediatrics and American Heart Association, 2006.

as possible. An infant often begins to cry at the touch of a cold stethoscope or cold hands, making the cardiopulmonary examination particularly difficult. The rest of the examination can then be completed in a calm and thorough manner.

As with the examination of adults and children, a complete history should be obtained on every patient. For the newborn, this includes the maternal history, antepartum course, course of delivery and any complications, and any postpartum complications. Specific attention to maternal medication and drug use, maternal medical conditions, traumatic events during delivery, neonatal resuscitation measures required, and maternal postpartum course assist in developing an appropriate assessment and plan for the neonate.

General Appearance

After collecting the history, it is important to observe the calm newborn. The normal term newborn rests with all extremities in some degree of flexion. Breathing should be quiet and effortless, but it can be very irregular. Episodes without breathing lasting 5 to 10 seconds are common and normal in newborns. Skin should be warm to the touch, soft, and smooth. Table 22-2 lists normal vital signs in the first days of life. Box 22-3 lists some common benign findings on the newborn examination. These are generally self-limited and require no further evaluation or treatment in the otherwise asymptomatic newborn.

Infants typically lose up to 10% of their birth weight in the first few days but should regain this weight by 2 weeks of age (Thureen et al., 2005). Excessive weight loss can indicate systemic disease or feeding difficulties and should be evaluated before discharge.

Skin

Examination of the skin should identify signs of systemic illness, signs of trauma from delivery, and birthmarks. Pallor, mottling, and central cyanosis can be signs of infection or respiratory distress. Petechiae on the face, scalp, and upper chest can occur as a result of a compressed nuchal cord during delivery. Bruising on the face and molding of the cranium are common in vaginal deliveries and often resolve in the first few days of life.

Several common benign skin conditions in the newborn period often cause significant worry for parents and caregivers. Accurate diagnosis and reassurance can be an important part of the physician-patient relationship. *Macular hemangiomas* (also known as "stork bites" and "salmon patches") are extremely common, particularly on the forehead and eyelids, and usually disappear before 1 year of age. *Milia* are tiny epidermoid cysts on the face that disappear within a few weeks. *Erythema toxicum* is a benign rash of yellowish papules on an erythematous base and resolves spontaneously in 4 to 5 days (Thureen et al., 2005).

Neurologic Examination and Newborn Reflexes

The neurologic examination of the newborn begins with the general appearance of the infant. The newborn should have a strong cry and exhibit symmetric movements; a high-pitched or weak cry can be associated with current illness or neurologic deficits. Asymmetric movements can indicate musculoskeletal or focal neurologic injury. Complete absence or asymmetry of any newborn reflex can indicate neurologic deficit or injury. The following developmental reflexes are present at birth in the normal newborn (Thureen et al., 2005):

Rooting reflex: When the cheek is stroked, the infant turns the head toward the stimulus and opens the mouth as if preparing to feed.

Sucking reflex: Stroking the lips causes the infant to open the mouth and begin to make sucking movements. The strength and coordination of suck can be assessed using a gloved finger placed in the mouth.

Moro reflex (or *startle reflex*): The infant's head is raised several centimeters above the examination table while supporting the head and neck. The head is allowed to drop a short distance into the examiner's other hand, and the infant responds by abduction and extension of the arms and opening of the hands. The infant then flexes arms and closes the fists and brings them back in toward the body.

Tonic neck reflex: With the infant lying supine, the head is turned to one side. The infant's arm on the side where the face is directed extends, and the opposite arm flexes.

Table 22-2 Vital Signs in the First Days of Life

Vital sign	Normal value
Heart rate	100-180 beats/min
Respiratory rate	24-60 breaths/min
Systolic blood pressure	65-90 mm Hg
Diastolic blood pressure	50-70 mm Hg
Temperature	<101.4° F (38.0° C) >96.8° F (36.0° C)

Data from Gunn VL, Nechyba C. The Harriet Lane Handbook, 16th ed, St Louis, Mosby, 2002; Rudolph AM. Kamei RK, Sagan P. Rudolph's Fundamentals of Pediatrics, 2nd ed. Norwalk, Conn, Appleton & Lange, 1998.

Box 22-3 Common Benign Findings in the Newborn (Partial List)

Caput succedaneum (edema crossing suture lines)
Epstein's pearls (retention cysts) on hard palate
Erythema toxicum
Enlarged breasts (male or female)
Hydrocele
Mild diastasis recti
Mild esotropia/exotropia
Milia
Miliaria
Mongolian spots
Nasolacrimal duct blockage (usually spontaneously resolves)
Neonatal pustular melanosis
Petechiae on presenting part (nonprogressive)
Protruding xiphoid
Salmon patches
Shortened tongue frenulum (does not need cutting)
Subconjunctival hemorrhage at birth
Umbilical hernia
Vaginal discharge or bleeding

Palmar and plantar grasp: Stroking the palm of the hand causes the infant to grip the examining finger. This grip tightens as the examiner pulls away. When firm pressure is placed on the plantar surface of the foot, the toes curl in toward the examining thumb.

Stepping reflex: The infant is held with both feet touching the examination table. The infant should exhibit alternating stepping movements.

Truncal incurvation (Galant reflex): The infant is held in the prone position above the examination table. Stroking one side of the spine with a finger or cotton swab should cause the infant to flex the pelvis toward the side of the reflex.

Head, Face, and Neck

Examination of the head and neck should include evaluation of cranial sutures, anterior and posterior fontanelles, facial symmetry, hard and soft palate, patency of the ear canal, patency of both nares, position of the nasal septum, placement of the ears, and intercanthal distance of the eyes.

The fontanelles should be flat and soft, and cranial sutures should be slightly mobile. The cranial sutures may override each other, and there may be temporary skull asymmetry after prolonged labor or vaginal delivery. Caput succedaneum and cephalohematoma (subperiosteal hemorrhage) are also common complications of labor and vaginal delivery. A *cephalohematoma* is a result of bleeding in the subperiosteal space and does not extend across a suture line, whereas caput succedaneum is caused primarily by subcutaneous edema and can involve any amount of the scalp. *Caput succedaneum* is present at delivery, and cephalohematoma is not evident until a few hours of age.

Many infants have transient skin lesions on the face and neck, and these should be noted and discussed with caregivers. Some birthmarks, however, can be a sign of underlying disease. For example, a port-wine stain occurring in the distribution of the first branch of the trigeminal nerve may be associated with Sturge-Weber syndrome. Hemangiomas are not always present at birth and might not be visible until 1 month of age. Most hemangiomas spontaneously regress during childhood and need no specific management. Periocular hemangiomas, however, should be managed with ophthalmologic consultation and aggressive therapy (Thureen et al., 2005).

The eyes, nose, mouth, and ears should be symmetric. Using a gloved finger, the hard and soft palate should be palpated and found to be fully merged. The oropharynx should be visualized, and the uvula should be single and midline. The ear canals should be inspected with an otoscope and found to be patent, and a small nasogastric tube should pass freely through each nare to the oropharynx. The helix of the ear (top portion) should be above the position of the inner canthi of the eyes.

Eyes

The newborn eye examination can be difficult immediately after birth, when the face may be edematous, and an assistant may help to hold the eyelid open. The sclera should be white but may appear a faint blue in premature infants. The pupils should be symmetric and reactive. A red reflex (reflex off the retina as viewed through ophthalmoscope) should be present bilaterally. In dark-skinned infants the retinal reflex can appear pale or grayish white (Tappero and Honeyfield,

2003). Absence of a retinal reflex can indicate a congenital cataract, and a bright white or asymmetric reflex may be seen with retinoblastoma. Subconjunctival hemorrhage can be seen, more frequently with traumatic labor or delivery, and often clears within the first few days of life. Prominent epicanthal folds over the medial upper aspect of the eye can be seen in Down syndrome but can also be a familial trait.

Chest and Lungs

Initial observation of the quiet infant should include assessment of respiratory rate and effort. Skin retraction between the ribs during inspiration is abnormal and usually indicates respiratory distress. The abdomen may move with each breath, but it should appear effortless. Breath sounds should be equal and clear in all lung fields. Fine crackles (wet lungs) can be normal, particularly in the infant who was delivered by cesarean section, as the infant is trying to clear the interstitial fluid left over from intrauterine life. This can also be associated with a transient tachypnea that resolves spontaneously.

Heart

The newborn cardiac examination should include inspection for adequate perfusion and palpation of the radial, brachial, and femoral pulses. Capillary refill time in the neonate is normally less than 2 seconds, and all pulses should be strong and equal bilaterally. Cyanosis or diaphoresis with crying, feeding, or Valsalva maneuver can be a sign of congenital heart disease and should be evaluated further. On auscultation, the heart rate should be regular and without murmur, and both heart sounds should be heard distinctly.

In the first 24 hours of life, the continuous rumbling murmur of a patent ductus arteriosus (PDA) is often heard in the second left intercostal space (Tappero and Honeyfield, 2003). In an otherwise asymptomatic infant, PDA can be observed and should resolve quickly. Coarctation of the aorta often produces a systolic ejection murmur radiating to the cardiac apex and to the back and may also be associated with asymmetric or absent femoral pulses.

Abdomen

The infant abdomen is normally round, soft, and symmetric. Abdominal masses, hepatomegaly, duodenal atresia, and other intra-abdominal abnormalities can cause asymmetry. Bowel sounds should be heard in all quadrants. The umbilical cord should be clamped and should be dry, showing no signs of infection. The abdomen should be palpated when the infant is not crying or upset, and the liver, kidneys, and spleen should be normal in size. The normal infant liver is 1 to 3.5 cm below the costal margin, and the left lobe often crosses the midline. The normal spleen should be slightly below the left lateral costal margin and should feel firm and small. The kidneys are felt with deep palpation as small, firm, lobular masses on either side of the abdomen.

Genitalia and Anus

The genitalia of the female child should have a visibly patent vaginal orifice, with the labia majora covering the labia minora, clitoris, and vaginal opening. The labia majora should be completely separate from each other (ensuring the absence of labioscrotal fusion). The labia majora should be palpated to evaluate the presence of inguinal hernia or ectopic gonads.

The male infant should have two palpable testicles of similar size within the scrotum. If the infant is cold during the examination, the testicles may be retracted and might even be found at the distal end of the inguinal canal. Each testicle, however, should be able to be easily brought down into the scrotum. The testicles should be similar in size and shape, although presence of significant hydrocele is a common transient finding in newborns. A hydrocele should transilluminate, and any testicular mass that does not transilluminate should be further evaluated.

The glans of the penis is normally covered completely by foreskin, and the urethral meatus should be located at the tip of the glans. A child with the urethral meatus opening on the ventral (hypospadias) or dorsal (epispadias) surface of the penis *should not be circumcised* until pediatric urologic consultation has been completed.

Most male and female infants urinate within the first 24 hours of life. Delay in urination should prompt an evaluation of the kidneys, bladder and urethra (Tappero and Honeyfield, 2003).

The anus should be inspected for patency during the initial examination, and the infant should pass stool within the first 24 hours of life. The first several bowel movements are meconium stools, dark and black with a tarry consistency. These eventually change to the thin, yellowish stools of the newborn.

Muscles, Skeleton, and Hips

The initial musculoskeletal examination should be the observation of the infant. All limbs should appear symmetric and move equally, and any deficit should lead to further evaluation.

Palpate both clavicles to evaluate for fracture or dislocation that might have occurred during delivery. In the event of a traumatic vaginal delivery, it is important to pay special attention to the potential for a brachial plexus injury. An infant with brachial plexus injury often has the affected arm straight down at the side and might have the wrist slightly bent, the fingers straight, and the forearm pronated (Thureen et al., 2005). Inspect hands and feet for syndactyly (fusion of fingers or toes), polydactyly (extra digits), clubfoot, and other congenital anomalies.

The incidence of *developmental dysplasia of the hip* (DDH) is estimated to be between 1.5 and 20 cases per 1000 infants (Shipman, 2006). Female gender, breech position, and family history are all reported risk factors for DDH; however, only a minority of cases of DDH are found in infants with identifiable risk factors (Shipman, 2006). In addition, as many as 80% of infants with an abnormal hip examination at birth resolved by 6 weeks, and 90% of mild dysplasia identified by ultrasound resolved between 6 weeks and 6 months (Shipman, 2006). The U.S. Preventive Services Task Force concluded that there was insufficient evidence to recommend routine screening for DDH in newborns (USPSTF, 2006). AAP (2000b) continues to recommend serial clinical examinations of the hip for the first 12 months of life.

There are two maneuvers in the neonatal hip examination: the Ortolani maneuver and the Barlow maneuver (Fig. 22-2). Each hip should be examined separately using gentle but firm pressure. Too much force can injure the hip in a normal infant.

The *Barlow maneuver* begins with flexion and adduction of the hip. The examiner should place the palm of the hand just below the infant's knee and the fingertips over the greater trochanter of the femur. The examiner exerts gentle pressure toward the examination table, and in a positive test the examiner can feel and often hear the femur slip posteriorly out of the acetabulum (Weinstein et al., 2004). This is often

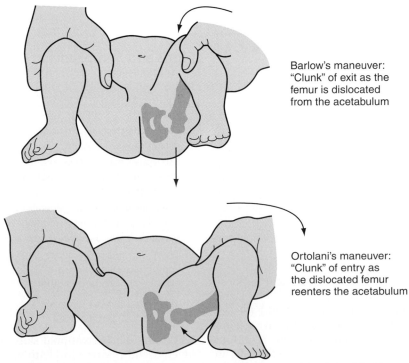

Barlow's maneuver: "Clunk" of exit as the femur is dislocated from the acetabulum

Ortolani's maneuver: "Clunk" of entry as the dislocated femur reenters the acetabulum

Figure 22-2 Physical examination maneuvers for developmental dysplasia of the hip.

called the "clunk of exit" or "click of exit" (Vain et al., 2004). The terminology used to describe the positive test can cause confusion to the inexperienced examiner. Benign adventitial sounds and high-pitched clicks often occur with flexion and extension of the extremities in a normal newborn and are mistaken for hip dysplasia (AAP, 2000b). If the newborn hip is already dislocated, the Barlow test will be negative because the femur is already outside the acetabulum.

The *Ortolani maneuver* is performed by abducting the hip and firmly pressing the greater trochanter up away from the examination table. In a positive test, a "clunk of entry" is heard and felt as the head of the femur reenters the acetabulum (Weinstein et al., 2004).

Newborn infants with any positive or equivocally positive result should be reexamined at 2 weeks of age. If at 2 weeks the examination remains positive, pediatric orthopedic consultation should be considered. Some newborns have ligamentous laxity that can be mistaken for hip dysplasia, but this should resolve in the first 2 weeks of life. A child with a history or physical examination suspicious for developmental dysplasia of the hip can be evaluated with serial hip examinations, hip ultrasound at 6 weeks of age, or pelvic radiographs at 4 months of age, and pediatric orthopedic referral should be considered (AAP, 2000b).

Postnatal Assessment of Gestational Age

Before delivery, gestational age is estimated using the date of the last menstrual period or obstetric ultrasound measurements. After birth, however, physical and neurologic criteria should be used to estimate the gestational age of the infant. The *new Ballard score* accurately estimates gestational age within 2 weeks for infants older than 20 weeks' gestation (Ballard et al., 1991). Identifying the preterm (less than 37 weeks) and post-term (more than 42 weeks) infant is important for appropriate risk management and observation after delivery.

The assessment of gestational age should be performed within 96 hours of birth by two separate examiners to ensure objectivity (Thureen et al., 2005). Box 22-4 and Figure 22-3 describe the new Ballard score and examination.

Audiology Screening

Congenital hearing loss affects approximately 1 to 3 infants per 1000 live births. At least 37 states and the District of Columbia have legislatively mandated universal newborn hearing screening programs in the United States (National Center for Hearing Assessment and Management [NCHAM], 2005). In a 2008 update, USPSTF changed its recommendation on newborn hearing screening to a B recommendation, indicating that the evidence shows moderate certainty that there is a moderate net benefit to universal newborn hearing screening.

There are three acceptable screening tests to detect congenital hearing loss: automated auditory brainstem response (AABR), transient evoked otoacoustic emissions (TEOAE), and distortion product otoacoustic emissions (DPOAE) (Hayes, 2002; NCHAM, 2006). The AABR is a more expensive test but has a lower audiology referral rate than testing for TEOAE or DPOAE. TEOAE might have higher false-negative results in particularly vulnerable populations such as premature infants

---

Box 22-4 Examination Technique for the New Ballard Score

Neuromuscular maturity

Posture: Assign score when infant is relaxed and quiet.

Square window: Measure the angle of the wrist in flexion, between the hypothenar eminence and the forearm.

Arm recoil: Score the position of the arm after flexing the forearms for 5 seconds, fully extending the arm and releasing quickly.

Popliteal angle: Measure the angle of the popliteal fossil with the hip fully flexed and the knee extended with gentle pressure.

Scarf sign: Maneuver arm over opposite shoulder keeping scapulae on the exam table.

Heel to ear: Keeping the pelvis on the exam table and without forcing the leg, move the infant's foot toward the head.

Physical maturity

Skin: With increasing gestational age, the skin becomes thicker, tougher, and less transparent.

Lanugo: Describe the fine, downy lanugo hair as seen over the infant's back and scapulae.

Plantar surface of foot: Measure from the tip of great toe to the back of the heel.

Breast tissue: Describe nipple size, stage of development, and amount of breast tissue.

Eye/ear: Loosely fused eyelids open with gentle traction; the pinna in a term infant is well formed and quickly recoils after bending.

Genitalia: Describe the development of the external genitalia.

Modified from Thureen PJ, Deacon J, Hernandez JA, Hall DM. Assessment and Care of the Well Newborn. 2nd ed. Philadelphia, Saunders, 2005.

---

or those hospitalized in the intensive care unit (Hayes, 2002). Many screening programs using TEOAE or DPOAE employ a two-stage screening program, where an infant who fails the initial screen will be tested with AABR before discharge (NCHAM, 2006). Infants who fail a hearing screening program should be promptly referred to a pediatric audiologist for further diagnostic testing.

Signs and Symptoms of Concern

Key Points

- The inability to maintain body temperature may be an early sign of sepsis in the newborn.
- Tachypnea, expiratory grunting, intercostal retractions, subcostal retractions, apnea, and cyanotic spells are signs of respiratory distress in the infant.
- Petechiae that become generalized or develop hours after delivery should prompt further evaluation.
- Most infants will pass urine and meconium stool by 24 hours of age.
- Group B streptococcal sepsis can be prevented through appropriate antepartum antibiotic use and appropriate management of the infant born to a high-risk mother.

General Observation

Using careful observational skills, the examiner can obtain much useful information without even touching the infant. One can assess the infant's skin color, respiratory effort, and

NEUROMUSCULAR MATURITY

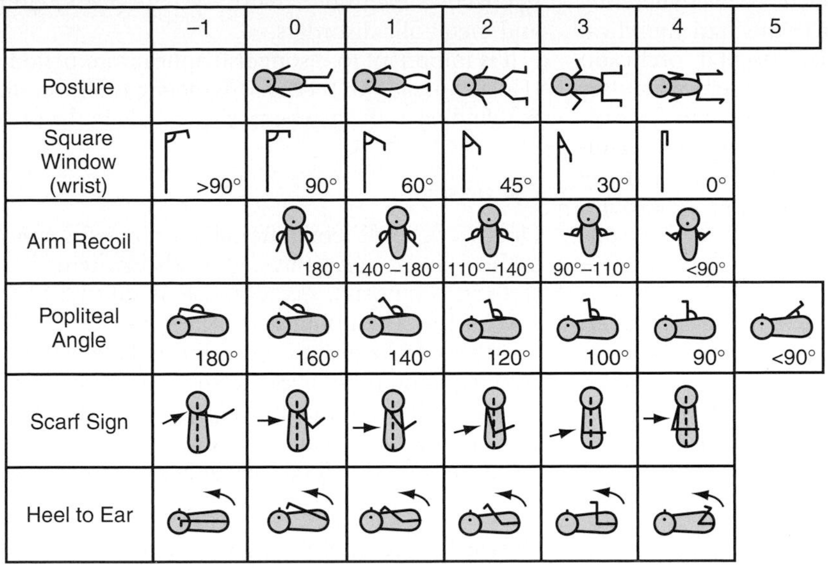

	−1	0	1	2	3	4	5
Posture							
Square Window (wrist)	>90°	90°	60°	45°	30°	0°	
Arm Recoil		180°	140°–180°	110°–140°	90°–110°	<90°	
Popliteal Angle	180°	160°	140°	120°	100°	90°	<90°
Scarf Sign							
Heel to Ear							

MATURITY RATING

Score	Weeks
−10	20
−5	22
0	24
5	26
10	28
15	30
20	32
25	34
30	36
35	38
40	40
45	42
50	44

PHYSICAL MATURITY

Skin	sticky; friable; transparent	gelatinous; red; translucent	smooth; pink; visible veins	superficial peeling and/or rash; few veins	cracking; pale areas; rare veins	parchment; deep cracking; no vessels	leathery; cracked; wrinkled
Lanugo	none	sparse	abundant	thinning	bald areas	mostly bald	
Plantar surface	heel-toe 40-50 mm: -1 <40 mm: -2	>50 mm; no crease	faint red marks	anterior transverse crease only	creases ant. 2/3	creases over entire sole	
Breast	imperceptible	barely perceptible	flat areola; no bud	stippled areola; 1-2 mm bud	raised areola; 3-4 mm bud	full areola; 5-10 mm bud	
Eye/ear	lids fused loosely: -1 tightly: -2	lids open; pinna flat; stays folded	sl. curved pinna; soft; slow recoil	well-curved pinna; soft but ready recoil	formed & firm; instant recoil	thick cartilage; ear stuff	
Genitals male	scrotum flat; smooth	scrotum empty; faint rugae	testes in upper canal; rare rugae	testes descending; few rugae	testes down; good rugae	testes pendulous; deep rugae	
Genitals female	clitoris prominent; labia flat	prominent clitoris; small labia minora	prominent clitoris; enlarging minora	majora & minora equally prominent	majora large; minora small	majora cover clitoris & minora	

Figure 22-3 Maturational assessment of gestational age (new Ballard score). See Box 22-4 for a description of the technique. *(From Ballard JL, Khoury JC, Wedig K, et al: New Ballard score, expanded to include extremely premature infants. J Pediatr 1991;119:417-423.)*

activity state; the muscle tone can be assessed by observing whether the infant lies in a flexed position and spontaneously moves the extremities.

Vital Signs

Heart Rate

Variations of the heart rate (HR) or rhythm are relatively common in the newborn period and, if isolated, are usually benign. HR abnormalities fall into one of two main categories: *tachycardia* (HR >180 beats/min) and *bradycardia* (HR <80 beats/min). Persistent tachycardia is abnormal and should be evaluated for conditions such as sepsis, anemia, hypoxemia, hypovolemia, and hyperthermia. Persistent bradycardia is abnormal and may be associated with sepsis, asphyxia of the fetus, hypoxemia, congenital heart block, increased intracranial pressure, and hypothyroidism (Hoekelman, 2001, Thureen et al., 2005).

Blood Pressure

It is unusual for blood pressure (BP) abnormalities to be isolated findings in the newborn. *Hypotension* (systolic BP <60 mm Hg in term infant) is usually accompanied by tachycardia and a physical examination consistent with poor perfusion. Hypotension usually is a complication of some other serious underlying problem, such as overwhelming sepsis or acute hemorrhage. In infants who had umbilical arterial catheters, occasionally a renal vascular occlusion leads to hypertension. A combination of poor femoral pulses and elevated pressures in the upper extremities calls for evaluating for coarctation of the aorta (Hoekelman, 2001; Thureen et al, 2005). Normal BP ranges for term infants vary by method obtained and birth weight (Versmold et al., 1981).

Temperature

An infant who is ill is more likely to have *hypothermia* than a fever. The newborn a few hours old often has difficulty maintaining body temperature and should not be allowed to become cold. This is particularly true in the delivery room when the infant is still wet. The newborn is particularly susceptible to environmental conditions. An infant who becomes cold-stressed has increased metabolic demands that could lead to metabolic acidosis, pulmonary hypertension, and hypoxemia. One of the early signs of sepsis is an inability to maintain body temperature. Hypothermia can also quickly lead to hypoglycemia. The infant's body temperature must be stable before giving the first bath (Hoekelman, 2001).

Respiratory Symptoms

Tachypnea

Tachypnea is a persistent respiratory rate greater than 60 breaths per minute. The respiratory rate should be determined while the infant is quiet, and the examiner should observe chest excursions for a full 60 seconds because newborns tend to be periodic breathers (Thureen et al., 2005). Tachypnea may be associated with cardiovascular, pulmonary, or metabolic diseases. Tachypnea is also often associated with other respiratory symptoms, as discussed later.

Expiratory Grunting

Audible expiratory grunting may be present during the first hour of life as lung fluid is cleared. Grunting can occur in association with intercostal or substernal retractions. However, if the grunting persists beyond the first hour of life, it can signal a significant pulmonary problem and should be promptly evaluated.

Retractions

Retractions (intercostal or substernal) are a common finding in newborns with respiratory problems. Retractions are seen in the preterm infant with *respiratory distress syndrome* (RDS) and in term infants with conditions such as GBS pneumonia and MAS. Retractions indicate that the infant is having difficulty breathing, and the cause should be defined and promptly treated.

Apnea

Episodes of apnea persisting for longer than 20 seconds are abnormal and should be promptly investigated. There might or might not be associated bradycardia and cyanosis. Apnea can have several causes, including medications administered to the mother during labor, sepsis, airway obstruction, severe hypoxemia, central nervous system (CNS) abnormalities, and metabolic disorders.

It is important to distinguish apnea from periodic breathing (Hoekelman, 2001). *Periodic breathing* is almost always a normal finding in the newborn, particularly in the preterm infant.

Cyanosis

One needs to differentiate *central* cyanosis, which is always pathologic, from *peripheral* cyanosis involving the hands and feet (acrocyanosis). Acrocyanosis is normal in the first few days of life. The infant with true generalized or central cyanosis should be given oxygen immediately and the cause of cyanosis should be investigated. The major causes of cyanosis are cardiac anomalies, respiratory problems, and sepsis. The approach to evaluation and management of cyanosis has been well described (Sasidharan, 2004).

Other Signs and Symptoms that Should Raise Concern

Refusal to Feed or Intolerance to Feedings

Most infants with a serious illness do not feed well. They might refuse to nurse or to take a bottle of formula, or they take much longer than usual to feed. One should be concerned about the infant who is vomiting, particularly if projectile, or if the vomitus is bilious. Most infants regurgitate or spit up, and this normal finding needs to be distinguished from true vomiting. Normal regurgitation is effortless, but vomiting is more forceful. In an infant who is septic, intolerance to feedings is very common. One of the early signs of congestive heart failure in a newborn is a change in ability to feed. The infant will tire during feeding and may also become diaphoretic.

Lethargy

Lethargy is a decrease in activity. Infants born to mothers who were given certain medications during labor may be quite inactive until the drug effect dissipates. Magnesium sulfate and narcotics have this potential effect on the newborn. Most infants who develop sepsis become lethargic, so this possibility needs to be considered in any infant who has prolonged lethargy. Some inborn errors of metabolism also manifest with persistent lethargy.

Hypotonia

Any acutely ill infant can demonstrate some degree of decreased muscle tone. Infants with trisomy 21 typically have decreased muscle tone. Magnesium sulfate given to the mother during labor can lead to a transient state of hypotonia in the newborn. An infant with low muscle tone usually has little to no resting limb flexion.

Hypertonia

Increased muscle tone is usually a manifestation of a CNS abnormality, such as hypoxic-ischemic brain injury, intracranial hemorrhage, or infection (meningitis). Persistent arching of the back may be a manifestation of hypertonia.

Jitteriness

Jitteriness is defined as rhythmic tremors of equal amplitude and is frequently seen in the healthy infant. These tremors can be easily initiated in the susceptible newborn by external stimuli such as handling or loud noise. One can stop the tremor by gently holding the affected extremity. Although jitteriness often occurs in the healthy infant, tremors may be a manifestation of a variety of neonatal problems, including hypoglycemia, hypocalcemia, drug withdrawal from maternal drug use, and perinatal asphyxia. In the infant with persistent or exaggerated tremors, possible causes must be investigated (Hoekelman, 2001).

Pallor

Pallor is skin color that is paler than normally expected in an infant of that race. Pallor can be secondary to vasoconstriction or significant anemia.

Petechiae

Petechiae are pinpoint hemorrhages into the skin that do not blanch when pressure is applied. Petechiae are typically seen on the presenting part of the infant after a vaginal delivery, and these are of no concern. If the petechiae later become generalized, however, platelet abnormalities should be considered and a platelet count obtained. Petechiae can be seen in a variety of scenarios, including sepsis and hematologic and immunologic conditions.

Absence of Femoral Pulses

Femoral pulses should be palpated in all newborns because absent or delayed femoral pulses are often associated with coarctation of the aorta. It is important to obtain four extremity BP readings in this situation. If BP is greater in the arms than in the legs, a coarctation is likely present.

Abdominal Distention

Abdominal distention may be an isolated finding, or it may be associated with emesis. Abdominal distention may be present because of a septic ileus, obstruction in the gastrointestinal (GI) tract, or enlargement of an abdominal organ. It is important to diagnose and treat the underlying cause. Infants with diaphragmatic hernias can present with a *scaphoid abdomen* (abdomen seems empty of much of its contents) because much of the bowel is in the chest cavity.

Delayed Passage of Meconium or Urine

More than 90% of term infants pass their first meconium stool by 24 hours of age, and 99% pass one by 48 hours of age (Hoekelman, 2001). Delay in passage of meconium can be caused by Hirschsprung's disease, meconium plug, or meconium ileus. When the infant has not passed a stool by 24 to 48 hours of age, a plain radiograph of the abdomen, taken with the infant in the prone position, often reveals the source of the problem. The absence of intraintestinal air in the pelvis suggests Hirschsprung's disease, and air trapped within meconium (characteristic soap bubble appearance) is highly suggestive of meconium ileus (Rudolph et al., 1998). Meconium ileus has a high association with cystic fibrosis. Early recognition of Hirschsprung's disease is essential to reduce the morbidity and mortality associated with late diagnosis.

More than 90% of newborns void by 24 hours of age, and 99% by 48 hours of age (Hoekelman, 2001). Failure to pass urine by 48 hours of age should lead to evaluation of the kidneys, ureters, and bladder, including renal sonography.

No infant should be discharged from the nursery without documentation of voiding and stooling. Before initiating any evaluation, however, talk with parents and with nursing staff to make certain that the infant did not have a stool or a wet diaper that was not recorded.

Differential Diagnosis of Concerning Signs and Symptoms

Group B Streptococcal Sepsis

Group B *Streptococcus* is a leading cause of neonatal morbidity and mortality in the United States (Schrag et al., 2002b). Newborns with GBS sepsis can present with respiratory symptoms (tachypnea, grunting, or retractions) or with symptoms such as poor feeding, intolerance to feeds, lethargy, or inability to maintain body temperature. If this disease is in the differential, prompt evaluation and treatment are necessary to prevent severe morbidity or mortality. Treatment protocols are available to manage the at-risk pregnant patient and evaluate and manage the newborn infant (Figs. 22-4 and 22-5).

Other Neonatal Infections

Newborns can be infected with organisms other than GBS, and thus blood cultures are an integral part of the diagnostic evaluation. These organisms include *Listeria monocytogenes*, *Chlamydia* species, and *Escherichia coli*. Infants with these diseases can present with respiratory symptoms or other symptoms depending on whether the infection is localized to the lungs or generalized.

Respiratory Distress Syndrome

Respiratory distress syndrome, sometimes referred to as "hyaline membrane disease," is seen in the surfactant-deficient preterm infant. RDS is also seen in the infant of a diabetic mother delivered before 38 weeks' gestation. These infants present with respiratory distress, including tachypnea, grunting, and retractions. They often become cyanotic as the disease worsens. The preterm infant is at higher risk for developing GBS sepsis, and the symptoms of both diseases are similar, as are the early radiographic findings. Thus, if symptomatic, the preterm infant should receive antibiotic therapy.

Pneumonia

The infant with pneumonia generally presents with respiratory symptoms, particularly with tachypnea. Pneumonia has various causes, including aspiration and infection. Meconium aspiration syndrome can lead to severe pneumonia, with subsequent development of persistent pulmonary hypertension. It becomes difficult to oxygenate

Vaginal and rectal GBS screening cultures at 35-37 weeks' gestation for *all* pregnant women (unless patient had GBS bacteriuria during the current pregnancy or a previous infant with invasive GBS disease, in which case intrapartum prophylaxis is automatically indicated).

Intrapartum prophylaxis indicated

• Previous infant with invasive GBS disease
• GBS bacteriuria during current pregnancy
• Positive GBS screening culture during current pregnancy (unless a planned cesarean delivery, in the absence of labor or amniotic membrane rupture, is performed)
• Unknown GBS status (culture not done, incomplete, or results unknown) and any of the following:
  • Delivery at <37 weeks' gestation
  • Amniotic membrane rupture ≥18 hours
  • Intrapartum temperature ≥100.4°F (≥38.0°C)

Intrapartum prophylaxis not indicated

• Previous pregnancy with a positive GBS screening culture (unless a culture was also positive during the current pregnancy)
• Planned cesarean delivery performed in the absence of labor or membrane rupture (regardless of maternal GBS culture status)
• Negative vaginal and rectal GBS screening culture in late gestation during the current pregnancy, regardless of intrapartum risk factors

Figure 22-4 Indications for intrapartum antibiotic prophylaxis to prevent perinatal group B streptococcal (GBS) disease under a universal prenatal screening strategy based on combined vaginal and rectal cultures collected at 35 to 37 weeks' gestation from all pregnant women. *(Modified from Schrag S, Gorwitz, R, Fultz-Butts K, Schuchat A. Prevention of perinatal group B streptococcal disease: revised guidelines from CDC. MMWR 2002;51(RR-11);1-22.)*

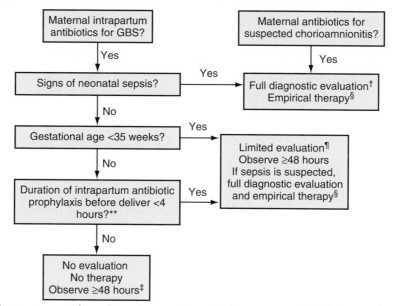

Figure 22-5 Sample algorithm for management of a newborn whose mother received intrapartum antimicrobial agents for prevention of early-onset group B streptococcal disease* or suspected chorioamnionitis. This algorithm is not an exclusive course of management. Variations that incorporate individual circumstances or institutional preferences may be appropriate.
*If no maternal intrapartum prophylaxis for GBS was administered despite an indication being present, data are insufficient on which to recommend a single management strategy.
†Includes complete blood cell count (CBC) and differential, blood culture, and chest radiograph if respiratory abnormalities are present. When signs of sepsis are present, a lumbar puncture, if feasible, should be performed.
§Duration of therapy varies depending on results of blood culture, cerebrospinal fluid findings, if obtained, and the clinical course of the infant. If laboratory results and clinical course do not indicate bacterial infection, duration may be as short as 48 hours.
¶CBC with differential and blood culture.
**Applies only to penicillin, ampicillin, or cefazolin and assumes recommended dosing regimens.
‡A healthy-appearing infant who was ≥38 weeks' gestation at delivery and whose mother received ≥4 hours of intrapartum prophylaxis before delivery may be discharged home after 24 hours if other discharge criteria have been met and a person able to comply fully with instructions for home observation will be present. If any one of these conditions is not met, the infant should be observed in the hospital for at least 48 hours and until criteria for discharge are achieved.
(Modified from Schrag S, Gorwitz R, Fultz-Butts K, Schuchat A. Prevention of perinatal group B streptococcal disease: revised guidelines from CDC. MMWR 2002;51(RR-11);1-22.)

and sufficiently ventilate the most severely affected infants. Infants with pneumonia should be treated with appropriate antibiotics and respiratory support. Meconium aspiration often requires endotracheal intubation and prolonged ventilatory support in addition to antimicrobial treatment.

Transient Tachypnea of the Newborn

The most common cause of tachypnea in the term newborn is transient tachypnea of the newborn (TTN). It likely represents delayed clearing of the fetal lung fluid and is particularly common in the infant who is delivered by cesarean section without labor. The symptoms are present from birth and can persist for up to 72 hours. TTN can be difficult to differentiate from other respiratory entities such as pneumonia; however, infants with TTN rarely exhibit signs of serious illness other than tachypnea.

Congenital Heart Disease

In an infant who is tachypneic and cyanotic, it may be difficult clinically to distinguish between cardiac and pulmonary disease. The physical examination is important, but an infant can have a congenital heart lesion and not have an audible murmur. The oxygen challenge test (OCT) can help to distinguish between pulmonary and cardiac causes. The OCT helps determine whether a significant cardiac anomaly is causing a right-to-left shunt, or whether oxygenated blood is mixing with unoxygenated blood. Arterial blood gases (ABGs) are tested while the infant is breathing room air and after the infant has been breathing 100% oxygen for at least 15 minutes. On 100% oxygen, the Po_2 should increase to greater than 150 mm Hg in the infant without cardiac disease (Sasidharan, 2004). If congenital heart disease is strongly suspected, the infant should be readily transferred to a facility with pediatric echocardiography and neonatal intensive care facilities.

Common Problems Encountered in the Term Newborn

Key Points

- The incidence of hypoglycemia in the infant of a diabetic mother is 25% to 40%.
- About 50% of healthy term newborns develop visible jaundice.
- Unconjugated (indirect) hyperbilirubinemia is caused by increased bilirubin production, decreased hepatic uptake of bilirubin, and increased enterohepatic circulation.
- Bilirubin levels should be interpreted according to the age of the infant, measured in hours.
- Breastfeeding should be encouraged throughout phototherapy if clinically possible, regardless of the cause of hyperbilirubinemia.

In the newborn, certain signs and symptoms of illness are readily apparent while others are much subtler. It is important to detect the subtle signs in an infant's illness to initiate early therapy. This section discusses many of the signs and symptoms in a newborn that may indicate potential disease processes.

Hypoglycemia

Hypoglycemia is relatively common in the newborn infant. In the healthy term newborn, low blood glucose concentrations are often encountered and usually reflect normal metabolic adaptation to extrauterine life. However, with prolonged or recurrent hypoglycemia, the newborn risks neurologic sequelae (Fluge, 1975).

The blood glucose level that defines clinically significant hypoglycemia is controversial. Cornblath and associates (2000) believe that a plasma glucose concentration less than 36 mg/dL warrants close monitoring. If the plasma glucose remains below this level or does not rise after a feeding, intervention is recommended. Liver glycogen stores are rapidly depleted within a few hours after birth. In the newborn, serum glucose levels decline after birth until 1 to 3 hours of age, when levels tend to begin spontaneously rising.

Serum glucose levels are higher than whole-blood glucose levels. Whole-blood measurements of glucose (bedside testing using finger or heel stick) often underestimate the plasma glucose concentration by as much as 10% to 15%.

Infants who are known to be at higher risk for hypoglycemia should have blood glucose concentrations routinely measured. Infants at high risk for hypoglycemia include infants of diabetic mothers (IDMs), small-for-gestational-age (SGA) newborns, infants with a history of perinatal hypoxia or ischemia, and infants who become hypothermic from cold stress. Infants who become septic are also at higher risk for hypoglycemia. For infants at risk, glucose monitoring should be initiated as soon as possible after birth, and within the first hour of life in IDMs. Healthy term newborns delivered after a normal pregnancy, with no known risk factors for hypoglycemia and with no clinical signs of low blood sugar, do not need monitoring of blood glucose concentrations (Cornblath et al., 2000). Routine blood glucose monitoring of large-for-gestational-age (LGA) infants who have no additional risk factors is not necessary (de Rooy and Hawdon, 2002).

If the infant is asymptomatic and alert, low blood sugar can be treated by breastfeeding or by giving formula and repeating the serum glucose concentration after the feeding. If the infant is symptomatic, intravenous (IV) glucose is recommended. The exact concentration and amount of IV glucose to deliver depends on the amount of decrease in the serum glucose concentration. Guidelines for management can be found in the *Harriet Lane Handbook* (Robertson and Shilkofski, 2005).

Infant of a Diabetic Mother

About 6% of pregnancies are complicated by maternal diabetes mellitus, and about 80% of these women have gestational diabetes. Almost 100,000 infants are born to diabetic and gestational diabetic women in the United States each year, and IDMs account for 5% of all neonatal intensive care unit (NICU) admissions (Tyrala, 1996).

Many IDMs are macrosomic. *Macrosomia* is defined as a birth weight of more than 4000 grams or greater than the 90th percentile for gestational age. The problems associated with being an IDM relate to the effects of hyperinsulinism and macrosomia. IDMs have higher rates of perinatal mortality and morbidity. Macrosomia is a predisposing factor for a variety of birth trauma–related injuries, including shoulder dystocia, clavicle fracture, facial nerve palsy, and brachial plexus injury. Poor intrauterine growth occurs at a higher incidence in diabetic pregnancies than in the nondiabetic pregnancy. Women with severe preexisting diabetic vascular disease and decreased uterine blood flow are at significant risk to deliver a growth-retarded infant (Tyrala, 1996).

The incidence of hypoglycemia in the IDM ranges from 25% to 40%. Many nurseries have protocols for the IDM that include checking a bedside whole-blood glucose measurement at 30 minutes of age and again at 1 and 2 hours of age. If the whole blood cell glucose value is reported as less than 40 mg/dL, a serum glucose should be obtained and the infant fed. If the infant is unable to feed orally, IV glucose should be initiated (Tyrala, 1996).

Polycythemia and hyperviscosity are more common in the IDM because of increased erythropoiesis secondary to fetal hypoxia related to hyperinsulinism. A greater amount of blood is shifted from the placenta to the fetus during hypoxia. *Polycythemia* is defined as a venous hematocrit of 65% or greater (Tyrala, 1996).

The risk of RDS in an IDM is five to six times greater than in the infant of the nondiabetic mother before 38 weeks' gestation. Animal studies have implicated hyperglycemia and hyperinsulinemia within the uterine environment as causing the delay of pulmonary maturation (Tyrala, 1996). Lung maturation studies (e.g., lecithin/sphingomyelin ratio by amniocentesis) should be considered before an elective cesarean section in a diabetic mother.

Poor blood sugar control during the early weeks of pregnancy can result in a fourfold to eightfold increase in congenital malformations, such as cardiac defects and CNS anomalies. The higher the hemoglobin A_{1c}, the greater is the incidence of congenital anomalies (Tyrala, 1996). There are no anomalies that are found only in the offspring of diabetic women. The most common cardiac malformations include transposition of the great vessels, ventricular septal defect, coarctation of the aorta, hypoplastic left ventricle, and pulmonic stenosis. CNS malformations include anencephaly, microcephaly, holoprosencephaly, and neural tube defects. Caudal regression syndrome is 600 times more common in IDMs. The IDM is also at increased risk for developing hyperbilirubinemia.

Jaundice

Jaundice is the most common condition requiring medical attention in the term newborn. *Hyperbilirubinemia* is one of the primary reasons for hospital readmission during the first week of life (Brown et al., 1999). Visible jaundice refers to a yellow coloration of the skin and sclera in infants with elevated levels of bilirubin and may be difficult to detect in infants with darker skin. Visible jaundice occurs in more than 50% of healthy term newborns. Although rare, high levels of bilirubin occurring in the first week of life can cause *kernicterus*, a permanent and devastating form of brain damage (Palmer et al., 2003). Neonatal hyperbilirubinemia results from the accelerated production of bilirubin in newborns and their limited ability to excrete it. The newborn liver has limited ability to conjugate bilirubin, and unconjugated bilirubin is not readily excreted.

The primary concern regarding exaggerated levels of bilirubin is the potential for neurotoxic effects. The concentration of bilirubin in the brain and the duration of exposure to bilirubin are important determinants of the neurotoxic effects. Bilirubin can enter the brain if it is not bound to albumin, if it is unconjugated, or if there has been damage to the blood-brain barrier (Dennery et al., 2001). Increased production of bilirubin, deficiency of hepatic uptake, impaired conjugation of bilirubin, and increased enterohepatic circulation of bilirubin account for most cases of pathologic jaundice in newborns.

Increased production of bilirubin can result from hemolytic and nonhemolytic causes. Examples of hemolytic causes include Rh incompatibility, ABO incompatibility, red blood cell membrane defects, and enzyme disorders. Nonhemolytic causes are conditions such as resolving cephalohematoma and polycythemia. The propensity toward hyperbilirubinemia in certain racial groups is not well understood (Dennery et al., 2001).

Deficient hepatic uptake of bilirubin is seen in certain inborn errors of metabolism such as Gilbert's syndrome, Crigler-Najjar syndrome, tyrosinemia, and galactosemia. The result is decreased clearance of bilirubin, which can also be seen with hormone deficiencies such as hypothyroidism.

Increased enterohepatic circulation of bilirubin can lead to hyperbilirubinemia. Newborn infants who are not feeding well or who are exclusively breastfed have low levels of the intestinal bacteria that are needed for the conversion of bilirubin to nonresorbable derivatives, and the enterohepatic circulation of bilirubin may be increased in these infants (Dennery et al., 2001).

Compared to *unconjugated* (indirect) hyperbilirubinemia, *conjugated* (direct) hyperbilirubinemia is rare and is usually caused by obstructed bile flow or hepatocyte injury with normal bile ducts. Hepatocyte injury may be seen in infectious causes, such as intrauterine viral infections. Obstructed bile flow occurs with biliary atresia and biliary stenosis.

The AAP Subcommittee on Hyperbilirubinemia established a clinical practice guideline in 2004. The guideline recommendations have 10 key elements. One recommendation is to establish nursery protocols for identifying and evaluating hyperbilirubinemia. Another key recommendation is to interpret all bilirubin levels according to the infant's age in hours. All infants should be assessed for the risk of severe hyperbilirubinemia before discharge. Factors that put the infant at high risk include jaundice in the first 24 hours of life, blood group incompatibilities, other known hemolytic diseases, prematurity, exclusive breastfeeding when feeding is going poorly, cephalohematoma, and extensive bruising. The history of a previous sibling requiring treatment with phototherapy also places the infant at higher risk (AAP, 2004b). The recommended method for assessing the risk of subsequent hyperbilirubinemia is to measure the total serum bilirubin or transcutaneous bilirubin and plot the results on a nomogram, as provided in Figure 22-6.

Guidelines for treatment with phototherapy are described in Figure 22-7. In breastfed infants who require phototherapy, the AAP recommends that, if possible, breastfeeding should be continued. Home phototherapy devices do not deliver the same degree of irradiance of surface-area exposure as hospital models. Therefore, home phototherapy should be used only for infants whose bilirubin levels are in the optional phototherapy range, according to the clinical guideline; home phototherapy is not appropriate for infants with higher bilirubin concentrations (AAP, 2004b). The infant must have bilirubin levels monitored even while receiving home phototherapy. The total serum bilirubin level at which one can discontinue phototherapy depends on the age of the infant when the treatment began and the cause of the hyperbilirubinemia (Maisels and Kring, 2002). For infants who can be safely discharged before 48 hours of age, the AAP guidelines recommend follow-up with the postdischarge physician within 48 to 72 hours of discharge (AAP, 1994).

Birth Trauma

Infants who present with shoulder dystocia are at risk for clavicle fracture during delivery. The fracture is usually at the midclavicle and may first be noticed when the infant does

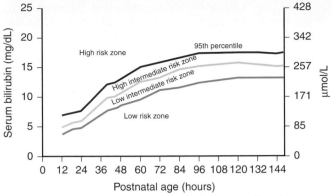

Figure 22-6 Nomogram for designation of risk in 2840 well newborns at 36 or more weeks' gestational age with birth weight of 2000 g or more or 35 or more weeks' gestational age and birth weight of 2500 g or more based on the hour-specific serum bilirubin values. The serum bilirubin level was obtained before discharge, and the zone in which the value fell predicted the likelihood of a subsequent bilirubin level exceeding the 95th percentile (high-risk zone). This nomogram should not be used to represent the natural history of neonatal hyperbilirubinemia.

(From American Academy of Pediatrics, Subcommittee on Hyperbilirubinemia. Management of hyperbilirubinemia in the newborn infant 35 or more weeks of gestation. Pediatrics 2004;114:297-316.)

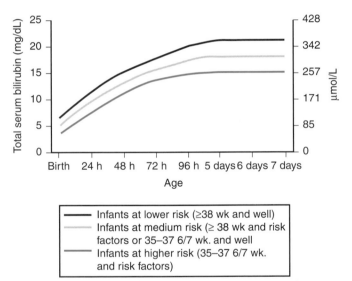

Figure 22-7 Guidelines for phototherapy in hospitalized infants of 35 or more weeks' gestation. For list of guidelines, see Box 22-5.

(From American Academy of Pediatrics, Subcommittee on Hyperbilirubinemia. Management of hyperbilirubinemia in the newborn infant 35 or more weeks of gestation. Pediatrics 2004;114:297-316.)

Box 22-5 Guidelines for Phototherapy in Hospitalized Infants ≥35 Weeks' Gestation (see Fig. 22-7)

- Use total serum bilirubin (TSB). Do not subtract direct-reacting or conjugated bilirubin.
- Risk factors: isoimmune hemolytic disease, glucose-6-phosphate dehydrogenase (G6PD) deficiency, asphyxia, significant lethargy, temperature instability, sepsis, acidosis, or albumin <3.0 g/dL (if measured).
- For well infants at 35 to 37 6/7 weeks, can adjust TSB levels for intervention around the medium-risk line. It is an option to intervene at lower TSB levels for infants closer to 35 weeks and at higher TSB levels for those closer to 37 6/7 weeks.
- It is an option to provide conventional phototherapy in hospital or at home at TSB levels of 2 to 3 mg/dL (35-50 mmol/L) below those shown, but home phototherapy should not be used in any infant with risk factors.

Note: These guidelines are based on limited evidence, and the levels shown are approximations. The guidelines refer to the use of intensive phototherapy, which should be used when the TSB exceeds the line indicated for each category. Infants are designated as "higher risk" because of the potential negative effects of the conditions listed on albumin binding of bilirubin, the blood-brain barrier, and the susceptibility of the brain cells to damage by bilirubin.

"Intensive phototherapy" implies irradiance in the blue-green spectrum (wavelengths of approximately 430-490 nm) of at least 30 $\mu W/cm^2$ per nm (measured at infant's skin directly below center of phototherapy unit) and delivered to as much of the infant's surface area as possible. Note that irradiance measured below the center of the light source is much greater than that measured at the periphery. Measurements should be made with a radiometer specified by the manufacturer of the phototherapy system.

If total serum bilirubin levels approach or exceed the exchange transfusion line, the sides of the bassinet, incubator, or warmer should be lined with aluminum foil or white material. This will increase the surface area of the infant exposed and increase the efficacy of phototherapy. If the TSB does not decrease or continues to rise in an infant who is receiving intensive phototherapy, this strongly suggests the presence of hemolysis.

From American Academy of Pediatrics, Subcommittee on Hyperbilirubinemia. Management of hyperbilirubinemia in the newborn infant 35 or more weeks of gestation. Pediatrics 2004;114:297-316..

not move the arm on the involved side as much as the opposite arm. A fracture can also be detected when an asymmetric Moro reflex is found on neurologic examination. Most of these fractures heal rapidly and normally and do not require specific therapy.

Brachial plexus injuries usually result from pulling on the arm at delivery. Injuries can be caused by stretching of the nerve, hemorrhage within a nerve, or tearing of the nerve or nerve root. *Erb's palsy* is an upper brachial plexus (C5-6) injury that leads to adduction and internal rotation of the shoulder with resulting pronation of the forearm. Erb's palsy can also be accompanied by an ipsilateral paralysis of the diaphragm. *Klumpke's palsy* is a lower plexus

(C7-8 and T1) injury leading to paralysis of the hand and the wrist. Neither of these conditions is usually associated with demonstrable sensory loss more suggestive of a tear or avulsion. Both conditions usually improve rapidly, and in most patients, no deficits persist (Beers and Berkow, 1995). If a significant neurologic deficit persists for longer than 3 months, magnetic resonance imaging (MRI) may be helpful to determine the extent of injury to the plexus, roots, and cervical spinal cord.

Bleeding beneath the periosteum of the skull (cephalohematoma) is often seen with minor trauma sustained during labor and delivery. Cephalohematomas usually have a parietal location on the right or left side of the head and are unilateral in most cases. Treatment is not required, but the infant needs to be watched for signs of anemia or hyperbilirubinemia. Infants with a large cephalohematoma are more likely to develop hyperbilirubinemia as the blood cells within the hematoma break down and are reabsorbed.

Parental Education and Anticipatory Guidance before Discharge

Key Points

- Parental education before discharge should include infant feeding, safety at home, tobacco exposure, and recognizing neonatal illness.
- Breastfeeding support should be provided throughout hospitalization and continuing after discharge.
- All infants should be secured in a rear-facing car seat, with accessibility of the car seat verified before hospital discharge.
- Parents should be encouraged to place their children in the supine position while sleeping to prevent sudden infant death syndrome.

Caring for an infant can seem like an overwhelming task for new parents. Complete and accurate parental education can help alleviate parental stress. Often, parents are particularly concerned with feeding and elimination habits, how to tell if their baby is sick or needs medical attention, and how to ensure safety for their baby. It is difficult to anticipate all upcoming questions, but thorough anticipatory guidance before hospital discharge can help alleviate some of the natural anxiety of caring for an infant.

Feeding and Elimination Habits

Breastfeeding support should be provided throughout hospitalization, beginning in the first several hours of the infant's life. Assisting the mother in holding the baby at the breast and establishing a good latch-on are important in facilitating successful breastfeeding (Sinusas and Gagliardi, 2001). Trained obstetric nurses, lactation consultants, or other trained providers should be available to help the nursing mother begin breastfeeding.

Breastfeeding mothers are often worried that they will not produce enough milk for their baby. In the first 2 or 3 days, as milk production is being established, the infant is primarily receiving low volumes of high-calorie colostrum, and mothers may think their baby is not receiving enough from the breast. Parents should be reassured that the normal newborn does not need supplementation with formula unless there is a specific medical indication (e.g., true dehydration, sepsis) (AAP, 1997b). A trained professional should observe the breastfeeding mother and baby before discharge from the hospital to help correct any problems.

All infants should be fed whenever they are hungry, and for the first few weeks of life, this may be every 1 to 3 hours for breastfed infants and slightly less frequently for those receiving formula. The infant should feed a minimum of every 4 hours and should be awakened from sleep if necessary (AAP, 1997b). Infants may lose up to 10% of their birth weight in the first few days of life, but they should be back to birth weight within 2 weeks of life. In the first few weeks of life the formula-fed infant should take 1 to 2 ounces per feeding, approximately 12 to 24 ounces per day. Formula and expressed breast milk should never be warmed in a microwave oven because hot spots can develop within the milk and burn the newborn's oropharynx. Expressed breast milk or liquid formula that has been at room temperature for more than 1 hour should be discarded (Thureen et al., 2005). Formula should always be mixed strictly according to the manufacturer's instructions, never diluted or concentrated.

After the first 48 hours, the normal infant has 6 to 8 wet diapers and 1 to 2 stools per day. The infant may appear to be uncomfortable as he or she has a bowel movement, possibly straining or turning red in the face. If the stool remains soft, parents should be reassured that the baby is not constipated (Thureen et al., 2005). Normal infant stools are soft, loose, and yellow or yellow-green, and they may be confused with diarrhea. Diarrheal stools are more watery and often leave a water ring in the diaper surrounding the more solid parts of the stool. Parents should be instructed to contact the family physician for true constipation (firm, small, pellet-like stools), diarrhea lasting more than 1 day, and blood or mucus in the stool.

Safety at Home

Sleep Position

Since the implementation of the AAP's Back to Sleep program, the incidence of sudden infant death syndrome (SIDS) has decreased by 40% (AAP, 2000a). Infants should be put to sleep on the back, on a firm mattress, in a crib without any soft or compressible structures (stuffed toys, crib bumpers, bedding) within the sleeping space to help prevent accidental suffocation, which is one cause of SIDS. Sleeping on quilts, comforters, waterbeds, sheepskin, pillows, or any other compressible surfaces increases the risk for SIDS.

Bed Sharing

Cosleeping of infants with other family members can be hazardous and can increase the risk of infant death (AAP, 2000a). Specifically, the risk of SIDS associated with cosleeping is significantly increased when the caregiver is a smoker (AAP, 2000a). Parents should be encouraged to move the bassinette or crib into their room to have the infant close by, but should be strongly discouraged from having the infant sleep in the same bed. Also, adults who smoke or use sedating substances (alcohol or other drugs) should not share a bed with an infant.

Car Seats

Every infant should be secured in a rear-facing car seat whenever riding in a moving vehicle. An infant car seat should never be placed in a seat equipped with an air bag, including front passenger-side and side-impact air bags (AAP Committee on Injury and Poison Prevention, 2002). In many vehicles, therefore, the safest place for the infant is the middle portion of the rear seat. Parents should be given information on how to secure the seat in their vehicle and how to secure the baby into the seat before discharge from the hospital.

Bathing

Parents should be particularly conscientious of safety while bathing the newborn. The infant (and toddler) should never be left unattended near standing water, to prevent accidental drowning. As long as the infant's face and diaper area are kept clean, the infant does not require daily bathing. Frequent bathing with soap can dry out sensitive newborn skin, and creams, lotions, and powders can irritate a baby's skin. If the infant has unusually dry skin, unscented, non-alcohol-based lotions can be used (Thureen et al., 2005). The parent can test the bathwater by dipping an elbow in the water. The water should be comfortably warm and not hot to the touch. The temperature of the water heater within the home should be kept below 120° F (49° C) to prevent accidental scalding injuries (Consumer Products Safety Commission, 2005).

Tobacco Exposure

Children exposed to environmental tobacco smoke are at higher risk for SIDS, otitis media with effusion, and lower respiratory illness in the first year of life (AAP, 1997a). Family physicians should encourage all adults to quit smoking, particularly when children may be exposed to tobacco smoke.

Shaken Baby Syndrome

All parents should be informed of the serious problem of shaken baby syndrome. A baby should never be shaken for any reason. The most common reason for shaking a baby is inconsolable crying (National Exchange Club Foundation, 2005). Discussing normal crying behavior and giving some suggestions for how to calm the baby and how parents can calm themselves is an important part of anticipatory guidance. A parental time-out is one suggestion for parents who find themselves angry, frustrated, or having thoughts about hurting their baby. After placing the infant in a safe place such as a crib or bassinet, parents can leave the room for a few minutes, sit down, close their eyes, and count to 20. After they have calmed themselves, they can once again try to calm their baby using one of many techniques (e.g., feeding, diaper change, rocking, stroller or car ride, soft music).

The symptoms of shaken baby syndrome are caused by the trauma to the brain during the forceful back-and-forth movement of the skull. Vomiting, irritability, and poor feeding can be signs of mild to moderate brain damage, and more severe injury can manifest with seizures, a bulging fontanelle (secondary to significant intracranial hemorrhage), or other CNS deficits (National Center on Shaken Baby Syndrome, 2005).

Circumcision

Parents and guardians of male infants are faced with the decision of whether or not to circumcise their infant. For some families, this is an easy decision based on culture, tradition, or specific preferences. Others, however, might not have strong opinions and might look to the family physician for information on the risks and benefits of this procedure. Epidemiologic studies have shown some potential medical benefits to circumcision, but real risks are associated with the surgery itself. Parents and guardians should be given full information on the risks and benefits before making a decision (AAP Circumcision Policy Statement, 1999).

The circumcised penis can take 7 to 10 days to heal. Parents should gently clean the penis with each diaper change, being careful not to be too aggressive and reopen the wounded glans. Any new or significant bleeding from the penis should be reported to the family physician. Bleeding from the circumcision site occurs in about 0.1% of cases and often can be treated in an office setting with local pressure, chemical cautery (silver nitrate), or sutures (AAP, 1999).

The uncircumcised penis does not require any particular care. Many parents may be anxious to retract the foreskin and clean between the glans and the foreskin. Early retraction, however, is unnecessary and can lead to paraphimosis. The foreskin should not be retracted until it can be retracted easily, without any force and without causing pain to the child. This can take 3 to 5 years, and at that time parents can teach the boy to clean under the foreskin daily (Thureen et al., 2005).

Preventing and Recognizing Illness

Before discharging the infant from the hospital, it is helpful to discuss with caregivers specific examples of when to be concerned about serious illness and how they can reach their family physician for questions or concerns during and after normal business hours. Parents should be encouraged to limit exposure of the infant to adults or children who are sick, especially in the first few months of life. It is good practice to ask family and friends to wash their hands before handling the newborn infant to prevent the spread of disease.

Parents can learn to take an infant's axillary temperature, recognize respiratory retractions, identify infection around the umbilicus or circumcision, and tell the difference between normal and abnormal muscle tone. Some normal infant behavior, such as sneezing, hiccups, effortless regurgitation after feeding, the startle reflex, and irregular breathing, can cause concern in parents. Anticipating and discussing these concerns can help put parents at ease.

See discussions of the following areas online at www.expertconsult.com:

- Early Care of the Well Newborn after Hospital Discharge
- Postpartum Major Depression
- Care of the Neonatal Intensive Care Unit Graduate

References

The complete reference list is available online at www.expertconsult.com.

Web Resources

www.cdc.gov/ncbddd/folicacid/index.html
Information on folic acid supplementation from the Centers for Disease Control and Prevention (CDC).

www.cdc.gov/groupBstrep/guidelines/summary.htm
Information from the CDC on perinatal screening for group B *Streptococcus* spp.

www.youtube.com/watch?v=OV8wtPYGE-I
Video describing fetal circulation before birth and immediately after delivery.

www.aap.org/nrp/nrpmain.html
Information on the Neonatal Resuscitation Program from the American Academy of Pediatrics and American Heart Association.

http://dermatlas.med.jhmi.edu/derm/cd_lists.cfm
Collection of dermatology images available on the Internet.

www.pediatriccareonline.org/pco/ub
A website offering multiple resources, including Point of Quickcare Reference, AAP Textbook of Pediatric Care, Bright Futures, Antimicrobial Therapy Guide, and a Visual Library. Other tools include Pediatric Care Updates, Algorithms, a Signs and Symptoms Search, and Patient Handouts.

http://aappolicy.aappublications.org/cgi/content/full/pediatrics;114/1/297
The full clinical practice guideline regarding the management of hyperbilirubinemia from the American Academy of Pediatrics.

http://newborns.stanford.edu/Gomco.html
Video from Stanford University showing penile circumcision using the Gomco technique.

www.cdc.gov/vaccines/recs/schedules/child-schedule.htm
Current childhood immunization schedule from the CDC.

www.marchofdimes.com/home.asp
The March of Dimes has excellent resources for parents and families of premature infants.

CHAPTER 23

Growth and Development

Sanford R. Kimmel and Karen Ratliff-Schaub

Chapter contents

Children are distinguished from people in other age groups by physical growth and developmental changes that are ongoing, normative, and expected. These changes usually proceed in an orderly progression that allows for individual variation. The family physician must be familiar with the range of normal physical and developmental changes that occur in the process of providing health supervision to children.

Growth is a dynamic process in which increasing cell size and number in various tissues result in a physical increase in the size of the body as a whole. Simultaneously, development occurs as tissues differentiate in form and mature in function, reflecting the person's genetic heritage and environmental interaction. Nutritional, family, emotional, sociocultural, and community influences as well as physical factors play a role in shaping the child's psychological and physiological development (Vaughan and Litt, 1992). The child responds emotionally to a particular stimulus in an apparently innate and characteristic style that reflects his or her temperament.

Knowledge of normal as well as abnormal patterns of growth and development enables the physician to assist the child in maximizing his or her fullest potential. Growth in height and weight is a sensitive reflection of a child's general health. Deviations from normal can reflect the presence of physical illness or a disturbance in the child's environment. Box 23-1 lists some significant causes of growth abnormalities.

Care of Children in Family Medicine

Family physicians have the opportunity to provide family-centered pediatric care in the context of the child's family and community. The office should be "child friendly" and child safe with at least one room equipped to evaluate the child's physical growth. Blood pressure cuffs should be available to measure a child's blood pressure, at least from age 36 months and older. Electrical outlets and cords should be secured and potentially hazardous chemicals and biohazard

Box 23-1 Significant Causes of Growth Abnormalities in Children

Short stature
Familial

Constitutional growth delay

Familial (genetic) short stature

Genetic

Down syndrome

Noonan's syndrome

Russell Silver syndrome

Skeletal dysplasia (dwarfism)

Turner's syndrome

Virilizing congenital adrenal hyperplasia (tall child, short adult)

Systemic disorders

AIDS

Asthma (poorly controlled)

Cancer, caused by poor nutrition, chemotherapy, or radiotherapy

Celiac disease

Chronic heart failure

Congenital heart disease

Cushing's syndrome

Cystic fibrosis

Diabetes mellitus (poorly controlled)

Endocrine disease

Gastrointestinal disease

Growth hormone deficiency, congenital or acquired

Heart disease

Hypopituitarism

Hypothyroidism

Immunologic diseases

Inflammatory bowel disease (Crohn's disease)

Malabsorption syndromes

Pulmonary disease

Renal disease, chronic renal failure, renal tubular acidosis

Severe combined immunodeficiency

Environmental

Malnutrition

Psychosocial deprivation

Toxin or drug exposure (e.g., lead)

Tall stature*
Familial

Constitutional acceleration of growth

Familial tall stature

Genetic

Beckwith-Wiedemann syndrome

Cerebral gigantism (Soto's syndrome)

Homocystinuria

Marfan's syndrome

Systemic disorders

Endocrine disease

Pituitary gigantism (acromegaly)

Thyrotoxicosis

*Data from Bell J. Tall stature. In Finberg L (ed). Saunders Manual of Pediatric Practice. Philadelphia, Saunders, 1998, pp 728-730.

bins stored either out of reach or under lock and key from curious young toddlers. Guidelines for the frequency of "well child" or "well teen" visits are available from the American Academy of Pediatrics (AAP) *Bright Futures: Guidelines for Health Supervision of Infants, Children, and Adolescents* (Hagan et al., 2008).

Initial history for a new infant or child includes the birth history, nutritional history (e.g., breastfed vs. bottle-fed), developmental milestones achieved, immunization record, and environmental history (e.g., do parents smoke?) Later, the physician or staff will also perform anticipatory guidance, including injury prevention and the need to immunize against vaccine-preventable diseases.

Observation of the parent-child interaction informs the physician about the relationship between parent(s) and the child, especially with infants and young children. The parent sitting in a chair reading a magazine while her young infant teeters on an exam table engenders more concern than the parent who is standing next to the child or has him in her lap. Observation of the child's appearance, alertness, muscle tone, state of hydration, and respiratory status also raise or lower the index of concern about a child. The cardiorespiratory examination is often done best if the child is sitting or lying on a parent's lap, whereas examination of the abdomen, genitalia, and hips is generally done on the exam table. The HEENT examination is often done last because it is the most likely to provoke discomfort.

Blood Pressure Monitoring

Hypertension has become increasingly common in children and adolescents. Since 1988, the prevalence of high blood pressure has increased, especially for certain populations, such as Mexican-Americans and blacks (Din-Dzietham et al., 2007). The rising rate of obesity, particularly truncal obesity, at least partly accounts for this. Because of potential end-organ damage and cardiovascular risk in adulthood, auscultatory monitoring of blood pressure (BP) is recommended during health care visits for all children 3 years and older and for younger children with certain high-risk features (Box 23-2). Automatic devices may be needed to measure BP in young infants. Elevated BP should be confirmed on repeat visits. The guidelines define *hypertension* as average systolic or diastolic BP of 95% or higher for gender, age, and height on three or more occasions. *Prehypertension* is defined as values of 90% or greater and less than 95%. For adolescents, BP greater than or equal to 120/80 mm Hg but less than 95% is defined as prehypertensive. Because of the inclusion of a diverse population, these guidelines and tables appear applicable to all ethnic groups (see **eTables 23-1** and **23-2** online at www.expertconsult.com).

The approach to confirmed hypertension in children should be individualized and should consider variables such as comorbidities and family history. In overweight or obese children, the possibility of metabolic syndrome should be investigated. Lifestyle changes, including diet and exercise, may be sufficient for overweight children with stage 1 hypertension (BP at 95% to 99% plus 5 mm Hg). Children with stage 2 hypertension (BP >99% plus 5 mm Hg) and those with end-organ damage likely require medical therapy (National High Blood Pressure Education Program Working Group, 2004).

Box 23-2 Indications for Blood Pressure (BP) Measurement in Children Under 3 Years Old

History of prematurity, very low birth weight, or other neonatal complication requiring intensive care

Congenital heart disease (repaired or nonrepaired)

Recurrent urinary tract infections, hematuria, or proteinuria

Known renal disease or urologic malformations

Family history of congenital renal disease

Solid-organ transplant

Malignancy or bone marrow transplant

Treatment with drugs known to raise BP

Other systemic illnesses associated with hypertension (e.g., neurofibromatosis, tuberous sclerosis)

Evidence of elevated intracranial pressure

Data from National High Blood Pressure Education Program Working Group on High Blood Pressure in Children and Adolescents: The Fourth Report on the Diagnosis, Evaluation, and Treatment of High Blood Pressure in Children and Adolescents. Pediatrics 2004;114:555-576.

Measuring Physical Parameters of Growth

Key Points

- Measure height and weight at all well-child visits.
- Measure head circumference in children up to 24 months of age and blood pressure in children 3 years and older.
- Plot measurements on NCHS growth charts to demonstrate normal growth.
- Investigate significant deviations if the child's growth crosses multiple percentile lines on the growth chart.

Weight, length, and head circumference are the most useful routine measurements in infants. Total body length in children up to age 2 is obtained most accurately by placing them in the recumbent position and measuring from crown to heel. The child's head is placed perpendicular to the surface touching a fixed plate, the hips and knees are fully extended, and the soles of the feet are placed against a sliding board. Older children should have their shoeless standing height measured with a stadiometer with their heels and back touching the wall. Regardless of age, the head should be positioned so that the outer canthus of the eye is aligned with the external auditory canal and perpendicular to the measuring surface (Halac and Zimmerman, 2004). Children should ideally be weighed on the same scale at each visit. Infants should preferably be weighed nude; older children may wear light clothing but not shoes. Height and weight are then plotted on age- and gender-appropriate growth charts developed by the National Center for Health Statistics (NCHS) (see **eFig. 23-1,** *A-H,* and Web Resources).

Body mass index (BMI) is a reliable indicator of body fatness for most children and teenagers that is age and gender specific. A BMI less than the 5th percentile for age is *underweight,* from the 5th to 85th percentile is *healthy weight,* from the 85th up to 95th percentile is *overweight,* and the 95th percentile or greater is considered *obese* (CDC, 2009). BMI charts are also available from the same website.

Head circumference reflects the growth of the cranium and its contents. It should be determined and recorded at all routine physical examinations during the first 2 years of life. This also may be done as part of the initial examination at any age. A nonstretchable measuring tape (usually paper or flexible plastic) is used to obtain the greatest circumference encompassing the occipital, parietal, and frontal prominences. A small head circumference (microcephaly) may be familial; caused by craniosynostosis, congenital viral infections, fetal drug syndromes, or underlying structural abnormalities; or secondary to trauma, infection, or dysmorphic syndromes. A large head circumference (macrocephaly) most often is caused by hydrocephalus, but it may be familial, caused by intracranial bleeding or masses or thickening of the skull, or associated with fragile X syndrome and other conditions (Green, 1986).

Proper Use and Interpretation of Growth Charts

The growth charts shown in **eFigure 23-1** online were revised by NCHS (2000) from surveys of generally well-nourished children representing a cross section of ethnic and economic groups in the United States. These graphs provide a normal range of weight and length or height for a given chronologic age. Recumbent length is recorded on the chart for children from birth to 36 months, and standing height is recorded on the chart for children from 2 to 18 years. Premature infants should have their chronologic age adjusted according to their degree of prematurity up to age 2 years, because most catch-up growth is complete by this time. Although a height or weight above the 95th percentile or below the 5th percentile should alert the physician to a possible problem, these can represent the outer fringe of the normal range.

Linear growth in infants has been shown to occur in incremental bursts rather than continuously (Lampl et al., 1992). A growth curve constructed by a series of heights and weights taken over time allows the physician to compare current growth with the child's previous pattern. The *linear growth velocity,* or rate of gain in height, decreases from 25 cm per year during the first year of life to a prepubertal rate of 5 to 6 cm/yr by age 6 or 7 years (Miller and Zimmerman, 2004). The rate accelerates during puberty. A child whose growth curve parallels the normal curve regardless of the child's absolute percentile has a normal rate of growth for that particular child. In comparison, a child whose height or weight crosses multiple percentile lines or whose linear growth rate drops below 4 cm/yr requires further evaluation for nutritional, psychosocial, or organic problems that could impede or accelerate growth (Lipsky and Horner, 1988). Children with genetic short stature have normal length and weight at birth, but their growth percentiles decline within the first 2 to 3 years of life as they reach their genetic potential (Halac and Zimmerman, 2004).

Although careful measuring and plotting of growth parameters is the most accurate method by which to follow a child's physical growth, approximate growth guidelines are helpful to the physician in remembering and forming an overall impression of the child's progress (Table 23-1).

Familial Short Stature and Constitutional Growth Delay

Each child has a different rate of maturation, or what Boas termed "tempo of growth" (Tanner, 1986). Persons with *short stature* are more than 2 standard deviations (SD) below the

Table 23-1 Approximate Growth Guidelines for Children

Age	Length or Height (ht)	Weight (wt)
Newborn	50 cm (20 inches) average	3.4 kg (7.5 pounds) average
Newborn to 3 months	—	1 kg/month (1 oz/day) average wt gain
3-12 months	—	Wt (kg) = [Age (mo) + 9] ÷ 2 Wt (lb) = Age (mo) + 11*
12 months	75 cm (30 in) average	Triples birth weight
12-24 months	Increases by >10 cm/yr	0.25 kg/month
>5 years	>5 cm (2 in)/yr until adolescent growth spurt	2.3 kg (5 lb)/yr until adolescent growth spurt
2-12 years	Ht (cm) = [Age (yr) × 6] + 77 Ht (in) = [Age (yr) × 2.5] + 30* (e.g., 4-year-old = 40 inches)	Ages 1-6: Wt (kg) = [Age (yr) × 2] + 8 Wt (lb) = Age (yr) × 5 = 17* Ages 7-12: Wt (kg) = [Age (yr) × 7 − 5] ÷ 2 Wt (lb) = Age (yr) × 7 + 5*
Puberty	8-14 cm/yr	

*Modified from Needleman RD. The first year. In Behrman RE, Kliegman RM, Jenson HB (eds). Nelson Textbook of Pediatrics, 17th ed. Philadelphia, Saunders, 2004, p 31.

Box 23-3 Causes of Short Stature and Relationship to Bone Age and Growth Rate

Bone age less than chronologic age
Growth rate normal or slightly decreased
Constitutional growth delay
Growth rate decreased
Endocrine disorders
Cushing's syndrome
Growth hormone deficiency
Chronic systemic disease
Crohn's disease
Heart failure
Renal failure
Severe malnutrition
Severe psychosocial deprivation

Bone age equals chronologic age
Growth rate normal or slightly decreased
Familial short stature
Skeletal dysplasias
Rickets
Growth rate decreased
Chromosomal disorders
Down syndrome
Turner's syndrome

Bone age greater than chronologic age
Growth rate initially increased but short adult
Congenital adrenal hyperplasia
Exogenous androgenic steroids
Precocious puberty

mean in height and constitute approximately 2.5% of children (Miller and Zimmerman, 2004). If a child's growth falls outside the range of normal, it is useful to obtain a bone-age radiograph, usually of the left hand and wrist, and compare it to age-specific standards. Children must be at least 2 years of age to reliably identify epiphyseal ossification centers. Box 23-3 lists some causes of retarded or accelerated bone age. Calculation of mean predicted adult height is also useful in determining whether a child is fulfilling her or his genetic potential. The mean predicted adult height is calculated as follows (Rogol, 2004):

> Boy's mean height =
> [Father's height + (Mother's height + 13 cm)] ÷ 2
> Girl's mean height =
> [(Father's height - 13cm) + Mother's height] ÷ 2

Children and adolescents of short stature whose bone age is delayed relative to their chronologic age have more growth potential than do children with a skeletal age appropriate for their chronologic age. If an organic cause of short stature has been excluded, children with delayed bone age are likely to have *constitutional growth delay*. The majority of these children are boys who were of normal length and weight at birth. Their growth rate decelerates during the first 2 years of life and subsequently returns to normal. The children then follow a lower percentile on the growth curve until the onset of their pubertal growth spurt and development, which often

occurs later than their peers. There is usually a family history of delayed growth and development (Bareille and Stanhope, 1998). The bone age of these children equals their height age, which is the age at which their height plots on the 50th percentile of the growth chart.

Children with familial short stature usually have parents or close relatives who are short. They often have normal birth weight and length, but their growth rate declines during the first 2 to 3 years of life. Their growth curve subsequently parallels the normal curve but falls below the fifth percentile (Bareille et al., 1998). Their bone age is approximately equal to their chronologic age but less than their height age. These children usually enter puberty at the appropriate age. The U.S. Food and Drug Administration (FDA) has approved the use of recombinant growth hormone for the treatment of idiopathic short stature. This can result in an increase of predicted height of more than 7 cm (Miller and Zimmerman, 2004). Because of potential side effects and the high cost, treatment should be undertaken in consultation with a specialist in pediatric growth disorders.

Pubertal Growth and Development

All children grow at a different tempo, with some maturing earlier than others and some later. This difference is most apparent during puberty. The NCHS growth charts now extend to age 20 years. Tanner and Davies (1985) took the

Table 23-2 Sexual Maturity Stages in Boys and Girls

Stage	Male genitalia	Pubic hair	Female breasts
1	Preadolescent: testes, scrotum, and penis are childlike in size.	None; may be vellus hair, as over abdomen.	Preadolescent: elevation of papilla only.
2	Slight enlargement of scrotum with reddening of skin; little or no enlargement of penis.	Sparse growth of long, slightly pigmented, downy hair, straight or slightly curled, primarily at base of penis or along labia.	Breast bud stage; breast and papilla form a small mound; areolar diameter enlarges.
3	Further enlargement of scrotum; penis enlarges, mainly in length.	Hair considerably darker, coarser, and more curled; spreads sparsely over junction of pubes.	Further enlargement of breast and areola with no separation of their contours.
4	Further enlargement and darkening of scrotum; penis enlarges, especially in breadth; glans develops.	Adult-type hair that does not extend onto thighs, covering a smaller area than in adult.	Areola and papilla project to form a secondary mound above the contour of the breast; stage 4 development of the areolar mound does not occur in 10% of girls and is slight in 20%; when present, it may persist well into adulthood.
5	Adult in size and shape.	Adult in quantity and type with extension onto thighs but not up linea alba.	Mature female; papilla projects and areola recesses to general contour of breast.
6	—	Spreads up linea alba (80% of men, 10% of women).	

Modified from Tanner JM. Normal growth and techniques of growth assessment. Clin Endocrinol Metab 1986;15:436.

earlier NCHS data and constructed height and weight velocity curves for American boys and girls that account for those groups who mature earlier and later. These charts also allow for notation of the various stages of puberty described by Tanner (1986) (Table 23-2).

The onset of puberty generally occurs at age 9 in American girls, with the peak height velocity occurring at age 11.5 years (range, 9.7 to 13.5 years for early to late maturers). American boys have onset of puberty at age 11 and peak height velocity at 13.5 years (range, 11.7 to 15.3 years) (Tanner and Davies,

1985). Because boys have two additional years of prepubertal growth and a peak height velocity greater than that of girls, their ultimate height is usually taller. Head, hands, and feet are first to reach their adult size, followed by leg length, trunk length (which accounts for much of the spurt), and body breadth. Pubertal boys develop greater shoulder breadth than do pubertal girls, who develop wider hips. Adolescents can be reassured that their bodies eventually will become more proportionate with their hands and feet. Boys ultimately gain greater muscle size and strength than do girls, while losing limb fat. This results from their increased secretion of testosterone, which also increases red cell mass and hemoglobin (Tanner, 1986).

The adolescent growth spurt in skeletal and body dimensions is associated closely with the development of the reproductive system. Although the onset and rate of maturation vary according to the individual, the sequence is usually the same within genders (Figs. 23-1 and 23-2). Girls who demonstrate signs of puberty before 7 to 8 years of age and boys who show signs before 9 years should be evaluated for *precocious puberty*. Conversely, girls who do not show signs of puberty by age 13 and boys by age 14 should be evaluated for *pubertal delay* (Plotnick, 1999).

The first sign of puberty in boys is an increase in growth of the testes and scrotum, with reddening and wrinkling of the scrotal skin. Pubic hair appears within 6 months, followed by phallic enlargement in 12 to 18 months and peak height velocity 2 to 2.5 years after testicular enlargement (Copeland, 1986). Axillary hair usually appears 2 years after the beginning of pubic hair growth (stage 4 pubic hair), but there is considerable variability. Some boys may have enlargement of the breasts midway through adolescence. Following the attainment of peak height velocity, boys develop mature spermatozoa, full facial hair, and voice change. However, breaking of the voice is a late and often gradual process.

In girls, the breast bud is the first sign of puberty, and the pubertal growth spurt typically occurs concurrently, peaking at stage 3 breast and pubic hair. The uterus and vagina develop simultaneously with the breast, but menarche usually does not occur until stage 4 breast and pubic hair. Although the peak height velocity has been passed, girls may grow an average of 6 cm more after menarche. Early cycles may be irregular and anovulatory, but early sterility should never be presupposed (Tanner, 1986).

Screening Healthy Children

Key Points

- All newborns should have a hearing screen within the first month of life.
- Examine eyes at all well care visits; screen vision beginning at age 3 years.
- Provide anticipatory guidance regarding discipline starting at 15 months of age.

Preventive care services for children often include screening for health conditions in which early detection and early treatment can prevent or ameliorate more serious disease in the future. Screening tests should detect most persons with the condition *(sensitivity)* while excluding most persons who do not have the condition *(specificity)* in a cost-effective manner. In an inner-city Medicaid population, high continuity of care in infancy was associated with improved screening for anemia, lead, and tuberculosis (Flores et al., 2008).

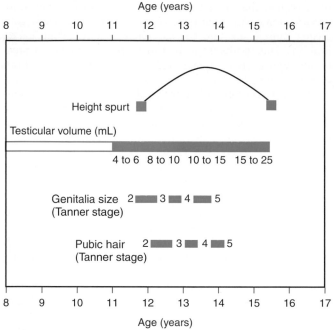

Figure 23-1 Sequence of pubertal events in average American boys. *(Modified from Brookman RR, Rauh JL, Morrison JA, et al: The Princeton Maturation Study; 1976, unpublished data for adolescents in Cincinnati, Ohio. In Copeland KC, Brookman RR, Rauh JL [eds]: Assessment of Pubertal Development. Columbus, Ohio, Ross Products Division, Abbott Laboratories, 1986, p 4.)*

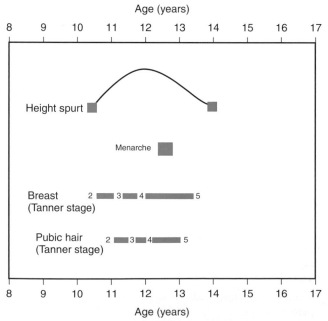

Figure 23-2 Sequence of pubertal events in average American girls. *(Modified from Brookman RR, Rauh JL, Morrison JA, et al: The Princeton Maturation Study, 1976 unpublished data for adolescents in Cincinnati, Ohio. In Copeland KC, Brookman RR, Rauh JL [eds]: Assessment of Pubertal Development. Columbus, Ohio, Ross Products Division, Abbott Laboratories, 1986, p 4.)*

Hearing and Vision Screening

Early detection and intervention for hearing and vision deficits are important for maximal long-term functioning. Without appropriate opportunities to learn language, children with significant hearing deficits fall behind peers in terms of communication, cognition, reading, and social-emotional development, with long-term effects on educational attainment and adult employment (AAP Joint Committee on Infant Hearing, 2007). It is now recommended that all infants be screened for hearing loss by 1 month of age, regardless of risk factors. Those who do not pass the screening should have a complete audiologic evaluation by 3 months of age, and those with confirmed hearing loss should receive appropriate treatment by 6 months to ensure optimal outcome. Regardless of the outcome of newborn screening, ongoing surveillance of hearing status is recommended. Developmental delays and other risk factors (Box 23-4), particularly in language, as well as the presence of parental concern about hearing, should prompt referral for a complete audiologic evaluation, even if the newborn screen was normal and there are no risk factors for hearing impairment (Hagan et al., 2008). Gradations of hearing loss are presented in Table 23-3.

Eyesight evaluation is a recommended part of routine health maintenance examinations in children beginning in the newborn period. In young children (<3 years) the

---

Box 23-4 Risk Factors for Delayed Onset of Hearing Loss in Young Children

Caregiver concern regarding hearing, speech, language, or developmental delay

Family history of permanent childhood hearing loss

Neonatal intensive care longer than 5 days

In utero infections (e.g., cytomegalovirus)

Craniofacial anomalies (e.g., ear pits, ear canal defects)

Syndromes known to be associated with hearing loss (e.g., neurofibromatosis)

Neurodegenerative disorders (e.g., Friedreich's ataxia)

Postnatal infections (e.g., meningitis)

Head trauma (e.g., basal skull/temporal bone fracture)

Chemotherapy

Modified from Hagan JF, Shaw JS, Duncan PM (eds). Bright Futures: Guidelines for Health Supervision of Infants, Children, and Adolescents, 3rd ed. Elk Grove Village, Ill, American Academy of Pediatrics, 2008, p 232.

Table 23-3 Hearing Loss Scale

Hearing impairment	Hearing threshold (dB)
None	10-25
Mild	26-40
Moderate	41-55
Moderate to severe	56-70
Severe	71-90
Profound	>91

evaluation, besides the actual eye examination, is somewhat subjective and based on parental history. Children with risk factors, such as prematurity, family history of retinoblastoma or glaucoma, or significant developmental delays or neurologic difficulties, should be referred to an experienced pediatric ophthalmologist. More formal testing of visual acuity should begin at age 3 years, using standardized systems such as the Allen Cards, which have easily recognized pictures (AAP Committee on Practice and Ambulatory Medicine, 2003). Normal visual acuity is in the 20/30 to 20/40 range for children 3 to 4 years old, but increases to 20/20 by early school age. Eye-specific screening should be attempted in an effort to detect amblyopia (more than one line difference on the chart) (SOR: B). The suspicion of amblyopia or strabismus requires further evaluation to prevent long-term visual loss (AAP Committee on Practice and Ambulatory Medicine, 1996). Routine screening should be done at least through early school age, at puberty and whenever there are other signs, such as squinting or complaints of inability to see the board at school (Hagan et al., 2008).

Screening for Iron Deficiency Anemia

The U.S. Preventive Service Task Force currently has found insufficient evidence to recommend for or against routine screening asymptomatic infants age 6 to 12 months for iron deficiency anemia (USPSTF, 2006). Venous hemoglobin is more accurate than capillary hemoglobin for detecting anemia; however, true iron deficiency is much more common than iron deficiency anemia. In addition, there is evidence that even children with severe anemia who are treated with iron supplementation continue to demonstrate behavioral and developmental deficits 10 years afterwards (Lozoff et al., 2000). Nevertheless, the AAP Committee on Nutrition presents two options for screening for iron deficiency anemia. If a community has a significant level of iron deficiency anemia or infants who are at risk by virtue of their diet, universal screening is recommended for all full-term infants between 9 and 12 months old, with a second screening 6 months later at 15 to 18 months old. Selective screening may be done on a similar schedule only for children deemed to be at risk for iron deficiency anemia, including low-birth-weight infants, infants not receiving iron-containing formula, or breastfed infants over 6 months old who lack adequate iron in their diet.

Screening for Lead Toxicity

Lead is neurotoxic and affects both intellectual and behavioral function, even below the 10 µg/dL level established by the U.S. Centers for Disease Control and Prevention (CDC) and World Health Organization (WHO) (Canfield et al., 2003). Federal Medicaid law has required lead screening of young children eligible for Medicaid at ages 12 months and 24 months, and for children ages 36 to 72 months not previously tested. However, 1999–2004 NHANES data demonstrate that the percentage of children with blood lead levels of 10 µg/dL or higher had decreased to 3.4% for black and 1.2% for white children age 1 to 5 years. The USPSTF finds insufficient evidence to recommend for or against screening asymptomatic children 1 to 5 years old who are at increased risk. The CDC recommends targeted screening of specific groups of children, except in areas where universal screening is still recommended because of a prevalence of elevated lead levels. Specific state information can be obtained at http://www.cdc.gov/nceh/lead. Children considered at risk who require screening include (1) those suspected by a parent or health care provider to be at risk for exposure; (2) those with a sibling or frequent playmate with an elevated blood lead level; (3) those with a parent or caregiver who works professionally or recreationally with lead; (4) a household member uses traditional folk or ethnic remedies or cosmetics; or (5) family designated at increased risk for lead exposure by the health department because of local risk factors for lead exposure, such as residing in a high-risk zip code (Wengrovitz and Brown, 2009).

Screening for Tuberculosis

In 2007, there were approximately 10 million cases of new and recurrent tuberculosis (TB) and 1.8 million deaths worldwide, with the highest rates occurring in low-income countries (Marais et al., 2009). The incidence of active TB is much lower in the United States, but an estimated 10 to 15 million persons have *latent tuberculosis infection* (LTBI). Six groups considered at high risk are children, foreign-born persons, HIV-infected persons, homeless persons, detainees and prisoners in correctional facilities, and close contacts of infectious persons (CDC, 2005). Targeted rather than universal testing of children for TB is now recommended. Risk factors for LTBI include (1) previous positive tuberculin skin test; (2) birth in foreign country with high prevalence of TB (e.g., China, India, Mexico, Philippine Islands, Vietnam, certain African countries); (3) nontourist travel to a high-prevalence country for more than 1 week; (4) contact with TB-infected person, and (5) presence in the household of another person with LTBI (CDC, 2005). The Mantoux TB skin test is recommended for children because its correlation with results of interferon-γ release assays is often discordant in children (Connell et al., 2008).

Discipline

Parents frequently ask their primary care physician about discipline. Discipline should be a priority topic for anticipatory guidance at 15 months and 18 months (Hagan et al., 2008). Effective discipline requires three essential components: (1) a positive, loving relationship between the parent(s) and child, (2) positive reinforcement strategies to increase desired behaviors, and (3) punishment or removal of reinforcement to reduce or eliminate undesired behaviors (AAP Committee on Psychosocial Aspects, 1998). Although often confused with punishment, discipline actually means to *teach*. All children benefit from guidance and structure, and most children require occasional discipline. The best discipline is consistent and considers the child's developmental level as well as the child's point of view. Effective strategies include environmental modifications (e.g., childproofing the house), distraction, redirection, giving appropriate choices, and time-out. Although many parents spank (Regalado et al., 2004), corporal punishment is controversial and has potential long-term negative effects (Smith, 2006). Other methods of discipline are more effective over time and should be used. Some families may require more intensive assistance, and clinicians should be aware of local resources for teaching parents.

Nutrition

Key Points

- Breast milk is the recommended food for infants and the standard to which infant formulas are compared.
- Give vitamin D supplements to all breastfed infants and those taking less than 1 L of vitamin D–fortified milk or formula per day.
- Begin iron-fortified cereal for infants older than 4 to 6 months or low-birth-weight infants older than 2 weeks.
- Obtain a fasting lipid profile in children with a family history of dyslipidemia, premature atherosclerotic vascular disease, or personal risk factors such as overweight, hypertension, smoking, and diabetes mellitus.

Infancy through Adolescence

Proper physical growth and appropriate cognitive development depend on adequate nutrition. Infants and young children with severe iron deficiency anemia were found to have significantly lower verbal and full-scale IQ scores and lower achievement test scores in arithmetic and writing than non-iron-deficient infants, even 10 years after treatment (Lozoff et al., 2000). An increase in behavioral problems was also reported, although this could not be directly linked to the preceding iron deficiency. In the Third National Health and Nutrition Examination Survey (NHANES III, 1988–1994), 7.2% of 12- to 16-year-old girls had iron deficiency, but only 1.5% demonstrated anemia (Halterman et al., 2001). Adolescent iron-deficient girls scored significantly lower math scores compared with non-iron-deficient girls. Vitamin D deficiency and insufficiency in children and adolescents has been reported worldwide, including North America (Wagner and Greer, 2008). Mealtime also represents a time for social interaction within the family unit, whether this is the bonding of mother and child during breastfeeding or discussion of the day's events during dinnertime.

Although malnutrition is still a problem in the United States, *inappropriate nutrition,* especially calorie-nutrient imbalance leading to overweight and obesity, has become commonplace. Recent NHANES studies demonstrate that the prevalence of overweight (BMI ≥95%) in girls 2 to 19 years old increased from 13.8% in 1999–2000 to 16% in 2003–2004, and the prevalence of overweight in boys 2 to 19 years old increased from 14% to 18.2% (Ogden et al., 2006). Increased pediatric BMI is associated with high blood pressure, sleep apnea, asthma, polycystic ovarian syndrome, type 2 diabetes, gastroesophageal reflux, and orthopedic problems (Benson et al., 2009). A nationwide survey of more than 6000 children and adolescents found that at least 30% consumed "fast food" on a typical day. These children consumed more total fat, total carbohydrate, more added sugars and sugar-sweetened beverages, less milk, and fewer fruits and nonstarchy vegetables than children who did not eat fast food (Bowman, 2004). The odds of having a BMI of 85th percentile or higher was more than four times that for 10- to

15-year-old children viewing more than 5 hours of television per day compared with those watching for 0 to 2 hours (Gortmaker et al., 1996). A survey of low-income preschool children in New York State found that children with a TV set in their bedroom watched 4.8 hours more TV/video than those without a bedroom TV. In this group the prevalence of child overweight (BMI >85%) was associated with an odds ratio of 1.06 for each additional hour per day of TV/video viewed (Dennison et al., 2002). Frequent television viewing can lead to decreased activity, excessive snacking on high-calorie junk foods, and subsequent obesity (Dietz and Gortmaker, 1985). In contrast, dieting in pursuit of the media's representation of the ideal woman can lead to eating disorders, such as bulimia or anorexia. The CDC has proposed 24 strategies to prevent obesity in the United States, including increasing the availability of healthier food and beverage choices, restricting the availability of less healthy foods and beverages in public service areas, and increasing the amount of physical activity in schools (Khan et al., 2009).

Infants and Toddlers

Infants require approximately 120 kcal/kg/day to meet basal metabolic requirements and the energy demands of growth and activity during the first 6 months of life. Low-birth-weight (LBW) newborns may require 130 to 150 cal/kg/day for catch-up growth (Klish, 2009). Weight gain should be 25 to 30 g/day during the first 3 months of life, decrease to 15 to 20 g/day between 3 and 6 months of age, and decrease to 10 to 15 g/day between 6 and 12 months (AAP, 2009). Energy requirements are increased by greater physical activity, stress imposed by disease processes (e.g., cystic fibrosis), or symptoms (e.g., fever). Fever can increase the fluid requirements of infants younger than 6 months beyond the usual 130 to 190 mL/kg/day (Barness and Curran, 1996).

The composition of human milk varies by time, day, and maternal nutrition and from woman to woman. Infant formulas contain about 50% more protein than human milk and, like breast milk, provide 40% to 50% of energy as fat (Table 23-4). Beginning at 2 years of age, fat calories should decrease to approximately 30% of total energy consumption, with less than 10% of calories from saturated fat, and dietary cholesterol less than 300 mg/day (AAP, 2009).

The ideal food for full-term infants during the first 12 months of life is human milk. Oliver Wendell Holmes once noted, "A pair of substantial mammary glands has the advantage over the two hemispheres of the most learned professor's brain in the art of compounding a nutritious fluid for infants" (Cone, 1979, p. 138). Human milk is fresh, readily available at the proper temperature, and generally free of contaminating bacteria. Its acid-resistant whey proteins include secretory immunoglobulin A (sIgA), α-lactalbumin, and lactoferrin, a whey protein that transports iron and inhibits the growth of a range of organisms in the intestine. The protein in human milk consists predominantly of whey proteins that are of higher nutritional quality and digested and absorbed more easily than cow's milk proteins (AAP, 2009).

Commercial cow's milk and soy-based formulas must contain higher levels of protein to compensate for their lower quality (see Table 23-4). However, they are quite acceptable for mothers who are unable to nurse their infants or for parents who wish to bottle-feed their children. Soy formulas are

Table 23-4 Comparison of Common Milks and Infant Formulas

Milk/ formula	kcal/30 mL	Protein (g/dL)	CHO (g/dL)	CHO type	Fat (g/dL)	Iron (mg/L)	comments
Human milk	20	1.0	6.9	Lactose (primary), glucose, oligosaccharides	4.4	<0.1	Small flocculent curd is easily digestible, and iron is absorbed.
Whole cow's milk	19	3.3	4.7	Lactose	3.7	Trace	Curd is less easy to digest. Can cause intestinal blood loss. Do not use before age 12 months.
Evaporated whole milk	43	6.9	10.0	Lactose	7.6	Trace	Curd is softer, smaller and may be less allergenic. Dilute and add dextrose to make 20 kcal/oz formula.
Prepared formula, cow's milk based	20	1.4-1.7	6.9-7.5	Lactose	3.4-3.8	4.7-12.2[*]	AAP recommends only iron-fortified formulas.
Prepared formula, soy based	20	1.7-1.8	6.8-7.4	Corn syrup, corn syrup solids, sucrose, corn maltodextrin	3.4-3.7	12-12.2	May use if lactase-deficient vegetarian, galactosemic, or allergic to cow's milk.[†]

Modified and compiled from Kleinman RE (ed). Pediatric Nutrition Handbook, 6th ed. Elk Grove Village, Ill, American Academy of Pediatrics (AAP), 2008, pp 1250-1265.
[*]Iron-fortified formula.
[†]However, cross-reactivity with cow's milk protein sometimes occurs.
CHO, Carbohydrate.

recommended for infants with hereditary lactase deficiency or galactosemia and may be tried in infants intolerant to cow's milk, but soy formula should not be used in preterm infants. Because some infants allergic to cow's milk protein will develop an allergy to soy protein, it is advisable to use an extensively hydrolyzed protein formula in cases of true milk allergy or malabsorption. These are lactose free and may contain medium-chain triglycerides to improve fat absorption (AAP, 2009).

Human breast milk or iron-fortified infant formula is recommended for the first 12 months of life. Cow's milk is not suitable for infants because the higher intake of protein, sodium, potassium, and chloride increases renal solute load. In addition, the lower concentrations of iron, zinc, essential fatty acids, vitamin E, and other micronutrients can result in deficiencies. Significant intestinal blood loss can occur in infants younger than 12 months of age receiving cow's milk. Very-low-fat milks lack adequate calories for growth despite promoting excessive volume ingestion. Breastfed full-term infants seldom develop iron deficiency anemia before 4 to 6 months of age because the iron present in breast milk is well absorbed. Iron-fortified infant cereal or meats are then good sources of the 1 mg/kg/day of elemental iron required by full-term infants. All preterm or LBW infants should receive at least 2 mg/kg/day of elemental iron from 2 weeks until 12 months of age (AAP, 2009). Parents should be warned that iron is toxic in excessive amounts, and appropriate precautions should be taken.

Children 6 months to 3 years old who do not drink fluoridated water or other beverages may be given 0.25 mg/day of supplemental fluoride. Human milk contains only small amounts of biologically active vitamin D, and rickets has been reported in breastfed infants, infants with darker skin pigmentation, and even older children with minimal exposure to sunlight. Consequently, all breastfed infants, partially breastfed, non-breastfed infants, and older children ingesting less than 1000 mL/day of vitamin D–fortified formula or milk should receive 400 IU/day of supplemental vitamin D daily beginning within the first few days of life until the infant or child is ingesting 1000 mL/day of vitamin D–fortified formula or milk (AAP, 2009). Higher doses of vitamin D may be required in children with chronic fat malabsorption. Vitamin B_{12} supplementation should be given to breastfed infants whose mothers are strict vegetarians.

Both WHO and AAP promote exclusive breastfeeding for the first 6 months of life. However safe, nutritious solid foods may be introduced between 4 and 6 months of age, when the infant is developmentally ready. The order of introduction of solid foods is generally not critical; however, single-ingredient foods should be tried for 1 week at a time to observe for possible allergic reactions before introducing another food or mixtures of foods. Single-grain infant cereals such as rice (which lacks gluten) are usually well tolerated and provide a source of fortified iron. Homemade infant foods should not have added salt or sugar. Honey is associated with infant botulism and should not be given to infants younger than 1 year. Teething biscuits or finely chopped foods may be given by 8 to 10 months of age. However, foods such as popcorn, nuts, or rounded candies should not be offered to infants or toddlers because of the risks of choking, aspiration, and even death. Potentially hazardous foods such as hot dogs and grapes must be cut into small pieces, and the caregiver should always be present during mealtime. Children should be weaned from the bottle to a "sippy cup" by 12 to 15 months of age and bedtime bottles discouraged because they are associated with dental caries (AAP, 2009).

A toddler's food intake may be quite variable from day to day or even meal to meal. Because young children cannot choose a well-balanced diet, parents must provide nutritious, safe, developmentally appropriate foods at regular meals and snacks. Children should be sitting in a designated area for mealtime, without distractions such as television (AAP, 2009). Small portions of food should be offered to preschool children, allowing the child to determine how much he or she will eat and offering more as necessary. Excessive portion sizes can contribute to obesity later in life. Guidelines about types and quantities of foods from the basic food groups are available from the U.S. Department of Agriculture (USDA) MyPyramid website (www.mypyramid.gov), which provides recommendations on the amount of grain products, vegetables, fruits, and milk products based on the person's age, gender, and activity level.

Parents should be counseled that toddlers and preschool children are often picky eaters but generally grow well despite this. Parents need to guide children in their selection of food by offering a variety of nutritious items such as fruits and vegetables, keeping in mind that it can require 8 to 10 exposures to a new food before a child accepts it (AAP, 2009). Mealtime should not turn into a battleground because forcing a child to clean the plate can lead to specific food dislikes or promote obesity in later life. Snacking or eating while watching television should be discouraged, and physical activity should be encouraged.

Healthy children eating a varied diet usually do not require a multivitamin supplement. Children who do not eat dairy products, meat, or eggs require supplemental vitamin B_{12} and are at risk for vitamin D deficiency, especially if they lack adequate sunlight exposure or have darkly pigmented skin. Children following strict vegetarian diets often have low intakes of iron and calcium that can require supplementation. They often have a low intake of zinc that may be obtained from zinc-fortified infant and adult cereals. The recommended fiber intake is 19 g/day for children 1 to 3 years old and 25 g/day for those 4 to 8 years old. Excessive fiber consumption may decrease the intake of energy-dense foods and inhibit the absorption of some minerals (AAP, 2009).

Children with malabsorption or hemolytic anemia can require additional folic acid. Parents who insist on using a vitamin supplement without any obvious deficiency on the part of the child should be counseled to use a preparation that does not exceed the dietary reference intakes (DRIs) established by the Institute of Medicine and the National Academy of Sciences. In particular, vitamins A and D can produce toxicity if given in excessive doses.

Adolescents

Adolescents are at greater risk than other age groups for nutritional deficiencies because they may skip meals, snack more, eat more fast foods, and follow fad diets for reasons ranging from weight loss to cultural differentiation. Teenage boys and girls often replace milk and juice with soft drinks, coffee, tea, and alcoholic beverages, thereby lowering their intake of calcium as well as vitamins A and C. Adolescents' iron intake may be lower than required for their rapid increases in lean body mass and hemoglobin mass in addition to menstrual blood loss in girls. Zinc is also required for growth and

sexual maturation. Most teenagers do not ingest the recommended 1300 mg of calcium daily (AAP, 2009).

Energy requirements vary greatly in teenagers, depending on their gender, activity, and stage of adolescence. Sedentary adolescent girls require 1600 to 1800 cal/day and sedentary boys 1800 to 2200 kcal/day. As much as 200 kcal/day may be added for moderate physical activity and 200 to 400 kcal/day added for those who are very active (Daniels and Greer, 2008). Healthy pregnant women of normal BMI should tailor their prenatal diet to achieve a total weight gain of 11.5 to 16 kg (26-35 lb), or an additional 300 kcal/day during the second and third trimesters. Additional protein requirements are about 15 and 27 g/day during the second and third trimesters, respectively. Most will require some form of iron supplementation, about 30 mg/day during the second and third trimesters. Because zinc deficiency has potential teratogenic effects, pregnant adolescents should receive about 13 mg/day of zinc supplementation along with 1 mg/day of copper supplementation. All women of childbearing potential should take 400 to 600 μg of folic acid supplement per day in addition to 400 μg of dietary folate to decrease the risk of giving birth to children with neural tube defects. Pregnant women also require 1300 mg/day of calcium in their diet (AAP, 2009).

Universal screening for hypercholesterolemia in children is not currently recommended. A fasting lipid profile should be obtained in children who have a family history of dyslipidemia or premature (men ≤55 years, women ≤65 years) coronary heart disease or peripheral vascular or cerebrovascular disease. Children for whom the family history is not known or who have other risk factors such as overweight (BMI ≥85% and <95%), obesity (BMI ≥95%), hypertension (BP ≥95%), cigarette smoking, or diabetes mellitus should also be screened. This screening should be done between 3 and 10 years of age. The National Cholesterol Education Program (NCEP) guidelines indicate that a total cholesterol less than 170 mg/dL is acceptable, 170 to 199 mg/dL is borderline, and 200 mg/dL or greater is high. Similarly, a low-density lipoprotein (LDL) level less than 110 mg/dL is acceptable, 110 to 129 mg/dL is borderline, and higher than 130 mg/dL is elevated (Daniels and Greer, 2008). The American Heart Association has designated triglyceride (TG) levels greater than 150 mg/dL and high-density lipoprotein (HDL) level less than 35 mg/dL as abnormal. If initial lipid values are within acceptable levels, retesting should be done in 3 to 5 years.

It is recommended that all healthy children older than 2 years follow a diet in which a wide variety of foods provide adequate caloric intake to achieve proper growth and development as well as desirable weight. Total fat and saturated fat intake should be no more than 30% and 10%, respectively, of total calories; dietary cholesterol should be less than 300 mg/day. Children who are overweight or obese and have a high TG or low HDL level should be counseled regarding proper diet and increased physical activity. Children at especially high risk based on familial hyperlipidemias or premature cardiovascular disease may undertake a diet restricting saturated fat to 7% of total calories and cholesterol to 200 mg/day (Daniels and Greer, 2008). Children 10 years and older may be considered for pharmacologic therapy with LDL of 190 mg/dL or higher without additional risk factors, 160 mg/dL or greater with a family history of early heart disease or two or more other risk factors, or 130 mg/dL or higher if diabetes mellitus is present (AAP, 2009).

KEY TREATMENT

Ensure vitamin D intake of at least 400 IU/day, either by diet or supplementation (Wagner and Greer, 2008) (SOR: A).

Children 2 years and older should follow a diet with less than 30% of calories from total fat and 10% from saturated fat (Daniels and Greer, 2008) (SOR: B).

Communities should improve the availability of affordable healthier food and beverage choices and restrict the availability of less healthy choices in public service areas, by decreasing the cost of healthy foods and increasing the cost of less healthy foods (Khan et al., 2009) (SOR: B).

Behavior and Neurodevelopment

Key Points

- Development is a product of factors intrinsic and extrinsic to the child.
- Basic knowledge of child development enables clinicians to guide and educate families.
- Development proceeds in a basic sequence.
- Delays in one area of development may affect another.
- In preterm infants, correct for prematurity until age 2 years.

One of the rewards of providing primary care for a child is sharing with the family in the development of cognitive, motor, social, and language skills. Clinicians need to understand the theoretic framework on which the scientific understanding of child development is based in order to individualize the approach to the unique needs and concerns of each family. Physicians should develop strategies for clinically assessing child development and managing identified developmental abnormalities.

Theories of Development

Child development was widely studied in the 20th century. A general understanding of the common theories can enrich the clinician's relationship with young patients. Most researchers in child development believe that developmental outcomes are a product of intrinsic child factors, including genetic potential and temperament, and extrinsic environmental factors, such as intrauterine, infectious, traumatic, chemical, and sociocultural factors (Vaughan and Litt, 1992). The relative weights of each of these factors vary considerably among persons, thus frustrating the attempts of researchers to develop a formula for predicting developmental outcome for any individual person.

A clinician who is familiar with the key elements of theoretic models can develop expertise in applying them appropriately to meet the needs of countless clinical scenarios. For example, a physician might use Erikson's theory of psychosocial stages to explain to a vexed parent of a 2-year-old that the child's constant temper tantrums represent a normal expression of the child's need to exert autonomy over the environment. In the next room, the physician might refer to Piaget's concept of concrete operational thought to explain why a 10-year-old might not be capable of considering remote consequences of present actions (e.g., "If I don't study for my science test, I might not meet my goal of becoming an astronaut").

Features of the most widely accepted developmental theories are found in many pediatric references (Dixon and Stein, 2000). A summary of the salient features of each theory and potential clinical applications is presented in Table 23-5.

Erikson's psychosocial stages theory is particularly relevant (Table 23-6). According to his theory, at each discrete life stage, persons are confronted with a crisis requiring integration of personal needs with sociocultural demands. Successful integration of needs and development indicates normal adaptation. A practitioner who is familiar with these stages can counsel families about the emotional needs of children at different ages and explain the appropriateness of challenging but normal childhood behavior.

The concept of temperament is also clinically relevant for primary care. *Temperament* is a set of consistent, inborn characteristics that influence how people interact with and learn from their environment (Thomas et al., 1968). The person's temperament characteristics are innate to his or her personality. Three basic temperament profiles based on nine separate infant characteristics are outlined in Table 23-7. These are broad generalizations, and not all infants fit easily into one of these three categories.

Each family's personal value system influences their reaction to a child of a particular temperament. For example, a highly competitive, athletically oriented family may view high-energy, high-intensity characteristics more positively than a family who values studiousness. Qualities such as introversion or extroversion are often based on characteristics of temperament and are not modified readily by the environment. In a family in whom "goodness of fit" between individual members' temperaments does not exist, knowledge of the inborn nature of temperament can help the family accept a child's unique characteristics. Anticipatory guidance can then focus on achieving a better relationship between family and child.

Guidelines for Clinical Assessment

Although individual children develop at their own rate, with great variability in the normal range, general rules for neurodevelopmental maturation can serve as guidelines to help practitioners formulate a developmental trajectory for each child (Sturner and Howard, 1997). The developmental trajectory can be envisioned as an individualized growth chart of anticipated developmental progress based on normal neurodevelopmental milestones and moderated by child, parent, and environmental factors such as temperament, parental mental health, and exposure to lead.

Development usually is categorized into the domains of language, fine motor, gross motor, personal-social, and cognitive. Delays can occur in one or any combination of these domains. For example, a child with mental retardation is likely to have delays in all domains, although gross motor skills may be fairly well preserved. Conversely, a child with cerebral palsy may have normal or near-normal cognitive development with significant delays in gross and fine motor function. Many of the neurodevelopmental rules of thumb address the relationships among these domains.

Children acquire developmental tasks in a predictable sequence. For example, children typically do not learn to walk until they have mastered crawling and then standing.

Table 23-5 Summary of Developmental Theories of Child Development

Theory (proponents)	Key features	Potential clinical applications
Normative approach: development as maturation (Gesell)	Behavior depends on neurologic and physical maturation. Universal progression of developmental sequence. Minimal rule of environment/temperament.	Basis for age norms for developmental milestones typically used in clinical setting.
Psychosexual and psychoanalytic theory: development as resolution of conflict (Freud, Erikson)	Emotional life exerts strong influence on development and behavior. Unconscious conflicts between biologic drive and social expectations continuously shape behavior and self-concept. Parents are primary interactors with child, influencing behavior into adulthood. Mastery of major developmental tasks at different stages is required for emotional growth.	Interpersonal relationships, especially with primary caregivers, influence present and future adjustment, functioning, and self-concept. Importance of "bonding."
Behaviorism and social learning: development as learning (Pavlov, Skinner, Bandura)	Behavior, but not its underlying influences and motives, can be studied and changed. Environmental stimuli are the major forces shaping development and behavior. Environmental stimuli act as positive and negative reinforcements to existing behavior.	Children imitate what they see, so environmental models are important to learning (e.g., influences of media). Basis for behavioral management approaches.
Constructivist views: development as cognitive change (Piaget)	Cognitive development depends on both nature and nurture. Child uses physical and mental abilities to observe and act on the environment. Observation and action advance cognitive development. Child's mental processing develops with age, influencing how child perceives and interacts with the world.	Children possess an innate drive to learn. Play is the medium by which children learn and develop. Parents can be guided in choosing appropriate playthings/settings to allow their children to learn.
Ecologic system: development as cultural and ecologic adaptation (Bronfenbrenner)	A set of interrelated systems (e.g., family, school, community, health services) influences development. These systems exert reciprocal influence on one another. Development is determined by interactions of child and family.	Child's needs must be considered in context of the family and the environment.

Table 23-6 Using Erikson's Psychosocial Stages to Guide Development

Psychosocial Stage	Guidance
Basic trust and mistrust (0-2 years; infancy)	Parent can provide consistent nurturing to aid development of attitude of trust.
Autonomy vs. shame and doubt (2-4 years)	Parent should allow safe exploration of environment and encourage decision making.
Initiative vs. guilt (5-7 years)	Limits on child should be for protection of child, family, and society, and not random or condemning.
Industry vs. inferiority (8-12 years)	Caregiver must work with the school to ensure that child is achieving to his or her abilities and feeling sense of competence vs. inferiority.
Identity vs. role confusion (13-17 years)	Selection of career goal; establishment of relationship with opposite sex; independence from family should be encouraged by caregiver; failures to adapt in previous stages make this stage more difficult.
Intimacy vs. isolation (18-22 years)	Need to make personal and occupational commitment.

Although most children are able to crawl by 9 months of age and walk by 14.5 months, even severely delayed children follow the sequence of crawl, stand, and walk (Milani-Comparetti and Gidoni, 1967). This predictable sequence is dictated by building on previously learned skills, as well as by maturation of the central nervous system (CNS) (Springate, 1981). Before a critical stage in the maturation of the CNS, certain skills cannot be learned regardless of the intellectual potential or will of the child or parent. For example, because CNS control of the external anal sphincter is incomplete before 18 to 24 months of age, it is impossible to toilet-train even the most precocious toddler before this age.

Responses to stimuli proceed from generalized, symmetric, whole-body reflexes to discrete, cortically controlled, voluntary actions. Newborn reflexes can be thought of in terms of their role in survival of the individual; an example is the rooting reflex, which helps the newborn seek out nutrition. Voluntary movements develop as the child learns to control the environment.

Development proceeds in head-to-toe (cephalocaudal) and proximal-to-distal directions. Therefore, the infant bears weight on the arms before bearing weight on the legs. As proximal-to-distal progression occurs, the infant becomes more precise in fine-tuning the smaller muscles involved in reaching, grasping, and manipulating an object with his or her hand. Vocalization skills follow this pattern as well. A newborn infant vocalizes with "grunts" originating in the

Table 23-7 Temperament Characteristics and Profiles

Feature	Description
Characteristics	
Activity	Frequency and speed of involvement
Rhythmicity	Regularity of physiologic functions (e.g., hunger, sleep, elimination)
Approach/withdrawal	Immediate reaction of child to new stimuli
Adaptability	Degree of ease or difficulty with which child adjusts to new stimuli
Intensity	Energy level of responses, without regard to positive or negative quality of the response
Mood	Predominance of pleasant and friendly versus unfriendly behavior during waking
Attention span/persistence	Length of time the child will engage in a single activity with or without interruption
Distractibility	Degree of ease with which extraneous stimuli interfere with child's task performance
Sensory threshold	Amount of external stimulation required to evoke a response
Profiles	
Easy (40% of children)	Regularity of biologic functions; positive approach responses to new stimuli; high adaptability to change; mild to moderately intense mood that is predominantly positive
Difficult (10% of children)	Irregularity of biologic functions; negative withdrawal responses to new stimuli; no or slow adaptability to change; intense expressions of mood that are predominantly negative
Slow to warm up (15% of children)	Negative responses of mild intensity to new stimuli, with slow adaptability with repeated contact; mild intensity of reactions

Modified from Chess S, Thomas A. Dynamics of individual behavior development. In Levine MD, Carey WB, Crocker AC (eds). Developmental-Behavioral Pediatrics. Philadelphia, Saunders, 1992, p 86.

chest. As proximal-to-distal maturation develops, vocalizations originate more distally in the larynx (cooing), glottis (guttural syllables, "ga"), tongue ("da"), and lips ("ba").

Delays in one developmental domain can impair development in another domain. For example, an 18-month-old infant with motor impairments secondary to spina bifida lacks the freedom to explore the environment to learn how two pieces of furniture are oriented in space. Likewise, delays in one developmental domain can impair the practitioner's ability to evaluate skills in other domains. A 4-year-old toddler with cerebral palsy might understand the concept of sorting by shape but lack the motor control to manipulate the shapes to pass a standardized test.

An outline of salient features of development in each domain based on age is presented in Table 23-8. This guide to normal development should be considered by the physician along with past history, parental concerns, clinical observations, and developmental screening in the ongoing surveillance of child development. Until chronologic age 2 years, the development of a premature infant should be judged on corrected age, that is, the chronologic age minus the number of weeks premature.

Developmental Screening in Young Children

Key Points

- Always refer the child to audiology if language is delayed.
- Never ignore parents' concerns.
- Suspect delays and refer early.
- Developmental screening, using parent report measures, is more accurate than clinical judgment.
- Autism usually manifests as language delay.

Every encounter between a physician and child involves developmental and behavioral issues. Attention to such matters can benefit every child. By monitoring development, the primary care physician has the opportunity to customize anticipatory guidance based on the child's current abilities and temperament (Sturner and Howard, 1997).

Additionally, the family physician has a responsibility to identify children with delayed development. Federal law (Individuals with Disabilities Education Act [IDEA]) mandates physicians to refer children with suspected delays to early intervention (birth to 3 years) or early childhood services (3 to 5 years). The specifics of these services vary from state to state but are free and individualized according to the child's and family's needs (AAP Committee on Children with Disabilities, 1999). As the professional with the most frequent—and sometimes only—contact with young children, the family physician is in the ideal position to detect possible developmental problems. Additionally, parents may feel more comfortable sharing concerns and seeking advice from a trusted physician.

Early detection of delays is important, because brain development is most malleable in the early years of life (Shonkoff and Phillips, 2000). Early intervention has been shown to be cost-effective, resulting in better intellectual, social, and adaptive behavior, increased high school graduation and employment rates, and decreased criminality and teen pregnancy (Gomby et al., 1995; Reynolds et al., 2001). Unfortunately, less than half of children with developmental difficulties are identified before kindergarten (Pelletier and Abrams, 2002).

Research shows that clinical impression alone is quite poor at detecting developmental delays (Glascoe, 2000). This has led the AAP to recommend routine monitoring (surveillance) at all preventive care visits and use of standardized developmental screening tests at 9, 18, and 24 or 30 months of age, with the addition of autism-specific screening at 18 and 24/30 months (AAP Council on Children with Disabilities, 2006). Newer screening tools based on parent report can facilitate fulfilling this recommendation. Parent report has been found to be a reliable way to identify children in need of further developmental assessment, particularly if the concerns are elicited and interpreted in a standardized manner (Glascoe, 2003).

Table 23-8 Developmental Milestones in Young Children

Age	Gross motor	Fine motor/Reflex motor	Social/Adaptive/Cognitive	Language
Neonate	Flexed attitude, turns head side to side when prone without lifting, head sags if unsupported, body sags on ventral suspension	*Reflex:* Moro symmetric, grasp reflex, stepping reflex, suck reflex, placing reflex	Fixates on face or light, moves in cadence with sound	Alerts to voice
1 mo	Extends legs more, holds chin up briefly when prone, head lag persists	*Reflex:* Persistence of neonatal reflexes, tonic neck posture	Watches person, visually tracks to midline, begins to smile, body moves in cadence with voice	Throaty noises, range of cries to signal hunger, pain, etc.
2 mo	Raises head from prone position, sustains head in plane with body or ventral suspension, head lag on pull to sit	*Reflex:* Stepping reflex fades	Smiles on social contact, attracts to voice	Coos
4 mo	Head up to vertical axis in prone position, bears weight on arms, extends legs, symmetric posture with hands in midline in supine position, no head lag on pull to sit, pushes with feet in standing position, holds head erect in sitting position	*Fine:* Grasps and attains object, brings to mouth *Reflex:* Grasps, Moro, tonic neck fade; downward parachute present	Laughs out loud, voices displeasure if contact is broken, excites at sight of food, regards a small pellet	Vowel sounds, visually searches for speaker
6 mo	Sits alone with rounded back, rolls over, pivots, creeps	*Fine:* Rakes at pellet, transfers, turns body to reach *Reflex:* Sideways parachute present	Prefers mother, responds to emotion, imitates banging, visually follows dropped objects	Polysyllabic babble, blows bubble ("raspberry"), laughs
9 mo	Sits with erect back, crawls, walks holding both hands, pulls to stand, can get to sitting position	*Fine:* Pokes with forefinger, uses assisted pincer grasp Reflex: Forward (7 mo) and backward parachute present, plantar grasp fades	Plays "peekaboo," "pat-a-cake"; waves bye-bye; finds an object after watching it hidden; may cry at sight of unfamiliar person	Responds to some verbal commands: "no"; imitates some sounds; uses "mama," "dada" nonspecifically
12 mo	Cruises holding on, stands alone, may take several steps, walks holding hand	*Fine:* Neat pincer grasp, releases on request; puts 2 cubes in cup, pellet in bottle	Plays ball, adjusts posture when dressing, drinks from a cup, imitates activity (talks on toy phone)	1-2 true words, symbolic gestures (e.g., shakes head "no"), points to indicate wants
15 mo	Walks alone, crawls up stairs, walks backward, rises after stooping	*Fine:* Dumps pellet from bottle or draws line with crayon when demonstrated, scribbles spontaneously, stacks 2 cubes	Feeds self with utensils, performs simple household tasks (pick up toys), hugs parent	Points to body parts, jargons, follows 1-step command without gestures
18 mo	Runs stiffly, sits on small chair, walks up stairs with hand holding rail	*Fine:* Tower of 4 cubes, dumps pellet on request, imitates line with crayon	Feeds self with utensils; kisses parent with pucker; explores drawers, wastebaskets; removes garment; seeks help when in trouble	10 words, says "no," names pictures, points to 1 body part
24 mo	Runs well; walks up and down stairs, one at a time; jumps in place, climbs on furniture; kicks ball	*Fine:* Tower of 7 cubes, "train" of 4 cubes; imitates vertical and circular crayon stroke; imitates folding paper	Listens to story with pictures, helps to undress, dresses with help, parallel play, uses spoon well	30-50 words; 2- or 3-word sentences; uses pronouns, sometimes incorrectly; relates recent experience; speech 50% intelligible
36 mo	Alternates feet climbing stairs, stands on one foot briefly, broad jumps with both feet, pedals tricycle, throws ball overhand	*Fine:* Tower of 10 cubes, imitates "bridge" of 3 cubes, imitates cross, copies circle, attempts to draw person	Knows age and gender, counts 3 objects, repeats 3 serial numbers, understands turn-taking, washes and dries hands, helps with dressing	States full name; uses complete sentences; speech 75% intelligible to stranger; uses plurals, past tense, pronouns correctly

Continued

Table 23-8 Developmental Milestones in Young Children—cont'd

Age	Gross motor	Fine motor/Reflex motor	Social/Adaptive/Cognitive	Language
48 mo	Hops on one foot, throws ball overhand, balances on each foot 2-3 seconds	*Fine:* Uses scissors to cut out pictures; copies cross, square; draws man with head and 2-4 body parts (pairs count as 1 part); tells a story	Counts 4 objects correctly, group play with role playing, toilets independently, dresses with little supervision	—
60 mo	Skips, balances on each foot 4-5 seconds	*Fine:* Copies triangle, 8- to10-part person	Counts 10 objects, prints first name, domestic role playing, asks meaning of words, dresses and undresses independently	Uses complete sentences, names 4 colors, repeats 10-syllable sentence, follows 3-stage command

Compiled from Vaughn VC, Litt IF. Growth and development. In Behrman RE, Kliegman RM, Nelson WE, Vaughn VC (eds): Nelson Textbook of Pediatrics, 14th ed. Philadelphia, Saunders, 1992, pp 41-42.

Parent report measures can be used in a variety of ways. They can be completed in the waiting room, sent out to be returned at the next appointment, or completed via an interview, either in person or by telephone with a staff member. It is helpful to have a staff member routinely inquire if the parents would like someone to go over the measure with them; this ensures that literacy or language issues are not barriers to screening. Even if staff administer the parent report, parent report measures are the most accurate and time-effective and cost-efficient method of developmental screening currently available. Accurate screening tools with acceptable sensitivity and specificity (70%-80%) are listed in Table 23-9. Physicians can bill for screening, although reimbursement varies widely (Glascoe, 2003). More information regarding developmental screening, including coding and billing aspects, can be found at the Developmental Behavioral Pediatrics website.

Table 23-9 Developmental Screening Tools

Tool	Age range	Time	Source
Ages and Stages Questionnaire	0-60 mo	~7 min	Paul H. Brooks, Publishers www.pbrookes.com
Child Development Inventories	3-72 mo	~10 min	Behavior Science Systems*
Parents' Evaluations of Developmental Status (PEDS)	Birth-8 yr	~2 min	Ellsworth & Vandermeer www.pedstest.com

*PO Box 580274, Minneapolis, MN 55458.

Evaluation of Developmental Delay

The estimated prevalence of developmental delay is 10%. Some children present with delays in multiple areas, or global developmental delay. *Global developmental delay* is defined as significant delay in two or more areas of development (gross or fine motor, speech and language, cognition, social and personal, and activities of daily living). The more severe the delay, the more likely a cause can be determined (Roberts et al., 2004). Once significant delay is recognized, parents are often eager to know the cause. The family physician can be instrumental in referring for appropriate intervention, as well as overseeing an initial workup.

Although many physicians refer to specialists (e.g., developmental pediatricians, neurologists) for further evaluation, these specialists may have long waiting lists. Some aspects of the workup can easily be ordered by the family physician. Guidelines from the American Academy of Neurology and Child Neurology Society for the workup of the child with global developmental delay are shown in Table 23-10 (Shevell et al., 2003). The guidelines listed in the table are evidence based and could be readily used by family physicians to start the workup while waiting for a specialist appointment. Results of the workup may facilitate more specific referrals. Even if not globally delayed, all children with language delay should have a formal audiology assessment to rule out hearing impairment.

Autism Screening

Autism is a developmental disability involving difficulties with communication and social interaction as well as unusual and restricted behavior. The prevalence of autism appears to be rapidly increasing, for reasons not yet clear (Fombonne, 2003; Yeargan-Allsopp et al., 2003). The latest prevalence estimates are 1.1 per 100 children (Kogan et al., 2009). This makes it essential that any primary care physician seeing children be able to recognize signs and symptoms suggesting autism and refer for further evaluation promptly. Early diagnosis allows earlier initiation of intensive behavioral intervention, which has been shown to be very helpful (Butter et al., 2003). Table 23-11 lists "red flags" that should prompt referral for further evaluation

Table 23-10 Evaluation of Global Developmental Delay

Indication	Workup
Everyone	
First-line workup	Comprehensive history and physical Hearing and vision screening Metabolic studies and T_4 (if newborn screen results not known) EEG if symptoms of seizures Screen for autism if language delayed
Positive family history	
Genetic, metabolic, or CNS disorder	Test for specific condition
Nonspecific developmental delays	Chromosomes and fragile X
Signs or Symptoms present	
Specific genetic disorder	Specialized genetic testing
Hypothyroidism	Thyroid studies
CNS abnormality	MRI
Other	
Possible lead exposure	Lead level
Regression of skills or parental consanguinity	MRI, chromosomes, fragile X, metabolic testing, EEG, genetics evaluation
No specific signs/symptoms (stepwise in order)	MRI, chromosomes, fragile X, metabolic testing, Rett's syndrome testing

Data from Roberts G, Pafrey J, Bridgemohan C. A rational approach to the medical evaluation of a child with developmental delay. Contemp Pediatr 2004;21:76-100; and Shevell M, Asheval S, Donley D, et al: Practice parameter: evaluation of the child with global developmental delay. Neurology 2003;60:367-380.
CNS, Central nervous system, *EEG,* electroencephalogram; *MRI,* magnetic resonance imaging.

Table 23-11 Red Flags and Absolute Indications for Immediate Evaluation

Age	Sign
12 months	No babbling No pointing No gestures
16 months	No single words
24 months	No 2-word phrases
Any age	Loss of language or social skills

Modified from Filipek PA, Accardo PJ, Ashwal S, et al. Practice parameter: screening and diagnosis of autism. Neurology 2000;55:468-479.

(Filipek et al., 2000). A formal audiology evaluation is also indicated, as well as lead screening if the child has pica. It is important to keep in mind that most young children with autism are presented to their physician with the chief complaint of language delay. The physician should consider autism in the differential diagnosis for a child with language delay.

Assessing Development in the School-Age Child

Developmental surveillance in a school-age child should focus on identification of unsuspected learning problems, including attention-deficit/hyperactivity disorder (ADHD), mild mental retardation, and learning disabilities, as well as detection of emotional problems such as anxiety, depression, or school phobia. Emotional problems can be screened for using the Pediatric Symptom Checklist (PSC). The PSC is a one-page questionnaire that is relatively easy to administer and interpret during routine well-child care. Positive results should prompt the physician to probe

further with questions regarding school, friends, family, moods, and activities. Referrals to other professionals can then be made if necessary. More information regarding the PSC is available on the Massachusetts General Hospital PSC website.

Asking the child and parent about school progress and reviewing report cards and standardized testing results are simple ways for the physician to monitor school progress. Checklists completed by the parent and teacher can provide further information about specific issues (e.g., attention) or behavior in general (Table 23-12).

Federal law (IDEA) mandates a free and appropriate education for all children, regardless of handicapping condition. Therefore, if a child is suspected to have a learning disability, the school is obligated to evaluate and provide necessary services, free of charge (AAP, 1999). The parent should be advised to request the evaluation, called the Multi-Factored Evaluation (MFE), in writing. Federal law requires the MFE be done within 60 days. The MFE consists of standardized assessments of various aspects of learning. Once the MFE is completed, school personnel meet with the parents to review testing results and determine if the child is eligible for special education services. These services may occur in the regular classroom or in a separate one, although the law requires that services be provided in the least restrictive environment. The goal is to keep children with their typical peers as much as possible.

Once a child is deemed eligible for services, an individualized education plan (IEP) is developed. Parent input is required as part of the process. If the parent disagrees with the suggested IEP, the parent has the right to due process. An explanation of due process must be given to all parents at the beginning of the MFE/IEP process. Once developed, the IEP is updated annually. Parents should receive progress reports throughout the school year. They may request interim changes to the IEP if needed. Reevaluations are conducted at least every 3 years (Henderson, 2001).

All this is often overwhelming for families. The physician can assist by providing simple explanations of the process as well as periodically reviewing the IEP and helping parents understand it. The physician should also encourage parents to become knowledgeable advocates for their child.

Some children have conditions that can benefit from extra assistance but that do not qualify as handicaps according to

Table 23-12 School-Age Checklists

Purpose	Ages	Description	Website/Contact
Pediatric symptom checklist			
Brief screening for behavioral concerns	4-16 years	35 items completed by parents	psc.partners.org
Child behavior checklist			
In-depth screening for behavioral/emotional problems	Separate forms for 1-5 years and 6-18 years	Parents, teachers, caregivers, youth (11-18 yr); 99-118 items depending on form used	www.aseba.org
Conners scales			
More specific for ADHD and learning difficulties	3-17 years	Parent, teacher, youth (12-17 yr); short and long forms, 27-87 items	www.pearson assessments.com
Clinical attention problem scale			
Brief, specific for attention and overactivity symptoms	6-12 years	24-item checklist Teacher version	www.dbpeds.org/handouts
Vanderbilt			
Symptoms of ADHD; common comorbidities	6-12 years	Teacher/parent; initial (43-55 items) and follow-up (26 items) forms	http://www.nichq.org/NIaCHQ/Topics/ChronicConditions/ADHD/Tools/

ADHD, Attention-deficit/hyperactivity disorder.

the IDEA. Conditions such as ADHD are covered by Section 504 of the Rehabilitation Act of 1973 (Henderson, 2001). The qualifications are broader under this law, allowing children with less serious issues to still receive special services. This assistance, though helpful, is often less extensive than if the child qualified for an IEP.

Regardless of the issues, communication with school personnel is often helpful. Teacher rating scales (general or specific for certain concerns) may be useful, as well as direct communication, either verbally or in writing. Such dialogue also illustrates for families the advantages of cooperative teamwork with school personnel. It is always important for physicians to follow the Health Insurance Portability and Accountability Act (HIPAA) guidelines, obtain written permission from parents, and show discretion ("need to know") when sharing information with schools.

Immunizations

Key Points

- Avoid missed opportunities to vaccinate by reviewing the child's immunization record at every visit.
- Schedule adolescents for an immunization visit at age 11 to 12 years to catch up on missed vaccines and administer new ones.
- Provide current vaccine information statements to parents or guardians for each vaccine given during the visit.

Indications and Contraindications

Routine immunizations are essential for the control and prevention of previously common childhood infectious diseases. During 2008, more than 76% of U.S. children age 19 to 35 months received 4 or more doses of diphtheria, tetanus toxoids, and pertussis vaccines (DTP/DT/DTaP); 3 or more doses of poliovirus vaccine; 1 or more doses of any measles-containing vaccine; at least 3 doses of *Haemophilus influenzae* type b (Hib) vaccine; at least 3 doses of hepatitis B vaccine; and at least 1 dose of varicella vaccine (CDC, 2009). However, there is still considerable disparity in immunization rates among states and communities. Young children might not be immunized at the recommended age because of missed opportunities to vaccinate, deficient health care delivery in the public sector, lack of insurance, inadequate access to medical care, lack of public awareness about the necessity for immunizations, or concern about potential or alleged adverse effects of immunizations. Both AAFP and AAP endorse the Childhood and Adolescent Immunization Schedules (see **eTables 23-3** to **23-5** online) (SOR: A).

Parents or guardians should be questioned about possible contraindications, precautions, and any previous adverse events in response to vaccine administration (see **eTable 23-6**). They should be informed about the potential benefits and risks of the vaccine and the risks of the natural disease should the immunization not be given. Health care providers administering any vaccine covered by the National Vaccine Compensation Injury Act or purchased by federal contract must provide the most current *vaccine information statements* (VISs) detailing the potential benefits and risks of each vaccine to the parents or guardians each time that vaccine is given (AAP Red Book, 2009, 5-6). Copies of VISs may be obtained from the CDC (www.cdc.gov/vaccines/pubs/VIS/default.htm), the Immunization Action Coalition (www.immunize.org), or state health departments.

Vaccines have become "victims of their own success" (Cooper et al., 2008). Because they no longer are confronted with the presence of vaccine-preventable diseases, some individuals, parents, and groups have become more concerned about the alleged adverse effects of immunization. A Danish study is one of many that has confirmed the effectiveness of vaccines such Hib and pertussis and did not find an association of MMR or thimerosal-containing vaccines with autism spectrum disorders (Hviid, 2006). Physicians serve as the primary source of information about immunizations, and the family physician should explain the potential benefits and risks of immunizations to parents and older patients such as adolescents (Gellin et al., 2000). If parents still do not wish to have their child vaccinated, further information and documentation may be obtained at http://www.aap.org/immuniz ation/pediatricians/pdf/RefusaltoVaccinate.pdf.

Before administering vaccines, the physician should ask about the child's current state of health, as well as that of other family members. An immunosuppressed member of the household might contraindicate the administration of certain live-virus vaccines, such as nasal live, attenuated influenza vaccine (LAIV). Minor febrile illnesses are not contraindications to vaccine administration. General contraindications are a previous anaphylactic reaction to the specific vaccine or a severe hypersensitivity reaction to vaccine constituents such as gelatin or antibiotics such as neomycin, streptomycin, or polymyxin B. Latex allergy may also be a contraindication if the vaccines are supplied in vials or syringes containing natural rubber (AAP Red Book, 2009, 848-853).

Vaccine Administration

Most immunizations must be given by deep intramuscular (IM) or subcutaneous (SC) injection. IM injections should be given in the anterolateral thigh for infants or the deltoid muscle of the arm for older children. The sciatic nerve may be injured by deep intragluteal injections. Although acetaminophen (paracetamol) administered for 24 hours has been demonstrated to decrease mild to moderate reactions, such as temperature of 38° C (100.4° F) or greater, it may reduce antibody responses to some vaccine antigens (Prymula et al., 2009). Topical local anesthetics, sweet-tasting solutions, and breastfeeding may decrease injection pain for childhood immunizations (HELPinKIDS, 2009).

Immune responses may be impaired if two live-virus vaccines are given within 28 days of each other. Live-virus vaccines must be given simultaneously or at least 4 weeks apart (AAP Red Book, 2009, 22). If immune globulin (IG) is given, live-virus vaccine administration should be delayed for up to 3 to 6 months to allow optimal antibody production (AAP Red Book, 2009, 448). An even longer period may be required if high doses of intravenous (IV) gamma globulin have been given.

Schedule of Immunizations

The recommended schedule for childhood and adolescent immunizations are given online in **eTables 23-3 to 23-5.** A lapse in the immunization schedule does not require starting over the entire series. Doses of any vaccine should not be divided or reduced, because this can result in an inadequate response. Premature infants should receive the same vaccine dose, usually at the same chronologic age as full-term infants. Most vaccines can be administered simultaneously using separate syringes at separate sites (AAP Red Book, 2009, 33).

Poliovirus Vaccine

The last indigenous case of wild-type poliomyelitis in the United States occurred in 1979, and the last identified imported case occurred in 1993. From 1980 to 1996, there were approximately eight cases per year of vaccine-associated paralytic poliomyelitis (VAPP) caused by oral poliovirus vaccine (OPV) in the United States. In 2000, inactivated

poliovirus vaccine (IPV) was recommended for all routine childhood polio vaccinations in the United States, and only one case of VAPP was imported from Central America in 2005 (AAP Red Book, 2009, 541).

Measles, Mumps, and Rubella Vaccine

The measles-mumps-rubella (MMR) vaccine should be given to children 12 to 15 months of age. The second MMR or measles-mumps-rubella-varicella (MMRV) vaccine is recommended before school entry at 4 to 6 years of age, but it can be given earlier in the event of an outbreak or as a requirement for travel, provided the second dose is given at least 28 days after the first. Physicians should review their records to ensure that all children receive the second MMR or MMRV by 11 to 12 years of age. Children may be immunized with MMR even if there is a pregnant or immunosuppressed family member, because the vaccine viruses are not transmitted (AAP Red Book, 2009, 47).

Haemophilus Influenzae Type b Conjugate Vaccine

The use of *H. influenzae* type b (Hib) conjugate vaccines has lowered the U.S. incidence of invasive Hib disease in children younger than 5 years of age by 99%. Vaccines currently available in the United States, such as HbOC (HibTITER), PRP-OMP (PedvaxHIB), and PRP-T (ActHIB, OmniHIB), are given beginning at age 2 months. ActHIB reconstituted with Tripedia as Trihibit is licensed only for the fourth dose of Hib and DTaP, while PRP-T (Hiberix) is licensed for use as a booster in children 15 months through 4 years of age (CDC,2009). PRP-OMP-HepB (Comvax) is administered at 2, 4, and 12 to 15 months of age and DTaP-IPV/PRP-T (Pentacel) at 2, 4, 6, and 15 to18 months of age (AAP Red Book, 2009, 318-321).

The schedule of administration varies according to the type of vaccine, as shown in **eTables 23-3** and **23-4.** Children age 15 to 59 months of age usually need only 1 dose of any Hib conjugate vaccine. Children with conditions predisposing to invasive Hib disease, such as sickle cell anemia, asplenia, human immunodeficiency virus (HIV) infection, chemotherapy for malignancies, and immunologic impairment, are given 2 doses of vaccine 2 months apart. Children age 60 months or older are generally not vaccinated unless they also have a chronic illness associated with an increased risk of Hib disease and require 2 doses of Hib conjugate vaccine 1 to 2 months apart (AAP Red Book, 2009, 321).

Acellular Pertussis Vaccine

Acellular pertussis vaccines combined with diphtheria and tetanus toxoids (DTaP) are used in the United States for the primary and booster doses in children. These vaccines (DAP-TACEL, Infanrix, Tripedia) are immunogenic and produce fewer adverse local and systemic reactions, such as fever and irritability, than do whole-cell pertussis vaccines. Whenever possible, the same DTaP vaccine should be used throughout the entire vaccination series, because there are no data on safety or efficacy when different formulations of these vaccines are interchanged. However, if the previously used vaccine is not known or is unavailable, any of the DTaP vaccines licensed for use in children may be given to complete the immunization series. Combination vaccines such as DTaP-IPV-HepB (Pediarix) and DTaP-IPV-Hib (Pentacel) are licensed for use as the first 3 doses and first 4 doses, respectively, of their components, whereas DTaP-IPV (Kinrix) is licensed only as the booster fifth dose of DTaP and fourth dose of IPV at ages 4 to 6 years (AAP Red Book, 2009, 508, 510).

Two vaccines containing reduced concentrations of diphtheria toxoid and pertussis antigens combined with tetanus toxoid (Tdap) are now licensed for use in adolescents and adults (Boostrix and ADACEL). The vaccines are recommended for adolescents 11 to 18 years of age in place of the Td booster to decrease the reservoir of *Bordetella pertussis* in this population. Increasing reports of pertussis in many U.S. states has led to a recent recommendation to give one dose of these vaccines to children 7 to 10 years of age who are incompletely immunized against pertussis.

Rotavirus Vaccine

Rotavirus is responsible for up to 500,000 deaths from diarrhea worldwide and 20 to 60 U.S. deaths in each year. Before the introduction of rotavirus vaccines (RV1 or Rotarix, RV5 or RotaTeq), rotavirus caused 3 million infections per year in the United States, resulting in more than 400,000 physician visits and 55,000 to 70,000 hospitalizations per year (CDC Pink Book, 2009, 245-256). RV1 is given as 2 oral doses at 2 and 4 months of age, and RV5 is given as 3 oral doses at 2, 4, and 6 months of age. The minimum interval between doses of either vaccine is 4 weeks. Neither vaccine should be started for infants age 15 weeks, 0 days or older, and all doses must given by 8 months, 0 days of age. The vaccine-specific package insert should be seen for full prescribing indications and contraindications.

Varicella Vaccine

Two SC doses of monovalent varicella (VZV) vaccine or MMRV are indicated in children age 12 months through 12 years. The doses should be separated by at least 3 months, with the second dose routinely recommended at age 4 to 6 years before kindergarten or first grade. Persons 13 years or older who do not have evidence of immunity to varicella should receive 2 doses of VZV vaccine at least 28 days apart because MMRV is not licensed in this age group. A second dose of varicella vaccine should be given to people who previously received only 1 dose. The vaccine is generally contraindicated in pregnant women, immunodeficient persons, or those receiving high doses of systemic corticosteroids (≥20 mg/day of prednisone or equivalent) for 14 days or more. However, VZV vaccine may be considered for HIV-infected patients with a CD4+ T-lymphocyte count of 15% or greater. Vaccine-strain VZV has been rarely transmitted, and vaccinated patients who develop a rash should avoid contact with immunocompromised persons (AAP Red Book, 2009, 724-726). Zoster vaccine is not interchangeable with varicella vaccine and is not used in children.

Hepatitis A Vaccine

Hepatitis A virus (HAV) is usually transmitted person to person through the fecal-oral route and by ingestion of contaminated food or water, but it has rarely been transmitted by transfusion of blood or blood products. Two HAV inactivated vaccines, HAVRIX and VAQTA, are licensed in the United States for use in children age 1 year and older. TWINRIX is a combined hepatitis A and hepatitis B vaccine licensed for use in persons at least 18 years old. Physicians should consult the package insert for proper dosing because there are different formulations of these vaccines.

Childhood vaccination against HAV is recommended for all U.S. children 12 to 23 months of age and should be considered for unimmunized children ages 2 to 18 years old. Indications for immunization with hepatitis A vaccine include travel to or residence in countries or areas endemic for hepatitis A, residence in Native American or Alaskan Native communities with high rates of HAV infection, persons who receive clotting-factor concentrates, persons with chronic liver disease, injection drug users (IDUs), men who have sex with men (MSM), and people at risk of occupational (e.g., handlers of primates), household, and sexual exposure (AAP Red Book, 2009, 329-337).

Hepatitis B Vaccine

Hepatitis B virus (HBV) is endemic in Southeast Asia, the Pacific Islands, China, Africa, parts of the Middle East, and the Amazon Basin. More than 350 million people worldwide have chronic HBV infection. Although transmission in U.S. children is less likely because of high coverage with HBV vaccine, the risk of perinatal transmission of HBV from an infected mother to her infant varies from 10% to as high as 90%, depending on whether the mother is negative or positive for hepatitis B e antigen (HBeAg) (CDC Pink Book, 2009, 99-122).

Immunization with the pediatric formulations of hepatitis B vaccine is recommended for all infants soon after birth or before hospital discharge. HBV vaccine should be given to newborns of mothers positive for hepatitis B surface antigen (HBsAg) or infants of mothers whose HBsAg status is unknown. An infant born to an HBsAg-positive mother should receive an initial dose of 5 μg Recombivax HB or 10 μg Engerix-B and 0.5 mL of hepatitis B immune globulin (HBIG) IM at separate sites within 12 hours of birth. Repeat vaccine doses should be given at ages 1 month and 6 months. For infants of HbsAg-negative mothers, the combination DTaP-HBV-IPV (Pediarix) or PRP-OMP-HBV vaccine (Comvax) may also be used, beginning at 6 to 8 weeks of age. Practitioners should consult the package insert for the appropriate dose according to the formulation and intended use. Any adolescents who have not yet received HBV vaccine should also be immunized with 2 doses at least 4 weeks apart, with a third dose 4 to 6 months after the second dose (CDC Pink Book, 2009, 99-122).

Hepatitis B vaccine should be given to susceptible high-risk children or adults who are institutionalized; those who have end-stage renal disease, chronic liver disease, or HIV infection; those who receive clotting-factor concentrates; those who have an HIV-infected household or sexual contact; MSM; IDUs; and adoptees from or long-term travelers to countries endemic for hepatitis B (AAP Red Book, 2009, 337-356).

Conjugate Pneumococcal Vaccine

The 13-valent conjugate pneumococcal vaccine (PCV13) covers 64% of the serotypes that cause invasive pneumococcal disease in children younger than 5 years old. The vaccine stimulates effective antibodies to all 13 serotypes in over 90% of recipients after three doses and is given to infants at 2, 4, 6, and 12 to 15 months of age. Children 7 to 11 months old require 2 doses 2 months apart, followed by a third dose at 12 to 15 months of age (2 or more months later). Children 12 to 23 months old require 2 doses 2 months apart. Only 1 dose is required for all healthy children 24 to 59 months of age. Children age 24 to 71 months at high risk for invasive pneumococcal disease should receive 2 doses of vaccine at least 8 weeks apart if they have not been previously immunized (CDC, 2010).

Influenza Vaccine

Routine annual immunization with trivalent inactivated influenza (TIV) vaccine is now recommended for all persons 6 months of age and older, including these with high-risk conditions such as HIV, chronic pulmonary (including asthma), cardiac, renal, or metabolic diseases; those receiving immunosuppressive or long-term aspirin therapy; those who have hemoglobinopathies, and those with any condition (e.g., cognitive dysfunction, seizure disorder, neuromuscular disorder) that could compromise respiratory function. TIV vaccine is also recommended for pregnant women and persons who are household contacts of high-risk patients, including health care workers. Several TIV products are now available, and providers should read the prescribing information regarding the appropriate age and dosing of these vaccines. Live, attenuated influenza vaccine (LAIV) is approved for use in healthy persons age 2 through 49 years and not pregnant. LAIV should not be used in persons with asthma or those in close contact with severely immunosuppressed hospitalized patients receiving care in a protected environment. Neither vaccine should be given to persons with a history of severe allergy to egg or any other vaccine component (CDC Pink Book, 2009, 141-154).

Conjugate Meningococcal Vaccine

Tetravalent meningococcal polysaccharide-protein conjugate vaccine (MCV4, Menactra, Sanofi Pasteur; and Menveo, Novartis) has been licensed in the United States for use in persons 2 to 10 years old and 11 to 55 years old. Routine immunization of all children age 11 to 18 years and especially 11 to 12 years at a health-care visit is recommended. The vaccines contain serogroups A, C, Y, and W-135, as does the current meningococcal polysaccharide vaccine (MPSV4). Serogroups C, Y, and W-135 cause 75% of all cases of meningococcal disease in persons older than 11 years in the United States (Bilukha and Rosenstein, 2005). Neither vaccine is protective against serogroup B, which accounts for most of the remaining cases. Persons 2 to 55 years with terminal complement or properdin deficiencies, anatomic or functional asplenia, and HIV should receive two doses 2 months apart (CDC, 2011). Travelers to countries with hyperendemic or epidemic *Neisseria meningitidis* (e.g., sub-Saharan Africa, Mecca during the Hajj) should also be immunized with MCV4 (CDC Pink Book, 2009, 177-188). College freshmen students living in dormitories have a higher risk of meningococcal infection than students living off campus and should be immunized with MCV4. MCV4 is given to all U.S. military recruits (AAP Red Book, 2009, 461-463). Revaccination is recommended for persons at prolonged increased risk who were vaccinated at age 7 years or older and were vaccinated 5 years previously, or for those at ages 2 to 6 years old and vaccinated 3 years previously (CDC, 2009). A booster dose of MCV4 is also recommended for adolescents at age 16 years who received their previous dose at age 11 or 12 years and at age 16 through 18 years for those who received their first dose at age 13 through 15 years (CDC, 2011).

Human Papillomavirus Vaccine

Although most human papillomavirus (HPV) infections spontaneously resolve, high-risk HPV types are found in 99% of cervical cancers with types 16 and 18, accounting for about 70% of cervical cancers worldwide. HPV is also believed to account for 90% of anal cancers; 40% of vulvar, vaginal, or penile cancers; and 12% of oral and pharyngeal cancers. Types 6 and 11 HPV account for 90% of genital warts and laryngeal papillomatosis. The bivalent HPV (types 16, 18) vaccine (Cervarix) and the quadrivalent HPV (types 6, 11, 16, 18) vaccine (Gardasil) are licensed for use in U.S. females age 10 to 25 and 9 to 26 years, respectively. Both are recommended for routine vaccination at age 11 or 12 years and are ideally given before onset of sexual intercourse. The bivalent HPV vaccine is given in a 3-dose series at time 0, 1, and 6 months and the quadrivalent HPV vaccine in a 3-dose series at time 0, 2, and 6 months, with the third dose following the first dose by at least 24 weeks (CDC Pink Book, 2009, 123-133). These vaccines are prophylactic only for the HPV types they contain and do not treat preexisting infection with these HPV types. They may be given at the same visit at different sites with the MCV4 and Tdap vaccines. The FDA (2009) has also approved the quadrivalent HPV vaccine for use in males 9 to 26 years old to prevent genital warts.

Special Clinical Situations

Children who are immunocompromised or infected with HIV usually should not be given live-virus vaccines. However, measles can cause severe disease and death in symptomatic HIV-infected patients. MMR (but not MMRV) is recommended at age 12 months for HIV-infected children with CD4+ T-lymphocyte counts of 15% or greater. The second dose can be given 28 days later to improve the immune response. Children with age-specific low CD4+ counts should not be given measles virus–containing vaccine (AAP Red Book, 2009, 447-455) All HIV-infected children or children of unknown status born to HIV-infected women should receive immune globulin at 0.5 mL/kg to a maximum dose of 15 mL, regardless of vaccination status, if exposed to wild-type measles. HIV-infected children are also at increased risk from complications of chickenpox and zoster, and those children with CD4+ counts of at least 15% should receive two doses of varicella vaccine 3 months apart. The MMRV vaccine is not used in this situation (AAP Red Book, 2009, 726).

Conjugate pneumococcal vaccine (PCV13) is recommended for all children younger than 60 months and children 24 to 71 months who have high-risk conditions such as sickle cell disease, functional or anatomic asplenia, HIV infection, other immune deficiencies or immunosuppressive therapies, chronic cardiac or pulmonary disease, chronic renal insufficiency, diabetes mellitus, cerebrospinal fluid leaks, or cochlear implants. High-risk children who have received 4 doses of PCV13 should also receive 1 dose of the 23-valent polysaccharide pneumococcal vaccine (PPSV23, Pneumovax-23) at 24 months. Children 24 to 71 months old who have received less than 3 doses of PCV13 should receive 2 doses of PCV13 followed by 1 dose of PPSV23 at 8 weeks later. Immunosuppressed children and those with sickle cell disease or functional asplenia should receive a second dose of PPSV23 vaccine 5 years after the first dose (AAP Red Book, 2009, 524-535).

National Childhood Vaccine Injury Act

The National Childhood Vaccine Injury Act of 1986 was passed to provide compensation for children inadvertently injured by any of the routinely recommended childhood vaccines and to provide liability protection for manufacturers and for health care providers who administer the vaccines. The intent of the law is to ensure a stable supply of vaccine and allow routine immunizations to continue. The physician or other health care provider must maintain permanent documentation of the date, vaccine type, manufacturer, lot number, and name, address, and title of the person administering the vaccine. A list of reportable but not necessarily compensable events is available from the Health Resources and Services Administration. Significant adverse events should be reported to the Vaccine Adverse Event Reporting System (VAERS) at 1-800-822-7967 or www.vaers.hhs.gov.

Acknowledgment

This chapter incorporates some material that was written by Lorraine M. Fay, MD, for this chapter in the 6th edition of *Textbook of Family Practice*.

KEY TREATMENT

Administer all recommended or required immunizations, except when true contraindications or precautions are present or the immunizations are refused by the parent or patient (AAP Red Book, 2009; Hviid, 2006) (SOR: A).

Key Resource

Centers for Disease Control and Prevention. Atkinson W, Wolfe S, Hamborsky J, McIntyre L (eds). Epidemiology and Prevention of Vaccine-Preventable Diseases. Pink Book. 11th ed. Washington, DC, Public Health Foundation, 2009, pp 123-133, 141-154, 177-188. Inexpensive reference from CDC that is updated yearly, covering nuts and bolts of vaccine-preventable diseases and immunizations.

References

The complete reference list is available online at www.expertconsult.com.

Web Resources

www.aan.com
American Academy of Neurology; practice parameters for screening and diagnosis of autism and evaluation of developmental delay.

www.aap.org
American Academy of Pediatrics; good general information regarding health care for children and access to guidelines for developmental screening and other topics.

www.cdc.gov/growthcharts/clinical_charts.htm
National Center for Health Statistics; growth charts for female and male development.

www.cdc.gov/ncbddd/child/screen_provider.htm
Centers for Disease Control and Prevention; developmental screening for health care providers; excellent information about child development and screening with helpful links and patient material.

www.cdc.gov/vaccines/pubs/VIS/default.htm
Centers for Disease Control and Prevention, National Immunization Program; vaccine information statements.

www.dbpeds.org
Developmental Behavioral Pediatrics; wealth of information about developmental screening and other topics related to child development and behavior.

www.hrsa.gov/vaccinecompensation/table.htm
Health Resources and Services Administration, National Vaccine Injury Compensation Program, National Childhood Vaccine Injury Act; vaccine injury table lists potentially compensable vaccine adverse events.

www.immunize.org/vis
Immunization Action Coalition; vaccine information statements.

http://psc.partners.org
Massachusetts General Hospital, Pediatric Symptom Checklist; free access and instructions for use and scoring.

www.mypyramid.gov
US Department of Agriculture MyPyramid; allows development of a personalized meal plan based on age, gender, and activity level.

www.hhs.gov/ocr/hipaa/US Department of Health and Human Services, Office for Civil Rights, Health Insurance Portability and Accountability Act (HIPAA).

www.vaers.hhs.gov Vaccine Adverse Event Reporting System (VAERS); individuals, health care providers, and manufacturers may report vaccine-associated adverse events; this does not prove causation.

24 CHAPTER

Behavioral Problems in Children and Adolescents

Scott E. Moser and John F. Bober

Behavioral problems are common reasons for parents to bring their child to see the family physician. In addition, addressing behavioral issues is an important component of the well-child visit. Childhood behavioral problems are a complex assortment of individual mental disorders, genetic and medical disorders, family interaction difficulties, social and school problems, and combinations of these. The rates of many psychosocial problems in children and adolescents, including depression, suicide, conduct disorders, and drug and alcohol abuse, have been rising in recent years throughout Western culture (Fombonne, 1998). This increase is only partly explained by changes in diagnostic criteria and reporting. The trend is particularly troubling when economic conditions and physical health of the population have been improving. The implication for office physicians is that psychosocial problems will encompass a growing proportion of patient care both as presenting problems and as cofactors in other medical conditions.

This chapter is arranged in problem-focused fashion along a developmental continuum from infancy through adolescence based on when various problems are most frequently encountered in practice. For conditions encountered at different developmental stages, discussions include similarities and differences in recognition and treatment at different ages. Management focuses on early, brief interventions the physician can make with the patient and family as well as suggestions about referral.

Regardless of the behavioral concern or the child's age, general principles for evaluation and management include the following:

1. Obtain specific examples of the problem behaviors rather than general conclusions. For example, "Child is out of his seat, walking around the classroom every few minutes," rather than, "Disruptive in class"; and "Screams inconsolably at 2 AM," rather than, "Doesn't sleep well."

2. Obtain as complete information from as many observers as possible. Unusual seizure disorders and other neurologic problems are included in the differential diagnosis of many behavioral disorders. Keys to their diagnosis are found in a careful history.

3. For the same reason just stated, include a careful neurologic and age-appropriate mental status examination.

4. Emotional stressors and abuse, whether physical, verbal, or sexual, can be important precipitators or exacerbators of behavioral problems. Therefore, explore these, including an interview of the child apart from their parents once the child is verbal.

5. Consider multiple diagnoses simultaneously. Multifactorial etiologies are common for many behavioral complaints, and many psychiatric diagnoses carry a high risk of comorbid conditions. Therefore, avoid a linear approach of working up one potential diagnosis at a time.

6. Use a multidimensional treatment approach. Many behavioral problems respond best to combinations of psychotherapy, medication, parent and teacher education, and other therapies, rather than only one of these at a time.

7. Familiarize yourself with the mental health regulations for the various insurance plans in which you participate. Many plans have "carve-outs" (separately contracted providers) for mental health services. If you are the initial contact regarding a concern, you may either assist or hinder your patient obtaining the appropriate assistance based on your knowledge of available service channels. This is particularly important in crisis situations; know the services in your area, including specific providers available on various insurance plans, and how to access them during evenings and weekends.

Sleep Problems

Key Points

- Many sleep problems can be prevented with good sleep hygiene.
- For obstructive sleep apnea syndrome, criteria to order a sleep study in the evaluation of a child are similar to criteria for adults, but interpretation of the results requires special pediatric expertise.
- The most common cause of obstructive sleep apnea in children is adenotonsillar hypertrophy, and the treatment of choice is surgery.

Normal sleep has a well-characterized pattern of rapid eye movement (REM) and non-REM sleep that changes with age. Non-REM sleep is further categorized into stages 1, 2, 3, and 4, on the basis of electroencephalographic (EEG) characteristics, with the deepest non-REM sleep occurring in stages 3 and 4. A normal nighttime sleep cycle is about every 90 minutes, with multiple brief arousals and quick returns to sleep without memory of having awakened. Deep non-REM sleep predominates in the first several hours of sleep, and REM is most prominent in the last few hours. Children have substantial periods of very deep sleep that lessen with age. There is a gradual decrease in the amount of REM sleep and a significant decrease in deep non-REM sleep, especially in adolescence.

Children and adolescents in American society sleep less than those in other societies and less than children in the past (Dahl, 1998). Because of the wide variations in normal sleep patterns and development, the physician should avoid rigid expectations in counseling parents, but the following are some useful guidelines. A typical infant is able to sleep 6 to 8 hours through the night by age 2 months and 10 to 12 hours by age 6 months. The child usually no longer requires a morning nap by about 1 year of age and outgrows the afternoon nap around age 3. The total daily sleep requirement decreases with age, from 16 $\frac{1}{2}$ hours at 1 week of age to 14 hours by age 1 year, 13 hours by age 2 years, 12 hours by age 3 years, 11 hours by age 5, and 10 hours by age 9 years (Blum and Carey, 1996).

An important aspect of preventing sleep problems is guidance regarding good sleep hygiene (Box 24-1). *Sleep hygiene* refers to the conditions that are most conducive to healthy, restorative sleep. Some children are reassured by a low-wattage night-light, but more light than that may disturb sleep. Parents of newborns should be counseled to put their infant to sleep supine rather than prone, unless

there is a specific medical indication to the contrary. This results from the association of the prone sleeping position with sudden infant death syndrome (SIDS) in young infants (Guntheroth and Spiers, 1992) (SOR: A). Many children rest better with a "transitional object," a favorite blanket or toy. However, parents should avoid putting the child to bed with a bottle left in the mouth because it may lead to severe dental caries. Finally, the child should be put to bed awake, so that the child develops self-soothing skills to initiate sleep and resume sleep after nighttime disruptions.

About 20% to 30% of children and adolescents have sleep problems that are a serious concern to them and their families (Dahl, 1998). Problems with sleep initiation and nighttime awakenings are most common during infancy. Parasomnias and obstructive sleep apnea syndrome are most common in the 3- to 8-year-old group. Sleep deprivation, delayed sleep-phase syndrome, and narcolepsy are important considerations in the adolescent age group (Carskadon and Roth, 2000).

Besides sleep problems being common, family physicians need to be alert to these conditions because they have such a negative impact on many aspects of physical, mental, and social well-being. Sleep problems early in life are predictive of many later behavioral and emotional problems (Dahl, 1998). Children with frequent nighttime awakenings are at increased risk for physical abuse, perhaps because parents of these children show increased levels of fatigue, irritability, and depression.

The assessment and management of sleep problems in general should include consideration of potential sleep interrupters as primary causes or as exacerbators. One important category of interrupters is conditions that cause pain or itching (e.g., juvenile rheumatoid arthritis, migraine, atopic dermatitis). Another category is problems that lead to respiratory symptoms, including nocturnal asthma, gastroesophageal reflux (GERD), and obstructive sleep apnea.

Box 24-1 Good Sleep Hygiene

Environment

Dark

Quiet

Cool

Schedule

Regular morning waking time

Consistent nap length

Regular bedtime

Activities

No frightening TV or stories

No vigorous physical activities in the hour before bedtime

Consistent bedtime routine

Consistent soothing methods

Child put into bed awake

From Blum NJ, Carey WB. Sleep problems among infants and young children. Pediatr Rev 1996;17:87-92.

Sleep Refusal

Toddlers often resist going to bed when their parents want them to go. Parents may have difficulty recognizing whether the resistance is related to true needs and fears or whether it is attention seeking or oppositional. The resistance often takes the form of repeated requests for a snack, a drink, or a trip to the toilet and may include fears of noises, shadows, or imaginary monsters.

A sleep diary can be helpful to sort out the etiology for the sleep refusal and direct management efforts. The parents record bedtimes and waking times for 2 weeks and indicate specific problem behaviors and their responses to each situation. Parents are often able to recognize patterns and problems themselves as they review the diary.

Many common refusal patterns can be addressed by focusing on the problem aspects of good sleep hygiene (Box 24-1). If the problem seems to be oppositional, the best approach is for parents to ignore it. If the child gets out of bed, a parent should place the child back in bed without conversation other than a firm, "It's time for bed." When the parents actively ignore their child's efforts to get attention, the behaviors often get worse before they improve. However, even persistent children eventually respond (Blum and Carey, 1996). If standard ignoring is too stressful on the family, a "gradual ignoring" technique is also effective (Reid et al., 1999) (SOR: B). This involves briefly checking on the child every few minutes until they are asleep and gradually lengthening the interval between checks.

For a child who is fearful, having parents ignore them may make the fears worse. A gradual withdrawal of the parent's presence after the bedtime routine works better. The parent may sit in the room while the child falls to sleep but should avoid lengthy discussion of the child's fears. Once the child is able to get to sleep without fear, the parent begins to move their chair closer to the child's door and eventually outside the bedroom. Fearful children who do not respond to this technique should be considered for referral for more intensive treatment similar to that applied toward phobias.

Night Waking

Most children wake up in the night but are able to get back to sleep without arousing their parents. The exceptions can have a serious impact on the entire family, as previously noted. As with sleep refusal, a sleep diary can help, and parent education regarding good sleep hygiene is beneficial. However, two common problems deserve particular attention: night terrors and nightmares (Table 24-1).

Night terrors come about as a sudden partial arousal from the deepest non-REM sleep. Essentially, part of the brain snaps into wakefulness, but part remains soundly asleep. Because deep non-REM sleep predominates in the first four hours of sleep, night terrors usually happen during the early part of the night. The child bolts upright in bed, screaming, sweating, tachycardic, and tachypneic. The episodes usually last only a few minutes, ending as abruptly as they began, with the child falling back to sleep quickly unless fully awakened by the parents. Not fully awake, these children do not respond to the parents' efforts to comfort them. The child appears disoriented and confused, often with a blank stare, and has no recall of the event the next morning. Night terrors

Table 24-1 Diagnostic Features of Night Terrors vs. Nightmares

Feature	Night Terrors	Nightmares
Time of night	Early; usually within 4 hours of bedtime	Late
State on waking	Disoriented or confused	Upset or scared
Response to parents	Unaware of presence; not consolable	Comforted
Memory of event	None, unless fully awakened	Vivid recall of dream
Return to sleep	Usually rapid, unless fully awakened	Often delayed by fear
Sleep stage	Partial arousal from deep non-REM sleep	REM sleep

From Blum NJ, Carey WB. Sleep problems among infants and young children. Pediatr Rev 1996; 17(3):87-92.
REM, Rapid eye movement.

usually occur in children ages 2 to 6 years and are more common during times of illness, stress, or sleep deprivation. A nocturnal seizure should be considered in the differential diagnosis if the events are more likely right at sleep onset or if there is a personal or family history of seizures (Dahl, 1998).

Nightmares, on the other hand, are frightening dreams that awaken the child from REM sleep. Therefore, they tend to occur during the second half of the night, leaving the child upset or scared with a vivid recall of the dream. The child responds to comforting efforts by the parent but may be slow to go back to sleep because of fear. As with night terrors, nightmares occur most often during the toddler to preschool years and are more common during stressful times.

Management

In general, sedative medications are not indicated for night waking. Instead, behavior management techniques similar to those outlined for sleep refusal are appropriate for most cases.

There is no specific treatment for night terrors. Parents should be reassured with the explanation that the problem is common and self-limited. They should not try to wake the child up because this may only frighten the child or slow the child's return to sleep. For children who thrash violently, the parent should take precautions to provide protection for them. If the child sleepwalks into potentially dangerous situations, the parents can hang a bell or electronic movement alarm on the child's bedroom door to warn them. Because overtiredness is a major factor in the tendency to have night terrors, increasing the total amount of sleep and keeping a consistent sleep-wake cycle should be emphasized.

Because nightmares tend to occur at times of emotional stress, the focus of treatment should be on assisting parents with effective ways to manage the underlying stress. When a nightmare has occurred, the child is awake and frightened. The parent should comfort the child *without* a detailed review of the nightmare contents or "flashlight searches for monsters" (Blum and Carey, 1996) which can further increase the child's fears.

Obstructive Sleep Apnea Syndrome

Habitual snoring occurs in 3% to 12% of preschool-age children. The childhood incidence of obstructive sleep apnea syndrome (OSAS) is estimated to be 2%. The American Academy of Pediatrics has published an evidence-based guideline for the diagnosis and management of OSAS (AAP, 2002).

In children, OSAS is most often associated with large adenoids and/or tonsils, as well as specific facial features such as micrognathia, macroglossia, and Down syndrome. Unlike adults with sleep apnea, children can be affected without large drops in blood oxygen levels, because children can have frequent brief awakenings to quickly reestablish their airway. Thus, the primary clinical issue may be sleep fragmentation. In the context of a child with snoring and restless sleep, OSAS should be considered any time there are symptoms or signs suggesting sleep deprivation, such as difficulty paying attention, emotional lability, partial arousals during the night (night terrors, sleepwalking), or difficulty waking up in the morning (Dahl, 1998).

Because only a portion of children with snoring and adenotonsillar hypertrophy have OSAS, a sleep study is recommended to avoid unnecessary surgery. A caution, however, is that sleep studies in children require special expertise that may not be available at an adult sleep center.

Treatment of a child with OSAS on the basis of adenotonsillar hypertrophy is surgery. Continuous positive airway pressure (CPAP) is effective in children but is reserved for when adenotonsillectomy is contraindicated or unsuccessful (AAP, 2002) (SOR: A).

Sleep Deprivation and Delayed Sleep-Phase Syndrome

Sleep deprivation and delayed sleep-phase syndrome are common problems in adolescents for several reasons. The total sleep requirement is as much or more in adolescence as in pre-adolescence (Carskadon and Roth, 2000), but adolescents tend to receive less sleep for both biologic and cultural reasons. School-age children are more likely to be "larks," preferring to wake up early even if they are up late at night. At puberty, a circadian rhythm change occurs that results in a switch from larks to "owls," the preference for a late-night bedtime and late-morning awakening. This biologic tendency is encouraged by the availability of stimulating activities late into the night, whether social events, part-time jobs, or technologic advances (e.g., TV, Internet). Stimulants such as caffeine and tobacco also act to delay sleep. Despite these factors that act to delay sleep, school schedules often require the adolescent to awaken early. Thus, sleep deprivation develops. Also, jet lag–like shifts often develop between the weekday and weekend or holiday schedule. These schedule shifts probably play a role in the most common adolescent sleep problem, delayed sleep-phase syndrome (Dahl, 1998).

The assessment is by history. The main differential diagnosis to consider from delayed sleep-phase syndrome is the teenager who is choosing a late-night schedule for some secondary gain. This person is not distressed by the dysfunctional sleep pattern and is unmotivated to change it. Therefore, the adolescent with secondary gain requires treatment directed at the underlying school or family issues rather than the sleep disturbance.

Treatment of the cooperative adolescent involves attempting a schedule shift and consistently maintaining it. Those with marked difficulty initiating timely sleep may respond to staying awake through an entire night, then reestablishing a regular schedule. Mindell and Owens (2009) provide a practical clinical guide for pediatric sleep.

Narcolepsy

Although rare, narcolepsy is an important cause of daytime sleepiness because it can affect personal safety and school performance but is readily treatable. Normally, REM sleep only occurs when a person has been asleep for 60 to 90 minutes and follows all four stages of non-REM sleep. Narcoleptic patients, on the other hand, experience sudden episodes of REM sleep in the middle of a wakeful state or immediately after falling asleep.

The key feature of narcolepsy is recurrent *sleep attacks:* sudden, unintentional, irresistible bouts of sleep that occur in inappropriate situations, such as during conversations or while driving. Other common findings include *cataplexy* (sudden bilateral loss of muscle tone without loss of consciousness), *hypnagogic hallucinations* (vivid dreamlike imagery just before falling asleep), and *sleep paralysis* (inability to move or speak just after morning awakening). Any child or adolescent with unexplained daytime sleepiness who does not respond to initial management with good sleep hygiene, or who has a family history of narcolepsy, should be considered for evaluation. A sleep study is required to make the diagnosis.

Narcolepsy treatment combines behavioral approaches with medications. The patient should adhere to good sleep hygiene. Therapeutic naps enhance daytime alertness and reduce the necessary dose of stimulants. Stimulant medications, such as methylphenidate, dextroamphetamine, or modafinil are very helpful for daytime sleepiness (Vgontzas and Kale, 1999) (SOR: A). The antidepressants are REM suppressants that help prevent cataplexy or hypnagogic hallucinations. The nonsedating antidepressants, especially the selective serotonin reuptake inhibitors (SSRIs), work synergistically when combined with stimulants (Vgontzas and Kale, 1999) (SOR: B).

Autism

Key Points

- Autistic disorder has onset before age 3 years and is characterized by impaired social interaction, impaired communication, and repetitive, stereotyped patterns of behavior.
- Autism is *not* caused by thimerosal-containing vaccines.
- Standard developmental screening tests have poor sensitivity for autism.
- Early intervention with a multidisciplinary approach improves autism outcomes.

The term *autism* refers to a spectrum of pervasive developmental disorders characterized by various degrees of impaired social interaction and communication and repetitive, stereotyped patterns of behavior. Patients may have relatively good skills in one area and very poor skills in others. The specific diagnosis of "autistic disorder" has an onset before 3 years of age and requires the presence of impairments in all three categories, whereas "Asperger's disorder" includes impaired social interaction and autistic behaviors but excludes language delay. The incidence of autistic disorder is 5 to 20 per 10,000 persons, with a much higher occurrence among siblings of affected patients (3%-7%) (Schaefer and Mendelsohn, 2008). Mental retardation, typically in the moderate range (IQ 35-50), accompanies the disorder in 75% of affected children (DSM-IV-TR, 2000).

Evidence is mounting that both genetic and environmental factors influence the etiology of autism (Kolevzon 2007; Schaefer and Mendelsohn, 2008). Assertions that autism is caused by thimerosal-containing vaccines have been discounted by a comprehensive meta-analysis (Parker et al., 2004) (SOR: A).

Assessment

Developmental screening should be part of each well-child examination. The Denver Developmental Screening tools have often been used for this purpose but they lack sensitivity and specificity for autism. The AAP provides a thorough examination of screening instruments for autism (Johnson and Myers, 2007). A variety of screening tools aimed specifically at autism are available but also lack sensitivity (Bryson et al., 2003). Therefore, physicians should take parental concerns about delayed speech and language development seriously, especially beyond 18 months of age, even in the context of normal screening. In addition to delayed speech development, the other common presenting symptom is *challenging behavior*. The behaviors may include a violent reaction to minor changes in the environment or routine, stereotypic movements such as clapping or rocking, and preoccupation with narrow interests or inanimate objects.

When autism is suspected, a thorough evaluation should be performed, including appropriate intellectual testing, speech-language assessment, Autism Diagnostic Interview–Revised (ADI-R) (Western Psychological Services [WPS], 2003) and the Autism Diagnostic Observation Schedule (ADOS) (WPS, 2001). Because hearing loss can mimic autism, the evaluation should also include formal audiologic testing. Common comorbidities include anxiety, depression, and obsessional behavior (Prater and Zylstra, 2002). Many autistic patients develop *infantile spasms* in the first year of life, a severe seizure disorder.

Management

Early intervention is important because the younger children are treated, the better the outcome. The most successful programs utilize a multidisciplinary approach that includes behavior modification, development of social communication, active involvement of parents and families, and use of psychotropic medications for dangerous behaviors that do not respond to behavior modification (Myers et al., 2007). Referral to an established program is recommended. Despite anecdotal reports of efficacy of alternative and complementary treatments, none of these has shown benefit in clinically controlled trials. Less than 5% of autistic people become self-sufficient adults, although one-third achieve some degree of independent living (Prater and Zylstra, 2002). Clear gain in language is the most important predictor of adult outcomes (Bryson et al., 2003)

KEY TREATMENT

Comprehensive treatments that address both the autistic child and the child's parents are "possibly efficacious" per meta-analysis (Rogers and Vismara, 2008) (SOR: B).
Risperidone effectively treats irritability, repetition, and social withdrawal in autism, with weight gain as the most prominent side effect (Jesner et al., 2007) (SOR: A).

Encopresis and Enuresis

See the discussion online at www.expertconsult.com.

Attention-Deficit/Hyperactivity Disorder

Key Points

- Consider ADHD in a child presenting with hyperactivity, impulsivity, inattentiveness, academic underachievement, or behavior problems.
- Use the DSM-IV-TR diagnostic criteria when assessing for ADHD.
- Obtain information from the parents, child, and teacher, using standardized behavior reports, if possible.
- When planning treatment, recognize that ADHD is a chronic condition for which medication only temporarily decreases symptoms and improves functioning.
- Stimulants are the first and second lines of medication treatment.

Attention-deficit/hyperactivity disorder (ADHD) is the most frequently diagnosed behavioral disorder of childhood, with a prevalence of 4% to 12% (DSM-IV-TR, 2000). At least 10% of behavior problems seen in a general pediatric practice are caused by ADHD. Boys are seen more frequently than girls. ADHD should be considered and assessed in a child who presents with inattention, hyperactivity, impulsivity, academic underachievement, or behavior problems (AAP, 2000; AHCPR, 1999). ADHD is a chronic disorder persisting from childhood into adolescence and adulthood. In general, symptoms decrease by half every 5 years between ages 10 and 25 (Goldman et al., 1998). Obvious hyperactivity disappears while inattention persists.

Research suggests that ADHD has a central nervous system (CNS) basis; however, no specific etiology has been discovered. Family genetic studies have shown up to 92% concordance in monozygotic twins and 33% concordance in dizygotic twins. Clinicians should keep in mind that the child's parents may also have ADHD. Various brain imaging studies of ADHD patients have demonstrated abnormalities of brain metabolism, supporting the validity of ADHD as a disorder. However, the strongest evidence of validity has been course prediction and treatment response to medication.

Box 24-2 DSM-IV-TR Diagnostic Criteria For Attention-Deficit/Hyperactivity Disorder

A. Either (1) or (2)

1. Inattention: six (or more) of the following symptoms of inattention have persisted for at least 6 months to a degree that is maladaptive and inconsistent with developmental level:
   (a) Often fails to give close attention to details or makes careless mistakes in schoolwork, work, or other activities
   (b) Often has difficulty sustaining attention in tasks or play activities
   (c) Often does not seem to listen to what is being spoken to directly
   (d) Often does not follow through on instructions and fails to finish schoolwork, chores, or duties in the workplace (not due to oppositional behavior or failure to understand instructions)
   (e) Often has difficulties organizing tasks and activities
   (f) Often avoids, strongly dislikes or is reluctant to engage in tasks (such as schoolwork or homework) that require sustained mental effort
   (g) Often loses things necessary for tasks or activities (e.g., school assignments, pencils, books, tools, or toys)
   (h) Is often easily distracted by extraneous stimuli
   (i) Often forgetful in daily activities
2. Hyperactivity-impulsivity: six (or more) of the following symptoms of hyperactivity-impulsivity have persisted for at least 6 months to a degree that is maladaptive and inconsistent with developmental level:

   Hyperactivity
   (a) Often fidgets with hands or feet or squirms in seat
   (b) Often leaves seat in classroom or in other situations in which remaining seated is expected
   (c) Often runs about or climbs excessively in situations where it is inappropriate (in adolescents or adults, may be limited to subjective feelings of restlessness)
   (d) Often has difficulty playing or engaging in leisure activities quietly
   (e) Is often "on the go" or often acts as if "driven by a motor"
   (f) Often talks excessively

   Impulsivity
   (g) Often blurts out answers to questions before the question has been completed
   (h) Often has difficulty awaiting turn
   (i) Often interrupts or intrudes on others (e.g., butts into conversations or games)
B. Some hyperactive-impulsive or inattentive symptoms that caused impairment were present before seven years of age.
C. Some impairment from the symptoms is present in two or more settings (e.g., at school [or work], and at home).
D. There must be clear evidence of clinically significant impairment in social, academic, or occupational functioning.
E. The symptoms do not occur exclusively during the course of a pervasive developmental disorder, schizophrenia or other psychotic disorder, and are not better accounted for by a mood disorder, anxiety disorder, dissociative disorder, or a personality disorder.

From American Psychiatric Association. Diagnostic and Statistical Manual of Mental Disorders, 4th ed, Text Revision (DSM-IV-TR). Washington, DC, American Psychiatric Association, 2000.

Comorbidity is common in ADHD; 65% of children diagnosed with ADHD have more than one psychiatric diagnosis (Biederman et al., 1991), including about 30% with more than one comorbid condition. Of children diagnosed with ADHD, 35% also have oppositional defiant disorder; 25% have conduct disorder; 18% have a depressive disorder; 25% have an anxiety disorder; and 12% to 60% have a learning disorder (AHCPR, 1999).

Assessment

There is no independent valid test to determine that a child has ADHD. The diagnosis can only be obtained reliably by using well-established diagnostic assessment methods. This involves using the standardized diagnostic criteria of the American Psychiatric Association's *Diagnostic and Statistical Manual of Mental Disorders* (DSM-IV-TR; Box 24-2), rather than the clinical description of the World Health Organization's *International Classification of Diseases* (ICD-9) (AHCPR, 1999). Unfortunately, only 30% of family physicians routinely use the DSM criteria (Rushton et al., 2004). This must be part of a comprehensive diagnostic evaluation that involves obtaining information from the parents, child, and teacher. The baseline assessment of target ADHD symptoms can be assisted by using standardized behavior reports, such as the Conners Rating Scales (1997 revision), NICHQ Vanderbilt forms, or the SNAP checklist. Broadband behavioral rating scales, such as the Child Behavior Check List (CBCL, Achenbach), do not effectively discriminate between ADHD and non-ADHD children but do assist in identifying comorbid disorders (AAP, 2000). Because of the significant prevalence of comorbid psychiatric disorders, the assessment should include inquiring about these conditions (AHCPR, 1999). In addition to psychiatric symptoms, the ability of the child to function normally in different domains must also be assessed. These domains include family relationships with adults, sibling relationships, peer social relationships, community behavior, school academic performance, school behavior, interests and play activities, and subjective psychological distress.

The physician should conduct a medical screening examination, including hearing and vision tests, if this has not already been done. Other diagnostic tests, including laboratory screening tests for lead intoxication, abnormal thyroid function, neuroimaging for brain tumor, or seizure disorder, should be conducted when indicated by the history and physical examination (AHCPR, 1999). Computerized continuous performance tests should not be used as a clinical screening or diagnostic tool for ADHD.

Management

The clinician should establish a comprehensive management program that recognizes ADHD as a chronic condition and works with the parents, child, and teachers to identify the most important problems as targets of treatment (AHCPR, 1999). Indications for referral to a specialist include (1) children with ADHD plus a comorbid psychiatric disorder and (2) children with ADHD who do not respond to initial treatment. More specific guidance in assessment and management may be obtained by consulting practice guidelines or parameters (AAP, 2000; McDonagh et al., 2009;

Pliszka et al., 2007) and health care guidelines (Moore, 2007; O'Brien, 2005). An initial effort must be made to educate the parents and child about ADHD (see Web Resources).

Psychosocial Therapy

The physician or staff should review techniques of parent behavioral management to assess how well they are understood and effectively implemented. This includes the proper use of positive reinforcers and punishment. A structured and standardized system, called the "token economy," can be very effective but requires considerable time and effort by the parents. Common mistakes made by parents include too much punishment versus positive reinforcement, too long a delay in receiving a reward, making the system too difficult initially so that the child never achieves success, inconsistent implementation, and poor supervision.

Assessing for proper educational placement is important. At a minimum, the parents should consult with the child's classroom teacher and confirm close supervision of the child, a structured classroom, good behavioral management, and good communication with parents. If this effort is not sufficient, the parents can request educational accommodations under Section 504 of the 1973 Rehabilitation Act. This federal law provides for special accommodations and services in a person with a chronic handicapping condition, including psychiatric disorder. The request must be accompanied by a physician statement documenting the handicapping condition and directed to the building principal or school district "Section 504 compliance officer." If this is not enough and the child is failing in one or more subjects, the parents can request a comprehensive evaluation by the Child Study Team for possible Special Education placement ("Other Health Impaired" eligibility condition—Federal Public Law 94-142, currently the Individuals with Disabilities Education Act, IDEA). The request should be in writing and directed to the building principal. The evaluation may take up to 85 school days but could result in an *individualized education program* (IEP), a description and contract of what special services the school will provide.

For children with ADHD alone, other psychosocial treatments have not been shown to be more effective than aggressive use of stimulant medication, or even to provide an additional benefit (MTA Cooperative Group, 1999). However, psychosocial treatments are beneficial in children with ADHD and other comorbid disorders or those from families with chaotic functioning.

Pharmacotherapy

The stimulants are the medications of first choice at any age (AHCPR, 1999); they do not have a paradoxical reverse effect at puberty. Methylphenidate was also shown to be beneficial for very young children with ADHD through the National Institutes of Mental Health (NIMH) Preschoolers with ADHD Treatment Study (PATS); however, the benefit was not as robust as in older children, and adverse effects were more prominent (Abikoff et al., 2007; Gleason et al., 2007). Table 24-2 provides measures for successful stimulant administration, and Table 24-3 lists specific dosing recommendations. Of ADHD children, 70% show significant

Table 24-2 Keys to Successful Pediatric Stimulant Administration

Recommendation	Comment
Be aggressive with titration of medication.	Increase dose until benefit clearly seen or side effects prevent further dose increases.
Frequency of doses: cover the day as much as possible and normalize functioning as much as possible.	Give doses at breakfast, lunch, and after school, depending on duration of benefit of the specific stimulant.
Monitor closely the beneficial and adverse effects of medication.	Obtain information from both parents and teachers. Use standardized behavior report.*
See patients at least every 3 months for maintenance treatment.	Try to head off problems before they develop into serious ones.
Consider annual discontinuation of medication to see if it is still needed.	However, this is unnecessary if parents still see a clear worsening when medication wears off.

*For example, NICHQ Vanderbilt Assessment Follow-up forms.

improvement on the first trial of a stimulant, and 85% to 90% improve significantly taking at least one of the listed stimulants. When the medication is in effect, motor activity decreases, certain cognitive processes improve, motivation improves, academic performance improves, and oppositional and aggressive behaviors decrease. However, the medication works only for as long as it is given, with no long-lasting or curative effect.

The physician should use a systematic approach. If the first stimulant is not effective after an adequate trial of maximum doses, a sequential trial of each available stimulant is appropriate before moving to another class of medication. At a minimum, at least one methylphenidate preparation and one amphetamine preparation should be tried. Follow-up appointments should be regular and scheduled and should include information from the parents, teachers, and child (AHCPR, 1999). Adverse effects are similar for all stimulants and can affect up to 20% of children. Important side effects include anorexia, weight loss, irritability (more likely in younger children), abdominal pain, insomnia (only if given after 5 PM), dysphoria (more likely in younger children), "behavioral rebound" after wearing off, impaired cognitive performance on laboratory tests (methylphenidate at single doses >1 mg/kg), tachycardia, and increased tic symptoms (if patient has tic disorder). In general, growth suppression is not a concern, except in children with dramatic anorexia. There is no evidence that the legitimate prescribed use of stimulants by ADHD children and adolescents lead to future drug abuse, and proper use may actually have a protective effect. Sudden death in children taking stimulant medication was recently a concern (Gould 2009). The U.S. Food and Drug Administration (FDA) issued a 2009 communication recommending caution but not stopping the use of stimulants for ADHD. A more definitive study involving 500,000 stimulant medication users is expected soon.

Table 24-3 Stimulant Medications Used in Treatment of Attention-Deficit/Hyperactivity Disorder (ADHD)

Drug	Brand Name	Dosage Forms	Duration of Behavioral Effects	Suggested Dosage
Methylphenidate	Ritalin regular Methylin	5-, 10-, 20- mg tablet Methylin also in chewable tablet and solution	1-4 hours	0.6-2.0 mg/kg/day in divided doses FDA approved for use in children age ≥6 years PDR: 60 mg max dose
	Ritalin SR	20-mg tablet	3-9 hours	Titrate quickly up to 0.5 mg/kg in a single dose. Observe for benefit and titrate to max dose if necessary.
	Methylin ER	10-, 20-mg tablet	—	—
	Ritalin LA	10-, 20-, 30-, 40- mg tablet	10-12 hours	—
	Metadate ER	10-, 20-mg tablet	—	
	Metadate CD	10-, 20-, 30-, 40-, 50-, 60-mg capsule	8-12 hours	—
	Concerta	18-, 27-, 36-, 54-mg tablet	12 hours	Child: up to 54 mg daily Adolescent and adult: 72 mg daily
	Daytrana skin patch	10-, 15-, 20-, 30-mg patch	9 hours while patch applied	—
Dexmethyl-phenidate	Focalin	2.5-, 5-, 10-mg tablet	—	0.3-1.0 mg/kg/day
	Focalin XR	5-, 10-, 15-, 20-, 30-mg capsule	—	PDR: 30 mg max daily dose
Amphetamine salts	Adderall	5-, 7.5-, 10-, 12.5-, 15-, 20-, 30-mg scored tablet	6-8 hours	0.3-1.0 mg/kg/day
	Adderall XR	5-, 10-, 1-, 20-, 25-, 30-mg capsule	10-12 hours	PDR: Max daily dose — child: 30 mg; adolescent/adult: 40 mg
Dextro-amphetamine	Dexedrine	5-mg tablet	1-8 hours	0.3-1.0 mg/kg/day FDA approved for use in children age ≥3 years
	Dexedrine SR	5-, 10-, 15-mg Spansule	8-9 hours	PDR: 40 mg max dose
Lisdexamfetamine	Vyvanse	20-, 30-, 40-, 50-, 60-, 70-mg capsule	—	Up to 70 mg daily
Methamphetamine	Desoxyn	5-mg tablet	—	0.3-1.0 mg/kg/day, typically 20-25 mg daily
		CR tablets are no longer available.	—	Up to 40 mg in morning

FDA, U.S. Food and Drug Administration; *PDR*, *Physicians' Desk Reference; CR*, controlled-release.

The third line of treatment (after two trials of stimulants) is atomoxetine, which has an FDA indication for the treatment of ADHD. It is initially given at 0.5 mg/kg/day, either in the early morning or as a divided dose (morning and late afternoon). It is titrated up to a maximum dose of 1.4 mg/kg/day (or 100 mg maximum). The full benefit may not be seen for 4 weeks (ICSI, 2005). Common adverse effects include nausea, vomiting, gastrointestinal pain, anorexia, headache, fatigue, and sleepiness. Atomoxetine is not a U.S. Drug Enforcement Administration (DEA) scheduled medication, has no potential for abuse, and therefore can be written with refills.

Bupropion, tricyclic antidepressants (TCAs, e.g., imipramine, nortriptyline), and the alpha-adrenergic agent clonidine do not have an official FDA indication for the treatment of ADHD. The evidence for their benefit is based on randomized controlled trials (RCTs) and nonrandomized trials with controls (ICSI, 2007). Two alpha agents, guanfacine and clonidine, in extended-release forms, have received FDA approval for treatment of ADHD. Further information can be found by referring to the Texas Children's Medication Algorithm Project (most recent algorithms, May 2006; see Web Resources), developed by expert consensus (Pliszka 2000). Atypical antipsychotic medication (i.e., risperidone), mood stabilizers (lithium,

KEY TREATMENT

The stimulants are the medications of first choice for ADHD at any age (AHCPR, 1999) (SOR: A)

Although not a first-line drug, atomoxetine is effective for treatment of ADHD (Hammerness et al., 2009) (SOR: A).

Behavioral treatments for children with ADHD are effective adjuncts to pharmacologic therapy (Fabiano et al., 2009) (SOR: A).

valproic acid), or clonidine can be used in children with comorbid severe aggression or suspected bipolar disorder after an adequate trial of a standard ADHD medication (Barzman and Sorter, 2009).

Oppositional Defiant Disorder

Key Points

- The provider must establish a therapeutic alliance with both the child and the family to be successful in treating oppositional defiant disorder.
- The diagnosis of ODD is based on reports from the parents and child; carefully consider the possibility of comorbid conditions.
- The best treatment of ODD usually is parent training in behavior management techniques.
- Medication may be helpful in treating the symptoms of comorbid conditions.

The prevalence of oppositional defiant disorder (ODD) in children under 18 years old is widely reported as 2% to 16%. Before puberty, males outnumber females, but after puberty the rates are more equal. The disorder is usually evident by 8 years of age (APA, 2000). ODD is a chronic persistent disorder; however, approximately 67% of childhood cases have resolved 3 years later. About 30% of children with early-onset ODD develop conduct disorder (Connor et al., 2002).

The characteristics predisposing to ODD are biologic, social, and psychological, involving the parents and child. The parents usually employ poor, ineffective, inconsistent, and indiscriminate behavioral management methods, which are often combined with unusually harsh but inconsistent discipline and poor monitoring of activities. These children are usually temperamental, impulsive, active, and inattentive. The parents themselves are frequently immature, temperamental, and impulsive. The family members usually experience significant marital, financial, health, and personal distress (Barkley, 1997).

Assessment

There are two periods of developmentally normal oppositional behavior: the "terrible twos," between 18 and 24 months of age, when the toddler behaves negatively as an expression of developing autonomy, and sometimes in adolescence, when the teenager is trying to separate from the parents and establish an autonomous identity. Unlike ODD, these stages usually last less than 6 months (see **eBox 24-1**).

A child with ODD reported by the parents may not show much oppositional behavior while being examined in the office. The symptoms of ODD that these children display are much more evident in interactions with people and situations that they know well. The child takes a self-defeating position in arguments with adults. The struggle becomes more important than the reality of the situation, such that the child may be willing to risk losing the object or activity rather than lose the argument. Even a significant delay by the child in complying with a parental request is seen as a victory by the child. The assessment of ODD should include direct information from the child and parents regarding symptoms, age of onset, duration, and degree of functional impairment.

If oppositional behavior is confined mostly to school and not much at home (except as it relates to schoolwork), additional diagnoses must be considered in the differential, including mental retardation, borderline intellectual functioning, a specific developmental disorder (e.g., learning disability), and most often, ADHD. No specific laboratory tests or pathologic findings can assist the clinician in making the specific diagnosis of ODD.

Management

With methodologically sound RCTs lacking and recommendations based on clinical consensus, the appropriate psychosocial interventions for ODD include parenting training in behavior management techniques: improved parent/child relationship, positive reinforcement, closer supervision, giving more effective commands, time-out, and token economies. Despite the usually chaotic family situation and high emotions involved, the family physician needs to establish a therapeutic alliance with both the child and the family to have the best chance of success (Steiner and Remsing, 2006). Interventions should be family based, targeted to specific concerns, and oriented to problem solving. Traditional individual psychotherapy, unstructured/nondirected family therapy, or short-term treatment is usually not helpful. Psychoactive medications are used to treat comorbid conditions and targeted symptoms but have not demonstrated benefit for ODD alone. Intense and prolonged treatment may be necessary for severe and persistent ODD. One-time crisis interventions (e.g., "scared straight" attempts) are not effective.

Conduct Disorder

Key Points

- Poorer prognosis for conduct disorder is associated with earlier age at onset, lower IQ, more conduct symptoms, greater frequency, and severity of symptoms.
- Suspect alcohol and drug use in a teenager with conduct disorder.
- Talking to the CD adolescent is not sufficient; collateral sources of information (parents, teachers, courts) are essential.
- Diligently search for another, more treatable condition, if it exists, because CD does not have effective treatment.
- Involvement by the juvenile court or placement outside the home may be the best option for some patients.

The prevalence of conduct disorder (CD) in children under 18 years old is 6% to 16% in males and 2% to 9% in females. At all ages, boys outnumber girls. Males usually exhibit more aggression, whereas females usually commit more covert crimes and prostitution. CD is more common in urban than rural settings and is one of the most frequent diagnoses in outpatient and inpatient psychiatric facilities for children. The mortality rate for seriously disturbed delinquents is 50 times higher than for normal youths. Adolescents with CD are more likely to die by homicide, suicide, violent accident, or drug overdose.

Generally, the natural history of children with severe CD is marked by the development of ADHD at a very early age, followed by ODD, then finally the onset of CD. In adolescence, alcohol and substance abuse occur. The factors that determine a poorer prognosis in the patient with CD are an early age of onset of symptoms, greater number of symptoms, and greater frequency of expression of these CD symptoms. The factors that determine a better prognosis are minimum number of CD symptoms, absence of comorbid psychiatric diagnoses, and normal intellectual functioning. Characteristics more common in childhood-onset versus adolescent-onset CD are greater frequency of neuropsychiatric disorders, lower IQ, higher levels of aggression, male gender, and greater frequency of externalizing behavior disorders in other family members. From 25% to 40% of children with CD go on to develop *antisocial personality disorder*, a chronic pattern of lawlessness.

Current views posit an interaction among genetic, biologic, and environmental factors (i.e., parental, sociocultural, psychological, prolonged abuse). No single factor accounts for more than 50% of the variance in the occurrence of CD, and no combination of factors accounts for more than 70% of the variance. Many children with risk factors do not develop CD.

Assessment

The diagnostic criteria for CD are summarized in **eBox 24-2**. The clinician should not quickly accept the diagnosis of CD in a youth, because no specific effective treatment exists, and instead should diligently search for other, more treatable psychiatric conditions. Other psychiatric diagnoses that should be considered as the primary disturbance in a child presenting with CD symptoms include ADHD, ODD, intermittent explosive disorder, psychoactive substance use disorder, mood disorders (bipolar and depressive disorders), posttraumatic stress disorder (PTSD), dissociative disorder, borderline personality disorder, and adjustment disorder with disturbance of conduct. A manic episode must be seriously considered in a teenager presenting with frequent lying, physical aggression against others, impulsive sexual activity, stealing, sneaking out in the middle of the night, grandiosity, and persistent pervasive irritability.

The interview of an adolescent with CD is not sufficient, in itself, for the psychiatric evaluation. Lying is a common problem for these teenagers, as is conscious and unconscious underreporting of their problem behaviors. Other sources of information, including parents, teachers, other professionals, past records, and court personnel, are essential to obtain a valid evaluation. Complications seen in association with CD symptoms include impairment in school performance, poor social and family relationships, problems with the legal system, poor work performance, physical injuries from fighting or carelessness, sexually transmitted diseases, teenage pregnancy, drug problems, suicide, and homicide. Common examples of interpersonal impairment in these children include suspiciousness or paranoia, misperception of others' actions as hostile, difficulty relating to peers and adults, lack of guilt, and lack of empathy.

Children with CD respond differently to punishment than normal children. The frequency of negative behavior of normal children decreases when they are punished, whereas the negative behavior of children with CD increases when they are punished.

There are no specific laboratory tests that assist in making the diagnosis of CD. However, the differential diagnosis for CD symptoms includes conditions for which tests may be important. These include head trauma, seizure disorder, birth injury to the brain, and encephalitis.

Management

One-time interventions affecting a single domain will be ineffective in treating CD. Interventions need to target all affected domains in a naturalistic setting for a long period in a consistent manner. Family interventions (parenting training/guidance, functional family therapy) and social skill training with a behavioral approach seem to be the most effective treatments for the CD patient (Dillon et al., 2007, Steiner, 1997). The focus should be on the child and the family. Individual therapy that focuses on problem-solving skills can also be useful. An environment with consistent rules and consequences is helpful. Proper school placement using behavioral techniques to encourage prosocial behavior and discourage antisocial incidents is appropriate.

Factors that can cause a cognitive-behavioral treatment program to fail include the following: the situation is "too hot to handle"; the youth is "too brittle"; the parents covertly support the youth's behavior; the parents have given up on the youth; the parents are inconsistent and are unable to supervise adequately; the program is poorly designed; rewards are too costly; or the parents have little social support. Factors that can interfere with limit setting of the child or adolescent at home include parental conflict, parental absence, parental psychiatric illness, inconsistent discipline, and vague or minimal expectations regarding appropriate behavior.

Several legal options are available if parents are unable to control their children. Most state laws have a special status that can be petitioned by the county district attorney to the juvenile court judge (i.e., Child/Person in Need of Care laws), that can allow the court to supervise the child by having hearings, placing a child on probation, mandating treatment and monitoring, or eventually taking the child away from the parents and placing the child in a residential treatment facility. However, some dangers must be kept in mind when teenagers with CD are confined to a juvenile detention facility. These patients prefer to be unrestricted and active; they can become depressed and at risk for impulsively attempting suicide when placed in confinement. Inpatient psychiatric hospitalization can be used to assess and initiate treatment for comorbid psychiatric disorders. A homicidal or suicidal patient can be stabilized and then moved to a less restrictive long-term setting. However, the stay is usually too brief to effectively treat CD itself.

Medications used as the sole treatment for conduct disorder have not been demonstrated to be effective. Psychoactive medications are used for the treatment of concurrent psychiatric disorders and concurrent target symptoms (aggression, impulsiveness, mood instability). Some of these medications are lithium, antidepressants, carbamazepine, propranolol, stimulants, clonidine, and antipsychotics (usually haloperidol). The physician should be cautious when prescribing medication to a youth with CD. Medication can be "cheeked," sold or traded, hoarded, and taken all at once in an impulsive suicide attempt.

Eating Disorders

Key Points

- When considering a diagnosis of feeding disorder, consultation with a physician familiar with growth problems in children may be necessary because of the extensive differential diagnosis.
- Long-term mortality for anorexia nervosa is 6% to 20%, the highest rate for any psychiatric disorder.
- The most useful measure to assess for extreme weight loss in adolescents is age-adjusted BMI less than the fifth percentile.
- For anorexia nervosa, vomiting is a poor prognostic feature, as is purgative use for bulimia nervosa.
- Patients with eating disorders should be managed by a multidisciplinary team that includes a primary physician, mental health professional, and nutritionist.

The most common and most serious eating disorders, anorexia nervosa and bulimia nervosa, typically have their onset in adolescence. However, several eating problems are associated with infants and children as well.

Feeding and Eating Disorders of Infancy and Early Childhood

Feeding difficulties are common in infants and young children. Most are minor and self-limited and can be addressed through education and reassurance of caregivers. However, physicians must be alert for specific feeding and eating disorders that can lead to malnutrition or chronic toxicity from ingested substances. The most important of these are listed in DSM-IV-TR as "Feeding Disorder of Infancy or Early Childhood." The diagnosis has previously been described as "psychosocial failure to thrive" and "psychosocial dwarfism." The key feature of the diagnosis is that the child fails to gain weight appropriately over a prolonged time, which is not fully explained by a gastrointestinal, endocrinologic, or neurologic condition. Of children admitted to the hospital for failure to thrive, as many as half have a psychosocial etiology.

The other important consideration in this category is *pica*, the persistent eating of nonnutritive substances, such as hair, soil, paint, animal droppings, or sand. Pica can result in vitamin deficiencies, lead or other heavy metal intoxication, phytobezoars, and other complications. The prevalence of pica is not certain, but it is probably fairly common in preschool children, especially those with mental impairment.

The most important aspect in assessing feeding difficulties in infants and children is tracking height and weight with each office visit. Children who are not maintaining expected gains should be observed more closely, keeping in mind that a significant proportion of these children have a psychosocial basis. The diagnosis of feeding disorder is suggested by improvement in feeding and weight gain following a change in caregivers. When a diagnosis of feeding disorder is entertained, consultation with a physician familiar with growth problems in children should be considered, because the differential diagnosis for growth problems is extensive, and diagnostic implications include child abuse and neglect.

The important aspect to assessment of pica is to *ask*. Evaluation and treatment then depend on the specific substance ingested and symptoms the child exhibits, if any.

Anorexia Nervosa and Bulimia Nervosa

In adolescent girls, eating disorders are the third leading chronic illness, after obesity and asthma. The number of young people diagnosed with eating disorders (anorexia nervosa or bulimia nervosa) and eating disturbances (some but not all criteria for diagnosis of a "disorder") is increasing, the result of a combination of improved recognition and reporting, as well as an apparent true increased incidence. About 95% of cases are female, and the prevalence of eating disorders has been directly correlated to the rates of dieting behavior. High-risk groups include female athletes and diabetic patients.

An individual with anorexia nervosa refuses to maintain a minimally normal body weight, is fearful of gaining weight, and exhibits a distorted body self-image. If she is postmenarchal, she is amenorrheic. The long-term mortality rate for anorexia nervosa is 6% to 20%, the highest rate for any psychiatric disorder (Roerig et al., 2002), often as an acute suicidal act rather than slow bodily destruction alone (Pompili et al., 2006). Bulimia nervosa is characterized by binge eating and inappropriate compensation attempts to avoid weight gain, such as self-induced vomiting, misuse of laxatives or diuretics, fasting, or excessive exercise. The prevalence of bulimia nervosa is 1% to 3% in adolescent and young adult women, more common but less often fatal than anorexia nervosa (DSM-IV).

Assessment

A prime objective in assessment is to distinguish "normal dieters" from individuals with eating disorders. In addition to the characteristics outlined in Table 24-4, patients with eating disorders have a pathologic reaction to weight gain. To explore this possibility, a useful question to ask is, "What would it be like to find you weighed one pound more next week when you get on the scales?" This may provoke an overly emotional response in a person with an eating disorder (Selzer et al., 1995).

Another important aspect to evaluation is to exclude certain medical conditions in the differential diagnosis as the primary cause of the symptoms. This includes such diverse problems as inflammatory bowel disease, hyperthyroidism, chronic infections, diabetes mellitus, and Addison's disease. The erythrocyte sedimentation rate (ESR) and serum albumin tend to remain normal in patients with eating disorders,

Table 24-4 Characteristics of Normal Dieting vs. Eating Disorders

Feature	Normal dieting	Eating disorder
Communication with others	Dieters tell those around them that they are dieting, seeing it as "something to be proud of."	Dieters are reluctant to discuss their diets even when it is obvious to those around them that they are restricting their intake.
Intake regulation	They use internal cues and the rules of their diet plan.	They often use external cues, such as eating less than the person at the table who eats the least, to avoid feeling selfish or gluttonous.
Behavior	When weight loss goal achieved, they want to show off their "new body," often in new and more revealing clothes or situations (e.g., new swimsuit, sunbathing).	They usually avoid exposing their bodies, often with baggy clothing, or regard their physical dimensions with disgust, no matter how much weight they lose.
Self-esteem	They exhibit a feeling of accomplishment and increased self-esteem when they achieve planned weight loss.	They tend to become self-critical, often depressed or irritable, and avoid social occasions.

so an elevated ESR or a reduced albumin suggest an organic cause for weight loss (Selzer et al., 1995).

It is important to assess the acuteness and severity of malnutrition or fluid and electrolyte abnormalities. Indications for immediate referral include any patient with abnormal findings on physical examination or laboratory studies because these indicate severe and entrenched eating disorders. Laboratory studies should include a complete blood count, electrolytes, magnesium, calcium, phosphorus, urea nitrogen, creatinine, glucose, albumin, and electrocardiogram (Walsh et al., 2000).

Extreme weight loss is difficult to define in growing adolescents. The usual criteria of less than 85% of average body weight (ABW) and body mass index (BMI) less than 17.5 kg/m^2 used to diagnose anorexia nervosa in adults can be misleading. The most clinically useful measure is BMI percentile adjusted for age (Hebebrand et al., 1996). A reading less than the fifth percentile is considered extreme (Selzer et al., 1995). Finally, for anorexia nervosa, the presence of vomiting is a poor prognostic feature, as is the use of purgatives for bulimia nervosa (Wilhelm and Clarke, 1998).

Management

Indications for inpatient management include "extremely low weight ($\leq$75% of expected body weight) or rapid weight loss; severe electrolyte imbalances, cardiac disturbances, or other acute medical disorders; severe or intractable purging; psychosis or a high risk of suicide; and symptoms refractory to outpatient treatment" (Becker et al., 1999).

Patients with eating disorders should be managed by a multidisciplinary team that includes a primary physician, mental health professional, and nutritionist. Family physicians should be aware of the resources available in their area and should be prepared to refer any adolescent suspected of an eating disorder or with abnormal eating behaviors who does not respond to initial efforts at diet education. A valuable resource for developing a treatment plan is a practice guideline published by the American Psychiatric Association (Yager, APA Work Group, 2006).

Various antidepressants are effective for treatment of bulimia nervosa but have not shown definite benefit for anorexia nervosa. Cognitive-behavioral therapy has been shown to be the most effective psychological approach to bulimia nervosa (Berkman et al., 2006).

KEY TREATMENT

Primary prevention programs have greatly improved knowledge, but with "small net effects on reducing maladaptive eating attitudes and behaviors." Studies targeted at high-risk groups produced greater benefits. "Concerns about iatrogenic effects of including psychoeducational material on eating disorders were not supported by the data" (Fingeret et al., 2006) (SOR: A).

"Anorexia nervosa (AN): The literature regarding medication treatments for AN is sparse and inconclusive. . . . Cognitive behavioral therapy may reduce relapse risk for adults with AN after weight restoration. Family therapy focusing on parental control of renutrition is efficacious in treating AN in adolescents" (Berkman et al., 2006) (SOR: B).

"Bulimia nervosa (BN): Fluoxetine (60 mg/day) reduced core bulimia symptoms in the short term. . . . The optimal duration of treatment is unknown. Cognitive behavioral therapy is effective in both short and long term" (Berkman et al., 2006) (SOR: A).

References

The complete reference list is available online at www.expertconsult.com.

Web Resources

www.dshs.state.tx.us/mhprograms/adhdpage.shtm
Texas Children's Medication Algorithm Project; most recent algorithms May 2006.

Sleep Disorders

www.nlm.nih.gov/medlineplus/sleepdisorders.html
National Institutes of Health (NIH)–sponsored patient-oriented site with extensive background information and links to recent research and ongoing clinical trials.

www.sleepfoundation.org/
Sponsored by the National Sleep Foundation, an advocacy group; a patient-oriented site with direct answers to frequently asked questions.

www.aasmnet.org/ Sponsored by the American Academy of Sleep Medicine, a professional society, with public access to patient information and referral centers.

Autism

www.ninds.nih.gov/disorders/autism/detail_autism.htm
NIH-sponsored patient-oriented site with extensive background information and links to other valuable sites.

www.autism-society.org
Sponsored by the Autism Society of America, a national advocacy group, with good general information and networking opportunities.

Encopresis and Enuresis

www.lpch.org/diseaseHealthInfo/healthLibrary/growth/encopres.html
Sponsored by the Lucile Packard Children's Hospital at Stanford, answers patients' frequently asked questions, including diet and activity recommendations.

http://familydoctor.org/online/famdocen/home/children/parents/toilet/366.html
Sponsored by the AAFP, with general patient recommendations; less commercialized than many other sites.

Attention-Deficit/Hyperactivity Disorder

www.chadd.org/
Resources from the national support group for children and adults with ADHD.

www.nichq.org/adhd_tools.html#adhd_parent
Resources for clinicians and parents on ADHD from the National Initiative for Children's Healthcare Quality, including a number of assessment forms.

www.add.org/
Resources from the ADD Association, a national ADHD adult support group.

www.nimh.nih.gov/health/topics/attention-deficit-hyperactivity-disorder-adhd/index.shtml
Information on ADHD from the National Institutes of Mental Health, including a link to current ADHD clinical trials.

Oppositional Defiant and Conduct Disorders

www.aacap.org/cs/ODD.ResourceCenter
Resource Center on ODD by the American Academy of Child and Adolescent Psychiatry.

http://jamesdauntchandler.tripod.com/ODD_CD/oddcdpamphlet.htm
Detailed assessment and treatment information on ODD and CD from a physician; includes case examples.

www.adhd.com.au/conduct.html
Information on CD from an Australian clinic.

Eating Disorders

www.nationaleatingdisorders.org
Sponsored by the National Eating Disorders Association, an advocacy group, with general information and networking opportunities.

www.anad.org
Sponsored by the National Association of Anorexia Nervosa and Associated Eating Disorders, an advocacy group with general information and networking opportunities.

CHAPTER 25

Gynecology

Sarina B. Schrager, Heather L. Paladine, and Kara Cadwallader

Patient-Centered Approach to the Well-Woman Examination

The well-woman examination is an opportunity for the family physician to promote health, prevent disease, and strengthen the physician–female patient relationship. Although women have traditionally been advised to see their doctors for an "annual examination," which includes a Papanicolaou smear, new screening guidelines have widened the scope of the visit and deemphasized the Pap smear (which may not be needed on an annual basis). Building a trusting relationship is important because women may be more likely to volunteer sensitive problems with a physician they trust. In addition, some women may have had previous negative experiences with pelvic examinations.

Evidence-Based Screening Guidelines

Screening guidelines published by the U.S. Preventive Services Task Force (USPSTF) provide an evidence-based guide for family physicians to follow. Recommendations with A and B levels of evidence for adult women are included in Table 25-1. Unfortunately, many established components of the well-woman examination are not supported by evidence. Screening for intimate-partner violence, routine breast self-examination, testing for lipid disorders in average-age-risk women, type 2 diabetes screening, and physical activity counseling are examples of "uncertain" recommendations, according to the USPSTF. A physician may choose to cover these areas in a well-woman visit, but it is important

to ensure that the areas with stronger evidence of benefit are thoroughly discussed. USPSTF also lists areas of screening that have the potential to cause harm and therefore are not recommended. These include cervical cancer screening in women with previous hysterectomy for benign causes, screening for gonorrhea in low-risk women, and screening for ovarian cancer.

Immunizations are an important part of well-woman care. All patients benefit from disease prevention, and women are often caregivers for children or elderly persons, who are at higher risk from vaccine-preventable illnesses. Vaccines recommended by the U.S. Centers for Disease Control and Prevention (CDC) Advisory Committee on Immunization Practices (ACIP) include tetanus/diphtheria/pertussis (Tdap), herpes zoster, and influenza for adults over age 50 and human papillomavirus vaccine for women 26 and younger.

Pap Smear Guidelines

Key Points

- Pap screening should begin at age 21. Women should have Pap smears every 2 years.
- Women who have had a hysterectomy for benign disease should not have Pap smear screening.
- Women are not required to have a Pap smear before starting hormonal contraception.
- Women do not need a pap smear over age 65 if they have had normal results in the past.

Although the Pap smear is still the mainstay of cervical cancer screening, recent advances in the understanding of human papillomavirus (HPV) have revolutionized this field. HPV is the most common sexually transmitted infection (STI), with its highest prevalence among the 20- to 24-year-old age group (44.8%) (Dunne et al., 2007). Although HPV is typically spread through sexual activity, 5.2% of women in this study who reported that they had never had sex were infected with HPV. Physicians should keep in mind that some of these women may have been uncomfortable disclosing their sexual activity, even on an anonymous survey, whereas others may have had sexual contact they did not consider intercourse. Risk factors for HPV infection include lifetime number of sexual partners, age at first intercourse, smoking, and lack of condom use (Burchell et al., 2006).

Strength of recommendation taxonomy (SORT) level A recommendations for cervical cancer screening include starting Pap test screening at age 21 and repeating every 2 years. "Low-risk women" are defined as those with three consecutive normal Pap tests, no history of cervical intraepithelial neoplasia type II (CIN-II) or higher, and no immunocompromise. A screening option for women age 30 and older is to perform Pap smear and HPV testing together, with repeat Pap tests every 3 years if both are normal. The recommendations for fewer Pap tests in women under 21 and over 30 are consistent with the epidemiology of HPV. Younger women acquire HPV infections more frequently, but most will clear the infection without intervention. Older women are less likely to develop new HPV infections, and only persistent HPV is a concern for cervical cancer. Women are not required to have a Pap smear before starting hormonal contraception. Physicians can use visits when a Pap test is not needed as an opportunity to educate female patients about STIs and reproductive health, as well as perform the other, evidence-based screening recommendations previously cited (ACOG, 2003).

Abnormal Pap Smear Management

Guidelines for management of abnormal Pap tests have also been updated to reflect understanding of the epidemiology of HPV infection (Wright et al., 2007). These guidelines include recommendations for the management of special populations, such as adolescents, pregnant women, and postmenopausal women, and are available online at the American Society for Colposcopy and Cervical Pathology (ASCCP) at www.asccp.org. Most women with low-grade squamous intraepithelial lesions (LSIL), atypical squamous cells of undetermined significance (ASCUS) with positive HPV testing, and high-grade SIL (HSIL) should have colposcopy.

Abnormal Vaginal Bleeding

Table 25-1 USPSTF Level A and B Recommendations for Adult Women

Condition	Recommendation	SORT*
Alcohol misuse	Screening and behavioral counseling	B
High blood pressure	Office sphygmomanometry	A
Breast cancer	Mammogram, with or without clinical breast exam, every 1-2 years for women 40 and older	B
Pap smear	Screening at least every 3 years, starting within 3 years of sexual activity or at age 21	A
Chlamydia	Women age 24 and younger who have ever been sexually active	A
Lipid disorders	Women age 45 and older at increased risk for heart disease	A
	Women age 20-45 at increased risk for heart disease	B
Colorectal cancer	Adults age 50-75, using fecal occult blood testing, sigmoidoscopy, or colonoscopy	A
Depression	Screening in adults as part of clinical practices with systems to ensure accurate diagnosis, effective treatment, and follow-up	B
Type 2 diabetes	Adults with blood pressure >135/80 mm Hg	B
Obesity	Screening adults; behavioral and counseling interventions	B
	Routine screening of women age 65 and older	B
Osteoporosis	Screening of women age 60 and older at increased risk	B
Tobacco use	Screening adults; cessation interventions	A

US Preventive Services Task Force recommendations, available at www.ahrq.gov/clinic/uspstfix.htm.
*Strength of recommendation taxonomy (level of evidence).

Key Points

- Anovulation is common in adolescents.
- Bleeding disorders typically present as menorrhagia in adolescence.
- Anovulation is the most common cause of abnormal vaginal bleeding in reproductive-age women.
- The four most common causes of secondary amenorrhea are pregnancy, hyperprolactinemia, thyroid disorders, and iatrogenic.
- Evaluation of abnormal bleeding in women over age 35 should include an endometrial biopsy.
- Anovulatory women are at risk for endometrial hyperplasia or carcinoma from unopposed estrogen and should have regular progesterone-induced withdrawal bleeds.
- Any bleeding after menopause in a woman who is not taking hormone therapy is abnormal.
- Evaluation with an endometrial biopsy or a pelvic ultrasound can exclude endometrial cancer.

Normal menstrual bleeding is defined as regular vaginal bleeding that occurs at intervals from 21 to 35 days. A normal menstrual cycle begins with the follicular phase before ovulation and then the luteal phase after ovulation. Abnormal vaginal bleeding is a common complaint in primary care. The prevalence of some type of abnormal bleeding is 10% to 30% among women of reproductive age. The estimated annual direct and indirect costs of abnormal bleeding are $1 and $12 billion, respectively (Liu et al., 2007). Abnormal bleeding is also a common reason for women to be referred to gynecologists and is an indication for up to 25% of all gynecologic surgery (Goodman, 2000). A life cycle approach to abnormal vaginal bleeding is helpful in determining etiology and treatment options.

Adolescents

In adolescents the three most common presentations of abnormal vaginal bleeding are anovulation, menorrhagia, and amenorrhea. It is normal for menstrual cycles to be anovulatory for an average of 18 months after menarche in adolescents while the hypothalamic-pituitary axis matures. *Menorrhagia* (heavy bleeding) is quite common in adolescent patients and is most often caused by anovulation (Rimsza, 2002). In some young women, however, menorrhagia at menarche can be a sign of a bleeding disorder. Up to 24% of adolescents with menorrhagia may have an undiagnosed bleeding disorder (Strickland, 2004). Evaluation of menorrhagia in adolescents includes a complete blood count (CBC), coagulation profile, and von Willebrand's screening test if clinically indicated. Treatment of both anovulation and menorrhagia in adolescents is usually hormonal contraception for cycle control.

The most common causes of primary amenorrhea include pregnancy, chromosomal abnormalities, (e.g., Turner's or Sawyer's syndrome); hypothalamic hypogonadism; congenital absence of the uterus, cervix, or vagina; and structural abnormalities (e.g., transverse vaginal septum or imperforate hymen). Evaluation of primary amenorrhea includes a careful history, pelvic examination, pelvic ultrasound to document the presence of pelvic organs, and chromosome analysis if clinically indicated.

Reproductive-Age Women

The most common causes of abnormal bleeding in reproductive-age women are pregnancy complications, anovulatory disorders, and benign pelvic pathology. Characteristics of ovulatory cycles include regular cycle length, presence of premenstrual syndrome (PMS) symptoms, and changes in cervical mucus. In contrast, anovulatory cycles tend to be unpredictable, with varying bleeding amounts and intervals.

Abnormal bleeding in ovulatory cycles includes menorrhagia, polymenorrhea, oligomenorrhea, and intermenstrual bleeding. Menorrhagia can be associated with structural lesions (uterine leiomyomas, endometrial polyps or hyperplasia), coagulation disorder, liver failure, or chronic renal failure. *Polymenorrhea* (bleeding at short intervals) can be caused by a luteal-phase disorder (not enough progesterone is produced after ovulation to stabilize the endometrium) or a short follicular phase. *Oligomenorrhea* (infrequent bleeding) is usually caused by a prolonged follicular phase.

Intermenstrual bleeding can be caused by cervical pathology (dysplasia or infection) or an intrauterine device (IUD). Evaluation of a woman with abnormal bleeding is based on the type of bleeding (Box 25-1).

Anovulation is the most common cause of abnormal vaginal bleeding in reproductive-age women. The majority of anovulation is related to hypothalamic abnormalities or polycystic ovarian syndrome (PCOS) (Box 25-2). By definition, anovulatory cycles are unpredictable and cannot be classified by any one type of vaginal bleeding pattern. A woman may experience 14 days of heavy bleeding one month, light spotting intermittently for the next month, and then go for 3 months without a cycle. The pathologic abnormality in these cycles is a lack of ovulation, which produces an unopposed-estrogen state. The lack of progesterone

---

Box 25-1 Clinical Evaluation of Reproductive-Age Woman with Abnormal Bleeding

Ovulatory abnormal bleeding

History, physical exam, pregnancy test

Menorrhagia

Consideration of liver function tests, BUN/Cr, CBC, coagulation profile

Pelvic ultrasound to exclude uterine fibroids

Endometrial biopsy (especially if over 35) to exclude endometrial hyperplasia

Intermenstrual bleeding

Pap smear, cervical cultures

Basal body temperature chart to determine length of follicular and luteal phases

Anovulatory bleeding

History, physical exam, pregnancy test

Laboratory studies

Thyroid-stimulating hormone level

Prolactin level

CBC (if acute bleeding episode or frequent heavy bleeding)

Fasting glucose and insulin levels

Screening for eating disorder, stress, and female-athlete triad

BUN/Cr, Blood urea nitrogen/creatinine; *CBC,* complete blood count.

Box 25-2 Causes of Anovulatory Cycles

Hypothalamic

    Weight loss

    Eating disorders

    Female-athlete triad

    Chronic illness

    Stress

    Excessive exercise

Polycystic ovarian syndrome

Thyroid disorders

Hyperprolactinemia

Idiopathic chronic anovulation

Medication induced (discontinuation of hormonal contraceptives)

production resulting from no ovulation contributes to irregular endometrial growth and non-uniform bleeding. In a normal cycle, the entire endometrium sloughs off during menstruation. In an anovulatory cycle, different sections of endometrium outgrow their blood supply at different times and bleed erratically.

Treatment of women with either ovulatory bleeding or anovulatory bleeding is not necessary unless the woman wants to become pregnant, is bothered by her bleeding pattern, or has systemic symptoms from anemia. However, anovulation is an unopposed-estrogen state, and treatment with some type of progesterone is necessary to reduce the risk of endometrial hyperplasia or carcinoma. *Unopposed estrogen* is a risk factor for endometrial cancer, along with obesity, diabetes, nulliparity, and age over 35. To protect against the development of endometrial hyperplasia, a precursor to endometrial cancer, all women with chronic anovulation should have a progesterone-induced withdrawal bleed at least four times a year (Albers et al., 2004). Women may take medroxyprogesterone acetate, 10 mg daily for 10 days, and then expect a withdrawal bleed within a few days of stopping the medication.

Treatment of abnormal bleeding consists of ovulation induction if pregnancy is desired or cycle control with hormonal contraceptives if it is not. In women who are not candidates for estrogen-containing contraceptives, a monthly cycling of progesterone or continuous administration of progestin contraception (e.g., depot medroxyprogesterone acetate or levonorgestrel IUD) can also be an effective treatment. For women who do not want to take hormonal medications, some nonsteroidal anti-inflammatory drugs (NSAIDs) can decrease the amount of bleeding (Ely et al., 2006) (Box 25-3).

Another common presentation of abnormal bleeding is an *acute bleeding* episode. In this situation, a woman is most likely anovulatory. Evaluation in an acute bleeding episode should include hemoglobin (Hb) and hematocrit (Hct), assessment of volume status, and an endometrial biopsy in women over 35.

If a woman presents with heavy bleeding and exhibits any signs or symptoms of *hypovolemia*, she should be admitted to hospital and either treated with intravenous (IV) estrogen to stop the bleeding or have a surgical procedure, such as dilation and curettage (D&C). If the woman is stable and her Hb and Hct are near normal, outpatient treatment with high-dose oral contraceptives (OCs), estrogen, or progesterone may be attempted (Ely et al., 2006).

A woman may also present with *amenorrhea*. The four most common causes of secondary amenorrhea (when a woman who previously had normal menses stops having menses for at least 6 months) are pregnancy, hyperprolactinemia, thyroid disorders, and iatrogenic (from medications). Other reasons for amenorrhea include outflow obstruction (e.g., Asherman's syndrome, caused by scarring of uterus from instrumentation, or cervical stenosis) and primary ovarian failure. Evaluation of a woman with amenorrhea begins with a history and physical examination. Laboratory studies should include a pregnancy test and thyroid-stimulating hormone (TSH) and prolactin levels. The next step is an induced withdrawal bleed after administering progesterone for 10 to 14 days. If a woman has a menstrual bleed after the progesterone, outflow obstruction and low estrogen state

---

Box 25-3 Treatment Options for Abnormal Vaginal Bleeding

Pregnancy desired

Ovulation induction with clomiphene citrate.
Referral to gynecologist.

Contraception desired

Cycle control with estrogen/ progestin method, depot medroxyprogesterone acetate, or levonorgestrel intrauterine device (IUD).

Acute bleeding episode

Outpatient

Administration of high-dose oral contraceptives (OCs), up to 4 pills daily for 5 to 7 days, with subsequent continuous OC cycling for at least a month.

Administration of oral estrogen or oral progesterone to stop the bleeding acutely.

Inpatient

IV fluids, supportive care, IV estrogen therapy.
Consultation for surgical intervention.

Contraception regimen used

Estrogen/Progestin

Supportive care for first 3 months.
Assessment of adherence to OC regimen.
Add supplemental estrogen.
Change to method with higher dose of estrogen or different class of progestin.

Progestin only

Add supplemental estrogen or combination OC.
Administer NSAID to decrease bleeding.

Modified from Ely JW, Kennedy CM, Clark EC, Bowdler NC. Abnormal uterine bleeding: a management algorithm. J Am Board Fam Med 2006;19:590-602; and Schrager S. Abnormal uterine bleeding associated with hormonal contraception. Am Fam Physician 2002;65:2073-2080.
IV, Intravenous; *NSAID*, nonsteroidal anti-inflammatory drug.

(as in primary ovarian failure) are excluded as the causes of amenorrhea. If a woman does not have a withdrawal bleed after progesterone administration, a trial of estrogen supplementation for 3 weeks should be given before another course of progesterone is attempted. In this situation, if a woman has a withdrawal bleed, the diagnosis of primary ovarian failure is considered, and levels of gonadotropins (FSH, LH) should be obtained. If a woman does not have a withdrawal bleed after estrogen and progesterone administration, a hysterosalpingogram (radiograph of uterus and ovaries after dye injection) should be obtained to evaluate for outflow obstruction.

Perimenopausal Women

Abnormal bleeding in the 5 to 10 years before menopause is very common. The most common pathology is anovulation caused by declining numbers of ovarian follicles and decreasing inhibin B levels (Jain and Santoro, 2005). Perimenopausal women may also bleed from structural lesions (most often uterine fibroid tumors) or bleeding disorders. Evaluation of a perimenopausal woman with abnormal

KEY TREATMENT

Unstable women with acute heavy vaginal bleeding should be admitted to hospital for IV estrogen therapy or surgical intervention.

Treatment of abnormal bleeding includes ovulation induction if a woman desires pregnancy and hormonal cycle control if she does not.

To protect against the development of endometrial hyperplasia, a precursor to endometrial cancer, all women with chronic anovulation should have a progesterone-induced withdrawal bleed at least four times a year (Albers et al., 2004).

If hemoglobin and hematocrit are near normal, outpatient treatment with high-dose oral contraceptives, estrogen, or progesterone may be attempted (Ely et al., 2006).

SOR: C.

bleeding should include an endometrial biopsy to exclude endometrial hyperplasia or cancer. The risk of endometrial cancer increases in women who are nulliparous, diabetic, or obese (Espindola et al., 2007). Nonsmoking women in this age group can be effectively managed with hormonal contraception for cycle control. Smokers can use cyclic progestin to provide a monthly withdrawal bleed.

Postmenopausal Women

Menopause is defined as 12 months without a menstrual period. After that 12-month period, any bleeding is abnormal. A large Danish study found a 10% prevalence of postmenopausal bleeding (Astrup, 2004). Bleeding episodes decreased as the time since menopause increased. The main concern in a postmenopausal woman with bleeding is endometrial carcinoma. Between 10% and 20% of all postmenopausal bleeding will be caused by malignancy (Hale and Fraser, 2007). Evaluation of postmenopausal bleeding can be done effectively with either a pelvic ultrasound or an office endometrial biopsy. A pelvic ultrasound can assess the thickness of the endometrium, the *endometrial stripe*. A stripe less than 4 mm in diameter is the cutoff to exclude endometrial cancer (Tabor et al., 2002). An office endometrial biopsy is an excellent diagnostic test to evaluate endometrial tissue (Dijkhuizen et al., 2000). In some postmenopausal women, however, cervical stenosis precludes a successful biopsy. In this situation, if the ultrasound is nonreassuring, a surgical procedure may be indicated.

Pelvic Mass

Key Points

- Pelvic examination is not sensitive or specific for the diagnosis of a pelvic mass.
- Initial evaluation of a pelvic mass should include a focused history, physical exam, and pelvic ultrasound.
- Pelvic ultrasound with cyst morphology and Doppler flow studies can distinguish benign cysts from ovarian carcinoma, especially in postmenopausal women.
- Although combination oral contraceptives can reduce the risk of functional ovarian cysts, OCs are not useful for treatment.

Diagnosis

A patient may report a symptomatic pelvic mass, or it may be discovered as part of a pelvic examination or ultrasound done for other reasons. A pelvic mass can be associated with the uterus, ovaries, or nongynecologic organs. The first step in evaluation is to review the patient's age, history, and risk factors. For example, an ovarian cyst is more likely to be a functional cyst in a younger woman, but it has a higher potential to be ovarian cancer in postmenopausal women. Additional historical details include menopausal status, menstrual history, family history, STI risk, symptoms of hyperandrogenism, and dysmenorrhea.

Pelvic examination is not sensitive or specific for diagnosis of a pelvic mass, especially as body mass index (BMI) increases (Myers et al., 2006). However, pelvic examination can provide other information helpful in the diagnosis, such as location of the mass, mobility of the mass, cervical motion tenderness, pelvic tenderness, and vaginal discharge. Initial evaluation of a pelvic mass should include a pelvic ultrasound, which can be transabdominal or transvaginal, depending on the size and location of the mass. Premenopausal women should be tested to exclude pregnancy. Doppler ultrasound, cyst morphology, and CA-125 testing are useful in ruling out ovarian cancer in a postmenopausal woman with an adnexal mass. Table 25-2 lists the differential diagnosis and common features of pelvic masses.

Uterine Fibroids

Uterine fibroids are present in approximately one third of reproductive-age women (Viswanathan et al., 2007). Although often asymptomatic, fibroids may cause pelvic pain, pressure, and heavy or irregular vaginal bleeding and are the most common reason for hysterectomy in the United States. Treatment options for fibroids include watchful waiting, since most fibroids will decrease in size after menopause. Although hysterectomy is definitive treatment, it carries the risks of major surgery. Myomectomy and other uterine-sparing procedures have a high rate of symptom recurrence (up to 50% within 5 years) and may be more effective for symptom control in perimenopausal women. Women with fibroids are more likely to be infertile, although it is not clear if the association is causative. Removal of fibroids has not been shown to improve fertility (Grifiths et al., 2009). Medical treatments such as NSAIDs and OCs have not been well studied. The levonorgestrel intrauterine system (Mirena) has been shown to prevent hysterectomy in women with heavy vaginal bleeding related to fibroids, but women with more than three fibroids or with one fibroid larger than 3 cm were excluded from this study (Lahteenmaki et al., 1998). Low-dose mifepristone (5 mg daily for 26 weeks) was found to decrease symptoms and improve quality of life (Fiscella et al., 2006).

Ovarian Cysts and Carcinoma

As mentioned, the initial evaluation of an ovarian cyst includes a transvaginal ultrasound. Premenopausal women should have pregnancy testing, and postmenopausal women should have CA-125 testing. Simple cysts are more likely to be benign, whereas complex cysts (with thick walls, irregularity, papillations, septa, and echogenicity) have a higher risk of

Table 25-2 Differential Diagnosis of Pelvic Mass

Diagnosis	Features
Uterus	
Uterine fibroid	Pelvic pressure, heavy vaginal bleeding
Intrauterine pregnancy	Positive pregnancy test, amenorrhea
Fallopian tubes	
Ectopic pregnancy	Positive pregnancy test, adnexal pain or tenderness, hemodynamic instability
Tubo-ovarian abscess	STI risk, pelvic pain, cervical motion tenderness, vaginal discharge, fever
Ovaries	
Simple cysts	More common in premenopausal women; sharp, may have pelvic pressure
Endometriomas	Dysmenorrhea
Dermoid cysts (teratomas)	Pelvic pressure
Ovarian carcinoma	Postmenopausal women
Polycystic ovarian syndrome	Hyperandrogenism, irregular menses, multiple cysts on ultrasound
Germ cell tumors	Pelvic pressure, chromosomal abnormalities, younger women (teens and 20s)
Intestines	
Appendicitis	Anorexia, right lower quadrant pain/tenderness, elevated white blood cell count, fever
Diverticulitis	Left lower quadrant pain/tenderness, cramping, constipation, older age, fever
Urinary tract	
Bladder tumor	Hematuria
Pelvic kidney	Usually asymptomatic

STI, Sexually transmitted infection.

malignancy. Malignant neoplasms also display increased vascularity on Doppler ultrasound. Women with complex cysts, cysts larger than 10 cm in diameter, or elevated CA-125 levels should have a surgical referral (Modesitt et al., 2003). Although combination OCs can reduce the occurrence of functional ovarian cysts, OCs are not helpful for treatment (Grimes et al., 2007).

KEY TREATMENT

Most simple ovarian cysts can be managed expectantly (Modesitt et al., 2003) (SOR: B).

The levonorgestrel intrauterine system can avoid hysterectomy in some women with fibroids and heavy vaginal bleeding (Lahteen-maki et al., 1998) (SOR: B).

Low-dose mifepristone decreases symptoms and improves quality of life (Fiscella et al., 2006) (SOR: B).

Vaginal Discharge

Key Points

- Douching is not helpful for prevention or treatment of vaginitis.
- Signs and symptoms of vaginitis are not specific, but a cause can usually be diagnosed on office microscopy.
- Speculum exam is not necessary for diagnosis of vaginitis; a blind swab in the vaginal vault is equally sensitive
- Self-diagnosis of vaginal infection by the patient is unreliable.

Vaginitis is the most common gynecologic diagnosis made in the primary care setting. Common symptoms include increased vaginal discharge without pelvic pain or systemic symptoms, vulvar itching and burning, dysuria, and possible odor. Physiologic leukorrhea varies and may change with a woman's menstrual cycle. If purulent cervicitis is present on examination, testing for *Chlamydia* and *Neisseria gonorrhoeae* should be performed (French et al., 2004). In postmenopausal women, vaginal irritation, dryness and superficial bleeding are often caused by atrophic vaginitis (see Menopause). A medication history is important because isotretinoin and some contraceptives may also cause dryness and itching. Personal hygiene habits of excessive washing with soap and use of highly absorbent panty liners may cause irritation. If a woman has self-diagnosed and treated with an antifungal and symptoms persist, a clinical examination should be encouraged (ACOG, 2006). Table 25-3 and Box 25-4 review differential diagnosis and findings in vaginitis.

Office microscopy is used most often to make a diagnosis of vaginitis. A finding of many leukocytes is uncommon in candidiasis or bacterial vaginosis (BV) and suggests trichomoniasis. If trichomonads are not present, consider gonorrhea or chlamydial infection (Anderson et al., 2004). Fem V, an over-the-counter (OTC) diagnostic kit, can be used; a positive test suggests BV or trichomoniasis; a negative test is likely a yeast infection (Prescriber's Letter, 2006).

Bacterial Vaginosis

Bacterial vaginosis is caused by a shift from the normal lactobacilli-dominated vaginal flora to a polymicrobial flora dominated by gram-positive anaerobes. Although BV is the most common cause of vaginal discharge and foul odor, more than half of women with BV are asymptomatic (CDC, 2006). BV is associated with postoperative infection, pelvic inflammatory disease (PID), premature delivery in women with certain risk factors (French et al., 2004), and an increased risk of human immunodeficiency virus type 1 (HIV-1) transmission (Oduyebo et al., 2009). Risk factors for acquisition of BV include tobacco use, intrauterine contraception (IUC) use, new male sexual partner, sex with another woman, and use of vaginal foreign bodies, perfumed soaps. or douching (Allsworth and Peipert, 2007).

The diagnosis of BV can usually be made by history and laboratory microscopy (Fig. 25-1). Self-diagnosis by the patient is unreliable (ACOG, 2006). A strong "musty cheese" odor predicts BV, whereas lack of a perceived odor makes BV unlikely (Anderson et al., 2004). Use of the Amsel criteria on a vaginal (not cervical) sample can be used to diagnose BV in clinical practice (Box 25-5).

Table 25-3 Comparison of Findings for Vaginitis

Type	Symptoms	Signs	pH	KOH	Saline Wet Mount
Bacterial vaginosis	Malodorous discharge	Thin, gray adherent discharge	>4.5	Amine/fishy odor	Clue cells
Vulvovaginal candidiasis	Itching, burning pain	Curdlike discharge, vulvar erythema	3.8-4.5	Pseudohyphae; budding yeast	Occasional hyphae; yeast
Trichomoniasis	Fish-odor discharge	Erythema, tenderness	6-7	Negative	Trichomonads, many WBCs
Atrophic vaginitis	Dryness, pain	Pale, friable	>4.5	Negative	RBCs, WBCs; many bacteria
Aerobic vaginitis	Foul odor	Heavy purulent discharge	>4.5	Negative	Cocci or coarse rods
Irritant/allergic vaginitis	Itching, swelling	Erythema	Any	Negative	Negative

WBCs, White blood cells; *RBCs,* red blood cells.

Box 25-4 Differential Diagnosis of Vaginal Discharge: Vaginitis

Candida spp. *(C. albicans, C. glabrata)*

Bacterial vaginosis (anaerobic bacteria: *Gardnerella vaginalis, Bacteroides* spp.)

Desquamative inflammatory vaginitis (DIV): aerobic bacteria

Trichomonas vaginalis

Allergic vaginitis/contact dermatitis

Chlamydial infection/gonorrhea

Erosive lichen planus vaginitis

Actinomyces Behçet's syndrome (associated with IUC use)

Vulvar vestibulitis

Physiologic (leukorrhea)

Atrophic vaginitis

IUC, Intrauterine contraceptive.

Box 25-5 Amsel Criteria for Bacterial Vaginosis*

1. Vaginal pH >4.5 (most sensitive) (89% sens, 74% spec)
2. Clue cells >20% on wet-mount (74% sens, 86% spec)
3. Homogeneous discharge, gray, adherent, but wipes off easily (79% sens, 54% spec)
4. Whiff test (amine odor when KOH added; 67% sens, 93% spec)

Modified from Gutman RE et al. Evaluation of clinical methods for diagnosing bacterial vaginosis. Obstet Gynecol 2005;105:551-556.
*A score of 3 of 4 is diagnostic.

sens, Sensitivity; *spec,* specificity; *KOH,* potassium hydroxide.

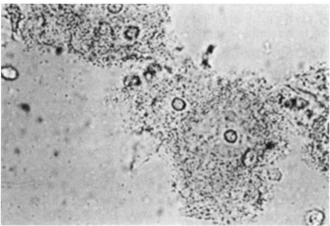

Figure 25-1 Bacterial vaginosis. Typical clue cells of vaginal epithelium are heavily covered by coccobacilli, with loss of distinct cell margins. (Magnification ×400.) *(From Holmes KK. Lower genital tract infections in women: cystitis/urethritis, vulvovaginitis, and cervicitis. In Holmes KK, Mårdh PA, Sparling PF, et al [eds]. Sexually Transmitted Diseases. New York, McGraw-Hill, 1984.*

There are many effective options for the treatment of BV. A 2009 Cochrane review states that clindamycin and metronidazole have equivalent efficacy, regardless of regimen. The standard oral dose of metronidazole for BV is 500 mg twice daily for 7 days. Both metronidazole and clindamycin vaginal cream are dosed daily. Clindamycin has lower adverse event rates. Intravaginal lactobacilli gelatin tablets are also effective (Oduyebo et al., 2009). The 2006 CDC guidelines do not recommend treatment with single-dose metronidazole. Tinidazole is effective with no serious side effects but is more expensive (Livengood et al., 2007). The FDA has recently approved metronidazole, 750 mg daily for 7 days, and a single dose of intravaginal clindamycin for treatment of BV, but only limited data are available on efficacy (CDC, 2006). Hydrogen peroxide douching and triple-sulfonamide cream are considered ineffective (Oduyebo et al., 2009).

Recurrent BV can present a treatment challenge. If recurrence is suspected, the diagnosis should be confirmed, risk factors identified and controlled, and other causes considered while re-treating BV (Alfonsi et al., 2004). Metronidazole gel used twice weekly reduces recurrence of BV but is offset by increased vaginal candidiasis and pain complaints. (Sobel et al., 2006). If re-treatment fails, suppressive therapy with metronidazole 0.75% gel for 10 days, then twice weekly for 4 to 6 months, should be tried. There is no evidence that treatment of sexual partners (BASHH, 2006) or using oral or vaginal *Lactobacillus acidophilus* is effective to prevent recurrence (Alfonsi et al., 2004).

Candidal Vaginitis

Vulvovaginal candidiasis (VVC) is the second most common cause of vaginitis after BV, with a lifetime prevalence in women of 70% to 75% (Spence, 2007). *Candida albicans* is the most common etiology (80%-90%). Type 1 diabetes

KEY TREATMENT

All symptomatic women with BV should be treated (BAASH, 2006).
Asymptomatic women undergoing abortion or hysterectomy should be treated to decrease the risk for infectious complications (BAASH, 2006).
Oral or vaginal metronidazole (BAASH, 2006) and vaginal clindamycin are effective and equivalent in nonpregnant women (Kane, 2001).
Treatment of male partners does not decrease relapse rates (BASHH, 2006).
Tinidazole is effective with no serious side effects but is more expensive than metronidazole (Livengood et al., 2007) (SOR: A).
In recurrent BV, suppressive therapy with metronidazole 0.75% gel for 10 days then twice weekly for 4 to 6 months may be successful (Alfonsi et al., 2004) (SOR: C).

is the strongest risk factor for VVC; other risk factors include recent antibiotic use, condom and diaphragm use, spermicide use, receptive oral sex, OC use, pregnancy, and immunosuppression. Patient self-diagnosis of VVC is incorrect 50% of the time and is therefore unreliable. Asymptomatic treatment of VVC is *not* recommended, even in women who have a positive swab for *Candida* (Spence, 2007). Because VVC is not sexually transmitted, routine partner treatment is also not recommended. Recurrent VVC is defined as four or more symptomatic episodes in a year. Rare complications of VVC include vulvar vestibulitis and chorioamnionitis (French et al., 2004).

The most common complaint associated with culture confirmed VVC is burning or pruritus. A thick, curdled-appearing discharge, signs of inflammation, and lack of odor all have high positive predictive value for diagnosing VVC (Anderson et al., 2004). In one study, however, a thin discharge was present in about half of women, later found to have VVC (French et al., 2004).

Although office microscopy is the first line for diagnosis of VVC, culture is the "gold standard" (Fig. 25-2) (ACOG, 2006). With *Candida albicans,* the vaginal pH is usually 5.0 or less but may be higher with non-*albicans* species. A wet mount should be performed to exclude trichomoniasis or BV. Potassium hydroxide (KOH) examination should also be performed, but it has a wide range of sensitivity. Thus, if candidiasis is suspected in a patient with persistent or recurrent symptoms and a wet mount and KOH are negative, a culture should be performed (French et al., 2004). The use of rapid antigen testing to detect vaginal yeast is more sensitive than a wet mount and is feasible for office practice. However, a negative result lacks sensitivity to rule out yeast, and a culture needs to be sent (Chatwani et al., 2007).

The imidazoles are the cornerstone of VVC treatment. Intravaginal OTC imidazoles (e.g., clotrimazole, miconazole, tioconazole) come in 1-, 3-, and 7-day therapy regimens and are equivalent to oral therapies for treatment, and single-dose therapy seems as efficacious as multidose therapy over days. The comparative efficacy of different azoles and of different durations of multidose regimens is unclear (Spence, 2007). *Lactobacillus,* administered vaginally, orally, or both, does not prevent postantibiotic-associated vaginal candidiasis (Priotta et al., 2004).

Recurrent VVC occurs in 5% to 8% of women. The Infectious Diseases Society of America recommends treating recurrent VVC for 10 to 14 days, followed by suppressive therapy using fluconazole, a single 150-mg dose weekly for

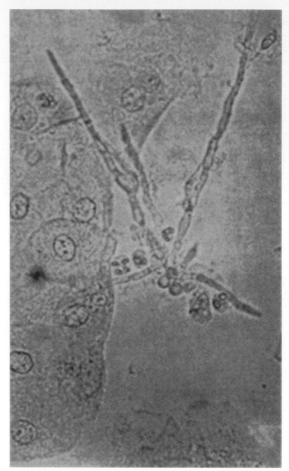

Figure 25-2 Candidal vaginitis (vulvovaginal candidiasis). Candidal organisms in a saline wet-mount preparation clearly demonstrate hyphae and conidia under high-power magnification.
(From Kaufman RH, Faro S: Benign Disease of the Vulva and Vagina, ed 4. St. Louis, Mosby, 1994.)

6 months (Pappas et al., 2009). It is unclear if oral regimens are better than intravaginal administration. In preventing recurrence, there is no evidence of benefit with intravaginal boric acid, tea tree oil, garlic, oral yogurt, douching, or treating a woman's male sexual partner. Douching is associated with increased pelvic infections (Spence, 2007). For specific treatment regimens: see http://www.cdc.gov/std/treatment/.

KEY TREATMENT

Oral fluconazole and itraconazole are both effective for vulvovaginal candidiasis (Spence, 2007) (SOR: A).
Oral and intravaginal regimens are equivalent, so cost and patient preference should guide choice (Nurbhai et al., 2009) (SOR: B).
Intravaginal imidazoles are equivalent to oral therapies for VVC treatment, and single-dose seems as efficacious as multidose therapy (Spence, 2007) (SOR: B).
Treat recurrent VVC for 10 to 14 days, followed by suppressive therapy using fluconazole, single 150-mg dose weekly for 6 months (Pappas et al., 2009) (SOR: A)

Trichomoniasis

Trichomoniasis is caused by a motile protozoan and affects 120 million women worldwide every year. It is usually sexually transmitted and is associated with transmission of other

STIs (Forna, 2009). Risk factors for acquisition include multiple sexual partners and possibly a decrease in the normal vaginal acidity. Men are usually asymptomatic carriers, but 10% of nongonococcal urethritis in men is caused by *Trichomonas* (French et al., 2004).

Up to 50% of women with trichomoniasis are asymptomatic. Symptomatic women may complain of a yellow-green, malodorous discharge, vaginal burning, and dysuria. On physical examination, hemorrhagic, punctate cervical lesions are pathognomonic but are only present in 2% of cases (French et al., 2004). More common signs are foul-smelling purulent discharge, vaginal tenderness, vulvar erythema and edema. The vaginal pH is usually basic. Office microscopy is first line for diagnosis of trichomoniasis (ACOG, 2006). The sample should be taken from the posterior vault, diluted in 2 drops of saline, and assessed quickly because motility of the protozoa diminishes rapidly (Fig. 25-3). Although microscopy has good specificity (99%), motile trichomonads are seen in only 50% to 80% of culture-proven cases. Thus, culture is the gold standard. Trichomonads can be reported on a Pap smear, but it is not recommended as a diagnostic test because of the low sensitivity (58%) (French et al., 2004). In men the wet prep has poor sensitivity, so culture of both a urethral sample and a first-voided urine sample is necessary to increase the diagnostic rate.

Metronidazole or tinidazole single-dose therapy is effective for treatment of trichomoniasis. An alternative effective regimen is metronidazole, 500 mg orally twice daily for 7 days. Metronidazole gel is less effective (<50% cure rate) as compared to oral metronidazole (CDC, 2006). Desensitization is recommended for patients allergic to metronidazole. Avoidance of alcohol is important with all nitroimidazoles. Metronidazole is not teratogenic in the first trimester (BASHH, 2007). Because most male sexual partners have asymptomatic trichomoniasis, simultaneous treatment is recommended.

If treatment fails with a 2-g single dose of metronidazole, a trial of metronidazole, 500 mg twice daily for 7 days, or a single 2-g dose of tinidazole is recommended (CDC, 2006). If this fails, a trial of tinidazole or metronidazole, 2 g orally once daily for 5 days, is recommended. Referral is advised for persistent failure. A test of cure is unnecessary if symptoms resolve (BASHH, 2007).

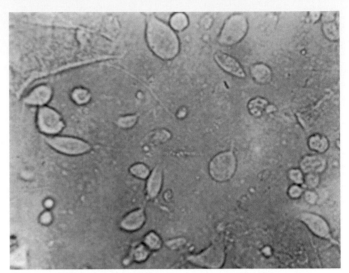

Figure 25-3 Trichomoniasis. Trichomonads are seen under high-power magnification in a wet mount prepared with physiologic saline. Usually, more immature epithelial cells are seen in the secretions of active trichomoniasis. *(From Kaufman RH, Faro S. Benign Disease of the Vulva and Vagina, 4th ed. St Louis, Mosby, 1994.)*

KEY TREATMENT

Women with trichomoniasis should abstain from intercourse until both she and her partner have been treated and are asymptomatic (ACOG, 2006) (SOR: A).

A single dose of a nitroimidazole can achieve parasitologic cure; tinidazole as a single 2-g dose may be most efficacious (CDC, 2006; Forna, 2009) (SOR: A).

If treatment fails with a single 2-g dose of metronidazole, a trial of metronidazole, 500 mg twice daily for 7 days, or a single 2-g dose of tinidazole is recommended (CDC, 2006) (SOR: B).

Other Forms of Vaginitis

Aerobic vaginitis is characterized by purulent vaginal discharge with a dominant abnormal aerobic flora. Patients experience a foul-smelling nonfishy discharge, and examination may reveal erythema, inflammation, and ulcers of the posterior fornix. Although culture is the gold standard, the diagnosis is usually one of exclusion, with pH greater than 6.0, white blood cells (WBCs) on microscopy, and absence of hyphae or clue cells. Treatment with topical clindamycin has a good response (French et al., 2004). The addition of a topical estrogen may increase treatment success.

Irritant and allergic vaginitis should be considered in the differential diagnosis of vaginal complaints. Common etiologies include spermicidal products, douching solutions, diaphragms, latex condoms, and topical medications. The treatment is discontinuation of intravaginal products (French et al., 2004).

Cytolytic vaginitis is caused by an overgrowth of lactobacilli and cytolysis of squamous epithelial cells. Although it may be related to intravaginal products or other medication use, its etiology remains unclear. It can mimic VVC with a white, curdled-cheese discharge, and the pH range is typically 3.5 to 5.5. Treatment is discontinuation of intravaginal medications. Baking soda douches or sitz baths have been used, but minimal data exist to support this recommendation (French et al., 2004).

Desquamative inflammatory vaginitis (DIV) is characterized by copious purulent discharge with squamous epithelial cell exfoliation. The etiology is unclear but likely multifactorial. Some cases may be linked to lichen planus spectrum. Laboratory evaluation reveals a negative wet mount, KOH, and cultures. Treatment options include a trial of local or systemic corticosteroids (French et al., 2004) or clindamycin suppositories.

Vulvar Lesions

Key Points

- Visible condyloma should be treated.
- Biopsy is indicated for treatment-resistant warts, chronic symptomatic lesions, and nevus-like, pigmented lesions.
- Biopsy of lichen sclerosus is recommended to rule out vulvar squamous cell carcinoma.
- Topical corticosteroids are the cornerstone of management for nonneoplastic epithelial disorders of the vulva.

The differential diagnosis of vulvar lesions includes external genital warts (EGWs), *Candida*, herpes simplex, lichen sclerosus et atrophicus, lichen planus, psoriasis, and eczema.

EGWs are caused by HPV, which is primarily transmitted through sexual contact. Although exophytic warts are usually diagnosable with the naked eye, application of acetic acid can make flat warts visible. Biopsy is indicated for treatment-resistant warts, chronic symptomatic lesions, and nevus-like, pigmented lesions. For EGWs, cryotherapy is as effective as trichloroacetic acid and more effective than podophyllin. Podophyllotoxin and podophyllin are equally effective for clearance of EGWs and useful for small, solitary lesions. Imiquimod cream is also effective and should be applied to intact skin. Topical interferon is effective and preferable to systemic interferon. Electrosurgery is at least as effective as cryotherapy and more effective than podophyllin (Buck, 2006).

Nonneoplastic epithelial lesions of the vulva include lichen sclerosus, lichen planus, and lichen simplex chronicus. *Lichen sclerosus* is most common in postmenopausal women and presents with intense vulvar pruritus. Physical examination initially reveals thickened, white skin not involving the vagina, which progresses to a thin, wrinkled, "cigarette paper" appearance. High-potency topical steroids are effective in alleviating symptoms and preventing progressive architectural damage. *Lichen planus* is an autoimmune disorder that may involve the vagina as well as vulva. High-potency topical steroids or hydrocortisone suppositories are effective for treatment. *Lichen simplex chronicus* presents as lichenified, erythematous plaques resulting from chronic itching and scratching. Breaking the itch-scratch cycle is the cornerstone of treatment (O'Connell et al., 2008).

> **KEY TREATMENT**
>
> For external warts, cryotherapy is as effective as trichloroacetic acid and more effective than podophyllin; electrosurgery is at least as effective as cryotherapy and more effective than podophyllin (Buck, 2006) (SOR: B).
> For lichen sclerosus, high-potency topical steroids are effective in alleviating symptoms and preventing progressive architectural damage (O'Connell et al., 2008) (SOR: B).
> For lichen simplex chronicus, breaking the itch-scratch cycle is primary treatment (O'Connell et al., 2008) (SOR: C).

Acute Pelvic Pain

Key Points

- Acute pelvic pain can be related to multiple organ systems.
- Gynecologic pain typically includes pregnancy complications, infection, and ovarian cysts.
- Clinicians should have a low threshold for treating pelvic inflammatory disease because of the potential for long-term complications.

Acute lower abdominal pain can be caused by multiple organ systems. Urinary tract infections (UTIs) are often associated with pain over the bladder related to dysuria, frequency, and urgency of urination. Gastrointestinal causes of lower abdominal pain include acute appendicitis, diverticulitis, irritable bowel syndrome, and ischemic bowel.

Gynecologic causes of acute pelvic pain are usually related to complications of pregnancy, infections, or ovarian pathology. *Ectopic pregnancy* is a serious cause of acute pain in the context of an early pregnancy. Ectopic pregnancy should be suspected when the quantitive human chorionic gonadotropin (hCG) level does not increase appropriately, or if hCG level is greater than 1500 mIU and transvaginal ultrasound does not show an intrauterine gestational sac. The dilation of the fallopian tube caused by the growing embryo is the etiology of the pain. Emergent treatment with either medication or surgery is necessary to prevent rupture of the tube. Ectopic pregnancy is usually diagnosed by ultrasound. Treatment of an ectopic pregnancy can be surgical or medical. Single-dose methotrexate is the most frequently used regimen, 50 mg/m^2 of body surface intramuscularly, but no studies have compared efficacy between single-dose and multidose therapies (Lozeau and Potter, 2005). Degenerating fibroid tumors may also cause pain as a result of ischemia during pregnancy, usually in the second trimester.

Pelvic infections such as acute cervicitis and *pelvic inflammatory disease* (PID) can cause pain associated commonly with abnormal vaginal discharge and systemic symptoms of infection. On examination, most women will have a purulent cervicitis, a tender uterus, and cervical motion tenderness. Both outpatient and inpatient treatment options are available from the CDC STI treatment guidelines, at www.cdc.gov (2006). Outpatient treatment of PID usually includes intramuscular (IM) ceftriaxone and doxycycline for 10 days to cover both *Neisseria gonorrhoeae* and *Chlamydia*. Untreated PID can lead to an abscess or scarring that can cause infertility. Clinical diagnosis of PID has a positive predictive value of 65% to 90% (BAASH, 2005). Therefore, clinicians should have a low threshold for treating women with suspected PID.

Ovarian cysts are common and often cause no pain. When cysts rupture, however, women will experience acute pelvic pain from peritoneal irritation. Large ovarian cysts are more likely to undergo torsion and can cause pain from ischemia.

> **KEY TREATMENT**
>
> Medical and surgical treatments for ectopic pregnancy are equivalent when patient selection is appropriate (Lozeau and Potter, 2005) (SOR: B).
> Single-dose methotrexate is the most common regimen (50 mg/m^2 body surface IM) for ectopic pregnancy (Lozeau and Potter, 2005) (SOR: C).
> Clinicians should have a low threshold for treating women with suspected PID because of potential long-term consequences (BAASH, 2005) (SOR: C).

Chronic Pelvic Pain

Key Points

- Chronic pelvic pain is an indication for 40% of the laparoscopies in the United States.
- The four most common causes of chronic pelvic pain are endometriosis, pelvic adhesions, interstitial cystitis, and irritable bowel syndrome.
- Up to 70% of women with chronic pelvic pain have more than one cause for their pain.

Chronic pelvic pain is defined as noncyclic pain that lasts longer than 6 months. It occurs frequently, affecting up to 15% of all women at some point in their reproductive years. Chronic pelvic pain is a diagnosis associated with up to 10%

of all outpatient gynecologic consultations, 40% of all laparoscopies, and 18% of all hysterectomies performed each year in the United States (Zondervan and Barlow, 2000). In 1990 the estimated cost of services related to chronic pelvic pain was $2 billion (Reiter, 1990).

Almost half of all women with chronic pelvic pain have a history of past sexual abuse or depression (Latthe et al., 2006). Women with a history of trauma have more severe symptoms (Meltzer-Brody et al., 2007). A recent meta-analysis of women with a history of abuse found an increased prevalence of functional bowel disorders, nonspecific chronic pain, and chronic pelvic pain (Paras et al., 2009). Drug and alcohol abuse are associated with an increased likelihood of pain (Latthe et al., 2006). There is no difference in prevalence based on race, ethnicity, education, or socioeconomic status (ACOG, 2004).

The etiology of chronic pelvic pain is frequently multifactorial and comes from multiple organ systems. Up to 70% of women have more than one cause of pain (Butrick, 2007). The most common gynecologic causes of chronic pelvic pain are endometriosis and pelvic adhesions. The most common gastrointestinal cause is irritable bowel syndrome, and the most common urologic cause is interstitial cystitis (Bordman and Jackson, 2006). In addition, many women who have chronic pelvic pain also have some myofascial pain from the pelvic floor muscles (Box 25-6).

Initial evaluation of a woman with chronic pelvic pain includes a careful history to determine any pattern of the pain that would lead to a possible diagnosis. For example, history of abdominal surgery increases the risk of pelvic adhesions. A complete medical, surgical, family, sexual, and psychological history should also be completed. It is important to determine how the pain is affecting the woman's daily life. The physical examination should include a general exam in addition to a thorough pelvic assessment. Every effort should be made to replicate the pain through a bimanual or rectovaginal examination.

Laboratory evaluation is focused on the likely diagnosis. Many women have a pelvic ultrasound for further evaluation of the pelvic anatomy. Ultimately, many women undergo a diagnostic laparoscopy to evaluate the etiology of the pain. Laparoscopy is normal in 35% to 40% of these women. Endometriosis is diagnosed in about 30% of women at laparoscopy, and adhesions are diagnosed in about 25% (Howard, 2000).

Treatment of a woman with chronic pelvic pain should be multimodal to address the multifactorial nature of her pain (ACOG, 2004; Stones et al., 2009). A strong physician-patient relationship is imperative as a basis for successful treatment. First-line treatment includes pain control with nonnarcotic medication. Hormonal manipulation with medroxyprogesterone acetate, combined hormonal contraception, or gonadotropin-releasing hormone (GnRH) analogues can be effective treatments for endometriosis-related pain. GnRH analogues can only be used for up to 6 months because of side effects (e.g., menopausal symptoms, osteoporosis).

Laparoscopic treatment of endometriosis and lysis of dense adhesions are helpful in a subset of women. Lysis of adhesions that are not severe has not consistently decreased pain (ACOG, 2004). Hysterectomy is performed in women with untreatable pain and is most effective if accompanied by bilateral oophorectomy. Hysterectomy is major surgery with many potential complications but can cure some cases of pain related to endometriosis. Uterosacral nerve ablation

is not an effective method for treating idiopathic chronic pelvic pain (Daniels et al., 2009).

None of the above treatment modalities addresses the *physiology* of chronic pain. Several newer anticonvulsants (gabapentin, topiramate, valproic acid, pregabalin) and antidepressants, such as tricyclic antidepressants and selective serotonin reuptake inhibitors, have been successful in treating neuropathic pain from other sources. However, limited data are available in women with pelvic pain. Trigger point injections and botulinum toxin (Botox) injections in pelvic floor muscles show promise for treating myofascial pain (Gomel, 2007). Multidisciplinary treatment teams should include mental health professionals and physical therapists as well as physicians.

Box 25-6 Common Causes of Chronic Pelvic Pain

Gynecologic

Endometriosis
Pelvic adhesions
Pelvic congestion
Pelvic inflammatory disease
Adenomyosis
Vulvodynia
Uterine myomas

Gastrointestinal

Irritable bowel syndrome
Inflammatory bowel disease
Chronic constipation
Colitis
Diverticulitis

Urologic

Interstitial cystitis
Chronic urinary tract infections
Urethral syndrome
Radiation cystitis
Urinary calculi

Musculoskeletal

Myofascial pain (abdominal wall or pelvic floor muscles)
Fibromyalgia
Coccygeal or low back pain
Nerve pain

Modified from Bordman R, Jackson B. Below the belt: approach to chronic pelvic pain. Can Fam Physician 2006;52:1556-1562; and Reiter RC. Chronic pelvic pain. Clin Obstet Gynecol 1990;33:117-118.

KEY TREATMENT

Treatment of chronic pelvic pain should be multidisciplinary and include a mental health professional (Stones et al., 2009) (SOR: A).
Uterosacral nerve ablation is not an effective method for treating idiopathic chronic pelvic pain. (Daniels et al., 2009) (SOR: A).
First-line treatment includes pain control with nonnarcotic medication (ACOG, 2004) (SOR: A).
Hormonal manipulation with medroxyprogesterone acetate, combined hormonal contraception, or GnRH analogues can be effective treatments for endometriosis-related pain (ACOG, 2004) (SOR: A).

Menopause

Key Points

- The average age of menopause is 52.
- Vasomotor symptoms are the most common menopausal sign.
- The Women's Health Initiative showed that hormone replacement therapy did not prevent cardiovascular disease in postmenopausal women and in fact increased the risk of breast cancer.

Menopause is defined as the cessation of menstruation. It is a retrospective diagnosis that comes after a woman has not menstruated for 12 months. The menopausal transition occurs over several years as the number of ovarian follicles slowly decreases. This period in a woman's life can include menstrual cycles of variable lengths and durations, called the *perimenopause*. Because of the waxing number of follicles, the ovaries require higher levels of estrogen to stimulate a luteinizing hormone (LH) surge and subsequent ovulation. Consequently, serum levels of estrogen can vary substantially from one cycle to the next. The first physiologic change noted is a decrease in inhibin B levels (Burger et al., 1999). Subsequently, follicle-stimulating hormone (FSH) level will increase in response to lower estrogen levels. An FSH level greater than 40 U/L on two separate occasions at least 1 month apart is diagnostic of menopause. The main pathologic cause of abnormal vaginal bleeding during this period is anovulation in those cycles when estrogen did not reach target levels.

The average age of menopause in the United States is 52 years old. The majority of women will go through menopause between ages 40 and 58. Menopause before age 40 is defined as premature ovarian failure and may be related to other autoimmune disease. Factors associated with age at menopause include smoking and family history (Nelson, 2008).

Vasomotor symptoms, including hot flashes and night sweats, are the most common symptoms of menopause. Some women may begin to experience these symptoms years before their final menstrual period, during those months where their estrogen levels are lower. Many women will experience symptoms for several years. Up to 10% of women will continue to experience vasomotor symptoms into their 70s (Politi et al., 2008). Symptoms are worse in women who experience premature ovarian failure, have a premenopausal oophorectomy, are overweight or obese, or are depressed (Hendrix, 2005). Treatment of vasomotor symptoms begins with lifestyle changes and also can include pharmacologic treatment with hormonal or nonhormonal medications. Women may be able to manage their vasomotor symptoms by wearing natural-fiber clothing in layers, avoiding spicy foods, avoiding hot environments (e.g., saunas, hot tubs), avoiding alcohol, exercising, and maintaining a healthy weight.

Pharmacologic treatment of vasomotor symptoms includes hormone therapy (HT) at the lowest effective doses orally or transdermally (Bachmann et al., 2007). HT should include both estrogen and progestin in women who have a uterus and estrogen alone in women who have had a hysterectomy. HT should be used in women at the lowest possible doses to treat symptoms for as short a time as possible (NAMS, 2004). In women for whom HT is contraindicated or who are worried about the risks, several nonhormonal options have been studied. Antidepressant medications such as fluoxetine, paroxetine, and venlafaxine have been shown to be better than placebo. Gabapentin, 900 mg daily, is also better than placebo in treating hot flashes (Grady, 2006).

Many women use complementary therapies to treat vasomotor symptoms. Various herbal preparations (e.g., black cohosh) have been used to treat vasomotor symptoms with varying success. Many women also obtain relief from soy products or other isoflavones. None of these treatments has consistently been more effective than placebo in randomized trials (Nelson et al., 2006). Stress management and meditation show promise in controlling these troublesome symptoms (Tremblay et al., 2008).

Atrophic vaginitis, or thinning of the vaginal epithelium caused by a lack of estrogen stimulation after menopause, is common, affecting 10% to 40% of all postmenopausal women. Women complain of vaginal dryness, irritation, and pain with intercourse. Unlike vasomotor symptoms, atrophic vaginitis does not develop immediately after menopause but causes symptoms months to years after the withdrawal of estrogen. Left untreated, atrophic vaginitis is progressive and is unlikely to improve spontaneously. Treatment of atrophic vaginitis begins with use of appropriate water based lubricants to make intercourse more comfortable. The mainstay of treatment is vaginal estrogen (Castelo-Branco et al., 2005). Several preparations of vaginal estrogen are available in the United States. Estrogen cream, tablets, and a slow-release silicone ring are all well tolerated and are equally effective in reducing symptoms of atrophic vaginitis. Because the vaginal estrogen has limited systemic absorption, a concomitant dosing with progestin is not necessary (Suckling et al., 2006).

Other common menopausal changes include memory difficulty (mostly with word finding), mood lability, and decreased libido (from decreased testosterone levels after menopause).

Before the Women's Health Initiative (WHI), HT was the most common treatment for menopausal symptoms. HT was also used for prevention of heart disease and osteoporosis. WHI was a large (>16,000 participants) population-based study of women between 50 and 79 years studying the effectiveness of estrogen plus progestin on congestive heart disease (CHD) prevention. The trial was stopped early because of excess cardiovascular and breast cancer events. There was an excess of 7 CHD events, 8 strokes, 8 breast cancers, and 14 venous thromboembolic events per 10,000 women. The estrogen-only arm of the study was stopped 2 years later due to excess strokes (12 per 10,000 women). There was no statistically significant increase in breast cancer incidence in the estrogen-only group (Anderson et al., 2004). The HT group in both arms of the study had fewer hip fractures. The estrogen-plus-progestin group also had fewer cases of colon cancer (Roussouw et al., 2002).

KEY TREATMENT

Hormone therapy can be used for treatment of menopausal symptoms but should be used at the lowest possible dose for the shortest time possible (NAMS, 2004) (SOR: C).

Atrophic vaginitis is treated most effectively by vaginal estrogen cream or tablets, usually three times a week initially and titrated down based on symptoms (Castelo-Branco et al., 2005) (SOR: A).

Antidepressant medications (fluoxetine, paroxetine, venlafaxine) are better than placebo in treating hot flashes (Grady, 2006) (SOR: A).

Gabapentin (900 mg daily) is also better than placebo in treating hot flashes (Grady, 2006) (SOR: A).

Stress management and meditation show promise in controlling troublesome menopausal symptoms (Tremblay et al., 2008) (SOR: B).

References

The complete reference list is available online at www.expertconsult.com.

Web Resources

www.ahrq.gov/CLINIC/uspstfix.htm
U.S. Preventive Services Task Force screening recommendations, includes the Electronic Preventive Services Selector (enter a patient's age and gender and receive a list of evidence-based recommendations) and the option to sign up for e-mail updates on preventive services.

www.cdc.gov/vaccines/recs/ACIP/default.htm
Centers for Disease Control and Prevention and Advisory Committee on Immunization Practices immunization guidelines, including tables for adults, adolescents, and pregnant women; e-mail updates also available.

www.asccp.org/consensus/cytological.shtml
www.asccp.org/pdfs/consensus/algorithms_cyto_07.pdf
American Society for Colposcopy and Cervical Pathology guidelines for management of abnormal Pap tests; provides detailed algorithms describing how to manage each specific Pap smear abnormality.

www.cdc.gov/std/treatment
The 2006 sexually transmitted infection (STI) treatment guidelines provide detailed recommendations for treatment of all sexually transmitted diseases (STDs) as well as other types of vaginitis.

Contraception

Adriana C. Linares and Ann I. Schutt-Ainé

Among U.S. women, the prevalence of ever using a contraceptive method is almost 98% (Chandra et al., 2005). By addressing issues related to contraception at each visit, an informed family physician can help prevent complications stemming from interactions with prescribed and over-the-counter medications, as well as from the use of the contraceptive method itself.

Use of Contraception

History

Humans have tried to control fertility since ancient times. Egyptian papyruses describe methods to avoid pregnancy (Benagiano et al., 2006). The ancient Greeks sought to control the birth of animals using herbs, barrier methods, and other remedies (Riddle, 1999), and evidence of use of barrier methods to prevent pregnancy is found among prostitutes in France (Head, 1961). The approval of the oral contraceptive pill in the second half of the 20th century marked a great revolution in the development and widespread use of contraception methods (Winter, 1970).

Prevalence

The National Survey of Family Growth found the most frequent contraception method used during the first sexual intercourse for men and women was the male condom, which is openly available in pharmacies, supermarkets, and medical offices (Chandra et al., 2005). When asked about use of current contraceptive methods, 62% of women report using a method, and in never-married cohabiting women, the most common method is the oral contraceptive pill (49%).

Impediments to Access

Lack of access is an important impediment to the use of contraception. With the exception of emergency contraception, all hormonal methods in the United States are available by prescription only. More than 47 million Americans (2010) do not have health insurance and have problems accessing primary care, and even with health insurance, access to contraception may be hampered by lack of coverage. For example, in a Washington state study comparing the 91 top-selling insurance plans, almost half did not cover any contraceptive method; 37% of women had no access to sterilization; and 53% had no access to pregnancy termination (Kurth et al., 2001). Another important impediment to the use of contraception can be physician difficulty in being reimbursed for contraception services. Therefore, Table 26-1 lists common *International Classification of Diseases* (ICD-9) codes for contraception counseling, prescriptions, and follow-up.

Counseling

When counseling patients about the use of contraception, nonjudgmental, impartial communication is best. Patients often bring experience, opinions, and some knowledge

Table 26-1 ICD-9 Codes Used for Contraception Reimbursement

Code	Description
V25.0	General counseling and advice on contraceptive management
V25.01	Oral contraceptive initiation or counseling
V25.02	Initiation of other contraceptive method (diaphragm fitting, foam, etc)
V25.03	Encounter for emergency contraceptive counseling and prescription
V25.04	Counseling and instruction on natural family planning to avoid pregnancy
V25.09	Other family planning advice
V25.1	IUD, insertion
V25.2	Sterilization
V25.3	Menstrual extraction/regulation
V25.4	Surveillance of previously prescribed contraceptive methods
V25.40	Contraceptive surveillance, unspecified
V25.41	Repeat prescription/surveillance of OCPs
V25.42	IUD check, re-insertion or removal
V25.43	Surveillance of implantable subdermal contraceptive
V25.49	Surveillance of other prescribed contraceptive method
V25.5	Insertion of implantable subdermal contraceptive
V25.8	Post-vasectomy sperm count
V25.9	Unspecified contraceptive management
V26.4	General and counseling and advice on procreative management
V26.41	Procreative counseling and advice using natural family planning
V26.42	Other procreative management and advice
V26.5	Sterilization status
V26.51	Tubal ligation status
V26.52	Vasectomy status
V26.9	Unspecified procreative management
57170	Diaphragm/cervical cap fitting
58300	IUD insertion
58301	IUD removal
99070	Supply, diaphragm, IUD
J7300	IUD, copper (supply)
J7302	IUD, levonorgestrel (supply)

From World Health Organization (WHO). International Classification of Diseases (ICD-9).
IUD, Intrauterine device; *OCPs*, oral contraceptive pills.

about contraception that are easily elicited by open-ended questions. From this information, counseling can be customized to fit their specific needs. Use of their own words, frequent questions and answers, and feedback from patients play an important role in future compliance with medical advice.

An important consideration in contraceptive counseling is age because fertility among women varies with age. Barrier methods and some hormonal contraceptives can have low compliance in adolescents (ACOG, 2009). Older women can have more complications during pregnancy, making contraception an important component of health maintenance. Older women who are obese, smoke, or have comorbidities (e.g., hypertension, diabetes, migraines) are not good candidates to take combined hormonal contraceptives; progestin-only methods, intrauterine devices (IUDs) and sterilization may be good alternatives (Kaunitz, 2008). Women who use combined hormonal contraceptives after age 40 can be encouraged to stop in their early to mid-50s, when the likelihood of ovulation is low (ACOG, 2006).

Smoking is another important variable to consider when counseling patients. All patients should be encouraged to avoid smoking or to quit if they are smoking. The use of combined hormonal contraceptives in women over age 35 who smoked more than 15 cigarettes per day is contraindicated due to the increased risk of serious cardiovascular effects (Kroon, 2007). All women should be encouraged to use condoms consistently to reduce risk of sexually transmitted infections (STIs), especially in younger women with an increased risk of STI exposure.

Contraception Methods

Contraception is defined as the intentional prevention of conception or impregnation through the use of various devices, agents, drugs, sexual practices, or surgical procedures. The many methods available vary in efficacy, contraindications, and ease of use. Table 26-2 lists preferred contraceptive methods by patient type.

Failure Rates

Failure rates are typically described as percentage of women experiencing an unintended pregnancy within the first year of use (Zeiman et al., 2007). Two failure rates are measured, as follows (Table 26-3):
Perfect-use failure rate refers to the percentage of women who become pregnant during the first year of use when the method is used correctly and consistently according to instructions.
Typical-use failure rate refers to the percentage of women who become pregnant during the first year of use, which includes both those who use the method correctly and consistently and those who do not.

Medical Eligibility Criteria

The World Health Organization (WHO) periodically convenes an Expert Working Group to make evidence-based recommendations for who can safely use a

Table 26-2 Preferred Contraceptive Options for Select Patient Groups

Patient type	Preferred options	Comments
Adolescent	DMPA, implant, COC, or IUC *plus* condoms	IUCs are excellent option currently underused in adolescents.
Potentially noncompliant	DMPA, implant, patch, ring, IUC	—
HIV and STD risk	Condom *plus* any other form of contraception	—
Postpartum and lactating	DMPA, implant, POP, IUC, LAM up to 6 months if specific criteria met	COCs can decrease quality and quantity of breast milk, but only if started before establishment of lactation.
Smoker >35 years old	DMPA, implant, POP, IUC, barrier methods	ECs contraindicated.
Diabetic	DMPA, implant, IUC, barrier methods	ECs appropriate in young normotensive well-controlled diabetic women.
Hypertensive	DMPA, implant, POP, IUC barrier methods	ECs appropriate in young well-controlled nonsmoking hypertensive women.
History of stroke/TIA	IUC, barrier methods	ECs contraindicated; may consider progestin-only methods.
History of thromboembolism	IUC, barrier methods	ECs contraindicated; may consider progestin-only methods.
Coronary artery disease	IUC, implant, barrier methods	ECs contraindicated, may consider progestin-only methods.
Mitral valve prolapse	DMPA, implant, IUC. COC; patch or ring if asymptomatic	—
Polycystic ovarian syndrome	COC, ring, patch, levonorgestrel IUC	COCs best shown to suppress androgen excess; levonorgestrel IUC provides excellent endometrial protection.
Sickle cell disease	DMPA, barrier methods	DMPA shown to decrease frequency of crises.
Gallbladder disease	DMPA, implant, IUC	COCs may accelerate progression.
Taking anticonvulsants or other hepatic inducers	DMPA, IUC	Efficacy of COCs, POPs, and implants may be reduced.
Desires long-term reversible contraception	DMPA, implants, IUC	—
Desires short-term reversible contraception	COC, POP, patch, ring, barrier methods	—
Desires convenience	DMPA, implant, IUC	—
Desires permanent contraception; no interest in future fertility	Vasectomy or tubal ligation	—

Data from World Health Organization. Medical eligibility criteria for contraceptive use 2004, and 2008 Update of the Guide (WHO website).
COC, Combined (combination) oral contraceptive; *DMPA*, depot medroxyprogesterone acetate; *IUC*, intrauterine contraceptive; *POP*, progestin-only pill; *LAM*, lactational amenorrhea method; *ECs*, estrogen-containing contraceptives.
STD, Sexually transmitted disease; *HIV*, human immunodeficiency virus; *TIA*, transient ischemic attack.

contraceptive method. These criteria can be found on the WHO website.

Barrier Contraceptives and Spermicides

Key Points

- Barrier contraceptives and spermicides create a physical barrier to fertilization.
- Many of these methods are available over the counter, increasing access.
- Some barriers can provide protection against cervical infections; condoms also offer protection against HIV.

Mechanism of Action

Barrier contraceptives provide a physical barrier that prevents sperm from accessing the upper reproductive tract. They are often used in conjunction with spermicides, which act to destroy sperm and prevent fertilization.

Male Condom

Materials

Male condoms have been used since ancient times, with early condoms made from animal intestine. Mass production began in the 1840s with the advent of vulcanized

Table 26-3 Failure Rates for Contraceptive Methods: Percentage of Women who Become Pregnant during First Year of Use

Contraceptive method	Women pregnant in first year	
	Perfect Use (%)	Typical Use (%)
No method	85	85
Barrier contraceptives and spermicides		
Male condom	2	15
Female condom	5	21
Cervical cap, nulliparous	9	16
Cervical cap, parous	26	32
Diaphragm	6	16
Contraceptive sponge, nulliparous	9	16
Contraceptive sponge, parous	20	32
Nonoxynol-9	18	29
Fertility awareness methods		
Standard Days	4.75	12
TwoDay	3.5	14
Symptomothermal	2	
Postovulation	1	
Lactational amenorrhea	0.45	2.45
Coitus interruptus/withdrawal	4	27
Combined hormonal contraceptives		
Combined oral contraceptives (OCs)	0.3	8
Contraceptive patch	0.3	8
Vaginal contraceptive ring	0.3	8
Progestin-Only contraceptives		
Progestin-only pills (POPs)	0.3	8
Depot medroxyprogesterone acetate	0.3	3
Contraceptive Implant	0	0.1
Intrauterine contraceptives		
Copper-T380A	0.6	0.8
Levonorgestrel intrauterine system	0.1	0.1
Sterilization		
Tubal ligation	0.5	0.5
Essure	0	<1
Vasectomy	0.10	0.15

Data from Arevelo et al., 2002, 2004; Harrison-Woolrych and Hill, 2005; Palmer and Greenberg, 2009; Perez et al., 1992; Trussel, 2004; and van der Wijden et al., 2003.

rubber. Modern condoms are most often made of latex or polyurethane, but those made from animal intestine do still exist. Polyurethane condoms provide increased sensitivity for male partners, but the breakage and slippage rates are significantly higher (relative risk, 6.6 for breakage and 6.0 for slippage) compared with latex condoms (Frezieres et al., 1998) (Level of evidence: A). This suggests that latex condoms should be encouraged except for those with latex allergy/sensitivity.

Advantages

Male condoms can decrease the transmission of STIs, including human immunodeficiency virus (HIV), when used correctly and consistently.

Disadvantages

To obtain maximum protection from pregnancy and STIs, condoms must be used correctly with every act of intercourse. Those individuals with an allergy or sensitivity to latex should avoid these condoms. Some men report decreased sensitivity with condom use. A new condom must be used for each act of intercourse.

Female Condom

The female condom is a thin polyurethane sheath with a ring on each end. It can be inserted into the vagina up to 8 hours before intercourse. It should not be used simultaneously with a male condom because of possible breakage or slippage of either device.

Advantages

Female condoms can decrease the transmission of STIs, including HIV, when used correctly and consistently. Many women prefer having direct control over a barrier device. The female condom can be placed in advance of intercourse, increasing spontaneity.

Disadvantages

To obtain maximum protection from pregnancy and STIs, condoms must be used correctly with every act of intercourse. Some women may experience vaginal irritation. A new condom must be used for each act of intercourse.

Cervical Cap and Diaphragm

Diaphragms are dome-shaped devices made from silicone or latex. Diaphragms come in a range of sizes and require a fitting and prescription from a health care provider. Diaphragms are used in conjunction with spermicide, can be placed in the vagina up to 6 hours before intercourse, and should be left in place for at least 6 hours after the last act of intercourse, but no longer than 24 hours. Subsequent acts of intercourse require insertion of additional spermicide without device removal.

A silicone cervical cap (FemCap) was approved by the U.S. Food and Drug Administration (FDA) in 2003. It is reusable, and the design includes a domed cap that completely covers the cervix and a brim that forms a seal against the vaginal wall, funneling the ejaculate into a groove between the dome and the brim that faces the vaginal opening, storing the spermicide and trapping sperm. It comes in three sizes: for nulliparas, for women who have been pregnant but did not deliver vaginally, and for women who have delivered a full-term infant vaginally. It requires a fitting and prescription from a health care provider. The cervical cap is used in conjunction with spermicide and should be left in place for at least 6 hours after the last act of intercourse, but no longer than 48 hours. Subsequent acts of intercourse require insertion of additional spermicide without device removal.

Advantages

Many women prefer having direct control over a barrier device. Diaphragms and cervical caps can be placed in advance of intercourse, increasing spontaneity. These methods may offer some protection against cervical infections and pelvic inflammatory disease (PID) but offer no protection against HIV.

Disadvantages

Diaphragms and cervical caps should be used in conjunction with spermicide, which may cause irritation in some individuals. Those individuals with an allergy or sensitivity to latex should avoid those diaphragms. The incidence of urinary tract infections (UTIs) may increase.

Contraceptive Sponge

The Today sponge was reintroduced to the U.S. market in 2005. It is a polyurethane sponge that contains 1 g of nonoxynol-9 spermicide. There is a dimple on one side that fits over the cervix and a loop on the opposite side to aid in removal. It is available over the counter (OTC) and is effective for up to 24 hours, regardless of the number of times intercourse takes place. It should be left in place for at least 6 hours after intercourse, but no longer than 30 hours. Each sponge can be used only once.

Advantages

Many women prefer having direct control over a barrier device. The contraceptive sponge may offer some protection against cervical infections and PID but offer no protection against HIV.

Disadvantages

Some individuals may experience sensitivity to the spermicide. Some women may experience vaginal dryness or an increased incidence of yeast infections, particularly if the sponge is left in place for longer periods.

Spermicides

Mechanism of Action

Nonoxynol-9 is a nonionic detergent that disrupts the membranes of epithelial cells, bacteria, and viruses. It reduces sperm motility and reduces nourishment by disrupting fructolytic activity. It is available OTC in many forms, including gels, foams, and film. Although shown to inactivate many sexually transmitted pathogens in vitro, in actual use, nonoxynol-9 does not reduce rates of HIV, gonorrhea, or chlamydial infections when used with latex condoms (Roddy et al., 1998) (Level A).

Advantages

Many women prefer having direct control over contraception. Spermicides may be placed in advance of intercourse, increasing spontaneity, and can be used with barrier devices to increase efficacy.

Disadvantages

Some individuals may experience sensitivity to spermicide. Fresh spermicide should be placed with each act of intercourse.

Fertility Awareness Methods

Fertility awareness methods (FAMs) rely on a woman's awareness of when she is most likely to conceive, with abstinence or use of barrier contraceptives during that time.

Advantages

Women with religious or cultural reasons for not using contraception can use FAMs to avoid intercourse during fertile times. There are no medical contraindications to using these methods, and when used in reverse, FAMs can help a couple conceive a wanted pregnancy.

Disadvantages

A couple must be highly motivated to avoid intercourse during fertile times, which can also be a time of increased libido. The signs of ovulation/fertile periods can be subtle, so it may take time to master these methods. Even women with regular cycles experience cycle variability, and these methods are not reliable in women with irregular cycles.

Calendar Method

A woman records her cycles prospectively for 6 to 12 months to determine her cycle length. Using the longest and shortest cycle lengths during this time, and assuming that ovulation occurs 14 days before menses and that sperm can survive for 2 to 3 days, the fertile period is calculated. A simplified version of the calendar method, the Standard Days Method, eliminates the need for extended cycle evaluation before use. For women in whom most cycles are 28 to 32 days long, intercourse is avoided on cycle days 8 to 19 (Arevelo et al., 2002). CycleBeads are a set of color-coded beads that can be used to help a woman keep track of her cycles.

Ovulation Method

The ovulation method requires a woman to check her cervical mucus manually to detect the changes that occur during fertile periods, then avoid intercourse during these times. A simplified, TwoDay method requires that a woman ask herself two questions: "Did I notice secretions today?" and "Did I notice secretions yesterday?" If the answer is "no" for 2 consecutive days, it is safe to have intercourse (Arevelo et al., 2004).

Basal Body Temperature

Women must take their temperature each morning before arising and record it on a chart. This temperature can increase noticeably (by 0.4°-0.8° F) with ovulation and indicates times when intercourse should be avoided or barrier contraceptives used.

Symptomothermal Method

The symptomothermal method combines fertility awareness indicators (basal body temperature, changes in cervical mucus, libido, or cervical texture) to help a woman recognize her fertile days and avoid intercourse or use barrier methods during that time.

Postovulation Method

The postovulation method allows intercourse only after signs of ovulation have resolved.

Lactational Amenorrhea Method

The lactational amenorrhea method (LAM) refers to a specific set of circumstances under which a lactating woman does not ovulate and thus cannot conceive. This method is extremely effective, but only if all the following conditions exist (Kennedy and Visness, 1992; LevelA):

1. The woman is exclusively breastfeeding an infant with both day and night feedings, so that 90% or more of the infant's nutrition is from breast milk.
2. The infant is less than 6 months old.
3. The woman is amenorrheic (except for spotting during first 8 weeks postpartum)

Once these specific conditions no longer exist, other contraceptive methods should be considered.

Mechanism of Action

Lactation causes a surge in prolactin, which inhibits ovulation.

Advantages

Breastfeeding provides excellent nutrition for infants and can aid in maternal weight loss, as well as decrease the risk for endometrial, ovarian, and possibly breast cancer.

Disadvantages

It is important to understand that ovulation will often precede the first menses in postpartum women, leaving them susceptible to pregnancy. This risk increases with time since delivery (Zieman et al., 2007). Some women may find long-term breastfeeding difficult or inconvenient.

Coitus Interruptus/Withdrawal

The male partner completely removes the penis from the vagina before ejaculation. Withdrawal reduces or eliminates sperm introduction into the vagina and thus the upper reproductive tract. Unless two acts of intercourse are close together, there is little concern for the presence of sperm in preejaculatory secretions (Zeiman et al, 2007).

The advantages are affordability and ready availability. The disadvantages are that coitus interruptus relies on the male partner to predict imminent ejaculation and quickly and completely remove the penis from the vagina and introitus. Withdrawal also may limit orgasmic pleasure and spontaneity.

Combined Hormonal Contraceptives

Key Points

- When used correctly and consistently, CHCs are very effective in preventing pregnancy.
- CHCs offer many noncontraceptive health benefits, such as increased cycle regularity, decreased risk of endometrial and ovarian cancers, and decreased PMS/PMDD.
- CHCs have not been shown to cause significant weight gain.
- The contraceptive patch and vaginal contraceptive ring can increase perfect-use compliance by decreasing dosing frequency.
- Ethinyl estradiol levels are higher in women using the contraceptive patch than in those using OCs or the ring, but there is no evidence of increased risk of venous thromboembolism.
- The patch may have decreased efficacy in women weighing more than 90 kg.

Mechanism of Action

Combined (or combination) hormonal contraceptives (CHCs) contain both an estrogen (ethinyl estradiol) and one of many progestins, which act in concert to suppress ovulation. This is achieved through negative feedback on the hypothalamic-pituitary system, leading to decreased gonadotropin-releasing hormone (GnRH) pulsatility, decreased pituitary responsiveness to GnRH stimulation, suppression of luteinizing hormone (LH) and follicle-stimulating hormone (FSH) production, and inhibition of the midcycle LH surge (Nelson et al., 2007). In addition, the progestin component causes thickening of the cervical mucus, which can inhibit sperm access to the upper genital tract.

Oral Contraceptives

Combined oral contraceptives (COCs, OCs), often referred to as "the pill," are the most common form of reversible contraception used in the United States (Chandra et al., 2005). Many formulations exist, with varying amounts of ethinyl estradiol and differing progestins. Newer formulations with 4-day pill-free intervals (vs. traditional 7 days), can offer increased relief from hormonal side effects (Sulak et al., 2000) and increased suppression of ovarian activity (Spona et al., 1996).

Advantages

The CHCs are very effective in preventing pregnancy when used correctly and consistently. OCs help to regulate menses, decrease menstrual flow and dysmenorrhea, and eliminate mittelschmerz. Certain formulations can be used to treat *premenstrual dysphoric disorder* (PMDD) (Lopez et al., 2009). Rapid return to fertility follows discontinuation of OCs. No

---

Box 26-1 Contraindications to Estrogen Use

- Smoker (≥15 cigarettes/day) ≥35 years old
- Active liver disease
- History of breast cancer
- Breast feeding (<6 weeks postpartum)
- Migraine with aura
- Uncontrolled hypertension
- History of clotting disorder
- Known thrombogenic mutations
- SLE with positive or unknown antiphospholipid antibodies
- Diabetes with vascular disease/retinopathy/neuropathy/nephropathy
- Major surgery with prolonged immobilization
- Multiple risk factors for CV disease/stroke
- DVT/PE (history of, acute, or established on anticoagulant therapy)
- Complicated valvular heart disease
- History of COC-related cholestasis or current gallbladder disease

---

evidence exists for significant weight gain in women taking CHCs. OCs may help reduce acne and may be used as emergency contraception with alternate dosing. Use of CHCs decreases benign breast disease, risk of ovarian and endometrial cancers, and risk of death from colorectal cancer (Zieman et al., 2007).

Disadvantages

Women must remember every day to follow the regimen for OCs to be effective. CHCs may cause spotting, breast tenderness, nausea, or headaches, especially in the first few months of use, as well as decreased libido. OCs offer no protection against STIs and cannot be used by women with contraindications to estrogen use (Box 26-1).

Contraceptive Patch

The contraceptive patch (OrthoEvra) is a 4.5-cm² adhesive patch placed on the upper arm, abdomen, back, or buttocks that provides 20 μg of ethinyl estradiol and 150 μg of norelgestromin daily. The patch is changed every 7 days for 3 weeks, with a patch-free week during which a woman is expected to menstruate. Steady-state hormone levels are achieved after 3 days, and there is enough hormone for up to 10 days' use (Abrams et al., 2002).

Advantages

Weekly dosing may offer increased compliance with correct use compared with COC use (Lopez et al., 2008). Sustained therapeutic hormone levels past the recommended 7 days for each patch give women leeway if they forget to change the patch on time. Other advantages are similar to those for COCs, although data on cancer and other noncontraceptive health benefits are not yet available.

Disadvantages

Overall, the contraceptive patch is similar to COCs, although the rate of side effects may be higher (Lopez et al., 2008). Localized skin reactions may occur. Decreased efficacy is noted in women weighing more than 90 kg (198 lb) (Nanda, 2007). Ethinyl estradiol concentrations are higher in women using the contraceptive patch than in those using either COCs

or the vaginal ring (van den Heuvel et al., 2005), raising concern for an increased risk of venous thromboembolism (VTE) or other cardiovascular events. However, the risk of nonfatal VTE for the contraceptive patch is actually similar to that for COCs with 35 μg of ethinyl estradiol (odds ratio 0.9; 95% CI 0.5-1.6) (Jick et al., 2006; Level A). Also, the risk of VTE with pregnancy remains much higher than with CHC use.

Vaginal Contraceptive Ring

NuvaRing is a flexible, colorless ring 4 mm thick and 5.4 cm in diameter. It is placed into the vagina and provides 15 μg of ethinyl estradiol and 120 μg of etonorgestrel daily. Each ring is left in place for 3 weeks, followed by a ring-free week during which a woman is expected to menstruate. Ovulation suppression begins within 3 days of use and continues for up to 35 days while the ring is in place (Nanda, 2007).

Advantages

Monthly dosing with the vaginal ring may increase compliance with correct use compared with COCs (Nanda, 2007). Sustained therapeutic hormone levels past the 21-day recommendation for each ring give women leeway if they forget to change the ring on time. The ring may be removed for up to 3 hours for intercourse, although this is not recommended because most women and their partners are not bothered by its presence. Other advantages are similar to those for COCs, although again, data on cancer and other noncontraceptive health benefits are not yet available.

Disadvantages

Overall, drawbacks to vaginal ring use are similar to COC use. Although rates of breast discomfort, nausea, and vomiting may be decreased, rates of vaginitis and leukorrhea may increase compared with COCs (Lopez et al., 2008).

Progestin-Only Contraceptives

Key Points

- Progestin-only contraceptives are very effective in preventing pregnancy when used correctly and consistently.
- Women with contraindications to estrogen use may safely use POPs.
- Overall, menstrual blood loss is decreased, but bleeding may be unscheduled or irregular.
- Longer-acting formulations may increase perfect-use compliance by decreasing dosing frequency.
- The effect of DMPA on weight gain is variable.
- Although prolonged DMPA use may decrease bone mineral density, this is reversible after discontinuation, and it is not associated with future fractures or osteoporosis.

Mechanism of Action

All progestin-only contraceptive methods act to thicken cervical mucus, thereby inhibiting sperm access to the upper genital tract. They also cause slowing of tubal motility and atrophy of the endometrium. Some methods act to suppress LH and FSH surges, inhibiting ovulation (Zieman et al., 2007).

Progestin-Only Pills

The sole progestin-only pill (POP, often called the "minipill") currently available in the United States contains 35 mg of nor-ethindrone. This pill is taken daily, without a pill-free interval. The main contraceptive effect is through thickening of cervical mucus; ovulation suppression occurs in only 50% of cycles.

Advantages

The POP is very effective in preventing pregnancy when used correctly and consistently. Benefits include decreased menstrual flow and dysmenorrhea, with rapid return to fertility. POPs may be used by women who desire an OC but have a contraindication to estrogen use.

Disadvantages

Main contraceptive effect begins to wane after 22 hours and is gone by 27 hours, so women who are more than 3 hours late with dosing need to use backup contraception. Although overall blood loss is decreased, bleeding or spotting may be irregular or unscheduled. POPs offer no protection against STIs, although infections of the ascending genital tract may be decreased because of thickened cervical mucus (Zieman et al., 2007).

Depot Medroxyprogesterone Acetate (DMPA)

A crystalline suspension, DMPA is injected every 3 months either intramuscularly (150 mg) or subcutaneously (104 mg). Its main contraceptive effect is through ovulation suppression.

Advantages

The convenient dosing schedule of DMPA can increase perfect-use compliance. Advantages include decreased menstrual flow, dysmenorrhea, and elimination of mittelschmerz. DMPA can improve pain from endometriosis and may be used by women with contraindications to estrogen use. It reduces the risk of endometrial and possibly ovarian cancer, as well as significantly decreasing sickle cell crises. DMPA can reduce the number of seizures in women with seizure disorders (Westhoff, 2003). No evidence indicates decreased efficacy in obese women (Goldberg and Grimes, 2007).

Disadvantages

Although overall blood loss is decreased, bleeding and spotting may be irregular or unscheduled. The high amenorrhea rate (>50%) may concern some women. Return to fertility may be delayed (average, 10 months from last injection). Patients often express concerns about weight gain, which is actually quite variable, with no studies showing a consistent impact on weight (Westhoff, 2003) (Level A). Although osteoporosis may develop with prolonged DMPA use because of decreased estradiol levels, bone mineral density (BMD) appears to recover completely after discontinuation, and BMD changes during DMPA therapy have not been linked to fractures or postmenopausal osteoporosis (Goldberg and Grimes, 2007).

Contraceptive Implant

The only contraceptive implant currently available in the United States is Implanon, a single rod 4 cm long and 2 mm wide made of ethylene vinylacetate (EVA) co-polymer and containing 68 mg of time-release etonogestrel. It is placed subdermally by a health care provider and acts primarily by ovulation inhibition. Although FDA approved for 3 years' use, the implant has proven efficacy to at least 4 years (Isly and Edelman, 2007).

Advantages

The contraceptive implant is one of the most effective forms of available contraception, with rapid return to fertility; most women ovulate within 4 weeks of removal (Isly and Edelman, 2007). Benefits include decreased menstrual flow, dysmenorrhea, and elimination of mittelschmerz. The implant can improve pain from endometriosis and may be used by women with contraindication to estrogen use. No effect on BMD is seen.

Disadvantages

The woman must see a health care provider for implant initiation and discontinuation. Although overall blood loss is decreased, bleeding and spotting may be irregular or unscheduled. Amenorrhea may concern some women. The implant provides no protection against STIs and may be associated with headaches or increased acne.

Intrauterine Contraceptives

Key Points

- IUCs are among the most effective forms of contraception available.
- Although preventing fertilization, IUCs are not abortifacients.
- Adolescents can safely use IUCs but underuse this method.
- The levonorgestrel IUC is an effective treatment for menorrhagia and can decrease the risk of ascending genital tract infections.
- IUCs do not increase the risk of PID outside the first 20 days after insertion.
- The copper-T380A IUD can be used as emergency contraception.

Intrauterine contraceptives (IUCs) are small, T-shaped devices inserted into the uterine cavity by a medical provider. IUCs provide excellent long-term, reversible contraception. The two IUCs currently available in the United States are the copper-T380A intrauterine device (IUD) (TCu380A, Paragard) and the levonorgestrel intrauterine system (LNG-IUS, Mirena). In 2007 the American College of Obstetricians and Gynecologists (ACOG) concluded that modern IUCs are an excellent contraceptive choice for adolescents and are underused by this population. Contrary to popular belief, both IUCs act by inhibiting fertilization and are not abortifacients (Grimes, 2007; WHO, 1987) (Level A).

Copper-T380A Intrauterine Device

The TCu380A (Paragard in U.S.) is a polyethylene IUD with copper wire wound on the stem and copper sleeves on each of the arms, for a total of 380 mm^2 of exposed copper surface area. Although FDA approved for 10 years' use, it has proved efficacious for at least 12 years (UN/WHO, 1997) (Level A).

Mechanism of Action

Copper ions released from this IUD act as a spermicide to inhibit sperm motility and the acrosomal enzyme reaction. In addition, increased macrophages in tubal and uterine fluids act to phagocytize sperm.

Advantages

Among the most effective forms of contraception available, IUCs are long acting but easily reversible, with rapid return to fertility. Nonhormonal methods may be preferable to some women. IUCs may be used by those with a contraindication to estrogen use. IUDs decrease the risk of endometrial and possibly cervical cancer (Hubacher and Grimes, 2002). IUCs can be used as emergency contraception.

Disadvantages

The IUC must be placed and removed by a health care provider. IUCs may cause increased menstrual bleeding and dysmenorrhea. The IUD does not offer protection against STIs. There is increased risk of upper tract infection the first 20 days after insertion, but otherwise no increased risk of PID (Grimes and Schulz, 1999) (Level A).

Levonorgestrel Intrauterine System

The LNG-IUS (Mirena in U.S.) contains a steroid reservoir around the stem that releases 20 µg of levonorgestrel per day into the uterine cavity. Although FDA approved for 5 years' use, it has proven efficacy for at least 7 years (Sivin et al., 1991) (Level A).

Mechanism of Action

The main mechanism of action of the LNG-IUS is thickening of the cervical mucus, which blocks sperm access to the upper genital tract. In addition, changes in tubal fluid can impair both sperm and egg motility. There is occasional inhibition of ovulation (~20% of cycles).

Advantages

Among the most effective forms of contraception available, the LNG-IUS is long acting but easily reversible, with rapid return to fertility. Benefits include decreased menstrual flow and dysmenorrhea and effective treatment for menorrhagia. Thickened cervical mucus may contribute to decreased risk of ascending cervical infections (decreased rates of PID), especially in patients under 25 years old (Toivonen et al., 1991). The IUS may be used by women with contraindication to estrogen use. It decreases the risk of endometrial and possibly cervical cancer (Hubacher and Grimes, 2002).

Disadvantages

The LVG-IUS must be placed and removed by a health care provider. Amenorrhea may concern some women. It offers no protection against cervicitis or viral STIs. Risk of upper tract infection is increased in the first 20 days after insertion, but otherwise there is no increased risk of PID (Grimes and Schulz, 1999) (Level A). Some women may experience mild hormonal side effects, including headaches, breast discomfort, and acne.

Sterilization

Key Points

- Sterilization is one of the most effective forms of contraception but is permanent.

- Regret rates are higher for men and women who are young at sterilization, so counseling is key.
- Tubal ligation increases the risk of ectopic pregnancy if it fails; vasectomy does not.

Sterilization is the most common form of contraception in the United States, relied on by 23% of contraceptive-using women (Chandra et al., 2005).

Mechanism of Action

Sterilization creates a physical disruption in either the male (vas deferens) or female (fallopian tube) reproductive tract, thereby preventing fertilization.

Tubal Ligation

Traditional tubal occlusion can be accomplished by the laparoscopic placement of clips or Silastic bands or by tubal cautery. Alternatively, a mini-laparotomy may be performed for a partial salpingectomy. The Essure device was approved for use in the United States in 2002. This is a coil device made of stainless steel and nickel-titanium that is inserted transcervically into the tubal ostia, avoiding the need for general anesthesia. Placement causes an inflammatory response in the tubes, leading to dense fibrosis and tubal occlusion (Ogburn and Espey, 2007).

Advantages

Tubal ligation is a permanent, highly effective form of contraception that requires little to no follow-up.

Disadvantages

Tubal ligation requires a surgical procedure; some women may be poor surgical candidates. It does not protect against STIs and carries an increased risk of ectopic pregnancy if ligation fails. It is irreversible; achieving pregnancy after sterilization is costly and involves either additional surgery or in vitro fertilization. The Essure device requires use of another contraceptive for 3 months, or until tubal occlusion is confirmed by hysterosalpingogram. Regret rates are 20% for women 30 and younger at the time of sterilization, but only 6% for those over 30 (Pollack et al., 2007). Counseling is key.

Vasectomy

Vasectomy is a quick procedure, usually performed under local anesthesia in 5 to 10 minutes. The no-scalpel technique involves puncturing the scrotum to deliver the vas deferens, which is then ligated or cauterized.

Advantages

Vasectomy is a permanent, highly effective form of contraception that requires minimal follow-up. It is safer and more effective than female sterilization and does not increase risk of ectopic pregnancy if it fails. Vasectomy allows the male partner to have a role in contraception.

Disadvantages

A surgical procedure is required. Vasectomy does not protect against STIs and requires use of another contraceptive method for about 12 weeks, until azoospermia is confirmed. It is irreversible; achieving pregnancy after sterilization requires additional surgery and can be hampered by the development of antisperm antibodies. Regret rates are highest in men who, at sterilization, are less than 31 years old, are in an unstable marriage, have no or very young children, and are in a time of financial crisis (Pollack et al., 2007). Vasectomy rarely leads to chronic testicular pain.

Emergency Contraception

Emergency contraception refers to methods a woman can use after unprotected intercourse to decrease the chance of pregnancy. There are two categories: emergency contraceptive pills (ECPs) and the copper-T380A IUD. The only contraindication to emergency contraception is pregnancy. ECPs are ineffective once pregnancy is established, but will not harm an existing pregnancy. IUD placement may disrupt a pregnancy or increase the risk of serious infection and septic abortion.

Emergency Contraceptive Pills

Modern emergency contraception began with the Yuzpe regimen in the 1970s. This regimen consists of 100 μg ethinyl estradiol and 0.5 mg of levonorgestrel or 1 mg norgestrel taken within 72 hours of unprotected intercourse, followed by a repeat dose 12 hours later. This was initially accomplished by taking high doses of COCs, but began to be marketed as a specific product, Preven, in 1998 (Stewart et al., 2007). This method has a failure/pregnancy rate of 2-3%, with an average 74% reduction in the number of expected pregnancies when used (Trussel et al., 1996). Side effects are common, with about 50% of women experiencing nausea and 20% vomiting from the high doses of estrogen. Subsequent research has led to the preferred use of other EC methods, and Preven was pulled from the market in 2004.

A 1998 study by the WHO Task Force on Postovulatory Methods of Fertility Regulation compared two doses of 0.75 mg of levonorgestrel given 12 hours apart to the Yuzpe regimen. The levonorgestrel-only method was both better tolerated and more effective than the Yuzpe regimen, with a failure/pregnancy rate of 1.1% and an 85% reduction in the number of expected pregnancies. In 1999 the FDA approved Plan B, which contains two 0.75-mg tablets of levonorgestrel. A single 1.5-mg dose of levonorgestrel taken up to 5 days after unprotected intercourse seems to be equally effective at pregnancy prevention (von Hertzen et al, 2002) (Level A). Plan B One-Step, a single pill containing 1.5 mg of levonorgestrel, is currently available.

Mechanism of Action

Treatment with levonorgestrel before ovulation inhibits the LH surge and therefore ovulation. If taken after ovulation, ECPs have little effect on hormone production and only a limited effect on the endometrium (Marions et al., 2002). Therefore, levonorgestrel for emergency contraception works by inhibiting ovulation; *it is not an abortifacient.*

Copper-T380A Intrauterine Device

The TCu380A IUD can be inserted up to 8 days after unprotected intercourse, and is the most effective form of emergency contraception, with a failure/pregnancy rate of about 0.1% (Zieman et al., 2007). Its mechanism of action likely involves the spermicidal activity seen in contraception, but the very high efficacy suggests that it may also interfere with implantation of a fertilized egg (Stewart et al., 2007). Insertion of the TCu380A IUD offers the additional benefit of providing continued contraception.

Conclusion

Many contraceptive methods are available to patients, and physicians should routinely counsel patients interested in contraception. Information and facts should be provided in an impartial, culturally sensitive, and customized manner, with the final decision made by the patient with support from the physician. Frequent follow-up and questioning about side effects and satisfaction with the chosen contraceptive method ensure an informed and involved patient.

References

The complete reference list is available online at www.expertconsult.com.

Web Resources

www.acog.org/publications/patient_education/
> Good examples of educational pamphlets for patients that providers can order. Can be ordered from providers

http://oregon.gov/DHS/ph/fp/edmat.shtml
> Posters, brochures and fact sheets on contraceptive methods. Sent for free to offices. Can be downloaded

www.apgo.org/elearn/modules/cpcm/
> Monograph and learning module about counseling on and management of contraception from the Association of Professors of Obstetrics and Gynecology

www.arhp.org
> Website for the Association of Reproductive Health Professionals – an excellent source of information and references on many reproductive health topics.

www.who.int/reproductivehealth/publications/family_planning/en/index.html
> World Health Organization website featuring publications in the area of family planning.

www.cdc.gov/mmwr/pdf/rr/rr59e0528.pdf
> The document on this website provides the latest (2010) U.S. medical eligibility criteria for contraceptive use.

Cardiovascular Disease

Peter P. Toth, Nicolas W. Shammas, Eric J. Dippel, and Blair Foreman

Chapter contents

Cardiovascular disease (CVD) is the leading cause of morbidity and mortality for both men and women in the United States. Enormous efforts are being made to stem the physical, emotional, and socioeconomic costs associated with the epidemic of cardiovascular diseases throughout the world. Almost 80,000,000 Americans have some form of CVD, and it was responsible for 34% of all mortality in 2006 (American Heart Association, 2010). Approximately 2300 people die from CVD daily in the United States (1 death every 38 seconds). The prevalence of various cardiovascular diseases in the U.S. is impressive, with 74 million people afflicted with *hypertension* (HTN); more than 16.8 million with *coronary artery disease* (CAD); 5.7 million with *congestive heart failure* (CHF); 6.5 million having a history of *stroke* (CVA); 1 million patients with a history of congenital heart disease; 8 to 12 million with *peripheral arterial disease* (PAD); and 2.2 million with atrial fibrillation. Unfortunately, 20.8% of the American population (47.1 million people) still smokes. Two thirds of the American population is afflicted with being overweight or obese. It is estimated that in 2009 the direct and indirect costs associated with the management of CVD will exceed $475 billion. In addition to the costs of pharmacologic intervention and lost productivity, some of this cost is also driven by a large number of cardiovascular procedures, including: 1,313,000 angioplasties; 1,115,000 diagnostic cardiac catheterizations; 448,000 coronary artery bypass graft (CABG) procedures; and the implantation of 199,000 pacemakers and 63,000 implantable defibrillators.

Detailed guidelines by professional societies and national commissions are being issued and continuously reevaluated and updated so as to optimize the management of risk factors and established forms of disease. Despite these efforts, compliance with guidelines remains relatively low throughout the world. As populations age worldwide, as more patients survive acute cardiovascular and cerebrovascular events, and as the incidence of hypertension, dyslipidemia, metabolic syndrome, diabetes mellitus, obesity, and other risk factors continues to increase, the burden on family physicians to identify and effectively manage CVD will continue to escalate dramatically. This chapter addresses issues related to CVD prevention; diagnosing and managing the various manifestations of atherosclerotic disease, valvular dysfunction, congestive heart failure, and cardiomyopathy; pericardial disease; and arrhythmia identification and management.

Atherosclerosis

Atherosclerosis is a complex, multifactorial disease highly prevalent throughout the world. Atherosclerotic disease is etiologic for acute coronary syndromes such as myocardial infarction (MI) and unstable angina, ischemic stroke, renal arterial stenosis, and peripheral vascular disease (Libby, 2001). The development and progression of atherosclerosis is driven by a variety of risk factors, including dyslipidemia, hypertension, impairments in glycemic control, age, family history, cigarette smoking, obesity, and systemic inflammation. Novel risk factors are being recognized and their utility for identifying patients at risk for disease tested in epidemiologic and clinical trial settings. Evaluating patients for global cardiovascular risk burden and aggressively treating modifiable risk factors are a significant focus of any primary care setting.

Atherogenesis is no longer viewed as an inevitable consequence of passive, progressive lipid accumulation within the arterial wall, gradually resulting in symptomatic reductions in blood flow and oxygen delivery. Instead, *atherosclerosis* is a dynamic process encompassing a diverse array of biochemical and histologic changes that continuously modulate the establishment and evolution of atheromatous plaque (Libby et al., 2002; Hansson, 2005). Atheromatous plaque is modifiable, and therapeutic interventions can stabilize and even regress plaque, resulting in reductions in risk for cardiovascular morbidity and mortality.

Endothelial cell dysfunction is an early hallmark of atherogenesis (Toth, 2009). The endothelium is now viewed as an organ system. Endothelial cells line the luminal surface of blood vessels and mediate vascular tone and molecular trafficking into the vessel wall. When endothelium is stressed by rheologic disturbances, increased inflammatory or oxidative insult, glycemic injury, hyperlipidemia and hypertension, its functional characteristics change. Dysfunctional endothelium has less vasodilatory capacity, is more thrombogenic, and upregulates the expression of a variety of *cell adhesion molecules* (CAMs), such as vascular cell adhesion molecule-1 (VCAM-1) and intercellular adhesion molecule-1 (ICAM-1) (Lusis, 2000). CAMs promote the binding of monocytes, T cells, and mast cells to the endothelial surface. Bound inflammatory white blood cells (WBCs) then follow a gradient of monocyte chemoattractant protein-1 and other cytokines by intercalating between endothelial cells and ultimately transmigrate into the subendothelial space. Once in the subendothelial space, these WBCs take up residence, creating an inflammatory nidus. Monocytes can convert to macrophages in response to macrophage colony-stimulating

factor. Inflammatory WBCs are potent sources of oxygen free radicals such as superoxide anion, peroxide, and hydroxyl radicals. These reactive oxygen species can oxidize phospholipids within lipoproteins, rendering them more atherogenic. When exposed to oxidatively modified atherogenic lipoproteins, macrophages upregulate the expression of cell surface scavenger receptors (e.g., CD36, scavenger receptor A), which promote the internalization of cholesterol and cholesterol esters, resulting in the formation of foam cells. *Foam cells* coalesce to form fatty streaks, the histologic precursor to atheromatous plaques. Resident macrophages, T cells, and mast cells facilitate additional WBC recruitment and progression of atherosclerotic disease by producing a variety of cytokines, interleukins, and oxidative enzymes that adversely impact endothelial, smooth muscle cell, and fibroblast function and proliferation.

With disease progression, the molecular and histologic dynamics of *atheromatous plaque* remain in continuous flux. As foam cells die, cellular debris accumulates and further potentiates the inflammatory response (Tabas, 2005). Matrix metalloproteinases are expressed, which degrade the collagen, elastin, and proteoglycan extracellular matrix of plaque. When this occurs in the shoulder region of a plaque, acute rupture or plaque fissuring can result. Sudden plaque rupture exposes collagen, tissue factor, and the thrombogenic lipid core to platelets and coagulation factors, ultimately resulting in overlying thrombus formation, luminal obstruction, acute ischemia, and possible infarction if tissue blood flow is not rapidly reestablished. Atheromatous plaques that are highly inflamed and contain concentrated macrophage infiltrates or large lipid cores are particularly vulnerable to architectural destabilization and acute plaque rupture. Plaque can also suddenly distend and reduce coronary luminal diameter from sudden intraplaque hemorrhaging if the delicate vasa vasorum feeding the surrounding vascular tissue is injured.

In the majority of cases, culprit lesions giving rise to acute MI are not flow limiting. Any atheromatous plaque identified on coronary angiography should be viewed as a potential cause of an *acute coronary syndrome* (ACS). Patients with evidence of atherosclerotic disease in any portion of the vascular tree require rigorous evaluation of all risk factors and the appropriate institution of lifestyle and pharmacologic intervention to reduce risk for both disease progression and cardiovascular morbidity and mortality.

Dyslipidemia

Key Points

- Patients undergoing screening for dyslipidemia should have a complete fasting lipid profile.
- LDL and non-HDL (total cholesterol – HDL) are atherogenic and have defined targets for therapy based on global risk factor burden.
- LDL-C is currently the primary target of therapy in patients with dyslipidemia, although non-HDL-C or apoB100 may become the next primary target of therapy.
- HDL is antiatherogenic, and when less than 40 mg/dL in men and 50 mg/dL in women, therapeutic effort should be made to raise HDL.
- Therapeutic lifestyle changes are an important component of any regimen designed to treat dyslipidemia.

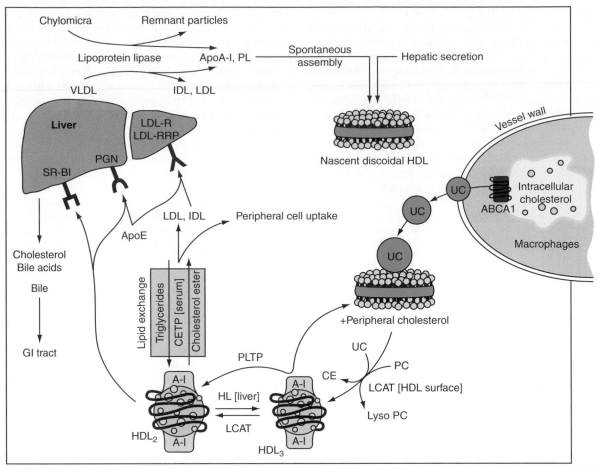

Figure 27-1 Molecular and histologic pathways for reverse cholesterol transport. To deliver peripheral cholesterol back to the liver or steroidogenic organs such as the adrenal glands, placenta, or ovaries, apoA-I and nascent discoidal HDL interact with cells such as macrophages and foam cells within blood vessel walls. The HDL undergoes a series of cell receptor–dependent and serum enzyme–dependent maturation and speciation reactions (HDL speciation). HDL can interact directly with a variety of hepatocyte surface receptors, including SR-BI. The cholesterol esters in HDL can also be transported back to the liver by an indirect pathway for reverse cholesterol transport that depends on CETP and the LDL and LDL-RRP receptors. *ABCA1*, ATP-binding membrane cassette transporter A1; *apoA-I*, apoprotein A-I; *ApoE*, apoprotein E; *CE*, cholesteryl ester; *CETP*, cholesterol ester transfer protein; *GI*, gastrointestinal; *HDL*, high-density lipoprotein; *HL*, hepatic lipase; *IDL*, intermediate-density lipoprotein; *LCAT*, lecithin:cholesterol acyltransferase; *LDL*, low-density lipoprotein; *LDL-R*, low-density lipoprotein receptor; *LDL-RRP*, low-density lipoprotein receptor–related protein; *Lyso PC*, lysophosphatidylcholine; *PC*, phosphatidylcholine; *PGN*, proteoglycan; *PL*, phospholipid; *PLTP*, phospholipid transfer protein; *SR-BI*, scavenger receptor BI; *UC*, unesterified cholesterol; *VLDL*, very-low-density lipoprotein. *(Reproduced with permission from Toth PP. High-density lipoprotein as a therapeutic target: clinical evidence and treatment strategies. Am J Cardiol 2005;96:50K-58K.)*

Causes

Although it is pathogenic, *cholesterol* is also an important modulator of cell membrane fluidity and is a substrate for hormone biosynthesis by steroidogenic organs. There is an unequivocal relationship between dyslipidemia and risk for atherogenesis within the coronary, peripheral, renal, and cerebral vasculature. *Dyslipoproteinemias* develop in response to genetic and environmental factors and are modifiable through lifestyle modification and pharmacologic intervention. As demonstrated in the Framingham Study, Multiple Risk Factor Intervention Trial, and the Seven Countries Study, as serum levels of cholesterol increase, the risk for developing CAD increases. The identification and treatment of dyslipidemia lowers the prevalence of atherosclerotic disease and its various clinical manifestations.

Serum very-low-density lipoprotein (VLDL) and low-density lipoprotein (LDL) particles deliver cholesterol to peripheral tissues and blood vessel walls. These lipoproteins can cross the endothelial barrier and induce atherogenesis. Atherogenic lipoproteins not taken up by peripheral tissues are cleared from the circulation by hepatic LDL receptors.

Therapies targeted at the upregulation of hepatic LDL receptors are antiatherogenic by virtue of their ability to reduce circulating levels of atherogenic lipoproteins.

High-density lipoprotein (HDL) particles are antiatherogenic. With few exceptions, epidemiologic investigation has shown that high HDL levels reduce risk for the development of CAD (Toth, 2001, 2009). Consistent with this finding, patients with familial hypo-α-lipoproteinemia (low HDL) have increased risk for premature CAD, whereas patients with familial hyper-α-lipoproteinemia (high HDL) are relatively resistant to CAD (Toth, 2003, 2004). HDL extracts excess intracellular cholesterol from macrophages and delivers it back to the liver for elimination as bile salts through the gastrointestinal tract in a process referred to as "reverse cholesterol transport" (Fig. 27-1). HDL has also been shown to reduce endothelial CAM expression, augment endothelial nitric oxide and prostacyclin production, reduce oxidized LDL, decrease platelet aggregability, and inhibit endothelial cell apoptosis (programmed cell death). An HDL greater than 60 mg/dL is a "negative" risk factor. In general, the more

Table 27-1 Low-Density Lipoprotein (LDL) Cholesterol Goals and Thresholds for Initiating Therapeutic Lifestyle Change (TLC) and Pharmacologic Intervention

Risk Category*	LDL Goal	LDL Level to Initiate TLC	LDL Level to Consider Drug Therapy
CHD or CHD risk equivalents (10-year risk >20%)	<100 mg/dL (optional goal <70)†‡	≥100 mg/dL All patients regardless of LDL	≥130 mg/dL (100-129 mg/dL: drug optional) ≥100 mg/dL‡ (<100 mg/dL: drug optional)
2+ risk factors (10-year risk: 10%-20%)	<130 mg/dL (optional goal <100)	≥130 mg/d All patients regardless of LDL	≥130 mg/dL (> 100 mg/dL: drug optional‡)
2+ risk factors (10-year risk ≤10%)	<130 mg/dL	≥130 mg/dL	≥160 mg/dL
0-1 risk factor†	<160 mg/dL	≥160 mg/dL	≥190 mg/dL (160-189 mg/dL: LDL-lowering drug optional)

Based on Grundy SM, Cleeman JI, Merz CN, Brewer HB, et al. Implications of recent clinical trials for the National Cholesterol Education Program Adult Treatment Panel III guidelines. Circulation 2004;110: 227-239.

*Coronary heart (artery) disease (CHD, CAD) risk equivalents include diabetes mellitus, peripheral vascular disease, carotid artery disease, and abdorninal aortic aneurysm. Risk factors included in Framingham risk evaluation are age, systolic blood pressure, total cholesterol, HDL-C, and smoking status.

†The optional goal of less than 70 mg/dL is particularly targeted at patients who are "very high" risk (e.g., recent acute coronary syndrome, poorly controlled diabetes with multiple risk factors).

‡When initiating statin therapy in these patients, the goal for LDL-C reduction should be 30% to 40% from baseline.

Box 27-1 National Cholesterol Education Program Risk Factors

Negative

High-density lipoprotein cholesterol (HDL-C) >60 mg/dL

Positive

Cigarette smoking

HDL <40 mg/dL

Hypertension (BP >140/90 mm Hg, or use of antihypertensive agents)

Family history of premature coronary artery disease (CAD)

    CAD in male first-degree relative <55 years

    CAD in female first-degree relative <65 years

Age

    Men ≥45 years

    Women ≥55 years

elevated the level of serum HDL, the lower is the risk for CAD. Therapeutic interventions should not be targeted at reducing serum HDL. Although emerging evidence suggests that some patients may harbor HDL species that appear to be proinflammatory and pro-oxidative because of alterations in their protein and enzyme cargo (Ansell, 2006), treatment with some types of lipid-modifying agents appears to restore normal functionality to these HDL particles (Heinecke, 2009).

Dyslipidemia can be the result of abnormalities in gastrointestinal nutrient absorption, serum and intracellular enzyme activities, and/or cell surface receptor expression. A complete fasting (12-14 hours) lipoprotein profile (including LDL, triglyceride, and HDL) should be obtained on anyone screened for dyslipidemia. Because of the relationship between specific lipoprotein fractions and risk for CAD, measuring total cholesterol levels has little clinical relevance.

Risk Factors

The National Cholesterol Education Program Adult Treatment Panel III (NCEP ATP-III, 2001) has defined risk-stratified, evidence-based target levels for atherogenic serum lipoproteins (Table 27-1). CAD risk is stratified by evaluating a patient's cardiovascular risk factor burden (number of risk factors) and, if two or more risk factors are present, calculation of the Framingham risk score. In the setting of primary prevention, low risk is defined as 0-1 risk factor. Moderate and moderately high risk are defined as 2 or more risk factors with a 10-year Framingham risk of 5% to 10% and 10% to 20%, respectively. Patients who are in the high risk category either have CAD (previous history of MI, stable/unstable angina, revascularization with CABG or percutaneous coronary angioplasty) or a CAD *risk equivalent*, defined as diabetes mellitus, abdominal aortic aneurysm, peripheral vascular disease, significant carotid artery disease (transient ischemic attack or stroke from carotid origin, >50% obstructive atheromatous plaque in carotid artery), or a 10-year Framingham risk that exceeds 20%. The American Heart Association (AHA) also defines chronic kidney disease (glomerular filtration rate [GFR] <60 mL/min/1.73 m^2) as a CAD risk equivalent. It is important to calculate the Framingham risk score so as to differentiate moderate, moderately high, and high risk among patients with multiple risk factors and no history of CAD or a CAD risk equivalent. An electronic Framingham risk calculator can be downloaded at www.nhlbi.nih.gov/guidelines/cholesterol. Box 27-1 summarizes established CAD risk factors.

Targets

In ATP-III the NCEP implemented these conceptual changes: (1) an optimal LDL-C is defined as less than 100 mg/dL for all patients independent of race or gender; (2) an HDL less than 40 mg/dL is now defined as a categorical risk factor for CAD; and (3) it defined target levels for non-HDL-C. *Non-HDL-C* is defined as total cholesterol minus HDL-C and is an estimate of atherogenic lipoproteins in serum (VLDL + LDL). The risk-stratified target for non-HDL-C is the LDL-C target plus 30 (see Table 27-1). LDL-C reduction is the primary goal of therapy in patients with dyslipidemia. However, in patients with fasting *triglyceride* (TG) levels greater than 200 mg/dL, non-HDL reduction is the secondary priority of therapy. There is currently no specified target for HDL-C elevation. However, in patients with low HDL-C, it is important to try to raise HDL-C as much as possible. According to a recent AHA Consensus Statement, an HDL-C less than 50 mg/dL in women is now considered low (Mosca et al., 2004). The American Diabetes Association (ADA) advocates

Table 27-2 Dietary Recommendations for Therapeutic Lifestyle Change

Dietary Component	Recommended Allowance
Polyunsaturated fat	Up to 10% of total calories
Monounsaturated fat	Up to 20% of total calories
Total fat	25%-35% of total calories
Carbohydrate	50%-60% of total calories
Dietary fiber	20-30 g/day
Protein	About 15% of total calories
Dietary cholesterol	<200 mg/day

HDL-C goals of 40 mg/dL or higher for men and 50 mg/dL or higher for women with diabetes mellitus.

Based on such trials as the Heart Protection Study (Heart Protection Study Collaborative Group, 2002), Treating to New Targets study (LaRosa et al., 2005), and the Pravastatin or Atorvastatin Evaluation and Infection Therapy–Thrombolysis in Myocardial Infarction trial (Cannon et al., 2004), in regard to LDL-C reduction and reducing risk for CAD-related morbidity and mortality, "the lower the better" (Toth, 2004). The NCEP "white paper" recommended that physicians consider treating LDL-C to less than 70 mg/dL and non-HDL-C to less than 100 mg/dL in very-high-risk patients (e.g., recent ACS, diabetic patient with multiple, poorly controlled risk factors) (Grundy et al., 2004). Other therapeutic options include initiating antilipidemic medication with therapeutic lifestyle change if baseline LDL-C is greater than 100 mg/dL in patients with moderately high and high risk; in patients at high risk with baseline LDL-C less than 100 mg/dL, a further reduction of LDL-C by 30% to 40% with medication is a therapeutic option. AHA recommends LDL-C less than 70 mg/dL as a reasonable option for any patient with CAD (Smith et al., 2006).

Nonpharmacologic Interventions

Therapeutic lifestyle change (TLC) is first-line therapy for patients at risk for cardiovascular events. Patients who smoke should stop. The amount of daily consumed cholesterol should be less than 200 mg. Table 27-2 summarizes the distribution of calories from nutrients. Reduced saturated fat and increased consumption of mono- and polyunsaturated fats promote serum LDL-C reduction. The ingestion of viscous fiber and plant stanols decrease cholesterol absorption. Ideally, patients should exercise for 20 to 30 minutes five times per week. Regular exercise promotes weight loss and relieves visceral adiposity and insulin resistance.

Pharmacologic Interventions

Statins

The statins are reversible, competitive 3-hydroxy-3-methylglutaryl coenzyme A (HMG-CoA) reductase inhibitors. HMG-CoA reductase is the rate-limiting step for cholesterol biosynthesis in the liver and systemic tissues. Statins are the most potent agents for reducing serum levels of LDL-C. The statins augment the elimination of atherogenic apoB100-containing lipoproteins (VLDL, VLDL remnants, and LDL) from plasma by upregulating the LDL receptor on the surface of hepatocytes. The statins also reduce VLDL secretion and stimulate apoprotein-AI expression and hepatic HDL secretion.

Many prospective, placebo-controlled clinical trials have shown that the statins significantly reduce rates of MI, stroke, and coronary and all-cause mortality in the primary prevention (Downs et al., 1998) and secondary prevention settings (Scandinavian Simvastatin Survival Study Group, 1994). Statins reduce the frequency of stable and unstable angina and decrease atheromatous plaque progression and, based on intravascular ultrasound measurement (Nissen et al., 2004), quantitative coronary angiography, and high-resolution magnetic resonance imaging (Corti et al., 2002), even stimulate some degree of plaque resorption. The statins reduce cardiovascular events in men and women, blacks and Hispanics, hypertensive and diabetic patients, smokers, and patients over age 70.

Seven statins are currently available. These drugs differ by potency and a number of pharmacokinetic properties. The choice of statin and its dosing depend on the magnitude of LDL-C and non-HDL-C reduction required (baseline vs. risk-stratified NCEP target). The LDL-C–lowering efficacy of the statins is as follows (e.g., Jones et al., 2003):
Rosuvastatin (Crestor): 45%-63% (5-40 mg daily)
Atorvastatin (Lipitor): 26%-60% (10-80 mg daily)
Simvastatin (Zocor): 26%-47% (10-80 mg daily)
Lovastatin (Mevacor): 21%-42% (10-80 mg daily)
Fluvastatin (Lescol): 22%-36% (10-20 mg daily)
Pitavastatin (Livalo): 32%-43% (1-4 mg daily)
Pravastatin (Pravachol): 22%-34% (10-80 mg daily)

Each doubling of a statin's dose yields an additional 6% reduction, on average, in serum LDL-C ("rule of 6s"). Patients who are heterozygous or homozygous for familial hypercholesterolemia frequently require high potency statins at their highest doses coupled to stringent restriction in dietary lipid ingestion and the addition of one or more other lipid-lowering agents. The statins induce significant reductions in serum TG levels (typically 10%-25%) and modest elevations in serum HDL-C (2%-14%). Unlike the other statins, atorvastatin therapy is associated with decreasing capacity for raising HDL-C as a function of increasing doses. In patients with high baseline serum TG levels (>300 mg/dL), simvastatin and rosuvastatin raise HDL-C up to 18% and 22%, respectively.

The statins display significant differences in their pharmacokinetic profiles. Because of their relatively short half-life (1-4 hours), lovastatin, fluvastatin, pravastatin, and simvastatin should be taken after the evening meal in order to intercept the peak activity of HMG–CoA reductase, which occurs around midnight. Rosuvastatin and atorvastatin can be taken at any time during the day or night because of their long half-life (~19 and 14 hours, respectively). The coadministration of drugs or compounds that inhibit cytochrome P450 3A4 (macrolide antibiotics [erythromycin, clarithromycin], azole-type antifungals [ketoconazole, itraconazole], cyclosporine, HIV protease inhibitors, nefazodone, >1 qt grapefruit juice daily) with atorvastatin, simvastatin, and lovastatin is contraindicated because these statins depend on this P450 isozyme for oxidative modification and elimination (Neuvonen et al., 1998). CYP3A4 inhibition is associated with increased risk for myopathy and hepatotoxicity. The dose of

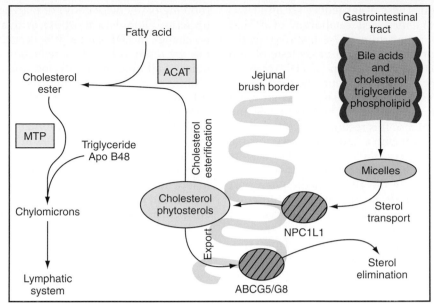

Figure 27-2 Gastrointestinal absorption of dietary and biliary lipid and cholesterol. In the gastrointestinal tract, cholesterol and triglycerides arising from biliary and dietary sources are assimilated with bile salts and phospholipids to form micelles. Micelles transport cholesterol and lipid to the jejunal brush border. Along the enterocyte surface, the sterol transporter known as Niemann Pick C1 Like 1 *(NPC1L1)* protein is responsible for importing cholesterol and phytosterols into the neurocyte. Once internalized, the cholesterol is esterified to cholesterol esters via the activity of acyl-CoA acyltransferase *(ACAT)*. The esterified cholesterol is packaged with triglycerides, phospholipids, and apoprotein B48 *(ApoB48)* to form chylomicrons in an assimilation reaction catalyzed by microsomal transfer protein *(MTP)*. The chylomicrons are released into gastrointestinal lacteals which conduct these lipoproteins into the central circulation. Excess intracellular sterols can be excreted back into the GI tract via the activity of the sterol exporter complex ABCG5/G8 (ATP-binding membrane cassette transporter G5/G8). *(Reproduced with permission from Toth PP, Davidson MH. Cholesterol absorption blockade with ezetimibe. Curr Drug Targets Cardiovasc Haematol Disord 2005;5:455-462.)*

simvastatin should be 20 mg or less daily in patients being treated with amiodarone or verapamil.

Although there is some concern about the potential toxicity of statins, their benefits significantly outweigh their risks. Liver toxicity can occur and is defined as an alanine transaminase (ALT) elevation of three times or more the upper limit of normal (ULN) on two occasions at least 1 month apart. The average risk of hepatotoxicity from statin therapy is approximately 1%, but risk increases as a function of increasing doses. Mild elevations in serum transaminase levels early during the course of therapy are relatively common and usually resolve spontaneously. If hepatotoxicity develops, statin therapy should be discontinued until transaminase levels normalize and therapy with a different statin can be initiated. There is no documented evidence that the statins increase risk for liver failure. The most important adverse event associated with statin therapy is rhabdomyolysis, myoglobinuria, and renal failure. The risk for rhabdomyolysis is less than 0.1%. Symptoms of rhabdomyolysis include worsening muscle pain, proximal weakness, nausea and vomiting, and brownish-red discoloration of urine. The statins can cause myalgia. If a patient develops myalgia or muscle weakness, a serum creatine kinase (CK) level can be obtained. The diagnosis of myopathy is made when CK levels exceed 10 times ULN. When assessing myalgia, it is important to evaluate patients for pain caused by arthritis, tendinopathy, fibromyalgia, and muscle strain induced by exertion.

Ezetimibe

Dietary and biliary sources contribute significantly to serum levels of cholesterol (Fig. 27-2). Although plant sterols and stanols block gastrointestinal (GI) cholesterol absorption,

ezetimibe (Zetia) is the first member of a class of lipid-lowering drugs known as cholesterol absorption inhibitors. Mechanistically, ezetimibe inhibits the Niemann-Pick C1 Like-1 protein, which mediates cholesterol and phytosterol transport along the brush border of the jejunal enterocyte (Altmann et al., 2004; Davis et al., 2004). After glucuronidation, ezetimibe undergoes enterohepatic recirculation with negligible systemic exposure. The half-life of ezetimibe is approximately 22 hours. When dosed at 10 mg once daily, ezetimibe reduces serum LDL-C on average by 20%, but up to 24% of patients experience a reduction of 25% or greater (Ballantyne et al., 2004; Davidson et al., 2002). Ezetimibe also decreases TGs by up to 8% and raises HDL-C by up to 4%. Ezetimibe does not decrease the absorption of bile acids, steroid hormones (ethinyl estradiol, progesterone), or such fat-soluble vitamins as vitamins A, D, E, or α- and β-carotenes.

The risk of hepatotoxicity with ezetimibe is almost identical to placebo (0.5% vs. 0.3%), and there is no documented evidence of increased risk for myopathy. Fixed-dose ezetimibe is also available in combination with increasing doses of simvastatin (Vytorin; 10/10, 10/20, 10/40, 10/80 mg daily). Ezetimibe can also be safely used in combination with other statins (Toth and Davidson, 2005). The ezetimibe provides additive changes in lipoprotein levels to that observed with statin therapy. The addition of ezetimibe to a statin regimen substantially reduces the likelihood of needing to titrate the statin.

Bile Acid–Binding Resins

The bile acid sequestration agents (BASAs) are orally administered anion-exchange resins that bind bile acids in the GI tract and prevent them from being reabsorbed into the enterohepatic circulation. These drugs reduce serum LDL-C by two mechanisms: (1) increased catabolism of cholesterol secondary to the upregulation of 7-α-hydroxylase, the rate-limiting enzyme for the conversion of cholesterol into bile acids; and (2) increased expression of LDL receptors on the hepatocyte surface, which augments the clearance of apoB100-containing lipoproteins from plasma. At maximum doses, the BASA can reduce serum LDL-C by 15% to 30% and increase HDL-C by 3% to 5%. It is recommended that these drugs be used in conjunction with a statin whenever possible because BASA therapy increases HMG-CoA reductase activity in the liver, which leads to increased hepatic biosynthesis of cholesterol, thereby offsetting the effects of the BASA over time. The BASAs are contraindicated in patients with serum TG levels greater than 400 mg/dL because these agents can exacerbate hypertriglyceridemia.

There are currently three different BASAs available: cholestyramine (Questran; 4-24 g in 2-3 divided doses daily), colestipol (Colestid; 5-30 g in 2-3 divided doses daily), and colesevelam (Welchol; 1250 mg 2-3 times daily). The development of constipation, flatulence, and bloating is relatively frequent, although colesevelam has the most favorable side-effect profile of the three available BASAs. Increasing water and soluble-fiber ingestion ameliorates some of the difficulty with constipation. The BASA bind negatively charged molecules in a nonspecific manner. Consequently, they can decrease the absorption of warfarin, phenobarbital, thiazide diuretics, digitalis, β-blockers, thyroxine, statins, fibrates, and ezetimibe. These medications should be taken 1 hour before or 4 hours after the ingestion of BASA. The BASA can reduce the absorption of fat-soluble vitamins. Colesevelam also has an indication to reduce serum glycated hemoglobin levels in patients with diabetes mellitus.

Fibrates

The fibrates are fibric acid derivatives that exert a number of effects on lipoprotein metabolism. These agents reduce serum TG levels by 25% to 50% and raise HDL-C by 10% to 20%. Fibrates activate *lipoprotein lipase* (LPL) by reducing levels of apoprotein CIII (inhibitor of LPL) and increasing levels of apoprotein CII (activator of LPL) (Fruchart et al., 1999). This stimulates TG hydrolysis in chylomicrons and VLDL. Fibrates increase HDL-C by two mechanisms. First, the fibrates are PPAR-α agonists and stimulate increased hepatic expression of apoproteins AI and AII. Second, by activating LPL, surface coat mass derived from VLDL is ultimately used to assimilate HDL in serum. In some patients, fibrate therapy may be associated with an increase in serum LDL-C ("β" effect) secondary to increased enzymatic conversion of VLDL to LDL. This effect may diminish over time as the patient increases the expression of hepatic LDL receptors.

The fibrates are particularly valuable for treating dyslipidemia in patients with a combination of hypertriglyceridemia and low HDL-C. In this patient type, post hoc evaluations of data from two studies (Helsinki Heart Study and Bezafibrate Infarction Prevention Study) have demonstrated substantial cardiovascular event rate reductions using fibrate therapy (Bezafibrate Infarction Prevention Study Group, 2000; Manninen et al., 1988). In the Veterans Affairs High-Density Lipoprotein Intervention Trial (VA-HIT), men with CAD and low HDL (mean, 31 mg/dL) were treated with either gemfibrozil (600 mg orally twice daily) or placebo over a 5-year follow-up period (Robins et al., 2001). With a 6% elevation in HDL, no change in LDL, and a 31% decrease in TGs, gemfibrozil therapy resulted in a 22% reduction in the composite end point of all-cause mortality and nonfatal MI versus placebo (Rubins et al., 1999). Gemfibrozil therapy also reduced the risk of stroke and transient ischemic attacks by 31% and 59%, respectively (Rubins et al., 2001). Diabetic patients in VA-HIT treated with gemfibrozil had a 32% reduction in the combined end point (41% in CHD death and 40% in stroke) (Rubins et al., 2002). Fibrates have been shown to exert many of the same pleiotropic effects as statins and to reduce atheromatous plaque progression in native coronary vessels and in coronary venous bypass grafts (Diabetes Atherosclerosis Intervention Study Investigators, 2001; Ericsson et al., 1996).

As with the statins, fibrates are associated with a low incidence of myopathy and mild elevations in serum transaminases. Fibrate therapy can increase the risk for cholelithiasis and elevate prothrombin time by displacing warfarin from albumin-binding sites. The periodic monitoring of serum transaminases (6-12 weeks after initiating therapy and twice annually thereafter) is recommended. The two most common fibrates are gemfibrozil (Lopid; 600 mg twice daily) and fenofibrate (Tricor; 54 or 160 mg daily). Bezafibrate is available in Europe and is dosed at 400 mg daily. The use of therapies combining a statin and fibrate is becoming more commonplace in clinical practice, especially as the incidence of complex dyslipidemias increases (Davidson and Toth, 2004). Gemfibrozil significantly reduces the glucuronidation of statins, which decreases their elimination (Backman et al., 2002; Prueksaritanont et al., 2002a, 2002b). This increases the risk for myopathy/rhabdomyolysis and hepatotoxicity. When used in combination with gemfibrozil, the doses for simvastatin and rosuvastatin should not exceed 10 mg daily. In general, when embarking on combination therapy, fenofibrate is a safer choice because it does not adversely impact the glucuronidation of the statins (Bergman et al., 2004). Fenofibric acid (Trilipix) is indicated for use in combination with statin therapy. Although there are no clinical trial data yet available to assess the effect of statin-fibrate combination therapy on cardiovascular morbidity and mortality, the efficacy of fenofibrate used in combination with simvastatin compared with simvastatin monotherapy is being tested in diabetic patients in the Action to Control Cardiovascular Risk in Diabetes Trial (http://www.nhlbi.nih.gov/health/prof/heart/other/accord/).

When serum TGs do not normalize in response to a low-fat diet and fibrate therapy, the physician should consider adding other agents. Patients with severe hypertriglyceridemia frequently possess mutations in LPL that reduce its lipolytic activity. The addition of orlistat (Xenical; 120 mg with meals) can reduce the absorption of dietary fat and thus the circulating levels of chylomicrons and TGs. The addition of fish oil should also be considered.

Fish Oils

Fish oil capsules enriched with omega-3 (eicosapentaenoic acid) and omega-6 (docosahexaenoic acid) fatty acids can reduce serum triglyceride and VLDL levels and raise HDL-C in a dose-dependent manner. The omega-3 fatty acids inhibit the enzyme diacylglycerol acyltransferase-2, thereby reducing intrahepatic TG biosynthesis. They also stimulate mitochondrial beta-oxidation of fatty acids, decrease VLDL production and biosynthesis, and stimulate TG hydrolysis by LPL (Toth et al., 2009). Dietary supplementation with the *n-3* polyunsaturated fatty acids (PUFAs) eicosapentaenoic acid (EPA) and docosahexaenoic acid (DHA) has also been shown to lower the risk of death, nonfatal coronary events, and stroke after MI (GISSI-Prevenzione Investigators, 1999). In several clinical trials, PUFAs have been shown to reduce TG levels by 20% to 30%, and up to 50% in patients with severe hypertriglyceridemia (TG >500 mg/dL) (O'Keefe and Harris, 2000).

The Japan EPA Lipid Intervention Study (JELIS) evaluated whether the addition of fish oils to patients already taking a statin would provide incremental risk reduction. Approximately 19,000 Japanese men and women with hypercholesterolemia were prospectively randomized to statin therapy with or without 1800 mg/day of EPA (Yokoyama et al., 2007). Combination therapy resulted in an additional 19% reduction in major coronary events at 4.6 years of follow-up compared to statin monotherapy.

Niacin

Niacin, or nicotinic acid, is a B vitamin that exerts multiple beneficial effects on lipoprotein metabolism. In contrast to statins and fibrates, niacin does not stimulate hepatic biosynthesis of HDL. Niacin appears to block HDL particle uptake and catabolism by hepatocytes without adversely impacting reverse cholesterol transport. This helps to increase circulating levels of HDL. Niacin reduces hepatic VLDL and TG secretion according to two mechanisms: (1) it decreases the flux of fatty acids from adipose tissue to the liver by inhibiting lipase activity; and (2) it inhibits TG formation within hepatocytes by inhibiting diacylglycerol acyltransferase. Niacin also reduces serum LDL-C concentrations by increasing the catabolism of apoB100. Consequently, niacin beneficially impacts all components of the lipoprotein profile.

When used as monotherapy at 3.0 g daily, crystalline niacin significantly reduced the incidence of MI and stroke in patients with established CAD in the Coronary Drug Project (1975). In the HDL-Atherosclerosis Treatment Study (HATS), combinations of high-dose niacin (2-4 g with simvastatin) reduced cardiovascular morbidity and mortality by up to 90% compared to placebo (Brown et al., 2001). This combination therapy also induced atheromatous plaque stabilization over a 3-year follow-up. Niacin should be started at a low dose and gradually titrated upward based on the results of follow-up lipid panels. When evaluated as a function of dose (500-2000 mg daily), Niaspan induces the following changes in serum lipid levels: LDL-C, 3% to 16% reduction; TGs, 5% to 32% reduction; HDL-C, 10% to 24% elevation (Capuzzi et al., 1998).

Niacin therapy is associated with a number of side-effects. The most common side-effect with niacin is cutaneous flushing; its incidence can be reduced by taking a 325-mg tablet of aspirin 1 hour before taking niacin. The flushing is prostaglandin mediated. Limiting fat intake for 2 to 3 hours before taking niacin also helps as fat is a source of

arachidonic acid, the substrate for cyclooxygenase. Niaspan is a sustained-release preparation of niacin associated with less flushing. Other side effects include bloating, pruritus, acanthosis nigricans, transient disturbances in glycemic control, and increased serum concentrations of uric acid. Niacin appears to increase rates of proximal tubular reuptake of urate from the glomerular ultrafiltrate. Niacin is available as a combination pill with lovastatin (Advicor; 500/20, 1000/20, and 2000/40 mg) or simvastatin (Simcor; 500/20, 750/20, and 1000/20 mg) with the two drugs in each combination pill providing additive changes in serum lipoprotein levels.

KEY TREATMENT

Statins, fibrates, niacin, omega-3 fish oils, and bile acid sequestration agents to treat dyslipidemia reduce cardiovascular morbidity significantly (SOR: A).

Statins are the most efficacious drugs currently available for reducing serum levels of LDL and significantly impact risk for both cardiovascular morbidity and mortality (SOR: A).

The omega-3 fish oils also appear to impact cardiovascular mortality, although the evidence is not as strong as with statins (SOR: A). Fibrates have the greatest capacity to reduce serum TGs and reduce cardiovascular morbidity (MI and stroke). The fibrates have not yet been shown to beneficially impact mortality as an independent end point in clinical trials. The fibrates have been shown to reduce rates of atherosclerotic disease progression in both diabetic and nondiabetic patients with CAD (SOR: A).

Niacin raises serum levels of HDL significantly better than other currently available antilipidemic medications, and it also reduces LDL, TGs, and lipoprotein(a) (SOR: A).

Therapy with combinations of drugs (statin-fibrate, statin-niacin, fibrate-niacin, statin-ezetimibe) is frequently required in patients with mixed forms of dyslipidemia and increases the likelihood of therapeutic success. The addition of niacin or omega-3 fish oils to statin therapy does provide incremental cardiovascular risk reduction over statin therapy alone (SOR: A).

The impact of fibrate and ezetimibe adjuvant therapy with a statin is currently being evaluated in prospective, randomized clinical trials.

POTENTIAL FOR HARM

Antilipidemic agents can induce hepatotoxicity and myopathy (SOR: A).

Statins and fibrates may induce transient elevations in serum transaminases and should be discontinued if levels exceed three times ULN. If levels are below this threshold, monitor liver function tests because transaminase levels usually decrease and trend toward normal spontaneously. Often, these drugs are discontinued prematurely to the detriment of patient care (SOR: A).

When combining a statin with a fibrate, use of gemfibrozil should be discouraged because it impairs the glucuronidation and elimination of the statins to varying degrees. This can result in increased risk for hepatotoxicity and rhabdomyolysis (SOR: A). Fenofibrate and fenofibric acid are safer choices in this context.

Patients complaining of myalgias or weakness, especially if escalating, should be monitored for myopathy. The statins and fibrates should be discontinued if serum CK levels exceed 10 times ULN (SOR: A). However, myalgias are common and not necessarily attributable to statin and fibrate use.

In patients presenting with rhabdomyolysis, antilipidemic medications should be discontinued immediately. Patients should be hospitalized, hydrated with intravenous fluids, and provided supportive care.

Table 27-3 JNC-7 Blood Pressure (BP) Classification

Classification	Systolic (mm Hg)	Diastolic (mm Hg)	Lifestyle Modification	Drug Therapy
Normal	<120	and <8	Yes	Usually no treatment
Prehypertension	120-139	and 80-89	Yes	Yes, for compelling JNC-7 indications
Stage 1 hypertension	140-159	or 90-99	Yes	Yes
Stage 1 hypertension	≥160	or ≥100	Yes	Yes

From Seventh Report of the Joint National Committee on Prevention, Detection, Evaluation, and Treatment of High Blood Pressure (JNC-7).

Hypertension

Key Points

- Hypertension is highly prevalent in men and women and people of all ethnic and racial groups
- Hypertension tends to be undertreated in patients with both complicated and uncomplicated forms.
- In uncomplicated HTN the specific choice of drug is less important than the attainment of goal blood pressure.

Hypertension (HTN) is highly prevalent and is a significant risk factor for CAD, left ventricular hypertrophy (LVH), CHF, PVD, stroke, sudden death, nephropathy, and diabetes mellitus. The incidence of HTN increases as a function of age; patients who are normotensive at age 55 have a 90% risk of developing HTN at some point in their lives. Risk for hypertension is regulated by genetic background (e.g., mutations in cell membrane cation transporters in the renal proximal tubular epithelium and vasculature, cell surface receptors, endocrine influences, calcium handling in smooth muscle cells) and environmental factors. The Seventh Report of the Joint National Committee on Prevention, Detection, Evaluation, and Treatment of High Blood Pressure (JNC-7) provides the current framework for defining and managing HTN in the U.S. population (Chobanian et al., 2003). Table 27-3 summarizes the JNC-7 classification of blood pressure (BP), soon scheduled for revision. The reduction of BP to guideline-specified targets in patients with complicated and uncomplicated HTN substantially reduces risk for acute cardiovascular events, progression of atherosclerosis, and end-organ injury.

As demonstrated by the Framingham Study, BP is a continuous risk factor for CVD, with no threshold effect yet identified (Vasan et al., 2002). For every increase of 20/10 mm Hg in BP above 115/75 mm Hg, risk for CVD increases twofold. Contrary to a widely held misconception in medicine, among patients older than 50 years, the treatment of systolic blood pressure (SBP) reduces risk for CVD and renal disease significantly more than diastolic blood pressure (DBP). Despite the recognized dangers of HTN and the large number of medications available, only one third of patients are treated to target levels in the United States (Whelton et al., 2002). Hypertension is a defining feature of the metabolic syndrome and usually suggests that the patient has some degree of underlying endothelial dysfunction, with an imbalance between vasodilatory and vasoconstrictive influences impacting the arterial wall.

Recommendations

In response to recent epidemiologic and clinical trial data, JNC-7 made a series of new recommendations for addressing the HTN epidemic, which now includes more than 73.6 million patients in the U.S. alone. Patients with SBP of 120 to 139 mm Hg and DBP of 80 to 89 mm Hg are defined as "prehypertensive" and warrant aggressive lifestyle modification to prevent progression to HTN. It must be assumed that even in this BP range, changes in vessel wall histology and physiology are inducing elevations in BP. Weight reduction, moderation of alcohol intake (2 drinks per day for men, 1 for women), reducing daily sodium intake to 2.4 g/day, increasing aerobic exercise, and the Dietary Approaches to Stop Hypertension (DASH) regimen are all associated with significant reductions in BP (Chobanian et al., 2003). Thiazide diuretics such as hydrochlorothiazide or chlorthalidone, alone or in combination with other antihypertensives, should be used to treat most patients with HTN.

If baseline BP is more than 20/10 mm Hg above target level, initial therapy should consist of two antihypertensive agents (one of which should be a thiazide diuretic unless there is a contraindication) started simultaneously. The majority of patients with HTN will need two or more drugs to achieve adequate control of BP. As demonstrated in the Hypertension Optimization Trial (Hansson et al., 1998), diabetic patients require, on average, 3.4 medications to achieve adequate control. In uncomplicated HTN the BP target is less than 140/90 mm Hg. In patients with diabetes or chronic kidney disease (GFR <60 mL/min/1.73m², baseline serum creatinine >1.5 mg/dL in men or >1.3 mg/dL in women, or albuminuria defined as >300 mg/day on 24-hr urine specimen or 200 mg albumin/g creatine on urine spot check), the BP target is less than 130/80 mm Hg.

A large number of antihypertensive medications are available (Table 27-4). Prevailing expert opinion now contends that, unless there are compelling indications for the use of a specific drug class because of background cardiovascular or renal disease, it makes little difference whether a calcium channel blocker (CCB), beta blocker, angiotensin converting enzyme inhibitor (ACEI), or angiotensin receptor

Table 27-4 Oral Antihypertensive Drugs (Usual Dose Range)

Drug	Trade Name	Total mg/day (Freq/day)	Select Side Effects and Comments
Diuretics* (partial list)			
Chlorthalidone (G)	Hygroton	12.5-50 (1)	
Hydrochlorothiazide (G)	HydroDIURIL, Microzide, Esidrix	12.5-50 (1)	
Indapamide	Lozol	1.25-5 (1)	Less or no hypercholesterolemia
Metolazone	Mykrox Zaroxolyn	0.5-1.0 (1) 2.5-10 (1)	
Loop Diuretics			
Bumetanide (G)	Bumex	0.5-4 (2-3)	Short duration of action; no hypercalcemia
Ethacrynic acid	Edecrin	25-100 (2-3)	Only nonsulfonamide diuretic; ototoxicity
Furosemide (G)	Lasix	40-240 (2-3)	Short duration of action; no hypercalcemia
Torsemide	Demadex	5-100 (1-2)	Hyperkalemia
Potassium-Sparing Agents			
Amiloride (G)	Midamor	5-10 (1)	
Spironolactone (G)	Aldactone	25-100 (1)	Gynecomastia
Triamterene (G)	Dyrenium	25-100 (1)	
Adrenergic Inhibitors			
Peripheral Agents			
Guanadrel sulfate	Hylorel	10-75 (2)	Postural hypotension, diarrhea
Fanethidine monosulfate	Ismelin	10-150 (1)	Postural hypotension, diarrhea
Reserpine (G)	Serpasil	0.05-0.25 (1)	Nasal congestion, sedation, depression, activation of peptic ulcer
Central Alpha-Agonist†			
Clonidine (G)	Catapres	0.2-1.2 (2-3)	More withdrawal hypertension
Guanabenz acetate (G)	Wytensin	8-32 (2)	Less withdrawal hypertension
Guanfacine (G)	Tenex	1-3 (1)	
Methyldopa (G)	Aldomet	500-3000 (2)	Hepatic and "autoimmune" disorders
Alpha Blockers			Can elevate high-density lipoprotein cholesterol (HDL)
Doxazosin mesylate	Cardura	1-16 (1)	
Prazosin (G)	Minipress	2-30 (2-3)	
Terazosin	Hytrin	1-20 (1)	
Beta Blockers			
Acebutolol	Sectral	200-800 (1)	Bronchospasm, bradycardia, heart failure; may mask insulin-induced hypoglycemia *Less serious:* impaired peripheral circulation, insomnia, fatigue, decreased exercise tolerance, hypertriglyceridemia (except agents with intrinsic sympathomimetic activity), reduced HDL, impaired glycemic control
Atenolol (G)	Tenormin	25-100 (1-2)	
Betaxolol	Kerlone	5-20 (1)	

Continued

Table 27-4 Oral Antihypertensive Drugs (Usual Dose Range) —Cont'd

Drug	Trade Name	Total mg/day (Freq/day)	Select Side Effects and Comments
Bisoprolol fumarate	Zebeta	2.5-10 (1)	
Carteolol	Cartrol	2.5-10 (1)	
Metoprolol tartrate (G)	Lopressor	50-300 (2)	
Metoprolol succinate	Toprol XL	50-300 (1)	
Nadolol	Corgard	40-320 (1)	
Penbutolol sulfate	Levatol	10-20 (1)	
Pindolol (G)	Visken	10-60 (1)	
Propranolol (G)	Inderal Inderal LA	40-480 (2) 40-480 (1)	
Timolol maleate (G)	Blocadren	20-60 (2)	
Nebivolol	Bystolic	2.5-5-10 (1)	
Combined Alpha/Beta Blockers			**Postural hypotension, bronchospasm**
Carvedilol	Coreg	12.5-50 (2)	
Labetalol (G)	Normodyne, Trandate	200-1200 (2)	
Direct Vasodilators			Headaches, fluid retention, tachycardia
Hydralazine (G)	Apresoline	50-300 (2)	Lupus syndrome
Minoxidil	Loniten	5-100 (1)	Hirsutism
Calcium Antagonists			Conduction defects, worsening of systolic dysfunction, gingival hyperplasia
Nondihydropyridines			
Diltiazem	Cardizem SR Cardizem CD, Dilacor XR, Tiazac	120-360 (2) 120-360 (1)	Nausea, headache
Verapamil	Isoptin Sr, Calan SR Verelan, Covera-HS	90-480 (2) 120-480 (1)	
Dihydropyridines			Edema of the ankle, flushing, headache, gingival hypertrophy
Amlodipine besylate	Norvasc	2.5-10 (1)	
Felodipine	Plendil	2.5-10 (1)	
Isradipine	DynaCirc DynaCirc CR	5-20 (2) 5-20 (1)	
Nicardipine	Cardene SR	60-90 (2)	
Nifedipine	Procardia XL, Adalat CC	30-120 (1)	
Nisoldipine	Sular	20-60 (1)	
Angiotensin-Converting Enzyme Inhibitors			
Benazepril	Lotensin	5-40 (1-2)	Common: cough; rare: angioedema, hyperkalemia, rash, loss of taste, leukopenia
Captopril (G)	Capoten	25-150 (2-3)	
Enalapril maleate	Vasotec	5-40 (1-2)	

Table 27-4 Oral Antihypertensive Drugs (Usual Dose Range)—Cont'd

Drug	Trade Name	Total mg/day (Freq/day)	Select Side Effects and Comments
Fosinopril sodium	Monopril	10-40 (1-2)	
Lisinopril	Prinivil, Zestril	5-40 (1)	
Moexipril	Univasc	7.5-15 (2)	
Quinapril	Accupril	5-80 (1-2)	
Ramipril	Altace	1.25-20 (1-2)	
Trandolapril	Mavik	1-4 (1)	
Angiotensin II Receptor Blockers			
Losartan potassium	Cozaar	25-100 (1-2)	Angioedema (very rare); hyperkalemia
Valsartan	Diovan	80-320 (1)	
Irbesartan	Avapro	150-300 (1)	
Telmisartan	Micardis	20-80 (1)	
Olmesartan	Benicar	20-40 (1)	
Candesartan	Atacand	8-32 (1-2)	
Direct Renin Inhibitor			
Aliskiren	Tekturna	150-300	Angioedema (very rare); hyperkaliemia
Combination Formulations			
Enalapril/felodipine	Lexxel	5/5 (1)	Angioedema (very rare); hyperkalemia; edema from CCB component
Trandolapril/verapamil	Tarka	2/180, 1-4/240 (1)	
Amlodipine/benazepril	Lotrel	2.5-10/10-20	
Amlodipine/valsartan	Exforge	5-160/10-160/ 5-320/10-320	

*Drug class side effects—*short term:* increases cholesterol and glucose levels; biochemical abnormalities; decreases potassium, sodium, and magnesium levels, increases uric acid and calcium levels; *rare:* blood dyscrasias, photosensitivity, pancreatitis, hyponatremia.

†Sedation, dry mouth, bradycardia, withdrawal hypertension.

(G), Generic agent available.

blocker (ARB) is used to initiate therapy in the setting of uncomplicated HTN (Blood Pressure Lowering Treatment Trialists wwwwCollaboration, 2003; Julius et al., 2004; National Institute of Clinical Excellence Guideline 18, 2004; Pepine et al., 2003; Williams, 2005). Risk reduction is predominantly driven by the magnitude of BP reduction, rather than the specific mechanism by which it is achieved. Ideally, pharmacologic intervention will be coupled to lifestyle modification in order to achieve lasting and consistent reductions in BP reduction. If a patient's BP is greater than 20/10 mm Hg above goal, initiating therapy with a combination preparation increases the likelihood of therapeutic success and patient compliance. The use of combination therapy is also associated with reduced cost. Many ACEI, ARBs, CCBs, centrally acting drugs (e.g., reserpine, methyldopa), and β-blockers are available in combination with fixed doses of hydrochlorothiazide (12-25 mg) and, less often, chlorthalidone. Box 27-2 summarizes combinations of drugs that are efficacious and those associated with undesirable side effect profiles. Box 27-3 summarizes recommendations for attaining BP targets in the more challenging patient.

Patients with BP poorly responsive to even aggressive intervention should be evaluated further for etiologies such as renal arterial stenosis, adrenal and pituitary tumors, poor compliance, thyroid "storm," and volume overload from acute or chronic renal disease. A broad range of clinical trials have demonstrated that the rate of progression of certain cardiovascular and renal disease states is slowed by the use of particular antihypertensive agents (Chobanian et al., 2003). These constitute "compelling indications" (Table 27-5). In patients requiring inhibition of the renin-angiotensin-aldosterone (RAAS) axis (CHF, CAD, post-MI, nephropathy, LVH), an elevation in serum creatinine of up to 35% is tolerable and is not an indication for discontinuing an ACEI or an ARB. In patients who develop

Box 27-2 Sample Antihypertensive Drug Combinations

Desirable

Thiazide diuretic *plus:*

ACE inhibitor

Aldosterone antagonist

Angiotensin receptor blocker

Beta blocker

Calcium channel blocker

Calcium channel blocker *plus:*

ACE inhibitor

Angiotensin receptor blocker

Beta blocker

NDHPCCB (with refractory hypertension; preserved systolic heart function)

Not Desirable

Beta blocker *plus:*

Central adrenergic inhibitor

Rate-lowering CCB (NDHPCCB)

Alpha blocker *plus:*

Central adrenergic inhibitor

ACE, Angiotensin-converting enzyme; *NDHPCCB,* nondihydropyridine calcium channel blocker.

Box 27-3 Ten Tips for Attaining Goal Blood Pressure (BP)

1. Establish minimum goal BP; when >15/10 mm Hg above goal, BP monotherapy is unlikely to be effective.
2. In most situations, wait 4-6 weeks before titrating BP medications upward.
3. Realize that most hypertensive patients will ultimately require more than one (>1) drug to attain goal BP, especially those with diabetes, obesity, decreased kidney function, or proteinuria.
4. Initiate lifestyle modifications; diet should limit sodium (<2 g/ day), saturated fat, cholesterol, and alcohol intake (<2 drinks/ day); appropriate aerobic exercise; and weight loss (if indicated).
5. Remember that hypertension is *not* asymptomatic and that BP medications alleviate more side effects than they cause.
6. Minimize exposure to nonsteroidal anti-inflammatory drugs, including COX-2 inhibitors, when kidney function is reduced (<60 mL/min/1.73m2).
7. A diuretic appropriate to the level of kidney function is essential to the multidrug regimen when more than two (>2) antihypertensives are prescribed.
8. Consider using a dihydropyridine and a rate-lowering calcium antagonist in combination when BP is refractory to treatment.
9. Diuretic doses may need to be relatively high (e.g., furosemide, 160 mg/day in divided doses, or metolazone, 10-20 mg/day) when kidney function is <30 mL/min/1.73m2.
10. If BP remains above goal on three or more (≥3) antihypertensives (one of which is a diuretic) at near-maximal doses, consider referral to a hypertension specialist or nephrologist.

Modified from Flack JM, Nasser SA. Hypertension Pocket Guide. New York, McMahon, 2005.

hyperkalemia in response to an ACEI or ARB therapy, consideration should be given to reducing their dosage, adding a thiazide diuretic to promote potassium excretion, reducing potassium intake, or, when necessary, discontinuing the drugs and arranging referral to a nephrologist. Acute hyperkalemia can be managed with oral or rectal Kayexalate, a resin that binds and promotes the excretion of GI potassium. Men with HTN and benign prostatic hypertrophy or low serum HDL can be treated with an alpha-adrenergic blocker. In contrast to α-blockade, which can raise HDL levels by up to 20%, β-blockade is associated with reductions in serum HDL. Beta blockers and thiazide diuretics are both associated with the antagonism of glycemic control. Potassium balance should be monitored regularly in patients receiving combinations of ACEI/ARB with aldosterone antagonists. Blood pressure management should be individualized, with providers paying close attention to potential unwanted side effects that may dampen the benefit of BP reduction.

Hypertensive emergencies increase risk for acute MI, hemorrhagic stroke, encephalopathy, and other adverse events. Table 27-6 summarizes intravenous (IV) medications that can be used to reduce BP rapidly in the acute, emergent setting.

The results of two prospective trials may impact JNC-8 recommendations. In the Anglo-Scandinavian Cardiac Outcomes Trial (ASCOT) an atenolol/hydrochlorothiazide (A/H) regimen was compared to amlodipine/perindopril (A/P) in 19,257 subjects with HTN and three other cardiovascular risk factors. Despite nearly identical BP control, the patients randomized to A/P experienced a 23% lower incidence of fatal/nonfatal stroke, 16% fewer cardiovascular events and procedures, 11% lower all-cause mortality, and 30% less new-onset type 2 diabetes mellitus compared to the

Table 27-5 JNC-7–Defined Compelling Indications for Use of Specific Antihypertensive Agents in Complicated Hypertension

Indications	Diuretic	BB	ACEI	ARB	CCB	AA
Heart failure	✓	✓	✓	✓		✓
Post-MI		✓	✓			✓
CAD risk	✓	✓	✓		✓	
Diabetes mellitus	✓	✓	✓	✓	✓	
Renal disease			✓	✓		
Recurrent stroke prevention	✓		✓			

From Seventh Report of the Joint National Committee on Prevention, Detection, Evaluation, and Treatment of High Blood Pressure (JNC-7).

BB, Beta blocker; *ACEI,* angiotensin-converting enzyme inhibitor; *ARB,* angiotensin receptor blocker; *CCB,* calcium channel blocker; *AA,* aldosterone antagonist; *MI,* myocardial infarction; *CAD,* coronary artery disease.

A/H regimen over a median follow-up of 5.5 years (Dahlof et al., 2005). In the Avoiding Cardiovascular Events through Combination Therapy in Patients Living with Systolic Hypertension trial, 11,506 hypertensive patients were randomized to treatment with either benazepril/amlodipine (B/A) or

Table 27-6 Parenteral Drugs for Treatment of Hypertensive Emergencies

Drug	Dose	Onset of Action	Duration of Action	Adverse Effects	Special Instructions
Vasodilators					
Sodium nitro-prusside	0.25-10 µm/kg/min as IV infusion (max dose, 10 min only)	Imme-diate	1-2 min	Nausea, vomiting, muscle twitching, sweating, thiocyanate and cyanide intoxication	Most hypertensive emergencies; caution with high intracranial pressure or azotemia
Nicardipine	5-15 mg/hr IV	5-10 min	1-4 hr	Tachycardia, headache, flushing, local phlebitis	Most hypertensive emergencies except acute heart failure; caution with coronary ischemia
Fenoldopam mesylate	0.1-0.3 µm/kg/min as IV infusion	<5 min	30 min	Tachycardia, headache, nausea, flushing	Most hypertensive emergencies; caution with glaucoma
Nitro-glycerin	5-100 µm/min as IV infusion	2-5 min	3-5 min	Headache, vomiting, methemoglobinemia, tolerance with prolonged use	
Enalaprilat	1.25-5 mg q6h IV	15-30 min	6 hr	Precipitous fall in pressure in high-renin states; response variable	Acute left ventricular failure; avoid in acute myocardial infarction
Hydralazine	10-20 mg IV	10-20 min	3-8 hr	Tachycardia, flushing, headache, vomiting, aggravation of angina	Eclampsia
	10-50 mg IM	20-30 min			
Diazoxide	50-100 mg as IV bolus, repeated, or 15-30 mg/min as infusion	2-4 min	6-12 hr	Nausea, flushing, tachycardia chest pain	Now obsolete; when no intensive monitoring available
Adrenergic Inhibitors					
Labetalol	20-80 mg as IV bolus every 10 min 0.5-2.0 mg/min as IV infusion	5-10 min	3-6 hr	Vomiting, scalp tingling, burning in throat, dizziness, nausea, heart block, orthostatic hypotension	Most hypertensive emergencies except acute heart failure
Esmolol	250-500 µm/kg/min for 1 min, then 50-100 µm/kg/min for 4 min; may repeat sequence	1-2 min	10-20 min	Hypotension, nausea	Aortic dissection; perioperative
Phentol-amine	5-15 mg IV	1-2 min	3-10 min	Tachycardia, flushing, headache	Catecholamine excess

benazepril/hydrochlorothiazide (B/H). The primary and secondary composite end points comprised (1) nonfatal MI and stroke, hospitalization for angina, resuscitation after sudden cardiac arrest, coronary revascularization, and cardiovascular mortality; and (2) nonfatal MI and stroke and cardiovascular mortality, respectively (Jamerson et al., 2008). The primary and secondary end points were both reduced more with B/A compared to B/H by 19.6% and 21%, respectively. These trials strongly support the use of ACE inhibition therapy combined with the dihydropyridine amlodipine when managing

hypertension. Among patients with established vascular disease or high-risk diabetes mellitus without heart failure, the ONTARGET trial demonstrated that the incidence of cardiovascular events was identical in groups treated with either telmisartan or ramipril (Yusuf et al., 2008). The incidence of angioedema in the telmisartan group was approximately one third of that observed in the ramipril group. Consequently, in patients such as those studied in ONTARGET, it is therapeutically legitimate to treat ACEI-intolerant patients with an ARB.

KEY TREATMENT

If BP is greater than 20/10 mm Hg above target level, two antihypertensives should be started simultaneously, usually including hydrochlorothiazide, although amlodipine is also used with an ACE inhibitor (SOR: A).

The use of combination therapy to treat HTN allows for the interception of multiple mechanisms etiologic for this disorder and increases the likelihood of therapeutic success (SOR: A).

JNC 7 encourages the use of specific antihypertensive agents in the setting of HTN complicated by CHF, CAD, MI, nephropathy, and other forms of CVD (SOR: A).

Lifestyle modification is an important component of HTN management (SOR: A).

Treatment with ACEI and ARBs is associated with decreased risk for new-onset diabetes mellitus in patients with HTN (SOR: A).

The majority of health care providers believe that diastolic BP impacts CVD more than systolic BP; the opposite is true (SOR: A).

POTENTIAL HARM

The CCBs (both dihydropyridines and nondihydropyridines) tend to be underused because of peripheral edema (SOR: A). Combining these drugs with a low dose of hydrochlorothiazide or an ACEI reduces the incidence of edema.

ACEI and ARBs tend to be withheld in patients with mild to moderate renal insufficiency. Such patients benefit significantly from these drugs. An increase in serum creatinine of up to 35% is acceptable, and patients should be monitored for hyperkalemia (SOR: A).

Beta blockers and thiazide diuretics can antagonize glycemic control in patients with insulin resistance and impaired glucose tolerance and are associated with increased risk for diabetes mellitus (SOR: A).

Metabolic Syndrome

Key Points

- Metabolic syndrome is an insulin-resistant state associated with visceral adiposity, hypertension, hyperglycemia, dyslipidemia, and a proinflammatory and pro-oxidative state.
- Metabolic syndrome is not a CAD risk equivalent but is associated with heightened risk for CVD and diabetes mellitus.
- Metabolic syndrome should be treated with aggressive lifestyle modification, including weight loss, exercise, smoking cessation, and dietary modification.

Causes and Incidence

The incidence of obesity is rising worldwide. With increased mechanization and changes associated with increased food availability and lower average daily caloric expenditure, people are experiencing continuous weight gain with aging. Being overweight and the development of obesity now constitute the second most important preventable cause of mortality. In the United States, 30% of the population is obese, and 70% is overweight. The incidence of obesity is rising among both genders as well as all racial and ethnic groups. An important consequence of obesity is the development of insulin resistance and the metabolic syndrome (Haffner et al., 1990; Haffner and Taegtmeyer, 2003). The metabolic syndrome (or "syndrome X") is defined by a constellation of cardiovascular risk factors and is associated with heightened risk for cardiovascular morbidity and mortality. A variety of definitions of the metabolic syndrome have been developed,

Table 27-7 NCEP ATP-III Criteria for Diagnosing Metabolic Syndrome

Risk Factor	Defining Level
Abdominal obesity	Men: waist >40 inches Women: waist >35 inches
Triglycerides	≥150 mg/dL
High-density lipoprotein cholesterol (HDL-C)	Men: <40 mg/dL Women: <50 mg/dL
Blood pressure	≥130/ ≥85 mm Hg
Fasting glucose	≥100 mg/dL

From Third Report of the Expert Panel on Detection, Evaluation, and Treatment of High Blood Cholesterol in Adults (Adult Treatment Panel III) (NCEP ATP-III).

*Patients having any three of the above five risk factors meet criteria for the diagnosis of the metabolic syndrome.

but the one with the greatest clinical utility is that defined by the NCEP ATP-III (Grundy et al., 2004a, 2004b; Eckel et al., 2005). Waist circumference, blood pressure, fasting blood sugar, and serum TG and HDL levels are used to make the diagnosis (Table 27-7). Once three of the five criteria are met, the diagnosis of metabolic syndrome can be made.

Based on data from the Third National Health and Nutrition Examination Survey (NHANES-III), the incidence of metabolic syndrome increases linearly in both men and women as a function of age (Alexander et al., 2003; Ford et al., 2002). Hispanic and Native Americans are disproportionately affected. Current estimates suggest that 24% of the U.S. population have metabolic syndrome. In the Kuopio Ischaemic Heart Disease Risk Factor Study, patients with metabolic syndrome experienced a 3.77- and 2.43-fold increase in risk for coronary heart disease mortality and all-cause mortality, respectively, over 12-year follow-up compared to patients without the metabolic syndrome (Lakka et al., 2002).

Cardiovascular Risk Factors

As waist circumference increases, visceral adiposity increases. Visceral adipose tissue is metabolically highly active. An important conceptual shift has occurred in recent years with respect to how adipose tissue is viewed. It is no longer seen as a passive storage site for excess caloric ingestion. Instead, it is clear that visceral adipose tissue displays many features of an endocrine organ (Bradley et al., 2001; Toth, 2005a) (Fig. 27-3). Visceral adipose tissue produces a variety of inflammatory cytokines (tumor necrosis factor, transforming growth factor-β), interleukins (IL-1, IL-6), and effector molecules that regulate appetite (leptin) as well as insulin sensitivity and resistance (e.g., adiponectin, resistin). As the mass of visceral adipose tissue increases, adiponectin production decreases, which is associated with increased insulin resistance in adipose tissue, skeletal muscle, and the hepatic parenchyma (see Fig. 27-3). As adipose tissue becomes more insulin resistant, the capacity to regulate the catabolism of stored TGs becomes progressively more dysregulated and unresponsive to systemic tissue

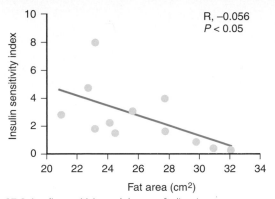

Figure 27-3 Insulin sensitivity and degree of adiposity. *(From Fujimoto WY, Abbate SL, Kahn SE, et al. The visceral adiposity syndrome in Japanese-American men. Obes Res 1994;2:364-371.)*

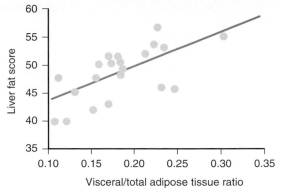

Figure 27-5 Severity of hepatic fat deposition as visceral adiposity worsens. *(From Banerji MA, Buckley MC, Chaiken RL, et al. Liver fat, serum triglycerides and visceral adipose tissue in insulin-sensitive and insulin-resistant black men with NIDDM. Int J Obes 1995;19:846-850.)*

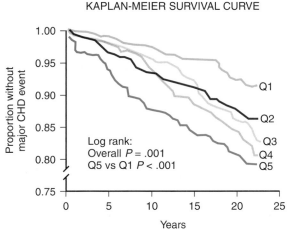

Figure 27-4 Risk of a major coronary heart disease (CHD)–related event associated with quintile of insulin levels in nondiabetic men enrolled in the Helsinki Policemen Study. *(From Pyorala M, Miettinen H, Laakso M, Pyorala K. Hyperinsulinemia predicts coronary heart disease risk in healthy middle-aged men: the 22-year follow-up results of the Helsinki Policemen Study. Circulation 1998;98:398-404.)*

needs. Serum levels of free fatty acids (FFAs) rise. The portal circulation becomes flooded with FFAs, resulting in both increased TG deposition within the liver (nonalcoholic steatohepatitis [NASH] or fatty liver) (Banerji et al., 1995) and increased VLDL secretion resulting in hypertriglyceridemia. A fatty liver in the absence of excessive alcohol intake is an important marker for insulin resistance and is highly correlated with the magnitude and severity of adiposity (Fig. 27-4). Elevation in FFAs induces progressive deterioration in glycemic control by (1) interfering with normal phosphorylation of the insulin receptor, resulting in less expression of a glucose transporter (GLUT 4) necessary for the internalization and oxidation of serum glucose (Dresner et al., 1999), and (2) the induction of "lipotoxicity," the process by which FFAs induce premature apoptosis and dropout of pancreatic β-islet cells. Patients experiencing concomitant worsening insulin resistance and progressive loss of insulin-producing capacity experience a continuum of glycemic disturbance, beginning with impaired fasting glucose, then impaired glucose tolerance, and ultimately diabetes mellitus. As serum levels of insulin rise, risk for CAD-related

events increases precipitously (Pyorala et al., 1996) (Fig. 27-5). Patients with metabolic syndrome have a threefold to fivefold increased risk for developing diabetes compared to patients without metabolic syndrome.

Insulin resistance and increased visceral adiposity in the setting of metabolic syndrome are associated with changes in multiple risk factors (Lamon-Fava et al., 1996) (Fig. 27-6). Insulin-resistant adipose tissue is a potent source of angiotensinogen, the precursor to vasoconstrictor angiotensin II. The BP in these patients also increases because (1) insulin stimulates increased sodium reabsorption at the level of the proximal tubular epithelium, which increases intravascular volume; (2) there is reduced endothelial nitric oxide production (Caballero, 2003); and (3) there is increased vascular sympathetic tone. In the face of insulin resistance, obesity can steadily worsen as a result of dysregulation of central centers transducing the signals for appetite and satiety. Serum HDL levels decrease for three principal reasons (Fig. 27-7). First, as the liver becomes insulin resistant, the capacity for insulin to stimulate the hepatic production of apo AI and AII is compromised, resulting in less HDL secretion. Second, in patients with insulin resistance, lipoprotein lipase is relatively inhibited. This reduces the hydrolysis of triglycerides in VLDL and chylomicrons. These large lipoproteins remain incompletely catabolized and form atherogenic remnant particles. Unless broken down further, they cannot release many of the surface-coat constituents used to assimilate HDL in serum. Third, as HDL particles become more enriched with TGs, they become a better substrate for *hepatic lipase,* an enzyme that catabolizes HDL and promotes its clearance from serum (Toth, 2005b). Patients with metabolic syndrome also tend to have smaller, denser LDL particles. These small LDL particles are believed to be more atherogenic than the larger, more buoyant variety because they are more easily oxidized, have reduced affinity for the hepatic LDL receptor resulting in less systemic clearance, and appear to more easily access the subendothelial space because of their smaller volume (St. Pierre et al., 2001). Visceral adipose tissue promotes increased systemic inflammation by secreting inflammatory mediators and by stimulating hepatic production of C-reactive protein (CRP) through IL-6. As serum levels of such acute-phase reactants as fibrinogen, CRP, and plasminogen activator inhibitor-1

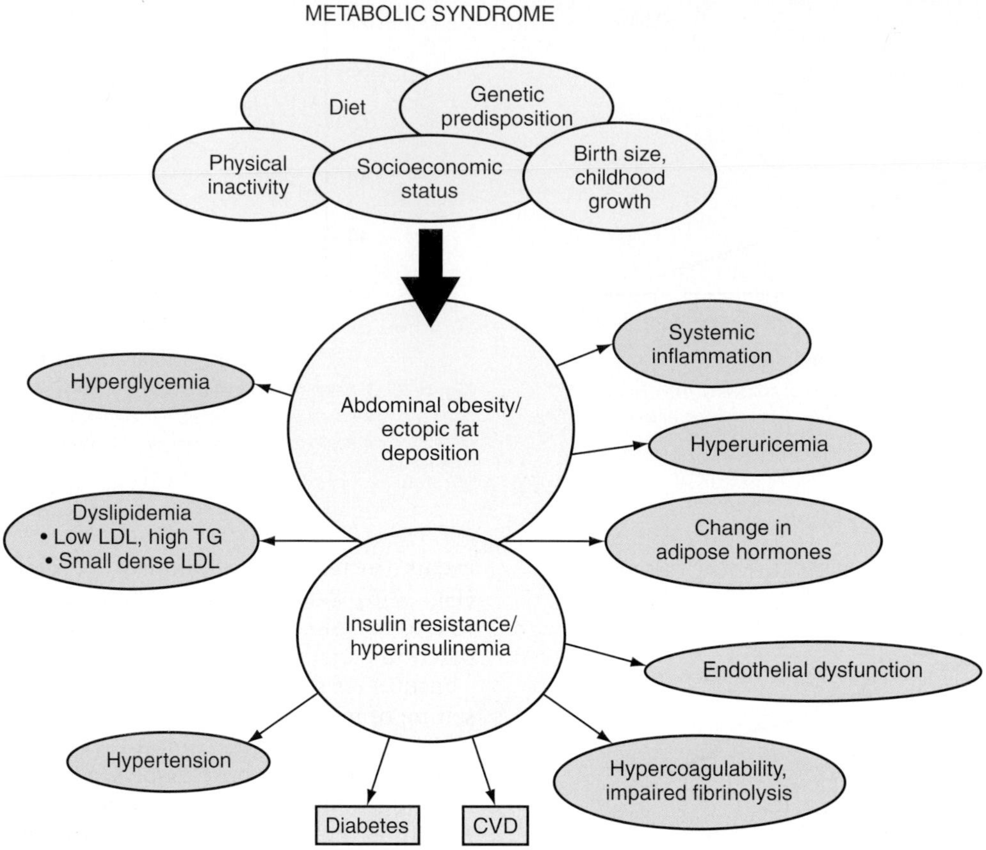

METABOLIC SYNDROME

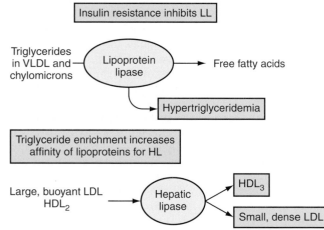

Figure 27-6 Complex interactions among genetic, environmental, and socioeconomic factors increase risk of developing visceral adiposity, insulin resistance with risk factor generation and clustering, and ultimately, diabetes mellitus with atherosclerotic disease. *CVD,* Cardiovascular disease; *LDL,* low-density lipoprotein; *TG,* triglyceride.

Figure 27-7 Molecular mechanisms that cause the atherogenic lipid triad in patients with insulin resistance. As a patient becomes insulin resistant, the activity of lipoprotein lipase *(LL)* decreases. This can occur secondary to reduced apoprotein CII and/or increased apoprotein CIII production. With reduced capacity to hydrolyze the triglycerides in such large lipoproteins as very-low-density lipoprotein *(VLDL,* derived from liver) and chylomicrons (derived from gut), triglycerides and large remnant particles accumulate in serum. In this scenario, low-density lipoprotein *(LDL)* levels in serum tend to be relatively low because less VLDL is being converted to LDL. As high-density lipoprotein *(HDL)* and LDL particles become progressively more enriched with triglycerides, these lipoproteins become better substrates for the enzyme hepatic lipase *(HL)*. HL catabolizes these lipoproteins to form small, dense LDL and HDL. The small HDL particles can be further degraded to their phospholipid and apoprotein constituents, thereby reducing circulating levels of this beneficial lipoprotein. *(Based on Toth PP, Davidson MH. Comparative effects of lipid-lowering therapies. Prog Cardiovasc Dis 2004;47:73-104.)*

(PAI-1) rise, the risk for metabolic syndrome and diabetes increases (Dandona et al., 2005; Festa et al., 2002). As shown in the Women's Health Study, as serum CRP levels increase in women with metabolic syndrome but no prior history of CAD, the risk for an acute cardiovascular event increases significantly (Ridker et al., 2003). As insulin resistance worsens, risk for nonalcoholic hepatic steatosis increases steadily (see Fig. 27-6).

Treatment

Metabolic syndrome is not defined by NCEP as a CAD risk equivalent. It is crucial that these patients undergo comprehensive evaluation of their global cardiovascular risk factor burden. Aggressive lifestyle modification with weight loss, increased exercise and physical activity, smoking cessation, and reductions in carbohydrate and saturated fat intake constitute front-line therapy for patients with the metabolic syndrome (Grundy et al., 2003b; Liu and Manson, 2001; Salmeron et al., 2002). Referral to a dietitian is frequently helpful. Weight loss and aerobic exercise are associated with improved insulin sensitivity and significant improvements in blood pressure and lipid levels (DeFronzo et al., 1987; Franssila-Kallunki et al., 1992). As shown in the Diabetes Prevention Project, aggressive lifestyle modification reduces risk for new-onset diabetes mellitus in obese middle-aged patients by 58% (Tuomilehto et al., 2001). In motivated patients unable to achieve adequate weight loss, pharmacologic intervention is an option. Orlistat (Xenical) is a GI lipase inhibitor that reduces the absorption of dietary fat from the gut. It facilitates weight reduction and should be taken with meals; its major side-effect is fatty, oily stools that can precipitate diarrhea. Bariatric surgery for morbidly obese patients has been shown to relieve insulin resistance, promote substantial weight loss, reduce BP, and improve dyslipidemia. The Mediterranean diet (increased consumption of fish, legumes, whole grains, olive oil) is associated with weight loss and improvements in lipid, insulin sensitivity, and inflammatory indices.

Serum LDL-C and non-HDL-C should be treated to NCEP-defined targets. Therapeutic effort should be expended to raise HDL-C. The choice of whether a statin or fibrate should be used as initial therapy should be dictated by the specific features of a patient's lipid profile. In post hoc analyses of the Helsinki Heart Study (Manninen et al., 1992), VA-HIT (Robins et al., 2002) and Bezafibrate Infarction Prevention trials (BIP Study Group, 2000), fibrate therapy significantly improved lipid profiles and reduced cardiovascular morbidity and mortality in patients with insulin resistance and the metabolic syndrome. Many of these patients will require combinations of antilipidemic medications to normalize their lipid profiles. Since patients with the metabolic syndrome have activation of the RAAS axis, many authorities on hypertension believe it is reasonable to treat the hypertension of these patients with ACEI and ARBs as first-line therapy (Grundy et al., 2004a, 2004b). However, no clinical trials help to establish whether this is the optimal approach compared to other available classes of antihypertensive medication. On the other hand, a number of studies, including the HOPE (Heart Outcomes Prevention Evaluation Study Investigators, 2000), VALUE (Julius et al., 2004), Captopril Prevention Project (Hansson et al., 1999) and LIFE (Dahlof et al., 2003) trials, among others, have shown that ACEI and ARBs can reduce the onset of diabetes mellitus by 20% to 34% compared to non-RAAS-affecting comparative antihypertensives. Aspirin prophylaxis should be considered in patients with a 10-year Framingham risk that exceeds 10%.

KEY TREATMENT

In metabolic syndrome, comprehensive risk factor evaluation should be undertaken in all patients at risk for diabetes and CVD (SOR: A).

Lifestyle modification can reduce risk of developing diabetes mellitus by 58% (Diabetes Prevention Project) (SOR: A).

Weight loss can be achieved through caloric restriction, exercise, and when indicated, pharmacologic intervention or bariatric surgery (SOR: A).

Diabetes Mellitus

Key Points

- Diabetes mellitus is a CAD risk equivalent.
- Blood sugar should be regulated aggressively and patients initially treated with a combination of insulin sensitizers, including metformin and thiazolidinediones.
- More than three fourths of diabetic patients will die of complications of macrovascular disease.

Incidence

According to statistics compiled by the U.S. Centers for Disease Control (CDC, 2003), approximately 18.2 million people in the United States had diabetes mellitus (DM). Of these, 13 million are diagnosed, but approximately 5.2 million or more go undiagnosed. Almost all adult patients with DM (90%-95%) have type 2. Based on recent demographic trends, an estimated 1.3 million or more new cases of DM will be diagnosed annually. The World Health Organization (WHO) estimates that by 2025, more than 300 million people will have DM worldwide (King et al., 1998; see also Amos et al., 1997). Diabetes significantly magnifies the risk for MI, sudden death, stroke, CHF, adult-onset blindness and loss of lower extremities, and end-stage renal disease (ESRD). Given its burgeoning incidence, complications of DM will likely incur a level of human suffering unprecedented outside of wartime. This is an issue that must be addressed directly by family physicians worldwide.

Cardiovascular Effects

Diabetes induces diffuse atherosclerotic disease throughout the vascular tree. Almost 80% of diabetic patients will die of cardiovascular disease. The hyperglycemic, insulin-resistant milieu of type 2 DM initiates a broad-ranging cascade of pathophysiology that accelerates atherogenesis. Unfortunately, because of increasing obesity and metabolic syndrome in adolescents and young adults, type 2 DM is becoming relatively common in those younger than 21. Diffuse endothelial dysfunction, the accumulation of damaging advanced glycation end products in the vasculature, and a heavy risk factor burden typify the patient with DM. Diabetes induces a prooxidative and proinflammatory state. Diabetic patients also tend to have hypercoagulability (Meigs et al., 2000), likely from (1) increased hepatic production of coagulation factors; (2) increased platelet reactivity and aggregability; and (3) as endothelial dysfunction progresses, the endothelium produces less tissue plasminogen activator (tPA) and more PAI-1, rendering the surface of the vascular lumen more prothrombotic. This hypercoagulability and disordered fibrinolysis increases the likelihood that acute plaque rupture will result in greater and perhaps complete vascular luminal obstruction with acute ischemia and infarction.

Management

It is critical for diabetic patients to be diagnosed early and their risk factors evaluated and treated comprehensively. In addition to monitoring indices of glycemia, BP, serum lipids, smoking, and obesity status, baseline renal function should be evaluated. Hypertension, dyslipidemia, and albuminuria or proteinuria require aggressive management. Based on the East-West (Haffner et al., 1998) and OASIS (Malmberg et al., 2000) studies, the NCEP has defined DM as a CAD risk equivalent. As shown in the EPIC-Norfolk Study, as hemoglobin A_{1c} (HbA$_{1c}$) levels steadily rise above 5.0, risk for coronary events rises continuously (Khaw et al., 2004). The ADA recommends that HbA$_{1c}$ be less than 7.0, although the American College of Endocrinology endorses a level less than 6.5. With more aggressive diabetes management, the risk for vascular disease development decreases, but the risk for episodic hypoglycemia increases (Diabetes Control and Complications Trial Research Group, 1995). The United Kingdom Prospective Diabetes Study (UKPDS 35) demonstrated that for every 1% drop in HbA_{1c}, diabetic patients experience a 21% reduction in any diabetes-related end point, 14% drop in MI, 12% reduction in stroke, and a 37% reduction in risk of microvascular disease (Stratton et al., 2000). In the STENO-2 Study, intensive therapy of blood sugars, BP, and serum lipids resulted in a 50% lower incidence of the primary composite cardiovascular end point compared to "conventional" therapy, which was substantially less aggressive (Gaede et al., 2003). The UKPDS showed that metformin therapy reduces the risk for acute cardiovascular events by 38%. The thiazolidinediones (pioglitazone, rosiglitazone) exert multiple beneficial effects within the vasculature, improve glycemic control and reduce insulin resistance, and improve lipid profiles. In the Prospective Actos Clinical Trial in Macrovascular Events (PROACTIVE) (Dormandy et al., 2005), carotid intima-media thickness in atherosclerosis using pioglitazone (CHICAGO) (Mazzone et al., 2006) and the Pioglitazone Effect on Regression of Intravascular Sonographic Coronary Obstruction Prospective Evaluation (PERISCOPE) trials (Nissen et al., 2008), pioglitazone had demonstrable capacity to reduce risk for stroke and MI and stabilize carotid intima media thickness and coronary atheroma in patients with DM, respectively. Both rosiglitazone and pioglitazone have "durability of effect" relative to metformin and the sulfonylureas, helping to stabilize glycemic control for longer periods without the need for additional antiglycemic medication, possibly because they preserve islet cell insulin secretory capacity (Kahn et al., 2006). Unless there is a contraindication, diabetic patients should take prophylactic aspirin therapy. When initiating therapy for non-insulin-dependent DM (NIDDM), strong consideration should be given to using combination therapy with metformin and a thiazolidinedione to ensure insulin sensitization in the liver, skeletal muscle, and adipose tissue.

Hypertension typically accompanies diabetes. Diabetic patients require, on average, three or more antihypertensive medications to meet BP targets. Based on NHANES-III, 65% to 80% of diabetic men and women (Caucasian, Hispanic, or African-American) either have HTN or BP greater than 130/80 mm Hg. In diabetic hypertensive patients with and without nephropathy, the percentage reaching BP goals is 11% and less than 10%, respectively. Clinical trials have unequivocally demonstrated that BP control decreases risk for acute cardiovascular events and the development of nephropathy in patients with type 2 DM. The Hypertension Optimal Treatment trial evaluated the effect of BP reduction on cardiovascular event rates in 1501 diabetic patients (Hansson et al., 1999). There were increasing, statistically significant differences in the triple composite end point (MI, stroke, and mortality) as diastolic BP was reduced from 90 to 85 to 80 mm Hg. When comparing patients in the groups whose DBP was treated to 80 or less and 90 or less, the more intensively treated group had 51% fewer acute cardiovascular events and 43% less cardiovascular mortality. Importantly, this trial found no confirmation of the "J curve" hypothesis (i.e., the incidence of cardiovascular events increases as DBP decreases secondary to a reduction in coronary perfusion pressure during diastole). There was no increase in adverse cardiovascular events; DBP was reduced to lower and lower levels. In the UKPDS (1998), 1148 type 2 diabetic patients were randomly assigned to one of two different BP target groups: less than 150/85 ("intensive" treatment) or less than 180/105 ("conventional" treatment). The average achieved BPs over 9 years of follow-up for the two groups were 144/82 and 154/87, respectively. The group that was more intensively treated experienced greater reductions in stroke (44%; $p = 0.01$), diabetes-related mortality (32%; $p = 0.02$), and microvascular complications (37%; $p = 0.009$), including nephropathy and retinopathy, compared to the group receiving conventional treatment. These studies endorse the need for aggressive pharmacologic intervention when treating HTN in diabetic patients.

In diabetic patients with nephropathy, ACEI and ARBs should be used as first-line therapy and titrated as tolerated so as to reduce BP and urinary albumin and protein excretion as much as possible (Brenner et al., 2001; Lewis et al., 1993 and 2001; Morgensen et al., 2000). It is recommended that 24-hour urine specimens be used to monitor the response to therapy and disease progression in patients with nephropathy (Cooper and Gilbert, 2000; Toth, 2003). In diabetic patients with albuminuria, both ACEI (HOPE Study Investigators, 2000) and ARBs (Parving et al., 2001) reduced the magnitude of albumin excretion and decreased the rates of progression to nephropathy. In the recent AMADEO trial, telmisartan was shown to be significantly more effective than losartan at reducing proteinuria in patients with diabetic nephropathy (Bakris et al., 2008). Nondihydropyridine CCBs (diltiazem, verapamil) have also been shown to reduce the magnitude of protein excretion in patients with diabetic nephropathy.

In diabetic patients, reductions in serum LDL and elevations in HDL are the first and the second priority of therapy, respectively, to reduce risk for acute cardiovascular events (Turner et al., 1998). Serum LDL and TG levels should be reduced to less than 100 mg/dL and less than 150 mg/dL, respectively. The ADA (2004) recommends that HDL be raised to 40 mg/dL or greater and 50 mg/dL or greater in men and women, respectively. The choice of antilipidemic medication should be dictated by the specific disturbances characterizing a lipid profile. In such studies as the Collaborative Atorvastatin Diabetes Study (Calhoun et al., 2004) and Scandinavian Simvastatin Survival Study (Pyorala et al., 1997), statin therapy was associated with a 37% and 42% reduction in the risk of cardiovascular events among diabetic patients in the primary and secondary prevention settings, respectively (Dunstan et al., 2002). Fibrate therapy has also been shown to reduce risk for cardiovascular events and rates of atheromatous plaque progression in patients with DM. The thiazolidinediones have also been shown to favorably impact lipoprotein levels (van Wijk et al., 2003).

KEY TREATMENT

Tight control of glycemia, dyslipidemia, and hypertension to nationally defined standards is tantamount to aggressive risk reduction for diabetes (SOR: A).

Treating diabetic patients with statins should be strongly considered regardless of lipid profile (SOR: A).

Nephropathy increases risk for CVD and should be screened for and treated with ACEI/ARB (SOR: A).

C-Reactive Protein

Key Points

- CRP can be measured in patients with a 10-year Framingham risk score of 10% to 20%.
- CRP helps further stratify patients into low-, moderate-, and high-risk groups.
- CRP should not be measured in low-risk or high-risk groups because it is unlikely to alter management.

Elevations in serum levels of C-reactive protein (CRP) have emerged as an important marker of systemic inflammation and increased risk for cardiovascular disease (Ridker, 2001; Ridker et al., 2002). CRP is a pentraxin molecule that, like other acute-phase reactants, is produced by the liver in response to increased levels of IL-6. Approximately one half of all strokes and acute MIs occur in people with normal cholesterol levels (Braunwald, 1997). Consequently, traditional risk factor evaluation does not always accurately identify patients at risk for acute cardiovascular events. Serum CRP levels measured with a high-sensitivity assay (hsCRP) add significant prognostic information when evaluating global cardiovascular risk factor burden at all levels of the calculated Framingham risk score and with all levels of severity of the metabolic syndrome.

Although not yet a therapeutic target, accumulating evidence suggests that CRP may play a direct role in atherogenesis (Ridker et al., 2003; Toth, 2005). CRP stimulates the expression of endothelial CAMs, monocyte chemoattractant protein-1, angiotensin type-1 receptors, endothelin-1 and promotes LDL oxidation. When bound to oxidized LDL, CRP can activate, complement, and promote formation of the cytotoxic membrane attack complex (Bhakdi et al., 1999; Torzewski et al., 1998). CRP induces endothelial cell dysfunction (Venugopal et al., 2002; Verma et al., 2002) and promotes the scavenging of LDL particles by macrophages. CRP is expressed by the cellular constituents of atheromatous plaque, further implicating its role in atherogenesis (Yasojima et al., 2001).

A number of studies have demonstrated a strong relationship between hsCRP and risk for cardiovascular disease. In the Physicians' Health Study, men in the highest quartile of CRP had a threefold higher risk for MI over 8 years of follow-up compared to men in the lowest quartile (Ridker et al., 1997). Similarly, the European Monitoring Trends and Determinants in Cardiovascular Disease (MONICA) study demonstrated a 2.6-fold increased risk for an acute cardiovascular event among men in the highest versus lowest quartiles of CRP over 8 years of follow-up (Koenig et al., 1999). CRP measurements also portend risk in women. Among women enrolled in the Women's Health Study, elevated CRP portends risk for cardiovascular disease and emerged as a better predictor of risk than serum LDL-C (Ridker et al., 2000, 2002). Elevated CRP levels are also associated with increased risk for stroke, metabolic syndrome, and new-onset DM (Pradhan et al., 2001; Ridker et al., 2003; Rost et al., 2001). Among patients with established CAD, a high CRP is associated with increased risk for recurrent ACS (Blake et al., 2003).

The AHA and CDC issued guidelines on the use of CRP for stratifying patients at risk for cardiovascular disease (Pearson et al., 2003). High-sensitivity assays for this analyte are highly reproducible and accurate. Although other inflammatory markers have demonstrated predictive value (e.g., VCAM-1, lipoprotein associated phospholipase A2), at present, CRP is the only such marker recommended for risk-screening purposes. Patients at low (10-yr risk <5%) and high (CAD, CAD risk equivalent, or 10-yr risk >20%) risk should not be screened for CRP. In the primary prevention setting, the target population consists of patients at moderate risk (10-yr risk 5%-20%). CRP levels less than 1.0, 1.0 to 3.0, and greater than 3.0 mg/L portend low, intermediate, and high risk, respectively, for cardiovascular disease. CRP should be measured twice over 2 weeks and the results averaged; hsCRP values that exceed 10 mg/L suggest acute inflammation and should not be used. The test should be repeated when acute infection or inflammation has resolved. Patients in the high-risk group should institute lifestyle modification. Weight loss, exercise, and smoking cessation reduce CRP significantly. Pharmacologic intervention should be instituted for dyslipidemia, hypertension, and impaired glycemic control as indicated. AHA and CDC do not recommend CRP screening in patients with established cardiovascular disease. These patients should already be receiving aggressive lifestyle and pharmacologic intervention to reduce risk for secondary events.

The Justification for the Use of Statin in Prevention: an Intervention Trial Evaluating Rosuvastatin (JUPITER) trial was a primary prevention trial performed in 26 countries (Ridker et al., 2008). The primary objective was to determine if statin therapy would reduce risk for first-time events in men and women at risk for CVD secondary to elevated hsCRP (>2.0 ng/L) but did not meet criteria for lipid-lowering statin therapy because of a low to normal LDL-C of less than 130 mg/dL, as set by the National Cholesterol Education Program. Men older than 50 and women over 60 were enrolled, had no evidence of atherosclerotic disease, and could not be diabetic. The combined primary end point included stroke, MI, cardiovascular mortality, need for revascularization, and hospitalization for unstable angina. Analysis was by intention to treat. The median age of subjects was 66.0 years. The median baseline lipid profile included: LDL-C of 108 mg/dL, TGs of 118 mg/dL, and HDL-C of 49 mg/dL. The median attained lipid values after 4 years of rosuvastatin therapy included LDL-C of 55 mg/dL, triglyceride of 99 mg/dL, and HDL-C of 50 mg/dL. The median achieved serum CRP level after 1 and 4 years of rosuvastatin therapy was 2.2 and 1.8 mg/L, respectively. Rosuvastatin therapy reduced the relative risk for the primary composite end point by 44% compared to placebo. Significant relative risk reductions with rosuvastatin were also achieved in multiple secondary end points, including nonfatal MI (65%), nonfatal stroke (48%), arterial revascularization (46%), and all-cause mortality (20%). The composite end points of MI, stroke, or hospitalization for unstable angina and MI, stroke, or cardiovascular death were both reduced by 47%. All prespecified subgroups (male/female, age >65 or <65, with or without hypertension, ±metabolic syndrome, smoking status, Framingham risk score >10% or <10%) derived significant benefit from rosuvastatin therapy. JUPITER is the first primary prevention trial with a statin to demonstrate statistically significant reductions in cardiovascular events for women (46%), elderly patients (>70 yr; 39%), and African American and Hispanic patients

(37%). Projected over 5 years, the number needed to treat (NNT) to prevent one vascular event is estimated at 25, a favorable figure for a primary prevention trial. In JUPITER, rosuvastatin therapy was also associated with reduced risk for thromboembolic phenomena.

Homocysteine

Although homocysteine is widely assumed to be an established risk factor for atherosclerotic disease, little prospective clinical trial or epidemiologic evidence supports this (Christen and Ridker, 2000). It has been known for decades that patients with homocystinuria have increased risk for CAD, stroke, PAD, and thromboembolic events (Handy and Loscalzo, 2003). Many documented enzyme mutations are etiologic for *hyperhomocysteinemia,* which is associated with increased endothelial dysfunction and hypercoagulability. Mutations in methylenetetrahydrofolate reductase, cystathionine-β-synthase, methionine synthase, and γ-cystathionase can lead to elevations in serum homocysteine levels. The supplementation of patients with folate and vitamins B_6 (pyridoxine) and B_{12} (cyanocobalamin) frequently helps to normalize the levels of patients with hyperhomocysteinemia. These three vitamins are available in a single combination formulation (Folbee, Foltx).

Two clinical trials evaluating folate/B_6/B_{12} supplementation in patients with CAD and undergoing percutaneous transluminal coronary angioplasty (PTCA) demonstrate the contradictory nature of some data in this field. In one study, triple-vitamin therapy resulted in reduced rates of atheromatous plaque progression, in-stent restenosis, and need for subsequent revascularization of the target lesion (Schnyder et al., 2001). In a subsequent study, triple-vitamin therapy showed increased rates of plaque progression as well as increased in-stent restenosis and need for target lesion revascularization (Lange et al., 2004). The AHA and American College of Cardiology (ACC) currently discourage widespread screening for hyperhomocysteinemia. Seven different randomized, placebo-controlled trials (RCTs) are prospectively evaluating whether treatment of homocystinemia reduces risk for cardiovascular morbidity and mortality.

Cigarette Smoking

Key Points

- Cigarette smoking is the single most preventable cause of mortality in the United States.
- Cigarette smoking cessation reduces risk for myocardial infarction and mortality by 36%.

On an annualized basis, cigarette smoking in the United States incurs over $193 billion in lost productivity and direct health care costs. Approximately 23.5% of American men and 20.9% of American women are smokers. Unfortunately, the incidence of smoking among adolescents and teenagers continues to rise despite legislation limiting some forms of advertising and the sale of cigarettes to minors. Smoking is the single most *preventable* cause of mortality in the United

States. In addition to increasing risk for developing pulmonary, oral, laryngeal, and bladder neoplasms, cigarette smoking significantly raises risk for developing all forms of atherosclerotic disease and potentiates myocardial ischemia, adverse structural damage to the lung parenchyma, and arterial aneurysm formation. More than 440,000 Americans succumb annually from tobacco-related disease. Smoking also increases risk for erectile dysfunction, osteoporosis, insulin resistance, poor wound healing, pneumonia, and other complications.

Cigarette smoke contains more than 4000 exogenous chemicals. Cigarette smoking is associated with increased intravascular oxygen free-radical production and induces diffuse endothelial dysfunction, resulting in marked reductions in nitric oxide and tissue plasminogen activator (tPA) production (Chia and Newby, 2002). These changes result in increased oxidative injury to cells and lipoproteins, vasoconstriction, and reduced capacity for fibrinolysis in the setting of plaque rupture and overlying thrombus formation. In addition to accelerating rates of atherogenesis in native arteries, continued smoking reduces rates of arterial and venous graft patency in the heart and peripheral vasculature. Cigarette smoking is associated with increased serum levels of multiple emerging risk factors, including CRP, fibrinogen, and homocysteine (Bazzano et al., 2003).

Achieving lifelong smoking cessation in patients who have, or are at risk for, cardiovascular disease is a critical therapeutic goal. Smoking cessation results in a 36% reduction in risk for MI and mortality (van Berkel et al., 1999). Bupropion (Zyban, 150-300 mg orally daily) reduces the intensity of withdrawal symptoms in patients trying to quit smoking by inhibiting the neuronal reuptake of norepinephrine, serotonin, and dopamine. These neurotransmitters are associated with central centers modulating addiction and craving/appetitive behaviors. After taking bupropion for about 2 weeks, patients can begin to wean themselves from cigarette smoke according to a plan established with their provider. Sustained smoking cessation is facilitated by continuing bupropion for 3 to 6 months after patients smoke their last cigarette. Continued counseling and encouragement are important. Smoking cessation classes are also usually available as part of community health awareness programs. Another approach involves the use of nicotine replacement therapies, such as NicoDerm CQ or Habitrol (transdermal delivery systems) and Nicorette gum. These therapies also control withdrawal and craving by providing an alternative source of nicotine that can be progressively weaned over weeks to months. One recommended regimen for the nicotine patch is to wear each dose (21, 14, and 7 mg) for 1 month in a stepped-down fashion. Patients wearing the patch should be counseled not to smoke because this can induce headache, nausea, flushing, and even angina. If a patient cannot achieve smoking cessation on single-agent therapy, the combination of bupropion and a transdermal nicotine patch has been shown to increase success rates compared to the use of either agent alone.

Another smoking-cessation agent, varenicline (Chantix), is a nicotinic acetylcholine receptor agonist that controls withdrawal symptoms during abstinence from nicotine. Treatment with varenicline at 1 mg orally twice daily is associated with a 44% smoking-discontinuation rate after 3 months of continuous therapy (Gonzales et al., 2006). However, side effects have been a concern.

KEY TREATMENT

Smoking cessation is facilitated by patient education about the dangers of smoking and pharmacologic intervention with nicotine replacement products, bupropion, and varenicline (SOR: A). Relapse rates are high in the absence of education, encouragement, and individualized courses of therapy and follow-up (SOR: A).

Coronary Artery Disease

Stable Angina

Angina pectoris can manifest as chest pain, chest pressure, or a heavy feeling or squeezing sensation. Angina is a symptom of myocardial ischemia. Stable angina is caused by a mismatch between coronary blood supply and myocardial oxygen demand. The latter is determined by several factors, including heart rate and left ventricular wall stress and contractility (Braunwald, 2000). Coronary supply is determined by oxygen transport capacity and delivery and conditions that regulate the coronary circulatory system (e.g., nitric oxide, endothelin), autonomic nervous system, metabolic activity, neural control, and perfusion pressure. Several pharmacologic interventions also affect the coronary circulation, including adrenergic receptor activation or blockade, adenosine, and acetylcholine. Most coronary flow occurs during systole, whereas only 25% of flow occurs in diastole (Feigl, 1998; Yada et al., 1999).

In stable angina, blood flow cannot meet myocardial oxygen demands because of an obstructive atherosclerotic plaque in one or more coronary arteries (Fig. 27-8). It typically occurs predictably with exertion and resolves within minutes of initiating rest. This stable angina pattern does not usually occur at rest. Nonatherosclerotic obstructive CAD can also cause angina. Although infrequent, it could be mediated by myocardial bridging, vasculitis, or congenital malformation of the coronary arteries. In addition, conditions without obstructive CAD (e.g., cardiomyopathies, valve disease) can trigger angina (Lee, 2000).

Symptoms of stable angina differ among patients. Angina can be perceived as a pressure, tightness, squeezing, or heaviness in the chest. This could radiate to the arm, jaw, shoulders, back, or abdomen. The pain can be associated with an increase in shortness of breath, a feeling of nausea, diaphoresis, or occasional vomiting. Lightheadedness and anxiety might accompany those symptoms. Patients might describe one or more of these symptoms, which can be very atypical in female and diabetic patients. Finally, as observed in patients with long-standing DM, myocardial ischemia can be silent with no angina reported. Dyspnea without chest pain can be an "anginal equivalent." Ischemia can induce stiffness in the myocardium and reduces ventricular relaxility, which in return raises left ventricular end-diastolic pressure and leads to dyspnea. Angina or anginal-equivalent symptoms typically resolve with rest or nitroglycerin.

Noncardiac chest pain typically occurs with certain maneuvers, such as taking a deep breath (e.g., sharp pleuritic pain), palpation of the chest wall (as in musculoskeletal pain, costochondritis), or after certain types of food ingestion (e.g., esophageal pain from refluxed acid). If chest pain is noncardiac in origin or the cause of pain cannot be easily identified, it is important to rule out pulmonary embolism (Lee, 2002) or aortic dissection (Collins, 2004) because these etiologies

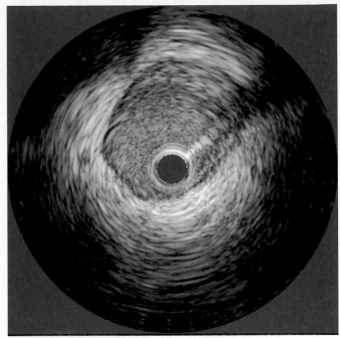

Figure 27-8 Glacov remodeling of the coronary lumen in response to early plaque formation.

can be fatal if missed. Pulmonary hypertension and pericarditis are also part of the differential diagnosis.

Several signs may be noted on examination in a patient with angina. Paradoxical splitting of the second heart sound (S2), systolic murmurs, and S3 or S4 can be appreciated during an anginal episode. Findings of cardiomyopathy or valvular disorders may help establish the diagnosis of a noncoronary cause of chest pain. Patients can also be hypertensive, have signs of hyperlipidemia (arcus cornea or xanthelasmas), or findings of diabetes (neuropathy or diabetic retinopathy).

Noninvasive Testing

Electrocardiogram

The electrocardiogram (ECG) often does not show ischemic changes in patients with stable angina who are at rest and have no symptoms. The resting ECG, however, might show nonspecific ST-segment and T-wave abnormalities in a patient with known severe CAD. False-positive results are common in patients with left ventricular hypertrophy (LVH), digoxin intake, electrolyte imbalances, or electrical conduction anomalies such as bundle branch blocks (BBBs) or preexcitation syndromes.

The ECGs need to be compared to previous readings. Frequently, new Q-wave abnormalities or the emergence of conduction disturbances might indicate an interval change in the patient's cardiac status. The ECG can be helpful during an episode of chest pain, when more than 50% of patients with normal resting ECG show new changes. Typically, these changes include the presence of ST-segment depression or elevation in two contiguous leads, new T-wave inversions or pseudonormalization of already-inverted T waves.

Exercise Treadmill Stress Testing

Exercise treadmill testing can be performed in patients who are able to exercise on a treadmill. Using different protocols (Bruce, Modified Bruce, Naughton), the patient exercises at

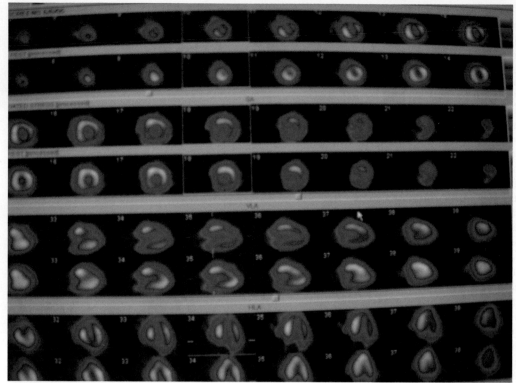

Figure 27-9 Myocardial perfusion scan shows reversible ischemia in the anterior wall, apex, and inferior wall.

different inclines and speeds until achieving 85% of peak predicted heart rate for age ([220 − age] × 85%). The test provides information about the presence of ischemic ST-segment changes, reproducibility of chest pain, arrhythmias, and changes in BP, heart rate, and functional capacity. Patients with good functional capacity generally have a good prognosis. An early positive stress test (in first two stages of exercise) can indicate a worse prognosis. The mean sensitivity of this test is 68% and specificity 77% (Gibbons et al., 2002). Some studies indicate that, when selection bias is removed, the sensitivity can be as low as 40% to 50%, but specificity as high as 85% to 90% (Detrano et al., 1989; Gianrossi et al., 1989).

The test specificity is reduced when baseline ECGs are abnormal with LVH, preexcitation syndrome, or BBB, or if the patient is taking digoxin (Sketch et al., 1981; Sundqvist et al., 1986) or has electrolyte abnormalities (Gibbons et al., 2002; Froelicher et al., 1999). Also, if a patient cannot reach target heart rate, the diagnostic accuracy of the test is diminished. If a patient experiences chest pain and 1 mm ST-segment depression during exercise, the test can be 90% predictive of the presence of CAD. A 2 mm ST depression accompanied by chest pain is almost pathognomonic of the presence of obstructive CAD. It should be noted that the presence of anti-ischemic agents (nitrates, β-blockers, calcium channel blockers) can reduce the sensitivity of the test and should be withheld for 2 to 3 days before the procedure for long-acting drugs and 24 hours for short-acting drugs, if the intent from the test is to diagnose the presence of obstructive disease (Gibbons et al., 2002).

A treadmill stress test can be a first choice test to diagnose CAD by the family physician, in both male and female patients, assuming the patient can exercise on a treadmill,

the baseline ECG has no indication of LVH or conduction abnormalities, and the patient has no electrolyte disturbances and is not taking digoxin (Melin et al., 1985). When adjusting for the pretest probability of disease, female patients have only a slightly reduced specificity on a regular stress than male patients. A baseline borderline ST-segment depression less than 1 mm is not an exclusionary criterion to perform a treadmill stress test.

The absolute contraindications to stress testing are decompensated CHF, symptomatic severe aortic valve stenosis, ongoing rest chest pain, a recent MI (in past week), severe hypertension, and intractable arrhythmias. When patients have conditions that reduce the specificity of a stress test, an imaging stress test (nuclear or echocardiographic) can more accurately evaluate for CAD.

Stress Myocardial Perfusion Imaging

Myocardial perfusion imaging (^{99m}Tc-sestamibi, ^{99m}Tc-tetrofosmin, or thallium-201) provides a more accurate modality to diagnose the presence of obstructive CAD than a treadmill ECG alone (Fig. 27-9). The sensitivity and specificity of this test have been reported to be 88% and 72%, respectively. When referral bias is accounted for, the specificity of this test is as high as 90%. In addition to myocardial perfusion, the test provides information about ejection fraction and wall motion abnormalities and is very valuable to predict a patient's prognosis (Klocke et al., 2003).

Nuclear stress testing is expensive, so regular treadmill testing is considered as the first diagnostic modality when possible. Nuclear stress testing is useful in patients with the likelihood of a low-specificity treadmill ECG. Nuclear imaging can provide information about prognosis and myocardial viability in regions of wall motion abnormalities, as well as help localize the area of myocardium in jeopardy. As with most stress tests, these are best ordered in patients with an intermediate likelihood of obstructive CAD.

Myocardial perfusion imaging can be also performed with the induction of pharmacologic stress, usually with adenosine or dobutamine. Adenosine is a vasodilator and stresses the heart by a "steal phenomenon." Adenosine and dipyridamole dilate normal coronaries, shunting blood from abnormal regions of the myocardium and creating a discrepancy in perfusion between normal and abnormal regions. Dobutamine increases heart rate and contractility and therefore increases myocardial oxygen demand.

Adenosine is typically infused over 4 or 6 minutes, depending on the protocol used. The infusion rate of 140 µg/kg/min starts with ECG monitoring. Usually halfway through the infusion, sestamibi (Myoview) or thallium is injected. Adenosine causes flushing, shortness of breath, nausea, chest pain, and a "strange" feeling in most patients that does not reflect the presence of CAD. Adenosine can also cause bradycardia and a high-degree atrioventricular (AV) block. Patients should not take any caffeinated beverages for at least 12 to 24 hours before the test. Also, adenosine can precipitate asthma and should not be used in patients with hyperreactive airway disease. Adenosine is an excellent choice for a test in patients who cannot exercise on a treadmill or those with a left BBB or a pacemaker rhythm. The sensitivity and specificity of adenosine stress imaging are 90% and 82%, respectively (Klocke et al., 2003).

Dobutamine is infrequently used and is reserved for patients who cannot exercise on a treadmill and have a contraindication to taking adenosine. Dobutamine is infused at 10 µg/kg/min for 3 minutes and then increased by increments of 10 µg/kg/min every 3 minutes to a maximum of 50 µg/kg/min, or if target heart rate has been achieved. If despite this high dose of dobutamine, target heart rate is not achieved, atropine is administered to a maximum of 1 to 2 mg. Cardiolite is injected typically at target heart rate, and the infusion is then terminated. Patients are generally observed for at least 10 minutes post-test or until the heart rate is below 100 beats/min. Dobutamine can cause a shaky feeling, nausea and arrhythmias. In general, it is well tolerated.

Although pharmacologic nuclear stress imaging provides similar diagnostic accuracy to treadmill nuclear stress testing, patients are best exercised on a treadmill. More information can be obtained from the treadmill test, including functional capacity, presence of arrhythmias with exercise, and hemodynamic response to physical exertion.

Stress Echocardiography

Stress echocardiography is an alternative imaging stress test to a nuclear stress test (Cheitlin et al., 2003). However, the sensitivity is slightly lower with an increase in specificity, making the overall accuracy of this test similar to stress nuclear imaging. Stress echocardiography is performed by obtaining an initial resting echocardiogram to assess a patient's left ventricular ejection fraction, wall motion characteristics, and cavity size. In about 25% of patients, it may be difficult to obtain optimal echocardiographic images for adequate interpretation of the test, and therefore an alternative stress testing is needed. This is particularly true in patients with severe chronic obstructive pulmonary disease (COPD) and patients with severe obesity. Patients are then exercised on a treadmill

using a symptom-limited protocol. Patients need to achieve the minimum target heart rate for age (85% of maximum predicted) but preferably a higher rate to allow ample time for the sonographer to obtain immediate post–stress echocardiographic images while the heart rate is still over target. Typically, the sonographer needs about 20 to 30 seconds to obtain these images. In patients who cannot exercise, dobutamine can be used as previously described to achieve the target heart rate, and then the infusion is discontinued when all echocardiographic images are acquired.

Regardless of the modality of stress testing, a test should be terminated when a patient displays significant arrhythmias, lightheadedness, a symptomatic drop in BP, or significant ischemic changes on the ECG, particularly if associated with anginal symptoms. Also, a stress test should not be performed in patients with unstable rest symptoms, frequent arrhythmia, known severe left main disease, severe symptomatic valvular disease, or decompensated CHF. The test needs to be closely monitored at all times by the technician, and a physician must always be nearby and frequently checking ECG changes and assessing the patient's symptoms and progress.

Computed Tomography of Heart

Multidetector computed tomography (MDCT) of the heart has recently emerged as an imaging modality for the diagnosis of coronary artery disease. As with the majority of noninvasive testing, MDCT is helpful in identifying CAD in patients with an intermediate pretest probability for CAD. Very-high-risk patients are not appropriate for this test and should undergo an invasive angiographic assessment. A negative MDCT result for CAD is helpful to exclude CAD, given the very high specificity of this test and thus low false-positive rate. Patients with equivocal noninvasive stress testing are ideal candidates, and if negative, MDCT can add to the reassurance of lack of significant obstructive CAD. CT angiography is not a screening tool in asymptomatic patients. Furthermore, MDCT is a reliable tool to evaluate bypass grafts and is an excellent test for identifying coronary anomalies (Cury et al., 2007). The test is not risk free, and the patient needs to be counseled on the risk of radiation exposure and contrast dye reactions.

Pharmacologic Management

Patients with stable angina have an imbalance between coronary blood supply and demand. Also, they are at increased risk of MI and arrhythmias. Medical therapies therefore should focus on alleviating angina, reducing plaque progression and rupture, and restoring a patient's functional capacity. Some reversible causes of angina need to be evaluated, such as conditions that increase myocardial oxygen demand. These include fever, thyrotoxicosis, anemia, and cardiac stimulants such as cocaine or amphetamines. Severe valvular dysfunction and CHF might also be precipitating factors.

Nitrate Therapy

Nitrate therapy reduces myocardial oxygen demand by increasing venous capacitance and therefore reducing venous return and ventricular wall stress. Also, nitrates increase coronary blood supply by dilating the coronary arteries (Parker and Parker, 1998). Administering nitrates to patients with stable angina increases their symptom-free walking distance and reduces the frequency and severity of their anginal episodes. Nitrates are not known to reduce risk for MI significantly or to prolong survival. On a chronic basis, nitrates can be administered orally or transdermally. Regardless of the mode of administration, it is important to have 8 to 10 hours of a nitrate-free period to avoid tolerance to this drug (Parker et al., 1995). Intravenous nitroglycerin is reserved for the unstable angina patient to reduce anginal pain and intracardiac filling pressures and to improve symptoms of heart failure.

Beta-Adrenergic Blockade

Beta-adrenergic blockers reduce myocardial oxygen demand primarily by reducing heart rate and contractility. Beta blockers are essential in patients with stable angina and a history of prior MI or reduced left ventricular function. In these conditions, β-blockers can prolong survival and should be administered to those patients unless absolutely contraindicated (Gottlieb et al., 1998).

It is unclear whether survival or serious arrhythmias are reduced in patients with stable angina and no prior MI or left ventricular dysfunction. Relative or absolute contraindications to beta-blocker therapy include patients with severe hyperreactive airway disease, heart block, severe bradycardia, or severe symptomatic peripheral vascular disease.

Calcium Channel Blockers

Long-acting CCBs are potent anti-ischemic drugs and also can be used to treat the patient with stable angina (Braunwald, 1982). Generally, short-acting CCBs need to be avoided because of the potential to increase adverse events. Dihydropyridines such as amlodipine (Norvasc) or nifedipine (Procardia XL) do not alter heart rate significantly and are primarily vasodilators. Diltiazem reduces heart rate but also increases coronary blood supply, whereas verapamil reduces oxygen demand primarily by reducing heart rate with less vasodilatory effects.

Ranolazine

Ranolazine (Ranexa) inhibits the cardiac late sodium current typically present in patients with ischemia. An increase in the late sodium current leads to excess entry of calcium into cardiomyocytes, which impairs cardiac relaxation. Ranolazine does not increase the rate pressure product, and its exact antianginal mechanism of action is unknown. In the Combination Assessment of Ranolazine in Stable Angina (CARISA) trial, patients were randomized to ranolazine and placebo added to standard antianginal therapy (Chaitman et al., 2004). Ranolazine increased exercise duration time and time to angina onset significantly, which was sustained at 12 weeks of therapy. Furthermore, in the Efficacy of Ranolazine in Chronic Angina (ERICA) RCT, ranolazine versus placebo was administered in patients with at least three anginal attacks per week despite high-dose amlodipine (10 mg/day). Over a 6-week period, ranolazine reduced anginal frequency by 23% and weekly nitroglycerin use by 25% compared to placebo (Stone et al., 2006).

Antiplatelet Agents

In high-risk patients, aspirin (81 mg) reduces vascular events by approximately 35% and is a prime therapy in patients with stable angina (Antiplatelet Trialists Collaboration, 1994). Aspirin is very effective in reducing MI in healthy subjects and elevated serum CRP levels (Ridker et al., 1997).

Aspirin resistance has been reported recently and can be present in approximately 25% of patients. Also, aspirin hypersensitivity is common and primarily related to GI side effects. Aspirin's side effects (e.g., bleeding, dyspepsia) can be reduced without compromising its effectiveness with the use of enteric-coated aspirin.

Clopidogrel (Plavix), an ADP-receptor antagonist, is a potent irreversible antiplatelet drug. In the Clopidogrel versus Aspirin in Patients at Risk of Ischaemic Events study (CAPRIE Steering Committee, 1996), Clopidogrel was slightly but statistically more effective than aspirin in reducing cardiovascular events in high-risk patients with a history of stroke, MI and peripheral vascular disease (8.7% relative risk [RR] reduction; $p = 0.043$). The combination of aspirin and clopidogrel in stable angina patients with no recent unstable coronary syndrome is unknown and currently being tested in the Clopidogrel for High Atherothrombotic Risk and Ischemic Stabilization, Management, and Avoidance (CHARISMA) trial (Bhatt and Topol, 2004). Clopidogrel is an effective alternative to patients who are unable to take aspirin.

In addition to the previous measures, aggressive management of dyslipidemia, hypertension, impaired glucose control, and smoking cessation are essential interventions to reduce future cardiovascular events in the stable angina patient. Cardiac rehabilitation is a critical therapeutic modality in patients with CAD, particularly after revascularization. The initiation of hormone replacement therapy in postmenopausal females is not indicated for cardiovascular risk reduction.

KEY TREATMENT

Beta blockers are recommended as initial therapy in the absence of contraindications in patients with or without prior myocardial infarction.

Aspirin is strongly recommended in patients with stable angina in the absence of contraindications.

ACC/AHA guidelines (Antman et al., 2008): SOR: A.

SECONDARY PREVENTION, CHRONIC STABLE ANGINA*

1. Comprehensive risk factor management and cardiac rehabilitation are essential in the management of the stable angina patients (SOR: A).
2. Recommended lipid management includes assessment of a fasting lipid profile. LDL-C should be less than 100 mg/dL (SOR: A).
3. Angiotensin-converting enzyme (ACE) inhibitors should be started and continued indefinitely in all patients with left ventricular ejection fraction (LVEF) of 40% or less and in those with hypertension, DM, or chronic kidney disease, unless contraindicated (SOR: A).
4. Angiotensin receptor blockers (ARBs) are recommended for patients who have hypertension, have indications for but are intolerant of ACE inhibitors, have heart failure, or have had an MI with LVEF of 40% or less (SOR: A).
5. Aldosterone blockade is recommended for use in post-MI patients without significant renal dysfunction or hyperkalemia who are already receiving therapeutic doses of an ACE inhibitor and a beta blocker, have LVEF of 40% or less, and have either diabetes or heart failure (SOR: A).
6. It is beneficial to start and continue beta-blocker therapy indefinitely in all patients who have had MI, acute coronary syndrome, or left ventricular dysfunction with or without heart failure symptoms, unless contraindicated (SOR: A).

*ACC/AHA quoted guidelines (Fraker, 2007).

Mechanical and Revascularization Strategies

Coronary Angioplasty and Bypass Surgery

Coronary angioplasty and stenting are currently reserved for patients who (1) are symptomatic and have failed optimal medical therapy with antianginal drugs or (2) have a moderate to large area of ischemia on nuclear scintigraphic imaging, severe proximal left anterior descending artery disease, single- or double-vessel CAD, or three-vessel CAD in nondiabetic patients with preserved left ventricular function.

Coronary artery bypass surgery is reserved for patients with (1) left main disease or severe three-vessel CAD, particularly diabetic patients or those with reduced left ventricular function, or (2) unsuitable anatomy for coronary angioplasty or those with disease in multiple CABGs, especially if the graft to the left anterior descending coronary artery is involved and can be considered for bypass surgery.

Enhanced External Counterpulsation (EECP)

Mechanical interventions such as EECP can be effective in the treatment of the patient with stable angina who is not a candidate for revascularization and has continued chest pain despite medical therapy (Michaels et al., 2005). This therapy requires about 32 sessions of 1-hour duration for 5 days a week. Although its functional mechanism is largely unknown, EECP improves exercise tolerance, reduces exercise-induced myocardial ischemia, and improves left ventricular diastolic filling in patients with CAD (Urano et al., 2001). Future therapies such as gene therapy to stimulate angiogenesis in the coronary arteries are being tested as an alternative to EECP in these patients.

Acute Coronary Syndromes

Key Point

- Patients with definite acute coronary syndrome should be evaluated for immediate reperfusion therapy (ACC/AHA guidelines; SOR: A).

Acute coronary syndromes (ACS) occur as a result of sudden atheromatous plaque rupture. Plaques with heightened inflammation, irrespective of severity, can rupture leading to overlying platelet and fibrin mesh formation, resulting in abrupt cessation of coronary blood flow. Patients might experience unstable angina or myocardial infarction (MI), depending on whether myocardial necrosis occurs. In the United States, 2.3 million people suffer an ACS annually.

Several crucial facts need to be considered by the practicing family physician. First, a large percentage of angiographically "normal" coronary arteries have significant plaque burden by intravascular ultrasound or magnetic resonance imaging (MRI), particularly in patients older than 40 years. Second, more than 60% of MIs are induced by culprit lesions that initially obstruct less than 50% of the arterial lumen. These lesions are generally not detected by stress testing. Third, when an ACS occurs, multiple vulnerable plaques generally coexist at the same time throughout the vascular tree. In an inadequately managed patient, any one of these lesions could suddenly rupture and precipitate an ACS. Therefore, a normal stress test does not necessarily exclude the possibility

of CAD and risk for MI. The prevention of MI should focus on reducing the chance of plaque rupture by controlling and normalizing, as much as possible, multiple cardiac risk factors, including hypertension, uncontrolled diabetes, dyslipidemia, obesity, lack of routine exercise, a heightened inflammatory state, and smoking.

Unstable Angina/Non–ST Segment Myocardial Infarction

Patients with unstable angina or a non–ST segment MI experience a partial occlusion to coronary flow as a result of plaque rupture and thrombus formation, microembolization, or the release of vasoactive substances leading to localized spasm. Patients typically have severe chest pain, with rest or minimal activity, which can be of sudden onset and with no preceding warnings and likely to last for more than 20 minutes unless treated with anti-ischemic agents. These patients are at high risk of ST-segment elevation MI and sudden death. Data from the Thrombolysis in Myocardial Infarction III (TIMI-III) registry indicated that death and MI could occur in these patients at a rate of 7.3% to 18.5%, depending on the severity of their symptoms, with postinfarction angina carrying the highest risk (Sharis et al., 2002). Patients might have electrocardiographic changes to indicate ischemia, mostly ST-segment depression in contiguous leads, T-wave inversion, or pseudonormalization of T waves. However, the electrocardiogram (ECG) could also be silent. Comparing the ECG to a previous one can be very helpful for detecting subtle but significant new changes.

Patients with suspected unstable angina should be referred to the emergency department (ED) or a specialized chest pain unit as soon as possible. They should be encouraged to call 9-1-1 and not drive themselves to the ED. A complete evaluation of their chest pain, including a comprehensive physical examination and history, obtaining an ECG within 10 minutes of arrival, chest radiograph and cardiac enzymes (e.g., troponin I, creatinine kinase MB), needs to be performed. Patients should be admitted to the hospital if they have ischemia on the ECG (ST-segment deviation or new T-wave abnormalities or new left BBB), ongoing chest pain, abnormal cardiac biomarkers, or develop CHF or hemodynamic instability.

Abnormal cardiac enzymes allow a definite diagnosis of MI. The most frequently used cardiac markers are myoglobin, creatinine kinase (CK) and CK-MB fractions, troponins T (TT) and I (TI). Myoglobin becomes abnormal in the first 1 to 2 hours following myocardial necrosis and remains abnormal for at least 7 to 12 hours. Its sensitivity is high for myocardial injury (83% within 6 hours of symptom onset), but it has a lower specificity. A positive myoglobin can result from muscle trauma, muscle disorders, rigorous exercise, and certain drugs such as statins. A more sensitive and specific marker than myoglobin is CK and its cardiac isoform CK-MB. This marker is 90% accurate for the diagnosis of MI at 6 hours from symptom onset. CK reaches its peak at about 24 hours of symptom onset and returns to normal or near normal by 72 hours. Troponin I is a very sensitive test for the diagnosis of MI at about 10 to 14 hours after onset of chest pain. Its sensitivity and specificity at 6 hours are approximately 58% and 94%, respectively, and 92% and 95% at 10 hours. TI levels remain abnormal for several days after myocardial injury.

Box 27-4 High-Risk Indicators in Patients with Unstable Angina*

1. New or presumably new ST-segment depression
2. Elevated troponin T or troponin I
3. Recurrent angina at rest or low level despite intense medical therapy
4. Reduced left ventricular function (ejection fraction <40%)
5. Recurrent angina or ischemia with congestive heart failure symptoms
6. Sustained ventricular arrhythmias
7. Hemodynamic instability
8. Recent history of coronary angioplasty or bypass surgery (past 6 months)
9. High risk based on noninvasive stress testing

*Level of evidence A, ACC/AHA guidelines (Braunwald, 2002).

Box 27-5 Acute Pharmacologic Therapy of Unstable Angina/Non–ST Elevation Myocardial Infarction*

1. Aspirin (or clopidogrel in patients who cannot take aspirin) should be administered as soon as possible after onset of symptoms and continued indefinitely.
2. Clopidogrel should be added to aspirin in the hospitalized patient and continued for a least 1 month whether patient will be undergoing percutaneous intervention or treated conservatively. Continuing clopidogrel and aspirin for up to 9 months is based on Level B evidence.
3. Antithrombin therapy with unfractionated heparin or low-molecular-weight heparin (preferred over unfractionated heparin unless bypass surgery is planned within 24 hours) should be started with clopidogrel and aspirin.
4. GpIIb/IIIa inhibitors should be added to aspirin, clopidogrel, and antithrombin in patients with planned revascularization, or those with no planned revascularization but who are undergoing ischemia or having abnormal cardiac biomarkers. However, abciximab should be avoided in patients with no planned revascularization.
5. Fibrinolytics are contraindicated in patients with unstable angina or non–ST segment elevation myocardial infarction.

*Level of evidence A, ACC/AHA guidelines (Braunwald, 2002)

Depending on the time of onset of chest pain, these markers have different levels of utility in the diagnosis of MI. For example, the diagnosis of MI in a patient who had chest pain more than 48 hours after presentation is best made with TI, whereas a recent onset MI of less than 6 hours' duration can best be made with myoglobin, CK and CK-MB. A negative TI after 12 hours of chest pain indicates a low risk for a cardiac event in the immediate future (<1 month). Therefore, patients who present with chest pain and have a negative TI at 12 hours after onset of chest pain can undergo a stress test either in the ED or as an outpatient, as long as the test has been scheduled within a few days of discharge.

Patients with suspected unstable angina/non–ST segment MI benefit significantly from an early aggressive therapy with angiography and revascularization, particularly when early high-risk indicators exist (Box 27-4).

The Treat Angina with Aggrastat and Determine Cost of Therapy with an Invasive or Conservative Strategy (TACTICS TIMI-18) study randomized unstable angina/non–ST elevation MI patients to an early aggressive therapy with revascularization (within 48 hours of presentation) versus an early conservative therapy in which patients were treated medically and then risk-stratified with exercise stress testing (Cannon et al., 2001). A significant reduction in the primary combined end point of death, MI, and rehospitalization for ACS was noted at 6 months (odds ratio [OR] 0.78, 95% CI [0.62, 0.97], p = 0.025). Other high-risk features include advanced age (>70), history of vascular disease, diabetes, and elevated hsCRP, WBC count, and B-type natriuretic peptide (BNP). Furthermore, based on data for the TIMI11B trial (1999), Antman and co-workers (2000) predicted that the risk of death, reinfarction, or recurrent severe ischemia requiring revascularization increased from 5% to 41% depending on the sum of the following individual prognostic variables: age greater than 65 years, more than three coronary risk factors, prior angiographic coronary obstruction, ST-segment deviation, more than two angina events within 24 hours, use of aspirin within 7 days, and elevated cardiac markers.

Although most unstable coronary syndromes are caused by plaque rupture, thrombosis, and superimposed spasm, rapidly progressive plaques can infrequently lead to an unstable syndrome. In addition, unstable angina can be precipitated by secondary causes such as thyrotoxicosis, severe hypertension or valvular stenosis, tachycardia, anemia, hypotension, and hypoxia.

Pharmacologic Therapy

Pharmacologic management of the patient with unstable angina or non–ST segment MI can be divided into acute and chronic therapy. In the *acute* phase (Box 27-5), patients are typically treated with an antithrombin drug (unfractionated heparin or low-molecular-weight heparin), upstream use of intravenous (IV) GP2b/3a inhibitors such as tirofiban (Aggrastat) or eptifibatide (Integrilin) (upstream use of the monoclonal antibody abciximab should be discouraged unless patients are brought to the cardiac catheterization laboratory within few hours of starting this drug, because the resurfacing of GP2b/3a receptors occurs with prolonged infusion of abciximab leading to partial loss of its antiplatelet effect), aspirin, clopidogrel, beta blockers, statins, IV nitrate therapy, ACE inhibitors (in patients with left ventricular dysfunction and continued hypertension or in diabetic patients) and supplemental oxygen therapy (in patients with respiratory distress and hypoxemia).

Low-molecular-weight heparin (LMWH; e.g., enoxaparin or Lovenox) has been shown to have some advantages over unfractionated heparin (UFH). These include more reliable anticoagulation with predictable pharmacokinetics, resistance to inhibition by platelet factor 4, a lower risk of causing heparin-induced thrombocytopenia (HIT), greater anti-Xa activity, and possibly greater efficacy in reducing risk for ACS. In the Efficacy and Safety of Subcutaneous Enoxaparin in Non-Q-Wave Coronary Events (ESSENCE) trial, enoxaparin plus aspirin was more effective than UFH plus aspirin in reducing the incidence of the combined end points of death, myocardial infarction, and recurrent angina (19.8% vs. 23.3%, respectively; p = 0.016) in patients with unstable angina or non-Q-wave MI at 1 month of follow-up (Cohen et al., 1997). A recent meta-analysis of 22,000 patients also demonstrated that enoxaparin is more effective than UFH in preventing the combined end point of death or MI (Petersen et al., 2004). Currently, enoxaparin, 1 mg/kg subcutaneously twice daily, is preferred over UFH (70 U/kg bolus IV, then 1000 U/hr adjusted every 6 hours with PTT checks) in patients who present with unstable angina or non–ST segment elevation MI.

Continued chest pain in patients with unstable angina despite optimal medical therapy indicates that the patient should be brought to the cardiac catheterization laboratory for immediate angiography and revascularization to minimize the chance of irreversible myocardial damage and loss of function. As previously noted, even in the pain-free patient with high-risk features, an aggressive approach to therapy is indicated and needs to be implemented within 48 hours of symptom onset. Morphine sulfate can be used to treat the acute pain unresponsive to anti-ischemic therapy.

Optimal antiplatelet treatment is needed with antithrombin drugs in the management of the patient with an ACS. Vascular injury leads to platelet activation and aggregation with subsequent fibrin deposition and thrombosis. Antithrombin therapy alone without optimal platelet inhibition leads to an inferior outcome during *percutaneous coronary intervention* (PCI). Early experience with PCI was performed with UFH in patients pretreated with aspirin. Aspirin is only partially effective as an antiplatelet drug by inhibiting cyclooxygenase and therefore partially blocking thromboxane A2 and collagen-mediated platelet activation and aggregation (Shammas et al., 2005). Platelet inhibition with clopidogrel (Plavix) is dose and time dependent. After a single 400-mg dose of clopidogrel, maximum platelet inhibition is achieved in 2 to 5 hours. In contrast, clopidogrel at 75 mg daily requires 3 to 7 days to reach the same level of inhibition. Blocking the ADP receptor irreversibly with clopidogrel has become an important step before PCI to reduce intermediate and long-term cardiac events. In the Clopidogrel for the Reduction of Events during Observation (CREDO) study, pretreatment of patients with clopidogrel (300 mg) at least 15 hours preintervention reduced long-term adverse events (Steinhubl et al., 2002). In the ISAR-REACT trial, pretreatment with clopidogrel (600 mg) provided similar outcomes in low-risk to intermediate-risk patients, regardless of assignment to abciximab or placebo, with maximum antiplatelet effect seen within 2 to 3 hours of treatment before intervention (Kandzari et al., 2004). In the Antiplatelet Therapy for Reduction of Myocardial Damage during Angioplasty (ARMYDA-2) study, clopidogrel at 600 mg was more effective in reducing cardiac events than clopidogrel at 300 mg when given at a mean of 6 hours before PCI in both arms (Patti et al., 2005). ARMYDA-2 also did not exclude patients from receiving GPIIb/IIIa inhibitors, thereby also supporting the hypothesis that optimal ADP receptor antagonism before PCI might be essential even when intraprocedural inhibition of platelet aggregation is achieved with GpIIb/IIIa inhibitors.

Currently, clopidogrel is given to all patients with an ACS immediately on presentation at an oral loading dose of 300 mg, then 75 mg daily. If a patient is proceeding to the cardiac catheterization laboratory and has not been receiving clopidogrel, a total of 600 mg as a loading dose should be administered.

In the *chronic* phase, typically following a revascularization procedure, the mainstay of therapy is aspirin, clopidogrel for 9 to 12 months, statins, ACE inhibitors, and beta blockade.

The Heart Outcomes Prevention Evaluation (HOPE) trial showed that ramipril (10 mg daily) reduced cardiovascular events significantly, including cardiovascular and total mortality and strokes (Yusuf et al., 2000). Patients were 55 years or older, and the majority had a history of vascular disease (80% history of CAD and 42% with PAD). Similar data were seen in the European Trial on Reduction of Cardiac Events with Perindopril in Stable CAD (EUROPA), which included 13655 patients with previous MI (64%), angiographic evidence of CAD (61%), coronary revascularization (55%), or a positive stress test only (5%). The mean age was 60 years, and patients had no CHF and stable CAD (Fox, 2003). In this study, 10% of placebo and 8% of perindopril (8 mg once daily) patients experienced the combined primary end point of cardiovascular death, MI, or cardiac arrest (20% RR reduction; $p = 0.0003$; favoring perindopril therapy) at a mean follow-up of 4.2 years.

Patients will also need to quit smoking, exercise, adhere to a low-fat, low-carbohydrate diet, lose weight if obese, and if diabetic, achieve aggressive control of their blood sugar to keep their HbA_{1c} less than 7% and preferably less than 6.5%.

KEY TREATMENT

Aspirin (75-324 mg daily) or clopidogrel (75 mg daily, in patients with intolerance or hypersensitivity to aspirin), lipid-lowering drugs, and diet are recommended in patients with low-density lipoprotein greater than 130 mg/dL (or LDL >100 mg/dL) (ACC/AHA guidelines) (SOR: B).

ACE inhibitors in patients with left ventricular dysfunction (ejection fraction <40%), congestive heart failure, hypertension, or diabetes should be initiated in those with unstable coronary syndromes (ACC/AHA guidelines) (SOR: A).

ST Elevation Myocardial Infarction

ST–segment elevation MI (STEMI) occurs secondary to a sudden interruption of coronary blood supply to a part of the myocardium as a result of a complete thrombotic occlusion of a coronary artery (DeWood et al., 1980). Plaque rupture is the predominant mechanism of STEMI with subsequent platelet and fibrin deposition. It is estimated that half a million STEMIs occur in the United States every year (Fig. 27-10).

Emergent and complete revascularization is the most important goal in the acute STEMI therapy. Current guidelines indicate that a patient with symptoms and signs of STEMI should receive either thrombolytics within 30 minutes or angioplasty within 90 minutes of arrival to the ED (Antman et al., 2004). Based on a hospital multidisciplinary protocol preapproved by the cardiologists, ED physicians, primary care physicians, and allied health care professionals, the ED physician generally decides on the choice of therapy. Currently, angioplasty is considered the first choice because it leads to overall superior results (Magid et al., 2000), primarily reducing the rate of nonfatal MI, and fewer intracranial bleeds compared to thrombolysis. Stronger evidence exists for primary angioplasty in STEMI as the risk of fibrinolysis increases (Kent et al., 2002). Patients with cardiogenic shock or severe CHF benefit more from primary angioplasty (Hochman, 2001; Wu et al., 2002). To be effective, however, angioplasty should be performed in intermediate- and

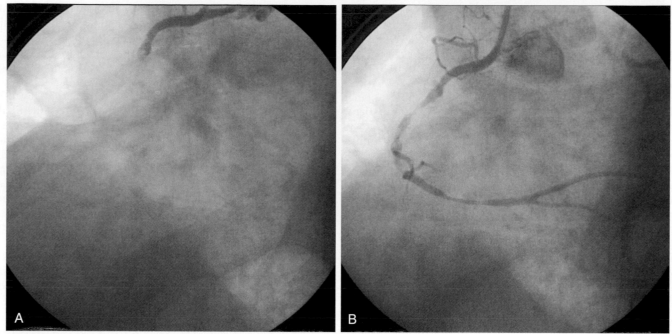

Figure 27-10 Acute inferior myocardial infarction. **A,** Sudden occlusion of the right coronary artery with a filling thrombus at the occlusion site. **B,** The same vessel after initial angioplasty showing multiple filling defects, indicating thrombus.

high-volume centers with an experienced catheterization team and interventional cardiologists on call and an multidisciplinary-approved hospital process (Canto et al., 2000). This MI "alert system" should be capable of effectively mobilizing all resources available to stay within the 90-minute period to first balloon inflation from arrival to the ED. Centers that do not have primary angioplasty capabilities should use fibrinolytic therapy as first-line therapy in STEMI. Box 27-6 lists contraindications to fibrinolysis.

Thrombolytic therapy has been shown to reduce mortality in patients with STEMI. Thrombolytics are contraindicated in patients with non–ST elevation MI because no clinical benefit has been shown and unwarranted risks exist. Thrombolysis enhances the body's fibrinolytic system by accelerating the formation of plasmin from plasminogen (Shammas, 1993). Plasmin degrades fibrin and several plasma proteins, including fibrinogen, prothrombin, and factors V and VIII, leading to a defective hemostasis. Thrombolytic agents are classified as clot-specific (alteplase [tPA], reteplase [recombinant-PA], and tenecteplase [TNK-tPA]) or non-clot-specific (streptokinase [SK], urokinase [UK], and anisoylated plasminogen activator complex [APSAC]). Clot-specific thrombolytics activate plasminogen at the site of the clot, whereas non-clot-specific ones act by generalized systemic lysis. In the United States, clot-specific thrombolytics are most often used (Table 27-8).

On arrival to the ED, patients with chest pain should have an ECG done within 10 minutes. If the ECG does not show ST-segment elevation, it is strongly advised that it be repeated within 5 to 10 minutes in patients with continued chest pain to rule out late appearance STEMI. It should be noted that ST-segment depression in the anterior leads with early precordial transition could indicate ST elevation posterior wall MI, particularly if associated with ST elevation in the inferior leads (inferoposterior MI). Right-sided precordial leads can be helpful in patients with acute inferior wall MI to

> **Box 27-6** Contraindication to Fibrinolytic Therapy*
>
> **Absolute**
> 1. History of intracranial hemorrhage
> 2. Known intracranial neoplasm or vascular lesions
> 3. Active bleeding or known bleeding disorder (exclude menses)
> 4. Embolic stroke within 3 months (exception: embolic stroke within 3 hours)
> 5. Suspected aortic dissection
> 6. Significant facial or head trauma within 3 months
>
> **Relative**
> 1. Uncontrolled severe hypertension (> 180 systolic, > 110 diastolic)
> 2. Prolonged CPR (> 10 minutes) or recent surgery (<3 weeks) or noncompressible vascular puncture
> 3. Recent internal bleeding or active peptic ulcer disease
> 4. Pregnancy
> 5. Currently anticoagulated with high INR
> 6. For streptokinase; prior exposure to the drug or history of allergic reaction
>
> *ACC/AHA guidelines (Antman, 2004).
> *CPR*, Cardiopulmonary resuscitation; *INR*, international normalized ratio.

determine right ventricular involvement (ST elevation will be seen in the right precordial leads) (Fig. 27-11).

Patients with STEMI should receive supplemental oxygen therapy, morphine sulfate for pain control, IV nitrate therapy if they are not hypotensive and have not ingested a phosphodiesterase inhibitor for erectile dysfunction, 162 mg of chewable aspirin, statins, ACE inhibitors (particularly in patients with CHF, reduced left ventricular function, hypertension, or diabetes), and clopidogrel (Box 27-7).

Hemodynamic instability should be aggressively treated with pressor agents, typically dopamine started at 5 µg/kg/min and titrated every 5 minutes to keep the systolic pressure above 90 mm Hg. Normal saline fluid boluses can be helpful, particularly in the inferoposterior MI patient with right-sided involvement. In these patients, bradycardia also needs to be aggressively treated if associated with hypotension, using either atropine (1 mg IV, can repeat twice) or a temporary pacemaker if there is inadequate response to atropine. Patients with right ventricular involvement usually respond well to a fluid challenge, correcting the bradycardia, administering dopamine, and maintaining sinus rhythm as they rely on a normal atrial kick for increasing their end-diastolic volume and cardiac output. If hypotension does not respond well to these conservative measures, patients need to have an intra-aortic balloon pump inserted. Typically, these patients should be brought emergently to the cardiac catheterization laboratory for more definitive management because their mortality is excessively high without immediate revascularization (Hochman et al., 2001).

The long-term management of these patients is similar to the unstable angina/non–ST elevation MI, with aggressive preventive measures and continued long-term aspirin, beta blockers, ACE inhibitors, statins, exercise, and low-fat diet. Smoking cessation, control of hypertension and diabetes, and achieving ideal body weight are paramount to prevent further progression of disease and MI. Preferably, clopidogrel needs to be continued for 12 months irrespective of whether the patient received a revascularization procedure with drug-eluting stents or was conservatively managed.

Prasugrel (Effient) is a new ADP-receptor antagonist, recently approved by the U.S. Food and Drug Administration (FDA) to treat ACS patients after coronary angioplasty. In the landmark Trial to Assess Improvement in Therapeutic Outcomes by Optimizing Platelet Inhibition with Prasugrel (TRITON-TIMI-38), in patients with acute coronary syndrome (unstable angina, non–ST elevation MI, and STEMI), prasugrel reduced the combined end point of death from cardiovascular causes, nonfatal MI, or nonfatal stroke at 450 days by 19% compared to clopidogrel (12.1% vs. 9.9%, p <0.001). Acute stent thrombosis was also reduced by 52% using prasugrel compared to clopidogrel (p <0.001) during the same time frame. Major bleeding, however, was increased with prasugrel (2.4% vs. 1.8%, p = 0.03) compared to clopidogrel, including life-threatening bleed (1.4% vs. 0.9%, p = 0.01) and fatal bleed (0.4% vs. 0.1%, p = 0.002). The net clinical benefit, however, favored prasugrel over clopidogrel for the combined end point of all-cause death, nonfatal MI,

Table 27-8 Common Thrombolytics in Treatment of Acute Myocardial Infarction

Drug	Dose	Cautions
Streptokinase	1.5 million IU intravenously (IV) Give infusion over 60 minutes.	Watch for hypotension, anaphylaxis, severe bleeding, and stroke.
Retavase	10 U IV over 2 minutes Give second dose of 10 U IV 30 minutes after first dose if no complications.	Watch for intracranial hemorrhage, arrhythmia, and hemorrhage.
Activase	15-mg bolus IV, then 0.75 mg/Kg (max 50 mg) over 30 minutes, then 0.5 mg/Kg (max 35 mg) over 60 minutes; give with heparin.	Watch for intracranial hemorrhage, arrhythmia, severe bleeding, and anaphylaxis.
Tenecteplase	Weight <60 kg: 30 mg IV, max 50 mg Wt 60-69 kg: 35 mg IV, max 50 mg Wt 70-79 kg: 40 mg IV, max 50 mg Wt 80-89 kg: 45 mg IV, max 50 mg Wt >90 kg: 50 mg IV, max 50 mg	Watch for intracranial bleeding, anaphylaxis, and reperfusion arrhythmias.

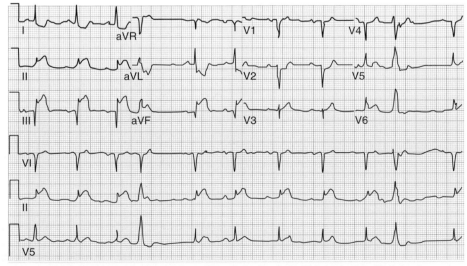

Figure 27-11 Acute inferior myocardial infarction with ST elevation in the inferior leads.

Box 27-7 Acute and Secondary Pharmacologic Therapy of ST Elevation Myocardial Infarction (STEMI)*

Acute Pharmacologic Therapy

1. Chewable aspirin (162 mg) in patients not previously taking aspirin.

2. Intravenous (IV) beta blockers should not be administered to STEMI patients who have (a) signs of heart failure, (b) evidence of a low-output state, (c) increased risk for cardiogenic shock, or (d) other relative contraindications to beta blockade (P-R interval >0.24 second; second-degree or third-degree heart block; active asthma; or reactive airway disease).

3. STEMI patients presenting to a hospital with percutaneous coronary intervention (PCI) capability should be treated with primary PCI within 90 minutes of first medical contact as a systems goal.

4. STEMI patients presenting to a hospital without PCI capability and who cannot be transferred to a PCI center and undergo PCI within 90 minutes of first medical contact should be treated with fibrinolytic therapy within 30 minutes of hospital presentation as a systems goal unless fibrinolytic therapy is contraindicated (Level B).

5. In the absence of arrhythmias, IV magnesium should not be administered.

Secondary Pharmacologic Therapy

6. For patients with BP of 140/90 mm Hg or greater (or ≥130/80 mm Hg for patients with diabetes or chronic kidney disease), it is useful as tolerated, to add BP medication, treating initially with beta blockers and/or ACE inhibitors, with the addition of other drugs such as thiazides as needed to achieve goal BP.

7. A fasting lipid profile should be assessed in all patients and within 24 hours of hospitalization for those with an acute cardiovascular or coronary event. For hospitalized patients, initiation of lipid-lowering medication is indicated as recommended before discharge. LDL-C should be less than 100 mg/dL.

8. If baseline LDL-C is 100 mg/dL or greater, LDL-lowering drug therapy should be initiated.

9. If on-treatment LDL-C is 100 mg/dL or greater, intensifying LDL-lowering drug therapy (may require LDL-lowering drug combination) is recommended.

10. Managing warfarin to INR of 2.0 to 3.0 for paroxysmal or chronic atrial fibrillation or flutter is recommended, and in post-MI patients when clinically indicated (e.g., atrial fibrillation, left ventricular thrombus).

11. ACE inhibitors should be started and continued indefinitely in all patients recovering from STEMI with left ventricular ejection fraction (LVEF) of 40% or less and for those with hypertension, diabetes, or chronic kidney disease, unless contraindicated.

12. Use of angiotensin receptor blockers (ARBs) is recommended in patients who are intolerant of ACE inhibitors and have heart failure (HF) or have had an MI (LVEF ≤40%).

13. It is beneficial to start and continue beta-blocker therapy indefinitely in all patients who have had MI, acute coronary syndrome (ACS), or LV dysfunction with or without HF symptoms, unless contraindicated.

*Level of evidence A. From Antman EM, Anbe DT, Armstrong PW, et al. ACC/AHA guidelines for the management of patients with ST-elevation myocardial infarction—executive summary: a report of the American College of Cardiology/American Heart Association Task Force on Practice Guidelines (Writing Committee to revise the 1999 guidelines for the management of patients with acute myocardial infarction). J Am Coll Cardiol 2004;44:671-719. Focused Update 2007. J Am Coll Cardiol 2008;51:210-247.

nonfatal stroke, and non-CABG TIMI major bleed (12.2% vs. 13.9%, $p = 0.004$). Physicians using prasugrel need to weigh its risks and benefits as they decide which drug to use when treating patients (Wiviott et al., 2007).

Congestive Heart Failure

Congestive heart failure (CHF) is a clinical syndrome resulting from the inability of the heart to meet the metabolic requirements of the body at normal filling pressures. Although heart failure can be precipitated by left ventricular systolic dysfunction, it can also be secondary to diastolic dysfunction. Occasionally, CHF can occur without impairment of myocardial function (Braunwald et al., 1976). CHF is highly prevalent in the United States, with more than 500,000 new cases diagnosed annually. Also, mortality remains very high, with over 300,000 people dying every year from this syndrome (Hunt et al., 2001). Hospitalization for CHF in the United States is rising in both men and women at a prohibitively high cost to the health care system (O'Connell and Bristow, 1993). It is important for family physicians to understand the pathophysiology of CHF and apply known effective therapies.

Pathophysiology

The hemodynamic model of CHF has been largely abandoned and replaced by the concept of left ventricular remodeling (Francis, 2001). Remodeling of the left ventricle indicates stretching and dilation with subsequent reduction in left ventricular function. The remodeling process can be triggered by a multitude of potential injuries (Levy et al., 1996; Kannel et al., 1994), including CAD, MI, hypertension, valvular heart disease, diabetes, congenital heart defects, anemia, and alcoholism. Regardless of the precipitating injury, neurohormonal mechanisms are activated and promote the remodeling process. These include the renin-angiotensin-aldosterone system (RAAS) and the sympathetic nervous system (SNS). A rise in endothelin-1 production, a product of dysfunctional endothelium, also occurs and contributes to vasoconstriction. In addition, inflammatory markers and cytokines are increased, further exacerbating endothelial dysfunction (Blum and Miller, 2001; Francis, 1998).

Pharmacologic interventions that block neurohormonal activation can reduce mortality and morbidity in patients with CHF (Fig. 27-12). A rise in angiotensin II (AII) promotes programmed cell death (apoptosis), hypertrophy, and fibrosis. AII also causes an increase in aldosterone secretion (Fig. 27-13), which in return augments the harmful effects of AII on myocardium and promotes adverse remodeling. Aldosterone, however, "escapes" angiotensin suppression (McKelvie et al., 1999) and, therefore, selective aldosterone blockade is needed in addition to therapy with ACEIs or ARBs (Pitt et al., 1999, 2001). A rise in circulating levels of catecholamines in response to SNS activation can lead to suppression of adrenergic receptors and has direct toxic effects on myocardium (Bristow et al., 1993). Catecholamines mediate toxicity as a result of beta-adrenoceptor-mediated cyclic adenosine monophosphate (cAMP)–dependent calcium overload of cardiac myocytes (Mann, 1998; Mann et al., 1992). Also, catecholamines increase myocardial oxygen consumption and coronary blood flow requirements and decrease myocardial

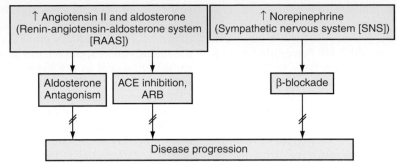

Figure 27-12 The renin-angiotensin-aldosterone system and the sympathetic nervous system are currently the target for treating patients with congestive heart failure. *ACE*, Angiotensin-converting enzyme; *ARB*, angiotensin receptor blocker.

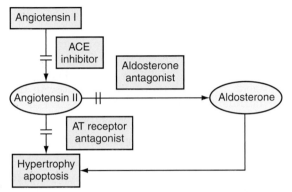

Figure 27-13 Various pharmacologic interventions to block the renin-angiotension-aldosterone system; *ACE*, angiotensin-converting enzyme; *AT*, angiotensin.

mechanical efficiency (Nikolaidis et al., 2004). Catecholamines also induce left ventricular hypertrophy (LVH) and can precipitate potentially debilitating and fatal arrhythmias.

American College of Cardiology/American Heart Association Classification

The newer ACC/AHA classification for CHF takes into account risk factors in addition to the presence of left ventricular dysfunction and symptoms (Hunt et al., 2001). This classification complements the New York Heart Classification (NYHC) and considers recent advances in pharmacologic and nonpharmacologic approaches to evaluate and treat the heart failure patient (Ahmed, 2003). The following four stages are proposed:

Stage A describes patients who are at risk of CHF but are asymptomatic and have no left ventricular dysfunction. More than 60 million people fall in this category and include those with CAD, hypertension, diabetes mellitus, and a family history of cardiomyopathy. Stage A is an additional classification that was not present in the prior NYHC.

Stage B describes patients with left ventricular dysfunction but no symptoms. This is equivalent to Class I of the NYHC. This includes about 10 million people in the United States.

Stage C describes patients with left ventricular dysfunction who are symptomatic with exertion. This is equivalent to the NYHC Class II and Class III. This includes about 5 million people in the United States.

Stage D describes patients with symptoms at rest. This is equivalent to Class IV of the NYHC. This includes about 200,000 people in the United States.

This classification reliably allows the physician to follow patients as their heart failure progresses from one stage to the next and offers a unique set of treatment appropriate to each stage.

Evaluation of the Patient

Patients with CHF need to have a complete history and physical examination with a focus on cardiovascular risk factors that lead to progression of failure. A careful documentation of their volume status, weight, and NYHC for symptoms needs to be done. Diagnostic tests should include a complete blood count (CBC), serum electrolytes, kidney and liver functions, urinalysis, blood glucose, thyroid function test, iron saturation test and ferritin, erythrocyte sedimentation rate (ESR), antinuclear antibodies to rule out connective tissue disease, 12-lead ECG, echocardiogram, and coronary angiogram, particularly in those with significant reduction in left ventricular function, to rule out underlying severe CAD. Brain natriuretic peptides (BNP and NT-proBNP) can be useful when a patient presents with symptoms of dyspnea of unclear etiology and the diagnosis of CHF is uncertain (de Lemos et al., 2003; Siebert et al., 2006).

Routine myocardial biopsy or Holter monitoring is not recommended. Levels of catecholamines might be obtained if clinically indicated in patients with severe episodic hypertension and tachycardia. The rapid development of CHF with reduced left ventricular function in the absence of a clear etiology should raise suspicion of a viral cardiomyopathy, especially in younger patients. This can be suspected if the patient had a recent viral syndrome over the past several weeks, followed by a progression of dyspnea and CHF. Findings on cardiac biopsy show mostly an acute inflammatory reaction, and since therapy is generally supportive, an endomyocardial biopsy will not alter treatment or prognosis. Therapy for viral cardiomyopathy and CHF consists of supportive therapy and the use of beta blockers, diuretics, ACE inhibitors, and if failure is advanced (class III and IV), spironolactone.

Risk Factor Modification

Patients with CHF should have their cardiovascular risk factors modified aggressively. Hypertension is strongly linked to the development of CHF and should be aggressively treated (Vasan and Levy, 1996). The target BP should be 130/85 mm

Hg or less, except in diabetic patients, in whom the target is lowered to 125/85 mm Hg or less.

Control of dyslipidemia and diabetes is also very important in the management of patients with CHF. Screening for sleep apnea and thyroid disease and aggressively treating these conditions need to be done. The avoidance of alcohol, illicit drug use, and smoking is strongly advised. Losing weight and establishing a routine exercise program are also important preventive measures in the CHF patient. Patients with a history of heart palpitations need to be evaluated for tachycardia because this is a well-established risk factor for cardiomyopathy and CHF. If patients have daily palpitations, a 24-hour Holter monitor is sufficient to help establish the type of arrhythmia. On the other hand, if palpitations occur infrequently (a few times per month), an "event care" monitor is more useful because patients can keep this type of monitor with them at home for a month and record the arrhythmia as it occurs. If palpitations are very infrequent, it is unlikely that they will be contributing to tachycardia-induced cardiomyopathy, but their diagnosis can be made with an implantable loop recorder, typically done by the electrophysiologist.

KEY TREATMENT

Control of systolic and diastolic hypertension in accordance with established guidelines is strongly indicated in the CHF patient (ACC/AHA guidelines; SOR: A).

Pharmacologic Therapy

Diastolic Dysfunction

Diastolic dysfunction is typically diagnosed by echocardiography. It is characterized by dyspnea and CHF with normal left ventricular systolic function but impaired relaxation. Conditions that increase left ventricular (LV) stiffness include CAD, hypertension, diabetes, valvular heart disease, and age (Ewy, 2004). Patients with LV diastolic dysfunction need to be treated with aggressive BP control and diuretics, beta blockade, or nondihydropyridine CCBs (diltiazem or verapamil). ACE inhibitors or ARBs can have long-term value in reducing LVH and theoretically may improve LV compliance (Mandinov et al., 2000).

Left Ventricular Systolic Dysfunction

Patients with *asymptomatic* LV dysfunction (Stage B, ACC/AHA classification) benefit significantly from ACE inhibitors and beta blockade. The correction of anatomic abnormalities that are linked to LV systolic dysfunction is also important, including severe mitral or aortic insufficiency and aortic stenosis. Periodic follow-up of these patients is indicated, with serial assessment of LV function using echocardiography or isotope ventriculography (IVG). Patients with familial LV systolic dysfunction need to have their immediate family members screened for asymptomatic cardiomyopathy.

Symptomatic LV systolic dysfunction (Stage C, ACC/AHA classification) requires intensive pharmacologic treatment and close follow-up. Echocardiography or IVG is typically done to monitor LVEF over time, generally every 6 months or less frequently if a patient is clinically stable. An IVG provides a more accurate assessment of ejection fraction (within ± 3%

variability in reading) than an echocardiogram but is more expensive. Whether an echocardiogram or an IVG is ordered depends on the patient's clinical presentation, history, and the management approach of the treating physician. Diuretics are important in the hypervolemic patient, and digoxin improves symptoms in patients with clinical evidence of CHF or symptomatic, severely reduced LV function. No data, however, support that a diuretic or digoxin alters a patient's long-term survival. Current therapies known to impact a person's mortality are summarized next (Cohn, 1996; Hunt et al., 2001; Packer et al., 1999). Table 27-9 lists drugs and dosages in treating patients with congestive heart failure.

Although there is no one way to start pharmacologic therapy for CHF patients, it is advisable that patients be started on a small dose of beta blockers, ACEI, or both. Diuretics are generally reserved for patients who are fluid overloaded. Caution needs to be exerted when a diuretic and an ace inhibitor are started simultaneously as hypotension could occur and serum creatinine levels can rise markedly. Beta blockers (Hori, 2004) and ACE inhibitors (Majumdar, 2004) need to be titrated to the maximum tolerated dose in order to achieve maximal therapeutic efficacy.

Angiotensin-Converting Enzyme Inhibitors

Angiotensin-converting enzyme inhibitors (ACEIs) reduce mortality by an absolute 4% and relative 15% to 20% in patients with LV systolic dysfunction (LVEF <40%). In addition, ACEIs reduce the combined end point of morbidity (heart failure hospitalizations) and mortality by 30% to 35%. Despite the benefits of ACE inhibitors (Wong et al., 2004), mortality from CHF remains at 50% within 5 years of the diagnosis and 30% of patients are rehospitalized within 3 months.

Several trials have noted a mortality reduction with ACEIs in patients with clinical evidence of CHF after sustaining an MI (Kober et al., 1995). The Acute Infarction Ramipril Efficacy Study (AIRE) showed a 27% ($p = 0.002$) reduction in the 30-month cumulative mortality with ramipril over placebo in post-MI CHF patients. Furthermore, trandolapril reduced mortality by 22% ($p = 0.01$) in patients with reduced left ventricular function after an MI (Kober, 1995). Guidelines also emphasize the use of ACEIs in patients with asymptomatic LV dysfunction and history of MI. These patients are at high risk of developing LV remodeling and CHF several months after the initial insult (Jessup, 2003).

KEY TREATMENT

ACE inhibitors are recommended in all patients with CHF and left ventricular dysfunction unless a contraindication exists.
ACEIs should be used in all patients with history of MI and asymptomatic reduced LV function regardless of ejection fraction.
ACC/AHA guidelines (SOR: A).

Angiotensin Receptor Blockers

Key Point

- Angiotensin receptor blockade can be used in patients being treated with digitalis, diuretics, and a beta blocker and who cannot be given an ACE inhibitor because of cough or angioedema (ACC/AHA guidelines; SOR: A).

Table 27-9 Selected Drugs and Dosages in Treatment of Congestive Heart Failure

Drug	Dosage
Angiotensin-Converting Enzyme Inhibitors	
Enalapril	2.5 to 20 mg PO bid, max 40 mg/day, start at 2.5 mg qd
Captopril	12.5 to 50 mg PO tid, max 150 mg/day, start 6.25 to 12.5 mg PO tid
Ramipril	5 mg PO bid, max 10 mg/day, start at 2.5 mg PO bid
Lisinopril	5-20 mg PO qd, max 40 mg/day, start 2.5 to 5 mg PO qd
Perindopril	4-16 mg PO qd, max 16 mg/day, start 2 mg PO qd
Monopril	10-40 mg PO qd/bid, max 80 mg/day, start 10 mg PO qd
Angiotensin Receptor Blockers (for ACE Inhibitor–Intolerant Patients)	
Losartan	25-100 mg PO qd, max 100 mg/day, start 25-50 mg PO qd*
Candesartan	8-32 mg PO qd, max 32 mg/day, start 16 mg PO qd*
Valsartan	40-160 mg PO bid, max 320 mg/day, start 40 mg PO bid
Irbesartan	75-300 mg PO qd, max 300 mg/day, start 75 mg PO qd*
Beta Blockers	
Carvedilol	3.125-25 mg PO bid, max 50 mg PO qd, start 3.125 mg PO bid
Metoprolol succinate	12.5 to 200 mg PO QD, max 200 mg/day, start 12.5 mg PO qd
Metoprolol	12.5-100 mg PO bid, max 100 mg PO BID, start 12.5 mg PO bid*
Aldosterone Antagonists	
Spironolactone	12.5-25 mg PO bid, max 50 mg/day, start 12.5 mg PO bid
Eplerenone	50 mg PO qd, max 50 mg/day, start 25 mg PO qd†

*Off-label use.

†For CHF patients post–myocardial infarction.

Early studies comparing ARBs and ACEIs in the management of CHF patients suggested that an ARB was as safe, effective, and tolerable as an ACEI. In the Randomized Evaluation of Strategies for Left Ventricular Dysfunction (RESOLVD) pilot study, 768 patients (NYHC II-IV, LVEF <40%) received candesartan, candesartan plus enalapril, or enalapril alone for 43 weeks (McKelvie et al., 1999). Left ventricular cavity size increased less and BNP levels decreased more with combination therapy compared to ARB or ACEI alone. In the Losartan Heart Failure Survival Study (ELITE II), 3152 patients (≥60 years old; NYHC II-IV; LVEF <40%) were randomly assigned to losartan (1578 patients) titrated to 50 mg once daily or captopril (1574) titrated to 50 mg three times daily (Pitt et al., 2000). There were no differences in all-cause mortality or sudden death between the two groups. In a subset of the Val-HeFT (Valsartan in Heart Failure Trial) trial of patients intolerant to ACEI, valsartan (titrated to 160 mg twice daily) reduced both all-cause mortality and combined mortality and morbidity compared with placebo (17.3% vs. 27.1%, $p = 0.017$; and 24.9% vs. 42.5%, $p < 0.001$, respectively) (Maggioni et al., 2002). In this trial, adding an ARB (valsartan) to an ACEI in CHF patients (LVEF<40%) did not reduce mortality further, whereas the combined end point of mortality and morbidity was reduced by about 27.5%, mostly from a reduction in CHF hospitalizations (Cohn et al., 2001).

In the Candesartan in Heart Failure Assessment of Reduction in Mortality and Morbidity (CHARM) trial, candesartan (titrated to 32 mg once daily) significantly reduced cardiovascular deaths and hospital admissions for CHF (Pfeffer et al., 2003). In the "overall programme" of this study, which included both preserved and reduced LV function, total mortality was not reduced compared to placebo. However, in a subset analysis, patients with symptomatic heart failure and reduced LV function (<40%), candesartan significantly reduced all-cause mortality, cardiovascular death, and CHF hospitalizations when added to standard therapies, including ACEIs, beta blockers, and aldosterone antagonists (Young et al., 2004). These patients should have their BP, creatinine, and serum potassium carefully monitored. The Valsartan in Acute Myocardial Infarction Trial (VALIANT) randomized patients 0.5 to 10 days after an acute MI with reduced LV function to valsartan (4909 patients) titrated to 160 mg twice daily, valsartan (80 mg twice daily) plus captopril (50 mg three times daily) (4885 patients), or captopril (4909 patients) titrated to 50 mg three times a day in addition to standard therapy (Pfeffer et al., 2003). Valsartan was equally effective as captopril in reducing all cause mortality. For reasons that remain unclear, combining valsartan with captopril did not improve survival compared to either captopril or valsartan alone but did increase adverse events.

Currently the recommendation is to use an ACEI as first line therapy to treat CHF patients. However, a growing body of evidence suggests that an ARB could be as effective as an ACEI in the treatment of heart failure patients with reduced left ventricular function.

Aldosterone Blockers

Aldosterone is secreted by the zona glomerulosa of the adrenal gland and is induced by AII, adrenocorticotropic hormone, and potassium. Aldosterone leads to sodium and water absorption and the excretion of potassium. Although AII is a dominant stimulus of aldosterone secretion (Weber, 2001), ACEI are not sufficient to block aldosterone secretion (McKelvie, 1999; Schjoedt, 2004). Until recently the role of aldosterone blockade in the management of patients with CHF has been unclear.

Two large trials investigated the role of aldosterone antagonists in CHF management. The Randomized Aldactone Evaluation Study (RALES) randomized patients with advanced CHF

(LVEF <35%) to spironolactone (25 mg daily) or placebo in addition to standard therapy (Pitt et al., 1999). After a mean follow-up of 24 months, spironolactone reduced mortality by 30% through reducing progression of CHF and sudden cardiac death. In addition, patients who received spironolactone had a significant improvement in the symptoms of heart failure as assessed by NYHA functional class (p <0.001). Recurrent hospitalization from worsening CHF was also reduced by 35% (p <0.001). The Eplerenone Post-AMI Heart Failure Efficacy and Survival Study (EPHESUS) randomized patients with CHF (LVEF<40%), 3 to 14 days post-MI, to eplerenone (25-50 mg daily) or placebo (Pitt et al., 2001). At a mean follow-up of 27 months, eplerenone, a competitive, relatively selective mineralocorticoid receptor antagonist, reduced total mortality by 15% (p = 0.008), cardiovascular mortality or cardiovascular hospitalizations by 13% (p = 0.002), and sudden cardiac death by 21% (p = 0.03). Based on these trials, aldosterone antagonists are now considered to be a primary therapy in patients with LV dysfunction and CHF.

Beta-Adrenergic Blockade in Heart Failure

The activation of the sympathetic nervous system in patients with CHF leads to excess catecholamine secretion, which adversely affects myocardium and contributes to left ventricular remodeling and CHF.

Multiple beta blockers have been tested in CHF. Beta blockers have been shown to reduce mortality by approximately 35% when added to an ACEI in mild to moderate CHF (MERIT-HF with metoprolol succinate, U.S. trials with carvedilol, and CIBIS-II trial with bisoprolol) or in very advanced CHF (Copernicus trial with carvedilol) (Packer et al., 2001). Beta blockers also reduce hospitalizations by 33% to 38% and work in synergy with ACEIs to reduce cardiac remodeling, reduce cavity size, and improve ejection fraction (CIBIS-II, 1999; Fowler et al., 2001; MERIT-HF, 1999; Packer et al., 1996; Remme et al., 2004).

There are differences in the antiadrenergic actions of β-adrenergic blocking drugs. The ratio of β_2- and α_1-adrenergic receptors in the damaged heart changes compared to the normal myocardium (Bristow, 1993). β_1 receptors are reduced and α_1 receptors increased with little change in the β_2 receptors. Almost 50% of the adrenergic receptors on the failing myocardium are β_2 and α_1, which are typically not affected by selective β_1 blockade. Norepinephrine is known to exert negative effects through β_1, β_2, and α_1 receptors. To test whether a nonselective β_1, β_2, or α_1 blocker yields better mortality reduction than a β_1 blocker alone, the Carvedilol or Metoprolol European Trial (COMET trial) recruited 3029 patients with NYHC II-IV heart failure at 317 centers in 15 European countries (Torp-Pedersen et al., 2005; Poole-Wilson et al., 2003). At 58 months, there was a 17% reduction in mortality with carvedilol compared to metoprolol tartrate (p = 0.0017). Despite the controversy about the adequacy of β-blockade and the use of the shorter-acting metoprolol tartrate instead of the long-acting metoprolol succinate in this study, the data seem to favor the theory that the nonselective adrenergic blockade is superior to the selective short-acting β_1-receptor blockade in reducing mortality in the CHF patient.

Carvedilol (6.25-25 mg twice daily) was shown in the Glycemic Effects in Diabetes Mellitus: Carvedilol-Metoprolol Comparison in Hypertensives (GEMINI) study not to alter glycemic control in diabetic patients compared with metoprolol tartrate (50-200 mg twice daily). Also, carvedilol did improve some components of the metabolic syndrome such as improving insulin sensitivity (Bakris et al., 2004). Carvedilol appears to be a favorable drug in diabetic patients, in contrast to other selective beta blockers.

Aggressive titration of beta blockers is needed in patients with CHF. Higher levels of β-blockade are associated with better improvement of ejection fraction and greater reductions in cardiovascular hospitalizations (Hori et al., 2004; Bristow et al., 1996). A stepwise approach in titration of beta-blockade is generally followed with an increase in the dose every 2 weeks as tolerated until achieving the maximum tolerable dose.

KEY TREATMENT

Beta blockers (bisoprolol, carvedilol, and sustained-release metoprolol succinate) should be used in asymptomatic patients with a recent MI regardless of ejection fraction (SOR: A).
Beta blockade should be used in all stable stage C patients unless contraindicated (ACC/AHA guidelines; SOR: A).

Miscellaneous Pharmacologic Therapy

Patients receiving ACE inhibitors might benefit from the addition of the combination of hydralazine and nitrates. ACC recommendations indicate that this treatment is likely to benefit African American patients with advanced CHF symptoms.

In addition to pharmacologic therapy, CHF patients should be instructed on dietary salt restriction (2 g sodium/day), daily weight monitoring (with reporting of 3-lb/wk weight increase to their physician), free water restriction to 1 L daily, smoking cessation, regular exercise, avoidance of alcohol intake, and aggressive treatment of hypertension and lipid disorders. Supplemental oxygen is needed in patients with oxygen saturation less than 92% on room air after ambulation. Finally, sleep apnea has been associated with CHF, and these patients need to be screened and aggressively treated for moderate to severe apnea. Patients with symptomatic CHF are best treated at a heart failure clinic to ensure appropriate therapy is administered by a specialized provider, to increase patient compliance, and to reduce recurrent hospitalization. A heart failure clinic will also ensure that national benchmarks in management of CHF patients are met. These include the optimal utilization of ACEIs and beta blockers, documentation of LV function, and smoking cessation.

KEY TREATMENT

The combination of a fixed-dose of isosorbide dinitrate and hydralazine to a standard medical regimen for heart failure (HF), including ACE inhibitors and beta blockers, is recommended to improve outcomes for patients self-described as African Americans, with NYHA functional class III or IV HF. Others may benefit similarly, but this has not yet been tested (ACC recommendations; Jessup, 2009) (SOR: A).
Referral of patients with refractory end-stage HF to a HF program with expertise in the management of refractory HF is useful (ACC/AHA guidelines; Jessup, 2009) (SOR: A).

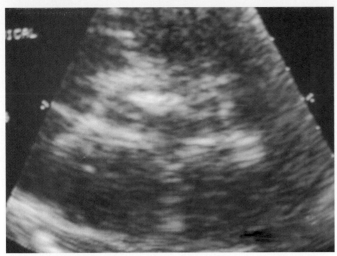

Figure 27-14 Aortic valve stenosis with calcification as seen with two-dimensional Doppler echocardiography.

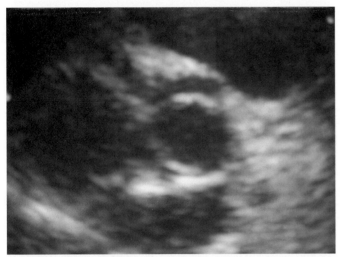

Figure 27-15 Bicuspic aortic valve.

Valvular Heart Disease

Aortic Stenosis

Aortic stenosis is defined as an obstruction that impedes blood flow from the left ventricle to the aorta and is mostly secondary to aortic valvular disease. Other, less common etiologies of aortic stenosis include supravalvular and membranous subvalvular stenosis, which are generally congenital.

Aortic valvular stenosis is the most common valvular abnormality in the United States. It can be congenital, rheumatic, or calcific and degenerative. *Calcific* aortic valve stenosis is most prevalent in patients over 70 years of age (Fig. 27-14), whereas *congenital,* mostly bicuspid valve disease is more common in younger patients (Fig. 27-15). A bicuspid aortic valve leads to flow turbulence and valve trauma, which in return precipitates fibrosis, stiffness, and calcification. A third of bicuspid valves will become stenotic between the fourth and sixth decades of life and account for half of all surgical cases. Age-related calcific valves are affected by the same risk factors as in atherosclerosis, with inflammatory

cells (macrophages, T lymphocytes), lipid and calcium deposits, and development of fibrosis. *Rheumatic* aortic valve stenosis is now uncommon in developed countries and is mediated by adhesion and the fusion of cusps.

The aortic valve surface area is normally 3.0 to 4.0 cm². Symptoms typically do not appear unless the valve is narrowed to at least a fourth of its normal surface area. Stenosis is graded as *mild* (valve area >1.5 cm²), *moderate* (>1.0 to 1.5 cm²), or *severe* (≤1 cm²) (Rahimtoola, 1989). The valve area narrows at an average rate of 0.12 cm² per year (Otto et al., 1997). As the valve narrows, cardiac output remains stable at rest but diminishes with exercise. As disease progresses, LV mass increases and diastolic dysfunction becomes evident with an increase in LV filling pressure. Myocardial oxygen demand typically increases, and even in the absence of CAD, patients may experience angina. Patients with aortic stenosis have a good prognosis if they do not have symptoms of angina, CHF, or syncope/near-syncope, particularly with activity. Surgical management of the valve becomes necessary in symptomatic patients because of the increased incidence of sudden cardiac death.

Patients with severe aortic valve stenosis describe progressive dyspnea, chest pain and syncope with exertion, and symptoms of CHF, including orthopnea, paroxysmal nocturnal dyspnea, and edema. Syncope at rest is typically induced by arrhythmia. Patients with severe aortic valve stenosis have a 5% history of sudden cardiac death. In addition, these patients may give a history of rheumatic fever or rheumatic heart disease, transient ischemic attacks from calcium deposit systemic embolization, and intermittent GI bleeding from an increased incidence of arteriovenous malformations.

The typical physical signs of severe aortic valve stenosis are diminished carotid pulses (delayed and weak), a sustained apical impulse, a single second heart sound, an S4 gallop, and midsystolic crescendo-decrescendo murmur with late peaking best heard at the base of the heart, although in elderly patients it might be heard only at the apex.

Diagnostic tests include a chest radiograph, which could show a calcified valve, pulmonary venous congestion, or an increase in ascending aortic root size secondary to post–stenotic dilation. Also, a 12-lead ECG may show LVH and conduction abnormalities. An echocardiogram typically confirms the diagnosis. Valve structure can be assessed, including the presence of calcification, reduction in cusp motion, and congenital abnormalities such as a bicuspid or abnormal tricuspid valve. A gradient can be measured across the valve (Fig. 27-16), and valve area can be determined using Doppler flow with reasonable accuracy (Currie et al., 1986). The presence of concomitant aortic valve insufficiency can also be visualized using color Doppler flow characteristics. Other important findings on echocardiography include the presence or absence of LVH and assessment of LV compliance, atrial size, and associated other valvular abnormalities. If noninvasive findings support the diagnosis of severe aortic stenosis and the patient is symptomatic, then diagnostic angiography is indicated to confirm the presence of severe aortic valve stenosis and assess the coronary arteries. Combined valve surgery and CABG can then be considered as indicated. Stress testing is absolutely contraindicated in the setting of symptomatic, severe aortic valve stenosis.

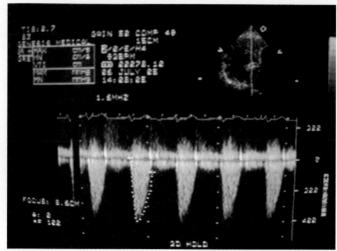

Figure 27-16 Velocity gradient across a calcified stenotic aortic valve, as seen with Doppler echocardiography.

Table 27-10 Prophylaxis for Bacterial Endocarditis[*]

Drug	Adult Dose	Pediatric Dose[*]	Time before Procedure
General Prophylaxis			
Amoxicillin	2 g PO 2 g IV or IM	50 mg/kg PO 50 mg/kg IM or IV	1 hour 30 minutes
Penicillin-Allergic Patients			
Clindamycin	600 mg PO	20 mg/kg PO	1 hour
Clarithromycin	500 mg PO	15 mg/kg PO	1 hour
Azithromycin	500 mg PO	15 mg/kg PO	1 hour
Clindamycin	600 mg IV	20 mg/kg IV	30 minutes
Cefazolin	1 g IV or IM	25 mg/kg IM or IV	30 minutes

From Dajani AS, Taubert KA, Wilson W, et al. Prevention of bacterial endocarditis: recommendations by the American Heart Association. Circulation 1997;96:358-366.

[*]Should not exceed adult dose

The treatment of aortic valve stenosis depends on the presence or absence of symptoms. Symptomatic, severe aortic valve stenosis carries a poor prognosis, with the average life expectancy of patients being 2 to 3 years (Ross and Braunwald, 1968). The 5- and 10-year mortality is approximately 52% to 80% and 80% to 90%, respectively (Horstkotte and Loogen, 1988; Turina et al., 1987). Aortic valve surgery with or without CABG is the treatment of choice (Lund, 1990; Schwarz et al., 1982). Aortic valvuloplasty carries a poor outcome and is reserved as a palliative therapy for inoperable patients. Typically, the improvement in the aortic valve gradient is mild with valvuloplasty, and a recurrence of severe stenosis can be expected within 6 months (Block and Palacios, 1988; Davidson et al., 1990). Surgery is typically not advised for asymptomatic severe valvular stenosis. Patients with dyspnea and indication of progressive LV dysfunction need to be considered for valve replacement. However, most patients with asymptomatic, severe aortic valve stenosis will develop symptoms within 5 years of follow-up. The 1-, 2-, and 5-year event-free probabilities were 80%, 63%, and 25%, respectively. Independent predictors of all-cause mortality include age, chronic renal failure, inactivity, and aortic valve velocity (Pellikka et al., 2005). A low threshold to intervene in patients with asymptomatic severe aortic stenosis needs to be considered, particularly when peak systolic velocity is 4.5 m/sec or greater on Doppler echocardiography, if associated with moderate or severe valvular calcification (Rosenheck et al., 2000).

Patients need to be advised on antibiotic prophylaxis to prevent endocarditis, especially with rheumatic valve disease (Dajani et al., 1997) (Table 27-10). Patients with moderate to severe aortic valve stenosis need to avoid moderate to severe physical exertion (Cheitlin et al., 1994). Arrhythmias need to be corrected promptly in patients with severe aortic stenosis. Follow-up echocardiography is indicated every year in patients with asymptomatic, severe aortic stenosis and every other year in those with moderate stenosis (Bonow et al., 1998).

Aortic valve replacement can be performed with a mechanical valve or a tissue valve depending on the clinical situation. For example, patients who have a contraindication to

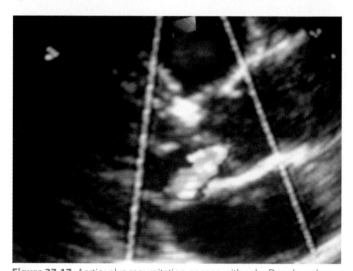

Figure 27-17 Aortic valve regurgitation, as seen with color Doppler echocardiography. Note the blue turbulent jet into the left ventricle in diastole.

anticoagulation with warfarin should receive a bioprosthetic valve. These valves typically do not require anticoagulation with warfarin, and patients generally receive only an aspirin subsequent to the procedure. Patients in their 60s or 70s with no contraindication to warfarin (Coumadin) are best served with mechanical valves because these last longer and may obviate the need for another valve surgery. Very elderly patients (80s) are typically given a tissue valve to obviate the need for anticoagulation. Antibiotic prophylaxis to prevent endocarditis is strongly recommended in patients with prosthetic valves.

Aortic Valve Regurgitation

Aortic valve regurgitation (AR) is defined as blood flow from the aorta to the left ventricle in diastole because of an incompetent aortic valve (Fig. 27-17). Aortic valve insufficiency is

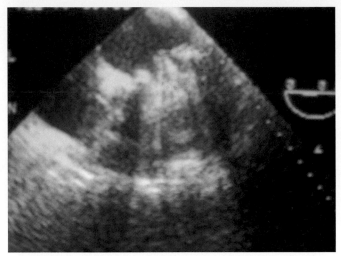

Figure 27-18 Mechanical prosthetic valve. Note the acoustic shadowing generated by the mechanical prosthesis.

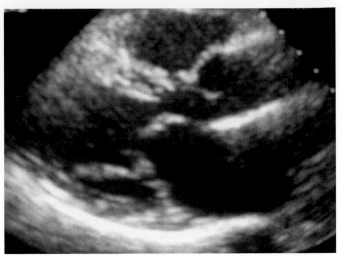

Figure 27-19 Rheumatic mitral valve stenosis. Note the doming of the stenotic mitral valve with thickening of the anterior leaflet.

generally acquired through valve infection, dilation and dissection of the aortic root, trauma, or long-term degenerative change of the valve, particularly in the setting of hypertension. Patients with a history of prosthetic valves can also have aortic valve insufficiency (Fig. 27-18). Aortic insufficiency can also be caused by a congenital bicuspid aortic valve.

Aortic regurgitation leads to volume overload of the left ventricle and an increase in left ventricular end-diastolic pressure (LVEDP). In chronic AR, symptoms might not appear before LV cavity dilation and reduced LV function develop. In acute AR, a sudden rise of LVEDP occurs because of the inability of the left ventricle to dilate acutely in response to a sudden volume overload. Patients are generally acutely symptomatic with CHF. Patients with severe AR will eventually become symptomatic, displaying symptoms of dyspnea and CHF. Angina is less common but can result from a reduction in coronary perfusion pressure. Physical signs of severe AR include a rapid, quick arterial pulse (Corrigan's pulse), a wide pulse pressure, an early high-pitched, blowing diastolic murmur heard best over the left sternal border, an S3 gallop, and a low-pitched diastolic murmur at the apex (Austin-Flint murmur).

The ECG shows LVH and possibly conduction abnormalities. Echocardiography can help make the diagnosis accurately and also provides information about LV function and cavity size. Other associated valvular abnormalities can also be assessed by the echocardiogram. Aortic root and left atrial sizes can be measured (Zoghbi et al., 2003). Stress testing can provide information about functional capacity and hemodynamic response to exercise. Diagnostic angiography allows the verification of the severity of the AR and helps in the assessment of the aortic root size, cavity size, and the presence or absence of CAD.

The surgical treatment of AR is indicated in symptomatic patients with dyspnea, angina, or CHF (Bonow, 2000). Asymptomatic patients should undergo surgery if LVEF is 55% or less, or left ventricular end-systolic dimension approaches 5.5 cm. Patients with moderate to severe AR should avoid competitive sports, heavy workloads, and weightlifting. Patients with severe AR may benefit from long-acting vasodilators such as nifedipine XL. This treatment

before aortic valve replacement may improve postoperative ejection fractions and improve long-term outcomes (Scognamiglio et al., 2005). Following valve replacement for AR, the use of beta blockers may improve cardiac performance (Matsuyama et al., 2000).

Mitral Stenosis

Mitral stenosis is defined as the reduced ability of the blood to move from the left atrium to the left ventricle in diastole. It is mostly caused by dysfunction in the mitral valve, which lacks the ability to open its leaflets in diastole (Fig. 27-19). Mitral valve stenosis (MS) is predominantly caused by rheumatic carditis and is more prevalent in female patients (Bonow et al., 1998). Acute rheumatic carditis leads to valvular disease in approximately 50% of affected patients. The mitral valve is the most often affected by rheumatic heart disease, followed by the aortic valve, then combined aortic/mitral valves. MS is considered severe if the valve area is less than 1 cm^2; normal mitral valve area is 4 to 6 cm^2. A valve area of 1.5 cm^2 or less associated with severe dyspnea (NYHC III or IV) or severe pulmonary hypertension (pulmonary pressure >50 mm Hg at rest and ≥60 mm Hg with exercise) is also considered clinically significant and warrants therapy.

The main symptom of MS is slowly progressive dyspnea and fatigue. In advanced MS, left atrial pressure develops with a redistribution of blood to the chest. Patients might complain of orthopnea and paroxysmal nocturnal dyspnea. Pulmonary hypertension can become severe, and right-sided ventricular failure can then lead to dependent edema, hepatomegaly, and right upper quadrant pain. An increase in left atrial size can lead to palpitations secondary to atrial fibrillation, as well as subsequent cardioembolic strokes if not recognized in a timely manner.

Most auscultatory signs of MS are missed if not performed in the left lateral decubitus position. Typically, the first heart sound (S1) is accentuated. A low-pitched diastolic rumble, heard with the bell of the stethoscope over the apex, is also present. The high-pitched *opening snap* (OS), caused by the abrupt stopping of the domed mitral valve into the left ventricle, is also appreciated in most patients midway between the left sternal border and apex. A shorter A2-OS distance indicates a more severe MS. Signs of pulmonary hypertension such as a loud P2 and right ventricular hypertrophy can also be present as MS becomes more severe.

The ECG findings in MS might show a biphasic P wave in V1, a large P wave in lead II, and possibly atrial fibrillation. A chest radiograph may show evidence of an enlarged left atrium and an increase in pulmonary congestion with interstitial edema. An echocardiogram can accurately diagnose MS and assess valvular and subvalvular structure and valve area (Rahimtoola et al., 2002). In addition, an echocardiogram can help distinguish the cause of MS, whether valvular or from different etiologies such as tumors, vegetations, extreme calcification of the annulus, left atrial myxoma, cor triatriatum, or presence of a large thrombus. An echocardiogram can also help estimate pulmonary pressures and assess for right-sided enlargement. Typically, LV function is preserved in MS. In addition, echocardiography can help in calculating a mitral valve score that takes into account leaflet mobility, thickening, valve calcification, and distortion of the subvalvular apparatus. The interventional cardiologist typically uses the valve score to determine the feasibility of balloon valvuloplasty. A score less than 8 generally indicates a good prognosis from mitral valvuloplasty. Furthermore, a transthoracic echocardiogram is not well suited to see the left atrial appendage, so transesophageal echocardiography (TEE) becomes necessary to rule out the presence of an atrial thrombus prior to valvuloplasty, because this can be a significant risk for an embolic stroke. Finally, a left- and right-sided heart catheterization remains the best modality to assess mitral valve severity and full hemodynamics and determine coronary anatomy before contemplated corrective surgery.

Treatment

All patients with rheumatic mitral valve disease require bacterial endocarditis prophylaxis before dental, genitourinary, or GI procedures. Increasing diastolic filling time is important in the treatment of moderate to severe MS. Therefore, drugs such as β-blockers or verapamil might be used. Maintaining sinus rhythm can also reduce symptoms because loss of atrial contraction reduces ventricular emptying. Patients with atrial fibrillation need to be aggressively treated with rate control and anticoagulation with warfarin to reduce embolic strokes. *Chemoversion* (with amiodarone or other antiarrhythmics) or cardioversion can be performed after the patient has been anticoagulated for at least 3 weeks. Anticoagulation should be maintained for a minimum of 1 month after the procedure. Generally, anticoagulation is maintained long term because the recurrence of atrial fibrillation can be unpredictable. TEE can be performed before cardioversion to rule out the presence of a left atrial thrombus (Fig. 27-20). Even when a thrombus is excluded, patients need to be heparinized for at least 48 to 72 hours before cardioversion, then maintained on warfarin. The target international normalized ratio (INR) in patients with atrial fibrillation needs to be 2.0 to 3.0.

Patients with moderate to severe symptoms (NYHC II-IV) or asymptomatic patients with severe MS (valve area <1.5 cm²) and pulmonary hypertension (pulmonary pressure >50 mm Hg at rest and ≥60 mm Hg with exercise) will require percutaneous valvuloplasty, mitral valve repair, or mitral valve replacement. Balloon valvuloplasty leads to

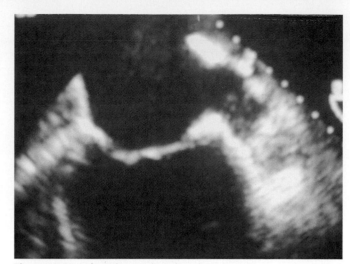

Figure 27-20 Left atrial appendage thrombus seen on transesophageal echocardiography.

Box 27-8 Common Contraindications for Mitral Balloon Valvuloplasty

1. Presence of left atrial thrombus seen on transesophageal echocardiography
2. Associated severe mitral regurgitation
3. Associated coronary artery disease that requires bypass surgery
4. A high valve score as determined by echocardiography (unfavorable valve morphology)
5. Associated other valvular pathology or aortic pathology that will require surgical interventions
6. Difficulty in obtaining access

---

commissural separation as the main mechanism that leads to an improvement in valvular function. Mitral valvuloplasty is currently the preferred method of treating severe MS when no contraindications exist (Box 27-8). The procedure carries an exceedingly low risk of mortality, with an acute success rate over 95% and very good long-term results similar to surgical commissurotomy (Rahimtoola et al., 2002). Patients who are qualified for valvuloplasty (favorable valve score) can undergo valve repair if balloon valvuloplasty is not available or left atrial thrombus persists despite anticoagulation. Mitral valve surgery is reserved for patients with a calcified valve and a high valve score on echocardiography who are essentially excluded from balloon valvuloplasty.

Mitral Regurgitation

Mitral regurgitation (MR) is defined as an abnormal blood flow into the left atrium in systole as a result of an abnormal closing of the mitral valve. In chronic mitral insufficiency, the LVEF and cavity size may remain preserved for several years. However, LV remodeling eventually occurs, cavity size begins to dilate, ejection fraction becomes reduced, and patients enter a decompensated state. In acute MR, the left atrium and left ventricle have no chance for gradual dilation, and therefore a sudden rise in LV and pulmonary venous pressure occurs, leading to pulmonary edema.

Chronic MR is generally asymptomatic or associated with minimal symptoms of dyspnea or generalized fatigue. When

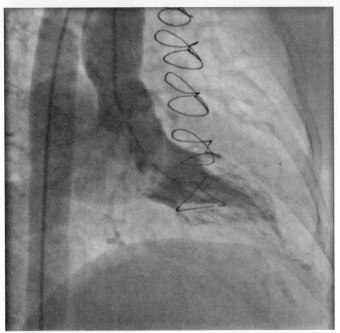

Figure 27-21 Left ventriculogram in the right anterior oblique (RAO) projection showing severe mitral insufficiency.

LV function declines severely, patients can become symptomatic with symptoms and signs of CHF. Patients might provide a history of rheumatic fever, endocarditis, CAD, or CHF. Acute MR needs to be in the differential diagnosis of a patient with sudden-onset pulmonary edema.

On examination, patients will display a systolic murmur, most often holosystolic, high-pitched and present at the apex with radiation to the axilla, left scapula, middle back, or left sternal border, depending on the direction of the regurgitant jet. A midsystolic click is often heard if associated mitral valve prolapse is seen. Occasionally a low-pitched diastolic rumble and an S3 sound can be heard.

The ECG often displays an enlarged left atrium (biphasic P wave in V1), large QRS complex secondary to LV enlargement, possible atrial fibrillation, and in ischemic MR, evidence of old or acute inferior infarcts can be seen. The chest radiograph may show an enlarged cardiac silhouette, calcified mitral valve, or increased pulmonary vascular congestion. Echocardiography provides the diagnosis by assessing the presence of the MR, its severity, and its etiology, such as severe prolapse, endocarditis, calcification, papillary muscle or chordae rupture, or a degenerative valve. Left- and right-sided heart catheterization is indicated before corrective surgery to determine the presence of CAD and confirm the diagnosis of MR with the use of left ventriculography. MR is graded based on the amount of contrast seen in the left atrium in systole: *grade I*, contrast does not opacify entire left atrium; *grade II*, contrast opacifies all left atrium but less dense than the contrast in the left ventricle; *grade III*, contrast equally opacifies left atrium and left ventricle; and *grade IV*, contrast in the left atrium is darker than the left ventricle with opacification of pulmonary veins (Fig. 27-21). Also, the angiogram can quantitatively determine the regurgitant fraction (RF). An RF greater than 50% generally indicates severe MR that requires corrective surgery.

Treatment

Patients with a history of mitral insufficiency need to have bacterial endocarditis prophylaxis. Chronic MR benefits from long-term afterload reduction, although this remains controversial. Aggressive treatment of atrial fibrillation with rate control and warfarin anticoagulation is needed. Patients with moderate to severe MR need to be closely monitored for LVEF and LV cavity size. A lower threshold for surgical intervention is generally agreed on when compared to AR. Symptomatic patients (NYHC II-IV) or asymptomatic patients with LV end-systolic dimension approaching 4.5 cm or LVEF of 60% or less should be treated. Patients with lower ejection fraction and a larger cavity size carry a poorer outcome after surgery. However, those with LVEF of 30% to 50% and LV cavity size in systole of 50 to 55 mm also benefit from surgery. Asymptomatic patients with preserved LV function and cavity size but with atrial fibrillation might benefit from surgery.

Acute MR should be treated aggressively with afterload reduction (e.g., sodium nitroprusside). These patients generally require immediate surgery but will do best if they can be initially treated medically and enter a compensated state before surgery. Most regurgitant mitral valves can now be repaired instead of replaced. Techniques for percutaneous repair of the mitral valve are now being tested and hold significant promise.

Mitral Valve Prolapse

Mitral valve prolapse (MVP) is described as bulging of one or more of the mitral leaflets into the left atrium in systole (see Fig. 27-21). Although the most common cause of significant MR (Cheng and Barlow., 1989), it can be isolated without valvular insufficiency. MVP with MR is a strong indication for prophylaxis against bacterial endocarditis during dental, GI, and genitourinary procedures. MVP carries a benign course (Freed et al., 2002). On rare occasions it may be associated with significant arrhythmias and sudden cardiac death. When associated with MR, patients need to be carefully monitored for progressive left atrial and left ventricular cavity dilation and atrial fibrillation.

Primary MVP might be familial and is inherited as an autosomal dominant trait with different rate of penetrance and typically found in patients with connective tissue disease, cardiomyopathies, and Marfan's syndrome (Pyeritz and Wappel, 1983). Secondary MVP is generally seen in patients with CAD and rheumatic heart disease.

Patients with MVP are often asymptomatic. However, some patients describe palpitations, chest pain, dyspnea, and fatigue with or without MR. Although previously thought that strokes occur more frequently in patients with MVP, recent data do not support this conclusion (Gilon et al., 1999). Panic attacks have been frequently described. A high-pitched midsystolic click is often heard that occurs shortly after S1 and can be associated with a systolic murmur. Baseline electrocardiography is often unrevealing, and routine stress testing carries a high false-positive rate. Stress imaging is more accurate in evaluating these patients for myocardial ischemia. An echocardiogram is the most helpful methodology for making the diagnosis of MVP. A displacement of the leaflets beyond the mitral annulus on a parasternal short axis is strongly suggestive of MVP. Cardiac catheterization is generally not needed for diagnosis.

Asymptomatic patients with MVP generally do not require treatment unless they have severe associated MR (Devereux et al., 1989). Symptomatic patients with MVP can be treated with beta blockers. Flail mitral leaflets caused by chordae rupture or severe MR associated with MVP needs to be followed and mitral valve repair becomes indicated if patients develop symptoms of dyspnea (NYHC III or IV), the ejection fraction and cavity size become adversely affected, or atrial fibrillation appears.

Tricuspid Valve Disease

Tricuspid regurgitation (TR) is commonly present on echocardiography in the majority of patients and therefore, when mild, is considered a normal variant. Severe TR can occur, however, and can create significant symptoms of right-sided CHF (cor pulmonale) and dyspnea. Isolated TR is most often seen in drug addicts secondary to tricuspid valve endocarditis but can also be caused by carcinoid syndrome, trauma, right ventricular (RV) infarction, and certain congenital anomalies. The most common etiology of TR, however, is annular dilation from RV cavity dilation.

Patients with TR present with various symptoms depending on the etiology of the valvular abnormalities. Typically, dyspnea, right- and left-sided failure, and in the case of endocarditis, fever and night sweats may be present. The right ventricle is generally dilated, and a precordial lift is present. The jugular veins are pulsatile and increased. A systolic murmur is generally heard along the left sternal border that increases with respiration.

Patients with severe TR are treated with diuretics and digitalis to treat the associated right-sided failure. ACE inhibitors are indicated if left ventricular dysfunction is present. Treatment of associated valvular abnormalities is typically indicated, such as severe MR or MS. Tricuspid valve annuloplasty is generally done, particularly when the symptoms are severe and long-standing and secondary to mitral valve disease. Tricuspid valve replacement is reserved for those patients with abnormal tricuspid valves not amenable to annuloplasty or tricuspid valve repair.

Tricuspid valve stenosis (TS) is mostly caused by rheumatic heart disease and is typically associated with other valvular involvement. TS can also be caused by the carcinoid syndrome (most frequently causes TR) and certain connective tissue diseases. Secondary causes of TS (e.g., tumors, thrombi) can also precipitate secondary TS. Patients can be dyspneic with activity. Typically, there is an increase in the jugular vein with a large *a* wave, indicating atrial contraction against a stiff tricuspid valve. TS is usually treated with percutaneous valvular commissurotomy, unless unfeasible. Open commissurotomy is then performed, or valve replacement if the leaflets and subvalvular structures are not reparable. Bioprosthetic valves are typically used, and patients generally start warfarin therapy after tricuspid valve replacement.

Pulmonic Valve Disease

Pulmonic valve regurgitation (PR) is typically acquired from increased pulmonic pressures (pulmonary hypertension). PR can also result from primary valve abnormalities caused by endocarditis. PR causes a diastolic murmur along the left sternal border. Surgery for patients with acquired PR is rarely performed.

Pulmonic valve stenosis (PS) is mostly congenital, although secondary causes include tumors, endocarditis, and carcinoid. PS is best treated with percutaneous valvuloplasty, with good long-term results.

Prevention of Endocarditis

To prevent adverse complications from infective endocarditis, recent guidelines indicate that only high-risk cardiac patients should receive bacterial endocarditis prophylaxis when undergoing dental procedures that involve manipulation of gingival tissue or periapical teeth or perforation of oral mucosa. The routine use of infective endocarditis prophylaxis before GI or genitourinary (GU) tract infections is not recommended, except in patients with GI or GU infections. Cardiac patients at high risk for complications of infective endocarditis include those with prosthetic cardiac valves or prosthetic material used for cardiac valve repair, prior history of infective endocarditis, unrepaired congenital heart disease, or repaired congenital heart defect with a prosthesis during the first 6 months after the procedure. Residual defects at the repair site and valvular regurgitation secondary to structural valvular disease in a cardiac transplant patient are also considered high risks (Nishimura et al., 2008).

Peripheral Arterial Disease

Key Points

- Patients must be encouraged and supported to stop smoking and to avoid secondhand smoke (Smith et al., 2001) (SOR: A).
- Nicotine replacement therapies to prevent withdrawal symptoms (bupropion, varenicline) are useful aids for tobacco cessation (SOR: A).
- Patients should participate in regular aerobic exercise for at least 30 minutes a day three or four times weekly. Walking improves claudication (SOR: A).
- Patients should receive dietary counseling and be encouraged to achieve an ideal body weight (SOR: A).
- Pedal pulses should be palpated as part of the routine physical examination in all patients at risk for atherosclerosis (SOR: A).
- Diabetic patients should undergo yearly foot examinations that consist of vascular, neurologic, musculoskeletal, and skin evaluation (SOR: A).
- Patients with absent pulses or symptoms suggestive of intermittent claudication should undergo a noninvasive vascular study. For patients with calcified, noncompressible vessels, the toe-brachial index can be used instead of the ankle-brachial index (ABI).
- Patients with an abnormal resting ABI, or postexercise ABI less than 0.9, should have CTA or MRA

Epidemiology

Atherosclerotic peripheral vascular disease (PVD) is an underdiagnosed, undertreated, age-dependent disease that profoundly impacts patient quality of life, and is an independent predictor of mortality (Criqui et al., 1992; Nikolsky et al., 2004; Vogt et al., 1993). On average the mortality rate of claudicant patients is 2.5 times higher than nonclaudicant patients (Fig. 27-22).

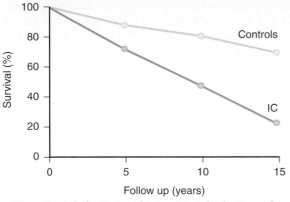

Figure 27-22 Survival of patients with intermittent claudication and matched controls. *(Reprinted with permission from the Society of Vascular Surgery. Dormandy JA, Rutherford RB. Management of peripheral arterial disease (PAD). TransAtlantic Inter-Society Consensus (TASC). J Vasc Surg 2000;31:S1–S296, Figure 12.)*

Atherosclerosis is a ubiquitous process of chronic low-grade inflammation with superimposed acute thrombotic events (Libby, 2001) that affects the entire arterial tree in the coronary, cerebral, visceral, and upper and lower extremity circulation. Patients with PVD are at increased risk of cardiovascular and cerebrovascular events, including death, MI, and stroke. The clinical continuum of PVD ranges from asymptomatic stenosis to limb-threatening ischemia. *Intermittent claudication* (IC) is defined as ischemic limb pain in one or both legs that occurs with exertion and is alleviated with rest. IC is associated with marked limitations in walking ability, which translates into a considerable negative impact on occupational, social, and leisure activities (Regensteiner et al., 1990; Olsen et al., 1988; Vogt et al., 1994).

Atherosclerosis begins in childhood and evolves over decades (Freedman et al., 1988), affecting more than 85% of adults over age 50 (Tuzcu et al., 2001). However, many patients remain entirely asymptomatic; thus estimating the true prevalence of PVD is difficult and highly dependent on the definition of disease. Most epidemiologic studies only report symptomatic disease; therefore the true incidence of PVD is not accurately known and underestimated. In addition, published reports on the incidence and prevalence of PVD vary greatly because the true occurrence of disease is directly related to the risk group of the population studied, and the sensitivity and specificity of the diagnostic testing methodology (Criqui et al., 1985).

Intermittent Claudication

Intermittent claudication is only a symptom of PVD and can be misleading in measuring the prevalence of PVD. For example, a patient with advanced PVD may not have significant IC due to functional decline and inactivity, whereas those who are very active may have significant IC even if they only have mild disease. Several questionnaires, such as the World Health Organization (WHO)/Rose, Edinburgh Claudication, and Walking Impairment questionnaires, have been developed to identify patients with IC. The prevalence of IC based on the Rose criteria ranged from 0.4% to 14% of the adult population (Dormandy and Rutherford, 2000). Although these questionnaires are typically highly specific in excluding healthy patients, as assessed by

a physician, they are only moderately sensitive in detecting disease. Only about one third of patients with PVD have typical symptoms of IC (Schroll and Munck, 1981; Zheng et al., 1997). Furthermore, asymptomatic patients are not at all detected by questionnaire screening. These individuals can only be diagnosed with noninvasive or invasive imaging. Therefore, epidemiologic studies based solely on the use of questionnaires significantly underestimate the true prevalence of disease.

Asymptomatic Disease

More than 50% of patients with PVD are asymptomatic and only identified by noninvasive testing, such as the ankle-brachial index (ABI). Most epidemiologic studies have used a resting ABI less than 0.9 as the criterion for the diagnosis of PVD. However, this definition has several limitations and also leads to an underestimation of the true prevalence of disease. For example, this definition will miss mild to moderate disease in patients with normal resting ABIs, but who may have a considerable ischemic drop in the ABI with exercise. Furthermore, heavily calcified vessels, particularly in diabetic patients, will have falsely elevated ABIs from inability to compress the vessel. Nonetheless, the Systolic Hypertension in the Elderly Program (SHEP) found a prevalence of asymptomatic PVD in 25.5% of 1537 patients (Newman et al., 1993), using a resting ABI <0.9 as the diagnostic criteria. The Peripheral Arterial Disease Detection, Awareness, and Treatment in Primary Care (PARTNERS) program evaluated 6979 patients age 70 years and older, or age 50 to 69 with a history of either diabetes or cigarette smoking, by history and ABI. The diagnosis of PVD was made based on a resting ABI <0.9, a documented medical history of PVD, or a prior lower extremity revascularization. The PARTNERS program found a prevalence of PVD in 29% of patients. More concerning, however, is that 83% of patients with a known prior history of PVD were aware of their diagnosis, whereas only 49% of their physicians were aware of this diagnosis (Hirsch et al., 2001).

Critical Limb Ischemia

Critical limb ischemia (CLI) is defined by the presence of ischemic resting pain in the distal foot, ischemic nonhealing ulcerations, or gangrene, and represents less than 10% of patients with PVD (Hiatt, 2001). Although this subset represents the smallest percentage of patients with PVD, these patients have tremendous disease burden and are clearly the highest risk subset for morbidity and mortality, with up to 73% to 95% progressing to limb loss or death at one year if left untreated (Wolfe and Wyatt, 1997). Each year 150,000 to 200,000 nontraumatic lower extremity amputations are performed in the United States, 85% to 90% of which could be avoided through early revascularization and aggressive risk factor management. Amputation carries a high rate of long-term morbidity and mortality. The fate of the amputee is poor, particularly in the elderly. The level of amputation also dictates the overall prognosis; two to three times as many below-the-knee (BK) amputees achieve full mobility compared to above-the-knee (AK) amputees, but the initial rehabilitation may take up to 9 months. In addition, 5 years after a BK amputation, 30% of patients will have had a major contralateral amputation, 50% will be dead, and only 20% will be alive with one leg intact (Dormandy and Rutherford, 2000).

Pathophysiology

Peripheral arterial insufficiency is caused by hemodynamically significant narrowing of the arterial circulation, usually from atherosclerosis, which clinically reduces blood flow to the affected limb. Longitudinal epidemiologic studies such as the Framingham Heart Study (Murabito et al., 1997), and INTERHEART study (Yusuf et al., 2004) have defined the risk factors for PVD.

Traditional Risk Factors

Age

The prevalence of PVD increases with age. The incidence of IC in five large population-based studies is four times higher and prevalence eight times higher comparing the 35-39 to the 70-74 age group (Dormandy and Rutherford, 2000).

Smoking

Smoking is a very strong independent cause of atherosclerotic PVD. The severity of PVD increases with the number of cigarettes smoked (Cronenwett et al., 1984; Powell et al., 1997) and the amount of exposure to second-hand smoke (Barnoya and Glantz, 2005). In a series of epidemiologic studies, the incidence of developing IC among smokers is twofold to threefold higher than in nonsmokers (Dormandy and Rutherford, 2000). Smokers develop IC approximately a decade before nonsmokers (Kannel and Shurtleff, 1973), and the association between smoking and PVD may be stronger than the association between smoking and CAD (Fowkes et al., 1992; Kannel, 1994). Moreover, smokers are much more likely to progress to CLI than nonsmokers. Smokers with IC have an 11-fold greater amputation rate than nonsmokers (Dormandy et al., 1999a).

Smoking cessation slows the progression of disease, improves the symptoms of IC, decreases the likelihood of amputation, improves the patency of revascularization procedures (Krupski, 1991), and improves overall longevity (Taylor et al., 2002). Finally, all-cause mortality is significantly reduced by smoking cessation, but not by smoking reduction (Godtfredsen et al., 2002). It is imperative that patients entirely cease smoking and not just reduce their consumption of tobacco products.

Diabetes Mellitus

Diabetes/glucose intolerance is one of the most powerful independent modifiable risk factors that contributes to the development of PVD, IC, and CLI (Murabito et al., 1997; Fowkes et al., 1992; Kannel and McGee, 1979). The incidence of IC in diabetic patients is approximately two times higher than in nondiabetic patients (Dormandy and Rutherford, 2000). Diabetes not only has a significant effect on the larger-vessel arterial circulation, but also directly causes microangiopathy as well. Therefore, in conjunction with diabetic peripheral neuropathy, these patients are particularly vulnerable to amputation.

Approximately 60% of all nontraumatic amputations performed in the United States each year are in diabetic patients (ADA Fact Sheet, 2005). The diabetic patient with PVD has approximately a 10-fold higher amputation rate than a nondiabetic patient (Da Silva et al., 1979). There does not appear to be any significant difference in microvascular or macrovascular comorbidity between type 1 and type 2 diabetics (Zander et al., 2002). However, there is a dose-response relationship between the HbA_{1c} level and the risk of amputation (Lehto et al., 1996). Therefore, patients with diabetes should be aggressively treated to normalize glycemic control. In addition, diabetic patients should be instructed on good foot hygiene, such as proper-fitting shoes and foot hygiene, to avoid skin breakdown and ulcer formation.

Hyperlipidemia

As in CAD, low-density lipoprotein cholesterol (LDL-C) and triglyceride (TG) levels are directly related, while high-density lipoprotein cholesterol (HDL-C) levels are indirectly related, to the progression of PVD, and the observed risk seems to demonstrate a linear relationship (Fowkes et al., 1992; Murabito et al., 2002). Most data on lipid-lowering therapy are from patients with CAD. However, several studies specifically demonstrate an improvement in the relative risk of an abnormal ABI, walking distance on a treadmill, frequency and severity of claudication, and limb loss (Blankenhorn et al., 1991; Buchwald et al., 1996; Mohler et al., 2003; Pedersen et al., 1998), suggesting that all patients with PVD should be treated with lipid-lowering therapy regardless of baseline LDL-C.

Hypertension

Hypertension is a major risk factor for PVD and carries a 2.5-fold age-adjusted risk for men and a 3.9-fold age-adjusted risk for women (Kannel and McGee, 1985; Murabito et al., 1997). There have been concerns, based on early case reports, that beta-blockade therapy may worsen the symptoms of IC. A meta-analysis on this subject and critical review of these studies concluded that beta blockers are safe and do not worsen IC (Radack and Deck, 1991). ACE inhibitors (ACEIs) may offer significant benefits for the prevention of atherosclerotic vascular disease beyond that expected from a reduction in blood pressure alone However, there remains considerable debate as to whether or not the data from the HOPE (Heart Outcomes, 2000) and EUROPA (Fox et al., 2003) studies can be generalized to all ACEIs.

Gender

The initial data from Framingham suggested that men develop IC approximately 10 years before women (Kannel et al., 1970). More recent data do not support this observation (Hirsch et al., 2001; Murabito et al., 2003; Reunanen et al., 1982). In light of these data, patients should be screened for PVD regardless of gender.

Obesity

Obesity, as measured by an increased body mass index (BMI) greater than 30, has long been recognized as a risk factor for atherosclerotic disease. It is now recognized that adipocytes, particularly visceral adipocytes, contribute to a proinflammatory state by generating a variety of cytokines (e.g., IL-6, TNF-α, CRP), which play a direct role in the development of atherosclerosis (Hansson, 2005). As further support, liposuction does not seem to lower risk for CAD, because it reduces subcutaneous fat mass but has no effect on lowering visceral fat mass (Klein et al., 2004).

Nontraditional Risk Factors

High-Sensitivity C-Reactive Protein

Atherosclerosis is a disease of chronic low-grade inflammation. High-sensitivity CRP is a nonspecific marker of inflammation emerging as a simple but powerful marker of atherosclerotic risk. Prospective data from the Physicians' Health Study demonstrate that baseline levels of hsCRP independently predict future risk of developing symptomatic PVD (Ridker et al., 1998).

Lipoprotein(a)

Lipoprotein(a) [Lp(a)] is an atherogenic subspecies of LDL that is covalently linked to apoprotein(a). Apo(a) is homologous to plasminogen. Lp(a) may exacerbate risk for ACS by inhibiting endogenous fibrinolysis (Hajjar et al., 1989). Furthermore, Lp(a) may augment the release of endothelial plasminogen activator inhibitor-1 (PAI-1), which further impairs fibrinolysis (Etingin et al., 1991). The net result is that Lp(a) contributes to atherogenesis and a prothrombotic or hypercoagulable state.

Lipoprotein(a) has been implicated as an independent predictor of PVD (Cheng et al., 1997; Prior et al., 1995). However, many of these studies are cross-sectional or retrospective and cannot establish causal relationships between risk factors and disease. Prospective data from the Physicians' Health Study did not show a significant relationship in baseline Lp(a) levels and the future development of PVD (Ridker et al., 2001). Widespread screening of Lp(a) levels in the general population is not recommended. However, this should be considered in patients who present with premature vascular disease and few traditional risk factors. Niacin can modestly reduce Lp(a) levels. There is no clinical trial evidence to prove that reducing serum levels of Lp(a) reduces risk for the development or progression of PVD.

Fibrinogen

Fibrinogen has been implicated in atherogenesis by early epidemiologic studies (Kannel et al., 1987). However, fibrinogen is an acute-phase reactant, with considerable intrapatient variability in its expression over time. Other markers of inflammation, such as hsCRP, have a more powerful association in predicting PVD. Furthermore, fibrinogen levels are directly related to age, obesity, cigarette smoking, diabetes, and LDL-C, and inversely related to HDL-C, physical activity, alcohol use, and estrogen levels. Controversy surrounds the independent predictive value of hyperfibrinogenemia. Therefore, routine fibrinogen level screening is not recommended, unless there is suspicion of a hypercoagulable state.

Natural History

Atherosclerosis is an age-dependent disease that begins in childhood and progresses throughout adulthood, particularly if the risk factors are left unchecked. However, early studies suggested that PVD led a contrary, benign course

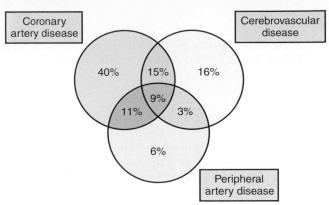

Figure 27-23 Overlap of atherosclerotic disease. Patients often manifest symptoms in more than one vascular bed. *(Modified from Ness J, Aronow WS. Prevalence of coexistence of coronary artery disease, ischemic stroke, and peripheral arterial disease in older persons, mean age 80 years, in an academic hospital-based geriatrics practice. J Am Geriatr Soc 1999;47:1255-1258.)*

that was not progressive (Imparato et al., 1975; McAllister, 1976). However, in most of these studies, IC was used as an end point, not ABI or even a patient functional assessment. Intermittent claudication is a relatively insensitive marker of PVD presence. Those studies typically reported a stabilization or improvement in IC over time, which does not necessarily indicate stabilization or improvement in the disease process, ability to ambulate, or functional status. Early authors suggested that relief of IC over time was a sign of improved collateral flow, but to experience IC, a patient must be physically active. Stabilization or improvement of IC was strongly related to functional decline (i.e., patients walked at a slower pace and for shorter distances to avoid experiencing IC) (McDermott et al., 2004). Thus, PVD is a progressive disorder that leads to a significant decline in quality of life.

Coexisting Vascular Disease

The most important fact regarding the diagnosis and management of PVD is that PVD is a powerful, independent predictor of mortality (Criqui et al., 1992). Intermittent claudication and/or CLI can have a significant impact on quality of life. Many patients may accept their physical limitations as a consequence of aging and tolerate this morbidity. Less than 5% of patients with IC will ever progress to amputation. Much more significant, however, is that PVD is a systemic disorder, and it has considerable overlap with CAD and cerebrovascular disease, ultimately leading to an increase in mortality. Approximately 40% of patients with atherosclerotic vascular disease manifest symptoms in more than one vascular bed (Fig. 27-23) (Ness and Aronow, 1999). Compared to people without PVD, patients with PVD are about four times more likely to have an MI (Criqui et al., 1992) and two to three times more likely to have a stroke (Wilterdink and Easton, 1992). The all-cause mortality rate in patients with PVD is about equal between men and women and is elevated even in asymptomatic patients (Hiatt, 2001). The lower the ABI, the greater is the risk for cardiovascular events. Patients with CLI, who typically have the lowest ABI, have an annual mortality rate of 25% (Dormandy et al., 1999b; McKenna et al., 1991; Vogt et al., 1993b).

Diagnosis

A thorough history and physical examination can accurately suggest a diagnosis of PVD 80% to 90% of the time.

History

The vast majority of disorders related to the peripheral vascular system are (1) atherosclerosis involving the arterial tree or (2) thrombophlebitis involving the venous circulation—both predominantly affecting the lower extremities more so than the upper extremities or viscera. Patients with suspected vascular disease typically present for evaluation with varying types of limb pain or discomfort, ulcerations or gangrene of the extremities, or swelling of the affected limb.

Most limb pain or discomfort typically falls into three etiologies: vascular, musculoskeletal, or neuropathic. Most limb swelling is caused by venous obstruction or insufficiency, increased venous pressure (e.g., CHF), decreased oncotic pressure (e.g., hypoproteinemia, hypoalbuminemia), lymphedema, or lipedema. Many patients, particularly the elderly, have multifactorial etiologies of pain or swelling that can usually be distinguished by a thorough history and physical examination. Using a systematic approach with key pointed questions, a presumptive diagnosis can often be deduced on clinical grounds and subsequently confirmed with noninvasive testing. The history should focus on identifying risk factors for atherosclerosis. The past medical history should concentrate on prior vascular events such as MI, stroke, amputation, DVT and revascularizations in any vascular bed either percutaneously or surgically, as well as, but not limited to, a history of CHF, back problems, osteoarthritis, inflammatory conditions (e.g., rheumatoid arthritis, plantar fasciitis, polymyalgia rheumatic), gout, varicose veins, and lymphatic obstruction (e.g., after surgery or radiation therapy).

The etiology of leg pain can be determined by the characteristics, severity, location, duration, frequency, and precipitating or alleviating factors of the discomfort. *Claudication* is typically described as a cramping or aching discomfort in the muscle associated with exertion and alleviated with rest. Most often this occurs in the calf, but it can occur in the hip and buttocks if there is occlusive disease in the aortoiliac segment. Nocturnal cramping of the calf and foot is not typically vascular in etiology and is most likely caused by an exaggerated neuromuscular response to stretch that occurs while sleeping.

Critical limb ischemia can cause resting pain that is constant throughout the day and night. A classic description of nocturnal pain from CLI is a moderate to severe aching paresthesia/dysesthesia while lying horizontal that is alleviated by dangling the leg over the side of the bed. Pain from CLI can be so severe that it may not be relieved by narcotic analgesia. On the other hand, diabetic patients with severe peripheral neuropathy may be completely insensate despite significant tissue loss. Distinguishing the etiology of constant resting limb pain between a vascular and nonvascular etiology can be done by physical examination and noninvasive testing. Pain that occurs at rest may be caused by CLI if other findings in the history and examination support the diagnosis of advanced atherosclerosis. Otherwise, pain that occurs at rest, with change in position, or simply standing without exertion, is more typically musculoskeletal or neuropathic in nature. Tables 27-11 and 27-12 list the distinguishing features and differential diagnosis of the most common types of leg pain and swelling, respectively.

For example, acute loss of motor and sensory function in the distal extremities, particularly with associated acute severe pain, pallor, and coolness of the limb, is a sign of acute arterial occlusion. However, chronic motor and sensory loss may be vascular in etiology but more likely is neuropathic. Several standardized classification schemes exist for categorizing the severity of both acute and chronic limb ischemia. Table 27-13 is the revised Rutherford-Baker classification for acute limb ischemia, and Table 27-14 is the combined Fontaine classification (more popular in Europe) and the Rutherford-Baker scheme for CLI (Dormandy and Rutherford, 2000; Rutherford et al., 1997).

Physical Examination

The physical examination in patients with PVD should consist of inspection, palpation, auscultation, and even percussion. Observations should note any asymmetry between the limbs, joint deformities, varicose veins, skin discoloration, absence of hair, swelling, ulcerations, tissue loss, and gangrene. Acute CLI from embolism or thrombosis typically causes pallor with decreased capillary refill that eventually leads to mottling unless adequate collateral flow can be recruited. Chronic ischemia may have a normal skin color with relatively normal or slightly delayed capillary refill, particularly if collateral flow has developed. Chronic advanced CLI can lead to dependent rubor due to chronic dilation of the postcapillary venules. The toes of the dependent limbs can become red with brisk capillary refill. This is often mistaken for hyperemia rather than a sign of severe ischemia. A cadaveric pallor on elevating the limb to greater than 45 degrees above the horizontal for 1 to 2 minutes, followed by slow venous filling with rubor after returning to a dependent position (Buerger's sign), also signals advanced CLI.

Ulcerations may be caused by chronic venous insufficiency or edema and arterial insufficiency. Chronic venous disease typically causes pigmentation of the lower legs from extravasation of red blood cells with superficial ulcers in the calves, more often medially than laterally. Arterial ulcerations are characteristically distal, involving the toes and even forefoot in advanced disease.

Palpation of the pedal pulses should be a mandatory part of the routine physical examination. Notably, even in healthy individuals, the dorsalis pedis (DP) pulse, the posterior tibial (PT) pulse, or both are unable to be palpated 8.1%, 2.9%, and 0.7% of the time, respectively (McGee and Boyko, 1998). This results from normal anatomic variation. Wide and prominent femoral or popliteal pulses may be a sign of an aneurysm. A significant temperature gradient from proximal to distal and between ipsilateral and contralateral limbs often is a sign of advanced disease. The abdomen should be palpated to assess for the presence of an abdominal aortic aneurysm. Reproduction of pain with palpation over joints is not caused by vascular disease and seems to be a sign of such orthopedic conditions as degenerative joint disease, sacroiliitis, gout, trauma, or plantar fasciitis. Reproduction of pain with palpation of muscle groups may be vascular in etiology if there is severe ischemia, but the clinician should also

Table 27-11 Differential Diagnosis of Claudication

Diagnosis	Location of Discomfort	Features of Discomfort	Onset Relative to Exertion	Onset Relative to Standing	Effect of Rest	Effect of Body Position	Other Features
Arterial claudication	Depends on level of stenosis (occlusion): aortoiliac disease affects hip/thigh/buttock, can affect entire limb Infrainguinal disease affects calf and foot	Aching, cramping, weakness	Consistently reproduced with same degree of activity	Unrelated to standing	Relieved promptly	None	Gradual onset of discomfort with exercise Very reproducible
Venous claudication	Entire limb, usually worse in thigh and groin	Tight, tense sensation	After exercise	Unrelated to standing	Relieved slowly	Relieved more quickly with elevation	History of DVT, edema, or venous congestion
Chronic critical limb ischemia	Always involves foot; symptoms may be more proximal with more proximal disease	Severe burning, aching, but may be asymptomatic in patients with profound neuropathy	Worse with minimal activity	Unrelated to standing	Improved, but incompletely	Symptoms may be improved with dangling foot over side of bed while sleeping	Gradual or subacute onset Dependent rubor Elevation pallor Gangrene
Acute critical limb ischemia	Always involves foot; symptoms may be more proximal with more proximal disease	Severe aching, cramping, painful	Worse with minimal activity	Unrelated to standing	Improved, but incompletely	Symptoms may be improved with dangling foot over side of bed while sleeping	Acute onset Pale, cold Loss of motor/ sensory functions is an emergency
Arthritis	Joints	Aching, may be sharp with position change	Variable	Weight bearing reproduces pain	Variable, may be present with rest	Less pain in non-weight bearing position	Variable, may be related to weather May have effusion
Lumbar back pain (e.g., herniated disc, nerve root compression)	Lumbar region; may radiate down dermatomes if there is nerve root compression	Sharp, stabbing, shooting	Immediate	Weight bearing reproduces pain	Variable, may be present at rest	Certain positions exacerbate or alleviate pain	History of back problems Worse with lifting May have motor/ sensory deficits Reproducible with percussion
Sacroiliitis	Sacroiliac region	Sharp, stabbing, shooting	Immediate	Weight bearing reproduces pain	Variable, may be present at rest	Certain positions exacerbate or alleviate pain	Inflammatory disorder Reproducible with palpation
Plantar fasciitis	Plantar region	sharp, stabbing, searing	Immediate	Weight bearing reproduces pain	Immediate relief with non-weight bearing	Less pain in non-weight-bearing position	Reproducible with palpation

Continued

Table 27-11 Differential Diagnosis of Claudication—Cont'd

Diagnosis	Location of Discomfort	Features of Discomfort	Onset Relative to Exertion	Onset Relative to Standing	Effect of Rest	Effect of Body Position	Other Features
Peripheral neuropathy	Stocking glove distribution	Paresthesia, dysthesia, may be quite severe	Unrelated to activity	Unrelated to standing	Usually a constant sensation, unrelated to rest	Unrelated to change in position	Common in diabetics Present 24 hours a day, may interrupt sleep
Myopathy	In the muscle groups, may be systemic	Dull, aching, weakness	Immediate	Variable	Improved with less physical activity	May exacerbate discomfort	Reproducible with palpation Statin myopathy not uncommon Inflammatory disorders rare

DVT, Deep venous thrombosis.

Table 27-12 Differential Diagnosis of Chronic Leg Swelling

Clinical Feature	Venous	Lymphatic	CardiacOrthostatic	"Lipedema"
Consistency of swelling	Brawny	Spongy	Pitting	Noncompressible (fat)
Relief by elevation	Complete	Mild	Complete	Minimal
Distribution of swelling	Maximal in ankles and legs, feet spared	Diffuse, greatest distally	Diffuse, greatest distally	Maximal in ankles and legs, feet spared
Associated skin changes	Atrophic and pigmented, subcutaneous fibrosis	Hypertrophic, lichenified skin	Shiny, mild pigmentation, no trophic changes	None
Pain	Heavy, ache, tight or bursting	None or heavy ache	Little or none	Dull ache, cutaneous sensitivity
Bilaterality	Occasionally, but usually unequal	Occasionally, but usually unequal	Always, but may be unequal	Always

From Rutherford RB. Basic approaches to vascular problems. In Vascular Surgery, 5th ed, vol 1, p 10. Philadelphia, Saunders, 2000.

Table 27-13 Clinical Categories of Acute Limb Ischemia

Category	Description/ Prognosis	Findings		Doppler Signals	
		Sensory Loss	Motor Weakness	Arterial	Venous
I. Viable	Not immediately threatened	None	None	Audible	Audible
II. Threatened					
a. Marginally	Salvageable if promptly treated	Minimal (toes) or none	None	Inaudible	Audible
b. Immediately	Salvageable with immediate revascularization	More than toes, associated with rest pain	Mild, moderate	Inaudible	Audible
III. Irreversible	Major tissue loss, or permanent nerve damage inevitable	Profound, anesthetic	Profound, paralysis (rigor)	Inaudible	Inaudible

From Rutherford RB, Baker JD, Ernst C, et al. Recommended standards for reports dealing with lower extremity ischemia: Revised version. J Vasc Surg 1997;26:517-538, Table 1. Reprinted with permission from The Society of Vascular Surgery.

Table 27-14 Clinical Categories of Chronic Limb Ischemia: Fontaine's stages and Rutherford's categories

Fontaine		Rutherford		
Stage	Clinical	Grade	Category	Clinical
I	Asymptomatic	0	0	Asymptomatic
IIa	Mild claudication	I	1	Mild claudication
IIb	Moderate-severe claudication	I	2	Moderate claudication
		I	3	Severe claudication
III	Ischemic rest pain	II	4	Ischemic rest pain
		III	5	Minor tissue loss
IV	Ulceration or gangrene	III	6	Major tissue loss

From Dormandy JA, Rutherford RB. Management of peripheral arterial disease (PAD). TransAtlantic InterSociety Consensus (TASC). J Vasc Surg 2000;31:S1-S296, Table 9. Reprinted with permission from The Society of Vascular Surgery.

consider other causes of myopathy, such as fibromyalgia, polymyalgia rheumatica, drug-induced myalgia, and trauma.

The carotid arteries, abdomen, and femoral arteries should be auscultated for *bruits*. Only gentle pressure should be applied with the stethoscope over the carotid and femoral arteries because pseudobruits can be created by compression of the underlying vessel. Finally, percussion over the lumbar spine may be useful in eliciting pain from sacroiliitis, lumbar disk disease, or nerve root compression.

Noninvasive Testing

Noninvasive vascular testing is useful to confirm clinical suspicion of PVD in patients with leg discomfort and to screen asymptomatic patients at risk for vascular disease, particularly diabetics. Noninvasive testing is also very helpful for the surveillance of vessel patency after percutaneous or surgical intervention.

Noninvasive Vascular Study

A complete noninvasive vascular study (NIVS) consists of the ABI, segmental BPs, and pulse-volume recordings (PVR) obtained at rest. When physically possible, the ABIs should also be ordered with exercise to assess for an ischemic response (Fig. 27-24).

The ABI is defined as the highest systolic blood pressure (SBP) of either the DP artery or PT artery divided by the higher of the SBP from either the right or left brachial artery (Table 27-15). Segmental BPs provide more specific information as to the location of the stenosis/obstruction. BP readings are obtained at the high-thigh, low-thigh, calf, ankle, metatarsal, and toe level, specifically looking for pressure gradients proximally to distally. Pulse-volume recordings

are plethysmographic measurements that detect changes in the blood volume flowing through the limb. A normal PVR tracing resembles a normal arterial pulse wave tracing with a rapid upstroke, prominent dicrotic notch, and rapid downstroke. As the severity of the disease increases, the waveforms become more blunted, the dicrotic notch disappears, and ultimately the waveforms become flat.

The standard exercise protocol of walking on a treadmill for 5 minutes at 2 mph at a 12% grade (Rutherford et al., 1997) is quite modest in comparison to the workload involved in a routine Bruce protocol that is typically employed for cardiac stress testing. The purpose of the Rutherford protocol is not to induce coronary ischemia and thus is typically well tolerated from a cardiopulmonary standpoint. Relative contraindications to walking on a treadmill include severe symptomatic CAD (Canadian Cardiovascular Society Class 3 or 4), severe decompensated CHF (NYHA Class III or IV), severe symptomatic COPD, orthopedic or balance disorders that preclude safe ambulation on a treadmill, or severely depressed resting ABI (<0.5). If patients are unable to walk on a treadmill, other means of exercise may suffice, such as stationary bicycling, walking in the hallway, or toe lifts. However, these alternative forms of exercise are not standardized and may impact the diagnostic sensitivity and specificity of the study.

Some patients with mild PVD may have an ABI that is normal at rest but significantly decreased with exercise (Fig. 27-25). In fact, comparing angiography, which is the "gold standard" for diagnosing PVD, to ABIs, there actually needs to be a rather severe single stenosis, or moderate diffuse multilevel disease, to have a depression in the resting ABI. Even a mildly depressed resting ABI implies there is a considerable burden of disease. Therefore, ABIs done at rest only and not with exercise will have a relatively high false-negative rate, and many patients with a normal resting ABI will be misdiagnosed as having nonvascular limb pain when the true etiology of their discomfort is PVD. A corollary to this is that many epidemiologic studies use only resting ABI as a diagnostic criterion for PVD, which leads to underestimation of the true incidence of PVD. In fact, obtaining ABIs at rest only without exercise is similar to performing a nuclear myocardial perfusion imaging study at rest only and trying to establish a diagnosis of coronary artery disease—this is impossible. The myocardial perfusion may be normal at rest, but it is the stress images that allow one to determine whether there is reversible ischemia.

Another potential pitfall of ABIs is vascular calcification. Severe calcification of the arterial wall eventually leads to an inability to compress the blood vessels despite cuffs inflated to suprasystolic pressures. Consequently, ABIs can be falsely elevated, and caution should be used in interpreting an ABI greater than 1.3. This is particularly common in patients with diabetes and patients on chronic hemodialysis. In this case the toe-brachial index has been established as an adequate surrogate to the ankle-brachial index (Sahli et al., 2004).

An NIVS can provide a general region (e.g., femoropopliteal segment) that is diseased. However, the NIVS is not precise enough to determine the exact location of the stenosis or occlusion. In other words, NIVS provides physiologic information with limited anatomic localization of disease. Arterial duplex Doppler ultrasound, computed tomography

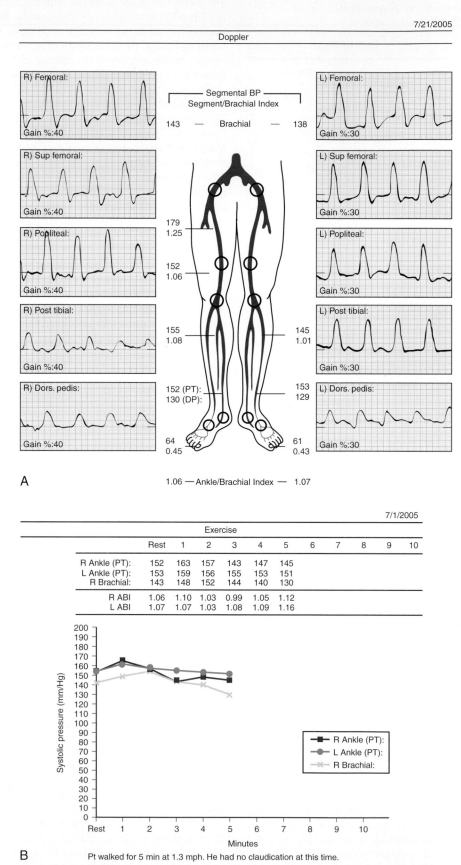

Figure 27-24 A, Normal pulse volume recording demonstrates triphasic waveforms with normal segmental pressures. No pressures were obtained in the left thigh because of previously placed stent. **B,** Normal ankle-brachial indexes at rest, with a normal response to exercise. The red lines and green lines are essentially flat throughout exercise.

angiography (CTA), or magnetic resonance angiography (MRA) are more suited to proven detailed anatomic information and complement the NIVS data.

Doppler Ultrasound

Arterial duplex Doppler sonography utilizes high-frequency sound waves (typically 5.0-7.5 MHz) to provide real-time vascular images that can accurately localize atherosclerotic disease. Color-flow encoding is useful to localize vessels quickly and determine the presence or absence of blood flow. Doppler technology uses the physical principles of the reflected sound wave frequency in relation to the transmitted frequency to determine the velocity of blood flow. As the severity of stenosis increases, the peak systolic velocity (PSV) of flow increases. By using established criteria of the absolute PSV and the ratio of PSV in the normal reference segment compared to the PSV in the diseased segment, the overall range of stenosis can be determined.

Ultrasound is particularly useful for assessing stent or graft patency after a revascularization procedure. Potential pitfalls of ultrasound include visualizing the tibial vessels, which are relatively small and deep in the calf, and visualizing highly calcified vessels, which are acoustically shadowed by the calcium.

Computed Tomography and Magnetic Resonance Angiography

The noninvasive imaging modalities CTA and MRA have essentially replaced traditional invasive diagnostic angiography. Both CTA and MRA produce similarly accurate anatomic information and provide highly detailed images that can be used to plan revascularization procedures, assess the size and location of aneurysms, and occasionally find incidental pathology such as occult malignancy. These two technologies are fundamentally very different.

Traditional CT has evolved by the addition of multiple detectors, now up to 64 per machine. MDCT allows much shorter acquisition times and submillimeter resolution; thus an entire body scan can be performed in seconds to minutes with excellent spatial resolution. By adding three-dimensional reconstruction software, the bone, soft tissue, and organs can be virtually removed, and the vasculature reconstructed and viewed from multiple projections. Figure 27-26 provides examples of normal and abnormal CT angiograms. CTA utilizes ionizing radiation and iodinated contrast. Therefore, multiple scans (cumulative radiation dose)

Table 27-15 Ankle-Brachial Index (ABI) and Severity of Disease

ABI	Disease Classification
>1.30	Noncompressible
0.90-1.30	Normal
0.80-0.89	Mild
0.60-0.79	Moderate
0.40-0.59	Severe
<0.40	Critical ischemia

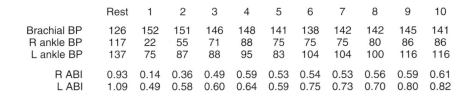

	Rest	1	2	3	4	5	6	7	8	9	10
Brachial BP	126	152	151	146	148	141	138	142	142	145	141
R ankle BP	117	22	55	71	88	75	75	75	80	86	86
L ankle BP	137	75	87	88	95	83	104	104	100	116	116
R ABI	0.93	0.14	0.36	0.49	0.59	0.53	0.54	0.53	0.56	0.59	0.61
L ABI	1.09	0.49	0.58	0.60	0.64	0.59	0.75	0.73	0.70	0.80	0.82

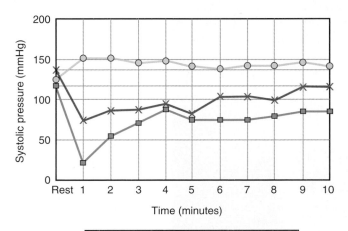

■ = R ankle BP ISCHEMIC WINDOW; 444
X = L ankle BP ISCHEMIC WINDOW; 393
◉ = Brachial BP

Figure 27-25 Normal noninvasive vascular study at rest. The right ankle-brachial index *(ABI)* is 0.93, and the left ABI is 1.09. However, there is a marked ischemic response to exercise. Note the pronounced drop of the red and blue lines with exercise and the severe drop of the right ABI to 0.14 and the left ABI to 0.49. This patient had bilateral, focal, 95% to 99% stenoses in the superficial femoral arteries, which were successfully stented. This example clearly demonstrates the importance of obtaining ABIs at rest and with exercise. Failure to obtain ABIs with exercise, particularly when the resting values are normal, often fails to diagnose the disease. *BP,* Blood pressure.

and renal insufficiency are relative contraindications to CTA. Other limitations include severe vascular calcifications and prosthetic joints, which cause scatter artifact. The lumen of a stented vessel can be visualized with CTA, although a mild to moderate degree of scatter artifact makes accurate assessment of in-stent restenosis difficult.

Traditional MRI has also evolved through the development of more powerful magnets and improved scanning algorithms. MRA can also produce submillimeter spatial resolution. In contrast to CTA, however, the scanning time for MRA can be up to an hour per patient. In a busy practice or hospital, this can lead to problems with patient throughput. Software can also reconstruct MRA images into three dimensions. MRA utilizes magnetic fields and variable-frequency radio waves to detect changes in alignment and distribution of protons in a given tissue. The obvious advantage over CTA is that MRA does not use ionizing radiation or iodinated contrast. Thus, there is practically no risk of stochastic injury or contrast nephropathy. Patients with pacemakers or defibrillators cannot undergo MRA because the magnet can interfere with device function. Severely calcified vessels can be adequately imaged with MRA, but stents appear as voids and thus falsely give the impression of a totally occluded artery even if the stent is widely patent.

The false-positive rate for detecting a hemodynamically significant stenosis is considerably higher with MRA than CTA. With CTA the lumen of the vessel visualized is essentially a column of contrast; thus a precise assessment of the

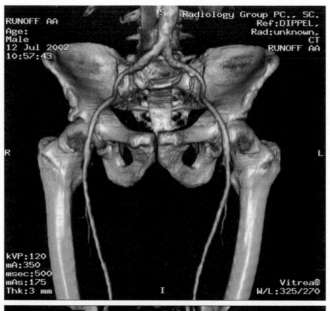

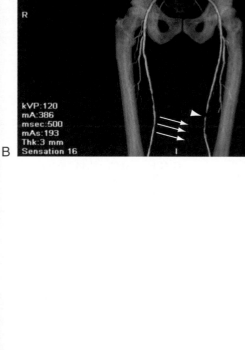

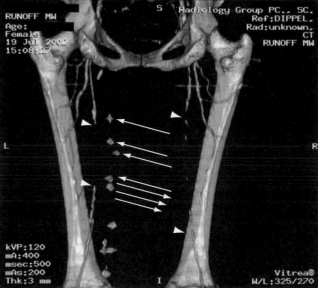

Figure 27-26 A, Anteroposterior (AP) view of a multidetector computed tomography angiogram (CTA) reconstructed with three-dimensional imaging software. This image shows the distal aorta, iliac arteries, common femoral arteries, and proximal superficial femoral arteries. There are minimal plaques in the distal aorta, common iliac arteries, and superficial femoral arteries. **B,** AP view of a multidetector CTA demonstrating a short total occlusion of the distal left superficial femoral artery *(arrowhead)*. Note surgical clips from prior saphenous vein harvest *(thin arrows)*. Note absence of the left kidney. **C,** Posterior view of a multidetector CTA demonstrating a long total occlusion of superficial femoral arteries (between *arrowheads*). These were successfully stented. Again, note vascular clips from prior saphenous vein harvest *(thin arrows)*.

degree of stenosis is usually possible. However, MRA technology requires flow through the vessel to determine where the lumen exists. The pitfall occurs when the vessel runs through the same plane as the frequency of the radio wave. This leads to flow voids, which appear as gaps in the vessel and are frequently overdiagnosed as stenoses. This phenomenon is particularly common at the origin of the renal arteries and throughout the tortuosity of the carotid arteries.

Invasive Imaging

Traditional invasive diagnostic angiography has been the gold standard for diagnosing PVD since the 1950s. This technique involves the percutaneous placement of catheters within the vessel, injecting iodinated contrast through the catheters, and recording fluoroscopic and cineographic images. As with CTA, conventional angiography uses ionizing radiation, and the same relative risks apply. The potential complications include vascular access site injury, pseudoaneurysm or arteriovenous fistula formation, bleeding, dissection, and atheroembolization. For these reasons, and with the advances in noninvasive CTA/MRA imaging, routine diagnostic standalone invasive angiography is not routinely recommended. The only remaining indications for a conventional diagnostic angiogram are an inconclusive or indeterminate CTA/MRA and at a planned endovascular intervention.

Therapy

Therapy for PVD should involve a patient care plan consisting of (1) patient education on pathophysiology of atherosclerosis, risk factors that contribute to disease, and prognosis; (2) encouragement of lifestyle changes that emphasize risk factor modification and routine exercise; (3) pharmacologic therapy to relieve symptoms and treat risk factors; and (4) revascularization procedures to relieve IC and limb salvage in CLI. The goals of therapy are to improve the patient's functional status by relieving symptoms, improving the quality of life, and improving exercise capacity; preserve the limb via revascularization and decrease or limit the extent of amputation; prevent the progression of atherosclerosis by aggressive risk factor modification; and reduce cardiovascular and cerebrovascular mortality and nonfatal events such as MI and stroke.

Risk Factor Management

By far the most important therapy for both primary and secondary prevention of PVD is aggressive management of the risk factors for atherosclerosis. Both the American Heart Association (AHA) and the National Cholesterol Education Program (NCEP) recommend the same level of risk factor modification in patients with PVD as in patients with known CAD (Grundy et al., 2004; Smith et al., 2001). Despite the growing recognition that PVD is associated with a higher mortality rate, the risk factors in patients with PVD have historically been grossly undertreated. This is exemplified by data on a cohort of 1733 patients with known PVD and no overt CAD. Of these patients, only 33.1% were receiving beta-blockade therapy, 28.9% were receiving ACEIs, and 31.3% were treated with a statin. Furthermore, 92% had a recent BP measurement, but 56% had SBP greater than 130 mm Hg, 45.5% had DBP >80 mm Hg, and 13.6% had DBP >90 mm Hg. In addition, only 62.6% had a screening lipid profile, yet 56% had an LDL-C >100 mg/dL, and 21% had an LDL-C >130 mg/dL. Finally, in patients with diabetes, HbA_{1c} was >7.0% in 54.2% of patients (Rehring et al., 2005). Unfortunately, such data are representative of current practice patterns. The risk factors of atherosclerosis must be aggressively identified and treated to reduce risk for disease progression.

Exercise

Routine aerobic exercise is recommended for all patients with PVD. The benefit of walking programs has been clearly established to increase time-to-claudication and maximal walking distance (Hiatt and Regensteiner, 1990; Hiatt et al., 1994). Regular exercise will have a strong impact on improving functional capacity and quality of life. A minimum of 30 to 60 minutes of exercise is recommended preferably daily, but at least three or four times a week. This should be supplemented by an increase in daily lifestyle activities, such as walking breaks at lunch, gardening, or household chores (Smith et al., 2001).

Weight Management

Obesity is at epidemic levels, which ultimately contributes to the progression of atherosclerosis. Patients should be counseled on weight loss strategies with a target body mass index (BMI) of 18.5 to 24.9 kg/m^2 (Smith et al., 2001).

Pharmacologic Therapy

Pharmacologic treatment can be divided into two separate but equally important components: therapy for the control of risk factors and therapy for the relief of symptoms of ischemia or claudication.

Pharmacologic therapy for risk factor modification is the same as for any other forms of atherosclerotic vascular disease, such as coronary or cerebrovascular disease. The most important consideration is that the mortality of patients with PVD is high, and thus they should be treated aggressively. Current national guidelines should be adhered to for the primary and secondary prevention of atherosclerotic vascular disease (ADA, 2005; Grundy et al., 2004; Seventh Report, 2004; Smith et al., 2001). The four primary categories of pharmacologic therapy include antiplatelet therapy, lipid-lowering therapy, antihypertensive therapy, and glycemic-lowering therapy, as discussed earlier. These therapies are complementary and confer additive benefit. From a practical standpoint, patients with several comorbidities may be taking multiple medications daily, so to ensure compliance, they should be repeatedly educated as to the importance of risk factor control.

The only FDA-approved pharmacologic therapy that has a consensus of benefit for the relief of claudication is cilostazol (Pletal). Cilostazol is a phosphodiesterase III inhibitor, which increases the intracellular concentration of cAMP, leading to significant antiplatelet and vasodilatory properties and possibly antiproliferative properties (Tsuchikane et al., 1999). Cilostazol undergoes extensive metabolism by the hepatic cytochrome P4503A4 (CYP3A4) isoform enzyme, and to a lesser extent the 2C19 and 1A2 isoforms. Although cilostazol does not inhibit the CYP450 system, drugs that inhibit CYP3A4, 2C19, and 1A2 can lead to increased levels of cilostazol in serum.

Pentoxifylline (Trental) is another drug FDA approved for claudication. However, no randomized data demonstrate

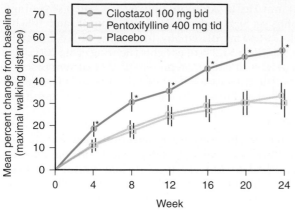

Figure 27-27 Mean percentage change from baseline maximum walking distance on a treadmill for patients with intermittent claudication randomly assigned to cilostazol, pentoxifylline, or placebo. *$p <0.05$ at each 4-week time point for cilostazol versus placebo and pentoxifylline. *(Reprinted with permission from Exerpta Medica. Dawson DL, Cutler BS, Hiatt WR, et al: A Comparison of cilostazol and pentoxifylline for treating intermittent claudication. Am J Med 2000;109:523-530, Figure 2.)*

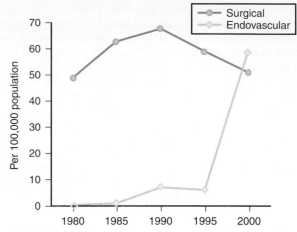

Figure 27-28 Volume trends for percutaneous revascularization and surgical revascularization for the lower extremities from 1980 through 2000. Data obtained by reviewing ICD-9 codes for all vascular procedures using the National Hospital Discharge Survey of nonfederal U.S. hospitals. *(Modified from Anderson PL, Gelijns A, Moskowitz A, et al. Understanding trends in inpatient surgical volume: vascular interventions, 1980-2000. J Vasc Surg 2004;39:1200-1208.)*

that it is better than placebo, so there is no recommendation to use this agent for the treatment of claudication. Eight RCTs compared cilostazol to placebo and pentoxifylline (Smith, 2002). In all studies, cilostazol demonstrated a statistically significant improvement in objective and subjective end points compared to placebo. In one study, comparing cilostazol (100 mg twice daily) with pentoxifylline (400 mg three times dally) or placebo, the maximal walking distance on a treadmill increased by 54% from baseline in the cilostazol group, versus 30% increase in the pentoxifylline group ($p <0.001$), and 34% increase in the placebo group (Fig. 27-27) (Dawson et al., 2000).

Revascularization

Peripheral arterial revascularization is indicated for relief of ischemic symptoms, including intermittent claudication and resting ischemic pain, and limb preservation in the setting of critical limb ischemia. Historically, revascularization has been performed surgically; however, with advances in endovascular technology, a percutaneous approach is now considered first-line therapy. From 1995 to 2000, the number of percutaneous revascularizations performed in the United States increased by almost 1000%, compared to a 30% to 35% decrease in the number of surgical revascularizations (Fig. 27-28) (Anderson et al., 2004).

An endovascular approach confers a similar acute procedural success rate and similar long-term results, with considerably less periprocedural morbidity, shorter recovery time, shorter hospitalization time, and less pain than a surgical procedure. In addition, failure of the two therapies is completely different. With surgical therapy, graft closure is often sudden without sufficient time to develop collateral flow, leaving the limb in an acutely ischemic situation that frequently results in major amputation. Furthermore, surgical therapy can only be repeated a limited number of times, as dissection planes, surgical targets, and anastomosis sites become obliterated by repetitive surgery and conduit becomes exhausted. On the other hand, restenosis by neointimal hyperplasia of an endovascular procedure is a well documented, slow process that occurs over weeks to months, and thus gives the limb ample

time to develop collateral flow. Patients returning with failure of an endovascular procedure rarely do so in a limb-threatening situation. Moreover, an endovascular procedure can be repeated as often as necessary to maintain vessel patency.

The appeal of a minimally invasive approach for revascularization is that it significantly lowers the threshold of when to treat patients. Traditional surgical dogma has reserved revascularization until there is a limb-threatening situation. However, this leaves many patients left to face debilitating IC inadequately treated. Endovascular therapy offers a paradigm shift in this philosophy. Because it is safer, effective, and reproducible, patients can be treated earlier in the disease process during the claudication stage, with marked improvement in quality of life (Dippel et al., 2004). Figure 27-29 shows an artery before and after an endovascular revascularization.

From 150,000 to 200,000 nontraumatic amputations are done annually (ADA Fact Sheet, 2005). The alarming statistic is that 40% to 50% of limbs are amputated without a presurgical angiogram. It is estimated that more than 90% of these limbs could be salvaged, or converted to a lesser amputation, with revascularization. Another advantage of an endovascular approach over a surgical approach is that totally occluded arteries can be revascularized endovascularly with a high acute procedural success rate, even when no distal targets are available to bypass and surgery is not technically feasible. Therefore, it is recommended that patients with CLI or claudication not adequately alleviated with medical therapy be referred for endovascular revascularization. If an endovascular approach is not viable, surgical therapy should be considered as a second-line alternative.

Conclusions

Peripheral vascular disease is an underdiagnosed, undertreated, highly prevalent, age-dependent condition associated with a high mortality rate because of cardiac and cerebrovascular events. Furthermore, PVD has a very strong negative impact on quality of life, and patients have a functional status similar to NYHA Class III symptoms of CHF.

Clinicians must be more diligent in diagnosing and treating PVD. The diagnosis consists of a goal-directed history and physical examination, non-invasive vascular studies, and CTA or MRA. Therapy consists of routine exercise, smoking cessation, treating the appropriate risk factors to their target goals, and relief of ischemic symptoms either pharmacologically or through a revascularization procedure. Patients with CLI, with or without tissue loss, should be referred urgently for revascularization. Figure 27-30 provides an algorithm for management.

KEY TREATMENT

Risk factors for atherosclerosis should be identified and treated to their target goals (SOR: A).

Patients should take aspirin (81-325 mg/day) unless there is a contraindication to aspirin therapy, such as active GI bleeding or a history of allergy to aspirin (SOR: A).

Clopidogrel (75 mg/day) can be used as an alternative to aspirin. Patients at high risk for vascular events may take both clopidogrel (75 mg/day) and aspirin (81 mg/day). Avoid aspirin (325 mg) when used in combination with clopidogrel because of a higher incidence of GI bleeding (SOR: A).

Ticlopidine (250 mg twice daily) may be used as an alternative to clopidogrel for patients with intolerance or allergy to clopidogrel, but routine blood counts must be performed to assess for bone marrow suppression (SOR: A). The safety of long-term combination ticlopidine-aspirin therapy has not been assessed (SOR: C).

LDL-C should be lowered to less than 100 mg/dL, or less than 70 mg/dL if the patient has concomitant CAD. A statin should be considered first-line pharmacologic therapy, in addition to diet and exercise. Ezetimibe and/or colesevelam may be added to statin therapy to achieve the target goal (SOR: A).

Blood pressure should be lowered to less than 130/80 mm Hg. For patients with vascular disease, ACEIs or ARBs have a vasculoprotective effect and should be considered first-line agents (SOR: A).

Diabetic patients should have HbA_{1c} lowered to less than 7%, preferably closer to 6.5%.

Cilostazol (50-100 mg twice daily) is recommended for symptomatic relief of claudication (SOR: A).

Pentoxifylline is not recommended for the treatment of PVD because of a lack of benefit versus placebo (SOR: A).

Because of its minimally invasive nature, an endovascular procedure should be considered first-line therapy for revascularization. Surgery is now second-line therapy, when an endovascular approach is not technically feasible (SOR: A).

Patients should be referred for a revascularization procedure when an exercise program and cilostazol therapy fail to alleviate ischemic symptoms.

All patients with critical limb-threatening ischemia with or without tissue loss should be urgently referred for a revascularization procedure (SOR: A).

Cardiac Electrophysiology and Arrhythmias

Key Points

- Treatment of patients with symptoms referable to an arrhythmia is possible for many physicians.
- Accurate diagnosis of the arrhythmic event may prove difficult, and additional diagnostic tests not readily available to the family physician may be needed.
- More conscientious use of antiarrhythmic drugs is necessary as their proarrhythmic effects become known.
- Implantable devices continue to evolve and promise to alter the natural history of many malignant cardiac disease states.

The accurate understanding and interpretation of electrocardiograms (ECGs), rhythm strips, and unusual cardiac beats is a rewarding practice. Understanding is based not only on recognition of patterns but also on knowledge of electrical activation and repolarization of individual cells alone and in the aggregate. Anticipation of what *should be* happening will aid in determining what *is* happening during any particular beat. Appreciation of the history of electrophysiology and arrhythmology further aids in rhythm management.

Normal cardiac cellular actions may include automaticity, rhythmicity, conductivity, and contractility. Specialized cardiac cells may perform one of these functions better than a prototypical myocyte, thus facilitating organ function. Clinical arrhythmias result from disorders of impulse formation, abnormal impulse conduction, or a combination of these events (Akhtar et al., 1988; Zipes and Jalife, 1990).

The correct action of all cardiac cells depends on a normally functioning cell membrane or sarcolemma. As with central and peripheral neurons, cardiac cells have bilayer cell membranes composed of phospholipid molecules with specialized channels or pores that function as a semipermeable membrane to a variety of molecules. Sodium (Na^+), potassium (K^+), calcium (Ca^{++}), chloride (Cl^-), and other ions move across the cell membrane in an organized fashion, resulting in depolarization of the cell from a resting electronegative state. Specialized structures along both the long axis and the short axis of cardiac cells facilitate in the coupling of mechanical and electrical action (Hoyt et al., 1989).

Two specialized electrical cell types with different permeability characteristics for Na^+ and Ca^{++} give rise to specialized action. Slowly depolarizing and conducting calcium-dependent cells are more abundant in the sinus node and the atrioventricular junctional area. Rapidly depolarizing, fast-conducting sodium-dependent cells are more widespread and include atrial and ventricular myocytes and specialized His-Purkinje fibers, as well as abnormal cardiac structures such as bypass tracts, as discussed later. Medications, ischemia, injury, fibrosis, and external stimulation affect these cells differently, allowing for treatment and diagnosis of a variety of arrhythmias.

Cardiac Conduction System

The normal heartbeat results from a series of electrical and mechanical actions that result in forward output of blood. Alterations in cardiac performance occur from changes in heart rate and contractility in response to variation in autonomic tone and metabolic stress. To carry this out, the heart has developed a specialized conduction system.

Sinus Node Complex

Arising in the right atrium in the superior septal aspect at the junction of the lateral margin of the superior vena cava with the right atrium and the atrial appendage, the sinoatrial (SA) node extends laterally into the crista terminalis

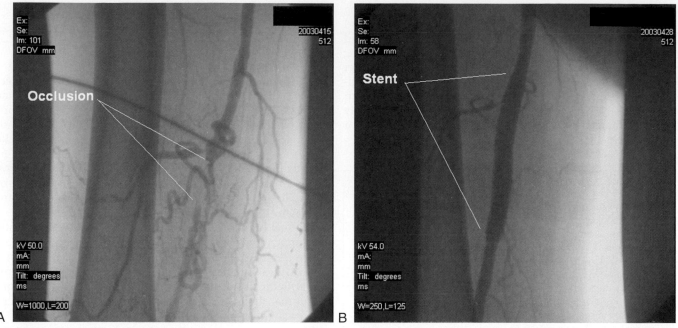

Figure 27-29 A, Baseline angiogram of the right superficial femoral artery demonstrates a short, chronic total occlusion. **B,** Angiogram of the same artery 2 weeks after stent placement.

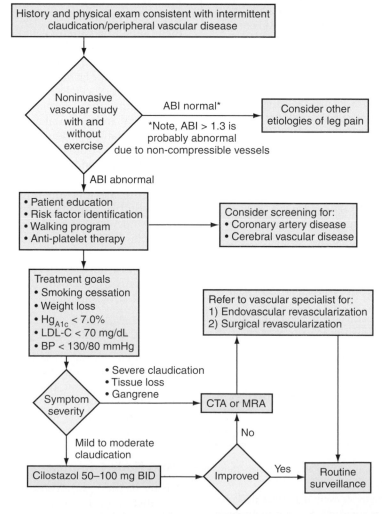

Figure 27-30 Management algorithm for patients with peripheral vascular disease. *ABI,* Ankle-brachial index; *BP,* blood pressure; *CTA,* computed tomographic angiography; *HbA1c,* hemoglobin A1c; *LDL,* low-density lipoprotein cholesterol; *MRA,* magnetic resonance angiography.

(Schlant et al., 1994). The sinus node includes three types of cells: nodal cells, transitional cells, and atrial muscle cells. Impulse formation and rhythmicity in primates are influenced by rich innervation with postganglionic adrenergic and cholinergic nerve terminals (Billman et al., 1989). Impulses leaving the sinus node complex travel through the right and left atria and converge on the atrioventricular node. Controversy still exists as to whether conduction spreads preferentially through specialized internodal and interatrial conduction pathways of the anterior, middle and posterior internodal pathways or simply through atrial myocytes (Racker, 1989). Regardless, right and left atrial depolarization occurs over 55 to 100 milliseconds (ms), resulting in the surface P wave. Cells residing in the SA node complex are predominantly Ca^{++} dependent, slow conducting, and have a higher resting membrane potential than atrial or ventricular myocytes and Purkinje tissue (Sperelakis, 1979).

Atrioventricular Node Complex

The atrioventricular (AV) node lies at the apex of the triangle of Koch. This is formed by the septal leaflet of the tricuspid valve and the tendon of Todaro (Anderson et al., 1988). The AV node is subendocardial and is not visible on gross inspection. The node extends through the AV groove into the ventricle as the His bundle, before branching into the right and left bundle branches of the His-Purkinje system. The AV node contains cells similar to the sinus node P cells. These cells and the associated transitional cells comprise a slow-conducting structure richly innervated with cholinergic and adrenergic fibers. Automaticity and conduction speed are influenced by this innervation. Slow, calcium-dependent cells predominate in the AV node. Conduction time through the AV node is approximated from the end of the P wave to the onset of the QRS complex.

Bundle Branch Network/His-Purkinje Tissue

The distal portion of the AV node becomes the His bundle. These cells have fast-conducting, sodium channel–dependent cells with more negative resting potentials. Branching off into the right and left bundle branches and finally the endocardial Purkinje network, these fibers transmit impulses 10 times faster than atrial or ventricular myocytes and 50 to 60 times faster than sinus or AV nodal cells (Sperelakis, 1979). Rapid activation of the His-Purkinje network results in global, nearly simultaneous activation of the right and

left ventricular myocytes. Purkinje activation results in a narrow QRS complex (<120 msec) noted on the surface ECG. Abnormalities of the right or left bundle braches result in slower activation of myocardium through cell–cell activation and thus the typical wide bundle branch block QRS on the surface ECG (>120 msec).

Atrial and Ventricular Myocytes

Myocardial cells are specialized cells designed to shorten when activated by a threshold electrical stimulus, thus providing mechanical force to produce contraction. The cell membrane is characterized by fast, sodium channel activation. Depolarization of the cell results in release of sarcoplasmic calcium and cardiac cell contraction. Conduction velocities are intermediate between SA and AV nodal cells and the Purkinje cells. Cell death, injury resulting in scarring or functional conduction slowing, or changes in cellular automaticity may result in clinical arrhythmias (Zipes, 1992).

The Action Potential

Diagrams of action potentials of cardiac tissue cause considerable consternation in student and physician alike. However, understanding a few simple concepts on the microscopic or cellular level facilitates arrhythmia evaluation and treatment.

Figure 27-31 is a schematic representation of the transmembrane action potentials of the fast, Na^+ inward current cell and the slow, Ca^{++} inward current cell. In the left panel, *Phase 4* represents the resting transmembrane potential and is –90 mV, with the intracellular area being negative. This membrane potential difference is maintained by a sodium/potassium pump utilizing energy to maintain the difference. The membrane is permeable to potassium (K^+) and impermeable to Na^+ at rest. By expending energy, 3 Na^+ ions are pumped out of the cell in exchange for 2 K^+ ions into the cell. Positive K^+ ions flow across their chemical gradients out of the cell, thus leaving the intracellular space electronegative.

Phase 0 is characterized by the rapid influx of Na^+ ions into the cell, thus depolarizing the cell. Sodium influx is gated. When a sufficiently large depolarization occurs, ion channels are recruited and open, allowing for more influx of ions. Conductance declines as the channel is open and the equilibrium potential for the ion is reached. The channel closes, and Na^+ is again impermeable to influx. *Phase 1* represents a

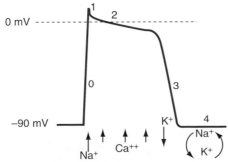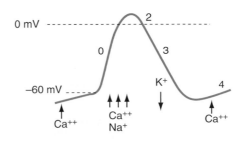

Figure 27-31 Currents and channels involved in generating the resting and action potential: *left,* time course of a stylized action potential of atrial and ventricular cells; *right,* time course of sinoatrial node cells. Above are the various channels and pumps that contribute the currents underlying the electrical events.

rapid repolarization of the cell through transient K^+ outward currents and beta-adrenergic, adenosine monophosphate (AMP), and histamine activated chloride (Cl^-) inward current restoring the membrane potential toward 0 mV.

Phase 2 or the plateau phase is a long phase that may last several hundred milliseconds. Conductance to all ions falls dramatically. Continued Na^+/K^+ pump activity reduces the membrane potential slightly. An *inward* rectifying K^+ current further depolarizes the cell along with continued Ca^{++} influx through the slow inward calcium channels. *Phase 3* represents the final rapid repolarization of the cell membrane. This occurs from inactivation of the slow inward calcium current and from activation of an *outward* K^+ current. The intracellular space becomes more negative, and potassium conductance increases in a regenerative manner.

Phase 4 resumes at the end of phase 3. In portions of the heart, however, a small depolarization current occurs and may result in threshold being reached and depolarization of the cell. This inward depolarizing current is noted in the SA node, distal AV node, and His-Purkinje fibers. This results in automaticity. The rate of depolarization is greater in the SA node than in other structures and thus results in the SA node as the dominant pacemaker. Adrenergic and cholinergic modulation further results in the SA node as the faster pacemaker, subordinating the automaticity of other pacemaker-like tissues. More frequent stimulation results in shortening of phases 2 and 3 of the action potential, resulting in unchanged or slightly increased conduction velocity.

In the right panel of Figure 27-31, the action potential of the slow inward current type of cells is shown. In these cells, C^{++} and K^+ play a greater role in setting the resting membrane potential slightly less negative than in Purkinje or myocytes (phase 4). Phase 0 occurs through activation of slow Ca^{++} current. No phase 1 is noted, and the plateau phase is not as prolonged because of the relative importance of the Ca^{++} and K^+ currents dominated by the slow activating and inactivating C^{++} current. More frequent stimulation leads to a decrease in the resting membrane potential, lower peak phase 0 velocity, slower phase 3 repolarization, and ultimately slower overall conduction velocity (Rosen and Schwartz, 1991).

Antiarrhythmic drugs have differential effects on the Na^+, K^+, and Ca^{++} channels or on receptors that mediated the channels. By slowing or enhancing cellular membrane pore activity, one observes changes in either conduction or repolarization characteristics. This may be reflected in changes in the surface ECG as well.

Surface Action Potential (Electrocardiogram)

The surface action potential can be thought of as a series of discrete electrical events occurring over time. Figure 27-32 schematically demonstrates cardiac events with the surface ECG. The P wave begins with spontaneous depolarization of the SA node with propagation throughout the right and left atrium. This is upright in the inferior leads as depolarization occurs from the topmost portion of the atrium and converges on the atrial septum at the AV node. The depolarization of and conduction through the AV node results in no surface activity, causing an isoelectric portion beginning at the end of the P wave and continuing to the onset of the QRS complex. The PR interval is the total time from SA node activation through the AV node until the beginning of ventricular depolarization. The His-Purkinje network is activated, rapidly depolarizing the large mass of ventricular myocardium. This results in the large QRS complex. The Q-T interval represents myocardial repolarization and may be prolonged in the setting of bundle branch block, drug effect, and genetic disorders causing abnormal ion channel function.

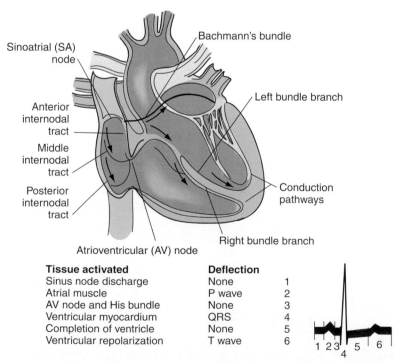

Tissue activated	Deflection	
Sinus node discharge	None	1
Atrial muscle	P wave	2
AV node and His bundle	None	3
Ventricular myocardium	QRS	4
Completion of ventricle	None	5
Ventricular repolarization	T wave	6

Figure 27-32 Schematic diagram of the cardiac chambers and the associated surface electrocardiogram findings.

Mechanisms of Arrhythmias

Two main mechanisms for the initiation and perpetuation of arrhythmias have been proposed. Putative mechanisms include disorders of *impulse formation* and disorders of *impulse conduction*. These may occur alone or in combination and result in isolated electrical events and sustained arrhythmias. Alterations in automaticity or triggered activity are two main areas of disordered impulse formation. Clinical examples of *abnormal automaticity* include inappropriate sinus tachycardia, multifocal atrial tachycardia, sinus pauses, idioventricular rhythm post-MI, and ectopy in heart failure. *Triggered activity*, or spontaneous depolarization dependent on prior stimulation, is characterized as early or late after depolarizations. This mechanism may be responsible for arrhythmic events during hypoxia, use of sotalol or the metabolite of procainamide, or in patients with idiopathic and acquired long QT syndrome and digitalis toxicity.

Changes in impulse conduction can be clinically divided into *block* with or without *reentry*. Simple block occurs when the propagation of the impulse results in an inadequate depolarization stimulus to the adjacent tissue and the impulse terminates. Clinical examples include SA or AV block or simple bundle branch block. In SA block, normal depolarization of the SA node is inadequate to excite adjacent tissue, resulting in absence of a P wave. In AV block, block may occur within the AV node or as it attempts to depolarize His tissue, resulting in a P wave followed by a delayed or absent QRS complex. On the surface ECG, differentiation between block in the AV node or His bundle is only a guess. Bundle branch block or hemiblock is a result of block in a specific branch of the specialized conduction tissue. Activation of tissue beyond the bundle branches must then occur through slower myocyte-to-myocyte activation.

In *block with reentry*, unidirectional block within a tissue results in activation of adjacent tissue (Fig. 27-33). Tissue not initially activated then becomes excited by the conducting tissue. Tissue that has had time to recover excitability may then be activated again in a single or perpetual event. Clinical examples may occur within the SA node, AV node, within the atrium such as atrial flutter, and in Purkinje and myocardial tissue as ventricular tachycardia. Additional macroreentrant rhythms include atrial reentry and preexcitation with orthodromic and antidromic reciprocating tachycardias.

Electrocardiographic Evaluation of Arrhythmias

The basic single-lead rhythm strip is still used in many offices as a quick verification of ongoing abnormal rhythms. New or used, inexpensive equipment can be found through many equipment vendors. This allows for rapid evaluation of symptoms reported during an office visit. Slightly more expensive, 12-lead ECG machines provide not only useful information on the ongoing rhythm but may demonstrate ischemic changes or prior or ongoing injury pattern. Multiple lead analyses help discern difficult-to-see P waves during arrhythmia evaluation as well.

The single-lead and 12-lead ECGs are helpful only for ongoing arrhythmia analysis. Obviously, short-lived events or events that occur unpredictably are rarely identified by these simple techniques. Ambulatory 24-hour recording of a single or multiple leads is performed through Holter monitoring. Small patches or electrodes are placed on the skin and are attached to a digital or analog recording device, usually worn on the belt. Off-line data analysis is performed and relayed to the interpreting provider. Monitoring over 24 to 48 hours allows for increased sensitivity in ambulatory screening. Longer periods of monitoring can be performed using small, 30-day recorders. By recording and repeatedly overwriting the last several minutes of a rhythm, individuals with very infrequent events can lock in a symptomatic event and then transmit the information over the phone. This method may also be helpful in monitoring response to pharmacologic therapy such as rate control in atrial fibrillation. However, prolonged electrode contact can result in skin irritation and poor patient acceptance.

Newer, implantable loop monitors became available in the early 1990s. Devices smaller than a disposable lighter are implanted under the skin overlying the chest wall. Lasting 18 to 30 months, these loop recorders have automatic and activated memory. Evaluation of the recorded events is performed in the clinician's office, remote from the clinical event. Implantation is usually performed by a cardiologist or an electrophysiologist when other recording efforts have failed.

Exercise testing may also be useful for clinical events that occur during activity or stress. Elevations in adrenergic state facilitate conduction and repolarization. Sinus node, AV node, or His-Purkinje disease resulting in block may be revealed. Initiation of various supraventricular or even ven-

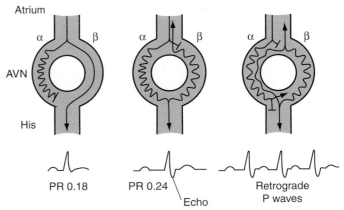

Figure 27-33 Mechanism of typical atrioventricular (AV) nodal reentry. The AV node *(AVN)* is drawn schematically with fast and slow pathways. Differential conduction and refractoriness is noted between the two pathways. The β pathway (fast pathway) has fast conduction and long refractoriness; the α pathway has slower conduction and shorter refractoriness. *Left,* The depolarization wave front from the atrium penetrates both pathways. The β pathway conducts the wave front faster than the slow pathway, and the P-R interval is normal. *Center,* Block occurs in the fast pathway. The slow pathway conducts the wave and depolarizes the ventricle. The β pathway (fast pathway) has time to recover, and conduction proceeds retrograde up the fast pathway and depolarizes the atrial tissue once again, resulting in an AV node echo beat. *Right,* Continuation of the reentry can occur. As the fast pathway is activated in the retrograde fashion during an echo beat, the slow pathway, with a shorter refractory period, is able to recover. The excitable tissue can then be activated, and conduction again proceeds back down the slow pathway (α pathway), and the cycle continues.

tricular tachycardias may also occur. Ischemia as a trigger for arrhythmias may be detected. Exercise testing should be considered in patients with reproducible, activity-associated arrhythmias and in those suspected of long QT syndrome or who manifest preexcitation.

Inpatient evaluation of arrhythmias is seldom needed. However, patients with clinical syncope or transient loss of postural control thought to be arrhythmic, patients in whom ischemia-induced arrhythmias is a concern, and those with a clinical history concerning for a life threatening ventricular arrhythmia should be considered for inpatient evaluation. In this setting, an organized testing regimen may be employed during continuous ECG monitoring.

A comprehensive discussion of rhythm and 12-lead ECG findings is beyond the scope of this chapter. However, using a standard, stepwise approach to all rhythm strips can be easily learned. Keeping in mind the changes in impulse formation and impulse propagation, the correct ECG diagnosis can usually be made. Clinical information such as drug therapy or prior myocardial injury can be equally useful. Each rhythm analysis should address the following questions:

- What is the origin of the impulse? In essence, determine the P-QRS relationship. Determine if the P wave is the initial event or the secondary event and if it is associated with neighboring depolarizations. If P waves exist, examine the morphology and determine if it is appropriate for the lead reviewed. If the rhythm is irregular, do the irregular beats look the same? These steps will help decide if the rhythm comes from the atrium, AV junction, or the ventricle. Further differentiation into irregular atrial events such as atrial fibrillation (AF) or multifocal atrial tachycardia can be made. Wide QRS beats may arise from premature ventricular contractions (PVCs), bundle branch block, or preexcitation.
- What is the basic heart rate? Is the rate appropriate for the origin of the impulse? This will distinguish tachycardias from bradycardias or normal rates for the rhythm (e.g., sinus arrhythmia).
- Is the rhythm regular? Is this appropriate? A fixed, regular ventricular response in the setting of AF suggests third-degree AV block and may be caused by digitalis toxicity if the rate is greater than expected for a junctional escape.
- *Are intervals appropriate and constant?* Changes occur in setting of altered origin of impulse, basic heart rate, and with varying degrees of block (e.g., type I second-degree SA or AV block).
- Are QT, ST segments, or T waves helpful? Are Q waves present? This may give clues to ongoing metabolic, ischemic or drug effects that cause common arrhythmias.

With these few questions in mind, most rhythm strips can be interpreted correctly.

Basic interpretation begins with a rhythm strip of good quality, typically representing lead I, II, or V1. Multiple leads aid in the diagnosis but are not always necessary. Evaluation of heart rate, intervals, and axis is necessary. Regularity of the rhythm, consistency of the P waves, QRS complexes, and T waves and abnormalities of the ST segment should be characterized.

Pattern Recognition of Arrhythmias

Atrial Rhythms

| Key Points |

- Treatment of asymptomatic or minimally symptomatic, non-life-threatening atrial rhythms should be less risky than no treatment at all.
- The proarrhythmic side effects of drug therapy, including ventricular fibrillation, should be carefully weighed before initiation of drug therapy.

Sinus rhythm is a regular, organized atrial rhythm between 60 and 100 beats/min at rest in healthy individuals. Slower rates as low as 40 to 50 beats/min may be normal in some individuals. Originating high in the right atrium, sinus P waves should be positive in limb leads I and II. *Sinus bradycardia* originates in the sinus node with a P wave indistinguishable from the normal sinus beat, but at a rate slower than the established lower limit of 60 beats/min. This is physiologically normal in patients during sleep, in athletic individuals, and as a consequence of many adrenergic blocking drugs (e.g., β-blockers). Excessive bradycardia may come as a consequence of changes in vagal tone in sleep apnea, during painful stimuli, or mesenteric stretch. There are typically no significant changes in the P-QRS-T intervals with resting sinus bradycardias. During vagal-mediated sinus slowing, associated prolongation in the P-R interval may give a clue as to the etiology. Typically, no treatment is necessary in this benign condition. If the heart rate slowing is excessive or symptomatic, acute atropine administration, epinephrine and dopamine may be used acutely. Over the long term, pacemaker implantation may be necessary.

Sinus arrhythmia is the normal variation of heart rate, likely caused by changes in volume and vagal tone as a consequence of respiration. Occasional slowing below 60 beats/min at rest is considered acceptable. Patients with high adrenergic tone such as heart failure often lose normal variations in heart rate and a reduction in the degree of sinus arrhythmia. A *wandering atrial pacemaker* occurs if, at normal heart rates, there is significant variation in the P wave morphology and regularity. Associated P-R and R-R intervals are variable because of the different atrial origin and variations in the prematurity of the atrial beat. It is more frequent in young persons and as a result of changes in vagal tone. The origin of the impulse may arise from within the sinus node complex but at distant sites within the right atrium, giving rise to the changes in P-wave morphology.

A *sinus pause* and the more extreme case of *sinus arrest* are demonstrated as a sudden change in the heart rate, often proceeded by mild slowing in the general sinus rate. A sinus pause is typically caused by changes in vagal tone such as gagging, carotid sinus stimulation, pain, and as a consequence of neurocardiogenic activation (Fig. 27-34). Very long episodes of no surface atrial activity are considered to have *sinus arrest*. This may result from atrial tissue disease, drug therapy, metabolic derangements, and significant vagal activation. Figure 27-35 demonstrates a long pause noted during neurocardiogenic reflex activation during a tilt-table test in the evaluation of syncope. The pause was approximately 50 seconds and resulted in loss of consciousness. Typically, withdrawal of the offending agent, improvement in cardiac

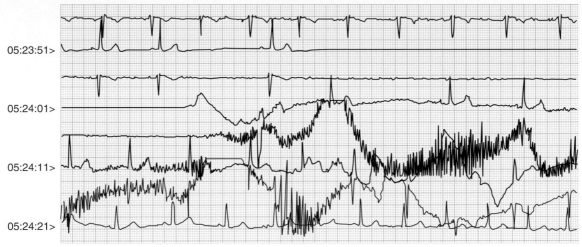

Figure 27-34 Sinus rhythm is followed by sinus arrest and motion artifact during a seizure. Sinus rhythm then resumes.

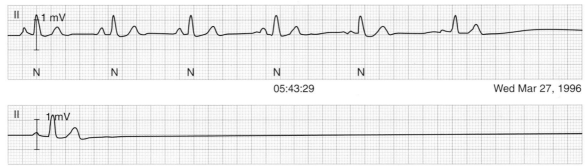

Figure 27-35 Sinus rhythm slows slightly before sinus arrest occurs for 50 seconds. Return of sinus rhythm is not shown.

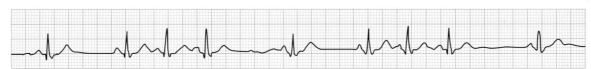

Figure 27-36 Sinus rhythm with type I Wenckebach sinoatrial block. Note shortening of the P-P interval before the dropped P wave and the pause of less than twice the shortest P-P interval. The return cycle length is longer than the cycle length before the pause.

function, and elimination of stimuli causing reflex vagal activation help ameliorate symptoms. In difficult symptomatic cases and in patients without a reversible cause, pacemakers may be necessary. Demonstration of sinus pauses and sinus arrest as a cause of dizziness or syncope may be difficult and requires prolonged ambulatory monitoring.

A pause may also result from sinus node disease. In patients with atrial disease, myofibrosis, and atrial pressure overload, changes in the automaticity and rhythmic depolarization of the SA node may be affected. Regular impulses may fail to exit the sinus node complex and depolarize the atrium, resulting in no P wave on the surface ECG and no atrial mechanical contraction. This may occur in regular patterns, such as in *type I SA block*, characterized by sequential shortening of the P-P interval and then absence of a P wave. The return cycle length is less than twice the shortest cycle length, and the next cycle is longer than the cycle length just before the dropped P wave (Fig. 27-36). *Type II SA block* is characterized by constant P-P intervals followed by a missing P wave. The pause is twice the cycle length of the P-P interval, and the return cycle length is the same as the sinus rate (Fig. 27-37).

Premature atrial contractions (PACs) or depolarizations may occur frequently in normal patients. The ECG finding is that of an abrupt early P wave that may or may not be followed by a QRS complex. PACs may occur as isolated events, couplets, or as sequential events. Most individuals are minimally symptomatic if at all. Benign causes include exogenous stimulants such as tobacco, caffeine, alcohol excess, and sympathomimetic drugs. Digitalis toxicity should be considered in patients receiving digitalis treatment. Patients with underlying heart or lung disease or ectopy from extrinsic compression on the atrium and adjacent abnormal structures may become symptomatic. Reducing automaticity or triggered activity through antiarrhythmic therapy and treating hypoxia and ischemic heart disease may reduce patient symptoms. In asymptomatic patients, no specific therapy is necessary. Beta blockers and calcium channel blockers may reduce ectopy rates and slow or block the ventricular response to the PACs, thus reducing symptoms. Potent antiarrhythmic medications (class Ia, Ic, or III) may occasionally be necessary.

An *ectopic atrial rhythm* is said to occur when the P wave does not have the normal upright morphology in limb leads

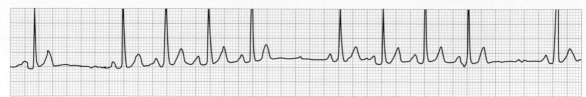

Figure 27-37 Sinus rhythm with type II second-degree sinoatrial block. Note the almost constant P-P interval before loss of P-wave activity. The pause is twice the cycle length of sinus rhythm. The return cycle length is the same as before the pause.

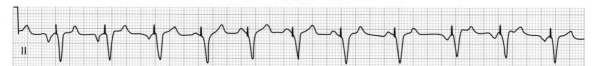

Figure 27-38 An ectopic atrial rhythm at 85 beats/min with negative P waves in lead II is replaced by slower sinus rhythm with upright P waves and then returns at the end of the rhythm strip. A dual-chamber pacemaker senses and tracks both types of P waves and paces the ventricle accordingly.

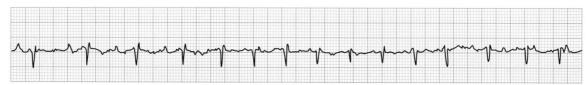

Figure 27-39 Ectopic atrial tachycardia is initiated by a premature atrial complex. Note the P-wave morphology change of the faster ectopic atrial rhythm.

I, II, and III. Heart rate during the rhythm can be slower than, equal to, or greater than normal sinus rhythm. Ectopic rates greater than 100 beats/min are termed *ectopic atrial tachycardia* (Figs. 27-38 and 27-39). The morphology of the ectopic P wave should be consistent and the P-P intervals approximately equal. This helps to distinguish this from sequential PACs. Asymptomatic ectopic atrial rhythms are usually benign and do not require therapy. Patients with incessant, rapid tachycardias may eventually develop rate-related cardiomyopathy. Treatment for or prophylaxis against this type of cardiomyopathy is warranted.

Several additional atrial tachyarrhythmias deserve attention. *Sinus tachycardia,* or sinus rhythm at a rate greater than expected for the physiologic state, may be seen. Atrial wave morphology is normal. However, sustained increased rates may be related to failure of autonomic regulation, metabolic stress, drug use (prescribed or illicit), or idiopathic causes. Inappropriate sinus tachycardia syndrome is usually a self-limited problem of young people and may be caused by a variety of factors. *Positional orthostatic tachycardia syndrome* (POTS) is a condition of marked increases in heart rate with upright posture, not always associated with a fall in blood pressure. Volume status is usually normal and differentiates this from simple orthostatic hypotension with reflexive tachycardia. Treatment of these disorders using beta blockers and serotonin antagonists has been helpful in some individuals. Expansion of plasma volume may also be helpful (http://home.att.net/~potsweb/POTS.html).

Multifocal atrial tachycardia is characterized as irregular atrial activity at rates greater than 100 beats/min. Three or more P waves are present as the driving force of the tachycardia. Patients in metabolic stress and with hypoxia are prone to this arrhythmia. Treatment is usually supportive, but verapamil helps some patients. Treatment with digoxin is rarely helpful, and upward titration may result in toxicity

indistinguishable from the original rhythm disorder (Hazard and Burnett, 1987).

The ECG findings of *atrial fibrillation* (AF) are the absence of organized atrial activity with an irregular, usually rapid ventricular response (Fig. 27-40). Atria are depolarized from widespread regions of both the left and right atrium and result in chaotic activation at rates exceeding several hundred beats per minute. AF may be asymptomatic or highly symptomatic, ranging from simple palpitations to MI and heart failure. Recognition of the arrhythmia is the first step in good care. Treatment using an appropriate anticoagulation strategy, ventricular rate control, and consideration of sinus rhythm restoration is necessary even in asymptomatic patients (see later discussion).

Atrial flutter (AFL) is also a rapid rhythm of the atrium, usually at a rate near 300 beats/min. The ventricular response may be fixed or variable. Sawtooth flutter waves are usually noted in the inferior limb leads (Fig. 27-41). Misidentification of atrial flutter with 2:1 conduction as sinus tachycardia is common and should be considered in all regular tachycardic rhythms. Similar to AF, treatment strategies should include anticoagulation with warfarin (Coumadin). In contrast to AF, atrial activation in flutter is organized and frequently caused by macroreentry. The wave front ascends the right atrial septum, crosses the roof of the right atrium, and extends down the lateral wall along the cristae. The wave front then extends between the inferior vena cava and the tricuspid annulus along the isthmus and proceeds to the atrial septum. Targeting the isthmus is often done with linear radiofrequency (RF) lesions to effect cure (Fig. 27-42).

Junctional Rhythms

Similar to PACs, earlier-than-expected depolarization arising from the AV node complex results in a QRS without a preceding P wave, termed a *premature junctional complex* (PJC).

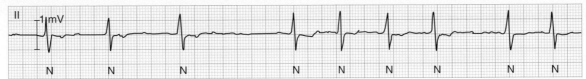

Figure 27-40 The rapid, irregular nature of atrial fibrillation and its chaotic activation of atrial tissue results in no discrete P waves. Conduction through the atrioventricular node is variable, resulting in the irregular ventricular response.

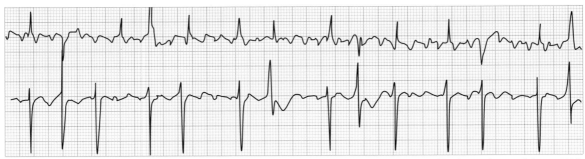

Figure 27-41 Atrial flutter is more organized, resulting in a sawtooth appearance in the limb leads and precordial leads. Atrial rates of almost 300 beats/min are noted, with variations in the ventricular response.

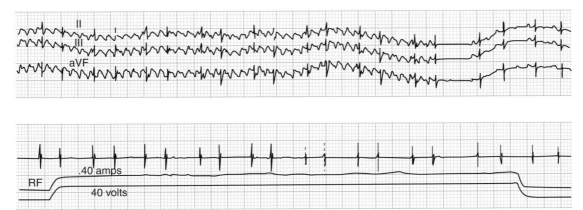

Figure 27-42 Atrial flutter waves noted in leads II, III, and aVF terminate abruptly, and sinus rhythm is restored. An intracardiac ventricular recording and output from a radiofrequency (RF) generator are shown in the lower portion of the diagram. RF application was made at the tricuspid–inferior vena cava isthmus. *(From Feld GK, Fleck P, Chen PS, et al. Radiofrequency catheter ablation for the treatment of human type I atrial flutter: identification of a critical zone in the reentrant circuit by endocardial mapping techniques. Circulation 1992;86:1233-1240.)*

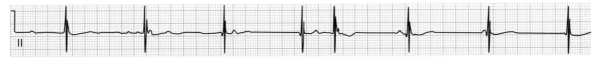

Figure 27-43 Junctional rhythm at a rate greater than the sinus node dominates the rhythm. Conduction through the atrioventricular node occurs with the fifth QRS complex and resets the junctional rhythm. Excessive bradycardia and the associated junctional rhythm may be associated with digoxin toxicity.

Retrograde, inverted P waves may be seen within the early portion of the QRS or following the QRS complex. These are usually benign but may be an early sign of occult cardiac disease. Drugs, adrenergic stimulants, and metabolic stress may be associated with PJCs. In the absence of heart disease or underlying medical condition, these usually asymptomatic beats do not require treatment.

When the AV junction has rhythmic spontaneous depolarization, a *junctional* or *nodal rhythm* occurs (Fig. 27-43). The normal pacemaker function of the AV node cells occurs at a rate of 35 to 50 beats/min. In sinus node failure, the junctional pacemaker rate may be higher than the sinus rate, resulting in junctional bradycardia. Abnormal reentry within the AV node results in *junctional tachycardia*, usually at a rate between 120 and 190 beats/min, and is considered a form of supraventricular tachycardia. Differentiation of accelerated junctional tachycardia from more typical supraventricular tachycardias is not possible by surface ECG. Because of simultaneous activation of the ventricle and retrograde activation of the atrium, junctional rhythms may be more symptomatic than their rate would predict.

Disorders of Atrioventricular Node Conduction

Key Points

- Atropine may worsen AV block if block occurs at the level of the Purkinje system. Increased sinus rates conducting through the AV node will be blocked from the refractory His-Purkinje tissue.

- In contrast, epinephrine may enhance both AV conduction and shorten Purkinje refractoriness, resulting in decreased block. Atropine delivery thus may help distinguish the level of AV block and determine the urgency of permanent pacing.

- The atrial rate must be faster than the escape rate to confirm complete heart block.

- Digoxin toxicity and ischemia may cause accelerated junctional rhythm and should be considered when this rhythm is seen.

First-degree AV block is demonstrated as a P-R interval of greater than 200 milliseconds (Fig. 27-44). Persistent AV delay is usually noted, but variations may be seen depending on heart rate. Adrenergic tone shortens the AV delay, whereas drugs such as beta blockers and calcium channel blockers may worsen AV conduction, leading to more progressive types of AV block. First-degree AV block is almost always at the level of the AV node. Except for very long AV intervals resulting in atrial contraction while the prior ventricular beat is maintaining AV valve closure, first-degree AV block typically does not require treatment. Advanced age is often associated with this conduction disorder.

Second-degree AV block is separated into type I (Wenckebach), type II, 2:1, and high-grade AV block. *Type I* second-degree AV block is characterized by a progressive prolongation of the P-R interval followed by failure to conduct and depolarize the ventricle. The P-R interval on the return beat will be shorter than the P-R just before the block

(Fig. 27-45). Similar to first-degree AV block, this typically does not require treatment with a pacemaker and does not predict life-threatening complete heart block. In patients with concomitant BBB, the clinician should question if block is actually occurring at the level of the His-Purkinje system. Withdrawal of drugs indicated in AV block is indicated. Dual-chamber pacing in symptomatic patients may be necessary.

Type II second-degree AV block is the abrupt failure of conduction through the AV node and absence of a QRS complex. The P-R intervals should be similar before and after block. Atrioventricular block may occur both at the level of the AV node and His-bundle complex and is indistinguishable without invasive electrophysiology study. Pacing is usually indicated to avoid unpredictable progression to complete heart block. Withdrawal of AV conduction blocking drugs is indicated. *Two-to-one* (2:1) AV block can result in very low heart rates and considerable symptoms, including syncope and low-output heart failure. Loss of ventricular activation every other beat typifies this rhythm. Block at the level of the AV node is suggested by preexistent PR prolongation, but block at the level of the His-Purkinje system cannot be excluded by surface ECG.

High-grade AV block or *intermittent complete* AV block is similar to type II second-degree AV block. However, more than one consecutive QRS complex is absent with the block. This degree of AV block strongly suggests significant AV nodal disease or distal Purkinje disease, and the physician should strongly consider permanent pacemaker implantation. The one exception may be high-grade AV block occurring at night in the setting of sleep apnea.

Third-degree AV block results from failure of atrial impulses from the sinus node to conduct down to the ventricle (Fig. 27-46). The finding on a rhythm strip or ECG indicates serious cardiac disease and may be related to significant valvular or coronary disease. An escape rhythm that is narrow suggests that the level of block is above the His-bundle complex and may be more stable. Adrenergic stimulation or atropine may result in an accelerated junctional escape. A slow, wide QRS escape suggests the level is below the His-bundle system, and atropine is unlikely to help. Adrenergic stimulation may help increase the escape rate. Urgent temporary or permanent pacing is indicated. Transcutaneous pacing may be used temporarily but is unreliable and poorly tolerated by the patient.

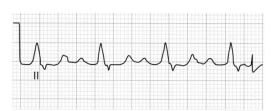

Figure 27-44 Sinus rhythm with first-degree atrioventricular block and bundle branch block.

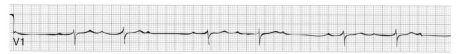

Figure 27-45 Sinus rhythm with type I (Wenckebach) second-degree atrioventricular block. There is prolongation of the P-R interval, then a dropped QRS.

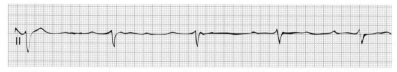

Figure 27-46 Sinus rhythm with third-degree (complete) atrioventricular block. There is complete dissociation of atrial and ventricular activity. The escape rate is less than 30 beats/min, and QRS complex is wide, suggesting a ventricular escape.

Ventricular Rhythms

Key Points

- Determination of the site of pacing is important.
- A bundle branch block pattern on surface ECG contralateral to the site of pacing should occur.
- Inappropriate left ventricular endocardial lead placement delivered across a patent foramen ovale can be detected before serious consequences of embolic stroke.
- Appropriate left ventricle epicardial pacing can be confirmed through paced right BBB morphology. Right ventricular endocardial pacing results in a left BBB pattern on surface ECG.

The presence of a wide QRS is usually caused by (1) normal AV conduction with bundle branch block (BBB) aberrancy, (2) presence of preexcitation, or (3) origin of the beat within the ventricle as a *premature ventricular contraction* (PVC) or consecutive ventricular activation, as seen in *ventricular tachycardia* (VT). A PVC is noted as an early beat, arising before normal atrial activation through the AV node can activate the His-bundle system and depolarize the ventricle. PVCs occur as single beats and couplets but may consecutively appear much like VT. Unifocal PVCs are typically seen as more benign than multifocal PVCs. The origin of the abnormal beats is usually enhanced automaticity or triggered activity. Cardiac literature has demonstrated higher mortality rates in patients with ischemic heart disease with decreased ejection fraction and increased rates of ventricular ectopy. Suppression of these ectopic beats with Class I or Class III antiarrhythmic medicines, however, has not significantly improved mortality (Cardiac Arrhythmia Suppression Trial, 1992; Echt et al., 1991).

Ventricular ectopy in patients with a normal heart is not correlated with significant increases in mortality. Patients are usually asymptomatic, although even low-frequency ectopy may bother some individuals. Beta-blocker therapy for these patients often results in symptomatic improvement. In highly symptomatic patients, membrane-active drugs (Class I or III) may occasionally be required. Electrophysiologist referral should be made if antiarrhythmics are used. Some symptomatic patients may also be treated with RF ablation of the arrhythmic focus.

Ventricular tachycardia is clinically divided into two main categories: In *monomorphic* VT, QRS complexes are nearly identical, and the R-R interval is typically regular. Slight variations at the beginning and end of a run of VT tend to show greater fluctuations in rate. This tends to occur more frequently in scar-related reentry in patients with prior MI and in patients with "normal heart" VT, such as right ventricular outflow tract tachycardia and idiopathic left ventricular tachycardia (Fig. 27-47). In *polymorphic* VT (PMVT), QRS morphology is constantly changing, and the R-R intervals are often inconsistent. Torsades de pointes is a specific clinical PMVT and is characterized by a long QT interval in the first beat of the tachycardia and a twisting about the axis on a rhythm strip (Fig. 27-48). In almost all cases, referral to a cardiologist or electrophysiologist is indicated. Frequently, inpatient evaluation is necessary.

Ventricular fibrillation (VF) is a disorganized electrical rhythm of the ventricle and leads to no meaningful ventricular contraction. Without cardiac resuscitation and electrical cardioversion, the individual will die. Figure 27-49 demonstrates a patient hospitalized with a myocardial infarction. Immediate hospitalization is recommended in patients who have had prior episodes of near syncope or syncope in which VT is suspected due to known underlying ischemic or nonischemic heart disease. Patients suspected of long QT syndrome or VT associated with clinically significant *hypertrophic obstructive cardiomyopathy* (HOCM) should be considered for inpatient or invasive evaluation. Patients who are resuscitated from an out-of-hospital VF arrest must be referred to a cardiac specialist for further evaluation and treatment because of the high rate of recurrence (Huikuri et al., 2001). Inpatient evaluation may include invasive coronary angiography or electrophysiology testing.

Paced Rhythms

Temporary or permanent pacemaker implantation is now performed at almost all hospitals in which a cardiologist practices. Activation of myocardium results in a nearly

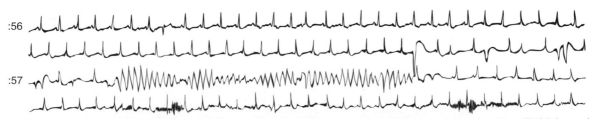

Figure 27-47 Nonsustained monomorphic tachycardia is seen in the setting of underlying atrial fibrillation with increased ventricular response. This terminates spontaneously.

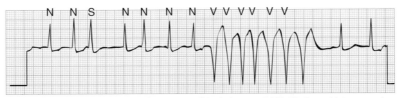

Figure 27-48 Torsades de pointes polymorphic ventricular tachycardia is initiated by sequential premature ventricular contractions (PVCs) that prolong the Q-T interval in a rate-dependent manner. An early PVC landing in the long Q-T interval results in the characteristic twisting about the axis. Spontaneous termination is seen.

normal P wave but with a notable BBB pattern of ventricular capture on the surface ECG. The ECG recorder may amplify the energy from the pacemaker pulse, resulting in a pacing artifact on the surface 12-lead or rhythm strip to aid in interpretation. Knowledge of the type of pacemaker and the current programming may be necessary for complete analysis. The pacing morphology can be reviewed to confirm consistent and appropriate lead placement. Sensed cardiac events may result in pacemaker inhibition and masking of its presence. Evaluation of unexpected events on the ECG may identify abnormal pacemaker operation (Fig. 27-50). Detailed pacemaker ECG interpretation is beyond the scope of this chapter.

Special Clinical ECG Syndromes

Sick sinus syndrome (SSS) is a group of electrocardiographic and clinical findings. Patients often have symptoms of fatigue, palpitations, and heart racing and may suffer from dizzy spells or even syncope. The findings of paroxysmal atrial tachycardia, atrial fibrillation (AF), or atrial flutter result in tachypalpitations and heart racing. Excessive SA

node suppression often occurs with drugs used to slow AV conduction or reduce atrial arrhythmias. Figure 27-51 demonstrates typical ECG findings seen in SSS. Pharmacologic treatment to reduce symptoms is often problematic, and permanent pacing is often required. Anticoagulation with warfarin in patients with documented AF should be considered. Patients without documented AF should be considered for aspirin anticoagulation because of the high frequency of asymptomatic AF in this patient population (Myerbaurg, 1994).

There are at least two types of *supraventricular tachycardia* (SVT) that should be routinely considered for referral. Patients with *preexcitation syndrome* (Wolfe-Parkinson-White, WPW) or *atrioventricular reciprocating tachycardia* (AVRT) and paroxysmal, symptomatic *atrioventricular node reentrant tachycardia* (AVNRT) may benefit from drug therapy or RF ablation therapy. The ECG signature of WPW is the delta wave. Atrial activation of the ventricle is through the AV node–Purkinje system and is activated through a bundle or bypass tract of muscle inserting along one of the AV valves. The combined activation pattern results in the delta wave. Figures 27-52 and 27-53 demonstrate presence and absence of the delta

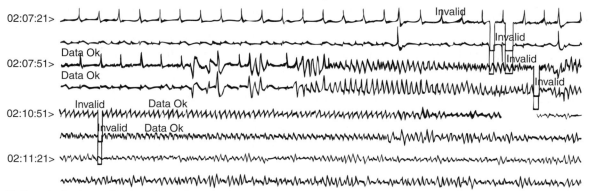

Figure 27-49 Sinus rhythm is noted to degrade initially to a polymorphic ventricular tachycardia and then organizes for about minutes (not shown in entirety). A premature ventricular contraction during ventricular tachycardia results in ventricular fibrillation, to which the patient ultimately succumbed.

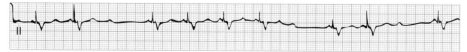

Figure 27-50 Dual-chamber pacing with loss of ventricular output.

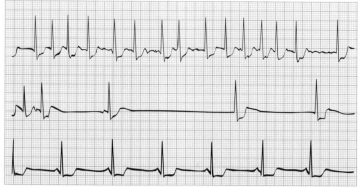

Figure 27-51 Sick sinus syndrome is characterized by rapidly conducted atrial fibrillation, pauses during restoration of sinus rhythm, and excessive bradycardia in normal rhythm.

wave before and after RF therapy for SVT associated with the bypass tract. SVT results from a macroreentrant circuit where conduction proceeds down the AV node into the ventricular myocardium and retrograde up the bypass tract to activate the atrium. The circuit is completed as the AV node is again activated. Tachycardias moving in the opposite direction are identified as wide QRS tachycardias and may be indistinguishable from VT by surface ECG. Adenosine administration during tachycardia may terminate WPW tachycardia but is unlikely to terminate VT. Caution to avoid hypotension or ventricular fibrillation during diagnostic atropine administration in nonhypotensive wide-complex tachycardia is recommended. Advanced cardiac life support equipment should be available during administration.

Sudden, rapid onset and offset of narrow-complex tachycardia occurs in AVNRT. Either an inverted P wave immediately follows the QRS complex, or it may not be visible at all. Termination of the arrhythmia using vagal maneuvers (e.g., carotid sinus massage, Valsalva, stimulation with ice-cold water) may be used clinically. Treatment with AV node–blocking agents can be successful in most patients. Safe, highly effective treatment with invasive electrophysiology study and RF therapy is common at most larger centers. Figures 27-53 and 27-54 illustrate the mechanism and ECG findings.

Long QT syndrome, a disorder of myocardial repolarization, results from abnormalities in membrane ion channels. Syncope and life-threatening polymorphous VT and VF may result. Autosomal dominant inheritance patterns and variable phenotypic penetrance may be seen. Diagnosis in affected individuals is difficult because the QT interval may occasionally be normal. Provocative maneuvers by a trained specialist may be necessary. Genetic testing for some but not all of the genetic abnormalities is available for confirmation.

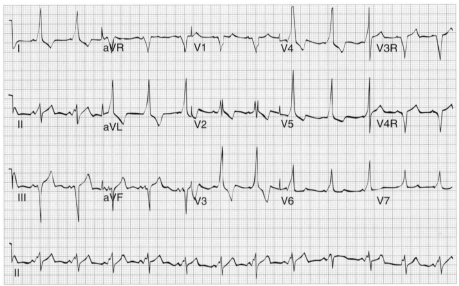

Figure 27-52 Sinus rhythm with obvious delta waves consistent with a right-sided septal or posteroseptal origin. Twelve-lead electrocardiography is performed before radiofrequency ablation.

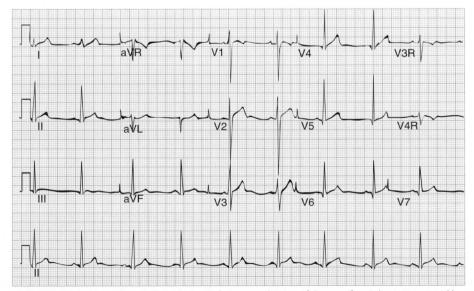

Figure 27-53 Normal electrocardiogram following radiofrequency ablation of the manifest right posteroseptal bypass tract.

Families with a history of sudden cardiac death or syncope should be evaluated carefully to determine the need for treatment, including beta blockers and implantable defibrillators (Priori et al., 2003).

Atrial fibrillation is the most frequent arrhythmia requiring treatment. In America, 2.2 million people have persistent or permanent AF (Feinberg et al., 1997). A basic understanding to the approach of AF can render most patients asymptomatic and dramatically reduce their risk of stroke. The AFFIRM trial represents a landmark study treating all AF patients with warfarin (Coumadin). Patients were then randomized to either (1) *control of heart rate* utilizing AV nodal blocking agents, or if necessary, AV junction ablation and pacemaker therapy, or (2) *maintenance of sinus rhythm* utilizing antiarrhythmic drug therapy and repeated direct-current (DC) cardioversion. Patients were followed for up to 5 years and had similar mortality. Patients randomized to rhythm control had more hospitalizations and adverse drug effects, mostly related to antiarrhythmic therapy. Stroke events were similar but were higher in patients who discontinued warfarin, regardless of treatment arm (AFFIRM Investigators, 2002). Based on this study, patients who are candidates for either heart rate control or rhythm control can pursue either treatment strategy with similar efficacy. In patients undergoing restoration of sinus rhythm, the use of DC cardioversion is safe and effective. Anticoagulation with an INR goal of 2 to 3 in nonvalvular AF is recommended for a minimum of 3 weeks before a cardioversion.

Conscious sedation with short-acting narcotics and intravenous benzodiazepines allows for synchronized shock delivery in ASA class I and II patients by experienced physicians. In patients adequately anticoagulated with warfarin, DC cardioversion can restore sinus rhythm at least transiently in 70% to 90% of patients (Lundstrom and Ryden, 1988; Sodermark et al., 1975; Van Gelder et al., 1991). Maintenance of sinus rhythm at 12 months on antiarrhythmic medications may be as low as 40% depending on drug selection and the patient population (Van Gelder et al., 1996). Despite this, the practicing physician may elect to gain expertise in conscious sedation and cardioversion when referral electrophysiologists are not readily available and in patients not requiring or intolerant to drug therapy. Prior recommendations for discontinuation of warfarin after 6 weeks in sinus rhythm (SR) are being scrutinized because of the high stroke rate in patients in the AFFIRM trial that discontinued warfarin despite being in SR. Caregivers may treat patients long term, even after SR is restored, or in patients with asymptomatic AF. Because of the high 6-month recurrence rate after cardioversion, many maintain patients on anticoagulation for 6 or more months before considering stopping it. Recommendations for anticoagulation are certain to change as new drugs become available.

Syncope is the sudden loss of postural tone and may be caused by both cardiac and noncardiac causes; up to 30% of patients may ultimately have no explanation. A detailed history that includes dietary and fluid intake, personal and family history, medication use and timing, and precipitating factors will aid in the diagnosis. The best single determinant of an etiology is likely the history. Additional testing depends on the presence or absence of structural heart disease. Invasive electrophysiology study in the setting of structural heart disease may identify the cause of syncope in up to one half of patients (Linzer et al., 1997). In the absence of structural heart disease, tilt-table testing may identify the cause in 11% to 87% of patients (Kapoor, 1990, 1992). Referral to an electrophysiologist should be considered in the setting of structural heart disease.

Treatment of Cardiac Arrhythmias

An organized approach to the treatment of cardiac arrhythmias is paramount. Initial steps include identification and verification of the arrhythmia type and an assessment of potential harm to the patient. Box 27-9 outlines various rhythms categorized by their cardiac chamber of origin. As previously described, inpatient evaluation is recommended in some patients. When pharmacologic therapy is recommended, the side-effects and proarrhythmia potential must be known. Table 27-16 outlines antiarrhythmic agents according to the Vaughan-Williams classification system. A newer classification based on channel effects and mechanisms of arrhythmogenesis, the Sicilian Gambit system, although helpful, is too complex for most individuals to use and has not gained favor in the current era of invasive arrhythmia therapy (Rosen and Schwartz, 1991).

Evaluation and treatment of patients with arrhythmias is a rewarding practice. Many arrhythmias can be symptomatically improved through use of medications, lifestyle changes, and reassurance. However, meta-analysis of antiarrhythmic drug trials and the Cardiac Arrhythmia Suppression Trial (CAST) demonstrated the potential dangers of drug therapy in the treatment of cardiac arrhythmias (Echt et al., 1991; Sodermark et al., 1975). In addition, invasive evaluation and treatment of common bothersome or malignant arrhythmias is carried out by cardiac specialists trained in electrophysiology. In addition to drug therapy, an electrophysiologist may offer invasive techniques to treat arrhythmias. Arrhythmia ablation, implantation of pacemakers and defibrillators, and cardiac resynchronization therapy are all techniques to help reduce morbidity and mortality.

Electrophysiology Study and Ablation

Patients recommended for invasive arrhythmia therapy are evaluated in special catheterization suites. During an electrophysiology study (EPS), several electrodes or wires are inserted through the femoral vein or jugular vein and advanced to the right atrium, right ventricle, coronary sinus,

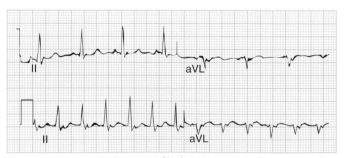

Figure 27-54 Sinus rhythm is noted in the upper strip. In the lower panel, supraventricular tachycardia consistent with atrioventricular nodal reentrant tachycardia is seen. Retrograde (inverted) P waves immediately following the QRS complex during tachycardia are evident. During the tachycardia at almost 150 beats/min, the normal P-R interval is no longer seen.

Box 27-9 Classification of Rhythms

Atrial

Sinus rhythm
Sinus bradycardia
Sinus pause
Sinus node exit block (type I and type II)
Sinus arrest
Sinus tachycardia
Premature atrial contraction
Wandering atrial pacemaker
Ectopic atrial rhythm
Ectopic atrial tachycardia
Multifocal atrial tachycardia
Atrial fibrillation
Atrial flutter

Junctional Rhythms

Premature junctional beat
Junctional rhythm
Accelerated junctional tachycardia
Atrioventricular nodal reentrant tachycardia

Atrioventricular (AV) Conduction Block

First-degree AV block
Second-degree AV block (types I and II; 2:1; high grade)
Third-degree AV block (complete AV block)

Ventricular Rhythms

Premature ventricular contractions
Accelerated idioventricular rhythm
Ventricular tachycardia (monomorphic and polymorphic)
Ventricular fibrillation

Special Rhythms

Preexcitation
AV reciprocating tachycardia
Long QT interval
Paced rhythms

and in the region of the AV node/His-bundle complex. Special pacing sequences and premature beat delivery are used to initiate arrhythmias. The wires may then be moved to different sites within the heart. Application of radiofrequency current through the tip of the catheter electrode results in elimination of the arrhythmia focus. Variations in duration and power of the current are used to alter lesion size. Studies may last less than an hour to several hours depending on the nature of the arrhythmias treated. This essentially painless method replaced the traditional technique of direct-current lesion application, which was poorly controlled and quite painful and required general anesthesia. Radiofrequency ablation is now used as the standard technique is treatment of AV node–dependent arrhythmias, including AVNRT, AV reciprocating tachycardia, and junctional tachycardia. Atrial flutter is successfully cured in most cases (see Fig. 27-42), and even paroxysmal atrial fibrillation may be suppressed or cured by RF ablation. Future refinements of this technique may be used to cure many more patients with bothersome atrial fibrillation.

Alternate energy sources, including microwave, ultrasound, and cryotherapy, are being investigated and used. Radiofrequency, however, remains the energy source in almost all cases for the routine treatment of supraventricular arrhythmias treated with ablation. Treatment of arrhythmias through open-chest procedures was once the only method to cure arrhythmias. Considered high risk in most patients and too invasive for nonlethal arrhythmias in the era of RF ablation, surgical ablation for AF has enjoyed a resurgence as adjunct therapy during valvular heart surgery with cryotherapy and RF therapy of pulmonary veins (Todd et al., 2003).

Pacemakers and Defibrillators

Significant development in the area of pacing has occurred since transvenous pacemakers were first produced and implanted. Once able to pace only in a single chamber at a preset rate and without the ability to detect underlying rhythms, current pacemakers are more sophisticated. A pacemaker in its simplest form is a battery, pulse generator, and a lead to deliver an impulse. The use of sensing and

Table 27-16 Common Antiarrhythmic Drugs

Type of Drug	Typical Indications	Route	Considerations, Contraindications, and Complications	Frequency of General Use
Class I				
Class Ia				
Disopyramide (Norpace)	PACs, AF, SVT, PVCs	PO	Useful in normal hearts without ischemia; prolongs QT; atropine effect	Atrial arrhythmias only
Procainamide (Procan, Procanbid)	AF, PAC, PVC, VT	PO, IV	Wider range of use in mild LV dysfunction; lupus side effect; prolongs QT and QRS; best used in normal hearts only. Renal excreted with active metabolite (class III)	Atrial arrhythmias Acute suppression of VT post-CABG
Quinidine (Quinidex, Quinaglute)	AF, PACs, PVC, VT	PO, IV	Marked QT prolongation, myasthenia, idiosyncratic blood defects; may enhance AV conduction	Limited use; mostly AF, AFL

Continued

Table 27-16 Common Antiarrhythmic Drugs—Cont'd

Type of Drug	Typical Indications	Route	Considerations, Contraindications, and Complications	Frequency of General Use
Class Ib				
Lidocaine	VT, torsade	IV	Rapid onset; may cause CNS changes and seizures	Acute VT termination and suppression Being replaced by IV amiodarone
Mexiletine (Mexitil)	PVCs, VT	PO	Significant GI upset, mild proarrhythmia, mild effect Can be used carefully in setting of LV dysfunction	PVC suppression when other agents fail
Phenytoin (Dilantin)	VPB, VT	PO, IV	CNS effects, rash, blood dyscrasias	Rarely used; minimal effect
Tocainide (Tonocard)	VT	PO	CNS, blood dyscrasias, GI upset, pneumonitis	Rarely used
Class Ic				
Flecainide (Tambocor)	AF, AFL, PACs, EAT, WPW	PO	Well tolerated; may increase conduction of slowed atrial flutter; contraindicated in CHF	Frequently used for AF, AFL
Propafenone (Rhythmol)	PACs, EAT, AF, AFL, PVC	PO	Contraindicated in CHF	Frequently used for AF, AFL
Class II				
Beta Nonselective				
Propranolol	ST, AT, IST, PVCs, VT, AF*	PO, IV	Excess bradycardia, hypotension, CNS effects Negative inotrope Pulmonary bronchospasm	Short acting, rapid onset; increased replacement by longer-acting cardiac selective agents
Beta Selective				
Atenolol	ST, AT, IST, PVCs, VT, AF*	PO, IV	Excess bradycardia, hypotension, CNS effects Negative inotrope	Inexpensive, resulting in frequent use
Metoprolol (Lopressor, Toprol)	ST, AT, IST, PVCs, VT, AF*	PO, IV	Excess bradycardia, hypotension, CNS effects Negative inotrope	Frequently used, long-acting preparation with infrequent side effects
Pindolol	ST, AT, IST, PVCs, AF*	PO	Excess bradycardia, hypotension, CNS effects Negative inotrope	Intermediate-frequency use
Timolol	ST, AT, IST, PVCs, AF*	PO	Excess bradycardia, hypotension and CNS effects Negative inotrope	Low-frequency use
Esmolol (Brevibloc)	ST, AT, IST, PVCs, AF*	IV	Short acting Excess bradycardia and nonselective at high doses	Low-frequency use caused by IV form only
Mixed Alpha/Beta				
Carvedilol (Coreg)	CHF, PVCs, AF*	PO	Excess bradycardia, hypotension, exacerbation of CHF, fatigue	Infrequent as first choice for arrhythmias but primarily indicated for systolic heart failure
Class III				
Ibutilide (Corvert)	AF, AFL	IV	Proarrhythmia frequent including PVCs, VT, and torsades; prolongs QT and slows heart rate; requires acute monitoring	Intermediate use; high efficacy in acute AF/AFL but with potential serious acute side effects
Dofetilide (Tikosyn)	PACs, AF, AFL	PO	High efficacy; prolongs QT and QRS; proarrhythmic including torsades; requires training to prescribe (Is mortality neutral in CHF and MI patients?)	Low-frequency use caused by inpatient initiation and potentially dangerous proarrhythmia

Table 27-16 Common Antiarrhythmic Drugs—Cont'd

Type of Drug	Typical Indications	Route	Considerations, Contraindications, and Complications	Frequency of General Use
Sotalol (Betapace)	ST, AT, IST, PVCs, VT, AF*	PO	Excess bradycardia; prolongs QT with potential torsades	Moderate-frequency use; reasonably safe in setting of mild LV dysfunction in absence of ischemia
Amiodarone (Pacerone, Cordarone)	ST, AT, AF, AFL, PVCs, VT, AF*	PO, IV	Class I, II, III, and IV effects Very well tolerated but may produce serious thyroid dysfunction and lethal pulmonary and liver dysfunction Close monitoring for side effects mandatory	High-frequency use caused by very low acute side effect profile and very high efficacy in variety of arrhythmias Indiscriminate use discouraged
Class IV				
Diltiazem (Cardizem, Cartia)	AF*,PVCs, calcium dependent VT,	PO, IV	Bradycardia, hypotension, exacerbation of systolic heart failure Continuous infusion available	Used frequently for AVN slowing in setting of AF with or without LV dysfunction
Verapamil (Calan, Isoptin)	AF*,PVCs, calcium dependent VT	PO, IV	Bradycardia, hypotension, exacerbation of systolic heart failure	Used frequently for AVN slowing in setting of AF
Class V (Other)				
Adenosine (Adenocard)	SVT	IV	Acute onset with very powerful AV node block and to less extent SA block, producing marked bradycardia and transient asystole; temporary pulmonary symptoms	Agent of choice for abrupt termination of most AV node–dependent arrhythmias
Digoxin	AF*	PO, IV	Proarrhythmic, including heart block and enhancing bypass tract conduction, GI side effects	Frequent adjuvant drug for slowing ventricular response in AF
Atropine	SB	IV	Avoid in patients with acute-angle glaucoma	Acute treatment for sinus bradycardia and heart block not caused by Purkinje failure
Magnesium sulfate	Torsades, PVC and VT suppression	PO, IV	Caution in renal failure	Frequent adjuvant drug for VT suppression

Drugs organized according to the Vaughan-Williams classification scheme. Indications represent both approved and nonapproved indications.

PO, Oral (per os); *IV,* intravenous; *SA,* sinoatrial; *ST,* sinus tachycardia; *AT,* atrial tachycardia; *IST,* inappropriate sinus tachycardia; *AF,* atrial fibrillation; *AFL,* atrial flutter; *AF*,* AV node blockade in atrial fibrillation; *PACs,* premature atrial contractions; *PVCs,* premature ventricular contractions; *SB,* sinus bradycardia; *VT,* ventricular tachycardia; *torsades,* torsades de pointes; *LV,* left ventricular; *GI,* gastrointestinal; *CNS,* central nervous system; *CHF,* systolic congestive heart failure; *CABG,* coronary artery bypass graft.

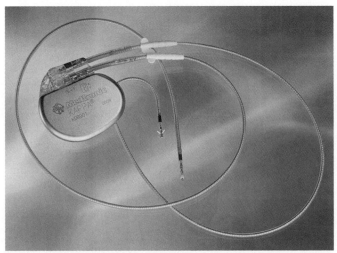

Figure 27-55 Dual-chamber pacemaker with endocardial passive and active fixation leads. *(Courtesy Medtronic, Minneapolis).*

timing circuits coupled with motion detectors within the pacemaker allows inhibition of pacing when sensed events occur and an increase in paced rate with motion or activity. As technology advanced, pacemakers were able to pace effectively in the atrium and ventricle and AV node, or P-R intervals could be adjusted. Telemetry through the skin using proprietary programming devices allow adjustment in the physician's office. Miniaturization has now resulted in sophisticated pacemakers able to pace the heart when necessary, detect rapid rhythms, and attempt to pace terminate the arrhythmia in a package about the size of a half-dollar coin (Fig. 27-55) (Furman et al., 1993). Implantable defibrillators with endocardial leads were developed in the early 1990s, allowing for a safer and less invasive procedure. These devices are now able to identify and attempt to terminate ventricular arrhythmias through painless overdrive pacing or using an endocardial shock that can be uncomfortable if the patient is not syncopal (Figs. 27-56 and 27-57).

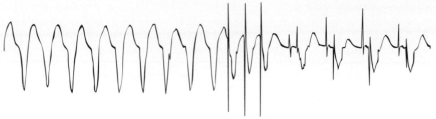

Figure 27-56 Ventricular tachycardia is pace terminated by three rapid ventricular pulses from the implanted pacemaker-defibrillator. Atrioventricular sequential pacing resumes following termination of the ventricular tachycardia.

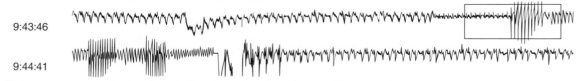

9:43:46

9:44:41

Figure 27-57 Attempt at pace termination of ventricular tachycardia with acceleration of the ventricular tachycardia into ventricular fibrillation. The transient of the endocardial shock is noted, and pacing resumes with organized cardiac activity.

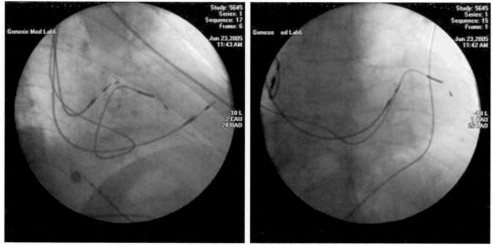

Figure 27-58 Radiographs from a dual-chamber biventricular defibrillator. Right and left anterior oblique views are shown in a patient treated for left ventricular systolic dysfunction and NYHA Class III heart failure. Standard leads terminate in the right atrium and the right ventricular septum. A third lead enters the coronary sinus from the right atrium and extends into a branching vein to provide synchronous left and right ventricular activation.

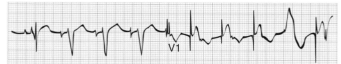

Figure 27-59 Left bundle branch block and right BBB are produced from contralateral ventricular pacing. Right ventricular pacing with left BBB morphology is noted on the left. Pacing activates one side of the ventricle earlier and therefore results in a BBB pattern of the opposite side of the chamber paced. On the right, inappropriate left ventricular endocardial lead placement delivered across a patent foramen ovale was detected before serious consequences of embolic stroke. Epicardial pacing of the left ventricle is also accomplished through lead placement through the coronary sinus.

Cardiac Resynchronization and Defibrillator Therapy

Patients with refractory clinical congestive heart failure have a sixfold to ninefold increase in sudden cardiac death compared to the general population (AHA, 2002). Despite therapy with beta blockers, ACE inhibitors, angiotensin II receptor blockers, diuretics, spironolactone, digoxin, and invasive revascularization strategies, patients continue to have significant morbidity and mortality from systolic CHF.

Electrophysiologists have been impacting mortality and morbidity for over a decade through cardiac pacing resynchronization therapy and defibrillator placement.

The slowing of conduction through the left ventricle in the setting of BBB or significant scarring leads to asynchronous lateral and septal contraction. This dyssynchrony (asynchrony) results in excess energy expenditure and decreases cardiac performance. Placement of a pacing device capable of pacing in the right ventricle as well as at the lateral left ventricle has significantly reduced morbidity and mortality. The addition of a defibrillator further decreases mortality (Bristow et al., 2004; Cleland et al., 2005; Young et al., 2003). Figure 27-58 shows the radiographic appearance of a biventricular system. Pacing in both ventricles demonstrates a shortening of the QRS complex and is associated with improvements in cardiac contractility and over time, reduction in LV chamber size, reduction in mitral valve regurgitation, and improvements in 6-minute walk test, quality of life, and NYHA classification (Abraham et al., 2002). Changes in the QRS morphology depend on the site of electrical stimulation (Fig. 27-59). During right and left ventricular activation, the QRS morphology in lead V1 is shown.

Patients suffering from lethal tachycardia events such as ventricular tachycardia and ventricular fibrillation have been extensively studied. For much of modern electrophysiologic history, the EPS was used to induce VT in patients with syncope and structural heart disease, in patients with symptomatic stable VT, and in patients resuscitated from arrhythmic sudden cardiac death. Drugs were then initiated and repeat testing performed to test the success of the antiarrhythmic drug. More recent studies have challenged this approach. Drug versus implantable defibrillator therapy trials have demonstrated mortality benefit as secondary prevention of syncopal VT or resuscitated sudden cardiac death with structural heart disease (AVID Investigators, 1997; Connolly et al., 2000; Kuck et al., 2000). Further studies have demonstrated mortality benefit from implantable defibrillators compared to drug therapy in primary prevention trials. Specific groups demonstrating superiority of device therapy over drugs include patients with asymptomatic ventricular ectopy with inducible VT, those with prior MI and ejection fraction less than 30%, and those with LVEF less than 35% with NYHA II or III heart failure for longer than 3 months (Bardy et al., 2005; Buxton et al. 2000; Moss et al., 1996, 2002). Patients fulfilling these criteria should be referred to an electrophysiologist.

References

The complete reference list is available online at www.expertconsult.com.

Web Resources

www.diabetes.org/
    American Diabetes Association site with information for patients and health professionals.
www.americanheart.org/
    American Heart Association site provides valuable range of Internet resources on a wide variety of cardiovascular diseases, including statistics on heart disease prevalence.
www.legdisorders.org/
    Comprehensive resource of peripheral arterial disease and other leg disorders; excellent resource for slides and current literature.
www.cardiosource.com/
    Journal of the American College of Cardiology site; outstanding functionality and features; requires subscription.
www.clinicaltrialresults.org/
    Outstanding resource on cardiovascular clinical trials with videos of principal investigators discussing results and slide decks.
www.dashdiet.org/
    Practical instructions on using diet to reduce blood pressure.

www.fammed.wisc.edu/integrative/modules/hypertension
    Summary for clinicians and patients on how to lower blood pressure without medications.
http://hypertensiononline.org/
    Slide resource on hypertension management.
www.lipidsonline.org/
    Slide resource on dyslipidemia management.
www.theheart.org/
    Excellent resource with coverage of all areas of cardiology.
www.nhlbi.nih.gov/guidelines/hypertension/index.htm
    Joint National Commission guidelines on treating hypertension.
http://hp2010.nhlbihin.net/atpiii/calculator.asp?usertype=prof
    Calculator based on Framingham data to calculate 10-year cardiovascular risk.
www.vbwg.org/
    Slide resource for management of dyslipidemia, hypertension, insulin resistance, and diabetes mellitus; updated regularly.

CHAPTER 28

Common Office Procedures

J. Mark Beard and Justin Osborn

Safe approaches to common surgical procedures can be performed by primary care providers in an outpatient setting without significant sedation. This chapter provides the foundation to build skills of competency in common procedures, including adequate preparation, appropriate setup, informed consent, good technical skills, and knowledge of how to handle potential complications. Discussions of the basic surgical skills and setup required, patient consent, and local anesthesia are followed by a review of common office procedures in family medicine, with tips to perform these successfully and methods to prevent complications.

As the U.S. health care system grapples with medical home concepts, family medicine providers must develop proficient skills to carry out common procedures in primary care clinics. The health care system may continue to provide high remuneration for procedural medicine but may change to a system driven by outcomes, competency, and ability to provide competent procedural services in the medical home. Comprehensive patient care will return to the primary care realm, where it is more cost-effective.

For a brief history of surgery, see the online discussion at www.expertconsult.com.

Basic Skills

The Patient History

Before undertaking any procedure, the physician must begin with a pertinent comprehensive health history and thorough understanding of the patient and their current health condition. Preexisting diagnoses, such as diabetes or hemophilia, may affect wound healing or bleeding.

Allergies to medication, tape, or preparation agents should be elicited along with any personal or family history of bleeding or thrombosis. Anticoagulant use, including aspirin, clopidogrel, warfarin, nonsteroidal anti-inflammatory drugs (NSAIDs), ticlopidine, dipyridamole, and fish oil may affect bleeding and hemostasis during any procedure. Short-acting NSAIDs should be held for 1 or 2 days before surgery based on their antiplatelet effect and drug half-life. Aspirin, dipyridamole, ticlopidine, and long-acting NSAIDs should be stopped 7 to 10 days before surgery if the benefit of improved hemostasis during the procedure outweighs the risk of complications from the underlying medical condition for which the medication is prescribed. Warfarin (Coumadin) should be stopped based on risk profiles. Low-risk patients with no thrombotic history who are taking anticoagulants for atrial fibrillation may have their warfarin stopped 3 to 4 days before surgery and may have no "bridging" heparin. If a patient has a high risk for thromboembolism, such as past pulmonary embolism, mechanical valve, or current treatment for deep vein thrombosis, a "bridge" with low-molecular-weight heparin or regular heparin should be given. Warfarin may be resumed immediately after surgery, and then the heparin may be discontinued once the international normalized ratio (INR) is therapeutic (Singer et al., 2008b).

Aspirin and other antiplatelet medications may be resumed 24 hours after surgery. If the patient is high risk and receiving a superficial procedure, the physician should continue the blood-thinning agent and consider using local anesthesia with epinephrine. Local cautery, direct ligation of bleeding vessels, and direct pressure are used as needed for hemostasis. Fish oil taken with aspirin or warfarin may potentiate the antiplatelet effects (Ramsay et al., 2005).

A history of delayed healing or keloid (thick scar) formation should be elicited. A prior vasovagal event or fainting episode warrants preventive measures to reduce the potential risk of complications should a patient faint during or after a procedure.

KEY TREATMENT

Anticoagulant agents should be stopped 7 to 10 days before surgery if there is no contraindication (SOR: A).
Warfarin should be stopped based on risk profiles (SOR: A).
(Singer et al., 2008b.)

Skin Preparation

Prepare the skin with an appropriate antiseptic solution starting in the middle of the surgical site and going outward in concentric circles in aseptic fashion. Alcohol, chlorhexidine, povidone-iodine (Betadine), or a combination may be used as an antiseptic cleansing agent (Mangram et al., 1999).

The U.S. Centers for Disease Control and Prevention (CDC) and Healthcare Infection Control Practices Advisory Committee (HICPAC) updated guidelines in 2002 on skin preparation related to reducing central line infections. The CDC issued additional guidelines for the prevention of surgical site infection in 1999. The U.K. National Institute for Health and Clinical Excellence–Surgical Site Infection guidelines from 2008 agreed with each of these groups as well. Skin aseptic preparation with chlorhexidine 2% plus 70% isopropyl alcohol was the best at preventing surgical site infections as it achieves greater reductions in skin microflora and has greater residual activity after a single application (Mangram et al., 1999).

Chlorhexidine gluconate is effective even in the presence of blood or serum proteins, whereas blood and serum proteins may inactivate povidone-iodine. However, conflicting data show that a combination of iodine povacrylex in isopropyl alcohol may reduce infection rates greatest in general surgery patients (Swenson et al., 2009). Isopropyl alcohol 70% is effective immediately, but the antiseptic effect is not sustained. Combinations are superior to isopropyl alcohol or chlorhexidine alone (Adams et al., 2005; Hibbard, 2005).

Many surgical site infections are from endogenous staphylococcal skin flora. An increasing number are also resistant to antibiotics, such as methicillin-resistant *Staphylococcus aureus* (MRSA). No clear guidelines exist on how best to reduce MRSA infections, but good handwashing and aseptic technique are a part of the prevention of MRSA-related surgical site infections (Siegel et al., 2006).

KEY TREATMENT

Chlorhexidine plus alcohol-containing skin preparations provide the best reduction in skin flora in the perioperative period (Murkin, 2009) (SOR: A).
Do not remove hair preoperatively unless the hair is at or around the incision site and would interfere with the procedure. If hair removal is required, clip immediately before surgery, and do not shave it (Mangram et al., 1999) (SOR: A).

Bites

Bites represent special risks for laceration repair. Cat bites often involve deep puncture wounds and should be cleaned and irrigated thoroughly and not closed but allowed to heal by secondary intention. Untreated cat bite infection rates are 18% to 33% (Dire, 1991). Treating cat bites with prophylactic antibiotics significantly reduces infection rates. Dog bites may be more lacerated and after high-pressure flushing at greater than 7 psi (obtained using 50-cc syringes and saline or iodine in water in 1:10 ratio) may be closed primarily in the first 6 hours after the injury. Infection rates for dogs are less than 20% (Dire, 1992).

Primary closure by suturing is not generally recommended for nonfacial bite wounds, especially deep punctures, bites to the hand, and clinically infected wounds. Anecdotal data suggest an increased risk of infection after closure of these wounds. Sterile skin closure strips or delayed closure may be appropriate (Singer et al., 2008a).

Human bites on the hands and specifically overlying the metacarpophalangeal joints are problematic because of potential damage to underlying tissue, tendons, and joint spaces. Hand injuries may therefore lead to aggressive secondary infections of these structures. Profuse flushing of human hand bites or lacerations, prophylactic antibiotics, and consultation are advised. These wounds may need to be surgically opened under anesthesia to flush adequately.

Wounds to both the hands and face need immediate care because infection rates almost double to 29% if not treated within 12 hours. Prophylactic antibiotics should be used with hand and facial bite wounds. Facial wounds may be flushed and closed primarily because of the good blood supply and a risk for poor cosmesis if left open (Henry et al., 2007).

> ### KEY TREATMENT
>
> A review of Cochrane data suggests that antibiotics should be used prophylactically in human bites to the hand (NNT = 4) (Medeiros and Saconato, 2008) (SOR: A).

Immunizations

With any laceration or open skin injury, tetanus immunizations should be updated if indicated. If patients have received 3 or more primary tetanus immunizations, they should receive an update if their last immunization was more than 10 years ago for a clean wound and if more than 5 years ago with a dirty wound. Patients should receive tetanus immune globulin (TIG) and begin their tetanus immunization series if they have had less then 3 immunizations in the past. Diphtheria toxoid and pertussis antigens with tetanus toxoid (Tdap) should replace a single dose of Td for adults age 19 through 64 years who have not received a dose of Tdap previously and require a booster. Tdap may be given as close as 2 years after a Td. Td can be given every 10 years when needed after one Tdap is received (CDC, 2009; see Web Resources).

Patients should begin the hepatitis B immunization series for any human bite wounds or for mucus membrane blood exposure. Patients should be offered and consented for baseline testing for hepatitis B virus (HBV) and C virus (HCV) and human immunodeficiency virus (HIV). Appropriate follow-up based on test results must be arranged. HBIG is indicated if the patient has injuries from a person known to be positive for hepatitis B surface antigen (HBsAg); however, needle stick guidelines suggest that the injured patient receive only a hepatitis B immunization series and not HBIG if the contact person has an unknown or negative carrier status. In the case of a needle stick, HIV prophylaxis with three drugs is recommended if the contact person is a known HIV positive. If the source patient has an unknown HIV status, postexposure prophylaxis (PEP) generally is not indicated, unless there is concern that the source is higher risk, in which case two-drug PEP is offered.

Procedure Room

A clean procedure room with a table that elevates and an overhead surgical light that can be adjusted and focused gives the provider the best environment to carry out procedures. An adjustable and mobile mayo stand allows the most comfortable access to sterile trays and instruments during a procedure. Surgical instruments should be stored in sterile packs, ideally set up for specific procedures. Extra equipment may be in individual sterile packs and should be readily available. Check sterility date expiration for all packaged equipment.

Patients should be made comfortable for the procedure with use of an adjustable bed and pillows as needed. Open, supportive conversation with an empathetic approach encourages relaxation and reassurance before, during, and after the procedure. An assistant is helpful in setup and during the procedure and provides support for the patient during care. In children undergoing general surgery, a family-focused dialog and ongoing conversation were similar to using midazolam in reducing anxiety and speeding recovery (Kain et al., 2007).

Equipment

The most basic sterile pack for skin procedures contains a needle driver, Adson tissue forceps with teeth, iris or suture scissors, and a scalpel handle with blade. The instruments should comfortably fit the physician's hands.

There are three primary scalpel blade styles used in the outpatient setting. A #10 blade has a large, rounded cutting surface and may be used for longer, straight incisions on larger areas with thicker skin, such as the trunk or limbs. A #15 blade has a smaller, rounded cutting surface to allow more mobility and may be used on most skin procedures, particularly those with nonlinear incisions. A #11 blade has a pointed blade without a curve and is better used for paring superficial lesions, such as warts or calluses, or puncturing skin abscesses. The Adson forceps with teeth has one side with one tooth and the other side with two teeth. Less tissue trauma occurs using the single tooth on the external tissue while everting the skin edges or using a skin hook (Fig. 28-1).

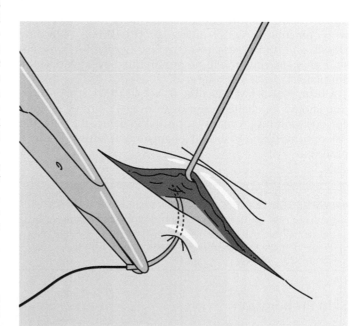

Figure 28-1 Use of a skin hook to evert wound edge. This technique allows the operator to see the needle path, ensuring that the proper depth has been reached, and promotes eversion of the skin edges.
(From Lammers RL. Methods of wound closure. In Roberts JR, Hedges JR [eds]. Clinical Procedures in Emergency Medicine, 5th ed. Elsevier, Philadelphia, 2010.)

Needle drivers should fit the physician's hand; the ring finger fits in the lower circle of the handle, and the thumb may fit in the top circle of the handle with the index finger extended along the shaft to stabilize the needle driver. Load the needle by locking the needle driver about three-quarters the way up the shank of the needle, with the needle held perpendicular to the needle driver. Sharps are kept in the same area of the sterile field to develop a system for reducing needle stick injuries.

Suture

Three basic types of suture exist: natural absorbable, synthetic absorbable, and nonabsorbable. Sutures are sized according to the 1937 *U.S. Pharmacopeia* classification system. Smaller suture has a higher number of zeroes (2-0 is 00 and 4-0 is 0000). The physician should use the smallest size that provides adequate tensile strength initially to close the wound and not to fail during the healing process. The clinician should use deep sutures to reduce surface tension if the wound is deep and there is high skin surface tension. Ideally, skin sutures gently approximate the skin edges with minimal tension.

Absorbable types of suture include plain gut, chromic gut, and synthetic sutures made of polyglycolic acid, polylactic acid, polydioxanone, and caprolactone. Plain gut suture used externally has a tensile strength lasting 5 to 7 days, whereas chromic gut used internally has a tensile strength lasting 10 to 14 days. The synthetic absorbable types of suture vary in length of tensile strength and rate of absorption. Nonabsorbable suture is made of nylon, special silk, polypropylene, or polyester. These sutures are made in different colors and are inert. Most have long-lasting tensile strength. Non-absorbable sutures are used externally but can be used internally for prolonged tissue reinforcement. Nonabsorbable sutures cause less immune response and therefore less scarring. Frequently, they are used superficially when cosmetic outcome is critical.

Traditionally, it was advised that absorbable suture be used only if it is placed below the skin's surface because of its porous structure and a possible wick for bacteria on the skin surface. However, this recommendation is not evidence based. A meta-analysis of two randomized, controlled trials (RCTs, Jadad scores 3) comparing absorbable versus nonabsorbable sutures in the management of traumatic lacerations and surgical wounds showed no changes in infection rates, scar appearance, patient satisfaction, or dehiscence. In children, the benefit is not requiring suture removal (Al-Abdullah et al., 2007).

Plain gut sutures last intact for 5 to 7 days and may be used to close small mucosal lacerations or excisions. Plain gut sutures do not survive long enough for use on deep tissue reapproximation. Use 5.0 to 6.0 nylon suture on the face, and remove in 3 to 5 days. If the wound is elsewhere on the trunk, extremities, or other areas with tension, use 3.0 to 4.0 nylon sutures and remove in 10 to 14 days.

Needles

Suture needles are classified by the geometry of their points. Taper needles have a round body that tapers smoothly to a point. Cutting needles are triangular with a sharp cutting edge on the inside curve of the needle; reverse cutting needles have the cutting edge on the outside of the curve. A taper-cut needle is round but ends in a short, triangular cutting point. Some needles are attached permanently to suture and others, called "pop offs" separate from the suture with a sharp pull. With a wide range of needle types, the physician should be familiar with supplies and examine the outside of the package closely before opening. Reverse cutting needles are stronger than conventional cutting needles; both minimize trauma to the skin and so are appropriate for most skin closure.

Anesthesia

Topical Anesthesia

An equal mixture of prilocaine 2.5% and lidocaine 2.5%, EMLA cream may be used as a topical anesthetic. EMLA works best if applied to the dermal site at least 1 hour before the procedure and covered with an occlusive dressing. It is not used more often because of the time needed for onset of anesthesia, increased expense, and risk of methemoglobinemia in susceptible individuals such as those with congenital disease, pyruvate kinase–deficient and glucose-6-phosphate dehydrogenase (G6PD)–deficient patients, and those with rare, acquired forms resulting from medications (e.g., prilocaine, antimalarials, sulfonamides). Patients under 3 months of age are vulnerable to developing methemoglobin because the breakdown product ortho-toluidine can produce methemoglobinemia following systemic doses of prilocaine approximating 8 mg/kg. A rectangle measuring 1.5 × 0.2 inches is about 1 g of EMLA or 25 mg of prilocaine. The maximal area of application is age and weight dependent (Table 28-1).

Other topical anesthetics are used in some circumstances. Ethyl chloride cools the skin superficially and works well for needle punctures. Unfortunately, it is flammable and has a brief action, limiting its usefulness. A 30% lidocaine cream

Table 28-1 EMLA Dosing

Age/Weight requirements	EMLA cream (max total dose)	Maximum application area	Maximum application time
0-3 months *or* <5 kg	1 g	10 cm²	1 hour
3-12 months *and* >5 kg	2 g	20 cm²	4 hours
1-6 years *and* >10 kg	10 g	100 cm²	4 hours
7-12 years *and* >20 kg	20 g	200 cm²	4 hours

Developed from EMLA drug information. In Facts and Comparisons, 2010. http://online.factsandcomparisons.com/MonoDisp.aspx?monoID=fandc-hcp14927&quick=341644%7c5&search=341644%7c5&isstemmed=true .
EMLA, Eutectic mixture of local anesthetics.

must be applied with an occlusive patch at least 45 minutes before any procedure. Liposomal encapsulation forms of topical tetracaine and lidocaine are as efficacious as EMLA (Eidelman et al., 2005). Lidoderm patches are a 5% concentration and are not potent enough for surgical skin anesthesia. (**See Tuggy Video: Topical Anesthesia.**)

Local Anesthesia

For most office procedures, a local injection is a quick and easy way to provide anesthesia, by blocking the fast sodium channels and stopping pain fiber neurotransmission. However, an injection of local anesthetic may distort skin edges and adversely affect skin anatomy and alignment. Consider marking incisions and vital alignment before infiltrating with a local anesthetic. Anesthetize before flushing the wound in repair of contaminated lacerations. Infiltration of 1% lidocaine does not damage local defenses, promote infection, or exhibit antimicrobial activity that would obscure a culture from a wound (Edlich et al., 2010).

There are two groups of local anesthetics: amides and esters. Allergies are more common to the esters. Allergy to an amide is usually caused by the preservative methylparaben. If a patient has an ester allergy, use an amide; no cross-reactivity occurs between classes (Archar an Kundar, 2002) (Box 28-1).

The most common locally injected anesthetic is lidocaine, with or without epinephrine; 1% lidocaine contains 10 mg/mL of lidocaine. Lidocaine dosing should not exceed 4.5 mg/kg without epinephrine (maximum 300 mg in adults, or 30 mL of 1% lidocaine) or 7 mg/kg of lidocaine with epinephrine (maximum 500 mg in adults, or 50 mL of 1% lidocaine with epinephrine) (Tetzlaff, 2000). Others list the recommended safe dose of infiltrated lidocaine as 200 mg or less in an adult, which is 20 mL of 1% lidocaine (Rosenberg et al., 2004). If doing a paracervical or pudendal block, the maximum total dose over 90 minutes is 200 mg of lidocaine, or 20 mL of 1% lidocaine

total (10 mL per side). Lidocaine has an elimination half-life of 1.5 to 2.5 hours in most patients, and average infiltrative anesthesia lasts 2 to 6 hours. Bupivacaine has a longer onset and length of action and an elimination half-life of 2.7 hours in adults and 8 hours in neonates. Data on mixing lidocaine and bupivacaine are limited.

Some local anesthetics have epinephrine as an additive to help with hemostasis in very vascular locations. Buffering any local anesthetic containing epinephrine with a 1:10 ratio of sodium bicarbonate to anesthetic before injection helps reduce discomfort during the injection by neutralizing the acidic properties of the fluid. The current dogma is to avoid the use of epinephrine on end-artery areas, including fingers, ears, nose, lips, penis, and toes. However, a recent review on the use of local anesthesia with epinephrine in a digital block challenges this dogma (Mohan and Cherian, 2007). To be safe, epinephrine should not be used in distal-end vascular beds until the data are more conclusive. (**See Tuggy Video: Local Anesthesia.**)

Local Ring Anesthesia Block

For anesthesia around a superficial skin lesion, a ring block can be placed with good results. Use a larger needle to draw up the anesthetic and a 25- to 30-gauge needle to infiltrate the tissues. Insert the needle into the subcutaneous skin a few millimeters outside the planned incision line, and advance along that circular line around the lesion. Aspirate intermittently to ensure no flashback of blood, to avoid direct instillation of anesthetic into a vein or artery. Infiltrate the local anesthetic as the needle is advanced. Use anesthetized areas to puncture the skin, and inject more distal areas as needed around the planned surgical field until the lesion is fully circumscribed. Slow instillation with the anesthetic solution and warming the syringe by holding in the hand can make the infiltration more comfortable for the patient. Local anesthesia may be instilled through the subcutaneous tissue through a laceration side wall and may be less painful than going through intact skin.

Digital Block

A digital block can be an effective method for providing anesthesia for fingers and toes. A dorsal or interdigital approach is used to provide anesthesia to the digit. The digital nerves are 3 to 5 mm under the skin at the 2, 4, 8, and 10 o'clock positions around the digit. Each location can be infiltrated with 1 to 2 cc (mL) of 1% lidocaine without epinephrine. It may take 5 to 30 minutes for distal anesthesia to develop after injection. Occasionally, local anesthesia is needed at the base of the digit circumferentially if achieving complete anesthesia becomes difficult (Fig. 28-2). Patients may continue to feel pressure and motion but should not feel sharp pain when the anesthesia is effective. (**See Tuggy Video: Digital Block.**)

Complications with Local Anesthesia

Recognizing the various side effects and reactions to local anesthesia is critical to prevent serious complications. The most common complication with the use of local infiltrative anesthesia is a vasovagal episode. The patient may look pale, begin to sweat, and then feel faint or even fall unconscious.

> **Box 28-1** Local Anesthetic Classifications
>
> ### Amides
>
> Lidocaine (Xylocaine)
> Bupivacaine (Marcaine)
> Prilocaine (Citanest)
> Etidocaine (Duranest)
> Mepivacaine (Carbocaine)
> Articaine (Septocaine, Zorcaine)
> Ropivacaine (Naropin)
> Dibucaine (Nupercainal)
>
> ### Esters
>
> Procaine (Novocain)
> Tetracaine (Pontocaine)
> Chloroprocaine (Nesacaine)
> Cocaine
> Benzocaine (Lanocaine, Americaine)
> Proparacaine (Alcaine, Ophthetic, Paracaine)
>
> Expanded from Archar S, Kundar S. Principles of office anesthesia. Part I. Infiltrative anesthesia. Am Fam Physician 2002;6:91-94.

Although accompanied by one or two tonic-clonic beats in some cases, this is not considered a seizure. Lying the patient down in reverse Trendelenburg positioning with both legs elevated can increase blood return to the heart and improve vagally depressed cardiac output. Atropine can reverse vagal bradycardia but is rarely needed. Recovery occurs spontaneously within minutes, but the queasiness may persist for 30 to 60 minutes.

Inadvertent instillation of an anesthetic into a blood vessel may cause seizures, jitteriness, or palpitations and may be avoided by always aspirating before infiltrating the local anesthetic. If a flash of blood is obtained on aspiration, pull the needle back partially, aspirate again, and instill only if no blood return occurs. Other reactions to local anesthesia are discomfort, bruising, and edema of the injection site. True anaphylaxis to lidocaine is estimated to occur in less than 1% of injections (Haugen and Brown, 2007). Administer diphenhydramine (Benadryl), 25 to 50 mg orally, intravenously, or intramuscularly in adults and 1 mg/kg in children, and epinephrine 1:1000 subcutaneously every 5 minutes as needed. The adult dose of epinephrine 1:1000 is 0.3 to 0.5 mL/kg and the pediatric dose 0.01 mL/kg at the same intervals. Emergency response personnel should be notified, and prolonged observation may be warranted.

Sedation

Some patients may require minimal to mild conscious sedation during a procedure in the outpatient clinic setting. Use of a low-dose benzodiazepine, such as 1 to 2 mg of lorazepam or 0.5 to 1 mg of alprazolam, may be appropriate for light conscious sedation. Sedation may also be accomplished with a dose of an oral opioid, such as hydrocodone or oxycodone. These patients should not operate a car or heavy machinery, and another person should provide their transportation. Use of an opioid in combination with a benzodiazepine may cause significant respiratory depression.

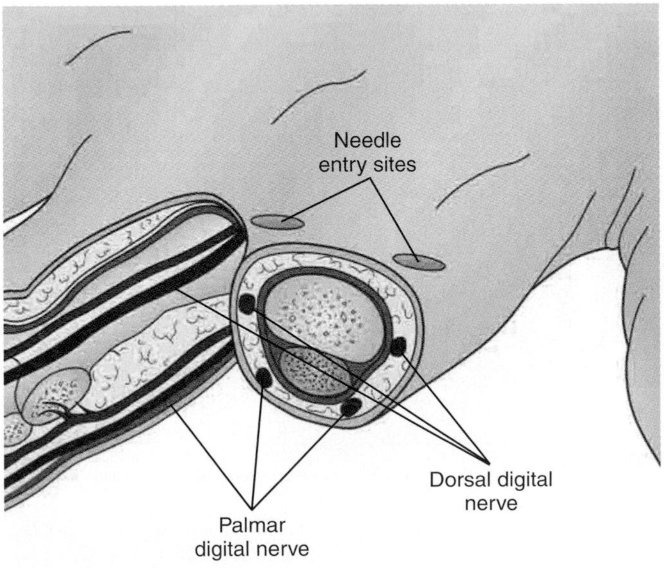

Figure 28-2 Digital nerve anatomy.
(From Frank BL. Principles of pain management. In Auerbach PS. Wilderness Medicine, 5th ed, Mosby-Elsevier, Philadelphia, 2007.)

This mixture is usually considered moderate to heavy sedation and requires additional constant monitoring of cardiac and oxygenation status, which may not be available in some ambulatory clinical practices.

Wound Irrigation

Wound healing is affected by infection, tension, perfusion, and alignment. Cleaning a wound with tap water or isotonic saline removes debris and bacteria mechanically from the wound and reduces infection rates. One study found no clinically important differences in infection rates between wounds irrigated with tap water or a normal saline solution (Valente et al., 2003).

Many studies recommend 7 psi (lb/in^2) or greater for adequate irrigation of dirty wounds and 0.5 psi for clean wounds. Irrigation of the wound with a 35-mL syringe and a 19-gauge needle produces 7 psi, whereas using a bulb syringe only produces 0.5 psi, which is inadequate to flush and decontaminate a dirty wound. The potential for lateral subcutaneous dissemination with use of high-pressure irrigation can make a clean wound more susceptible to infection, so it should be reserved for contaminated wounds where benefits are greater than the risk of dissemination. The low-pressure bulb syringe is used for clean lacerations. The pressure is more important in dislodging adherent bacterial and small particles than the amount of solution used. Splash protection should be used by all health care personnel (Edlich et al., 2010).

There is debate on using povidone-iodine (Betadine) to cleanse dirty wounds. In general, avoid Betadine surgical scrubs within the laceration because it can be toxic to tissue. If used, dilute Betadine 1:10 with water. Chlorhexidine and hydrogen peroxide may also be toxic to tissue inside a laceration and should be used with care. Poloxamer-188 solutions are safe to use within wounds and are even used on ophthalmologic skin surgeries to cleanse the conjunctiva and by dentists to cleanse oral mucosa.

> **KEY TREATMENT**
>
> Studies recommend 7 psi or greater for adequate irrigation of dirty wounds (Edlich et al., 2010) (SOR: A).

Debridement

A dirty, uneven wound may benefit from direct sharp debridement back to clean viable tissue. Obtaining clean, even skin edges may improve healing, facilitate repair, and reduce scarring. If road grit is present, it must be removed to avoid infection and tattooing and may also need to be scrubbed. Generally, unless high-pressure irrigation is not removing grit, scrubbing is avoided because it may disrupt clotting along the skin edges. High-velocity trauma, soiled deep wounds, and fecal contamination represent wounds best cleaned in the operating room and allowed to heal open by secondary intention, as primary closure is contraindicated (Edlich et al., 2010).

Good anesthesia is critical to appropriate irrigation and debridement. If significant debridement is planned, the physician should document neurologic function in the injured area and distally before infiltration of the anesthetic.

Principles of Healing

Wound healing begins immediately after the initial trauma or cut. Traditional descriptions of wound healing use three distinct but overlapping phases (inflammatory, proliferative, remodeling), whereas others use four phases to better describe the healing process. Surgical technique and smoking are modifiable risk factors for poor wound healing. Other factors affecting wound healing include anemia, diabetes, malnutrition, HIV infection, and cancer.

Trauma to surrounding tissue by the injury and surgical techniques (e.g., too much tension on sutures) may affect healing. Adequate oxygenation and blood flow are critical to good healing. Medications that affect healing include steroids, NSAIDs, and immunosuppressive medications.

Stages of Healing

Exudative or Inflammatory Phase

Immediately after a laceration, fibrin deposits with an influx of platelets, forming a visible clot. The platelets secrete various wound-healing growth factors that activate macrophages and fibroblasts. These growth factors and more then 30 cytokines cause an influx of cellular structures. This phase occurs from 0 to 72 hours (Fig. 28-3).

Resorptive Phase

After 24 to 72 hours, the degradation products of fibrin lead to activation of chemotaxis in the resorptive phase. Leukocytes and macrophages migrate into the wound, causing inflammation. The cellular components then begin autolysis and remove injured tissue by a fermentative process. This process creates an effective phagocytosis, a sterilizing defense, and an activation of the immune system.

Proliferative Phase

Between 72 hours and day 7, fibroblasts migrate into the wound, and vascular proliferation occurs. Granulation tissue formation marks the proliferative phase. Epidermal cells begin to grow at the edges of the wound. A delicate balance of cytokine systems leads to new capillary formation to feed and oxygenate the budding granulation tissue. Extracellular matrices form and act as struts to support the new tissue. The primary clots are broken down by naturally developing fibrinolytic compounds (Fig. 28-4).

Regenerative or Remodeling Phase

The remodeling stage is a continuation of the proliferative phase, with ongoing maturation of collagen. The thickening collagen leads to an increased resistance to shearing and tearing forces. The regenerative phase is characterized by epithelialization and scar formation. This last phase may take up to 1 year. Collagen type III is converted into the mature type I collagen (Fig. 28-5). The extracellular matrix and cells within the wound are regulated by cytokines and integrins (transmembrane cell receptors) (Fig. 28-6).

Keloids

Keloids are fibrous elevated scars that extend outside wound margins. Keloids are unlikely to regress, are likely to recur if excised, and are most likely to occur in patients with darker skin (relative risk [RR] 15-20). Keloids are frequently located over the midline chest, cheeks, and earlobes, and peak incidence is age 10 to 20 years. Wounds that heal by secondary intention and burn wounds are high risks for developing keloids. Keloids may be painful as well as cosmetically unacceptable (Juckett and Hartman-Adams, 2009) (Fig. 28-7).

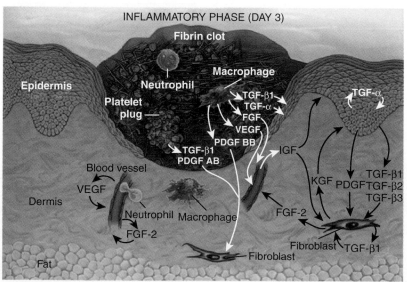

Figure 28-3 Cutaneous wound 3 days after injury. The cells and growth factors necessary to facilitate cell migration into the wound are shown. *FGF,* Fibroblast growth factor; *IGF,* insulin-like growth factor; *KGF,* keratinocyte growth factor; *PDGF,* platelet-derived growth factor; *TGF,* transforming growth factor; *VEGF,* vascular endothelial growth factor.
(From Singer AJ, Clark RAF: Mechanisms of disease: cutaneous wound healing. N Engl J Med 1999;341:738; and Ethridge RT, Leong M, Phillips LG. Wound healing. In Townsend CM, Beauchamp RD, Evers BM, Mattox KL [eds]. Sabiston Textbook of Surgery, 18th ed. Saunders-Elsevier, Philadelphia, 2008.)

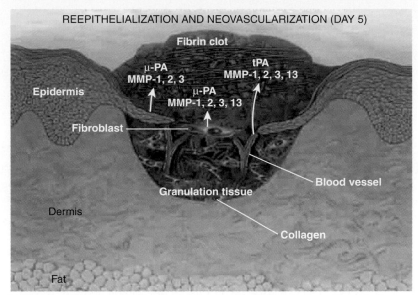

Figure 28-4 Cutaneous wound 5 days after injury. Blood vessels are seen sprouting into the fibrin clot as epidermal cells resurface the wound. Some of the proteinases involved in cell movement at this point are shown. *MMP*-1, 2, 3, and 13, matrix metalloproteinases 1, 2, 3, and 13 (collagenase 1, gelatinase A, stromelysin 1, and collagenase 3, respectively); *t-PA*, tissue plasminogen activator; *u-PA*, urokinase-type plasminogen activator.
(Modified from Singer AJ, Clark RAF. Mechanisms of disease: cutaneous wound healing. N Engl J Med 1999;341:738; and Ethridge RT, Leong M, Phillips LG. Wound healing. In Townsend CM, Beauchamp RD, Evers BM, Mattox KL [eds]. Sabiston Textbook of Surgery, 18th ed. Saunders-Elsevier, Philadelphia, 2008.)

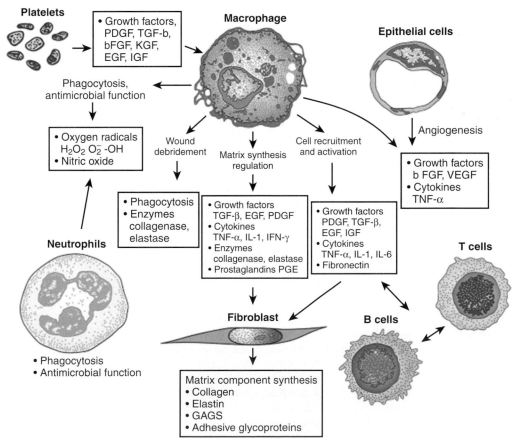

Figure 28-5 Interaction of cellular and humoral factors in wound healing. Note the key role of the macrophage. *bFGF*, Basic fibroblast growth factor; *EGF*, epidermal growth factor; *GAGs*, glycosaminoglycans; H_2O_2, hydrogen peroxide; *IFN-γ*, interferon gamma; *IGF*, insulin-like growth factor; *IL*, interleukin; *KGF*, keratinocyte growth factor; O_2^-, superoxide; *PDGF*, platelet-derived growth factor; PGE_2, prostaglandin E_2; *TGF*, transforming growth factor; *TNF*, tumor necrosis factor; *VEGF*, vascular endothelial growth factor.
(Modified from Witte MB, Barbul A. General principles of wound healing. Surg Clin North Am 1997;77:513; and Ethridge RT, Leong M, Phillips LG. Wound Healing. In Townsend CM, Beauchamp RD, Evers BM, Mattox KL [eds]. Sabiston Textbook of Surgery, 18th ed. Saunders-Elsevier, Philadelphia, 2008.)

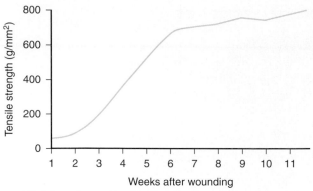

Figure 28-6 Rate of wound healing. Based on the rate of maximum collagen strength, limitation of strenuous activity after 6 weeks of wound healing is not indicated.
(From Lawrence WT, Bevin AG, Sheldon GF. Acute wound care. In Emergency Care. Chicago, Scientific American, American College of Surgeons, 1998; and Chavez MC, Maker VK. Office surgery. In Rakel RE. Textbook of Family Medicine, 7th ed. Saunders-Elsevier, Philadelphia, 2007.)

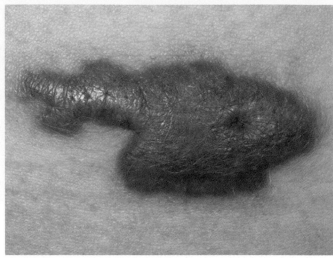

Figure 28-7 Skin keloid.
(From Habif TP. Clinical Dermatology, 5th ed. Elsevier, Philadelphia, 2010.)

Hypertrophic Scars

Hypertrophic scars are limited to the wound edges and tend to regress over the first year. The treatment of both keloid and hypertrophic scars is similar, except hypertrophic scars have better outcomes. Genetic expression of various cytokines and inflammatory pathways may affect the myofibrocytes in granulation tissue to continue producing scar; the exact causes are being investigated. Pressure dressings and colloidal silicone placed on scars after suture removal or on burn scars may reduce the incidence of both keloids and hypertrophic scars, whereas onion-skin extract (Mederma) alone is not effective (Karagoz et al., 2009).

Hypertrophic scar fibroblasts exhibit resistance to a specific form of apoptosis, or cell death, elicited by contraction of collagen matrix gels. This phenomenon depends on excess activity of cell surface tissue transglutaminases (Linge et al., 2005).

KEY TREATMENT

Cryotherapy is useful for smaller lesions such as acne and keloids (SOR: B).
Pressure dressings in burns help prevent hypertrophic scars (SOR: B).
Intralesional corticosteroid injections are first-line primary care therapies for keloids; surgery is a second-line option (SOR: B).

Juckett and Hartman-Adams, 2009.

Wound Dressings

Covering the wound with an occlusive dressing prevents drying and allows the wound to be moist, promoting healing with collagen synthesis and angiogenesis (Field, 1994). Using a topical antibiotic reduces infection only in wound laceration repairs (Dire et al., 1995), not in elective hospital or office surgical procedures (Smack et al., 1996). Studies show no dressing preference for burn wound care (American Burn Association, 2001), although it should be based on wound origin, depth, size, location, exudate, and degree of contamination (Singer et al., 2008a). Wounds closed with tissue adhesives provide their own protection and require no additional dressing. Review warning signs of infection with the patient, and advise on standard postoperative wound care and timing of suture removal.

Nonhealing Wounds

Patients underlying healing status may be affected by nutritional status and underlying medical conditions such as diabetes, cancer, and anemia. Healing may be slowed by smoking as well as age. Surgical repairs with too much tension on skin closure increase the chance of dehiscence and nonhealing. In the United States, chronic wounds affect 6.5 million patients. More than $25 billion is spent annually on treatment of chronic wounds, and the burden is rapidly growing because of increasing health care costs, an aging population, and a sharp rise in the incidence of diabetes and obesity worldwide (Sen et al., 2009).

Principles of Skin Closure

Closure techniques should minimize skin trauma, result in good skin-edge approximation without undue tension, and result in a cosmetically pleasing appearance (Fig. 28-8). The best cosmetic results can be achieved by using the finest suture possible, depending on skin thickness and tension. Generally a 3-0 (000) or 4-0 (0000) suture is appropriate on the trunk, 4-0 or 5-0 on the extremities and scalp, and 5-0 or 6-0 on the face. Forceps with teeth and skin hooks should be used to reduce crush injury to wound edges. Use the least amount of sutures to close the skin with good approximation and without deep, open space. Sutures on the face should be removed about day 3 to day 5, wounds not under tension on day 7 to 10, and wounds under tension, on the hands, or over joints on day 10 to 14. If you remove a suture and the wound opens up, cease removing the other sutures and place a sterile strip while asking the patient to return in 2 days.

Sutures are an option along with staples, tissue adhesives, and use of hair to tie edges together on some scalp wounds. Avoid staples in the scalp if computed tomography (CT) or magnetic resonance imaging (MRI) is planned. Expedient cleaning, debridement, and closure with the least trauma to the wound and patient should be the goal.

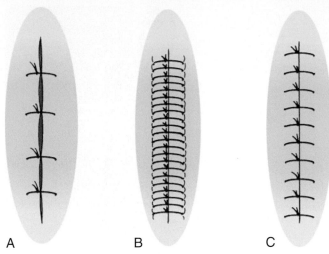

Figure 28-8 Wound repair: skin closure. **A,** Too few stitches used. Note gaping between sutures. **B,** Too many stitches used. **C,** Correct number of stitches used for a wound under an average amount of tension. *(From Lammers RL. Methods of wound closure. In Roberts JR, Hedges JR [eds]. Clinical Procedures in Emergency Medicine, 5th ed. Elsevier, Philadelphia, 2010.)*

Skin Tension Orientation

Surgeons searching for an ideal guide for elective incisions have developed 36 named guidelines. Karl Langer (1819–1887) studied and drew skin lines of cleavage after noting that round punctures in cadaveric skin produced ellipses. The topographic orientation of these lines coincides with the dominant axis of mechanical tension in the skin. Langer lines were developed by studying skin tension in cadavers with rigor mortis and therefore may not be representative of a living human's skin tension lines. Kraissl noted tension lines in living tissue and developed lines oriented perpendicular to the contraction of the underlying muscles. Later, Borges described *relaxed skin tension lines* (RSTLs), which follow furrows formed when the skin is relaxed and are produced by pinching the skin. These are only guidelines, however, and many factors contribute to the camouflaging of scars, including wrinkles and contour lines. RSTLs are formed by the natural tension on the skin from underlying soft tissue and rigid bony or cartilaginous substructure.

Superior results in scar revision arise from making incisions parallel or nearly parallel to RSTLs. The Borges RSTLs and Kraissl lines may be the best guides for elective incisions of the face and body and are often mislabeled "Langer lines." Cosmetic appearance is best if RSTLs are used on the face. The face can be divided into parallel variations of the four main facial lines: the facial median, nasolabial, facial marginal, and palpebral lines. When doing punch biopsies, stretch the skin 90 degrees perpendicular to follow the RSTLs so that the resulting ellipse-shaped wound and closure are parallel. This also improves cosmesis (Fig. 28-9).

Skin Tension on Closure

Ideally, any wound, excision, or repair should be designed so that the skin edges approximate under minimal tension. If not, and it is a clean laceration or elective excision, the surgeon may undermine tissue and trim to make edges approximate. Debridement or excision of the edges of dirty wounds may improve alignment and allow closure. Placement of tension-relieving sutures or deep sutures should always be considered to facilitate direct closure of noninfected wounds under tension. If a suture is less than ideal, it is best to remove and replace it.

Tips and beveled lacerations are challenges because too much tension on the narrowest edges may contribute to necrosis or wound breakdown. Ideally, the skin sutures are used to approximate slightly everted edges and not to pull primary deep tissue under high tension. If the wound or excision has a clean approximation under minimal tension, a single-layer repair is preferred. If not, consider deep interrupted sutures to close the potential space (Fig. 28-10). The goal is also to avoid deep pockets where hematomas, infection, or abscesses could develop. **(See Tuggy Video: Inverted Subcuticular Stitches.)**

Tissue Adhesive

On clean lacerations under low tension in dry areas, skin adhesives are an appropriate substitute for standard suturing materials and methods. Adhesives may also work on shallow, irregular, beveled lacerations and are useful on pediatric scalp lacerations. Since 1998, the long-chain medical tissue adhesive, 8-carbon 2-octylcyanoacrylate (OCA), has been available in the United States for tissue adhesive closure of wounds. OCA is more durable and flexible than the short-chain butylcyanoacrylates. The long-chain cyanoacrylates create less dehiscence in wounds longer than 8 cm. Avoid adhesive use in moist or hairy areas, on mucous membranes, if hemostasis is required, over joints or highly mobile tissue, and in bite wounds or dirty lacerations. Consider the adhesives to have about the same strength as 5.0 sutures. If OCAs are used, the patient may shower immediately, but if the butylcyanoacrylates are used, the repaired wound should be kept dry for at least 48 hours. Moisture exposure increases dehiscence risk (Singer and Dagum, 2008). If the area to repair is under higher tension, deep sutures to approximate the skin edges before closing with a superficial adhesive results in better outcomes (Singer and Thode, 2004).

Tissue adhesive agents form their own bandage, and no additional care is needed. Full tensile strength is achieved after $2\frac{1}{2}$ minutes. Because antibiotic and white petrolatum ointments can remove tissue adhesive, patients must be instructed to avoid using these on the repaired wound (Forsch, 2008).

Dehiscence occurred on 2.5% of wounds closed with tissue adhesives in an animal study comparing 2-cm and 10-cm laceration repairs with adhesive versus various suture types and different stitches. In the 2-cm wounds, results were identical. The 10-cm wounds favored deep suturing even if tissue adhesive was used. The final decision on the method and materials used for wound closure depends on the length and location of the wound as well as the time for closure and efficiency of closure (Zeplin et al., 2007). **(See Tuggy Video: Tissue Glue.)**

KEY TREATMENT

Wound closure of superficial lacerations by tissue adhesives is quicker and less painful compared with conventional suturing, with similar outcome on appropriate wounds (Aukerman et al., 2005) (SOR: A).

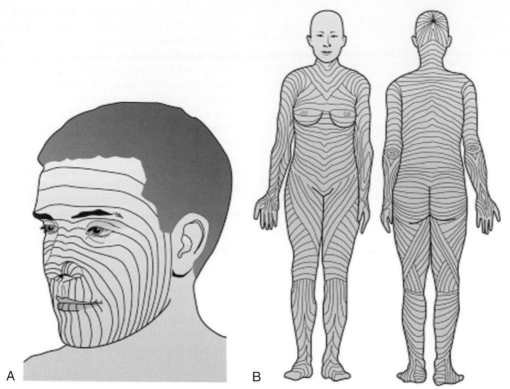

Figure 28-9 A, Facial relaxed skin tension lines (RSTLs). **B,** RSTLs of the entire body.
(From Trott A. Wounds and Lacerations: Emergency Care and Closure, 2nd ed. St Louis, Mosby, 1997; and Burns JL, Blackwell SJ. Plastic surgery. In Townsend CM, Beauchamp RD, Evers BM, Mattox KL [eds]. Sabiston Textbook of Surgery, 18th ed. Saunders-Elsevier, Philadelphia, 2008.)

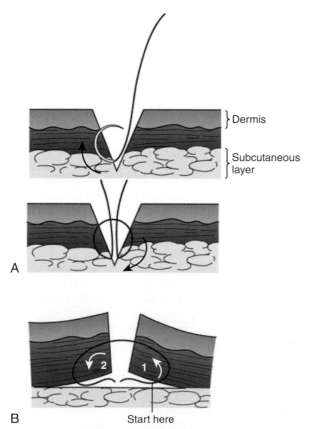

Figure 28-10 Inverted subcutaneous stitches.
(From Lammers RL. Methods of Wound Closure. In Roberts JR, Hedges JR [eds]. Clinical Procedures in Emergency Medicine, 5th ed. Elsevier, Philadelphia, 2010.)

Suture Placement

Interrupted Sutures

Individually placed single sutures are the most common form of closure. Although slower than using a running suture, single sutures usually appear better cosmetically and have a reduced risk for dehiscence. Slightly everting skin edges will result in the best wound appearance. Enter the skin 2 to 3 mm from the skin edge with the needle perpendicular to the skin plane, and rotate the wrist smoothly. Go an equal distance in depth as the horizontal distance from the wound edge. If unable to obtain an equidistant bite on the opposite side in one step, use an additional step. Bring the needle out through the laceration, then enter at the same level within the laceration, and come out through the skin at a symmetric distance from the wound's edge (Fig. 28-11). **(See Tuggy Video: Instrument Tie.)**

One may reduce the risk for dog-ears by placing a suture in the middle of a laceration and then another in the middle of the remaining gaps until equal tension and alignment approximate the skin edges in a cosmetic and hemostatic fashion. If bleeding persists, ligate or cauterize the vessel before further closing. If suturing a landmark such as vermillion borders on lip edges, consider marking opposing points before instilling anesthesia, then place an aligning suture there first.

Planning excision of an ellipse with a 3:1 to 4:1 length/width ratio has been the standard recommendation, but recent data suggest less tissue removal and better healing if a round excision is used, with adequate margins and repair of any subsequent dog-ears that develop. With this technique, 59% of the repairs required dog-ear repair (Seo et al., 2008).

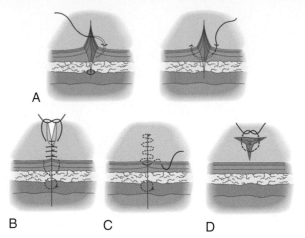

Figure 28-11 Suture technique and methods. **A,** Sutures are placed through the entire thickness of the dermis at right angles to the skin and suture line while everting the wound edge. **B,** Sutures are placed 2 to 3 mm apart and 2 to 3 mm from the wound edge. **C,** The subcuticular stitch prevents crosshatch scarring. **D,** Intradermal sutures help preserve peninsular flaps in this stellate wound.

(Modified from Wright CV, Ronaghan JE: Office surgery. In Rakel R. Textbook of Family Practice, 5th ed. Philadelphia, Saunders, 1995.)

Running Sutures

If rapid suture placement is needed and an area is not over a joint with movement, the physician can use a running suture. If the suture breaks, however, the entire wound would open up. If the running sutures are left too long, "baseball lacing" tracks may remain visible on the skin. In one study (not funded by manufacturers), deeply buried absorbable suture used along with running subcuticular polyglactin 910 (Vicryl) suture left in place resulted in the best results on trunk and extremity scar healing from elective excision of atypical moles (Alam et al., 2006).

Subcuticular Sutures

Halstead first described the subcuticular suturing technique in 1889 as a way to approximate wound edges with the least scarring. A running intradermal, buried subcuticular suture is useful in places where the dermis is shallow and when skin edges are well approximated under minimal tension, such as on the face. Placing subcuticular sutures on the back, chest, and other areas under tension without deep interrupted sutures may give poor results.

For subcuticular suture placement, use either absorbable or nonabsorbable 4-0 suture and anchor it on one end external to the wound. Enter the skin and come out in the apex of one end of the wound. Place horizontal subcuticular zigzagging sutures with symmetric bites and level entry and reentry sites on each side of the wound. If using absorbable suture, tie and bury a knot at the end of the wound by tying the knot and then placing a stitch to come out through the skin near the wound, then cut the suture flush with the skin while pulling upward on the suture. The knot will be retracted below the skin. Alternatively, with either absorbable or nonabsorbable suture, enter and exit the skin away from the wound, and tie off the suture externally. A nonabsorbable suture may be removed after 1 to 3 weeks by cutting one end of suture and gently pulling with countertraction from the other end of the wound. **(See Tuggy Video: Subcuticular Running Stitches.)**

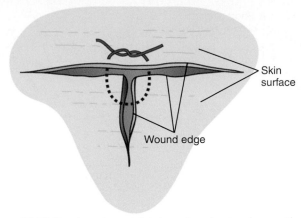

Figure 28-12 View from above stellate laceration, showing closure with half-buried mattress stitches. For some stellate lacerations, it is best to cover with Steri-Strips and revise the scar later or, if small, excise the laceration and convert it to a linear repair.

(From Lammers RL. Methods of wound closure. In Roberts JR, Hedges JR [eds]. Clinical Procedures in Emergency Medicine, 5th ed. Elsevier, Philadelphia, 2010.)

Half-Buried Mattress or Tip Sutures

Half-buried mattress sutures can be used on stellate edges and on triangular defects to reapproximate the skin edges with reduced tension on the tips (Fig. 28-12). Tip sutures are similar and used to secure a laceration tip with minimal tension. This tension can reduce blood and oxygen flow to the distal tip. **(See Tuggy Video: Mattress Stitches.)**

Pulley Sutures

The far-near, near-far pulley sutures are a modification of the vertical mattress suture and may be used as a temporary measure to reduce tension and approximate skin edges to place interrupted sutures. These sutures are used for longer repairs, but do not leave them in too long or place them too tightly because cross-hatching scars may occur. Enter with the needle 4 to 6 mm back from the wound edge, come out on the opposite side 2 mm from the wound, and loop back across the wound opening, then enter the skin 2 mm from the edge and come out on the opposite side 4 to 6 mm back from the edge (Wu, 2006).

Modified pulley sutures offer some mechanical advantage in vitro by requiring less force to achieve closure compared with horizontal mattress or single interrupted sutures. These pulley sutures are generally used when a wound is under moderate tension (Austin and Henderson, 2006).

Z-Plasty

The Z-plasty technique is used to improve the appearance of long scars, correct contractures over joints, and change the orientation of the scar line to align better with RSTLs. The key is to measure the laceration, then draw a line of the same length as the laceration on each side of the laceration at 60-degree angles for proper alignment on the repair (Fig. 28-13).

Complications

Dog-ear formations occur when the two edges of a wound are not equal length. Tissue may be trimmed before suturing. An ellipse can be cut around the dog-ear, or an

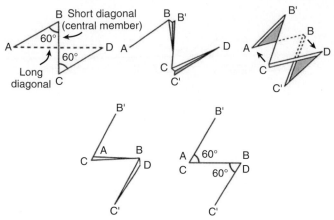

Figure 28-13 Classic equilateral triangle 60-degree Z-plasty.
(Modified from Thomas JR, Holt GR. Facial Scars, Incisions, Revision, and Camouflage. St Louis, 1989, Mosby; and Thomas JR, Mobley SR. Scar revision and camouflage. In Cummings CW, Flint PW, Haughey BH, et al. Otolaryngology: Head and Neck Surgery, 4th ed. Mosby-Elsevier, Philadelphia, 2005.)

extension laterally at an angle, and then repaired (Fig. 28-14). Another technique is called "leashing the dog-ear." Tie off the repair near the start of the dog-ear. Place a single, interrupted suture by diving through the wound along the axis of the wound and out behind the dog-ear. When tied down, this suture may flatten a small dog-ear (Khachemoune et al., 2005).

Excisions

Incisions should be made perpendicular to the skin with symmetric edges and no angulation. Poor technique may jeopardize healing. For best results, the physician should make an ellipse with the length three to four times the width. If a portion of a pigmented lesion has a worrisome appearance, complete excision is recommended. The American Cancer Society uses the ABCDE mnemonic to recognize lesions of most concern: *A*, asymmetry; *B*, border irregularity; *C*, more than one color; *D*, diameter greater than 6 mm; and *E*, increased elevation or enlargement. If a lesion has one or more of these concerns, an excisional biopsy should be considered. In other lesions, the clinician may consider a shave biopsy or punch biopsy. **(See Tuggy Videos: Excisional Skin Biopsy, Punch Biopsy, Shave Biopsy.)**

Atypical Moles and Pigmented Lesions

Elliptic full-thickness excisional biopsies are preferred for any suspicious pigmented mole. Punch biopsies can easily miss a high number of positive findings because of fusiform invasion of the margins (Chang et al., 2009).

Management of dysplastic nevi with positive margins remains controversial. Although a National Institutes of Health (NIH) Consensus Conference established margin guidelines for reexcision of dysplastic nevi (0.2-0.5 cm), it did not specify indications for reexcision. No clear guidelines exist regarding whether an incompletely removed nevus with a mild or moderate degree of dysplasia should be reexcised. Dermatopathologists are discordant in identifying dysplasia and differing degrees of atypia, further complicating

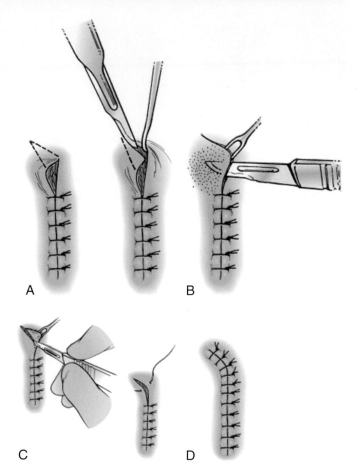

Figure 28-14 Dog-ear repair.
(Modified from Simon BC. Skin and subcutaneous tissue. In Rosen P et al [eds]: Atlas of Emergency Procedures. St Louis, Mosby, 2001; and Simon B, Hern HG. Soft tissue injuries. In Marx JA. Rosen's Emergency Medicine, 7th ed. Philadelphia, Mosby-Elsevier, 2009.)

decision making. Most dermatologists recommend that nevi with severe atypia should be reexcised because they may represent early melanoma or a lesion evolving into melanoma (Goodson et al., 2009).

Despite recurrence rates of 8% to 20% and a growing body of literature suggesting the inadequacy of a 5-mm marginal excision, a definitive change has not been made in recommended guidelines. In 2008 the National Cancer Comprehensive Network published guidelines indicating that a 5-mm excisional margin may be inadequate for lentigo maligna and lentigo maligna melanoma (Bosbous et al., 2009).

Melanomas account for 90% of the deaths associated with cutaneous tumors. Confirmed melanomas are initially excised with 10–to 20–mm safety margins both in depth and laterally if possible. Full-thickness depth is therefore important in diagnosis and prognosis of melanomas. Unsuspected melanomas found in excisional biopsies should have their bases reexcised for appropriate 1– to 2–cm margins as a second procedure. Sentinel lymph node dissection is routinely offered as a staging procedure in patients with tumors more than 1 mm in thickness, although there is as yet no resultant survival benefit. Interferon-α can be offered as adjuvant therapy to patients with melanoma more than 1.5 mm thick and stage II to III because it increases relapse-free survival.

KEY TREATMENT

Elliptic full-thickness excisional biopsies are preferred for suspicious pigmented moles (Chang et al., 2009) (SOR: A).
A 5-mm excisional margin may be inadequate for lentigo maligna and lentigo maligna melanoma (Bosbous et al., 2009) (SOR: A).
Confirmed melanomas are initially excised with 10– to 20–mm safety margins (SOR: A).

Basal Cell Cancer

The excision of small basal cell cancers (BCCAs) of less than 20 mm with well-defined borders and a 3-mm peripheral surgical margin will remove the tumor in 85% of cases. A 4– to 5–mm peripheral margin will increase the clearance rate to approximately 95%. Approximately 5% of small, well-defined BCCAs extend more than 4 mm beyond their apparent clinical margins. Morpheic (morpheaform) and large BCCAs require wider surgical margins to maximize the chance of complete histologic removal. On initial removal of morpheic lesions, the rate of complete excision with a 3-mm margin is 66%; 5-mm margin, 82%; and 13– to 15–mm margin, over 95% (Telfer et al., 2008).

Standard vertical-section processing of excision specimens allows the pathologist only to examine representative areas of the peripheral and deep surgical margins, and at best an estimated 44% of the entire margin can be examined in this manner. Therefore, tumors that appear fully excised occasionally recur (Telfer et al., 2008). If the BCCA is on an area with little excisable tissue, consider Mohs microscopic surgery to obtain adequate margins and minimize tissue removal.

If the BCCA lesion is completely excised, the recurrence rate is about 1%. If not completely excised, BCCAs have recurrence rates of 17% to 35% for lateral-margin positivity and 33% for deep-margin positivity. Only a third of positive-margin BCCA lesions recur, so the physician might reexcise the margins or consider reexcision only if a recurrence develops, with the following exceptions: lesions of long duration, size greater than 2 cm, previous recurrence, and aggressive histologic features, including perineural and perivascular invasion and infiltrative, morpheaform, or micronodular appearance. If marginal positivity is detected in such cases after excision, reexcision and removal of the residual tumor is advised over watchful observance (Ünlü et al., 2009). **(See Tuggy Video: Basal Cell Curettage and Cautery.)**

KEY TREATMENT

A 4– to 5–mm peripheral margin will increase the cure rate of BCCAs to approximately 95% (Telfer et al., 2008) (SOR: A).
Morpheaform and large basal cell cancers require wider surgical margins (Telfer et al., 2008) (SOR: A).

Cryotherapy

Cryotherapy can be easily mastered for treatment of many skin lesions. Cryotherapy is well tolerated and results in minimal to no scar. It is best used in those with lighter skin and in non-hair-bearing areas because of occasional pigment changes or hair loss with deeper treatments. Liquid nitrogen, the most widely available, cost-effective cryogen for medical therapy,

boils at $-196°$ C, and temperatures of $-25°$ to $-50°$ C can be achieved in 30 seconds of appropriate skin application. Destruction of benign lesions occurs at $-20°$ to $-30°$ C, and malignant lesions often require temperatures of $-40°$ to $-50°$ C for destruction (Andrews, 2004). Correct use of cryotherapy results in selective cell destruction while sparing the tissue matrix of collagen and fibroelastic tissue and reducing the risk of scar formation. Repeated freeze-thaw applications can increase tissue damage.

Indications and Contraindications

Cryotherapy can be an important treatment option for many lesions commonly encountered in a primary care clinical practice. It can be used in all age groups to treat a number of dermatologic lesions. Even though well tolerated, cryosurgery also has contraindications (Box 28-2). Some body areas or conditions should be approached with prudence because of increased complication risks. Basal cell cancers, particularly in the nasolabial fold or periauricular area, tend to be

---

Box 28-2 Cryotherapy: Indications and Contraindications

Indications

Verruca (warts)
Condylomata acuminata
Papular nevi
Selected basal cell cancer
Seborrheic keratosis
Molluscum contagiosum
Granulation tissue
Selected squamous cell cancer
Actinic keratosis
Acrochordons (skin tags)
Cervical intraepithelial neoplasia

Contraindications
Absolute
Prior cryotherapy sensitivity
Vascular compromise
Complication nonacceptance
Steroid therapy
Melanoma
Invasive skin cancer
Need for tissue diagnosis
Expected poor wound healing

Relative*
Hepatitis B and C
Mononucleosis
Leukemia
Lymphoma
Myeloma
Systemic lupus
Nephritic syndrome
Nephrotic syndrome
Macroglobulinemia
Rheumatoid arthritis

*High-risk of cryoglobulins.

more extensive than expected and more likely to recur. The vermillion border, periorbital area, and areas overlying cutaneous nerves present confounding variables to safe application of a cryogen for therapy.

Equipment and Technique

Liquid nitrogen can be applied with a regular or modified cotton-tipped applicator, cryogen spray device, or cryoprobe, all readily available to providers. The cotton-tipped applicator is the least expensive and can be modified to hold more cryogen or to match the size or shape of the lesion with a cotton ball. Liquid nitrogen can be stored in an insulated device in the office and taken out in small aliquots in a polystyrene cup for individual use with patients.

Handheld cryogen spray devices have recently been improving. Traditional cryotherapy systems provide a reservoir for the liquid nitrogen and an applicator tip to dispense the cryogen. The applicator tip can have a varying aperture for altering cryogen dispersion. Some providers use an otoscopy cone to protect surrounding skin and direct the spray onto a small central lesion. The unit is generally held 1 to 2 cm above the lesion and the spray directed at a 90-degree angle and aimed at the lesion center. Newer spray devices use a continuous infrared sensing device to determine the treatment site skin temperature and ensure consistent freeze times. These modifications can improve accuracy and assist in achieving optimum cryotherapy results (Cry-Ac Tracker, www.brymill.com).

Prior to cryotherapy, the depth and diameter of the freeze must be anticipated to minimize injury to surrounding tissues. Mark the skin to ensure adequate treatment in critical cryotherapy sessions. Keratin layers are very resistant to cryotherapy and can be treated for 1 to 2 weeks with topical 40% salicylic acid plaster or mechanically pared away before freezing. Application of salicylic acid alone is equally efficacious to cryotherapy of warts for many patients (Gibbs and Harvey, 2006). A well-hydrated skin lesion can increase cryotherapy success rates.

For superficial benign skin lesions, the cryotherapy applicator should almost cover the lesion and should be applied for 20 to 40 seconds to create an ice ball edge 2 to 3 mm beyond the edge of the lesion. In contrast, deeper or premalignant lesions should be treated with an applicator smaller than the lesion to ensure a depth more equal to the radius of treatment. It should be applied for 40 to 90 seconds to form an ice ball 3 to 4 mm outside the lesion. Superficial malignant lesions also require a smaller applicator, but applied for 1 to 3 minutes for an ice ball 5 to 8 mm beyond the lesion. Malignant cells are more resistant to cryotherapy, and destruction requires temperatures at −40° to −50° C. In most cases the depth of a freeze is similar to the radius of the superficial ice ball formed. The lethal zone for tissue destruction is 2 to 3.5 mm inward from the outer margin of the ice ball (Pfenninger, 2003).

Complications

Cryotherapy results in minimal scarring. Vascular or hypertrophic lesions are resistant and sometimes require multiple treatments 2 to 3 weeks apart. Most patients may experience pain and burning for 1 to 2 days. During these first days, the skin may be red and sensitive and may form a hemorrhagic bulla followed by sloughing. Infection and pyogenic granuloma formation are rare complications. In deeper cryotherapy,

the potential damage to underlying neural structures must be considered. **(See Tuggy Video: Wart Treatment.)**

KEY TREATMENT

A significant keratin layer is resistant to cryotherapy (SOR: B).
The lethal zone for cryogen tissue destruction is 2 to 3.5 mm inward from the outer margin of the ice ball (Pfenninger, 2003) (SOR: A).
Salicylic acid application alone to warts is equally efficacious to cryotherapy (Gibbs and Harvey, 2006) (SOR: A).

Incision and Drainage of Cutaneous Abscess

A cutaneous abscess is identified by a fluctuance or compressible softness in skin surrounded by induration, inflammation, warmth, and tenderness. *Furuncles* are superficial and result from abscess formation in a sweat gland or hair follicle. *Carbuncles* are deeper and extend into the subcutaneous tissue. Offending bacteria include *Staphylococcus aureus*, streptococci, and occasionally gram-negative rods. These infections can be severe in patients with diabetes or vascular disease. Primary treatment of an abscess is surgical drainage. An area of induration alone with no fluctuance indicates isolated cellulitis and is treated with antibiotics and warm compresses.

When performing an incision and drainage of an abscess, the skin is prepared with a sterilizing and cleansing agent. Local anesthetics do not work well in the acidic environment of an abscess, so a ring or field block can be infiltrated around the periphery of the lesion. Superficial cooling of the surface of the skin with ethyl chloride or liquid nitrogen can also provide brief anesthesia for a stab incision.

A linear incision is made over the area of maximal fluctuance and has been shown to heal in a shorter time than deroofing procedures used in the past (Sørensen et al., 1987). Once the incision is made into the center of the abscess with a #11 blade, the abscess cavity is probed with a curved hemostat to disrupt any loculations. The abscess cavity is packed with ¼- to 1-inch gauze to prevent early superficial wound closure and allow secondary healing. Primary closure is not recommended (Korownyk, 2007). A bulky sterile dressing can be applied to absorb any drainage and the packing and dressing changed every 1 to 2 days or when soiled. Evidence does not support using oral antibiotics after surgical drainage. Routine swabbing for culture in immunocompetent individuals is not recommended (Korownyk, 2007). Patients are educated on wound care and return in 2 to 7 days for follow-up. **(See Tuggy Video: Abscess Incision and Drainage.)**

Recurrent skin abscesses should be investigated based on location. Crohn's disease, subcutaneous fistulas, and pilonidal cysts can present as recurrent cutaneous abscesses. MRSA should be suspected in recurrences as well.

KEY TREATMENT

Primary treatment of an abscess is surgical drainage (SOR: A).
Incision and drainage of an uncomplicated abscess does not require oral antibiotic treatment (SOR: A).
Routine culture of abscess drainage in immunocompetent individuals is not recommended (SOR: A).

Korownyk, 2007.

Lipomas

Lipomas are mature adipose tissue arranged in a nodular formation surrounded by a capsule and commonly located in the subcutaneous tissues. Lipomas can be diagnosed by clinical examination and identification of their unique, well-circumscribed, round, mobile character with a doughy consistency. Although most do not require it, excision may be considered for large tumors, rapidly growing lipomas, and those causing pain. Lipomas can occur in isolation or with other systemic diseases, as a component of genetically inherited disorders, or in other connective tissue layers.

A steroid injection or liposuction can be used to treat select lipomas. Steroid injections can be used to treat painful lipomas less than 1 inch (2.5 cm) in size and in which pathologic examination is likely unnecessary. An injection of 1 to 3 mL of triamcinolone diluted with 1% lidocaine to a 10 mg/mL concentration can be performed into the center of the lipoma monthly to shrink the tumor to the desired size. Formal liposuction can be done with cannula or 16-gauge syringe under local anesthesia (Salam, 2002). Neither of these procedures is likely to eliminate the lipoma in its entirety, and recurrences are frequent.

Surgical excision of a lipoma removes the neoplasm from the tissue and allows for pathologic examination. Marking the boundaries of the lipoma is helpful for identification of the tumor edges before a local anesthetic field block is placed. The skin is prepared with a povidone-iodine or chlorhexidine solution. Small lipomas can be enucleated with their capsule using blunt dissection through a small incision. Larger lipomas require excision through a linear or elliptic incision. Blunt and sharp dissection can be used to free the mass from the surrounding tissues using hemostats or clamps for traction. Hemostasis should be confirmed and cautery or ligature placement used to ensure a dry wound base. The remaining dead space is closed with buried, interrupted, dissolvable subcutaneous sutures and the skin closed with interrupted sutures or staples depending on location and cosmetic need. A compression dressing should be used for 1 to 2 days to prevent formation of a hematoma, and sutures are removed in 5 to 10 days depending on location. Submit any specimen for pathologic examination. **(See Tuggy Video: Lipoma Removal.)**

Surgery of the Nail and Digits

Ingrown Nail (Onychocryptosis)

The great toe's lateral and distal nail beds are the most common locations for ingrown nails. Poorly fitting shoes, poor nail-trimming techniques, and trauma can result in their formation. Most ingrown nails respond to conservative local treatment of warm soaks and elevation of the distal nail with cotton to allow unobstructed nail growth. If poor toenail trimming is the cause, a shard of nail is impaling the distal lateral nail groove and can be simply trimmed and removed for resolution of pain with standard curved or straight iris scissors.

When conservative measures fail, a partial or complete nail excision is performed to remove the portion of offending nail. The digit is prepared and a digit block placed using 1% lidocaine. A tourniquet at the base of the toe can help with hemostasis. A nail elevator is used to separate the section of nail to be removed from the underlying nail bed down to the base of the nail and germinal matrix and from the cuticle. Once elevated, an iris or bandage scissors can be used to cut the nail longitudinally to the matrix. A straight hemostat is used to grasp the nail, and the nail is rolled laterally for removal. Hemostasis can be obtained with compression or silver nitrate. A bulky tube-gauze dressing can be placed for protection. Recurrent ingrown nails unresponsive to conservative measures can be ablated after nail removal. A phenol solution is applied to a hemostatic germinal nail matrix under the proximal nail fold for 30 to 60 seconds before neutralizing the phenol with rubbing alcohol. **(See Tuggy Video: Ingrown Toenail Removal.)**

Nail Plate Avulsion for Onychomycosis

Conservative treatment of onychomycosis is the first-line choice for management. A fungal culture of nail clippings can be done to confirm the diagnosis but may take up to 1 month for growth and identification. There is good evidence that oral terbinafine, 250 mg daily for 3 months, is the most effective oral treatment for fungally infected toenails (Crawford et al., 2002). Even with terbinafine, failure rates can reach 50%. When onychomycosis causes dystrophic nails resulting in pain or toe dysfunction, a complete nail plate avulsion can be performed, with high patient satisfaction (see Ingrown Nail).

KEY TREATMENT

Oral terbinafine, 250 mg daily for 3 months, is the most effective oral treatment for fungally infected toenails (Crawford et al., 2002) (SOR: A).

Paronychia

An *acute* paronychia is caused by a bacterial infection of the lateral or proximal nail folds after minimal to significant trauma, whereas a *chronic* paronychia results from an inflammatory condition caused by repetitive irritant contact exposure. Acute paronychia can be treated conservatively with warm soaks, gentle compression, topical steroid creams, and topical or oral antibiotics (Rigopoulos et al., 2008). Chronic paronychias respond to removal of the offending agent or treatment of the underlying condition or inflammatory cause.

When the local cellulitis of an acute paronychia develops into an abscess, drainage is indicated. If the fluctuant pocket of the abscess is superficial and underlying the cuticle or nail fold, a 23-gauge needle or #11 blade tip can be used to lift the edge of the fold and allow drainage without local anesthesia. A digital nerve block can be performed if the infection is deeper and requires more extensive drainage or for patient comfort. Once anesthetized, an incision can be placed parallel to the nail fold with a stab incision using a #11 bladed into the abscess with subsequent drainage and exploration to break up loculations as needed. Warm soaks should follow with oral antibiotics for the cellulitis (Fig. 28-15).

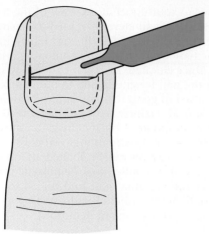

Figure 28-15 Incision and drainage of paronychia. The tip of a #11 scalpel is advanced just under the cuticle and parallel to the nail. The size of the incision should be large enough to include all fluctuant areas and no more. *(From Chavez MC, Maker VK. Office surgery. In Rakel RE. Textbook of Family Medicine, 7th ed. Saunders-Elsevier, Philadelphia, 2007.)*

Evacuation of Subungual Hematoma

Trauma to the nail causing bleeding between the nail plate and nail bed can be excruciatingly painful. Subungual hematomas can be drained easily in an office setting by creating a 2-mm hole in the nail and draining the blood, using a handheld cautery unit or heated end of a metal paper clip. If trauma was significant, with the hematoma involving more than 50% of the nail, the provider should consider a nail bed laceration requiring primary closure, and this should be radiographically evaluated. Frequently, phalanx tuft fractures can underlie the hematoma after significant trauma (Wang and Johnson, 2001).

Anorectal Disease

Bleeding, pain, discharge, or change in bowel habits can indicate active anorectal disease, and all warrant medical evaluation. The patient history and a complete anorectal examination lead to a clear diagnosis in most complaints. Inflamed internal hemorrhoids or rectal polyps typically cause painless rectal bleeding. Painful anal bleeding can result from anal fissures, proctitis, thrombosed external hemorrhoids, or a draining perianal abscess. Palpable chronic masses can indicate an anal skin tag, polyp, or prolapsed rectal mass, and acute masses are usually caused by abscesses or thrombosed hemorrhoids. More than 90% of anorectal complaints can be managed in the primary care physician's office using simple techniques (Pfenninger and Zainea, 2001).

Anoscopy

Anoscopy is performed easily in the office to evaluate and treat many anorectal conditions. Scopes can be 7 to 10 cm long and 2 to 3 cm wide and range from a slotted or beveled metal version to a disposable plastic tubular version. The tubular version can be used for diagnosis, whereas the slotted style allows for ease in treating most anorectal conditions.

For a thorough examination, the patient can be placed in a comfortable lateral decubitus position with hips flexed. The examiner may require nonpermeable protective clothing and eyewear. The anal tissues should be examined for tags, hemorrhoids, fissures, dermatitis, condylomata, and masses. A digital rectal examination should precede anoscopy to assess for internal pain or mass.

During examination the thumb can be pressed against the internal index finger to determine tenderness, induration, or abscess formation in the perianal tissues in all quadrants. The lubricated anoscope with obturator is introduced fully into the anal canal with gentle, constant pressure. Once fully inserted, the obturator is removed and the anorectal mucosa visualized through 360 degrees during gradual withdrawal. Adequate lighting is essential. Valsalva maneuver may distend vascular lesions for ease in visibility. Anal Pap smears can be obtained if warranted for anorectal cancer concerns and biopsies performed using a Kevorkian or Tischler biopsy forceps. Hemostasis is obtained using silver nitrate sticks. **(See Tuggy Video: Anoscopy.)**

Hemorrhoids

Hemorrhoids are submucosal vascular beds located in the anal and rectal canal that assist with defecation and the sensation of anorectal fullness. These vascular beds can occur in insensate areas above the dentate line as *internal* hemorrhoids or below the dentate line as *external* hemorrhoids in exquisitely sensitive areas. Hemorrhoid development may result from genetic factors, aging or serial local trauma. One study found that 4.4% of the U.S. population, or 10 million people, complain of hemorrhoid disease (Reese et al., 2009).

Internal Hemorrhoids

Internal hemorrhoids are classified according to the severity of prolapse. No rectal prolapse occurs with first-degree hemorrhoids, and spontaneously reducible prolapse occurs with second-degree disease. These can be treated with conservative or surgical methods. Third-degree hemorrhoids prolapse and require manual reduction, and fourth-degree hemorrhoids have irreducible prolapse. As the prolapse progresses, surgical treatment becomes a more common treatment.

Painless, bright-red rectal bleeding is the primary symptom of internal hemorrhoids. Anoscopy can be used for identification of the site of bleeding acutely. Internal hemorrhoids typically occur in three locations in the anal canal: right anterior, right posterior, and left lateral. A flexible sigmoidoscopy or colonoscopy is performed if the patient's symptoms or history warrant more extensive colonic evaluation, or if the site of colorectal bleeding is not easily identified or persists after treatment. Patients over age 40 who have hemorrhoidal bleeding may have other colorectal pathology and should have further colorectal evaluation (Chong and Bartolo, 2008).

Dietary management consisting of adequate fluid and fiber intake is the primary noninvasive treatment of symptomatic hemorrhoids (Cataldo et al., 2005). Persistent hemorrhoid symptoms decreased by 53% in those receiving dietary fiber for hemorrhoid care (Alonso-Coello et al., 2005). Conservative therapy can be offered for mild first- and second-degree hemorrhoids, but more advanced disease may require surgical management. Rubber band ligation or hemorrhoid banding is known to be highly effective in outpatient treatment of first-, second-, and some third-degree internal hemorrhoids (Reese et al., 2009). Other options include sclerotherapy, infrared coagulation, radiofrequency coagulation, and cryotherapy (Cataldo et al., 2005).

Prolapsing internal hemorrhoids can be easily treated in the office with *rubber band ligation* using a McGilvney ligator or similar device. After appropriate consent is obtained, a slotted or beveled anoscope is inserted into the anus. The hemorrhoid is then identified, and with the circular McGilvney ligator in place within the anoscope, the hemorrhoid is grasped with a forceps and drawn into the ligator cylinder. Sensation of the hemorrhoid is assessed to prevent ligation of a high external hemorrhoid. Care is taken not to draw too much tissue into the ligator to avoid denuding the anal lining. Once the base of the hemorrhoid is in the ligator, two rubber bands are released from the ligator by one cylinder sliding over the other. The bands cause ischemic necrosis of the hemorrhoid, and the tissue sloughs over days. Bleeding can occur for up to 1 to 2 weeks and is occasionally significant. Patients may feel some rectal fullness, a spasm, or dull ache for a few days after banding. Rare episodes of pelvic cellulitis have been reported. Only one site should be treated per patient visit (Fig. 28-16). **(See Tuggy Video: Internal Hemorrhoid Banding.)**

Sclerotherapy can be performed on first- and second-degree hemorrhoids using a sclerosant of 5% phenol or saline. The base of the hemorrhoid is injected with 1 to 2 mL of the sclerosant through a syringe while viewed through an anoscope. More late complications can be seen with sclerotherapy when compared to banding. In a recent systematic review, sclerotherapy had unknown effectiveness in treating hemorrhoids. Infrared photocoagulation was found to be likely beneficial and as effective as rubber band ligation in the same review. The infrared coagulator light is fired three to five times at the base of the hemorrhoid through an anoscope for 1.5 seconds during one treatment session. Multiple sessions may be required for infrared treatment of first-degree through small third-degree hemorrhoids. Radiofrequency coagulation is performed with a Bicap probe placed at the base of the hemorrhoid above the dentate line and activated four to six times for 2 seconds, forming a white coagulum.

Because of prolonged healing after cryotherapy, it is no longer recommended (Reese et al., 2009).

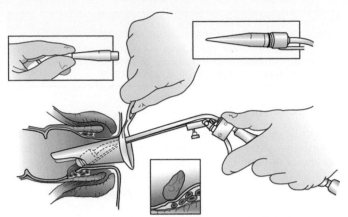

Figure 28-16 Rubber band ligation for internal hemorrhoid. The band is advanced onto the end of the ligator instrument using a conical attachment *(insets)*. The hemorrhoid is identified at a level proximal to the dentate; this area is tested for sensation before banding. Occluding the suction port of the ligator instrument draws the hemorrhoid into the open end of the ligator, and the instrument is fired. The banded hemorrhoid typically sloughs in 1 week. *(Courtesy Mayo Foundation; and Nelson H, Cima RR. Anus. In Townsend CM, Beauchamp RD, Evers BM, Mattox KL [eds]. Sabiston Textbook of Surgery, 18th ed. Saunders-Elsevier, Philadelphia, 2008.)*

> **KEY TREATMENT**
>
> Patients over the age of 40 who have hemorrhoidal bleeding cannot be assumed to have no other colorectal pathology and should have further colorectal evaluation. (Chong and Bartolo, 2008) (SOR: B).
> Dietary management of symptomatic hemorrhoids consists of adequate fluid and fiber intake (Alonso-Coello et al., 2005) (SOR: B). Rubber band ligation is known to be highly effective outpatient treatment for first-, second-, and some third-degree hemorrhoids (Reese et al., 2009) (SOR: B).

External Hemorrhoids

A nonpainful or painful anal swelling can represent an external hemorrhoid. Hemorrhoids should be differentiated from anal skin tags, condylomata, fissures, and abscesses on anal examination. Symptomatic external hemorrhoids can be excised if conservative treatment fails. The patient is placed in the lateral decubitus position with hips flexed. The external hemorrhoid or tag is identified and anesthetized at its base with buffered 1% lidocaine with epinephrine. The area is cleansed with povidone-iodine or chlorhexidine. A radially oriented elliptic incision is made around the hemorrhoid or tag and the center removed with the hemorrhoid vein. The resulting defect is frequently left open and allowed to heal. Stool softeners and topical anesthetics may be very beneficial. Because of the vascularity, healing can occur in 5 to 10 days. **(See Tuggy Video: External Hemorrhoid Excision.)**

Thrombosed External Hemorrhoids

An external hemorrhoid can become thrombosed and may be identified by an acute onset of perianal pain and development of a purplish nodule with or without bleeding. Thrombosed hemorrhoids can be managed conservatively with avoidance of constipation, patient analgesia, and ice or sitz baths (Cataldo et al., 2005). Office surgical excision, not incision, of a thrombosed external hemorrhoid results in a lower recurrence rate and earlier resolution of symptoms (Greenspon et al., 2004). Simple incision of the thrombosed hemorrhoid may not remove multiple clots and can result in higher recurrence rate and even extension.

To excise a thrombosed hemorrhoid, the patient is placed in the lateral decubitus position with buttocks separated for visualization. The surface can be cleansed and anesthesia provided with a local injection of buffered lidocaine or bupivacaine with epinephrine at the base of the hemorrhoid. Once anesthetized, an elliptic incision is made in a radial orientation over the hemorrhoid, and all thrombus is removed with excision of the hemorrhoidal vein at its base. Bleeding can be controlled with pressure, Monsel's solution, or careful electrocautery. More complex hemorrhoids or those associated with partial rectal prolapse should be referred to a colorectal specialist.

KEY TREATMENT

Office surgical excision, not incision, of a thrombosed external hemorrhoid results in a lower recurrence rate and earlier resolution of symptoms (Greenspon et al., 2004) (SOR: B).

Anorectal Abscess

An anorectal abscess can lead to severe pain and disability in patients. Abscesses occur most often in the third or fourth decade of life and in a 3:1 to 2:1 male/female ratio (Hebra, 2009). An anorectal abscess develops from an infection originating in the anal glands and crypts at the level of the dentate line and tracking along the lines of least resistance. This tracking results in up to 50% of abscesses being associated with simultaneous fistula development. Locations of the abscess can vary and may be located in the perianal area (60%), ischiorectal area (20%), intersphincter region (5%), supralevator region (4%), and submucosal location (1%) (Fig. 28-17). Abscesses can result from other anorectal infections or pathology such as Crohn's disease fistulas, adenocarcinoma, trauma, immunosuppression, and sexually transmitted diseases. A thorough anorectal examination, frequently under anesthesia, is required for complete evaluation. Most abscesses can be localized by physical examination. Deep or large abscesses require a pelvic CT scan to determine the extent of tracking and to plan surgical intervention.

An anorectal abscess should be treated by incision and drainage. The lack of fluctuance should not delay a timely drainage procedure. Antibiotics are an unnecessary addition to routine incision and drainage of uncomplicated perianal abscesses (Whiteford et al., 2005). No conclusive evidence exists for a simple drainage versus sphincter-cutting procedure in the treatment of anorectal abscess (Quah et al., 2006). Antibiotics should be considered only as an adjunct to drainage in patients with immunosuppression, diabetes, prosthetic devices, or significant systemic illness.

Before surgical decompression, an anoscopy should be performed to identify a potential internal draining fistula source at the dentate line. Injecting an agent over or under the mass can provide local anesthesia, although rarely patients may need spinal or general anesthesia. Incision and drainage of superficial abscesses can be accomplished with use of an 11 blade over the area of maximal fluctuance or swelling in a radial orientation. Loculations can be broken by probing with a forceps or gloved finger. A Penrose drain or gauze packing can be placed for continued drainage with appropriate follow up in 1 to 2 days. Recurrent abscesses can occur when there is an unrecognized and untreated underlying fistula. A fistulotomy must be performed in these cases.

KEY TREATMENT

About 50% of perirectal abscesses are associated with simultaneous fistula development.

The lack of fluctuance should not delay a timely drainage procedure for perianal abscesses (Whiteford et al., 2005) (SOR: B).

Antibiotics are an unnecessary addition to routine incision and drainage of uncomplicated perianal abscesses (Whiteford et al., 2005) (SOR: A).

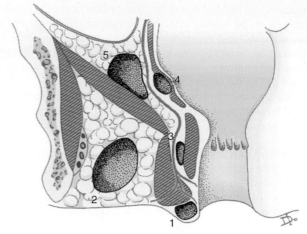

Figure 28-17 Classification of perirectal abscesses: *1*, perianal; *2*, ischiorectal; *3*, intersphincteric; *4*, high intramuscular; and *5*, pelvirectal. *(From Hill GJ II [ed]. Outpatient Surgery, 3rd ed. Philadelphia, Saunders, 1988; and Coates WC. Anorectal procedures. In Roberts JR, Hedges JR [eds]. Clinical Procedures in Emergency Medicine, 5th ed. Elsevier, Philadelphia, 2010.)*

Anal Fissure

An anal fissure is a tear in the anal mucosa that can cause severe anal pain and rectal bleeding and results from local stool trauma. Most occur posteriorly in the midline. Other causes or locations should prompt a more complete anorectal evaluation. On examination, the anus is exquisitely tender and may demonstrate internal anal sphincter spasm. Evaluation can occur with gentle spreading of the anus, but some require anoscopy to assess their extent. A radial tear is seen that can be bleeding and very tender.

Most *acute* anal fissures can be managed conservatively with dietary fiber, prevention of constipation, adequate hydration, and stool softeners. Sitz baths may provide symptomatic improvement. Topical anesthetics such as 5% lidocaine ointment or gel can be used for comfort or before defection until healing. No surgical treatment is warranted in uncomplicated occurrences. *Chronic* anal fissures do not resolve after the 3-month acute phase and are generally less tender. Chronic fissures are still associated with significant internal sphincter spasm and may present with a large, protuberant sentinel tag, sometimes confused with a hemorrhoidal tag.

Conservative therapy includes continued constipation prevention. Other therapeutically equal treatment options include topical nitroglycerin ointment, botulinum toxin injections, or calcium channel blockers such as diltiazem or nifedipine for 30 days. However, no conservative medical therapy approximates the efficacy of surgical sphincterotomy for chronic fissures (Nelson, 2006). An open or closed partial lateral internal sphincterotomy appears to be equally efficacious as surgical treatment (Nelson, 2008). An experienced specialist in the technique and anorectal anatomy should perform this procedure.

KEY TREATMENT

No conservative medical therapy approximates the efficacy of surgical sphincterotomy for chronic fissures (Nelson, 2006) (SOR: A).

Pilonidal Cyst and Abscess

Pilonidal disease may manifest itself as a chronically draining sinus or fistula at the base of the spine in the intergluteal crease 5 to 10 cm from the anus. Pilonidal cysts can also become infected and may lead to extensive presacral abscess formation. Multiple hair shafts may be seen within the cyst. Incision and drainage or an elliptic incision under local anesthesia over the sinus track is performed. Drainage is the preferred office management technique and is similar to standard abscess treatment. Packing of the wound should be done, and referral is recommended for excision of the extensive presacral complex. Recurrence is common without excision.

Gynecologic Office Procedures

See also Chapters 25 and 26.

Paracervical Block

A paracervical block can be placed before any uterine procedure requiring instrumentation of the cervix or cervical dilation. Contraindications include current desired pregnancy, infection, and bleeding disorders. The local anesthetic used is determined by the length of anesthesia required, most often 0.5% lidocaine or bupivacaine for injection.

The patient is placed in a dorsal lithotomy position and a vaginal speculum placed to allow adequate visualization of the cervix. Two 10-mL syringes are drawn up of a 1:1 ratio of 1% lidocaine or bupivacaine and sterile saline. The cervix and vaginal canal is cleansed with chlorhexidine or povidone-iodine. An injection of 1 to 2 mL of this mixture is placed in the anterior cervical lip, where a single-toothed cervical tenaculum is placed. The cervix is lifted upward and deviated laterally to obtain access to the lateral posterior fornix. The 4 and 8 o'clock positions are identified on the cervix, and 8 to 10 mL of the mixture is injected at each site. This injection starts into the cervicovaginal reflection at the apex of the posterior fornix at these positions and is advanced 2 to 5 cm in depth along the external serosa of the uterus, to provide anesthesia to the uterine plexus of nerves near the uterine arteries. Intravascular injection is avoided by pulling back on the syringe plunger before infiltration.

Women have less pain during uterine intervention with paracervical block than with placebo injections (SOR: B).

Contraceptive Devices

Diaphragms

Diaphragms have an arcing, coil, or flat spring with the latex brands and a wide-seal rim, arcing or coil spring with the silicone devices. The arcing spring diaphragm is used most often because it is easier to place in the posterior fornix without an introducer. When fitting a diaphragm, the size can be determined with a simple pelvic examination.

With the patient in a dorsal lithotomy position, the provider inserts the lubricated and gloved index and middle finger straight into the vagina to the posterior fornix. Once there, the spot where the inferior pubic arch impacts the index finger is noted. The fingers are withdrawn, and the distance from that point on the index finger to the end of the middle finger is noted; this is about the diameter of diaphragm needed. Diaphragms come in 5-mm increments from 60 to 90 mm, with 75 and 80 mm most common. The diaphragm is then inserted and size confirmed with placement posteriorly in the posterior fornix behind the cervix and anteriorly behind the pubic arch. Removal of the diaphragm can be accomplished by hooking the anterior rim with a finger and gently extracting. Women should be given an opportunity to remove and replace the diaphragm to confirm placement before use.

The diaphragm can be placed in the posterior vagina covering the cervix up to 6 hours before intercourse. Generally, women have used 5 mL of spermicide within the diaphragm at insertion, although a Cochrane review failed to prove its contribution to contraceptive effectiveness (Cook et al., 2003). Additional spermicide can be inserted in front of the diaphragm before each act of intercourse without dislodging the diaphragm. The diaphragm is removed at least 6 hours and not more than 24 hours after the last intercourse. An increased risk of urinary tract infections exists with diaphragm use and risk of toxic shock syndrome if the diaphragm is left in place more than 24 hours. The diaphragm size needs to be reestablished after a weight change of 10 to 15 pounds, pregnancy, or pelvic surgery. Failure rate for the diaphragm is 18% but may be better with perfect use.

Cervical Caps

Two brands of cervical caps are currently approved and marketed in the United States. Although neither requires specific fitting by a practitioner, both require a prescription for pharmacy or manufacturer dispensation. FemCap comes in three sizes and is ordered based on pregnancy history, whereas Lea's Shield comes in one size for all women with normal anatomy.

The FemCap is a silicone rubber nonhormonal intravaginal contraceptive (IVC). The smaller rim size (22 mm) is for women who have never been pregnant. The medium size (26 mm) is intended for women who have been pregnant, even for up to as little as 2 weeks with no vaginal delivery. The larger-diameter cap (30 mm) is for women who have had a full-term vaginal delivery. When in doubt of prior pregnancy, the 26-mm cap should be used. The patient places the cap over the cervix with up to ¾ tsp of 2% nonoxynol-9 spermicide used around the outside groove at least 15 minutes before sexual arousal. Placement over the cervix is critical and accomplished best while squatting. Once in place, the cap should be pushed in opposition to the cervix for at least 10 seconds to ensure firm placement against the vaginal wall, because it does not fit snug against the cervix. Additional spermicide should be placed with each act of intercourse without removing the cap. Hooking a finger under the removal strap in a squatting position and withdrawing gently removes the cap. The cap must be removed at least 6 hours but not longer than 48 hours after the last act of intercourse. During a 6-month clinical trial for approval, the FemCap was 86.5% successful in preventing pregnancy (FemCap, 2010). The device is washed and dried thoroughly between uses.

Lea's Shield is a silicone rubber IVC placed vaginally at any time before intercourse. It is inserted with spermicide to the depth of the vagina, and any trapped air is vented through a one-way valve, creating a tight fit between the vaginal wall and the device. The Shield is removed using the incorporated removal loop with a finger more than 8 hours after intercourse. Women had an 8.7% chance of becoming pregnant within 6 months when using the Lea's Shield (Yama, 2010). The shield is cleaned with warm soapy water and dried for reuse.

KEY TREATMENT

Failure rates for the diaphragm are 18% but may be better with perfect use (Cook et al., 2003) (SOR: A).
FemCap was 86.5% successful in preventing pregnancy over 6 months of use (FemCap, 2010) (SOR: B).
Women have an 8.7% chance of becoming pregnant within 6 months when using Lea's Shield (Yama, 2010) (SOR: B).

Intrauterine Devices

Insertion

Long-acting reversible contraception has become increasingly popular in the form of intrauterine devices (IUDs). IUDs are T-shaped devices that are very easy to place in an office setting and have a failure rate less than 1% to 2% per year. They can be used in nulliparous and parous women and have a high continuance rate after 1 year of use (78%-81%). Both device types have attached strings at the end for removal in the office, and pregnancy rates return to normal soon afterward. IUDs are contraindicated in women with a current or suspected pregnancy, abnormal uterine cavity, pelvic inflammatory disease or endometritis, known endometrial or cervical malignancy, genital bleeding of unknown etiology, artificial heart valve placement, or allergy to IUD components.

A pregnancy during use of an IUD is more likely to be ectopic, but the overall rate of ectopic pregnancy is less than in sexually active women who use no contraception. Complications of IUD placement include pelvic infection, embedment in the uterine wall, IUD migration or expulsion, and perforation of the uterus. Unlike oral contraceptives, IUDs can be used during lactation and are not contraindicated in women with a history of venous thromboembolic events, those at increased risk of myocardial infarction or stroke, or those who smoke. Perforation rates are 0.6 to 1.6 per 1000 insertions but are higher in the 6 to 8 weeks after delivery, so postpartum placement is delayed until a later visit (McCarthy, 2006).

Prior to placement of an IUD, the federally mandated patient information included with the IUD should be fully reviewed with the patient and formal written consent obtained after discussion of risks and benefits. Confirm a pregnancy test is negative, and consider placement during the first 5 to 7 days of her menstrual cycle. A pelvic examination must be performed before insertion to assess the uterine size and location and evaluate for current cervical infection. A prescription dose of an NSAID (e.g., ibuprofen 600-800 mg) should be provided 30 to 60 minutes before placement to help with analgesia. After placement, the patient may continue to use an NSAID for cramping and can expect to have some spotting for a few days. She should be willing to check for the IUD strings monthly to confirm proper retention.

KEY TREATMENT

IUDs have a failure rate less than 1% to 2% per year (SOR: A).
IUDs (e.g., Mirena) can be used during lactation and are not contraindicated in women with a history of venous thromboembolic events, those at increased risk of myocardial infarction or stroke, or those who smoke (SOR: A) (McCarthy, 2006).

Mirena

The Mirena IUD is a levonorgestrel-releasing IUC system placed for up to 5 years for extremely effective contraception. The levonorgestrel is released into the uterus, with minute amounts entering systemic circulation. Variable to no menstrual bleeding is the norm for patients after 3 to 6 months.

The Mirena device is supplied in its own delivery system aiding with placement. The patient is placed in a dorsal lithotomy position and a sterile speculum introduced into the vagina. The cervix and vaginal mucosa is cleansed with a chlorhexidine or povidone-iodine solution. A paracervical block can be placed as described earlier. The anterior or posterior cervix is grasped with a single toothed cervical tenaculum for stabilization of the cervix during the procedure. If normal, the uterus should be sounded to depths of 6.5 to 8.5 cm. If the uterus is sounded to a different depth, consider misplacement, cervical stenosis, or uterine perforation. The cervix can be dilated for placement, if significant stenosis is present.

Open the Mirena package, release the IUD threads, position the IUD arms, and position the flange at the proper sounded depth. Once in the same plane as the inserter system, retract the arms into the inserter by pulling on the strings at the end of the system and pushing forward on the green thumb slider. Lock the strings into the cleft at the end of the inserter. Insert the IUD system gently through the cervix into the uterus, but stop 1.5 to 2 cm before the fundus. Pull back on the thumb slider to the designated mark, and release the arms outward. Wait for 10 to 15 seconds to allow the arms to fully extend. Hold the slider with the thumb and advance the system fully forward to place the IUD arms against the uterine fundus. Now pull only the slider all the way outward to release the threads at the proximal end of the inserter, then remove the entire inserter system from the cervix, leaving behind the IUD with threads. Cut the two threads to a length of 3 to 5 cm. Remove the tenaculum and observe for any significant bleeding. Monsel's solution or pressure can be used for hemostasis. Remove the speculum, and give the patient instructions for follow-up visits and postinsertion care. **(See Tuggy Video: IUD insert.)**

Paragard T380A

The Paragard can be placed for up to 10 years and in a similar manner as the Mirena IUD. Patients should receive counseling and informed consent for the Paragard IUD, with specific warnings about contraindications in patients with Wilson's disease because of the copper content of the Paragard. Positioning of the patient, placement of the speculum, cleansing of the vagina and cervix, placement of the tenaculum, and uterine sounding are the same as described for the Mirena. However, the IUD arms are loaded differently into the Paragard inserter, folded backward with the distal arms inserted into the end of the inserter tube to lie next to the IUD shaft.

The IUD system is then inserted through the cervix to the uterine fundus. The white inserter plunger is held steady and the outside clear tube retracted 1 to 2 cm to release the arms. The clear tube is then advanced back to the fundus to assist in extending the arms and placing them in the apex of the fundus. The central plunger is then removed before the outside tube to prevent inadvertent removal of the IUD (Fig. 28-18). Once the inserter is removed, the two threads can be cut to 3 to 5 cm in length and the tenaculum and speculum removed, with hemostasis as needed. The patient is instructed in post-placement care and subsequent monthly cervical thread checks. Warning signs for infection, perforation, and bleeding are given. **(See Tuggy Video: IUD Insertion.)**

Removal

Removal of an IUD is quite simple for the majority of devices. An oral NSAID is beneficial to assist with analgesia. The patient is placed in a dorsal lithotomy position and a speculum placed in the vagina. The two IUD strings are identified and grasped with a ring forceps. The strings are gently pulled on, and the IUD should easily follow for removal. If the strings are not present, the IUD strings are generally just inside the cervical os. One can use a Cytobrush to dislodge the strings, attempt to grasp the strings in the os with a straight hemostat, or consider cervical dilation and use of an IUD hook or extractor for removal of the IUD. In some women the IUD may be malpositioned, and an ultrasound or plain abdominal film can locate the system for removal. If the IUD does not come out easily or is disconnected from the strings with the initial traction, hysteroscopy-assisted IUD removal may be necessary in a few rare cases.

Intradermal Contraceptive Device

Implanon is a device 4 cm long and 2 mm wide containing 68 mg of etonogestrel. It is inserted on the inner side of the nondominant upper arm above the medial epicondyle in a subdermal location for up to 3 years of contraception. Insertion should occur during the first week of a patient's menstrual cycle. The site for insertion is selected, marked, and locally anesthetized. The device is placed using a subdermal insertion trochar. Complications from insertion are 1% and from removal 1.7%. Irregular bleeding is the most common side effect (11% of patients). The manufacturer requires providers to complete a 3-hour comprehensive training program, which should be completed before device placement (www.implanon-usa.com).

Bartholin's Gland Abscess or Cyst

The Bartholin's glands are located between the hymen and labia minora bilaterally at the 4 and 8 o'clock positions. *Cysts* occur when the duct is blocked from trauma or edema, and *abscesses* occur when retained secretions become infected. Abscesses are frequently surrounded by some level of cellulitis of the tissues and can be very painful and indurated. Treatment relies on drainage of the cyst or abscess, treatment of any associated cellulitis with oral antibiotics if indicated, and creation of a track that eventually epithelializes, allowing normal gland drainage and reduced recurrence.

For drainage, the patient is placed in the dorsal lithotomy position and the cyst or abscess identified in the introitus in

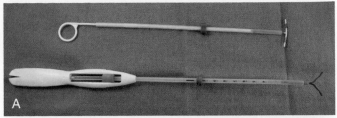
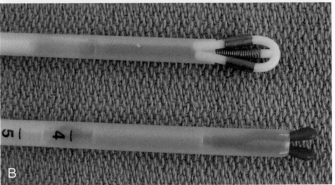

Figure 28-18 A, Paragard T380A is displayed above Mirena. Note that both intrauterine devices have IUD arms extended. **B,** End of Paragard T380A is displayed above end of Mirena with both IUDs having arms fully retracted in opposite directions and ready for placement.

the area of maximal swelling and fluctuance. Topical anesthesia can be used on the surface or a local anesthetic injected under the mass for patient comfort. The cyst wall is grasped through the mucosal surface with two clamps 3 to 5 mm apart and a #11 blade used to puncture and open the site. The contained fluid is removed and cultured. The cyst can be packed with gauze, but recurrence is frequent. To prevent recurrence, a Word catheter can be placed into the open cyst or abscess. The catheter is a latex stem attached to an inflatable balloon. The catheter is inserted into the incision between the clamps, with care taken to place it in the center of the cyst wall. The balloon is then filled with 2 to 3 mL of normal saline and left in place for 4 to 6 weeks until epithelialization of the track occurs. The catheter can then be removed. If the incision was done inside the hymen ring, the catheter end can be tucked into the vagina for comfort during the healing process. **(See Tuggy Video: Bartholin's Cyst Word Catheter Placement.)**

Colposcopy

Colposcopically directed cervical biopsy and cervical curettage is primarily used to investigate abnormal findings on routine pelvic examination or an abnormal Pap smear. Consensus guidelines for the management of cervical intraepithelial neoplasia (CIN) have been developed (Wright et al., 2007). Colposcopy requires diligent record keeping and patient communication with follow-up arranged pending pathologic results. Contraindications to colposcopy are current infection and delivery within the preceding 6 weeks. Pregnancy does not preclude colposcopy but may impact the decision to biopsy the cervix or perform endocervical curettage based on increased bleeding and miscarriage risks. A pregnancy test is best performed before a biopsy is contemplated. Patients should receive informed consent and understand the risk and benefits as well as their responsibility to follow up based on exam findings.

Colposcopy is performed with a stereoscopic operating microscope with correct focal length. The patient is placed in the dorsal lithotomy position. The vulva and introitus are inspected for lesions. A speculum is placed in the vagina, with the size selected to maximize visualization of the cervix and minimize patient discomfort. The vaginal canal and cervix are visualized and any abnormal lesions of concern noted. Acetic acid (3%-5%) is applied to the vaginal canal and cervix liberally with a cotton swab. Abnormal areas will display as acetowhite or leukoplakia with the acetic acid and may also show signs of punctation, mosaicism, or frank abnormal changes of superficial vessels. A green light filter can assist with visualizing atypical vascular changes. Lugol's solution can also be applied to improve identification of abnormal tissue, taken up by glycogen in normal mature squamous cells and not by dysplastic, metaplastic, or columnar epithelial tissues. Any findings are recorded in a drawing to correlate with biopsy sites or abnormal pathology. Satisfactory examination includes full visualization of the entire transformation zone between squamous and columnar epithelium at the cervical os. Most pathology is located in this zone. An endocervical speculum can be used to assist in visualization. Types of future treatment for any lesion seen should be considered and noted for ease in planning future management.

Endocervical Curettage

Endocervical curettage frequently precedes external cervical biopsies so as not to cross-contaminate the specimens. Endocervical lesions can require much more extensive and invasive treatment. Endocervical sampling is done if the cause for the abnormal Pap smear is not identified or if an ectocervical lesion extends into the cervical canal. An endocervical curette is placed into the cervix with the sharp edge against the wall of the canal. The curette is then drawn back and forth against the cervical canal in a 360-degree sampling twice around. The sample removed can be retrieved with an endocervical brush and sent for pathologic assessment separate from any other specimens. Endocervical curettage is contraindicated in pregnant patients. (**See Tuggy Video: Colposcopy.**)

Cervical Biopsy

If abnormal areas are identified on the ectocervix, a correlation for consistency with Pap results is required. A biopsy of the abnormal areas identified by the colposcope can be undertaken using a Kevorkian or Tischler biopsy forceps. To aid in visualization and prevent cross-contamination, biopsies are done on the posterior cervix first, followed by the anterior aspect. The fixed end of the biopsy forceps is usually placed into the cervical os, and biopsies are done in a radial orientation to obtain a sampling of the squamocolumnar transition zone in the area of concern. Samples should be deep enough to include the epithelial surface and a small amount of underlying stroma.

Once biopsies are completed, hemostasis is best achieved with use of a Monsel's paste applied with a cotton applicator or silver nitrate sticks. The vagina is wiped of remaining debris and the speculum withdrawn. The patient is instructed to use analgesics as needed, to abstain from intercourse or tampon use for 10 to 14 days, and to expect some intermittent spotting. Any excessive bleeding, fever, discharge, or significant pelvic pain should warrant a return visit and assessment and treatment of the cause. Confirm a method of contact with the patient and relay the results and treatment recommendations when the pathologic results return.

Endometrial Biopsy

An endometrial biopsy can be performed to evaluate abnormal uterine bleeding in women who are premenopausal or postmenopausal in conjunction with ultrasound. It can also be used to assess for a short luteal phase in infertility and abnormal or atypical glandular cells seen on Pap smear in women over 40. Women with spontaneous postmenopausal bleeding and an endometrial thickness greater than 5 mm should be further evaluated with an endometrial biopsy (Amann et al., 2006).

A number of endometrial biopsy devices are available; the disposable flexible plastic aspirator is easiest to use. This aspirator can be used with most women and even those with mild cervical stenosis. Before biopsy, a pregnancy test should be completed if the patient is of childbearing age and an oral NSAID given. The patient is placed in the dorsal lithotomy position, and uterine size and location and any pelvic abnormalities are assessed. A speculum is placed to allow full visualization of the cervical os. The vaginal canal and cervix are cleansed with a chlorhexidine or povidone-iodine solution, and a single-toothed tenaculum is placed on the anterior cervix to aid in stabilization later. A paracervical block can be placed for patient comfort.

Once the preparation is complete, the aspirator is inserted into the cervical os using the tenaculum to straighten the cervical canal as needed. It is advanced to the fundus, and then the central plunger is retracted to create intrauterine negative pressure for suction of endometrial contents. The aspirator catheter is then withdrawn to the lower uterine segment and advanced again repetitively to the fundus and rotated to sample all aspects of the uterine body cavity. The catheter is then removed from the uterus. Endometrial cells and blood will have entered the aspirator catheter and can be sent for pathologic examination. The tenaculum and speculum are then removed and withdrawn. The patient may experience uterine cramping and bleeding for a few days and should refrain from intercourse until this resolves. Excessive bleeding, fever, or pelvic pain warrants immediate evaluation in the postoperative period. Pathology results are discussed with the patient when available and any treatment arranged as needed. If the sample is insufficient, the patient should be triaged to a transvaginal ultrasound in a low-risk group, with full dilation and curettage for any high-risk patients (Brand et al., 2000). (**See Tuggy Video: Endometrial Biopsy.**)

KEY TREATMENT

An endometrial biopsy can be performed with ultrasound to evaluate abnormal uterine bleeding in premenopausal or postmenopausal women.

Women with spontaneous postmenopausal bleeding and an endometrial thickness >5 mm should be further evaluated with an endometrial biopsy (Amann et al., 2006) (SOR: B).

If the endometrial sample is insufficient., the patient should be triaged to a transvaginal ultrasound in a low-risk group, with dilation and curettage for high-risk patients (Brand et al., 2000) (SOR: B).

Cervical Polyp Removal

Cervical polyps are generally benign, asymptomatic, and noted most often during a routine gynecologic examination. Most polyps arise from the endocervical mucosa, and most occur in perimenopausal women age 30 to 50. For their removal, the patient is placed in the dorsal lithotomy position and a speculum inserted vaginally. A Pap smear should be obtained and the base of the polyp identified to prevent inadvertent removal of a prolapsed endometrial polyp. The polyp is then grasped as close to its base as possible with a ring forceps and twisted. This twisting motion will dislodge the polyp, which should be sent for pathologic assessment. Hemostasis is obtained with Monsel's solution or silver nitrate sticks if direct pressure is not sufficient. (See Tuggy Video: Polyp Removal.)

Uterine Aspiration for Biopsy or Miscarriage Management

Manual vacuum aspiration (MVA) can be used in the office setting for easy sampling of the uterine endometrium with a 4-mm or 5-mm cannula when a small endometrial biopsy catheter is insufficient (Fig. 28-19). The MVA can also be used in the office for removal of retained products of conception after an incomplete or missed miscarriage up to 12 weeks without the added cost of an emergency room visit, surgical suite, and general anesthesia. The MVA device is a hand-held plastic aspirator syringe attached to a plastic cannula of varying sizes. The cannula can be flexible or rigid to allow for provider preference. Vacuum aspiration is safe, quick to perform and less painful than sharp curettage and should be recommended for use in the management of incomplete abortion (Forna and Gulmezoglu, 2001).

Confirmation of a non-viable pregnancy or incomplete abortion is verified with a falling serum β-hCG level, an appropriately timed ultrasound, or by clinical findings of uterine bleeding in pregnancy with significant cervical dilation in the first trimester. A blood type is obtained to determine if Rho-GAM is necessary. A hematocrit may be obtained if bleeding has been significant. Once informed consent outlining the risks of bleeding, pelvic infection, uterine perforation, Asherman's adhesions, and possible need for reaspiration is obtained, the patient may receive a sedative, analgesia, or anesthesia. Most women do well with an oral NSAID for analgesia and a paracervical block for local anesthesia. For comfort, the patient should void before the procedure.

The patient is placed in the dorsal lithotomy position, and uterine size, location, and shape are assessed. A transvaginal or transabdominal ultrasound can be performed at this time to confirm findings but is not required. A speculum is placed intravaginally, vagina and cervix are cleansed, and a paracervical block is placed before the procedure. A single-toothed tenaculum is placed on the anterior cervix.

The uterus is sounded to the fundus to determine intracavitary size and position. If not already dilated, the cervical os is successively dilated to a size in millimeters corresponding to the gestational age, using Denniston, Pratt, or Hegar dilators. The MVA curette is generally chosen in millimeters to correspond to the gestational age in weeks as well. Thumb buttons are used to occlude the opening to the MVA barrel, and the plunger is retracted and allowed to snap into place

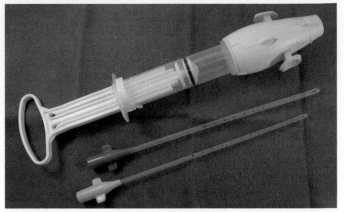

Figure 28-19 The Ipas manual vacuum aspirator (MVA) is displayed with 4-mm and 5-mm cannulas used for miscarriage management in outpatient setting. Note thumb buttons that close the barrel entrance to hold negative pressure in the canister when the plunger is retracted. The buttons are then released to transfer the suction pressure to the cannula once in place.

to develop the negative pressure for suction. The cannula is attached to the MVA and placed through the cervix to the uterine fundus. The thumb buttons on each side are released, and the negative suction from the syringe is transferred to the endometrial cavity. The MVA barrel can be rotated and then brought in and out in a piston motion to dislodge the remaining products of conception. These can be observed passing through the cannula and can be evaluated fully by visual or pathologic examination after the procedure. The syringe may need to be emptied and the negative pressure reapplied based on the volume of the uterine contents. A sensation of grittiness is present in the fundus and all four uterine quadrants when the products of conception are completely removed and the cannula makes contact with the myometrium.

On completion, the MVA cannula is removed from the uterus, tenaculum from the cervix, and speculum from the vagina. The patient is observed for 15 to 30 minutes to assess for excessive bleeding, hemodynamic stability, and unusual pain. Intrarectal or intravaginal misoprostol, intracervical or intramuscular methylergonovine, and intramuscular carboprost may be used for excessive bleeding. The patient may be discharged and instructed to refrain from intercourse for 2 weeks or until the bleeding resolves. She should return for excessive bleeding, significant pelvic or abdominal pain, and fever. A form of contraception is provided if the patient desires.

Breast Mass

In a patient who presents with a breast mass, a careful clinical and family history with focused physical examination, a mammogram or ultrasound, and fine-needle aspiration of the mass is termed a *triple test*. Most primary care physicians can perform the triple test with radiologic assistance for the evaluation of a breast mass. A positive triple test (indeterminate, suspicious, or malignant) was found in 99.6% of breast cancers. On the other hand, if all three test components are negative and the patient is deemed low risk by personal or family history, the patient requires no further workup and has a less than 1% risk of cancer (National Breast Cancer Centre, 2006).

Breast Cyst Aspiration

When a discrete breast mass is first discovered, a determination of solid or cystic must be made to assist with further evaluative decisions. A rapid determination can be made with one of two methods. Ultrasound can be used to identify a cystic or solid mass rapidly with minimal discomfort to the patient. If ultrasound is not available or if a therapeutic intervention is needed for drainage of a palpated cyst, a breast cyst aspiration can be performed.

The patient can be placed in a recumbent position and the skin over the breast cleansed. The mass is stabilized between the thumb and index and middle fingers on the nondominant hand. Anesthesia can be used locally, but most women feel minimal discomfort. A 1.5-inch, 20- to 23-gauge needle is attached to a 10- to 30-mL syringe. The skin is punctured and the end of the needle directed into the mass with continuous suction on the syringe. The fluid of a cyst is aspirated completely before the needle is removed. Fluid should be sent for pathologic evaluation. Straw- to green-colored fluid is usually benign, and bloody brown to red fluid is more suspicious for malignancy. If bloody fluid is obtained in an atraumatic aspirate or if a lump remains, the patient should be referred for a core needle or open biopsy. (**See Tuggy Video: Breast Cyst Aspiration.**)

KEY TREATMENT

Vacuum aspiration is safe, quick to perform, and less painful than sharp curettage and recommended in the management of incomplete abortion (Forna and Gulmezoglu, 2001) (SOR: B).

The triple test of (1) careful clinical examination, (2) mammogram or ultrasound, and (3) fine-needle aspiration of a breast mass approaches the false-negative rate of surgical breast biopsy and the false-positive rate of frozen section (National Breast Cancer Centre, 2006) (SOR: B).

If bloody fluid is obtained on an atraumatic breast mass aspirate or if a lump remains after drainage, the patient is referred for surgical consult for core or open biopsy (National Breast Cancer Centre, 2006) (SOR: B).

Fine-Needle Aspiration Cytology or Biopsy

Fine-needle aspiration (FNA) can be performed in the office with minimal equipment for diagnosis of a discrete, solid breast mass. FNA testing results in a sensitivity of 90% and a false-negative rate of 3% to 10% in experienced hands (Valea and Katz, 2007). Contraindications include an overlying skin infection, underlying pulsatile mass, and a history of bleeding disorders.

The patient is properly given informed consent. She is recumbent in position, and the area of puncture is identified, marked, and cleansed. A local injection of 1 to 2 mL of anesthetic is infiltrated into the skin over the mass. The mass is stabilized with the three-finger technique previously mentioned. A 10- to 20-mL syringe with 18- to 22-guage needle attached is advanced into the mass. Full aspiration suction is performed, and the needle is passed through the mass in different planes three to five times for an adequate sample. The suction is released and the needle removed. The cell sample, frequently only in the needle itself, is placed on a cytology slide and fixed for proper pathologic assessment.

FNA provides histologic diagnosis but cannot determine architectural features. FNA should not be used to investigate microcalcifications, and it cannot distinguish ductal carcinoma in situ from invasive cancer. A core or open biopsy should be performed in these patients for more definitive diagnosis before excision or definitive treatment. (**See Tuggy Video: Needle Aspiration.**)

Neonatal Circumcision

Circumcision has been used in religious rites for centuries and was used in ancient Egypt as a method for hygiene. Modern data in the United States is conflicting as to the benefits versus risks. By age 5 years, 90% of boys have a spontaneously retractable foreskin. The incidence of phimosis decreases with age and may be treated with a steroid cream. The medical approach to phimosis is initially successful in about 80% of cases and a year later 60% had no phimosis (Ku and Huen, 2007). Many parents still elect to have their male infants circumcised.

The American Urological Association revised their policy to say that circumcision should be presented for health benefits (Tobian et al., 2010). The American Academy of Pediatrics, American Medical Association, and American College of Obstetrics and Gynecology all consider the procedure elective with minimal benefits (Lannon et al., 1999). The WHO–United Nations program on HIV/AIDS concluded that male circumcision is efficacious in reducing sexual transmission of HIV from women to men. In Africa, circumcision decreased HIV acquisition by 53% to 60%. Herpesvirus type 2 is decreased by 28% to 34% and HPV prevalence by 32% to 35% in circumcised men. Among female partners of circumcised men in these African studies, the incidence of bacterial vaginosis was reduced by 40% and *Trichomonas vaginalis* by 48%; genital ulcers decreased as well (Tobian et al., 2010).

The incidence of urinary tract infection (UTI) is reduced with circumcision in some populations. If a population has a baseline UTI incidence of 3% or higher and circumcision complication rate less than 2%, circumcision is helpful in reducing UTIs. In normal infants the risk of UTI is 1% or less, in those with prior UTI 10%, and in those with vesicoureteral reflux 30% (Singh-Grewal, 2005). The main risk is bleeding, followed by infection. Actual rates of hemorrhage in medically indicated or ritual hospital-based circumcision range from 0.2% to 3% (Bocquet et al., 2010).

Although numbers may be declining in some U.S. areas, circumcision remains one of the most common procedures performed. A neonatal circumcision is normally performed at 12 to 48 hours old once the infant has stabilized after birth, but may be performed up to 4 to 6 weeks of age. Before the procedure, each patient should be examined thoroughly for signs of congenital anomalies of the penis, urethra, or urinary tract. If hypospadias is present, circumcision is stopped or not performed, to allow the tissue to be used in a corrective surgical procedure to repair the urethra and glans.

Many locations recommend no oral intake for 1 hour before the procedure to prevent aspiration. Oral sucrose can be used to reduce pain during the procedure (Gatti, 2003). A dorsal penile block or penile ring block is more effective then EMLA cream or sucrose. EMLA cream provides anesthesia but has a risk of methemoglobinemia (Brady-Fryer et al., 2010).

Inspect first to make sure there is no hypospadias or hidden penis. If the penis is normal and parental consent has been obtained, the infant is placed on a circumcision restraint board and the skin prepared. A dorsal block is achieved by injecting 0.4 to 0.5 mL of 1% lidocaine without epinephrine at the base of the penile shaft at both the 10 and 2 o'clock positions and 5 mm distal to the skin reflection onto the pubic area. Inject 1 to 3 mm deep under Buck's fascia after aspirating to ensure you are not in a blood vessel. A ring block can also be done, slightly higher on the penile shaft circumferentially in the subcutaneous tissues, taking care to avoid injury to the urethra or vasculature (Fig. 28-20).

Once anesthesia is complete, grasp the foreskin distally at 3 and 9 o'clock with two hemostats. All techniques require freeing of adhesions with blunt dissection, usually done with a straight Kelly clamp inserted between the foreskin and glans in a superior direction to avoid the urethra. Open the clamp and sweep laterally. Avoid the highly vascular frenulum. Free the adhesions to the coronal sulcus of the glans. Use a straight hemostat to clamp the free dorsal foreskin, again making sure the tip is held up and away from entering the urethra. Clamp three-fourths the length of the foreskin dorsally. Insert iris scissors and carefully cut the foreskin along the crushed line. Peel the foreskin back to reveal the glans. Avoid degloving the shaft and damage to the frenulum.

Gomco Clamp

The Gomco is the most common circumcision clamp. Test the clamp's fit with the base before use. Estimate the correct size so that the bell covers at least seven-eighths of the glans (1.1, 1.3, and 1.5 sizes available). The glans is then covered with the Gomco bell and the foreskin pulled over it, sometimes with the aid of a clamp or safety pin. The bell and foreskin are then pulled through the hole in the base plate and the foreskin is arranged to ensure even tissue removal. The clamp is than placed on the base plate and the bell stem hooked over the clamp bar. Once positioning is confirmed, the clamp is tightened for 5 to 10 minutes and the remaining foreskin removed with a #10 scalpel. If hemostasis is confirmed, the clamp is removed and the glans is covered regularly with petroleum jelly at each diaper change. Healing should take 4 to 10 days. Complications include bleeding, infection, and trauma to the penis. Bleeding can be controlled with silver nitrate or a simple suture if not resolved with pressure. **(See Tuggy Video: Neonatal Circumcision.)**

Plastibell

The Plastibell device is a plastic ring on the end of a central removable post. The ring is placed between the glans and foreskin. A tight ligature of moistened suture is placed around the foreskin and tightened into a sulcus on the ring. Foreskin distal to the ring is excised and the handle of the device broken off. The plastic ring stays in place, with the ligature tied tightly around the protective ring, for 5 to 10 days and falls off spontaneously. The appearance of the small amount of necrotic skin may worry parents, and it may be

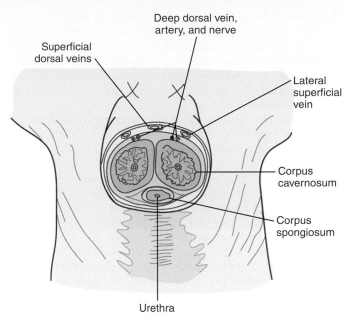

Figure 28-20 Dorsal penile block. The dorsal penile nerve is anesthetized using no more than 1.0 mL total of 1% lidocaine without epinephrine. The anesthetic is administered at the dorsum of the penis approximately 0.5 cm distal to the penile root at the 12 and 2 o'clock positions.
(From Pfenninger JL, Fowler G [eds]: Procedures for Primary Care Physicians, 2nd ed. St Louis, Mosby, 2003; and Chavez MC, Maker VK. Office surgery. In Rakel RE. Textbook of Family Medicine, 7th ed. Saunders-Elsevier, Philadelphia, 2007.)

complicated with incomplete or irregular skin edges if the ligature is not tied tightly enough.

Mogan Clamp

The Mogan clamp is used in traditional Jewish circumcisions and may cause less pain by being faster. The foreskin is grasped with the nondominant hand and the glans pushed downward. The foreskin is slid into the clamp from anterior to posterior, taking care not to trap the glans. The clamp opens only 3 mm to prevent major glans entrapment. Once in place and the glans is confirmed below the plate, the clamp is closed and the distal foreskin removed. The clamp is left in place for a few minutes, then removed, and the foreskin retracted over the glans.

KEY TREATMENT

Oral sucrose reduces painful procedures in infants (Gatti, 2003) (SOR: A).

Dorsal penile block or penile ring blocks are more effective than EMLA cream or sucrose (Brady-Fryer et al., 2010) (SOR: A).

EMLA cream provides anesthesia but has a risk of methemoglobinemia (Brady-Fryer et al., 2010) (SOR: A)

Musculoskeletal Office Procedures

Aspiration of Knee Joint (Arthrocentesis)

The knee is one of the largest and most accessible joints for arthrocentesis or joint injection. Aspiration of joint fluid from the knee is performed to assess for infection, inflammation, crystal deposition, or traumatic complications. Infections may show a significantly high white blood cell infiltrate with visible organisms on Gram stain. Inflammation may show the same without organisms seen. Crystal disease may show urate or calcium pyrophosphate crystals. Trauma may produce a bloody aspirate with tears of a ligament or cartilage and fat lobules with an intra-articular fracture.

Prior to the aspiration, the patient is consented and placed in a recumbent position with the knee flexed slightly with a rolled towel. The knee is assessed for effusion and the aspiration site marked and cleansed with a sterilizing wash. The knee joint space can be entered with a 22-gauge needle on a syringe on either side, but usually from the lateral aspect 1 cm lateral and superior to the patella, and directed 45 degrees downward angling under the patella, with aspiration done during insertion. When the joint space is entered, fluid should enter the syringe rapidly. Milking the lateral and medial recesses of the knee toward the needle tip will remove more fluid. The needle is removed after aspiration, or it is left in place and the syringe changed under sterile conditions for a steroid injection to follow, if necessary. Large joints can be injected with 20 to 40 mg of triamcinolone or 6 to 12 mg of betamethasone with 3 to 6 mL of 1% lidocaine for inflammatory conditions unrelated to infections. Procedural risks include septic arthritis, mild injury to the articular cartilage, and hemarthrosis. **(See Tuggy Video: Knee Aspiration.)**

Shoulder Injection

The subacromial bursa is another location frequently treated with steroid injection for bursitis or tendonitis. Injections of 10 to 20 mg of triamcinolone with 2 to 4 mL of lidocaine can be performed into the subacromial bursa. The easiest approach to the subacromial space is with the patient seated comfortably and arms resting at the side. The lateral shoulder is prepared with a sterile solution after palpating landmarks. The acromial process is identified on the lateral shoulder above the humeral head. In the sulcus between the humeral head and the acromial process lies the subacromial bursa. Marking the lateral border of the acromial process can provide some assistance. A 22- to 25-gauge needle on a syringe with the injection is then aimed directly into the sulcus between the bones 1 cm below the acromial process perpendicularly through the deltoid muscle. Ligamentous or muscular structures will resist injection, but the bursa should allow free infusion. Relief of pain may be noted in a few minutes if lidocaine is used and confirms the injection was placed appropriately. **(See Tuggy Video: Joint Injection—Shoulder.)**

References

The complete reference list is available online at www.expertconsult.com.

Web Resources

www.cdc.gov/rabies/exposure/postexposure.html
    Centers for Disease Control and Prevention website has advice on rabies prophylaxis for animal bites.
www.cdc.gov/mmwr/preview/mmwrhtml/rr5011a1.htm#tab3
    CDC website has details from the 2001 postexposure prophylaxis (PEP) guidelines.
www.mdconsult.com/das/book/body
www.npinstitute.com
    Postgraduate procedural skills training.

www.proceduresconsult.com/medical-procedures/
    Procedural training and videos.
www.nejm.org/multimedia/medical-videos
    Procedural education and videos.
http://emedicine.medscape.com/clinical_procedures
    Information on additional procedures, including those covered in this chapter
www.mpcenter.net/
    Excellent patient education materials.

CHAPTER 29

Sports Medicine

Jonathan A. Drezner, Kimberly G. Harmon, and John W. O'Kane

Chapter contents

Sports medicine involves the care of patients with illnesses and injuries related to sports and exercise. Both orthopedic and medical conditions affect a wide spectrum of patients during sports and recreational activities. The field of primary care sports medicine has emerged over the last 30 years as a leader in the comprehensive care of athletes, teams, and exercising individuals. Although sports medicine is often viewed in the context of professional and elite athletes, the principles and practice of sports medicine apply to athletes of all levels and ages.

The role of a sports medicine physician is to promote the health and safety of exercising individuals, prevent injury and illness, optimize function, and minimize disability that would preclude sports participation. Sports medicine physicians work closely with a multidisciplinary team of health care providers (specialty physicians and surgeons, athletic trainers, physical therapists, nutritionists, psychologists, and conditioning coaches) to satisfy the complete medical needs of athletes.

Sports medicine includes a rapidly expanding core of knowledge related to medical issues in sports and exercise for which the primary care sports medicine physician is uniquely trained. *Primary care sports medicine* is a subspecialty designation obtained through completion of an accredited sports medicine fellowship and passing the Certificate of Added Qualification examination. Many practicing primary care providers also gain vast experience in sports medicine through office treatment of orthopedic injuries, event coverage, and preparticipation screening evaluations.

Musculoskeletal problems account for up to 20% of all primary care office visits (Urwin et al., 1998; Woodwell and Cherry, 2004), and approximately 90% of all sports injuries are treated nonsurgically. Thus, a sound clinical foundation in the evaluation and treatment of musculoskeletal disorders is critical to primary care providers and helps guide appropriate referral to orthopedic and rehabilitative specialists.

This chapter focuses on both the medical aspects of sports medicine and common orthopedic injuries in athletes. Detailed reviews cover the preparticipation physical evaluation, cardiac disorders in athletes, concussion assessment and management, cervical spine injuries, on-the-field assessment of the injured athlete, facial trauma, environmental influences such as exertional heat illness, common infections in athletes, and a systems-based review of dermatologic, pulmonary, hematologic, gastrointestinal, and genitourinary disorders in athletes. Orthopedic areas common in primary care sports medicine are also included, such as athletic low back pain, muscle strains, tendinopathy, shin pain, stress fractures, and issues unique to the pediatric or female athlete. See Chapters 30 and 31 for a comprehensive review of additional musculoskeletal problems relevant to sports medicine and the care of exercising individuals.

Preparticipation Physical Evaluation

Key Points

- The primary objective of the preparticipation physical evaluation is to detect preexisting medical or musculoskeletal conditions that predispose an athlete to injury, disability, or catastrophic injury.
- Syncope that occurs during exercise is a serious warning sign and warrants a comprehensive cardiology evaluation to rule out an underlying cardiac disorder that predisposes to sudden death.
- Any athlete with a systolic murmur of grade 3/6 in severity, a murmur that gets louder with a Valsalva maneuver or on standing (suspicious for hypertrophic cardiomyopathy), a diastolic murmur, a family history of premature sudden cardiac death, or concerning exertional symptoms should be further evaluated by a cardiovascular specialist.

A preparticipation physical evaluation (PPE), or "sports physical," is frequently required for medical clearance before participation in organized sports. The *Preparticipation Physical Evaluation* monograph, first introduced in 1992, provides recommendations for the content and format of the evaluation (AAFP et al., 2005). The third edition of the monograph, updated in 2005, is supported by six national medical societies: American Academy of Family Physicians (AAFP), American Academy of Pediatrics, American College of Sports Medicine, American Medical Society for Sports Medicine, American Orthopaedic Society for Sports Medicine, and American Osteopathic Academy of Sports Medicine. The fourth edition published in 2010 also includes collaboration with the American Heart Association (AHA) regarding the preparticipation cardiovascular evaluation.

The primary objectives of the PPE include the following:
1. Detection of potentially life-threatening or disabling medical or musculoskeletal conditions before athletic clearance.
2. Identification of preexisting conditions that may predispose athletes to injury.

3. Satisfying legal or administrative requirements.

Secondary objectives of the PPE include the following:
1. Promoting the health and safety of athletes in training and competition.
2. Serving as an entry point into the health care system for adolescents.
3. Providing an opportunity for a general health assessment.

The recommended frequency of the PPE varies widely according to the requirements of the specific school, organization, or state. AHA first published consensus recommendations for cardiovascular screening in athletes in 1996 and reaffirmed these recommendations in 2007, which have influenced the format and timing of the PPE (Maron et al., 1996b, 2007). A comprehensive PPE is recommended on entry into middle school, high school, and college before participation in competitive sports. For youth and high school athletes, a comprehensive PPE should be repeated every 2 years. For years not requiring a comprehensive PPE, annual updates consisting of a comprehensive history and determination of height, weight, and blood pressure, along with a problem-focused evaluation of new concerns, illnesses, or injuries, should occur on interval years for youth and high school athletes and on all subsequent years for college athletes.

The PPE history focuses on symptoms related to exercise, such as exertional syncope, lightheadedness, chest pain, palpitations, dyspnea, wheezing, or fatigue with less than expected activity (Box 29-1). A past medical history of preexisting cardiac or pulmonary conditions, murmurs, hypertension, coronary artery disease risk factors, asthma, concussions, illicit drug use, prior orthopedic injuries, or other medical conditions that place an athlete at risk of injury should be noted. Specific questions to identify a family history of premature death, cardiovascular disease, and hereditary cardiac disorders, such as hypertrophic cardiomyopathy, Marfan's syndrome, and long QT syndrome, are also recommended.

The PPE examination consists of both medical and musculoskeletal components. The cardiovascular examination is a major focus of the medical evaluation and consists of a blood pressure measurement, palpation of the radial and femoral artery pulses, cardiac auscultation with the patient both supine and standing, and recognition of the physical manifestations of Marfan's syndrome (Maron et al., 1996b; Maron et al., 2007). Any heart murmur detected should be further assessed during the Valsalva maneuver or while moving the patient from a squatting to a standing position. These maneuvers decrease venous return and may accentuate the murmur of hypertrophic cardiomyopathy, the leading cause of sudden cardiac death in young athletes. However, hypertrophic cardiomyopathy is difficult to detect on examination alone because outflow tract obstruction, which causes the harsh systolic murmur, is present in only about 25% of patients with the disorder (Maron, 1997) (Fig. 29-1).

The musculoskeletal assessment serves as a screening evaluation of the spine and upper and lower extremities. Joint range of motion, strength, and stability should be tested. Several functional tests, such as hopping, squatting, and "duck walking," assess many anatomic areas at once and make the evaluation more efficient. Previous orthopedic injuries can also be evaluated in more detail to detect problems that require further rehabilitation or protective bracing before sports participation.

Box 29-1 Prepartication Physical Evaluation (PPE): Cardiovascular History Questions

- Have you ever passed out or nearly passed out during or after exercise?
- Have you ever had discomfort, pain, pressure, or tightness in your chest during exercise?
- Do you get lightheaded or feel more short of breath than expected during exercise?
- Does your heart ever race or skip beats (irregular beats) during exercise?
- Has a doctor ever told you that you have a heart problem, high blood pressure, high cholesterol, a heart murmur, a heart infection, Kawasaki's disease, or an unexplained seizure disorder?
- Has a doctor ever ordered a test for your heart, for example, an ECG or echocardiogram?
- Has any family member or relative died of heart problems or had an unexpected or unexplained sudden death before age 50 (including drowning, motor vehicle crash, or sudden infant death syndrome)?
- Has anyone in your family had unexplained fainting, seizures, or near-drowning?
- Does anyone in your family have a heart problem, pacemaker, or implanted defibrillator?
- Does anyone in your family have hypertrophic cardiomyopathy, Marfan's syndrome, arrhythmogenic right ventricular cardiomyopathy, long QT syndrome, short QT syndrome, Brugada syndrome, or catecholaminergic polymorphic ventricular tachycardia?

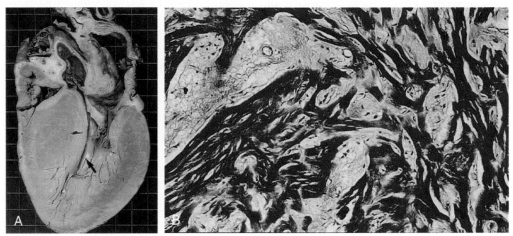

Figure 29-1 Hypertrophic cardiomyopathy. **A,** Gross appearance; **B,** histologic appearance. Note the myocardial fiber disarray. *(From Braunwald E. Essential Atlas of Heart Diseases, 3rd ed. Philadelphia, Current Medicine, 2000.)*

Warning Symptoms in Athletes

Warning or "red flag" symptoms that may indicate the presence of an underlying cardiovascular disorder should be recognized and further assessed before medical clearance. Syncope that occurs during but not after exercise is of great concern and warrants a comprehensive cardiology evaluation to rule out the presence of an occult cardiac disorder that may lead to sudden death. Other worrying symptoms include palpitations, chest pain, lightheadedness, and fatigue or dyspnea greater than expected for the level of activity. Athletes with warning symptoms should be evaluated by an electrocardiogram (ECG), echocardiogram, and exercise stress test and referred to a cardiologist. In addition, systolic murmurs of grade 3/6 in severity, all diastolic murmurs, any murmur that becomes louder with a Valsalva maneuver or on standing (suspicious for hypertrophic cardiomyopathy), and a concerning family history of premature sudden cardiac death or hereditary cardiac disorder should be further evaluated by a cardiovascular specialist.

If a cardiac abnormality is identified, the decision to withhold medical clearance for participation in competitive sports is difficult and should be carefully considered on an individual basis. The American College of Cardiology 36th Bethesda Conference defined eligibility recommendations for athletes with cardiovascular abnormalities (Maron and Zipes, 2005).

Limitations of Cardiovascular Screening

Despite efforts to standardize the format and approach to the PPE, several limitations of the screening process still exist. In 2007, only 19% of U.S. states used forms that were considered adequate by AHA, and 35% of states allowed practitioners with limited cardiovascular training to perform the evaluation (Glover et al., 2007). Unfortunately, recommendations to use a comprehensive personal and family questionnaire to guide the PPE are not widely adopted, and recommended screening protocols are often incompletely or inadequately implemented. In addition, the PPE is screening for medical conditions that place an athlete at increased risk of sudden death, and no outcomes-based research has demonstrated that the PPE is effective in preventing sudden death or potentially catastrophic events, or for identifying athletes at risk. A complicating feature of the screening process is that athletes who harbor underlying structural heart disease may be asymptomatic until the sudden cardiac arrest. In a review of 134 cases of sudden cardiac death, only

18% of athletes had symptoms of cardiovascular disease in the 3 years before their death, and only 3% were suspected of having a cardiovascular condition after PPE (Maron et al., 1996a).

Limitations in the traditional screening process have led to widespread debate regarding the addition of noninvasive cardiovascular screening techniques, such as electrocardiography (ECG), to the PPE. In 2007, AHA reaffirmed recommendations against universal ECG screening in athletes, citing a low prevalence of disease, poor sensitivity, high false-positive rate, poor cost-effectiveness, and a lack of clinicians to interpret the results (Maron et al., 2007). In contrast, the European Society of Cardiology, International Olympic Committee, and the governing associations of several U.S. and international professional sports leagues endorse the use of ECG in the screening of athletes (Corrado et al., 2006; Ljungqvist et al., 2009). These recommendations are supported by studies showing that ECG is more sensitive than history and physical examination alone in identifying athletes with underlying cardiovascular disease, including a 77% greater power to detect hypertrophic cardiomyopathy (Corrado et al., 1998).

In 2006, Corrado and associates reported results from screening 42,386 athletes over 25 years from the national PPE program in Italy. Disqualification on the basis of a screening protocol using history, physical examination, and ECG produced a 10-fold reduction in the incidence of sudden cardiac death in young competitive athletes and an 89% reduction of sudden death from cardiomyopathy. Although only 0.2% of athletes were disqualified for potentially lethal cardiovascular conditions, the study reported a 7% false-positive rate and a 2% overall disqualification rate. This raised concerns that adopting such a program in the United States would lead to an unacceptable number of disqualifications in athletes with a low risk of sudden death.

Complex issues regarding feasibility, cost-effectiveness, appropriate physician, and healthy system infrastructure remain before large-scale implementation of ECG screening in the United States can be considered. However, some physicians are using ECG during PPE to improve detection of potentially lethal cardiovascular abnormalities. When used, ECG interpretation must be based on modern criteria to distinguish abnormal findings from physiologic alterations in athletes, to ensure acceptable accuracy and a low false-positive rate (Drezner, 2008). In a study of 2720 competitive athletes and physically active schoolchildren, a U.K. study reported a false-positive rate of 3.7% using history, physical examination, and ECG, with only 1.9% of false-positive results determined by ECG alone (Wilson et al., 2008). Nine athletes (0.3% of those screened) were found to have a cardiovascular condition known to cause sudden cardiac death in young persons, and all athletes were detected by ECG, not by history or physical examination. Physicians interpreting ECGs in athletes should be familiar with common training-related ECG alterations that are normal variants. In contrast, training-unrelated ECG changes suggest the possibility of underlying pathology, require further diagnostic workup, and should be considered abnormal. Current recommendations for ECG interpretation in athletes to distinguish pathologic ECG abnormalities from physiologic ECG alterations have been recently provided (Corrado et al., 2009).

Cardiac Disorders in Athletes

Key Points

- Bradyarrhythmias caused by increased resting vagal tone are common in athletes and include sinus bradycardia, sinus arrhythmia, first-degree atrioventricular block, and Wenckebach (Mobitz I) second-degree AV block.
- Mobitz II second-degree and complete third-degree AV blocks are always pathologic and warrant cardiologic evaluation.
- Supraventricular tachyarrhythmias in the athlete are abnormal and require further evaluation and treatment, often with radiofrequency ablation, before participation in strenuous exercise.
- Ventricular arrhythmias are life-threatening events and usually occur in the presence of structural heart disease or ion channel disorders.
- Hypertrophic cardiomyopathy, coronary artery anomalies, and commotio cordis are the most common causes of sudden cardiac death in young U.S. athletes.

Arrhythmias

Cardiac arrhythmias in athletes range from benign to life threatening. Bradyarrhythmias are more common in athletes than in the general population because of an increase in resting vagal tone as a response to regular strenuous exercise. Common bradyarrhythmias include sinus bradycardia, sinus arrhythmia, first-degree atrioventricular (AV) block, and Wenckebach (or Mobitz I) second-degree AV block (Huston et al., 1985; Link et al., 2001). These bradyarrhythmias are usually asymptomatic and should resolve during exercise by the withdrawal of vagal tone and associated catecholamine influx.

Athletes with symptomatic Wenckebach block, such as presyncope or syncope during exertion, require further evaluation by a cardiologist and often placement of a permanent pacemaker and restriction of activities. Higher degrees of heart block, such as Mobitz II second-degree and complete third-degree AV blocks, are always pathologic in any individual, including athletes (Fig 29-2). Mobitz II and complete heart blocks signify marked disease in the His-Purkinje system and are generally accepted as a class I indication for permanent pacemaker placement, even in the absence of symptoms (Link et al, 2001).

Tachyarrhythmias in the athlete are abnormal and require further evaluation and treatment before participation in strenuous exercise. The treatment of many supraventricular

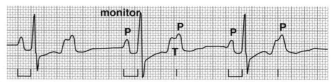

Figure 29-2 Mobitz II second-degree atrioventricular block. Note that every alternate P wave is blocked.
(From Goldberger E. Treatment of Cardiac Emergencies, 5th ed. Philadelphia, Saunders, 1990.)

tachyarrhythmias has been greatly advanced by the use of radiofrequency (RF) ablation, which might offer an actual cure and obviate the need for lifelong pharmacologic treatment.

The most common tachyarrhythmia in athletes is *atrial fibrillation* (AF). Studies have suggested that AF occurs more frequently in athletes than in the general population (Furlanello et al., 1998; Huston et al., 1985). This might be a consequence of increased vagal tone and bradycardia in athletes, which allows dispersion of atrial repolarization and results in a higher susceptibility to AF. Radiofrequency ablation is curative in most cases of paroxysmal AF (Link et al., 2001). If pharmacologic treatment is needed, rate control can be accomplished with beta-adrenergic blockers or calcium channel blockers, and anticoagulation should be considered with aspirin or warfarin, depending on the frequency of AF and other risk factors for thromboembolism. Any athlete receiving anticoagulation therapy with warfarin should be restricted from sports involving collision or bodily contact.

Atrioventricular nodal reentrant tachycardia (AVNRT) is characterized by abrupt onset and termination of symptoms, a narrow QRS complex, and no evidence of atrial activity on the ECG during the tachycardia. AVNRT caused by an accessory bypass tract, known as Wolff-Parkinson-White (WPW) syndrome, may be evident on the ECG by the characteristic delta wave (slurred upstroke of QRS complex), short PR interval, and prolonged QRS complex (Fig. 29-3). Athletes with WPW may be at risk of sudden death and should be strongly considered for RF ablation. Radiofrequency ablation for both AVNRT and WPW offers cure rates higher than 95% (Link et al., 2001; Manolis et al., 1994).

Atrial flutter is an unusual arrhythmia in trained athletes and typically results from an underlying cardiomyopathy.

Ventricular tachyarrhythmias in athletes are life threatening and usually the result of structural heart disease such as hypertrophic cardiomyopathy, anomalous coronary artery, dilated cardiomyopathy, arrhythmogenic right ventricular dysplasia (ARVD), or atherosclerotic coronary artery disease (CAD). Ventricular arrhythmias and sudden death may also occur in individuals with structurally normal hearts. This may occur from ion channel disorders, such as long QT syndrome, catecholaminergic polymorphic ventricular tachycardia (CPVT), and Brugada syndrome, or from commotio cordis. Long QT syndrome is characterized by a prolonged QTc interval, and Brugada syndrome is suggested by an incomplete right bundle branch block and ST-segment elevation in the precordial leads. Exercise may provoke ventricular arrhythmias because of high catecholamine levels and make ventricular fibrillation more difficult to terminate. Athletes who experience a resuscitated sudden death should undergo an extensive workup and treatment with an implantable cardioverter-defibrillator (Link et al., 2001).

Sudden Cardiac Death

Sudden cardiac death in athletes is a catastrophic event and the leading cause of death in exercising young athletes (Maron et al., 2009) The estimated incidence of sudden cardiac death in high school and college athletes is 1 in 100,000 to 200,000 athletes per year (Maron et al., 2009; van Camp et al., 1995). However, these studies are limited by the lack of a mandatory reporting system for juvenile sudden death and their reliance on electronic databases and media reports to identify cases of sudden death. Thus, current reports likely underestimate the true incidence of sudden cardiac death in athletes.

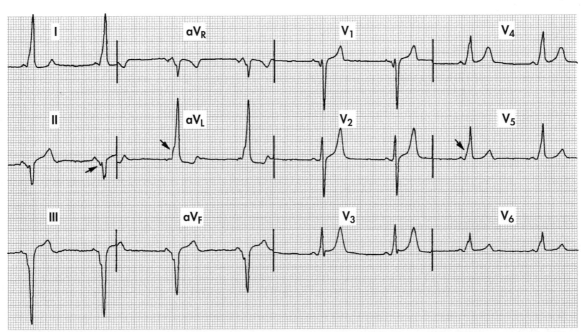

Figure 29-3 Atrioventricular nodal reentrant tachycardia. Notice the characteristic triad of the Wolff-Parkinson-White (WPW) pattern: wide QRS complexes, short PR intervals, and delta waves *(arrows)* that are negative in some leads (e.g., II, III, aV$_R$) and positive in others (aV$_L$ and V$_2$ to V$_6$). The Q waves in leads II, III, and aV$_F$ are the result of abnormal ventricular conduction (negative delta waves) rather than an inferior myocardial infarction. This pattern is consistent with a bypass tract inserting into the posterior wall of the left ventricle.
(From Goldberger AL. Clinical Electrocardiography: a Simplified Approach, 7th ed. Philadelphia, Saunders-Elsevier, 2006.)

Box 29-2 Causes of Sudden Cardiac Death in Young Athletes

Structural

Hypertrophic cardiomyopathy (HCM)*
Coronary artery anomalies
Aortic rupture/Marfan's syndrome*
Dilated cardiomyopathy (DCM)*
Myocarditis
Left ventricular outflow tract (LVOT) obstruction
Mitral valve prolapse (MVP)
Coronary artery [atherosclerotic] disease (CAD)*
Arrhythmogenic right ventricular cardiomyopathy (ARVC)*
Postoperative congenital heart disease

Electrical

Long QT syndrome (LQTS)*
Wolff-Parkinson-White syndrome (WPW)
Brugada syndrome*
Catecholaminergic polymorphic ventricular tachycardia (CPVT)*
Short QT syndrome*
Complete heart block (CHB)

Other

Drugs and stimulants
Commotio cordis
Primary pulmonary hypertension (PPH)*

*Familial/genetic etiology.

The cause of sudden cardiac death in young athletes (<35 years) is usually a structural cardiac abnormality, with hypertrophic cardiomyopathy and coronary artery anomalies representing 36% and 17% of U.S. cases, respectively (Box 29-2) (Maron et al., 2009). *Commotio cordis,* involving a blunt, nonpenetrating blow to the chest that leads to a ventricular arrhythmia, accounts for approximately 3% of cases. Commotio cordis is most common in younger athletes (mean age, 13 years) with compliant chest walls (Maron et al., 2002). Commotio cordis occurs most often in sports using a firm projectile, such as baseball, softball, hockey, and lacrosse, but can also occur from contact with stationary field equipment, the ground, or another player. In older athletes (>35), atherosclerotic CAD accounts for more than 75% of cases of sudden cardiac death.

Automated External Defibrillators in Athletic Medicine

Limitations of the cardiovascular screening process, the overwhelming desire to protect young athletes from a tragic event, and the success of early defibrillation programs (Caffrey et al., 2002; Page et al., 2000; Valenzuela et al., 2000) using accessible automated external defibrillators (AEDs) have propelled the placement of AEDs into the athletic setting (Drezner et al., 2005). Recent research suggests an improved survival rate for young athletes with sudden cardiac arrest if early defibrillation is achieved. A retrospective cohort of 1710 U.S. high schools with an on-site AED program found 14 cases of sudden cardiac arrest in high school student-athletes and a 64% survival rate if early cardiopulmonary

resuscitation (CPR) and prompt defibrillation with an AED were provided (Drezner et al., 2009).

Comprehensive emergency response planning is needed to ensure an efficient and structured response to sudden cardiac arrest in the athletic setting. This includes establishing a communication system to activate the emergency medical services (EMS) system and alert any on-site response team, training of anticipated responders (e.g., coaches) in CPR and AED use, access to an AED, and practice and review of the response plan. High suspicion of sudden cardiac death should be maintained in any collapsed and unresponsive athlete, with application of an AED as soon as possible for rhythm analysis and defibrillation if indicated (Drezner et al., 2007).

KEY TREATMENT

High suspicion of sudden cardiac arrest should be maintained in any collapsed and unresponsive athlete, with application of an automated external defibrillator (AED) as soon as possible for rhythm analysis and defibrillation if indicated (Drezner et al., 2007, 2009) (SOR: B).

Concussion in Sports

Key Points

- Concussion is a neurologic disturbance with variable symptoms, including confusion, headache, vision problems, nausea, balance problems, amnesia, and loss of consciousness.
- Concussion assessment includes evaluation of cranial nerves, pupillary dilation and reactivity, balance and coordination, motor strength, and cognitive function.
- A player should never return to play while symptomatic from a concussion.
- Once asymptomatic, athletes should follow a stepwise and graded exercise program before return to play.
- Neuropsychological testing can aid return-to-play decisions for complex concussions.

In 1966 the Congress of Neurological Surgeons proposed a consensus definition of concussion. Since then, both the definition and our understanding of concussion have been evolving. A concussion is defined as a traumatically induced transient disturbance in neurologic function, usually caused by a direct blow to the head, neck, or face (Aubry et al., 2002).

Symptoms and Incidence

A concussion usually results in the rapid onset of brief neurologic impairment that resolves spontaneously. Symptoms of concussion include loss of consciousness, amnesia, confusion, headache, vision problems, nausea, and balance problems (Box 29-3). A concussion may or may not be associated with a loss of consciousness. Over 90% of concussions are not associated with a loss of consciousness, and unconsciousness is not a marker of the severity of the injury (Lovell et al., 1999). *Amnesia* can include loss of memory of the events before (retrograde amnesia) or

Box 29-3 Signs and Symptoms of Concussion

Disorientation	Feeling "foggy" or "dazed"
Confusion	Inability to focus
Amnesia	Difficulty concentrating
Loss of consciousness	Irritability
Headache	Emotional lability
Dizziness	Excessive drowsiness
Balance problems	Delayed verbal or motor response
Poor coordination, gait	Vacant, "glassy" stare
Nausea, vomiting	Slurred, incoherent speech
Visual problems (flashing lights)	Decreased playing performance
	Seizure (rare)
Hearing problems (tinnitus)	

after (posttraumatic amnesia) the concussion, or both, and amnesia appears to be the best predictor of severity in athletic concussion (Collins et al., 2003). Conventional imaging studies such as computed tomography (CT) or magnetic resonance imaging (MRI) are normal in concussion, indicating that concussion is a *functional* rather than a structural injury (McCrory, 2001).

An estimated 300,000 concussions occur each year from sports-related activity (Centers for Disease Control and Prevention [CDC], 1997). In high school football, there are 40,000 concussions per year, for a 3% to 5% incidence (Powell and Barber-Foss, 1999). High-risk sports include contact and collision sports such as football, ice hockey, rugby, wrestling, and to a lesser extent, soccer and basketball. Women may be more prone to concussion in some sports (Tierney et al., 2005), for unclear reasons, with further research needed. Younger players also may be more prone to concussion because of less developed neck muscles and the higher relative weight of the head compared with the rest of the body. In addition, children may sustain more serious concussions because of their immature nervous system.

Sideline Management

When attending to an athlete on the field with a suspected concussion, attention must first be given to basic first aid. Airway, breathing, and circulation (ABCs) and level of consciousness should be initially assessed, followed by an evaluation for potential cervical spine injuries. If loss of consciousness has occurred, the duration of unconsciousness should be determined. A brief loss of consciousness is generally defined as less than 30 to 60 seconds. If a player is unconscious for more than 30 to 60 seconds or still unconscious by the time a physician reaches the athlete on the field, most would consider this "prolonged." Patients with concussions involving prolonged loss of consciousness, suspected cervical spine injuries, or gross neurologic impairment should be stabilized and transported to a hospital for further evaluation (see Cervical Spine Injuries: On-the-Field Assessment).

After it is determined that the athlete is stable and safe to be moved, further assessment can take place on the sideline. Physical examination should include evaluation of cranial nerves, pupillary dilation and reactivity, balance and coordination, motor strength, and cognitive function. Orienta-

tion to time, place, and person is an incomplete assessment of cognitive function in the sports setting. Memory and recall testing, serial 7s (counting backward by 7 from 100), serial 3s (counting backward by 3 from 100), and listing the months of the year backward and forward are simple sideline tests of cognitive function. Several sideline assessment tools exist to aid medical professionals in the evaluation of an athlete with concussion. The Standardized Assessment of Concussion (SAC) is a validated sideline assessment tool, and the most recent consensus conference on concussion recommended a modified and expanded tool, the Sport Concussion Assessment Tool (SCAT2) (McCrea et al., 1997; McCrory et al., 2009). This includes a symptom scale, standard cognitive assessment, and guided physical examination. Such standardized examinations are useful for serial follow-up and if different medical personnel will be evaluating the athlete. It is important to reassess concussed athletes frequently to monitor for resolution of symptoms or signs of deterioration.

Return to Play

Return-to-play decisions are driven by the concern of preventing potential complications, primarily second-impact syndrome and permanent neurologic deficit. *Second-impact syndrome* occurs when a player returns to play following a first concussion before the symptoms have completely resolved, and a second, often minor, blow to the head is sustained, which leads to diffuse cerebral swelling, brainstem herniation, and death. The risk for catastrophic injury in athletes returned to play while still symptomatic is of particular concern in children and adolescents.

Long-term cognitive deficits from concussion or repetitive blows to the head are also a concern. Repetitive concussions, especially if severe, might put athletes at risk for permanent neurologic deficits (Guskiewicz et al., 2003). However, no evidence indicates that repetitive nonconcussive blows, such as those sustained from heading a soccer ball, lead to short-term or long-term neurologic impairment.

Most concussion guidelines designed to facilitate return-to-play decisions rely on loss of consciousness and the presence of amnesia to grade the severity of the concussion. This approach makes their usefulness limited because most sports-related concussions do not involve loss of consciousness or amnesia. Current recommendations suggest that management of concussion be based on symptoms and severity. The mildest concussion is one that involves transient symptoms that resolve quickly. More severe concussions involve persistent or prolonged symptoms and cognitive deficits on neuropsychological testing. Management of concussion includes both physical and mental rest, until all symptoms have cleared, and the neurologic examination, followed by a graded and stepwise program of exertion before return to sport (Box 29-4). *Repetitive concussions,* which take longer to return to baseline or that occur with progressively less trauma, are also considered of greater severity. Complex or recurrent concussions with persistent cognitive impairment, neurologic findings on examination, or prolonged symptoms may warrant advanced imaging and formal neuropsychological testing and should be managed by physicians with specific expertise in sports-related concussion.

Box 29-4 Graded Return to Play after Concussion[*]

1. Rest until asymptomatic
2. Light aerobic exercise (stationary cycling, slow jogging)
3. More strenuous aerobic training (running, sprinting)
4. Sport-specific training
5. Noncontact drills
6. Full contact drills
7. Return to competition

Modified from McCrory P, Johnston K, Meeuwisse W, et al. Summary and agreement statement of the 2nd International Conference on Concussion in Sport, Prague, 2004. Br J Sports Med 2005;39:196-204.

[*]A player should never return to play while symptomatic from a concussion. In this supervised stepwise progression, the athlete can proceed to the next level if asymptomatic at the current level. If any postconcussion symptoms occur, the athlete should return to the previous asymptomatic level and try to progress again after 24 hours. Athletes with simple concussions may progress through these stages over several days. In cases of complex concussion, recovery is more prolonged.

Neuropsychological testing in concussion, initially a comprehensive battery of conventional written tests administered by a trained neuropsychologist, has evolved into a variety of computer assessment tools. These neuropsychological assessment tools are gaining acceptance in high-risk sports at the collegiate and professional levels and are most useful when there is a baseline assessment done before injury. Widespread use of these tests in youth and high school sports with limited budgets and medical personnel might not be practical.

In summary, concussion is a common injury in sport, and athletes sustaining a concussion should be medically evaluated by a physician. No symptomatic athlete should be allowed to return to play, and an athlete should not be allowed to return to play in the same game or practice during which an injury has occurred. Once asymptomatic, athletes should follow a graded program before return to play. Referral should be considered in complex or complicated concussions. Further research is needed to provide evidenced-based return-to-play guidelines and preventive strategies.

KEY TREATMENT

A player with a concussion who is still symptomatic should be held from practice and competition and should not return to the field of play.
Once asymptomatic, athletes should follow a stepwise and graded exercise program before a return to sport.
(SOR: C; McCrory et al., 2009).

Cervical Spine Injuries

Key Points

- "Stingers" result from a blow to the neck and shoulders with transient unilateral upper extremity pain and paresthesias resolving in minutes.

KEY TREATMENT

Axial loading is the most common mechanism for catastrophic injury to the cervical spine during sports competition.
Any athlete with significant neck or spine pain, diminished level of consciousness, or significant neurologic deficits should be immobilized and prepared for transport.
Unconscious athletes are presumed to have unstable spine injuries until proven otherwise.
The football helmet in a downed player wearing shoulder pads should not be removed to avoid hyperextension of the neck and secondary injury to the cervical spine.

Strains and Sprains

Most sports-related neck injuries are mild and self-limiting. Patients with muscle strains and ligament sprains typically present with minor complaints and no neurologic symptoms. More significant injury should be suspected in the presence of significant cervical muscle spasm, tentative active range of motion (ROM), severe pain, or abnormal neurologic signs. Evaluation includes active cervical ROM and strength testing of the neck and upper extremities. Manual compression and axial loading to the cervical spine (Spurling's maneuver) should not cause pain or radicular symptoms and is helpful in ruling out more significant injury (Magee, 1997). The athlete is cleared to return to play when full pain-free ROM and normal strength of the cervical spine are restored.

Stingers

Stingers or "burners" are characterized by transient unilateral upper extremity pain and paresthesias resulting from a blow to the neck and shoulders. Stingers are common in American football and have been reported in up to 50% to 65% of college players (Clancy et al., 1977; Sallis et al., 1992). Stingers are peripheral nerve injuries and are considered a transient neurapraxia of the cervical nerve roots, usually involving the upper trunk of the brachial plexus (C5-C6). Stingers typically manifest with dysesthesia (burning pain) that begins in the shoulder and radiates down the arm. They often are associated with transient numbness or weakness, and all symptoms typically resolve in minutes.

Stingers can occur from a tensile or compression overload (Watkins, 1986). In most high school athletes, the mechanism of injury involves a tensile or traction injury when the involved arm and the neck are stretched in opposite directions. This occurs when the neck is forcibly flexed away while the shoulder is depressed. In college and professional athletes, who have a higher likelihood of degenerative changes of the cervical spine, a compression mechanism is more likely. This involves a pinch of the cervical nerve root within the neural foramen as the neck is forcibly extended in a posterolateral direction (Levitz et al., 1997).

Stingers are always unilateral, a distinguishing feature from spinal cord injuries, which involve symptoms in multiple limbs. Athletes are safe to return to play when symptoms have fully resolved and the athlete can demonstrate full cervical ROM and a normal neurologic examination.

Radiography and MRI should be considered in athletes with recurrent stingers to evaluate for cervical degenerative disk disease (Levitz et al., 1997). Rarely, more significant nerve injury involving *axonotmesis* (axon disruption) occurs, causing persistent weakness. Athletes with significant weakness 24 to 48 hours after injury may benefit from treatment with a short burst of oral corticosteroids. If weakness persists, electromyography performed 2 weeks or more after the injury will assess the distribution and degree of injury. Fortunately, most cases of axonotmesis recover within 1 year (Clancy et al., 1977).

Cervical Cord Neurapraxia

Cervical cord neurapraxia is characterized by an acute, transient sensory or motor change, or both, to more than one extremity. Symptoms include burning pain, numbness, and tingling with or without paresis or complete paralysis. *Transient quadriplegia* is a type of neurapraxia characterized by temporary paralysis and loss of motor function in all four limbs (Torg et al., 1986). *Burning hands syndrome* is characterized by burning dysesthesias of the hands and associated upper extremity weakness (Maroon, 1977). Episodes of cervical cord neurapraxia usually resolve within 10 to 15 minutes, although gradual resolution may take more than 24 to 48 hours.

Congenital or degenerative narrowing of the anteroposterior (AP) diameter of the cervical spinal canal is an established risk factor for cervical cord neurapraxia (Torg et al., 1997). Athletes with an episode of cord neurapraxia should be held from competition and undergo radiographic evaluation and MRI. Return to play after an episode of cervical cord neurapraxia is a highly controversial area in sports medicine. Several cases of permanent neurologic injury following cervical cord neurapraxia associated with cervical spinal stenosis have been reported (Brigham and Adamson, 2003; Cantu, 1993, 2000). Functional spinal stenosis on advanced imaging in an athlete with a history of cervical cord neurapraxia is an absolute contraindication to return to play in contact and collision sports (Cantu, 2000).

Catastrophic Cervical Spine Injury

Injury to the spinal cord resulting in temporary or permanent neurologic injury is a rare but potentially catastrophic event during sports competition. Cervical spine trauma is most common in contact and collision sports such as American football, rugby, ice hockey, gymnastics, skiing, wrestling, and diving (Cantu and Mueller, 1999; Carvell et al., 1983; Tator and Edmonds, 1984; Wu and Lewis, 1985). Cervical spinal cord injuries are the most common catastrophic injury in American football and the second leading cause of death attributable to football. The National Center for Catastrophic Sports Injury Research reported that the incidence of cervical spinal cord injury in American football between 1977 and 2001 was 0.52, 1.55, and 14 per 100,000 participants in high school, college, and professional football, respectively (Cantu and Mueller, 2003).

Axial loading is the most common mechanism for catastrophic injury to the cervical spine during sports competition (Torg et al., 1979, 1990). Axial loading occurs when a player strikes another player with the top of the head as the point of initial contact ("spear tackling"). In athletes with cervical spinal stenosis, axial loading followed by forced hyperextension or hyperflexion can further narrow the AP diameter of the spinal canal, resulting in compression of the spinal cord and transient or permanent neurologic changes (Eismont et al., 1984; Penning, 1962; Torg et al., 1993).

Recognition of the axial load mechanism as the major cause of catastrophic cervical spine injury in American football resulted in rule changes that banned "spearing," defined as intentionally striking an opponent with the crown of the helmet, as well as other tackling techniques in which the helmet is used as the initial point of contact. In 1976 the incidence of quadriplegia was 2.24 and 10.66 per 100,000 in high school and college athletes, respectively. In 1977, only 1 year after rule changes that banned spear tackling, the incidence decreased to 1.30 and 2.66 per 100,000 in high school and college athletes (Torg et al., 2002).

On-the-Field Assessment

Medical providers at sporting events must be prepared to assess, stabilize, and transport athletes with suspected cervical spine injuries. Adequate preparation of and anticipation in required personnel and equipment and a well-designed emergency response are critical to the management of catastrophic neck injuries. In general, any athlete with significant neck or spine pain, diminished level of consciousness, or significant neurologic deficits should be immobilized and prepared for transport.

Guidelines for the prehospital care of the spine-injured athlete were established by the Inter-Association Task Force for Appropriate Care of the Spine-Injured Athlete (2001). The initial assessment of an injured athlete begins with a basic assessment of the ABCs and level of consciousness. EMS personnel should be contacted for any concerns regarding basic life support. Unconscious athletes are presumed to have unstable spine injuries until proven otherwise.

The face mask of a protective helmet should be removed as soon as possible, regardless of respiratory status (Inter-Association Task Force, 2001). In football the face mask can be removed with screwdrivers or the loop straps cut with various cutting tools such as pruning shears or a Trainer's Angel (Knox and Kleiner, 1997). Football helmets and chin straps should be left in place. If the helmet is removed from a downed player wearing shoulder pads, the athlete's head will hyperextend, which may result in secondary injury to the cervical spine. If the athlete is not breathing, an adequate airway can be established by the jaw thrust maneuver, which allows opening the airway while maintaining the cervical spine in a stable position. Rarely, assisted ventilation may be necessary.

If transport is indicated, the athlete should be immobilized to a spine board. A supine athlete can be transferred to a spine board using a six-plus person lift technique, with one person responsible for stabilization of the head and neck (Inter-Association Task Force, 2001). To transfer an athlete who is facedown, a logrolling technique is recommended. Transport of a spine-injured athlete should be directed to a trauma center or medical facility with diagnostic and surgical capabilities for spinal injury.

KEY TREATMENT

Athletes with an episode of cervical cord neurapraxia involving sensory or motor changes, or both, to more than one extremity should be held from competition and undergo radiographic evaluation and MRI to rule out functional spinal stenosis.

In an athlete with a history of cervical cord neurapraxia, functional spinal stenosis on advanced imaging is an absolute contraindication to return to play in contact and collision sports (SOR: C; Cantu, 2000; Inter-Association Task Force, 2001).

Environmental Influences

Exertional Heat Illness

Key Points

- Hydration sufficient to replace fluid lost in sweat is essential to prevent heat stroke.
- Athletes exercising in the heat who exhibit mental status changes must be immediately removed from competition and cooled.
- Ice-water immersion produces the most rapid decrease in core body temperature.

Heat stroke is the third leading cause of death in high school athletes (Lee-Chiong and Stitt, 1995). This is tragic because these deaths should be largely avoidable.

The exercising human is an engine operating at about 25% efficiency, resulting in 3 W of heat production for every watt of work, and requires a biologic radiator to avoid overheating. Humans dissipate heat through convection, conduction, radiation, and evaporation, with evaporative sweat loss being the most significant. Higher temperatures limit heat dissipation from convection and conduction, warm sunny days elevate body temperature through radiant heating, and higher humidity decreases evaporative cooling. Thus, the combination of high ambient temperature, radiant heat from the sun, and high humidity works synergistically to create dangerous playing conditions that promote the development of heat illness.

The wet bulb globe temperature (WBGT) index incorporates ambient temperature, relative humidity, and the amount of radiant heat coming from the sun to provide a measure of the risk of overheating. The American College of Sports Medicine Inter-Association Task Force on Exertional Heat Illnesses Consensus Statement (2006) recommends that WBGT readings from 18° to 23° C (64.4°-73.4° F) result in moderate risk, 23° to 28° C (73.4°-82.4° F) in high risk, and more than 28°C (82.4° F) in extreme risk. The cumulative effect of successive days of exercise in the heat must also be considered. In a U.S. Marine Corps, investigators demonstrated that the risk of exertional heat illness was best predicted by considering the current and the previous day's WBGT index (Wallace et al., 2005).

Because evaporative cooling is the primary mechanism for heat dissipation, adequate hydration is essential to keep the biologic radiator functioning. Losses of 2% to 3% of body weight are common with high-intensity exercise in the heat (Galloway, 1999). Below 5% fluid losses, performance and thermoregulation are impaired, and thirst is an inconsistent

stimulus to rehydrate, so regular, planned fluid consumption is essential. Fluid recommendations vary, but experts have suggested about 500 mL of fluid intake 2 hours or less before exercise and then about 250 mL every 20 minutes during exercise (Convertino et al., 1996). Because of differences in sweat rate, acclimatization, intensity of exercise, clothing, protective equipment, and environmental factors, individual fluid requirements vary. Thus, recording an athlete's nude weight in the morning and evening is an effective method for determining adequate rehydration. If athletes are losing more than 2% to 3% of their body weight with training, they need to consume more fluids during training. If they cannot regain the lost weight before the next morning's training, they need to consume additional fluids after training and during recovery time. For every kilogram of body weight lost, 1 L of fluid should be consumed. Cooler, flavored fluids are recommended to increase palatability and absorption.

Heat illness is classified as heat edema, heat cramps, heat syncope, heat exhaustion, and heat stroke (Table 29-1) (Binkley et al., 2002; Eichner, 1998). Heat stroke is of the greatest concern, with hallmark features of an elevated core temperature higher than 40.5° C (105° F) and associated mental status changes. Any athlete exhibiting mental status changes and participating in an environment conducive to heat illness requires immediate removal from participation and active cooling. An ice-water tub should be prepared in advance if rapid cooling may be necessary in high-risk events, and an affected athlete should be fully submerged, with only the head above water (Smith, 2005). Other methods of cooling, such as applying ice bags to the neck, axilla, and groin, or using cold-water spray combined with fanning, can be effective, but the rate of core body temperature loss is slower than in ice-water immersion. Close monitoring of mental status and vital signs (e.g., core temperature) is indicated, and athletes should be transported to the hospital if they do not exhibit improving mental status with normalization of vital signs. The National Athletic Trainers' Association Exertional Heat Illness Position Statement is an excellent reference regarding proper preparedness for heat illness (Binkley et al., 2002).

Exertional Hyponatremia

Key Points

- Life-threatening hyponatremia develops when excessive hypotonic fluid is consumed, with concomitant sodium sweat loss.
- Exertional hyponatremia most often occurs in women completing endurance races in over 4 hours who drink copiously throughout the race.
- Symptoms of exertional hyponatremia include mental status changes and peripheral edema, without significant elevation in core temperature.

Exertional hyponatremia (serum sodium <130 mmol/L), once considered a rare complication of exercise in the heat, is now recognized as more common and responsible for a number of exercise-related deaths (Almond et al., 2005). Controversy surrounds the exact pathophysiology, but the condition develops in the setting of excessive hypotonic fluid replacement while sodium is progressively lost in

Table 29-1 Exertional Heat Illness

	Definition	Management	Prevention
Heat edema	Dependent edema usually occurring before acclimation.	Elevation of swollen extremity, rest, cooling. Diuretics contraindicated.	Gradual acclimation to heat.
Heat (exercise associated) muscle cramps	Painful spasms of single or multiple muscles. Likely sodium deficiency and salty sweaters most prone.	Rest, stretching, cooling, oral hydration with hypertonic sodium drink. Intravenous fluids (normal saline) if oral treatment limited or to expedite recovery.	Maintain hydration and increase salt intake. Add salt to fluids, especially for those with predisposition based on past history.
Heat syncope	Orthostatic dizziness at cessation of exercise, with prolonged standing, or after assuming upright posture.	Rest, cooling, place supine with legs elevated, monitor vital signs, and mental status. Oral fluid hydration.	Adequate hydration and acclimation. If occurs during exercise, requires cardiovascular evaluation.
Heat exhaustion	Inability to continue exercise in heat. Symptoms: weakness, fainting, dizziness, headache, nausea, vomiting, cramps, dehydration with low urine output. Minimal mental status symptoms; core temperature <40° C.	Immediate rest, rapid cooling (ice bath), close monitoring of mental status, vital signs (e.g., core temperature). Serum sodium if hyponatremia considered. Oral fluid hydration with IV fluids (normal saline) if hypotension present.	Adequate acclimation, monitor hydration, adjust training to climate, follow player's weight, and close monitoring for symptoms of heat illness.
Heat stroke	Heat exhaustion with core temperature >40° C and mental status alteration or central nervous system collapse.	As for heat exhaustion, with hospitalization as soon as possible.	As for heat exhaustion, be prepared with ice baths, monitoring equipment, and access to emergency medical services.

sweat (Levine and Thompson, 2005; Noakes, 2002). Typical victims are relatively inexperienced female marathon runners who tend to be light sweaters, finish in over 4 hours, and drink copiously throughout the race. Nonsteroidal anti-inflammatory drugs (NSAIDs) taken before the race may be a contributing factor (Hsieh, 2004). Athletes with a history of exercise-induced hyponatremia do not seem to be predisposed to water overload at rest, although there may be some physiologic mechanism beyond pure water overload that accounts for the condition in some susceptible individuals (Speedy et al., 2001). Symptoms are similar to those of heat exhaustion, including weakness, dizziness, headache, nausea, vomiting, and cramping, but the headache is more prominent and progressively severe, extremity swelling may be noted, and progressive mental status changes occur despite a core temperature lower than 40° C (104° F). Cerebral edema underlies the mental status changes, and pulmonary edema may also occur.

The serum sodium level must be assessed in athletes in whom the diagnosis is suspected, to differentiate hyponatremia from heat stroke. Intravenous (IV) fluids, often indicated in heat stroke, can actually worsen hyponatremia if related to excessive hypotonic fluid intake. Prompt hospitalization is indicated for any athlete with mental status changes or persistently altered vital signs once the diagnosis of hyponatremia has been established. Exertional hyponatremic encephalopathy is treated with 3% hypertonic saline boluses (100 mL) (Hew-Butler et al., 2008). Prevention includes following an athlete's weight change with exercise to understand the fluid requirements more precisely, not deviating from established fluid intake on race day to avoid overhydration, incorporating sodium/electrolyte-containing fluids, and limiting fluid intake to 1 L/hr unless higher fluid requirements have been established (Gardner, 2002).

KEY TREATMENT

Any athlete exhibiting mental status changes and participating in an environment conducive to heat illness requires immediate removal from participation and active cooling (American College of Sports Medicine, 2006) (SOR: B).
Exertional hyponatremic encephalopathy is treated with 3% hypertonic saline boluses (100 mL) (Hew-Butler et al., 2008) (SOR: B).

Cold Injury

Key Points

Cold-weather exercise requires proper layering of synthetic clothing with a waterproof, breathable outer layer to maintain body temperature, but excessive sweating or environmental dampness should be avoided.

Hypothermia victims should be sheltered, dried, and warmed, and resuscitation attempts should continue until body temperature is higher than 32° C.

Outdoor sports participation, particularly winter sports, places athletes at risk for cold-induced injury. Two problems commonly encountered are frostbite and hypothermia.

Frostbite most frequently affects the toes, fingers, and exposed skin of the face. As tissue cools, a progressive cell membrane leak results initially in increased extracellular fluid, with progression to extracellular ice crystal formation and then ischemic necrosis. Prevention includes dry layering of clothing that is not constricting; avoidance of skin exposure, especially in windy, cold conditions; and maintaining the core temperature, because hypothermic shunting of blood centrally promotes distal extremity freezing. Treatment involves warming, although this is not recommended until the victim has been safely evacuated—warming and then refreezing is more damaging. Antibiotics, tissue debridement, and possibly amputation may be required, depending on the extent of injury. Sallis and Chassay (1999) provide a more in-depth discussion of frostbite and other cold-induced injuries.

Hypothermia is defined as a core temperature at or below 32° C (90° F). Lower ambient temperatures and longer exposure times increase the risk for hypothermia, but *moisture* is the most dangerous variable that must be controlled. Wet clothing results in significant increases in conductive heat loss, which is made worse in the wind. Prevention of hypothermia requires proper clothing for outdoor exercise in the cold. Clothing should be layered so that with increased exertion and endogenous heat production, layers can be removed to avoid excessive sweating. Underlayers should consist of breathable wicking fabrics that move sweat moisture away from the skin. Outer layers should be windproof, waterproof, and breathable. Midlayers, which can be added depending on the temperature and exertion level, should provide loft (synthetic pile or down) to trap air; this provides a temperature gradient between the warm underlayers and cold outer layers, much like the blubber on a marine mammal. Heat loss from the head is significant, so a hat or hood that wicks moisture is necessary, and mittens are warmer than gloves for very cold weather. Dehydration must be avoided, because low plasma volume results in peripheral vasoconstriction and increases the risk of frostbite.

Treatment of mild hypothermia involves finding warm shelter away from the wind, removing wet outer layers, and covering with dry blankets. Sharing a sleeping bag with a warm climbing partner can be lifesaving in a desperate situation. In the setting of severe hypothermia, warm IV fluid (40° C), warm humidified oxygen, and warming lamps are indicated, if available. The adage "one is not dead until warm and dead" applies, and ventricular fibrillation or asystole in the settling of hypothermia should be treated with advanced cardiac life support (ACLS) protocols until the patient has a core temperature above 32° C (Sallis and Chassay, 1999; Tom et al., 1994).

Altitude Illness

High-altitude medicine, once the preoccupation of research pulmonologists and physicians practicing at high altitude or caring for climbers, has become essential for many primary care providers because of increasing numbers of recreational athletes engaging in skiing, hiking, trekking, and other high-altitude pursuits.

Acute mountain sickness (AMS) and its two most significant manifestations, high-altitude pulmonary edema and high-altitude cerebral edema, are complications of travel to higher altitude with insufficient acclimatization. Symptoms of AMS include headache, sleep difficulty, and gastrointestinal (GI) upset, including loss of appetite, nausea, and vomiting. Symptoms occur a few hours after rapid ascent in 25% of individuals at as low as 8500 feet (Harris et al., 1998), with a higher percentage being affected at higher altitudes. Individuals vary in their susceptibility to AMS, and a high level of physical fitness is not protective. Gradual ascent, allowing acclimatization, will prevent symptoms. If symptoms occur, delaying any further ascent with relative rest for 1 to 3 days usually results in improvement. More significant symptoms respond to decreasing altitude. Individuals with a history of AMS are likely to have it recur when they return to a higher altitude.

Planning time for acclimatization and avoiding excessive exercise when first arriving at a higher altitude are helpful. Nocturnal periodic breathing probably contributes to worsening hypoxia and subsequent AMS symptoms, so avoiding alcohol or other sedatives is also helpful. Acetazolamide, 125 to 250 mg twice daily, started the day of initial ascent and continuing for 48 hours, has been shown to decrease AMS symptoms and hasten acclimatization, possibly by decreasing nocturnal periodic breathing (Bartsch et al., 2004).

High-altitude cerebral edema (HACE) is defined as a progression of AMS symptoms to include ataxia, mental status changes, lassitude, and eventual coma. HACE is fatal if untreated. Treatment requires immediate descent. Hyperbaric treatment can be lifesaving if immediate descent is not possible; portable hyperbaric chambers are available for mountaineering expeditions. In addition to immediate descent, treatment includes oxygen at 2 to 4 L/min and dexamethasone, 4 to 8 mg orally, followed by 4 mg every 6 hours.

High-altitude pulmonary edema (HAPE) is the development of pulmonary edema, dyspnea, and hypoxemia in the setting of AMS. Rapid descent to lower altitude is also the primary treatment. The administration of supplemental oxygen, 4 to 6 L/min, and nifedipine, 10 mg once, followed by 30 mg of sustained-release nifedipine every 12 to 24 hours, is helpful if immediate descent is not possible (Rodway et al., 2003).

KEY TREATMENT

Hypothermia victims should be sheltered, dried, and warmed and resuscitation attempts continued until body temperature is higher than 32° C (90° F) (Sallis and Chassay, 1999; Tom et al., 1994) (SOR: B).

Pharmacologic prophylaxis can be helpful, but definitive treatment of high-altitude pulmonary or cerebral edema (HAPE, HACE) requires descent to lower altitude as rapidly as possible (Rodway et al., 2003) (SOR: B).

Sports Trauma to the Teeth, Face, and Eyes

Key Points

- Dental trauma is common in many sports and can be largely prevented with a custom-molded mouth guard.

- Avulsed teeth or tooth fragments should be wrapped in saline-soaked gauze, with urgent transport to a dentist and luxated teeth repositioned if possible.

- Facial and nasal injuries requiring immediate referral include those with prolonged loss of consciousness, visual abnormalities suggesting orbital fracture, malocclusion of the teeth suggesting maxillary or mandibular fracture, facial paresthesias suggesting infraorbital nerve injury, open or significantly displaced nasal fractures, and uncontrollable epistaxis.

- Acute auricular hematomas should be fully evacuated to avoid chronic fibrosis and deformity (cauliflower ear).

- Eye trauma is usually preventable using appropriate eye protection.

- Loss of visual acuity, evidence of globe rupture or leaking aqueous humor, limitation or asymmetry of extraocular movements, persisting pupil abnormalities, and evidence of hyphema all require urgent ophthalmologic consultation.

Dental Trauma

Dental trauma is common, with one third of all dental injuries in the United States occurring with sports activities (Honsik, 2004). Mouth guards are recommended by the American Dental Association for participation in all collision and contact sports as well as weightlifting, skydiving, skateboarding, gymnastics, racquetball, squash, and skiing. Dental injury is especially common in sports combining collision and a hard ball or puck, such as ice hockey or field hockey. A study of college basketball found a significant decrease in tooth injuries in participants using custom-fitted mouth guards; however, there was no decrease in oral soft tissue injury or concussion (Labella et al., 2002). Sports physicians and dental professionals agree that although off-the-shelf molded mouthpieces are less expensive and more readily available, they do not protect teeth as effectively as a custom mouthpiece (Honsik, 2004).

Teeth rest in a bony socket, each with a neurovascular root connected to the socket by a periodontal ligament. Above the gum the tooth consists of three layers: dentin, pulp, and superficial enamel. Injuries involve fracture of the tooth or some degree of luxation. *Fractures* range from an enamel chip to those involving the deeper components. *Luxation* can result in a normally positioned loose tooth or a displaced tooth still positioned in the socket. Injury can also result in complete tooth avulsion.

After injury, tooth fragments or avulsed teeth should always be recovered, if possible, and transported to a dentist in saline-soaked gauze. Fractures involving only enamel and dentin can be managed by dental evaluation within 48 hours. Pulp involvement (visible pink or blood in center of the tooth) mandates urgent dental referral, and medical-grade cyanoacrylate (Super Glue) can be placed on the tooth acutely for pain and to prevent infection. Luxation without impaction can be reduced if jaw fracture is not suspected, and return to play with a custom mouth guard can be considered, depending on successful reduction, level of pain, and level of competition. If the tooth is easily repositioned, dental consultation can be delayed 24 hours. Players with impacted luxation or teeth that cannot be repositioned should not return to play, and dental consultation sought immediately. Avulsed teeth should be rinsed with sterile saline and replaced, if possible, taking care not to handle or damage the root, followed by immediate dental consultation (Honsik, 2004).

Facial Trauma

Nasal injuries are frequently encountered in sports. The higher the impact velocity, the higher is the probability of concomitant injury requiring urgent referral. Situations requiring emergency department (ED) evaluation include associated prolonged loss of consciousness, vision abnormalities suggesting orbital fracture, malocclusion of the teeth suggesting maxillary or mandibular fracture, facial paresthesias suggesting infraorbital nerve injury, open or significantly displaced nasal fractures, and uncontrollable epistaxis. Examination findings prompting early referral include clear rhinorrhea suggesting cribriform plate injury with cerebrospinal fluid (CSF) leak and impaired extraocular movements, especially unilateral limited upward gaze, which suggests an orbital fracture with inferior oblique or rectus muscle entrapment, or both. Nasal septal hematoma should be referred to an otolaryngologist expeditiously for incision and drainage. If left untreated, subsequent cartilage degeneration can result in a nasal saddle deformity (Stackhouse, 1998).

If initial assessment does not mandate immediate referral, subsequent management requires assessing the extent of deformity and controlling epistaxis. In the first few days, swelling can make assessment for bony deformity difficult, but close follow-up is helpful. Any persistent obstruction of the nares or cosmetic abnormality unacceptable to the patient should be referred to an otolaryngologist within 5 days, because reduction is best performed within 10 days of injury. Epistaxis is best managed with a topical decongestant such as oxymetazoline nasal 0.05% (Afrin) and compression of the anterior plexus by pinching the nose for 15 minutes. A short nasal tampon soaked with oxymetazoline can be placed into the bleeding nostril to assist with hemostasis and return to play, but anterior packing should only be performed with appropriate visualization, to avoid further injury.

Ear trauma in sports can result in auricular hematomas or injury to the tympanic membrane. *Auricular hematomas* mainly occur in wrestling, rugby, and boxing and result in hemorrhage between the perichondrium and the underlying cartilage. Failure to evacuate the hematoma can lead to fibrosis, necrosis, and a chronic deformity known as *cauliflower ear*. An acute auricular hematoma should be drained by needle aspiration under aseptic conditions, and a pressure dressing (using cotton wool soaked in collodion or a silicone splint) carefully applied against the contours of the outer ear and reexamined daily. Occasionally, incision and drainage are required.

Blows across the side of the head can also result in *tympanic membrane rupture*, marked by pain, bleeding, fluid drainage, and impaired hearing. Tympanic membrane ruptures usually heal spontaneously over 4 to 6 weeks. Antibiotic prophylaxis in the first week should be considered, especially if the rupture occurred in a contaminated environment. The ear canal should be kept clean and dry, and a cotton ball coated with petroleum jelly and placed gently into the ear canal can be helpful while showering.

Eye Trauma

Ocular injury is common in sports and largely preventable if athletes wear appropriate eye protection. The highest risk sports are those in which intentional injury can occur (e.g., boxing and combative martial arts) and those in which hard projectiles, sticks, or fingers are likely to encounter the eye. High-risk sports include basketball, baseball, softball, cricket, lacrosse, squash, racquetball, fencing, and all varieties of hockey. Squash and racquetball are particularly concerning because of the high likelihood of severe injury. Athletes with preexisting monocular visual impairment must understand the importance of protecting the good eye, and preparticipation visual acuity assessment of binocular and monocular vision is essential. The American Society for Testing and Materials (ASTM) is the primary U.S. organization for certifying eyewear for sports, and experts have provided recommendations for eye protection for different sports (Vinger, 2000).

Common sports-related eye injuries include presence of a foreign body and corneal abrasion. More significant impact results in possible iris injury, posttraumatic iritis, hyphema, or globe perforation or rupture. Athletes presenting with eye pain should be removed from participation and have a thorough eye examination, as follows:

1. Assessment and documentation of visual acuity
2. Inspection for evidence of globe rupture or leaking aqueous humor
3. Assessment of extraocular movements, limitation, or asymmetry suggesting orbital fracture
4. Assessment of pupil reactivity (A dilated, constricted, or sluggish pupil can be transient secondary to iris trauma or may indicate hyphema or globe injury.)
5. Inspection of anterior chamber for blood indicating hyphema

Abnormalities identified on this initial examination require consultation with an ophthalmologist. If the examination is normal, lid inversion should be performed, inspecting for a foreign body, with slit-lamp evaluation using fluorescein staining to assess for corneal abrasions. Anesthetic eyedrops may be required to facilitate the examination and for initial pain management but should not be used to allow return to play or for ongoing pain management (Moeller and Rifat, 2003).

Corneal abrasions are treated with antibiotic eyedrops to prevent infection and topical NSAIDs given for pain, if necessary (Weaver and Terrell, 2003). Once pain-free, with a normal follow-up examination, athletes might return to play. After ocular injury, an athlete is often more receptive to counseling on protective eyewear.

Infectious Disease

Key Points

- Upper respiratory infections are more common in heavily training athletes, and team physicians must consider both infection control measures and avoiding banned substances when treating high-level athletes.
- Infectious mononucleosis is associated with splenomegaly and a risk of splenic rupture. It requires that athletes avoid heavy exertion and contact sports until the spleen is of normal size, usually within 4 weeks.

Upper respiratory tract infection (URI) is a common complaint in primary care sports medicine. Regular, moderate exercise may decrease the risk for contracting a URI, but acute bouts of heavy exercise, such as running a marathon, and prolonged heavy training increase the risk for URI (Nieman, 2003). Treatment of URI is symptomatic, but health care providers of competitive athletes must consider which substances are banned by the governing body overseeing their sport. Banned substances are subject to change, and physicians must be aware of current regulations. For example, the World Anti-Doping Agency (WADA), responsible for drug regulation for many international sports organizations, bans stimulants and many sympathomimetics. Ephedrine is banned above a urine concentration threshold, and pseudoephedrine was banned until a rule change in 2005.

Most governing bodies, such as WADA (2009) and the National Collegiate Athletic Association (NCAA, 2009), have websites posting current banned substances (see Web Resources). These sites should be consulted before prescribing or recommending any medication for athletes subject to drug testing.

Physicians caring for teams must also consider infection control measures. URI, viral gastroenteritis, skin infection, and mononucleosis are of particular concern. Vectors that must be considered include common source spread (enteroviruses), person-to-person spread from sharing secretions (viral, fungal, bacterial skin infection), and airborne droplet spread (picornaviruses). Sharing of water dispensers, bottles, and towels should be eliminated. Handwashing must be encouraged and antibacterial soap or alcohol-based hand sanitizers provided. Shared equipment must be disinfected. Simple infection control measures are often not practiced in the setting of team sports, and educating athletes, coaches, and training staff is the responsibility of the team physician.

Mononucleosis

Infectious mononucleosis (mono) caused by Epstein-Barr virus (EBV) or occasionally by cytomegalovirus (CMV) deserves special mention. Splenomegaly and spleen fragility are often associated with mono and are a concern for team physicians because of the risk of splenic rupture. The prolonged fatigue accompanying mono is also especially difficult for athletes trying to return to training as soon as possible.

Epstein-Barr virus is prevalent and shed in saliva, thus, mono's reputation as the "kissing disease." About 50% of the U.S. population seroconverts by age 5 years, with a mild viral syndrome or asymptomatically. If an individual reaches college age (18-22) without infection, seroconversion results in a 30% to 70% incidence of mono (Schooley, 1999). Symptoms include 1 week of significant flulike symptoms with anterior and often significant posterior cervical lymphadenopathy and exudative pharyngitis. Splenomegaly occurs in 50% of cases during weeks 2 to 3 of illness and usually resolves by weeks 4 to 6. Splenomegaly is difficult to confirm on examination alone and should be suspected in all athletes with mono. Significant fatigue is often prevalent, and although most symptoms resolve by 4 weeks, fatigue can last 12 weeks or longer (Rea et al., 2001).

Once suspected, the diagnosis of mono should be confirmed because of the risk of splenic rupture and implications for withholding sports participation. The diagnosis can be confirmed by a positive EBV heterophile antibody (Monospot) with 90% sensitivity by 3 weeks. False-negative results are common in the first 2 weeks, with a positive test in only 40% of those infected during the first week of illness. Therefore, an initially negative Monospot test in a suspicious case should be repeated 1 week later. An EBV or CMV viral capsid antigen (VCA) immunoglobulin M (IgM) assay can also provide evidence of acute infection, with 90% sensitivity at the onset of symptoms (Cohen, 1998).

There is no clear evidence-based answer for when an athlete with mono can safely return to sports. The risk of splenic rupture associated with sporting activity occurs almost exclusively in the first 3 weeks of illness (Kinderknecht, 2002). Many authorities recommend restriction from noncontact sports for 3 weeks, until symptoms have largely resolved and the spleen is not palpable. Returning athletes to contact sports can be considered after 4 weeks of illness, when all symptoms have resolved and splenomegaly is absent (Auwaerter, 2004). The range for normal spleen size varies significantly, and splenic ultrasound is not necessary in most cases but can be considered before returning an athlete to contact sports. Larger-than-normal ranges for splenic size have been described for taller athletes (Spielmann et al., 2005).

KEY TREATMENT

For athletes with confirmed mononucleosis, return to sport can be considered after 3 weeks for noncontact sports and after 4 weeks for collision sports once symptoms have largely resolved and the spleen is not palpable (Auwaerter, 2004) (SOR: C).

Sports Dermatology

Key Points

- Fungal, viral, and bacterial skin infections are usually transmitted through person-to-person contact in sports activities.
- Management requires a high index of suspicion, prompt treatment, restriction of participation for contagious athletes, covering lesions when appropriate to allow participation, and appropriate prophylaxis and treatment.
- Skin problems are usually caused by laceration or abrasion, environmental exposure, inflammation, or infection.

Fungal Infections

Tinea (ringworm) is one of the most common fungal infections. Tinea pedis is frequently seen in athletes secondary to group showering, and it can be prevented to some extent by having athletes regularly change socks and use wicking materials in socks to keep feet dry, drying powders (many of which contain prophylactic topical antifungals), and shower shoes. Treatment with topical antifungals and oral therapy for severe cases are effective.

Fungal infections are spread directly from person to person through contact sports, with the type seen in wrestlers (tinea corporis gladiatorum) being the most problematic. Tinea tonsurans occurs most often, with infection rates in high school wrestlers of 24% to 75% (Adams, 2000; Beller and Gessner, 1994). Infection is caused by contact with an infected opponent and usually occurs on the arms, neck, or head. The lesions often appear initially as annular plaques with raised erythematous borders and may progress without the central clearing often appreciated with ringworm (Adams, 2002). Microscopic evaluation of skin scrapings with potassium hydroxide (KOH) may reveal fungal elements. Topical treatment with azole agents and oral treatment have been studied. A randomized prospective study of topical clotrimazole 1% cream twice daily versus oral fluconazole, 200 mg weekly, showed equal symptomatic improvement after 10 days and a similar 50% lesion reduction at 17 days. However, 50% culture eradication took 11 days with oral treatment and 22 days with topical treatment, leading to the conclusion that weekly fluconazole should be first-line treatment (Kohl et al., 1999). For

multiple lesions, a 3-week treatment course with an oral antifungal is recommended.

Return-to-play recommendations after tinea corporis gladiatorum infection vary. The NCAA requires 72 hours of topical therapy for skin lesions and 2 weeks of oral therapy for scalp lesions, and also stipulates that athletes may participate with an active lesion provided it is covered entirely by an adhesive nonpermeable dressing (NCAA, 2009). The National Federation of State High School Associations does not allow participation with communicable lesions even if covered (Landry and Chang, 2004). Prophylaxis using oral itraconazole every other week and oral fluconazole weekly has been shown to be effective (Hazen and Weil, 1997; Kohl et al., 2000), but the potential for exposure and time loss morbidity of an active infection must be weighed against the cost and potential side effects.

Viral Infections

Herpes gladiatorum, caused by herpes simplex virus (HSV), is highly contagious and spread by person-to-person contact, with a predilection for the face, arms, and upper trunk. As the name suggests, herpes gladiatorum is common in wrestling, although epidemics are also reported in other sports, such as rugby (Adams, 2002) (Fig. 29-4). Because herpes lacks definitive treatment, it is considered more serious than tinea. Herpes gladiatorum has a prevalence as high as 40% in collegiate wrestlers (Anderson, 1999). Outbreaks generally occur 2 to 5 days after exposure. Lesions typically manifest with prodromal pain or itching, followed by clear vesicles on an erythematous base. Primary infections may cause systemic flulike symptoms, and recurrent infections occur in the same dermatome. Often, the vesicles have been traumatized before evaluation, making the rash appear nonspecific, although the prodromal symptoms or history of previous outbreak in the same location suggests herpes. Traditionally, diagnosis was confirmed with Tzanck testing or culture, but the direct fluorescent antibody test is widely available and provides rapid detection of HSV in specimens with greater sensitivity than traditional methods.

The natural history of a herpes outbreak is to resolve and possibly recur, with frequency and severity dependent on both host and environmental factors. Treatment with oral antiviral agents can shorten the duration of the outbreak,

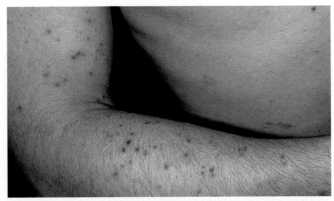

Figure 29-4 Herpes gladiatorum. Lesions may be numerous in wrestlers and involve a wide area of the skin surface.
(From Habif T. Clinical Dermatology, 5th ed. Philadelphia, Elsevier, 2009.)

decrease contagion, and prevent recurrent infection. No one agent has proved superior. The most cost-effective regimen is acyclovir, 400 mg three times daily for 10 days for primary infections and for 5 days for recurrent infections. Treatment is most effective when started at the first sign of infection. Prophylaxis with valacyclovir (500-1000 mg daily) limited herpes gladiatorum recurrence (Anderson, 1999), and acyclovir (400 mg twice daily) has demonstrated effectiveness comparable to valacyclovir, limiting recurrent genital herpes (Reitano et al., 1998). Research using antivirals for primary prevention is lacking, but entire teams may be placed on prophylactic doses if a team member or opposing team member has an outbreak. Some team physicians offer prophylactic treatment to the squad before large tournaments or for the entire competitive season.

Return to play after herpes infection is more conservative than with tinea infection. The NCAA requires that wrestlers be free of any systemic symptoms, have no new blisters for 72 hours, have all lesions crusted over, and have taken treatment doses of antiviral medication for 120 hours before competition (NCAA, 2009).

Bacterial Infections

Bacterial infections are common in sports, and treatment is similar for both athletes and nonathletes. Bacterial infections of the skin generally manifest as furuncles, carbuncles, impetigo, cellulitis, or erysipelas. Staphylococcal and streptococcal infections are most common, but community-acquired methicillin-resistant *Staphylococcus aureus* (CA-MRSA), first reported in the late 1990s, has become a significant problem in athletic training facilities (Lindenmighter et al., 1998; Nguyen et al., 2005).

Sports activities provide a favorable environment for the acquisition and spread of bacterial skin infection. Abrasive surfaces such as artificial turf can harbor bacteria and become a source of infection. Shared equipment, improperly laundered practice gear, person-to-person contact, and inadequate showering facilities without antibacterial soap have all been implicated in the spread of bacterial skin infections in athletes.

Controlling infection in athletes involves prevention, good surveillance, and prompt, appropriate treatment. Shared equipment requires regular cleaning with antibacterial disinfectant. Athletes should shower with antibacterial soap after practice and competition. Abrasions should be addressed expeditiously, scrubbed with antibacterial wash, and covered with sterile dressings, which are changed regularly. Athletes must be instructed to report suspected infections as soon as identified. Topical antibiotics are appropriate for mild infections, with oral or IV antibiotics required for more severe infections. Any significant abscess should have incision and drainage with bacterial culture, including MRSA. Thus far, most CA-MRSA infections in athletes have shown sensitivity to trimethoprim-sulfamethoxazole, with some isolates sensitive to macrolides and quinolones (Arnold and Wojda, 2005). The resistance patterns are susceptible to rapid change, however, making routine culture of these wounds essential. Athletes with recurrent MRSA infections should be assessed by nasal culture for colonization with MRSA and treated with topical mupirocin ointment if positive.

Pulmonary Problems

Key Points

- Exercise-induced bronchospasm is the transient narrowing of the airways in response to exercise.
- Symptoms of EIB include wheezing, coughing, dyspnea, and chest tightness.
- The diagnosis should be confirmed by spirometry testing before and after exercise showing a 10% to 15% reduction in FEV_1.

Exercise-Induced Bronchospasm

Exercise-induced asthma or, more accurately, exercise-induced bronchospasm (EIB) is a transient narrowing of the airways following vigorous exercise. Ninety percent of known asthmatics and 40% of patients with allergic rhinitis have bronchoconstriction caused or worsened by exercise (Feinstein et al., 1996). In some patients, the only manifestation of airway hyperresponsiveness is EIB, with up to 50% of athletes having EIB in some high-risk sports (Langdeau and Boulet, 2001).

The pathophysiology of EIB involves mucosal drying secondary to large volumes of dry (often cool) air, which causes changes in mucosal pH, osmolarity, and temperature and triggers the release of inflammatory mediators, leading to bronchoconstriction (Hallstrand et al., 2005). This osmotic hypothesis explains the relationship between the intensity and duration of exercise to EIB, the role of inflammation and bronchoconstriction in EIB, and the increased prevalence of EIB in outdoor winter sports, such as cross-country skiing. A refractory period typically follows EIB, in which the patient has fewer symptoms on reexercise. This probably occurs because of increased bronchial blood flow following exercise, which enhances water delivery to airway mucosa and makes it more resistant to osmotic changes. The mechanism of EIB in swimmers may be different and related to exposure to direct bronchial irritants, such as chlorine.

Symptoms of EIB include exercise-related wheezing, coughing, dyspnea, and chest tightness. The diagnosis of EIB, however, is difficult, and screening by medical history and physical examination alone is often inaccurate. In a study of 256 adolescent athletes participating in organized sports, 39.5% reported symptoms or a previous diagnosis suggestive of EIB, although only 9.4% were found to have EIB based on an exercise challenge test and serial spirometry (Hallstrand et al., 2002). Thus, any athlete with suspected EIB should be tested with an exercise challenge test. A decrease in forced expiratory volume in 1 second (FEV_1) greater than 10% to 15% is indicative of EIB.

Management of EIB involves both nonpharmacologic and pharmacologic methods. Nonpharmacologic treatment includes emphasis on a good warm-up to precipitate the refractory period, exercising in warm and humid environments, and covering the mouth and nose during cold weather. The goal of pharmacologic therapy is for the athlete to be asymptomatic during exercise. First-line pharmacologic treatment involves the use of an inhaled beta-2 agonist (e.g., albuterol metered-dose inhaler, 2 puffs) 15 to 30 minutes before exercise. If the athlete is still symptomatic, the addition of a leukotriene modifier (e.g., montelukast, 10 mg) taken at least 1 hour before exercise can provide additional relief (Coreno et al., 2000). Another treatment alternative is an inhaled mast cell stabilizer (e.g., cromolyn) before exercise. Inhaled corticosteroids are not as useful for acute prophylaxis because of their delayed onset of action, but can be very useful in patients with chronic persistent asthma and EIB. Any underlying chronic asthma or allergic rhinitis should also be optimally controlled.

Pneumothorax

Spontaneous and traumatic pneumothorax can occur in the setting of sports. Spontaneous pneumothorax should be suspected in tall, thin male athletes with the acute onset of dyspnea, pleuritic chest pain, and shortness of breath. Traumatic pneumothorax should be considered when an athlete is short of breath after sustaining a blow to the chest, particularly if a rib fracture is suspected (Partridge et al., 1997). Diagnosis is confirmed by chest radiograph, and treatment depends on the amount of lung involved. If the patient is stable and there is less than 15% to 20% volume loss, this can generally be treated with observation. Return to play after a pneumothorax can usually occur safely in 3 to 4 weeks (Putukian, 2004).

KEY TREATMENT

Treatment of exercise-induced bronchoconstriction involves an adequate warm-up and use of an inhaled beta-2 agonist 15 to 30 minutes before exercise, with the addition of montelukast or cromolyn, if needed (Coreno et al., 2000; Hallstrand et al., 2005) (SOR: B).

Hematologic Problems

Key Points

- Sports anemia is a dilutional anemia caused by the expansion of plasma volume in the trained athlete.
- Exertional hemolysis occurs from increased destruction of red blood cells, and diagnosis is confirmed by low hemoglobin or hematocrit and low haptoglobin level.
- Low iron stores, even in the absence of anemia, can adversely affect performance in endurance athletes.
- Athletes with sickle cell trait, especially if poorly hydrated, exercising in hot conditions, at altitude, or unconditioned, have a higher risk of exertional rhabdomyolysis and sudden death; screening at-risk populations should be considered.

There are several hematologic issues specific to athletes. This section reviews dilutional pseudoanemia or sports anemia, exertional hemolysis, iron deficiency anemia and low iron stores without anemia, and special considerations regarding athletes who are sickle cell trait–positive.

Sports Anemia

Sports anemia is not representative of true pathology. Rather, it represents an adaptive response to strenuous training and is caused by an expanded plasma volume. The degree of anemia typically correlates with the intensity of training. Plasma volume can expand by 5% to 20%. This adaptive response begins a few days after starting or intensifying training. Moderate exercisers may see a decrease in hemoglobin (Hb) of 0.5 g/dL, and elite athletes may have an apparent Hb decrease of 1 g/dL. Athletes with low Hb or hematocrit (Hct) value and a characteristic history should be checked for iron deficiency. A normal ferritin level, iron level, and total iron-binding capacity (TIBC) confirms the diagnosis of dilutional anemia, or sports anemia, which does not need to be treated (Eichner, 1992; Shaskey and Green, 2000).

Exertional Hemolysis

Exertional or "foot strike" hemolysis is another problem often encountered in athletes. Exertional hemolysis was initially described in endurance runners but is also seen in swimmers, rowers, and weightlifters. Hypothesized mechanisms for red blood cell (RBC) destruction include trauma secondary to impact, turbulence in the blood vessel, acidosis, and elevated temperature encountered in working muscles. Diagnosis is made with an elevated mean corpuscular volume (MCV) and reticulocyte count and a low haptoglobin level. Treatment consists of mitigating impact by having the athlete run in biomechanically correct shoes and on cushioned surfaces and by recommending slow, incremental increases in training (Telford et al., 2003).

Iron Deficiency Anemia

As in the general population, iron deficiency anemia is common in athletes, especially among female athletes. This is typically caused by low intake of dietary iron, but can also be caused by exertional GI or genitourinary bleeding or GI bleeding related to NSAID use. Iron requirements of athletes, particularly endurance athletes, may also be higher than for sedentary individuals (Beard and Tobin, 2000). The diagnosis of iron deficiency anemia is made by a low Hb or Hct level and a low ferritin or iron level. Treatment consists of increasing dietary iron, iron supplementation, and treating the underlying cause if present.

Low Ferritin in Nonanemic Athlete

The common belief among coaches and endurance athletes is that a low ferritin level can cause fatigue, poor recovery, and poor performance. The ferritin level generally reflects total body iron, and 82% of female endurance athletes have a low ferritin level (Shaskey and Green, 2000). Many studies have examined whether improvements in performance seen in nonanemic athletes are caused by small increases in Hb level (from a normal to a higher normal Hb level) or by an increase in iron alone (Garza et al., 1997). A review of eight randomized, controlled trials (RCTs) indicates that iron has a positive effect on performance in iron-deficient athletes without anemia, independent of Hb increases (Fogelholm et al., 1992; Friedmann et al., 2001; Hinton et al., 2000; Klingshirn et al., 1992; LaManca and Haymes, 1993; Newhouse et al., 1989; Rowland et al., 1988; Zhu and Haas, 1998).

Sickle Cell Trait and Sudden Death

Sickle cell trait occurs in 6% to 8% of the African American population (Kerle and Nishimura, 1996). Among black military recruits, the likelihood of sudden death is 28-fold higher in individuals with sickle cell trait than in those without (Kark et al., 1987). Most of these deaths are associated with *exertional rhabdomyolysis*. This typically occurs when the athlete is poorly hydrated, exercising in hot conditions, at altitude, or unconditioned. Athletes with sickle cell trait are generally not restricted from competition; however, consideration should be given to screening high-risk populations, with special precautions taken to ameliorate risk.

Gastrointestinal Problems

Key Points and Treatment

- Gastroesophageal reflux can be worsened by exercise; treatment with dietary modifications and proton pump inhibitors is usually successful.
- Exercise-induced diarrhea is common in endurance sports; treatment focuses on dietary manipulation before competition and antidiarrheal medications such as loperamide in refractory cases.
- Gastrointestinal bleeding in athletes ranges from microscopic blood loss to ischemic hemorrhagic gastritis or colitis, but pathologic causes of bleeding should be ruled out.

Gastrointestinal problems are common in the general population and in exercising individuals. Although diagnosis and treatment for many of these issues are similar, exercise may make some issues worse or may present special treatment challenges. See online discussions for the following at www.expertconsult.com.
- Gastroesophageal reflux
- Exercise-induced diarrhea
- Gastrointestinal bleeding

Genitourinary Problems

Hematuria and proteinuria are also common findings in athletes. They may be caused by repetitive mechanical trauma to the bladder or by exercise-related changes in renal physiology. Initial workup is to rule out infection, refrain from exercising for 48 to 72 hours, and retest. If hematuria or proteinuria persists, a full evaluation should be performed (Abarbanel et al., 1990).

Genitourinary problems in male cyclists are particularly common. Pressure from the bicycle saddle can cause compression neuropathies (pudendal nerve), impotence, urethritis, or prostatitis (Leibovitch and Mor, 2005). Pudendal neuropathy manifests with numbness or tingling in the scrotum or penile shaft. Treatment involves relieving pressure by changing seat type, proper bicycle fitting, and wearing padded shorts.

Low Back Pain

See the discussion online at www.expertconsult.com.

Spondylolysis

Spondylolysis, a stress fracture of the pars interarticularis, is a common cause of low back pain (LBP) in athletes and is the most common cause of athletic LBP in adolescents (Standaert and Herring, 2000; Standaert et al., 2000). Athletes who participate in sports involving repeated and forceful hyperextension of the spine (e.g., gymnastics, American football) are more likely to develop spondylolysis from the cumulative effect of repetitive loading of the bone imposed by physical activity. Athletes generally have an insidious history of increasing focal back pain reproduced by lumbar extension.

Spondylolysis can be identified by plain radiography in approximately 5% of the general population, but the vast majority of these lesions occur without associated symptoms. Identification of spondylolysis on radiographs in an athlete with LBP must be correlated with the clinical presentation and advanced imaging. Single-photon emission computed tomography (SPECT), high-resolution (thin-slice) computed tomography (HRCT), and MRI are helpful to determine the metabolic activity of the stress fracture, the acuity of the lesion, and potential for fracture healing, and to exclude other spinal pathology that may be present.

Conservative treatment is usually successful in controlling symptoms and restoring function. Treatment requires activity restriction and temporary discontinuation of the aggravating sport or activity. Some patients may require lumbosacral bracing to achieve treatment goals, and only a small percentage of patients require surgical intervention for pain or progressive spondylolisthesis (Standaert and Herring, 2000; Standaert et al., 2000).

Muscle and Tendon Injuries

Key Points

- Eccentric loading produced when the muscle is contracting and lengthening is a common mechanism for muscle and tendon injuries.
- Tendinosis is the predominant pathologic feature in painful overuse tendinopathies.

Mechanism of Injury

Muscle and tendon injuries occur from repetitive microtrauma or a single traumatic event that causes overload to the tensile strength of the myotendinous unit or muscle fiber itself. *Eccentric loads,* produced when the muscle is contracting and lengthening at the same time, are a common mechanism of injury and can produce higher forces compared with concentric contractions (Stanton and Purdam, 1989). Sports activities with repetitive eccentric demands place the athlete at higher risk of injury. In sprinters, for example, hamstring muscle strains typically occur during the late swing phase of the running cycle as the hamstring muscle contracts while lengthening in an attempt to decelerate the lower leg in preparation for foot strike (Stanton and Purdam, 1989). Achilles tendinopathy and patellar tendinopathy (jumper's knee) also result from repetitive eccentric loading of the tendons during running and jumping.

Histopathology

Acute muscle injuries go through a predictable cycle of healing and repair. Exercise-induced muscle injury first causes fiber disruption and local microhemorrhage, followed by extravasation of inflammatory cells and a phagocytic phase to remove injured tissue, and finally a regenerative phase of muscle fiber healing occurs (Armstrong et al., 1991). Limiting overall inflammation decreases pain and minimizes secondary tissue injury caused by hypoxia and inflammatory mediators. However, some amount of inflammation is required in the healing process to remove necrotic muscle fibers and allow scar tissue to bridge the defect (Almekinders and Gilbert, 1986), but how far to limit this inflammation through pharmacotherapy remains uncertain.

In contrast to acute muscle injuries, the pathologic findings in most tendon injuries are consistent with tendinosis, a degenerative condition of the tendon, and not a tendinitis involving inflammation, as was formerly believed. Healthy tendon contains parallel bundles of tightly packed collagen fibers, with little extracellular matrix (ground substance) and no fibroblasts or myofibroblasts. In contrast, symptomatic tendons contain disorganized collagen fibers, increased mucoid ground substance, prominent capillary proliferation, and increased numbers of fibroblasts and myofibroblasts (Khan et al., 1999). Histopathologic examination is notably devoid of inflammatory cells. Animal models have also suggested that inflammatory cells are absent by 1 week after induced overuse injury (Zamora and Marini, 1988). These findings are present in the most common tendon injuries, including the patella, Achilles, rotator cuff, and extensor carpi radialis brevis tendons, and have important implications in the treatment of tendon disorders (Khan et al., 1999). Use of the term *tendinopathy*, rather than tendinitis, is recommended to describe a painful tendon condition.

The generation of pain in chronic tendon injuries appears to involve more than just inflammation. A biochemical hypothesis to explain tendon pain states that biochemical agents are leaked from a degenerated tendon and irritate nociceptors (pain receptors) on adjacent structures (Khan and Cook, 2000). In patellar tendinopathy, higher levels of glycosaminoglycans have been found in the infrapatellar fat pad (Khan et al., 1996), and in patients with partial rotator cuff tears higher levels of substance P were found in the adjacent subacromial bursa and were significantly associated with pain (Gotoh et al., 1998).

Muscle Strains

Muscle injuries can be classified as *mild* (grade 1, strain), *moderate* (grade 2, partial tear of myotendinous units), or *severe* (grade 3, complete tear of myotendinous units). Mild injuries are tender and painful with active use but cause minimal strength loss. Moderate injuries demonstrate clear *weakness* with resisted muscle testing and *pain* with passive stretching. Severe injuries cause significant functional and strength deficits and may show ecchymosis and a palpable defect on examination.

In running and sprinting athletes, hamstring muscle strains are the most common muscle injury (Lysholm and Wiklander, 1987; Meeuwisse et al., 2000; Orchard and Seward, 2002). Other common muscle strains include those of the quadriceps (especially the rectus femoris) and the gastrocnemius. The most significant risk factor for a muscle strain is a recent or past history of that same injury, and incomplete rehabilitation may also contribute to recurrent injuries (Ekstrand and Gillquist, 1983; Orchard, 2001). Other risk factors for muscle injury include poor warm-up, muscle fatigue, and muscle imbalance (Agre, 1985; Croisier et al., 2002; Garrett, 1996; Safran et al., 1989).

Initial treatment of an acute muscle strain involves ice application to limit pain and swelling and relative rest to protect the muscle from more significant injury. A short 3- to 5-day course of NSAIDs can help limit overall inflammation and pain in acute muscle injuries. Gentle stretching to restore flexibility should begin when pain allows, and rehabilitation should progress through isometric, concentric, and finally eccentric strengthening exercises before returning to sports-specific activities.

Tendinopathy

Tendon injuries can involve acute overuse tendinopathy, chronic tendinosis, partial-thickness tears, or complete rupture of the tendon. The exact role of NSAIDs in the treatment of tendinopathy remains uncertain. NSAIDs are potentially helpful initially following acute tendon injury, when inflammation is most likely to be present. For tendinopathy of longer duration, use of NSAIDs, although an adjunct to pain control, does not contribute to tendon healing. The exact mechanism of action of corticosteroid injections, such as in the treatment of lateral epicondylosis and rotator cuff tendinopathies, is also unclear. Corticosteroid injections bathe the region of tendinosis, alter the chemical composition of the matrix, and may modify nociceptors on nearby structures (Khan and Cook, 2000). NSAIDs and corticosteroids also may have an effect on other biochemical irritants (yet to be defined) that play a role in the generation of tendon pain.

The use of therapeutic methods to stimulate collagen repair is also a major focus in the treatment of tendinopathy. Common strategies to induce collagen remodeling include manual therapies such as deep-friction massage, eccentric conditioning of the tendon, tenotomy (needling a degenerated tendon), and injection of autologous growth factors. Eccentric strengthening programs have shown favorable results for patients with chronic Achilles tendinopathy as well as for athletes with chronic patellar tendinopathy (Alfredson et al., 1998; Purdam et al., 2004). When conservative treatments such as physical therapy fail, treatment options are limited and often lead to either the discontinuation of exercise or surgery. In competitive athletics, chronic tendon injuries can lead to persistent pain, lost time from participation, and suboptimal performance. In occupational injuries, chronic tendon trauma leads to significant cost and morbidity.

With a better understanding of the pathogenesis of tendon injury and healing, newer therapies strive to stimulate the failed healing response in tendinopathies, including percutaneous tenotomy with or without injection of autologous blood or growth factor into the degenerative tendon

(McShane et al., 2006; Housner et al., 2009). The most common form of autologous growth factor therapy is platelet-rich plasma (PRP) and is increasingly used to treat tendinosis. Although a relatively novel option for sports-related injuries, PRP has been used in other medical conditions for two decades. The use of PRP migrated to orthopedic procedures, where it has been used effectively to augment bone and soft tissue healing in the operating room, especially in poorly healing fractures and those at high risk for nonunion. Most recently PRP has been used in the outpatient setting for a variety of sports-related soft tissue injuries, including the treatment of chronic tendinopathies, as well as moderate to severe acute ligament, muscle, and tendon injuries. Autologous growth factor therapy in the treatment of chronic tendinosis can initiate a stalled or failed healing response, leading to a healthier and less symptomatic tendon. In the management of chronic lateral epicondylosis (tennis elbow), injection of PRP demonstrated significant pain reduction at 6 months versus injection of anesthetic alone (Mishra and Pavelko, 2006). In the setting of acute soft tissue injury, it is hypothesized that PRP augments the healing response, leading to faster healing, more rapid recovery, and earlier return to sport or activity. In a series of acute muscle injuries in elite soccer players, PRP therapy was found to significantly shorten the time to return to play (Sanchez et al., 2009).

Although research is still needed to understand the optimal indications and treatment protocols for autologous growth factor therapies, initial findings provide optimism that a new, minimally invasive therapeutic option is available in the management of chronic tendinopathies.

KEY TREATMENT

Treatment of an acute muscle strain involves ice application to limit pain and swelling, relative rest and protection from more significant injury, gentle stretching to restore flexibility, and progressive rehabilitation through isometric, concentric, and finally eccentric strengthening exercises before returning to sports-specific activities (SOR: C).

Eccentric strengthening programs can be effective for patients with chronic Achilles or patellar tendinopathy (Alfredson et al., 1998; Purdam et al., 2004) (SOR: B).

Novel therapies using autologous growth factor injections (platelet-rich plasma) show favorable results in the treatment of chronic tendinopathy (Mishra and Pavelko, 2006; Sanchez et al., 2009) (SOR: C).

Shin Pain

Key Points

- Medial tibial stress syndrome is the most common cause of lower leg pain in running athletes.
- Chronic exertional compartment syndrome is characterized by cramping or burning lower leg pain or numbness, which may radiate to the foot and ankle and resolves within minutes of rest.

Medial Tibial Stress Syndrome

Exercise-related lower leg pain is an extremely common condition among athletes. The most common presentation is shin pain exacerbated by exercise and diminished with rest. *Shin splints* is a nonspecific term used to describe shin pain in running athletes from almost any cause. *Medial tibial stress syndrome* (MTSS) is the most widely accepted term to describe pain along the medial border of the tibia experienced by running athletes and is considered to be the most common cause of athletic lower leg pain (Kortebein et al., 2000).

The pathogenesis of MTSS is not fully understood. Some support the concept of a traction periostitis along the posteromedial border of the tibia at the origin of the soleus, flexor digitorum longus, and posterior tibialis muscles (Beck and Osternig, 1994; Michael and Holder, 1985). Scintigraphic and biopsy studies, however, have not consistently shown an inflammatory process of the periosteum to support periostitis as the pathogenesis of shin pain. Others suggest that MTSS is caused by a traction fasciitis (involving the crural fascia) or possibly a bony stress reaction and precursor to stress fracture (Batt, 1995). Bone scan and MRI studies indicate that MTSS is part of a continuum of stress response in bone. Investigation of runners with medial tibial pain demonstrated a spectrum of bone injury, beginning with periosteal edema, progressive marrow edema, and finally frank cortical defects (Fredericson et al., 1995). The mechanism of injury in MTSS probably involves bony overload from the pull of muscle contraction and the impact forces with running.

Athletes with MTSS complain of shin pain that is aggravated with running. Examination reveals tenderness in a broad distribution along the medial border of the tibia, usually spanning the middle and distal thirds of the tibia. In contrast, tibial stress fractures manifest with a focal area of tenderness. Management of MTSS includes rest, activity modification, ice, and anti-inflammatory medications. Correction of biomechanical abnormalities is also helpful. Poor hip abductor and external rotator muscle function may contribute to internal femoral rotation and excessive stress on the medial tibia during running. Extreme foot types, both pes planus and pes cavus, may also contribute to impaired shock absorption and force distribution to the tibia and may improve with orthotic devices.

Chronic Exertional Compartment Syndrome

Chronic exertional compartment syndrome (CECS) is another cause of athletic lower leg pain. Patients with CECS complain of cramping, burning, or aching lower leg pain with pain or numbness that may radiate to the foot and ankle. The pain is clearly associated with exertion. Pain onset is characteristically at a fixed point in the patient's activity, with progressively increasing pain if the exercise continues and a dramatic reduction in pain within minutes of rest. The pathophysiology of CECS involves elevated intracompartmental pressure, which causes relative ischemia of the involved muscles and pressure on neurovascular structures. The diagnosis of CECS can be confirmed by compartment pressure testing after exercise demonstrating increased intracompartmental pressure correlated with symptom reproduction. Patients with CECS should be questioned about the use of nutritional supplements, such as creatine, that may increase muscle water content and overall muscle mass and contribute to the development of CECS. Surgical treatment by fasciotomy provides good functional improvement and symptomatic cure in a high proportion of cases (Blackman, 2000).

Stress Fractures

Key Points

- Stress fractures typically occur weeks after an abrupt increase in activity level, running distance, or training frequency.
- Navicular stress fractures, anterior tibial stress fractures with a "dreaded black line," and femoral neck stress fractures are high-risk stress fractures for nonunion or progression to a complete fracture and should be referred to an orthopedic specialist.

Stress fractures result from a failure of bone to adapt successfully to repetitive loads encountered during running. Wolff's law of adaptation suggests that a bone responds to external stress by mechanical remodeling. Bone strain may become excessive as a result of increases in load magnitude, rate of loading, or number of loading cycles (Crossley et al., 1999). Advances in imaging techniques and understanding of bone pathophysiology indicate that stress injury to bone occurs on a continuum, ranging from normal bone remodeling to bone strain, to stress reaction, to stress fracture, to frank cortical fracture (Fredericson et al., 1995).

A stress fracture, or *fatigue fracture*, occurs when abnormal stress is applied to normal bone. In contrast, an *insufficiency fracture* occurs when normal or physiologic stress is applied to abnormal bone. Female athletes with premature osteoporosis, as seen in the female athlete triad, may have stress fractures resulting from abnormal stress applied to abnormal bone (Callahan, 2000).

Most stress fractures occur in the lower extremities because of impact forces produced from weight bearing during exercise. Common locations for stress fractures include the metatarsals, navicular, tibia, fibula, femoral shaft, femoral neck, and sacrum. The tibia is the most common site of stress fractures in running and jumping athletes and represents about 50% of all cases (Matheson et al., 1987). Less frequently, stress fractures can occur in the upper extremities, ribs, and clavicle from repetitive activity such as throwing, rowing, or weightlifting.

Lower baseline conditioning and training errors are usually involved in the development of stress fractures. A careful history will often reveal an abrupt increase in activity level, running distance, or training frequency within the 2 or 3 months before symptom onset. Many studies have analyzed bone geometry as a risk factor for stress fracture. In male military recruits and runners, studies have demonstrated that a narrower tibia in combination with a smaller tibial cross-sectional area is a risk factor for tibial stress fractures (Beck et al., 1996; Crossley et al., 1999; Giladi et al., 1987).

Female athletes with a history of eating disorders, oligomenorrhea or amenorrhea, and delayed menarche are more likely to develop stress fractures (Arendt, 2000; Bennell et al., 1995). Inadequate caloric intake relative to energy expenditure, also known as a negative energy balance, has been implicated as the primary cause of menstrual dysfunction in young female athletes and is thought to be responsible in part for bone density changes.

Pain from a stress fracture begins with mild pain during activity that resolves with rest. As the stress fracture progresses, pain increases during activity and continues for hours afterward, usually forcing the athlete to stop exercising. With further progression, pain is present with walking and sometimes at rest. On examination, there is local tenderness at the site of the stress fracture. The hop test (asking the patient to hop on one leg) is a useful functional test for suspected lower extremity stress fractures. If a stress fracture is present, the athlete either is reluctant to hop or will have pain reproduction with hopping. Stress fractures may be seen on radiographs as an area of cortical thickening (periosteal reaction) and may have a linear fracture line visible. Radiographs are positive in only about 50% of cases, and an advanced imaging study such as MRI or bone scanning is often needed to confirm the diagnosis.

Stress fractures are treated with rest, activity modification, and avoidance of aggravating activities. Ambulation must be pain-free to allow for fracture healing. If the athlete cannot achieve pain-free ambulation, a period of non–weight bearing on crutches is indicated. Foot stress fractures may benefit from the use of a rigid walking boot, and tibial stress fractures may benefit from a compressive pneumatic leg brace (Swenson et al., 1997). The time for healing of a stress fracture can vary (range, 4-12 weeks), depending on the site and severity. To maintain overall conditioning, athletes can engage in nonimpact cross-training activities, such as swimming or cycling, assuming that the activity is performed without pain. Athletes with two or more stress fractures should be screened for osteopenia or osteoporosis with a bone density scan. Low bone density requires further investigation to rule out secondary causes of osteoporosis, such as vitamin D deficiency or thyroid abnormalities. Menstrual irregularities, disordered eating, and a negative energy balance in female athletes should also be corrected.

Some stress fractures are at higher risk for nonunion or progression to a complete fracture. High-risk stress fractures include navicular, anterior tibial (diagnosed by the "dreaded black line" on lateral radiograph), and femoral neck stress fractures (Fig. 29-5). Athletes with a confirmed or suspected high-risk stress fracture should be made non–weight bearing and referred to a sports medicine or orthopedic specialist.

> ### KEY TREATMENT
>
> Treatment of lower extremity stress fractures include rest, avoidance of aggravating activities, and pain-free ambulation with use of crutches or immobilizing walking boots if needed (SOR: C).

The Pediatric Athlete

Key Points

- Children are not "little adults." Sports competition and training must be age appropriate to prevent injury to developing bone and soft tissue and prevent psychological trauma, which could lead to an aversion to physical activity.
- Overuse injuries common in pediatric athletes include articular cartilage injuries (osteochondritis dissecans), chronic physeal injuries, and apophysitis.

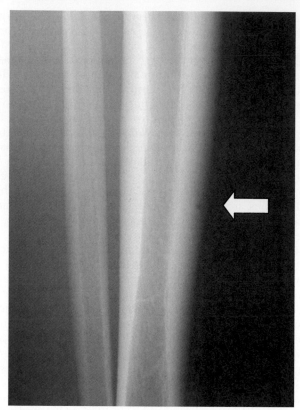

Figure 29-5 Stress fracture. Lateral tibial radiograph shows the "dreaded black line." Note cortical disruption on the anterior cortex.
(From Delee and Drez's Orthopaedic Sports Medicine, 3rd ed. Philadelphia, Elsevier, 2009.)

Pediatric sports injuries are increasing in frequency secondary to increased sports participation, prolonged and overlapping seasons, and children being subjected to adult levels of training and competition prematurely. Although the benefits of exercise and sports participation for children are well recognized, overtraining can have adverse physiologic and psychological consequences. In a review of age-appropriate sports participation from a neurodevelopmental and psychological perspective, Patel and colleagues (2002) suggested that children are not prepared for full competitive participation in complex sports before age 12 years. Children obtain the developmental tools to accomplish complex sports tasks at different ages, and future athletic talent cannot be predicted by childhood performance. Children subjected to age-inappropriate levels of competition or sports-specific skill development are likely to stop participating and create negative associations with sports and exercise, an unfortunate outcome that may affect them adversely for life. Primary care physicians must counsel parents to recognize these issues and not make physical activity and sports participation a negative experience for children.

Physeal and Apophyseal Injuries

The adage that "children are not little adults" applies when considering sports injuries. Open physes in long bones and apophyses at tendon attachments to bone provide weak links through which acute and repetitive overuse injury can occur. These growth centers usually close within defined age ranges throughout adolescence, but significant variation between individuals exists. Thus, physeal and apophyseal injury must always be considered when evaluating children or adolescents with musculoskeletal complaints.

Physeal fractures are common and must not be missed, because growth arrest can occur if they are not recognized and treated appropriately. The diagnosis of an ankle or knee sprain in a young adolescent with open physes should only be considered after physeal injury has been ruled out. Acute physeal injuries and the Salter-Harris classification system are addressed in greater detail in Chapter 30.

Overuse injuries are increasing in frequency in pediatric athletes, with the most common being articular cartilage injuries (osteochondritis dissecans), chronic physeal injury, and apophysitis. Osteochondritis dissecans (OCD) involves a focal loss of cartilage and the underlying bone fragment and may be idiopathic or associated with overuse activities. Apophysitis is the pediatric equivalent of tendinopathy in adults. The growth center at the tendon-bone interface is susceptible to injury similar to that sustained by the physes of long bones. Risk factors contributing to the development of pediatric overuse injuries include overtraining; strength and flexibility deficits somewhat inherent in bone and soft tissue development; prior injury with inadequate rehabilitation; faulty technique, often resulting from poor coaching; and excessive pressure from adults to train and perform. The diagnosis is usually straightforward and requires a familiarity with the demands and common overuse injuries of that sport (Lord and Winell, 2004; Thordarson and Shean, 2005). Table 29-2 lists common apophyseal injuries in pediatric athletes.

The treatment of OCD varies according to location, but the offending activity should be stopped immediately and the upper extremity joint immobilized or the lower extremity joint made non–weight bearing. The patient should be referred to an orthopedist for further management, which may involve prolonged rest with radiographic follow-up, reattachment of loose fragments, or removal of fragments with drilling or grafting of joint surfaces.

The treatment for chronic physeal injury or apophysitis consists of initial rest, followed by rehabilitation directed at improving flexibility and strength, then a gradual return to activity. Parents and young athletes should be counseled that low-level recurring symptoms can be expected until growth plates have closed, but that escalating symptoms should be managed with rest and physician follow-up. The most challenging aspect of treatment is ensuring proper coaching, educating parents regarding appropriate levels of participation and competition for children, and having adults accept reasonable limits for childhood participation in sports.

Special Concerns for the Female Athlete

Key Points

- An energy deficit is the primary cause of amenorrhea in athletic women, and treatment should focus on the restoration of a normal energy balance.

- Menstrual dysfunction or hypothalamic pituitary axis suppression caused by an energy deficit in exercising women is a diagnosis of exclusion, and workup should include evaluation for medical causes

Table 29-2 Common Apophyseal Injuries in Pediatric Athletes

Eponym/Common Injury	Body Part and Pathophysiology	Common Sports/Activity
Little League shoulder	Proximal humeral epiphysiolysis from repetitive microtrauma	Overhead sports: baseball, softball, tennis, swimming, volleyball
Little League elbow	Medial epicondylar apophysitis from traction to ulnar collateral ligament	Baseball (especially pitchers)
Lateral Little League elbow/osteochondritis dissecans (OCD)	OCD of capitellum or less likely radial head from repetitive compression-rotation forces	Baseball, gymnastics, overhead throwing and arm weight-bearing sports
Osgood-Schlatter's disease	Traction apophysitis of tibial tubercle	Soccer, basketball, running/jumping sports
Sinding-Larsen-Johansson disease	Traction apophysitis to distal patella	Soccer, basketball, running/jumping sports
Sever's disease	Calcaneal apophysitis from traction on Achilles insertion	Soccer, gymnastics, running/jumping sports
Pelvis-ASIS apophysitis	Traction from sartorius origin	Sprinting, kicking, jumping, hurtling
Pelvis-AIIS apophysitis	Traction from rectus femoris origin	Sprinting, kicking, jumping, hurtling
Buttock-ischial apophysitis	Traction from hamstring origin	Sprinting, kicking, jumping, hurtling
Spondylolysis	Stress fracture of vertebral pars interarticularis	Gymnastics, figure skating, football lineman, sports with spine loading in extension

of amenorrhea, including a pregnancy test and determination of prolactin, follicle-stimulating hormone (FSH), luteinizing hormone (LH), thyroid-stimulating hormone (TSH), dehydroepiandrosterone (DHEA), and testosterone levels.

- Bone mineral density is adversely affected by menstrual dysfunction and, although treatment with hormone replacement (e.g., oral contraceptives) should be considered, this does not fully address the mechanisms of bone loss.

Exercise results in many benefits for both male and female athletes. In female athletes, exercise coupled with low energy intake can lead to a spectrum of disorders, culminating in the *female athlete triad,* strictly defined as the presence of an eating disorder, amenorrhea, and osteoporosis. It is important to recognize the precursors to the development of the female athlete triad when they may be more amenable to treatment, resulting in less severe long-term sequelae.

The menstrual cycle in the female athlete represents a complex and delicate interplay of hormones. The array of menstrual function seen in athletes ranges from normal ovulatory cycles to luteal-phase defects, to anovulation, to oligomenorrhea, and to amenorrhea. Menstrual dysfunction can exist even in women with normal cycle length, and various types of cycles are common in an individual athlete (De Souza and Williams, 2004).

Athletic amenorrhea is caused by hypothalamic-pituitary axis suppression and is a diagnosis of exclusion. Other causes of amenorrhea must be ruled out, including pregnancy, hyperthyroidism, hyperprolactinemia, primary deficiency of gonadotropin-releasing hormone, and hyperandrogenic anovulatory syndrome (polycystic ovarian syndrome) (Ahima, 2004). When amenorrhea occurs in the setting of exercise or weight loss and initial hormonal testing is normal, a diagnosis of athletic amenorrhea can be made. Recent research has established that energy deficit is the primary cause of amenorrhea in athletic women

(De Souza and Williams, 2004). Strenuous exercise alone in the setting of adequate energy intake does not disrupt the menstrual cycle. An energy deficit results in low concentrations of leptin and in changes in the neuroendocrine axis, including low levels of reproductive hormones, thyroid, and insulin-like growth factor-1 (IGF-1) and an increase in cortisol and growth hormone levels. Similar changes can be seen with psychogenic stress in sedentary women, and stress-induced changes may also contribute to menstrual dysfunction in both normal and underweight female athletes (Ahima, 2004).

The attainment of peak bone mineral density is adversely affected in both the short term and the long term by menstrual dysfunction (Keen and Drinkwater, 1997). The degree of menstrual dysfunction is related to the severity of osteopenia or osteoporosis (Hartard et al., 2004). Initially, the low estrogen state associated with athletic amenorrhea was thought to be solely responsible for bone density problems similar to those seen in postmenopausal women. More recent research has indicated that micronutrient deficiency and low levels of leptin, IGF-1, and other bone trophic factors also contribute to bone mineral deficits (Chan and Mantzoros, 2005).

Treatment of menstrual dysfunction and low bone density has traditionally consisted of hormone replacement therapy, most often with oral contraceptives. Oral contraceptives are not associated with complete bone recovery, most likely because of the multifactorial nature of bone metabolism. Bisphosphonates can increase bone density in adolescents with anorexia, although not as effectively as weight restoration (Golden et al., 2005). Bisphosphonates have extremely long half-lives and remain in the skeleton for many years. Because of concern about potential teratogenicity, bisphosphonates should not be used in young women of childbearing age until further studies on their long-term safety.

The primary treatment for athletic amenorrhea should be restoration of a normal energy balance. Disordered eating patterns must be addressed. Anorexia nervosa and bulimia nervosa are common in women, particularly those competing in sports in which there is an emphasis on leanness or appearance, such as gymnastics, figure skating, and cross-country running. Eating disorders are best addressed with an interdisciplinary management team that includes both psychological and nutritional counseling (Otis et al., 1997).

Menstrual dysfunction, although common in female athletes, should prompt evaluation for medical causes and eating disorders. It is never normal or desirable for a female athlete to cease menstrual function, and this should not be seen as a marker of adequate training. Exercise alone should not be blamed for menstrual dysfunction. Treatment should focus on the restoration of energy balance and a safe continuation of activity.

KEY TREATMENT

The primary treatment for athletic amenorrhea should be restoration of a normal energy balance by addressing disordered eating and training patterns (Otis et al., 1997) (SOR: C).

References

The complete reference list is available online at www.expertconsult.com.

Web Resources

www.ncaa.org/wps/ncaa?key=/ncaa/ncaa/legislation+and+governance/eligibility+and+recruiting/drug+testing/drug_testing.html
National Collegiate Athletic Association (NCAA): Drug-testing program.

www.ncaa.org/wps/ncaa?key=/ncaa/NCAA/Sports%20and%20Championship/Wrestling/Playing%20Rules/index.html
National Collegiate Athletic Association (NCAA): Wrestling 2005: Rules and interpretation.

www.wada-ama.org/en/World-Anti-Doping-Program/Sports-and-Anti-Doping-Organizations/International-Standards/Prohibited-List/
World Anti-Doping Agency (WADA) list of prohibited drugs.

CHAPTER 30

Common Issues in Orthopedics

Jeffrey A. Silverstein, James L. Moeller, and Mark R. Hutchinson

Fractures

Key Points

- Always obtain two different radiographic perspectives of a bone or joint when evaluating for fractures.
- Always examine the joint above and below a fracture to look for associated injuries.
- Open fractures are orthopedic emergencies and need to be urgently washed out in the operating room.
- Be particularly alert for growth plate fractures in children.

The most common reason for not identifying a fracture is failure to examine or radiograph the area or extremity appropriately. When evaluating a patient for a fracture, the primary care physician must be sure to palpate and examine the joint above and below the fracture for potential concomitant injuries. Always obtain orthogonal views from at least two perspectives (e.g., AP and lateral). Additional radiographs are necessary only if a fracture is suspected. When communicating about fractures, health care professionals require a similar vocabulary to visualize the description accurately. This is especially true when family physicians and emergency physicians communicate with orthopedic consultants to make treatment decisions.

Fractures can be oriented in a variety of planes, and certain patterns are associated with greater risk of instability. Typical fracture orientations are transverse, spiral, oblique, compression, buckle, avulsion, stress, and greenstick. Additional features include the specific bone, region within the bone (diaphysis, metaphysis, epiphysis) (Fig. 30-1), and whether the fracture is complete or incomplete, open or closed, intra-articular or extra-articular, displaced or nondisplaced, angulated, shortened, or comminuted. In children, physeal involvement is a special concern.

Open fractures are surgical emergencies and require immediate irrigation and debridement, tetanus prophylaxis, and antibiotic coverage. Orthopedists typically refer to the Gustilo-Anderson classification for open fractures, which is based on the size of skin wound, soft tissue damage, and bone comminution (Box 30-1). Even a small puncture wound over a fracture may allow skin flora to infiltrate the fracture site and initiate an infection. Any open fracture warrants an immediate referral to an emergency department (ED) for orthopedic evaluation.

Growth Plate Fractures

The physeal plate is a cartilaginous plate present in ends of long bones, adjacent to the metaphysis. This is the area that provides longitudinal growth to bones and eventually matures into bone. During growth, the physeal cartilaginous plate is weaker than the surrounding bone and often weaker than the ligaments and tendons that attach nearby, causing it to fracture before other areas. The Salter-Harris classification system describes these injuries (Fig. 30-2).

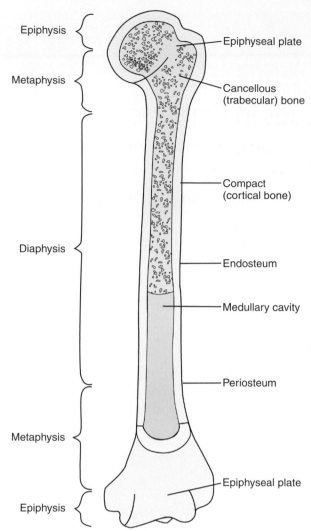

Epiphysis

Metaphysis

Diaphysis

Metaphysis

Epiphysis

Epiphyseal plate

Cancellous
(trabecular) bone

Compact
(cortical bone)

Endosteum

Medullary cavity

Periosteum

Epiphyseal plate

Figure 30-1 Bone regions: diaphysis, metaphysis, and epiphysis.

Box 30-1 Gustilo-Anderson Open-Fracture Classification

Type I

Wound is less than 1 cm, with minimal soft tissue injury.

Wound bed is clean.

Fracture is usually a simple transverse, short oblique fracture, with minimal comminution.

Type II

Wound is greater than 1 cm, with moderate soft tissue injury.

Fracture is usually a simple transverse, short oblique fracture, with minimal comminution.

Type III

Fracture involves extensive damage to the soft tissues, including muscle, skin, and neurovascular structures.

Fracture is often accompanied by a high-velocity injury or a severe crushing component.

Special patterns classified as type III:

    Open segmental fracture, regardless of the size of the wound

    Gunshot wounds: high-velocity and short-range shotgun injuries

    Open fracture with neurovascular injury

    Farm injuries, with soil contamination, regardless of size of wound

    Traumatic amputations

    Open fractures more than 8 hours after injury

    Mass casualties (e.g., war, tornado victims)

Subtype IIIA

Adequate soft tissue coverage despite soft tissue laceration or flaps or high-energy trauma, regardless of size of wound; includes segmental fractures or severely comminuted fractures.

Subtype IIIB

Extensive soft tissue lost with periosteal stripping and bony exposure; usually associated with massive contamination.

Subtype IIIC

Fracture with major arterial injury requiring repair for limb salvage.

Salter-Harris Type I

The epiphysis is separated from the metaphysis along the physis, without an associated fracture through the metaphyseal or epiphyseal bone. The injury goes directly through the cartilaginous physeal plate. These injuries can be displaced or nondisplaced. A nondisplaced Salter-Harris I fracture will have a normal-appearing growth plate on radiographs, but patients will have pain on palpation directly over the growth plate. Stress radiographs or magnetic resonance imaging (MRI) may be necessary to reveal the injury. Displaced type I injuries are typically easy to reduce because the periosteal attachment remains intact. These injuries have an excellent chance of normal healing with full growth of the injured bone. Despite this, growth delay and growth arrest are complications of growth plate injuries, which should be discussed with the patient and family.

Salter-Harris Type II

The fracture line incompletely extends through the physeal plate and then turns into the metaphysis in an extra-articular fracture pattern. The Salter-Harris II fracture is the most common type of growth plate fracture. The periosteum remains

intact on the concave side of the injury, creating a "hinge" and making reduction relatively easy. Prognosis is excellent for future growth when anatomically reduced, with only minor risk of angular deformity.

Salter-Harris Type III

The fracture line extends incompletely along the physis and then turns through the epiphyseal bone into the joint. Salter-Harris III fractures are intra-articular injuries that imply an increased risk of arthritis, especially if they are not anatomically reduced. Alignment of the joint surface is the top priority, and open reduction is often necessary. Prognosis is good, provided the blood supply to the fracture fragment remains intact.

Salter-Harris Type IV

This intra-articular fracture pattern extends from the epiphysis, across the physeal plate, and through a portion of the metaphysis. Open reduction with internal fixation is usually needed to ensure anatomic alignment of the joint surface and perfect alignment and apposition of the physeal plate.

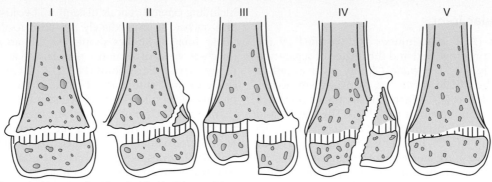

Figure 30-2 Types of growth plate injury (I to V) as classified by Salter and Harris. *(From Salter RB, Harris WR. Injuries involving the epiphyseal plate. J Bone Joint Surg (Am) 1963;45:587.)*

Premature growth arrest and angular deformities can occur with Salter-Harris IV fractures. Prognosis can be good but depends on ability to restore growth plate.

Salter-Harris Type V

Salter Harris V fractures are crushing injuries in which an axial load compresses the epiphysis into the metaphysis, squeezing the actively growing physis between them. Prognosis for future growth is poor, with a high rate of premature closure of the physis and resultant joint deformity. Fortunately, these are rare injuries.

Shoulder

Key Points

- Diagnosis of joint injuries is usually clinical based on the subcutaneous anatomy. Special care should be taken to rule out injury to associated neurovascular structures.
- Baseline imaging studies of the shoulder should *always* include a second tangential view of the scapula and glenoid. The best radiographic screening series is an anteroposterior view in internal rotation, AP view in external rotation, and axillary view of shoulder.
- Impingement, rotator cuff injuries, and shoulder instability are best diagnosed with a panel of clinical assessment tools rather than an isolated maneuver.
- Performance, injury prevention, and injury recovery of shoulder problems are optimized when the entire kinetic chain is addressed, including a sound base, core strength, scapular stability, antagonist capsular and muscle stretching, and classic rotator cuff–strengthening program.

The true functional shoulder joint comprises the glenohumeral joint, scapular thoracic joint, acromioclavicular joint, and sternoclavicular joint. Problems around the shoulder can be acute or chronic and include pain, weakness, dysfunction, stiffness, and instability. To ensure optimal outcome of treatment, an accurate, anatomic-based diagnosis is necessary. Less targeted treatment regimens tend to be less successful. Several evidence-based reviews remain inconclusive regarding specific interventions when a nonspecific diagnosis such as "shoulder pain" is targeted.

Injuries of Clavicular Complex

Key Points

- Most clavicle fractures can be definitively treated nonsurgically with a sling or a figure-eight dressing if they are minimally or nondisplaced.
- Grade 1 (tenderness) and grade 2 (tenderness and displacement with intact coracoclavicular ligaments) acromioclavicular injuries are managed conservatively with ice, pain control and a sling for comfort.
- Anterior shoulder dislocations are common, whereas posterior dislocations are less common but more dangerous with risk of compressing the great vessels.

The diagnosis of clavicle, acromioclavicular, and sternoclavicular injuries is straightforward; direct palpation along the clavicular complex should lead to an area of focal pain. Imaging studies should include the entire clavicle and a clear view of the targeted area from at least two planes. All injuries around the shoulder should include examination of the cervical spine and distal neurovascular evaluation. The brachial plexus, subclavian vein, and axillary artery lie immediately beneath the clavicle and can be at risk of injury.

Clavicle fractures account for 5% to 10% of all fractures and can be classified as either displaced or nondisplaced as well as by their specific location (proximal-distal) on the clavicle. Most fractures involve the midshaft (80%); however, distal third (15%) and proximal third (5%) fractures are also possible. Fortunately, most clavicle fractures can be definitively treated nonoperatively with a sling or a figure-of-8 dressing if they are minimally displaced or nondisplaced. Figure-of-8 bracing has been linked with skin necrosis over the fracture site, indicating the need for careful observation of skin integrity when used. In most cases, a simple sling for comfort is adequate over the first few weeks, followed by progressive range of motion (ROM) activities. More significant displacement (>100%), any tenting of the skin, significant comminution, or excessive shortening (>2 cm) may warrant surgical intervention, and referral to an orthopedist is recommended. Distal clavicle fractures have a higher rate of nonunion with nonsurgical treatment than midshaft or medial fracture patterns, so careful follow-up is necessary (Kahn et al., 2009; McKee et al., 2004).

Acromioclavicular Joint

Acromioclavicular (AC) joint injuries are classified by the ligamentous structures involved and the degree of separation of the AC joint (Fig. 30-3). A *grade 1* injury involves only a partial injury to the AC ligaments, no displacement occurs, and the coracoclavicular (CC) ligaments are intact. A *grade 2* injury involves the complete injury of the AC ligaments, and therefore mild superior translation of the distal clavicle occurs (<100% translation), and CC ligaments are intact. Both grade 1 and grade 2 injuries have an excellent prognosis with conservative treatment, which includes local application of ice, reduction of stresses, and a sling for comfort. Most patients will have substantial active motion and functional use of the arm within 6 weeks. A *grade 3* involves the complete rupture of both AC and CC ligaments. The distal end of the clavicle and acromion are now separated by more than a full clavicular width (>100% displacement). Stress radiographic views may magnify this separation even further; however, stress views rarely alter the treatment plan and are painful to patients and thus no longer considered required diagnostic images.

Treatment of grade 3 AC injuries is controversial and ranges from surgical to conservative treatment with a sling. With conservative treatment, the distal clavicle may ultimately heal in a superiorly translated position, leaving a prominent bump over the lateral aspect of the shoulder. However, nonelite athletes can function well and have a full return to activities. Acute repair of grade 3 injuries is suggested more for elite athletes, but has not been proved in randomized, controlled trials (RCTs) because subtle changes occur at this important point in the kinetic chain. Chronic reconstructions have been suggested in patients who have grade 3 injuries but with residual pain or dysfunction. The more severe injuries of the AC joint have significant posterior, superior, or inferior displacement and require surgical reduction and repair.

A *grade 4* AC separation is a complete injury of both AC and CC ligaments with a posterior subluxation of the distal clavicle relative to the acromion. These are frequently missed on routine anteroposterior (AP) radiographs but can be easily identified if routine axillary shoulder views are obtained. Fundamental management of bone and joint injuries requires a view from two perspectives. *Grade 5* injuries are basically equivalent to severe grade 3 injuries where the distal clavicle is riding so high that it either buttonholes through the fascia or tents beneath the skin (300% translation). The fascial injury prevents reduction, and the pressure on the undersurface of the skin risks skin slough or an open injury. Finally, *grade 6* AC injuries are extremely rare and are associated with an inferior dislocation of the distal clavicle beneath the coracoid.

Sternoclavicular Joint

Patient with sternoclavicular (SC) injuries present with a history of trauma (e.g., landing on lateral aspect of shoulder) or a history of chronic overuse that has led to popping and pain over the medial aspect of the clavicle (Matave et al., 2005). Acute SC joint dislocations can be identified clinically with localized tenderness over the medial clavicular aspect, and gross deformity may be present. More often, however, patients present with a subtle chronic situation caused by esthetic findings with a palpable or gross asymmetry. The examination should always include an assessment of the patient's airway and circulation, including cervical venous distention, because the great vessels and trachea lie immediately posterior to the SC joints (Fig. 30-4). Imaging studies should include an AP radiograph of the chest, views of the entire clavicle, and a tangential or serendipity view of the SC joint (Fig. 30-5). Because of overlapping shadows, these studies may be difficult to interpret. When suspicious, the best test is computed tomography (CT).

Traumatic SC joint dislocations can be either anterior or posterior. *Anterior dislocations* are generally easily palpated, with the proximal clavicle anteriorly displaced and painful. Anterior injuries may be reduced by placing a rolled towel or beanbag between the shoulder blades, then creating a distraction force along the arm in extension. Anterior dislocations tend to be unstable and to redisplace after attempted reduction. Fortunately, anterior injuries usually heal uneventfully, leaving an asymptomatic medial prominence and occasional popping, with minimal effect on the patient's activities of daily living. *Posterior dislocations* can be dangerous because of proximity to the great vessels posteriorly. If patients have venous engorgement in the neck and difficulty breathing, closed reduction may be attempted. A towel clip is used at the medial end of the clavicle, pulling anteriorly and creating the reduction. If this is attempted, a vascular surgeon should be available in case the proximal clavicle was actually tamponading an injury to the great vessels. This reduction should never be performed on the sideline in the absence of immediate cardiothoracic surgical response, unless the patient's life is at risk and there is no other option.

When treating injuries to the proximal clavicle, age of the patient and normal maturation of the proximal epiphysis are also important considerations. The medial clavicle epiphysis is one of the last to appear, at 19 to 23 years of age, and then the last to fuse, at 23 to 25 years of age. In patients younger than 23, these injuries are generally physeal injuries and not true dislocations, reducing the need for aggressive treatment (Fig. 30-6).

KEY TREATMENT

Subacromial injection for rotator cuff disease or intra-articular injection for adhesive capsulitis may be effective, although the effect may be minimal and not well maintained (Buchbinder et al., 2003) (SOR: A).

The use of some physiotherapy interventions is indicated in specific and circumscribed cases of shoulder pain (Green et al., 2003) (SOR: B).

Little evidence supports the benefit of manual therapy for adhesive capsulitis, shoulder pain, or subacromial impingement syndrome (Ho et al., 2009) (SOR: A).

The use of acupuncture for shoulder pain can be neither recommended nor refuted (Green et al., 2005) (SOR: A).

Shoulder Impingement and Rotator Cuff Disease

Key Points

- Tests to diagnose impingement syndrome include a positive Hawkins test, a painful arc of motion, and weakness with external rotation.
- Tests to diagnose a complete cuff tear include a positive drop-arm test, a painful arc of motion, and weakness to external rotation.
- Incomplete tears of the rotator cuff improve with physical therapy, anti-inflammatory medications, or subacromial injection.

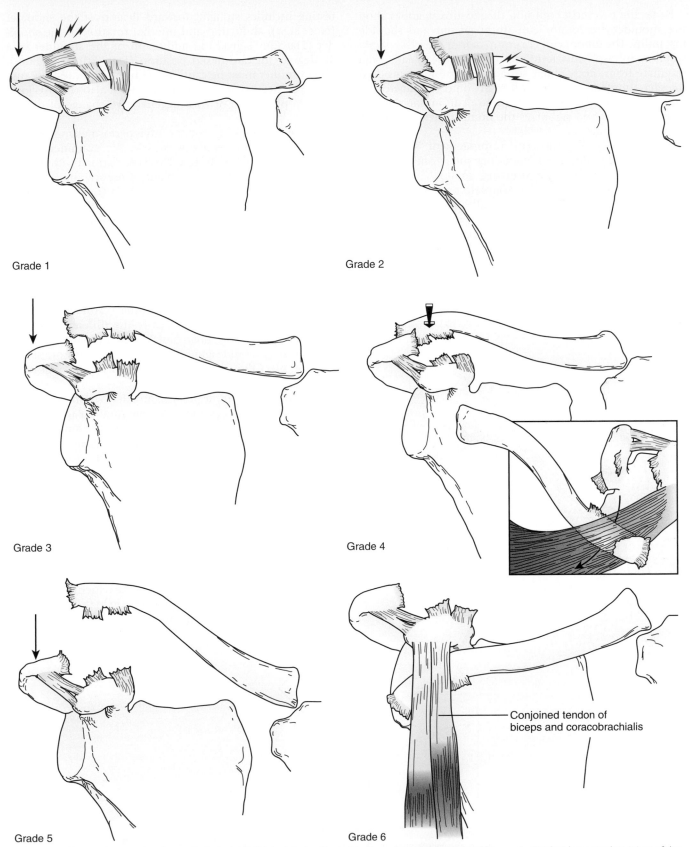

Grade 1

Grade 2

Grade 3

Grade 4

Grade 5

Grade 6

Conjoined tendon of
biceps and coracobrachialis

Figure 30-3 Progressive severity of acromioclavicular (AC) joint injuries. Grade 1 indicates incomplete injury of ligaments. Grade 2 has complete injury of the AC ligaments but intact coracoclavicular (CC) ligaments. Grade 3 injuries have complete injury of both AC and CC ligaments. Grade 4, 5, and 6 injuries are progressively severe, with posterior displacement of clavicle, severe superior displacement of clavicle, and inferior displacement of clavicle beneath the coracoid process.

By far the two most common diagnostic categories about the shoulder are rotator cuff impingement and shoulder instability. The rotator cuff is a group of four muscles—supraspinatus, infraspinatus, teres minor, and subscapularis—that originate from the scapular surface, traverse just outside of the glenohumeral capsule, and insert onto the tuberosities of the humerus (Fig. 30-7). The rotator cuff initiates motion in the shoulder and stabilizes the humeral head in the glenohumeral joint.

The diagnosis of rotator cuff impingement is actually a continuum of pathologies, including subacromial bursitis, AC joint hypertrophy and spurring, rotator cuff tendinosis, partial rotator cuff tears, complete or massive rotator cuff tears, and ultimately, rotator cuff arthropathy; that is, degenerative disease related to chronic rotator cuff insufficiency (Almekinders, 2001). Patients generally present with shoulder pain exacerbated by repetitive overhead activities, perhaps weakness, and occasionally difficulty sleeping on the shoulder. Physical examination of the shoulder includes provocative maneuvers that exacerbate impingement findings and evaluate the function of each rotator cuff muscle (Tennent et al., 2003a, 2003b). Impingement

testing includes straight, forward flexion of the shoulder (Neer sign), abduction and internal rotation of the shoulder (Hawkins sign), and adduction of the shoulder in a 90-degree, forward-flexed position (Figs. 30-8 and 30-9). The examiner must be cautious with the latter test because it may be positive with impingement but also with AC joint hypertrophy alone or with degenerative change of the AC joint.

Isolated testing of the rotator cuff is performed in sequence. To isolate the supraspinatus muscle, the examiner should perform the "empty can" test. This is performed with the arm slightly forward-flexed in the plane of the scapula, abducted to 90 degrees, with full internal rotation (i.e., with thumbs down, or empty can). The examiner should then place resistance on the patient's distal hand in an inferior direction. If this exacerbates pain, it is a positive finding of impingement or rotator cuff tendinopathy. If the patient has a positive "drop arm" sign, unable to maintain the arm in this position, a complete rotator cuff tear should be suspected. However, this does not confirm a complete rotator cuff tear because the patient may be guarding secondary to pain. Clinically, the examiner can clarify the difference by performing a diagnostic subacromial injection with lidocaine. The injection should significantly diminish pain complaints but not affect the motor function of an intact rotator cuff (Park et al., 2005).

To evaluate the infraspinatus and teres minor muscles, the examiner should evaluate external rotation against resistance. This is best done with the arm at the side, keeping the elbows near the torso, and asking the patient to rotate externally against resistance. Isolating the subscapularis muscle is more difficult. Resisted internal rotation with the arms at the side will recruit the pectoralis muscles and not isolate the subscapularis. To isolate the subscapularis, two tests have been described. In the *lift-off test*, the patient places the arm behind the back and lifts the hand into further internal rotation against resistance (Fig. 30-10). If able to do this, the patient's subscapularis muscle is likely intact. Modification of this test has been described as the "tummy pat" or the "Napoleon" test, in which the patient abducts the elbow, which must be away from the body in the plane of the torso, and is then asked to pat the stomach against resistance

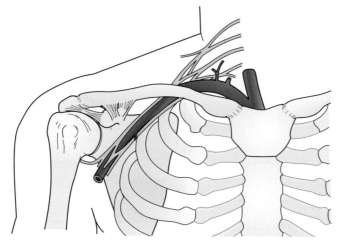

Figure 30-4 Drawing shows proximity of major neurovascular structures to sternoclavicular joint.

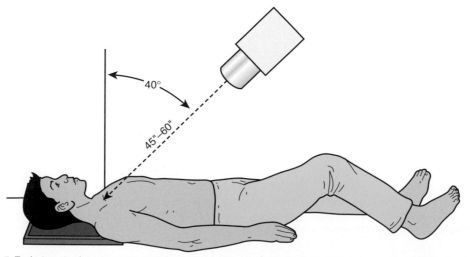

Figure 30-5 Technique in obtaining a tangential radiographic image, the serendipity view, to assess sternoclavicular joint injuries.

(Fig. 30-11). Weakness or inability to press against resistance is considered to be a positive test. Once the diagnosis is made clinically, AP and axillary shoulder x-ray studies can be obtained to evaluate the extent of injury further or assess for concomitant injuries. MRI is not routinely indicated with an intact rotator cuff clinically, and we usually recommend trying a course of physical therapy for 6 to 12 weeks before ordering MRI (Park et al., 2005).

If the patient has intact rotator cuff function on clinical examination and otherwise normal findings on radiographs, a conservative course of physical therapy is indicated for the impingement symptoms. From 90% to 95% of patients with incomplete tears of the rotator cuff improve with the course of physical therapy, anti-inflammatory medications, or a subacromial injection, although some may require surgery eventually (Matava et al., 2005). Physical therapy should focus on rotator cuff strengthening, ROM, posterior capsular stretching, and scapular stabilization. If patients fail a 6- to 12-week course of conservative treatment, a corticosteroid injection should be considered before surgery. If a patient is refractory to both corticosteroids and physical therapy, surgical intervention may be indicated. This is a more appropriate time to order an MR image because preoperative MR scanning can evaluate the extent of rotator cuff pathology, associated spurring, and degeneration within the shoulder joint. Although not necessary for making the diagnosis, MRI can assist the surgeon at surgery.

For incomplete rotator cuff tears (<50% of surface), a partial debridement and subacromial decompression using arthroscopy can provide effective, long-term relief of impingement pain. Management of rotator cuff tears greater than 50% or complete with clinical dysfunction is generally surgical. If the tear is identified before chronic retraction and muscle changes, primary arthroscopic or open repair has been effective in reducing pain and improving function. Rehabilitation after rotator cuff repair requires at least 6 weeks of passive ROM only, to protect the repair, followed by a gradual increase to resistance activities for the rotator cuff. Patients usually begin strengthening at 12 weeks. In patients with nonreparable chronic rotator cuff tears or those with advanced rotator arthropathy and degenerative disease, surgical interventions include muscle transfers, soft tissue grafts, hemiarthroplasties, and reverse shoulder hemiarthroplasties.

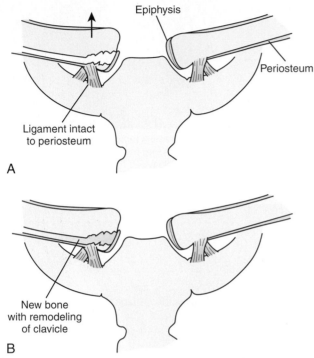

Figure 30-6 Medial clavicle injuries in patients younger than 23 to 25 years are likely physeal injuries and have the potential to remodel.

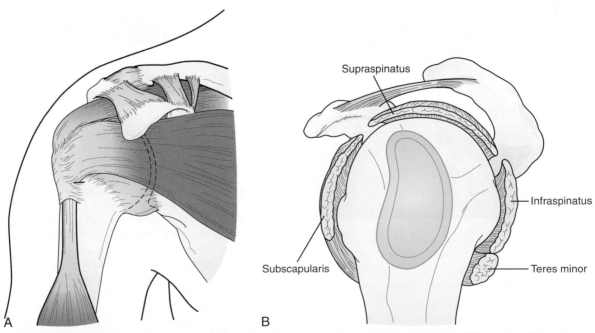

Figure 30-7 Anteroposterior **(A)** and lateral cross-sectional **(B)** drawings of the shoulder demonstrate the relationship of the rotator cuff muscles (supraspinatus, infraspinatus, teres minor, and subscapularis) to the bony structure of the shoulder.

EVIDENCE-BASED SUMMARY

- In a review of eight clinical trials (>390 patients), no definitive evidence supports or refutes the efficacy of common interventions, including physiotherapy, NSAIDs, corticosteroid injections, or open and arthroscopic surgery, for rotator cuff tears in adults (Ejnisman et al., 2003) (SOR: A).
- Based on limited data from two quality RCTs, no evidence supports the superiority of conservative versus surgical treatment for subacromial impingement syndrome (Dorrestijn et al., 2009) (SOR: B).
- Review of 14 RCTs evaluating rotator cuff surgery showed no long-term pain benefit of surgical decompression versus exercise programs (Coghlan et al., 2009) (SOR: A).

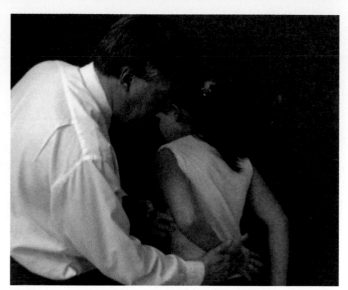

Figure 30-10 Lift-off test is used to assess subscapularis muscle function. Patients are asked to lift their hand off their back against resistance. Weakness or pain indicates subscapularis pathology. *(Courtesy Mark R. Hutchinson, MD.)*

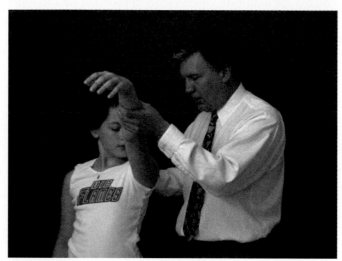

Figure 30-8 Hawkins test for shoulder impingement is performed by forward-elevating the humerus against the fixed scapula. Pain indicates anterior impingement. *(Courtesy Mark R. Hutchinson, MD.)*

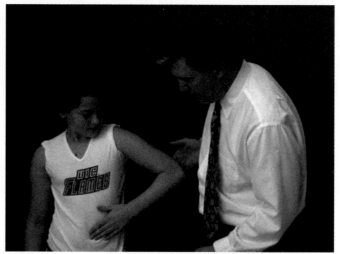

Figure 30-11 "Napoleon" or "tummy pat" test is a modified lift-off test to evaluate subscapularis function. Patients are asked to maintain their elbow laterally while pressing into their belly. (Ensure that patients do not drop their arm and use their humerus extensors to mimic subscapularis function.) *(Courtesy Mark R. Hutchinson, MD.)*

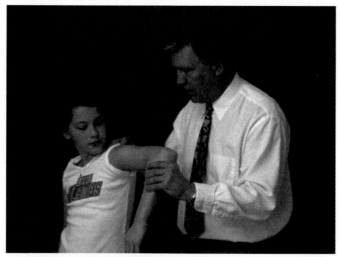

Figure 30-9 Neer test for shoulder impingement is performed with abduction and internal rotation of the shoulder. Pain indicates lateral impingement. *(Courtesy Mark R. Hutchinson, MD.)*

Shoulder Instability

Bony anatomy provides minimal stability to the glenohumeral joint; therefore the primary stability depends on both static and dynamic soft tissue structures. The static soft tissue structures include the fibrocartilaginous labrum, glenohumeral ligaments, and capsule. The labrum attaches to the periphery of the glenoid and serves to deepen the socket, reducing translation out of the socket. The glenohumeral ligaments attach to the labrum, are thickenings in the capsule, and connect to the humeral head. The intrinsic dynamic stabilizers are the rotator cuff and biceps, which help to maintain the humeral head in the glenoid socket. The extrinsic dynamic stabilizers include the rhomboid, levator scapulae, serratus, and trapezius muscles, which position the glenoid beneath the humeral head.

The diagnosis of shoulder instability begins with the patient's history and mechanism of injury, which often include episodes of subluxation, dislocation, or apprehension. Classically, anterior instability is appreciated when the arm is placed in abduction and external rotation (Tennent et al., 2003a, 2003b) (Fig. 30-12). *Inferior* instability is appreciated

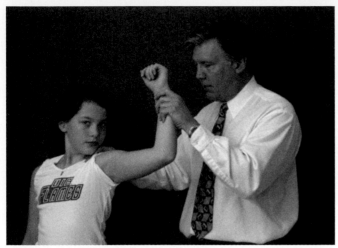

Figure 30-12 Apprehension test is performed with the arm in full abduction and external rotation. Sensation of impending subluxation is a positive finding. (*Courtesy Mark R. Hutchinson, MD.*)

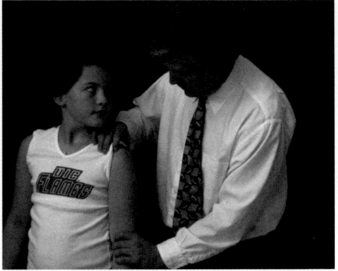

Figure 30-13 Presence or absence of a sulcus sign is evaluated by distracting the arm inferiorly to sublux the humeral head out of the socket. If a sulcus is appreciated as the glenoid is emptied of the humeral head, the clinician should suspect multidirectional instability. *(Courtesy Mark R. Hutchinson, MD.)*

when the patient tries to hold a heavy object and the shoulder subluxes inferiorly. *Posterior* instability is frequently associated with a fall on an outstretched arm, or occasionally with weightlifters who lock out their arms in extension while bench pressing. The clinical examination targets these specific pathologies with the classic *apprehension test* for anterior instability, performed with the arm in abduction and external rotation, and the patient having the sensation of the arm going out of place. In the *relocation test* the examiner then presses the humeral head back into a reduced position, thus eliminating the sensation of apprehension. Posterior instability is assessed in a supine position with the arm forward-flexed 90 degrees with a posteriorly directed force. Inferior instability is assessed by pulling inferiorly on the arm and looking for or feeling the humerus come out the socket and looking for a concavity just below the acromion, called the "sulcus sign" (Fig. 30-13).

Some patients may have generalized ligamentous laxity, but laxity itself is not a painful process and is therefore not pathologic. However, some patients with generalized ligamentous laxity do have symptoms of instability and pathology that can be assessed by comparison to the opposite side or looking at the elbows, fingers/thumb, or knees for excessive recurvatum, In general, patients with generalized ligamentous laxity should undergo an extensive course of conservative treatment because of the increased risk of failure associated with most surgical interventions compared to simple unidirectional instability.

The conservative treatment of shoulder instability is targeted at balancing the flexibility, optimizing the motor strength, and optimizing the function of the kinetic chain. The core component is rotator cuff–strengthening exercises as well as scapular stabilizer exercises. Controversy surrounds the ideal treatment for a first-time shoulder anterior dislocation. In young athletes or military populations, the risk of recurrence and future shoulder problems approaches 90%. Surgical treatment with repair of labral detachments has led to a high rate of return to play and return to performance, with a low risk (<10%) of recurrent instability for a first dislocation. Older nonathletic patients (>40) with first-time dislocation have a reduced risk of recurrent instability (<50%), so surgical treatment is unnecessary. However, if any patient has recurrent instability

or pain, surgery to repair the torn capsule or labral lesions is strongly recommended, with outcomes ranging from 75% to 95% good to excellent results. The Bankart procedure is most often performed and involves direct repair of the torn labrum back to the glenoid from which it was detached (Fig. 30-14). Classically, this procedure was performed open, although the current trend is toward arthroscopic assistance.

Posterior instability accounts for only 10% to 15% of isolated instability of the shoulder. The classic treatment for posterior instability is to initiate a course of conservative treatment focused on strengthening the posterior capsular muscles, including infraspinatus and teres minor. If a conservative course fails, surgical treatment can once again address either capsular laxity or posterior labral injuries.

Multidirectional instability is usually not secondary to a single acute traumatic event. More frequently, the patient will have underlying generalized ligamentous laxity that may or may not be exacerbated by a single traumatic event. These patients are generally loose jointed in all directions and in other joints. Initially, treatment is conservative, although in resistant cases, surgical capsular tightening can be successful in improving symptoms. A thorough history is necessary to rule out psychologic factors (e.g., voluntary dislocation for attention or party trick). These patients have an extremely high failure rate with surgical intervention.

KEY TREATMENT

Primary surgical repair is indicated for young athletes engaged in highly demanding physical activities who have sustained their *first* shoulder dislocation (Handoll et al., 2004) (SOR: A).

Surgical repair of shoulder instability from dislocation results in significantly lower recurrent instability than conservative treatment, especially for younger athletes and those in collision sports (Brophy and Marx, 2009) (SOR: B).

No significant difference exists between arthroscopic and open techniques in the surgical treatment of recurrent shoulder instability in adults (Pulavarti et al., 2009) (SOR: B).

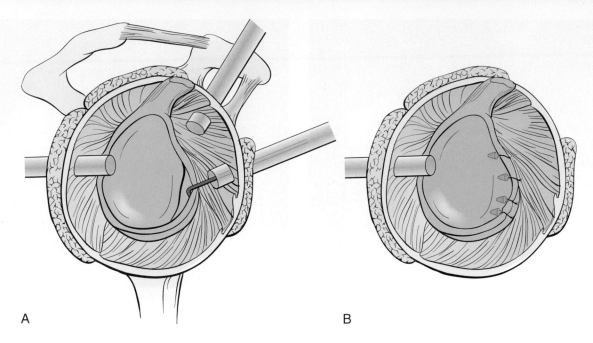

A   B

Figure 30-14 A, Detachment of the anterior inferior labrum (a Bankart lesion). **B,** Subsequent suture repair.

Elbow

Key Points

- Chronic lateral epicondylitis is more likely to be a degenerative process than an inflammatory process.
- Topical or oral NSAIDs and corticosteroid injections provide short-term relief of lateral epicondylitis pain.
- Steroids must not be injected into an infectious bursitis.

Lateral Elbow Tendinopathy

Lateral elbow tendinopathy or *lateral epicondylitis*, commonly called "tennis elbow," is caused by repetitive overuse of the wrist extensor and forearm supinator muscles that originate at the lateral epicondyle of the humerus—more specifically, the extensor carpi radialis brevis tendon. Once thought to result from inflammation, lateral elbow tendinosis is probably caused more by chronic changes in the musculotendinous matrix (Nirschl, 1992), with minimal inflammation present, particularly with symptoms present for more than 4 to 6 weeks. Microtears, chronic granulation tissue, and scar tissue formation are often seen in pathologic specimens of surgical cases of tennis elbow.

Patients present because of pain in the lateral aspect of the elbow and may complain of weakness or restricted elbow motion, but this is not as common. Pain is worsened by gripping, turning handles, and lifting activities, particularly with the hand in a palm-down position, as in lifting a suitcase, briefcase, or purse. Common positive physical examination findings include tenderness to palpation of the lateral epicondyle of the elbow and over the proximal wrist extensor and forearm supinator muscle tendons. Pain is intensified with resisted wrist extension and forearm supination. Pain can also limit patient strength. There should be no tenderness directly over the radial head, with normal ligamentous stability and neurovascular status.

Plain radiographs are not needed to make an accurate diagnosis of lateral epicondylitis but should be considered in patients with a history of trauma, motion loss, or locking or with a prolonged period of pain.

Management focuses on pain control and restoration of normal elbow function. Cryotherapy, ice massage, and nonsteroidal anti-inflammatory drugs (NSAIDs) or acetaminophen are excellent pain relievers. NSAIDs and corticosteroid injection have been mainstays of treatment, although they are now questioned because inflammation no longer seems a main factor in the injury process. Corticosteroid injections help quickly reduce the pain of lateral elbow tendinosis, but do not alter long-term outcome (Smidt et al., 2002). Cortisone injection may lead to a short-lived increase in pain in a large percentage of patients (Wang et al., 2003).

Counterforce straps can effectively reduce discomfort in some patients (Fig. 30-15). The strap is applied just distal to the area of maximal tenderness. The strap may relieve some of the tension exerted on the affected muscle tendon units during activities, thereby reducing pain. However, straps, medications, and injections should not replace therapeutic exercises, which include massage, stretching, and strengthening exercises. The most effective stretch is performed with the elbow extended, forearm fully pronated, and wrist flexed. From this position, gentle traction is applied to the middle and ring fingers toward the olecranon. Strengthening exercises with light weights for wrist extension and forearm supination can be done.

Most patients with lateral elbow tendinopathy will obtain excellent relief of symptoms with the program just described, although minimal evidence exists to support these plans (Bissett et al., 2005). If these measures do not lead to adequate relief, other protocols can be added. Formal physical therapy is often used in recalcitrant cases. Treatments such as

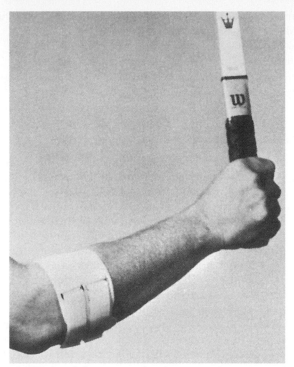

Figure 30-15 Lateral elbow counterforce brace. Note that wide, nonelastic support is curved to fit the conical forearm shape. This does not allow for full muscular expansion, thereby diminishing intrinsic muscular force on the lateral epicondyle.
(From Morrey BF [ed]: The Elbow and Its Disorders. Philadelphia, Saunders, 1985.)

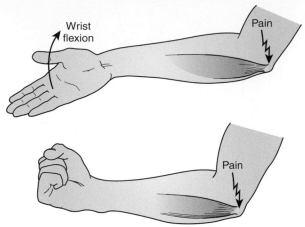

Figure 30-16 Medial epicondylitis may be diagnosed clinically by pain localized to the medial epicondyle during wrist flexion and pronation against resistance. There is often pain elicited after making a tight fist, and grip strength is usually diminished on the affected side.
(From Morrey BF [ed]: The Elbow and Its Disorders. Philadelphia, Saunders, 1985.)

prolotherapy, dry needling, platelet-rich plasma injections, and extracorporeal shock wave therapy are still experimental, and studies have not fully proved their effectiveness. Surgical intervention is sometimes needed and has excellent results.

KEY TREATMENT

No specific physical therapy modality is preferred over another in the treatment of lateral elbow tendinopathy (Smidt et al., 2003) (SOR: A).

Topical and oral NSAIDs are both effective in providing short-term pain relief from lateral epicondylitis; topical NSAIDs have fewer adverse effects (Green et al., 2002) (SOR: A).

Corticosteroid injections are helpful in reducing pain from lateral epicondylitis but do not alter the long-term outcome (Smidt et al., 2002) (SOR: A).

Little evidence exists to support the use of therapeutic exercises or braces in the treatment of lateral epicondylitis (Bisset et al., 2005) (SOR: A).

Extracorporeal shock wave therapy provides little or no benefit in terms of pain and function in lateral elbow pain (9 placebo-controlled trials, 1006 participants; Buchbinder et al., 2009) (SOR: A).

Medial Elbow Tendinopathy

Medial elbow tendinopathy or *medial epicondylitis,* commonly called "golfer's elbow," is caused by repetitive overuse of the wrist flexor and forearm pronator muscles that originate at the medial epicondyle of the humerus. Patients present due to pain in the medial aspect of the elbow, rarely weakness, and loss ROM. Pain is worsened by gripping and lifting activities, particularly with the hand in palm-up position. Common

positive findings include tenderness to palpation of the medial epicondyle of the elbow and over the proximal wrist flexor and forearm pronator muscle tendons. Pain is intensified with resisted wrist flexion and forearm pronation (Fig. 30-16). Patient discomfort often limits strength. Elbow motion, ligamentous stability, and neurovascular status are typically intact.

As with lateral elbow tendinopathy, plain radiographs are not needed to make an accurate diagnosis of medial elbow tendinopathy, but should be considered with a history of trauma, motion loss, locking, or chronic pain. Also similar to lateral epicondylitis, management of medial epicondylitis includes ice, medications, injections, and straps. However, corticosteroid injections are not recommended because of possible ulnar nerve injury. In medial elbow tendinopathy, the most effective stretch is performed with the elbow extended and the wrist and fingers gently pulled into full extension. The forearm can be pronated or supinated. Strengthening focuses on wrist flexion and forearm pronation exercises.

Olecranon Bursitis

Olecranon bursitis is a common cause of painless elbow swelling from repetitive friction of the olecranon against a firm surface or traumatic impact. Patients most often present with a painless swelling at the dorsal tip of the elbow, described as "a golf ball" or "goose egg" (Fig. 30-17). With trauma-induced swelling, pain and a hematoma may be present. Pain, redness, warmth, and lymphadenopathy may accompany septic bursitis. ROM loss, instability, neurovascular compromise, and strength loss are uncommon. On examination, there is a soft, fluctuant area of swelling directly over the olecranon. Diagnostic studies are generally not necessary to make a diagnosis of olecranon bursitis. However, plain radiographs should be obtained if trauma preceded the bursitis or fracture or dislocation is suspected.

Treatment includes compression, ice, and avoidance of impact at the olecranon. NSAIDs may help to reduce swelling. If the fluid collection is large or infection is suspected, aspiration of the bursa can be done in the office with a large-bore needle under sterile conditions. The bursa fluid should be clear and straw colored but may be bloody in a

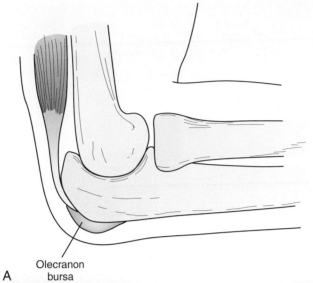

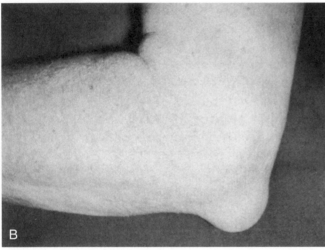

A
Olecranon
bursa

B

Figure 30-17 A, Relation of the olecranon bursa to the skin and olecranon.
B, Photograph of an enlarged olecranon bursa.
*(From Singer KM, Butters KP: Olecranon bursitis. In Delee JC, Drez D [eds]. Orthopedic Sports
Medicine: Principles and Practice, vol 1. Philadelphia, Saunders, 1994, pp 890, 892.)*

traumatic injury. If an infection is not suspected clinically
once the fluid is withdrawn, a corticosteroid can be injected.
Corticosteroids should never be injected if infection is a possibility. Oral antibiotics can be started if an infection is present. A local incision and drainage (I&D) may be required
in the presence of an infection and abscess. Aspiration does
not replace compression wrap, ice, and avoidance of impact.
Fluid may reaccumulate but should decrease. Serial aspirations are an option in a recurrent aseptic bursitis, but bursec-
tomy is occasionally needed for definitive treatment.

Wrist and Hand

Key Points

- Both bracing and cortisone injection may reduce carpal tunnel
  syndrome pain in the short term.
- Surgical treatment of carpal tunnel syndrome leads to better
  symptom relief than bracing.

- Immobilization of suspected scaphoid injuries should be instituted
  while workup is completed.
- Initial immobilization of any scaphoid fracture should be in a
  thumb spica cast.
- Proximal pole and displaced scaphoid fractures should be treated
  by an orthopedic surgeon.

Carpal Tunnel Syndrome

Carpal tunnel syndrome (CTS) is the most common nerve
entrapment syndrome encountered in primary care. CTS is
more common in women than men and affects about 3% of
the adult American population. Of the many possible etiologies, the most common is tenosynovitis of the hand flexors,
leading to median nerve compression. CTS can develop during pregnancy as well. Nine flexor tendons course through
the carpal tunnel along with the median nerve (Fig. 30-18).

Patients typically present due to pain, numbness, paresthesias, and loss of grip strength in the wrist and hand.
Symptoms may even radiate into the shoulder region. Symptoms usually involve the radial 3½ digits as supplied by
the median nerve and are noted more with repetitive hand
motion activities and at night. Physical examination may
reveal thenar atrophy and decreased sensation over the radial
3½ digits. These two clinical findings, along with a history
of pain in the distribution of the median nerve, are highly
suggestive of CTS and correlate to positive nerve conduction
study findings (D'Arcy and McGee, 2000).

Tinel's test (sign) at the wrist is performed by tapping over
the wrist flexor retinaculum and having increased or reproducible symptoms of pain, numbness and tingling in the
radial 3½ digits. The most sensitive test is the carpal compression test, in which direct compression over the tunnel elicits
the symptoms. Phalen's maneuver is performed by having
the patient flex the wrists to a 90-degree position, holding the
dorsal aspects of the hands back-to-back. The patient maintains this position up to 1 minute, until symptoms develop.

Diagnostic imaging is not necessary to make a diagnosis of
CTS. Electrodiagnostic tests can be used to confirm the diagnosis but are not needed to initiate or direct early treatment
in most patients. Although up to 25% are false negative in
patients with clinical CTS, electrodiagnostic tests should be
done before surgery.

Treatment begins with attempts to avoid or at least modify activities known to cause pain for the patient. This may
include ergonomic changes in the workplace, such as wrist
support pads for computer use. Wrist splinting, particularly
at night, may prove helpful. Nerve gliding exercises are routinely prescribed and can provide relief (Fig. 30-19). Oral
analgesic and NSAID use may also lead to relief, although
studies show these are no more effective than placebo. Corticosteroid injection is a helpful adjunct in many patients
and may relieve symptoms better than placebo (Germisten et
al., 2002). A majority of patients will experience good relief
of symptoms if these conservative measures are followed.
Unfortunately, most of these patients will have a return of
symptoms in 1 year (Kanaan and Sawaya, 2001). Surgery is
considered in patients who have recurrence of symptoms
despite adequate conservative measures, and outcomes are
excellent. Both open and endoscopic techniques are available, with equivalent long-term results.

KEY TREATMENT

Oral analgesic and NSAID use to treat symptoms of CTS are no more effective than placebo (Gerritsen et al., 2002) (SOR: A).

Corticosteroid injection is more effective than placebo in relieving symptoms (short term) (Gerritsen et al., 2002) (SOR: A).

Bracing for CTS may lead to significant short-term pain reduction (O'Connor et al., 2003) (SOR: A).

Surgery relieves CTS symptoms significantly better than bracing (Verdugo et al., 2005) (SOR: A).

DeQuervain's Tenosynovitis

DeQuervain's tenosynovitis is a painful repetitive and over-use condition of the abductor pollicis longus and extensor pollicis brevis along the dorsal radial aspect of the wrist. Patients present due to pain and swelling along the dorsal radial side of the wrist, which is worsened with activities. Physical examination reveals tenderness with palpation, and the classic clinical finding is a positive Finkelstein test. This is performed by having the patient flex and adduct the thumb to the palm, then close the remaining fingers over the thumb. The examiner then passively takes the patient's wrist into ulnar deviation. Pain along the tendons with this

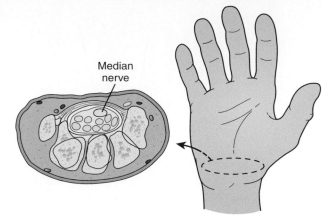

Figure 30-18 Cross-sectional anatomy of the carpal tunnel, bounded on three sides by the carpal bones and volarly by the transverse carpal ligament. Nine flexor tendons and the median nerve pass through the tunnel. Anything that causes increased pressure in this canal can produce the symptoms of carpal tunnel syndrome.
(From McCue FC, Bruce VF: Hand and wrist. In Delee JC, Drez D [eds]. Orthopedic Sports Medicine: Principles and Practice, vol 1. Philadelphia, Saunders, 1994, p 997.)

Starting position 1

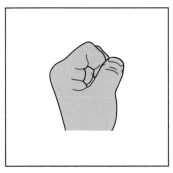

Wrist in neutral,
fingers and thumb in flexion

Position 2

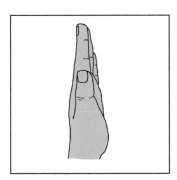

Wrist in neutral,
fingers and thumb extended

Position 3

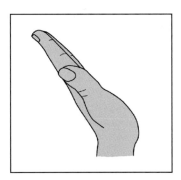

Thumb in neutral,
wrist and fingers extended

Position 4

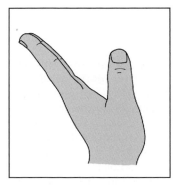

Wrist, fingers and thumb extended

Position 5

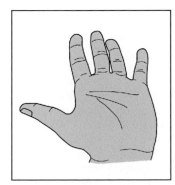

Same as in position 4,
with forearm in supination
(palm up)

Position 6

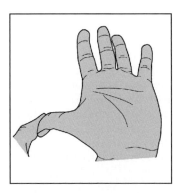

Same as in position 5,
other hand gently stretching
thumb

Figure 30-19 Carpal tunnel nerve glide exercises.

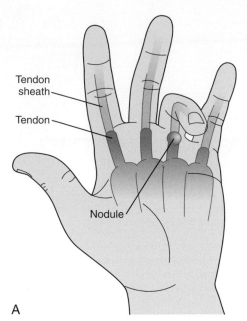

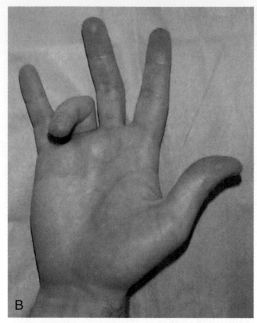

Figure 30-20 Flexor tendon nodule.

maneuver is considered a positive test (Finkelstein, 1930). Radiographic tests are not necessary to make an accurate diagnosis.

Treatment begins with avoidance of the inciting activities. Ice may reduce pain and swelling, and analgesic medications are often used as well. Thumb spica splinting is very helpful, allowing the irritated tendons to rest (Winzeler and Rosenstein, 1996). Prolonged splinting may be needed to reduce pain significantly. Corticosteroid injection along the tendon sheath is often used to reduce pain more acutely (Peters-Veluthamaningal et al., 2009a; Wood and Dobyns, 1986). In refractory cases, surgical decompression of the tendons can be performed.

Digital Flexor Tenosynovitis

Tenosynovitis of a digital flexor tendon, also called "trigger finger," is quite common. Patients present with the complaint of a finger that "sticks" with motion, primarily flexion, and they must painfully force the finger back into extension. Usually, a painful palpable nodule on the flexor tendon is present along the distal palmar crease or at the base of the thumb, at the level of the metacarpophalangeal (MCP) joint (Fig. 30-20). Motion and activities may be associated with pain. Radiographs and other diagnostic tests are not needed to make an accurate diagnosis.

Treatment options for digital flexor tenosynovitis include anti-inflammatory medications, modification of activities, ice, massage, stretching of the flexor tendons, and gentle-grip strength exercises, although these usually provide little relief. Corticosteroid injections are often used to relieve pain and triggering symptoms (Marks and Gunther , Peters-Veluthamaningal et al., 2009b). Symptoms may return, and repeat injections are considered if the first injection provided reasonable pain relief. However, surgery may be needed in patients with frequent recurrence.

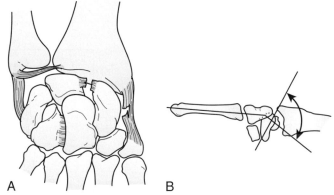

Figure 30-21 A, Disruption of scapholunate and radiocarpal ligaments leads to progressive dissociation between scaphoid and rest of carpal bones. This injury is frequently mistaken for a persistent wrist sprain. **B,** Chronic dissociation of scapholunate joint allows scaphoid to rotate downward toward the palm. This increases the angle between scaphoid axis and radiolunate-capitate axis. The capitate then slowly migrates toward the radius, and osteoarthritis rapidly develops.

(From Connolly JF: DePalma's The Management of Fractures and Dislocations: an Atlas, 3rd ed. Philadelphia, Saunders, 1981.)

Scapholunate Sprains

Ligament sprains of the wrist usually result from falls on an outstretched hand. Most are mild and resolve with splinting and symptomatic treatment. However, the clinician must be careful not to miss potentially catastrophic injuries that could compromise a patient's hand and wrist function, including carpal dislocations, carpal instability (more specifically, scapholunate ligament instability), scaphoid fractures, and displaced intra-articular distal radius fractures. Injury to the scapholunate joint may be missed by physicians who do not consider it in their differential diagnosis of wrist injuries (Fig. 30-21).

Patients with scapholunate sprains have pain in the wrist with motion, gripping, and lifting and along the dorsal aspect

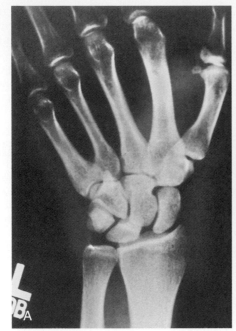

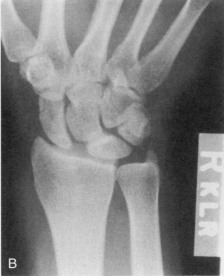

Figure 30-22 A, Posteroanterior radiograph of left wrist in 27-year-old soccer player who fell, landed on his left palm, and complained of pain. Note the abnormal widening of the scapholunate interval. **B,** Comparison view of the uninjured right wrist demonstrates the same scapholunate separation (>3 mm) ("David Letterman" sign). Patient recovered with only splint support.
(From Nicholas J, Hershman E. The Upper Extremity in Sports Medicine, 2nd ed. St Louis, Mosby, 1995, p 456.)

of the wrist at the scapholunate joint just distal to Lister's tubercle (bump on distal radius) on the dorsal aspect of the wrist. Physical examination typically reveals no gross deformities, although dorsal swelling may be noted. The pain may be exacerbated by flexion and extension while palpating directly over the scapholunate joint on the dorsal aspect of the wrist.

Impacts strong enough to cause scapholunate sprain are sufficient to cause fracture. Therefore, plain radiographs should be obtained in all patients with suspected scapholunate sprain to look for associated fracture or avulsion. The series should include a standard AP view, AP with a clenched fist (accentuates scapholunate joint widening), standard lateral view, and posteroanterior (PA) view in ulnar deviation (assess scaphoid bone better for fracture). It is often helpful to obtain a comparison AP view of the opposite wrist. An increased gap between the scaphoid and lunate bones of 2 to 3 mm on the AP projection (e.g., "Terry Thomas" [U.K.] or "David Letterman" [U.S.] sign, for their gapped-tooth grin) is indicative of scapholunate dissociation (Fig. 30-22).

Patients with a "simple" scapholunate sprain require protection and rest with a period of splinting. This can be accomplished with a custom fiberglass or plaster splint, or a prefabricated cock-up wrist splint until the patient is asymptomatic. After initial treatment, the patient is weaned from the wrist splint and begins active ROM and hand-strengthening therapy. In patients with scapholunate dissociation, surgical consultation should be considered early, and referral to a hand specialist is encouraged. Fixation of the joint is often needed to maximize future wrist function (Fig. 30-23).

Distal Radius Fractures

Patients with distal radius fractures most often present with wrist pain and deformity immediately after a fall. All patients with wrist pain after a fall should have AP, lateral,

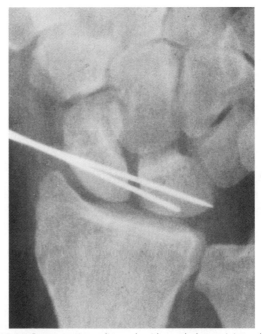

Figure 30-23 Postoperative radiograph with scapholunate joint reduced and two K wires properly positioned to stabilize the joint.
(From Nicholas J, Hershman E. The Upper Extremity in Sports Medicine, 2nd ed. St Louis, Mosby, 1995, p 393.)

and oblique radiographs of the wrist. Deformity may or may not be present, and some patients may complain of paresthesias in the affected extremity. A patient's ability to move the wrist does not rule out fracture. It is important to palpate the entire extremity to assess any injury above or below the primary injury site for concomitant fractures. If suspected, radiograph those areas as well. Neurovascular status should always be evaluated and documented.

Treatment is based on fracture type, patient age, and demand. A nondisplaced or minimally displaced fracture can be initially treated in a splint for 5 to 7 days until swelling subsides, then casted in a short-arm cast. Average healing time is 4 to 8 weeks, and repeat radiographs should be obtained during the healing process at an interval of every 2 to 3 weeks. An extra-articular, angulated fracture is initially treated with closed reduction with block (lidocaine injection into fracture hematoma). If postreduction alignment is adequate, a splint can be placed for 5 to 7 days to maintain the alignment pending casting. Because displacement or angulation of fracture fragments is a high risk even when appropriately splinted or casted, radiographic follow-up is important, and distal radius fractures are often treated by an orthopedic surgeon. Comminuted or displaced intra-articular fractures usually require closed reduction with percutaneous pinning or open reduction, internal fixation to maintain position and articular surface integrity; orthopedic surgery referral is recommended.

Scaphoid Fracture

Patients typically present after a fall onto an outstretched hand and complain of pain and swelling in the radial aspect of the wrist, worsened by motion. Gross deformity is not usually seen. The most common physical examination finding is tenderness with palpation over scaphoid tubercle or in the anatomic snuffbox. Radiographs should be obtained in all patients with suspected scaphoid injury, including AP, lateral, and oblique views, as well as PA ulnar deviation or scaphoid views (Fig. 30-24). Importantly, radiographs are often negative shortly after immediate injury and up to 14 days; radiographs should be repeated in 2 weeks if suspicion remains high. Because a fracture is suspected, interim splinting or casting is necessary. Other diagnostic tests may be obtained if repeat x-ray films are negative after 2 weeks and the patient is still symptomatic, or if definitive diagnosis is needed sooner than the planned 2-week follow-up. These tests may include radionuclide bone scan (usually positive within 2-3 days of injury), CT, or MRI.

Treatment of scaphoid fracture is initiated if suspicion is high, even though radiographs are initially negative. If fracture is ruled out at follow-up visits, treatment is adjusted accordingly. Nondisplaced scaphoid fractures are treated with cast immobilization. Thumb spica casting is essential, but whether the initial cast needs to be a long-arm or short-arm variety is controversial. Studies have shown decreased time to union and reduced rates of delayed union and nonunion with a long-arm thumb spica cast (Gellman et al., 1989). However, union rates of up to 95% with short-arm casting have been reported. A combination, with a long-arm cast for the initial 6 weeks followed by short-arm casting from 6 weeks until radiographic healing is present, addresses both these key issues.

Healing rates and average healing time depend on location of the fracture because the blood supply differs throughout the scaphoid. Nondisplaced distal pole fractures tend to receive a better blood supply and have a healing rate of close to 100%, with average healing time of 10 to 12 weeks. Scaphoid waist fractures have a healing rate of 80% to 90%, with average healing also 10 to 12 weeks. Proximal pole fractures have a healing rate of only 60% to 70%, with average healing time of 12 to 20 weeks. Poor outcomes (i.e., nonunion,

malunion) in any scaphoid fracture are more likely to occur if the diagnosis or appropriate treatment is delayed; this is why it is important to initiate treatment based on suspicion of injury with normal radiographs.

Fractures that are displaced (≥1 mm) can be treated with closed immobilization, but the risk of poor outcome is high. These fractures should be referred to an orthopedic surgeon for consideration of surgical fixation.

EVIDENCE-BASED SUMMARY

- One controlled study showed significant benefit of steroid injections for DeQuervain's tenosynovitis. Because of a limited number of patients and limited quality supportive studies, however, definitive recommendations cannot be made (Peters-Veluthamaningal et al., 2009a) (SOR: B).
- Pain and symptoms of people with "trigger finger" may improve with a corticosteroid injection (Peters-Veluthamaningal et al., 2009b) (SOR: A).
- Bone scintigraphy and MRI have equally high sensitivity and high diagnostic value for excluding scaphoid fracture. However, MRI is more specific and better for confirming scaphoid fracture (Yin et al., 2009) (SOR: A). We believe additional studies are needed to assess diagnostic performance of CT.

Knee

Key Points

- In clinical examination of ligament injuries about the knee, the Lachman test is the most sensitive for anterior cruciate ligament (ACL) instability.
- The clinician should maintain a high level of suspicion of associated ligament injuries, especially the lateral collateral ligament (LCL) and posterolateral corner. Acute surgical intervention (within 3 weeks) of LCL and posterolateral corner injuries significantly improves prognosis.
- Viscosupplementation, therapeutic exercise, and oral supplementation with glucosamine and chondroitin sulfate may all provide some symptomatic relief and functional improvement for generalized knee arthritis. Arthroscopic debridement alone (in the absence of loose bodies, cartilage flaps, and meniscus tears) may not provide relief.
- Vertical, peripheral meniscus tears in the vascular zone of the meniscus of young patients should be treated with meniscus repair whenever possible to avoid focal increased pressures in the articular surface and future risk of degenerative joint disease.
- In older patients with degenerative meniscus pathology and no locking, prevention of arthritic progression may be surgical or nonsurgical. When performed, partial is preferred to complete meniscectomy.

Degenerative Osteoarthritis

Degenerative osteoarthritis (OA) of the knee is caused by loss of the hyaline cartilage along the knee joint surfaces. This can occur in an isolated compartment or diffusely throughout all three compartments of the knee. OA more often develops in the medial side or medial compartment of the knee, first

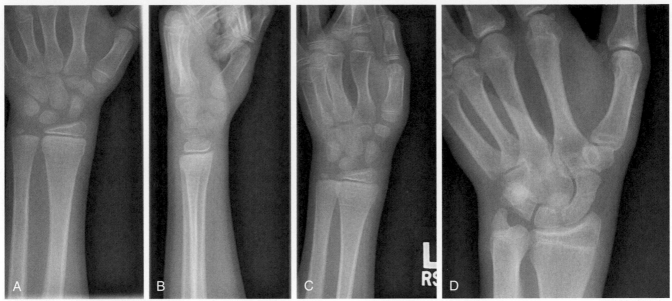

Figure 30-24 24 Transverse fracture through waist of scaphoid.
(Courtesy James L. Moeller, MD.)

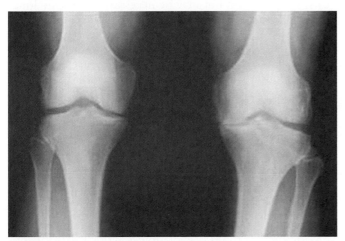

Figure 30-25 Weight-bearing knee radiographs showing osteoarthritis.

leading to joint space narrowing and varus or bowleg deformity. Loss of articular cartilage and joint space on the lateral aspect of the knee leads to valgus or knock-knee deformity. Weight-bearing (standing flexed-knee PA) radiographs are strongly recommended to evaluate joint space narrowing and OA extent. Lateral and patella sunrise tangential views complete the study (Fig. 30-25). MR images are not routinely required and should not be ordered instead of plain x-ray films. MRI is best reserved for mechanical pathology or preoperative planning. X-ray findings include loss of the joint space, presence of osteophytes, subchondral sclerosis, and cysts.

Patients with OA typically complain of knee pain and stiffness with walking, after prolonged sitting, descending stairs, and early in the morning. Swelling of knees and worse symptoms are typical with weather changes. Physical exam findings often reveal decreased ROM (flexion contractures), knee varus or valgus deformity, joint line tenderness, and crepitus with palpation during ROM.

Treatment of OA is based on the patient's age, demand, comorbidities, and severity of osteoarthritis. Conservative treatment for knee arthritis should include a generalized conditioning program, weight loss, a knee sleeve to improve the proprioceptive control, cushioned shoes, and NSAIDs. Oral supplementation with glucosamine and chondroitin sulfate may also be considered. If these do not provide relief after 4 to 6 weeks, corticosteroid or viscosupplement injections can be administered, typically with variable pain relief and duration. Injections may be repeated depending on patient response. In resistant cases, total or partial knee replacement can provide excellent pain relief and improve function. The effect of arthroscopy in patients with degenerative arthritis remains controversial (Hunt et al., 2002; Mosely et al., 2002). However, arthroscopy in the absence of loose bodies, cartilage flaps, or meniscal pathology is unlikely to be unsuccessful.

EVIDENCE-BASED SUMMARY

- The short-term benefit of intra-articular corticosteroid in treatment of knee osteoarthritis is well established; however, longer-term benefits have not been confirmed, and the response to hyaluronic products appears to have more durability (Bellamy et al., 2005a) (SOR: A).
- Based on a single RCT, bracing for OA may provide additional benefit compared to medical treatment alone (Brouwer et al., 2001) (SOR: B).
- Land-based therapeutic exercise programs reduce pain and improve physical function for patients with OA of the knee (Brosseau et al., 2003; Fransen et al., 2001) (SOR: A).
- Viscosupplementation (injection of hyaluronate) is an effective treatment for OA of the knee, with beneficial effects on pain and function (Bellamy et al., 2005b) (SOR: A).
- Nonglucosamine preparations failed to show benefit, whereas glucosamine preparations were superior to placebo in the treatment of pain and functional impairment resulting from symptomatic OA (Towhead et al., 2009) (SOR: A).
- Arthroscopic debridement has no benefit for undiscriminated OA with mechanical or inflammatory causes (Laupattarakasem et al., 2009) (SOR: A).
- In OA patients, exercise results in a modest reduction in pain and a modest improvement in physical function (Fransen and McConnell, 2009) (SOR: B).

Infections

Intra-articular joint infections are orthopedic emergencies and require urgent surgical irrigation and debridement as well as long-term antibiotic therapy. The most common source of infection is *Staphylococcus aureus,* which aggressively and quickly destroys cartilage and leaves the patient with permanent OA. Patients with a knee joint infection present with increased pain, swelling, warmth, redness, fever, and decreased ability to ambulate on that leg. Most patients will not want to move their knee at all. The knee should be aspirated and the fluid inspected and sent for laboratory analysis (Gram stain, cell count, culture, crystal evaluation). Crystalline arthropathy such as gout should always be considered because the aspirated fluid often appears cloudy and may mimic a joint infection. C-reactive protein (CRP) and erythrocyte sedimentation rate (ESR) should also be obtained. Appropriate antibiotic treatment is initiated based on the offending organism. Although proposed in the medical literature for low-virulent organisms, serial aspiration is discouraged in the orthopedic literature, with surgical irrigation the preferred treatment.

Inflammatory Conditions

Bursae are synovial fluid–filled structures or "cushions" that pad bony prominences as protection against repetitive impact from external forces or snapping anatomic structures, such as ligaments or tendons. Several bursae around the knee can become inflamed, irritated, and rarely, infected, including the prepatellar bursa, infrapatellar bursa, pes anserine bursa, and iliotibial (IT) band bursa (beneath IT band laterally). Knowing their anatomic location is important so that these bursae can be palpated directly (Fig. 30-26).

Treatment of *bursitis* includes compression, ice, protective padding, and avoidance of impact on the bursa. NSAIDs may help to reduce swelling. If the fluid collection is large or an infection is suspected, aspiration of the bursa can be performed in the office with a large-bore needle under sterile conditions. The bursa fluid should be clear and straw colored or may be bloody in a traumatic injury. If an infection is not suspected clinically once the fluid is withdrawn, a corticosteroid can be injected. Corticosteroids should never be injected if infection is a possibility. Oral antibiotics can be started if an infection is present. Local I&D may be required with infection and abscess. Aspiration does not replace compression wrap, ice, and avoidance of impact. Reaccumulation of fluid may occur, but total volume usually decreases. Serial aspirations are an option in patients with recurrent aseptic bursitis.

Extensor Mechanism Problems

The extensor mechanism comprises the quadriceps muscle, quadriceps tendon, patella, and patellar tendon. Differential diagnosis of problems in the extensor mechanism is broad, including muscle or tendon rupture, patellar fracture, patellar tendinopathy, patellofemoral syndrome, patellar instability, Osgood-Schlatter's disease, and symptomatic medial plica. Examination of patients with anterior knee pain or extensor mechanism problems should always include a careful evaluation of the lumbar spine and hip to rule out referred pain, as well as assessment of the antagonist hamstring muscles posteriorly. Hamstring tightness can exacerbate problems of tendinosis, patellofemoral syndrome, and instability.

If the patient presents with focal tenderness over the patellar tendon at the distal pole of the patella, or potentially at the quadriceps insertion onto the patella, the likely diagnosis is tendinosis. Numerous studies show that chronic repetitive overuse does not actually lead to inflammation of the tendon itself, but rather to a central degeneration or tendinosis of the fibers of the tendon (Fithian, 2002). Steroid injections into patellar tendinosis are highly discouraged because they may predispose the tendon to complete failure. Treatment protocols for patellar tendinosis, or "jumper's knee," should include hamstring stretching, quadriceps strengthening with eccentric loading, and occasionally the use of a counterforce brace such as a Cho-Pat strap (Fig. 30-27).

Alternative treatments, including deep friction massage, prolotherapy, platelet-rich plasma injections, topical anti-inflammatory drugs, ultrasonic waves, and radiofrequency (RF) probes, show mixed results. Although no RCTs have yet proved their efficacy, these modalities have had some success. Surgical intervention for debridement of the tendinosis is uncommon but may be necessary to provide long-term relief. In the skeletally immature patient, tenderness at the distal pole of the patella may represent an avulsion apophysitis called Sinding-Larsen-Johansson disease. If the skeletally immature patient has pain at the insertion of the patellar tendon on the tibia, the most likely diagnosis is an apophysitis of the tibial tubercle, or Osgood-Schlatter's disease. Both problems are more common during active phases of growth and are generally treated conservatively with rest, flexibility exercises, and gradual return to activity. Complete failure or rupture of the extensor mechanism at the patellar or quadriceps tendon requires surgical repair (Ilan et al., 2002).

Patellofemoral Syndrome

Anterior knee pain has been variously termed patellofemoral syndrome and chondromalacia patellae. When treating anterior knee pain, the physician should identify the specific pathology to initiate targeted treatment. *Chondromalacia patellae,* or degenerative changes on the undersurface of the patella, is more common in young females. Pain complaints related to chondromalacia are exacerbated by sitting for an extended period with a flexed knee, doing deep squats, or going up and down stairs. Each of these activities increases the posteriorly directly forces of the patella, directing increased pressure onto the chondral surfaces.

Treatment of these early arthritic changes is typically rehabilitation. Surgical intervention, such as cartilage scraping and debridement, has not been shown to provide long-term relief or benefit. In rare patients who have associated tight lateral retinacular structures and patellar tilt, surgical release of the lateral retinaculum can provide benefit. Conservative treatment of patellofemoral syndrome includes cushioned shoes, rehabilitation focused on the vastus medialis obliquus muscle, reductive taping techniques, hamstring stretches, and NSAIDs. Correction of the foot alignment with orthotic devices is also a treatment option, but supportive evidence is limited. From

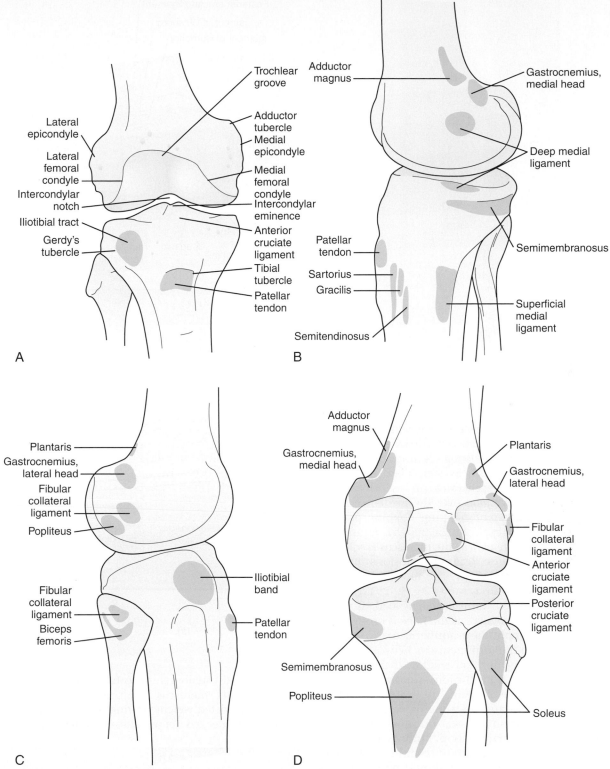

Figure 30-26 Line drawing shows anatomic sites of bursae around the knee.

70% to 80% of patients will improve with this conservative treatment. Unfortunately, the remaining patients with resistant symptoms can have a frustrating long-term therapeutic course, with guarded prognosis for any surgical intervention. Ultrasound therapy had no clinically important effect on patients with patellofemoral pain syndrome (Brosseau et al., 2001).

Meniscus Injuries

The menisci are fibrocartilaginous structures situated on the tibial plateau both medially and laterally that help disperse the weight-bearing contact forces across the knee joint cartilage surfaces (Fig. 30-28). In the presence of a meniscus tear or the complete absence of a meniscus, focal stresses

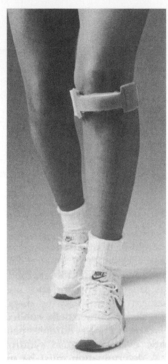

Figure 30-27 Counterforce brace (Cho-Pat strap) can be effective in reducing symptoms of patellar tendinosis (jumper's knee).

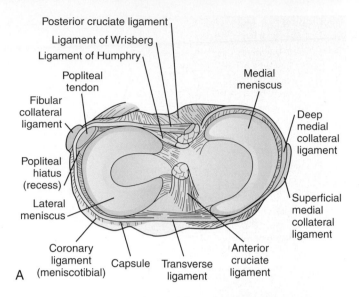

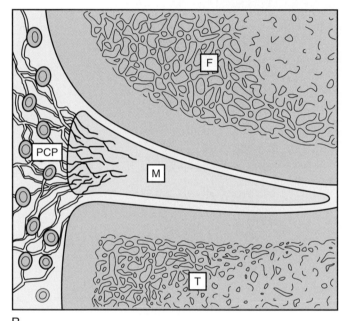

Figure 30-28 Medial and lateral meniscus anatomy as viewed from above **(A)** and via cross section **(B)**. Note the circulation provided to the peripheral third of the meniscus only.

increase. This in turn increases the loading of the hyaline cartilage and early progressive degenerative arthritis (Sherman, 1996). Meniscus tears can occur with axial loading but primarily occur because of twisting, cutting, or rotational forces. In older patients, meniscus tears may simply be a progression of the normal degenerative process. On physical examination, patients have pain over the medial or lateral joint line and may complain of snapping, popping, or catching within the knee (Greis et al., 2002a, 2002b). Varus or valgus loading may exacerbate pain as the meniscus is squeezed between the bony structures. Recurrent effusions may also represent intra-articular pathology. The most common test for meniscus injury is McMurray's test (Fig. 30-29). The knee is hyperflexed, stressed with varus or valgus load, as well as internally and externally rotated, as the knee is brought into full extension. More simply, the examiner uses the lower leg and tibia to try to trap the torn meniscus between the tibia and the femur through a full knee ROM. If the examiner feels a snapping or a pop along the joint-line and the patient simultaneously complains of pain, the test is considered positive and highly indicative of a meniscus tear. A single finding may raise suspicion of a tear but does not confirm its presence. Indeed, sensitivity of both findings, the pop and pain, is over 90%. MRI can be used to confirm the diagnosis or assist preoperative planning but should never replace a thorough physical examination.

Definitive treatment of meniscus pathology depends on the actual damage and pattern of the meniscus injury on MRI (Sherman, 1996; Greis et al., 2002a, 2002b) (Fig. 30-30). Depending on the pattern, the meniscus can either be reparable or nonreparable. Because of its essential role in sharing load and preventing the progression of degenerative arthritis, salvageable meniscus tears should always be repaired if possible. After debridement, patients can bear weight as

tolerated and usually return to full activities by about 3 or 4 weeks. With meniscus repair, recovery is extended and requires restricted weight bearing for 3 to 6 weeks, with 2 to 3 months needed before return to unrestricted activities.

EVIDENCE-BASED SUMMARY

- With no RCTs, no conclusions about surgical or nonsurgical treatment of meniscal injuries can be drawn, or about meniscal tear repair versus excision. Partial meniscectomy seems preferable to total removal and improves overall recovery in the short term (Howell and Handoll, 2005) (SOR: B).
- In a meta-analysis, sensitivity and specificity were 70% and 71% for McMurray's test, 60% and 70% for Apley's test, and 63% and 77% for joint line tenderness; no single test appears to diagnose a torn tibial meniscus accurately (Hegedus et al., 2007) (SOR: A).

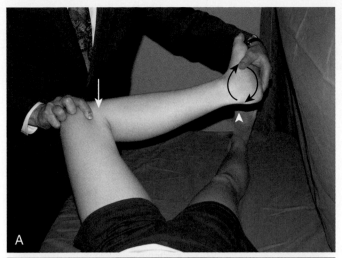

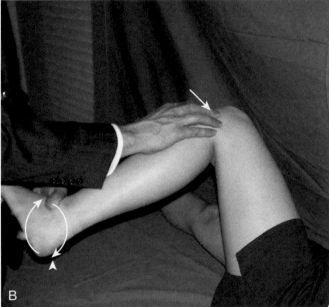

Figure 30-29 Classic examination for meniscal pathology. **A,** Medial McMurray's test is performed by palpating along the medial joint line *(thin arrow)* while creating a varus force *(solid triangle)*, ranging the knee through flexion and extension, and internally and externally rotating the leg *(yellow arrows)*. A positive finding is noted when the maneuver recreates the symptoms *and* the examiner feels a palpable click. **B,** Lateral McMurray's test is done in a similar manner with valgus stress.

(Courtesy Mark R. Hutchinson, MD.)

Ligamentous Injuries

Four major ligaments keep the knee stable: anterior cruciate ligament (ACL), posterior cruciate ligament (PCL), medial collateral ligament (MCL), and lateral collateral ligament (LCL). They can be injured in isolation or in combinations related to knee dislocations. Most ligament injuries about the knee are not urgent. However, the primary care physician must remember (1) always to look out for the potential of a multiligament knee injury and the possibility of an arterial injury and (2) always to assess the LCL, based on the significantly poorer prognosis if the diagnosis and treatment are delayed beyond 4 to 6 weeks. Early identification and surgical repair of acute LCL injuries improve patient outcomes from 50% to 90%.

Medial Collateral Ligament

The MCL is the most frequently injured ligament of the knee and often associated with concomitant ligamentous injuries; 95% are associated ACL ruptures. The MCL is the primary knee restraint to valgus loads. The MCL is tested in isolation at 30 degrees of knee flexion with a valgus load (Fig. 30-31); at 0 degrees, bony constraints contribute to stability. Valgus laxity at near or full extension implies concurrent injury to the posteromedial capsule and/or cruciate ligaments. Grade 1 injuries have pathologic laxity, indicated by increased medial joint space widening, of 1 to 4 mm; grade 2, laxity of 5 to 9 mm; and grade 3, more than 10 mm of increased laxity compared to the contralateral side.

Imaging studies should include AP and lateral radiographs looking for associated bone injury or avulsions. MR scans may be of benefit in more severe injuries to look for additional associated soft tissue injuries. Initial treatment is nonsurgical for grade 1, 2, and 3 ligament sprains. Protected weight bearing is allowed with crutches and a hinged knee brace until pain resolves medially. Unrestricted ROM is allowed and encouraged. Most patients with MCL injuries do well with conservative treatment. Occasionally, patients with grade 3 injuries who do not respond to nonoperative treatment may require surgery. Timing of return to sport or function is related to severity of injury: grade 1 injuries, usually 1 week; grade 2, 2 to 4 weeks; and grade 3, 4 to 8 weeks.

Lateral Collateral Ligament and Posterolateral Ligament Complex

When evaluating the lateral side of the knee, the physician should evaluate the function of the LCL but also the stability of the knee to posterolateral rotation. The LCL is assessed with the knee unlocked at about 20 to 30 degrees of flexion with varus stress (Fig. 30-32). The posterolateral corner is tested by externally rotating the tibia when the knee is flexed at 30 and 90 degrees. If an increased spinout to external rotation is visualized compared with the opposite knee at 30 and 90 degrees, the patient has a posterolateral corner and PCL injury. If the knee spins out only at 30 degrees compared with the opposite side, an isolated posterolateral corner injury is present (Fig. 30-33). Imaging usually includes AP/lateral radiographs and MR image. Perhaps the simplest rule for primary care physicians is that any patient with acute varus instability (injury of LCL) should be referred to an orthopedic surgeon as soon as possible.

Treatment is based on the severity of the injury. Nonsurgical treatment with protected weight bearing and protected ROM early for a few weeks is recommended for isolated grade 1 or 2 LCL; grade 1 is an opening of the lateral joint line less than 5 mm, and grade 2 is an opening of 6 to 10 mm. Progressive ROM and functional rehabilitation are initiated. Return to sports can be expected in 6 to 8 weeks. Surgical indications are recommended for isolated grade 3 LCL injuries (>10 mm gapping) and any rotator instability of the posterolateral corner. Acute surgery has more favorable outcomes, and early referral to an orthopedic surgeon is recommended.

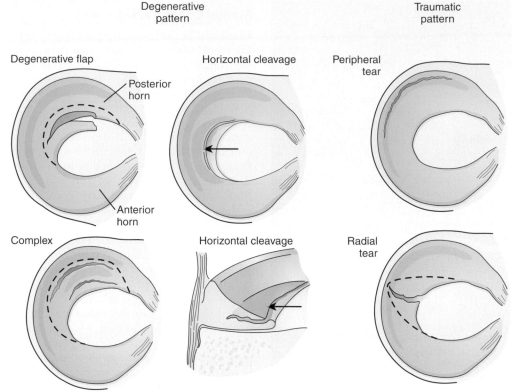

Degenerative
pattern

Traumatic
pattern

Degenerative flap

Horizontal cleavage

Peripheral
tear

Posterior
horn

Anterior
horn

Complex

Horizontal cleavage

Radial
tear

Figure 30-30 Representations of meniscus pathology. Degenerative tears tend to be complex, fibrinous, and horizontal. Acute tears that are vertical in the periphery may be reparable.

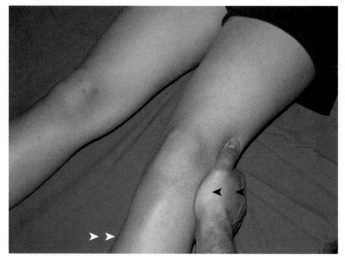

Figure 30-31 Valgus stress is used to assess function of the medial collateral ligament. To best isolate the MCL, the knee is unlocked to 30 degrees of flexion when stress is applied. If the knee is still unstable in full extension, other structures (PCL, ACL, posterior capsule) have been injured.
(Courtesy Mark R. Hutchinson, MD.)

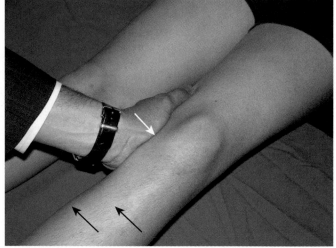

Figure 30-32 Varus stress is used to assess function of the lateral collateral ligament. Varus laxity noted in an acute knee injury should *always* be referred to an orthopedic surgeon; urgent primary repair of injured structures has a better prognosis than delayed reconstruction.
(Courtesy Mark R. Hutchinson, MD.)

Posterior Cruciate Ligament

The PCL is the primary restraint to posterior tibial translation in the knee. The most sensitive test for the PCL is the posterior drawer, which is a posterior-directed force on the knee with the knee flexed to about 90 degrees (Fig. 30-34). The PCL is usually injured secondary to a posteriorly directed force on the tibia, from a fall or potentially from a dashboard injury during a motor vehicle crash. Grading of the PCL

injury is based on the posterior drawer test and the relationship of the proximal tibia to the femoral condyles. In grade I PCL injuries, the tibial plateau is slightly anterior to the femoral condyles; in grade II, plateau and condyles sit flush at the same level; and in grade III the tibia is posterior to the level. Treatment of a PCL injury is guided by injury severity and associated ligamentous injuries (Cosgarea and Jay, 2001; Wind et al., 2004). Typically, grades I, II, and III are treated nonsurgically with bracing and functional rehabilitation, to

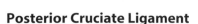

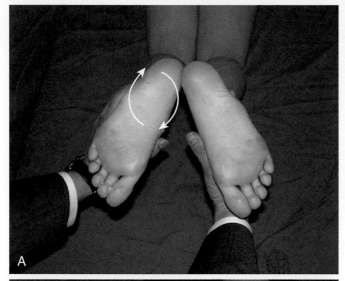

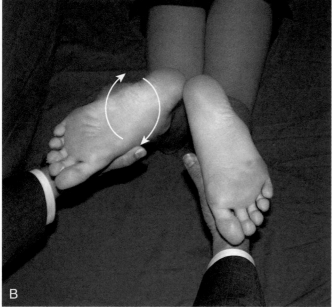

Figure 30-33 Dial test is used to assess the posterior cruciate ligament (PCL) and posterolateral corner and is best done with patient prone and knees together. **A,** Normal examination should reveal symmetry with forced external rotation. **B,** If increased external rotation is identified with knee flexed 30 degrees, an injury to the posterolateral corner is identified. If asymmetry persists as knee is flexed to 90 degrees, the PCL is likely also involved. *(Courtesy Mark R. Hutchinson, MD.)*

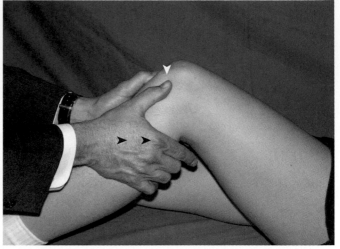

Figure 30-34 Posterior drawer is the most sensitive test for evaluating posterior cruciate ligament function. Place thumbs on femoral condyles, feeling the tibial offset at the level of the joint line *(black arrow).* Then create a posteriorly directed force *(white arrows)* and reassess the tibial step-off. *(Courtesy Mark R. Hutchinson, MD.)*

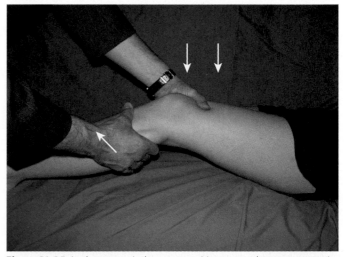

Figure 30-35 Lachman test is the most sensitive approach to assess anterior cruciate ligament function. The femur is stabilized *(white arrows)* with the knee flexed about 15 to 20 degrees and the tibia drawn anteriorly *(yellow arrow).* Comparison to the opposite side and assessment of a ropelike end point are key.

focus on quadriceps strengthening. PCL ruptures, unlike ACL ruptures, tend to heal, and often a grade III will heal as a grade II, and a grade II as a grade I, with appropriate bracing and protection. Mild PCL laxity is usually not symptomatic for patients. If the knee becomes unstable, however, reconstruction can be delayed.

Anterior Cruciate Ligament

The ACL is perhaps the most famous of knee ligaments because of its notoriety in twisting and cutting sports. The common presentation of an ACL injury is an athlete landing in a twisting and cutting sport, feeling a pop, and having an acute hemarthrosis within 24 hours. The most sensitive test

for ACL rupture is a Lachman test, which is basically an anterior translation of the tibia on the femur with the knee flexed 20 to 30 degrees (Fig. 30-35). The anterior drawer test is also used but is less sensitive (Fig. 30-36). The most specific test is the "pivot shift."

Initial treatment of ACL injury focuses on rehabilitation to regain ROM and strengthen the knee. Surgical indications are based on patient's function as well as future demands (Beynnon et al., 2005). For young athletes who want to play a twisting or cutting sport more than two or three times per week, ACL reconstruction is strongly recommended. The key reason for that indication is the absolute requirement to avoid the current instability or pivoting. Recurrent wobbling or pivoting of the knee leads to an increase in stress along the meniscus, meniscal failure, meniscal degeneration, hyaline cartilage degeneration, and degenerative changes in

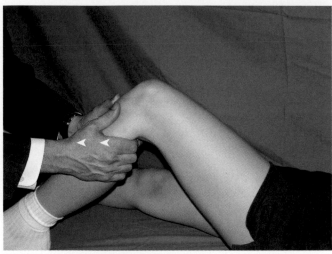

Figure 30-36 Anterior drawer test is less sensitive for isolating anterior cruciate ligament injuries but may assist in diagnosing associated pathology. The knee is flexed 90 degrees and the tibia drawn anteriorly. *(Courtesy of Mark R. Hutchinson, MD.)*

the knee. If the athlete is willing to give up his sport, with no complaints of instability performing activities of daily living, surgical ACL reconstruction is not always necessary.

Skeletally immature athletes pose a unique challenge because of their open growth plates. Treatment options include delay of definitive surgical reconstruction until maturity, extra-articular reconstruction, and reconstruction with soft tissue across the physis (Bates et al., 2004). Most studies have shown that children are not fully cooperative with programs that have them reduce activities until skeletal maturity. This leads to recurrent episodes of instability with associated meniscal and cartilage damage. Based on this there has been a strong trend to surgically stabilize these young athletes to reduce the risk of arthrosis at a young age.

EVIDENCE-BASED SUMMARY

- No RCTs have compared surgical and nonsurgical outcomes in reduction of future osteoarthritic change for PCL injuries (Peccin et al., 1995) (SOR: A).
- Based on two clinical trials in the 1980s and insufficient RCTs, no conclusions can be drawn about conservative versus surgical treatment of ACL ruptures in adults (Linko et al., 2005).
- Surgical stabilization should be considered for skeletally immature patients with ACL injuries because they carry a high risk of recurrent instability and subsequent injury and damage to the meniscus (Bates et al., 2004) (SOR: B).

Ankle and Foot

Key Points

- Radiographs for foot and ankle imaging should be weight bearing if a fracture does not preclude it.
- Radiographs are not necessary in all cases of suspected ankle sprain.

- Early mobilization with external supportive device usually leads to a quicker recovery from ankle sprain, although it may not affect the long-term outcome.
- Surgical repair of Achilles tendon tears leads to a reduced risk of rerupture, although surgical complications exist.
- Although corticosteroid injections can provide short-term relief of plantar fasciitis pain, no single intervention appears superior to another.
- Fractures through the watershed area of blood supply in the proximal fifth metatarsal (Jones' fracture) has a high risk of nonunion/malunion and is often best treated surgically.

The foot and ankle are complex structures that provide the foundation to the musculoskeletal system and are intimately related to a person's ability to ambulate, run, jump, and traverse unstable and variable terrain. Optimal foot and ankle function implies a higher level of function for activities of daily living. Thorough examination and imaging should consider a broad differential diagnosis of common problems, ranging from ligament sprains, stress fractures, fractures and avulsions, chronic tendinopathies, and tendon ruptures. A more expansive differential diagnosis includes nerve entrapment, circulatory dysfunction, and systemic disease, as well as congenital and developmental problems. All x-ray imaging of the foot and ankle for pain should be weight-bearing views in the absence of suspicion of a fracture, to allow a more accurate clinical picture because the patient usually experiences pain when weight bearing and not at rest (Stiell et al, 1992, 1993).

Ankle Sprains

Sprains are injuries to the ligamentous structures of the ankle. About 85% of ankle sprains involve the lateral ligaments; medial and syndesmosis sprains make up the remaining 15%. Diagnosis is based primarily on history and physical examination, although radiographs are often helpful. Advanced diagnostic testing is not usually necessary. The family physician must be aware of the many potential pitfalls in the diagnosis of ankle sprain as well.

Lateral Ankle Sprains

The anterior talofibular ligament (ATFL), calcaneofibular ligament (CFL), and posterior talofibular ligament (PTFL) are the three ligaments of the lateral ankle (Fig. 30-37). The ATFL primarily restricts anterior motion of the talus within the ankle mortise; the CFL restricts inversion; and the PTFL restricts posterior translation. The most common mechanism of lateral ankle sprain is an *inversion* ankle injury. Inversion events with the ankle in a plantar-flexed position often lead to ATFL injury (Fig. 30-38), whereas inversion events with the ankle in a dorsiflexed position more often lead to CFL injury (Fig. 30-39). Patients present due to ankle pain that may be associated with swelling, bruising, decreased motion, and increased pain with weight bearing, if able.

Examination begins with observing the patient's gait; a limp is often noted. Gross observation of the foot and ankle often reveals lateral edema and ecchymosis. Active motion may be severely restricted. Neurovascular structures are usually normal. Along with palpation of the ATFL, CFL, and PTFL, important structures to palpate on the lateral aspect

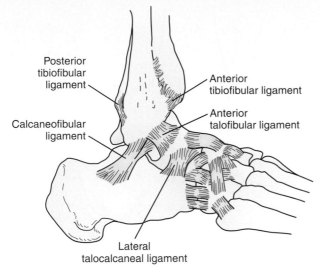

Figure 30-37 Anatomy of lateral ankle ligaments.
(From Nicholas J, Hershman E. The Lower Extremity and Spine in Sports Medicine, vol 1, 2nd ed. St Louis, Mosby, 1995, p 424.)

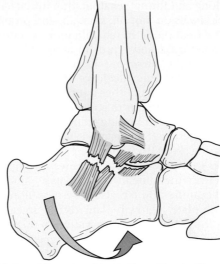

Figure 30-39 Forceful inversion of the hindfoot with a dorsiflexed ankle, possibly tearing the calcaneofibular, cervical, and interosseous talocalcaneal ligaments. (From Meyer JM, Garcia J, Hoffmeyer P, et al. The subtalar sprain: a roentgenographic study. Clin Orthop 1988;226:169-173.)

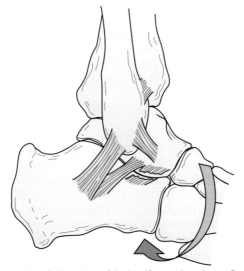

Figure 30-38 Forceful inversion of the hindfoot with a plantar-flexed ankle, possibly tearing the anterior talofibular and interosseous talocalcaneal ligaments.
(From Meyer JM, Garcia J, Hoffmeyer P, et al. The subtalar sprain: a roentgenographic study. Clin Orthop 1988;226:169-173.)

of the ankle include the fibula (entire length), peroneal tendons, lateral process of the talus, neck of the talus, cuboid, and base of the fifth metatarsal. Stress testing is performed to assess the integrity of ligamentous structures. The anterior drawer test translates the talus within the mortise and assesses the ATFL, performed with the ankle in slight plantar flexion to place the ATFL under tension while decreasing CFL tension. Both the amount of excursion compared to the opposite side and the end-point feel to the test are important determinants in the evaluation. The CFL is tested by the talar tilt. The ankle is placed in a neutral position, putting tension on the CFL and decreasing tension on the ATFL. The talus is then inverted within the mortise while the examiner assesses excursion and end-point feel. Once again, these findings are compared to the opposite side to determine severity of injury.

In the United States, patients presenting for ankle injury often undergo radiographic evaluation, but the utility of routine radiographs to evaluate ankle injury is under debate. Well-designed studies from Canada have shown that many patients with ankle injury can be managed safely without routine radiographs. Indications for lateral ankle radiograph include age under 18 or over 55; inability to bear weight for four consecutive steps, either immediately after injury or in the examination room; and pain over the posterior portion of the distal 6 cm or at the tip of the fibula (Stiell et al., 1992, 1993). If pain is noted in the proximal or midshaft fibula, tibia/fibula films should be obtained, and pain over the base of the fifth metatarsal indicates the need for foot radiographs.

Various scales are available to grade ankle injuries, and interexaminer variability is high. The most common scale is mild (grade 1), moderate (grade 2), and severe (grade 3). However, grading does not significantly affect treatment, complication rates, or long-term outcomes. Grading may have a predictive role in duration of recovery.

Treatment of lateral ankle sprains has changed drastically over the past 25 years. Complete immobilization and rest were once thought to be important initial components of treatment. Currently, early mobilization with an external support device and rehabilitation are common therapies. Early immobilization may lead to greater stability and patient compliance, and the risk for early reinjury is low. In the early mobilization and rehabilitation plan, recovery tends to occur slightly quicker (based on full return to work), and early discomfort may be decreased (Eiff et al., 1994; Karlsson et al., 1996). With immobilization, the ankle joint can become stiff and lead to muscle atrophy. This may require a prolonged postimmobilization program focused on regaining motion and strength. Long-term outcomes of early mobilization and immobilization treatment plans are not significantly different.

Basic stages of treatment include early external support and, depending on severity, limited weight bearing, pain control, reducing swelling with ice and elevation, and maintaining motion. Once the initial acute injury subsides, weaning from supportive devices such as crutches, walking boots or casts should be done and formal rehabilitation initiated. Rehabilitation should focus on motion, strength, and proprioception activities. The final phase of rehabilitation is reintroduction of sport-specific tasks and return to sport. Participation in a prevention training program with a focus on balance and proprioception reduces the incidence of ankle sprain without increasing the incidence of other injuries (Bahr et al., 1997). Bracing the ankle on return to sport may reduce the risk of recurrent injury. Whether bracing reduces the risk of an initial sprain is under debate (Sitler et al., 1994; Surve et al., 1994).

When treating skeletally immature patients, it is important to remember that physeal plate fractures through the distal fibula result from the same mechanism as an ankle sprain. If the physical examination reveals tenderness along the distal fibular growth plate, a growth plate fracture must be considered, even if the radiographs are negative. In this case, a short period of immobilization followed by repeat imaging in 2 weeks is appropriate.

Medial Ankle Sprains

The main ligament on the medial side of the ankle is the deltoid ligament (Fig. 30-40). Deltoid injuries are typically caused by an eversion mechanism. Medial ankle examination is similar to that of the lateral ankle. Observation of gait usually reveals a limp, and gross observation of the ankle often reveals medial edema but no other deformity. Active motion may be severely restricted, and neurovascular status should be normal. Careful palpation of bony, tendinous, and ligamentous structures of the medial ankle include the deltoid ligament, medial malleolus, medial process of talus, neck of talus, medial cuneiform, cuboid, navicular, and medial ankle tendons (posterior tibialis, flexor digitorum longus, and flexor hallucis longus).

Stress testing of the deltoid ligament is performed by an eversion stress test, usually performed with the ankle in neutral position. Amount of excursion compared to the opposite side and the end-point feel determine the severity of the injury. Deltoid function can also be assessed by stressing the ankle, translating it from medial to lateral and assessing for instability or mortis widening. Any offset increases the stresses on the articular cartilage and increases the risk of arthritis. Obtaining radiographs in the patient with medial ankle injury is decided on a case-by-case basis but should be done more readily than for the typical lateral ankle sprain. Treatment plans are similar to those for lateral ankle sprains. It is widely believed that medial sprains take longer to heal than their lateral counterparts.

Syndesmosis Ankle Sprains (High Ankle Sprains)

The ankle *syndesmosis* is the area of the distal tibia-fibula joint. The five soft tissue structures in the syndesmosis region include the anterior tibiofibular, posterior tibiofibular, transverse tibiofibular, and interosseous ligaments and the interosseous membrane; of these, the anterior tibiofibular ligament is most often injured. Syndesmosis sprains account for 1% to 18% of ankle sprains, with a higher incidence in high-level athletes. Syndesmosis sprains are generally thought to take longer to heal than lateral or medial sprains (Hopkinson et al., 1990), and persistent ankle pain and persistent dysfunction are more common (Gerber et al., 1998);

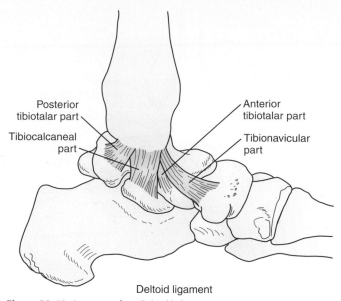

Figure 30-40 Anatomy of medial ankle ligaments.
(From Nicholas J, Hershman E. The Lower Extremity and Spine in Sports Medicine, vol 1, 2nd ed. St Louis, Mosby, 1995, p 424.)

syndesmosis injuries are often associated with fractures. The mechanism of injury is different than for the more common lateral and medial sprains; syndesmosis sprains are most often caused by forceful external rotation and hyperdorsiflexion injuries.

Physical examination often reveals an antalgic gait limp and anterolateral ankle swelling over the anterior tibiofibular ligament just proximal to the joint line. Ecchymosis is often a delayed finding and is usually noted proximal to the ankle joint, in contrast to that noted in lateral and medial sprains, which is often below the ankle and occasionally throughout the foot. Careful palpation reveals tenderness directly over the anterior tibiofibular ligament. Syndesmosis injuries may be present along with medial ankle injury, so tenderness over deltoid ligament may be noted as well. Be sure to palpate the proximal fibula, because extreme forced external rotation may lead to Maisonneuve's fracture (proximal fibular fracture). Strength testing is often limited by pain, and neurovascular status remains intact.

Special stress tests to evaluate the syndesmosis include the squeeze, external rotation, and dorsiflexion-compression tests. The squeeze test is performed by compressing the fibula and tibia above the midpoint of the calf (Hopkinson et al., 1990) (Fig. 30-41). The test is positive if compression causes pain in the region of the syndesmosis ligament. The external rotation test is performed with the knee at 90-degree flexion and the ankle in neutral position. An external rotation force is applied to the foot while stabilizing the remainder of the leg. Pain in the anterior tibiofibular region is a positive test. The external rotation test is thought to be the most reliable of the common clinical tests used to diagnose syndesmosis sprains.

Because of the risk of concurrent fracture with syndesmosis sprains, radiographs should be obtained. Plain radiographs are adequate to assess for frank *diastasis* (widening between fibula and tibia). Stress radiographs may be necessary to discover latent diastasis. The three major radiographic considerations are the (1) *tibiofibular clear space*, the distance between medial border of fibula and lateral border of posterior tibia,

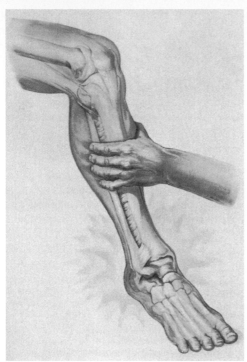

Figure 30-41 Squeeze test.
(From Hopkinson WJ, St. Pierre P, Ryan IB, et al. Syndesmosis sprains of the ankle. Foot Ankle Int 1990;10:325-330. Copyright American Orthopedic Foot and Ankle Society, 1990.)

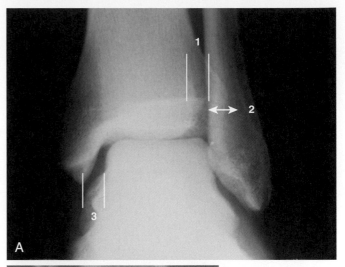

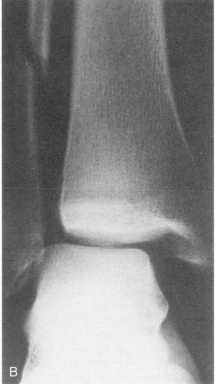

Figure 30-42 Normal anteroposterior radiograph of the ankle revealing a normal tibiofibular clear space *(1)*, normal tibiofibular overlap *(2)*, and normal medial clear space *(3)*. Significant mortise widening is noted with widening of all three of these parameters. Note the distal fibula fracture. This injury is best treated with internal fixation of the fracture and stabilization of the ankle mortise with a syndesmosis screw. **B,** Football eversion injury shows widening medial mortise with associated deltoid tear, widening distal tibiofibular syndesmosis, high fibular fracture, and small posterior malleolus fracture (not seen here).
*(**A** courtesy James L. Moeller, MD; **B** from Nicholas J, Hershman E. The Lower Extremity and Spine in Sports Medicine, vol 1, 2nd ed. St Louis, Mosby, 1995, p 465.)*

measured 1 cm above tibial plafond; (2) *tibiofibular overlap,* the maximum amount of overlap of distal fibula and anterior tibial tubercle; and (3) *medial clear space,* the distance between medial malleolus and medial border of talus, measured 1 cm below tibial plafond (Fig. 30-42).

Additional testing such as CT scan can be helpful early in the workup to look for occult fracture and later to assess for heterotopic ossification, a common complication of syndesmosis sprains. MR scan is sometimes used and has a high sensitivity and specificity for detecting anterior and posterior tibiofibular ligament injuries (Oae et al., 2003).

Initial treatment begins with protection of the joint, relative rest, ice, compression, and elevation. Various modalities to reduce swelling and inflammation can be used. Rehabilitation includes ROM exercises, strengthening and balance exercises, and proprioception training. Activities can be advanced when pain is reduced, and rehabilitation exercises can be performed pain-free. Return to full activities can be entertained when the patient has full motion, full strength, no tenderness on examination, and no functionally limiting pain.

Latent diastasis can be treated nonoperatively if reduction can be achieved. Therapy includes immobilization with non–weight bearing followed by progressive weight bearing beginning at about 4 weeks and full weight bearing by 2 months. Surgery is needed if reduction cannot be achieved or if diastasis recurs despite immobilization. Frank diastasis is treated surgically.

A common adverse outcome of syndesmosis sprain is heterotopic ossification. Plain radiographs are adequate to make the diagnosis in patients with persistent pain (Fig. 30-43). Affecting 25% to 90% of patients, heterotopic ossification may or may not be symptomatic. Ossification may cause pain without causing frank synostosis. The discomfort comes from an inflammatory response in early stages, then from pressure on adjacent bones. Fracture of the ossification is also a potential cause of pain. Frank synostosis can occur. Pain typically results from restricted tibiofibular motion, particularly during full ankle dorsiflexion. Conservative treatment may reduce the pain, but surgical excision may be required (Hopkinson et al., 1990; Taylor et al., 1992).

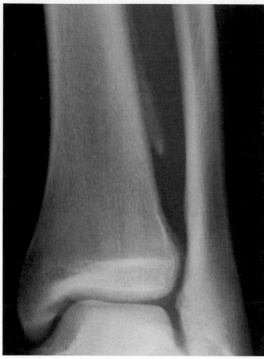

Figure 30-43 Heterotopic ossification noted after syndesmosis ankle sprain. *(Courtesy James L. Moeller, MD.)*

Achilles Tendinopathy

Achilles tendinopathy is a common problem, especially in running and jumping athletes. The Achilles tendon consists of the distal ends of the gastrocnemius and soleus muscles and attaches broadly across the posterior aspect of the calcaneus. Contraction of the Achilles results in plantar flexion of the ankle. Activities that cause eccentric loading of the tendon may result in tendonitis. Achilles tendonitis is considered an overuse injury.

Patients present with pain in the posterior aspect of the distal lower leg or heel. Pain is worsened with push-off activities, such as walking up hills or stairs, running, or jumping. Examination reveals tenderness to palpation of the distal portion of the tendon. A palpable area of swelling and firmness may be noted as well as "wet crepitus" from fluid in the peritenon. Strength may be limited because of discomfort. This can be assessed by direct manual testing or by having the patient perform repeated single-foot toe-raise exercises.

Assessment of the integrity of the Achilles tendon is essential and best done by the Thompson test. Asking the patient simply to plantar-flex the ankle actively is not sufficient because there are several secondary plantar flexors. Lay the patient prone on the examination table with the knee flexed to 90 degrees and the ankle in neutral position. Squeeze the midgastrocnemius area and observe for passive ankle plantar flexion. If the Achilles is intact, the ankle will plantar-flex (negative test). If the Achilles is torn, the ankle will remain in neutral position (positive test).

Radiographs generally are not necessary to make an accurate diagnosis of Achilles tendinopathy or to initiate treatment. X-ray films are considered in chronic cases, primarily to rule out calcific tendinopathy and Haglund deformity (bump on back of calcaneus near Achilles insertion).

Ultrasound and MRI are not routinely needed early on but may be used to assess for partial tears, as well as assess the vascular integrity of the injured area. Ultrasound and MR changes in the tendon can persist even after functional recovery (Khan et al., 2003).

Treatment of Achilles tendinopathy is similar to that for other forms of tendinopathy and includes ice treatment, relative rest, NSAIDs, stretching and strengthening programs, and proprioception exercises. An exercise program focused on eccentric training has been described and renders promising results in many cases (Alfredson et al., 1998). Most experts agree that corticosteroid injection should not be considered due to the risk of tendon rupture. For recalcitrant cases, treatments such as prolotherapy and extracorporeal shock wave therapy have been studied, but short-term follow-up and isolated reports of effectiveness are mixed. Platelet-rich plasma injections for chronic Achilles tendinopathy have no benefit over saline injections. Surgical debridement is reserved for chronic cases and involves debridement of the diseased tendon and may require tendon transfers for grafting.

Achilles Tendon Rupture

Tears of the Achilles tendon are most often encountered in males 40 to 60 years old. The most common mechanism of injury is sudden, forceful eccentric loading of the tendon. This can occur from a sudden forceful push-off from a single foot, or landing on a single foot. Patients present due to sudden onset pain in the posterior heel and decreased push-off strength. Patients often describe a feeling of being kicked or hit in the heel, often hearing or feeling a pop at the time of injury. Examination may reveal a palpable gap in the tendon, usually distally. Thompson's test is positive, with no ankle plantar flexion when the examiner squeezes the calf. Imaging studies are not typically needed to make an accurate diagnosis of Achilles tendon rupture.

Both surgical and nonsurgical treatment options exist (McComis et al., 1997; Weber et al., 2003). Patient selection and including the patient in the decision-making process are important. Generally, younger patients who desire or require greater posttreatment push-off power are likely to be good surgical candidates, whereas older patients or patients who require less push-off power are nonsurgical candidates. Nonoperative risk of repeat rupture is as high as 10%, versus up to 2% with surgery. Skin necrosis of the surgical wound occurs in 5% to 10% of patients.

Conservative treatment entails a period of immobilization accomplished through casting or brace use, usually 8 to 10 weeks; early weight bearing is controversial. After immobilization, progressive rehabilitation to regain motion, strength, and proprioception is initiated. Surgery is associated with improved push-off power and reduced rate of repeat rupture and generally allows for the best functional recovery (Wong et al., 2002).

Plantar Fasciitis

Plantar fasciitis is the most common cause of plantar heel pain in active individuals. The plantar fascia is a fibrous band of tissue that originates at the medial calcaneal tubercle, fans out across the plantar aspect of the foot, and then splits before inserting into the plantar aspects of the proximal phalanges. Plantar fasciitis is an overuse injury often seen in people who stand for prolonged periods, as well as in runners and regular exercisers. Many believe plantar fasciitis is an inflammatory condition, but it is more likely caused by chronic changes and microtears of the fascia.

Patients present with plantar heel pain. Pain has often been present for several months before presentation. The pain is often described as sharp and stabbing and tends to be worst in the morning, on arising from prolonged sitting, and after standing for prolonged periods. Other symptoms, such as bruising, swelling, weakness, numbness, and tingling, are uncommon. The primary finding on physical examination reveals tenderness over the origin of the plantar fascia.

Treatment protocols are variable, and it may take several months for the patient to feel significant pain relief. Most treatment plans include plantar fascia stretching, ice or ice massage, heel cushioning, and analgesic medication. NSAIDs are often used, but are helpful most likely because of their analgesic, not anti-inflammatory, effects. Other common treatment options include night splints, physical therapy, orthotic devices, and cortisone injection. Cortisone injection reduces pain from plantar fasciitis, but the mechanism is unclear (Hunt and Sevier, 2004). Cortisone is a potent anti-inflammatory, but as previously stated, chronic plantar fasciitis is probably not an inflammatory problem. Risks with cortisone injection include plantar fascia rupture and necrosis of the plantar fat pad, the natural heel cushion. These adverse outcomes should be reviewed with patients before injection.

New modalities for the treatment of plantar fasciitis are under investigation. Extracorporeal shock wave therapy has shown mixed results (Rompe et al., 2002, 2003). Prolotherapy and autologous blood injection involve injecting substances into the area of pathology. Dry needling is also being studied. None of these options has proved to be consistently helpful. Surgical intervention is sometimes needed in recalcitrant cases.

Metatarsal Fractures

Nondisplaced fractures of the midshaft and distal portions of the metatarsals are treated with immobilization. Short-leg casting and immobilizer boots can lead to adequate healing in 6 to 8 weeks in most cases. Postoperative shoe use without formal immobilization can also lead to adequate healing of metatarsal fractures, although the risk of adverse outcome is higher. Displaced, angulated, and rotated fractures may require operative fixation.

Fractures of the proximal portion of the metatarsal (first through fourth metatarsals) should be approached with great care. Nondisplaced fractures may be associated with injury to the intermetatarsal ligaments, leading to widening of these joints; surgical consultation is recommended in these cases. If there is no apparent injury to the tarsometatarsal (Lisfranc) joint, cast immobilization typically leads to adequate fracture healing.

Fractures of the base of the fifth metatarsal deserve special discussion. A watershed area of blood flow in the proximal portion of the fifth metatarsal puts it at particular risk for malunion and nonunion. Avulsion fractures off the most proximal portion of the bone have an opportunity to heal with conservative management. Fractures that occur in the watershed area, so-called Jones fractures, have a high chance for malunion and nonunion that should be discussed with the patient. Jones fractures occur in the proximal one third of the metatarsal and do not involve the tarsometatarsal joint. Screw fixation of Jones fractures often leads to more acceptable outcomes.

EVIDENCE-BASED SUMMARY

- Early mobilization with an external support device after ankle sprain leads to better short-term outcomes (reduction of pain and return to work/sport activities) compared to early immobilization; long-term outcomes are similar (Eiff et al., 1994; Karlsson et al., 1996; Kerkhoffs et al., 2004) (SOR: A).
- Use of an external ankle brace after ankle sprain reduces the risk of recurrent sprain. Evidence also supports balance and proprioception training for reducing risk of recurrent sprain (Bahr et al., 1997; Surve et al., 1994) (SOR: B).
- An eccentric training program is effective in treating chronic Achilles tendinopathy (Alfredson et al., 1998) (SOR: B).
- Surgery for acute Achilles tendon ruptures reduces the risk of repeat rupture compared to nonsurgical treatment but produces a significantly higher risk of other complications, including wound infection (Khan et al., 2004) (SOR: A).
- Corticosteroid injection can reduce plantar fasciitis pain in the short term (Hunt and Sevier, 2004) (SOR: B).
- For acute Jones fractures in recreationally active patients, early intramedullary screw fixation results in lower failure rates and shorter times to both clinical union and return to sports than non-weight-bearing short-leg casting (Vu et al., 2006) (SOR: B).

References

The complete reference list is available online at www.expertconsult.com.

Web Resources

Shoulder
www.shoulderdoc.co.uk/article.asp?section=497
    Review of the shoulder exam with specific instructions on physical exam.

http://emedicine.medscape.com/article/1260953-overview
http://orthoinfo.aaos.org/topic.cfm?topic=A00072 Clavicle fracture
http://orthoinfo.aaos.org/topic.cfm?topic=a00033
www.eorthopod.com/node/10838 AC sprain.

www.eorthopod.com/node/10847 SC sprain.

http://emedicine.medscape.com/article/92974-overview

http://orthoinfo.aaos.org/topic.cfm?topic=A00032 Shoulder impingement.

www.emedicinehealth.com/rotator_cuff_injury/article_em.htm

http://orthoinfo.aaos.org/topic.cfm?topic=A00406
Rotator cuff tear.

http://orthoinfo.aaos.org/topic.cfm?topic=A00529
Shoulder instability.

Elbow

http://emedicine.medscape.com/article/1231903-overview

http://orthoinfo.aaos.org/topic.cfm?topic=A00068
Lateral tendinopathy

http://emedicine.medscape.com/article/327860-overview

www.mayoclinic.com/health/golfers-elbow/DS00713
Medial tendinopathy

Wrist and Hand

www.mayoclinic.com/health/carpal-tunnel-syndrome/DS00326
Carpal tunnel syndrome.

www.mayoclinic.com/health/de-quervains-tenosynovitis/DS00692

www.handuniversity.com/topics.asp?Topic_ID=45
DeQuervain's tenosynovitis.

www.mayoclinic.com/health/trigger-finger/DS00155
Trigger finger.

http://orthoinfo.aaos.org/topic.cfm?topic=a00412
Distal radius fracture.

http://orthoinfo.aaos.org/topic.cfm?topic=A00012

www.handuniversity.com/topics.asp?Topic_ID=30
Scaphoid fracture.

Knee

http://orthoinfo.aaos.org/topic.cfm?topic=A00212
Degenerative osteoarthritis.

http://orthoinfo.aaos.org/topic.cfm?topic=A00197
Joint infection.

www.mayoclinic.com/health/patellar-tendinitis/DS00625
Patellar tendinitis.

www.webmd.com/a-to-z-guides/patellofemoral-pain-syndrome-topic-overview
Patellofemoral pain.

http://orthoinfo.aaos.org/topic.cfm?topic=a00358
Meniscus tear.

www.webmd.com/a-to-z-guides/anterior-cruciate-ligament-acl-injuries-topic-overview

http://orthoinfo.aaos.org/topic.cfm?topic=A00297 Ligament injury.

Ankle and Foot

www.emedicinehealth.com/ankle_sprain/article_em.htm

http://orthoinfo.aaos.org/topic.cfm?topic=a00150
Ankle sprain.

www.mayoclinic.com/health/achilles-tendinitis/DS00737
Achilles tendinitis.

www.emedicinehealth.com/achilles_tendon_rupture/article_em.htm

www.mayoclinic.com/health/achilles-tendon-rupture/DS00160 Achilles tendon rupture.

www.mayoclinic.com/health/plantar-fasciitis/DS00508
Plantar fasciitis.

http://emedicine.medscape.com/article/399372-overview
Metatarsal fracture.

Splinting and Casting

http://intermed.med.uottawa.ca/procedures/cast/#02

CHAPTER 31

Back: Cervical and Thoracolumbar Spine

Minal Patel and Krupa Shah

Cervical Spine

The cervical spine provides support and stability for the head. Articulation at the joints of the vertebrae allows for the range of motion of the head. The spine is also the route through which the nerve roots travel out from the spinal canal to the extremities. As with back pain, chronic neck pain or disorders related to limited function from neck problems are common reasons for office visits. A careful history and examination help elucidate the cause and the level and extent of compromise affecting cervical function.

Anatomy

The cervical spine is made up of seven vertebrae (C1-C7). A typical vertebra has a body and neural arch. The neural arch is made up of two pedicles and two vertebrae; the laminae meet at the spinous process posteriorly. A transverse process projects out laterally on each side of the pedicle and lamina (Fig. 31-1). The articular processes on the superior and inferior parts of each vertebra at the junction of the pedicle and lamina meet at the facet joints. The first two vertebrae have distinct features. The atlas, C1, articulates with the occipital bone and has no spinous process or body. The axis, C2, has an odontoid process that articulates with C1 (Fig. 31-2); much of the rotational function of the neck occurs at this joint. C7 has a long spinous process, resulting in a palpable prominence below the skin in the lower neck.

Several ligaments stabilize the neck. The anterior and posterior ligaments support the entire vertebral column (Fig. 31-3). The spinous process of each vertebra is attached by the nuchal ligament to the neck and the interspinous ligaments. Intervertebral disks separate each vertebra. Their function is to distribute the pressure over a wider area of the vertebra and allow mobility. Each disk consists of a gelatinous central nucleus and outer fibrous annulus fibrosus. Eight pairs of nerves originate from the cervical spine. The first seven nerve roots exit the spinal canal above the corresponding vertebra, and the eighth nerve root exits from below C7 (Fig. 31-4).

History

The relevant history includes age of the patient, location of any pain, acute or gradual onset, radiation and duration of pain, and any related associated symptoms that indicate whether the pain is of cervical origin or referred from another condition. An older patient is more often affected by arthritis and a younger person by musculoskeletal pain. Rest or nighttime pain may be a symptom of a tumor or infection. Other symptoms include neck stiffness, headache, and symptoms of radiculopathy such as tingling, numbness, and loss of strength in the upper extremities. Where the pain is caused by nerve entrapment, the pain may radiate along the distribution of the involved nerve. Events leading up to the presentation may also give clues to the problem.

Physical Examination

The neck examination includes inspection for any neck lesions, masses, or scars as well as posture and normal cervical lordosis, characterized by a slight anterior curvature (Fig. 31-5). The neck is palpated for points of tenderness.

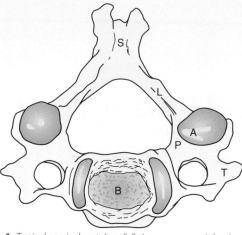

Figure 31-1 Typical cervical vertebra. *S,* Spinous process; *L,* lamina; *A,* articular facet; *P,* pedicle; *T,* transverse process; *B,* body. *(Redrawn from Mercier L. Practical Orthopedics, 5th ed. St Louis, Mosby, 2000, p 27.)*

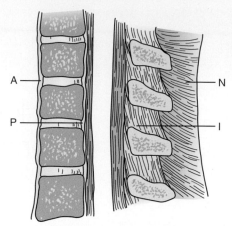

Figure 31-3 Ligaments of the cervical spine. *A,* Anterior longitudinal ligament; *P,* posterior longitudinal ligament; *N,* nuchal ligament; *I,* interspinous ligament. *(Redrawn from Mercier L. Practical Orthopedics, 5th ed. St Louis, Mosby, 2000, p 27.)*

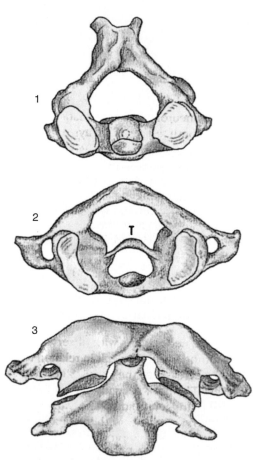

Figure 31-2 **1,** Axis. **2,** Atlas and transverse ligament *(T).* **3,** Articulation of the atlas and axis. *(Redrawn from Mercier L. Practical Orthopedics, 5th ed. St Louis, Mosby, 2000, p 27.)*

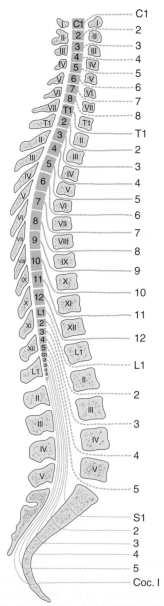

Figure 31-4 Spinal cord and nerve roots in relation to the vertebrae. *(Redrawn from Brinker MR, Miller MD. Fundamentals of Orthopedics. Philadelphia, Saunders, 1999, p 242.)*

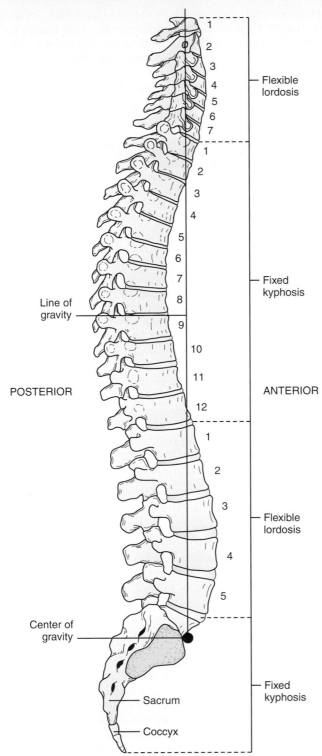

1
2
3
4
5
6
7

Flexible lordosis

1
2
3
4
5
6
7
8
9
10
11
12

Fixed kyphosis

Line of gravity

POSTERIOR

ANTERIOR

1
2
3
4
5

Flexible lordosis

Center of gravity

Fixed kyphosis

Sacrum

Coccyx

Figure 31-5 Vertebral spine. Note that thoracic spine has relatively fixed kyphosis and lumbar spine relatively flexible lordosis. *(Redrawn from Brinker MR, Miller MD. Fundamentals of Orthopedics. Philadelphia, Saunders, 1999, p 241.)*

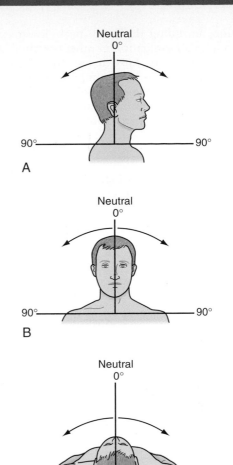

Neutral
0°

90°   90°

A

Neutral
0°

90°   90°

B

Neutral
0°

90°   90°

C

Figure 31-6 Range of motion. **A,** Flexion. **B,** Lateral flexion. **C,** Rotation. *(Redrawn from Carr AJ, Harnden A. Orthopedics in Primary Care. Newton, Mass, Butterworth-Heinemann, 1997, p 56.)*

Table 31-1 Normal Range of Movement: Neck (Cervical Spine)

Motion	Range
Flexion	0-45 degrees
Extension	0-45 degrees
Lateral flexion	0-45 degrees
Rotation	0-60 degrees

Modified from Carr AJ, Harnden A. Orthopedics in Primary Care. Newton, Mass, Butterworth-Heinemann, 1997.

The range of movement is assessed by observing *forward flexion* with chin tilted down toward the chest and *backward extension* with the head tilted backward so that the eyes are looking toward the ceiling (Fig. 31-6). Lateral flexion to the right and left is the lateral bending of the neck, pointing the ear toward the shoulder on the same side. Lateral rotation to the right and left is the chin turned toward each shoulder while the head is kept upright (Table 31-1).

Examination should also include examination of the extremities. Inspection of the upper limbs may reveal muscle wasting or fasciculations. A detailed examination of the nervous system includes assessment of the power and tone of the muscles, reflexes, and sensory system, using sharp and light touch. Mapping the sensory loss by dermatomes and demonstrating asymmetry of deep tendon reflexes may show the cervical level with nerve compression. A complete general examination, including the head, neck, lower extremities, and gait, allows for evaluation of other potential causes and effects of neck problems. Specific tests to evaluate the cervical spine also include the axial compression test, which may increase symptoms of radicular pain. The distraction test may relieve radicular symptoms. Spurling's test may produce pain on the same side as nerve root encroachment.

Diagnostic Tests

Diagnostic tests include radiographs of the cervical spine. Computed tomography (CT) may assess the bone further, and magnetic resonance imaging (MRI) is useful to assess the soft tissue, especially with associated neurologic symptoms.

Torticollis

Key Points

- Torticollis may be congenital or acquired.
- Congenital torticollis may be characterized by a palpable tumor in the sternomastoid muscle in some cases.
- Acquired torticollis may be caused by a spinal tumor.
- Traumatic injury and retropharyngeal abscess require emergency treatment.
- Management of acquired torticollis includes treating the underlying cause.

Torticollis, also called *wry neck,* is characterized by contraction of the sternomastoid muscle on one side of the neck, in which the head is tilted to the same side as the contracted muscle, and the chin is rotated to the opposite side. The condition may be congenital or acquired.

Congenital torticollis is caused by the contraction of the sternomastoid muscle. The cause is unclear but may be associated with birth trauma or an abnormal fetal uterine position causing local muscle ischemia. Children with hip dysplasia and breech delivery have a higher incidence of torticollis. Also, delayed development of the face on the affected side may result in facial asymmetry and changes in the cervical vertebrae. On examination, a small lump may be palpable in the muscle, known as a *sternomastoid tumor.*

In mild cases, treatment is initiated early and includes gentle stretching exercises several times daily. Supervised physical therapy may be considered. Surgery may be considered in special circumstances with patients who do not respond to conservative treatment. The procedure includes surgical release of the sternomastoid muscle, followed by corrective exercises.

Acquired torticollis usually does not involve contraction of the sternomastoid on the same side of the neck. The torticollis has a particular cause, such as upper respiratory tract infections, cervical lymphadenitis, trauma minor neck injury, unilateral subluxation of the vertebrae, or fractures, as well as unusual causes such as spinal tumor or retropharyngeal abscess. Torticollis may also be seen in relation to ocular disturbance, such as strabismus, known as *ocular* torticollis.

History includes duration and onset of symptoms, whether sudden or gradual, associated symptoms (e.g., fever, sore throat), and history of injury. Clinical examination, in addition to the clinical appearance of torticollis, requires careful general examination of the head and neck, looking for a cause. Diagnosis may be apparent from the history and physical examination. Radiographs of the cervical spine may be obtained, if indicated, to rule out a vertebral cause.

Management includes referral for emergency evaluation and treatment of traumatic injury and retropharyngeal abscess. Pain is relieved and the underlying cause treated. Persistent pain requires further evaluation.

> ### KEY TREATMENT
>
> Treatment of congenital torticollis includes gentle stretching exercises; surgical treatment may be considered in special circumstances (Do, 2006) (SOR: C).

Whiplash

Whiplash is a hyperextension injury. The injury is caused by abnormal stretching of the muscles and soft tissue structures. There may be an associated disk herniation and tracheal and esophageal injury, resulting in hoarseness and dysphagia. Clinical features are pain in the lower neck and shoulders radiating to the occipital area, which may cause headaches. The neck pain may continue for weeks to months. The patient may have tenderness on palpation of the neck, perhaps some limitation in range of movement, and usually a normal neurologic examination. Radiographs are usually normal. Treatment is conservative with rest, a cervical collar, cold compresses, and pain relief, followed by simple range of motion (ROM) exercises. If symptoms improve, structured physical therapy may be considered.

Cervical Strains and Sprains

Cervical strains and sprains are characterized by pain in the neck because of irritation and spasm of muscles at the back of the neck. Common related factors are poor posture (e.g., while working or studying), carrying heavy bags on one shoulder, emotional or physical stress, and trauma. The patient has a history of pain in the lower neck and upper back; stiffness in the neck, back, and shoulders; and perhaps a new work environment, working in a certain posture (e.g., at computer), and trauma. Clinical findings include tenderness posterior to neck, with or without ROM limitation. Diagnosis may be apparent from the history and physical examination. Uncomplicated pain is managed by conservative treatment and correction of causative factors, such as changes in associated environmental factors (e.g., adjustment of height of desk or chair, avoiding straps on shoulders). Stress reduction is beneficial to aid reduction of muscle tension. Warmth applied to the neck is helpful, as are ROM exercises, pain relief, and referral to physical therapy. Persistent symptoms, history of trauma, or neurologic signs in the extremities require further evaluation with radiography.

Cervical Radiculopathy

Radiculopathy occurs when nerve root compression at the neck or spine results in pain, tingling, and numbness, with or without loss of function in the area supplied by the affected nerve. Common causes of cervical radiculopathy are neural foramen narrowing, usually caused by cervical arthritis in older adults, and cervical disk lesion caused by disk degeneration or herniation. *Disk degeneration* results in loss of disk space, with closer approximation of the vertebrae on either side of the involved disk space and subsequent impingement on the neural foramen (Fig. 31-7). The decrease in size of the neural foramen results in nerve root compression. The C5-C6 and C6-C7 disk spaces are more often affected. *Disk herniation* also occurs more often in these disks (Fig. 31-8). Some of the gelatinous pulp protrudes through the annulus fibrosus at the weakest point, usually where the posterolateral longitudinal ligament crosses the disk. In a smaller disk herniation, mild local pain may be caused by pressure on

the posterior ligament. A larger disk herniation may impinge on the nerve and may be posterolateral or central herniation with resultant radicular symptoms.

The patient has a history of pain radiating to the shoulder or down the upper extremity, which may be aggravated by coughing, sneezing, or straining; paresthesias of the fingers; and less often, weakness in the extremity. There may be a history of prior trauma. Cervical radiculopathy on examination may reveal tenderness on the neck, limitation in certain movements of the neck, focal neurologic findings such as sensory loss in the dermatome pattern corresponding to the distribution of the affected nerve root, and asymmetric tendon reflexes in the upper extremities (Fig. 31-9).

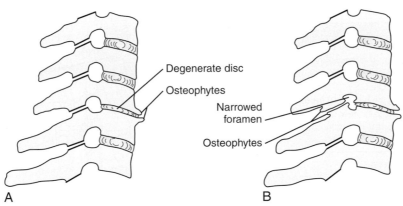

Figure 31-7 Osteoarthritis of cervical spine. **A,** Initial degeneration and narrowing of intervertebral disk, with formation of osteophytes anteriorly. **B,** Later, posterior or facet joints are affected; articular cartilage is worn away, and marginal osteophytes may encroach on the intervertebral foramen. *(Redrawn from Adam JC, Hamblen DL. Outline of Orthopedics, 13th ed. New York, Churchill Livingstone, 2001, p 159; and Anderson BC. Office Orthopedics for Primary Care: Diagnosis and Treatment, 2nd ed. Philadelphia, Saunders, 1999, p 266.)*

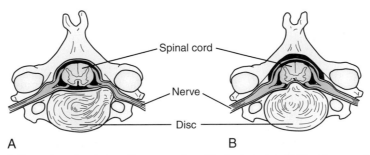

Figure 31-8 Prolapsed cervical disk**. A,** Posterolateral prolapse, with compression of the issuing nerve. **B,** Much less common central prolapse, with impingement on the spinal cord. *(Redrawn from Adam JC, Hamblen DL. Outline of Orthopedics, 13th ed. New York, Churchill Livingstone, 2001, p 163.)*

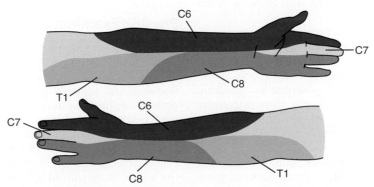

Figure 31-9 Volar and dorsal dermatome patterns of the forearm and hand. Pain and paresthesias may radiate into these areas when the affected nerve root is compressed. Note that extremity symptoms as a result of disk disease are almost always unilateral. *(Redrawn from Mercier R. Practical Orthopedics, 5th ed. St Louis, Mosby, 2000, p 29.)*

General examination should include the lower extremities and gait. Axial compression testing may reproduce the pain.

Diagnostic tests include radiographs of the cervical spine, which may appear normal or may show loss of normal cervical lordosis, narrowing of the disk space, and bone spurs with foramen encroachment. If the patient has neurologic symptoms, MRI identifies soft tissue structures and may show displacement of the disk. CT may also be performed.

Treatment relieves pressure on the affected nerve and is mainly conservative, including rest, pain relief, stress reduction, and short-term muscle relaxants. Patients with persistent symptoms may need structured physical therapy and referral for specialist evaluation. Neurologic signs and symptoms and loss of strength are also indications for referral to neurosurgery. A few patients require surgical intervention.

KEY TREATMENT

Whiplash is usually managed conservatively (Binder, 2007) (SOR: C).
Uncomplicated pain in cervical strains and sprains is managed conservatively (Binder, 2007) (SOR: C).
Range of motion exercises may be beneficial for uncomplicated cervical strain or sprain (Cochrane Review, 2005) (SOR: A).
Treatment of cervical radiculopathy is usually conservative (Binder, 2007) (SOR: C).

Thoracolumbar Spine

The thoracolumbar spine is the cause of frequent patient visits to a family physician. Back pain is the most common and expensive diagnosis of patients age 30 to 60 years. It is responsible for lost time at work, lost wages, increased surgeries, litigation expenses, and economic and psychosocial burden. Appropriate and timely diagnosis and treatment can prevent most of the sequelae of back pain.

Anatomy

The back is supported by 12 thoracic vertebrae (T1-T12) and five lumbar vertebrae (L1-L5). The lumbar vertebrae are larger and thicker than the cervical and thoracic vertebrae because they carry the most amount of body weight and are subject to the largest forces and stresses along the spine (see Fig. 31-5). The alignment of thoracolumbar vertebrae with their disk and ligament is similar to the cervical spine. The joints between the vertebrae, ligaments, and muscles of the back stabilize the vertebral column.

The major longitudinal ligaments connecting the vertebrae are the anterior and posterior ligaments (connect vertebral bodies), ligamentum flavum (between adjacent laminae), and supraspinous and interspinous ligaments (connect spinous processes). The anterior and posterior longitudinal ligaments and supraspinous ligament run along the entire length of the vertebral column and support the spine. The interspinous ligament and ligamentum flavum provide additional posterior stability to the spine (Fig. 31-10).

Intervertebral disks make up about one third of the length of the spine. The normal movements of thoracolumbar spine are forward flexion (by asking the patient to touch toes), extension, lateral bending, and symmetric rotation (Fig. 31-11

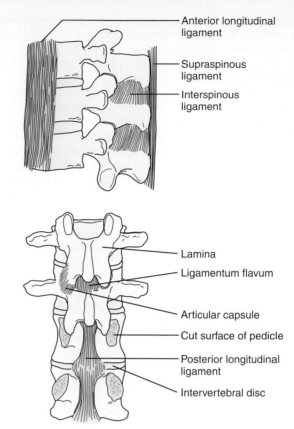

Figure 31-10 Supporting ligaments of the spine. *(Redrawn from Brinker MR, Miller MD. Fundamentals of Orthopedics. Philadelphia, Saunders, 1999, p 242.)*

and Table 31-2). Flexion and extension are limited in the thoracic region because of the rib cage.

History

The patient history of conditions in the thoracolumbar spine is similar to the cervical spine. A complete description of the onset, duration, nature, severity of symptoms, and aggravating and relieving factors should be obtained. Other important history includes medical history (including previous injuries) and psychosocial stressors at work or home. Symptoms may require urgent referral and workup and include unremitting back pain, urinary or bowel paralysis, weakness, fever, and weight loss.

Physical Examination

The physical examination should begin with observing the patient in the sitting and standing positions from the back as well as the front. Observing the patient moving around, dressing, and undressing may also help in confirming the severity of the symptoms. Muscle spasms, swellings, deformities, unusual markings, redness, and hair patches should be noted. The patient's posture and gait should be observed. The area palpated includes soft tissues and bone structures for tenderness and swellings. It helps to isolate the level of the lesion. ROM should be observed. A thorough neurologic examination should be performed to assess for sensations, deep tendon reflexes, and muscle strength. Examining the

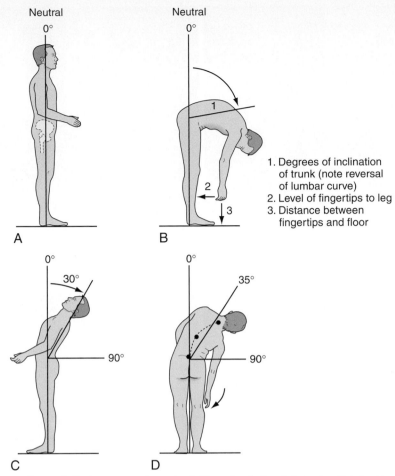

1. Degrees of inclination of trunk (note reversal of lumbar curve)
2. Level of fingertips to leg
3. Distance between fingertips and floor

Figure 31-11 Methods of measuring flexion. **A,** Flexion, zero starting point. **B,** Measuring flexion. **C,** Extension. **D,** Lateral bend. *(Redrawn from Carr AJ, Harnden A. Orthopedics in Primary Care. Boston, Butterworth-Heinemann, 1997, p 70.)*

Table 31-2 Normal Range of Movement: Thoracolumbar Spine

Motion	Range
Flexion	0-80 degrees
Extension	0-20 degrees
Lateral bend	0-35 degrees
Rotation	0-45 degrees

Modified from Carr AJ, Harnden A. Orthopedics in Primary Care. Newton, Mass, Butterworth-Heinemann, 1997.

rectal tone, perineal sensations, and reflexes is essential if the patient has significant nerve root pain and weakness and chord compression is suspected.

Special tests are done for determining nerve root impingement. The straight-leg raise test is performed with the patient lying on the back on the examination table. Passive lifting of the leg with the knee extended produces pain radiating down the posterior or lateral aspect of the leg, distal to the knee and often into the foot. Dorsiflexion of the foot (Lasegue's test) will increase these symptoms (Fig. 31-12). The bowstring sign is performed after a straight-leg raising test by flexing the knee to reduce radicular pain. Compression is then applied to the popliteal fossa. Return of radicular pain is considered a positive sign (Fig. 31-13). Crossed straight-leg raise is done by performing a straight-leg raise of the unaffected extremity. If the symptoms are produced on the affected extremity, the test is positive for central disk herniation. Femoral nerve traction test aids in the diagnosis of disk herniation that affects the upper lumbar spine (L2, L3, and L4). The patient lies on the stomach on the examination table with the knee flexed to 90 degrees. The physician then extends the patient's hip by lifting it off the table (Fig. 31-14). The test is positive if it produces radicular pain.

The peripheral pulses are palpated, and any abnormalities in the vascular status of the extremities are noted.

Diagnostic Testing

Diagnostic testing for thoracolumbar conditions is similar to that for the cervical spine. Plain radiographs (AP, lateral, and oblique views) can be obtained (Fig. 31-15). CT, MRI, or myelography may be indicated in patients with worsening neurologic deficits or a suspected systemic cause of back pain, such as infection or neoplasm. These imaging studies are also useful when referral for surgery is considered.

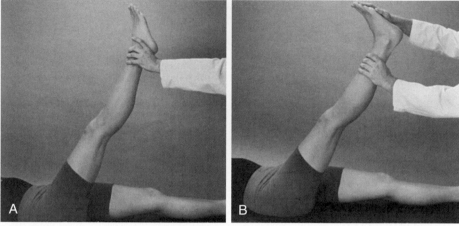

Figure 31-12 **A,** Straight-leg raising test. **B,** Lasegue's test. *(From Reider B. The Orthopedic Physical Examination. Philadelphia, Saunders, 1999, pp 364, 365.)*

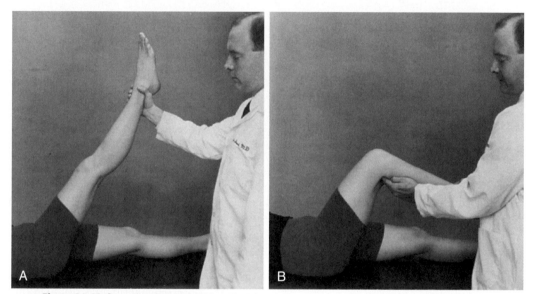

Figure 31-13 Bowstring sign. *(From Reider B. The Orthopedic Physical Examination. Philadelphia, Saunders, 1999, p 365.)*

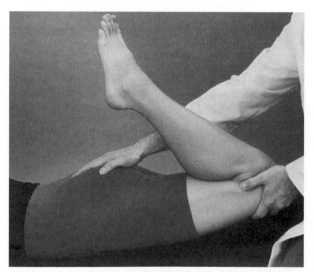

Figure 31-14 Femoral nerve stretch test. *(From Reider B. The Orthopedic Physical Examination. Philadelphia, Saunders, 1999, p 367.)*

Low Back Pain

Key Points

- A careful history and physical examination are essential in diagnosing any case of low back pain.
- Unremitting back pain and loss of bowel control require emergency assessment.
- Radiographs and laboratory tests are generally unnecessary with low back pain.
- With acute low back pain The therapeutic goal is to make the patient ambulatory and return to premorbid status.
- Recurrence of back pain and functional limitation can be prevented with appropriate conservative management, early mobilization, exercise, return to normal activity, and patient education.
- Exercise and physical therapy are the most effective treatment for chronic back pain.

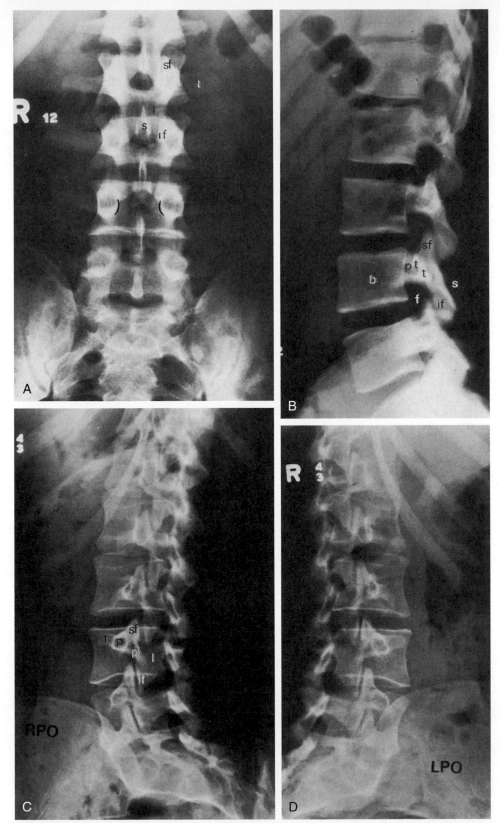

Figure 31-15 Plain radiographs of the lumbar spine. **A,** Anteroposterior view. **B,** Lateral view. **C** and **D,** Right posterior oblique (RPO) and left posterior oblique (LPO) views. *b,* Body of vertebra; *f,* intervertebral (neural) foramen; *if,* inferior facet; *l,* lamina; *p,* pedicle; *pi,* pars interarticularis; *s,* spinous process; *sf,* superior facet; *t,* transverse process (denotes interpedicular distance). *(From Brinker MR, Miller MD. Fundamentals of Orthopedics. Philadelphia, Saunders, 1999, p 249.)*

- With chronic low back pain, the therapeutic goal is to provide a long-term increase in function or a decrease in pain and disability.
- Psychological support and therapy may provide relief in chronic low back pain.

Low back pain is the most common cause of both acute and chronic pain. In the United States, approximately 90% of adults experience back pain at some time in their life, and 50% of working persons have back pain annually. As many as 90% of patients with acute back pain return to work within 3 months, but 10% experience symptom recurrence and functional limitations and eventually develop chronic pain. Low back pain is one of the leading causes of both disability and absenteeism from work. Less than half of patients out of work for more than 6 months secondary to low back pain will ever work again, creating an enormous financial strain on the patient, family, and community.

In primary care practice the specific anatomic cause of low back pain is usually not known; only a small percentage of patients have an identifiable underlying etiology. Less than 2% of patients have disk herniation, and only rarely do patients have a life-threatening condition. The most common cause of back pain is the lumbosacral strain following a single action or multiple lifting or twisting maneuvers. Factors that predispose to low back strain include repetitive use of poorly toned muscles, obesity, smoking, poor work habits, high-heeled shoes, and lack of physical activity. Most patients with acute low back pain improve in 2 to 4 weeks. Patients who progress to chronic back pain spend much time and money to become "pain free."

Assessment and Clinical Features

Most causes of low back pain are benign, but a thorough history and physical examination can identify a small percentage of patients with serious infection, malignancy, rheumatologic disease, or neurologic disorder. These serious conditions need immediate further evaluation. The review of systems includes constitutional symptoms, night pain, bone pain, morning stiffness, visceral pain, and claudication. The history includes exact location of the pain and the day, time, and activity involved in the initial back pain.

The patient's occupational risk assessment includes heavy lifting, prolonged sitting or standing, bending or twisting, and work with heavy, vibrating equipment. Patients often point to a well-localized area of the lower part of the back. Patients may have paraspinal muscle spasm and tenderness. Any movement may be painful, and the patient may walk in a slightly flexed position. Muscle spasm may be severe enough to cause loss of normal lumbar lordotic curve. If the strain is unilateral, the back may tilt to the affected side secondary to muscle spasm. The patient has reduced ROM, especially flexion and lateral bending secondary to pain. Neurologic examination should reveal no signs of radiculopathy in a normal back exam.

At subsequent visits, further assessment and evaluation are based on the history of persistence, recurrence of pain, and functional limitations. Functional overlay and signs of excessive pain behavior should be sought. Complaints without objective findings suggest a psychological role in symptom formation; psychological testing and behavior intervention may be needed. During further encounters, psychosocial obstacles to recovery should be explored. Patients whose work provides lower job satisfaction are more likely to report back pain and have a delayed recovery. Patients with affective mood disorders (e.g., depression) or substance abuse problems are more likely to have chronic pain and difficulty with pain resolution.

Diagnostic Testing

Radiographic imaging in uncomplicated cases of lumbosacral strain is rarely necessary and usually does not correlate with the patient's pain. Most people older than 40 years have anatomic defects on plain films of the spine. If the low back pain is probably more than a lumbosacral strain or has persisted for more than 6 weeks, radiographs may be helpful. CT or MRI should be reserved for low back pain accompanied by moderate to severe radicular symptoms, in the presence of motor weakness and neurologic deficits.

Treatment

Once it is determined that the patient has an uncomplicated lumbosacral strain, the goal of therapy for acute low back pain is to make the patient ambulatory and return to premorbid status. This goal should be explained to the patient, whose active participation is critical. Successful treatment depends on the patient's understanding of the disorder and the prevention of repeat injury. Patients should remain active to assist recovery, compared with short-term bed rest.

Family physicians should begin with conservative therapy. Most patients with acute low back pain improve with conservative management within 2 to 4 weeks. Early mobilization and return to normal activities should be encouraged. Nonsteroidal anti-inflammatory drugs (NSAIDs) and acetaminophen are mainstays of pharmacologic therapy for acute low back pain. Muscle relaxants are effective for short-term relief. Short-term use of a narcotic could be considered for relief of severe, acute pain. As the pain permits, gentle stretching exercises should be initiated (Fig. 31-16). Patients should taper use of the analgesics while gradually increasing their normal activities. Extremes of twisting, bending and tilting should be avoided. If these are work-related activities, the patient may require a change to "light duty." Teach techniques to lift heavy objects and educate patients about maintaining proper posture (Fig. 31-17).

Most patients recover and require no additional evaluation. Prevention of repeated back injuries is then the focus. The patient should be instructed on overall body conditioning. Exercises that do not stress lower back muscles include swimming, water aerobics, and low-impact walking. Rehabilitation exercises and aerobic conditioning for trunk extensors, abdominal muscles, and back strengthening (modified sit-ups, weighted side bends, gentle extensions) should become part of the patient's daily routine (Fig. 31-18).

The patient with chronic low back pain remains a challenge. The ultimate goal in chronic pain management is long-term increase in function or decrease in pain and disability. Typically these patients already had multiple therapies for acute back pain. Assessment of social and psychological factors may help identify a pain etiology that affects treatment.

Exercise is more effective for chronic low back pain than treatment with medication plus return to usual activity. Exercise is as effective as conventional physiotherapy. Exercise and physical modalities are the mainstays of therapy. Heat, cold, massage, ultrasound, and muscle stimulation

Back-stretching exercises play a vital role in the treatment of lumbosacral muscle spasms. The lower back is heated for 15 to 20 minutes. Sets of 10 to 20 stretches, each held for 5 seconds, are performed on each side. The muscles are kept relaxed. Rest for 1 to 2 minutes between exercises. Mild muscle soreness is to be expected. Severe pain, electric-like sharp pain, or severe muscle spasms suggest overstretching.

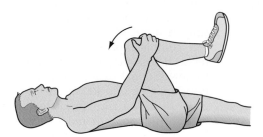

Knee-chest pulls
Bring your knee slowly up to your chest, holding it in place with your hands. Relax the buttock and back muscles. Do the left side, then the right side, and then both simultaneously (curling up in the fetal position).

Pelvic rocks
With knees bent, rotate your pelvis forward and then backwards. The abdominal muscles do the work, as the back muscles are relaxed.
Caution: Do not overextend when arching the back!

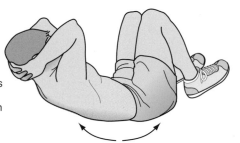

Side bending
While lying down, crawl your fingers down the side of your thigh. Hold in this tilted position for 5 seconds. Return to a neutral position. Repeat on the other side.

Initially, these exercises should be performed while lying down or floating in the bath or hot tub. With improvement, these exercises can be performed standing or sitting. Follow these movements with exercises to strengthen the back.

Figure 31-16 Back-stretching exercises. *(Redrawn from Anderson BC. Office Orthopedics for Primary Care: Diagnosis and Treatment, 2nd ed. Philadelphia, Saunders, 1999, p 266.)*

are effective modalities. NSAIDs or acetaminophen can be reinitiated. The need for prolonged narcotic therapy should prompt reevaluation of a patient's back pain. Reassurance and psychological support are also important. Often, depression accompanies the pain; addressing psychological issues may provide some relief. Patients often require referral to a specialized pain clinic or multidisciplinary back program. These clinics offer education, physical therapy, pharmacologic treatment, epidural steroid injections, chiropractic therapy, and psychological services.

Family physicians should emphasize the prevention of reinjury, review healthy lifestyle changes, and address weight loss, if indicated, as well as continue primary care for the patient.

KEY TREATMENT

Acetaminophen and NSAIDs are effective for pain relief in patients with acute low back pain; muscle relaxants are effective for short-term relief (Harwood and Chang, 2002) (SOR: A).
Remaining active speeds recovery from low back pain compared with short-term bed rest (Harwood and Chang, 2002) (SOR: A).
For chronic low back pain, exercise is more effective than treatment with medication plus return to usual activity. Exercise is as effective as conventional physiotherapy (Carter and Lord, 2002) (SOR: A).

Lumbar Disk Syndromes

Key Points

- Degeneration of the intervertebral disk can result in herniation, particularly at the L4-L5 and L5-S1 levels.
- The presence of pain, radiculopathy, and other symptoms depends on the site and degree of herniation.
- Initial screening for pathology and monitoring for complications (progressive neurologic defects, cauda equina syndrome, refractory pain) are essential in managing lumbar disk herniation.
- Most patients with herniated disk recover in 4 weeks.

The pattern of lumbar disk herniation is similar to that observed in the cervical spine. The most common levels for a herniated disk are L4-L5 and L5-S1. With aging and repetitive trauma, the disk undergoes significant changes in volume, shape, biochemical composition, and biomechanical properties. Lumbar disk herniations are believed to result from annular degeneration that leads to a weakening of the annulus fibrosus, leaving the disk susceptible to annular fissuring and tearing and subsequently allowing degenerated disk contents to herniate and impinge on adjacent structures (Fig. 31-19). Herniation usually occurs at the weakest area,

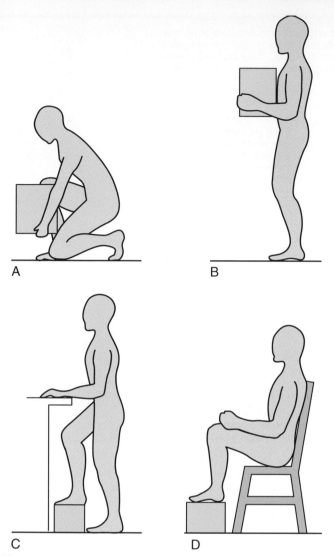

Figure 31-17 General postural instructions. **A,** Bend the knees and hips and keep the back straight when lifting. **B,** Hold objects close to the body when carrying. **C,** Place one foot on a stool when standing. **D,** Keep the knees higher than the hips when sitting, and keep the back straight when standing by tucking in the abdomen and tightening the buttocks to decrease sway-back. In addition, patients should avoid high-heeled shoes and sleeping on the abdomen, activities that increase lordosis. *(Redrawn from Mercier L. Practical Orthopedics, 5th ed. St Louis, Mosby, 2000, p 125.)*

the posterolateral aspect of the disk (Fig. 31-20). Disk herniation is most common in the third and fourth decades of life.

Clinical Features

The onset of symptoms is usually gradual; the most common complaint is low back pain. When the disk herniates, it impinges on adjacent structures, causing sharp, burning, stabbing pain radiating down the posterior or lateral aspect of the leg, to below the knee, and finally to the foot. Pain is generally superficial and localized, often associated with numbness or tingling along the dermatome. In more advanced cases, motor deficit, diminished reflexes, or weakness may occur. An occasional massive central herniated disk compresses the cauda equina, resulting in bilateral symptoms, weakness, numbness, difficult urination, incontinence,

or impotence, causing the cauda equine syndrome. Often the difficult aspect of evaluating patients with symptoms of a herniated disk is differentiation from low back strain. Pain caused by low back strain is exacerbated with standing or twisting motions, whereas pain caused by disk herniation, especially central, worsens with sitting or bending, Valsalva maneuver, coughing, or sneezing because of increased pressure on annular fibers.

A complete physical and neurologic examination can reveal defects at specific levels. The physician first assesses for any external manifestations of pain by inspecting body position, gait, and ROM. The patient may be bending laterally or listing away from the affected side, or may stand with the affected hip and knee slightly flexed to relieve the pain or nerve compression. Local guarding and muscle tenderness on palpation of the area may be present. Sensory examination may reveal deficits along the specific nerve root distribution (Fig. 31-21). Motor weakness should be tested to localize the nerve root. Nerve tension tests (straight-leg raising, crossed straight-leg raising, Lasegue's test, bowstring sign) are often positive.

Diagnostic Testing

The major finding on plain radiographs of patients with a herniated disk is decreased disk height. Radiographs have limited diagnostic value for herniated disk because degenerative changes are age related and equally present in asymptomatic and symptomatic persons. Therefore, patients with characteristic herniated disk or chronic disk degeneration usually do not require advanced imaging; it should be performed if suspicion is high for cauda equine syndrome, tumor, infection, progressive neurologic symptoms, trauma, or symptoms inconsistent with monoradiculopathy. CT and MRI should also be reserved for patients who fail conservative management and are being considered for surgery. With herniated disk, waiting 4 to 6 weeks is considered advantageous because herniations tend to reduce and most symptoms resolve. Both CT and MRI can identify disk herniations, but CT with myelography has increased sensitivity and specificity. CT also is less expensive and less sensitive to patient movement. However, MRI better visualizes the spinal chord (Fig. 31-22).

Treatment

Although low back pain and radiculopathy are common causes of disability, most patients experience resolution of their symptoms. Family physician is responsible to determine the goals and optimal management for each patient. The condition should be thoroughly explained to the patient, including the likely natural history and the potential forms of treatment.

First-line treatment of a patient with lumbar disk syndrome or herniation is conservative, with limited bed rest, adequate pharmacologic treatment, and exercise. Patients are advised to remain active to speed recovery; excessive bed rest can result in deconditioning, bone mineral loss, and economic losses. Pain should be treated with NSAIDs or narcotics, muscle relaxants, and moist heat; most patients begin to improve with this regimen. The patient should resume early ambulation and begin gentle stretching exercises (see Fig. 31-16).

Before starting a strengthening program for the back, flexibility must be restored with 3 to 6 weeks of daily back stretching. Strengthening exercises should be performed when the body is well-rested. First, the back muscles are stretched out for 5 to 10 minutes. Then sets of 15 to 20 of the following are performed daily for 6 weeks. As the strength of the back increases, the frequency can be reduced to three times a week.

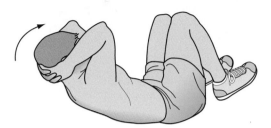

Modified sit-ups
The knees are kept bent. The lower back is kept flush with the ground. The hands can be kept either behind the neck or held over the chest. The head and neck are raised 3 to 4" and held for 5 seconds. The abdominal muscles will gradually strengthen.

Weighted side-bends
In a standing position, a 5- to 15-pound weight is held in the hand. The back is tilted to the weighted side and is immediately brought back to center. The back should be tilted only a few inches! The farther away from the body the weight is held, the greater is the amount of muscle work! After a set of 15 to 20, the weight is shifted to the opposite side.

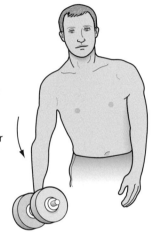

These specific exercises are complementary to a regular aerobic exercise program. No single exercise is better than another. If you are having problems doing any specific exercise, discuss it with your health care provider.

Figure 31-18 Back-strengthening exercises. *(Redrawn from Anderson BC. Office Orthopedics for Primary Care: Diagnosis and Treatment, 2nd ed. Philadelphia, Saunders, 1999, p 268.)*

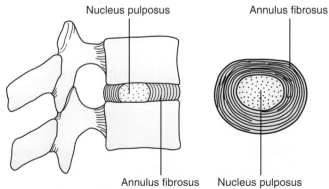

Nucleus pulposus   Annulus fibrosus

Annulus fibrosus   Nucleus pulposus

Figure 31-19 Normal intervertebral disk seen in sagittal section *(left)* and in horizontal section *(right)*. *(Redrawn from Adam JC, Hamblen DL. Outline of Orthopedics, 13th ed. New York, Churchill Livingstone, 2001, p 199.)*

treatment or have persistent symptoms are referred to specialists. Indications for referral include cauda equina syndrome, progressive and profound neurologic deficit, and disabling pain refractory to 4 to 6 weeks of conservative treatment. Any surgical decisions should be firmly based on the clinical symptoms, which are confirmed with results of diagnostic testing.

Percutaneous lumbar diskectomy, performed under local anesthesia, is a safe and effective noninvasive alternative to laminectomy. The percutaneous procedure is contraindicated in the presence of tumor, infection, foramina stenosis, loose disk fragments, spondylolisthesis, or severe facet joint arthritis. No long-term difference has been observed in the outcomes of patients treated conservatively versus surgically.

Caudal or epidural steroid injection is controversial. Patients who continue to improve should begin preventive therapy, including overall muscle toning such as swimming or water aerobics; specific toning of the muscles of the back should become part of the patient's daily routine. Lifestyle changes should be incorporated to reduce predisposing factors.

Most patients' disk problem may be effectively treated conservatively; those who do not respond to conservative

KEY TREATMENT

Conservative management is the initial approach in patients with low back pain with radicular symptoms, unless cauda equine syndrome is diagnosed (Snyder et al., 2004) (SOR: C).
Procedures for spinal decompression may be considered in patients who have failed conservative therapy (Cochrane Review, 2005) (SOR: C).

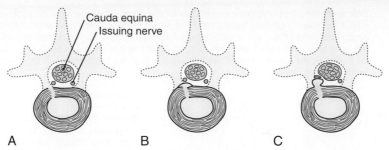

Figure 31-20 Stages in prolapse of an intervertebral disk. **A,** Annulus fibrosus is torn, but no extrusion of nucleus pulposus. **B,** Extrusion of nuclear material through the rent. Posterior longitudinal ligament is stretched, but protrusion has not reached the nerve. **C,** The protraction is larger, and the nerve is stretched over it. Sometimes, a fragment of the torn annulus itself protrudes backward. *(Redrawn from Adam JC, Hamblen DL. Outline of Orthopedics, 13th ed. New York, Churchill Livingstone, 2001, p 199.)*

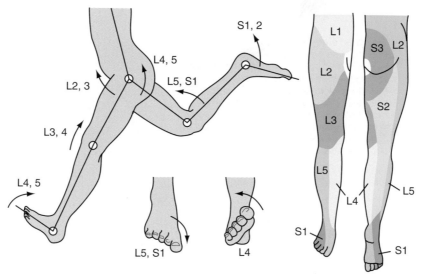

Figure 31-21 Root (segmental) distribution. Note that motion in each joint is controlled by four nerve roots running in sequence. Hip—flexion L2, L3, extension, L4, L5; knee—extension (and knee jerk) L3, L4, flexion L5, S1; ankle—dorsiflexion L4, L5, plantar flexion (and ankle jerk) S1, S2. (Inversion involves L4, and eversion L5, S1.) A useful mnemonic for the low limb dermatomes is that "we kneel on L3, stand on S1, and sit on S3." *(Redrawn from McRae R, Kinninman AWG. Orthopedics and Trauma. New York, Churchill Livingstone, 1997, p 26).*

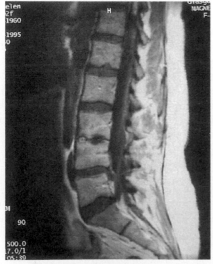

Figure 31-22 MR scan showing inflammatory changes in the L3-L4 disk (diskitis) and an L4-L5 prolapse. *(From McRae R, Kinninman AWG. Orthopedics and Trauma. New York, Churchill Livingstone, 1997, p 52.)*

Thoracolumbar Vertebral Compression Fractures

Key Points

- Vertebral compression fractures are common, especially in the elderly. Causing significant disability, deconditioning, and pain.
- The most common site for fractures is thoracolumbar junction (T12-L1).
- Family physicians can prevent compression fractures and sequelae by identifying high-risk patients, educating patients, and encouraging lifestyle modification.

Vertebral compression fractures are common, especially in elderly persons. Vertebral fractures can cause significant pain and impairment in activities of daily living, leading to potentially life-threatening disability and deconditioning in the elderly patient. Patients with preexisting vertebral fractures have greater risk of future vertebral as well as nonvertebral (especially hip) fractures than those without prior fractures.

The most common site for fractures is the thoracolumbar junction (T12-L1) because the change in facet provides poor resistance to anteroposterior displacement. The other common location is the midthoracic region (T7-T8). Osteoporosis is the most frequent cause of vertebral compression fractures in the elderly population. Other causes should be suspected if fracture occurs in a person neither elderly nor postmenopausal or if solitary fracture higher than T7 is seen, ruling out osteomalacia, hyperparathyroidism, granulomatous disease, and hematologic disease.

Clinical Features

Most thoracolumbar compression fractures are asymptomatic, diagnosed as incidental findings on chest or abdominal plain radiographs. Patients with symptomatic fractures usually have no preceding history of trauma, and even minimal trauma (coughing, sneezing) can cause the fracture. The pain from a vertebral compression fracture is variable in quality and sharp or dull. Movements aggravate the pain. The classic patient presents with acute back pain radiating to the anterior abdomen, unlike radiation into the legs seen in herniated disk. Physical examination may reveal tenderness directly over the area of fracture. Thoracic kyphosis and lumbar lordosis may be noted secondary to vertebral height lost. Straight-leg raise and neurologic exam are normal in uncomplicated fractures. Acute episodes usually resolve after 4 to 6 weeks; if pain lasts longer, the physician should suspect more fractures, with chronic pain or other diagnosis.

Diagnostic Testing

A complete blood count, erythrocyte sedimentation rate, and alkaline phosphatase, serum calcium, phosphorus, vitamin D, and parathormone levels should be obtained to rule out malignancy, hyperparathyroidism, or infection, if a cause other than osteoporosis is suspected. Plain radiographs are obtained if compression fracture is suspected. Radiographic characteristics of compression fractures include anterior wedging of one or more vertebrae, with vertebral collapse, demineralization, and vertebral end-plate irregularity. Advanced imaging is not routinely necessary unless the patient has a neurologic abnormality, which may indicate fracture fragments in the spinal canal. Imaging also helps rule out other causes of back pain.

Treatment

Initial management involves pain control and resumption of exercise as early as possible. When osteoporosis is present, inactivity could lead to further bone loss and subsequent fractures. Nonnarcotic analgesics should be used for pain relief. If narcotics are required, laxatives should be used because straining with defecation can cause further fractures. Nasal calcitonin may be a useful adjunct to these analgesics for acute pain relief. Treating the underlying disease is important. Muscle relaxants, external back braces, and physical therapy also may help. Immediate surgical referral should be made if fracture fragments are impinging on the chord and causing neurologic symptoms, or if the fracture is unstable.

Most patients respond to conservative treatment, with significant improvements or full recovery after 6 to 12 weeks. Patients who do not respond to conservative treatment may be candidates for percutaneous vertebroplasty or kyphoplasty.

The family physician can help patients prevent compression fractures and the sequelae by identifying high-risk patients, educating patients about measures to prevent falls, and encouraging lifestyle modifications. A regular weight-bearing exercise program, adequate calcium and vitamin D supplement intake, smoking cessation, and medications to treat osteoporosis may help prevent additional compression fractures.

KEY TREATMENT

Conservative management (pain management, back braces, physical therapy) is the first line of therapy for stable compression fractures (Old and Calvert, 2004) (SOR: B).

Patients nonresponsive to conservative treatment may be candidates for percutaneous vertebroplasty or kyphoplasty (Predley et al., 2002) (SOR: B).

Diagnosing and treating osteoporosis reduces the incidence of compression fractures of the spine (Old and Calvert, 2004) (SOR: A).

Regular activity and muscle-strengthening exercises have been shown to decrease vertebral fractures and back pain (Sinaki et al., 2002) (SOR: B).

Spinal Stenosis

Spinal stenosis is the narrowing of the spinal canal and neural foramina. Spinal stenosis has been classified into congenital and acquired types. The more common acquired spinal stenosis is caused by degenerative changes in the intervertebral disks, ligaments, and facet joints surrounding the lumbar canal. These degenerative changes can be caused by disk or joint disease, back surgery, and repetitive trauma. Stenosis initially becomes symptomatic at 40 to 50 years and older. Congenital narrowing of the spinal canal causes symptoms earlier in life and is uncommon.

Spinal stenosis usually occurs at cervical and lumbar segments. Patients with cervical stenosis present with radiating arm pain, numbness, paresthesia, and motor weakness. The common symptoms with lumbar stenosis are insidious low back pain, leg pain, and numbness. The pain is most often bilateral, involving the buttocks and thighs and spreading distally toward the feet. The classic presentation is radiating leg pain (burning or cramping) that begins or worsens with walking and standing and is relieved by sitting or lying down with hips and knees drawn up in a sitting posture (*neurogenic claudication*). Bending forward diminishes pain. The signs and symptoms of neurogenic claudication should be differentiated from the leg claudication produced by vascular claudication. Vascular disease pain is exercise induced, is localized to the affected group of muscles, and is relieved rapidly with rest in any position. Neurologic symptoms are absent, and vascular disease is associated with skin and trophic changes (pallor, cyanosis, nail dystrophy, decreased or absent pulse).

Severity of symptoms in spinal stenosis may not necessarily be associated with the degree of compression seen on imaging studies. Rarely, patients with spinal stenosis present with

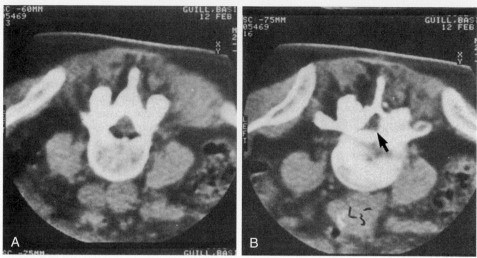

Figure 31-23 Normal **(A)** and abnormal **(B)** CT scans of the lumbar spine. Marked narrowing *(arrow)* is present in **B** because of hypertrophic spurring. *(From Mercier R. Practical Orthopedics, 5th ed. St Louis, Mosby, 2000, p 129.)*

signs or symptoms of muscle atrophy and loss of bowel and bladder control. Physical examination is frequently normal but may include loss of lumbar lordosis, impairment of spinal mobility, asymmetric knee or ankle reflexes, and muscle weakness. Results of straight-leg raising are characteristically negative.

Advanced imaging studies are obtained to establish and confirm the diagnosis of spinal stenosis when surgery is considered. Plain spine radiographs often reveal degenerative changes. MRI is currently the preferred modality, followed by CT scan (Fig. 31-23).

Conservative treatment is the first line of therapy for spinal stenosis, including adequate pain management, physical therapy, exercise, and weight loss. Progressive symptoms or intractable pain warrant surgical intervention. Wide decompression at the level of stenosis can relieve the symptoms.

KEY TREATMENT

Patients with mild to moderate symptoms of spinal stenosis are managed conservatively (pain/physical therapy, exercise, weight loss) (Snyder et al., 2004) (SOR: C).

Patients with severe symptoms of spinal stenosis benefit from surgery (Amundsen et al., 2000) (SOR: B).

Scoliosis

Scoliosis is characterized by the lateral deviation of the spine from its normal position and is associated with rotation of the vertebrae. Scoliosis may be caused by a structural spine deformity or another problem (e.g., unilateral leg shortening) or may be a protective reaction of muscle spasm in the back for lumbar disk disease or inflammation. Of the structural causes, *idiopathic* scoliosis is most common, affects women more frequently, and is often asymptomatic in young people. Other causes include neurologic deficit,

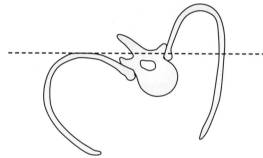

Figure 31-24 Scoliosis with rib prominence resulting from vertebral rotation is best exhibited on forward bending (Adams position). Cross section of the chest shows rib distortion resulting from vertebral rotation. *(Redrawn from Mercier R. Practical Orthopedics, 5th ed. St Louis, Mosby, 2000, p 132.)*

myopathy, and neurofibromatosis; presence of pain may signify another cause.

The patient with scoliosis may present with apparent deformity, pain, symptoms of difficult movement, or neurologic deficits. The examiner stands behind and observes the patient bending forward at the waist with arms loosely directed toward the feet, which may reveal a prominence of the ribs on one side of the back of the chest and abnormal curvature of the spine (Fig. 31-24). Worsening scoliosis may result in pain, progressive deformity, disability, and cardiopulmonary compromise.

Radiographs aid in the diagnosis and also allow measurement of the angle of curvature of the spine (Fig. 31-25). MRI may be indicated if there are additional symptoms, such as pain or neurologic problems. Early detection is important, and prompt referral to specialists is indicated in certain cases. Spinal growth continues until bone growth has been completed, and serial radiographs are useful to monitor the condition.

Treatment of scoliosis is primarily based on severity and angle of curvature. Braces may be recommended and in special cases, surgery (Janicki and Alman, 2007; SOR C, 3).

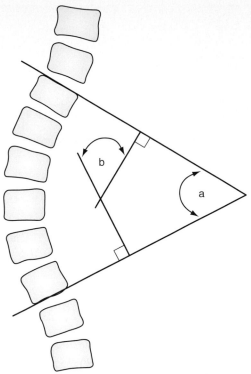

Figure 31-25 Cobb method of measuring the severity of a curve. Upper and lower end vertebrae are identified. Upper end vertebra is higher, its superior border converging toward the concavity of the curve, and lower end vertebra has inferior border converging toward the concavity. Lines are drawn along these borders, and the curve is measured directly *(a)* or geometrically *(b)*. *(Redrawn from Mercier R. Practical Orthopedics, 5th ed. St Louis, Mosby, 2000, p 132.)*

References

The complete reference list is available online at www.expertconsult.com.

Web Resources

www.ninds.nih.gov/disorders/backpain/backpain.html
   Information on back pain with links to other sites, including clinical trials in the U.S. and worldwide.
www.aaos.org/research/research.asp
   American Academy of Orthopedic Surgeons site that includes Clinical Practice Guidelines, Research News, and information about common musculoskeletal disorders.

www.nlm.nih.gov/medlineplus/neckinjuriesanddisorders.html
www.familydoctor.org
   Consumer health information on a variety of disorders, provided by the American Academy of Family Physicians.

Rheumatology and Musculoskeletal Problems

Douglas Comeau, Kevin Heaton, and Andrea Gordon

Chapter contents

Arthritis is the most common health complaint in the United States and a common reason for an office visit to the family physician, despite the numerous over-the-counter treatments for joint pain and other musculoskeletal problems. In a Center for Disease Control and Prevention (CDC) National Ambulatory Medical Care Survey, 49 million American adults reported physician-diagnosed arthritis, 21 million of whom reported chronic joint symptoms (Hootman and Helmick, 2006). The 30-year projection rate of patients age 65 and older will increase from 21.4 million to 41.4 million. These statistics lead to 75,000 hospitalizations and 36 million outpatient visits annually.

The term *arthritis* actually applies to more than 180 different disorders, all with pain in or around one or more joints, some with an inflammatory component. Although patients and physicians refer to this collection of diseases as arthritis or "rheumatism," the family physician must attempt to identify the disease process more precisely because of the many treatments available. Musculoskeletal symptoms might be harbingers of other, serious diseases affecting other organs. Patients should know their prognosis, whether their symptoms will most likely be self-limited, chronic, or progressive.

Rheumatic diseases greatly impact the U.S. health care system and society. Approximately 1% of the U.S. gross national product is spent each year on rheumatic diseases alone. Work absences, lost wages, and long-term disability also impact the quality of life of patient and family. Family physicians must be knowledgeable about new treatment options in the evaluation, assessment, and treatment of these conditions.

Evaluation of Joint and Other Musculoskeletal Symptoms

Precise anatomic localization of pain is the first task of the physician caring for a patient presenting with joint pain, while also evaluating stiffness, redness, warmth, or swelling in the absence of trauma. It is important to distinguish pain that is truly articular from *periarticular* pain. Causes of *localized* periarticular pain include bursitis, tendonitis, and carpal tunnel syndrome, whereas fibromyalgia, polymyalgia rheumatica, and polymyositis all can cause *diffuse* periarticular pain.

The number of involved joints and presence or absence of symmetry are criteria for further diagnosis of articular pain (Figs. 32-1 and 32-2). Monoarticular (one joint) or *oligoarticular* (several joints) arthritides can be caused by conditions such as *osteoarthritis* (OA), gout, pseudogout, or septic arthritis. Asymmetric polyarthritis occurs in ankylosing spondylitis, psoriatic arthritis, Reiter's disease, and spondyloarthropathies. *Symmetric* arthritis, meaning that the same joint is affected on the contralateral side but not necessarily to the same degree, is characteristic of *rheumatoid arthritis* (RA), *systemic lupus erythematosus* (SLE), Sjögren's syndrome, polymyositis, and scleroderma. Fibromyalgia, reflex sympathetic dystrophy, and predominantly psychological

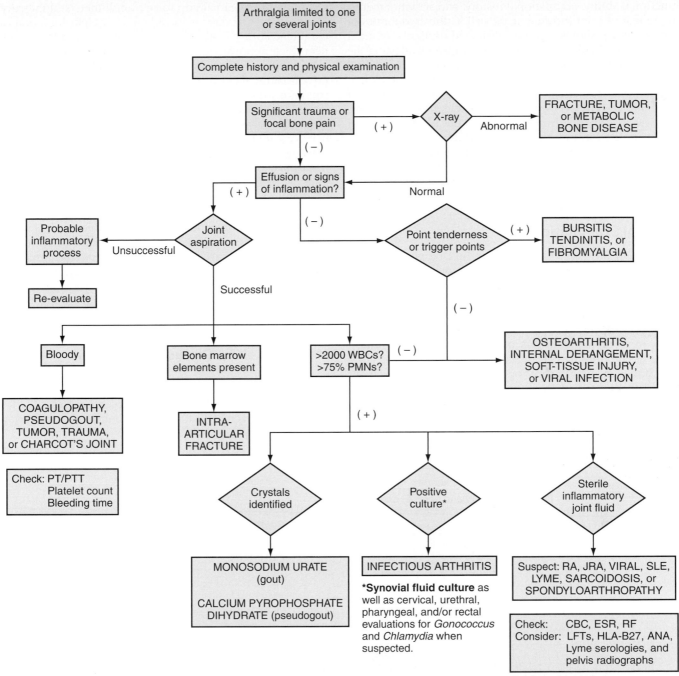

Figure 32-1 Evaluation of monoarticular or pauciarticular symptoms. *ANA,* Antinuclear antibodies; *CBC,* complete blood cell count; *ESR,* erythrocyte sedimentation rate; *JRA,* juvenile rheumatoid arthritis; *LFTs,* liver function tests; *PMNs,* polymorphonuclear (leukocyte) neutrophils; *PT,* prothrombin time; *PTT,* partial thromboplastin time; *RA,* rheumatoid arthritis; *RF,* rheumatoid factor; *SLE,* systemic lupus erythematosus; *WBCs,* white blood cells. *(From American College of Rheumatology Ad Hoc Committee on Clinical Guidelines. Guidelines for the initial evaluation of the adult patient with acute musculoskeletal symptoms. Arthritis Rheum 1996;39:1.)*

factors must be considered when pain is diffuse, not relatable to specific anatomic structures, or described in vague terms. (See also Chapter 30.)

Other differentiating criteria include the correlation with activity or rest and the character of the pain. Mechanical causes tend to be more directly related to the joint's activity than inflammatory conditions. Neuropathies tend to cause burning or prickling sensations, whereas arthritides often cause an aching pain. The presence of joint stiffness after a period of inactivity might also aid in diagnosis; RA is characterized by morning stiffness lasting 30 to 60 minutes or longer, whereas OA-related morning stiffness lasts a shorter period, typically less than 30 minutes, but stiffness might also occur during the day. In neurologic conditions such as Parkinson's disease, stiffness might be relatively constant. Vascular pain, such as intermittent claudication, is felt with activity, relieved quickly by rest, and described as a "deep, aching" sensation.

Constitutional symptoms such as fatigue, weakness, malaise, and weight changes are common chief complaints heard in a primary care office practice and often associated symptoms of specific rheumatic diseases. The patient's functional ability, occupational history, and activities requiring repetitive joint movement, as well as the ergonomics of such activities, should also be considered routinely in initial and serial evaluations. How are the symptoms affecting the patient's ability to perform self-care activities of daily living (ADLs) such as bathing, dressing, and eating? Is the patient able to do instrumental activities of daily living (IADLs) such as buying groceries, cooking, using the telephone, and opening jars? Rheumatic disease can have a devastating effect on quality of life for both the patient and the family, with serious psychosocial and economic consequences. Therefore the physician should address effects on occupational, recreational, and sexual activities in the context of family and other support systems.

Physical Examination

A thorough physical examination should be performed on all patients presenting with joint pain, including examination of asymptomatic joints and other organ systems that might be involved. Joints should be examined for swelling, tenderness, deformity, instability, and limitation of motion. Comparisons with the patient's contralateral side can be made in all these parameters, as well as with the physician's joints as a control. Instability can be tested by moving adjacent bones in the direction opposite to normal movement and observing for greater-than-normal motion. Serial grip strength measurements can be made by asking the patient to squeeze a blood pressure (BP) cuff inflated to 20 mm Hg and

recording the maximal grip force in millimeters of mercury. Signs of systemic disease include fever; weight loss; oral or nasal ulcerations; liver, spleen, or lymph node enlargement; neurologic abnormalities; rashes; subcutaneous nodules; eye iritis; conjunctivitis or scleritis; and pericardial or pulmonary rubs. Because of circadian changes in patients with RA, serial comparisons of the physical examination are more accurate if the time of day is also recorded. Using skeleton diagrams of joint involvement facilitates the recording of a comprehensive joint examination (Fig. 32-3).

Myalgias can be caused by localized trauma or overuse, systemic infection, metabolic disorder, or primary muscle disease. Multiple tender sites in an otherwise healthy patient suggest fibromyalgia. An elevated creatine kinase (CK) level with proximal weakness may be caused by an inflammatory myopathy.

Rheumatic and other musculoskeletal problems are properly diagnosed by careful history and physical examination rather than by just ordering many laboratory tests, the results of which might actually confuse diagnosis. Laboratory tests and radiologic imaging help confirm a presumptive clinical diagnosis made from a careful history and physical examination.

Pathogenesis of Rheumatic and Other Musculoskeletal Diseases

As with most disease, research into the causes of rheumatologic and musculoskeletal diseases shows that the cause for each disease is actually multifactorial. Further identification

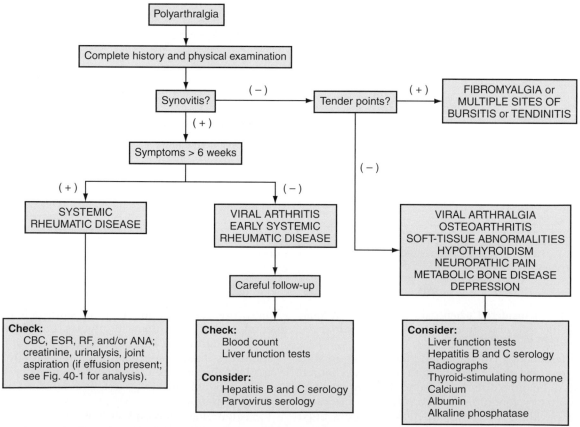

Figure 32-2 Evaluation of polyarticular symptoms. *ANA,* Antinuclear antibodies; *CBC,* complete blood cell count; *ESR,* erythrocyte sedimentation rate; *RF,* rheumatoid factor. (*From American College of Rheumatology Ad Hoc Committee on Clinical Guidelines: Guidelines for the initial evaluation of the adult patient with acute musculoskeletal symptoms. Arthritis Rheum 1996;39:1.*)

of these factors will help the family physician and rheumatologist modify the course of disease and eventually perhaps even prevent them.

Genetic factors have been identified for several arthritides. Presence of the human leukocyte antigen (HLA) system's HLA-DR4 antigen is associated with increased incidence and severity of RA. The HLA-B27 antigen is found in a higher percentage in patients with ankylosing spondylitis and other spondyloarthropathies than in the general population. Other factors are apparently involved, however, because its presence or absence neither guarantees nor excludes development of arthritis testing for these antigens if not routinely performed. A National Institutes of Health (NIH) study found that genetic factors contributed 39% to 65% of OA variance. About 80% of patients with chondrodysplasias were found to have a type II collagen gene mutation likely linking these findings to OA (Prockop, 1998).

Inborn errors of metabolism are well known to cause diseases such as gout, in which uric acid is overproduced or underexcreted by the kidneys. Poorly controlled metabolic diseases such as diabetes or hemochromatosis might lead to arthropathies. Mechanical or traumatic factors cause OA in soccer players but not in long-distance runners, indicating that the type and direction of joint stress might be more important than the stress itself. Adduction moment is associated with OA disease severity. Obesity is also an identified factor in OA of the knee, possibly because of metabolic influences as well as mechanical forces (Eaton, 2004).

Infectious agents such as parvovirus B19, human immunodeficiency virus (HIV), *Neisseria gonorrhoeae*, *Borrelia burgdorferi* (Lyme disease), and streptococci (rheumatic fever) are all well-known causes of arthritides. Some speculate that dietary factors might contribute to autoimmune syndromes, and fasting or a vegan diet (or both) can lead to improvement in RA (Kjeldsen-Kragh et al., 1991; McDougall et al., 2002). The imbalance of omega-6 and omega-3 fatty acids in the standard American diet (a ratio of 30:1, as opposed to the ratio of 1:2 that is thought to have been present in Paleolithic diets) is also postulated to contribute to a more inflammatory state. Omega-6 fatty acids are preferentially converted to more inflammatory prostaglandins such as arachidonic acid, whereas omega-3 fatty acids can be converted into eicosapentaenoic acid (EPA) and docosahexaenoic acid (DHA), which contribute to anti-inflammatory series-3 prostaglandin production (Fig. 32-4). Omega-3 fatty acids are useful in RA, showing a decrease in use of nonsteroidal anti-inflammatory drugs (NSAIDs) and decreased levels of pain (Oh, 2005).

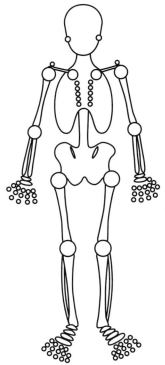

Figure 32-3 Skeleton diagram for recording joint examination findings. *(From Polley HF, Hunder GG. Rheumatologic Interviewing and Physical Examination of the Joints, 2nd ed. Philadelphia, Saunders, 1978.)*

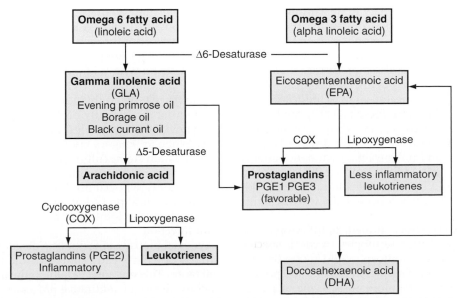

Figure 32-4 Influence of omega-6 fatty acids and omega-3 fatty acids on inflammation. *(From Rakel R. Integrative Medicine. Philadelphia, Saunders-Elsevier, 2007.)*

Other medical systems, such as traditional Chinese medicine (TCM), may have completely different explanations for the changes seen in rheumatologic conditions. Although a conventional practitioner may not be aware of these, it is helpful to know about complementary modalities that may be beneficial (e.g., acupuncture helping patients with OA and fibromyalgia).

Laboratory Studies

A complete cell count (CBC) with differential, urinalysis, and renal and liver function tests should be performed if asymptomatic rheumatic disease is suspected. Importantly, the frequency of abnormal laboratory results increases with increasing age in the normal population, even in the absence of disease, including common tests such as erythrocyte sedimentation rate (ESR), uric acid, antinuclear antibodies (ANAs), and rheumatoid factor (RF). Thus, arthritis panels can confuse the situation and should not be performed routinely. For example, only 80% of patients with RA have a positive RF. RF is a serum autoantibody against immunoglobulin G (IgG). Up to 4% of the healthy population has a positive RF, which is also frequently positive in patients with *chronic obstructive pulmonary disease* (COPD), viral hepatitis, and sarcoidosis, and can also be positive in malignancy, and primary biliary cirrhosis and other autoimmune diseases. The higher the RF titer, however, the more likely it is caused by RA. ANA test results are positive in 95% of patients with lupus, and the test is often used to screen for SLE, but the result is also positive in 5% of the normal population. Drug use, age, and other factors might also cause a positive ANA test result. ANA titer also does not correlate exactly with changes in disease activity, so it should not be ordered in the absence of systemic symptoms. A patient with a positive ANA without clinical features is unlikely to have SLE. However, higher titers of ANA make it more likely that the result is related to lupus or another rheumatologic disorder.

Laboratory studies can be helpful in monitoring disease activity and drug toxicity as well as in establishing a diagnosis. CBC can detect anemia secondary to the chronic disease of RA or from NSAID-induced gastrointestinal (GI) blood loss. Patients with SLE can have hemolytic anemia, thrombocytopenia, or lymphopenia. Urinalysis can detect renal disease secondary to SLE, NSAIDs, or disease-modifying antirheumatic drugs (DMARDs) being used to treat RA. An elevated uric acid level can suggest gout. Acute-phase reactants such as ESR and C-reactive protein (CRP) can be useful to monitor disease activity but are nonspecific; they can also be negative in the presence of active disease. Patients with temporal arteritis and polymyalgia rheumatica almost always have a greatly elevated ESR. With weakness or muscle pain, CK level should be measured and arthralgias with abnormal liver enzyme levels followed up with hepatitis viral serologies.

Other tests, such as HLA-B27, antineutrophil cytoplasmic antibody, Lyme or parvovirus serologies, myositis-specific antibodies (anti–Jo-1), and antiphospholipid antibodies, are useful only when the clinical suspicion is high for spondyloarthropathies, Wegener's granulomatosis, Lyme or parvovirus infection, inflammatory myositis, or antiphospholipid antibody syndrome, respectively (American College of Rheumatology, 1996).

Synovial Fluid Analysis

Synovial fluid analysis can be helpful in evaluating a febrile patient with an acute joint to rule out septic arthritis or acute monoarthritis. Synovial fluid should be analyzed for white blood cell (WBC) count differential, cultured, and tested with polarized light microscopy for crystals. Purulent synovial fluid with greater than 90% polymorphonuclear leukocytes (PMNs), low viscosity, and turbid clarity can be caused by infection or crystal arthropathy (gout or pseudogout). Urate crystals are needle-shaped and negatively birefringent; calcium pyrophosphate dihydrate crystals are rhomboidal and weakly positively birefringent. Noninflammatory fluids generally have a clear appearance, normal viscosity, fewer than 2000 WBCs/mm³, and less than 75% PMNs (Table 32-1).

Synovial fluid analysis should always be performed on freshly obtained fluid. A simple bedside test is to attempt to read newsprint through the synovial fluid; newsprint can be read through noninflammatory fluid (Fig. 32-5). Traditional tests on synovial fluid that are of limited or no value include measurement of glucose, lactate, and protein levels; subjective determination of viscosity; mucin clot test (examining the friability of the precipitate formed by mixing synovial fluid with dilute acetic acid); and immunologic tests. When looking for crystals and infection, direct examination, Gram stain, culture, and WBC count with differential are the only tests worth performing on synovial fluid. Inflammatory synovial fluid must be considered secondary to infection until proved otherwise by culture. The presence of crystals in the joint does not exclude the possibility of joint infection.

Synovial biopsy can facilitate a diagnosis in some settings. Arthroscopy has greatly simplified the acquisition of synovial tissue. This might be helpful in the diagnosis of granulomatous disease or infiltrative processes such as lymphoma, metastatic disease, or amyloidosis (Klippel, 2001).

Table 32-1 Interpretation of Synovial Fluid Cell Count

Leukocyte Count (WBCs/mm³)	Interpretation
<200	Normal synovial fluid
<2000	Noninflammatory fluid
>2000	Inflammatory fluid
2000-20,000	Mild inflammation (e.g., SLE)
20,000-50,000	Moderate inflammation (e.g., RA, reactive arthritis)
50,000	Severe inflammation (e.g., sepsis, gout)
>100,000	Sepsis, until proved otherwise

From Towheed TE, Hochberg MC. Acute monoarthritis: a practical approach to assessment and treatment. Am Fam Physician 1996;54:2239.

WBCs, White blood cells; *SLE*, systemic lupus erythematosus; *RA*, rheumatoid arthritis.

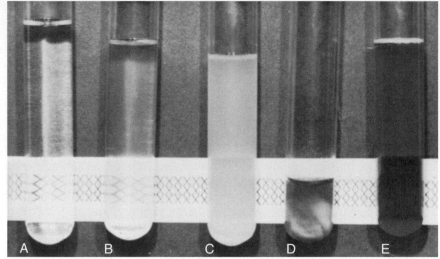

Figure 32-5 Synovial effusions. **A,** Normal or edema fluid is clear, pale yellow, or colorless. Print is easily read through the tube. **B,** Fluid from noninflammatory joint disease is yellow and clear. **C,** An inflammatory effusion is cloudy and yellow. Print may be blurred or completely obliterated, depending on the number of leukocytes. The effusion is translucent. **D,** A purulent effusion from septic arthritis contains a dense clump that does not even allow light through the many leukocytes. **E,** Hemorrhagic fluid is red. The supernatant may be darker yellow-brown (xanthochromic). A traumatic tap is less uniform and often has blood streaks. *(From Schumacher HR. Synovial fluid analysis and synovial biopsy. In Kelley WN, Harris ED, Ruddy S, et al [eds]. Textbook of Rheumatology, 5th ed, vol 1. Philadelphia, Saunders, 1997, pp 609-625.)*

Imaging Studies

Plain radiographs are still the most common imaging studies done for evaluation and management of rheumatic diseases. Techniques such as magnetic resonance imaging (MRI) and radionuclide scintigraphy (bone scan) are being used more often, although costly and often unnecessary. Many arthritides have characteristic radiographic findings, but these techniques are not indicated for most patients with acute and new symptoms of SLE, gout, mechanical lower back pain, or RA, because radiographs are usually normal early in the course of the disease. Normal radiographs also do not rule out OA. In established RA, the physician might see periarticular osteoporosis, soft tissue swelling, and marginal erosions. Gouty erosions cause characteristic overhanging edges because of reparative changes. (See also Chapter 31.)

The severity of radiographic changes in association with severe symptoms can help guide the aggressiveness of treatment. Overreliance on radiographs, however, can lead to undertreatment or overtreatment of disease. Treatment of RA with a DMARD should usually be initiated long before severe radiographic abnormalities are present. The near-ubiquitous presence of osteophytes on the lumbar vertebrae should not be used to justify aggressive surgical treatment for low back pain; on the other hand, many patients with chronic lower back pain have normal lumbar radiographs. Radiographs for acute joint symptoms might be helpful to rule out fractures, metastases, or infection, especially in older patients. If symptoms persist for more than 10 days, the physician should consider repeat radiography, looking for callus formation.

Besides rotator cuff injuries, MRI studies are particularly useful for possible cruciate ligament, complete lateral collateral ligament (LCL), and meniscal tears in the knee for potential surgical candidates. Although expensive, MRI shows soft tissue destruction long before plain radiographs. Bone scans also are costly and are nonspecific but demonstrate RA changes before radiographs.

Functional Assessment

Instruments such as the Arthritis Impact Measurement Scale and the Health Assessment Questionnaire Disability Index can quantify the impact of the rheumatic disease process on quality of life, pain, physical function, and psychosocial adaptation. However, these tools are more useful in clinical research studies than a busy family physician's office practice. A functional assessment screen is a practical tool for the family physician and takes only minutes (see **eTable 32-1** online). Focusing on disease impact on the patient as well as on the patient's joints can be an important contribution by the family physician. Functional assessment helps the primary care physician determine the role of other team physicians (rheumatologist, orthopedic surgeon, physical therapist, occupational therapist, mental health professional). Assessment of function can also lead to a discussion of disease impact on the family and help them deal with this chronic, possibly progressive condition.

Arthrocentesis

Arthrocentesis is most helpful in diagnosing crystal-induced and septic arthritis. Synovial fluid analysis can also be helpful in ruling out the coexistence of two or more types of arthritis in a single patient and even in a single joint. RA might coexist with a septic joint, secondary OA, hemarthrosis, or calcium pyrophosphate dihydrate (CPPD) disease. Hemarthrosis and bacterial infections usually occur in joints already damaged by arthritis. Arthrocentesis is a simple office procedure that can rule out bacterial infection in an acutely inflamed joint. Untreated or delayed treatment of infectious arthritis can cause rapid joint destruction, necessitating prompt diagnosis. A second line of treatment for RA should generally not be started until crystal arthropathy first has been ruled out. A physician is much more likely to harm a patient by not obtaining synovial fluid analysis when needed to make an accurate diagnosis. This is more common than the relatively rare occurrence of iatrogenic infection (particularly if proper sterile technique is used) or hemarthrosis (usually seen in patients with coagulopathies). The iatrogenic infection rate is generally estimated at 1 in 10,000, much less common than missed diagnosis of a septic joint. Anticoagulation therapy is not an absolute contraindication in the setting of acute arthritis.

The preferred route of entry for arthrocentesis traverses the shortest distance through tissue and avoids major vessels, tendons, and nerves. The knee, ankle, wrist, and elbow are the easiest joints to aspirate, and aspiration can be performed with only a moderate amount of trauma. Other joints normally require more extensive experience. Sterile technique normally does not require draping, but the same needle should not be used to aspirate the joint and to transfer the aspirated fluid to collection bottles.

The knee is the easiest joint to aspirate, best done with a medial or lateral approach at the superior third of the patella between it and the femur. Ankle arthrocentesis entry is midline, equidistant from the medial and lateral malleoli. A lateral entry between the olecranon process and the lateral epicondyle is best for the elbow. The shoulder can be approached posteriorly below the posterolateral aspect of the acromion process or anteriorly just lateral to the coracoid process.

A local anesthetic can be used but might distort landmarks; ethyl chloride spray immediately before needle insertion is usually sufficient. An 18-gauge needle is used for the knee and a 20-gauge needle for other joints; only 1 to 5 mL of synovial fluid is needed for diagnostic purposes. Fluid aspiration by itself is often therapeutic because it reduces articular pressure. Cartilage puncture should be avoided, if possible, by inserting the needle only as deeply as needed to obtain fluid, obtaining as much fluid as possible without risking unnecessary trauma by trying to aspirate every last drop, and avoiding side-to-side needle movement.

Therapeutic Corticosteroid Injection

Arthrocentesis can also be a therapeutic technique to deliver local corticosteroid to a joint that has not responded to systemic therapy and after infection has been excluded. Synovial fluid is first aspirated to ensure proper positioning in the joint space, followed by 1 to 2 mL of corticosteroid to large joints (knees, hips, shoulders); 0.5 to 1 mL to wrists, elbows, and ankles; and 0.25 to 0.5 mL to small joints and soft tissue sites. A 1:2 dilution with lidocaine can be used to provide instant relief, although many believe lidocaine adds to the risk of infection (e.g., requiring a more complex procedure, changing needles) with limited benefit and therefore do not use it. After injection, the joint should be moved through its passive range of motion (ROM), followed by at least 24 hours of rest. Steroid injections should be limited to no more than three to four times per joint per year because of concerns about possible cartilage and ligamentous damage from repeated injections.

Nonsteroidal Anti-Inflammatory Drugs

The NSAIDs are among the most frequently prescribed drugs and are used by family physicians for almost all rheumatic and musculoskeletal pain conditions. By suppressing the synthesis of prostaglandins, NSAIDs reduce inflammation and therefore pain but do not prevent tissue injury or joint damage. Cyclooxygenase-2 (COX-2) inhibitors are used for rheumatologic and musculoskeletal pain because of decreased GI side effects. The VIGOR (Bombardier et al., 2000) and CLASS (Silverstein et al., 2000) studies

for rofecoxib and celecoxib, respectively, showed that the decreased GI effects outweighed any cardiovascular risk. The APPROVe study linked rofecoxib (Vioxx) to an increased risk of cardiovascular disease (Bresalier et al., 2005). An unpublished trial studying celecoxib (Celebrex) and naproxen (Naprosyn, Aleve) in Alzheimer's disease prevention was stopped secondary to a 50% increase in cardiovascular events in subjects not taking placebo (NIH, 2004). Overall, COX-2 inhibitors have produced minimal decrease in GI bleeding and thus should be used cautiously for rheumatologic and musculoskeletal pain because the cardiovascular risk outweighs the GI benefit. Currently, celecoxib has a "black box" warning; rofecoxib was removed from the market.

Patients respond to different classes of NSAIDs for unknown reasons, and no NSAID appears superior to others in efficacy. Treatment is largely empiric. Most clinicians start with a low dose and titrate upward if needed. An adequate trial of an NSAID requires that the patient take a maximum dose for 3 weeks before changing to a different NSAID, although many patients will expect a change in medication before this. It is usually best to switch to an NSAID from a different class. There is no benefit to combining nonsalicylate NSAIDs. All COX-1 NSAIDs can cause dyspepsia and GI toxicity, interfere with platelet function, and prolong bleeding times. Other common side effects include renal toxicity and central nervous system (CNS) symptoms such as drowsiness, dizziness, and confusion. A 2004 Cochrane review of NSAIDs for lower back pain concluded that the various types of NSAIDs (e.g., COX-2 inhibitors) are equally effective, and selection of an NSAID for OA should be based on relative safety and patient acceptability.

Combining NSAIDs with misoprostol (Cytotec), 100 to 200 mg four times daily with meals, or omeprazole (Prilosec), 20 mg daily (Hawkey et al., 1998) has been shown to decrease the incidence of gastric and duodenal ulcers. A meta-analysis of 112 randomized controlled trials (RCTs) found no evidence supporting the effectiveness of H_2 receptor antagonists, while the risk of symptomatic ulcers was significantly reduced by proton pump inhibitors (PPIs), misoprostol, and COX-2 inhibitors (Koch et al., 1996). Omeprazole and other PPIs are better tolerated than misoprostol and famotidine (Hawkey et al., 1998). The physician should monitor for decreased renal function, interaction with antihypertensives, and transaminase (ALT, AST) elevations when starting NSAID therapy or increasing dosage, or when the patient's condition changes.

A common issue for the family physician is whether a patient prescribed aspirin for cardiac prophylaxis needs to stop the aspirin when prescribed a traditional NSAID. Patients taking both do not appear to be at significantly increased risk of GI toxicity. However, the aspirin might not yield any additional cardioprotective benefit, because these patients already benefit from the traditional nonselective NSAID antiplatelet effect. If taking both aspirin and NSAID, it is best to take the aspirin at least 4 hours before the NSAID for its full protective effect.

Arthritis of Systemic Disease

Arthritis can be a component of many systemic diseases, including metabolic disorders, infections, malignancies, and various endocrine, hematologic, and GI diseases. Parvovirus

B19 is responsible for erythema infectiosum and can also cause polyarthritis, especially in the hands, knees, and ankles. HIV infection sometimes causes symmetric polyarthritis, spondylitis, or acute oligoarthritis. Hepatitis B and C can cause acute symmetric polyarthritis in large and small joints. Inflammation in a few large joints and back pain are among the earliest symptoms of infective endocarditis in about 25% of patients with this disorder (Totemchokchyakarn and Ball, 1996).

Lyme arthritis caused by *Borrelia burgdorferi* can cause migratory monoarthritis or oligoarthritis in the knees or shoulders weeks to months after the rash of erythema chronicum migrans has developed. Poorly controlled *diabetes* (affecting foot, ankle, and knee), *hyperthyroidism* (affecting fingers and toes), *hypothyroidism* (causing noninflammatory effusions in knees, wrists, and hands), and *parathyroid disease* (causing chondrocalcinosis) are all endocrine disorders that can cause arthritis.

Metabolic disorders can cause degenerative arthritis. *Hemochromatosis* (caused by iron deposition) typically affects the second and third metacarpophalangeal (MCP) joints, wrists, knees, hips, and shoulders. *Wilson's disease* (caused by copper deposition) can cause premature OA in wrists and knees. Sickle cell disease can be complicated by knee arthritis; arthritis is also often seen in patients with hemophilia and leukemia. Arthritis is associated with inflammatory bowel disease and primary biliary cirrhosis. Reactive carcinoma synovitis can be the presenting symptom of an underlying malignancy, particularly of the breast or the prostate.

Referral to the Rheumatologist

As for all types of disease conditions, referral to the subspecialist largely depends on the family physician's knowledge, interest level, and logistical ability to provide state-of-the-art care to a given patient for a given disease entity at a given time in the disease course. Specific conditions, such as suspected septic arthritis, acute myelopathy or mononeuritis multiplex, suspected acute tendon or muscle rupture, or acute internal derangement, should probably be referred. In addition, referral should be considered for patients without a specific diagnosis after 6 weeks; those with difficulty in symptom control, systemic symptoms in pregnancy, or severe symptoms; patients requiring steroid, immunosuppressive, or other drugs unfamiliar to the primary care physician; or those with end-stage joint disease. The often nonspecific nature and psychosocial impact of rheumatic symptoms require continued active involvement of the family physician in the patient's care, regardless of referral.

Rheumatic Diseases

Osteoarthritis

Key Points

- Osteoarthritis affects 20% of the U.S. population; 44% of OA patients are not active.
- Primary and secondary OA must be differentiated.
- NSAIDs, not COX-2 inhibitors, are still the pharmacologic treatment of choice for OA.

Osteoarthritis, also known as "degenerative joint disease," is the most common form of arthritis and causes more work disability in the United States (17%) than any other disease. Arthritis affects 20% of the U.S. population, about half of whom primarily have OA. Long thought to result from "wear and tear," OA is now known to have genetic, traumatic, metabolic, and developmental causes, which complicates prevention and treatment. OA is found radiographically in almost all 75-year-old patients, most of whom are asymptomatic. OA occurs about equally in men and women ages 45 to 55 but after 55 is more common in women (CDC, 2005). Most OA patients are not seriously affected and are asymptomatic. Others, however, require joint replacement surgery because of its severity.

Although OA is considered a noninflammatory type of arthritis affecting primarily the cartilage, it actually involves active biochemical disease processes as well as mechanical forces that affect the entire synovial joint. An OA variant affecting primarily the hands runs in families and is inflammatory. Women are more prone to this inflammatory variant of OA of the hands that causes Heberden's nodes (in distal interphalangeal [DIP] joints) and Bouchard's nodes (in proximal interphalangeal [PIP] joints). The articular cartilage may not even be involved, with the disease process centered more on subchondral bone turnover (Peterson et al., 1998). Quadriceps muscle weakness might precede the onset of knee OA, indicating the importance of biomechanical factors (Slemenda et al., 1997).

Osteoarthritis can be separated into primary (idiopathic), hereditary (resulting from collagen gene defects), and secondary. Secondary OA results from previous cartilage damage. Occupations causing repetitive joint trauma predispose a patient to OA. Episodic trauma, congenital anatomic abnormalities (slipped capital femoral epiphyses, congenital hip dysplasias), neuropathies, and endocrine-metabolic causes (obesity, hemochromatosis, Wilson's disease, CPPD disease, Paget's disease, acromegaly) all might lead to OA. Inflammatory arthritides such as RA, infections, or gout damage cartilage and are often followed by the development of OA.

Occupational kneelers (e.g., shipyard workers, miners, carpet or floor layers) have a significantly higher incidence of knee OA than control groups of clerical workers (Maetzel et al., 1997). However, repetitive sports activities such as long-distance running are unlikely to cause OA in the absence of joint injury or antecedent joint abnormality (Panush and Lane, 1994). More than 44% of patients with diagnosed OA are inactive (Gordon et al., 1998). Low-impact activity in normal joints is not associated with OA, but high-intensity and high-impact activity resulting in injury is associated with OA. Mechanical risk factors might affect the initiation more than the progression of OA. Most mild OA does not progress to severe joint damage. Mild OA might be a different disease than severe OA, which depends on processes other than early OA.

Clinical Findings

Most OA is asymptomatic, an incidental finding on radiographs performed for other reasons. No treatment or further evaluation is indicated for asymptomatic OA. Early symptomatic OA is characterized by local pain of gradual onset exacerbated by using the involved joint. Pain typically worsens as the day progresses and is relieved by rest. There is less than 30 minutes of localized morning stiffness and no constitutional or systemic symptoms, and the gel phenomenon (stiffness after periods of rest and inactivity) resolves within several minutes of activity. Damp, cool, rainy weather often exacerbates symptoms because of changes in intra-articular pressure associated with changes in barometric pressure. Patients with OA of the knees might complain of buckling or instability, especially when descending stairs. OA of the hip can manifest as pain radiating from the groin and down the anterior thigh. OA of the neck might be felt in the neck, back, or upper extremities, causing pain, weakness, or numbness. As OA progresses, pain can become continuous, including at night.

Primary OA can be divided into three classifications: generalized OA, large-joint OA, and erosive OA. *Generalized* OA involves five or more joints, most often the DIP joints of the hand (Herberden's nodes), the PIP joints of the hand (Bouchard's nodes), the first carpometacarpal joint, the first MTP joint of the feet, and the knee, hip, and spine. There is a significant familial component. *Large-joint* OA of the knees and hips might occur as part of generalized OA or alone. OA of the knees often occurs in the medial and patellofemoral compartments. OA of the hips can be characterized in two subsets, central and superior poles. Central or medial involvement of the hip joint space occurs in the setting of generalized OA, is usually bilateral, and is seen in women more than men. Most hip OA is superior pole, usually unilateral, seen more in men, and occurs without other joint involvement. As many as 40% to 90% of cases of adult hip OA might arise from subtle developmental abnormalities of the hip, including acetabular dysplasia, developmental (formerly "congenital") hip dislocation, Legg-Calvé-Perthes disease, and slipped capital femoral epiphysis (Brandt and Slemenda, 2004).

A rare form of primary OA known as *erosive* OA involves the hand's PIP and DIP joints equally, with significant inflammation. Other joints are often not involved, although 15% of erosive OA cases might subsequently evolve into seropositive RA (Kujala et al., 1995).

Physical Findings

Physical findings of OA typically include joint swelling, tenderness, crepitus, and enlargements at joint margins, causing deformity. The location of pain should be precisely localized as to whether it is truly articular or periarticular; if pain is located in the joint, an inflammatory or infectious cause should be ruled out first. Patients might have reduced ROM or, in severe cases, joint instability, resulting in excess motion or locking because of loose cartilage fragments. Warmth and soft tissue swelling because of joint effusion might be present, but a markedly swollen, hot, erythematous joint suggests a septic or microcrystalline disease rather than OA.

Laboratory Studies

Clinical study criteria for OA classification are helpful as a means to standardize the diagnosis (see **eTables 32-2** and **32-3** online). Although the diagnosis of OA can almost always be made by history and physical examination, definitive diagnosis can be helped by synovial fluid analysis, radiography, and normal ESR, ANA, and RF during symptomatic periods. Synovial fluid analysis of large-joint effusions can

be used to exclude other processes. Joint effusions in OA typically show leukocyte counts lower than 1000 WBCs/mm³, predominantly lymphocytes (Table 32-2). Serum tests might be misleading because ESR rises with age and 20% of healthy older adults have positive RF levels. A greatly elevated ESR suggests a process other than OA. Although many have been identified, biochemical markers of OA are not generally useful to the practicing clinician at this time.

Imaging Studies

Radiographs are generally the first-line confirmation of the presence of OA. Treatment should not be based solely on radiographic abnormalities, however, given the frequency of asymptomatic joints demonstrating radiographic OA changes. OA changes include osteophyte formation, asymmetric joint space narrowing (defined as <3 mm on a weight-bearing knee), and subchondral bone sclerosis (Figs. 32-6 and 32-7). Later in the disease process, subchondral cysts with sclerotic walls might develop. Periarticular osteoporosis and marginal erosions suggest RA or some other inflammatory arthritis rather than OA. Patients with OA involving atypical joints (MCP joints, wrists, elbows, shoulders, or ankles) should be evaluated for an underlying disorder such as CPPD or hemochromatosis.

Treatment

Treatment of OA includes pharmacologic therapy, nonpharmacologic therapy, and surgery. Before initiating treatment, a definitive diagnosis of OA must be made by careful history and

Table 32-2 Criteria for Classification of Idiopathic Osteoarthritis (OA) of Knee

Clinical and Laboratory	Clinical and Radiographic	Clinical*
Knee pain *plus* at least five of nine:	Knee pain *plus* at least one of three:	Knee pain *plus* at least three of six:
Age >50 years Stiffness <30 minutes Crepitus Bony tenderness Bony enlargement No palpable warmth ESR <40 mm/hr RF <1:40 SFOA	Age >50 years Stiffness <30 minutes Crepitus *plus* Osteophytes	Age >50 years Stiffness <30 minutes Crepitus Bony tenderness Bony enlargement No palpable warmth
92% sensitive	91% sensitive	95% sensitive
75% specific	86% specific	69% specific

From Altman R, Asch E, Bloch G, et al. Development of criteria for the classification and reporting of osteoarthritis: classification of osteoarthritis of the knee. Arthritis Rheum 1986;29:1039-1049, with permission of the American College of Rheumatology.

*Alternative for the clinical category would be four of six, which is 84% sensitive and 89% specific.

ESR, Erythrocyte sedimentation rate (Westergren); *RF*, rheumatoid factor; *SFOA*, synovial fluid signs of OA (clear, viscous, or white blood cell count <2000/mm³).

physical examination. No currently available treatment has been shown to alter the natural history of the disease. Therefore, the goal of management of OA is primarily to relieve pain, stiffness, and swelling. The physician seeks to reduce limitation of motion and disability without causing iatrogenic side effects. Patients and their families must also be educated about the disease and their treatment options (Box 32-1).

Nonpharmacologic therapy includes rest during pain episodes, exercise, weight control, avoidance of trauma, patient and family education, and assistive devices. The patient's ability to perform both self-care ADLs and IADLs requiring higher functioning (e.g., shopping, driving, writing) should be assessed. Physical and occupational therapists can provide great benefit by offering an exercise program and assistive devices to maintain independence and minimize symptoms (Fransen et al., 2001). Patients benefit from the use of canes, walkers, bathtub and toilet wall bars, and dressing sticks for socks and from the other methods of joint protection and symptom relief, such as heat massage. Rest is important for patients with acute pain. Otherwise, helpful exercise programs include swimming, other aerobic conditioning, and walking (van Baar et al., 1999). Weight control and weight reduction have also been shown to improve symptoms (Messier et al., 2004).

First-line pharmacologic therapies for symptom control include acetaminophen, up to 1000 mg four times daily in the absence of liver disease, and traditional NSAIDs, beginning with ibuprofen. Because few RCTs studied differences in efficacy of NSAIDs, the initial choice is empiric. Therefore, relative safety, patient adherence, and cost should determine selection. Risk factors for upper GI bleeding with NSAIDS include age over 65, history of peptic ulcer disease or upper GI bleeding, concurrent use of oral corticosteroids and anticoagulants, and possibly smoking and alcohol consumption. Evidence suggests that NSAIDs are superior to acetaminophen for improving knee and hip pain from OA. No significant difference in overall safety was found, although patients taking NSAIDs were more likely to experience an adverse GI event (Towhead et al., 2006). Capsaicin (Zostrix) topical cream four times daily, formerly a first-line agent, now has been shown to have minimal benefit, especially when considering side effects that impair compliance (Mason et al., 2004). Combination therapy (NSAIDs with

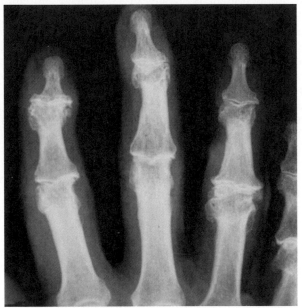

Figure 32-6 Osteoarthritis in the hand. *(From Resnick D, Yu JS, Sartoris D. Imaging. In Kelley WN Harris ED, Ruddy S, et al [eds]. Textbook of Rheumatology, 5th ed, vol 1. Philadelphia, Saunders, 1997, pp 626-686.)*

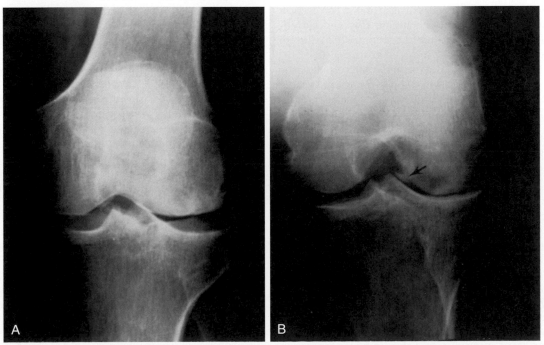

Figure 32-7 Osteoarthritis in the knee. **A,** Anteroposterior radiograph of knee showing asymmetric joint narrowing. **B,** Anteroposterior radiograph showing osteophyte formation in knee *(arrow)*. *(From Resnick D, Yu JS, Sartoris D. Imaging. In Kelley WN Harris ED, Ruddy S, et al [eds]. Textbook of Rheumatology, 5th ed, vol 1. Philadelphia, Saunders, 1997, pp 626-686.)*

Box 32-1 Options in the Management of Patients with Osteoarthritis

Nonpharmacologic Therapy

Patient education and self-management programs
Social support through telephone contact
Physical and occupational therapy
Range of motion (ROM) and strengthening exercises
Aerobic conditioning
Weight loss
Assistive devices for ambulation and activities of daily living

Pharmacologic Therapy

Oral nonopioid analgesics (e.g., acetaminophen)
Topical analgesics (e.g., capsaicin cream)
Nonsteroidal anti-inflammatory drugs (NSAIDs)
Intra-articular steroid injections
Opioid analgesics

Surgical Therapy

Closed tidal joint lavage
Arthroscopic debridement and joint lavage
Osteotomy
Total joint arthroplasty

From Hochberg MC. Osteoarthritis: clinical features and treatment. In Klippel JH (ed). Primer on the Rheumatic Diseases, 12th ed. Atlanta, Arthritis Foundation, 2001, pp 293-295.

analgesics) may also be helpful. The addition of tramadol (Ultram, 200 mg/day) in patients responding to 1000 mg/day of naproxen has been shown to allow significant reduction (by half) in the naproxen dose needed without compromising pain relief (Schnitzer et al., 1999).

Misoprostol (Cytotec) was the first U.S. Food and Drug Administration (FDA)–approved drug for GI protection when used with NSAIDs, although higher doses of famotidine (Pepcid), nizatidine (Axid), and omeprazole (Prilosec) also decrease the risk of NSAID-induced gastric ulcers. Currently, NSAIDs plus a PPI such as omeprazole remains the treatment of choice for prevention of NSAID-induced gastric ulcers. Opioid analgesics and limited intra-articular corticosteroid injections (up to 4 injections per joint per year) are the remaining traditional choices. Opiates should generally be avoided for long-term use but might be helpful for acute exacerbations. It is unclear whether the risks of long-term NSAID use outweigh the addiction potential of chronic opiate use.

Intra-articular glucocorticoids are often used and are particularly useful in patients with contraindications or continued pain despite NSAIDs. This modality is postulated to work by decreasing cartilage catabolism and osteophyte formation. A meta-analysis found that patients receiving intra-articular steroid injections for OA of the knee were twice as likely to have short-term improvement as controls (Arroll et al., 2004). Data on injection of the hip and knee joint show the most promise, but efficacy at other sites is less certain. Aseptic technique should be used to prevent iatrogenic complications of infection. Patients should be counseled on postinjection complications such as bleeding, infection, skin hypopigmentation, fat necrosis, and steroid flare.

Because OA is a common incurable disease that causes pain, many other treatments, including dietary supplements and other alternative therapies, have been tried for centuries. Balanced hormone therapy, copper bracelets, bee venom, vitamins, herbs, homeopathic remedies, and certain types of foods are promoted as effective treatments or cures for OA. Family physicians should be aware of proven and unproven remedies used by their patients. One therapy shown to be efficacious is glucosamine sulfate.

Glucosamine and chondroitin sulfates both stimulate the production of proteoglycan in cartilage and inhibit its breakdown. Over-the-counter formulations vary in the amount of glucosamine (made from crab shells) and chondroitin (processed from cow cartilage). Research has shown that patients have moderately benefited from glucosamine and chondroitin supplements over 3 years with less knee joint space narrowing on radiography, significant reduction of symptoms, and no adverse effects (Richy et al., 2003). The major studies of glucosamine used two different formulations of the supplement, which yielded different results, the Rotta brand and non-Rotta formulations. A 2005 Cochrane review found that a non-Rotta preparation failed to show benefit in pain and function, whereas the Rotta preparation showed that glucosamine was superior to placebo in the treatment of pain and functional impairment resulting from symptomatic OA. Studies for chondroitin are less convincing, with no consistent improvement in pain or functional status (AAFP, 2006). The safest daily intake is 1500 mg/day of glucosamine and 1200 mg/day of chondroitin. Most capsules containing both minerals are also formulated with manganese, theorized to assist in proteoglycan metabolism but not studied (Richy et al., 2003).

A meta-analysis of 11 studies found that S-adenosylmethionine (SAMe) was as effective as NSAIDs at reducing pain and functional limitations, with a somewhat better adverse effect profile (Soeken et al., 2002).

A Cochrane review of herbal therapies for OA found two studies demonstrating that avocado-soybean unsaponifiables showed beneficial effects on function, pain, intake of NSAIDs, and global evaluation (Little et al., 2004). Another beneficial intervention is transcutaneous electrical nerve stimulation (TENS) for OA of the knee; electrical stimulation has been shown to improve knee OA moderately by 25% and cervical OA by 12% (Osiri et al., 2004).

Studies comparing acupuncture with a sham control found greater improvement in those receiving the actual treatment (Berman et al., 2004; Ezzo et al., 2001; Vas et al., 2004). A meta-analysis found that acupuncture was more effective than placebo in pain reduction in peripheral OA (Kwon et al., 2006). Two studies found that therapeutic touch, an energy modality, showed benefit in OA (Gordon et al., 1998). Although previously cited as beneficial for OA secondary to antioxidants, the literature reports an increased risk of cardiovascular disease with vitamins C and E (Alkhenizan and Palda, 2003).

Other, less traditional therapies have received much media attention but not shown effectiveness. Cycles of three or more weekly intra-articular injections of hyaluronic acid (viscous substance in synovial fluid that lubricates and protects joints) have been used, with partial success (Abramowicz, 1998a). Hyaluronate sodium (Hyalgan) and hylan G-F 20 (Synvisc) are FDA approved for OA of the knee. Onset of pain relief can take several weeks and can last for 6 months or longer. Meta-analyses of hyaluronic acid have shown minimal effectiveness versus placebo. The cost/benefit ratio favors therapies other than joint injection (Lo et al., 2003).

Other largely unproven therapies include doxycycline, diathermy (deep heat using ultrasound), iontophoresis with dexamethasone, and intra-articular therapeutic gene therapy before joint replacement. Although diathermy and iontophoresis are widely used and have widespread anecdotal reports of subjective relief of pain, there is no definitive proof of benefit.

KEY TREATMENT

Treatment of osteoarthritis begins with nonpharmacologic modalities, including weight loss (Messier et al., 2004), physical therapy (Fransen et al., 2001), exercise (van Baar et al,, 1999), and orthotics if needed (SOR: A).

Acetaminophen and NSAIDs are both first-line pharmacotherapy for pain associated with OA, although NSAIDs appear to be more effective (Towhead et al., 2006) (SOR: A).

Intra-articular glucocorticoids show short-term improvement in pain associated with OA of the hip and knee (Arroll et al., 2004) (SOR: B).

Treatments such as Synvisc (Lo et al., 2003), glucosamine (Richy et al., 2003), and acupuncture (Kwon et al., 2006) are often used for OA relief before surgical measures (SOR: B).

Rheumatoid Arthritis

Key Points

- Rheumatoid arthritis affects women 3:1 over men, with 70% having an insidious onset.
- Symmetric synovitis with morning stiffness longer than 1 hour is the hallmark of RA.
- Constitutional symptoms are common in patients with RA.

Rheumatoid arthritis is a chronic inflammatory systemic disease in which cellular and autoimmune mechanisms result in destruction of tissues, primarily the synovium. Genetic predisposition appears to be important, but a specific inciting infectious agent or other cause has still not been found. RA manifestations vary from very mild, self-limited disease to multiorgan destruction and early death. Increasing knowledge of the modulating factors in disease progression is transforming the treatment of RA. Without treatment, the normally fluctuating disease course results in progressive joint destruction. Patients with active, polyarticular, RF-positive RA have more than a 70% chance of developing joint damage or erosion within 2 years (Fuchs et al., 1989). Because RA is relatively uncommon compared with OA and is now treated quite differently, the family physician must be able to make the correct diagnosis and initiate disease-modifying therapy early, before joint destruction.

Epidemiology

Rheumatoid arthritis affects women more frequently than men (about 3:1 ratio) and occurs in all age groups but has a peak incidence between 20 and 50 years. Prevalence is 1% to 2% of adults, ranging from 0.3% of the population younger than 35 to about 10% of those older than 65. There is a higher concordance of RA in monozygotic twins than in dizygotic twins because of gender differences and differences in major histocompatibility complex (MHC) class II gene products (HLA-DR). Combinations of different genes most likely predispose patients to the disease. The HLA-DR antigen appears to be triggered by many stimuli. After this inciting event, the synovial lining cells and subsynovial vessels proliferate, forming a pannus. Leukocytes invade, followed by a further inflammatory cascade involving proteases and cytokines. RF produces autoantibodies to IgG Fc fragment, influenced by HLA-DR polymorphism and associated with more severe, extra-articular disease. Again, RF is not specific to RA and can be detected in normal persons.

Diagnosis

Rheumatoid arthritis is a clinical diagnosis made by careful history and physical examination. Laboratory testing can be confirmatory but is also misleading if not interpreted in context. Radiographic evidence of erosions appears only several months to a year after disease onset. The American College of Rheumatology (ACR) published useful criteria in 1987 for the diagnosis of RA (Table 32-3). Symptoms must be present for at least 6 weeks for initial diagnosis.

Symmetric synovitis is the hallmark of RA and can be suggested by joint aspiration of synovial fluid, yielding over 2000 WBCs/mm^3 without crystal, or by radiographic evidence of erosions. Because the cause of synovitis cannot be differentiated clinically, extra-articular manifestations can help distinguish RA from other inflammatory conditions.

History

Approximately 70% of patients with RA experience an insidious onset over weeks to months, 10% have an acute abrupt onset, and 20% have an intermediate onset, with increasing symptoms for days to weeks. Morning stiffness occurring for more than 1 hour is suggestive of RA. Morning stiffness results from joint immobilization during sleep and is not related to time of day. As opposed to patients with OA, patients with RA have constitutional symptoms such as fatigue, malaise, weight loss, low-grade fever, and anemia. Small joints in hands and feet (PIP, MCP) are typically involved first, with larger joints involved later. The joints themselves might be warm to the touch but are usually not erythematous. A pannus of inflamed synovium palpable as a rubbery mass of tissue strongly suggests RA.

The presentation of exacerbations of chronic rheumatoid synovitis might differ from those of early acute synovitis. Chronic inflammation causing fibrosis decreases synovial vascularity, reducing the amount of swelling from previous episodes. Although the frank swelling of burned-out RA appears less severe, the amount of pain, morning stiffness, constitutional symptoms (fatigue, malaise), and joint destruction on radiography shows this physical finding to be misleading. These episodes in patients with chronic, long-term RA should therefore not be considered improvement over more visible, earlier episodes of synovitis.

Less common presentations of RA include acute onset (which has the best prognosis) and palindromic RA, which

Table 32-3 American College of Rheumatology Revised Criteria for Classification of Rheumatoid Arthritis (Traditional Format)

Criterion*	Definition
1. Morning stiffness	Morning stiffness in and around the joints lasting at least 1 hour before maximal improvement.
2. Arthritis of three or more joint areas	At least three joint areas with simultaneous soft tissue swelling or fluid (not bony overgrowth alone) observed by physician. The 14 possible joint areas are right or left PIP, MCP, wrist, elbow, knee, ankle, and MTP joints.
3. Arthritis of hand joints	At least one joint area swollen as above in a wrist, MCP, or PIP joint.
4. Symmetric arthritis	Simultaneous involvement of the same joint areas on both sides of the body; bilateral involvement of PIP, MCP, or MTP joints is acceptable without absolute symmetry.
5. Rheumatoid nodules	Subcutaneous nodules over bony prominences or extensor surfaces or juxta-articular nodules regions, observed by physician.
6. Serum rheumatoid factor	Demonstration of abnormal amounts of serum rheumatoid factor by any method that has been positive in less than 5% of normal control subjects.
7. Radiologic changes	Radiologic changes typical of rheumatoid arthritis on posteroanterior hand and wrist radiographs, which must include erosions or unequivocal bony decalcification localized to, or most marked adjacent to, the involved joints (osteoarthritis changes alone do not qualify).

From Arnett FC. Revised criteria for the classification of rheumatoid arthritis. Bull Rheum Dis 1989;38:1. Used with permission.

*Four or more criteria are needed for the diagnosis of rheumatoid arthritis (RA). Criteria 1 through 4 must be present for 6 weeks or longer. Presence of criteria is not conclusive evidence for the diagnosis of RA. Absence of criteria is not conclusively negative.

MCP, Metacarpophalangeal; *MTP*, metatarsophalangeal; *PIP*, proximal interphalangeal.

of the transverse ligament of the first cervical vertebra (C1, which stabilizes odontoid process of C2), as well as disease of the apophyseal joints.

Neck pain without neurologic features tends to be self-limited and usually improves, but neck pain and neurologic symptoms often do not correlate well. A neurologic examination, even in the absence of neck pain, is therefore prudent in patients with RA. Radiographs of the cervical spine in flexion and extension might be needed to detect C1-C2 involvement, which necessitates caution during surgical procedures requiring intubation.

Physical Examination

Upper Extremity

Shoulder RA usually manifests as decreased ROM. Elbow RA is more accessible than shoulder RA for physical examination and joint aspiration. Elbow involvement can manifest with elbow pain and swelling; ulnar compression syndrome (paresthesia and weakness of fourth and fifth digits) can develop from the synovitis. The wrists are affected in most RA patients, in contrast to OA patients; carpal tunnel syndrome is seen frequently. RA usually involves the MCP and PIP joints rather than the DIP joints. Classic late changes such as swan neck and boutonnière deformities and ulnar deviation of the MCP joints caused by ligamentous laxity might occur. The swan neck deformity is characterized by flexion of the DIP and MCP joints and hyperextension of the PIP joint, probably resulting from shortening of the interosseous muscles and tendons and shortening of the dorsal tendon sheath. The boutonnière deformity results from avulsion of the extensor hood of the PIP because of chronic inflammation. This causes the PIP to pop up in flexion while the DIP stays in hyperextension.

Lower Extremity

Hip involvement in RA might be difficult to detect on physical examination and might manifest as only a small decrease in ROM. If pain develops, it can be felt in the buttock, lower back, groin, thigh, or medial aspect of the knee. RA of the knee is usually easily apparent on examination. A *Baker's cyst* (posterior herniation of the joint capsule to the popliteal area) might occur and can be diagnosed by ultrasound. Rupture of a Baker's cyst into the posterior leg might mimic thrombophlebitis. RA might involve the MTP, talonavicular, and ankle joints, causing gait problems. The tarsal tunnel containing the posterior tibial nerve can be compressed by synovitis, causing burning paresthesias on the sole of the foot made worse by weight bearing.

Joint Deformities

The synovitis of RA has many effects on cartilage, bone, muscles, tendons, and ligaments. Cartilage and bone erode, and muscles and tendons shorten in response to chronic inflammation. Ligaments are weakened by collagenases released by inflamed synovium and pannus. Upper extremity joints (shoulder, wrist, elbow) are prone to more severe deformities, as previously noted, than knees and ankles because splinting (avoiding joint motion to minimize pain) is easier in these lower extremity joints. The decreased use of these joints leads to more destruction by tendon shortening and contraction of the articular capsule.

is characterized by brief episodes of swelling of a large joint such as a knee, wrist, or ankle. Palindromic RA can therefore be easily misdiagnosed as gout.

Approximately 20% of patients with RA have intermittent symptoms. The remainders have progressive disease of varying severity. from slowly to rapidly progressive. In addition to morning stiffness, synovitis, and structural damage, RA exhibits classic manifestations in specific joints. Cervical spine involvement is common, whereas thoracic and lumbar spine involvement is rare. Early symptoms are neck stiffness and decreased motion, which can lead to neurologic complications from C1-C2 instability resulting from tenosynovitis

Extra-Articular Manifestations

Systemic constitutional symptoms such as fatigue, malaise, anorexia, weight loss, and fever occur in addition to joint inflammation and destruction in RA. Significant inflammation of almost all organ systems occurs. Patients have an increased incidence of renal, cardiac, pulmonary, and neurologic disorders, serious infections, and hematologic malignancies such as non-Hodgkin's lymphoma. Subcutaneous rheumatoid nodules occur frequently in RA patients, usually in areas subject to pressure such as the elbows and sacrum. Their onset can be abrupt or gradual, and they might also resolve spontaneously. Biopsies are sometimes required to differentiate these from a gouty tophus or xanthoma. Rheumatoid nodules can also occur throughout the body, including (rarely) organs such as the lungs and heart.

Pulmonary involvement can include pleural effusions, interstitial fibrosis, solitary or multiple nodular lung disease, and pleurisy. Asymptomatic pericarditis diagnosed by echocardiography during RA exacerbations is relatively common but rarely results in cardiac-related sequelae. Nodules can occur rarely in the myocardium, heart valves, and aorta. Renal and GI complications are generally secondary to the treatment of RA rather than arising from the disease itself. Eye dryness from keratoconjunctivitis sicca, episcleritis, or scleritis is associated with RA. Hematologic complications of RA include a hypochromic microcytic anemia with a low serum ferritin level and low or normal iron-binding capacity. Because many RA patients are taking NSAIDs, it can be difficult to distinguish anemia associated with their RA from NSAID-induced GI blood loss. *Felty's syndrome* (RA, splenomegaly, leukopenia, leg ulcers, lymphadenopathy, thrombocytopenia, HLA-DR4 haplotype) is most common in patients with severe, nodule-forming RA.

Laboratory Studies

Arthritis panels should not be routinely performed and might only confuse the diagnosis. RF, ESR, uric acid level, ANA, and radiographic abnormalities all increase with age in the general population, even in the absence of disease. Therefore, laboratory studies should be reviewed as confirmatory of the clinical diagnosis made by careful history and physical examination.

Rheumatoid factor, ANA, and ESR are normally the most helpful tests to diagnose RA. RF is present in 80% to 90% of patients with RA. Therefore, 10% to 20% of patients with RA never have a positive RF. Also, up to 4% of normal young persons have low levels of RF. Moreover, RF titers are not helpful in following disease progression; when a patient is discovered to have a positive RF, repeating the test is of no value. Repeating an RF 6 to 12 months later for patients with initially negative RF may be useful when RA is still being strongly considered. RF can be increased in other diseases, mainly chronic infections (Lyme disease, subacute bacterial endocarditis, tuberculosis, syphilis), viral infections (infectious mononucleosis, cytomegalovirus, influenza), parasitic infections, and other chronic inflammatory diseases such as sarcoidosis, pulmonary interstitial disease, and noninfectious hepatitis.

Anti–cyclic citrullinated peptide (anti-CCP) antibody is another laboratory test useful in the diagnosis of RA when the diagnosis is in question or the RF is negative. Anti-CCP is more specific than rheumatoid factor for RA with 95% specificity and 69% sensitivity. Positive anti-CCP serology has also been linked with more severe radiologic progression of joint erosions from RA (Nishimura at el., 2007). Anti-CCP can also be positive in patients with active tuberculosis or other autoimmune diseases.

Other serum tests include ANA titers, complement, ESR, and CBC. Abnormal ANA titers indicate SLE, Sjögren's syndrome, and scleroderma, but up to 30% of RA patients also have abnormal ANAs. Complements (CH50, C3, and C4) are decreased in SLE but are normal or increased in RA. The ESR, a nonspecific marker of inflammation, might help differentiate RA from other noninflammatory diseases. C-reactive protein (CRP), an acute-phase reactant, is also nonspecific but increases more rapidly than the ESR in early inflammation. A CBC showing a mild normochromic, normocytic anemia and a normal WBC count suggests RA. Thrombocytosis might also mimic disease activity as another acute-phase reactant, and eosinophilia might be seen.

Synovial fluid analysis in RA shows a yellow-white, turbid, but sterile fluid without crystals. WBC counts of synovial fluid in RA are typically 10,000 to 20,000 cells/mm^3 but are at least higher than 2000/mm^3, with more than 75% PMNs. Synovial CH50 is lower than serum levels, and the serum and synovial glucose difference is usually higher than 30 mg/dL.

Imaging Studies

Radiography is indicated early when infection or fracture must be ruled out, the patient has a history of malignancy, the physical examination fails to localize the source of pain, or pain persists despite conservative treatment. Early RA might show only soft tissue swelling. Advanced destruction on radiographs should not be required to initiate disease-modifying therapy if a diagnosis of RA is strongly suspected clinically. In late-stage disease, radiographs might show marginal bony erosions, periarticular osteoporosis, and joint space narrowing, especially in the hands and feet (Figs.32-8 and 32-9).

Course

Almost 90% of joints ultimately affected in a given patient are involved during the first year of the disease, allowing the family physician to alert the patient with chronic RA about which joints will ultimately be affected (Anderson, 2004). Rate of spontaneous remission is extremely low, usually occurring within 2 years of disease onset. The presence of RF, nodules, extra-articular manifestations, and HLA-DR4 haplotype is associated with a more severe course. Mortality rates for patients with severe RA are higher secondary to infections; cardiovascular, pulmonary, and renal disease; GI bleeding; and excess malignancy. The strongest predictors of survival appear to be extra-articular manifestations of the disease and comorbidities (Gabriel et al., 2003).

Treatment

Initiation of early aggressive treatment of RA is essential to achieve the best prognosis in an individual patient. An integrated approach using up-to-date pharmacotherapy, patient

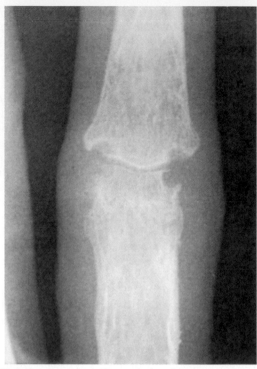

Figure 32-8 Rheumatoid arthritis marginal erosions and joint space narrowing. *(From Resnick D, Yu JS, Sartoris D. Imaging. In Kelley WN Harris ED, Ruddy S, et al [eds]. Textbook of Rheumatology, 5th ed, vol 1. Philadelphia, Saunders, 1997, pp 626-686.)*

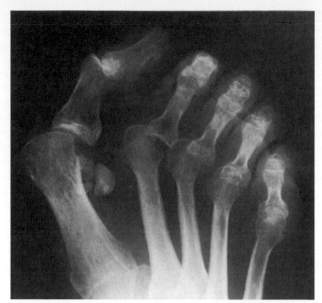

Figure 32-9 Classic forefoot deformities of rheumatoid arthritis. *(From Resnick D, Niwayama G. Diagnosis of Bone and Joint Disorders. Philadelphia, Saunders, 1988.)*

education, physical and occupational therapy, and surgery is optimal. The family physician's role in early diagnosis of RA and subsequent initiation of DMARDs gives patients the best chance for minimizing joint destruction. The early aggressive treatment of RA begins with initial sign and symptom onset through the first 1 to 2 years of the disease. Considering symptomatology such as the patient's overall function, fatigue, inflammation and erosion of joints, and extra-articular symptoms can lead to an early diagnosis.

Although long used as the mainstay of pharmacologic therapy, NSAIDs provide only symptomatic relief without improving prognosis. Therefore, almost all patients should start taking a DMARD as soon as the diagnosis of RA has been made (Fig. 32-10). Many DMARDs are no more toxic than high-dose NSAIDs. Treatment options include DMARDs (hydroxychloroquine, sulfasalazine, and methotrexate) and minocycline. After 1 to 2 years of this therapy, the disease will have progressed to established RA. For moderate signs and symptoms, single and combination therapy is applicable, with options such as methotrexate, anti-TNF (tumor necrosis factor), anti–K-1, leflunomide, azathioprine, gold, cyclosporine, and other medications for mild RA (Osiri et al., 2003; Wells et al., 2004). The disease progresses to severe rheumatoid arthritis if the treatment options for established rheumatoid arthritis have failed. Therapy such as cyclophosphamide (Cytoxan), a different DMARD selection, pulse steroids, and Prosorba Column (protein A) could then be considered. Along with prescribing the DMARD, the family physician must educate the patient and family about the importance of DMARD compliance. Physical and occupational therapy are important for joint protection during exacerbations, as is exercise to improve function and ROM. Early consultation with a rheumatologist is generally recommended.

Disease-Modifying Antirheumatic Drugs

Although traditional first-line therapy has included aspirin and NSAIDs, DMARDs are now used more frequently in early RA (Table 32-4). Because of the potential for toxicity, it is important to differentiate RA from other causes of synovitis as well as from OA. The 2008 ACR recommendations identified four adverse prognostic factors that would encourage use of DMARDs: functional limitation, extra-articular disease, RF positivity or presence of anti-CCP antibodies, and bony erosions documented on radiographs. Hydroxychloroquine appears to be the least toxic of the DMARDs, followed (in order) by sulfasalazine (Azulfidine), methotrexate (Rheumatrex), intramuscular (IM) gold sodium thiomalate (Myochrysine), and aurothioglucose (Solganal). Hydroxychloroquine is dosed at 200 mg orally once or twice daily; however, patients need ophthalmologic follow-up in 6 months (Carmichael et al., 2002; Wassenberg and Rau, 2003). Hydroxychloroquine is generally only used for patients with milder RA symptoms. Significant improvement was seen in patients with mild RA taking hydroxychloroquine compared with those taking placebo (Davis et al., 1991).

Sulfasalazine is given at 2 to 3 g/day in two divided doses (Suarez-Almazor et al., 2000a). Before prescribing sulfasalazine, a sulfa drug, the physician must be aware of potential allergy and check CBC and liver function tests (LFTs) weekly for 1 month, then every 4 to 6 weeks. Using sulfasalazine use as the sole DMARD for treatment should be limited to those patients lacking the poor prognostic factors noted earlier or those with contraindications to methotrexate. A meta-analysis of 15 trials showed that sulfasalazine was effective for treatment of RA (Weinblatt et al., 1999b). Oral gold, or auranofin (Ridaura), is not as effective as IM preparations and should be used only for early mild RA or in combination with other DMARDs (Suarez-Almazor et al., 2004a). Gold is given as 3 mg twice daily, and CBC must be done every 4 to 6 weeks. Diarrhea is a frequent side effect. The onset of action of most DMARDs is at least several months, so adequate

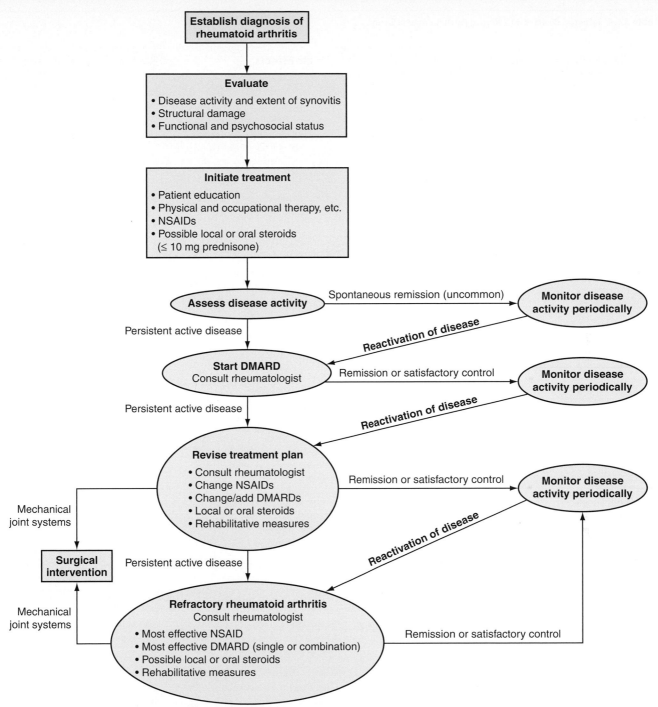

Figure 32-10 Algorithm for management of rheumatoid arthritis. *DMARD,* Disease-modifying antirheumatic drug; *NSAID,* nonsteroidal anti-inflammatory drug. *(From American College of Rheumatology Ad Hoc Committee on Clinical Guidelines. Guidelines for the initial evaluation of the adult patient with acute musculoskeletal symptoms. Arthritis Rheum 1996;39:1.)*

pain control with analgesics should be given and the patient counseled about realistic expectations.

Methotrexate

Many rheumatologists consider methotrexate to be the DMARD of first choice; it is the most frequently used DMARD in the United States. Methotrexate inhibits folic acid synthesis and is the primary choice for moderate to severe RA, showing significant short-term benefit but adverse effects on abrupt withdrawal (Suarez-Almazor et al., 2004a; Ortiz et al., 2000). Folic acid (1 mg/day) reduces methotrexate-induced mouth sores without decreasing the drug's efficacy. Patients cannot drink alcohol and must have LFTs every 4 to 6 weeks. Increasing the dose up to 25 mg/week and using the subcutaneous or IM route might enhance efficacy. Liver biopsies are no longer recommended during therapy unless abnormal alanine transaminase (ALT) or albumin levels persist (Kremer et al., 1994). Methotrexate toxicities include hepatotoxicity, bone marrow suppression, rare development of B-cell non-Hodgkin's lymphoma, subcutaneous nodules

Table 32-4 Selected Disease-Modifying Antirheumatic Drugs

Class/Drug (Brand)	Recommended Dosage	Toxic Effects	Recommended Monitoring
Gold Compounds			
Gold sodium thiomalate (Myochrysine)	IM: 10 mg followed by 25 mg 1wk later, then 25-50 mg weekly until there is toxicity, major clinical improvement, or cumulative dose of 1 g. If effective, interval between doses is increased.	Pruritus, dermatitis (frequent in one third of patients), stomatitis, nephrotoxicity, blood dyscrasias, "nitritoid" reaction: flushing, weakness, nausea, dizziness 30 min after injection	CBC, platelet count before every other injection U/A before each dose
Auranofin (Ridaura)	Oral: 3 mg bid or 6 mg qd; may increase to 3 mg tid after 6 mo	Loose stools, diarrhea (up to 50%), dermatitis	Baseline CBC, platelet count, U/A, renal, liver function at onset, then CBC with platelet count, U/A at 9 mo
Antimalarial			
Hydroxychloroquine (Plaquenil)	Oral: 400-600 mg qd for 4-12 wk, then 200-400 mg qd	Retinopathy, dermatitis, muscle weakness, hypoactive DTRs, CNS	Ophthalmologic examination every 3 mo (visual acuity, slit lamp funduscopic, visual field tests) neuromuscular examination
Penicillamine (Cuprimine)	Oral: 125-250 mg qd, then increasing doses by125-250 mg at monthly intervals to max 750-1000 mg	Pruritus, rash, or mouth ulcers; bone marrow depression; proteinuria, hematuria, hypogeusia myasthenia, myositis, GI distress, pulmonary toxicity, teratogenic	CBC every 2 wk until dose stable, then every month U/A weekly until dose stable, then every 9 mo hCG as needed
Methotrexate (Rheumatrex)	Oral: 7.5-20 mg weekly	Pulmonary toxicity, ulcerative stomatitis, leukopenia, thrombocytopenia, GI distress, malaise, fatigue, chills, fever, CNS, elevated LFTs or liver disease, lymphoma, infection	CBC with platelet count LFTs weekly for 6 wk, then monthly U/A periodically hCG as needed
Azathioprine (Imuran)	Oral: 50-100 mg qd, increase at 4-wk intervals by 0.5 mg/kg/day, up to 2.5 mg/kg/day	Leukopenia, thrombocytopenia, GI, neoplastic if previous therapy with alkylating agents	CBC with platelet count, weekly for 1 mo, twice monthly for 2 mo, then monthly hCG as needed
Sulfasalazine (Azulfidine)	Oral: 500 mg daily, then increase, up to 3 g daily	GI, skin rash, pruritus, blood dyscrasias, oligospermia	CBC, U/A every 2 wk for 3 mo, then monthly for 9 mo, then every 6 mo
Alkylating Agents			
Cyclophosphamide (Cytoxan)	Oral: 50-100 mg daily, up to 2.5 mg/kg/day	Leukopenia, thrombocytopenia, hematuria, GI, alopecia, rash, bladder cancer, non-Hodgkin's lymphoma, infection	CBC with platelet count, regularly hCG as needed
Chlorambucil (Leukeran)	Oral: 0.1-0.2 mg/kg/day	Bone marrow suppression, GI, CNS, infection	CBC with platelet count every wk WBC 3-4 days after each CBC during first 3-6 wk at therapy hCG as needed
Cyclosporine (Sandimmune)	Oral: 2.5-5 mg/kg/day	Nephrotoxicity, tremor, hirsutism, hypertension, gum hyperplasia.	Renal function, liver function
Pyrimidine Synthesis Inhibitor			
Leflunomide (Arava)	Loading dose: 100 mg/day for 3 days Maintenance therapy: 20 mg/day; if not tolerated, 10 mg/day	Hepatotoxicity, carcinogenesis Immunosuppression, long half-life	LFTs every month, drug levels after discontinuation (after 1-mo therapy, remains in blood for 2 yr without cholestyramine)

Table 32-4 Selected Disease-Modifying Antirheumatic Drugs — *cont'd*

Class/Drug (Brand)	Recommended Dosage	Toxic Effects	Recommended Monitoring
Tumor Necrosis Factor (TNF) Inhibitors			
Etanercept (Enbrel)	2-5 mg SC twice weekly *or* 50 mg SC weekly	Sepsis, opportunistic infections, congestive heart failure, injection site pain	PPD, CBC, ALT at baseline monthly until dose is stable; then every 2-3 mo
Infliximab (Remicade)	5 mg/kg IV on weeks 0, 2, 6; then biweekly	Sepsis, opportunistic infections, reactivation of hepatitis B and TB, pancytopenia	PPD, CBC, ALT at baseline monthly until dose is stable; then every 2-3 mo
Adalimumab (Humira)	40 mg SC every 2 wk	Sepsis, opportunistic infections, reactivation of TB	PPD, CBC, ALT at baseline monthly until dose is stable; then every 2-3 mo
Extracorporeal*			
Staphylococcal protein A immunoadsorption	IV weekly for 12 wk	Hypotension (especially with ACE inhibitor), injection site infection, anemia, flulike symptoms, joint pain	CBC routinely

*Use only in patients whose disease is refractory to disease-modifying antirheumatic drugs (DMARDs).

ACE, Angiotensin-converting enzyme; *ALT,* alanine transaminase; *bid,* twice daily; *CBC,* complete blood count; *CNS,* central nervous system; *DTRs,* deep tendon reflexes; *GI,* gastrointestinal; *hCG,* human chorionic gonadotropin; *IM,* intramuscular; *IV,* intravenously; *LFTs,* liver function tests; *PPD,* purified protein derivative; *qd,* once daily; *SC,* subcutaneously; *TB,* tuberculosis; *tid,* three times daily; *U/A,* urinalysis; *WBC,* white blood cell count.

(treated with colchicine), opportunistic infections, and hypersensitivity pneumonitis (treated with corticosteroids). It can be difficult to withdraw methotrexate once it has been started without causing a disease flare.

Other Disease-Modifying Antirheumatic Drugs

Azathioprine (Imuran) is used for moderate and severe RA as a second- or third-line drug after methotrexate, sulfasalazine, gold, and hydroxychloroquine have been tried. It suppresses bone marrow and can lead to infection. After the initial DMARD therapy, azathioprine can be tried in a 2- to 6-week course. No evidence has demonstrated increased effectiveness over other DMARDs (Suarez-Almazor et al., 2000d).

Cyclosporine (Sandimmune, Neoral) is used in combination with methotrexate and is given as a 2.5-mg/kg dose to prevent hypertension and renal disease. It has shown modest efficacy in short-term treatment with progressive RA (Wells et al., 2000). D-Penicillamine (Depen, Cuprimine) has unpredictable toxicity, making it a less attractive choice. The alkylating agents cyclophosphamide and chlorambucil, as well as cyclosporine, are effective but are reserved for refractory severe cases because of their toxicities. All second-line drugs are teratogenic, so a family physician must help the patient establish an effective means of birth control. The risk of toxic effects is an important factor in choice of these agents, and selection is generally best handled in consultation with the rheumatologist.

Leflunomide (Arava) inhibits pyrimidine synthesis, is given orally, and is considered a possible alternative to methotrexate for decreasing erosion and controlling inflammation, but it provides no apparent benefit over methotrexate and is expensive. Leflunomide has been shown not only to reduce symptoms but also to slow disease progression. The routine dosage is 100 mg daily for 3 days, followed by a maintenance dosage of 10 to 20 mg/day. LFTs must be ordered, and as

with methotrexate, levuflunomide is better for short-term therapy (Suarez-Almazor et al., 2000a). Research continues into combining DMARDs to lower drug resistance. DMARD combination therapy in early RA has shown minimal benefit (Mottonen et al., 1999).

Anticytokine Therapy

Cytokines such as interleukin-1, tumor necrosis factor alpha (TNF-α), granulocyte-macrophage colony-stimulating factor, interleukin-6, and chemoattractant cytokines (known as chemokines) are derived from macrophages and fibroblasts and appear to be the most important cytokines involved in RA treatment. TNF-α is produced by synovial macrophages and causes many destructive inflammatory actions in the rheumatoid joint. Synovial macrophages proliferate; synoviocytes (fibroblast-like cells lining the joint) produce prostaglandins and cytokines, continuing the inflammatory process. Administering monoclonal antibodies such as infliximab (Remicade) to bind TNF-α and block its activity and giving TNF-α receptors such as etanercept (Enbrel) are two approaches to decrease TNF activity. Patients with a suboptimal response to methotrexate at 25 mg/wk (maximum dose) are the best candidates for etanercept or infliximab. Before starting any anticytokine therapy, CBC and tuberculin test (PPD) are required.

Etanercept, a recombinant p75 TNF-α receptor–Fc fusion protein, is given subcutaneously once to twice weekly. It decreases binding of TNF-α to cellular receptors and avoids downstream inflammation. It is well tolerated and is indicated for use alone or with methotrexate for methotrexate-refractory disease (Blumenauer et al., 2003; Weinblatt, 1999). The most common side effect is injection site erythema, which must be carefully watched in RA patients with diabetes mellitus. Etanercept has significantly reduced disease activity in a dose-related manner over 6 months, with no laboratory abnormalities noted (Moreland et al., 1999).

Infliximab, an anti–TNF-α monoclonal antibody, is given intravenously for refractory disease every 4 to 8 weeks. It is 75% human and 25% mouse antibody to TNF-α. The primary mechanism is halting joint space narrowing, with subsequent decreased erosion. It is FDA approved only in combination with methotrexate. Again, caution is warranted in diabetic patients for skin ulcers. If the patient has a positive PPD, isoniazid and vitamin B_6 therapy must be given for 9 months with the treatment. Fewer appropriate trials exist for infliximab than etanercept; however, the benefit in refractory disease has been demonstrated (Blumenauer et al., 2004).

Adalimumab (Humira), 40 mg subcutaneously every other week, has a greater therapeutic potential when used with methotrexate (OnMedica, 2005). It is a full human anti–TNF-α. Fewer studies exist on its long-term efficacy, but short-term studies show a greater effect than infliximab or etanercept. Risk factors with this regimen include skin infection, malignancy, and demyelination.

Nonsteroidal Anti-Inflammatory Drugs

The NSAIDs improve inflammation and pain but do not alter disease progression. Therefore, most patients with RA should be taking a DMARD. NSAIDs are used for analgesia and to help control symptoms. DMARDs generally have a slow onset of action, necessitating use of other agents to help keep the patient comfortable while awaiting onset of the DMARD's action. NSAID-associated GI bleeding is a widespread problem; one in three RA patients will be hospitalized or will die from a GI bleed at some point. Selection of NSAID is largely empiric (Table 32-5). The least toxic NSAIDs are coated or buffered aspirin, salsalate (Disalcid, Mono-Gesic, Salflex), and ibuprofen (Advil, Motrin, Nuprin, Rufen). The most toxic are indomethacin (Indocin), tolmetin sodium (Tolectin), meclofenamate sodium (Meclomen), and ketoprofen (Orudis, Oruvail). High-toxicity NSAIDs provide no more clinical benefit than lower-toxicity drugs (Fries et al., 1991).

Misoprostol (Cytotec), a synthetic prostaglandin analogue, helps decrease NSAID-induced risk of gastric and duodenal ulceration. Although 30% to 40% of patients receiving 200 mg of misoprostol four times daily experienced diarrhea, lower doses (100 mg two or three times daily) cause less diarrhea, with most GI protection maintained. PPIs such as omeprazole used with the NSAID are better tolerated than misoprostol and are also efficacious. As mentioned, sucralfate and normal doses of H_2 blockers might help dyspepsia but have not prevented ulcer formation from NSAIDs such as PPIs and misoprostol. Patients receiving long-term nonselective NSAIDs should be monitored several times annually for hematocrit abnormalities and should undergo stool guaiac testing and have renal and liver function evaluated. There is no benefit to combining different NSAIDs.

Aspirin and Salicylates

High-dose aspirin (900-1050 mg four times daily) is as effective as much more expensive NSAIDs but is often less well tolerated and less convenient to take.

Glucocorticoids

Glucocorticoid articular injections are often used for temporary localized suppression of RA but are not recommended for use more than three times per joint per year. Common drugs for injection (used with lidocaine to minimize patient discomfort) include hydrocortisone, triamcinolone (Kenalog, Aristocort), methylprednisolone (Depo-Medrol), dexamethasone (Decadron-LA), and betamethasone (Celestone Soluspan), in ascending order of duration of action.

Systemic corticosteroids are used primarily as bridge therapy for several months when initiating DMARDs and awaiting their onset. Prednisone might be especially useful for constitutional symptoms such as fatigue and malaise. Low-dose prednisone (<7.5 mg daily) in a single morning dose might particularly be useful in older adult patients when other drugs have more potential for toxicity.

Surgery

Surgery is useful in RA patients with more severe disease who, despite optimal medical treatment, develop joint erosions and severe destruction resulting in pain and limitation of function. Surgical procedures range from carpal tunnel release to synovectomy, joint fusion, and arthroplasty. About 90% of older adult patients with severe incapacitating rheumatoid joint disease can expect excellent pain relief and increased ROM after total hip or knee replacement (Harris and Sledge, 1990).

Other Therapies

On the basis of the theory that persistent mycoplasma infection might cause RA, tetracyclines such as minocycline (Minocin) have been used by some physicians for years. Minocycline, 100 mg orally twice daily, has shown modest efficacy but can lead to dizziness and dosing sensitivity in early RA (O'Dell et al., 2001). A small study showed that use of minocycline (100 mg twice daily) in early RA (first 3 months after diagnosis) resulted in more frequent remissions, and the need for DMARD therapy was reduced after follow-up for 4 years (O'Dell et al., 1999). These antibiotics result in mild improvement in RA patients, and other actions may include inhibition of collagenase activity, direct anti-inflammatory effect, and interference with leukocyte function.

Stress management, cognitive-behavioral pain management techniques, relaxation training, biofeedback, and family-oriented behavior therapy have all been shown to improve daily functioning, pain reports, and disease activity in RA patients (Parker et al., 1995). A small RCT showed a 28% decrease in mean disease severity at 4 months using writing therapy (Smyth et al., 1999). Another study showed that 20% of the disability of RA was related to psychosocial factors (Escalante and del Rincon, 1999). Educating patients about methods to cope with their disease can significantly improve quality of life. Interventions shown to improve outcomes include tai chi (Han et al., 2004) and journaling (Smyth et al., 1999). A meta-analysis of psychological interventions (e.g., biofeedback, relaxation, cognitive-behavioral therapy) found significant effects on pain, disability, functional status, and coping, although these might be more effective for patients with RA of shorter duration (Astin et al., 2002). Experimental therapies include total lymphoid irradiation, interferon gamma (IFN-γ), high-dose prednisolone, and oral collagen. Oral collagen has thus far not been shown to cause statistically significant improvement, but better-designed studies might demonstrate a benefit. The theory is that collagen will induce regulatory T cells to be generated in the gut, which will then migrate to

Table 32-5 Selected NSAIDs Used in Rheumatoid Arthritis and Osteoarthritis

Class/Drug (Brand)	Usual Dosage Range for Arthritis
I. Arylcarboxylic acids A. Salicylic acids 1. Acetylated	
Aspirin, extended release	1600 mg bid
Aspirin, enteric coated	1000 mg qid
2. Nonacetylated	
Diflunisal (Dolobid)	250-500 mg bid, max 1500 mg/day
Choline-magnesium salicylate	3 g/day in 1-3 doses
Salsalate (Disalcid, Salflex)	3-4 g/day in 2-3 doses
B. Anthranilic acid	
1. Meclofenamate sodium	200-400 mg/day in 3-4 doses
II. Arylalkanoic acids A, Arylacetic acids	
1. Diclofenac (Voltaren	150-225 mg/day in 3-4 divided doses
2. Naproxen (Naprosyn)	250-500 mg bid-tid
3. Naproxen sodium (Anaprox)	275-550 mg bid
B. Arylpropionic acids	
1. Ibuprofen (Advil, Motrin)	300-800 mg/tid-qid
2. Ketoprofen (Oruvail)	100-200 mg daily
3. Fenoprofen (Nalfon)	300-600 mg tid-qid
C. Oxazolepropionic acid	
1. Oxaprozin (Daypro)	600-1800 mg/day in 1-2 doses
D. Heteroarylacetic acid	600-1800 mg/day in 3-4 doses
1. Tolmetin	
E. Indoleacetic and indeneacetic acids	
1. Indomethacin (Indocin, Indocin SR)	25-50 mg tid-qid 75 mg qd-bid
2. Sulindac (Clinoril)	150-200 mg bid
F. Pyranocarboxylic acid	
1. Etodolac (Lodine)	300-500 mg bid
III. Enolic acids-Oxicam	
1. Piroxicam (Feldene)	20 mg daily
IV. Nonacidic agent	
1. Nabumetone (Relafen)	1000-2000 mg divided qd-bid
2. Meloxicam (Mobic)	7.5-15 mg qd
V. Cyclooxygenase (COX-2) inhibitor	
1. Celecoxib (Celebrex)	100-200 mg bid

NSAID, Nonsteroidal anti-inflammatory drug; *qd,* once daily; *bid,* twice daily; *tid,* three times daily; *qid;* four times daily.

joints where a protein analogous to the orally dosed antigen resides, resulting in immune tolerance and reduced inflammation (Kalden and Sieper, 1998).

Nutritional changes are hypothesized to decrease RA signs and symptoms. A Cochrane review of herbs found that gamma-linolenic acid (GLA) resulted in some improvement in clinical outcomes (Little and Parsons, 2000; Zurier et al., 1996), consistent with other findings on essential fatty acids. Fish oil, high in omega-3 fatty acids, significantly improved the number of tender joints and morning stiffness (Fortin et al., 1995; Volker et al., 2000); the recommended dose would be 3 g/day, and symptom relief might not be evident until 12 weeks of use. Changes in the total diet have been studied as well. Fasting has anecdotal evidence for inducing remission of symptoms. A 7- to 10-day fast followed by a gluten-free vegan diet was found to sustain improvements (Kjeldsen-Kragh et al., 1991; McDougall et al., 2002). Proceeding immediately to a vegan gluten-free diet resulted in RA symptom improvement (Hafstrom et al., 2001). Symptoms were exacerbated with challenges of foods that patients had reacted to on skin-prick test (Karatay et al., 2004). Therefore, a trial of such a diet or an elimination diet would be reasonable options (Box 32-2).

Monitoring Arthritic Activity

Because RA is a chronic disease with significant psychosocial impact, the continuity that the family physician provides is crucial. Frequency of visits depends on disease activity, need for drug toxicity monitoring, and psychosocial functioning of the patient (see eTable 32-4 online). Periodic ESR/CRP levels, radiography, and functional status assessment are important, in addition to serial joint examination. A team approach using the expertise of a rheumatologist and physical and occupational therapists is generally indicated. Patients' ability to perform their job must be considered, and using modified work profiles or absences may be necessary. Osteoporosis resulting from RA should be monitored and prevented. The patient should also be monitored for infection, pulmonary disease, renal disease, or GI bleeding, taking a general health maintenance approach to this systemic disease.

KEY TREATMENT

The NSAIDS are the preferred treatment for pain in rheumatoid arthritis (SOR: C).

Treatment of RA with DMARDs should be started as soon as possible (SOR: C).

Methotrexate has substantial benefit in the treatment of RA and is generally the first-line DMARD (Suarez-Almazor et al., 2000a) (SOR: A).

Sulfasalazine has proven benefits on RA disease activity (Weinblatt et al., 1999) (SOR: A). However, it should be used as sole therapy only in patients with minor symptoms and no poor prognostic signs of RA.

Hydroxychloroquine has been shown to be effective in treatment of RA (Davis et al., 1991) (SOR: B). However, it is generally used with another DMARD or methotrexate in refractory cases when initial treatment fails. Biologic agents such as etanercept and infliximab reduce RA disease activity and are important treatment options in patients with moderate to severe RA who have failed treatment with methotrexate or combination therapy (Blumenauer et al., 2003; Weinblatt, 1999) (SOR: A).

Box 32-2 Elimination Diet: Patient Handout

Special diets called *elimination diets* are sometimes used to discover whether food allergies or sensitivities are related to symptoms you might be having. The goal of an elimination diet is to identify problem foods. The diet is temporary and must be followed very carefully so that a permanent diet to help you feel better can be planned. The steps in an elimination diet follow:

1. **Decide which foods might be causing problems.** This step involves describing your diet for your doctor and sharing your ideas about what foods might be causing problems. Sometimes, food allergy tests are used to help with the decision.

2. **Avoid the foods completely for 2 to 4 weeks.** This is the actual elimination step. This step involves the greatest restrictions in your diet.

   - The foods need to be avoided completely for symptoms to be noticeable when the foods are added back.
   - Foods should be avoided both in their whole form and as ingredients in food.
   - Keeping track of how you feel during this step is important. It is useful to keep a written record. You may feel worse before you feel better, but that should last only 1 or 2 days. If you feel worse for longer, please call your doctor.

3. **Add the foods back one at a time.** This is called the *challenge step*. It allows you to learn which foods, if any, are causing symptoms.

   - Decide with your doctor which food to add back first.
   - Keep track of how you feel throughout this step with a written record.
   - On the day a food is added, eat that food twice. For the next 2 days, do not eat that food again, but continue to follow the elimination diet. You can have a reaction up to 3 days after a food is eaten.
   - Add a new food every 3 days, because you can have a reaction up to 3 days after the challenge food is eaten.
   - If the food does not cause a reaction, that food "passes" and can be added back to your diet when the entire process is over. Do not eat the foods you have added back, even if they "passed," until you have tested all the foods.
   - After following the elimination diet carefully, you and your doctor will have a better picture of which foods, if any, are causing your problems. Remember that problems with foods can be intermittent, and it is sometimes difficult to tell exactly whether foods are a problem.

From Rakel D: Integrative Medicine. Philadelphia, Saunders, 2002.

Crystal Arthropathies

Gout and pseudogout are conditions caused by deposition of crystals of urate and calcium pyrophosphate dihydrate, respectively, with a resulting inflammatory response. These conditions can be distinguished from each other and from other causes of an acutely swollen joint or joints by synovial fluid examination, looking for crystals using polarized light microscopy.

Gout

Key Points

- Hyperuricemia is present (usually >8 mg/dL) in patients with gout.
- Gout affects more men than women.
- Negative birefringent crystals are seen on fluid analysis in gout.

Gout primarily affects middle-aged men (40-60 years) and postmenopausal women. It typically manifests as an acutely painful monoarticular arthritis, possibly becoming chronic after years of progressively more severe and frequent episodes, interspersed with variable symptom-free periods. *Hyperuricemia* is a marker for gout, but each can exist without the other. Asymptomatic hyperuricemia is not a disease. The risk of gout, however, is proportional to the degree and duration of hyperuricemia. Multiple genetic and environmental factors affect uric acid concentration. Uric acid is derived from ingestion of a diet rich in purines (e.g., typical American diet), as well as from endogenous production of purines. Inborn errors of metabolism, either reduced excretion (90% of patients) or increased production (10%) of uric acid, cause primary hyperuricemia. Secondary hyperuricemia results from diseases or drug therapies that raise uric acid levels.

In addition to attempting to prevent acute flares, the family physician's goal in treating patients predisposed to gout is to minimize the risk of developing other sequelae. These include interstitial nephropathy with renal function impairment; accumulation of urate crystal deposits in joints, soft tissue, cartilage, and bone, called *tophi*; and uric acid calculi in the genitourinary (GU) tract.

Clinical Presentation

The first MTP joint (great toe) is involved in 50% of initial acute gouty attacks (podagra) and is eventually affected in 75% to 90% of gout patients. This joint sustains more microtrauma and is relatively cool compared with the rest of the body. The heel, ankle, knee, midtarsal joints, and olecranon bursa can all be initially involved but are so less frequently than the first MTP joint. Gout severity ranges from vague aches and pains to severe pain, swelling, redness, and exquisite tenderness. Acute attacks resolve within several days to weeks, even in untreated gout.

In contrast to the typical middle-aged male presentation, gout in women and in older adult patients tends to be polyarticular. Because gout in these patient subgroups tends to involve more than one joint, it can often be misdiagnosed as RA (tophi are mistaken for rheumatoid nodules) or septic joint cellulitis, especially if low-grade fever, leukocytosis, redness, or desquamation is present. Synovial fluid analysis is necessary for definitive diagnosis.

Synovial Fluid Examination

A presumptive diagnosis of gout can be made by clinical signs and symptoms, a negative joint culture, response to NSAIDs or colchicine, and hyperuricemia. However, definitive diagnosis can be made only by finding needle-shaped, negatively birefringent urate crystals on synovial fluid examination or in tophi.

Clinical Stages of Primary Gout

Hyperuricemia is defined as two standard deviations (2 SD) above the individual laboratory's mean based on gender, usually 8 mg/dL in men and 7 mg/dL in women. Hyperuricemia is present in 5% of men, only 5% to 10% of whom develop acute gout. It normally takes at least 20 years of hyperuricemia before a patient has a first episode of gouty arthritis. Lowering the serum uric acid level does not decrease the risk of gouty nephropathy; chronic renal disease is almost always caused by

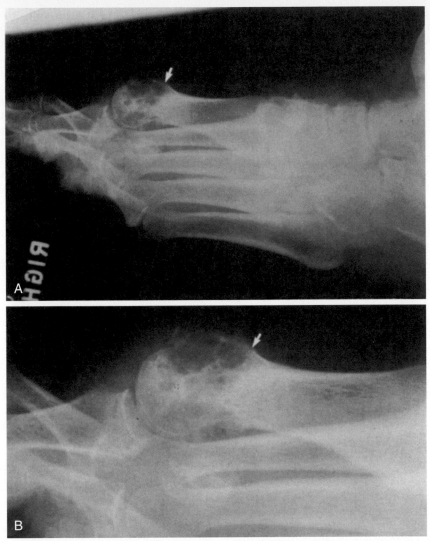

Figure 32-11 Advanced gout in the feet. **A,** Calcified tophi (*arrow*) of gout seen on x-ray. **B,** Osteophyte formation in knee (*arrow*). *(From Visual Aids, Subcommittee of the Professional Education Committee of the Arthritis Foundation. Clinical Slide Collection on the Rheumatic Diseases. New York, Arthritis Foundation, 1972, p 82.)*

concurrent diseases such as diabetes or hypertension. Because of expense and potential drug toxicity, treatment of asymptomatic hyperuricemia is therefore generally not recommended.

The two most important factors in the development of acute gouty arthritis are obesity and alcohol (Choi et al., 2005). Ethanol metabolism blocks renal excretion of uric acid, leading to gouty attacks. Studies have shown a 2.5-fold increase in the risk of gout in men who drink 2 or more beers per day. This risk was similar but slightly lower in men who drank the same amount of distilled alcohols. In contrast, two 4-ounce glasses of wine or more per day was not associated with an increased risk of gout (Choi at al., 2004). Other factors include rapid decrease or increase in serum urate level (thus a possible attack at start of allopurinol treatment), emotional stress, infection, and surgery. Dietary excesses of purine-rich foods (e.g., sweetbreads, sardines, anchovies, kidney, liver) have traditionally been mentioned but are in reality rarely responsible for acute gouty attacks. Diuretics, both hydrochlorothiazide and loop, have been associated with increased serum uric acid. Risks, benefits, and cost must be evaluated before deciding to change or stop these medications for hypertension.

After an initial gouty attack, more than half of patients will have a recurrent attack. The timing is highly variable, however, and the recurrent attack can be weeks or years later. As time passes, gouty attacks tend to become more frequent, more severe, and less responsive to therapy and to involve more joints. Between acute attacks, urate crystals can still be aspirated from asymptomatic joints, demonstrating that this so-called intercritical or interval gout represents a progression of disease. Chronic tophaceous gout occurs at least 10 years into the disease and is now seen infrequently because of more aggressive treatment of gout and hyperuricemia. Tophi can occur anywhere but tend to occur in the helix of the ear, on the proximal ulnar surface of the forearm, on the olecranon, on the Achilles tendon, on the prepatellar bursa, or near active joints. Tophi are not seen on plain radiographs unless they are calcified. The classic radiographic finding of chronic gout is sharply marginated erosions proximal to the joint space, with an overlying rim of cortical bone (Fig. 32-11).

Secondary gout is caused by drugs or disease processes affecting uric acid metabolism or excretion. Myeloproliferative and lymphoproliferative diseases, hemolytic anemia, multiple myeloma, and other malignancies result in overproduction. Renal disease, diuretics, salicylates, alcohol, nicotinic acid, and chronic lead intoxication (saturnine gout) all cause underexcretion. Chemotherapy for hematologic or myeloproliferative disorders can result in gouty nephropathy unless adequate hydration and possibly allopurinol prophylaxis are initiated before therapy.

Treatment of Gouty Arthritis

The NSAIDs are generally used first because of their efficacy and relative lack of toxicity. Indomethacin (Indocin) has been used for years for gouty arthritis attacks, but any NSAID can probably be used with similar efficacy, as long as an initial maximal dose is given. After 2 days of therapy at the maximal dose, the NSAID can be tapered over the next several weeks.

Colchicine decreases inflammation associated with lactic acid production and phagocytosis of urate; it terminates most gouty attacks within 6 to 12 hours but is limited by GI side effects (nausea, vomiting, abdominal cramps, diarrhea). Two 0.5- or 0.6-mg tablets are taken initially, then 1 tablet every hour, until clinical response has been achieved, GI side effects cause discontinuation, or a total of 6 mg has been given (Cox, 2004). Colchicine at 0.5 to 1 mg every 6 hours intravenously, up to 4 mg total, can also be given for a single attack, but the parenteral route is associated with increased bone marrow suppression, renal and hepatic toxicity, and myopathy. No additional colchicine should be given for at least 1 week if the patient is given the full 4-mg total dose.

When NSAIDs and colchicine are ineffective or contraindicated, corticosteroids might be used. Treatment options include oral corticosteroids using prednisone, 0.5 mg/kg, followed by tapering the dose by 5 mg/day. An intra-articular injection can be given using triamcinolone hexacetonide (Aristospan), triamcinolone acetonide, or methylprednisolone (Medrol); typical doses are 10 to 40 mg in large joints and 5 to 20 mg in small joints. Intra-articular injection is preferred for monoarticular episodes. Finally, adrenocorticotropic hormone (ACTH), 40 to 80 mg intravenously or intramuscularly every 8 to 12 hours, has been successful when all other therapies fail, but it is quite expensive.

Prophylaxis of Recurrent Gout

Asymptomatic hyperuricemia need not be treated, but after one episode of acute gouty arthritis or acute nephrolithiasis, patients should be offered the option of prophylaxis. Some choose not to take a daily drug, particularly if their gouty attacks are not severe or are infrequent. For patients with recurrent gouty attacks, renal damage, nephrolithiasis, or uric acid levels higher than 12 mg/dL, or those undergoing cancer chemotherapy, uric acid–lowering therapy should be initiated. Prophylaxis may be discontinued when uric acid levels are brought down to normal levels for 2 months. Patients should be instructed to avoid alcohol, aspirin, diuretics, prolonged fasting, and high-purine foods. Several days before initiating uric acid–lowering therapy, it is prudent to start colchicine, 0.5 mg twice daily, to avoid precipitating an acute attack. This therapy can continue for up to 6 months after the desired uric acid levels have been obtained.

Allopurinol (Zyloprim) is a xanthine oxidase inhibitor that decreases uric acid production but also produces a more soluble metabolite. Allopurinol is therefore effective regardless of the cause of the hyperuricemia. Allopurinol therapy

should never be initiated until an acute attack has subsided. Allopurinol is started at 100 mg/day with food, then increased at weekly intervals by 100 mg/day until the serum uric acid level is lower than 6 mg/dL. The usual effective dose is 200 to 300 mg/day, although some patients require up to 600 mg/day (Perez-Ruiz et al., 1998). Patients should ensure adequate fluid intake to produce more than 2 L of urine output daily. The dose needs to be adjusted for decreased creatinine clearance. If an acute attack occurs when the patient is taking allopurinol, the dose should be maintained and the attack treated as usual (NSAIDs, colchicine, corticosteroids). Allopurinol can cause rash, liver transaminase level elevations, and renal toxicity if used with thiazide diuretics. It might also potentiate the effect of anticoagulants and cause a rash if used with amoxicillin.

The uricosuric drugs probenecid and sulfinpyrazone (Anturane) block renal tubular reabsorption of uric acid. Probenecid is started at 250 mg twice daily for 1 week, then increased to 500 mg twice daily, and then increased by 500 mg/week, up to 3 g/day, until the urate level is normal. Sulfinpyrazone is started at 100 mg twice daily, increasing to 400 mg twice daily. These drugs should also never be started during an acute attack but should be maintained if the patient is already taking them. Urate stone formation risk can be minimized by a high fluid intake and alkalization of the urine. A 24-hour urine sample for determination of creatinine clearance and uric acid level should be obtained before starting these drugs, because GFR must be higher than 50 mL/min and uric acid excretion less than 800 mg/24 hr.

KEY TREATMENT

Patients with gout who are overweight should be instructed on weight loss (Choi et al., 2005) (SOR: B).

Patients with gout should limit intake of beer and distilled alcohol (Choi et al., 2005) (SOR: B).

Colchicine is an effective treatment for acute gout but should be used as second-line therapy when NSAIDs or corticosteroids are ineffective (SOR: C).

Allopurinol should be started for prophylaxis in patients with frequent severe attacks, nephrolithiasis, or gouty tophi (Perez-Ruiz et al., 1998) (SOR: B).

Antihyperuricemic therapy should be titrated to a dose that results in a serum urate level less than 6 mg/dL (slowly, <0.6 mg/dL/mo) (SOR: C).

Before starting allopurinol, colchicine prophylaxis can be used for up to 6 months after desired uric acid level is reached, to prevent acute attacks (SOR: C).

Pseudogout

Key Points

- Knees are the most common source of pain in pseudogout (CPDD).
- Genetic factors are present in calcium pyrophosphate deposition disease.
- Positive birefringent crystals are seen on fluid analysis in CPPD disease.
- Radiographic appearance of CPDD is punctate or linear densities in cartilage.

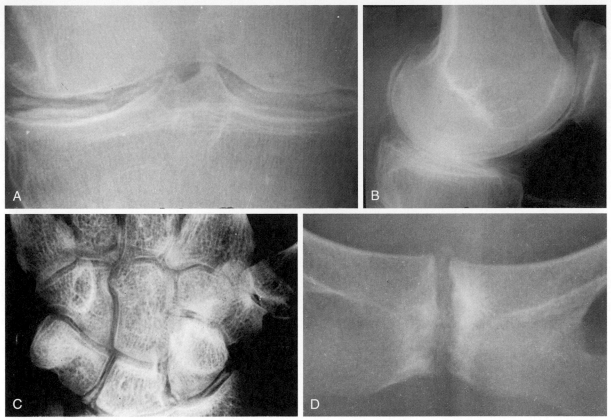

Figure 32-12 Chondrocalcinosis in calcium pyrophosphate deposition disease. **A,** Anteroposterior radiograph of knee. **B,** Lateral radiograph of knee. **C,** Anteroposterior radiograph of wrist. **D,** Radiograph of pelvis. *(From Reginato AJ, Reginato AM. Diseases associated with deposition of calcium pyrophosphate or hydroxyapatite. In Kelley WN Harris ED, Ruddy S, et al [eds]. Textbook of Rheumatology, 5th ed, vol 2. Philadelphia, Saunders, 1997, pp 1352-1367.)*

Calcium pyrophosphate deposition disease (CPDD) is known as pseudogout because of the acute goutlike attacks that CPPD crystals can cause. *Chondrocalcinosis* refers to radiographically detectable densities in cartilage and joint inflammation caused by these calcium-containing crystals. Calcium pyrophosphate (CP) crystals can be deposited not only on articular cartilage but also in ligaments, tendons, soft tissues, and synovium.

This arthritis is caused by genetic factors (autosomal dominant inheritance pattern) secondary to trauma and various metabolic diseases or is sporadic or idiopathic. CPDD is most often associated with aging, and about 4% of the adult U.S. population has articular CP crystal deposits at death (Agudelo and Wise, 2000). CPPD disease can be associated with hyperparathyroidism, hypothyroidism, hypomagnesemia, hypophosphatemia, hemochromatosis, and amyloidosis. Therefore, newly diagnosed CPDD should be followed up with serum measurements of calcium, magnesium, phosphorus, thyroid-stimulating hormone (TSH), ferritin, transferrin, serum iron, and alkaline phosphatase (ALP) levels.

The most common site is the knee, although the first MTP joint is also often affected, resulting in difficulty differentiating CPDD from gout. Any joint can be affected, however. Synovial fluid examination for rhomboid or rod-shaped, weakly positively birefringent crystals is diagnostic. Analysis needs to be done promptly after aspiration because identification of crystal diminishes over time. The crystals are also smaller and more difficult to detect, so careful preparation of the slide to avoid false-positive results must be taken. Pseudogout can also cause pseudo-RA. CPDD can be misdiagnosed as RA because of its often multiple joint involvement with symmetric distribution, morning stiffness, and elevated ESR, and because 10% of CPDD patients have positive RF tests. CPDD might also be confused with OA because of its knee and hip involvement, but it also often affects the wrists, MCP joints, elbows, and shoulders. An acute attack of CPDD can cause low-grade fever, leukocytosis (12,000 15,000/mm^3), and elevated ESR. The typical radiographic appearance of CPDD is punctate or linear densities in cartilage (chondrocalcinosis) (Fig. 32-12). Definitive diagnosis relies on either the typical radiographic signs or synovial fluid confirmation.

Treatment of acute pseudogout consists of removal of the crystals through joint aspiration, use of NSAIDs or colchicine during the acute inflammatory period, intra-articular joint injection with a glucocorticoid when possible, and a limited period of joint immobilization. No solid data support removal of crystals and prevention of crystal deposition, which are done only for diagnostic purposes and pain relief. If only one or two joints are involved, intra-articular injections may give the most symptomatic relief; if more joints are involved, a NSAID or colchicine is a better option. Because of severe pain associated with acute events, limited weight bearing may be needed for a short period while symptoms improve.

For patients with recurrent episodes of pseudogout, prophylaxis with colchicine, 0.6 mg twice daily, should be considered.

In 10 patients with recurrent attacks, colchicine was associated with a marked decrease in the number of episodes (10) in 1 year compared with the previous year (32 episodes) (Alvarellos and Spilberg, 1986).

KEY TREATMENT

Aspiration of knee joint for symptomatic relief and diagnosis of pseudogout (CPDD) (SOR: C).

The patient with CPDD receives intra-articular injection of glucocorticoid if septic joint has been ruled out and less than two joints are involved (SOR: C).

A NSAID or colchicine is prescribed for acute pain of pseudogout (SOR: C).

For recurrent pseudogout attacks, colchicine can be used for prophylaxis to decrease number of episodes (Alvarellos and Spilberg, 1986) (SOR: B).

Spondyloarthropathies

The spondyloarthropathies are a group of multisystem inflammatory disorders that affect predominantly the spine but also other joints and extra-articular tissues. Most are linked to the HLA-B27 gene, but HLA-B27 by itself does not explain the development of these diseases; pathogenesis of these conditions is still unknown. They include ankylosing spondylitis, reactive arthritis (Reiter's syndrome), psoriatic arthropathy, enteropathic arthropathy, juvenile-onset arthropathy, and undifferentiated spondyloarthropathy. Both genetic and environmental factors probably contribute to the onset and progression of these diseases. Most people with HLA-B27 do not develop these diseases, and these diseases occur in the absence of HLA-B27.

Ankylosing Spondylitis

Key Points

- Back pain and progressive stiffness are primary symptoms of this chronic inflammatory disease of axial skeleton.
- The male predominance for ankylosing spondylitis is 5:1.
- Clinical history, physical exam, and radiologic findings are key to AS diagnosis.

Primary or uncomplicated ankylosing spondylitis (AS) is a systemic inflammatory disorder predominantly affecting the sacroiliac joints and the spine. Patients with secondary AS have inflammatory bowel disease (IBD), psoriasis, or Reiter's syndrome in addition to their arthropathy. Hip and shoulder joints may also be involved in AS. Inflammation occurs at the intervertebral disk's annulus fibrosis–vertebral bone margin. This area is replaced by fibrocartilage and then ossified. Progression of this process results in the classic vertebral fusion known as *bamboo spine;* this ankylosis is a very late finding. Inflammation also occurs at the sites of ligament and tendon attachments (enthesitis) in the spine and pelvis, which become ossified.

Ankylosing spondylitis usually affects men (male/female ratio 5:1) in their 20s and 30s. It often manifests as vague, somewhat diffuse low back pain, felt generally in the buttocks or sacroiliac area but often in the lumbar area. Pain becomes more persistent and bilateral. Back stiffness after inactivity, such as on awakening, becomes more predominant and is relieved by activity or a hot shower. AS can also disturb sleep, leading to complaints of fatigue, and can be associated with systemic symptoms such as malaise, low-grade fever, and weight loss. Symptoms can be subtle, but AS should be considered if back stiffness or discomfort persists, is relieved by exercise, and occurs in a man younger than 40 years. In juvenile-onset AS, hip and shoulder symptoms might predominate first, whereas in adult AS the back is usually the first affected area. Disease progression is highly variable and can be mild and self-limited or can cause disability.

The two most common techniques to detect AS are palpation of the sacroiliac joints and assessment for spinal mobility. Decreased mobility early on is usually caused by pain and muscle spasm rather than by ankylosis. Flexion, hyperextension, axial rotation, and forward flexion should be assessed. Over time, the spine becomes increasingly stiff at an unpredictable rate, and stiffness might or might not eventually involve the entire spine.

Other extra-articular manifestations of AS include acute uveitis (iritis), aortitis, and neurologic complications resulting from cervical spine fractures from even minor trauma. Diaphragmatic breathing and limited chest excursion can be seen as a result of costovertebral involvement. The earliest radiographic abnormality can usually be seen in the sacroiliac joints, with sacroiliitis progressing to bony erosions and sclerosis (Figs. 32-13 and 32-14). These changes might also be seen at the sites of ligamentous attachments to bones. Bone scans, computed tomography (CT), and MRI should be used only if plain radiography does not confirm clinical suspicion of AS.

From 70% to 80% of AS patients report substantial relief of their symptoms with NSAIDs, the mainstay of AS therapy (Song et al., 2008). Continuous NSAID use may decrease radiographic progression of the disease (Ward, 2005). However, the benefits must be weighed against the risks associated with prolonged NSAID use. Corticosteroids have not been shown to be helpful. Physical therapy focusing on strengthening of back extensor muscles might improve functional status and, at the very least, help maintain an erect position if spinal ossification occurs (Dagfinrud et al., 2004). Patients should be encouraged to walk erectly and to keep the spine erect as much as possible, sleep on a firm mattress with the spine extended, and swim for exercise. Splints and braces do not help.

A home exercise program is better than no intervention for AS patients, and supervised group exercise is better than home exercise. Combined inpatient spa treatment and exercise (group physical exercises, walking, correction therapy, hydrotherapy, sports, sauna), followed by supervised outpatient weekly group physiotherapy, is better than weekly physiotherapy alone (Dagfinrud et al., 2004).

Second-line drug therapies include etanercept, sulfasalazine, and methotrexate, as well as topical or oral steroids for associated uveitis, in consultation with an ophthalmologist. Second-line drugs, however, have shown no clear effect on the progression of decreased spinal mobility (Dagfinrud et al., 2004). A meta-analysis indicated that all three of the anti-TNF agents were similar in efficacy for patients with AS, and that 80% of patients responded to treatment, with improved

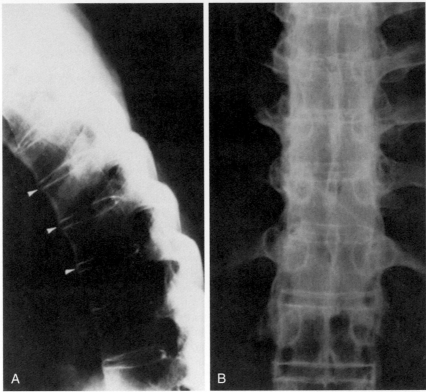

Figure 32-13 Ankylosing spondylitis. **A,** Bone erosion of dorsal aspect of thoracic spine. **B,** Classic appearance of bamboo spine. *(From Resnick D, Yu JS, Sartoris D: Imaging. In Kelley WN Harris ED, Ruddy S, et al [eds]. Textbook of Rheumatology, 5th ed, vol 1. Philadelphia, Saunders, 1997, pp 626-686.)*

global, pain, and functional assessment and reduced inflammation, based on morning stiffness (MacLeod et al., 2007). Sulfasalazine in general is only used for peripheral AS. Methotrexate, sulfasalazine, and leflunomide are ineffective for axial disease of AS.

KEY TREATMENT

NSAIDs are the recommended initial therapy for ankylosing spondylitis (Song et al., 2008) (SOR: A).

Patients with AS should initiate an exercise program (Dagfinrud et al., 2004) (SOR: B).

Systemic glucocorticoids are not recommended for AS therapy (SOR: C).

For AS patients with axial disease who do not respond to NSAIDs, anti-TNF therapy is recommended (MacLeod et al., 2007) (SOR: A).

Reactive Arthritis (Reiter's Syndrome)

Key Points

- Signs and symptoms of reactive arthritis develop within 1 month after a genitourinary or gastrointestinal infection.
- *Chlamydia* infection or common enteric bacterial infections are the primary cause of Reiter's syndrome.
- Only one third of patients with reactive arthritis will present with the classic triad of urethritis, conjunctivitis, and arthritis.

Reactive arthritis, or Reiter's syndrome, is characterized by asymmetric oligoarticular arthritis with other extraarticular manifestations within 1 month of GU or GI tract

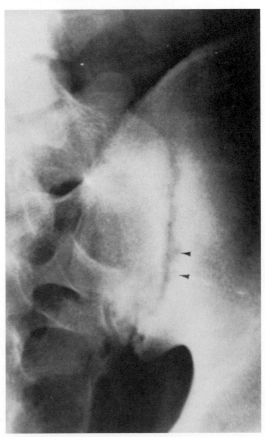

Figure 32-14 Ankylosing spondylitis. Arrows indicate sacroiliitis progressing to bony erosions and sclerosis. *(From Resnick D, Yu JS, Sartoris D. Imaging. In Kelley WN Harris ED, Ruddy S, et al [eds]. Textbook of Rheumatology, 5th ed, vol 1. Philadelphia, Saunders, 1997, pp 626-686.)*

(and possibly pulmonary) infection. The arthritis often occurs after the urethritis, uveitis, or gastroenteritis has resolved. The classic triad of nongonococcal urethritis, conjunctivitis, and arthritis is fully present clinically in only one third of patients.

Reactive arthritis occurs secondary to *Chlamydia trachomatis* and possibly *Ureaplasma urealyticum* urethritis. Urethritis is sometimes asymptomatic or, in male patients, might manifest not with a mucopurulent discharge but rather with gross hematuria secondary to a hemorrhagic cystitis. *Neisseria gonorrhoeae* infection does not cause reactive arthritis, but a septic joint, including that from gonococcal infection, must be ruled out. GI infections caused by *Shigella, Salmonella, Campylobacter, Klebsiella, Clostridium,* or *Yersinia* can all lead to reactive arthritis. By the time the gastroenteritis has resolved and arthritis has developed, the inciting bacterial agent cannot be cultured from the stool. Pulmonary infections with *Chlamydia pneumoniae* might also cause the disease (Braun et al., 1994). Conjunctivitis occurs at the same time or several days after the arthritis, if it occurs at all. The relationship between Reiter's syndrome and HIV infection is most likely caused by HIV's association with *Chlamydia* and enteric bacterial infections rather than by HIV itself. Two thirds of patients with reactive arthritis are HLA-B27 positive, indicating genetic factors as well as infectious causes.

Reactive arthritis usually affects several joints, most often in the lower extremity (knees, ankles, feet). Common sites are entheses (where ligaments attach to bones), in particular the Achilles tendon attachment, which causes heel pain. Extra-articular manifestations of reactive arthritis include oral ulcers, aortitis, keratoderma blennorrhagicum (a papulosquamous skin rash occurring most commonly on the palms and soles), and balanitis circinata.

Reactive arthritis usually resolves within 1 year. Although there is no cure, the underlying illness should be treated. When *Chlamydia* is suspected, patients might be given doxycycline or an analogue for up to 3 months, but the optimal duration of therapy is unknown (Mandell et al., 2004). Antibiotics might limit recurrences as well as shorten the course after an episode of urethritis; however, antibiotic use following enteric infections has not been shown to affect the course of reactive arthritis. Reactive arthritis is treated with NSAIDs or intra-articular corticosteroid injections acutely and subsequently with sulfasalazine, 1 g two or three times daily, or methotrexate, 7.5 to 25 mg weekly. No specific studies using anti-TNF therapy have been done, but antidotal research indicates it may be helpful. Long-term disability is uncommon but is usually caused by chronic foot or heel pain or vision problems.

> **KEY TREATMENT**
>
> NSAIDs are the mainstay of treatment for symptomatic reactive arthritis but do not alter or shorten its course (SOR: C).
> Intra-articular injections can be helpful and are not contraindicated in Reiter's syndrome (SOR: C).
> When there is unsatisfactory response to NSAIDs or steroid injections, a trial of sulfasalazine is suggested for patients with reactive arthritis (SOR: C).
> For patients with contraindications or intolerance to sulfasalazine, a trial of etanercept can be attempted (SOR: C).

Psoriatic Arthritis

> **Key Points**
>
> - Psoriatic arthritis affects 5% to 7% of psoriasis patients.
> - Arthritis can occur before or after psoriatic lesions.
> - Obtaining family history for psoriasis is important in those without current diagnosis and active psoriatic lesions.

Psoriatic arthritis is seen in approximately 5% to 7% of psoriasis patients, but it might affect up to 40% of hospitalized patients with extensive psoriatic lesions (Cuellar et al., 1994). The associated inflammatory peripheral arthritis might be monoarticular, asymmetric oligoarticular, or symmetric polyarticular, resembling RA. RF is usually absent. Psoriatic arthritis is associated with multiple HLA genes; environmental factors such as infections and physical trauma likely are also involved.

Psoriatic skin lesions predate arthritis in 70% of patients, occur with arthritis in 15%, and follow arthritis in 15%. Family history of psoriasis is therefore important for diagnosis in patients with an arthritis similar to psoriatic but without a known history. Psoriatic arthritis often manifests initially as an asymmetric monoarticular or oligoarticular arthritis of a large joint, such as a knee, evolving into asymmetric polyarticular arthritis. The distribution of involvement of psoriatic arthritis might resemble RA but involves the DIP joints more often, as well as causing enthesitis. Psoriatic arthritis might also cause spondylitis, sacroiliitis, chest wall pain from enthesitis, arthritis mutilans (destruction of phalanges and metacarpals, causing telescoping of fingers), conjunctivitis, and Achilles tendon and plantar fascia involvement. Radiographic abnormalities include marginal erosions at DIP and PIP joints, with new bone formation.

In addition to treating the psoriatic skin lesions, the arthritis is treated first with NSAIDs, followed by DMARDs for widespread disease and corticosteroid injections if only one or two joints are involved (Cuellar et al., 1994). A Cochrane analysis showed that high-dose methotrexate and sulfasalazine have efficacy in psoriatic arthritis (Jones et al., 2000). Azathioprine, etretinate, low-dose methotrexate, and colchicines all had some effectiveness versus placebo, but more studies are necessary. Anti-TNF medications are also used if patients continue to have symptoms despite DMARD treatment or if axial disease is present and NSAIDs have not worked. A meta-analysis of RCTs showed that anti-TNF drugs are effective against psoriatic arthritis (Saad et al., 2008). When contemplating local steroid joint injection the physician should keep in mind that bacterial colonization of psoriatic skin lesions with streptococcus or staphylococcus is common. Injecting through skin lesions should therefore be avoided.

> **KEY TREATMENT**
>
> NSAIDs are the first line of treatment for psoriatic arthritis (Cuellar et al., 1994) (SOR: B).
> Methotrexate and sulfasalazine have proven efficacy in the treatment of psoriatic arthritis (Jones et al., 2000) (SOR: B); used as second-line agents if inadequate response to NSAIDs.
> Patients with axial disease or who have peripheral disease without improvement to DMARD treatments are candidates for anti-TNF medications, which have proven efficacy (Saad et al., 2008) (SOR: A).

Enteropathic Arthropathy

There seems to be a connection between the gut and spondyloarthropathies. Of patients with inflammatory bowel disease (IBD; ulcerative colitis and Cohn's disease), 10% to 20% have a peripheral arthritis different from other defined arthritides. Migratory arthralgias, especially of the knees, ankles, and feet, often coincide with periods of GI disease flares. Other joints, including the spine and sacroiliac joints, might be involved but are seemingly less coincident with bowel exacerbations. HLA-B27 is found in 50% of patients with IBD-associated spondylitis but is not found in a higher percentage than in the general population for this type of spondylitis. RF and ANA are negative. NSAIDs are normally used but must be taken with caution given the patient's underlying GI disease. As noted earlier, dietary factors might increase the patient's baseline inflammatory state, so a trial of dietary manipulation or the addition of omega-3 fatty acids is reasonable.

Infectious Arthritis

Septic Arthritis

Key Points

- The knee is the most common source of infectious arthritic pain.
- Septic arthritis is a surgical emergency.
- *Staphylococcus aureus* and *Neisseria gonorrhoeae* are the two most common causes.

Acute bacterial arthritis is one of the few rheumatologic emergencies. Failure by the primary care physician to diagnose this entity and to initiate prompt antibiotic therapy results in significant morbidity (functional disability, joint destruction) and at least 5% mortality. Even in patients with known rheumatologic disease, a bacterial infection may cause an acutely inflamed joint. The three mechanisms of a septic joint are (1) hematogenous spread from a distant location, such as a urinary tract infection (UTI) or pneumonia; (2) contiguous spread from a wound infection, abscess, or osteomyelitis; and (3) direct introduction of bacteria through trauma, surgery, or arthrocentesis. Concern about the third mechanism should not prevent the family physician from ruling out bacterial infection by performing synovial fluid analysis in an inflamed joint if the diagnosis is unclear. As for lumbar puncture, if the physician thinks it should, arthrocentesis probably should be done.

From 80% to 90% of acute bacterial articular infections are monoarticular. In adults with nongonococcal bacterial arthritis, the most common sites are the knee (50%), hip (20%), shoulders (8%), ankles (7%), wrists (7%), elbow (6%), other (5%), and more than one joint (usually two; 12%) (Brusch, 2005). In children, the most common sites are the knee (40%), hip (28%), ankle (14%), shoulder (4%), wrist (3%), elbow (11%), other (3%), and more than one joint (7%) (Baker and Schumacher, 1993). About 20% of patients are afebrile. Septic joints are normally painful, swollen, red, and warm. Diabetes mellitus, malignancy, chronic liver disease, and other rheumatic diseases (e.g., RA, SLE) increase the risk of a septic joint and probably its severity. Other risk factors for a septic joint include advanced age, intravenous drug abuse, HIV infection, and having a prosthetic joint. Almost half of adults with septic arthritis are older than 60 years, and the condition usually affects an arthritic hip, knee, or shoulder. Septic arthritis in older adults causes a fever in only 10% of patients and a marked leukocytosis in only one third, although ESR elevation is usually marked. Joint and blood cultures are usually positive.

Most polyarticular disease is seen in immunosuppressed patients or those with underlying rheumatic disease. The causative organism is usually *Staphylococcus aureus*. The mortality rate in patients with polyarticular septic joints approaches 40% (Youssef and York, 1994).

Most cases of septic arthritis are secondary to hematogenous spread of infection. In drug abusers, the causative organism is usually *S. aureus* or gram-negative organisms and affects predominantly the joints of the axial skeleton (hip, shoulder, vertebrae, symphysis pubis, costochondral, sternoclavicular, sacroiliac). Iatrogenic septic arthritis is usually caused by *S. aureus*, *Staphylococcus epidermidis*, and gram-negative organisms. This complication might be difficult to recognize because the joint is already symptomatic (which prompted the arthroscopy or arthrocentesis) before infection. Bacterial infection after arthroscopy is 0.04% to 4% and after arthrocentesis, 0.01%. Septic arthritis complicating RA is polyarticular in 50% of patients, usually caused by *S. aureus*, and arises from pulmonary or UTIs, infected rheumatoid nodules, or foot infections. Prosthetic infections are from direct inoculation or hematogenous spread; the prosthesis often must be removed.

Septic arthritis in children normally involves the lower extremities (knee, hip, and ankle). An infant or child with a septic joint often presents with not moving the infected joint and being generally irritable. Septic arthritis can complicate otitis media, an umbilical catheter, meningitis, or osteomyelitis. *S. aureus* and group B streptococci are the most common organisms in infants and children, except ages 6 months to 2 years, when *Haemophilus influenzae* and *Kingella kingae* organisms predominate. *H. influenzae* septic arthritis is seen especially in partially immunized children.

The most common form of acute bacterial arthritis is disseminated gonococcal infection, which causes a migratory polyarthritis and tenosynovitis, affecting predominantly the small joints of the hands, wrists, elbow, ankles, and knees. Papules and vesicles are often apparent on the trunk and extremities, including the palms and soles. Patients usually do not have symptoms of urethritis, cervicitis, or pharyngitis. If gonococcal arthritis is suspected, empiric treatment should be initiated immediately while culture results are pending. *Neisseria meningitidis* can cause a similar arthritis-rash syndrome following an illness, ranging from a mild upper respiratory infection to a frank meningitis. In contrast to gonococcal infections, the meningococcus might cause oral mucosal lesions as well as skin lesions.

Acute gonococcal arthritis can be confirmed by Gram stain in only 25% of patients and by culture in 50%; nongonococcal bacterial arthritis can be confirmed in 50% and 90% of patients, respectively. It is therefore important to make a clinical diagnosis rather than rely solely on laboratory studies. Fever is often absent or of low grade. Blood cultures are also positive only approximately half the time but might be positive when synovial fluid cultures fail to identify an organism. Synovial fluid analysis usually shows WBC count over $50,000/mm^3$, with over 90% PMNs. Crystals can coexist with bacterial infections, and their presence should not rule out bacterial infection. Plain radiography might detect an osteomyelitis and should be done as a baseline study, because destruction can be seen on radiographs 10 to 14 days later. Air in the joint suggests an anaerobic infection, which accounts for 1% of septic joints.

The duration of appropriate intravenous (IV) antibiotic treatment depends on the presumptive or culture-identified causative organism. Initial therapy depends on the Gram stain result from synovial fluid. If gram-positive cocci are seen, IV vancomycin should be started empirically. If gram-negative bacilli are seen, a third-generation IV cephalosporin should be initiated. If Gram stain is negative, IV vancomycin should be considered. Once sensitivity data return, antibiotic therapy can be narrowed appropriately. Duration varies, but often the patient will receive 2 weeks of IV therapy followed by 2 weeks of oral therapy. Intra-articular antibiotic injections are unnecessary. A joint might need repeated needle aspirations or tidal lavage with arthroscopy to sterilize the joint space (Klippel, 2001).

KEY TREATMENT

Empiric treatment of infectious arthritis with appropriate IV antibiotics is based on Gram stain results; joint and blood culture sensitivities narrow the antibiotic regimen (SOR: C).
Joints may need drainage in patients with septic arthritis (SOR: C).

Viral Arthritis

See the discussion online at www.expertconsult.com.

Lyme Arthritis

Key Points

- *Borrelia burgdorferi* is the most common source of Lyme disease.
- Lyme titer is diagnostic but might have a high false-negative ratio.
- False-positive titers can be caused by RA or lupus.
- About 80% of Lyme disease patients have classic erythema migrans rash.

Lyme disease is caused by the *Ixodes* tick-borne spirochete *Borrelia burgdorferi* and was first described in 1975 after an apparent outbreak of juvenile RA in Lyme, Connecticut. The characteristic target rash of erythema migrans (EM) develops within 1 month (mean 1 week) of a tick bite and can be complicated by CNS disease (meningitis, neuritis), cardiac disease (atrioventricular conduction blocks), and arthritis. It occurs most often in northeastern states (New York, Connecticut, Massachusetts, New Jersey, Rhode Island, Pennsylvania) and upper midwestern states (Wisconsin, Minnesota). As with other rheumatologic diseases, Lyme disease is a clinical diagnosis, with laboratory tests used only to clarify the diagnosis.

Although most patients with Lyme disease do not recall an actual tick bite, most (80%) manifest the EM rash, which might be confluent or have central clearing or darkening. This rash may enlarge quickly and may be accompanied by arthralgia, myalgia, fatigue, fever, and chills. Weeks to months after the EM rash, neurologic involvement can occur. A facial nerve palsy is common, although most facial nerve palsies are not caused by Lyme disease, even in endemic areas. As with neurologic signs, carditis might be the first presenting symptom, often manifesting as a first-, second-, or third-degree atrioventricular block or bundle branch block. Cardiac symptoms normally do not occur for 1 to 2 months after onset of symptoms.

Arthritis can occur in approximately half of untreated Lyme patients but is rare in treated patients. Rheumatic symptoms occurring late in the clinical course include polyarthralgias, a migratory polyarthritis, or an oligoarticular arthritis with few systemic symptoms. In those untreated patients developing an arthritis, some develop a chronic arthritis resistant to antibiotics.

Laboratory Studies

The current recommended approach is a two-tier strategy using a sensitive enzyme-linked immunosorbent assay (ELISA) and, if positive, Western blot. ELISA is associated with a high false-positive rate, so all positive results must be confirmed with a positive Western blot. Western blot can test for both immunoglobulin M (IgM) and IgG antibodies to *B. burgdorferi*. IgM antibodies typically appear within 1 to 2 weeks and IgG in 2 to 6 weeks, after onset of EM rash. Only one third of patients with a single lesion of EM are seropositive at diagnosis (Verdon and Sigal, 1997). The presence of EM is itself enough to make the clinical diagnosis, and testing is not required. Negative serology in a suspected case should be followed by acute- and convalescent-phase samples (2-4 weeks after initial sample). False-positive ELISA test results can occur in RA, juvenile rheumatoid arthritis (JRA), SLE, and infectious mononucleosis. Serologic testing after treatment is not helpful because seroreactivity persists long after successful treatment.

Treatment

Treatment of early Lyme disease in adults includes doxycycline, 100 mg twice daily, or amoxicillin, 500 mg three times daily, for 21 days. Amoxicillin is first-line therapy in children less than 8 years old; cefuroxime axetil or erythromycin is used in cases of doxycycline or amoxicillin allergy (Worsmer et al., 2006). Oral therapy is as effective as IV therapy for patients with either early Lyme disease or Lyme arthritis and is less costly (Eckman et al., 1997). Concern about the risk of late neurologic sequelae should not lead to more aggressive treatment with IV antibiotics for these patients (Wormser et al., 2000). Early treatment prevents recurrent arthritis as well as neurologic and cardiac sequelae. IV therapy with ceftriaxone (Rocephin), cefotaxime (Claforan), or penicillin G is used for early disseminated and late Lyme disease. IV antibiotic therapy is preferable for patients with neurologic symptoms, with the possible exception of those with facial palsy alone (Steere, 1989). Most patients are symptomatically better with 20 days of treatment. Continued symptomatology in patients with treated infection does not respond to further antibiotics (Klippel, 2001). Antibiotic treatment failures can occur but are rare and usually associated with poor absorption. Antibiotic resistance to typically used agents has not been shown.

For preventive measures against Lyme disease, see the online discussion at www.expertconsult.com.

For preventive measures against Lyme disease, see the online discussion at www.expertconsult.com.

KEY TREATMENT

Adults and children 8 years and older should be treated with oral doxycycline for 21 days for early Lyme disease (Worsmer et el., 2006) (SOR: A).

Pregnant women and children younger than 8 years should be treated with oral amoxicillin or cefuroxime (SOR: C).

Patients with neurologic (excluding isolated facial nerve palsy) or cardiac manifestation are treated with IV antibiotic therapy for Lyme disease (Wormser et al., 2000) (SOR: B).

Other Infectious Arthritides

Although mycobacteria, parasites, and fungi rarely cause arthritis, incidence has increased with increasing numbers of HIV/AIDS and other immunosuppressed patients. *Mycobacterium tuberculosis* arthritis occurs by hematogenous spread from the lung and is diagnosed by synovial fluid culture. The classic tuberculosis infection involves the spine and is known as Pott's disease. Thoracic vertebrae are most often involved, but a monoarticular arthritis can also occur in large, weight-bearing joints. Mild arthritides might also be caused by *Giardia lamblia* infection, histoplasmosis, cryptococcosis, blastomycosis, sporotrichosis, coccidioidomycosis, actinomycetes, and atypical mycobacteria.

Rheumatic Fever

Key Points

- Rheumatic fever is seen 2 to 4 weeks after beta-hemolytic streptococcal pharyngitis.
- Antibiotic treatment for streptococcal infection can help prevent development of rheumatic fever.

The Jones criteria and antistreptolysin O titers are helpful in diagnosis of rheumatic fever.

Rheumatic fever is a systemic inflammatory process initiated by group A beta-hemolytic streptococcal pharyngitis. Often, younger children in particular do not recall antecedent pharyngitis, which usually occurs 2 to 4 weeks before symptom onset. Rheumatic fever appears to be linked only to pharyngitis; group A streptococcal (GAS) impetigo does not seem to be associated with rheumatic fever. Rheumatic fever most often affects children 4 to 9 years of age, and onset is usually characterized by an acute febrile illness that can cause large-joint migratory arthritis, CNS involvement (Sydenham's chorea), characteristic rash, and carditis with inflammation of heart valves and subsequent damage. Antibiotic treatment of GAS pharyngitis greatly reduces development of rheumatic fever. The 1992 revised Jones criteria are useful in the diagnosis of acute rheumatic fever (Table 32-6).

Rheumatic fever–related arthritis is often preceded by arthralgias out of proportion to frank swelling, lasting approximately 1 week. Arthralgias usually migrate to lower extremity joints and then to the upper extremities. Children experience this arthritis less frequently than adolescents and adults. The arthritis then resolves spontaneously. Carditis involving the valves, particularly the mitral valve, is the most severe sequela. Rheumatic heart disease is the most common serious sequela and usually occurs 10 to 20 years after the original attack. Patients might also have erythema marginatum, a rash with open or closed ring lesions with sharp outer edges or macular rings with pale centers, or both. The rash spreads centrifugally from the trunk to the extremities with lesions that come and go.

The antistreptolysin O (ASO) titer is the most useful laboratory test, because pharyngeal cultures are often negative by the time rheumatic fever develops. The ASO titer rises 4 to 5 weeks after the onset of GAS pharyngitis, or 2 to 3 weeks after development of rheumatic fever. Because only 80% of patients with rheumatic fever develop an increase in ASO titer, clinically suspicious rheumatic fever with a negative ASO titer should be followed up by testing for antistreptococcal antibody, such as anti-DNase, anti-DNase B, and anti-hyaluronidase antibody tests.

Aspirin is the drug of choice for acute rheumatic fever and usually results in a dramatic response. The usual dose is 80 to 100 mg/kg/day for children and 4 to 8 g/day for adults. Penicillin should also be given for a 10-day course whether or not pharyngitis is present, and family members and other close contacts should be cultured and treated if necessary. Intramuscular (IM) penicillin is more effective than oral (PO) penicillin in clinical trials. No benefit has been shown from IV immune globulin (IVIG) or corticosteroids for rheumatic fever, but studies continue (Manyemba and Mightosi, 2004).

Patients who have had documented rheumatic fever and who develop subsequent GAS pharyngitis are at high risk for a recurrent rheumatic episode and thus at increased risk for worsening rheumatic heart disease. For this reason, prevention of recurrent episodes requires continuous antimicrobial prophylaxis (Gerber et al., 2009). Before prophylaxis initiation, a full treatment course for GAS pharyngitis should be completed. In the United States,

Table 32-6 Revised Jones Criteria for Diagnosis of Acute Rheumatic Fever*

Major Manifestations	Minor Manifestations
Carditis	*Clinical:*
Polyarthritis	Arthralgia, fever
Chorea	*Laboratory:*
Erythema marginatum	Elevated acute-phase reactants (ESR, CRP)
Subcutaneous nodules	Prolonged PR interval

Plus:
Supporting evidence of antecedent group A streptococcal infection
   Positive throat culture or rapid streptococcal antigen test
   Elevated or rising streptococcal antibody titer

From Gibofsky A, Zabriskie JB. Rheumatic fever. In Klippel JH (ed). Primer on the Rheumatic Diseases, 12th ed. Atlanta, Arthritis Foundation, 2001, p 282.

*If supported by evidence of preceding group A streptococcal infection, the presence of two major manifestations or of one major and two minor manifestations indicates a high probability of acute rheumatic fever.

ESR, Erythrocyte sedimentation rate; *CRP,* C-reactive protein.

typical prophylactic therapy is with long-acting IM ben-zathine penicillin G every 4 weeks until early adulthood (about 18 years of age).

KEY TREATMENT

Patients with acute group A streptococcal pharyngitis should receive antibiotic therapy to help prevent the complication of acute rheumatic fever (Denny et al., 1950) (SOR: B).

Patients with acute rheumatic fever should receive appropriate antibiotic therapy to eradicate the GAS infection, regardless of whether pharyngitis is present at diagnosis (SOR: C).

Use of aspirin is the treatment of choice for the acute symptoms of acute rheumatic fever (SOR: C).

Prevention of recurrent acute rheumatic fever requires prophy-lactic treatment for GAS pharyngitis with antibiotics (Gerber et al., 2009) (SOR: A).

Systemic Lupus Erythematosus

Key Points

- The 5-year survival rate of SLE patients is 90%.
- The female/male ratio is 2:1 before and 4:1 after puberty.
- Four of 11 criteria are needed for SLE diagnosis.

Systemic lupus erythematosus is a generalized autoimmune disease of unknown cause characterized by the production of antibodies to numerous antigens. The most common antibodies found in SLE are those directed against the cell nucleus (ANAs). These antibodies bind DNA, RNA, nuclear proteins, and protein-DNA or protein-RNA complexes. Antibodies to double-stranded DNA and an RNA-protein complex called Sm are found almost exclusively in SLE. Immune complex deposition results in inflammation and vasculitis, causing multiorgan pathology.

Systemic LE is most common in women of reproductive age (15-40 years), and the female/male ratio is approximately 2:1 before puberty and 4:1 after puberty. However, SLE can be seen in all ages, including infants and older adults; in these two subpopulations, the female/male ratio is only 2:1. SLE affects approximately 1 in 1000 to 2500 in the general population, but disease incidence in African American and Latino women is much higher (up to 1 in 250 in African American women ages 18-65 years). The 5-year survival after diagnosis is 90%.

Systemic LE also shows a strong familial tendency. An association with MHC genes *DR2*, *DR3*, *DR4*, and *DR5* has been found. As with other rheumatologic diseases, SLE appears to result from a genetic abnormality that can be triggered by environmental factors. Some of these hypothesized factors include infections, stress (neuroendocrine changes), exposure to sunlight, diet, and toxins, including drugs. In addition to autoantibody production, SLE involves immune cell (B, T, monocyte) abnormalities. Because of the wide variety of presentations, ACR created a classification system to standardize the diagnosis of SLE (Box 32-3). To confirm a diagnosis of SLE, patients must have at least 4 of 11 criteria present either serially or simultaneously.

Box 32-3 Criteria for Classification of Systemic Lupus Erythematosus*

1. *Malar rash.* Fixed erythema, flat or raised, over the malar eminences, tending to spare the nasolabial folds.
2. *Discoid rash.* Erythematous raised patches with adherent keratotic scaling and follicular plugging; atrophic scarring may occur in older lesions.
3. *Photosensitivity.* Skin rash as a result of unusual reaction to sunlight, by patient history or physician observation.
4. *Oral ulcers.* Oral or nasopharyngeal ulceration, usually painless, observed by a physician.
5. *Arthritis.* Nonerosive arthritis involving two or more peripheral joints, characterized by tenderness, swelling, or effusion.
6. *Serositis*
   a. Pleuritis—convincing history of pleuritic pain or rub heard by a physician or evidence of pleural effusion *or*
   b. Pericarditis—documented by electrocardiogram or rub or evidence of pericardial effusion.
7. *Renal disorder*
   a. Persistent proteinuria higher than 0.5 g/day or higher than 3+ if quantitation not performed *or*
   b. Cellular casts: may be red cell, hemoglobin, granular, tubular, or mixed.
8. Neurologic disorder
   a. Seizures—in the absence of offending drugs or known metabolic derangements (e.g., uremia, ketoacidosis, electrolyte imbalance) *or*
   b. Psychosis: in the absence of offending drugs or known metabolic derangements (e.g., uremia, ketoacidosis, electrolyte imbalance).
9. *Hematologic disorder*
   a. Hemolytic anemia—with reticulocytosis *or*
   b. Leukopenia—less than 4000/mm3 total on two or more occasions *or*
   c. Lymphopenia—less than 1500/mm3 on two or more occasions *or*
   d. Thrombocytopenia—less than 100,000/mm3 in the absence of offending drugs.
10. Immunologic disorder
    a. Positive lupus erythematosus cell preparation *or*
    b. Anti-DNA: antibody to native DNA in abnormal titer *or*
    c. Anti-Sm: presence of antibody to Sm nuclear antigen *or*
    d. False-positive serologic test for syphilis known to be positive for at least 6 months and confirmed by *Treponema pallidum* immobilization or fluorescent treponemal antibody absorption test.
11. *Antinuclear antibody.* An abnormal titer of antinuclear antibody by immunofluorescence or an equivalent assay at any point in time and in the absence of drugs known to be associated with "drug-induced lupus" syndrome.

From Tan EM, Cohen AS, Fries JF, et al. The 1982 revised criteria for the classification of systemic lupus erythematosus (SLE). Arthritis Rheum 1982;25:1271-1277, with permission of the American College of Rheumatology.

*The proposed classification is based on 11 criteria. For the purpose of identifying patients in clinical studies, a person is said to have systemic lupus erythematosus if any four or more of the 11 criteria are present, serially or simultaneously, during any interval of observation.

Clinical Features

Constitutional symptoms found in patients with SLE include fatigue, malaise, fever, and weight loss. The family physician therefore has an important role to play in the diagnosis of this multisystem disease, which must be differentiated from infections such as HIV (which often is false positive in SLE) and subacute bacterial endocarditis; other connective tissue diseases such as vasculitis, RA, and mixed connective tissue disease; and malignancies such as lymphomas. SLE is characterized by specific organ system abnormalities. The disease most often affects the skin, joints, kidneys, CNS, GI tract, and lungs, with a spectrum of disease severity and an unpredictable course. SLE is truly systemic; other asymptomatic organ involvement must be searched for during active periods of disease, regardless of the presenting sign or symptom.

Mucocutaneous Manifestations

More than 90% of SLE patients eventually have a mucocutaneous manifestation. The classic malar butterfly rash gave lupus its name, because it was thought to resemble the bite of the wolf. This rash is present in only one third of patients; when it occurs, it is often after sunlight exposure. One third to two thirds of SLE patients are extremely photosensitive. Sun exposure not only can cause a maculopapular, erythematous rash but also can induce a flare of systemic symptoms. Other lesions can occur, such as bullae or generalized erythema.

Subacute cutaneous lupus erythematosus (SCLE) occurs in sun-exposed areas of the skin, particularly on the upper torso, in two forms—annular or papulosquamous lesions. The former variant might be confused with erythema annulare and the latter with psoriasis or lichen planus. About 70% of patients with photosensitivity have anti-Ro antibodies (Boumpas et al., 1995). SCLE lesions do not result in scarring. Discoid lupus lesions are raised plaques that often occur in the absence of any other systemic manifestations, most often on the face, neck, scalp, and external ears. Unlike SCLE lesions, these erythematous plaques with heavy scales can cause scarring, with a hypopigmented, atrophic central area. Other mucocutaneous manifestations of SLE include alopecia, which resolves when the acute SLE exacerbation ends, unless the alopecia is secondary to discoid scarring. Oral, nasal, and vaginal ulcerations as well as palpable purpura also occur.

Latent lupus refers to the condition of those patients who do not meet the ACR criteria for diagnosis of SLE but have many features consistent with lupus. This form is mild and is treated symptomatically. Many of these patients never develop classic SLE; there are no identifiable prognostic indicators of propensity for progression to frank lupus.

Drug-induced lupus occurs when a patient taking a drug develops clinical and serologically consistent lupus, which then resolves (clinically and then serologically) on discontinuation of the drug. Drugs known or suspected to cause lupus include *antituberculous* drugs (e.g., isoniazid, streptomycin), *antibiotics* (e.g., penicillin, tetracycline, sulfa, griseofulvin), *anticonvulsants* (e.g., phenytoin [Dilantin], ethosuximide [Zarontin], carbamazepine [Tegretol]), *phenothiazines* (e.g., perphenazine [Trilafon], promethazine [Phenergan], thioridazine [Mellaril]), and *antihypertensives* (e.g., hydralazine, methyldopa, reserpine), as well as oral contraceptives, lithium, propylthiouracil, and procainamide. Symptoms are usually mild and do not involve the CNS or kidneys.

Musculoskeletal Manifestations

Arthralgias and arthritis are the most common initial symptoms of SLE. The typical pattern is symmetric involvement of the hands, wrists, or knees, either migratory or persisting in an involved joint. There may be subcutaneous nodules similar to those of RA, but SLE usually does not cause RA-like erosions. Subluxations causing swan neck deformities and other deformities in the hands are known as *Jaccoud's arthropathy,* characterized by deformity without erosion of bone and cartilage. SLE patients sometimes experience myalgias but usually not to the degree seen in dermatomyositis.

Musculoskeletal complications of SLE also include osteoporosis and avascular necrosis of bone (osteonecrosis), especially in corticosteroid-treated children with SLE. In one study, 65% of premenopausal women with SLE had abnormal bone mineral density (Petri, 1995). Screening for osteoporosis, even in premenopausal women, and treatment, if indicated, are therefore prudent measures, as is minimizing the use of corticosteroids. Late SLE can cause osteonecrosis, particularly of the hip, independent of active SLE episodes. Major risk factors for osteonecrosis include a prednisone dosage higher than 20 mg/day for 1 month or longer and the presence of Raynaud's disease or vasculitis. Avascular necrosis of the hip is diagnosed early by MRI.

Renal Disease

Called *lupus nephritis,* SLE-induced renal disease is typically asymptomatic until relatively late. More than 50% of all patients and 75% of African American patients with SLE have renal involvement. Immune complex deposition along the glomerular basement membrane leads to the nephrotic syndrome or renal failure, which can be the presenting sign. An elevated serum creatinine level can be found, as well as proteinuria, hematuria, pyuria, and casts in the absence of infection. Definitively diagnosed by renal biopsy, lupus nephritis constitutes a spectrum of severity from mild to more severe that involves mesangial, focal proliferative, diffuse proliferative, and advanced sclerosing forms of glomerulonephritis (Petri, 1998). SLE patients should have an annual urinalysis and renal function test to rule out proteinuria. An elevated creatinine level (>2 mg/dL) is the best predictor of prognosis. Patients with SLE have had successful renal transplants, although lupus nephritis can recur.

Neuropsychiatric Disease

Neuropsychiatric symptoms are common when SLE is active but can occur in isolation. Manifestations include headache, generalized seizures (20% of SLE patients), stroke, cranial and peripheral neuropathies, psychosis, severe depression (40%), cognitive abnormalities, and organic brain syndrome. Cranial neuropathies may manifest as visual defects, tinnitus, vertigo, nystagmus, ptosis, or facial palsies. A migraine-type headache is common and can be intractable. *Neuropsychiatric lupus* is a diagnosis of exclusion, after other causes of the patient's symptoms have been ruled out. Electroencephalographic findings are often abnormal but nonspecific. MRI of the head can show diffuse, small focal areas of increased signal density on the cerebral white matter and cortical gray matter that clear with corticosteroid treatment. Cerebrospinal fluid (CSF) studies are important to rule out infectious causes. Even in long-term mild disease, neurocognitive abnormalities affecting memory or causing speech abnormalities often persist. Antiribosomal P antibody presence correlates with cognitive impairment in SLE (Hirohata and Nakanishi, 2001).

Cardiovascular Manifestations

Patients with SLE have an increased risk of premature atherosclerosis from the disease itself as well as from its treatment; up to 40% of SLE patients have been found to have this complication in screening studies. Corticosteroids increase cardiac risk factors such as weight, BP, cholesterol, and homocysteine levels, which the family physician must keep in mind. Primary coronary disease prevention monitoring and patient education plans for the SLE patient are important, because the mortality from myocardial infarction is approximately 10 times that in an age- and gender-matched population (Klippel, 2001). Myocarditis and endocarditis are rare, but pericarditis can occur in up to 45% of SLE patients (25% in most series). Symptoms might be mild or severe, but constrictive pericarditis and cardiac tamponade are rare.

Thrombosis is a major cause of morbidity and mortality in lupus patients. Between 30% and 50% of SLE patients make antiphospholipid autoantibodies to the phospholipid part of the normal cell membrane, although most people with these antibodies do not have lupus. Types of antiphospholipid antibodies include anticardiolipin antibody, β2-GP-I antibody and lupus anticoagulant. Lupus anticoagulant antibodies might result in prolonged partial thromboplastin time (PTT) and prothrombin time (PT) but paradoxically result in an increased risk of thrombotic events for these patients. This might be caused by an antibody-induced vasculopathy. Anticardiolipin and β2-GP-I antibodies can be detected using ELISA, but there is no direct testing for the lupus anticoagulant. If the lupus anticoagulant is clinically suspected but activated PTT is normal, more sensitive coagulation tests should be done, including kaolin clotting time (KCT), modified Russell viper venom time (RVVT), and platelet neutralization procedure (PNP) (Petri, 1994).

Antiphospholipid antibody syndrome is defined as the presence of lupus anticoagulant, β2-GP-I antibody or anticardiolipin antibody with one of these four entities: arterial thrombosis, venous thrombosis, recurrent first-trimester or one late (second- or third-trimester) spontaneous abortion, or thrombocytopenia. This acquired autoimmune hypercoagulability is more common in SLE patients than in the general population.

The incidence of spontaneous abortion, intrauterine death, and prematurity is also increased in women with SLE alone. Studies differ, but currently pregnancy is not thought to exacerbate SLE, as formerly thought. It is recommended that women be flare free for 6 months and do not have serious comorbidities such as renal disease before deciding to become pregnant. Fertility is apparently not affected by SLE. Women with either recurrent first-trimester or late pregnancy loss can reduce their risk of pregnancy loss with heparin and low-dose aspirin therapy.

Other Manifestations

Serositis that causes pericarditis, pleurisy, and peritonitis is common in SLE. Bilateral pleural effusions are usually small and are seen most often in drug-induced lupus patients and in older adult patients. Pleurisy is clinically more common than pericarditis, which rarely becomes severe enough to be constrictive.

Systemic LE can cause multiple GI symptoms such as nausea, vomiting, anorexia, and abdominal pain, often as a result of peritoneal inflammation. Mesenteric vasculitis can cause lower abdominal pain and rectal bleeding. Hepatomegaly with increases in liver enzyme levels and pancreatitis with amylase level elevations can occur with SLE. In addition to hepatomegaly, splenomegaly and lymphadenopathy can occur with lupus exacerbations.

Lung involvement can include pulmonary hemorrhage, pulmonary hypertension, and pneumonitis. *Lupus pneumonitis* often manifests as a diffuse interstitial disease. *Shrinking lung syndrome,* seen in late SLE, is a restrictive condition with decreased lung volumes resulting from abnormal musculoskeletal respiratory function.

Laboratory Abnormalities

There are no specific tests for lupus. The lupus erythematosus cell, formed when complexes of nuclei and antibodies are phagocytosed by PMNs, is highly specific but of low sensitivity. ANA, anti–double-stranded DNA, and antiphospholipid antibody are all markers for SLE, but antibody test results are misleading if not considered in the clinical context. From 2% to 5% of patients with SLE are ANA negative, whereas 5% of the normal population and up to 20% of healthy young women are ANA positive (Fritzler et al., 1985). Antibodies to an RNA-protein complex called Sm (anti-Smith antibody) and to double-stranded DNA (dsDNA) are almost unique for SLE, both being 95% specific. ESR is normally increased, whereas CRP is normal (Linares et al., 1986).

Autoantibodies in SLE include ANA and anticytoplasmic antibodies (including lipoproteins), antibodies against blood cells, antibodies against various organs and structures (e.g., gastric mucosa, neurons, muscle sarcolemma, thyroglobulin), and antibodies against collagen. Different antibodies against different parts of the cell nucleus appear as the four patterns of ANA staining. These include membranous antibodies against single-stranded DNA, speckled antibodies against extractable ribonucleoproteins, dsDNA antibodies against native dsDNA, nucleolar antibodies against nucleolar antigens and sometimes associated with scleroderma, and homogeneous antibodies against deoxyribonucleoproteins.

In active SLE, serum complement (C3, C4, and often CH50) levels are depressed. ESR is often elevated during active disease but is not a precise indicator of disease activity. DNA autoantibodies also do not correlate well with periods of active disease. A normochromic normocytic anemia, leukopenia (2500-4000 WBCs/mm^3), and thrombocytopenia are common because of bone marrow suppression or the autoimmune process, although other causes must be ruled out first. SLE can manifest as immune thrombocytic purpura years before the patient develops other symptoms of lupus.

The confirming tests for lupus (e.g., ANA, anti-DNA titers) are generally not helpful in follow-up. Monitoring for disease or treatment sequelae often involves serial CBC, renal function testing (creatinine), urinalysis, C3 and C4, and laboratory tests monitoring specific drug toxicities, including homocysteine and cholesterol levels for patients taking corticosteroids.

Treatment

The major goal of treatment is to treat the active disease without causing iatrogenic long-term complications and to be supportive of the patient and family. The family physician has a vital role in educating patients with SLE about signs and symptoms of disease flares. Continued monitoring, even when the disease appears inactive, is also important. General advice includes avoiding sun exposure or using potent sunscreens, early evaluation of unexplained fevers, annual influenza vaccine, adequate rest and exercise, and weight control. Other specific information tailored to the patient's needs is also important, such as SLE and its effect on pregnancy.

Vigilance for severe infections, particularly when corticosteroids are being used, should be continual. Proper monitoring for drug toxicities must include ophthalmologic examination with antimalarials and monitoring for corticosteroid-induced side effects. Treatment approaches for SLE emphasize using a drug combination to minimize corticosteroid use. Corticosteroids increase cardiovascular risk factors, including weight, BP, and cholesterol and homocysteine levels. Too-rapid steroid tapering should also be avoided. Immunosuppressive drugs are also being used more often, requiring careful monitoring.

The NSAIDs are still the drugs of choice for musculoskeletal manifestations, especially mild symptoms. The potential renal and GI toxicity of these drugs being used for a disease that in itself causes renal and GI damage must be kept in mind and monitored. Gastroduodenal cytoprotective therapy should be strongly considered for patients taking NSAIDs.

For minor polyarthritic disease activity, prednisone at 0.5 mg/kg/day in a single dose can be given, but many recommend other agents if the daily maintenance prednisone dose is 10 mg or more. Antimalarials such as hydroxychloroquine (Plaquenil) are often used for lupus arthritis but require ophthalmologic monitoring every 6 to 12 months. For severe arthritis or flare-ups, prednisone at 1.0 mg/kg/day, intra-articular injection with triamcinolone hexacetonide, or IV methylprednisolone sodium succinate (Solu-Medrol), 1000 mg over 90 minutes daily for 3 days, can be used, followed by oral prednisone. Methotrexate, 7.5 mg orally once weekly, along with folic acid supplementation or azathioprine, can also be used to minimize prednisone dosage, although methotrexate cannot be used during pregnancy.

Cutaneous lupus is treated with sunscreen and sun avoidance, topical or intralesional corticosteroids, topical cryotherapy with liquid nitrogen (less often), and antimalarials. The most common antimalarials are hydroxychloroquine, chloroquine (Aralen), and quinacrine. For patients who cannot take antimalarials, dapsone and retinoids such as etretinate (Tegison) or isotretinoin (Accutane) might be used with appropriate precautions. Fluocinonide cream has greater effect than hydrocortisone for discoid lupus (Jessop et al., 2001). Dapsone should not be used in patients with glucose-6-phosphate dehydrogenase (G6PD) deficiency, and retinoids should be avoided in pregnant patients. Severe cutaneous lupus can be treated with high-dose corticosteroids, but if the daily dose of prednisone exceeds 10 mg, methotrexate or azathioprine should be considered. Finally, thalidomide is effective for discoid lupus, but its use is limited by concerns about neuropathy and teratogenicity.

Lupus nephritis, once diagnosed by renal biopsy, can be treated with high-dose corticosteroids alone or with steroid-sparing drugs such as methotrexate or azathioprine. Cyclophosphamide for rapidly progressive or severe nephritis is effective but has substantial toxicities and is generally best left for the rheumatologist to prescribe. Toxicity can be minimized somewhat with prehydration and a mesna (Mesnex) injection, a cyclophosphamide metabolite binder, to avoid hemorrhagic cystitis. Later development of hematologic malignancies (rare) and premature ovarian failure (common) can result from cyclophosphamide use. If cyclophosphamide is indicated in a young woman, her family physician should raise options such as egg harvesting to preserve fertility.

Patients with SLE and antiphospholipid antibody syndrome who consequently have venous or arterial thrombosis can be treated with warfarin (Coumadin) to keep the international normalized ratio (INR) between 2 and 3. Although somewhat controversial, therapy should continue for at least 3 to 6 months, and often, lifelong anticoagulation is recommended based on high risk for subsequent events. Severe hemolytic anemia responds to IV methylprednisolone. Leukopenia rarely requires treatment. Severe thrombocytopenia with platelet counts below 50,000/mm^3 can be treated with methylprednisolone, danazol (Danocrine), immunosuppressive drugs, and possibly splenectomy.

Arthritis, serositis, and constitutional signs usually respond to 0.5 mg/kg/day of prednisone; nephritis and CNS disease usually require doses of 1 mg/kg/day. Patients who do not respond to high-dose steroids after 7 weeks should be considered for immunosuppressive drugs.

Rarely, plasma exchange is necessary for severe thrombotic thrombocytopenic purpura and pulmonary hemorrhage. Plasmapheresis has not shown long-term benefit for lupus nephritis. End-stage lupus nephropathy is treated with dialysis or kidney transplantation. Other experimental therapies for SLE include immunotherapy with anti-CD4, anti–TNF-α, and interferon-α.

Treatment of SLE has been successful in decreasing morbidity and mortality in what used to be considered a universally progressive, terminal disease. More than 90% of treated patients survive at least 15 years. SLE evolves over time with new manifestations and sometimes vague symptomatology arising unpredictably. Therefore, good communication in an ongoing physician-patient relationship and teamwork between the family physician and the rheumatologist are necessary for optimal care.

> **KEY TREATMENT**
>
> Cutaneous lupus should initially be treated with topical corticosteroids (Jessop et al., 2001) (SOR: B) and avoidance of precipitating factors such as sun exposure (SOR: C).
> Patients with persistent cutaneous lesions should be considered for treatment with antimalarials such a hydroxychloroquine (SOR: C).
> NSAIDs are the initial treatment for SLE-associated myositis, serositis, and arthritis. Refractory cases can be treated with 0.5 to 1 mg/kg/day of prednisone (SOR: C).

Sjögren's Syndrome

Sjögren's syndrome (SS) is an autoimmune disorder caused most likely by T-cell-mediated exocrine gland destruction characterized by dry eyes (keratoconjunctivitis sicca) and dry mouth (xerostomia). Patients with secondary SS have these symptoms in association with other autoimmune diseases such as RA, SLE, polymyositis, systemic sclerosis, or biliary cirrhosis.

Box 32-4 San Diego Criteria for Sjögren's Syndrome

I. Primary Sjögren's syndrome*

A. Symptoms and objective signs of ocular dryness
1. Schirmer's test <8 mm wetting per 5 minutes, *and*
2. Positive rose bengal staining of cornea or conjunctiva to demonstrate keratoconjunctivitis sicca

B. Symptoms and objective signs of dry mouth
1. Decreased parotid flow rate using a Lashley cup or other method *and*
2. Abnormal findings from biopsy of minor salivary gland (focus score of ≥1 based on average of four evaluable lobules)

C. Serologic evidence of a systemic autoimmunity
1. Elevated rheumatoid factor >1:320 *or*
2. Elevated antinuclear antibody <1:320 *or*
3. Presence of anti–SS-A(Ro) or anti–SS-B(La) antibodies

II. Secondary Sjögren's syndrome

Characteristic signs and symptoms of Sjögren's syndrome (described above), plus clinical features sufficient to allow a diagnosis of rheumatoid arthritis, systemic lupus erythematosus, polymyositis, scleroderma, or biliary cirrhosis

III. Exclusions

Sarcoidosis, preexisting lymphoma, HIV infection, hepatitis virus B or C infection, primary fibromyalgia, and other known causes of autonomic neuropathy, keratitis sicca, or salivary gland enlargement

*Definite Sjögren's syndrome requires objective evidence of dryness of eyes and mouth and autoimmunity, including a characteristic minor salivary gland biopsy (criteria IA, IB, and IC). Probable Sjögren's syndrome does not require a minor salivary gland biopsy but can be diagnosed by demonstrating decreased salivary function (criteria IA, IB-1, and IC).

From Fox RI, Saito I. Criteria for diagnosis of Sjögren's syndrome. Rheum Dis Clin North Am 1994;20:391.

A diagnosis of definite SS requires a minor salivary gland biopsy; a probable SS diagnosis can be based on demonstrating decreased salivary function. Exclusions to the diagnosis based on the San Diego Criteria include patients with HIV, primary fibromyalgia, sarcoidosis, preexisting lymphoma, keratitis sicca, hepatitis B or C, or salivary gland enlargement (Box 32-4). Objective evidence of ocular dryness can be obtained by the Schirmer II test, which involves stimulating the nasolacrimal reflex by inserting a cotton swab into the nostril; the increase in tear flow is then measured for both eyes (Tsubota, 1991). Rose bengal staining of the corneal or conjunctiva epithelial layer is another objective test. Serologic evidence of SS includes an elevated RF (>1:320), elevated ANA (>1:320), or presence of anti–SS-A (Ro) or anti–SS-B (La) antibodies.

Salivary secretions can be quantified by asking the patient to suck on a sugarless piece of candy for 3 minutes and then expectorate. If there is very little or no expectorant, a probable diagnosis of SS can be made; a follow-up minor salivary gland biopsy is definitively diagnostic. Patients not fitting these objective criteria can be reassured that their dry eyes or mouth is most likely not caused by an autoimmune disorder. Other manifestations of SS include constitutional symptoms such as fatigue, dry skin, vaginal dryness, upper respiratory tract dryness, and difficulty swallowing (caused by decreased saliva).

SS is not the only entity that can cause enlarged lacrimal and salivary glands and glandular dysfunction. SS needs to be differentiated from infiltrative processes (lymphoma, sarcoidosis, fatty infiltrates, hemochromatosis); infectious diseases (blepharitis, HIV, hepatitis B and C, tuberculosis, syphilis); neuropathic dysfunction of the glands caused by multiple sclerosis or Bell's palsy; autonomic neuropathy; and drug side effects.

Treatment of keratoconjunctivitis sicca consists of the use of artificial tears while monitoring for blepharitis caused by preservatives used in these preparations. Punctal plugs can be used to increase eye moisture, with either collagen plugs that dissolve after 2 days or silicone plugs, which are more durable but can be removed if excessive tearing occurs. If this is helpful, permanent punctal occlusion surgery might be considered. Humidifiers may also be helpful. Cyclosporine ophthalmic preparations are FDA approved for treatment of keratoconjunctivitis sicca, with objective and subjective improvement in dry eyes (Sall et al., 2000).

Dry mouth can be relieved by sugarless mints or gum. Frequent sips of water are also helpful. Those with continued symptoms may be candidates to try artificial saliva solutions (Salivart, Mouth Kote). Meticulous dental care should be encouraged because caries can occur more frequently with reduced salivary flow. Secretagogues such as pilocarpine or cevimeline can be used, but adverse effects such as flushing, increased perspiration, and increased bowel or bladder motility might outweigh their benefits. Topical antifungal troches are useful for low-grade oral infections.

Systemic treatment of SS is similar to that of SLE. NSAIDs and antimalarials, in particular, are useful for concomitant arthralgias and other systemic symptoms, but corticosteroids and immunosuppressants might be needed for refractory severe systemic disease.

KEY TREATMENT

Simple treatments such as the use of humidifiers, artificial tears, sugarless gums, and frequent sips of water are adequate in most patients with keratoconjunctivitis sicca and xerostomia of Sjögren's syndrome (SOR: C).

Vasculitic Syndromes

Vasculitis refers to a broad spectrum of conditions involving inflammation of blood vessels. Although many classification schemes have focused on the size of the vessels involved, this might not be very useful clinically because of the significant amount of overlap between these disorders. Many vasculitides characteristically affect certain age groups for unknown reasons: Kawasaki's disease in children, temporal arteritis in the elderly, and Henoch-Schönlein purpura with a bimodal distribution. Most vasculitic syndromes are of unknown cause. Pathologic findings are usually not diagnostic for a specific syndrome; diagnosis is still made primarily on clinical grounds. Most vasculitides tend to cause sporadic involvement of vessels with skip lesions. That is, they involve only part of the vessel wall for only part of the segmental length of the vessel and do not occur uniformly in other vessels of the same size.

Giant Cell Arteritis

Also known as *temporal arteritis,* giant cell arteritis (GCA) usually occurs in patients older than 50 years. It is most common in whites, particularly in people of northern European ancestry. Giant multinucleated cells are found in vessel walls, most frequently in the temporal arteries but sometimes in the vertebral or carotid arteries. The disease usually begins gradually with constitutional symptoms for weeks or even months, such as fatigue, malaise, fever, weight loss, and *polymyalgia rheumatica* (PMR, a separate entity characterized by proximal muscle pain and stiffness, elevated ESR, and constitutional symptoms). Specific symptoms then develop, such as jaw claudication (masticatory muscle discomfort with chewing); new-type or new-onset headache; scalp tenderness, particularly overlying the temporal arteries; diplopia; and visual loss secondary to retinal ischemia. Patients might also have loss of taste or hearing. About 30% of patients have neurologic symptoms such as peripheral neuropathies and transient ischemic attacks (TIAs). About 10% of patients have respiratory tract symptoms such as sore throat, cough, and hoarseness.

On physical examination, the temporal arteries might be tender, thickened, and erythematous. New carotid artery bruits should also raise suspicion. The aortic arch or its branches might be involved, manifested by reduced BP in one or both arms or arm claudication. Temporal artery biopsies confirm the diagnosis before initiating treatment, although the skip lesion nature of involvement means that a negative temporal artery biopsy does not rule out the diagnosis. The ESR tends to be high in GCA, usually 80 to 100 mm/hr, although in one small study, 25% of all patients with GCA on temporal artery biopsy had a normal ESR (Weyand et al., 2000). ALP and aspartate transaminase (AST) levels are mildly elevated in one third of patients. Serum IL-6 levels parallel inflammatory activity, and CRP may also be used to follow inflammation. The family physician should consider the diagnosis of GCA for any patient older than 50 years presenting with new-onset or new-type headache, elevated ESR, abrupt loss of vision, PMR, and prolonged fever.

The treatment for temporal arteritis or clinically suspected temporal arteritis with a negative biopsy is prednisone, 40 to 60 mg/day for 2 to 4 weeks. One should not wait for the biopsy results if clinical suspicion is high; treatment should start immediately. If symptoms and laboratory values suggest that the disease is under control, the dose is decreased 10 mg every 2 weeks for 1 month and then by 10% of the daily dose every 2 weeks (serum ESR and CRP levels are measured before decreasing the dose). Full courses often last 9 to 12 months. Prednisone often eliminates symptoms within 12 to 48 hours. GCA is usually self-limited, up to 2 years, at which time prednisone can be discontinued in most patients, although some still require small doses of corticosteroids for years to control symptoms. Because thoracic aortic aneurysms and renal artery stenosis are relatively common sequelae, the patient should be evaluated for these.

KEY TREATMENT

Prednisone is the treatment of choice in temporal arteritis (SOR: C).

Polymyalgia Rheumatica

As with GCA, polymyalgia rheumatica usually occurs in whites older than 50 years, especially those of northern European ancestry. Constitutional symptoms such as fever, fatigue, malaise, and weight loss occur early on, followed by neck and proximal upper extremity muscle aches. PMR is sometimes misdiagnosed as a frozen shoulder because of this. PMR later involves the lower extremity proximal muscles of the hips and thighs. Morning stiffness of large joints can make it difficult for the patient to perform ADLs, such as getting out of bed or combing the hair. The only typical physical finding is muscle tenderness, but without other objective signs. A transient mild synovitis of the knees, wrists, and sternoclavicular joints might occur. Diagnosis is made clinically by noting the combination of proximal extremity and truncal muscle pain and stiffness, increased ESR, and response to steroids.

Both PMR and GCA (temporal arteritis) are often seen together. PMR can precede, appear simultaneously with, or follow the onset of GCA symptoms. These two conditions might represent different manifestations of the same pathologic process. The best treatment for PMR is corticosteroids, with the dose determined by patient characteristics as well as by whether GCA is present. The typical dose is 15 to 30 mg/day of prednisolone; the daily dose is reduced by 5 mg/week until the dose is 15 mg/day, at which point the dosage is decreased by 2.5 mg/month.

Treatment can be stopped after 6 to 12 months if the ESR remains normal and the patient remains asymptomatic at a daily dose of 2.5 mg. Serial ESRs should be performed every 2 to 3 weeks, although following the patient's symptoms closely is more important than simply following laboratory values. For recurrences, 15 mg of prednisolone is restarted and gradually tapered. NSAIDs might help relieve symptoms but do not protect against vasculitis.

KEY TREATMENT

Prednisone is the treatment of choice in polymyalgia rheumatica (SOR: C).

Other Vasculitic Conditions

See the discussions of the following online at www.expertconsult.com.

- Takayasu's arteritis
- Polyarteritis nodosa
- Churg-Strauss syndrome
- Wegener's granulomatosis
- Cryoglobulinemia
- Hypersensitivity vasculitis
- Behçet's disease

Inflammatory Myopathies

This heterogeneous group of diseases causes inflammation of skeletal muscle, increases in levels of enzymes derived from muscle, and proximal muscle weakness or myopathy. The two most common myopathies are dermatomyositis and polymyositis. Inflammatory myopathies are classified by patient age at onset or by coexisting diseases, such as myositis associated with neoplasia or myositis associated with collagen vascular diseases (e.g., systemic scleroderma, SLE, SS). They have a bimodal distribution and are seen most often between age 10 to 15 and 45 to 60 years. Myositis is most common after age 50. The cause of inflammatory myopathies is unknown, but evidence suggests a genetic predisposition (associated with certain HLA markers) combined with an environmental insult, such as viruses, thereby initiating an autoimmune process.

Patients usually experience progressive, symmetric, proximal muscle weakness with fatigue, malaise, and morning stiffness. Muscles often affected are those of the shoulder, neck, and pelvic girdle. Pulmonary (interstitial pneumonitis or fibrosis), cardiac (cardiomyopathy, congestive heart failure, arrhythmias), pharyngeal (dysphagia), and musculoskeletal (myalgias, arthralgias) symptoms might occur, although most patients do not experience synovitis. CK as well as aldolase, alanine transaminase (ALT),AST, and lactate dehydrogenase (LDH) levels might be elevated, although ESR is elevated only half the time. Muscle biopsy can also be helpful in diagnosis. *Dermatomyositis* is characterized by all these manifestations plus a scaly, erythematous, or violaceous rash on the face and neck, upper back (shawl sign), and upper anterior chest and neck (V sign). Other signs include dystrophic cuticles, mechanic's hands (darkened or dirty-appearing horizontal lines across palmar aspect of fingers), and Gottron's papules, seen on dorsal aspects of the PIP, DIP, or MCP joints, elbows, patellae, and medial malleoli (Olsen and Wortmann, 2004). Disease in patients with skin changes but without muscle inflammation is termed *amyopathic dermatomyositis.*

Inflammatory myopathies can result from malignancies. Screening for malignancies common for the patient's gender and age should be undertaken, but further exploration is not indicated. However, ovarian cancer appears to be associated with dermatomyositis, so the family physician should consider evaluation for this.

Before treatment, a thorough motor neurologic examination is done, with muscle enzyme levels (CK, aldolase, ALT, AST, LDH) and cancer screening tests appropriate for patient age and gender. Prednisone, 1 mg/kg/day for up to several months, is the drug of choice; the earlier started in the disease process, the more effective it normally is. If prednisone is not sufficient, methotrexate, azathioprine, or another immunosuppressant is added.

Systemic Sclerosis

Key Points

- CREST syndrome and diffuse cutaneous systemic sclerosis are the primary manifestations of systemic sclerosis.
- Female/male predominance is 8:1 for sclerosis.
- The major ACR criterion for systemic sclerosis is skin thickening proximal to the MCP and MTP joints.

"Scleroderma," or hardening of the skin, is now recognized to be a disorder involving almost every organ system in the body and is therefore more appropriately referred to as *systemic sclerosis.* Systemic sclerosis is characterized by a progressive fibrosis of the skin, blood vessels, lungs, kidneys, heart, and GI tract. The degree of skin involvement (diffuse or limited) is useful for prognosis. *Diffuse cutaneous systemic sclerosis* (DCSS) involves almost the entire body, including the trunk, face, neck, and extremities. Cardiopulmonary disease is the leading cause of death in DCSS. Limited cutaneous systemic sclerosis has a more benign course and involves the face, neck, and distal extremities below the knee and elbow. CREST syndrome (calcinosis, Raynaud's phenomenon, esophageal dysmotility, sclerodactyly, and telangiectasias) is one of the limited forms of systemic sclerosis, characterized by cutaneous thickening of the distal limbs only. Skin biopsy showing subcutaneous fibrosis is helpful if the diagnosis is in doubt.

Systemic sclerosis affects women up to eight times more often than men; peak incidence is in the 40s and 50s. There is no significant familial connection, but systemic sclerosis patients typically have a family history of autoimmune disease. Many chemicals and toxins have been implicated, most clearly silica exposure in coal miners.

The major ACR classification criterion for systemic sclerosis is skin thickening proximal to the MCP or MTP joints. The three minor ACR criteria are involvement distal to the MCP joints (sclerodactyly), fingertip-pitting scars or loss of subcutaneous tissue, and chronic pulmonary interstitial changes. Patients with the major criterion or two of the three minor criteria are considered to have systemic sclerosis; however, many patients with clear-cut systemic sclerosis do not meet these criteria because their disease might be early or undifferentiated or in an overlap category with other connective tissue diseases. Ninety-five percent of patients have a positive ANA test result, most often nucleolar staining. Various serologic tests, including anti-RNA polymerase, anticentromere antibody, and antifibrillarin, can provide prognostic information.

The vast majority (>90%) of systemic sclerosis patients have *Raynaud's phenomenon,* which is the initial complaint in most patients, although some might complain first of puffy hands and fingers and of arthralgias. Raynaud's patients experience cold hands and feet, usually triggered by cold temperature or emotional stress. Vasospasm of the digital arteries and arterioles causes skin pallor, followed by cyanosis. With rewarming, the digits have a hyperemic or red color, thus completing this white, blue, and red phenomenon.

Scleroderma's skin changes result from inflammation and subsequent collagen deposition. The skin feels (and is) thickened, with decreased flexibility. As the skin becomes more fibrotic and thickened, it becomes very dry, causing pruritus. Late-stage skin changes include atrophy. Arthralgias and myalgias progress to muscle atrophy and weakness.

Scleroderma patients can develop two different pulmonary diseases, pulmonary hypertension and pulmonary fibrosis. Pulmonary hypertension (which can occur independently of fibrosis) is associated with a poor prognosis. Gastrointestinal symptoms include dysphagia with heartburn, dry mucosal membranes, esophageal reflux, and dysmotility. Cardiac manifestations are usually late and caused by coronary vasospasm, myocardial fibrosis, and pericardial effusions.

Scleroderma renal crisis is characterized by accelerated hypertension, rapidly progressive renal failure, or both (Steen, 1994). Depression is present in more than 50% of patients with systemic sclerosis and is often amenable to

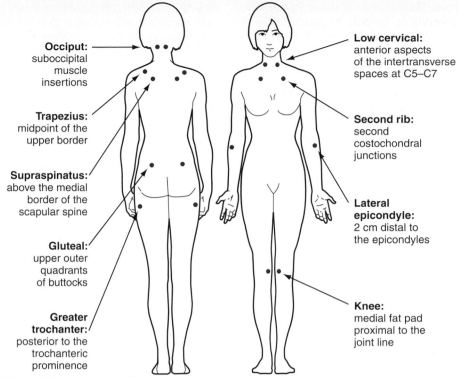

Occiput: suboccipital muscle insertions

Trapezius: midpoint of the upper border

Supraspinatus: above the medial border of the scapular spine

Gluteal: upper outer quadrants of buttocks

Greater trochanter: posterior to the trochanteric prominence

Low cervical: anterior aspects of the intertransverse spaces at C5–C7

Second rib: second costochondral junctions

Lateral epicondyle: 2 cm distal to the epicondyles

Knee: medial fat pad proximal to the joint line

Figure 32-15 Location of the specific tender points in fibromyalgia. *(From Freundlich B, Leventhal L. Diffuse pain syndromes. In Klippel JH [ed]. Primer on the Rheumatic Diseases, 11th ed. Atlanta, Arthritis Foundation, 1997, pp 123-127.)*

antidepressants. Thyroid fibrosis might lead to hypothyroidism; sicca syndrome can be treated with artificial tears and good dental care.

Treatment

Treatment for systemic sclerosis is difficult. Penicillamine, immunosuppressive drugs, and other agents have been used to treat scleroderma, but none has yielded dramatic results. Localized sclerosis can soften with ultraviolet-A (UVA) light therapy, with dramatic improvement in symptoms seen in two small, non-RCTs (Kreuter et al., 2004; Stege et al., 1997). Other options include high-dose topical corticosteroids and methotrexate. Treatments for calcinosis, including probenecid, colchicine, and warfarin, have not shown improvement. A five-patient study showed that the calcium channel blocker (CCB) diltiazem caused significant regression in calcinosis and clinical improvement (Palmieri et al., 1995); more studies are needed. Raynaud's phenomenon is treated by cold avoidance for the entire body (not only hands), tobacco avoidance, and biofeedback or other stress reduction techniques; pharmacologic therapy includes CCBs, topical nitroglycerin, and prazosin (Pope et al., 2004). A meta-analysis concluded that CCBs are efficacious for reduction in frequency and severity of attacks (Thompson et al., 2005). Skin care consists of avoiding excessive bathing and using moisturizers.

The NSAIDs are used first for musculoskeletal symptoms of systemic sclerosis, but low-dose corticosteroids or narcotic analgesics might be needed. No studies have been performed, but in general, acid-reducing medications such as PPIs or H$_2$ blockers are used to prevent the development of possible esophageal strictures, given the high rates of esophageal dysmotility in the systemic sclerosis. Delayed

small intestinal tract transit time may lead to bacterial overgrowth, causing GI symptoms; antibiotics might be effective. Angiotensin-converting enzyme (ACE) inhibitors are useful in the treatment of renal crisis manifested by hypertension and renal failure.

For *scleroderma-like disorders*, see the discussion online at www.expertconsult.com.

> ### KEY TREATMENT
>
> Systemic sclerosis is difficult to treat. UVA therapy is the most effective treatment for localized skin sclerosis (Kreuter et al., 2004; Stege et al., 1997) (SOR: B).
> Pharmacologic therapy with calcium channel blockers is effective at decreasing the frequency and severity of Raynaud's phenomenon (Thompson et al., 2005) (SOR: B).

Diffuse Fasciitis with Eosinophilia

See the discussion online at www.expertconsult.com.

Fibromyalgia Syndrome

Key Points

- Fibromyalgia syndrome accounts for 20% of visits to the rheumatologist.
- The diagnosis is confirmed by finding 11 of 18 areas of tender points over 3 months.
- The female/male predominance is 9:1 for FMS.

Fibromyalgia syndrome (FMS) is one of the most common rheumatic diseases, affecting up to 20% of patients seen in rheumatology practices (Keefe and Caldwell, 1997). Patients have fatigue, diffuse myalgias, poor sleep, and stiffness; the diagnosis is confirmed by finding at least 11 of 18 specific areas of point tenderness (Fig. 32-15). Pain must be present for more than 3 months to make a diagnosis of FMS. Psychological factors and comorbid conditions might aggravate symptoms. FMS is more common than RA and causes a comparable degree of disability and loss of family income. About 90% of FMS patients are women, and there is evidence of familial aggregation. Fibromyalgia might also be present in patients with autoimmune disorders such as SLE, RA, and AS and should be suspected when symptoms are unresponsive to anti-inflammatory therapies.

Fibromyalgia syndrome is probably caused by central pain mechanism dysfunction, possibly in neurotransmitters. Several studies have found that FMS patients have up to three times higher levels of substance P in CSF than normal controls (Russell et al., 1994). FMS can be initially triggered by trauma or peripheral inflammatory arthritis, but peripheral, ongoing inflammation is not present in this syndrome. Important secondary factors contributing to the patient's pain include nonrestorative sleep, muscle deconditioning secondary to pain, and psychological factors. Pain is most common in the neck, back, shoulders, pelvic girdle areas, and hands. Paresthesias in the extremities are also common, as are tension-type headaches, irritable bowel syndrome, primary dysmenorrhea, chronic fatigue syndrome, restless legs syndrome, temporomandibular joint (TMJ) dysfunction, and regional fibromyalgia (myofascial pain syndrome). Although some FMS patients have depression, most do not. Physical examination reveals tenderness with moderate pressure in 11 out of 18 defined points, although some patients might clinically have incomplete FMS, with fewer sites involved. Care must be taken on examination not to palpate too softly or too firmly. The proper amount of palpation pressure is about the amount of pressure required to blanch the nail of the examining finger when it is pressed against the patient's forehead (Yunus, 1996).

No laboratory tests are available to diagnose FMS. CBC results; tests for ESR, muscle enzyme, electrolyte, and ANA levels; and radiography are all normal in the absence of comorbid disease. Sleep electroencephalograms are often abnormal and should be considered if a history of particular sleep disturbances is suspected (see **eTable 32-5** online). Because FMS is often seen in association with other rheumatic diseases, the diagnosis is often missed because FMS symptoms might be mistaken for the comorbid disease. Conversely, patients presenting with FMS should be evaluated for an underlying condition.

The cause of fibromyalgia is unknown. Muscle biopsies reveal no apparent abnormalities. There is great overlap with chronic fatigue syndrome, but there is no evidence that an infection such as chronic Epstein-Barr virus (EBV) is associated with fibromyalgia. About 80% of fibromyalgia patients have sleep disturbances, particularly disrupted non–rapid eye movement (non-REM) sleep (stages 3 and 4, which is deep, restorative sleep). Non-REM sleep deprivation studies have reproduced the signs and symptoms of FMS, which make the sleep disturbance possibly an integral part on the pathogenesis and continuation of fibromyalgia. Patients with RA and other rheumatic diseases have disrupted sleep with nocturnal awakening and arousals to a lighter stage of sleep throughout the night. Sleep studies reveal that patients often cannot recall these episodes on awakening the next day but do feel fatigued or describe themselves as light sleepers.

Treatment

It is important to educate patients with FMS and to reassure them that FMS is a common disease, that it is not psychiatric, and that there are treatments available.

Tricyclic antidepressants (TCAs), selective serotonin reuptake inhibitors (SSRIs), and serotonin-norepinephrine reuptake inhibitors (SNRIs) help relieve pain associated with fibromyalgia. A meta-analysis (18 RCTs with a variety of antidepressants) concluded there was strong evidence of efficacy for antidepressants for relief of pain, fatigue, mood, sleep disturbance and health-related quality of life (Hauser et al., 2009). The effect size for pain reduction was large for TCAs and small for the SSRIs and SNRIs, although newer studies of SNRIs were not included. Studies of the SNRIs milnacipran (Savella) and duloxetine (Cymbalta) have show significant reductions in pain, and both have been FDA approved for the treatment of fibromyalgia. Amitriptyline doses are typically 25 to 50 mg at night, much lower than the doses used for the treatment of depression. The addition of amitriptyline to SSRIs or SNRIs showed a trend toward improvement versus medication alone, but results were not statistically significant (Goldenberg et al., 1996).

Cyclobenzaprine has a chemical structure similar to TCAs, and various dosing regimens have been studied in the treatment of fibromyalgia. A meta-analysis found that pain was significantly decreased in patients receiving cyclobenzaprine over placebo at 4 weeks, but not statistically significant at 8 or 12 weeks. Overall, patients treated with cyclobenzaprine were three times more likely to report subjective improvement, and five patients would need to be treated for one patient to experience symptom improvement (Tofferi et al., 2004).

Pregabalin (Lyrica), a second-generation anticonvulsant, was the first medication to be FDA approved for the treatment of fibromyalgia. As with gabapentin, pregabalin has effects on cellular calcium channels and may exert its analgesic effects by blocking various neurotransmitters. Multiple large studies have shown its efficacy for the treatment of pain, fatigue, and improvement in sleep (Mease et al., 2008). Gabapentin has not been FDA approved for this use but is efficacious for reducing pain in fibromyalgia (Arnold et al., 2007).

The NSAIDs and corticosteroids are usually not helpful because no evidence indicates FMS is an inflammatory disease, and NSAIDs are no better then placebo in the treatment of pain. Combination analgesic therapy with acetaminophen and tramadol was found to decrease pain significantly in these patients (Bennet et al., 2003). However, the long-term use of tramadol needs to be carefully considered, and this approach is best employed after other therapies (e.g., antidepressants) have failed.

At least two thirds of FMS patients use some type of complementary method, such as herbal supplements or acupuncture. A meta-analysis of acupuncture suggested benefit, but study quality was generally poor (Berman et al., 1999). Local anesthesia injected into tender points can sometimes relieve pain, and topical capsaicin (Zostrix) cream has helped some patients. Treatment of underlying depression is also important.

Daily exercise programs, particularly aerobic exercise, and physical therapy might also help FMS patients; it is important that exercise regimens begin at a low intensity and build up slowly. A review of controlled trials for aerobic exercise for fibromyalgia found beneficial effects in overall global function, physical function, and possibly in reduction of pain and tender points (Busch et al., 2008).

Cognitive-behavioral treatment (CBT) is promising for FMS patients, although there have been few controlled studies. There might be even more benefit if CBT is combined with physical exercise. Patients are often resistant to starting exercise programs such as walking or bicycling because they fear exacerbation of pain. CBT programs can overcome negative self-statements that prevent the initiation of exercise or limit the amount of exercise that can be done. An emphatic ongoing relationship with a caring physician is particularly important treatment for patients suffering from FMS. Although musculoskeletal rehabilitation has no effect by itself, physical therapy can help subacute low back pain and other comorbidities. Subacute aerobic exercise is also effective in decreasing symptoms but might need to begin at very low levels (Busch et al., 2004).

KEY TREATMENT

Aerobic exercise programs have positive effects for overall global function, physical function and pain (Busch et al., 2008) (SOR: A). Antidepressant therapy is effective for fibromyalgia patients; TCAs show the greatest improvements (Hauser et al., 2009) (SOR: A). Pregabalin improves pain, fatigue, and sleep in patients with fibromyalgia (Arnold et al., 2007; Mease et al., 2008) (SOR: A). Acetaminophen and tramadol significantly reduce pain associated with fibromyalgia (Bennet et al., 2003) (SOR: B), but prolonged use of tramadol should be considered only after inadequate response to antidepressant therapy (SOR: C).

Temporomandibular Joint Syndrome

See the discussion online at www.expertconsult.com.

Rheumatic Disease in Children

Juvenile Rheumatoid Arthritis

Juvenile rheumatoid arthritis (JRA), formerly known as Still's disease, is a heterogeneous group of diseases clinically distinct from adult RA. Although much less common than RA, JRA is four times more common than sickle cell anemia or cystic fibrosis and 10 times more common than other pediatric diseases, such as hemophilia, muscular dystrophy, acute lymphocytic leukemia, and chronic renal failure (Gortmaker, 1984). Fortunately, most children with JRA have long remissions without loss of function or significant residual deformity.

There are no specific laboratory tests to diagnose JRA. Other causes for arthritis must be excluded, including reactive arthritis from extra-articular infection, septic arthritis, neoplastic disorders, endocrine disorders (thyroid disease, type 1 diabetes mellitus), degenerative or mechanical disorders, and idiopathic pediatric joint pain. Diagnosis of JRA requires true arthritis (signs of inflammation rather than simply arthralgias) persisting for more than 6 weeks, with onset at or before age 16 years.

The three major subtypes of JRA are pauciarticular (40%-50%), polyarticular (30%), and systemic (5%-10%), all with different clinical presentations and courses; their differentiation determines treatment. *Pauciarticular* JRA involves four or fewer joints, usually large joints asymmetrically. Early-onset pauciarticular JRA affects mostly girls younger than 4 years and has a 30% risk of chronic iridocyclitis and a 10% risk of ocular damage. Late-onset pauciarticular JRA affects mostly boys older than 8 years, many of whom later develop spondyloarthropathies; 10% develop iridocyclitis. Slit-lamp ophthalmic examinations are recommended. *Polyarticular* JRA is defined as arthritis in five or more joints; patients are RF positive or negative. RF-positive patients usually are girls age 8 years or older, have symmetric small-joint arthritis, and have a worse functional prognosis than RF-negative patients. *Systemic-onset* JRA is characterized by high intermittent fevers (>38.8° C; 102° F), rash, hepatosplenomegaly, lymphadenopathy, arthralgias, pericarditis, pleuritis, and growth delay. Anemia, leukocytosis, and thrombocytosis are common laboratory findings. Extra-articular symptoms are usually mild and self-limited. Boys and girls are equally affected. The severity of the arthritis is a harbinger of prognosis.

The NSAIDs are the first-line treatment for JRA, but patience is necessary because clinical improvement might not be seen for up to 1 month. Approximately two thirds of patients need another agent in addition to NSAIDs; methotrexate is often used, particularly for systemic and polyarticular JRA. Corticosteroids are used orally for severe, life-threatening, systemic JRA and intra-articularly for pauciarticular JRA. Eye inflammation is best treated by an ophthalmologist.

Juvenile RA is an excellent example of a disease that significantly affects the entire family. JRA can actually have a greater negative psychological impact on siblings than on the patient (White and Shear, 1992). Most children with JRA require extensive physical as well as psychological support. Encourage families to receive support from social programs and JRA advocacy and support groups. The consulting rheumatologist and physical and occupational therapists are vital, but patients and families also benefit greatly from a continuous, supportive relationship with the family physician. Physical and occupational therapy are important because children often stop using painful joints, adding to disability.

Spondyloarthropathies

Four spondyloarthropathies are seen in children: juvenile AS, psoriatic arthritis, Reiter's syndrome (reactive arthritis), and IBD-associated arthritis. Definitive diagnoses of these conditions are often delayed. JAS patients must have their lumbar spine motion monitored. Plain radiographs often do not show the changes characteristic of adult AS. NSAIDs are used for treatment. Significant arthritis can be seen in 7% to 20% of IBD patients.

Systemic Lupus Erythematosus in Childhood

Systemic LE primarily affects adolescent girls, many of whom do not have the typical malar rash. The small joints of the hands or feet and the kidneys are typically affected; the

Box 32-5 Diagnostic Guidelines for Kawasaki's Syndrome*

Fever lasting >5 days *plus* four of the following five criteria:
1. Polymorphous rash
2. Bilateral conjunctival infection
3. One or more of the following mucous membrane changes:
   Diffuse infection of oral and pharyngeal mucosa
   Erythema or fissuring of the lips
   Strawberry tongue
4. Acute, nonpurulent cervical lymphadenopathy (one lymph node must be >1.5 cm)
5. One or more of the following extremity changes:
   Erythema of palms, soles, or both
   Indurative edema of hands, feet, or both
   Membranous desquamation of the fingertips
   Other illnesses with similar clinical signs must be excluded.

From Freundlich B, Leventhal L. Diffuse pain syndromes. In Klippel JH (ed). Primer on the Rheumatic Diseases, 12th ed. Atlanta, Arthritis Foundation, 2001, p 409.

*Based on the Centers for Disease Control and Prevention case definition.

patient should be monitored for proteinuria and hematuria. Because of steroid side effects, immunosuppressant drugs are often used for severe cases.

Henoch-Schönlein Purpura

Henoch-Schönlein purpura is a small-vessel vasculitis seen mostly in children. Immune complexes are deposited, causing petechiae, nephropathy, or renal disease (40%) and GI bleeding. The purpura is usually in dependent areas such as the buttocks and lower extremities. Affected children often present with abdominal pain after an upper respiratory infection. Symptoms typically resolve spontaneously without treatment within 2 weeks, but serious GI and renal involvement can occur, requiring steroids. NSAIDs might be helpful for arthralgias.

Kawasaki's Syndrome

Kawasaki's syndrome (KS), also known as Kawasaki's disease, is the leading cause of acquired heart disease in children. Prolonged high fever (up to 40° C [104° F]), with an urticaria-like rash and injection of mucous membranes, including a strawberry tongue, is followed by erythema of the palms and soles and desquamation of the fingertips. Most patients have cervical lymphadenopathy. A myocarditis is present in more than 50% of patients and is manifested by a tachycardia. Many other symptoms might also occur, such as respiratory, neurologic, and GI symptoms (Box 32-5). Because KS symptoms resolve spontaneously, cardiac manifestations might not be diagnosed. A coronary arteritis and even aneurysms might develop, with significant morbidity and mortality. Laboratory studies are not helpful. Serial electrocardiograms are recommended at diagnosis, 2 to 3 weeks into the illness, and 1 month after that.

Although KS's seasonal variation (winter and spring) and epidemics suggest an infectious cause, none has yet been identified. IV fluids, aspirin, and IVIG have been used most frequently for KS. Antibiotics are of no use unless there is a concomitant bacterial infection. Steroids might actually increase the incidence of aneurysms and should be avoided, if possible.

Nonarticular Rheumatism

Any pain and stiffness without true inflammation in the joint and with normal laboratory results in children is termed *nonarticular rheumatism,* or "growing pains." These usually occur at night, last several hours, and often resolve spontaneously or are helped by massage or analgesics. Pain is sometimes felt behind the knees. No further evaluation is indicated unless pain occurs during the day. Overuse or hypermobile joints are two possible explanations; nonarticular rheumatism does not normally cause any reduction in activity.

Rheumatology Information on the Internet

A great deal of information on rheumatic diseases for both physicians and patients can be found on the Internet. This can be a valuable tool for the family physician in this era of active research and new treatment modalities in rheumatology. Patients might receive online support from numerous advocacy and support groups for these conditions, although the Internet can also be a source of misinformation, with charlatans touting arthritis cures. Websites of the ACR, Arthritis Foundation, and Medline Plus are particularly good sources of information (see Web Resources).

References

The complete reference list is available online at www.expertconsult.com.

Web Resources

General Reference

www.rheumatology.org
American College of Rheumatology; Internet resources, academic and government sites, foundations/associations.

www.arthritis.org
Arthritis Foundation; excellent site, primarily for patients.

www.nlm.nih.gov/medlineplus/arthritis.html
Medline Plus.

www.curearthritis.org
Arthritis National Research Foundation—information on financial support for research.

www.nih.gov/niams
   National Institute of Arthritis and Musculoskeletal and Skin Diseases (NIAMS) and National Institutes of Health (NIH)—conducting research in these areas.

Disease-Specific Sites

www.aarda.org
   American Autoimmune Related Diseases Association—patient education.

www.rheumatology.org/public/factsheets/fibromya_new.asp
   American College of Rheumatology—fibromyalgia.

www.aldf.com
   American Lyme Disease Foundation.

www.lupus.org
   Lupus Foundation; patient advocacy, patient information, local chapters.

www.myositis.org
   Myositis Association of America—polymyositis, dermatomyositis.

www.risg.org
   Reiter's Information and Support Group; patient education.

www.sjogrens.com
   Sjögren's Syndrome Foundation.

www.spondylitis.org
   Spondylitis Association of America; patient education on ankylosing spondylosis, psoriatic arthritis, other types of spondylitis.

33 CHAPTER

Dermatology

Richard P. Usatine and Jennifer Krejci-Manwaring

Chapter contents

Principles of Diagnosis

Dermatologic diagnosis often begins with *pattern recognition*. Experts can look at most lesions and make an immediate and accurate diagnosis through pattern recognition. The basic terms used to describe lesion morphology and patterns provide the vocabulary to describe what is seen. The physician then combines keen observation of the lesions (including type and distribution) with a careful history to create an informed differential diagnosis. If the diagnosis is still not known, the physician can consult a dermatology atlas (online or print), textbook, or expert to complete the diagnosis. In some cases, further testing (scraping, culture, biopsy) may be needed.

Initial Evaluation

Although medical school teaches students to perform the history before doing the physical examination, this is not the most efficient way to approach the diagnosis of a skin condition. When the patient has a skin complaint, immediately look at the skin while asking your questions. Look carefully at the lesions and determine the lesion morphology. Table 33-1 provides definitions for the terms used to describe primary and secondary morphology. A magnifying glass and good lighting help to distinguish the morphology of many skin conditions. Next, touch the lesions, with gloves when appropriate. For some lesions, such as actinic keratosis with

Table 33-1 Primary and Secondary Skin Lesions

Lesions	Description
Primary (Basic) Lesions	
Macule	Circumscribed flat discoloration (up to 5 mm)
Patch	Flat nonpalpable discoloration (>5 mm)
Papule	Elevated solid lesion (up to 5 mm)
Plaque	Elevated solid lesion (>5 mm) (often a confluence of papules)
Nodule	Palpable solid (round) lesion, deeper than a papule
Wheal (hive)	Pink edematous plaque (round or flat), topped and transient
Pustule	Elevated collection of pus
Vesicle	Circumscribed elevated collection of fluid (up to 5 mm in diameter)
Bulla	Circumscribed elevated collection of fluid (>5 mm in diameter)
Secondary (Sequential) Lesions	
Scale (desquamation)	Excess dead epidermal cells
Crusts	Collection of dried serum, blood, or pus
Erosion	Superficial loss of epidermis
Ulcer	Focal loss of epidermis and dermis
Fissure	Linear loss of epidermis and dermis
Atrophy	Depression in skin from thinning of epidermis/dermis
Excoriation	Erosion caused by scratching
Lichenification	Thickened epidermis with prominent skin lines

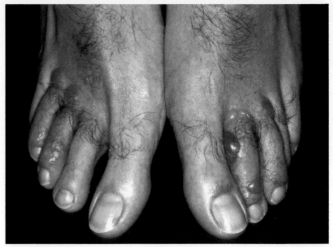

Figure 33-1 Vesicular tinea pedis leading to autosensitization reaction. *(© Richard P. Usatine.)*

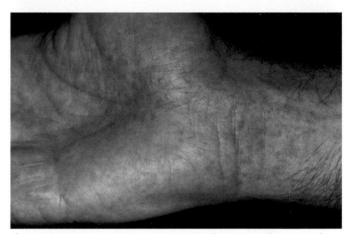

Figure 33-2 Autosensitization reaction secondary to vesicular tinea pedis (id reaction). *(© Richard P. Usatine.)*

scaling or the sandpaper rash of scarlet fever, lightly feeling the skin provides much information. For deeper lesions, such as nodules and cysts, deep palpation is needed. Observe the distribution of the lesions. Try to determine if the primary lesions are arranged in groups, rings, lines, or merely scattered over the skin.

Determine which parts of the skin are affected and which are spared. Be sure to look at the remainder of the skin, nails, hair, and mucous membranes. Patients often show only one small area and appear reluctant to expose the rest of their skin, especially their feet. With many skin conditions, it is essential to look beyond the most affected area because other areas may provide important clues (e.g., nail pitting when considering psoriasis). Patients may have lesions on their back or feet that they have not observed. For example, a patient may have a papular eruption on the hands or arms that represents an autosensitization reaction *(id reaction)* to a fungal infection on the feet; not looking for the fungus on the feet will lead to a missed diagnosis (Figs. 33-1 and 33-2). Some skin diseases have manifestations in the

mouth; finding white patches on the buccal mucosa may lead to the correct diagnosis of lichen planus (Fig. 33-3).

Once the physician starts to look at the skin, the patient history will be more focused, directed toward finding the correct diagnosis. The following information assists in making a dermatologic diagnosis and planning treatment:

- Onset and duration of skin lesions: continuous or intermittent?
- Pattern of eruption: Where did it start? How has it changed?
- Any known precipitants, such as exposure to medication (prescription, OTC), foods, plants, sun, topical agents, chemicals (occupation, hobbies)?
- Skin symptoms: itching, pain, paresthesia
- Systemic symptoms: fever, chills, night sweats, fatigue, weakness, weight loss
- Underlying illnesses: diabetes, thyroid disease, human immunodeficiency virus (HIV)
- Family history: acne, atopic dermatitis, psoriasis, skin cancers, dysplastic nevi

The most important in-office examinations of the skin are the following:

Microscopy. To diagnose a fungal infection, scrape some of the scale onto a microscope slide, add 10% potassium

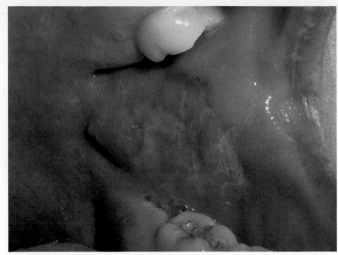

Figure 33-3 Oral lichen planus showing Wickham's striae. (© *Richard P. Usatine.*)

hydroxide (KOH) (best with dimethyl sulfoxide [DMSO] and fungal stain), and look for the hyphae of dermatophytes or the pseudohyphae of *Candida* or *Pityrosporum* species. *Wood's light examination.* This is helpful in diagnosing tinea capitis and erythrasma. Tinea capitis caused by *Microsporum* spp. produces green fluorescence, but *Trichophyton* spp. do not fluoresce. Erythrasma has a coral-red fluorescence. Wood's lamp also helps distinguish lesions of vitiligo in patients with fair skin.

Surgical biopsy. The biopsy can be used as a diagnostic and treatment tool. Having a reasonable differential diagnosis will help the physician choose shave, punch, or elliptic biopsy.

General Management

Topical Corticosteroids

The choice of a topical steroid involves maximizing benefit and minimizing adverse effects. Many skin conditions benefit greatly from topical steroids. However, local adverse effects of topical steroids are common with regular use over weeks to months. The most common adverse effect of topical steroids is skin *atrophy,* in which the epidermis becomes thin and the superficial capillaries dilate. Epidermal atrophy can be accompanied by hypopigmentation and telangiectasias. If atrophy involves the dermis, striae may occur. Although the epidermal atrophy may be reversible in months, striae are irreversible. When fluorinated steroids (the strongest steroids) are continuously applied to the face, perioral dermatitis, rosacea-like eruptions, and acneiform eruptions can occur.

Systemic adverse effects are rare and occur when large amounts of topical steroids are absorbed systemically. The risk of such absorption increases with stronger steroids, thinner skin, younger patients, longer duration of therapy, and the use of occlusion in therapy. Prescribing the minimum strength needed for the shortest duration required helps prevent adverse effects. In choosing the best topical steroid, consider the following factors:

1. **Skin disorder.** As the severity of the disorder increases, the need for higher-potency steroids increases. Also, thicker lesions (e.g., psoriatic plaques, lichen planus) need higher-potency steroids.

2. **Site.** Use only the weakest-potency steroids on the face, genitals, and intertriginous areas, where skin is thin or moist and skin atrophy and striae occur most rapidly. There are exceptions, however, as when clobetasol is needed to treat certain vulvar disorders. The skin on the palms and soles is so thick that the most potent steroids may be needed.

3. **Age.** Avoid the use of high-potency topical steroids in infants and children because they have greater surface area per body mass than adults and have greater risk and consequences of systemic absorption.

4. **Steroid potency** (strength and concentration). There are more than 50 types and brands of steroids; family physicians should know at least one steroid from each of four basic strengths (Table 33-2). Generic agents can be used from all the potency groups to save on costs.

5. **Vehicle.** The vehicle is the substance in which the steroid is dispersed. The most common vehicles are ointments, creams, gels, solutions, lotions, and foams. The choice of vehicle is determined by the characteristics of the lesion (dry or moist), the site involved, and patient preference. Further, the vehicle affects the potency of the steroid because it determines the rate at which the steroid is absorbed through the skin.

Most skin preparations can be applied two times a day (bid), conveniently in the morning and evening. Try to estimate and prescribe an appropriate amount; many topical products are supplied in 15-gram, 30-g, 60-g, and 80-g sizes; 80 g is about the size of a tube of toothpaste. Based on common practice, it is accepted that 2 g of cream is required to cover the face or one hand, 3 g for an arm, 4 g for a leg, and 12 to 30 g for an entire body. To avoid adverse effects of steroid overuse, do not prescribe large quantities for small lesions, and specify duration of use. On the other end of the spectrum, prescribing only 15 g of steroid for a large area of involvement will be frustrating to the patient when the steroid is depleted before completing the prescribed treatment. Generic triamcinolone comes in 1-pound tubs (454 g), extremely helpful for patients with inflammatory conditions covering much of the body.

The duration of therapy is usually the time required for resolution of symptoms or lesions. To avoid adverse effects, the highest-potency steroids should not be used for longer than 2 to 4 weeks continuously. However, these can be used intermittently for chronic conditions such as psoriasis in a pulse-therapy mode (e.g., apply every weekend, with steroid-sparing medication on weekdays). For conditions with dry skin, liberal use of emollients between steroid applications can minimize steroid exposure while maximizing the benefits of therapy.

Management of Pruritus

Often, patients present because of the pruritus associated with a skin condition rather than the skin condition itself. Itching associated with visible lesions often responds to relatively nonspecific antipruritic treatments. If the itching is generalized, patients may obtain temporary relief from cool or tepid baths with the addition of colloidal oatmeal (Aveeno). Soap should be avoided. Oral antihistamines can be given every 6 to 8 hours, especially at bedtime to promote sleep. Diphenhydramine (Benadryl) and hydroxyzine (Atarax, Vistaril) are first-generation antihistamines that are relatively

Table 33-2 Potency of Topical Corticosteroids

Potency	Generic Drugs	Brand Names
"Superpotent" (class 1)	Clobetasol, betamethasone dipropionate, halobetasol, fluocinonide	Clobex, Diprolene, Olux, Psorcon, Temovate, Ultravate, Vanos
High potency (classes 2 and 3)	Betamethasone dipropionate, mometasone, halcinonide, fluocinonide, desoximetasone, triamcinolone 0.1%, fluticasone, amcinonide	Diprolene, Elocon, Halog, Lidex, Psorcon, Topicort, Aristocort, Cutivate, Cyclocort
Midpotency (classes 4 and 5)	Prednicarbate, mometasone, betamethasone valerate, hydrocortisone probutate, fluocinolone, desoximetasone, hydrocortisone valerate, triamcinolone 0.025%	Dermatop, Elocon, Luxiq, Pandel, Synalar, Topicort, Westcort, Cordran, Cutivate, Locoid
Low potency (classes 6 and 7)	Alclometasone, desonide, fluocinolone, hydrocortisone	Aclovate, DesOwen, Synalar, Hytone, Desonate

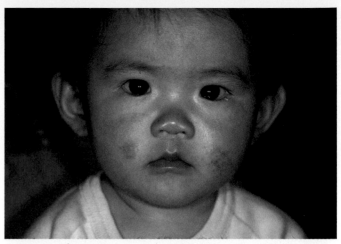

Figure 33-4 Atopic dermatitis. *(© Richard P. Usatine.)*

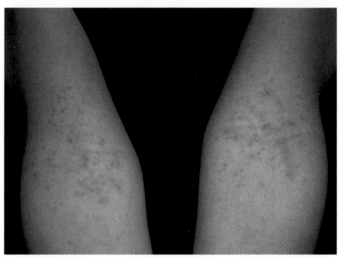

Figure 33-5 Atopic dermatitis in antecubital fossa. *(© Richard P. Usatine.)*

safe and effective, although caution should be used in older adult patients. Second-generation antihistamines are similarly effective for reducing pruritus in the daytime, and are less sedating for some patients. These include fexofenadine (Allegra), loratadine (Claritin), and cetirizine (Zyrtec). Usually, second-generation antihistamines are given once daily.

Skin Problems Beginning in Childhood

Atopic Dermatitis (Eczema)

Key Points

- Atopic dermatitis is a common inherited childhood disorder that may occur with other atopic conditions such as allergic rhinitis and asthma.
- Topical steroids and emollients are the mainstays of treatment for AD.
- Topical and systemic antibiotics are used for AD secondarily infected with bacteria.

Atopic dermatitis (AD) is a potentially debilitating condition that can compromise quality of life. Its most frequent symptom is pruritus. Pruritus leads to scratching, resulting in secondary skin changes such as lichenification, excoriation, and breakdown of the skin barrier. Consequently, atopic dermatitis has been referred to as "the itch that rashes."

Atopic dermatitis is a common problem affecting up to 15% of all children. In most cases, AD occurs before 5 years of age, frequently on the face in the first year of life (Fig. 33-4). As children grow, the antecubital and popliteal fossae are often involved (Fig. 33-5). The disease may occur intermittently between periods of complete remission. By adulthood, the incidence becomes less than 1%. Treatment should be directed at limiting itching, repairing the skin, and decreasing inflammation. Lubricants and topical corticosteroids are the mainstays of therapy. Topical pimecrolimus or tacrolimus are considered steroid-sparing agents and are effective for short-term use or in cases unresponsive to topical corticosteroids. These agents are only approved for second-line treatment in patients over 2 years of age. When required for severe cases, oral corticosteroids can be used. If pruritus does not respond to treatment, other diagnoses, such as bacterial overgrowth or viral infections, should be considered.

Always look for signs of bacterial superinfection, such as weeping of fluid and crusts (Fig. 33-6). Superinfection with *Staphylococcus aureus* may lead to worsening of atopic dermatitis as the bacteria functions as a super antigen. *S. aureus* superinfections are usually sensitive to methicillin, so oral cephalexin is frequently a good choice for treatment. Bleach baths are helpful to cut down on colonization. (Add ½ cup regular bleach per full tub of lukewarm water and soak for 5 to 10 minutes before washing off bleach water.)

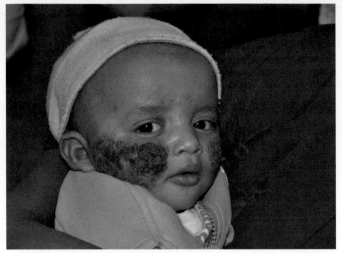

Figure 33-6 Impetiginized atopic dermatitis. *(© Richard P. Usatine.)*

KEY TREATMENT

Topical steroids and emollients are the mainstay of treatment for atopic dermatitis (Hanifin et al., 2004) (SOR: A).

Topical and systemic antibiotics are used for AD with secondary bacterial infection; weeping fluid and crusting during an exacerbation should prompt consideration of antibiotic use (Hanifin et al., 2004) (SOR: A).

Topical calcineurin inhibitors (immunomodulators such as pimecrolimus and tacrolimus) reduce the rash severity and symptoms of AD in children and adults (Hanifin et al., 2004) (SOR: A).

Dietary restriction is useful only for infants with proven egg allergies (Hanifin et al., 2004) (SOR: B).

The value of antihistamines in AD is controversial; if used, the sedating agents are most effective and can be given at night (Hanifin et al., 2004) (SOR: B).

Pityriasis Alba

Pityriasis alba is a common hypopigmented dermatitis that may affect nearly one third of school-age children in the United States. The condition is more common in patients with a history of atopic dermatitis. Patients present with numerous hypopigmented macules ranging from 1 to 4 cm in size on the face, neck, and shoulders (Fig. 33-7). The macules are poorly defined and may have fine scales. Occasionally, erythema and pruritus occur before the lesions. Generally, pityriasis alba is self-limited and asymptomatic, so therapy is typically unnecessary. Lesions usually fade by adulthood. Topical steroids, emollients, and phototherapy have limited efficacy. Hydrocortisone 1% cream or ointment may provide some benefit, and if used for no more than 2 weeks, the patients should be relatively safe from adverse effects.

Keratosis Pilaris

Keratosis pilaris is very common and presents as tiny (<1 mm) keratotic follicular papules found on extensor arms and thighs and occasionally the cheeks. The numerous papules give the skin a rough feeling. Often there is a ring of erythema around the follicle. Incidence of keratosis pilaris

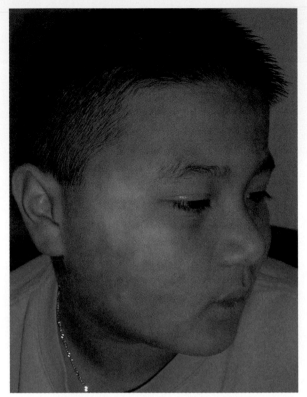

Figure 33-7 Pityriasis alba. *(© Richard P. Usatine.)*

is increased in AD patients. Treatment consists of emollients combined with keratolytic agents; common preparations are 5% or 12% ammonium lactate (AmLactin, Laclotion, Lac-Hydrin) and urea-based creams or lotions. Patient education should stress that keratosis pilaris is genetic and cannot be cured. Any smoothing with topical agents is temporary and will return if the treatment is stopped.

Melanocytic Nevi

Nevi (moles) are benign lesions composed of collections of nevus cells of neuroectodermal origin. They appear in childhood, tend to increase in number throughout the adult years, and then resolve with age. *Pigmented* nevi can be flat, raised, or pedunculated and have impressive variations in size, color, and surface characteristics. Histologically, *junctional* nevi are located in the epidermis, *intradermal* nevi in the dermis, and *compound* nevi in the epidermis and dermis. Junctional nevi are flat and pigmented, intradermal nevi are raised and often not pigmented, and compound nevi may be raised and pigmented (Figs. 33-8 and 33-9).

Unless they become suspicious for melanoma, nevi need not be removed except for cosmetic reasons or because of chronic irritation based on their location. Nevi should be examined frequently, however, for changes in color, shape, or size. These changes may herald the onset of a melanoma in a previously benign nevus and warrant excision with pathologic evaluation of the tissue.

Nevi that are present at birth and are visible shortly thereafter are considered *congenital* nevi. Although these nevi may have a slightly higher risk of developing melanoma than acquired nevi, it is not cost-effective or sensible to recommend the

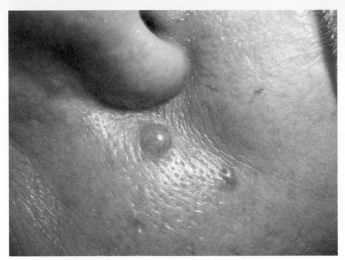

Figure 33-8 Intradermal nevi. *(© Richard P. Usatine.)*

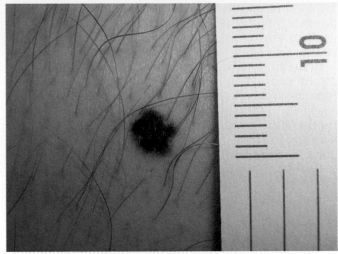

Figure 33-10 Dysplastic nevus. *(© Richard P. Usatine.)*

The presence of five or more dysplastic nevi should alert the patient and physician to this higher risk of melanoma, and therefore regular skin examinations should be performed, with sun avoidance and sun protection.

Infantile Hemangioma

A hemangioma is an extremely common type of benign tumor that occurs most frequently in infants and children. It is composed of newly formed blood vessels that result from malformation of angioblastic tissue during fetal life. The two main types are capillary (superficial) and cavernous (deep) hemangiomas (Figs. 33-11 and 33-12).

Hemangiomas undergo a growth phase before resolving spontaneously. Although some regression begins by the end of the first year of life, many hemangiomas do not completely resolve until the child is 10 to 12 years old. Although typically benign, rapidly proliferating hemangiomas can ulcerate. Those on the face may obscure vision and can cause blindness. Hemangiomas of the genital region are also problematic and may indicate other internal malformations. Persistent or obstructive hemangiomas have been successfully treated with propranolol, lasers, excision, systemic corticosteroids, interferon, imiquimod, and cryosurgery.

Acne Vulgaris

Acne is a disorder of the pilosebaceous follicles on the face, chest, and back. Follicular obstruction leads to comedones, and inflammation results in papules, pustules, and nodules. The four most important steps in acne pathogenesis are (1) sebum overproduction related to androgenic hormones and genetics, (2) abnormal desquamation of follicular epithelium (keratin plugging), (3) *Propionibacterium acnes* proliferation, and (4) follicular obstruction, which leads to inflammation and follicular disruption. These steps are stimulated by androgens, and strong genetic factors determine a person's likelihood of developing acne. Although common, acne can cause physical pain, psychosocial suffering, and scarring. Acne may be associated with fever, arthritis, and other systemic symptoms in acne fulminans (Fig. 33-13).

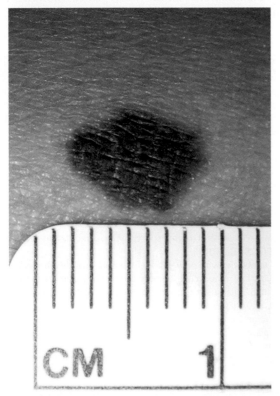

Figure 33-9 Compound nevus. *(© Richard P. Usatine.)*

removal of all congenital nevi. It is even controversial with regard to removal of large, "bathing suit" nevi, which have the highest risk of melanoma. Children born with these nevi are at risk for developing melanoma in the central nervous system (CNS) as well as subcutaneous melanoma, which is not visible and requires palpation in order to detect on routine skin examination.

Dysplastic nevi (atypical moles) are markers for increased risk of melanoma somewhere on the body. These nevi have more atypical features but are not at high risk of converting to melanoma (Fig. 33-10). Therefore, removing dysplastic nevi does not provide a survival benefit for patients.

Topical treatments include retinoids, antibiotics, benzoyl peroxide (BP), azelaic acid, and alpha or beta hydroxyl acid products. Topical retinoids are comedolytic and anti-inflammatory, normalize follicular hyperproliferation and hyperkeratinization, and reduce the numbers of microcomedones, comedones, and inflammatory lesions. The most frequently prescribed topical retinoids include tretinoin (Retin-A), adapalene (Differin), and tazarotene (Tazorac, Avage). Patients are frequently sensitive to topical retinoids and may have skin irritation, peeling, and redness. Mild cleansers and noncomedogenic moisturizers can reduce the inflammation, as does less frequent dosing of the retinoids. Glycolic acid (α-hydroxy acid) or salicylic acid (β-hydroxy acid) come in various products, are used in chemical peels, and are also effective for hyperkeratinization.

Topical antibiotics are effective against *P. acnes* and also act as anti-inflammatories. Erythromycin and clindamycin are frequently used once or twice daily. Topical dapsone (Aczone) was approved in 2008 for acne treatment. Benzoyl peroxide is also effective against *P. acnes* and is available over the counter (OTC) in various preparations. Combination products with antibiotics and BP are a convenient method of delivering synergistic medications in one preparation.

Oral medications used in acne treatment include antibiotics, hormone therapies, and isotretinoin. Isotretinoin is a known teratogen and should not be used in women of childbearing age unless avoidance of pregnancy is ensured. Contraception counseling is mandatory, and two negative pregnancy test results are required before initiation of therapy. The baseline laboratory examination should also include determination of cholesterol, fasting triglycerides, transaminase levels, blood urea nitrogen (BUN)/creatinine, and complete blood count (CBC). Pregnancy tests and laboratory examinations should be repeated monthly during treatment.

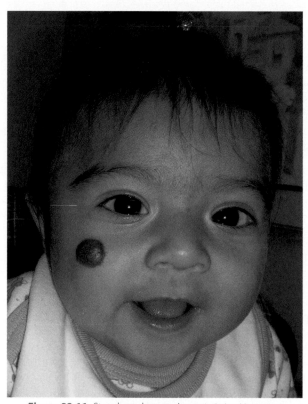

Figure 33-11 Strawberry hemangioma. *(© Richard P. Usatine.)*

KEY TREATMENT

Topical benzoyl peroxide (gel, cream, lotion, wash) has an antimicrobial effect in acne treatment. Higher-percentage products (10%) cause more irritation and are not more effective (Agency for Healthcare Research and Quality, 2001) (SOR: A).

Topical antibiotics such as clindamycin and erythromycin are beneficial treatments (AHRQ, 2001) (SOR: A).

Combination products with antibiotics and BP deliver synergistic medications in one preparation (AHRQ, 2001) (SOR: B).

Topical retinoids (tretinoin, adapalene, tazarotene) are excellent to treat all types of acne and the primary treatment in comedonal acne (AHRQ, 2001) (SOR: A).

Azelaic acid is useful to treat spotty hyperpigmentation and acne (AHRQ, 2001) (SOR: B).

Oral antibiotics with proven benefit in acne include tetracycline, doxycycline, minocycline, and erythromycin and are particularly useful for inflammatory acne and trunk acne (AHRQ, 2001; Strauss et al., 2007) (SOR: A).

Isotretinoin is the most powerful treatment for cystic and scarring acne that has not responded to other therapies (Fig. 33-14) (Strauss et al., 2007) (SOR: A).

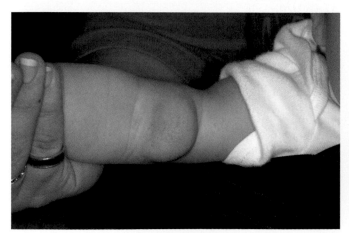

Figure 33-12 Cavernous hemangioma. *(© Richard P. Usatine.)*

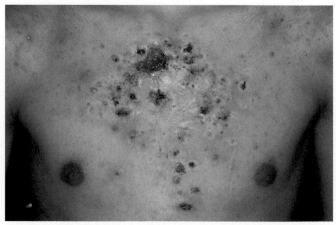

Figure 33-13 Acne fulminans. *(© Richard P. Usatine.)*

Viral Exanthems

Viral causes of rashes include varicella, rubeola, rubella, roseola, and erythema infectiosum (fifth disease). Treatment is aimed at symptoms using acetaminophen or ibuprofen for fever and diphenhydramine for pruritus.

Varicella

Varicella is now much less common with universal varicella vaccination of children. Occasionally the family physician sees a case of breakthrough chickenpox in a vaccinated child. Unvaccinated adults may also present with varicella. Patients with varicella have fever and general malaise as a mild prodrome lasting 1 to 2 days before the rash appears. The rash typically begins on the face, scalp, or trunk and then spreads to the extremities. The lesions appear as erythematous macules and progress to papules with an edematous base. The papules quickly evolve into vesicles, appearing as "dewdrop on a rose petal" (Fig. 33-15). The vesicles evolve into pustules, which become umbilicated and subsequently crust over in the ensuing 8 to 12 hours. A defining characteristic of varicella is that lesions may be present in all stages simultaneously.

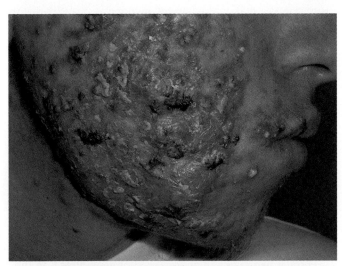

Figure 33-14 Acne conglobata. (© Richard P. Usatine.)

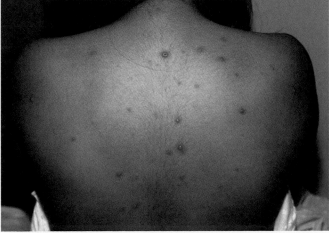

Figure 33-15 Chickenpox. (© Richard P. Usatine.)

In children the most common varicella complication is secondary bacterial infection of excoriated lesions. Other complications include cerebellar ataxia, encephalitis, meningitis, transverse myelitis, and rarely Reye's syndrome. Varicella pneumonia and encephalitis can be serious complications in adults. Because of the risk of Reye's syndrome, aspirin use should be avoided in patients with varicella. Acyclovir is recommended for adolescents, adults, and children with varicella who are taking steroids or otherwise immunocompromised.

Measles (Rubeola) and Rubella

Rubeola presents as maculopapular (morbilliform) eruption. It starts on the face and spreads centrifugally. It is associated with cough, coryza, conjunctivitis, fever, and Koplik spots (red-white-blue macules in mouth). As with varicella, rubeola is now uncommon because of vaccinations.

The exanthem of rubeola (measles) begins around the fourth febrile day, with discrete lesions that become confluent as they spread from the hairline downward, sparing the palms and soles. The exanthem typically lasts 4 to 6 days. The lesions fade gradually in order of appearance, leaving a residual yellow-tan coloration or faint desquamation. Rubeola is also distinguished by the presence of Koplik spots in the oral mucosa. These are usually small white or bluish macules with a ring of erythema on the buccal mucosa.

Rubella is similar to rubeola and is caused by a togavirus. It causes less severe symptoms, and its exanthem characteristically has a duration of 2 to 3 days. Rubella is associated with tender cervical lymphadenopathy, most notably in the posterior cervical and occipital areas. Another unique feature is Forchheimer spots, which are pinpoint red macules and petechiae over the soft palate and the uvula.

Hand, Foot, and Mouth Disease

This common childhood illness usually occurs in the summer or early fall and presents as flat-topped vesicles on hands, feet, and mouth, especially on the palms and soles. Every case may not involve all three sites. Hand, foot, and mouth disease is most often caused by coxsackievirus A16.

Erythema Infectiosum (Fifth Disease)

Erythema infectiosum is caused by human parvovirus B19 and primarily affects children 3 to 12 years old. The prodrome may consist of fever, anorexia, sore throat, and abdominal pain. Once the fever resolves, the classic bright-red facial rash ("slapped cheek") appears. The exanthem progresses to a diffuse, reticular or "lacy" pattern on the extensor extremities that may wax and wane for several weeks.

Roseola Infantum (Sixth Disease, Exanthem Subitum)

Roseola infantum, or exanthema subitum, is caused by human herpesvirus 6. This disease occurs in children younger than 3 years. As in fifth disease, the rash of sixth disease appears after the resolution of several days of high fever. The diffuse morbilliform eruption often spares the face and is of short duration, typically fading within 3 days.

Inflammatory Dermatologic Diseases

Seborrhea

Seborrheic dermatitis is a chronic inflammatory disorder affecting areas of the head (scalp, face) and body where sebaceous glands are prominent. The inflammation is thought to be caused by *Malassezia (Pityrosporum)* species. All age groups may be affected, and seborrhea can be chronic or intermittent. On the scalp, seborrhea can range from mild dandruff to thick, adherent plaques. Seborrhea on the face and body appears as greasy scales in skin folds and along hair margins, with a symmetric distribution bilaterally. On the face, two common locations are around the eyebrows and around the beard and mustache in men (Fig. 33-16 and 33-17).

Treatments are aimed at the inflammation and the *Malassezia* overgrowth and include shampoos containing selenium sulfide, ketoconazole, or pyrithione zinc that target the fungus. Topical antifungal lotions and corticosteroid preparations are also effective. Low-potency corticosteroids used intermittently are safe and effective. In infants, seborrheic dermatitis might only involve the scalp (cradle cap) or can be seen in other areas of skin folds such as the diaper area. If not treated prophylactically, seborrheic dermatitis has a tendency to recur.

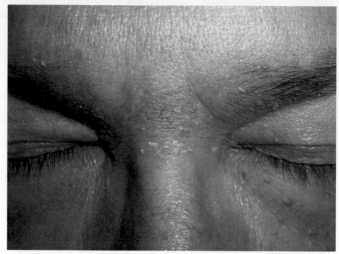

Figure 33-16 Seborrheic dermatitis. *(© Richard P. Usatine.)*

KEY TREATMENT

Shampoos containing ketoconazole, selenium sulfide or zinc pyrithione are effective for moderate to severe seborrhea capitis (Danby et al., 1993; Pierard-Franchimont, 2002) (SOR: A).

Ketoconazole 2% cream, gel, or emulsion is safe and effective for facial seborrheic dermatitis (Chosidow et al., 2003; Pierard et al., 1991) (SOR: B).

Oral terbinafine, 250 mg daily for 4 weeks, is effective for moderate to severe seborrhea (Scaparro, 2001; Vena et al., 2005) (SOR: A).

Hydrocortisone 1% cream or lotion can be used twice daily on face, scalp, or other affected area (Firooz et al., 2006) SOR: B).

Desonide 0.05% lotion is safe and effective for short-term treatment of seborrheic dermatitis of the face (Freeman, 2002) (SOR: B).

For moderate to severe seborrhea on the scalp, 0.05% fluocinonide solution once daily is affordably priced and beneficial (SOR: C).

Psoriasis

Psoriasis is a common skin disorder that most often appears as inflamed plaques covered with a thickened, silvery-white scale. Psoriasis is divided into the following nine categories, although a patient can have more than one type at the same time:

1. *Plaque* psoriasis accounts for 80% to 90% of patients with psoriasis (Fig. 33-18).
2. *Scalp* psoriasis causes plaques on the scalp (Fig. 33-19).
3. *Guttate* psoriasis appears as small, round plaques that resemble water drops (Fig. 33-20).
4. *Inverse* psoriasis causes inflammation in the intertriginous areas of the axilla, groin, inframammary folds, and intergluteal fold. Inverse psoriasis may not exhibit classic scaly plaques, and the erythema, scaling, or maceration in intertriginous areas is often mistaken for fungal infection (Fig. 33-21).
5. *Palmar-plantar* psoriasis occurs on the plantar aspects of the hands and feet (palms and soles) (Fig. 33-22).

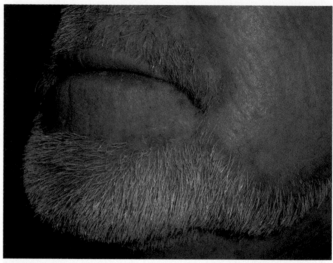

Figure 33-17 Seborrheic dermatitis around beard and mustache. *(© Richard P. Usatine.)*

6. *Erythrodermic* psoriasis is widespread erythema and scales.
7. *Pustular* psoriasis can be localized or generalized. In the generalized form, superficial pustules may appear and coalesce to form lakes of pus that dry and desquamate in sheets (Fig. 33-23).
8. *Nail* psoriasis causes the nails to develop pits, onycholysis, and oil spots and to thicken.
9. *Psoriatic* arthritis affects the joints of the hands, feet, and knees but can involve other joints as well.

From 1% to 2% of the U.S. population has plaque psoriasis. Genetic factors are involved; when both parents are affected by psoriasis, the rate of psoriasis may be as high as 50%; with one parent affected, the rate is approximately 16%. Psoriasis can appear at any age, but the two peak age ranges are 16 to 22 and 57 to 60. Guttate psoriasis often occurs after streptococcal pharyngitis or another upper respiratory infection. Pustular psoriasis may be provoked by the withdrawal of systemic steroids in a patient already diagnosed with psoriasis.

The most common areas involved include the elbows, knees, extremities, trunk, scalp, face, ears, hands, feet, genitalia, intertriginous areas, and the nails. In most cases,

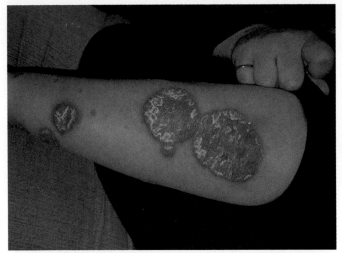

Figure 33-18 Psoriatic plaques. *(© Richard P. Usatine.)*

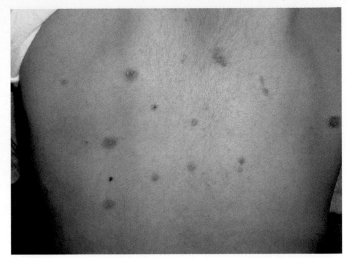

Figure 33-20 Guttate psoriasis after streptococcal throat infection in child. *(© Richard P. Usatine.)*

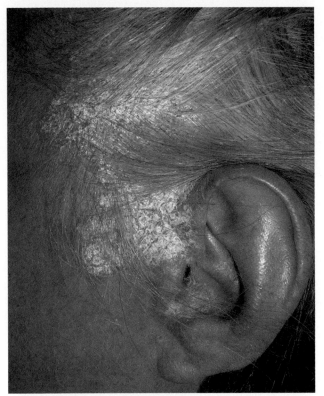

Figure 33-19 Scalp psoriasis. *(© Richard P. Usatine.)*

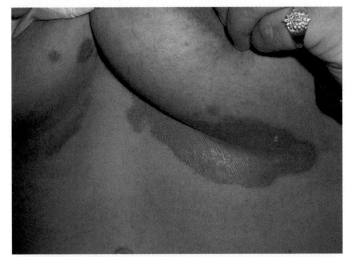

Figure 33-21 Inverse psoriasis under breasts. *(© Richard P. Usatine.)*

diagnosis of psoriasis is based on the clinical appearance. The differential diagnosis list is long, however, and a KOH preparation or skin biopsy may be needed. A biopsy may also be helpful to establish the diagnosis in less common types of psoriasis (pustular, palmar-plantar, inverse). Do not treat psoriasis with oral or systemic steroids; this can precipitate a life-threatening case of generalized pustular psoriasis.

A meta-analysis showed that 68% to 89% of patients treated with clobetasol (ultrahigh-potency steroid) had clear improvement or complete healing (Nast et al., 2007). Comparable efficacy was shown for topical calcipotriene (vitamin D analogue) and tazarotene (retinoid), with a slight increase in adverse effects for tazarotene (Afifi et al., 2005). Combination topical steroids and calcipotriene or tazarotene is the most promising

current topical treatment and seems to have increased efficacy and fewer side effects (Afifi et al., 2005; Nast et al., 2007). Clinical trials suggest that tacrolimus (0.1 %) ointment twice daily produces a good response in a majority of patients with facial and intertriginous (inverse) psoriasis (Brune et al., 2007; Lebwohl et al., 2004; Martin et al., 2006). Methotrexate as a weekly oral dose of 5 to 15 mg can be very effective for widespread psoriasis not responding to topical treatments (Saporito and Menter, 2004). Acitretin (Soriatane) is a potent systemic retinoid used for psoriasis that is widespread or palmar-plantar and not responding to topical treatments (Pearce et al., 2006)

Etanercept (Enbrel) is a subcutaneous biologic agent that is especially valuable in patients with psoriatic arthritis, as well as those with moderate to severe cutaneous psoriasis (Nast et al., 2007). Adalimumab (Humira), a subcutaneous biologic agent, and infliximab (Remicade), an intravenous biologic agent, are effective for patients with psoriatic arthritis as well as those with moderate to severe cutaneous psoriasis (Bansback et al., 2009). Ustekinumab (Stelara), the most recently approved subcutaneous biologic agent, significantly reduced signs and symptoms of psoriatic arthritis and diminished skin lesions compared with placebo (Gottlieb et al., 2009).

KEY TREATMENT

Potent topical steroid ointments are a good choice for first-line therapy of psoriasis (Afifi et al., 2005) (SOR: A).

Clobetasol successfully treated 68% to 89% of patients with psoriasis (Nast et al., 2007) (SOR: A).

Topical calcipotriene and tazarotene show comparable efficacy as clobetasol for psoriasis (Afifi et al., 2005) (SOR: A).

Topical steroids and calcipotriene or tazarotene show increased efficacy in psoriasis and fewer side effects (Afifi et al., 2005; Nast et al., 2007) (SOR: A).

Tacrolimus (0.1 % ointment bid) helps most patients with facial and inverse psoriasis (Brune et al., 2007; Lebwohl et al., 2004; Martin et al., 2006) (SOR: B).

Narrowband UVB is safer and more effective than broadband UVB for psoriasis (Ibbotson et al., 2004) (SOR: A)

Methotrexate (5-15 mg/wk) is effective for widespread psoriasis not responding to topical treatments (Saporito and Menter, 2004) (SOR: A).

Acitretin (Soriatane) is used for unresponsive widespread or palmar-plantar psoriasis (Pearce et al., 2006) (SOR: A).

Etanercept (Enbrel) is especially valuable in patients with psoriatic arthritis or cutaneous psoriasis (Nast et al., 2007) (SOR: A).

Pityriasis Rosea

Pityriasis rosea is a common acute eruption usually affecting children and young adults; the cause is unknown. It is characterized by the formation of an initial herald patch (Fig. 33-24), followed by the development of a diffuse papulosquamous rash. Pityriasis rosea is difficult to identify until the appearance of characteristic, smaller, secondary lesions that follow Langer's lines in a "Christmas tree" pattern (Fig. 33-25). The rash of pityriasis rosea typically lasts 5 to 8 weeks, with complete resolution in most patients. An important goal of treatment is to control pruritus, which may be

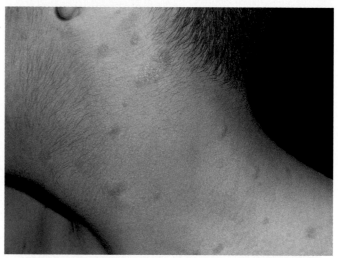

Figure 33-24 Pityriasis rosea with herald patch on neck. (© *Richard P. Usatine.*)

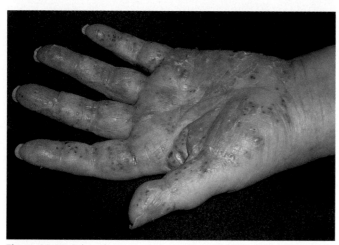

Figure 33-22 Palmoplantar psoriasis as a form of localized pustular psoriasis. (© *Richard P. Usatine.*)

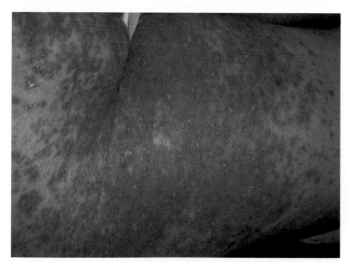

Figure 33-23 Generalized pustular psoriasis presenting as erythroderma. (© *Richard P. Usatine.*)

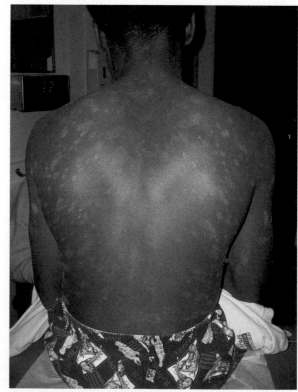

Figure 33-25 Pityriasis rosea with "Christmas tree" pattern on back. (© *Richard P. Usatine and E.J. Mayeaux, Jr. The Color Atlas of Family Medicine.*)

severe; zinc oxide, calamine lotion, topical steroids, and oral antihistamines are usually helpful. Systemic steroids are generally not recommended.

Ultraviolet (UV) radiation and erythromycin have been used with varying results. Because no bacterial cause has been associated with the disease, the likely effect of erythromycin is a result of its anti-inflammatory properties. Postinflammatory hyperpigmentation may occur with UVB radiation therapy, so some experts recommend against its use. High-dose acyclovir (800 mg qid) may help shorten disease, especially if instituted early in the disease course, but studies are limited.

Patients should be reassured about the self-limited nature of pityriasis rosea. Persistence of the rash or pruritus beyond 12 weeks should prompt reconsideration of the original diagnosis, consideration of biopsy to confirm the diagnosis, and questioning the patient again about use of medications that may cause a rash similar to that of pityriasis rosea.

Rosacea

Rosacea, sometimes called "acne rosacea," is an inflammatory disease with unknown etiology. Various facial manifestations occur, and symptoms differ from patient to patient. The four types of rosacea are erythematotelangiectatic, papulopustular, phymatous, and ocular. Patients may have overlapping features of more than one type. The predominant manifesting complaints of *erythematotelangiectatic* rosacea are intermittent central facial flushing and erythema. Itching is often absent; however, many patients complain of a stinging pain associated with flushing episodes. Common triggers include exposure to the sun, cold weather, sudden emotion including laughter or embarrassment, hot beverages, spicy foods, and alcohol consumption.

Papulopustular rosacea presents with acnelike papules and sterile pustules and can occur alone or in combination with the erythema and telangiectasias (Fig. 33-26). Intermittent or chronic facial edema may also occur in all forms. Some patients develop *rhinophyma*, a coarse hypertrophy of the connective tissue and sebaceous glands of the nose. This can be extremely disfiguring and even cause nasal airway obstruction. Approximately one third of patients with

rosacea develop ocular symptoms, including eyes that are itchy, burning, or dry; a gritty or foreign body sensation; and erythema and swelling of the eyelid. The ocular changes can become chronic. Corneal neovascularization and keratitis can occur, leading to corneal scarring and perforation. Episcleritis and iritis have also been reported to occur in patients with rosacea.

First-line treatment is avoidance of triggering or exacerbating factors. Although patients have different trigger(s), almost all patients benefit from strict sun avoidance and protection. Acnelike lesions respond well to long-term topical treatment using metronidazole, azelaic acid, erythromycin, and clindamycin. Oral tetracyclines used in antimicrobial (high) doses or anti-inflammatory (low) doses are helpful for moderate to severe rosacea. Oral or topical retinoid therapy may also be effective. Laser treatment is an option for progressive telangiectasia, erythema, or rhinophyma. Ocular symptoms generally require oral tetracyclines. Consultation may be required for the management of rhinophyma, ocular complications, or severe disease.

KEY TREATMENT

Best evidence supports the topical use of metronidazole (0.75% or 1%) and azelaic acid (15% or 20%) for rosacea (van Zuuren et al., 2005) (SOR: A).

If the skin lesions are more extensive, oral antibiotics, such as tetracycline and metronidazole, are recommended for rosacea (van Zuuren et al., 2005) (SOR: C).

Both anti-inflammatory (low-dose) doxycycline (40-mg delayed-release Oracea) and 100-mg doxycycline are equally effective once-daily treatments for moderate to severe rosacea; higher dosage (100 mg) is associated with a higher incidence of adverse effects (mostly GI symptoms) (Del Rosso et al., 2008).

Pulsed-dye laser and intense pulse light result in significant reduction in erythema, telangiectasia, and patient-reported associated symptoms (Neuhaus et al., 2009).

Lichen Planus

Lichen planus is a papular pruritic skin eruption characterized by its violaceous color and polygonal shape. Most frequently, flat-topped papules and plaques are found on the flexor surfaces of the upper extremities, on the genitalia, around the ankles, and on the mucous membranes (Figs. 33-27 and 33-28). Lesions can be intensely pruritic. Because lichen planus is thought to be immune-mediated, it may be

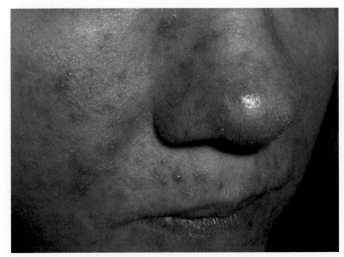

Figure 33-26 Rosacea. *(© Richard P. Usatine.)*

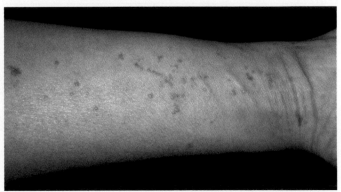

Figure 33-27 Lichen planus with linear papules. *(© Richard P. Usatine.)*

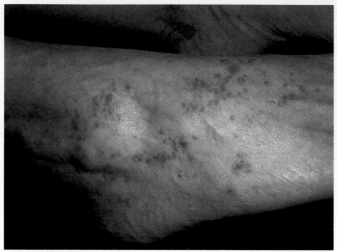

Figure 33-28 Lichen planus on lateral ankle. *(© Richard P. Usatine.)*

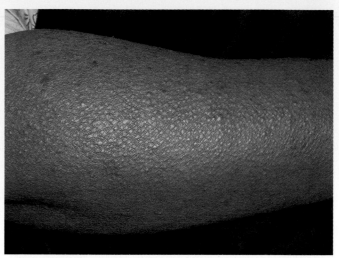

Figure 33-29 Lichen simplex chronicus. *(© Richard P. Usatine.)*

found in conjunction with ulcerative colitis, vitiligo, myasthenia gravis, dermatomyositis, and alopecia areata. Lichen planus is also associated with primary biliary cirrhosis, chronic active hepatitis, and hepatitis C infection.

Patients with lichen planus are usually between 30 and 60 years old, although the disorder may occur at any age. Men and women are equally affected, and there is no racial predisposition. The cutaneous form spontaneously resolves within 6 months in about half of patients, and most forms resolve within 18 months. Mucous membrane lesions may become chronic and persist for years. Mild cases can be treated symptomatically with antihistamines and topical steroids. More severe cases or those involving the mucous membranes can be treated with systemic steroids, oral acitretin, or UV light. Other immunosuppressants, such as mycophenolate mofetil and cyclosporine, have also been used with some success.

KEY TREATMENT

Treatment of lichen planus starts with high-potency topical steroids twice daily to the affected areas (SOR: C).
Intralesional triamcinolone (3 mg/mL) is considered for hypertrophic or mucous membrane lichen planus lesions (SOR: C).
Systemic treatment with oral steroids, acitretin, mycophenolate mofetil, and cyclosporine can be considered for severe cases of lichen planus that involve mucous membranes (Zakrzewska et al., 2005) (SOR: B).

Lichen Simplex Chronicus

Lichen simplex chronicus (LSC) is a secondary condition that results from repeated mechanical trauma to the skin, usually through rubbing and scratching, which causes lichenification (thickening of epidermis). Skin appears leathery, violaceous to hyperpigmented, and scaly (Fig. 33-29). Involved areas are within the patient's easy reach, such as arms, legs, posterior neck, upper back, buttocks, and scrotum. The cycle of pruritus, which is alleviated by scratching, perpetuates the condition. Pruritus is usually worse during periods of inactivity, usually at bedtime and during the night. Stress also may provoke pruritus, which

is relieved by rubbing and scratching and often becomes an unconscious behavior.

Treatment of LSC is aimed at treating existing lesions, reducing pruritus, providing insight into the itch-scratch cycle, and eliciting behavioral changes, Topical steroids decrease inflammation and pruritus and help "thin down" the hyperkeratosis. Because lesions are by nature chronic, long-term treatment should be stressed. Occlusion can be used to increase potency and enhance delivery of the topical steroid and also provides a barrier to scratching. Flurandrenolide tape (Cordran) is very effective and can be cut to fit each lesion of LSC. Anxiolytics and antihistamines such as diphenhydramine and hydroxyzine may be considered as adjunct treatments. In severe, debilitating cases, oral doxepin and clonazepam may be considered. For secondary infections, a topical or oral antibiotic is appropriate.

Contact Dermatitis

Key Points

- Contact dermatitis is classified as irritant (ICD) or allergic (ACD).
- Clinical findings of ICD and ACD can be identical, and both entities can be present simultaneously.
- Nickel is the most common cause of ACD.
- Avoidance of irritating substances or environments and allergens is key to therapy. Dry-skin care and topical corticosteroids are also helpful.
- Referral for patch testing can help identify the causative agent in ACD.

Contact dermatitis may be classified by cause into two subgroups: *irritant* contact dermatitis (ICD) and *allergic* contact dermatitis (ACD). ICD occurs when the skin is exposed to an environment or substance in a sufficient frequency, quantity, or duration that it overcomes the barrier function of the skin. Therefore, given adequate exposure, anyone may experience ICD. ACD is a delayed-type hypersensitivity (type 4) reaction to a topical agent and requires initial contact with a substance causing a T helper cell type 2 (Th2)–mediated immune response in a predisposed individual. Only with repeated exposure do the primed T cells cause the clinical response of dermatitis.

Findings of contact dermatitis can include erythema, vesicles, bullae, exudation, and crusting from breaking of blisters, swelling, and scaling. Common areas affected are the hands, neck, eyelids, face, genitalia, and legs. ICD and ACD can look identical and can present on similar body areas. Both may be intensely pruritic, further complicating the diagnosis. In addition, ACD and ICD can be present simultaneously, as with the health care worker allergic to latex who washes the hands repeatedly throughout the day. A careful history and patch testing are often the key to diagnosis.

Each year, millions of patients develop an allergic rash after contact with poison ivy, poison sumac, or poison oak, and contrary to popular belief, the fluid within these vesicles does not cause poison ivy "to spread." Nickel is the most common nonplant cause of ACD and historically more common in women because of costume jewelry and ear piercing (Fig. 33-30). With the increased popularity of jewelry and body piercing, the prevalence is rising in men. The 10 top causes of ACD in North America are nickel, neomycin, balsam of Peru (common fragrance), fragrance mix, thimerosal (preservative no longer used in vaccines but still found in eye preparations), sodium gold thiosulfate, quaternium-15 (preservative), formaldehyde (preservative), bacitracin, and cobalt (metal often in conjunction with nickel in silver-colored jewelry).

In the workplace, ACD is very common. For skin conditions, 90% of workers' compensation claims result from contact dermatitis. Common offenders in specific occupations are rubber or latex in health care workers, hair and clothing dyes in hairdressers, chromates in cement workers, and the Rhus family (poison ivy, oak, and sumac) in agricultural workers. ICD most often develops in response to excessive exposure to soaps, cleansers, hand sanitizers, and water. Therefore the primary treatment is avoidance of these irritating substances, application of a barrier ointment such as petrolatum, and protective equipment such as gloves.

For ACD caused by plants, the skin and clothes with soap and water should be thoroughly washed as soon as possible to minimize exposure to the antigen. Cool, wet soaks for 10 to 15 minutes may be soothing. Superpotent topical steroids, such as clobetasol propionate or betamethasone dipropionate applied twice daily for 1 to 2 weeks, are effective for treating small areas of moderate ACD. Systemic steroids are reserved for severe episodes of and should be continued for at least 2 weeks to prevent rebound dermatitis. In otherwise healthy persons, a tapering dose of prednisone is not required for short courses of systemic therapy. Severe pruritus may respond to antihistamines such as hydroxyzine, diphenhydramine, or a nonsedating H_2 blocker such as loratadine, cetirizine, or fexofenadine.

If ACD is suspected based on history, consultation for patch testing with a dermatologist can be customized to the patient's occupation or hobbies. Once the offending agent is identified, avoidance is crucial. When the offending agent is occupational, a change in jobs may be required. Alternative protective equipment can be sufficient in other cases, such as substituting nitrile gloves for latex. Generalized dry-skin care, topical steroids, or immunomodulators (pimecrolimus, tacrolimus) can help prevent recurrence and treat flares.

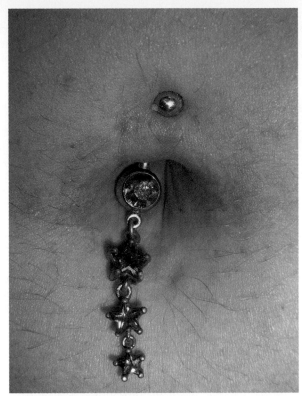

Figure 33-30 Contact dermatitis to nickel jewelry in umbilicus. (© *Richard P. Usatine.*)

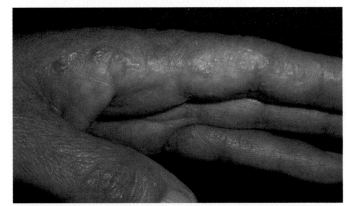

Figure 33-31 Dyshidrotic eczema with tapioca vesicles (pompholyx). (© *Richard P. Usatine.*)

Dyshidrotic Eczema (Pompholyx)

Dyshidrotic eczema is a form of dermatitis characterized by a pruritic vesicular eruption on the fingers, palms, and soles (Figs. 33-31). Patients may be affected at any age, with women affected twice as often as men. The condition may be acute, intermittent, or chronic. Eruptions occur with varying severity and can be mild or debilitating. Before the formation of vesicles, patients describe itching or burning of the hands and feet. Small vesicles appear along the lateral aspects of the fingers or feet, palms, and soles. Lesions may persist for weeks and may be accompanied by erythema of the palms and soles.

Treatment of dyshidrotic eczema includes high-potency topical steroids and cold compresses for symptomatic relief of the burning sensation. Greasy emollients are helpful to moisturize, protect, and prevent fissures. If fissures do occur, cyanoacrylate ("superglue") can be used to seal small cracks in the skin and decrease pain. Short courses of oral steroids may be used for acute flares.

Stasis Dermatitis

Stasis dermatitis occurs on the lower extremities in patients with chronic venous insufficiency (Fig. 33-32). Impaired function of the venous valves permits backflow of the blood from the deep venous system to the superficial system, causing increased venous hydrostatic pressure and increased permeability of dermal capillaries. The condition typically affects middle-aged and older-adult patients, except for patients with acquired venous insufficiency resulting from surgery, trauma, or thrombosis.

Stasis dermatitis can range from mild to severe. In all stages, reddish brown discoloration is caused by staining from hemosiderin that has leaked out of red blood cells in the overtaxed dermal capillaries. Pedal edema and scaling are also present in various degrees, and one leg can be more affected than the other. ACD is often superimposed on stasis dermatitis and can mislead the physician into suspecting cellulitis because of a sudden reddening, weeping, or induration of the area. Because of the impaired skin barrier and frequent use of OTC products and "home remedies," neomycin, lanolin, iodine, fragrances, and preservatives are common triggers for ACD in these patients.

Long-term treatment focuses first on reducing pedal edema with compression therapy, after assessing the integrity of the arterial circulation to prevent claudication or ischemic necrosis. Compression stockings are best applied early in the morning, before the patient rises from bed, when leg edema is at a minimum. For the pruritus and dermatitis, stasis dermatitis is treated in the same manner as other forms of acute eczematous dermatitis. Dry skin care with mild cleansers (Dove, Cetaphil) and bland emollients (petrolatum, Aquaphor or Absorbase) should be used liberally. Medium-potency topical corticosteroids (e.g., triamcinolone 0.1% ointment) should be used twice daily when inflammation and pruritus are present. If infection is suspected, mupirocin should be used preferentially over other topical antibiotics. For severe cases with exuberant purulent drainage and induration, oral antibiotics with activity against *Staphylococcus* and *Streptococcus* should be used.

Nummular Dermatitis (Nummular Eczema)

Nummular dermatitis consists of well-demarcated, coin-shaped lesions of eczema, typically on the extremities and less often the trunk (Fig. 33-33). Nummular dermatitis tends to worsen in dry, cold weather. Lesions may be mildly to severely pruritic and as a result become excoriated or even lichenified with scratching. Nummular dermatitis can be confused with plaques of psoriasis or tinea corporis but skin scrapings will not reveal hyphae on KOH preparation. Also, lesions lack the typical central sparing of tinea corporis. If necessary, a biopsy can help differentiate nummular eczema from psoriasis.

As with all eczematous dermatitis, general dry skin care is recommended with mild cleansers and bland emollients.

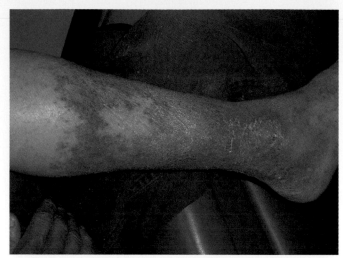

Figure 33-32 Stasis dermatitis. *(© Richard P. Usatine.)*

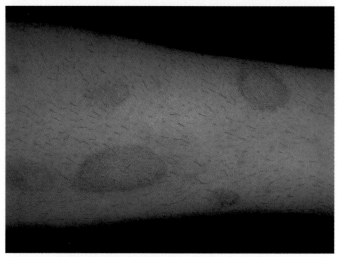

Figure 33-33 Nummular eczema. *(© Richard P. Usatine.)*

An intermediate to potent topical steroid may be applied two to four times daily to the affected areas. Once lesions improve, a lower-potency steroid should be used to minimize skin atrophy. Pruritus may be treated with an antihistamine if needed.

Generalized Exfoliative Dermatitis

Exfoliative dermatitis, also known as *erythroderma*, is an uncommon but serious skin disorder defined as erythema and scale covering over 90% of the body surface area (Fig. 33-34). The four most common causes of erythroderma are psoriasis, AD, cutaneous T-cell lymphoma (CTCL), and drug reactions. More than 60 drugs have been implicated in cases of exfoliative dermatitis; more often allopurinol, beta-lactam antibiotics, antiseizure medications, and sulfa drugs. More than half of patients will have a known underlying skin disease, but in up to 25% an etiology may never be determined and is termed *idiopathic* erythroderma. The majority of patients are adults over age 40.

The long-term prognosis is good in patients with drug-induced exfoliative dermatitis. The course tends to be remitting and relapsing in idiopathic cases. The prognosis of patients with associated malignancy usually depends on the

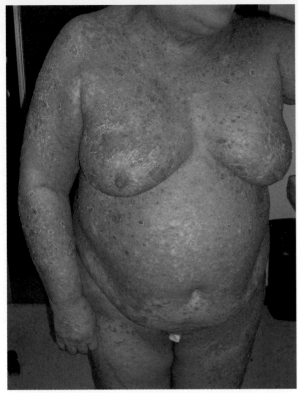

Figure 33-34 Erythroderma secondary to pustular psoriasis. *(© Richard P. Usatine.)*

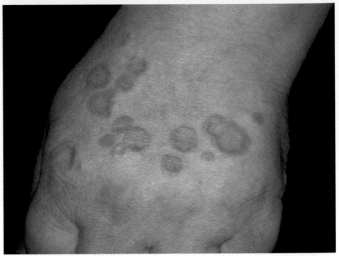

Figure 33-35 Granuloma annulare. *(© Richard P. Usatine.)*

outcome of the malignancy. A skin biopsy can help establish the diagnosis when the underlying skin disease is not known. The approach to treatment should include discontinuation of potentially causative medications and a search for any underlying malignancy. Initial evaluation and treatment usually require hospitalization for fluid and electrolyte replacement, temperature modulation, and prevention and treatment of secondary infection.

Erythema Nodosum

Erythema nodosum is an acute inflammatory process involving the fatty tissue layer underlying the skin (panniculitis). The condition is more frequently seen in women, and although often idiopathic, many cases are associated with streptococcal infections of the upper respiratory tract, drugs such as estrogens/oral contraceptives, sarcoidosis, and inflammatory bowel disease. Other, less frequent bacterial causes include tuberculosis, brucellosis, mycoplasma, and chlamydia. Fungal infections such as blastomycosis and histoplasmosis may also cause erythema nodosum. Rare causes are Behçet's disease, acute myelogenous leukemia, and Hodgkin's disease.

Patients present with tender red nodules, most frequently on the pretibial area or lower legs. The nodules may become fluctuant but do not suppurate or ulcerate. New lesions may continue to appear for several weeks. Additional symptoms may include fever, malaise, and arthralgia. Treatment is aimed at determining any underlying cause. Infectious processes should be evaluated and treated appropriately. Discontinuation of any possible offending agents is also advised. Bed rest, leg elevation, and nonsteroidal anti-inflammatory drugs (NSAIDSs) are the mainstays of therapy. Spontaneous

resolution occurs within 4 to 6 weeks in most patients, but residual leg pain and ankle edema can persist for weeks.

Granuloma Annulare

Granuloma annulare is a benign, self-limited dermatosis characterized by a raised annular distribution (Fig. 33-35). The condition may be localized, generalized, perforating, or subcutaneous. Except for subcutaneous granuloma annulare, the subtypes have similar appearances, but each follows a distinct clinical course. *Subcutaneous* granuloma annulare appears differently, with deep dermal or subcutaneous nodules. Patients with *localized* granuloma annulare present with groups of 1-mm to 2-mm papules in an annular arrangement over the distal extremities, ranging in color from skin tone to erythematous. Lesions most frequently appear on the dorsal surfaces of the hands and feet, fingers, and extensor aspects of the arms and legs. In *generalized* granuloma annulare, patients have a few to thousands of papules and rings that involve many body regions. The rings tend to be distributed symmetrically. Patients with *perforating* granuloma annulare present with up to hundreds of grouped 1-mm to 4-mm papules that may evolve into pustular lesions that drain and umbilicate, leaving atrophic scars. These lesions tend to appear on the extensor surfaces of extremities and the dorsa of the hands and fingers. Granuloma annulare may resolve spontaneously but can take several years. When patients request treatment, steroid injections are most effective.

Infectious Skin Diseases

Bacterial Infections

Key Points

- Most bacterial skin infections are caused by *Streptococcus pyogenes* or *Staphylococcus aureus*.
- Impetigo is the most superficial bacterial skin infection and often appears with honey-crusted lesions.
- Erysipelas is a superficial bacterial skin infection that extends into the cutaneous lymphatics, most often on the face or lower leg.

- Cellulitis is a deeper skin infection that requires oral antibiotics active against *S. pyogenes* and *S. aureus*.
- Abscesses often require incision and drainage to resolve completely.
- Community-acquired methicillin-resistant *S. aureus* is a common cause of abscesses and other bacterial skin infections.

Impetigo

Impetigo is a bacterial infection of the epidermis caused by *Staphylococcus aureus* and group A beta-hemolytic streptococci (GABHS). Both organisms may be present at the same time in the affected site. Community-acquired methicillin-resistant *S. aureus* (CA-MRSA) may cause impetigo. Impetigo is highly infectious and easily transmitted by hand contact. Various types of dermatitis can become secondarily infected with bacteria, and the skin is then called "impetiginized." About 30% of people are colonized in the anterior nares by *S. aureus*. The bacteria are transmitted from one person to another through hand contact, entering through broken skin created by cutaneous diseases, burns, surgery, trauma, radiation therapy, and insect bites.

Impetigo is a common condition that occurs in all age groups and in both genders equally. The incidence in those younger than 6 years is higher than in adults. Peak incidence occurs during the summer and fall. Most patients recover without complications. Individuals with impetigo from streptococcal infections can develop glomerulonephritis as a rare complication. Impetigo is usually diagnosed clinically based on its characteristic appearance of honey crusts and superficial ulcerations (Figs. 33-36). Exudate from beneath the skin crust should be obtained for culture and sensitivity testing if a community outbreak has occurred, MRSA is suspected, or poststreptococcal glomerulonephritis is present.

Mupirocin ointment is the treatment of choice for small areas of impetigo and is as effective as oral antibiotics, including cases caused by MRSA and GABHS. Mupirocin three times daily for 5 days each month is also recommended intranasally for patients found to be chronic nasal carriers. Oral antibiotics are used in patients with extensive impetigo or with refractory infection. A cephalosporin, semisynthetic

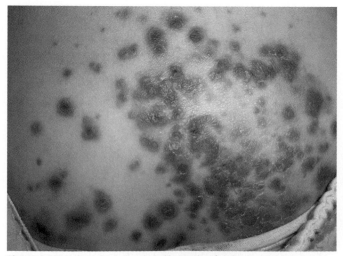

Figure 33-36 Impetigo on back and buttocks of child showing honey crusts. (© Richard P. Usatine.)

penicillin, or beta-lactam–beta-lactamase inhibitor is recommended. If bacterial cultures reveal MRSA, trimethoprim-sulfamethoxazole, doxycycline (over age 10), or clindamycin are appropriate. Gentle debridement of crusts using antibacterial soap and a washcloth is also recommended. Patients should be encouraged to use careful handwashing to prevent further spread of infection.

Erysipelas (St. Anthony's Fire)

Erysipelas is a superficial bacterial skin infection that extends into the cutaneous lymphatics. Usually, this infection is caused by *Streptococcus pyogenes* and occurs on the face or lower leg. Bacterial inoculation into an area of damaged skin is the initial event in developing erysipelas, although patients may not recall the precipitating event. The source of the bacteria is often from the host's nasopharynx. A history of recent streptococcal pharyngitis is reported in up to one third of patients.

The most common complaints during the acute infection are pain, fever, chills, and swelling of the skin. Infants, young children, and older adult patients are the groups most often affected, with a peak incidence at age 60 to 80. Erysipelas may become a red, indurated, tense, and shiny plaque with sharply demarcated margins. Local inflammatory signs, such as warmth, edema, and tenderness, are universal. Lymphatic involvement is manifested by a peau d'orange look to the skin, with sharp borders and regional lymphadenopathy. More severe infections may include numerous vesicles or bullae, petechiae, and even skin necrosis. Streptococci cause erysipelas in as many as 80% of cases, with two thirds of those caused by group A and 25% by group G streptococci. *S. aureus* has been implicated in cases of recurrent erysipelas secondary to lymphedema. Atypical forms have been caused by *Streptococcus pneumoniae*, *Klebsiella pneumoniae*, *Yersinia enterocolitica*, and *Moraxella* spp. and should be considered in cases refractory to standard antibiotic therapy.

In cases involving the extremities, elevation and rest of the affected limb are recommended to reduce local swelling and inflammation. Oral or intramuscular (IM) penicillin for 10 to 14 days is sufficient for many cases of erysipelas. A macrolide such as erythromycin or azithromycin may be used if the patient is allergic to penicillin. Hospitalization for close monitoring and intravenous (IV) antibiotics are recommended for severe cases and for infants, older adults, and immunocompromised patients. Facial erysipelas should be treated empirically with a penicillinase-resistant antibiotic such as dicloxacillin to cover for possible *S. aureus*. Predisposing skin lesions, such as tinea pedis and stasis ulcers, should be treated aggressively to prevent superinfection.

Cellulitis

Cellulitis is an acute infection of the skin and soft tissues, usually developing after a break in the skin. The condition is characterized by localized pain, swelling, tenderness, erythema, and warmth (Fig. 33-37). The vast majority of cases are caused by *Streptococcus pyogenes* or *S. aureus*. Other causes include *Vibrio vulnificus* and *Pseudomonas*. Cellulitis is generally localized and nonrecurrent when treated appropriately.

Mortality is extremely rare but may occur when the condition is neglected or caused by a highly virulent organism. Patients typically present with a red, hot, swollen, and tender area of skin. Unlike erysipelas, the borders are neither elevated nor sharply demarcated. Lymphangitis and local lymphadenopathy may be present. Fever is common, and patients with severe cases may develop hypotension. Those with mild cellulitis may be treated as outpatients. Oral antibiotics are usually effective for treatment of cellulitis in immunocompetent hosts. Severe cases or patients with comorbid conditions (e.g., cardiac, renal, or hepatic failure, immunosuppression) should be initially treated with IV antibiotics in the hospital setting. Elevation of affected limbs improves resolution of swelling.

Folliculitis

Folliculitis is caused by infection or irritation of individual hair follicles. Patients with folliculitis present with pustules at the bases of hairs, particularly on the scalp, back, legs, and arms (Fig. 33-38). Folliculitis occurs more often in obese, immunocompromised, or diabetic patients. *S. aureus* is the most common pathogen. A form of folliculitis

caused by *Pseudomonas*, "hot tub folliculitis," occurs when patients use poorly maintained hot tubs. The condition may be self-limited, requiring only the use of antibacterial soap, or may persist and require topical or systemic antibiotic therapy. If a pseudomonal infection is suspected and lesions persist for more than 5 days without treatment, an oral fluoroquinolone (e.g., ciprofloxacin) should be considered.

Abscesses: Furuncles and Carbuncles

Furuncles, or "boils," are small abscesses in the skin. Patients present with a painful, often fluctuant swelling in areas of friction, the nasal area, or the external ear. A *carbuncle* is a collection of furuncles and usually occurs on the back of the neck in middle-aged and older men. Treatment often requires drainage of the lesion. Antibiotic therapy should be considered if the furuncle is not yet fluctuant, there is evidence of surrounding cellulitis or lymphadenitis, or the lesion is on the face. Carbuncles have many interconnecting sinuses and tend to recur despite drainage and antibiotics. Surgical drainage and resection of the lesions are often necessary. Many abscesses are now caused by MRSA, but the primary treatment is still incision and drainage.

Erythrasma

Erythrasma is a superficial skin infection caused by *Corynebacterium*, a normal inhabitant of the skin. The infection typically occurs in intertriginous spaces, especially in obese, hyperhidrotic, or diabetic patients (Fig. 33-39). Moderate itching and discomfort may occur, and the infected skin is often reddish brown and may be slightly raised, with some central clearing. The lesions are largely confluent but may have poorly defined borders. Because of the production of porphyrins by the infecting corynebacteria, Wood's light demonstrates the lesions as a coral red. However, if the patient has recently washed the affected area, the coral-red fluorescence may be absent. Erythrasma is often confused with a fungal infection. Erythrasma may be treated with oral or topical erythromycin or clindamycin.

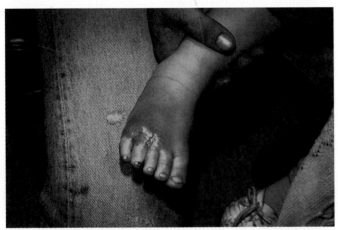

Figure 33-37 Cellulitis on foot of child after a break in the skin. *(© Richard P. Usatine.)*

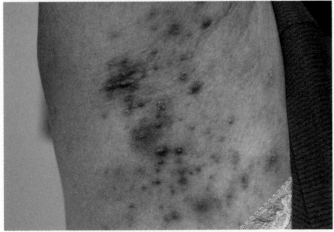

Figure 33-38 Folliculitis secondary to methicillin-resistant *Staphylococcus aureus* (MRSA). *(Courtesy of Alisha N. Plotner, MD, and Robert T. Brodell, MD, with permission from J Fam Pract 2008; 57(4):253–255.)*

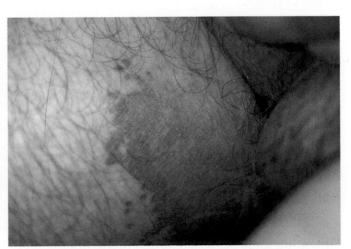

Figure 33-39 Erythrasma in groin. *(© Richard P. Usatine.)*

Fungal Infections

Key Points

- Tinea capitis should be treated with oral antifungal agents.
- Tinea infections may be transmitted from person to person by animals (pets, livestock) and through fomites.
- Over-the-counter topical antifungals are often effective for tinea pedis.
- Tinea versicolor is caused by *Malassezia* and can be treated by topical antidandruff shampoos or oral antifungal (ketoconazole, fluconazole).

Dermatophytosis (Tinea)

Mucocutaneous fungal infections are caused by dermatophytes (*Microsporum, Epidermophyton,* and *Trichophyton*) and yeasts. About 40 species in the three dermatophyte genera can cause tinea pedis and manus, tinea capitis, tinea corporis, tinea cruris, and onychomycosis. Yeasts of *Candida* can cause diaper dermatitis, balanitis, vulvovaginitis, and thrush (Fig. 33-40). The yeastlike organism of *Malassezia (Pityrosporum)* causes tinea versicolor and contributes to seborrhea. Although tinea versicolor has the name tinea in it, it is not a true dermatophyte.

The most important test for a suspected fungal infection is the KOH prep. Scrape the leading edge of the lesion onto a slide using the side of a #15 scalpel or another slide. Use the coverslip to push the scale into the center of the slide. Add 2 drops of KOH (with or without fungal stain) to the slide, and place coverslip on top. Examine with microscope starting with 10× and low light to look for the cells and hyphae. The fungal stain helps the hyphae to stand out among the epithelial cells. Look for groups of cells that appear to have fungal elements within them; don't be fooled by cell borders that look linear and branching. Switch to 40× to confirm any areas that appear to have fungal elements by looking for true fungal morphology. The fungal stains bring out these characteristics, including cell walls, nuclei, and arthroconidia (Fig. 33-41). KOH test characteristics without fungal stain are sensitivity, 77% to 88%, and specificity, 62% to 95% (Thomas, 2003).

Tinea Corporis

Tinea corporis is a superficial dermatophyte infection of the cornified layers of skin on the trunk and extremities. Lesions are typically annular with central clearing and a scaling border and may be pruritic (Fig. 33-42). Infection may be transmitted from person to person, by animals such as household pets or farm animals, and through fomites. Because the cornified layer of skin is involved, topical therapy is usually sufficient for localized cases. A topical antifungal should be applied to the lesion and proximal surrounding skin twice daily for a minimum of 2 weeks. Various agents have demonstrated effectiveness, including the azoles (miconazole, clotrimazole, ketoconazole, itraconazole) and the allylamines (naftifine, terbinafine). Terbinafine 1% cream (available OTC as Lamisil AF) produced a mycologic cure of 84.2%, versus 23.3% with placebo (Budimulja et al., 2001). In another study, patients with mycologically diagnosed tinea corporis and tinea cruris were randomly allocated

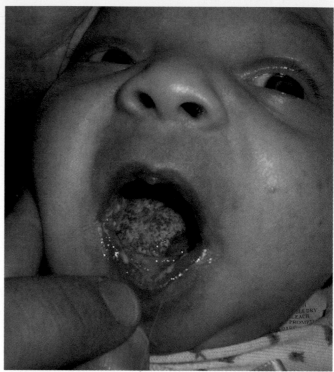

Figure 33-40 Thrush caused by *Candida albicans*. *(© Richard P. Usatine.)*

to receive either 250 mg of oral terbinafine once daily or 500 mg of griseofulvin once daily for 2 weeks. The cure rates were higher for terbinafine at 6 weeks (Voravutinon, 1993). Patients should be instructed to avoid direct contact with others and avoid sharing towels and clothing to prevent spread of the infection. Oral antifungal agents should be considered for first-line therapy for tinea corporis covering large areas of the body (Fig. 33-43).

> **KEY TREATMENT**
>
> All topical antifungal agents (not nystatin) may be effective, but evidence supports the greater effectiveness of the allylamines (e.g., terbinafine) over the less expensive azoles (e.g., clotrimazole) for tinea pedis and corporis (Crawford, 2000) (SOR: A).
> Terbinafine 1% cream or solution once daily for 7 days is highly effective for tinea corporis or cruris (Budimulja et al., 2001) (SOR: B).
> Oral terbinafine, 250 mg once daily, showed higher cure rates for tinea corporis and cruris than griseofulvin (Voravutinon, 1993) (SOR: B).

Tinea Pedis

Tinea pedis is most often caused by *Trichophyton rubrum*. Typically, patients describe pruritic scaly soles, often with painful fissures between the toes. Vesicular or ulcerative lesions may also be present. The most characteristic type of infection is interdigital (Fig. 33-44). Erythema, maceration, and fissuring occur between the toes and are accompanied by intense pruritus. Patients may also have chronic hyperkeratotic tinea pedis, characterized by plantar erythema and hyperkeratosis that may be completely asymptomatic or mildly pruritic. This is described as a moccasin distribution (Fig. 33-45). Inflammatory tinea pedis causes painful vesicles on the foot (see Fig. 33-1).

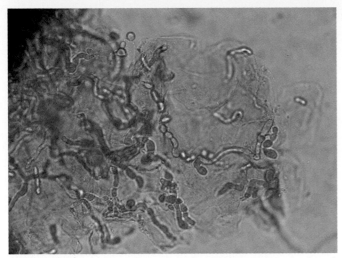

Figure 33-41 *Trichophyton rubrum* seen after KOH preparation using fungal stain. *(© Richard P. Usatine.)*

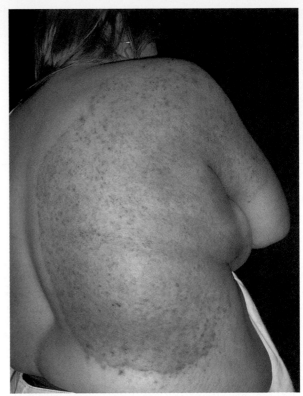

Figure 33-43 Tinea corporis covering half the body. *(© Richard P. Usatine.)*

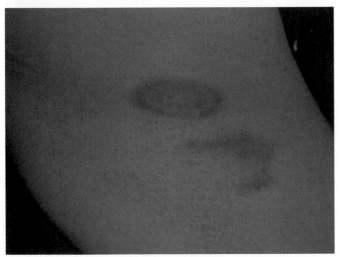

Figure 33-42 Tinea corporis showing concentric circles. *(© Richard P. Usatine.)*

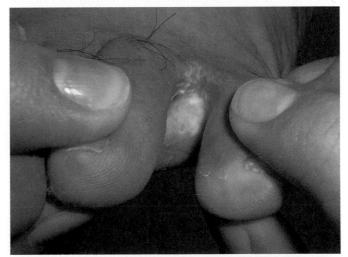

Figure 33-44 Tinea pedis between toes. *(© Richard P. Usatine.)*

Tinea pedis is more common in men than in women and rarely occurs in children. Infection can occur through contact with infected scales on bath or pool floors, so wearing protective footwear in shared areas may help decrease the likelihood of infection. Occlusive footwear promotes infection by creating warm, humid, macerating environments; therefore patients should try to minimize foot moisture by limiting the use of occlusive footwear and frequently changing socks.

The treatment of tinea pedis involves application of an antifungal cream to the web spaces and other infected areas. Topical antifungal agents containing allylamines (naftifine, terbinafine, butenafine) or azoles (clotrimazole, miconazole, econazole) all work to treat tinea pedis. Allylamines cure slightly more infections than azoles but are more expensive. No differences in efficacy were found between individual allylamines or individual azoles (Crawford et al., 2000) Infrequently, systemic therapy is used for refractory infections. Twice-daily application of the allylamine terbinafine has resulted in a higher cure rate than twice-daily application of the imidazole clotrimazole (Lotrimin AF), and more rapidly.

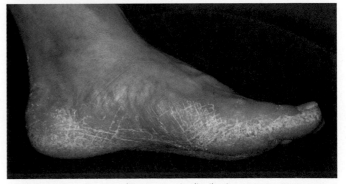

Figure 33-45 Tinea pedis in moccasin distribution. *(© Richard P. Usatine.)*

KEY TREATMENT

With topical antifungals to treat tinea pedis, allylamines cure slightly more infections than azoles but are more expensive (Crawford et al., 2000) (SOR: A).
Consider oral antifungals such as terbinafine, 250 mg daily for 2 weeks, when tinea pedis is severe or does not respond to topical agents (Bell-Syer et al., 2002) (SOR: B).
Oral itraconazole is equal to oral terbinafine in patient outcomes. Itraconazole can be prescribed as two 100-mg tabs daily for 1 week (Bell-Syer et al., 2002; Thomas, 2003) (SOR: B).

Tinea Cruris

Tinea cruris, commonly called "jock itch," is a dermatophyte infection of the groin. This dermatophytosis is more common in men than women and is frequently associated with tinea pedis. Tinea cruris occurs when ambient temperature and humidity are high. Occlusion from wet or tight-fitting clothing provides an optimal environment for infection. Tinea cruris involves the proximal medial thighs and may extend to the buttocks and lower abdomen (Fig. 33-46). The scrotum tends to be spared. Patients with this dermatophytosis frequently complain of burning and pruritus. Pustules and vesicles at the active edge of the infected area, along with maceration, are present on a background of red scaling lesions with raised borders. Care should be taken to evaluate the feet as a source of infection.

In addition to topical antifungals, treatment can include a low-dose corticosteroid for the first few days to reduce the inflammation of the involved skin. Oral antifungal therapy is needed if the tinea cruris has spread beyond the groin (Fig. 33-47). Inverse psoriasis may be mistaken for tinea cruris and will not respond to antifungal treatment (Fig. 33-48). The fungicidal allylamines naftifine and terbinafine and the allylamine derivative butenafine are more costly topical tinea treatments but allow for a shorter duration of treatment compared with fungistatic azoles (clotrimazole, econazole, ketoconazole, oxiconazole, miconazole, sulconazole) (Nadalo et al., 2006).

KEY TREATMENT

Tinea cruris may be treated with a topical allylamine or a topical azole (Nadalo et al., 2006) (SOR: B).
Fluconazole, 150 mg once weekly for 2 to 4 weeks, appears effective against tinea cruris (Nozickova et al., 1998) (SOR: B).

Tinea Capitis

Tinea capitis, the most common dermatophytosis in children, is an infection of the scalp and hair follicle. Transmission is fostered by poor hygiene and overcrowding and can occur through contaminated hats, brushes, and pillowcases. After being shed, affected hairs can harbor viable organisms for more than 1 year. Tinea capitis is characterized by irregular or well-demarcated alopecia and scaling (Fig. 33-49). Cervical and occipital lymphadenopathy may be prominent. When hairs fracture a few millimeters from the scalp, "black dot" alopecia is produced. Tinea scalp infection also may result in a cell-mediated immune response termed a *kerion*, which is a boggy, sterile, inflammatory scalp mass

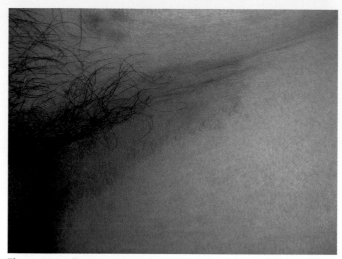

Figure 33-46 Tinea cruris in woman. *(© Richard P. Usatine.)*

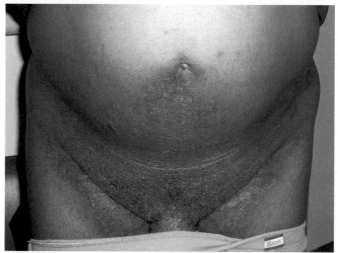

Figure 33-47 Tinea cruris that has spread up to umbilicus. *(© Richard P. Usatine.)*

(Fig. 33-50). A kerion does not require antibiotics or incision and drainage. If a kerion does not respond to oral antifungals alone, an oral steroid may be added for a short course.

Oral griseofulvin daily for 6 to 8 weeks is a proven treatment for tinea capitis, even if it requires a somewhat longer course than the newer antifungal agents (Fleece et al., 2004). It is available in a liquid form for children. Also, consider 4 weeks of oral terbinafine daily; it was as effective as 8 weeks of griseofulvin after 8 weeks, but at week 12 the efficacy of griseofulvin decreased to 44%, whereas the efficacy of terbinafine was 76% (Caceres-Rios et al., 2000). Consider oral fluconazole as an option because it is available in liquid form and appears to be effective and safe, but fewer clinical trials have been done (Foster et al., 2005).

KEY TREATMENT

Give oral griseofulvin daily for 6 to 8 weeks to treat tinea capitis (Fleece et al., 2004) (SOR: B).
Consider 4 weeks of oral terbinafine daily (Caceres-Rios et al., 2000) (SOR: B).
Consider oral fluconazole (available as liquid) as an option to treat tinea capitis (Foster et al., 2005) (SOR: B).

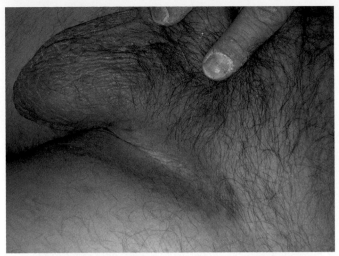

Figure 33-48 Inverse psoriasis that resembles tinea cruris. Note nail pitting of psoriasis. *(© Richard P. Usatine.)*

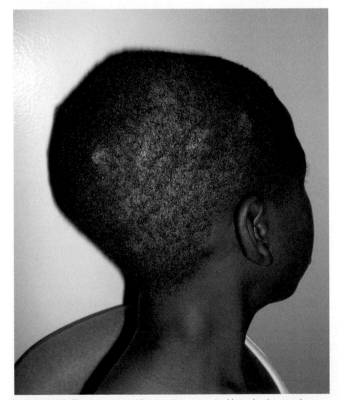

Figure 33-49 Tinea capitis with prominent cervical lymphadenopathy. *(© Richard P. Usatine.)*

Onychomycosis

Onychomycosis is a fungal infection that affects the toenails or fingernails. It may involve any component of the nail unit, including the nail matrix, nail bed, or nail plate. Onychomycosis may be unsightly but is often asymptomatic. In the worst cases, it causes enough discomfort and disfigurement to produce physical and occupational limitations. Use of topical agents should be limited to cases involving less than half the distal nail plate and patients unable to tolerate systemic treatment. Agents include ciclopirox 8% (Penlac), azoles, and allylamines. Topical treatments are poorly effective because of inadequate nail plate penetration. Oral antifungal agents such as terbinafine and itraconazole have replaced older therapies in the treatment of onychomycosis. Oral antifungals offer shorter treatment regimens, higher cure rates, and fewer adverse effects. Removal of the nail plate should be considered an alternative treatment in patients who cannot tolerate oral therapy and are having symptoms that interfere with their quality of life.

> ### KEY TREATMENT
>
> Terbinafine is more effective than griseofulvin, and terbinafine and itraconazole are more effective than no treatment (Cochrane review; Bell-Syer et al., 2004) (SOR: A).
>
> Two clinical trials of nail infections found no evidence of benefit for topical treatments (did not include ciclopirox) compared with placebo (Cochrane review; Crawford et al., 1999) (SOR: A).

Tinea Versicolor

Tinea versicolor presents with hypopigmented, pink/brown macules and patches on the trunk with fine scale. *Versicolor* means varied colors, and this tinea tends to be white, pink, and brown (Fig. 33-51). Tinea versicolor is found on the back, chest, abdomen, and upper arms, often in a capelike distribution. Tinea versicolor is caused by *Malassezia furfur (Pityrosporum)*, a lipophilic yeast that can be normal human cutaneous flora. Tinea versicolor is also called *pityriasis versicolor* after the causative organism. *Pityrosporum* is also associated with seborrhea, and thus antidandruff shampoos are effective in treating this tinea. *Pityrosporum* spp. thrive on sebum and moisture and tend to grow on the skin in areas where sebaceous follicles secrete sebum. Topical and oral treatments are effective, but tinea versicolor tends to recur, especially during the warmer months. The diagnosis can usually be made with the clinical examination, and if there is any doubt, a KOH prep can be examined for the typical "spaghetti and meatballs" pattern (Fig. 33-52). The spaghetti or "ziti" is the short mycelial form, and the meatballs are the round yeast of *Pityrosporum ovale*.

Patients may apply selenium sulfide 2.5% lotion or shampoo to the involved areas daily for 1 week. A double-blind study found that selenium sulfide (2.5%) lotion applied daily for 10 minutes for 7 consecutive days was effective in the treatment of tinea versicolor (Sanchez and Torres, 1984). A single oral dose of 400 mg of oral fluconazole or ketoconazole can also be used to treat tinea versicolor. Fluconazole provided the best clinical as well as mycologic cure rate, with no relapse during 12 months of follow-up (Bhogal et al., 2001). Oral itraconazole, 200 mg twice daily for 1 day a month, has been shown to be safe and effective as a prophylactic treatment for tinea versicolor (Faergemann et al., 2002).

> ### KEY TREATMENT
>
> Selenium sulfide 2.5% lotion (or shampoo) daily for 1 week is effective treatment of tinea versicolor (Sanchez and Torres, 1984) (SOR: B).
>
> Ketoconazole 2% shampoo (Nizoral) may be applied daily for 3 days to treat tinea versicolor (Lange et al., 1998) (SOR: B).
>
> Oral fluconazole or ketoconazole (400 mg) also treats tinea versicolor (Bhogal et al., 2001) (SOR: B).
>
> Oral itraconazole (200 mg bid 1 day a month) is effective prophylactic treatment for tinea versicolor (Faergemann et al., 2002) (SOR: B).

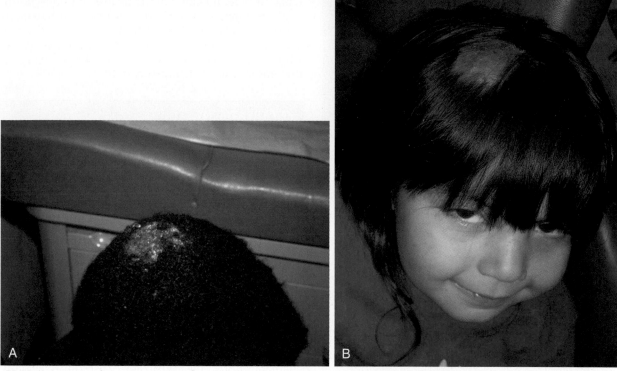

Figure 33-50 Kerions secondary to tinea capitis inflammation. *(© Richard P. Usatine.)*

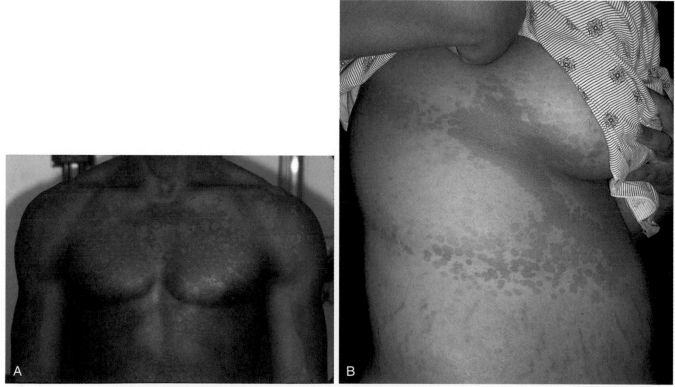

Figure 33-51 Tinea versicolor with hypopigmentation **(A)** and hyperpigmentation **(B)**. *(© Richard P. Usatine.)*

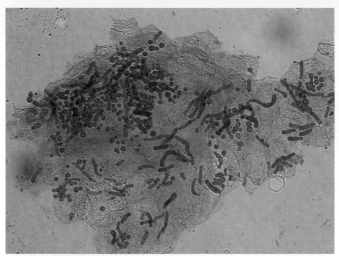

Figure 33-52 "Spaghetti and meatballs" pattern of tinea versicolor on microscopy (blue fungal stain, 40×). (© *Richard P. Usatine.*)

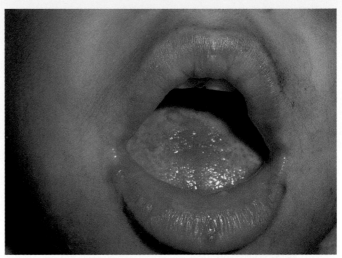

Figure 33-53 Oral herpes gingivostomatitis as primary infection in 2-year-old child. (© *Richard P. Usatine.*)

Viral Infections

Key Points

- Herpes simplex virus type 1 (HSV-1) is the most common cause of oral herpes infection (80%). HSV-2 is the primary pathogen in genital herpes (70%-90%). Both can cause oral or genital lesions.

- HSV-1 and HSV-2 are characterized by a primary infection, latent periods, asymptomatic shedding, and reactivation.

- Approximately 10% to 20% of the U.S. population develop zoster, but rates are likely to decrease with VZV vaccine for children.

- Corneal involvement should be suspected when herpes zoster involves the tip of the nose and is an ophthalmologic emergency because it can lead to blindness.

- For herpes zoster, antiviral therapy (acyclovir, valacyclovir, famciclovir) should by started within 3 days of onset of symptoms to reduce disease severity and postherpetic neuralgia.

- Human papillomavirus types 6 and 11 are associated with condylomata acuminata (genital warts); HPV types 16 and 18 are associated with carcinoma. The quadrivalent HPV vaccine is active against HPV types 6, 11, 16, and 18.

- Molluscum contagiosum is a common, self-limited viral infection most often affecting children. It is considered sexually transmitted in adults.

- Lesions of molluscum usually resolve spontaneously over months to years; with or without treatment, lesions can leave pitted scars.

Herpes Simplex

Herpes simplex virus types 1 and 2 (HSV-1 and HSV-2) are very common pathogens that cause orolabial and genital blisters or erosions. Seroprevalence of HSV-1 is estimated at 80% to 90% worldwide and is the most common cause of oral herpes infection (80%). HSV-2 is the primary pathogen in genital herpes (70%-90%) and is one of the most common sexually transmitted diseases (STDs). Approximately 50 million Americans have genital herpes, and an estimated 1 million new cases occur each year.

Herpes simplex infection can be characterized by an initial infection, episodes of latency, asymptomatic viral shedding, and recurrent activation. Spread of HSV-1 is primarily through direct contact with contaminated saliva or other secretions. Symptoms of primary orolabial herpes usually occur 3 to 7 days after exposure and include a prodrome of fever, sore throat, and lymphadenopathy. Localized pain, tingling, tenderness, or burning can occur before the eruption of the vesicles, which are usually grouped on a background of erythema and edema (Fig. 33-53). The lesions coalesce, ulcerate, and heal within 2 to 3 weeks.

Herpes simplex type 2 usually is transmitted through genital contact and must involve mucous membranes or open or damaged skin. Primary HSV-2 occurs up to 3 weeks after exposure to the virus and has more severe clinical manifestations. Systemic symptoms include fever, malaise, edema, inguinal lymphadenopathy, dysuria, and vaginal or penile discharge. These are more common in women. In men, painful vesicles and erosions usually occur on the penis but can also appear on the buttocks or perineum (Fig. 33-54). In women, lesions occur primarily on the labia but may also appear on the cervix, buttocks, or perineum. Symptoms of the primary episode typically last 2 to 3 weeks. Risk factors for genital herpes include age 15 to 30 (age of greatest sexually activity), increased number of sexual partners, black or Hispanic race, lower income levels and education, female gender, homosexuality, and HIV.

In both serotypes, HSV may be latent for months to years following the primary infection. During latency, the virus resides in the sensory nerve root ganglia. Recurrent outbreaks are often preceded by a prodrome of pain, itching, tingling, burning, or paresthesias and are usually less severe than the primary outbreak.

The diagnosis of herpes simplex is conveniently done with a direct fluorescent antibody test (DFA), and results may be obtained within hours. A viral culture can be performed, but results take 2 to 5 days. Serologic testing is also available and approved by the U.S. Food and Drug Administration (FDA) to establish serostatus, but this is not helpful for acute disease.

The treatment of HSV depends on whether the infection is a first episode or a recurrence. Many different dosing schedules are available with oral antivirals, including acyclovir

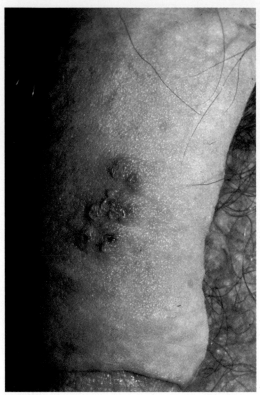

Figure 33-54 Herpes simplex type 2 (HSV-2) recurrence on penis with cluster of vesicles. *(Courtesy Jack Rezneck, Sr., and The Color Atlas of Family Medicine.)*

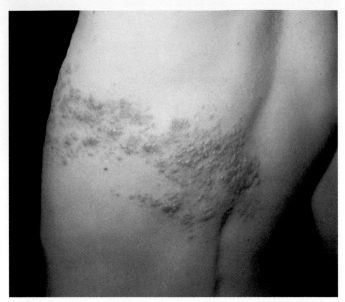

Figure 33-55 Herpes zoster in dermatomal pattern. *(© Richard P. Usatine.)*

(Zovirax), valacyclovir (Valtrex), and famciclovir (Famvir). Suppressive therapy may be considered in patients with recurrent genital herpes. Women who are pregnant or contemplating pregnancy should receive information regarding neonatal transmission and possible cesarean delivery if active lesions are present at the onset of labor. The risk of transmission is highest for women with a primary infection during the third trimester of pregnancy. Neonatal herpes infection can cause long-term CNS morbidity, such as mental retardation, chorioretinitis, seizures, and even death.

Herpes Zoster (Shingles)

Zoster is caused by the reactivation of the varicella-zoster virus (VZV, human herpesvirus 3, HHV-3, chickenpox). After the primary infection, VZV lies dormant in the dorsal root ganglia. The time between the onset of primary chickenpox and reactivation can be any time but usually decades later. Approximately 10% to 20% of the U.S. population eventually develop one or more cases of zoster in their lifetime. The incidence is much higher in immunocompromised patients and older adults. These rates are likely to decrease over time now that a VZV vaccine is given as part of the routine immunization schedule in children.

Patients typically experience pain and paresthesias, followed by the appearance of small groups of vesicles on an erythematous base in a dermatomal distribution (Fig. 33-55). The rash rarely crosses the midline of the body and is usually confined to a single dermatome. The eruption may be accompanied by a fever, headache, and malaise. Lesions usually resolve in 2 to 3 weeks. Pain can be severe and may persist long after skin lesions heal in a condition known as

postherpetic neuralgia. Corneal involvement should be suspected when lesions appear on the tip of the nose or in the distribution of cranial nerve VI and should prompt an emergency ophthalmology consultation because this can cause permanent blindness (Fig. 33-56).

Antiviral therapy such as acyclovir, valacyclovir, and famciclovir should be started within the first 3 days of onset of symptoms, to reduce the severity and duration of symptoms and skin lesions. Early treatment may also reduce the incidence and severity of postherpetic neuralgia. However, benefits can be seen even if started up to 7 days after onset of symptoms. Analgesics such as acetaminophen and even narcotics are sometimes required to control the pain caused by zoster. Cool compresses may also help soothe during the acute phase. Postherpetic neuralgia occurs in up to 40% of adult patients over age 60 but in less than 10% of patients less than 60. In 2006 the FDA approved a live, attenuated vaccine (Zostavax) for adults over 60 years who are immunocompetent and have not already had zoster. The vaccine decreased the burden of illness by 61% and decreased the incidence of postherpetic neuralgia by 67% in large clinical trials (Oxman et al., 2005).

Verruca (Warts)

Warts are common growths of skin and mucosa caused by the human papillomavirus (HPV). Currently, more than 100 types of HPV have been identified. Specific HPV types often correlate to the lesion location, morphology, or oncogenic potential. Although most are benign, warts can be disfiguring or can cause significant psychological distress, and some cause cancer.

Verruca vulgaris (common warts) are dome-shaped keratotic papules that usually develop on the dorsal hands, fingers, or other sites on the extremities (Fig. 33-57). *Palmoplantar* warts are on the palms or soles and are surrounded by hyperkeratotic calluslike skin. These can be painful when occurring on weight-bearing surfaces. Multiple plantar warts may combine to become a large mosaic wart. Both common

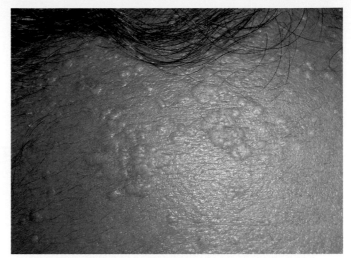

Figure 33-58 Flat warts on forehead. (© *Richard P. Usatine.*)

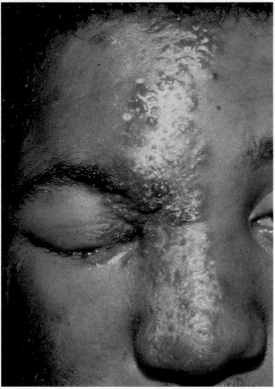

Figure 33-56 Herpes zoster on face with herpes ophthalmicus. (© *Richard P. Usatine.*)

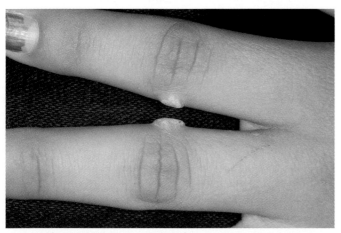

Figure 33-57 Kissing warts on fingers. (© *Richard P. Usatine.*)

warts and palmoplantar warts have characteristic punctuate black dots, mistakenly leading to the common term "seed warts," whereas these black dots actually represent thrombosed capillaries. *Filiform* warts have fingerlike projections and often appear on the face. *Verruca plana* (flat warts) are smooth, small (1-4 mm) flesh-colored papules, often occurring on the face or legs and often spread by scratching or shaving (Fig. 33-58). Although inconspicuous at first, flat warts propagate rapidly, often into the hundreds.

Condylomata acuminata (genital warts) occur on the external genitalia, perineum, perianal, or adjacent intertriginous regions but can also be found on the oral mucosa. These lesions are generally considered sexually transmitted, but it is usually impossible determine when the inoculation occurred. The lesions begin as small papules, which often become whitish with maceration and take on a cauliflower-like appearance as they grow (Fig. 33-59). Condylomata are associated with cervical carcinoma and penile cancer. Among the many subtypes of HPV, types 6 and 11 are most often associated with condylomata, whereas types 16 and 18 are most often associated with the development of carcinoma.

There is no standard treatment for warts. Most warts spontaneously regress over many months to years. Local treatments include cryotherapy, salicylic acid, imiquimod, podophyllin, 5-fluorouracil (5-FU), cantharidin, and duct tape. For physician-applied treatments such as cryotherapy or podophyllotoxin, patients should be seen every 3 to 4 weeks for repeat treatment as needed. For home treatments with salicylic acid, podofilox (Condylox), or imiquimod (Aldara), most are applied daily, and patients should be advised that treatment can take months of extreme persistence for resolution. Office and home treatment modalities can also be combined to hasten resolution, but studies are lacking.

Women with condylomata should have annual Papanicolaou tests to evaluate for cervical neoplasia. For both men and women, it is advisable to refrain from sexual activity while genital lesions are present, to prevent transmission. In 2006 the FDA approved an HPV vaccine (Gardasil), recommended for females age 11 to 26 regardless of abnormal Pap history, positive HPV status, or genital warts. It is active against HPV types 6, 11, 16, and 18. In clinical trials, Gardasil decreased the incidence of cervical intraepithelial neoplasia (CIN), cervical cancer, and anogenital warts by 90% (Villa et al., 2006).

Molluscum Contagiosum

Molluscum contagiosum is a common, self-limited viral infection seen most frequently in children and can occur anywhere on the body; most often on the trunk, face, and extremities. In adults, mollusca are considered sexually transmitted and occur in the genital region or lower abdomen. Infection occurs through direct skin-to-skin contact or indirect contact with fomites. The typical molluscum lesion is a pink to flesh-colored, firm, smooth, dome-shaped papule with central umbilication (Fig. 33-60). A white material

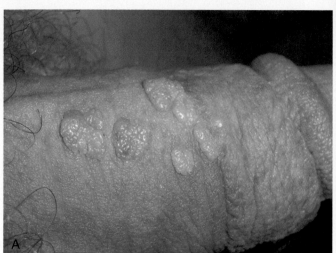

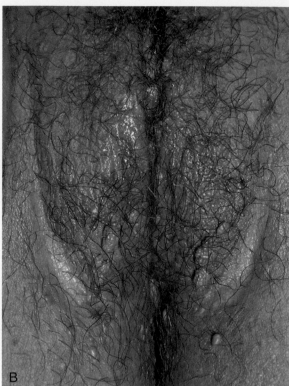

Figure 33-59 **A,** Condyloma acuminata on penis. **B,** Condyloma acuminata on vulva. *(© Richard P. Usatine.)*

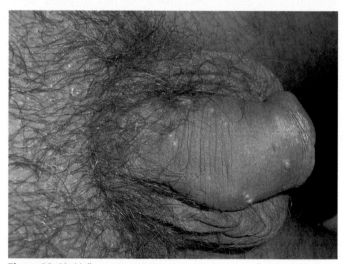

Figure 33-60 Molluscum contagiosum on penis as sexually transmitted disease. *(© Richard P. Usatine.)*

can sometimes be visualized in the umbilication and can be easily expressed. This caseous material is teeming with viral particles. Lesions are usually 2 to 5 mm in diameter and number less than 30, but can number in the hundreds. Particularly in immunocompromised patients, the infection may be much more extensive, may fail to resolve spontaneously, and may be resistant to treatment. Over months to years, lesions of molluscum normally resolve spontaneously.

Some patients or parents desire treatment, and cryotherapy, cantharidin, trichloroacetic acid (TCA), tretinoin (Retin-A), or imiquimod may be effective. Cantharidin is most easily given to young children because its application is painless.

Cryotherapy is another good option, but many young children will not willingly submit to this therapy, which is painful. Often it is best to reassure parents that molluscum is not harmful and will eventually resolve, although with or without treatment, lesions can leave pitted scars.

Infestations

Key Points

- Scabies is a pruritic rash involving interdigital spaces, wrists, ankles, waist, groin, and axillae.
- The three types of human lice infest the hair of the head, the body, or the pubic hair.

Scabies

Scabies is caused by the mite *Sarcoptes scabiei*, an obligate human parasite. Patients present with a pruritic rash that is often worse in the night. Skin findings include papules, nodules, burrows, and vesiculopustules (Fig. 33-61). The distribution includes the interdigital spaces, wrists, ankles, waist, groin, and axillae. Pruritic nodules around the axillae, umbilicus, or on the penis and scrotum are highly suggestive of scabies. In children the head can also be involved. Look for burrows because these are pathognomonic of scabies and will be the best site to find mites.

For the most part, scabies is a clinical diagnosis based on the typical rash and the history. It is often helpful if other family members have pruritus and a similar rash. In cases in which the diagnosis is in question or there appears to

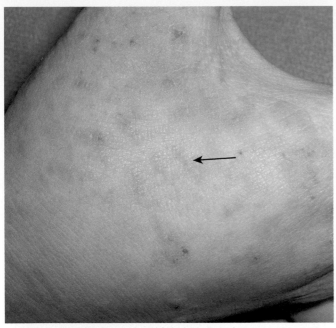

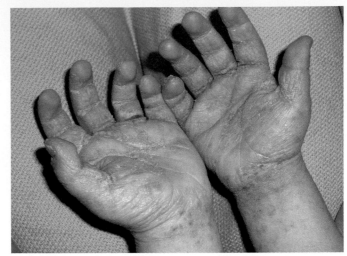

Figure 33-63 Crusted scabies on hands of 2-year-old child. (© Richard P. Usatine.)

Figure 33-61 Scabies with visible burrow (arrow). (© Richard P. Usatine.)

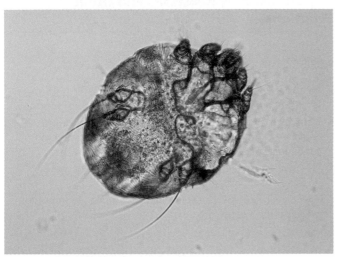

Figure 33-62 Scabies mite (40×). (© Richard P. Usatine.)

be multiple recurrences, the scraping is worthwhile to confirm the clinical impression. A dermatoscope or magnifying lens can be used to look for the small arrowhead-appearing mite at the end of a burrow. Scraping of active lesions can yield the identification of mites, eggs, or feces under the microscope (KOH or mineral oil can be used on the slide) (Fig. 33-62).

Crusted (Norwegian) scabies is a highly contagious form with a propensity for older adults and immunocompromised or physically debilitated patients (Fig. 33-63). Widespread, crusted lesions appear with thick, hyperkeratotic scales over the elbows, knees, palms, and soles. Infections may occur with thousands of mites at a time and can be especially problematic in nursing homes or assisted-living environments. Ivermectin is an oral treatment for resistant or crusted scabies with demonstrated safety and efficacy. Most studies used a single dose of ivermectin at 200 µg/kg (Strong and Johnstone, 2007).

Permethrin cream is applied from the neck down (include the head when involved) and rinsed off 8 to 14 hours later. Usually this is done overnight. Repeating the treatment in 1 to 2 weeks may increase the cure rate. Unfortunately, scabies resistance to permethrin is increasing. Antihistamines and midpotency steroid creams can be used for symptomatic relief of itching. It is important to note that pruritus may persist for 1 to 2 weeks after successful treatment because the dead mites and eggs still have antigenic qualities that may cause persistent inflammation. Environmental decontamination is a standard component of all therapies. Clothing, bed linens, and towels should be machine-washed in hot water. Clothing or other items (e.g., stuffed animals) that cannot be washed may be dry-cleaned or stored in bags for 1 week. All household or family members living in the infested home should be treated. Failure to treat all involved individuals often results in recurrences within the family.

KEY TREATMENT

Begin treatment of scabies with permethrin 5% cream (Strong and Johnstone, 2007) (SOR: A).

Oral ivermectin (200 µg/kg) is used to treat resistant or crusted scabies. (Strong and Johnstone, 2007) (SOR: A).

Antihistamines and steroid creams can be used for symptomatic relief of itching (SOR: C).

Environmental decontamination is a standard component of all scabies therapy (SOR: C).

All those living in the infested home should be treated to prevent recurrences (SOR: C).

Pediculosis Capitis (Head Lice)

Lice are obligate human parasites transmitted by person-to-person contact. Infestations are increasing in frequency because of the development of resistance to current treatments. The infestation is usually detected because of intense itching and the presence of eggs or nits adherent to the hair shaft (Fig. 33-64). Once the nit is attached to the hair shaft, the head louse develops over 3 to 4 days. Within 12 days of hatching, the nymph becomes a sexually mature adult capable of reproducing. After a single fertilization, each female lays up to 10 eggs a day during her 30-day life span. Typically, infestation occurs over a 2-week period, resulting in an allergic reaction to the louse saliva, causing the pruritus. Without frequent blood meals from the host, lice survive only 15 to 20 hours.

Detection of a single live louse is sufficient for diagnosis of infestation. Nits should be examined for viable embryo, which will show some movement under magnification. Because of the route of transmission, outbreaks are often seen in daycare centers, classrooms, and homeless shelters.

Effective eradication of pediculosis often requires two treatments given 7 to 10 days apart. Several OTC preparations are available, including 4% piperonyl butoxide with 0.33% pyrethrins (RID, Pronto, A-200) and permethrin (Nix). Malathion is available by prescription for treatment of resistant strains but should not be used in infants or children younger than 6 years. Instructions for use must be followed carefully, including treatment of all household contacts. Removal of all nits is not necessary following eradication but can be done with a fine-toothed comb, if desired. Schools often require no visible nits before permitting children to return to classes. Use of a 50% vinegar and water rinse after shampooing may help reduce adherence of nits to the hair shaft.

Bedding and clothing should be washed in the hottest water possible or dry-cleaned. Combs, barrettes, and hair ornaments may be soaked in hot water for 10 minutes. Items that cannot be otherwise cleaned, such as stuffed animals or decorative pillows, can be sealed in plastic bags for 2 weeks.

KEY TREATMENT

Pediculicides effective in the treatment of head lice include 1% permethrin cream rinse, pyrethrins with piperonyl butoxide shampoo and malathion cream; no evidence shows one is better than another (Cochrane review; Dodd, 2006) (SOR: A).

Pediculosis Corporis (Body Lice)

Body lice are most frequently seen in patients who live in environments that prevent regular changing of clothing and bedding, such as the homeless. Diagnosis should be suspected in patients with generalized itching and excoriations and poor hygiene. Body lice are more likely to be found in the seams of clothing than on the patient (Fig. 33-65). Initial treatment of body lice entails washing the entire body surface and wearing clean clothing. In severe infestations, topical use of permethrin, pyrethrin, or malathion may be indicated. Again, clothing and bedding should be washed in hot water or dry-cleaned. As an alternative to topical treatment, ivermectin may be given orally.

Phthirus Pubis (Pubic Lice, Crab Lice)

Pubic lice are sexually transmitted and may be transmitted through clothing and towels. Treatment is the same as for head lice and should include any sexual contacts. Additionally, the presence of pubic lice should prompt consideration of other STDs.

Hypersensitivity Reactions and Other Eruptions

Key Points

- Morbilliform drug reactions occur 1 to 2 weeks after initial exposure but occur much quicker (1-3 days) on repeat exposure.
- Urticaria can be acute or chronic and is triggered by drugs, infections, arthropods, autoimmune disease, food, and even emotional stress.
- The mainstay of therapy for urticaria is avoidance of known triggers and antihistamines.
- Oral corticosteroids for urticaria should be limited to short-term therapy of severe episodes.

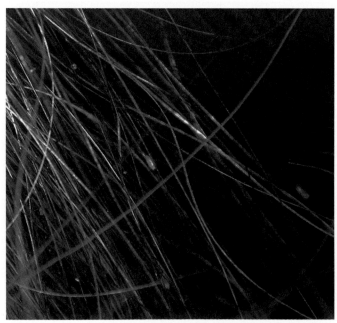

Figure 33-64 Pearly nits of head lice. (© Richard P. Usatine.)

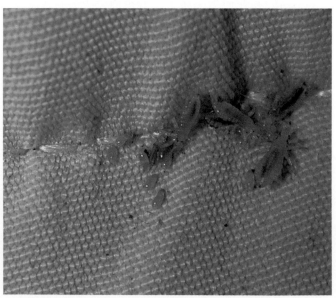

Figure 33-65 Body lice on seams of clothing. (© Richard P. Usatine.)

- Erythema multiforme is a reaction pattern secondary to a variety of etiologic agents and characterized by distinctive target lesions.
- Half of EM cases are caused by HSV; drugs and other infections are also common causes.
- Stevens-Johnson syndrome and toxic epidermal necrolysis typically occur 7 to 21 days after starting NSAIDS, antibiotics, or antiepileptics.

"Morbilliform" (Maculopapular, Exanthemlike) Reaction

Morbilliform eruption is by far the most common type of drug eruption, reported in response to almost every drug. Small, pink to red papules and macules usually start on the face or upper chest and can extend to limbs; resembling measles (Fig. 33-66). The rash may be relatively asymptomatic or extremely pruritic. The typical course begins 7 to 14 days after drug initiation if the first exposure. On reexposure to the same medicine, the eruption will occur much more quickly, within 1 to 3 days. Maculopapular reaction is not generally life threatening and does not proceed to anaphylaxis; therefore, when no alternative drug is available, the offending agent can be continued. The eruption can be treated symptomatically with antihistamines and midpotency topical corticosteroids.

Urticaria

Urticaria, commonly known as "hives," can be acute or chronic, and the numerous triggers include drugs, food, infections, arthropods, autoimmune disease, and stress. The wheals consist of circumscribed areas of raised erythematous plaques that are often annular and very pruritic (Fig. 33-67).

These wheals can occur on any skin area and are transient and migratory. The acute form of urticaria lasts less than 4 to 6 weeks, and the chronic form lasts more than 6 weeks. When there is an obvious new drug causing the eruption, the causation is easy to determine.

For patients on multiple medications and no evidence of infection or illness, diagnosis can be very difficult. Skin prick testing or radioallergosorbent assay testing (RAST) testing, typically done through an allergy specialist, may help determine the cause but may be elusive. Patients with chronic urticaria unresponsive to antihistamines require an extensive workup. In more than 50% cases of chronic urticaria, no etiology is found, and it is considered idiopathic or chronic "autoimmune" urticaria.

The mainstay of therapy for urticaria is avoidance of known triggering agents and antihistamines. Classic antihistamines are effective (diphenhydramine, hydroxyzine, doxepin), but sedation limits their use to primarily nighttime dosing. Second-generation and third-generation antihistamines are helpful for daytime use (cetirizine, loratadine, fexofenadine, desloratadine, levocetirizine). Oral corticosteroids are useful but should be limited to short-term therapy of severe acute urticaria. H_2-receptor antagonists (cimetidine, ranitidine, famotidine) and leukotriene antagonists are sometimes helpful as adjunctive therapy.

Erythema Multiforme

Erythema multiforme (EM) is a reaction pattern secondary to a variety of etiologic agents characterized by distinctive target lesions. About 90% of cases of EM are caused by infections, most often HSV (50%) and *Mycoplasma pneumoniae* (Fig. 33-68). The other 10% are caused by drugs, most often

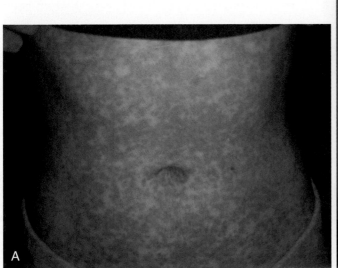
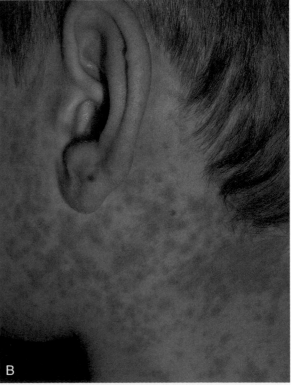

Figure 33-66 **A,** Amoxicillin drug eruption in young woman with mononucleosis. **B,** Amoxicillin rash in child with otitis media. *(© Richard P. Usatine.)*

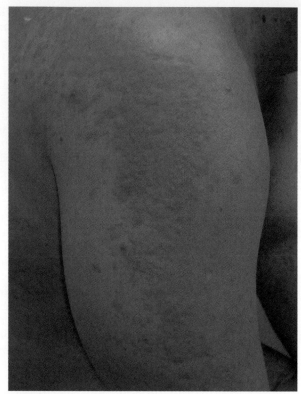

Figure 33-67 Urticarial drug eruption secondary to trimethoprim-sulfamethoxazole (TMP-SMX) therapy. (© Richard P. Usatine.)

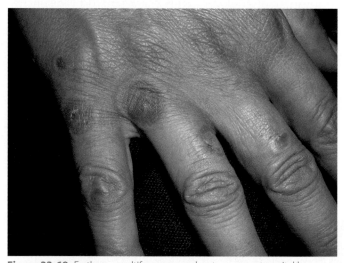

Figure 33-68 Erythema multiforme secondary to recurrent genital herpes simplex. (© Richard P. Usatine.)

NSAIDs, sulfonamides or other antibiotics, antiepileptics, and barbiturates.

Lesions begin as dull-red macules or urticarial plaques on the palms, soles, or extensor surfaces of the extremities and tend to expand in size. A small papule, vesicle, or bulla develops in the center with concentric rings forming around the blister. The center of the lesion becomes dusky or violaceous from necrosis of the epidermis. Most EM cases spontaneously subside within 3 weeks without sequelae.

Identification of the cause should be made, if possible. Patient should be queried for prescription and OTC medications and history of HSV. A thorough examination should

be performed, looking for oral or genital ulcers with Tzanck prep or DFA test for HSV. Cultures of the skin, nose, throat, and conjunctiva are indicated to evaluate for infections and treated appropriately.

Stevens-Johnson Syndrome and Toxic Epidermal Necrolysis

Both Stevens-Johnson syndrome (SJS) and toxic epidermal necrolysis (TEN) are rare, severe, life-threatening reactions that are almost always drug related. The most common offending medications are NSAIDS, antibiotics, and antiseizure medications. SJS or TEN typically occurs 7 to 21 days after the start of the medication.

Stevens-Johnson syndrome often presents with a prodrome of fever, painful swallowing, stinging eyes, and *painful* skin. Two or more mucosal surfaces eventually become involved (conjunctiva, oral mucosa, genitalia) with vesicles, bullae, erosions or hemorrhagic crusts. Skin lesions usually begin as dusky purpuric macules that progress to bullae or erosions on the trunk and spread centrifugally. *Targetoid lesions*, similar to EM, may also be present. By definition, less than 10% body surface area (BSA) is involved in SJS. A similar presentation occurs in TEN, but the bullae and erosions involve greater than 30% BSA. Also, the skin that initially appears normal may easily slide off with gentle tangential pressure (Nikolsky's sign), leaving more denuded skin. When skin and mucosal involvement is 10% to 30% BSA, it is considered SJS/TEN overlap.

Both SJS and TEN can be fatal; mortality is 1% to 5% for SJS and 25% to 35% for TEN, but may be even higher in elderly patients or those with comorbidities. Above all, removal of the offending agent is paramount. Most patients are treated in a burn unit because the skin is necrotic and no longer functioning as a barrier. Care is supportive and aimed at regulation of fluids, electrolytes, protein, temperature, and prevention of infection. Neither systemic steroids nor intravenous immune globulin (IVIG) demonstrate consistent clinical efficacy in clinical studies, which are limited because of the rarity of SJS and TEN.

Skin Signs of Systemic Disease

Lupus Erythematosus

Key Points

- Lupus erythematosus is an autoimmune disease of connective tissue that may be limited to the skin (cutaneous lupus), or the skin findings may indicate systemic disease.
- All LE variants are photosensitive, and primary treatment should include education in sun protection and avoidance.

Lupus erythematosus (LE) is an autoimmune disease of connective tissue that has frequent dermatologic manifestations. LE may be limited to the skin, or the skin findings may indicate systemic disease. For dermatologic purposes, there are three main variants:

Acute cutaneous (ACLE): exemplified by the malar rash, usually associated with systemic disease and positive antinuclear antibodies (Fig. 33-69).

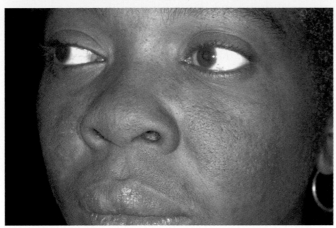

Figure 33-69 Systemic lupus erythematosus and with malar rash. *(© Richard P. Usatine.)*

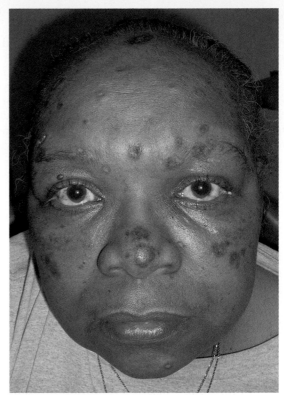

Figure 33-71 Discoid lupus with hyperpigmentation atrophy and scarring. *(© Richard P. Usatine.)*

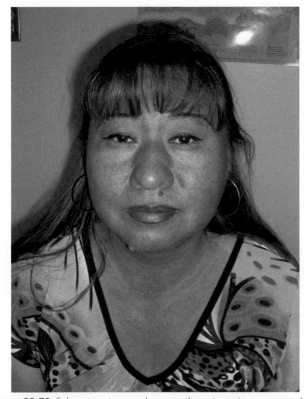

Figure 33-70 Subacute cutaneous lupus erythematosus in sun-exposed areas. *(© Richard P. Usatine.)*

Subacute cutaneous (SCLE): characteristic photosensitive papulosquamous annular lesions of the trunk and arms, associated with anti-Ro antibodies (70%); 10% to 15% will have systemic involvement (Fig. 33-70).

Discoid (DLE): inflammation involves deeper adnexal structures, with predilection for head and neck; results in scarring; less than 10% have systemic involvement (Fig. 33-71).

Acute cutaneous LE presents as the classic "butterfly rash" and tends to follow sun exposure. Erythema and edema may be mild to severe. The presence of *poikiloderma* (patches of hypopigmentation, hyperpigmentation, telangiectasias, and epidermal atrophy) may help to differentiate the malar rash of lupus from other skin diseases of the midface, such as rosacea

or seborrheic dermatitis, which are not poikilodermatous. There is sparing of the nasolabial folds and the skin under the nose and upper lip, areas that are shaded from the sun.

Lesions of SCLE are very photosensitive and appear as annular, scaly, erythematous patches or papulosquamous rings with central clearing. These usually affect the lateral face (instead of central face), upper chest, arms, and shoulders, areas that are sun exposed. Discoid lesions are somewhat photosensitive but also found on nonexposed skin and mucosal surfaces. Most often these present on the ears, face, and neck and appear as scaly, brightly erythematous to violaceous plaques. Because of the deeper involvement of inflammation, as DLE lesions resolve, they often leave behind hyper- or hypopigmentation, even depigmentation. Severe scarring and disfigurement may also occur. ACLE, or systemic lupus erythematosus (SLE), is more common in women, especially of childbearing age (female/male ratio 6-10:1), suggesting a hormonal factor in susceptibility. The female/male ratio for patients with only cutaneous forms of lupus is much lower (3-4:1 for SCLE; 2:1 for DLE). The prevalence of ACLE/SLE is also fourfold higher in African American women than Caucasian American women, and DLE is slightly more common in African Americans. However, SCLE is more prominent in Caucasians (80%).

Occasionally, drugs can induce ACLE or SCLE. Procainamide, hydralazine, isoniazid, quinidine, and phenytoin are most frequently reported for ACLE, whereas hydrochlorothiazide, calcium channel blockers (diltiazem), angiotensin-converting enzyme (ACE) inhibitors, terbinafine, NSAIDs, griseofulvin, and tumor necrosis factor (TNF) antagonists are most frequently reported for SCLE. Drug-induced ACLE usually fades once the drug is discontinued but may take many months. Drug-induced SCLE may or may not clear with cessation of the drug.

For skin lesions of lupus, sun protection and sun avoidance are crucial because all types are photosensitive. Although discoid lesions are not as photosensitive as the other variants, some patients with ACLE, SLE, or SCLE can even be triggered by indoor light. Topical corticosteroids and calcineurin inhibitors (pimecrolimus, tacrolimus) are the mainstay in treatment of skin lesions. If oral medications are required to control skin disease, antimalarials (most often hydroxychloroquine) are first-line therapy.

Dermatomyositis

Key Points

- Dermatomyositis, presumably an autoimmune disease, is triggered by malignancy, drugs, or infection.
- High-dose corticosteroids with a slow taper over 2 to 4 years are the primary treatment, and muscle disease usually responds more rapidly than skin disease.

Dermatomyositis is presumably an autoimmune disease that is triggered by an outside factor. Antinuclear antibodies or anticytoplasmic antibodies (antisynthetase) are found in up to 95% of patients. Clinically, dermatomyositis is characterized by a symmetric proximal inflammatory myopathy and distinct skin lesions. Proximal muscle weakness may precede the skin findings, may follow them, or may be absent ("dermatomyositis sine myositis"). Classic cutaneous lesions include the *heliotrope rash*, pink to lilac, poikilodermatous or edematous patches of the periocular skin (Fig. 33-72). The *shawl sign* consists of poikiloderma of the upper chest, shoulders, and upper back. Gottron's papules are erythematous, scaly or lichenified papules or plaques over the knuckles. Similar plaques may be seen on the elbows, mimicking psoriasis. Other common cutaneous findings are periungual telangiectasias (visible dilated capillary loops) and ragged cuticles (cuticular dystrophy).

Although the etiology of dermatomyositis is unknown, triggers may include malignancy, drugs, and infection. In adults with dermatomyositis, studies report a wide range of association with internal malignancy (10%-50%). Common malignancies include genitourinary, ovarian, colon, breast, lung, pancreatic, and lymphoma. The same association is not found in juvenile cases of dermatomyositis. Therefore, any adult with a new diagnosis of dermatomyositis should be screened with a chest-abdominal-pelvic CT scan with close surveillance for 2 to 3 years.

Double-blind, placebo-controlled trials are lacking for this rare disease, but the mainstay of treatment for dermatomyositis is high-dose corticosteroids with slow taper over 2 to 4 years. Other immunosuppressants used include methotrexate, azathioprine, cyclophosphamide, and cyclosporine. In general, the myopathy responds more rapidly and easily than the skin lesions, and severe pruritus can persist long after muscle disease is controlled. For skin lesions, sun protections, topical corticosteroids, or antimalarials may help.

Sarcoidosis

Sarcoidosis is a systemic granulomatous disease of unknown etiology that most often involves the lungs (90%). The skin is involved in about one third of patients with systemic sarcoidosis. In the United States, women and African Americans are more frequently affected. As with syphilis, sarcoidosis is considered a "great imitator" because it has widely variable presentations and may involve almost any organ system.

Classic skin lesions of sarcoidosis are red-brown, nonscaly papules and plaques appearing on the face, especially around the nose or mouth (Fig. 33-73). Color can vary significantly from yellow to red to brown, and lesions also occur on the trunk or extremities and tend to be symmetric. Lesions on the alar rim of the nose, also known as *lupus pernio*, are highly

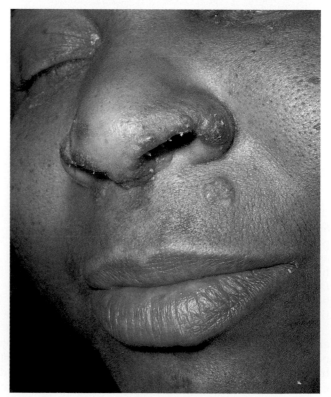

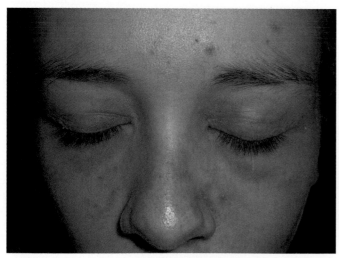

Figure 33-72 Heliotrope rash of dermatomyositis. *(© Richard P. Usatine.)*

Figure 33-73 Cutaneous sarcoidosis. *(© Richard P. Usatine.)*

associated with granulomatous infiltration of the upper airway. Patients with cutaneous sarcoidosis should have a complete evaluation for systemic disease, including history and physical examination, renal and hepatic function testing, chest radiograph, pulmonary function tests, electrocardiography, and ophthalmologic evaluation.

Lesions of cutaneous sarcoidosis are difficult to treat and tend to recur. The most effective therapy is intralesional injection of corticosteroids repeated at 2- to 4-week intervals. Topical corticosteroids are often ineffective because they do not penetrate the skin lesions adequately. Systemic corticosteroids are effective in treating lesions that are widespread or impairing function. In especially difficult cases, agents such as hydroxychloroquine or methotrexate may be used.

Benign Growths

Key Points

- The most important reason to be able to recognize benign skin growths is to differentiate them from skin cancers.
- Seborrheic keratoses, epidermal cysts, and dermatofibromas can be surgically excised if they are suspicious for cancer or causing symptoms.
- Pyogenic granulomas bleed easily and should be excised and sent for pathology to rule out amelanotic melanoma.
- Seborrheic keratoses and dermatofibromas have characteristic patterns with dermoscopy that can help guide the need for a biopsy.

Seborrheic Keratosis

Seborrheic keratoses (SKs) are hyperkeratotic lesions of the epidermis that often appear to be stuck on the surface of the skin (Fig. 33-74). SKs usually have a discrete border and vary in color from white or tan to dark brown and even black. Most lesions have a rough surface and usually range from 2 mm to 3 cm in diameter, but can be larger. Seborrheic keratosis may start as a hyperpigmented macule and progress to the characteristic plaque. The trunk is the most common site, but the lesions can be found on the extremities, face, and scalp.

The incidence of seborrheic keratosis increases with age in men and women. *Stucco keratoses,* a variant of seborrheic keratosis, are many skin-colored or white, dry scaly lesions often seen on the arms and legs. *Dermatosis papulosa nigra* is another type of seborrheic keratosis consisting of many small, brown or black papules on the faces of patients with highly pigmented skin.

Differentiating between seborrheic keratosis and melanomas can be a challenge, especially in patients with numerous lesions. Both have varying dark colors, the potential for large size, and irregularity. SKs have a rough surface, and the keratin can have horn cysts or look cerebriform. The best way to differentiate a seborrheic keratosis from a melanoma is with a dermatoscope. This special magnifying light can distinguish specific characteristics of the keratosis with higher specificity than with the naked eye. These characteristics are comedo-like openings and milia-like cysts (Fig. 33-74).

Some patients want their SKs treated for cosmetic reasons or to decrease irritation from abrasion on clothing.

Cryosurgery, curettage, and shave excision are the most frequently used methods of removal. Cryotherapy with liquid nitrogen is effective for most SKs, except for extremely thick lesions. Repeat treatments may be necessary. Curettage can be performed with or without electrocautery after administration of local anesthesia. Excisional biopsy should be used to remove lesions suspicious for melanoma.

Pyogenic Granuloma

Pyogenic granulomas (lobulated capillary hemangiomas) are benign vascular lesions that occur most often in young adults and children (Fig. 33-75). These rapidly growing hemangiomas may start at sites of trauma. Treatment is surgical removal. Pyogenic granulomas do not have malignant

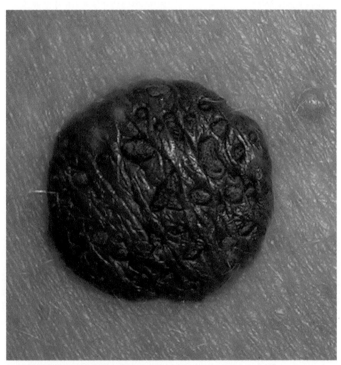

Figure 33-74 Seborrheic keratosis with horn cysts (comedo-like openings). *(© Richard P. Usatine.)*

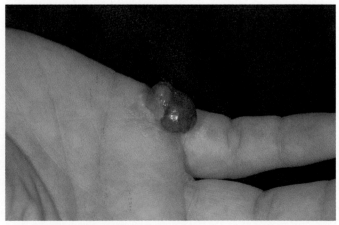

Figure 33-75 Pyogenic granuloma. *(© Richard P. Usatine.)*

potential, but it is important to send the tissue for pathology to rule out an amelanotic melanoma. Lesions most commonly occur on the fingers, head, neck, extremities, and on mucous membranes. Pyogenic granulomas frequently occur on the gingiva during pregnancy and regress spontaneously after childbirth. Patients usually are acutely concerned that the lesion has grown quickly and bleeds easily with little or no trauma.

Removal can be accomplished with shave excision and then curettage and electrodesiccation of the base to reduce chances of recurrence. Alternatively, the whole lesion can be cut out down to subcutaneous fat. Pyogenic granulomas will recur if any residual tissue remains after excision.

Epidermal Inclusion Cysts

Epidermal inclusion cysts, also known as *sebaceous cysts,* are filled with keratin and lined with stratified squamous epithelium. Epidermal cysts usually occur on the back, face, and chest and open to the skin through a small, central punctum or keratin-filled plug. On the back, these may be deep and barely palpable, whereas on the scalp an epidermal cyst (pilar cyst) can be elevated and freely movable. The cysts may remain small for years or may grow rapidly. Rupture of the cyst wall into the dermis initiates an inflammatory response.

Acutely inflamed, fluctuant cysts should be incised and drained. Destruction of the cyst wall at incision decreases the risk of cyst recurrence. Alternately, the cyst may be removed intact by excision and blunt dissection. Complete drainage is enhanced with gauze packing, changed frequently during wound healing. The use of antibiotics is unnecessary unless a concurrent cellulitis exists. If a patient requests removal of an epidermal cyst before an acute inflammatory event, the cyst wall can be more easily shelled out, minimizing risk of recurrence.

Dermatofibroma

Dermatofibromas (benign fibrous histiocytomas) are most likely fibrous reactions to minor trauma, insect bites, viral infections, ruptured cysts, or folliculitis. The nodules can be found anywhere on the body, but most often appear on the legs and arms. Dermatofibromas are firm, raised papules, plaques, or nodules that vary from 3 to 10 mm in diameter (Fig. 33-76). Dermatofibromas have a central fibrous scar and often have a hyperpigmented or pink halo around the central hypopigmented area. This has a characteristic pattern on dermoscopy.

Dermatofibromas dimple downward when compressed laterally, caused by tethering of the overlying epidermis to the underlying nodule (Fig. 33-77). Dermatofibromas are usually asymptomatic but may be tender or pruritic. Dermatofibromas can be confused with melanomas, and if growing rapidly, they could be a malignancy called a "dermatofibrosarcoma protuberans." An excisional biopsy can be used to determine the diagnosis. Because of the dermal location of the nodules, excision is superior to shave biopsy to ensure clear histology and complete removal. A punch biopsy can be used for smaller lesions. Dermatofibromas that are stable in size and asymptomatic can be left alone without treatment.

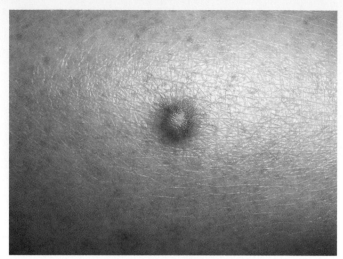

Figure 33-76 Dermatofibroma on leg with hyperpigmented halo. *(© Richard P. Usatine.)*

Premalignant and Malignant Skin Lesions

Key Points

- Actinic keratosis is a scaly macule on sun-damaged skin and often easier to feel than to see.
- Topical 5-FU therapy is used for patients with multiple AKs rather than treating each lesion with cryotherapy.
- Bowen's disease (squamous cell carcinoma in situ) and superficial basal cell carcinoma look more like patches of dermatitis than tumors.
- The typical nodular basal cell carcinoma presents as a pearly-colored papule with overlying telangiectasias and a central depression or ulcer.
- Left untreated, local destruction from BCC can be extensive.
- Most SCCs arise from AKs, radiation dermatitis, leukoplakia or erythroplakia, and burn scars or chronic ulcers.
- Organ transplant recipients have a 5% to 10% greater risk of developing BCC and a 40 to 250 times greater risk of developing SCC.
- Risk factors for melanoma include fair skin, red or blond hair, no tan/easily burns, freckles, excessive childhood sun exposure, blistering childhood sunburns (>3), moles (nevi) or dysplastic nevi, family or personal history of melanoma, immunosuppression, and older age.
- One third of melanomas arise in a preexisting nevus.
- Depth of tumor invasion is the most important prognostic indicator for melanoma; most patients with thin tumors (<1 mm) have over 90% 10-year survival.

Actinic Keratosis

Actinic keratoses (AKs) are also known as "solar keratoses" because of their relationship to chronic sun exposure. These lesions are most common on the dorsal surfaces of the hands and arms, neck, ears, bald scalp, and face, areas that are not covered by clothing on a daily basis (Fig. 33-78). AKs are usually scaly, pink to flesh-colored macules or papules and are often easier to feel than see. They have a rough texture as

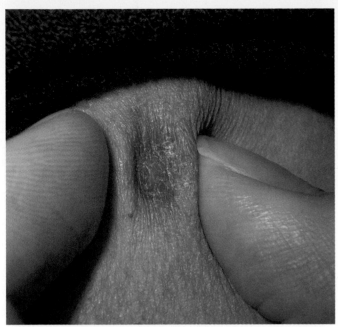

Figure 33-77 Dermatofibroma undergoing pinch test, in which lesion dimples downward. (© *Richard P. Usatine.*)

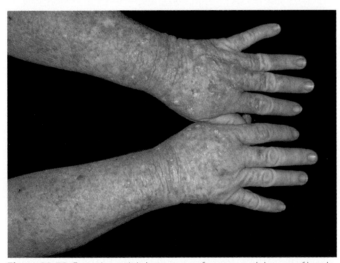

Figure 33-78 Extensive actinic keratoses on forearms and dorsum of hands. (© *Richard P. Usatine.*)

a bare finger slides over the skin. The lesions have malignant potential and can transform into squamous cell carcinoma at a rate of about 0.1% per lesion per year.

Cryotherapy with liquid nitrogen is the most effective and practical method for treating AKs when a limited number of lesions are present. For more extensive lesions, topical 5-FU (Efudex 5%, Carac 0.5%), diclofenac (Solaraze), or imiquimod (Aldara) is recommended. This treatment can be temporarily disfiguring with erythema, crusting, or ulcerations, but if the skin is kept lubricated with petroleum jelly during treatment, the process usually looks worse than it feels. Both 5-FU and diclofenac are applied daily for 4 weeks. Patients often will not tolerate the 4-week duration, but if erythema or crusting is achieved in 2 to 3 weeks, treatment may still be successful. Lesions will take another 2 to 4 weeks to heal. Treatment with imiquimod is once daily for 3 to 5 days of

the week (depending on irritation) and is continued for 12 to 16 weeks. Imiquimod is supplied in small, expensive packets, so it is less practical for treating larger surface areas. Lesions that are hyperkeratotic should be biopsied because they often recur with cryotherapy and may not be penetrated by topical therapies.

Treating AKs with liquid nitrogen using a 1-mm halo freeze demonstrated complete response of 39% for freeze times less than 5 seconds, 69% for times over 5 seconds, and 83% for more than 20 seconds (Thai et al., 2004). More hypopigmentation is caused by 20 seconds of freeze time. The physician should base duration of freeze time on the size and thickness of the lesion, using sufficient time for clearance while attempting to avoid hypopigmentation and scarring.

All patients with actinic keratosis or skin cancer should be educated on daily sun protection and sun avoidance. This includes sunscreen with a sun protection factor (SPF) of 30 or greater, wide-brimmed hats, long sleeves and pants, and avoiding peak hours of sunlight (10 AM to 4 PM).

> ### KEY TREATMENT
>
> Sunscreen twice daily for 7 months may protect against development of actinic dermatoses (de Berker et al., 2007) (SOR: A).
> Treating AKs with liquid nitrogen showed complete response of up to 83% for freeze times greater than 20 seconds (Thai et al., 2004) (SOR: A).
> Treat multiple AKs of the face, scalp, forearms, and hands topically with 5-FU, imiquimod, or diclofenac (de Berker et al., 2007) (SOR: A).
> Average complete clearance of AKs using 5-FU was 52% (±18%) and for imiquimod, 70% (±12%) (Gupta et al., 2006) (SOR: A).

Bowen's Disease and Erythroplasia of Queyrat

Bowen's disease (BD) is squamous cell carcinoma (SCC) in situ most often caused by chronic solar damage. Therefore, lesions are found most often on the dorsal hands and forearms, neck, ears, bald scalp, and face. HPV also has been documented as a cause of BD, especially HPV-16. Inorganic arsenic ingestion, radiation dermatitis (x-ray damage), immunosuppression or HIV, burn scars, and chronic ulcers are also associated with BD.

Bowen's disease often presents with an asymptomatic, slowly enlarging, erythematous, scaly patch on the skin that mimics an eczematous dermatitis (Fig. 33-79). The head and neck are most frequently affected, followed by the extremities. As they enlarge, lesions may become hyperkeratotic, crusted, fissured, or ulcerated. When BD occurs on mucous membranes, it is a white, red, or erosive patch. SCC in situ on the penis is referred to as *penile intraepithelial neoplasia* (erythroplasia of Queyrat).

Treatment of BD depends on the location, size, number of lesions, clinician's expertise, patient factors (age, immune status, concomitant medication, comorbidities, compliance), cosmetic outcome, and patient preference. For the trunk or extremities, electrodesiccation and curettage (ED&C) is practical. Cryotherapy is also an option but often results in poorer wound healing. One prospective study suggests a superiority of ED&C over cryotherapy in treating BD, especially for lesions on the lower leg. Curettage was associated with a significantly shorter healing time, less pain, fewer complications, and a lower recurrence rate (Ahmed et al., 2000).

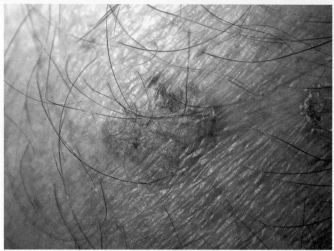

Figure 33-79 Bowen's disease (squamous cell carcinoma in situ) on arm. *(© Richard P. Usatine.)*

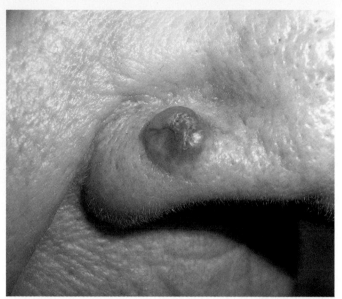

Figure 33-80 Nodular basal cell carcinoma on nasal ala. *(© Richard P. Usatine.)*

For larger or poorly defined lesions, topical therapy with 5-FU or imiquimod can be used, working best when the patient can see and reach the lesion. In a randomized, double-blind, placebo-controlled trial of imiquimod daily for 16 weeks, 9 of 12 patients (75%) in the imiquimod group and none in the placebo group had complete clearance of BD, with no recurrence in the 9-month follow-up (Patel et al., 2006). Lesions can also be excised with 4-mm margins or referred for Mohs micrographic surgery when tissue sparing is crucial. Mohs surgery is recommended for BD at sites such as digits or penis, where it is important to limit removal of unaffected skin. It is also useful for poorly defined or recurrent head and neck BD (Cox et al., 2007). Excision should be an effective treatment with low recurrence rates, but the limited evidence cannot address specific lesion sites (Cox et al., 2007).

The overall risk of progression of BD to invasive cancer is about 3% to 5%, However, risk is greater for patients with oral and genital lesions (about 10%), as well as those with a history of arsenic exposure or lesions located in a chronic scar or ulcer.

KEY TREATMENT

Curettage and electrodesiccation may be superior to cryotherapy in treating Bowen's disease, especially for lesions on the lower leg (Ahmed et al., 2000) (SOR: A).
Use of 5-FU is more practical than surgery for large BD lesions, especially at potentially poor healing sites (Cox et al., 2007) (SOR: B).
Imiquimod effectively clears BD lesions in most patients (Patel et al., 2006) (SOR: B).
Mohs surgery is recommended for BD at the digits or penis and is useful for poorly defined or recurrent head and neck BD (Cox et al., 2007) (SOR: B).

Basal Cell Carcinoma

Basal cell carcinoma (BCC) is the most common human malignancy. In the United States, BCC affects almost 1 million people per year, and this estimate is likely low because no national registry exists for nonmelanoma skin cancers.

BCC typically appears in areas of sun-exposed skin, is usually slow growing, and rarely metastasizes. Prognosis is excellent with proper therapy, but BCC can cause significant local destruction and disfigurement if neglected. The estimated lifetime risk in Caucasians approximately is 1 in 5 but increases to 1 in 3 in those over age 65 living in southern latitudes. The incidence is extremely low in those with highly pigmented skin. Organ transplant recipients have a 5 to 10 times greater risk of BCC.

Patients often present with a nonhealing sore on the face, ears, scalp, neck, or upper trunk. The most common type of BCC is *nodular,* which is usually a pink papule or nodule, with a central depression or ulceration and pearly, rolled borders with overlying telangiectasias (Fig. 33-80). *Superficial* BCC is the second most common type (Fig. 33-81). *Sclerosing* (morpheaform, infiltrating) BCC is the least common (Fig. 33-82). It is not unusual to see pigment in a nodular BCC (Fig. 33-83). A shave biopsy is usually adequate to confirm the diagnosis.

Superficial BCC can be treated with ED&C or topically with 5-FU or imiquimod. Imiquimod 5% cream once daily five times weekly for 6 weeks for superficial BBC produced an initial clearance rate of 90%, with 80% of subjects clinically clear at 2 years (Gollnick et al., 2005). In another study, superficial BBC lesions on the trunk or limbs were treated with 5-FU cream twice daily for up to 12 weeks. The histologic cure rate was 90%, and mean time to clinical cure was 10.5 weeks. 5-FU was generally well tolerated, with a good cosmetic outcome; most patients had no pain or scarring and only mild erythema (Gross et al., 2007).

Nodular BCC can be excised with 3 to 5–mm margins or treated with ED&C, depending on location and patient comorbidities and preference. Cryotherapy is another option but is infrequently performed due to poor wound healing. Tumors that are more aggressive by histologic pattern (sclerosing, morpheaform, or infiltrating) or those occurring near vital or cosmetically sensitive structures are best treated with Mohs micrographic surgery (MMS). This tissue-sparing method also allows for examination of almost 100% of the

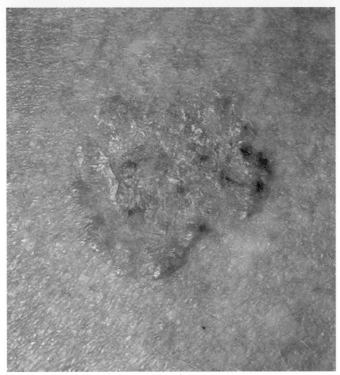

Figure 33-81 Superficial basal cell carcinoma on back. *(© Richard P. Usatine.)*

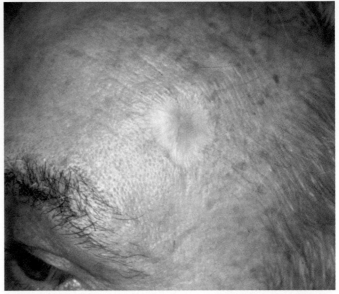

Figure 33-82 Sclerosing basal cell carcinoma. *(© Richard P. Usatine and The Skin Cancer Foundation)*

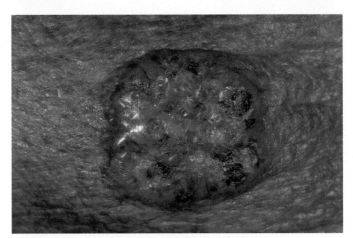

Figure 33-83 Pigmented nodular basal cell carcinoma. *(© Richard P. Usatine.)*

tissue margins. MMS is the removal of tumor by scalpel in sequential horizontal layers, in which each tissue sample is frozen, stained, and microscopically examined. This is repeated until all the margins are clear. MMS is the treatment of choice for BCCs greater than 2 cm, with poorly defined margins, with aggressive histology, involving areas of cosmetic or functional importance (mouth, ears, nose, eyelids), or recurrent lesions (Thissen et al., 1999).

Patients diagnosed with BCC have an approximately 30% higher risk than the general population of being diagnosed with another BCC unrelated to the previous lesion. Because BCC can recur, patients should have frequent full-body skin examinations at least twice yearly for the first 2 years, then yearly if no new lesions occur. As with all sun-related malignancies and precancerous lesions, patients must be instructed on sun protection and sun avoidance.

KEY TREATMENT

Mohs surgery (3 studies, *n* = 2660) is the "gold standard" but is not needed for all basal cell carcinomas. Recurrence rate was 0.8 to 1.1. Systematic review also showed the following (Thissen et al., 1999) (SOR: A):
Surgical excision (3 studies, *n* = 1303): recurrence rate was 2 to 8. Mean cumulative 5-year rate was 5.3. Recommended margins are 4 to 5 mm.
Curettage and desiccation (6 studies, *n* = 4212): recurrence rate was 4.3 to 18.1. Cumulative 5-year rate was 5.7 to 18.8. Three cycles of curettage and desiccation can produce higher cure rates then one cycle.
Cryosurgery (4 studies, *n* = 796): recurrence rate was 3.0 to 4.3. Cumulative 5-year rate (3 studies) was 0 to 16.5.
Superficial BCC is effectively treated with imiquimod 5% cream (Gollnick et al., 2005) or 5-FU cream (Gross et al. 2007) (SOR: B).

Squamous Cell Carcinoma

Cutaneous squamous cell carcinoma is the second most common form of skin cancer, also arising primarily on sun-exposed skin of middle-aged and older adults. Most SCCs arise from sun-induced precancerous lesions (actinic keratoses). As in BD, there is a higher risk of SCC in patients with radiation dermatitis (x-ray damage), leukoplakia or erythroplakia (in oral or genital mucosa), burn scars, and chronic skin ulcers. It is important to note that organ transplant recipients have a 40 to 250 times greater risk of developing SCC, purportedly from interaction of HPV and immunosuppression.

Lesions are typically pink to flesh-colored papules or nodules, often with crusting or ulceration (Fig. 33-84). They may also be keratotic or may develop a cutaneous horn. The most common locations include the face, scalp, lips, ears, neck, dorsal arms and hands, and genitalia (Fig. 33-85). Although many SCCs are asymptomatic, symptoms such as bleeding, pain, and tenderness, may be noted. SCC has an overall *metastasis* rate of 2% to 3%, but it is highly variable based on location, size, depth, invasion, and immunosuppression;

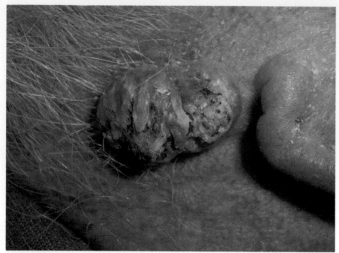

Figure 33-84 Squamous cell carcinoma under ear. *(© Richard P. Usatine.)*

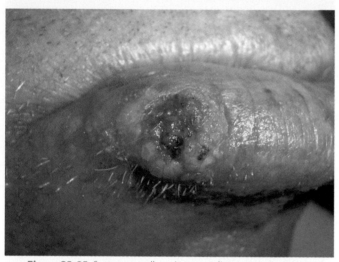

Figure 33-85 Squamous cell carcinoma on lip. *(© Richard P. Usatine.)*

rates can be as high as 30% to 40%. High-risk areas for metastasis include the ear, lip, genitalia, and areas of chronic inflammation (burns, scars, ulcers). A biopsy is required for diagnosis, which can be done with the shave or punch technique. Treatment of superficial SCC is covered under Bowen's disease.

Many SCCs can be excised with 4-mm to 5-mm margins. Smaller lesions may be amenable to ED&C. Several series report excellent cure rates with ED&C, and experience suggests that small (<1 cm), well-differentiated, primary slow-growing tumors arising on sun-exposed sites can be removed by experienced physicians with curettage (Motley et al., 2003). As with BCC, tumors of SCC that are large, invasive, recurrent, or near vital or cosmetically sensitive structures are best treated with Mohs surgery. Surgical resection with 4-mm margins should be adequate for well-defined low-risk tumors less than 2 cm in diameter. Such margins are expected to remove the primary tumor mass completely in 95% of cases. MMS should therefore be considered as first-line treatment of high-risk SCC, particularly at sites where wide surgical margins may be difficult to achieve without functional impairment (Motley et al., 2003). A prospective, multicenter case series of 1263 patients with SCC who

underwent MMS, recurrence after MMS was diagnosed in 15 of the 381 patients (3.9%) who completed the 5-year follow-up: 2.6% in patients with primary SCC, and 5.9% in patients with previously recurrent SCC (Leibovitch et al., 2005).

KEY TREATMENT

Surgical resection with 4-mm margins should remove small cell carcinoma (low risk, <2 cm) completely in 95% of patients (Motley et al., 2003) (SOR: A).

Mohs surgery (MMS) is considered first-line treatment of high-risk SCC (Motley et al., 2003) (SOR: B).

Experienced physicians can remove small (<1 cm) slow-growing SCC tumors on sun-exposed sites with curettage (Motley et al., 2003) (SOR: B).

Melanoma

Melanoma is the most lethal of the cutaneous malignancies, causing more than 77% of skin cancer deaths. In the United States, more than 62,000 new cases of invasive melanoma and almost 50,000 new cases of melanoma in situ were diagnosed in 2008. Melanoma arises from the pigment-producing cells (melanocytes) located predominantly in the skin, but it also found in the eyes, ears, GI tract, leptomeninges, and oral and genital mucous membranes. Early detection and treatment of melanoma are the best means of reducing mortality.

The development of melanoma is not completely understood and is not as directly linked to chronic sun exposure as is BCC or SCC. Risk factors include fair complexion, red or blond hair, inability to tan or predisposed to burn, freckles, excessive childhood sun exposure, more than three blistering childhood sunburns, an increased number of moles (nevi) or dysplastic nevi, family history of melanoma, personal history of melanoma, immunosuppression, and older age.

One third of melanomas arise in a preexisting nevus. A changing or newly acquired nevus in a person over age 20 is the most common warning sign for melanoma. Increase in size, change in color, asymmetry of borders, and variegated pigmentation are signs that warrant a biopsy. The mnemonic ABCDE (*a*symmetry, *b*order irregularity, *c*olor, *d*iameter, *e*volving) is helpful to assess lesions that may be melanocytic (Table 33-3). Symptoms such as bleeding, itching, ulceration, and pain in a pigmented lesion are less common but also warrant further evaluation.

The subtypes of melanoma include superficial spreading melanoma (60%-70%), nodular melanoma (15%-30%), lentigo malignant melanoma (5%-15%), and acral lentiginous melanoma (5%-10%). These are essentially histologic subtypes but do tend to favor certain areas or populations. Superficial spreading, the most common type usually occurs on the trunk or legs (Fig. 33-86). Lentigo maligna melanoma is an in-situ variant and usually found on the face in elderly persons (Fig. 33-87). Nodular melanomas often have a solid-black color, and their thickness predicts a worse prognosis (Fig. 33-88). Acral lentiginous melanoma is most often found on the great toe or thumb and is the most common type to occur in African Americans (Fig. 33-89).

Excisional biopsy, including 1 to 2 mm of normal skin surrounding the pigmented lesion, is optimal to provide

Table 33-3 Mnemonic for Signs and Symptoms of Melanoma

ABCDE	Description
Asymmetry	Half the mole does not match the other half.
Border irregularity	Edges of mole are ragged, blurred, or notched.
Color	Color over mole is not homogeneous; may be varying shades of tan, brown, or black; patches of red, blue, or white in some cases.
Diameter	Mole is larger than 6 mm.
Evolution	Previously stable mole that is changing (evolving) in color, size, or other signs or symptoms.

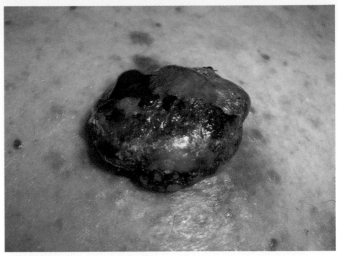

Figure 33-88 Nodular melanoma with 22-mm Breslow depth. *(© Richard P. Usatine.)*

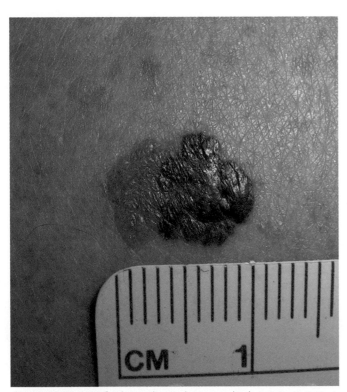

Figure 33-86 Superficial spreading melanoma on back. *(© Richard P. Usatine.)*

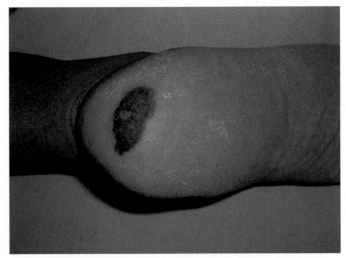

Figure 33-89 Acral lentiginous melanoma on heel of African American woman. *(© Richard P. Usatine.)*

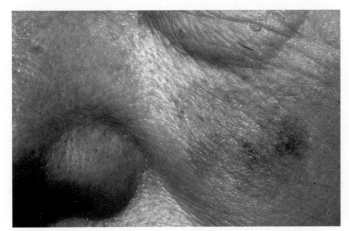

Figure 33-87 Lentigo maligna melanoma on the face. *(© The Skin Cancer Foundation.)*

accurate diagnosis and histologic staging. Referral for biopsy may be appropriate based on the location and size of the lesion. "Scoop shave" biopsies can be performed as long as the depth of the specimen obtained is greater than 1 to 2 mm. This is important because the depth of tumor invasion (Breslow depth) is the most important prognostic indicator and used in staging. Melanomas are also staged based on presence of ulceration (histologically), lymph node involvement, and location of metastasis. Diagnosing melanoma early is critical to a good prognosis. Most thin tumors (Breslow depth <1 mm) have a greater than 90% 10-year survival rate.

Treatment for melanoma is primarily surgical and depends on the depth of the tumor. Lesions with Breslow thickness less than 1 mm can be excised with 1-cm margins. Lesions with Breslow thickness of 1 mm or greater should be referred for sentinel lymph node biopsy to provide accurate staging. There is limited adjuvant therapy for melanoma that has spread to the lymph nodes, and at this time there is no standard chemotherapy for metastatic melanoma. Clinical trials are an option for patients with advanced-stage disease. Patients with advanced melanoma should be referred to a medical oncologist to consider adjuvant therapy with interferon-alpha. This may offer a small benefit in terms of recurrence-free and overall survival (Garbe and Eigentler, 2006).

For 2 to 3 years after any diagnosis of melanoma, patients should be seen every 3 to 6 months because most metastases occur in the first few years. If no new tumors are found, annual full-body skin examinations should be performed for life because of the higher risk of subsequent primary melanomas. Strict sun protection and sun avoidance should also be followed.

KEY TREATMENT

World Health Organization recommendations for excision margins are 5 mm for melanoma in situ lesions, 1 cm for lesions less than 1 mm, and 2 cm for melanomas 2 to 4 mm in thickness (Lens et al., 2002) (SOR: A).

Sentinel lymph node biopsies are recommended for melanomas 1 mm or greater in depth, although it is unclear whether this improves survival (Tanis et al., 2008) (SOR: B).

Interferon-α may offer some benefit in recurrence-free and overall survival of melanoma patients (Garbe and Eigentler, 2006) (SOR: B).

References

The complete reference list is available online at www.expertconsult.com.

Web Resources

http://dermatlas.org/
   DermAtlas; large international atlas of dermatology from Johns Hopkins University.
www.dermnet.com
   Dermnet skin disease atlas with over 23,000 images of skin diseases.
http://dermis.net
   DermIS (Derm Information Systems); large dermatology information service containing adult and pediatric dermatology atlases; founded at University of Erlangen.

www.dermatlas.net
   Interactive Dermatology Atlas; contains more than 1500 photographs, a sophisticated search tool, quiz mode, and over 60 interactive cases developed by Dr. Richard Usatine.
www.skinsight.com/
   Skinsight (Logical Images); contains free information for patients and professionals; although promoting their VisualDx product, the site has good information and images.

CHAPTER 34

Diabetes Mellitus

Louis F. Amorosa, Esther J. Lee, and David E. Swee

Definition and Pathogenesis

Diabetes mellitus is currently defined as a group of metabolic disorders characterized by hyperglycemia that result from defects in the secretion and action of insulin. Normally, plasma glucose, the primary substrate for brain function, is tightly regulated within a narrow fasting range of 60 to 100 mg/dL by insulin secreted from the beta cells of the pancreatic islets. Daily mean glucose values which exceed 100 mg/dL have been associated with the progression of diabetic complication. Over the long term, diabetic patients often develop complications such as retinopathy, neuropathy, nephropathy, and accelerated aging of the cardiovascular system.

Although elevated fasting glucose remains the earliest and most readily detectable sign of the onset of diabetes mellitus (DM), the metabolic errors of diabetes are likely disordering the utilization of all substrates long before hyperglycemia becomes apparent. Both glucose and fatty acids are energy substrates oxidized by muscles, including the myocardium, for adenosine triphosphate (ATP) generation. The relative lack of insulin in DM leads to lipolysis or the release of fatty acids stored in adipose tissue, resulting in increased free fatty acid (FFA) levels. FFAs then compete with glucose for oxidative disposal or storage in muscles. This substrate competition further promotes hyperglycemia. During conditions of marked insulin deficiency, a massive efflux of FFAs from adipose tissue can precipitate diabetic ketoacidosis because of the incompletely oxidized FFA degradation products β-hydroxybutyrate and acetoacidic acid. Defects in FFA removal from lipoproteins account for the dyslipidemias implicated in the acceleration of atherogenesis in the diabetic state. When fatty acids packaged into triglycerides are not properly degraded in tissues, their intracellular accumulation causes lipotoxicity, which in turn impairs cellular function, including the beta cell of the pancreatic islets.

Insulin is also important in maintaining the integrity of proteins, whose amino acids become substrates for hepatic gluconeogenesis when cortisol and glucagon's actions are unopposed by insulin. Insulin insufficiency of diabetic disorders has ubiquitous adverse effects on metabolism of all energy substrates, which contributes to the diverse complications challenging diabetic patients in their activities of daily living.

Classification and Diagnosis

Key Point

- Fasting serum glucose values of 100 to 125 mg/dL are considered to be *prediabetes* to indicate that these values have an increased risk of progressing to diabetes by various pathophysiologic processes.

Diabetes mellitus has been subdivided into four groups: type 1, type 2, other specific types, and *gestational diabetes mellitus* (GDM). The diagnosis of DM is made by finding any one of the following criteria subsequently confirmed on another day by any of the criteria:

1. Typical symptoms of hyperglycemia, such as weight loss, polyuria, and polydipsia, associated with a casually found serum glucose value greater than 200 mg/dL.
2. Fasting serum (blood) glucose (FSG, FBG) value of 126 mg/dL or greater.
3. An FSG value of 200 mg/dL or greater obtained 2 hours after a 75-g glucose challenge (after 72 hours of eating 300 g of carbohydrate daily).

The diagnosis of GDM is made during pregnancy using specific criteria discussed later.

Glucose circulating in the blood enters red blood cells (RBCs) and reacts with the amino acid sequence of hemoglobin (Hb), resulting in a glycosylated product called hemoglobin A_{1c}. The HbA_{1c} value reflects the average FSG value of the prior 3 months that hemoglobin circulated in RBCs (given that RBCs have a mean half-life of 90 days). The HbA_{1c} value has become extraordinarily useful in gauging the level of glycemic control, and values of 6.5% or greater are now being considered a level diagnostic of DM. However, the test has limitations as the result can be lowered by anemia, renal disease, and other disorders that shorten RBC survival (e.g., chronic disease, hemoglobinopathy). Some forms of hemoglobinopathy can also increase the HbA_{1c} test despite near-normal glycemic control. The fructosamine test measures the glycosylation of albumin, which has a shorter circulating half life than hemoglobin, and may be used to resolve inconsistencies between average glucose values and HbA_{1c} level, although this is related to the albumin concentration. Insulin and C-peptide levels are readily affected by the toxic effects of glucose and fatty acids on beta cells, making low levels difficult to interpret.

Fasting glucose values of 100 to 125 mg/dL are consistent with prediabetes and increase the risk of progressing

to diabetes through various pathophysiologic processes. Finding these values allows the family physician to initiate prospective and preventive interventions. Participants in the Diabetes Prevention Program had impaired glucose tolerance, and those randomized to metformin or intensive lifestyle modification had reduced incidence of diabetes compared to those randomized to placebo (Knowler et al., 2002). Predictors of prediabetes changing to normal glucose regulation over 3-year follow-up included lower baseline fasting and 2-hour glucose levels, younger age, intensive lifestyle modification, and greater weight loss (Perreault et al., 2009).

Epidemiology

Prevalence

Prevalence of diabetes has increased worldwide. In 1990 the prevalence of self-reported diabetes was 2.9% in the United States, increasing to almost 8% in the first decade of the 21st century. Because self-report misses persons with undiagnosed diabetes, the Centers for Disease Control and Prevention (CDC) estimates total prevalence of diabetes in adults 20 or older approaches 11% of the U.S. population, and those with impaired fasting glucose (prediabetes), about 26% (2003–2006).

In both men and women the prevalence of diabetes increases with age; the rate now is almost 1 in 4 for those 60 years and older. In those over 20, American Indians and Alaskan Natives have high prevalence rates (16.5%). Blacks (11.8%) and Hispanics/Latinos (10.4%) also have rates greater than whites (6.6%). Education is inversely proportional, with the highest prevalence among those not finishing high school. Perhaps because of its effect on weight, smoking reduces the prevalence of diabetes, although ex-smokers have an even higher prevalence. The Southeast has a much higher prevalence than other parts of the United States. Regional differences are probably explained by differences in the populations cited, as well as cultural factors.

The lifetime risk of acquiring diabetes is high and is climbing. More than one third of those born in the year 2000 will eventually become diabetic; risk for men is 32.8%, and risk for women is 38.5% and higher risk at all ages. The lifetime risk for Hispanics is about 50% (45.4% for men, 52.5% for women); for black women, 49.0%; and for black men, 40.2%.

Types

Patients with type 1 diabetes make up only 5% to 10% of the diabetic population; the remaining 90% to 95% have type 2. Usually, type 1 diabetic patients first manifest their illness in childhood or adolescence, with about 1 in 4000 children having DM; this includes a few young people with the increasingly prevalent *maturity-onset diabetes of the young* (MODY), although this form may not manifest until adulthood. MODY is classified under "other specific types," which include a heterogeneous group of conditions (specific genetic conditions, surgery, drugs, malnutrition, infections) that result in diabetic manifestations and symptomatology (Table 34-1). These other types are found in 1% to 5% of the diabetic population. GDM is by definition temporal and is categorized separately; 3% to 6% of all pregnant women

Table 34-1 Other Specific Types of Diabetes

Cause or Category	Examples
Genetic defects of beta-cell function	Maturity-onset diabetes of the young (MODY)
Genetic defects in insulin action	Lipoatrophic diabetes
Diseases of exocrine pancreas	Pancreatitis, cystic fibrosis
Endocrinopathies	Acromegaly, Cushing's syndrome, hyperthyroidism
Drug or chemical induced	Nicotinic acid, thiazides
Infections	Congenital rubella, cytomegalovirus
Uncommon forms of immune-mediated diabetes	Antibody against insulin receptor
Other genetic syndromes occasionally associated with diabetes	Down, Klinefelter's, Turner's

From Report of the Expert Committee on the Diagnosis and Classification of Diabetes Mellitus. Diabetes Care 2003;26(suppl 1):4-20.

develop GDM, and 40% to 60% of women with GDM develop diabetes, usually type 2, within a decade of the pregnancy.

Genetics

The exact nature of how diabetes or at least the risk of diabetes is transmitted is still not well understood. It is known that those with HLA DR3 and DR4 (human lymphocytic antigens that are cell surface markers) have a fourfold increased risk of developing type 1 diabetes. If a person has both antigens, the risk increases to 12 times normal. There is a very strong familial transmission, with concordance of type 2 in 90% of identical twins older than 40, compared with 50% in type 1 diabetes. Certain genetic types (e.g., MODY) may have different responses to medications than other types.

Complications

Mortality in diabetic adults with heart disease is two to four times higher than in nondiabetic persons, and strokes occur two to four times more often in diabetic patients. Approximately three quarters of diabetic adults have high blood pressure. Diabetic retinopathy is now the leading cause of blindness in adults, and DM is also the leading cause of end-stage renal disease (44% of all cases). About two thirds of diabetic patients have some form of neural damage (e.g., peripheral neuropathy, gastroparesis, carpal tunnel syndrome, erectile dysfunction). Younger diabetic adults are twice as likely to have periodontal disease, and all those with poorly controlled diabetes are three times more likely to have gum disease. GDM poorly controlled in the first trimester can cause major birth defects (5%-10% of pregnancies) and spontaneous abortions (15%-20%).

The total direct costs (costs of medical care and services) and indirect costs (disability, work loss, premature mortality) of diabetes in 2007 were an estimated $174 billion ($116 billion for direct, $58 billion for indirect).

Prevention

When diabetes is controlled, the risk of complications decreases. For example, for every 1% decrease in HbA_{1c}, there is a corresponding 40% decrease in the risk of microvascular complications. Similarly, for every 10–mm Hg drop in blood pressure, there is a 12% reduced risk of cardiovascular and microvascular complications; controlling LDL cholesterol reduces risks of large-vessel disease even further (20%-50%). Appropriate eye and foot programs (e.g., laser therapy, podiatry monitoring) can reduce the risk of loss of vision or amputation by 50% or more.

Pathophysiology

Common Mechanisms

The pathogenic mechanisms resulting in DM are generally divided into (1) primary defects in beta-cell function, causing variable insulin deficiency (type 1diabetes), and (2) defects in the peripheral action of insulin associated with a slowly evolving loss of the beta cells' ability to compensate (type 2 diabetes). The failure of beta cells in type 1 is most likely caused by autoimmunity, comparable to other disorders affecting endocrine gland function (e.g., Hashimoto's thyroiditis, Addison's disease). Anti–islet cell antibodies are markers of the ongoing process resulting in type 1 diabetes. Beta-cell failure of type 2 diabetes is thought to result from primary genetic defects or acquired dysfunction, as in mitochondrial metabolism that reduces the oxidation of glucose and fatty acids needed for insulin synthesis and secretion. Such defects in mitochondrial function may also account for the peripheral insulin resistance in skeletal muscle, liver, and adipose tissue at the onset of type 2 diabetes. The insulin secretory function of beta cells and muscle energy metabolism can be significantly improved by any intervention that reduces hyperglycemia and hyperfatty acidemia. These observations are the basis of reversible glucotoxicity and lipotoxicity. Thus any diabetic patient with type 1 or 2 diabetes may have similar mechanisms of both insulin deficiency and insulin resistance.

The clinical characteristics of type 1 and 2 diabetes are shown in Table 34-2. However, diabetic classification and nomenclature have required frequent revisions over the years as the pathogenesis of DM is better understood and changes in culture and human behavior continue to alter its clinical expression. The finding of hyperglycemia on routine examinations of apparently healthy individuals has resulted in a new DM subclass that does not lend itself to easy classification. The finding of anti–islet cell antibodies designates this group as *latent autoimmune diabetes of adults* (LADA). This group mostly consists of young adults who have a prolonged subclinical development of DM. The diabetes may remain indolent or more rapidly deteriorate into classic insulin-dependent type 1 diabetes, or it may continue to evolve into insulin resistance and dependency coincident with weight gain. In this case, LADA patients are clinically

Table 34-2 Characteristics of Types 1 and 2 Diabetes Mellitus

Sign	Type 1	Type 2
Age of onset	Usually childhood and adolescence	About 40 years, increasing with age; adolescence with childhood obesity
Family history, concordance in twins	Uncommon; 50% before age 40	Common, 95% after age 40
Diagnostic markers	Anti-GAD, undetectable C peptide	C peptide variable: high with insulin resistance; low values improve with glycemic control.
Other associated disorders	Primary hypothyroidism, celiac disease, other autoimmune endocrine disorders	Metabolic syndrome
Glycemic control, ketosis	Marked brittleness, ketosis prone with hyperglycemia	Stable hyperglycemia without ketosis
Treatment requirement	Absolute need for insulin; coincident genetic insulin resistance that might respond to oral drugs	Therapeutic lifestyle changes with and without oral agents; insulin is required when other measures fail.

GAD, Glutamic acid decarboxylase.

indistinguishable from type 2 patients but have continuing risk of deteriorating to insulin dependency. Thus a patient recognized to have DM may have diverse etiopathogenic mechanisms causing insulin dependency and resistance resulting in hyperglycemia.

Adolescents with significant obesity who develop type 2 diabetes are younger at presentation than usual, so age of onset of type 2 now overlaps with type 1 diabetes. Because their obesity is often intractable, their marked state of insulin resistance at DM onset eventually becomes a state of insulin deficiency. When DM patients develop marked hyperglycemia and dyslipidemia, the resulting glucotoxicity and lipotoxicity cause systemic cellular dehydration along with triglyceride accumulation in skeletal muscle. These acquired defects further accentuate defects in beta-cell insulin secretion and muscle insulin sensitivity. Pathogenic mechanisms may differ (Fig. 34-1), but the resulting glucotoxicity and lipotoxicity so impair insulin secretion and effectiveness that diabetes from any mechanism may lead to similar metabolic crises: diabetic ketoacidosis with or without hyperosmolality.

Mechanisms Underlying Other Specific Types of Diabetes

A diverse array of genetic defects or acquired clinical disorders can impair beta-cell function or insulin sensitivity, resulting in hyperglycemia and the diagnosis of diabetes mellitus (see Table 34-1). These patients generally appear to have type 2 diabetes at presentation and manifest varying degrees of diabetic severity during the course of their primary disorder.

Maturity-Onset Diabetes of Young

Genetic defects of beta-cell function involve genes coding for hepatic transcription factors and glucokinase. In the MODY variant, hyperglycemia is observed during childhood or adolescence and is caused by a diminution in beta-cell secretion without impairment in insulin action. The genetic disorders are autosomal dominant, and the glucokinase defect impairs the conversion of glucose to glucose-6-phosphate, which is involved in insulin secretion. This glucokinase dysfunction causes a loss of the beta-cell "glucose sensor." The resulting diabetes is generally not prone to ketosis. Many patients with milder forms of diabetes treated as type 1 eventually are found to have similar genetic defects.

Genetic Disorders of Insulin Resistance

These genetic defects may cause diabetes varying from mild to severe. Marked hyperinsulinemia activates epidermal growth factor receptors in skin, resulting in *acanthosis nigricans,* a darkening of skin folds at the nape of the neck or in the axilla. Marked hyperinsulinemia stimulates ovarian steroidogenesis, which can result in enlarged ovaries and a virilizing syndrome. This condition provided insight into the connection of insulin resistance to polycystic ovarian syndrome, which is now routinely treated with metformin to attenuate hirsutism and stimulate ovulation. The genetic defects in patients with generalized lipoatrophy have not been fully defined, but these patients are extremely insulin resistant because energy substrates can be stored only in liver and muscle. Impairment in fatty acid storage compromises muscle uptake and glucose oxidation.

Disorders of Exocrine Pancreas

Hemochromatosis, chronic pancreatitis, cystic fibrosis, and fibrocalculous pancreatopathy (observed in tropical countries) all cause decreased insulin release to varying degrees.

Other Endocrinopathies

Production of excessive counterregulatory hormones requires an increased insulin output. When increased insulin secretion cannot be maintained and hyperglycemia results, the physician can infer preexisting beta-cell abnormalities in insulin production and secretion.

Infectious Etiologies

Type 1 diabetes may result from viral destruction of beta cells, as in congenital rubella, mumps, cytomegalovirus, or coxsackievirus.

Other Syndromes

Syndromes involving chromosomes (Down, Klinefelter's), fat and muscle metabolism (Prader-Willi, myotonic dystrophy), and autoimmune mechanisms (stiff man syndrome) can affect insulin secretion or sensitivity.

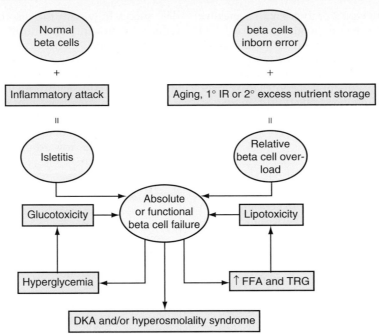

Figure 34-1 How normal or genetically impaired beta cells can be affected by inflammation and overnutrition, resulting in absolute or relative loss of insulin secretory reserve and the activation of the common mechanism leading to diabetic crisis. *1° IR*, Primary insulin resistance; *2° IR*, secondary insulin resistance; *DKA*, diabetic ketoacidosis; *FFA*, free fatty acids; *TRG*, triglycerides.

Presentation

Key Points

- Fasting glucose values of at least 200 mg/dL usually indicate significant beta-cell failure comparable to type 1 diabetes. Beta-cell loss in type 2 may still be reversible, however, even after long periods, if gluco/lipotoxicity is successfully treated.
- Hyperglycemia (even at prediabetes levels), dyslipidemia, and hypertension associated with increased abdominal girth are the cardinal signs of metabolic syndrome.
- Somatic symptoms and signs of type 2 diabetes usually take years to develop; the prolonged "latent" phase depends on the severity of hyperglycemia.

Type 1 Diabetes

The symptoms of type 1 diabetes may be indolent or precipitous, depending on the rate of decrease in insulin secretion. *Indolent* asymptomatic diabetes can decompensate as a result of a coincident illness. The resulting hyperglycemia causes polydipsia and polyuria from the osmotic effects of glycosuria. Weight loss, blurred vision, and fatigue occur as energy metabolism is disordered. Most patients become aware of a problem at this point, and the diagnosis is easily recognized if the patient seeks help.

If the insulin deficiency is allowed to become profound, the disorder in FFA metabolism results in *ketonuria*, which accentuates the osmotic diuresis. The stress of illness can increase counterregulatory hormones (epinephrine, cortisol, growth hormone) that antagonize the effects of already-reduced insulin. The result is increasing hyperglycemia and further osmotic diuresis. Progressive hyperglycemia causes intravascular and intracellular dehydration, which reduces beta-cell

function and insulin delivery to the periphery. Gastric dysfunction can occur under these conditions, further compromising fluid intake. The result is a "glucotoxic" state in which dehydration compromises the kidney's ability to excrete ketones, whose production is accelerated by insulin's failure to regulate FFA oxidation. Acidemia as a result of marked ketonemia causes hyperventilation and subsequent dyspnea. The increasing hyperglycemic state with dehydration causes brain *hyperosmolality*, producing lethargy, stupor, and if uninterrupted with insulin therapy, coma. This sequence is the description of the descent into diabetic ketoacidosis.

Diabetes mellitus may be discovered incidentally in an asymptomatic child or adult when hyperglycemia is noted on a comprehensive metabolic profile or glycosuria on routine urinalysis. Presuming that a lean child, adolescent, or adult has an autoimmune process leading to type 1 diabetes would be strongly supported by the finding of anti–islet cell antibodies. Asymptomatic patients with mild hyperglycemia thought to have an autoimmune pathogenesis require glucose monitoring to determine when therapeutic intervention is needed. Although these patients are likely to respond early to a variety of oral agents like any type 2 patient, no interventions have been effective thus far in slowing their progression to clinically overt type 1 requiring insulin. Prudent lifestyle measures, including exercise, dietary discretion, glucose monitoring, and oral therapies designed to reduce insulin secretion, may be efficacious over a surprisingly long period in deferring insulin therapy.

Type 2 Diabetes

The typical indolent course of type 2 diabetes can be further extended by a therapeutic lifestyle. However, this does not mean it is any less serious than type 1 as a state of accelerated vascular aging. Unfortunately, treating middle-aged and older patients with long-term type 2 diabetes with aggressive pharmacologic methods to correct hyperglycemia has failed to improve cardiovascular outcomes (ACCORD, 2008; VADT, 2009). Improved glycemic control in type 2 diabetes, as in type 1, has been shown to preclude progression of small-vessel disease and nerve function disorder to diabetic retinopathy, nephropathy, and neuropathy (UKPDS, 1998a).

Dyslipidemia, Hypertension, and Atherosclerosis

The unexpectedly negative outcomes of diabetic studies targeting hyperglycemia as a cardinal risk factor for progression of atherosclerosis emphasize the need to correct dyslipidemia and hypertension typical of the type 2 diabetic state. Dyslipidemia occurs chiefly when beta cells are unable to maintain the high insulin levels required to inhibit lipolysis from adipose cells. The resulting free fatty acidemia associated with high insulin levels causes the liver to repackage these energy substrates into more triglyceride-rich lipoproteins.

Hyperinsulinemia has also been associated with hypertension, changes in vascular responsiveness (endothelial dysfunction), and appearance of inflammatory proteins, especially C-reactive protein. The precise causal factor in these relationships and relative importance of these changes are not well understood.

Overt Type 2 Diabetes

Remarkably, only 20% to 25% of individuals with hyperinsulinemia and insulin resistance progress to overt type 2 diabetes. This progression begins when FSG becomes 100 mg/dL or greater, the threshold for the diagnosis of prediabetes. Type 2 diabetes may be diagnosed at this phase if a casual postprandial glucose of 200 mg/dL or higher is detected.

Most patients diagnosed with type 2 diabetes may not note the typical hyperglycemic symptoms described for type 1 diabetes. The difference may be that type 2 diabetes evolves over years below the symptomatic threshold because sufficient insulin is present to prevent the marked lipolysis and ketonemia more typical of type 1 diabetes, with its obligatory water and electrolyte losses. Most patients with type 2 diabetes are discovered incidentally, such as during routine risk factor assessment for cardiovascular disease or other work-up for various symptoms, including peripheral sensorimotor neuropathy, Bell's palsy, erectile dysfunction, visual changes, and gastrointestinal complaints, which may lead to finding an elevated FSG and the diagnosis of type 2 diabetes.

Management

Behavioral Therapy

> **Key Point**
>
> - Self-management is the essence of behavioral therapy for DM, consisting of daily glucose monitoring, diet, exercise, and insulin adjustment.

The diagnosis of diabetes mellitus requires lifestyle adjustments and enduring major inconveniences and sacrifices to deal successfully with the disorder. Behavioral adjustments reduce the difficulty of controlling type 1 diabetes, but their impact in a type 2 patient can be so powerful as to alter the course of the disorder. All patients receive rational treatment regimens, but those who consciously monitor their diet and glucose variations learn how to make daily adjustments to achieve near-normalization of glucose values. Positive daily outcomes usually stimulate a continuing self-managing effort. Thus the goal of diabetic treatment is to promote this "winning attitude" toward the disorder.

> **KEY TREATMENT**
>
> *Risk management:* A therapeutic lifestyle based on achieving weight control and maintaining physical fitness can delay the onset of diabetes mellitus in persons in the high-risk groups (ADA, 2009; Knowler et al., 2002; Tuomeilehto et al., 2001) (SOR: A).
> *Global risk management:* All patients should be advised not to smoke. Patients with blood pressure greater than 130/80 mm Hg should receive pharmacologic therapy in addition to lifestyle therapy. Even in patients without overt cardiovascular disease, the primary goal is LDL level less than 100 mg/dL (ADA, 2009; Haffner, 1998; Haire-Joshu et al., 1999; Hanson et al., 1998; UKPDS, 1998b; Vaccaro et al., 2004) (SOR: A).

Glucose Monitoring

Monitoring behavior is itself therapeutic because it warns of the risk of hypoglycemia or a shift to a hyperglycemic state caused by dietary indiscretion or a smoldering stress. Glucometers are now available that require less than 1 μL of blood (taken up by capillary action). A sample may be taken from a fingertip, earlobe, forearm, or thigh, with the result available in 5 to 15 seconds. Arm or thigh values are derived from interstitial glucose concentration and may be approximately 15 minutes "out of phase" with blood values if the patient is not in a fasting steady state. Average monitored values over 14 to 30 days correlate with HbA_{1c} values. Monitored glucose data are also the basis of formulating therapeutic targets. For a young girl with diabetes, the fasting target may be 150 mg/dL to avoid early-morning hypoglycemia. As she matures, the target becomes the current American Diabetes Association (ADA) goal of less than 120 mg/dL fasting and before meals. In elderly diabetic patients, glycemic targets again can be liberalized to preclude hypoglycemic risks.

Although costs of monitoring must be considered, frequent glucose monitoring usually indicates the patient is well motivated and is attempting to make the necessary adjustments that will improve their mean glucose value and impact favorably on the HbA_{1c}. In an informed patient with stable type 2 diabetes, there is less evidence that daily is any more effective than weekly testing.

> **KEY TREATMENT**
>
> Insulin treatment of type 1 and monotherapy or combination therapy of type 2 diabetic patients, when guided by self–glucose monitoring, can accomplish tight glycemic control to HbA_{1c} less than 7%, which reduces the occurrence and progression of the microangiopathic complications of DM (ADA, 2009; DCCT, 1993; UKPDS, 1998a) (SOR: A).

Nutrition and Diet

Key Points

- Intentional weight loss can help reverse hyperglycemia, dyslipidemia, hypertension, and other risk factors in patients with type 2 diabetic pathoetiologies.
- Caloric restriction without an accompanying exercise program is much less likely to succeed, although increased eating in compensation for exercise is a potential pitfall.

Dietary consistency will also ease the difficulties of living with diabetes. As with a regular exercise program, a stable diet will simplify insulin treatment schedules in type 1 patients but will not produce the marked effects observed in type 2 patients. Therefore, dietary manipulation should be directed toward ensuring content regularity rather than weight loss in type 1 patients.

Dietary Principles and Weight Loss

In terms of *medical nutrition therapy*, there is no longer a specific diabetic diet; all recommendations are individualized as part of a comprehensive plan that includes exercise and appropriate medical therapies. A meal plan that includes a variety of usual foods is recommended as long as the plan is healthy, with conscious control of carbohydrate intake. Weight loss will improve blood pressure control and, along with decreasing fat intake and increasing physical activity, will reduce fasting lipid levels.

It is not necessary to attempt weight loss before instituting medical therapy, especially since weight loss alone may not provide any glycemic control in highly insulin-deficient patients. However, a multifaceted approach with education, reduced energy, and fat-calorie intake, increased regular physical activity, and other lifestyle changes can produce long-term weight loss and glycemic improvement. Less need for calories in elderly patients leads to obvious dietary changes. Of note, patients should not avoid breads and other starches; in fact, complex carbohydrates are an important part of the modern approach to diabetes.

Dietary Details

The current dietary principles recommended by ADA are the same as those of the American Heart Association (AHA). The caloric content should be that which will permit a patient with type 2 diabetes to attain a body mass index (BMI) of 25 kg/m². With gender, height, weight, and age known, the basal daily caloric requirement and the desired weight can be obtained from standard online calculators. A simpler method, for patients with routine and not intensely physical activities, is to estimate the daily caloric expenditure by multiplying the ideal weight in kilograms by 30 calories/kg. Weight loss can be safely achieved if the patient is taught how to reduce caloric intake by 100 calories per day for each 10 pounds of desired weight loss over 1 year. National Institutes of Health guidelines advocate that weight changes be methodically accomplished over long periods. This will preclude acute energy shifts that could cause gallstones, gout, and depression and have 95% likelihood of recidivism. The guidelines suggest a weight loss goal of 7%, usually rounded

to 10%, per year until the patient attains ideal BMI. For example, for a patient with type 2 diabetes weighing 200 pounds, the advice should be to lose 20 pounds in 1 year by reducing dietary caloric intake by 200 calories per day and/or increasing energy expenditure by that amount.

If a new and reduced weight set point is achieved in the central nervous system, longitudinal studies have shown a reduction in the progression of prediabetes, which confirms widespread clinical experience that the weight loss has a reversal effect on type 2 diabetes.

Dietary Recommendations

The 2008 ADA guidelines considered the risk and advisable intake of carbohydrates, fats, proteins, and other food ingredients. Monitoring carbohydrate by counting, exchanges, or experience-based estimation remains a key strategy in achieving glycemic control. Saturated fat should be less than 7% of calories, and there should be minimal *trans* fat. Total cholesterol should be less than 200 mg daily. Higher fiber intake may improve glycemic control; thus fiber intake should be at least 14 g/1000 calories daily. Sugar, alcohols, and nonnutritive sweeteners are safe when consumed within daily levels established by the Food and Drug Administration (FDA). Usual dietary protein of 15% to 20% of calories is appropriate in diabetes in the absence of significant renal insufficiency. Reduction of protein intake to 0.8 to 1.0 g/kg/day in diabetic individuals with early stages of chronic kidney disease, and to less than 0.8 g/kg/day in later stages, may improve renal function. High-protein diets (>20% of calories) are not recommended for weight loss because the long-term effects on renal function are unknown. A reduced sodium intake of 2300 mg/day, with a diet high in fruits, vegetables, and low-fat dairy products, is prudent. For patients with diabetes and symptomatic heart failure, dietary sodium intake of less than 2000 mg/day may reduce symptoms.

Alcohol

The general consensus is that alcohol in moderation is appropriate for diabetic patients, if only for its protective cardiac effects. "Moderate drinking" means a glass of red wine daily, depending on body mass. Also, for accurate carbohydrate counting, the patient must include the amount in alcohol.

Exercise

Key Points

- Exercise is the single best broad-spectrum therapeutic activity to offset the age-related decline of lean body mass and the consequent loss of insulin sensitivity.
- Exercise does not always promote glucose utilization.
- Clinical prudence requires that cardiac risk be evaluated before a patient engages in a rigorous exercise regimen.
- A prudent guideline is to instruct a nonactive patient to stay within a pulse rate 60% of maximum heart rate for age, before progressing to 75% to 85%.

In addition to dietary guidelines, the U.S. Department of Agriculture (USDA, 2005) also recommends daily exercise activities for weight loss and health maintenance. The difference in these objectives is related to the duration and the intensity of exercise. The advocacy of exercise, as with dieting and food choices, has become an American industry. Exercise is an essential intervention in the diabetic lifestyle. Studies show that exercise activities even without weight loss result in consistently beneficial and safe outcomes. In type 2 diabetic patients with HbA$_{1c}$ of less than 9%, exercise can lower this indicator by 1%. A similar effect in type 1 diabetes has not been demonstrated, despite improved insulin sensitivity. However, both type 1 and 2 patients show improved serum lipid profile and increased fibrinolytic proteins after exercise. Based on its effects in improving athletic performance, exercise in a diabetic patient encourages good cardiac function with increased circulation to muscles and the periphery.

Risks

Hypoglycemia

As with other effective antidiabetic treatments, exercise has risks, especially in patients who maintain good glycemic control. These risks can be reduced, however, by applying increased care in exercising and its timing. Patients who engage in rigorous activities such as team sports can experience a dramatic hypoglycemic reaction either at the time of the activity or later that night. This risk can be prevented by anticipating and monitoring glucose during exercise. The hypoglycemia is a result of energy expended as oxidized glucose and fatty acids and the latent effects of exercise, which improve muscle blood flow and insulin sensitivity for hours, further facilitating glucose uptake. All these phenomena accelerate plasma glucose clearance, which may require decreasing antidiabetic therapies, especially insulin dosages, to prevent a late, insidious decline in glucose. Understanding all the effects of a particular exercise allows adjustments in treatment and nutrient supplementation.

Hyperglycemia

Rigorous exercise undertaken when insulin levels are insufficient and glycemic control is unsatisfactory will stimulate a stress reaction in which epinephrine activates glycogenolysis. If insulin is insufficient to signal muscle utilization of this hepatic outpouring of glucose, marked hyperglycemia results. Ketosis may also occur as lipolysis, stimulated by the sympathetic nervous system, is unregulated. To avoid this diametrically opposed reaction, rigorous exercises should be initiated only when the blood sugar is known to be under control. The more intense the activity, the more monitoring and nutritional supplementation are necessary. However, overeating in response to exercise is not appropriate.

Complications Associated with Heart and Microvasculature

There are also organ-specific risks of exercise in diabetes. Many cardiac patients are found to be unaware of their type 2 diabetes; almost all long-term patients with diabetes have cardiac dysfunction, often "silent ischemia."

Retinopathy and Neuropathy

Rigorous exercise that elevates blood pressure can exacerbate exudative and proliferative retinopathy. These findings may limit exercise to low-intensity activities such as walking,

which is safe and effective, even in patients with reduced cardiac function.

Walking

Walking improves peripheral perfusion and diverts blood volume to the lower extremities, where muscles have greater capacitance. Blood pressure and cardiac afterload are reduced. Regular walking can even overcome intermittent claudication by stimulating collateralization. With sufficient effort and duration, and even if done in short but repeated patterns as part of the activities of daily living, walking can facilitate weight loss. Postprandial walking may be more effective than preprandial walking (Colberg et al., 2009).

Walking can become hazardous, however, when the foot is affected by marked sensorimotor peripheral neuropathy. Exercise involving the feet requires that the patient is aware of risks and understands how to avoid them. Dry, thin skin lacking the cooling and lubricating effects of sweating is very susceptible to blistering when walking causes rubbing of the foot within the shoe. Prior foot injuries resulting from neuropathic trauma or the microfractures of diabetic osteonecrosis often cause foot deformities and uneven distribution of weight over the surface of the foot. The hyposensitive skin beneath bony deformities is at risk for ulceration. Prophylactic treatment requires orthotic devices, daily foot lubrication, and footwear that is soft with room to expand. Rather than contraindicating exercise of the foot and lower leg, advanced diabetic foot problems benefit from the increased perfusion accompanying non-weight-bearing exercise. Safe, effective exercise activities helpful in this situation use devices that "lock" the feet into the pedals of a stationary bicycle or an elliptical cycler.

Exercise Prescription

The type, duration, and intensity of exercise as therapy for diabetes is often decided by patient preference and common sense based on the patient's age and abilities and the previous considerations. As noted with walking, modest but periodic low-intensity efforts such as stationary cycling, arm conditioning with light weights, and dancing for 30 to 45 minutes with brief rest period, as often as daily, but at least three times per week, will achieve measurable improvement in HbA$_{1c}$ and lipid levels, indicative of the overall physiologic benefit.

For patients under age 40, the maximum heart rate (HR) is calculated simply by subtracting the patient's age from 220; for a 35-year-old patient, maximum HR would be 220 − 35, or 185 beats/min. Within a 30-minute exercise regimen, after a 5-minute warm-up, there should be 20 minutes of exercise in the pulse range of 111 to 124 beats/min (60%-67% of 185), followed by another 5 minutes of a cool-down phase. With more conditioning, the patient should aim to exercise in the range of 75% to 85% (139-157 beats/min). For patients over 40, the formula for maximum HR is 208 − (0.7 × age); for a 45-year-old patient, 208 − (0.7 × 45) = 208 − 32 = 176 beats/min, with the calculated HR guideposts of 106 (60%), 118 (67%), 132 (75%), and 150 (85%) beats/min.

Pharmacologic Therapies

Key Points

- The ongoing UKPDS combines oral agents and insulin to confirm that better glycemic control lessens microangiopathic complications in type 2 diabetes, independent of the agents used.
- Lowering blood glucose at any time will augment the action of oral medications, which are intended to take over control once the hyperglycemia is overcome.

Glycemic Targets

Since the publication of the Diabetes Control and Complication Trial (DCCT) in 1993, which demonstrated that improved glycemic control meant less neuropathy, retinopathy, and nephropathy in patients with type 1 diabetes, development of antidiabetic agents has accelerated. These include the α-glucosidase inhibitors, metformin, meglitinides, thiazolidinediones (also called glitazones), designer insulins, synthetic analogs of pancreatic peptides called amylin, and incretins, as well as antagonists of incretin degradation called dipeptidyl peptidase inhibitors. How intensely these agents should be used to limit the macrovascular complications of diabetes (coronary heart disease, peripheral vascular disease, stroke) requires continuing study.

Although the efficacy of attaining HbA_{1c} values in the low 7% range resulted in reduced microangiopathic complications, the DCCT and U.K. Prospective Diabetic Study (UKPDS) did not provide conclusive evidence of protection from macrovascular complications. In contrast, UKPDS demonstrated the efficacy of antihypertensive therapy given primarily as a beta blocker or angiotensin-converting enzyme (ACE) inhibitor in slowing the progression of proteinuria and reducing cerebrovascular and cardiac events. Other clinical trials of the statins showed that diabetic patients experience better cardiovascular outcomes with relatively brief treatment. Controlling other major cardiovascular risk factors in DM has a more readily apparent effect on improving diabetic macrovascular outcomes than correction of hyperglycemia.

Similar data from other large trials indicate that the difference in intensive efforts to lower HbA_{1c} to values below 6% versus conventional treatment was not associated with reduced cardiovascular events in middle-aged type 2 diabetic patients (ACCORD, 2008; VADT, 2009). This may have resulted from unawareness of hypoglycemia common in patients with HbA_{1c} values approaching 6%. Recurrent hypoglycemia may downregulate appropriate physiologic response to the stress of cardiac ischemia, which may be clinically silent in diabetic patients.

Considering these data, professional societies recommend that glycemic targets be applied with clinical judgment based on the patient's age and life expectancy, which would relate to the patient's risk of developing microangiopathic complications. Thus an HbA_{1c} target of about 6.5% is appropriate for a young diabetic patient with type 1 but inappropriate for 75-year-old woman with type 2 and cardiovascular disease. Hemoglobin A_{1c} values of less than 8% in type 2 patients are readily attainable and would likely slow the progression of retinopathy, neuropathy, and subtle renal loss while preventing an acute metabolic decompensation associated

with rapid onset of infection. Glycemic targets of 7% or less are ideal if attained without the risk of hypoglycemia unawareness.

Table 34-3 lists the classes of antidiabetic drugs, mode and duration of action, effectiveness, and side effects. The introduction of the newer agents now allows the clinician to consider drugs that address a specific etiopathogenic mechanism. If the patient is thought to have a type 1 presentation, insulin at the onset is the logical and safest treatment, as discussed later. Oral medications, at least in the short term, should be advised for type 2 diabetic presentations. Behavioral therapies can produce dramatic improvement even at higher HbA_{1c} values, but a FSG over 200 mg/dL indicates marked insulin insufficiency, and some form of drug therapy (including insulin) is necessary to reduce such values expeditiously. Instituting drug therapy should not deemphasize behavioral therapies; as noted, once the inertia of gluco/lipotoxicity is overcome with drugs, effective behavioral therapies could control DM indefinitely.

> ### KEY TREATMENT
>
> Management of either type 1 or type 2 diabetes should be continually modified to find the optimal therapeutic regimen yielding HbA_{1c} of less than 7% while avoiding the risk of hypoglycemia (ADA, 2009; DCCT, 1993; UKPDS 1998) (SOR: A).

Oral Agents

Metformin

With various oral medications available, the physician can choose different therapeutic protocols according to clinical factors. For an overweight patient with a FSG value in the mid–100 mg/dL range, current consensus recommends metformin as the first-line drug (ADA and European Association for the Study of Diabetes, 2009). Metformin blocks glucose production by the liver, which reduces insulin resistance. Metformin is available in generic form and generally does not cause further weight gain. The contraindication is renal insufficiency or the risk of renal impairment secondary to low renal perfusion from dehydration or heart failure. Lactic acidosis can occur if metformin is given in renal failure. Procedures with a risk of nephrotoxicity (e.g., x-ray contrast studies) may necessitate holding the metformin therapy, usually for 24 hours before and after the procedure.

Sulfonylureas and Meglitinides

The sulfonylureas are the oldest class of drugs and were found to be as safe and effective as insulin in the UKPDS. They shut down membrane potassium ion (K^+) channels, allowing membrane calcium (Ca^{++}) channels to open, thereby establishing a calcium gradient that stimulates insulin secretion. In the initial phase of treatment, insulin levels are higher than the previous state following the drug's stimulatory effects. As insulin resistance factors are improved by controlling hyperglycemia, insulin levels fall into a normal range. Treatment is usually effective for 5 to 10 years, depending on the efficacy of behavior treatment and the underlying diabetic progression. The therapeutic duration of sulfonylureas

Table 34-3 Classification of Noninsulin Antidiabetic Agents

Category/Drug	Action	Onset; Duration	Dosage	Clearance; Side Effects
Metformin (Glucophage)	Limits hepatic glucose output	1 hr; 4-6 hr	0.5-1 g bid 850 mg tid	Renal clearance GI upset, diarrhea (10%)
Sulfonylureas				
Glyburide (Micronase, Diabeta)	Increase insulin secretion	1 hr; 24 hr	5-20 mg/day	Hepatorenal clearance Hypoglycemia
Glipizide (Glucotrol)		1 hr; 12 hr	10-40 mg/day	
Glipizide, extended release (Glucotrol XL)		2 hr; 24 hr	5-20 mg/day	
Glimepiride (Amaryl)		2 hr; 24 hr	1-8 mg/day	
Nonsulfonylurea secretagogues				
Repaglinide (Prandin)	Increase insulin secretion	½ hr; 3 hr	0.5-4 mg*	Hepatic clearance Hypoglycemia
Nateglinide (Starlix)		½ hr; 3 hr	60 mg*	
Thiazolidinediones (Glitazones)				
Pioglitazone (Actos)	Express transcription factors promoting insulin sensitivity, secretion	3-6 hr; 24 hr	15-45 mg/day	Hepatic clearance Weight gain, edema, CHF
Rosiglitazone (Avandia)		3-6 hr; 24 hr	1-8 mg/day	
α-Glucosidase inhibitor				
Acarbose (Precose)	Inhibits intestinal digestion of disaccharides, slowing glucose absorption	½ hr; 2-4 hr	50-100 mg*	Intestinal clearance Flatulence, abdominal discomfort, diarrhea
Incretin (GLP) agonist				
Exenatide (Byetta) Liraglutide (Victoza)	Enhances postprandial insulin secretion Enhances postprandial insulin secretion	¼ hr 2-3 hr Max effect at 10-12 hr, up to 24 hr	5 or 10 µg SC bid* 0.6 to 1.8 µg SC/day	Hepatic clearance Nausea, sense of non-well-being
Dipeptidyl peptidase (DPP) inhibitor (Gliptin)				
Sitagliptin (Januvia)	Enhances postprandial insulin secretion	½ hr; 12-24 hr		

*At mealtime.
GI, Gastrointestinal; *bid*, twice daily; *tid*, three times daily; *CHF*, congestive heart failure; *SC*, subcutaneously; *GLP*, glucagon-like peptide.

can be prolonged if an overnight insulin preparation is added to control FSG level.

Sulfonylureas are insulin secretogogues that can be used as first-line drugs or in combination with any of the oral medications. An important advantage is their low cost. However, diabetic patients who do not demonstrate fasting hyperglycemia have an increased risk of hypoglycemia if HbA$_{1c}$ is being maintained below 7%. Another hypoglycemic risk is renal disease, which reduces gluconeogenesis and permits typical sulfonylureas such as glyburide and glipizide to accumulate. Glimepiride and the meglitinides may be used in mild azotemia because of their greater hepatic excretion. The meglitinides are nonsulfonylurea secretogogues that activate a different K$^+$ channel. The meglitinides are theoretically safer in elderly patients because of their short half-life, although treatment is required before all meals. Their disadvantage is that generic preparations are not yet available. Failure to respond to metformin is an indication for adding an insulin secretogogue and titrating the dosage to attain near normalization of HbA$_{1c}$.

Alpha-Glucosidase Inhibitors

The α-glucosidase inhibitors have been the least utilized of the oral medications available in the United States because of their side effects, not because of their lack of efficacy. The agents interfere with intestinal digestion of complex carbohydrates, slowing the absorption of glucose and limiting the beta-cell insulin response, thus lowering insulin levels. Their disadvantage is that they require administration with meals and often cause postprandial abdominal discomfort and flatulence. Patients who can tolerate these agents can experience HbA$_{1c}$ reductions comparable to other oral agents. However, most patients eventually request a change in medication. These drugs may be better tolerated at the onset of diabetes and prediabetic phase of diagnosis.

Thiazolidinediones (Glitazones)

Thiazolidinediones (TZDs) were developed as transcription factors that stimulate the induction of many cellular proteins facilitating insulin action in the cytosol and mitochondria. TZDs were frequently used as first-line treatment either alone or in combination with metformin because these glitazones can be dramatically effective, especially in overweight patients. Insulin resistance may be significantly improved. However, glitazones can cause unpredictable weight gain and development of peripheral edema, and some patients experience no response. In the presence of renal insufficiency and diastolic dysfunction, glitazones can cause an acute pulmonary edema or subtle congestive heart failure. In fact, a controversial meta-analysis indicated that rosiglitazone increased coronary events, but this was not confirmed in several other series, when patients receiving glitazones were carefully selected. However, these TZDs demonstrating efficacy in slowing the progression of diabetes have been associated with greater fracture risk. For these reasons and high cost, treatment with glitazones is now recommended only after careful deliberation in patients not achieving therapeutic glycemic targets with other agents; the patient and family must be fully informed about the risks before initiating therapy.

Dipeptidyl Peptidase Inhibitors (Gliptins)

The naturally occurring *incretins*, glucagon-like peptide (GLP) and glucoinsulinotropic peptide (GIP), enhance beta-cell insulin secretion after glucose ingestion. The *incretin effect* is the increase in insulin secretion after gastrointestinal (GI) absorption of glucose compared to the amount of insulin secreted in response to glucose infused intravenously. The augmentation of insulin secretion is secondary to a stimulatory effect of GLP and GIP on beta cells. The metabolic clearance of these hormones is governed by dipeptidyl peptidase (DPP), which enzymatically inactivates the incretins. Thus, inhibition of DPP by drugs known as *gliptins* causes a more sustained postprandial insulin secretion.

The prototype DDP inhibitor is sitagliptin, which is safe and generally very effective in the treatment of patients with HbA_{1c} values less than 8%. As with metformin, sitagliptin is not associated with weight gain. It maintains control in patients treated with metformin and sulfonylureas who are slipping out of control. Sitagliptin is rarely efficacious for patients with HbA_{1c} above 8%. Its safety makes sitagliptin a good choice for use alone or in combination with metformin in patients who have insulin secretion, but cost should relegate it to a tertiary role behind more potent sulfonylureas. Other DPP inhibitors are currently in development, and saxagliptin was recently approved as a once-daily tablet to treat type 2 diabetes in adults. Sitagliptin requires dose adjustments for renal failure.

Incretin Agonist (Exenatide)

The prototype GLP agonist is exenatide, which is structurally similar to GLP and was initially approved for use as the therapeutic effects of metformin and sulfonylurea diminished. Exenatide is given subcutaneously by fixed dosages of 5 or 10 μg, twice daily before meals. Its major side effect is nausea and a sense of non-well-being, which limits appetite and food intake. About 50% of patients are intolerant of treatment in the short term, although many adjust to the side effects, which lessen over time. Overweight patients who are able to take exenatide lose more than 10 pounds (4.5 kg) in the first year. Weight losses can be dramatic, with marked improvement in HbA_{1c} values. Significant weight loss without HbA_{1c} improvement in suggests that the patient has minimal insulin secretory reserve. Exenatide is a therapeutic consideration in overweight patients no longer or not responding to oral agents. Although experience combining exenatide with insulin is sparse, some clinicians report the combination of basal insulin to control fasting glucose with exenatide to be efficacious.

Amylin (Pramlintide)

Amylin is a peptide secreted normally from the pancreas in equimolar amounts with insulin after a meal. It is thought to regulate gastric motility and the release of carbohydrates into the absorptive surfaces of the gut. Pramlintide is an amylin mimetic injected subcutaneously with meals, initially approved to be given with insulin in type 1 diabetic patients. The effect is usually modest to negligible, but anecdotal experience indicates that an occasional brittle diabetic patient may experience dramatic improvement. Pramlintide is now also used in type 2 patients with or without insulin because of its mild effect in limiting food intake and causing weight loss. Pramlintide is therefore used as a tertiary agent when other, more widely used drugs are not fully efficacious.

Developing Therapies

New extended-release incretin agonists will be available soon in addition to other DPP inhibitors. Novel concepts in therapy include the dopamine agonist bromocriptine, shown to reduce FFA levels and improve glucose metabolism. The FDA has recently approved a new formulation of bromocriptine for antidiabetic therapy. Another novel class, the sodium glucose-linked transporter protein (SGLT) inhibitors, interfere with renal reabsorption of filtered glucose in the kidney. The prototype SGLT inhibitor is dapagliflozin, and investigational studies show favorably improved glucose control with modest weight loss.

Insulins

Key Points

- Thresholds for beginning supplemental insulin in type 2 diabetic patients vary depending on whether microangiopathic complications are likely to develop if glucose is not controlled over the patient's lifetime; the better the prognosis, the lower the threshold.
- For elderly patients, keeping fasting serum glucose (FSG) less than 150 mg/dL or HbA_{1c} less than 8% will attenuate the risk of dehydration and metabolic decompensation in the face of stress.
- Appropriate and frequent insulin is the essential therapy of type 1 diabetes and should be used more often in type 2 diabetes if the patient fails to achieve the glycemic goal.

The discovery of insulin by the Toronto group in 1921 has saved the lives of millions of type 1 diabetic patients who would have succumbed to diabetic ketoacidosis. The remarkable efficacy of insulin despite its nonphysiologic route of administration has stimulated the development of insulins with pharmacokinetic effects mimicking the beta-cell secretion pattern, from short-acting and long-acting beef, pork, and fish extracts, to genetically synthesized human insulins introduced in the 1980s, to biochemically designed insulins with more predictable onset and duration of action (Table 34-4).

Initiating Insulin for Type 2 Diabetes

The classic setting for the use of insulin is in a newly diagnosed type 1 diabetic patient. However, insulin is more frequently used in the treatment of type 2 diabetes to compensate for the secretory defect that often progresses to a profound loss of insulin secretory reserve. This is suggested when FSG or HbA$_{1c}$ continue to rise despite the patient's best behavioral efforts and multiple oral drugs. A patient with type 2 diabetes can also present late in its course with marked hyperglycemia and even ketosis. In these patients, insulin treatment protocols used in type 1 diabetes are appropriate until the type 2 pattern of glucose homeostasis is recognized. In most patients, convenience insulins such as human or synthetic 70/30 or 75/25 combinations can be used for several days until the effects of behavioral measures and oral agents "kick in." Dosage is usually from 0.2 to 0.5 units (U)/kg body weight/day (in elderly patients, consider 0.1 U/kg/day). The initial dosage selected is a probe of insulin sensitivity and responsiveness, which will be informative in advising further adjustments in therapy. The dosage can be given before meals to offset postprandial hyperglycemia and at bedtime to control inappropriate overnight hepatic glucose production.

The oral drugs frequently used with insulin are the insulin-stimulating agents and metformin. With multiple therapies, the duration and peak actions of long-acting insulin preparations must be considered to avoid an overlapping effect and precipitous decline in glucose. This phenomenon may occur if multiple doses of insulin are necessary. Once FSG falls below 200 mg/dL, insulin therapy should be decremented to determine if oral drugs are effective and beta-cell functioning is recovering; continued indefinite insulin therapy may be indicated. In this case, basal bolus insulin regimens as described later may be required as ineffective oral drugs are discontinued.

KEY TREATMENT

Early initiation of insulin therapy in type 2 diabetes is indicated when behavioral therapy and combined oral agents are not achieving near-normalization of HbA$_{1c}$ and FSG levels (ADA, 2009; Mayfield and White, 2004; UKPDS, 1998) (SOR: A).

Table 34-4 Common Insulin Preparations

Category/Preparation	Onset; Duration	Common Schedule	Advantage; Disadvantage
Short-Acting human insulin			
Human insulin (rDNA) (Humulin R, Novolin R)	1-2 hr; 6-8 hr; dose dependent	At mealtime	Less expensive Late action can cause nocturnal hypoglycemia.
Rapid-Acting synthetic insulins			
Insulin lispro (Humalog) Insulin aspart (rDNA) (Novolog) Insulin glulisine (rDNA) (Apidra)	½ hr; 2-4 hr; dose dependent	At mealtime, before or after meal, with 24-hr basal preparation coverage	Controls 2-hr postprandial glucose Cost
Intermediate-Acting human insulin			
Isophane human insulin (Humulin N, Novolin N)	2-3 hr; 10-14 hr; dose dependent	Overnight to limit hepatic glucose production or 12-hr basal action	Less expensive Hypoglycemic risk, especially nocturnal
Combination insulins			
Isophane human insulin (70/30 Humulin [N/R], Novolin 70/30)	1-2 hr; 10-14 hr	At breakfast and dinner	Convenience Nighttime hypoglycemia
70/30 Insulin aspart protamine, insulin aspart (NovoLog Mix 70/30)	½ hr; 8-10 hr	At breakfast and dinner	Convenience Nighttime hypoglycemia
75/25 Insulin lispro protamine, insulin lispro (Humalog Mix 75/25)	½ hr; 8-10 hr	At breakfast and dinner	Convenience Nighttime hypoglycemia
Long-Acting synthetic insulins			
Insulin glargine (Lantus)	2-3 hr; 24 hr	Basal coverage overnight or 24 hr	Less nocturnal hypoglycemic risk, convenience; cost
Insulin detemir (Levemir)	2-3 hr; 24 hr		

Subacute Presentation of Type 1 Diabetes

The management of type 1 diabetes will depend on the patient's age and the acuity of the diabetes at presentation. Since there is usually no family history of diabetes, or diabetic experience at home, and given the fragility of the new-onset diabetic state, many children or adolescents presenting with type 1 diabetes require hospitalization to initiate and teach glucose monitoring techniques and to begin insulin treatment. The indication for hospitalizing a newly diagnosed child who is not drifting into ketosis depends on the availability of outpatient educational resources and the clinical judgment that the patient can be closely monitored and the family appropriately advised while developing the capabilities of diabetic self-management.

Basal Bolus Insulin

Synthetic insulin preparations designed to achieve either a prolonged steady effect or an acute action, mimicking physiologic insulin secretion, have allowed patients to develop personal and flexible injection schedules. This is known as the basal bolus regimen and is indicated in the treatment of type 1 diabetes. It provides rapidly acting or bolus insulin to cover carbohydrate ingestion in meals and snacks, and basal insulins are usually given at bedtime to achieve a steady state at breakfast, with an ideal FSG target of 120 mg/dL or less. To a large extent, control of the important fasting blood (serum) glucose will depend on attaining an ideal bedtime value of 120 to 140 mg/dL, which is based on rapidly active insulin given at dinner. The authors' experience indicates that basal insulin is most predictable in patients who demonstrate overnight glucose production and have controlled glucose values at bedtime. However, an occasional patient will experience hypoglycemia at 4 AM, and therefore nighttime monitoring is necessary when increasing dosage. Hypoglycemia can also be seen before lunch with overnight basal insulinization.

The starting dosage of insulin as previously discussed is often a conservative approximation. In general, a type 1 diabetic patient requires approximately 0.5 U/kg, half of which is given as basal insulin and the other half in divided boluses before a meal. Experience and clinical judgment may suggest a lower starting dosage if the diabetes is mild, especially with children and elderly patients, who may receive a starting dose of 0.1 or 0.2 U/kg/day. However, hyperglycemia may have resulted in secondary insulin resistance caused by cellular dysfunction, and higher dosages may quickly become necessary. If the patient is not at risk of ketoacidosis, cautiously increasing the dosage from 0.5 U/kg/day is prudent (usually by 10% per day).

The effectiveness of a specific dose of most insulin preparations depends on local factors at the injection site related to capillary perfusion. Insulin uptake is enhanced when hydration is adequate and a patient is vasodilated after exercise or a warm shower (or has a fever). The effectiveness of short-acting preparation is also related to the carbohydrate load about to be consumed. Preprandial hyperglycemia may adversely affect the action of insulin and should be considered as well in deciding proper insulin dosage.

Patients using basal bolus regimens may be taught how to adjust dosage based on the preprandial glucose value, carbohydrate content of anticipated meal, and physical activity. If glucose monitoring indicates prebreakfast dosage is achieving postprandial glucose of 160 mg/dL or less, and subsequent premeal values are 120 mg/dL or less, the short-acting insulin dosage and the long-acting steady-state dosages are in perfect harmony with the patient's diet and lifestyle.

A long-acting insulin analog (e.g., glargine, detemir) can be used to provide the basal insulin, but in a dynamic situation, intermediate-duration insulin preparations such as N (formerly known as NPH) provides more short-term flexibility and "kick" in the first 12 to 24 hours (see Table 34-4). The short-acting insulin preparations available include R (formerly known as Regular), lispro, aspart, and glulisine. The latter three are synthetic insulins and are ideal for limiting postprandial glucose elevations. R insulin does not have a sharply defined absorption and may remain active for 4 to 6 hours. A patient with slow GI absorption may find the slower onset of action of insulin R more efficacious. However, R can have a delayed effect, putting a tightly controlled patient at hypoglycemic risk, especially if N insulins are also used, with their potential for peak action.

As with 70/30 human N/R insulin, lispro and aspart have been formulated as mixtures of 75/25 and 70/30, respectively, with acute and intermediate duration of action. These might be used to introduce insulin in a subacute presentation of type 1 diabetes to avoid deterioration to ketoacidosis, but these are not as safe and lack the fine-tuning potential of basal bolus regimens. Insulin combinations may promote hypoglycemia if insulin needs to be administered at intervals of less than 12 hours. The treatment of type 1 patients during illness or daily living requires insulins that minimize the risk of hypoglycemia and are therefore safe enough for multiple daily injections.

When glucose values of less than 200 mg/dL are achieved at bedtime, the patient is ready to begin long-acting basal insulin analogs to preclude early-morning hypoglycemia, more often seen with intermediate insulin. Basal insulin analogs are given either at a dosage of 80% of the total daily N requirement or at the calculated basal dosage of 0.25 U/kg/day. Clinical judgment and instinct may modify this recommendation because this dosage should be further titrated based on the agreed fasting glucose target level. Usually, daily bedtime insulin increments of 10% or 2 to 4 U are safe.

Estimating the correct insulin schedule provides goals for the patient. Unless the family physician is proficient and available, nutritionists who are certified diabetic educators should instruct patients on carbohydrate content of meals and insulin dosing. Motivated patients given proper diabetic education will eventually determine their ideal, safe insulin/carbohydrate ratios and corrections for other factors such as activity. Only patients capable of this self-management can successfully use the insulin pump (discussed later).

Supportive Care for Children and Adolescents Requiring Insulin

As subacute diabetes is stabilized, the patient and family require extensive formal diabetic education, support, and empathy to ease the anxieties associated with a new diagnosis of a long-term disorder. A maladjustment in the needed insulin therapy could adversely affect the patient's success in living with diabetes. Instruction in dietary principles includes carbohydrate counting and insulin coverage, correction and adjustment of the insulin dosages based on glucose variability and physical activities, and the standards of care to limit acute and long-term risks of diabetes, as detailed next. Following clinical stabilization, the family physician can further consider the etiology and alternative treatments according to ongoing diabetic manifestations.

Insulin Rebound

A diabetic complication that family physicians routinely manage is caused by nighttime or very-early-morning hypoglycemia, which leads to fasting hyperglycemia and sometimes ketosis, especially in children (Somogyi effect). If the patient and physician are not careful, they can get caught in a spiral of ever-increasing insulin doses in response to rebounding glucose values. When confronting persisting morning hyperglycemia, the first step is for the patient to monitor 3 AM glucose levels. If low, reduced dosage or timing change in evening insulin administration is necessary.

The Difficult Patient

Some patients cannot self-manage insulin therapy because of personality factors, family issues, or other difficulties of daily living, which can promote and exacerbate both type 1 and type 2 diabetes mellitus. Counseling is indicated for these patients, and insulin regimens may need to be simplified to ensure adherence. At the same time, these more fixed regimens indicate an increased need for a constant, regular diet and predictable behavior and activities. Difficulty achieving this means such patients often have marked glucose fluctuation and elevated HbA$_{1c}$ values. Many patients will eventually benefit from their repeated attempts and the physician's efforts, as their therapeutic behavior synergizes with newer therapies.

Insulin Pump Therapy

Motivated type 1 diabetic patients who are frequently monitoring and self-managing insulin dosages but have not attained their glycemic targets should be considered for an insulin pump protocol. Ideally in these patients, the target should be HbA$_{1c}$ less than 7%, with fluctuations in monitored FSG limited to ±50 mg/dL. A key requisite for pump therapy is the patient's willingness to monitor frequently (up to 6-8 times daily) to ensure a safe transition from the flexible insulin regimen and learn to adjust basal and bolus infusion rates.

Use of the insulin pump in type 2 diabetic patients who fail to achieve therapeutic targets is less clear-cut. Often, insulin resistance accounts for failed outcomes rather than beta-cell insufficiency in these patients. If planning to use the pump, patients need to maintain high daily basal rates of 3 to 5 units per hour, which would mean frequent reloading of the insulin reservoir. On a physiologic basis, pump therapy may or may not overcome insulin resistance. Also, subjective factors such as "winning" expectations and renewed motivation are associated with pump use. The resulting behavior changes along with pumping effects can alter the frustrating course of DM.

Using the insulin pump requires more detailed diabetic education, but starting principles are simple. A basal rate is programmed based on 50% of the day's daily insulin requirement. The other 50% is used as reactive therapy to cover meals or make corrections. This can be given as an acute bolus infusion or over 2 to 3 hours. Once patients become proficient in safely covering their ingested carbohydrates and determining their optimal basal rates, they require less professional guidance, and if stable with well-controlled HbA$_{1c}$ levels, they can revisit every 4 to 6 months for periodic organ monitoring and patient reeducation.

The insulin pump is not free of risk. Some patients never master self-monitoring and continue to experience marked swings in blood glucose. Although once thought to result from physiological factors (e.g., unpredictability of diabetic gastroparesis), essentially all patients can develop strategies to overcome such physiologic problems. Most patients have functional problems or some family, school, work, or other environmental issue causing their difficulty adjusting to DM. In these patients and tightly controlled patients, hypoglycemia will remain an ever-present risk until advances in real-time glucose monitoring provide early warning. At a minimum, the family physician should be alerted that issues outside diabetes management need to be addressed.

The other risk is pump failure or *catheter dissociation*, which halts insulin delivery. If the patient was tightly controlled and the insulin effect was countered by high levels of counter-regulatory hormone, a sudden drop in insulin could provoke a rebound in lipolysis leading rapidly to ketogenesis. If the patient is unaware of the pump failure (e.g., because of infrequent monitoring schedule), a rapid deterioration to diabetic ketoacidosis may occur in less than 24 hours. Another complication is localized infection at the injection site of the 3-day indwelling needle. These complications require local therapy but may become severe enough to require incision, drainage, and antibiotics. Family physicians should be able to treat such problems, but consultation is always an option.

Surgery as Therapy

The increasing prevalence of type 2 diabetes coincides with the epidemic of obesity in western and developing societies. As noted earlier, obesity has been an intractable medical problem (see also Chapter 36). One response has been a concomitant increase in gastric bypass surgery. In morbidly obese patients (BMI ≥40), diabetes may go into complete remission after successful surgery. Diversion of nutrients from absorptive surfaces may promote the secretion of antidiabetic factors as efficacious as caloric deprivation in counteracting type 2 diabetes. Less invasive techniques are making surgery an option in the treatment of type 2 diabetes. However, complication rates and calcium metabolism problems require that patients make individualized decisions with their physician about surgical risks and benefits.

Diabetic Ketoacidosis

Key Points

- Presentation in diabetic ketoacidosis always requires hospitalization for fluid resuscitation and insulinization.
- Fluid resuscitation is a critical part of treating DKA. Intravenous solutions replace extravascular and intravascular fluids and electrolyte losses.
- Protracted symptoms suggest hypokalemia and total-body potassium depletion.

- If diagnosis of DKA is made immediately by history, physical examination, or fingertip glucose determination, and confirmed with tests demonstrating metabolic acidosis, specific treatment should not be delayed by pending laboratory results.
- Sodium bicarbonate is safely delivered isotonically as 100 mEq or 100 mL added to 1 L of 0.45% normal saline.
- In a previously known diabetic patient, an episode of ketoacidosis results from the patient's inability to recognize deterioration in glucose control and react promptly with insulin.
- When transitioning to subcutaneous insulin from continuous infusion, basal SC insulin dose should precede cessation of insulin infusion by 4 to 6 hours to prevent recurrent ketosis.

In only a few emergencies in medicine has an understanding of the pathophysiology reduced mortality from 100% to less than 1% in less than 50 years. One example is the discovery and rapid clinical deployment of insulin in 1921 as the major intervention shutting down the diabetic ketogenic state and preventing profound acidosis with cerebral dehydration and edema. With the introduction of low-dose insulin infusion protocols in the early 1970s, the residual mortality of 6% to 8% associated with potassium and water shifts common with overaggressive insulin treatment was reduced to 1%. Cerebral edema and hypokalemic deaths from ketoacidosis in adults are now rare.

Pathogenesis and Presentation

Diabetic ketoacidosis (DKA) results when an absolute or relative lack of insulin allows hyperglycemia to become dehydrating and lipolysis to become ketosis. This progression occurs over several days in patients who are usually unaware of their DM diagnosis. As dehydration becomes more severe, the brain begins to experience an increase in osmolality. Altered mental status begins with lethargy and coincident metabolic acidosis. The patient may become dependent on others to secure medical care; if care is further delayed, lethargy becomes stupor and eventually coma. The pH falls to 7.00 or lower. The crisis has been defined.

Occasionally, acidosis rather than dehydration is the chief presenting system. Such patients are usually known diabetics who are alert, but with dyspnea stimulated by their acidosis. This could occur when a tightly controlled patient fails to take several scheduled insulin doses or after insulin pump failure or the stimulatory phase of overconsumption of alcohol. These circumstances result in a marked outpouring of counterregulatory hormones with their lipolytic and gluconeogenic actions.

Fasting serum (blood) glucose in DKA is usually greater than 450 mg/dL, but this is a function of dehydration, which will further elevate FSG. Awareness of the onset of acidosis might prompt the patient with lower glucose values to seek medical attention. If the development of acidosis is slow, the patient may not be seen until glucose approaches 1000 mg/dL. The severity of the symptomatology is also related to the patient's prior experience with DKA. Repeat offenders are patients who have problems with self-management, typically because of functional issues such as depression, alcohol, or other drug problems, rather than a physiologic disorder. These patients may have pH of less than 7.00 relatively asymptomatically. A patient who is aware of the diagnosis should be prepared to intervene quickly to block the descent to DKA and know when to seek professional help.

After the introduction of home glucose monitoring in the 1980s and the emphasis on self-management in the 1990s, DKA has become very uncommon among responsible patients. The occurrence of DKA in a patient known to be responsible indicates some failure in insulin administration or an occult or apparent stress, such as urinary tract infection, acute gastroenteritis, pneumonia, other viremia, or worse, a bacteremia.

The classic presentation of DKA is a child or adolescent who has become increasingly weaker over 3 to 5 days with dyspnea and lethargy. Vomiting and abdominal pain can result from gastric distention caused by marked hyperglycemia. Profound acidosis can cause Kussmaul's respirations, with retractions and lifting of the clavicle, to expand the chest fully for maximal hyperventilation and elimination of carbon dioxide (CO_2). Rarely, the odor of acetone may be perceived. The pulse rate may be rapid, with low blood pressure indicative of hypovolemia. Elevation of the temperature is not unusual, caused by a precipitating infection or the mechanical work of heavy breathing, because dehydration prevents normal sweating and cooling.

Laboratory Findings

The family physician should expect the hematocrit and hemoglobin to be elevated in these patients as a result of hemoconcentration. A low value with dehydration indicates a source of blood loss, such as a stress ulcer in the stomach. A white blood cell (WBC) count as high as 20,000 cells/mm^3 without other evidence of infection is not unusual but should trigger a thorough evaluation, especially of the chest, where the signs of pneumonia may be confounded by the dehydration. A reduction in oxygen partial pressure (Po_2) with marked hyperventilation is an ominous sign of lung compromise. Antibiotic coverage after appropriate cultures is indicated until the clinical situation is better defined.

The diagnostic hyperglycemia associated with reduced bicarbonate (HCO_3^-, usually designated "CO_2" on a basic metabolic profile [BMP]) is accompanied by hyperkalemia in approximately 30% of patients, normokalemia in 50%, and hypokalemia in 15% to 20%. To some extent, serum potassium depends on the severity of the acidosis and duration of the polyuria or vomiting. Hypokalemia is the most dangerous clinical scenario because insulin treatment can cause a precipitous decline in potassium, which may weaken the hyperventilatory effort, causing more profound acidosis and cardiopulmonary arrest. The finding of hypokalemia (and probably even normokalemia) on BMP or electrocardiogram (ECG) with good urine output indicates immediate potassium replacement. In general, hypokalemia on the initial BMP indicates a potassium deficit greater than 400 mEq. Hyperkalemia at the onset of DKA indicates a loss of about 200 mEq of potassium before presentation.

Serum sodium and chloride may also be affected by the extent of water depletion or urine losses caused by the osmotic diuresis or sodium bound to the ketonic anions. Thus, serum sodium of 145 mEq/L would indicate a predominant water deficiency, whereas 129 mEq/L suggests more significant sodium losses. In either case, water is always deficient despite dilutional changes in serum sodium caused by hyperglycemia, and patients require water and salt repletion therapies. Importantly, the anion gap indicates the severity of the acidosis. Values in the high 30s suggest tissue hypoxia and possible lactate production in addition to the ketonic anions. This could be a dangerous sign if no improvement is noted after fluid resuscitation and insulinization. Lactic acidosis accompanying DKA is rare unless there is an underlying serious diagnosis such as sepsis or a myocardial infarction. However, a patient who is near death before presenting may have perfusion failure initiating lactate production.

Other abnormalities in DKA include prerenal azotemia, although the serum creatinine can be elevated artifactually by ketones in the blood. If so, creatinine promptly normalizes as ketones are cleared with treatment. Phosphate may shift the same as potassium in metabolic acidosis. Total-body phosphate is depleted, but repletion is usually deferred to the subacute phase of treatment, unless extreme weakness does not improve and extremely low serum phosphates are found. If drawn, amylase may be elevated without specific signs of pancreatitis.

Initial Treatment

Insulin and Potassium

Management of DKA involves administration of insulin, water, and electrolytes safely to prevent marked fluid shifts into the brain and a precipitous drop in potassium, which would impair compensatory hyperventilation. Insulinization promptly blocks further liposis and shuts down ketogenesis. R insulin is given as an intravenous (IV) bolus of 0.1 U/kg with the start of saline administration. Some suggest the initial bolus should be as much as 20 U. The bolus infusion is followed by a continuous infusion of 0.1 U/kg/hr, with hourly adjustments based on decline in serum glucose and reversal of acidosis. Low-dose insulin infusions are safe if the potassium value is monitored, and improving metabolic parameters should be apparent in 1 or 2 hours. Some patients may be remarkably resistant, and a significant bolus adjustment of up to 20 units may be necessary in 1 hour, with modification of the infusion concentration. The objective is not to decrease glucose precipitously but to turn off ketosis. Rapid glucose reductions with more aggressive insulinization protocols have resulted in fluid shifts, especially in children, which may account for the most serious complication, cerebral edema.

The serum potassium value on presentation can be estimated by reviewing the ECG. Peaking of the T wave with P-wave flattening or worse, QRS widening, means that the full protocol should be instituted at once with continued ECG monitoring to prevent a hyperkalemic cardiac crisis. If there is no evidence of hyperkalemia, and certainly if there is flattening of the T wave with a U wave, indicating the opposite risk of hypokalemia, then potassium chloride or phosphate should be given as long as urine flow is apparent. This situation requires caution with fluid and insulin administration to avert a drop in potassium caused by a rapid intracellular glucose shift. Cardiac monitoring should be continued and renal function ascertained immediately by BMP or urine flow to assess the amount and speed of potassium replacement.

Water and Salt

Intravenous fluids are initiated to maintain and restore capillary perfusion. The first 1 to 2 L should be normal saline (NS), which is the best crystalloid volume expander. The rate of infusion depends on the patient's age and size. An otherwise healthy adolescent or young adult can tolerate 1 L/hr for 2 hours, but this will require clinical evaluation and judgment based on severity of presentation and patient response. A prompt urinary response to the first liter of NS ensures the safety of replacing potassium from the onset. Simply administering water and electrolytes will not turn off DKA but will help reverse the hyperosmolar state.

Crisis and Sodium Bicarbonate

Insulinization with saline infusion for 2 hours is usually sufficient to halt ketosis and gluconeogenesis and begin reversing metabolic acidosis. Rarely, life-threatening acidosis exists with pH below 6.90. Blood pressure and cardiac output may be compromised. The anion gap may be approaching 40 mEq/dL, suggesting a coexisting component of lactic acidosis. These are the extreme conditions that justify consideration of sodium bicarbonate ($NaHCO_3$) infusion. The concern involves the serum potassium, which could shift intracellularly with a rapid rise in pH. If present, hyperkalemia would be an overall benefit, but if the ECG is indeterminate or hypokalemia already exists, a further decline in serum potassium would be disastrous. Thus, administration of sodium bicarbonate should be done slowly with caution. Bolus therapy with 100 mEq $NaHCO_3$ can also cause a transient hyperosmolality. with a potentially deleterious water shift in the brain. Sodium bicarbonate is more safely delivered isotonically as 100 mEq or 100 mL added to 1 L of 0.45% NS. The addition of the sodium would make this almost an isotonic solution, and delivery of bicarbonate ions in the large volume would preclude any sudden pH shifts.

Further Treatment of the Acutely Ill Patient

After the first 2 L of NS, the patient is transitioned to 0.45% saline, delivered at 250 to 500 mL/hr with a continuous insulin infusion. FSG will usually begin to approach 200 mg/dL in about 4 hours, depending on the initial value. A safe rate of decline in glucose is approximately 150 ±50 mg/dL/hr. This may require hourly adjustments in the insulin infusion rates or repeated low-dose insulin boluses for refractoriness. Once the glucose level is approximately 200 mg/dL, the insulin infusion may need to be adjusted to 0.05 U/kg/hr and 5% dextrose with 0.45% saline administered. Insulin will promote glucose oxidation, generating CO_2, which becomes plasma bicarbonate and further normalizes the pH. In some cases, as the anion gap is close to normal, a hyperchloremic acidosis occurs with decreased CO_2. This should be of no concern because chloride given in saline replaced the ketonic anions before enough bicarbonate could be regenerated. Hyperchloremia will spontaneously improve as the patient advances to oral fluids.

Transitioning

When clinically appropriate, usually at 6 to 12 hours, the patient should be offered oral fluids to determine GI function. When the diet is advanced to solid food, the patient should be started on subcutaneous (SC) insulin, basal and reactive therapy, while still maintaining the insulin infusion. A common error at this phase is discontinuation of the insulin infusion before SC insulin achieves an adequate steady state to prevent recurrent ketosis. This takes 4 to 6 hours if the correct basal insulin dosage is given. Rebound hyperglycemia and ketosis are more likely with uncontrolled underlying infection.

Once oral fluid intake is adequate, the patient should be appropriately educated about self-management of insulin before being discharged. Even if previously trained to do this, the patient should receive a refresher on this important skill. Appropriate professional guidance can prevent progression of ketosis if obtained before the symptomatology becomes too profound. If patients are educated to avail themselves of this help in a timely manner, they will never again have to endure this potentially life-threatening emergency.

Nonketotic Hyperosmolality Syndrome

See the discussion online at www.expertconsult.com.

Diabetes and Pregnancy

Key Points

- Outcome of diabetic pregnancy depends on the mother's glucose levels, duration of DM before pregnancy, diabetic complications (nephropathy, retinopathy, vascular disease), and age at conception.
- Because of the increasing prevalence of DM, all pregnant women, except those in low-risk groups, should be screened for diabetes.
- Screening for gestational diabetes is performed at 24 to 28 weeks' gestation with 50-g oral glucose load and blood glucose measured 1 hour later (abnormal: >130 mg/dL).
- Diagnosis of GDM is confirmed by an oral glucose tolerance test. Glucose values are determined fasting and at 1, 2, and 3 hours (normal: <95, <180, <155, and <140 mg/dL, respectively; two higher values make diagnosis).
- The patient with GDM is advised of lifetime risk of diabetes and preventive effects of diet and exercise.

Diabetic pregnancies include gestational diabetes mellitus, which is the development of hyperglycemia during pregnancy, and pregnancy in women with prior history of type 1 or type 2 diabetes.

Gestational Diabetes Mellitus

In about 50% of women, GDM is reversible after pregnancy and does not inevitably evolve to type 2 diabetes. Asymptomatic type 1 or 2 diabetes or LADA existing before pregnancy may become clinical and irreversible. Women with no prior evidence of diabetes may demonstrate their type 2 diabetic gene during pregnancy and either remain diabetic postpartum or experience a long, normal latent period before the gene is expressed again. The expected conversion rate of women with GDM to type 2 diabetes after pregnancy can be reduced with therapeutic lifestyle changes.

Screening

Screening for GDM also identifies the woman at risk of having a macrosomic baby, the result of excessive glucose crossing the placenta. Non–low-risk pregnant women are routinely screened, usually before the mid–second trimester, with a 50-g glucose challenge test given under random conditions—not necessarily fasting. The "low-risk group" is defined as nonminority women younger than 25 years old with no suggestion of insulin resistance, that is, no prior history of glucose intolerance, obesity, hypertension, or family history of DM. A glucose value of 140 mg/dL after ingestion is positive and leads to a formal glucose tolerance test (GTT).

To prepare for GTT, the patient is asked to increase carbohydrate intake to about 300 g for 3 days. Although this is a diabetogenic stimulus, restricting carbohydrates can also downregulate the beta-cell response and result in a false-positive study. The fasting patient drinks 100 g of a glucose solution. Glucose values are determined fasting and at 1, 2, and 3 hours. Normal values are less than 95, 180, 155, and 140 mg/dL, respectively; two higher values make the diagnosis of GDM. However, GTT does not consider the woman's preconception weight. Small women, whose total daily carbohydrate intake may never exceed 250 g, may demonstrate positive results despite their fasting and postprandial glucose values during pregnancy (or later on their regular diet) remaining within normal range. The standard GTT using 75 g has now been standardized for pregnancy but is subject to the same criticism as the 100-g test.

Treatment

Many women who are diagnosed with GDM can be maintained within fasting and postprandial glycemic goals with dietary adjustments and exercise. When glycemic goals are not achieved with behavioral therapies, insulin has traditionally been given in increasing dosages. Although high concentrations of insulin overcome the characteristic insulin resistance of the second half of pregnancy, the result is often marked weight gain. This has been a dilemma. Also, human and lispro insulin are the only antidiabetic agents approved for treatment in pregnancy. Although there are no reports of risk to the fetus from any short- or long-acting synthetic insulin preparations, many experts have been reluctant to use long-acting synthetic basal insulin preparations, which mimic basal insulin secretion and limit weight gain, until more outcome data are available. Thus the role of oral agents in pregnancy has been reconsidered.

Comparable to insulin, *glyburide* is effective in treating GDM and increasingly used because of tight plasma protein binding with minimal transplacental transfer, although some glyburide crosses into the fetus. Theoretically, this might result in islet cell hyperplasia in the fetus, causing hypoglycemia in utero or in the neonatal period. *Metformin* is also known to cross the placenta, but metformin limits insulin secretion. Metformin and insulin treatment for GDM show comparable favorable outcomes. The long-term safety of glyburide and metformin has not been ascertained despite over 10 years of experience, and women should be counseled before receiving these oral agents.

Glitazones might be effective in overcoming the insulin resistance of pregnancy but are contraindicated. Their mechanism of action as transcription factors is a theoretic risk for teratogenesis.

Postpartum Gestational Diabetes

Some authorities recommend GTT at 3 months postpartum to detect evidence of persisting DM if fasting values have normalized. This nonpregnant GTT merely measures the 2-hour value after a 75-g glucose challenge. Values of 200 mg/dL or greater confirm type 2 diabetes; values of 160 to 200 mg/dL and higher indicate impaired tolerance consistent with insulin resistance.

Finding normal glucose values at 3 months does not preclude the onset of type 2 diabetes later, when further changes in body composition occur with aging. Thus a woman with a history of GDM should periodically self-monitor fasting and postprandial values to assess her inherent diabetic risk and demonstrate her motivation to suppress it indefinitely.

Type 1 Diabetic Pregnancy

> **Key Point**
>
> - Newborns of diabetic mothers always require intensive monitoring for hypoglycemia, even following ideal pregnancies.

In anticipation of pregnancy in a type 1 diabetic patient, insulin dosage schedules may need to be modified to flexible, intensive regimens. As mentioned, controversy surrounds continuing effective basal bolus regimens with synthetic insulins during pregnancy. If an insulin pump is being used, adjustments need to be made frequently to attain target HbA_{1c} values of less than 7%. The risk of diabetic embryopathy resulting in congenital anomalies has been directly related to the HbA_{1c} value in the first trimester. Unless the family physician has a particular interest and experience, maternal fetal medicine physicians and endocrinologist should provide counseling and insulinization schedules for type 1 diabetic women preparing for pregnancy.

Type 2 Diabetic Pregnancy

With type 2 diabetes being diagnosed at a younger age, more women will be diabetic and untreated at conception. However, they still require counseling on the risk of embryopathy, dietary considerations, and effects of their oral drugs in the first trimester and later. Some nutritionists argue that limiting calories rather than supplementing in patients with marked obesity will reduce the risk of exacerbating diabetes during pregnancy. Insulin treatment might still become necessary to maintain blood glucose within the acceptable postprandial range.

Hospital Care of Diabetic Patients

Achieving diabetic control under normal ambulatory conditions is difficult enough in most patients. When illness prevents a patient from utilizing diabetic survival skills, however, and the stress of illness overcomes the patient's available insulin, care of the patient becomes a professional challenge. In the past, lack of data often resulted in less-than-optimal diabetic care in favor of managing the primary illness. Recent observations, however, demonstrate the efficacy of glycemic control in critically ill surgical patients. As a result, intensive glucose management protocols with continuous insulin infusion are now being widely applied. Good glucose control in known diabetic patients and those with marked hyperglycemia and critical illness shortens intensive care unit (ICU) and respirator time and reduces associated polymyopathy while generally improving all outcome parameters. Many post–cardiothoracic surgery units have adopted these protocols to improve myocardial "energetics," limit infection, and discharge the patient sooner.

Similar studies of glycemic control have not been definitive in critically ill patients with sepsis to GI bleeding, although these varying diagnoses may have created methodologic issues. Thus, professional societies are recommending that critically ill patients be maintained with glucose levels less than 140 mg/dL (ADA, 2009). These therapeutic goals seem reasonable, until therapeutic methodology improves to limit hypoglycemia, which adversely affects outcomes associated with intensive insulin treatment protocols.

Preoperative Clearance and Treatment

In all types of procedures, the appropriate preparations begin weeks before surgery, when the family physician clears the patient for surgery. The physician ensures not only that the diabetes is under good control, but also that the patient has no asymptomatic cardiac or renal disease. Immediately before surgery, oral drugs as well as short-acting and intermediate-acting insulin are discontinued in favor of basal insulin coverage along with glucose to provide energy (75-100 mL/hr of dextrose 5%) and potassium (usually 10-20 mEq/L), assuming normal renal function and preoperative testing. If the glucose swings out of control (>200 mg/dL) perioperatively, IV insulin infused at a few units per hour will be more effective than the SC sliding-scale schedule, which can lead to erratic results. Although the ideal, IV insulin requires frequent monitoring by anesthesia and nursing. Alternatively, if this degree of monitoring is not available, no insulin is given or a conservative SC bolus provided, and appropriate adjustments are made immediately postoperatively.

Postoperative Care

Intensive insulinization should be maintained in the postoperative ICU, especially in patients with increased risk of ketoacidosis. Problems can occur when ICU patients transfer to step-down units, where tight control to achieve 120 to 180 mg/dL values depends on SC insulin delivery, which is inherently more unstable. The principles of adequate basal coverage and reactive bolus insulin apply, although frequent adjustments remain necessary because of altered insulin pharmacokinetics associated with bed rest and decreased peripheral perfusion. Sick or postoperative patients also have dietary instability from tests, missed meals, and insulin therapy. Basal and bolus dosages must be flexible and reconsidered daily. Bolus dosages may need to be given immediately after a meal, when the nurse is certain the patient has eaten.

No definite rules can be made, but several generalizations may apply. Basal insulinization can be provided once in 24 hours or 2 or 3 doses of intermediate insulin. Glargine and detemir dosages provide good control 12 hours later, but intermediate insulin dosages could overlap, causing hypoglycemic risk. Shorter-acting synthetic insulins are more safely used in the evening.

Appropriate Antidiabetic Protocols

The family physician must determine if it is appropriate to continue the outpatient treatment schedule in the hospitalized diabetic patient, depending mainly on the reason for hospitalization. If the patient can eat, the regular outpatient treatment (oral agents and/or insulin) should be continued with appropriate adjustments. Supplementing this with basal/bolus insulin may be appropriate if significant hyperglycemia (>200 mg/dL) occurs associated with the stress of illness and hospitalization. The outpatient regimen should not be discontinued in favor of a fixed sliding-scale insulin schedule, which will take days to titrate to the patient's needs and may result in erratic hyper- and hypoglycemic intervals. If the patient cannot be fed and glucose values are drifting above the 150– to 180–mg/dL range because of stress-mediated gluconeogenesis, treatment to prevent further hyperglycemia is appropriate.

Basal insulin can be given to fasting patients at starting dosages of 0.25 U/kg/day and further adjusted as the glycemic pattern becomes apparent. Periodic corrections in bolus insulin dosage may be necessary until titrated to levels achieving glucose values in the mid-100–mg/dL range. Once a safe basal dosage is determined, it should not be withheld if the patient is to be kept fasting for a procedure. Basal insulin will somewhat block hyperglycemic surges after catecholamine release in response to procedure stress. Patients with any remaining risk of hypoglycemia are given dextrose 5% at 75 to 100 mL/hr with continued basal insulin, which also blocks lipolysis from fasting, promoting gluconeogenesis and peripheral insulin resistance. After illness, diabetic patients not previously treated with insulin may require weeks before they can be titrated to their prior oral agents. This partly depends on regaining their lean body mass and state of fitness, which improves sensitivity to their endogenous insulin reserve. In some patients, insulin dependency becomes necessary indefinitely.

KEY TREATMENT

Diabetic care is best individualized for children, pregnant women, elderly patients, and hospitalized and seriously ill patients (ADA, 2009).

Children with type 1 diabetes are prone to hypoglycemia, which can cause apprehensive stress and result in maladjustment to diabetic treatment. Clinicians need to consider options as diverse as intensive insulin pump therapy to deferring tight glycemic goals until the child attains the maturity to participate in care (SOR: C).

In women with preconception diabetes, to lessen the risk of diabetic embryopathy, glycemic goals are to tighten HbA_{1c} within 1% of normal. Planning pregnancy appropriately motivates patients, and the goal can be attained with frequent glucose monitoring (Goldman et al., 1986; Kitzmiller et al., 1991) (SOR: B).

In patients older than 65, glycemic control has not been shown to reduce the risk of micro- and macroangiopathy. Clinical judgment suggests that geriatric patients with short-term life expectancy (<10 years) should be treated to a relaxed HbA_{1c} range of about 7.5% to 8.5%, which provides some reserve in preventing acute hyperglycemia and delaying dehydration associated with acute illness, while limiting the risk of hypoglycemia (Brown et al., 2003) (SOR: B).

In critically ill surgical patients, glucose level generally should be kept below 140 mg/dL to ensure better outcomes (Furnary et al., 2003; van den Berghe, 2001) (SOR: A).

Diabetic Complications

Key Points

- Normalization of glucose control as far as can be accomplished safely has become the objective of all diabetic therapy.
- Physical therapies should promote blood flow into the foot and nerve function and stimulate the patient's psyche.
- Examination of the retina is critical to determine changes requiring immediate attention.
- Angiotensin-converting enzyme (ACE) inhibitors and angiotensin receptor blockers (ARBs) are effective in reducing and reversing microalbuminuria and slowing the onset of diabetic nephropathy, independent of blood pressure (BP) control.
- Systolic BP should be less than 130 and diastolic less than 80 mm Hg, with HbA_{1c} as close to normal as possible considering the risk of hypoglycemia.
- Coronary heart disease is so problematic among diabetic patients that the National Cholesterol Education Panel (NCEP), in recommending guidelines for the treatment of hypercholesterolemia, considers DM equal to prior evidence of coronary artery disease.
- The more risk factors and signs of diabetes (dyslipidemia, microalbuminuria, erectile dysfunction), the more aggressively the patient should be monitored for occult heart disease.

The "Triopathy"

Before the landmark DCCT results in 1993, no definitive evidence showed that better control of type 1 diabetes slowed the progression of the common somatic complications of DM: neuropathy, retinopathy, and nephropathy. The DCCT showed that in 7 years, the average difference in HbA_{1c} between the conventionally treated diabetic patients and the intensive study cohort of 9.0% versus 7.0%, respectively, resulted in reductions of over 50% for each microangiopathic component of the "triopathy." In fact, the investigators discontinued their trial 2 years early to report these remarkable benefits. The UKPDS confirmed the preventive effects of intensive control on reducing diabetic microangiopathic complications in 1998 in patients with type 2 diabetes treated for as long as 15 years. Trials repeatedly reaffirmed that control of hyperglycemia can limit progression of the triopathy in both type 1 and type 2 diabetic patients.

How hyperglycemia causes microangiopathy is complex and not fully understood. Hyperglycemia is known to be associated with increased thickness of capillary basement membranes, and glycosylation is better defined because diabetic blood contains high levels of HbA_{1c}. Advanced glycosylated end products are present in diabetic tissues, and collagen in diabetic patients becomes glycosylated. This accounts for the thickened skin sometimes observed in fingers and hands of diabetic patients and the fibrosis of hand tendons causing Dupuytren's contractures. Albumin and circulating lipoproteins are also altered by hyperglycemia.

Paradoxically, the thickened capillary basement membranes of diabetic patients are known to be "leaky," which may explain capillary rupture or leakage in the retina initiating the beginning of diabetic retinopathy. The onset of nephropathy may be a similar leakage of plasma proteins and albumin into the glomerulus. Capillary thickening leads to closure of the blood vessel supplying the nerves in diabetic neuropathy. The pathoetiology of each of these common complications is complex; in short, hyperglycemia results in damage to the infrastructure of organ systems by altering the protein matrix and its function and by other mechanisms adversely affecting cellular function.

Diabetic Neuropathy

All components of the peripheral nervous system are susceptible, but nerves in the feet are often the first structures to signal the impact of DM. Typically, onset of symptoms occurs in the evening or at night, suggesting nerve dysfunction because capillary peripheral perfusion diminishes with reclining or sleeping. Paresthesias are perceived as numbness, burning, or "pins and needles" in the toes or the bottom of the foot. Massaging the foot, pushing against a bed board, or walking may help as the microcirculation improves. Remarkably, some patients demonstrate these classic symptoms of diabetic neuropathy even before hyperglycemia occurs in the blood.

Polymotor-Sensory Neuropathy

In the early phase of diabetic neuropathy, physical examination may be uninformative. Assessing the adequacy of perfusion is critical and easily accomplished by inspecting the toenails for capillary perfusion and palpating the tibialis posterior and dorsalis pedis arteries. As noted, a dry, cool foot with thickened or thin subcutaneous tissue and nonelastic skin is demonstrating microangiopathy, despite a palpable dorsalis pedis, indicating a likely positive result in decreased deep tendon reflexes at the ankle, vibratory sensation, position sense, hot-cold discrimination, or fine touch with monofilament test. Inability to perceive the monofilament indicates advanced neuropathy that would endanger the foot if injured. Peripheral neuropathic symptoms may also result from hyperglycemia-mediated nerve injury with no clinical evidence of loss of capillary density. Over time, paresthesias and burning pains usually improve, unless functional factors (endogenous or related to narcotic therapy) prolong or confound the symptomatology.

Loss of the ankle reflex with sensory abnormalities indicates that the classic diabetic polyneuropathy is fully defined, with probable coexisting microangiopathy in the foot. Preventive foot care needs to be practiced to prevent skin breakdown. Patients should never walk barefooted because sharp objects penetrating the diabetic foot are often not perceived, leading to foot-threatening infections. The patient may require professional advice on footwear, orthotic devices, and toenail care. For symptomatic relief of nocturnal paresthesias, including "charley horses," increasing doses of gabapentin or amitriptyline, with acetaminophen, or low-dose nonsteroidal anti-inflammatory drugs (NSAIDs) often provide some relief. The nutritional supplement αα-lipoic acid also can reduce neuropathic pain. New drugs such as duloxetine and pregabalin are approved for specific treatment of *diabetic neuritis*. Patients with these dyskinesias may require benzodiazepines or oxycodone,

although the use of drugs associated with dependency can lead to more difficulties.

KEY TREATMENT

Because the high-risk diabetic foot demonstrates deformities, loss of monofilament sensation, vascular impairment, and prior ulcer or amputations, foot care may require podiatric, orthopedic, and vascular consultation, in addition to optimal glycemic control, to attenuate the progression of diabetic neuropathy (Umpierrez et al., 2002) (SOR: A).

Mononeuropathies

An individual nerve may be affected, such as the peroneal, resulting in footdrop, the seventh cranial nerve causing Bell's palsy, or the extraocular nerves causing strabismus and diplopias. Similar to other causes of Bell's palsy, the pathogenesis of these large-nerve injuries is thought to result from vascular injury; the paralysis is usually self-limiting and spontaneously improves over several months. In general, all these neuropathies have become less common as average HbA_{1c} levels have fallen from above the 9% range over the last 10 years.

Occasionally, a diabetic mononeuritis with a localized region of pain can be misdiagnosed clinically as a mechanically mediated neuritis, such as a herniated intravertebral disk. If the appropriate imaging studies fail to demonstrate a mechanical etiology, a presumptive diagnosis of diabetes neuritis should be made and treatment aimed at glycemic control with physical therapy. On the other hand, diabetic neuritis of this type with constant pain may be initiated by mechanical factors. For example, a diabetic patient may acutely injure spinal nerves with a lifting maneuver, but this "neuromuscular pain" may become a continuing neuropathic pain as diabetic nerve fibers fail to heal in the presence of marked hyperglycemia. With no other etiologies evident, these patients eventually improve with more effective diabetic management.

Autonomic Neuropathies

See the discussion online at www.expertconsult.com.

Diabetic Retinopathy

Limiting the disability of diabetes mellitus has been greatly advanced with laser control of retinal disease. The onset of retinopathy is the appearance of *microaneurysms* indicative of diabetic angiopathy. Microaneurysms represent the beginning of a progression from background to proliferative retinopathy with neovascularization. Advanced retinopathy is caused by continuing capillary failure with leakage, hemorrhage, and closure, producing zones of retinal ischemia. The resulting compensatory capillary proliferation in the ischemic parts of the retina is prone to leak and rupture, causing gross hemorrhage. A reabsorbing hemorrhage in the vitreous can exert a pull on the retina resulting in retinal detachment with onset of blindness. Capillary hemorrhage can be detected by inspection or imaging modalities. Treatment by laser application decreases angiogenesis and further hemorrhagic risks. Vitreous hemorrhage can be removed, restoring vision and eliminating the risk of retinal detachment.

All type 1 diabetic patients should begin to have periodic dilated retinal examinations about 5 years after diagnosis. Because of the long asymptomatic latent period of type 2 diabetes, these formal eye evaluations should begin at the onset of type 2 diabetic management. In patients maintaining near normal HbA_{1c} of 7% or less, some authorities believe that formal dilated eye examinations can be deferred longer than 12 months.

Measures to prevent diabetic retinopathy include maintenance of glycemic control with avoidance of the stress of hypoglycemic reactions and control of blood pressure (BP). Aspirin therapy does not exacerbate or predispose to bleeding. However, intensive physical activity (exercise, sexual intercourse) can promote ocular bleeding.

KEY TREATMENT

Tight diabetic and optimal BP control reduces risks and progression of retinopathy (ADA, 2005, 2009; DCCT, 1993; UKPDS, 1998) (SOR: A).

Type 1 and 2 diabetic patients should be examined for retinopathy annually (Klein, 2003; Vijan et al., 2000) (SOR: B).

Preferably, a retinologist should follow patients with any degree of retinopathy, including marked nonproliferative change, proliferative change, or macular edema, because laser therapy reduces the risk of vision loss for these conditions (ETDRS, 1991) (SOR: A).

Diabetic Nephropathy, Diabetic Glomerulopathy, Renal Interstitial Syndromes

Before the DCCT, a patient with type 1 diabetes had a 30% to 40% likelihood of developing macroproteinuria (>300 mg/day), which would quickly progress to renal insufficiency and the need for renal dialysis. This process begins with proteinuria and increasing BP as early as 10-15 years after diagnosis of type 1 diabetes. In the early 1970s, when repeated studies showed that lowering of BP reduced cardiovascular events, diabetologists began to observe that good BP control, including use of diuretics, prolonged the interval from the onset of proteinuria to renal failure. The first studies of the angiotension-converting enzyme (ACE) inhibitor captopril suggested that treatment reduced macroproteinuria in patients with moderate renal insufficiency. Subsequent work in the 1990s indicated that reduced proteinuria impaired nephron loss and preserved renal function. The protein leak into the glomerular space may contribute to the mesangial proliferative reaction, starting a process that may end with nodular glomerulosclerosis.

Microalbuminuria

The introduction of the microalbuminuria assay lowered the threshold for the diagnosis of diabetic nephropathy to 20 to 200 µg/min, or 30 to 300 mg/day. Unlike smaller proteins that normally appear in the urine after exercise or fever, albumin does not appear in the urine without significant glomerular capillary leakage. Microalbuminuria can be detected before clinical signs of diabetic retinopathy; as a quantitative measure, it is the target of treatment protocols.

Although ACE inhibitors may exert a specific protective effect by relaxing transglomerular hydraulic pressure, the UKPDS observed that the use of atenolol achieved similar results in slowing proteinuria and renal loss. In fact, in longitudinal BP trials comparing multiple agents in diabetic patients, even diuretic therapy was as efficacious as newer drugs, without affecting mortality.

Renal protection afforded by BP-lowering drugs might be the consequence of decreasing renal perfusion. Patients with nephropathy and unilateral renal artery stenosis do not develop histologic evidence of diabetic glomerulosclerosis in the stenotic kidney. In contrast, hyperperfusion is deleterious to the diabetic kidney. Type 1 diabetic patients with the highest glomerular filtration rate (GFR) are most likely to develop proteinuria, possibly because of higher blood glucose causing an osmotic diuresis. Moreover, poorly controlled diabetic patients also have high levels of amino acids, some of which mediate renovasodilation and enhance GFR. Before the DCCT results, short-term studies confirmed that correction of glucose control with intensive insulin treatment reversed microalbuminuria.

Renal Protection

Renal protection, achieved with BP and glucose control, is a primary objective in diabetic care. The urine should be checked for microalbuminuria yearly. Finding marginal elevations indicates that control should be tightened and an ACE inhibitor or angiotensin receptor blocker (ARB) prescribed or increased. However, if BP is normal, pharmacotherapy can be difficult because of potential orthostasis. Another measure that could affect microalbuminuria is weight, which relates to the total-body water and the nitrogenous load the kidney must excrete. An appropriate weight reduction will decrease renal perfusion and microalbuminuria. If microalbuminuria increases, more aggressive BP drugs should be used. The onset of edema indicates advanced albumin losses or underlying renal or cardiac dysfunction. Diuretic management can significantly reduce micro- or macroalbuminuria, even though its effect on renal perfusion may cause a rise in serum creatinine (usually reversible when diuretic discontinued). Thus, diuretic therapy may need to be cyclic, depending on edema accumulation and renal function.

Screening for microalbuminuria is controversial because it fails traditional tests of acceptability, including agreement on diagnostic criteria (e.g., measurement of albumin/creatinine ratio in spot collection; 24-hour creatinine collection, with simultaneous measurement of creatinine clearance; time collection of 4-8 hours) and confusing rationale for ongoing testing when the patient is already taking an ACE inhibitor.

The development of significant *macroalbuminuria* above 300 mg/day despite treatment indicates significant glomerular changes with risk of progression to nephritic syndrome or renal failure. Evidence of the nephrotic syndrome may become apparent with hyperlipidemia and more hypertension. The objective of therapy at this point is to attenuate the slope of renal decline and prevent congestive symptoms associated with coincident cardiac dysfunction. Treatment is based on BP and volume control. Dietary limitation of salt, potassium, protein, and fluid intake will be helpful. We believe exposure to nephrotoxic agents can cause a quantum leap in the decline of the diabetic kidney at any stage of the pathophysiologic process. Unfortunately, nephrotoxicity is frequently the result of radiocontrast agents used repeatedly to detect and treat coronary artery disease or overexposure to antibiotics.

Diabetic Renal Interstitial Syndromes

See the discussion online at www.expertconsult.com.

KEY TREATMENT

To reduce the occurrence and slow the progression of renal disease that begins with microalbuminuria, attain tight glucose and blood pressure control (ADA, 2004, 2005; DCCT, 1995; Lewis et al., 1993; Reichard et al., 1993) (SOR: A).

ACE inhibitors and ARBs have the most favorable outcome data in patients with albuminuria (ADA, 2009; Lewis et al., 1993, 2001; Remuzzi et al., 2006) (SOR: A). In general, ACE inhibitors delay progression of nephropathy in type 1 with hypertension and any degree of albuminuria, and ARBs, in type 2 with renal insufficiency and macroalbuminuria. Both ACE inhibitors and ARBs have shown similar efficacy in type 2 patients with microalbuminuria (Andersen et al., 2000; Brenner et al., 2001; Lindholm et al., 2002; Molitch et al., 2003) (SOR: A).

Diabetic Macroangiopathy: Accelerated Atherosclerosis

Premature development of coronary heart disease (CHD) is the leading cause of morbidity among diabetic patients. Type 1 diabetic patients who are not troubled with diabetic nephropathy will likely experience CHD as early as their third or fourth decade, depending on the duration of their diabetes. The onset of renal disease in type 1 patients will further accelerate this timetable. Premenopausal status does not protect diabetic women from CHD.

The mechanisms causing accelerated atherosclerosis in DM are linked to the lipid and inflammatory pathogenic paradigms. Lipid abnormalities are not as common in type 1 patients, but long-term follow-up of the DCCT cohorts found thickening of large blood vessels related to their history of diabetic control. The disturbances in fatty acid metabolism in type 2 patients result in common dyslipidemias implicated in development of atherosclerotic plaque. Insulin resistance is associated with lipoprotein and coagulation abnormalities, hypertension, and evidence of endothelial dysfunction, all of which contribute to atherogenesis, even before the onset of hyperglycemia. These associations suggest that type 2 diabetes occurring as insulin levels decline is only one component of a larger pathophysiologic process.

KEY TREATMENT

ACE inhibitors reduce cardiovascular events in patients with known cardiovascular disease (ADA, 2009; HOPE, 2000) (SOR: A). Beta-adrenergic blockers reduce mortality in patients with prior myocardial infarction or other heart disease and those with cardiovascular risks undergoing major surgery (Foody et al., 2002) (SOR: A). No diabetic patients should smoke (Haire-Joshu et al., 1999) (SOR: A).

Hypertension

In recent years there has been a growing consensus that the control of high BP in diabetic patients may be more important than the control of hyperglycemia in terms of macroangiopathy. In UKPDS, captopril and atenolol were efficacious in preventing stroke and heart attacks despite less control of blood sugar. These agents were also equal to glycemic control in preventing proteinuria and nephropathy. Given these results, ACE inhibitors have often been recommended as first-line therapy for patients with high BP and diabetes. However, large hypertension trials such as ALLHAT continue to find that diuretics, ß-blockers, as well as ACE inhibitors have similar effectiveness in this population and any of these can be used as first-line therapy. Outcomes are also equivalent with ARBs and calcium channel blockers, although these are usually not recommended for initial anti-hypertensive therapy. As noted above, the current recommendation is for lower blood pressure targets in diabetic patients, specifically less than 130/80.

KEY TREATMENT

Blood pressure of 130 to 139 mm Hg systolic or 80 to 89 mm Hg diastolic following therapeutic lifestyle efforts must be lowered with drug therapy (ADA, 2009; UKPDS, 1998) (SOR: A). Pharmacologic therapy for patients with diabetes and hypertension should include an ACE inhibitor or ARB or thiazide diuretic (GFR >30 mL/min). (Loop diuretics are much weaker antihypertensives and should be reserved for patients requiring a diuretic and with estimated GFR <30.) ACE inhibitors, ARBs, beta and calcium channel blockers, and thiazide diuretics have all been shown to reduce cardiovascular events (ALLHAT, 2002; JNC-7, 2003) (SOR: C).

Coronary Artery Disease

Diabetic atherosclerosis in the coronary arteries is most deadly, but the same disease process is ongoing in the vessels of the central nervous system, lower extremities, and abdominal organs. The question is when to search for these problems in an asymptomatic diabetic patient; the recurring nightmare of a diabetologist is having sudden death as a patient's presenting symptom of diabetic heart disease. The cardiac risk of patients with long-term diabetes or middle-age onset of type 2 should be periodically considered.

The cholesterol threshold for using statins in diabetic patients has been lowered to low-density lipoprotein (LDL) cholesterol greater than 100 mg/dL, with a therapeutic target of 70 mg/dL. A large statin trial has shown that patients who demonstrate elevated C-reactive protein (CRP) with normal LDL cholesterol values will benefit from statin therapy (Ridker et al., 2008). Many patients had metabolic syndrome with elevated triglycerides, which raises non–high-density lipoprotein (n-HDL) cholesterol, a risk lowered by statin therapy and more pathologic than LDL cholesterol. Aspirin may not be efficacious in all patients because of genetic factors. However, considering the relative safety of low-dose aspirin, many clinicians think the potential benefits outweigh a possible lack of efficacy. As noted, UKPDS showed that beta blockers and ACE inhibitors were equally effective in protecting the heart, brain, and kidney. Beta blockers are known to protect the previously injured heart but have adverse effects on erectile dysfunction. Cardiac stress studies are indicated for multiple risk factors, new symptoms, and changes of ischemia on periodic ECG or echocardiogram. Once triple-vessel disease is excluded, repeat coronary angiography in asymptomatic patients to consider prophylactic stent placements is controversial. Stenting appears to be effective in improving angina and cardiac function, but no data yet demonstrate it prevents myocardial infarctions, probably because MIs are more likely to result from rupture of nonobstructing plaques. In 2009 the BARI 2D trial showed that in patients with type 2 diabetes, and stable coronary artery disease, there was no difference in mortality or major cardiovascular events based on randomization to prompt revascularization or medical therapy.

KEY TREATMENT

Reducing lipids is critical in attenuating diabetic macroangiopathy (ADA, 2009; Heart Protection Study, 2003; Pyorala et al., 1997) (SOR: A).

Therapeutic lifestyle changes focusing on reducing saturated fat and cholesterol intake, losing weight, and increasing physical activity will improve lipid profiles (ADA 2004, 2005; NCEP [ATP-III], 2002) (SOR: A). Regardless of LDL level, statin therapy should be added to lifestyle therapy in diabetic patients with overt cerebrovascular disease (CVD), or without CVD who are over 40 and have one or more CVD risk factors (ADA, 2009; Grundy et al., 2004b) (SOR: A).

Patients without overt CVD and diabetes should be treated to an LDL cholesterol of value < 100mg/dL. ADA Diabetes Care Supplements, January 2009 (NCEP [ATP-III], 2002) (SOR: A).

For antiprocoagulant therapy, aspirin (81-162 mg/day) should be used in patients with known CVD (Colwill, 1997; Hayden et al., 2002) (SOR: A).

Cerebral and Peripheral Vascular Disease

The diagnostic and therapeutic considerations discussed earlier apply to the carotid and peripheral vessels with other generalizations and exceptions. Beta-blocker therapy causing bradycardia could provoke neurologic and peripheral symptoms distal to a stenotic lesion. BP control appears to be more important than glycemic control in preventing cerebrovascular accidents (CVAs, strokes). Patients with claudication-like stable angina might respond to exercise. Vascular surgery is indicated for patients with nonhealing ulcers and pain at rest. Insulinization promotes vasodilation and improves perfusion and WBC function in patients treated for a nonhealing wound or foot ulcer.

Extrarenal Macrovascular Disease

The kidney is also susceptible to the accelerated atherogenic process affecting the blood vessels. Acute onset of hypertension or loss of BP control in a known hypertensive patient should suggest a vascular etiology. Accumulation or rupture of an atherosclerotic plaque in a renal artery may cause renal ischemia and secondary hyperaldosteronism through the renin response. Rarely, diffuse atherogenesis in the diabetic aorta can result in cholesterol emboli traveling into the renal microvasculature. The urine sediment can become active, indicative of glomerulonephritis.

The diagnosis of extrarenal macrovascular disease is also evident clinically by the appearance of distal microinfarcts in the toes. The renal arteries can be examined for stenosis using Doppler ultrasound. Magnetic resonance angiography (MRA) can provide high-resolution imaging of stenotic plaques and quality of the great vessels without the risks of contrast agents. Advances in endovascular surgery with stent placements have simplified renal artery repair and stabilized the aorta in the face of aneurysmal dilation and threatening rupture, which might be signaled by release of cholesterol-laden plaques. Early treatment with statins is thought to stabilize plaques and preclude devastating vascular complications.

Diabetic Dermopathy

See online discussion of dermopathy as an indicator of neuropathy and vascular impairment.

The Metabolic Syndrome

The Adult Treatment Panel (ATP), in recommending guidelines for the treatment of hypercholesterolemia, defined the components of metabolic syndrome as any three of the following (NCEP [ATP-III], 2002; Grundy et al., 2004a, 2004b):

1. Fasting serum glucose greater than 110 mg/dL, a prediabetic value but consistent with insulin resistance. The CDC (2005) recommends that prediabetes be defined by a serum glucose value of 100 mg/dL or greater and less than 126 mg/dL.
2. Systolic BP of 130 mm Hg or greater, or diastolic BP of 85 mm Hg or greater.
3. Fasting serum triglycerides greater than 150 mg/dL.
4. HDL cholesterol less than 40 mg/dL in men and less than 50 mg/dL in women.
5. Waist circumference of 102 cm (40 inches) or greater for men and 88 cm (35 inches) or greater for women.

Ruderman and colleagues (1981) defined the concept of metabolic obesity in type 2 diabetes by noting the association of diabetes with hypertriglyceridemia, low HDL, and hypertension, in patients who were not overtly obese. Prevalence of obesity associated with diabetes has greatly increased in the last 30 years, and obesity is now evident in at least 80% of patients with type 2 diabetes. Others noted the connection of high insulin levels with impaired glucose tolerance leading to type 2 diabetes, disordered fatty acid metabolism, hypertension, and increased abdominal fat deposition indicative of visceral obesity (Reaven, 2003). The linkage of these risk factors with insulin has become known as the *metabolic syndrome*, which is now considered the leading cause of atherosclerosis (Grundy et al., 2004a).

Besides lipoproteins, patients with metabolic syndrome may have high levels of plasminogen activator inhibitor 2, which results in impaired fibrinolysis. Other abnormalities promoting vascular injury in these patients include endothelial dysfunction and inflammatory proteins.

The Friedenwald equation is used to calculate the value of LDL cholesterol from the measured values of total and HDL cholesterol and triglycerides in the serum, as follows:

$$\text{LDL cholesterol} = (\text{Total cholesterol} - \text{HDL cholesterol}) - (\text{Triglycerides}/5)]$$

Because high triglycerides would lower the calculated LDL cholesterol value, the ATP recommends treatment for non–HDL cholesterol (total cholesterol – HDL cholesterol) to a target of 130 mg/dL or less. However, the diabetic, hypertensive, and coagulopathic disturbances of patients with metabolic syndrome also require intervention. Many drugs are needed to address these multiple risk factors, but restoring fitness through exercise redistributes abdominal fat stores, lowers insulin levels, and reverses to some extent several of the described abnormalities.

Office Management to Improve Diabetic Outcomes: Activating the Patient

Key Point

- A mainstay of modern diabetes management is the "activated" patient, who is educated and prepared and involved in care.

Over the last several years, there has been increasing evidence of the effectiveness of the "chronic care model" as developed by Wagner (1998). The essential elements of the model are divided into the *community* (resources and policies), *health system* (self-management support, delivery system design, decision support, clinical information systems), an *informed activated patient*, and a *prepared proactive practice team* (Fig. 34-2). Of note, community programs and organizations are often acknowledged but may not be used in a busy practice. Self-management support involves not only providing instructions but also facilitating the patient's acceptance of control over DM. The delivery system design means clarifying roles and responsibilities, as well as ensuring that the right care is delivered, with up-to-date information about the patient and appropriate follow-up. Currently, decisions need to be supported by evidence-based medicine and guidelines, and patients monitored for ongoing care and response. This approach should lead to a patient who is the true locus of control and a practice in which all the professionals and staff provide current and responsive care to their patients. The essential skills needed by the family physician are working in teams and facilitating teamwork in the office setting.

A 2004 Cochrane review found that a multifaceted approach can enhance management of patients with diabetes, such as regular prompted recall and review of patients and patient-oriented interventions, along with proactive, involved nursing. Other models, such as stages of readiness for change, have led to more effective counseling and intervention strategies. Studies have shown that without an organized approach, using the current system of care will not succeed in adequately controlling diabetes, and that simply introducing diabetic flow sheets or the concept of nonphysician personnel interacting with diabetic patients is not enough to change outcomes. Following guidelines, measuring performance, and working to improve the clinical practice are hallmarks of the modern family physician's approach to diabetes management (see Web Resources; Physician Consortium).

Diet, exercise, medications, foot care, and self-testing are under the patient's direct control ("locus of control"), as well as keeping appointments, seeing consultants (e.g., ophthalmologist), and participating in daily medical decision making. Self-help manuals and websites can assist the activated patient in self-care. In addition, psychosocial issues, ranging from developmental effects of adolescence to severe psychopathology or aberrant family interactions, can have serious consequences for diabetic control. For example, a well-controlled adolescent may not take her insulin or follow an appropriate diet. However, the effectiveness of treatments for adolescent diabetic patients still varies widely, even within a similar culture, possibly because of underlying

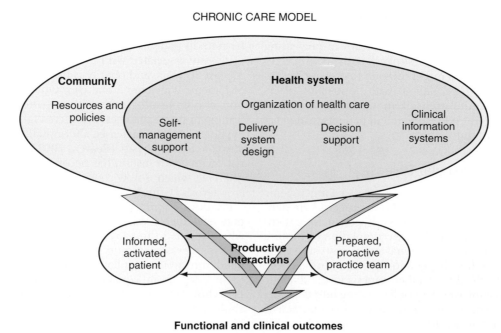

CHRONIC CARE MODEL

Figure 34-2 Model for improvement of chronic illness care. *(From Wagner EH. Chronic disease management: what will it take to improve care for chronic illness? Eff Clin Pract 1998;1:2-4.)*

psychopathology. A the extreme, eating disorders or severe depression can cause marked variations in the intake of essential nutrients, leading to either the dangers of hypoglycemia or the initiation of DKA. This is true among adults with diabetes as well as adolescents. Not surprisingly, therefore, diabetes has been associated with depression, at least in a Caucasian population, and as expected, those with such "dual diagnoses" tend to have more emergency room visits and inpatient hospitalizations.

Parents of a child with diabetes are less depressed or distressed than parents of a child diagnosed with cancer. Over time, however, parents of diabetic children can become more distressed, including their sense of control, self-esteem, and disease-related fears. If a family cannot be appropriately supportive, regardless of the patient's psychological state, the locus of control may need to be switched from the patient-family to the patient-physician relationship.

A major social issue is inequitable care for diabetic patients depending on their socioeconomic background. Thus, it is widely accepted that minority populations bear a disproportionate burden of diabetes, as do those with less education and lower earnings. Stereotyping and bias have long been part of the U.S. health care system, and the Institute of Medicine report Unequal Treatment: Confronting Racial and Ethnic Disparities in Health Care demonstrates that much needs to be done before resolving these issues. It is not only that minority patients have a higher prevalence of diabetes, or that these patients have more severe disease, more cardiovascular complications, and higher mortality, but also that these patients struggle with multiple barriers to adequate care. Access to any care is a perennial problem in many populations, so that for a chronic disease such as diabetes, which requires multiple visits and interventions, the automatic disparity in access leads to significant differences in outcome. In addition, cultural belief systems that lead to the use of alternative healers, distrust of traditional medicines, and misunderstanding of the disease process also serve as barriers to care. Given the complex interchange among culture, diet, body image, illness behavior, and the dynamics of race and gender, a family physician caring for a patient with diabetes must overcome not only the pathophysiology of the disorder but also these diverse barriers to care. The task is difficult, but diabetes control can be achieved when an "activated" patient and the physician confront these challenges together.

KEY TREATMENT

Both disease management and case management of diabetes improve the health and socioeconomic outcomes of patients. These approaches employ an organized, multimethod, responsive approach to delivering health care to diabetic patients (Systematic review; Task Force on Community Preventive Services, 2002) (SOR: A).

References

The complete reference list is available online at www.expertconsult.com.

Web Resources

www.ama-assn.org/ama1/pub/upload/mm/370/diabetesset.pdf
Physician Consortium for Performance Improvement; website provides free set of measures that can be used to monitor diabetes care.

www.cdc.gov/diabetes/pubs/factsheet07.htm
Centers for Disease Control and Prevention; National Diabetes Fact Sheet provides general information and national estimates on diabetes in the United States.

http://endotext.org
Endotext; up-to-date, comprehensive source of information on all topics in clinical endocrinology.

http://metabolicpulse.org
Metabolic Pulse; diabetes education for health care providers, including opportunities for continuing medical education (CME).

http://diabetes.niddk.nih.gov.libproxy2.umdnj.edu
National Diabetes Information Clearinghouse (NDIC).

Available at http://www.who.int/diabetes/facts/en
World Health Organization; diabetes program fact sheet.

35 CHAPTER

Endocrinology

George Wilson, Arshag Mooradian, Irene Alexandraki, and George Samrai

Chapter contents

Pituitary Disorders

Key Points

- The hypothalamic-pituitary axis orchestrates the hormonal secretions of the other endocrine glands.
- The pituitary is composed of the adenohypophysis (anterior lobe) and neurohypophysis (posterior lobe).
- The hormonal secretions of the anterior pituitary are regulated by hypothalamic releasing hormones and inhibitory molecules.
- The posterior pituitary lobe is where nerve endings, originating in the paraventricular and supraoptic nuclei, project as the supraopticohypophyseal tract.

Hypothalamic-Pituitary Axis

The hypothalamus affects several nonendocrine functions, including appetite, sleep, body temperature, and activity of the autonomic nervous system. In addition, the hypothalamus modulates the pituitary hormone secretions. The

pituitary gland is often referred to as the "master gland" in recognition of its role in orchestrating the hormonal secretions of the other endocrine glands (Mooradian and Korenman, 2007; Mooradian and Morley, 1988). The pituitary gland is located in the anterior fossa, in the sella turcica, close to the optic chiasm. The pituitary is composed of the adenohypophysis, or anterior lobe, and the neurohypophysis, or posterior lobe, and is connected to the hypothalamus by the pituitary stalk.

The hormonal secretions of the anterior pituitary (the adenohypophysis) are regulated by a number of hypothalamic releasing hormones and inhibitory molecules. These factors reach the pituitary through the portal circulation and, on interaction with specific receptors, either stimulate or inhibit the secretion of the anterior pituitary hormones. The main releasing hormones include thyrotropin-releasing hormone (TRH), gonadotropin-releasing hormone (GnRH), corticotropin-releasing hormone (CRH), and growth hormone–releasing hormone (GHRH). The two major inhibitory factors are *dopamine*, which principally inhibits prolactin release, and *somatostatin*, a potent inhibitor of growth hormone (GH), and to a lesser extent, thyrotropin (TSH). Other factors have an important regulatory effect on anterior pituitary function. The kisspeptin hormones are a family of peptides encoded by the KiSS-1 gene and are thought to play a critical role in reproduction. Kisspeptin receptors stimulate GnRH release and activation of the mammalian reproductive axis. Mutations in kisspeptin receptor GPR-54 cause idiopathic hypogonadotropic hypogonadism, characterized by delayed or absent puberty (Jayasena and Dhillo, 2009).

The portal circulation also allows pituitary hormones to flow backward to the hypothalamus and provide feedback on their own releasing hormones to create a short-loop regulatory system. The control of the pituitary hormonal secretion is the result of interplay between the effects of hypothalamic releasing hormones and the long-loop negative feedback on the pituitary and hypothalamus by hormones secreted by endocrine glands in the periphery. For example, a rise in plasma thyroid hormone level "feeds back" and suppresses pituitary TSH and hypothalamic TRH secretion.

The posterior lobe (pars nervosa) of the pituitary is essentially an extension of the hypothalamus where the nerve endings, originating in the paraventricular and supraoptic nuclei, project as the supraopticohypophyseal tract. The posterior pituitary hormones *vasopressin* and *oxytocin* are directly controlled by neural impulses and are released into the inferior hypophyseal veins and then into the systemic circulation (Mooradian and Morley, 1988).

Approach to Pituitary Disease

Key Points

- Pituitary disease may manifest with pituitary hormone excess or deficiency or symptoms of mass expansion, including headaches and visual disturbances.
- Pituitary adenoma is the most common cause of pituitary dysfunction in adults.
- Hypothalamic-pituitary axis function should be assessed in patients with a mass in the sella turcica.
- Evaluation of pituitary dysfunction involves serum measurements (prolactin, GH, IGF-1, FT_4, TSH), free cortisol or dexamethasone suppression test, and imaging.

The most common cause of pituitary disease is the development of benign tumors. Adenomas can cause symptoms because of excessive production of hormones such as prolactin, GH, or adrenocorticotropic hormone (ACTH), or can cause pituitary hormone insufficiency secondary to tissue destruction. The pituitary hormones that can be lost early during the gradual destruction of pituitary tissue include GH and GnRH, followed by TSH and lastly ACTH. Occasionally, however, the autoimmune destruction of the pituitary can be cell specific and cause selective pituitary hormone deficiency.

Pituitary tumors can expand into the optic chiasm and hypothalamus and cause visual field defects and symptoms of hypothalamic disease, respectively. The classic symptom of optic chiasm compression is *bitemporal hemianopsia* (inability to see either side). Early manifestations of optic chiasm impingement can be subtle and include seeing images that float apart or seeing one half of the face higher than the other half (Picasso effect, or hemifield slide phenomenon). These

symptoms emerge when the patient is tired or anxious and are the result of failure to fuse the images from both eyes because of the lack of nasal fields. Expansion of tumors into the hypothalamus can cause disturbances in sleep, appetite, temperature regulation, sweating, water balance, and memory (Mooradian and Morley, 1988).

In children, pituitary adenomas are less common, and hypothalamic pituitary dysfunction is typically the result of hypothalamic tumors, notably craniopharyngiomas.

When microadenoma (<10 mm) is discovered incidentally, the initial evaluation should seek hormone hypersecretion by measuring levels of serum prolactin, insulin-like growth factor type 1 (IGF-1), TSH, and free thyroxine (FT_4) levels and 24-hour urine free cortisol or a 1-mg overnight dexamethasone suppression test (Mooradian and Korenman, 2007). More extensive workup is required for pituitary masses larger than 10 mm (macroadenoma), regardless of symptoms. Overall workup and management of pituitary disease should include identifying and treating hormonal deficiency and excess as well as diagnosing and managing mass effects of the tumors.

Hypopituitarism

Key Points

- Hypopituitarism refers to total or partial deficiency of one or more pituitary hormones.
- Hypopituitarism can result from a genetic disorder or releasing factor deficiency but more often results from pituitary tissue destruction secondary to mass expansion, infiltrative process, autoimmune or infectious disease, vascular accidents, radiation injury, or trauma.
- Pituitary apoplexy may result in life-threatening hypocortisolism.
- Lymphocytic hypophysitis is a rare autoimmune pituitary disease occurring in women in late pregnancy or postpartum that may mimic pituitary tumor but does not require resection.
- Kallmann syndrome is characterized by an isolated defect in GnRH secretion.
- Approximately 10% of patients with empty sella syndrome have clinically apparent hypopituitarism, and some may have pituitary adenomas.
- Systemic disease, including end-stage liver disease or chronic renal failure, is associated with variable degrees of hypopituitarism without significant histopathologic changes in the pituitary.

Hypopituitarism refers to total or partial deficiency of one or more pituitary hormones resulting in end-organ changes or reduced hormonal secretion of target endocrine glands (Toogood and Stewart, 2008). The deficiencies could be the result of primary disease of the pituitary or could be secondary to failure of hypothalamic hormone synthesis or transport. There are no good estimates of the incidence of hypopituitarism because the disease is often subclinical.

Causes

Hypopituitarism may result from a genetic disorder or deficiency in hypothalamic releasing factor but more often is the result of pituitary tissue destruction secondary to mass expansion, infiltrative process, autoimmune or infectious disease, vascular accidents, radiation injury, or trauma. In some patients the etiology of hypopituitarism cannot be identified and is considered *idiopathic.* Most idiopathic cases are sporadic, although there are well-described familial causes of hypopituitarism.

The most common cause of hypopituitarism in the adult population is *intrasellar pituitary tumors.* Occasionally, hypopituitarism is resolved with surgical or medical treatment of the pituitary mass. Parasellar masses that cause hypopituitarism include craniopharyngiomas, meningiomas, optic nerve gliomas, teratomas, germinomas, chordomas, metastatic cancers, and lymphomas.

The second most common cause of hypopituitarism is *postpartum pituitary necrosis* (Sheehan's syndrome). The portal system of the anterior pituitary vascular supply, increased oxygen demand of an enlarged pituitary gland during pregnancy, excessive blood loss, and possibly increased intravascular coagulation combine to cause ischemic pituitary injury. Other ischemic causes of pituitary necrosis can occur in systemic vascular diseases such as diabetes mellitus, temporal arteritis, and sickle cell disease. These diseases can also result in hemorrhagic infarction *(apoplexy)* of the pituitary, with acute onset of severe headache, visual impairment, altered mental status, and hypopituitarism. The sudden decline in ACTH and thus hypocortisolism may be the most life-threatening consequence of hypopituitarism, requiring emergency treatment with corticosteroids. Although pituitary adenomas are the most common cause of pituitary apoplexy, it may often be related to complications of diabetes, radiotherapy, or open heart surgery (Toogood and Stewart, 2008).

Rarely, infectious diseases can lead to hypopituitarism. Examples include meningitis, intracranial abscess, septic shock, fungal infections of the central nervous system (CNS), tuberculosis (TB), malaria, and syphilis.

Infiltrative diseases of the pituitary, and more frequently of the hypothalamus, can cause hypopituitarism. Sarcoidosis can present with hypopituitarism along with polydipsia and polyuria. Histiocytosis X may present as a suprasellar tumor. Lipid storage diseases and hemochromatosis can cause hypopituitarism, often with hypogonadotropin deficiency.

Lymphocytic hypophysitis is a rare autoimmune disease of the pituitary occurring in women during late pregnancy or in the postpartum period. Lymphocytes and plasma cells infiltrate the pituitary gland, which results in the destruction of anterior pituitary cells. This disease may mimic pituitary tumor but does not require resection, making the correct diagnosis especially important. Lymphocytic hypophysitis cannot be distinguished from tumor except by biopsy. The diagnosis is suspected in women who develop hypopituitarism during or immediately after pregnancy, in the absence of a history of hemorrhage during delivery or previous history of infertility or menstrual disorders.

Mutations in the genes coding for specific anterior pituitary hormones have also been described, the most common being isolated GH deficiencies manifesting as short stature, beginning in infancy or childhood. *Kallmann syndrome* is characterized by an isolated defect in GnRH secretion. Young men develop a eunuchoid appearance and testosterone deficiency, and women have amenorrhea or oligomenorrhea. The syndrome may also be associated with hyposmia or anosmia (Oliveira et al., 2001). Mutations in the *PROP-1* gene

are the most common causes of congenital hypopituitarism and present as deficiencies of GH, prolactin, TSH, luteinizing hormone (LH), and follicle-stimulating hormone (FSH). Older adults with *PROP-1* gene mutations may present with ACTH deficiency (Wu et al., 1988). Iatrogenic causes of hypopituitarism include surgical ablation and radiotherapy. Hypothalamic and pituitary deficiency may occur after several years, with GH and gonadotropin deficiencies the most common. Prolactin level may be mildly elevated.

Approximately 10% of patients with *empty sella syndrome* have clinically apparent hypopituitarism, and some may have pituitary adenomas (Mooradian and Morley, 1988). The empty sella syndrome occurs when a defect in the sellar diaphragm allows the subarachnoid space to herniate into the pituitary fossa. It is a relatively common disorder found in 5% to 8% of autopsies.

Systemic disease, including end-stage liver disease and chronic renal failure, is associated with variable degrees of hypopituitarism without significant histopathologic changes in the pituitary (Mooradian, 2001; Nowak and Mooradian, 2007).

Clinical Manifestations

Key Points

- Progressive loss of hormones occurs in pituitary injury, starting with loss of GH and gonadotropin and followed by TSH and ACTH deficiency.
- ACTH deficiency results in cortisol deficiency, leading to hypotension, shock, and cardiovascular collapse.
- TSH deficiency results in signs and symptoms of hypothyroidism.
- Gonadotropin deficiency results in the signs and symptoms of hypogonadism.
- GH deficiency causes short stature in children and may be asymptomatic in adults.

The clinical manifestations of hypopituitarism are highly variable and depend on age and gender of the patient as well as on the etiology of the pituitary disease (Toogood and Stewart, 2008). Patients can be completely asymptomatic for many years or present with dramatic symptoms of nausea, vomiting, headache, and vascular collapse. Symptoms are more common in pituitary apoplexy, when the sudden withdrawal of ACTH and ensuing adrenal insufficiency cause hemodynamic instability. It is believed that at least 75% of the glandular tissue must be destroyed before an individual becomes clinically symptomatic. If the etiology is a space-occupying lesion, such as expanding adenoma or carotid aneurysm, the clinical manifestations will include headache and visual field defects, which are classically bitemporal hemianopsia. Other, subtle changes in vision involve color perception, patchy scotomas, and difficulty in passing a thread through the eye of a needle (Mooradian and Morley, 1988).

Failure to lactate may be the first clinical sign of Sheehan's syndrome (postpartum pituitary necrosis). Lethargy, anorexia, and weight loss; failure to resume normal menstrual periods; and loss of sexual hair may also be present later in the postpartum period. On the other hand, symptoms and signs of pituitary infarction may be subtle and not recognized for years.

Patients with *panhypopituitarism* (Simmonds' syndrome) are usually pale and lethargic, have dry skin and low blood pressure, and rarely may look cachectic (Toogood and Stewart, 2008). These patients have lost all the anterior pituitary hormones, and the clinical manifestations are caused by a mixture of hypogonadism, hypothyroidism, adrenal insufficiency, and GH deficiency. The clinical manifestations depend on whether the deficiency is partial or complete. Individual signs and symptoms reflect the biologic actions of various hormones secreted by the pituitary.

Growth hormone deficiency manifests as growth retardation in children. The body proportion and primary teeth are normal, but secondary tooth eruption is delayed. In up to 10% of children with GH deficiency, symptomatic hypoglycemia may occur. In adults, GH deficiency may be asymptomatic. Subtle changes may occur in insulin sensitivity, manifested by reduced insulin requirements in diabetic patients, decreased muscle and bone mass and increased adiposity, delayed wound healing, and fasting hypoglycemia, and may contribute to anemia of hypopituitarism. Additional adverse effects associated with GH deficiency in adults include increased low-density lipoprotein (LDL) and decreased high-density lipoprotein (HDL) cholesterol, decreased cardiovascular function and increased risk of cardiovascular events, and a diminished sense of well-being. Life expectancy is reduced in these patients compared with age-matched controls (Svensson et al., 2004).

Gonadotropin deficiency will result in *hypogonadotropic hypogonadism* (HH) or secondary hypogonadism. In prepubertal children, HH manifests as failure to achieve pubertal changes along with lack of pubertal growth spurt. Girls will have primary amenorrhea and lack of breast development or widening of the pelvis. In boys, testicular size will remain small, scrotal skin will not thicken, and penile growth, muscle development, and hoarseness of voice will not appear. In adults, HH presents as infertility, loss of libido, decreased facial hair and muscular mass in men and amenorrhea, and decreased breast size and atrophic vaginal mucosa in women. If left untreated, men and women with HH will develop osteoporosis.

A deficiency in TSH will cause secondary hypothyroidism unless the patient has concomitant Graves' disease or an autonomously functioning thyroid nodule. The classic clinical manifestations of hypothyroidism include lethargy, easy fatigability, dry skin, cold intolerance, constipation, fine silky hair, slow mentation, and slow relaxation phase of deep tendon reflexes. Other features include anemia and hyponatremia secondary to increased antidiuretic hormone (ADH) secretion. In general, these symptoms are less severe in patients with TSH deficiency compared with patients with primary thyroid failure, and other findings, such as hypercholesterolemia, hypercarotenemia, myxedema and effusions in body cavities, may occur less frequently (Toogood and Stewart, 2008).

A deficiency in ACTH will result in deficiency of cortisol secretion and is referred to as *secondary adrenal insufficiency*. The clinical features resemble primary adrenal disease, such as Addison's disease. In both entities, anorexia, lethargy, nausea, vomiting, abdominal pain, postural hypotension, and vascular collapse may occur. Hyponatremia is more common in ACTH deficiency, whereas hyperkalemia is seen only in primary adrenal insufficiency and loss of aldosterone secretion, primarily regulated by the renin-angiotensin system and serum potassium/sodium concentrations. Hyperpigmentation of the skin and vitiligo are features of primary adrenal insufficiency, whereas patients with ACTH deficiency have difficulty tanning on exposure to sunlight. Mild ACTH deficiency may be asymptomatic and may go undiagnosed for a long time.

Diagnosis

Key Points

- If one pituitary hormone insufficiency is documented, the other pituitary hormones should be tested.
- An 8 AM plasma cortisol level less than 5 μg/dL strongly suggests hypocortisolism; a level greater than 18 μg/dL excludes ACTH deficiency.
- Serum free T_4 must be used with serum TSH concentration in assessing thyroid function.
- Normal or subnormal LH level in menopausal or amenorrheic women, in the presence of a low estradiol level, indicates secondary hypogonadism (in men, low testosterone level).
- Diagnosis of GH deficiency requires provocative testing.

Since the presenting complaints can be subtle, clinicians should have a high index of suspicion to diagnose hypopituitarism (Toogood and Stewart, 2008). If the clinical manifestations fit hypogonadism, hypothyroidism, or adrenal insufficiency, those hormonal tests should be ordered to confirm the diagnosis. If one pituitary hormone insufficiency is documented, every attempt should be made to test the status of the other pituitary hormones as well. The underlying etiology of the disease should be determined by computed tomography (CT) or magnetic resonance imaging (MRI) of the hypothalamic-pituitary area. Occasionally, angiography is needed when carotid artery aneurysm is suspected, or to define the blood supply of the tumor. Formal ophthalmologic examination with visual field evaluation should be ordered if the patient is symptomatic or has a pituitary mass lesion.

Pituitary hormone secretion is episodic, and in general, dynamic testing is more valuable than single, baseline hormone measurements. For practical reasons, however, the screening can be done with pituitary hormone and target hormone measurements simultaneously. For evaluating suspected hypopituitarism, tests include thyroid function, LH, serum testosterone in men and estradiol in women, IGF-1 (because GH has a short half-life in blood), prolactin, and morning cortisol. Provocative testing for GH and ACTH reserve may be required as well. Patients with known pituitary disease and deficiency of ACTH, TSH, or gonadotropins have a 95% chance of a subnormal provocative stimulus for GH. Also, patients with known pituitary disease and a serum IGF-1 concentration lower than normal can be presumed to have GH deficiency (Gharib et al., 2003). Provocative tests for GH are either physiologic (sleep or exercise) or pharmacologic such as insulin-induced hypoglycemia, GHRH with arginine, and levodopa with arginine tests (Biller et al.,

2002). GH deficiency is diagnosed when GH does not rise above 5 ng/mL in response to two or more stimuli.

A plasma cortisol level less than 5 µg/dL at 8 AM on two occasions in the patient with a disorder known to cause hypopituitarism strongly suggests hypocortisolism, and in the presence of normal or low serum ACTH concentration, it establishes the diagnosis of secondary adrenal insufficiency. Conversely, a cortisol level of 18 µg/dL or greater virtually excludes the diagnosis of ACTH deficiency.

To evaluate ACTH reserve, insulin hypoglycemia test (0.1-0.15 U/kg IV) should be done. A normal cortisol response to adequate hypoglycemic stimulus (blood glucose <50 mg/dL) is either an incremental level of 6 to 10 µg/dL or an absolute level greater than 20 µg/dL. The test allows for concomitant evaluation of GH reserve; however, it is contraindicated in elderly patients and those with coronary artery disease or epilepsy (Nowak and Mooradian, 2007). An alternative is the metyrapone test, 750 mg orally every 4 hours for six doses, which assesses the sensitivity of the pituitary to the negative inhibition by cortisol. Metyrapone blocks 11β-hydroxylase, an enzyme that catalyzes the final step in cortisol biosynthesis. The decrease in cortisol secretion after metyrapone is given should result in a compensatory increase in the ACTH level. The level of the precursor steroid 11-deoxycortisol should also increase. A normal response is an increase in serum 11-deoxycortisol level greater than 10 µg/dL, when serum cortisol level is reduced to less than 8 µg/dL, indicating adequate suppression of glucocorticoid synthesis. In the more convenient overnight test, metyrapone, 30 mg/kg orally, is administered at midnight. An increase in the 8 AM serum 11-deoxycortisol level to more than 7 µg/dL is found in healthy persons. If symptomatic postural hypotension occurs after metyrapone administration, hydrocortisone should be administered exogenously.

Cosyntropin, 250 µg intramuscularly (IM) or intravenously (IV), should result in an increase in the serum cortisol level of 18 µg/dL or greater at 60 minutes in normal subjects. The test may not reliably determine the ACTH reserve, especially in those with recent ACTH deficiency, in whom the adrenal glands may not be sufficiently atrophied. Some controversy surrounds whether the 1-µg cosyntropin stimulation test (IV only) may be more sensitive for the diagnosis of subtle secondary adrenal insufficiency.

Thyrotropin (TSH) deficiency is diagnosed when low baseline free T_4 and low or normal TSH is documented on more than one measurement. Gonadotropin deficiency in men is tested with measurements of baseline LH, FSH, and total testosterone. Serum samples are drawn between 8 and 10 AM, and low concentrations should be confirmed with a second serum sample. The 8 to 10 AM serum testosterone concentration generally should be 300 to 1000 ng/dL. A low testosterone value (<200 ng/dL) with low or normal LH is indicative of hypogonadotropic hypogonadism. For serum total testosterone levels between 200 and 400 ng/dL, free testosterone level should also be ordered (Mooradian and Korenman, 2006). The presence of amenorrhea in premenopausal women, along with low estrogen level (<30 pg/mL), establishes the diagnosis of HH. In menopausal women the absence of elevated FSH and LH is sufficient for the diagnosis.

Elevated serum prolactin level in a hypogonadal patient suggests a pituitary adenoma. Prolactin deficiency often indicates severe intrinsic pituitary disease and is uncommon without concomitant deficiencies of other anterior pituitary hormones.

Conditions known to mimic hypopituitarism should be excluded when evaluating patients, including anorexia nervosa, protein-calorie malnutrition, systemic illness, chronic renal failure, and liver cirrhosis.

Treatment

Key Points

- Hydrocortisone is given to ACTH-deficient adults at 20 to 30 mg/day and increased twofold to threefold during times of illness and other stresses.
- The goal of thyroid replacement is to achieve a normal serum free thyroxine concentration and clinical euthyroidism.
- Thyroid replacement will increase the clearance of cortisol, so ACTH status is assessed; if deficient or uncertain, glucocorticoid replacement is indicated before replacing thyroid hormone.
- Treatment of secondary hypogonadism depends on gender and whether fertility is desired.
- Serum IGF-1 concentration and growth rate in children are used for monitoring the effectiveness of GH replacement.

The treatment of hypopituitarism depends on the etiology and the particular hormonal deficiency. Surgical and medical interventions may be necessary for treatment of pituitary masses, infiltrative diseases, and carotid aneurysms.

Growth hormone deficiency is treated with recombinant human GH (somatotropin) preparations (Gharib et al., 2003). The recommended GH dose in children with GH deficiency is 0.04 mg/kg/day. In adults, recombinant human GH is administered subcutaneously (SC) at 0.001 to 0.008 mg/kg/day. The usual starting dose is 0.1 to 0.3 mg/day for a 70-kg man, with a typical maintenance dose of 0.3 to 0.6 mg/day. In general, women require higher doses than men because estrogen increases GH resistance. Serum IGF-1 concentration should be monitored to maintain it at the mid-normal range. Side effects that should be monitored include edema, carpal tunnel syndrome, arrhythmias, paresthesias, and glucose intolerance.

Levothyroxine (L-thyroxine) is the hormone of choice for the treatment of patients with TSH-deficient hypothyroidism (Oiknine and Mooradian, 2006). A typical replacement dose in adults is approximately 1.6 µg/kg/day. The daily requirements should be individually determined based on clinical and biochemical evaluations. The free T_4 level should be in the middle to upper third of the normal range. Since thyroid replacement will increase the clearance of cortisol and uncover a subclinical adrenal insufficiency, the ACTH status should be assessed, and if deficient or uncertain, glucocorticoid replacement is indicated before thyroid hormone is replaced.

Treatment of secondary hypogonadism depends on the patient's gender and whether or not fertility is desired. Estradiol and progesterone replacement is the treatment of choice for secondary hypogonadism in premenopausal women who have an intact uterus and do not desire fertility. These hormones can be given cyclically or daily in fixed-dose combinations. In women with hysterectomy, estrogen replacement is sufficient, to maintain vulvar and vaginal lubrication, relieve symptoms of vasomotor instability, and reduce bone loss. Women wanting to restore fertility should be referred to specialized centers for pharmacologic induction of ovulation with exogenous pulsatile GnRH and exogenous FSH and LH treatment. GnRH can be used to restore fertility when hypothalamic disease and tertiary hypogonadism are present. Women over age 50 with secondary hypogonadism should be treated as menopausal, taking into consideration the risk/benefit ratio of estrogen replacement therapy in this age group.

Secondary hypogonadism in men is treated with testosterone replacement. Fertility can be restored in men with pituitary disease using gonadotropin replacement or human chorionic gonadotropin (hCG) therapy. GnRH can be used when hypothalamic disease is the cause of hypogonadism.

Many preparations are available for testosterone replacement. Traditional oral androgens, including 17α-methyltestosterone, fluoxymesterone, and other 17α-alkylated steroids, may cause hepatic toxicity and should be avoided. The current injectable testosterone esters, such as testosterone enanthate or testosterone cypionate, act similarly. The usual replacement dose is 200 mg IM every 2 weeks. In older men, it may be prudent to start at 50 to 75 mg weekly. Testosterone undecanoate is available as an oral preparation that does not have hepatotoxicity; because of its short half-life, however, it must be taken three times daily. Transdermal preparations can be given as patches or gels. Some androgen skin patches are associated with a high incidence of skin reactions. The commercially available transdermal gel preparations (Androgel 1%, Testim 1%) are applied over the trunk daily. Sublingual and buccal preparations of testosterone (e.g., Striant) are also available for replacement therapy (Mooradian and Korenman, 2006).

Side effects of testosterone replacement should be monitored carefully. Digital rectal examination (DRE), hematocrit (Hct), and prostate-specific antigen (PSA) should be measured at 3, 6, and 12 months follow-up, then annually or semiannually. Bone density measurements should be obtained at baseline and if low, at 2-year intervals to monitor improvement. In addition to monitoring clinical response, serum testosterone levels should be measured with the goal of achieving a midnormal range at 7 days after injection of testosterone enanthate or cypionate, at 3 to 10 hours after application of a testosterone patch, or at any time after application of a testosterone gel.

Absolute contraindications to testosterone therapy are prostate or breast cancer, Hct of 55% or more, or sensitivity to ingredients of the testosterone preparation (Mooradian and Korenman, 2006). Relative contraindications include obstructive sleep apnea, congestive heart failure, obstructive symptoms of prostatic hyperplasia, and Hct of 52% or greater. However, there are no data to suggest that testosterone replacement aggravates subclinical prostate cancer.

Patients with ACTH deficiency should be treated with glucocorticoids, preferably hydrocortisone, which the adrenals produce. Hydrocortisone replacement should be given orally as 20 to 30 mg/day divided into two doses, with two thirds of the daily dose given in the morning and one third given in the early afternoon or evening (Coursin and Wood, 2002; Toogood and Stewart, 2008). Alternatively, prednisone is given at a total daily dosage of 5 to 7.5 mg/m²/day in one to two doses. Clinical evaluation is the primary modality to assess the adequacy of cortisol replacement. It is important to increase the dose of hydrocortisone twofold to threefold during illness and other stresses. All patients should carry medical alert tags or cards to identify the need for high-dose glucocorticoids in an emergency. Those with secondary adrenal insufficiency usually do not require mineralocorticoid replacement because ACTH is not essential for aldosterone secretion.

Hyperfunctioning Pituitary Adenomas

Key Points

- Pituitary adenomas may present with visual impairment, headache, or hormonal abnormalities.
- Prolactinomas are the most common type of functioning pituitary adenoma and manifest with galactorrhea and hypogonadism.
- Nonpathologic causes of hyperprolactinemia are sought, and primary hypothyroidism is excluded.
- MRI is the imaging modality of choice for the anatomic evaluation of the hypothalamus and pituitary gland.
- Prolactin level over 150 ng/mL and pituitary adenoma not identified on imaging suggest macroprolactinemia.
- A dopamine agonist (bromocriptine or cabergoline) is first-line treatment of prolactinomas.

Pituitary adenomas can arise from any cell type and can be functioning or nonfunctioning. The precise pathogenesis of these adenomas is not known but mutations found in several genes can play a role in the development of many adenomas. With prolactinomas the most common type, other functioning pituitary adenomas include gonadotropic, thyrotropic, somatotropic, and corticotropic adenomas.

Hyperprolactinemia and Prolactinomas

Diagnosis

Prolactin is a polypeptide secreted from the lactotrophs of the anterior pituitary (Leung and Pacaud, 2004; Mancini et al., 2008). The main function of prolactin is the development of breast tissue in preparation for milk production and maintenance of lactation postpartum. Unlike other pituitary hormone regulation, prolactin release is predominantly under inhibitory control. Dopamine is the principal inhibitor, and prolactin stimulators such as TRH and estrogen have minor roles.

Hypersecretion of prolactin may be physiologic or pathologic in origin. Physiologic stimulators include exercise, pain, breast stimulation, sexual intercourse, general anesthesia, and pregnancy. Pathologic causes of hyperprolactinemia include prolactinomas, decreased dopaminergic inhibition of prolactin secretion through pharmacologic agents, and decreased clearance of prolactin. Early manifestation of prolactin hypersecretion is galactorrhea and menstrual irregularities, notably amenorrhea, in women and erectile dysfunction or loss of libido in men. Rarely, galactorrhea with gynecomastia can occur in men. These patients are at risk of developing osteoporosis secondary to hypogonadism as well as a result of the direct inhibitory effect of prolactin on bone formation. Galactorrhea is rarely found in postmenopausal women with hyperprolactinemia, in whom mass effect of prolactinomas may cause the principal presenting symptom, such as headache or visual disturbance (Mancini et al., 2008). Similarly, the diagnosis of prolactinomas in men is often delayed because the clinical signs and symptoms of hyperprolactinemia are less obvious.

Clinical evaluation of patients with suspected prolactinomas should include a thorough evaluation of medication history and presence of comorbidities. Many drugs are known to cause hyperprolactinemia, including phenothiazines, haloperidol, metoclopramide, H_2 antagonists, imipramines, selective serotonin reuptake inhibitors (SSRIs), calcium channel blockers, and hormones. The physical examination may reveal galactorrhea and visual field defects. Women may have mild hirsutism and men decreased facial hair growth.

Laboratory tests include serum prolactin and thyroid function. Primary hypothyroidism is associated with hyperprolactinemia secondary to elevated TRH that induces prolactin secretion. Testing should also seek systemic illnesses with increased prolactin levels, such as liver or renal failure. MRI is the imaging modality of choice for the anatomic evaluation of the hypothalamus and pituitary gland. Complete pituitary hormone evaluation should be performed when an adenomatous mass is noted in the region of the pituitary.

Features to distinguish hyperprolactinemia associated with pituitary tumors include (1) prolactin levels greater than 150 ng/mL, (2) loss of normal sleep-associated increases in prolactin levels, and (3) failure of prolactin levels to rise in response to exogenous TRH. No test is absolute, and diagnosis of prolactinoma depends on radiologic studies.

Clinicians should be aware of two prolactin assay–related conditions that may cause diagnostic confusion. In *macroprolactinemia*, large-molecular-weight prolactin, aggregated with globulins, is recorded as elevated levels of prolactin in the absence of any physiologic or pathologic cause of hyperprolactinemia (Mancini et al., 2008). Macroprolactinemia is suspected in the patient with very high prolactin level and no galactorrhea or tumor on pituitary MRI. The second area of confusion occurs when extremely high concentrations of serum prolactin overwhelm the assay reagents such that the measurements underestimate the true concentration of prolactin. This is referred to as the "hook effect."

Treatment

The treatment of hyperprolactinemia depends on the etiology, presence or absence of mass effects (e.g., visual changes), presence of bothersome galactorrhea or associated pituitary hormone deficiencies, and whether fertility is desired (Leung and Pacaud, 2004; Mancini et al., 2008). If possible, drugs known to cause prolactin elevation should be discontinued and serum prolactin concentration remeasured. Persistent hyperprolactinemia requires pituitary-hypothalamus imaging.

Treatment of prolactinomas includes dopamine agonists as first-line treatment. In select subgroups, surgical excision is recommended, usually through the transsphenoidal approach. Rare patients with large, residual tumor mass after surgery not responsive to medical therapy may be offered radiation therapy. Associated hormone deficiency should also be targeted. Often, as the prolactin levels are normalized, symptoms of hypogonadism can be reversed.

Bromocriptine and cabergoline are U.S. Food and Drug Administration (FDA)–approved dopamine agonists used to treat hyperprolactinemia. Cabergoline has greater tolerability than bromocriptine and is more effective in achieving

normalization of prolactin levels in 90% of patients with prolactinomas. Because of long-standing experience, however, bromocriptine is the preferred agent in women who want to become pregnant. Bromocriptine should be discontinued once pregnancy has been confirmed, even though the risk of teratogenicity is small. Pregnant women with prolactinomas should be warned to report any visual disturbances or headaches, because up to 10% of microprolactinomas and 30% of macroprolactinomas increase in size sufficient to cause symptoms. During pregnancy, prolactin levels should be monitored periodically, but interpretation of the results may be difficult. Pregnant women with macroadenomas should receive similar advice and have serial visual field testing.

Pergolide is an alternative but non-FDA-approved medication for hyperprolactinemia. Caution should be exercised with all these ergot derivatives because of rare case reports of valvular heart damage in patients taking the drug at very high doses for prolonged periods.

Withdrawal of the drug may lead to recurrent prolactin hypersecretion and adenoma growth, although the microadenomas have resolved after a few years of treatment in some patients. The dosage of the dopamine agonist may be reduced when prolactin levels have been normalized for 1 year and tumor size has been significantly reduced. Medication withdrawal may be considered after 2 years in those with normal prolactin levels and an MRI scan showing no tumor, or tumor reduction more than 50% and more than 5 mm from the optic chiasm, with no invasion of the cavernous sinus. Pituitary MRI and serum prolactin levels should be monitored closely thereafter.

Indications for transsphenoidal surgery in patients with prolactinomas include medical treatment failure or medication intolerance, very large tumors threatening visual pathways, or hemorrhagic infarcts (apoplexy). Approximately 30% of macroadenomas can be successfully removed surgically.

Acromegaly and Gigantism

See the discussion online at www.expertconsult.com.

Cushing's Disease

Key Points

- Cushing's syndrome is categorized into ACTH-dependent or ACTH-independent cases. Pituitary ACTH-dependent Cushing's syndrome is Cushing's disease.
- The diagnosis is established when the clinical findings of Cushing's syndrome are associated with laboratory documentation of excess cortisol production.
- Measurement of 24-hour urinary cortisol excretion is a good screening tool.
- Comparison of serum ACTH concentration with serum cortisol level can help determine the cause of hypercortisolism.
- Treatment of Cushing's syndrome is directed at the cause of hypercortisolism. The treatment of choice for Cushing's disease is selective transsphenoidal resection.

Hypercortisolemia (also hypercortisolism, hyperadrenocorticism), caused by either exogenous administration of cortisol or other synthetic glucocorticoids or endogenous overproduction of cortisol, leads to a constellation of clinical and biochemical findings referred to as *Cushing's syndrome* (Arnaldi et al., 2003; Findling and Raff, 2005). The multiple causes include pituitary adenomas, excess production of CRH leading to hyperplasia of corticotropes in the pituitary, ectopic production of ACTH and CRH, and adrenocortical adenomas and carcinomas. The term *Cushing's disease* specifically refers to pituitary-dependent cortisol hypersecretion (Biller et al., 2008). Pituitary, ACTH-dependent Cushing's disease accounts for at least 70% of endogenous cases, while the most common cause of ACTH-independent Cushing's syndrome is prolonged glucocorticoid therapy.

Patients who have undergone bilateral adrenalectomy for hypothalamic-pituitary–dependent Cushing's syndrome may develop pituitary tumors associated with marked skin pigmentation. This condition is known as *Nelson's syndrome.* The skin hyperpigmentation occurs because of excess production of melanocyte-stimulating hormone (MSH), a product of the gene that also encodes ACTH and beta endorphin.

Diagnosis

A high index of suspicion is required to make the diagnosis of Cushing's syndrome because manifestations of the disease are insidious and develop over months.

The clinical features include weight gain with centralized obesity distributed in the face, neck, trunk, and abdomen with facial rounding and plethora. The thinning of the skin and loss of subcutaneous tissue result in easy bruisability and violaceous abdominal striae. Patients with ectopic ACTH-dependent Cushing's syndrome have extreme ACTH increases that cause rapid hyperpigmentation and are more likely to demonstrate features of mineralocorticoid excess, such as hypokalemia and metabolic alkalosis. Gonadal dysfunction is associated with decreased testosterone levels in men and decreased serum estradiol levels and menstrual disorders, notably amenorrhea, in women. Virilization and androgen excess are more common in patients with Cushing's syndrome caused by adrenal carcinomas.

Glucocorticoid excess also interferes with calcium and bone metabolism and leads to osteoporosis. Catabolic effects of excess glucocorticoid on muscles cause proximal muscle weakness. Glucose intolerance is found in 30% to 60% of those with hypercortisolism. Other complications of hypercortisolism include risk of opportunistic infections, including *Pneumocystis jiroveci* (formerly *carinii*) pneumonia, hypercoagulable state, and thromboembolic events secondary to increased plasma concentration of clotting factors and neuropsychiatric changes (Arnaldi et al., 2003; Findling and Raff, 2005).

Establishing the Cause

The diagnosis is established when the clinical findings of Cushing's disease are associated with laboratory documentation of excess cortisol production, loss of diurnal variation of plasma cortisol level, and more than 50% suppression of plasma and urine cortisol after administration of 2 mg of dexamethasone every 6 hours (high-dose dexamethasone suppression test). Measurement of 24-hour urinary cortisol excretion is a good screening tool. Alternatively, impaired suppression of cortisol after an overnight 1-mg dexamethasone suppression test can be used as a screen in nonobese individuals. Plasma ACTH concentration less than 5 pg/mL

and serum cortisol concentration greater than 15 µg/dL suggest an ACTH-independent cause. Plasma ACTH concentration greater than 15 pg/mL in a patient with hypercortisolism likely indicates ACTH-dependent Cushing's syndrome (Arnaldi et al., 2003; Findling and Raff, 2005).

The vast majority of ACTH-dependent Cushing's syndrome patients have a pituitary adenoma as the cause. The few patients who have an ectopic source of ACTH must be identified with high-resolution CT scanning of chest, abdomen, and pelvis.

Suppression of urinary cortisol excretion, after administration of high-dose dexamethasone, is consistent with the diagnosis of Cushing's disease, whereas urinary cortisol excretion in cases of ectopic ACTH syndrome is usually not suppressible. When the high-dose dexamethasone suppression test fails to differentiate an ectopic source from a pituitary source of ACTH, and radiographic imaging is not conclusive, further CRH testing and petrosal sinus sampling of ACTH are indicated to localize the tumor to the pituitary.

Treatment

The treatment of choice for Cushing's disease is selective transsphenoidal resection of the pituitary adenoma. The cure rate for this procedure is 70% to 80% for microadenomas at experienced centers. In some patients, total hypophysectomy is considered when the disease recurs after transsphenoidal resection. Many postsurgical patients require low-dose cortisol replacement for up to 12 months, until their endogenous adrenal function recovers.

Bilateral adrenalectomy with or without pituitary irradiation is offered to patients who have recurrence of hypercortisolemia or severe disease. For poor surgical candidates, adjunctive medical therapy is offered and includes metyrapone (blocker of 11β-hydroxylase), mitotane (O'P'DDD), and cyproheptadine. These treatment options have variable efficacy.

Craniopharyngiomas; Thyrotropin-Secreting Pituitary Adenomas; Gonadotropic and Other Adenomas

See the discussions of these pituitary tumors online at www.expertconsult.com.

Posterior Pituitary Disorders

Arginine vasopressin (AVP) and oxytocin are the principal hormones secreted from the posterior pituitary. The two major stimuli of oxytocin secretion are suckling during lactation and dilation of the cervix during labor. Although not essential for initiation of labor, oxytocin can be used pharmacologically to initiate labor or control postpartum hemorrhage and uterine atony. Rarely, it has been used to induce milk ejection. The physiologic role of oxytocin in males is not known. AVP differs from oxytocin by only one amino acid. AVP is found in all mammals except pigs and related species, in which lysine vasopressin replaces AVP. In humans and many mammals, AVP and oxytocin are associated with two neurophysins, the exact roles of which are not known, except as carrier proteins in storage and transport of posterior pituitary hormones (Mooradian and Morley, 1988).

Antidiuretic hormone (vasopressin) is synthesized in the hypothalamus and migrates down into the posterior lobe of the pituitary to be stored and later secreted. Some ADH is secreted directly into the cerebrospinal fluid (CSF) rather than the posterior pituitary. Thus, pathologic lesions affecting the hypothalamus below the median eminence may preserve some functional ADH that migrates from the CSF into the systemic circulation. The half-life of AVP in circulation is only 20 minutes because of its susceptibility to peptidases. Loss of the terminal amino group in position 1 makes this peptide resistant to degradation, whereas substitution of the *levo* analog of arginine for dextroarginine in position 8 reduces presser effect without altering its antidiuretic properties. The resultant peptide deamino-8-D-argenine vasopressin (DDAVP) is currently the treatment of choice for central diabetes insipidus.

The biologic effects of AVP are initiated at two receptors, V1 and V2. The V1 receptors are located in the vascular system, and their stimulation results in vasoconstriction. The V2 receptors are located in the kidneys, and their stimulation results in free-water reabsorption (Korbonits and Carlsen, 2009). Plasma osmolality, blood volume, and blood pressure are the most important physiologic stimuli of AVP secretion. Other factors that modulate AVP secretion include pain, stress, nausea, hypoglycemia, hypercapnea, angiotensin II, atrial natriuretic hormone, and drugs. Many stimuli of AVP release also promote thirst. Thirst is less sensitive than AVP release in response to these stimuli and therefore is a second-line defense against dehydration.

Central Diabetes Insipidus

Key Points

- Diabetes insipidus is characterized by excessive dilute urine with thirst and polydipsia and results from decreased ADH secretion.
- Differential diagnosis of hypotonic polyuria includes neurogenic DI (vasopressin sensitive), nephrogenic DI (vasopressin resistant), and primary polydipsia.
- The water restriction test assists in diagnosis.
- Desmopressin is the primary treatment for central DI.

Clinical Features

Diabetes insipidus (DI) is characterized by the production of excessive dilute urine with secondary thirst and polydipsia. *Polyuria* is defined as 3 L or more of urine daily in adults and 2 L or more in children. Central DI may be familial or sporadic and is caused by head trauma, neurosurgery, neoplasms, granulomas, infections, inflammation, chemical toxins, vascular disorders, congenital malformations, and genetic disorders. Other causes include hypoxic encephalopathy; infiltrative disorders, notably *histiocytosis X* (Hand-Schuller-Christian disease); anorexia nervosa; acute fatty liver of pregnancy; and Wolfram syndrome (central DI, diabetes mellitus, optic atrophy, and deafness) (Reddy and Mooradian, 2009). An autoimmune process is probably the cause of idiopathic DI and accounts for 30% to 50% of cases of central DI (de Bellis et al., 1999).

Thickening or enlargement of the posterior pituitary on MRI may represent lymphocytic infiltration and inflammation. Classically, DI after head trauma or neurosurgery has three phases: polyuria in the first 1 to 2 days after surgery, oliguria for 3 to 4 days, and culminating in a polyuric phase. These phases reflect the early paralysis of vasopressin-producing cells, followed by neuronal degeneration and massive ADH release, with subsequent permanent loss of vasopressin production.

Vasopressin-resistant DI is usually a familial disorder, although sporadic causes are recognized, as in chronic medullary kidney disease associated with sickle cell disease, multiple myeloma, amyloidosis, Sjögren's syndrome, and renal medullary cystic disease. In addition, prolonged primary polydipsia can wash out the normal medullary concentration gradient and may mimic ADH-resistant nephrogenic DI.

Diagnosis

Although a variety of diseases may present as polyuria and polydipsia, thorough history and routine laboratory evaluation can narrow the differential diagnosis of hypotonic polyuria to three possibilities: neurogenic DI (vasopressin sensitive), nephrogenic DI (vasopressin resistant), or primary polydipsia (Mooradian and Morley, 1988).

Serum sodium concentrations less than 137 mEq/L and polyuria are usually manifestations of primary polydipsia. Patients with serum sodium concentration less than 143 mEq/L should have a water deprivation test after an overnight fast, with hourly measurement of body weight, urine volume, and osmolality. In severe cases the dehydration test can be started at 6 AM. When the urine osmolality remains constant during three consecutive measurements, or if the patient loses more than 5% total body weight, plasma osmolality, ADH, and sodium concentrations are determined, and aqueous vasopressin (0.1 U/kg SC) or 10 μg of nasal desmopressin is administered and the response evaluated. An increase in urine osmolality of 150 mOsm/kg above baseline will exclude nephrogenic DI. In central DI, 10 μg of nasal desmopressin will result in increases in urine osmolality of as much as 800%. The response to desmopressin in partial central DI may result in urine osmolality increases of 15% to 50%. Patients with nephrogenic DI continue to have urine osmolality levels that remain below isosmotic. Primary polydipsia responds to the water deprivation test with urine concentrating to 500 mOsmol/kg or higher, compared with urine osmolality increasing to 800 mOsmol/kg or higher in normal subjects. Administration of exogenous vasopressin produces no further concentration in cases of primary polydipsia.

When the water suppression test yields equivocal results, the serum AVP concentration at baseline and after the water restriction test should be measured. However, the results of these tests may still be misleading because primary polydipsia will result in submaximal secretion of AVP, mimicking the pattern of AVP secretion in partial central DI.

Treatment

The treatment of choice for central DI is desmopressin. DDAVP can be administered IV, SC, nasally, or orally. An initial nasal inhalation of 5 μg is given at bedtime and increased by 5-μg increments until nocturia is resolved, when a morning dose is given. The total daily dosage of nasal desmopressin is 5 to 20 μg daily. Oral desmopressin should be given on an empty stomach; absorption can be reduced by up to 50% when taken with food. A 0.1-mg tablet is equivalent to 2.5 to 5.0 μg of nasal spray (de Bellis et al., 1999).

Patients with partial DI will benefit from oral agents that potentiate AVP action or stimulate the release of AVP. These agents include chlorpropamide, carbamazepine, and clofibrate. In such cases, desmopressin requirements may be lower than available preparations can provide. Patients with nephrogenic DI benefit from thiazide diuretics or indomethacin. Patients with DI should wear a medical alert bracelet. When the ability to drink fluids is impaired, intravenous hydration will be required to avoid dehydration and hypernatremia.

Syndrome of Inappropriate Secretion of Antidiuretic Hormone

Key Points

- Laboratory evaluation of plasma osmolality, urine osmolality, and urine sodium concentration assist in determining the cause of hyponatremia.
- Water restriction and salt replacement are the most important treatments in hyponatremia. The underlying cause should be identified and treated, when possible.
- Vasopressin antagonists are currently indicated for the treatment of euvolemic and hypervolemic hyponatremia.

Syndrome of inappropriate secretion of antidiuretic hormone (SIADH) is associated with plasma ADH concentrations that are inappropriately high for the plasma osmolality. Laboratory and clinical features of SIADH include (1) euvolemic hyponatremia; (2) decreased measured plasma osmolality (<275 mOsm/kg); (3) urine osmolality >100 mOsm/kg; (4) urine sodium usually >40 mEq/L; (5) normal acid-base and potassium balance; (6) blood urea nitrogen (BUN) <10 mg/dL; (7) hypouricemia <4 mg/dL; (8) normal thyroid and adrenal function; and (9) absence of advanced cardiac, renal, or liver disease (Reddy and Mooradian, 2009). Conditions or factors associated with SIADH include CNS trauma and infections, tumors, drugs, major surgery, pulmonary disease (e.g., TB), hormone administration, human immunodeficiency virus (HIV) infection, hereditary SIADH, idiopathic causes, and cerebral salt wasting (Box 35-1).

In some cases it is difficult to differentiate SIADH from mild to moderate depletional hyponatremia. The response of urinary and plasma sodium concentration to an infusion of 1 to 2 L of 0.9% (isotonic) saline may help in the differential diagnosis. In the patient with SIADH who is at equilibrium, the saline will be excreted, and therefore urinary sodium will increase while plasma sodium concentration will either not change or decrease slightly. If the patient has depletional hyponatremia from renal losses, sodium from the administered saline is retained and the excess water excreted. Urinary sodium decreases, whereas plasma sodium concentration increases.

Box 35-1 Select Causes of Syndrome of Inappropriate Antidiuretic Hormone Secretion (SIADH)

Nonosmotic stimuli

Nausea, pain, stress
Human immunodeficiency virus (HIV)
Acute psychosis
Surgery
Pregnancy (physiologic)
Hypokalemia
Congestive heart failure exacerbation

Central nervous system lesions

Tumors (neuroblastoma)
Cerebrovascular accident (stroke)
Meningitis, encephalitis
Abscess
Guillain-Barré syndrome
Hydrocephalus
Pituitary stalk lesion
Delirium tremens
Demyelinating disease
Acute porphyria

Malignancies

Lymphoma, leukemia, Hodgkin's disease
Carcinoma of uterus
Ureteral, prostate, and bladder carcinoma
Carcinoma of duodenum and pancreas
Ectopic production of vasopressin by tumors (small cell lung carcinoma, carcinoids)
Cancers of head and neck and nasopharynx
Renal cell carcinoma
Osteosarcoma

Increased intrathoracic pressure

Mediastinal tumors (thymoma, sarcoma)
Positive-pressure ventilation
Infections (pneumonia, TB, aspergillosis, lung abscess)
Bronchogenic carcinoma, mesothelioma
Bronchiectasis, empyema
Chronic obstructive pulmonary disease
Pneumothorax

Drug induced

Antipsychotics

Phenothiazines
Haloperidol

Antidepressants

SSRIs, TCAs, MAOIs
Bupropion

Anticonvulsants

Carbamazepine, oxcarbazepine
Sodium valproate

Analgesics and recreational drugs

Morphine (high doses)
Tramadol
MDMA ("ecstasy")
Nonsteroidal anti-Inflammatory drugs
Colchicine, venlafaxine
Duloxetine (Cymbalta)

Continued

Box 35-1 Select Causes of Syndrome of Inappropriate Antidiuretic Hormone Secretion (SIADH)—cont'd

Cardiac drugs

Thiazides, clonidine

ACE inhibitors, aldosterone antagonists

Amiloride, loop diuretics

Methyldopa, amlodipine

Amiodarone, lorcainide

Propafenone, theophylline, terlipressin

Unfractionated heparin (aldosterone antagonist)

Antidiabetic drugs

Chlorpropamide

Tolbutamide, glipizide

Lipid-lowering agent

Clofibrate

Antineoplastic agents

Cyclophosphamide

Vincristine, vinblastine

Cisplatin, hydroxyurea

Melphalan

Immunosuppressives

Tacrolimus, methotrexate

Interferon α and γ, levamisole

Monoclonal antibodies

Antibiotics

Azithromycin, ciprofloxacin

Trimethoprim-sulfamethoxazole

Cefoperazone/sulbactam, rifabutin

Modified from Reddy P, Mooradian AD. Diagnosis and management of hyponatremia in hospitalized patients. Int J Clin Pract 2009;63:1494-1508.
TB, Tuberculosis; *SSRIs,* selective serotonin reuptake inhibitors; *TCAs,* tricyclic antidepressants; *MAOIs,* monoamine oxidase inhibitors; *ACE,* angiotensin-converting enzyme; *MDMA,* 3,4-methylenedioxymethamphetamine.

A *reset osmostat* may be suspected when mild hyponatremia persists despite changes in fluid and salt intake. A reset osmostat may be confirmed by giving the patient a fluid bolus of 10 to 15 ml/kg. Normal patients, or those with a reset osmostat, should excrete 80% of this bolus in 4 hours, which does not occur with SIADH. Cerebral salt wasting induces SIADH-like symptoms. Salt wasting, followed by volume depletion, occurs in some patients with cerebral disease. This leads to a secondary rise in ADH levels. The mechanism underlying cerebral salt wasting is unclear.

Treatment

Management of SIADH should begin with water restriction and treatment or elimination of the underlying etiology. In all patients with hyponatremia, free-water intake from all sources should be restricted to less than 1 to 1.5 L daily. In patients with mild symptoms, the rate of urinary solute excretion, the main determinant of urine output, can be increased by a high-salt, high-protein diet or supplementation with urea (30-60 g/day) or salt tablets (200 mEq/day) (Reddy and Mooradian, 2009). However, salt therapy is generally contraindicated in patients with hypertension and edema because it leads to exacerbation of both conditions. In addition, water restriction is contraindicated in subarachnoid hemorrhage with hypovolemia, in which water restriction may result in hypotension, creating a risk for cerebral infarction. This risk is more pronounced if the patient has cerebral salt wasting, which must be treated first, with isotonic or hypertonic saline solution, until adequate volume status is demonstrated.

In general, plasma sodium concentration should be corrected at a rate of 1 mEq/L/hr until the reversal of neurologic symptoms. The correction rate is then reduced to 0.5 mEq/L/hr until the plasma sodium has reached a level of 120 to 125 mEq/L. This approach effectively prevents the devastating neurologic consequences of acute hyponatremia and is associated with reduced risk of osmotic demyelination of pontine and extrapontine neurons.

The most specific treatment for SIADH is to block the V2 receptors in the kidney that mediate the diuretic effect of ADH.

Vasopressin antagonists are currently indicated for the treatment of euvolemic and hypervolemic hyponatremia (Loh and Verbalis, 2008). For hospitalized patients, conivaptan is given as an intravenous (IV) loading dose of 20 mg delivered over 30 minutes, then as 20 mg continuously over 24 hours. Subsequent infusions may be administered every 1 to 3 days at 20 to 40 mg daily by continuous infusion (Reddy and Mooradian, 2009). More recently, an orally active vasopressin receptor antagonist, tolvaptan, became available. Rapid correction of hyponatremia has been reported in patients receiving these agents; therefore, frequent checks of plasma sodium are needed. Chronic SIADH can occur in patients with ectopic ADH-producing tumors and in whom antipsychotic drugs cannot be discontinued. If water restriction and salt tablet therapy is ineffective, attempt (1) administration of loop diuretic along with salt tablets; (2) demeclocycline; (3) lithium carbonate; and (4) orally active vasopressin antagonists such as tolvaptan (cost limits its utility). Demeclocycline is nephrotoxic in patients with cirrhosis and is contraindicated in children because of interference with bone development and teeth discoloration. Lithium carbonate may induce interstitial nephritis and renal failure. Therefore, lithium should be considered for use only in patients in whom demeclocycline is contraindicated.

KEY TREATMENT

Hydrocortisone is given to ACTH-deficient adults at 20 to 30 mg daily, increased twofold to threefold during illness and other stresses (Coursin and Wood, 2002; Toogood and Stewart, 2008) (SOR: A).

The goal of thyroid replacement should be to achieve a normal serum free-thyroxine concentration and clinical euthyroidism (Oiknine and Moordian, 2006) (SOR: A).

A dopamine agonist is first-line treatment of prolactinomas (Mancini et al., 2008) (SOR: A).

Transsphenoidal surgery to remove the pituitary adenoma is usually the treatment of choice in individuals with acromegaly (Melmed et al., 2009) (SOR: A).

Octreotide (Sandostatin) is often effective in normalizing GH and IGF-1 levels. Pegvisomant is a GH receptor antagonist also approved for treatment of acromegaly (Melmed et al., 2009) (SOR: A).

Treatment of Cushing's syndrome should be directed at the cause of hypercortisolism. The treatment of choice for Cushing's disease is selective transsphenoidal resection (Biller, 2008) (SOR: A).
Desmopressin is the primary treatment for central diabetes insipidus (Loh and Verbalis, 2008; Reddy and Mooradian, 2009) (SOR: A).
Water restriction and salt replacement are the most important treatment modalities in hyponatremia. The underlying cause should be identified and treated, when possible (Reddy and Mooradian, 2009) (SOR: A).
Vasopressin antagonists are currently indicated for the treatment of euvolemic and hypervolemic hyponatremia (Loh and Verbalis, 2008; Reddy and Mooradian, 2009) (SOR: A).

Thyroid Disorders

Key Points

- Primary thyroid disorder is caused by abnormal function of the thyroid gland.
- Secondary thyroid disorder is the result of abnormalities at the level of the pituitary.
- Tertiary thyroid disorder results from malfunction at the level of the hypothalamus.

Thyroid disorders include processes that affect function (physiology) as well as structure (anatomy). Extraglandular causes include metastatic neoplasia, pituitary disorders, dietary issues, autoimmune diseases, infections, and genetic or familial diseases, such as multiple endocrine neoplasia IIA and familial medullary thyroid carcinoma. Other causes are intrinsic to the thyroid and include cysts, nodules, and goiter. In either case, all thyroid diseases exist in one of three functional states: euthyroid, hyperthyroid, or hypothyroid; each is defined by the level of total bound and free, circulating thyroid hormone. The presence of any one of these states in an individual can be transient, static, or progressing. Laboratory abnormalities of circulating thyroid hormone, at any point in time, do not prove disease and do not depend on the etiology of thyroid dysfunction. All three states may exist at different times during the course of an illness, and each state can exist with or without disease or clinical findings. In addition, the various thyroid structures can reflect disease independent of endocrinologic function.

Accurate assessment of thyroid function, with determination of presence or absence of disease, requires data in addition to levels of circulating thyroid hormones. These data include serum free and total thyroid hormone levels, thyrotropin (TSH) levels, and in some cases, antithyroid antibody (ATA) titers. This battery of tests will provide diagnosis in the majority of common thyroid disorders. When imaging studies and fine-needle aspiration are added, 90% to 95% of patients with thyroid disease who present in the primary care setting can be diagnosed and appropriately managed.

Thyroid disorders affect 60 to 80 per 1000 adults worldwide and up to 8.9% of the adult U.S. population (Bagchi et al., 1990; Vanderpump et al., 1995). Since most have an insidious onset or closely mimic other, more common disorders, thyroid disorders are easily missed and, although rarely fatal, can cause significant morbidity. Early recognition is critical to minimizing morbidity. With the exception of conditions such as simple goiter or visible nodule, patients who ultimately are diagnosed with thyroid disease rarely present to the family physician with complaints suggesting thyroid disorder.

Anatomy and Physiology

Key Points

- Thyroxine (T_4) is the major product of the thyroid gland.
- Triiodothyronine (T_3) is the active hormone at the cellular level.
- The majority of circulating T_3 is formed in the peripheral circulation by deiodination of T_4.
- Thyroxine serves as a reservoir (prohormone) for T_3.
- Serum thyrotropin (sTSH) is required in all evaluations of dementia or depression.

Histologically, the thyroid gland consists of five primary elements: follicular cells, colloid, interstitial tissue, "C" cells, and lymphoid cells. The most prominent element is the follicular cell, which produces colloid. The thyroid follicle is the functional unit of the gland and the site where colloid is stored. It is within the follicle where thyroid hormone (thyroxine, or T_4) synthesis occurs. The remaining cellular elements are C cells and lymphoid cells. The few C cells are located in the intrafollicular space and produce calcitonin. Lymphoid cells are found scattered throughout the gland stroma in small, isolated clusters.

Circulating Thyroid Hormones

Biosynthesis of thyroid hormone is unique among endocrine glands because final assembly occurs extracellularly in the follicular lumen. The source of thyroid hormones (T_4 and triiodothyronine, or T_3) is *thyroglobulin* (Tg), an iodoprotein produced by thyroid follicular cells. Thyroglobulin is the major portion of intraluminal colloid and is the most important protein of the thyroid gland (Kopp, 2005). Thyroglobulin provides a matrix for the synthesis of thyroid hormones and a vehicle for subsequent storage. Stored thyroglobulin is oxidized by thyroid peroxidase (TPO), adding an iodine molecule to tyrosine to form monoiodotyrosine (MIT) and diiodotyrosine (DIT). MIT and DIT are then assembled into the final products, tetraiodothyronine (T_4) and triiodothyronine (T_3), which are stored in the follicular colloid for future use. When stimulated by serum thyrotropin (sTSH), thyroglobulin within the colloidal space is internalized by thyroid cells and enzymatically degraded to release T_4 and T_3 into the peripheral circulation. Approximately one third to one half of T_4 released into the peripheral circulation is deiodinated to form T_3.

In the peripheral circulation, T_4 and T_3 are bound to thyroid-binding globulin (TBG). Thyroxine is bound to TBG in concentrations 10 to 20 times greater than T_3, and neither bound T_4 nor bound T_3 is directly available to tissues. Only unbound or "free" portions of T_4 and T_3 are metabolically available at the cellular level. The free portion of T_4 represents 0.02% to 0.05% of total serum T_4 and the free portion of T_3 represents 0.1% to 0.3% of total serum T_3 (Benvenga, 2005; Meier and Burger, 2005; Toft and Beckett, 2005). Most T_3 (>99.5%) is bound to TBG, but T_3 is not as tightly bound as T_4, allowing easier release into the free state.

Thyroid hormones exert their effect by binding to thyroid receptors (TRs) within cells. At the cellular level, T_3 is about

Table 35-1 Laboratory Tests for Evaluation of Thyroid Function

	Screening	Hyper	Hypo	Graves	CAT	Nodule	Thyroiditis	Other
TSH	Yes	Yes	Yes	Yes	Yes	Yes	Yes	No
T_4	No	No	No	No	No	No	No	No
T_3	No	Yes	No	Yes	No	No	No	No
FT_4	No	Yes	Yes	Yes	No	Yes	Yes	No
FT_3	No	No	No	No	No	No	No	No
Thyroglobulin	No	No	No	No	No	No	No	Yes
TSH-RS Abs	No	Yes	No	Yes	No	No	No	No
TPO Abs	No	No	No	No	Yes	No	No	No
Tg Abs	No	No	No	No	±	No	No	No
Thyroid microsomal Abs	No	No	No	No	No	No	Yes	±

TSH, Thyroid-stimulating hormone (thyrotropin); *CAT*, chronic autoimmune thyroiditis; *T_4*, thyroxine; *T_3*, triiodothyronine; *FT_4*, free thyroxine; *FT_3*, free triiodothyronine; *TSH-RS Abs*, TSH receptor-stimulator antibodies; *TPO Abs*, thyroid antiperoxidase antibodies; *Tg Abs*, thyroglobulin antibodies.

twice as biologically active as T_4, partly because T_3 binds to TRs 10 to 15 times more than T_4 (Yen, 2005). T_3 is the biologically active form of thyroid hormone. Thyroxine's role in this process appears to be that of a prohormone, providing a readily accessible reservoir for conversion to T_3; otherwise, its exact purpose is unknown (Bianco and Larsen, 2005).

Thyroid hormones (T_4 and T_3) regulate growth, development, and metabolism by affecting oxygen consumption and protein, carbohydrate, and vitamin metabolism. Around puberty, the effect on growth and development begin to wane, and in adults, thyroid hormones essentially affect only metabolism (Yen, 2005).

Normal thyroid function, in terms of circulating levels of T_4, T_3, free T_4 (FT_4), free T_3 (FT_3), and the thyrotropin feedback system, appears to remain stable throughout life. Without intrinsic disease of the hypothalamic-pituitary-thyroid axis, age does not appear to have an adverse effect on the function of the thyroid gland or its component parts, in terms of serum concentration of T_4 and T_3 (Oiknine and Mooradian, 2006). Although changes in measurable levels of total serum T_4 and T_3 do result from changes in transport protein concentrations, FT_4 and FT_3 levels remain mostly constant (Hassani and Hershman, 2006).

Laboratory Testing

Tests for thyroid disorders include laboratory, imaging, and biopsy. Before imaging or biopsy is undertaken, it is important to determine the functional state of the thyroid gland, even when the initial presentation is a thyroid mass or thyromegaly. This is accomplished via laboratory testing of a peripheral blood sample. These simple, and readily available, tests will provide direction for further workup.

The initial laboratory tests, regardless of the presenting complaint or finding, include sTSH and FT_4. The results of these initial studies help determine the functional state of the gland (hyperthyroid, euthyroid, or hypothyroid) and thus suggest which additional tests are required (Table 35-1).

Second-tier laboratory tests include thyroid antibodies and FT_3 if T_3 toxicosis is suspected. As noted previously, aging and comorbidities that affect circulating levels of thyroid transport protein can result in T_4 levels that appear abnormally low, suggesting a hypothyroid state. However, FT_4 and FT_3 will be normal, as will sTSH. Thyroid antibodies are useful in evaluating several disease states, primarily Graves' disease and chronic autoimmune thyroiditis (CAT, Hashimoto's thyroiditis). In Graves' disease the primary antibody class is TSH receptor-stimulator antibodies (TSH-RS Abs). In CAT the primary antibodies are thyroid antiperoxidase antibodies (TPO Abs) and thyroglobulin antibodies (Tg Abs). Patients with hypothyroidism occasionally exhibit TSH receptor-blocker antibodies (TSH-RB Abs), although the role this plays in the disease course is unclear. Thyroid microsomal antibodies (TPO Abs, Tg Abs) are occasionally seen in the self-limited processes of postpartum thyroiditis and silent thyroiditis.

Figure 35-1 provides an algorithm for diagnosing thyroid dysfunction.

Imaging

In the primary care office, ultrasonography is the first-line study for a palpable thyroid mass. The goal is to determine whether the mass is cystic, solid, or mixed. It is also used to provide a presumptive diagnosis of malignancy in the hands of an experienced radiologist, since malignant thyroid nodules have some very specific ultrasonographic characteristics. If the patient is hyperthyroid, with suppressed sTSH, ultrasound is done in conjunction with radioisotope scan.

Nuclear imaging utilizes iodine 123 (^{123}I) to evaluate gland activity. Patients with normal gland function will show homogeneity throughout the gland, with the exception of areas where cysts or nonfunctioning nodules are located. Patients with autonomously functioning nodules or multinodular goiter will show ^{123}I uptake in nodular areas,

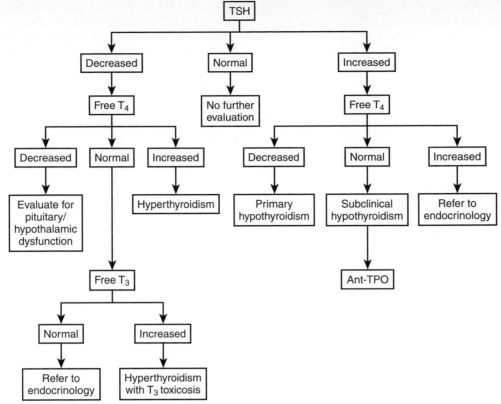

Figure 35-1 Algorithm for diagnosis of thyroid dysfunction, beginning with abnormal serum thyrotropin (sTSH) level.

with the remainder of the gland, under the control of sTSH, being hypoactive or inactive.

Computed tomography and MRI are not useful in diagnosis and treatment of nonmalignant diseases of the thyroid and thus are not recommended as initial studies. For biopsy-proven malignancy, CT and MRI can be useful preoperatively to define the area of involvement and for postoperative follow-up. CT and MRI should be reserved for the surgeon and oncologist.

Biopsy

Fine-needle aspiration (FNA) biopsy is a well-defined procedure for evaluating thyroid masses. It is safe and virtually painless in the hands of an experienced interventional radiologist, endocrinologist, or pathologist. When a definitive diagnosis cannot be made, and there is concern for possible malignancy, surgical referral is required. This usually results in a lobectomy or subtotal thyroidectomy.

Hyperthyroidism

Key Points

- Hyperthyroidism is diagnosed with a suppressed TSH and increased FT_4.
- Graves' disease is caused by abnormal response to circulating antithyroid antibodies.
- Serum TSH in Graves' disease is usually less than 0.1 mIU/L and may be unmeasurable.
- Diagnosis of Graves' disease in a patient without goiter and ophthalmic abnormality should be suspect.

Hyperthyroidism is a biochemical process represented by an increase in thyroid hormone biosynthesis and secretion (Toft, 2001). Diagnosis of hyperthyroidism is based on (1) sTSH level less than 0.1 mIU/L and (2) elevated FT_4 and/or T_3, and is often associated with symptoms consistent with a hypermetabolic state (Box 35-2). Determining the exact etiology requires further testing that includes laboratory studies and imaging (Box 35-3).

Graves' Disease

Graves' disease is the most common cause of hyperthyroidism and results from the development of TSH-RS Abs. These antibodies attach to TSH receptors in the thyroid gland and "mimic" action of TSH, stimulating production and release of T_4. Because of excess circulating T_4, the pituitary feedback loop for TSH production is suppressed, resulting in sTSH levels significantly less than 0.01 mIU/L. Serum TSH levels greater than 0.05 mIU/L, although not impossible with Graves' disease, should make the diagnosis suspect.

Graves' disease can present at the family physician's office as thyrotoxicosis or thyroid storm, but more often it presents with hypermetabolic symptoms or goiter. How it is treated initially will be determined by age, comorbidities, and acuity of symptoms. The primary symptomatic treatment is directed toward the cardiovascular responses of tachycardia, systolic hypertension, and volume depletion. Concurrent with this is the administration of antithyroid medication (propylthiouracil or methimazole). Once the patient's symptoms have been controlled, and there is evidence the hyperthyroid state is resolving, planning for long-term treatment can ensue.

Box 35-2 Symptoms Consistent with Hypermetabolic state

Tachycardia, wide pulse pressure

Systolic hypertension

Fever, tremor

Warm moist skin

Anxiety, hyperactivity

Diarrhea, weight loss

Modified from Braverman LE, Utiger RD. Introduction to thyrotoxicosis. In Braverman LE, Utiger RD [eds]. The Thyroid: a Fundamental and Clinical Text. 9th ed. Philadelphia, Lippincott, Williams & Wilkins, 2005.

Box 35-3 Common Causes of Hyperthyroidism

Autonomous functioning (toxic) nodule

Toxic multinodular goiter (TMNG, Plummer's disease)

Factitious disorder (Munchausen's disease)

Iatrogenic disease

TSH receptor-stimulator antibody production (Graves' disease)

Acute thyroiditis

TSH-producing pituitary tumor (adenoma)

TSH, Thyroid-stimulating hormone (thyrotropin).

Two courses of action can be followed for long-term treatment of Graves' disease. The goal is to maintain a euthyroid state. This can be accomplished with continued use of antithyroid medication, adjusting dose to maintain sTSH in a normal range. The alternative treatment is ablation of the thyroid gland using ^{131}I, usually requiring postradiation thyroid hormone replacement. Either is appropriate, and usually the patient must take some medication on a permanent basis. Occasionally, a patient will undergo spontaneous remission, so a trial of antithyroid medication for 6 months to 1 year may be worthwhile. This requires close follow-up, however, once the antithyroid medication is discontinued, in case the patient rebounds. The majority of patients elect radioactive ablation and long-term treatment with thyroxine replacement.

Intervention in hyperthyroidism begins with a β-adrenergic receptor blocker as a temporizing agent to control sympathetically mediated symptoms. Specific therapy is deferred pending confirmation of etiology. For Graves' disease, autonomously functioning nodule, or toxic multinodular goiter (TMNG), specific intervention includes propylthiouracil (PTU) or methimazole (MMI) to control thyroxine synthesis and, with PTU, to reduce conversion of T_4 to T_3 in the peripheral circulation. Once the patient is converted to a euthyroid state, specific treatment based on cause can be instituted.

With treatment of Graves' disease, the goiter found in more than 90% of these patients may shrink. However, large goiters often require surgery for satisfactory cosmetic appearance.

Thyroxine-Producing Nodules

Autonomously functioning thyroid nodules are found occasionally during workup for a hypermetabolic state or palpation of a thyroid mass. Autonomous nodules have a much higher incidence of occurring in iodine-deficient areas, accounting for approximately 60% of cases of thyrotoxicosis.

Autonomous functioning nodules and TMNG (Plummer's disease) result in sTSH and FT_4 values similar to those in Graves' disease, although sTSH is generally not less than 0.05 mIU/L. In both cases, one would expect the TSH-RS Abs to be negative or, at most, an extremely low titer. Evaluation includes radioisotope scan with ^{123}I, which will demonstrate the nodule(s). These tumors are rarely malignant, and treatment is surgical after appropriate thyroid suppression. Long-term results are excellent, with no expectation of recurrence.

For patients with TMNG and those with autonomous nodules who cannot tolerate surgery, ^{131}I ablation can be used. The ^{131}I is picked up by the most active portion(s) of the gland, so residual normally functioning thyroid gland often remains. However, iatrogenic hypothyroidism is always possible. After ^{131}I treatment of an autonomous nodule or TMNG, sTSH levels are required to determine if the gland can provide sufficient T_4 to meet physiologic requirements.

Other

See online text for other forms of hyperthyroidism (fictitious/iatrogenic thyrotoxicosis).

Thyrotoxicosis

Thyrotoxicosis is a physiologic process manifesting as hypermetabolism and hyperactivity that is caused by high serum concentrations of T_4, T_3, or both (Braverman and Utiger, 2005). It is not necessarily caused by excess hormone production and therefore may not represent a true hyperthyroid state. The cause of thyrotoxicosis in 2% to 4% of patients is elevated T_3 levels, with concomitant upper-limit normal T_4 levels (Meier and Burger, 2005).

Thyrotoxicosis has a predilection for female patients, tends to be more common in persons of northern European extraction, and is rare in blacks. Spontaneous thyrotoxicosis is most often caused by Graves' disease, accounting for 60% to 90% of all cases, followed by *silent,* or postpartum, thyroiditis caused by the sudden spike of circulating T_4, although it is transient and usually not clinically significant. Other less common, but not rare, causes of thyrotoxicosis include TMNG, autonomous functioning adenoma, and ingestion of exogenous thyroid hormone. Acute onset of thyrotoxicosis is almost always caused by thyroiditis. Thyrotoxicosis associated with Graves' disease has a more insidious course, evolving over a more protracted period. If a patient is thyrotoxic and the thyroid gland is not palpable, consider painless thyroiditis, unsuspected Graves' disease, or exogenous thyroxine. A thyrotoxic patient with a goiter or ophthalmopathy has Graves' disease until proven otherwise. Treatment of hypermetabolic symptoms should not be delayed pending further testing or referral.

Symptoms of hyperthyroidism in younger individuals are usually the result of sympathoadrenal activity, whereas elderly patients have an age-related desensitization of β-adrenergic receptors, which probably accounts for a blunting of some symptoms usually associated with hyperthyroidism (Oiknine and Mooradian, 2006; Trivalle et al.,

1996). In older individuals with altered sympathetic and parasympathetic function, symptoms of thyrotoxicosis tend to include cardiovascular dysfunction, dyspnea, weight loss, and proximal muscle weakness. Cardiovascular symptoms in elderly patients usually consist of resting tachycardia, wide pulse pressure, exercise intolerance, and dyspnea on exertion. Atrial fibrillation is uncommon but occurs more often in older individuals (5%-15%) (Franklyn and Gammage, 2005). Other cardiovascular effects that affect both young and old patients are decreased peripheral resistance, decreased cardiac filling times, increased blood volume, and fluid retention. Individuals with preexisting coronary artery disease (CAD) may have ischemic congestive heart failure (CHF) as a result of their hypermetabolic state, but this generally improves with appropriate antithyroid therapy. Atrial flutter, paroxysmal supraventricular tachycardia, premature ventricular beats, and ventricular fibrillation are rare as complications of thyrotoxicosis and may be a sign of unsuspected CAD.

Signs and symptoms of CHF are common in both young and old patients with thyrotoxicosis (Trivalle et al., 1996). Because of decreased effective circulating arterial volume, aldosterone secretion increases, with a concomitant increase in sodium retention that results in dependent edema. After thyrotoxicosis is effectively treated, all CHF symptoms quickly resolve. When present, periorbital edema is caused by Graves' disease. TSH-RS Abs needs to be checked.

Apathetic thyrotoxicosis is an uncommon presentation but represents the most common mental disorder associated with excess thyroid hormone production and release. Symptoms include apathy, lethargy, pseudodementia, weight loss, and depressed mood. It usually occurs in older patients without symptoms of tachycardia, hyperphagia, sweating, warm skin, or goiter (Wagle et al., 1998). This syndrome is easily confused with depression or dementia and, unless specifically sought, is easy to miss. A screening sTSH should be included in every depression or dementia workup.

Treatment of thyrotoxicosis is straightforward with three objectives: ameliorate acute symptoms, suppress synthesis and secretion of thyroid hormones, and treat the primary cause to prevent recurrence. Acute symptoms respond readily to beta-receptor blockers, which should be continued until FT_4 levels have returned to the normal range. Calcium channel blockers (CCBs) can be used in patients who cannot tolerate beta blockers. Inhibition of synthesis of thyroid hormones is achieved with PTU or methimazole. Adjunct therapies include fluid resuscitation with 5% dextrose or 10% dextrose in normal saline and administration of steroids. Fever generally responds satisfactorily to acetaminophen. The high fevers associated with thyroid storm may require cooling blankets. Nonsteroidal anti-inflammatory drugs (NSAIDs) and salicylates should be avoided in the acute phase due to competition for thyroid hormone–binding sites on transport proteins. This can cause release of bound thyroid hormone into the peripheral circulation. With aggressive therapy, acute symptoms of thyrotoxicosis should improve within 12 to 24 hours.

Once acute symptoms are controlled, treatment of the primary cause can be considered. This could include watchful waiting in the case of thyroiditis, surgery for an autonomously functioning adenoma, or ^{131}I in Graves' disease.

Thyroid Storm

Key Points

- Unrecognized thyroid storm has mortality as high as 75%.
- Thyroid storm is usually the result of another disorder that unmasks a preexisting but unidentified hyperthyroid state.
- Thyroid storm is a clinical diagnosis not defined by levels of TSH, T_4, or T_3.
- Suspicion of thyroid storm is a medical emergency with close monitoring (ICU) and appropriate consultation (endocrinologist).

Thyroid storm is a severe variant of thyrotoxicosis in which the metabolic state is sufficiently increased such that organ system failure can occur. It represents a rare complication of thyrotoxicosis and has a mortality rate as high as 75%, depending on how quickly it is recognized and treated (Tiegens and Leinung, 1995; Trzepacz et al., 1989; Wartofsky, 2005). Diagnosis of thyroid storm is based on clinical findings, not measured levels of circulating T_4 or sTSH. Thyroid storm is often precipitated by infection, which can cause symptoms that mask a thyrotoxic state. Clinical findings in thyroid storm include hyperpyrexia (>38.8° C [102° F]), tachycardia out of proportion to temperature, gastrointestinal (GI) dysfunction (nausea, vomiting, diarrhea, jaundice), and CNS dysfunction (marked hyperirritability, anxiety, confusion, apathy, coma) (Wartofsky, 2005). There is usually pronounced decompensation of one or more organ systems. Any patient presenting with goiter, fever, and marked tachycardia should be considered to be in thyroid storm and treated accordingly. Admission to the MICU and consultation with an endocrinologist is appropriate.

Treatment of thyroid storm includes beta blockers, antithyroid drugs, antipyretics, aggressive fluid replacement, and identification and treatment of any precipitating process. For patients with severe symptoms, Lugol's solution or potassium iodide (SSKI) will help inhibit release of T_4 into the peripheral circulation. If either is used, it should only be given after loading doses of antithyroid drugs, to block iodine-induced synthesis of T_4. Lithium also has an antithyroid effect and can be used in severe cases of thyroid storm. Severe thyrotoxic symptoms, unresponsive to all these regimens, may respond to sodium ipodate at 500 mg/day.

Hypothyroidism

Hypothyroidism is a hypometabolic state resulting from levels of circulating thyroid hormone insufficient to meet body requirements. Primary causes are listed in Box 35-4.

Chronic Autoimmune Thyroiditis (Hashimoto's Thyroiditis)

Key Points

- Hashimoto's thyroiditis is an autoimmune disorder that results in fibrosis of the thyroid gland.
- Hashimoto's thyroiditis is the most common cause of hypothyroidism in the United States.
- Diagnosis of Hashimoto's thyroiditis is based on an elevated TSH, low FT4, and antithyroid peroxidase antibodies (TPO Abs).

Box 35-4 Causes of Hypothyroidism

Insufficient intake of dietary iodine (uncommon in U.S.)
Autoimmune disease (primarily Hashimoto's thyroiditis)
Surgery (thyroid surgery)
Radiation exposure (head and neck)
Viral infection
Central disease (primary pituitary failure)

The most common cause of hypothyroidism worldwide is inadequate dietary intake of iodine. Because of the addition of iodine to table salt, however, this is a rare cause in the United States. In the U.S. and the rest of the developed world, the most common cause of hypothyroidism is chronic autoimmune thyroiditis (Hashimoto's disease). CAT is caused by the development of antithyroid antibodies that attack the thyroidal struma, causing progressive fibrosis; TPO Abs and Tg Abs appear to be responsible, with TPO Abs considered the primary cause (Dayan and Daniels, 1996). Diagnosis is based on elevated sTSH (>10.0 mIU/L), low-normal or low FT_4, and presence of TPO Abs.

Hashimoto's thyroiditis occurs most often in women, with a female/male ratio of 10:1 to 14:1. CAT is usually diagnosed in the fifth decade and is progressive (Vanderpump, 2005). As it progresses, more functioning thyroid gland will become fibrotic, and less endogenous T_4 will be produced. After diagnosis, replacement doses of T_4 should be used. In adults, average replacement dose of L-thyroxine is 1.6 µg/kg daily. Serum TSH is followed annually to ensure adequate control.

Other Forms of Hypothyroidism

Central hypothyroidism is caused by pituitary failure and is rare. The diagnosis is suggested with low to nonexistent sTSH levels in a patient without symptoms of hypermetabolism (thyrotoxicosis) and with low circulating FT_4. Generally, when presented with these data, further evaluation to determine the etiology of the hypothyroidism is not necessary. However, the patient should be evaluated for pituitary failure if not already done (see Pituitary Disorders).

Depending on the degree of injury to the thyroid gland, thyroiditis (postpartum, sporadic, and subacute) can result in a transient hypothyroid state, with eventual recovery. Subacute thyroiditis is more likely to undergo this process, with insufficient T_4 production for 3 to 6 months. Treatment is usually unnecessary, but low-dose thyroxine replacement can be used on a temporary basis for patients who become symptomatic.

Other causes of hypothyroidism include dietary iodine deficiency, surgery, ^{131}I radiation therapy, and nonthyroid head and neck cancer treatment.

Hypothyroidism is typically treated with L-thyroxine replacement alone. However, some believe that patients occasionally have T_4-resistant disease and recommend mixed T_4/T_3 replacement. Although true T_4 resistance is controversial, if a patient receiving replacement T_4 has sTSH in the therapeutic range but continues to complain of hypothyroid symptoms, combination T_4/T_3 can be tried to alleviate these symptoms.

Initial doses of L-thyroxine depend on the patient's age, duration of hypothyroid state, and comorbidities. The starting dose is generally 0.05 mg (50 µg) in a healthy young adult, with increases of 0.025 to 0.05 mg weekly, depending on clinical response. If the patient becomes tachycardic, is tremulous, or sweats, the increases are reduced to every 2 to 3 weeks. Once the patient is stabilized on 0.1 to 0.125 mg of L-thyroxine daily, further increases are made based on sTSH response. Serum TSH needs to be checked only every 4 to 6 weeks. More frequent testing does not allow sufficient interval for developing homeostasis and can result in overdosing. Once the patient is receiving a steady dose, further treatment is adjusted so that sTSH remains at 0.5 to 4.5 mIU/L (mean, 2.5). Doses of L-thyroxine resulting in sTSH less than 0.1 mIU/L indicate iatrogenic hyperthyroidism and should be avoided.

Thyroiditis

Forms of thyroiditis include postpartum (silent); sporadic, which is a variant of postpartum but outside the postpartum period; subacute (granulomatous); chronic autoimmune (Hashimoto's); and "other," which includes bacterial or pyogenic (Farwell, 2005; Lazarus, 2005). The forms usually encountered in primary care are postpartum, sporadic, and chronic autoimmune, which are all autoimmune diseases, and subacute, which is thought to be viral in etiology.

The mechanism of injury to the thyroid gland is disruption of thyroid architecture caused by lymphocytic infiltration, resulting in leakage of colloid-stored thyroxine into the peripheral circulation. This nonphysiologically triggered leakage of stored T_4 causes a spike in peripheral circulating T_4 and transient hypermetabolic symptoms. Early testing in the disease can demonstrate an elevated FT_4 level, although not necessarily outside the normal range. Depending on duration of the destructive process and degree of injury, sTSH may be normal, low normal, or low. If the cause of this variability is not appreciated, it could lead to the erroneous initial diagnosis of Graves' disease (increased FT_4 and low sTSH). With protracted acute thyroiditis, however, sTSH is not as low as in Graves' disease and TSH-RS Abs titers are low to absent. In addition, patients with acute thyroiditis will lack the optic findings and goiter of Graves' disease.

As a general rule, acute thyroiditis is a short-lived process, with T_4 stores being rapidly depleted. This represents a case of thyrotoxicosis (increased circulating T_4) but not hyperthyroidism (increased production of T_4). Follow-up testing over the next few weeks demonstrates progressively lower T_4 levels, which eventually return to normal. As T_4 levels return to normal (and below), the acute hypermetabolic symptoms will begin to decline. Duration of T_4 elevation determines how low the sTSH value will go and how quickly it will return to normal.

Subclinical Thyroid Disease

Key Points

- Subclinical thyroid disease is based on TSH levels only marginally outside the normal reference ranges in an asymptomatic patient with normal FT_4.
- Screening for subclinical thyroid disease is *not* recommended by the American Association of Clinical Endocrinologists (AACE), U.S. Preventive Services Task Force (USPSTF), or American Academy of Family Physicians (AAFP).

- The American Thyroid Association (ATA) recommends screening all adults for thyroid disorder beginning at age 35 and then every 5 years.
- Treatment of subclinical hyperthyroid disease is not recommended, although follow-up should occur every 6 months.
- Treatment of subclinical hypothyroid disease is recommended by the American College of Physicians (ACP) for women over 50 with symptoms consistent with hypothyroidism.

Discussion about subclinical thyroid disease has focused on whether it is a real clinical entity. Subclinical thyroid diseases are defined as (1) subclinical hyperthyroidism (or subclinical thyrotoxicosis) with sTSH less than 0.1 mIU/L and normal circulating FT$_4$ and FT$_3$ or (2) subclinical hypothyroidism with sTSH greater than 4.5 mIU/L but less than 10.0 mIU/L with normal circulating FT$_4$. Both entities assume a patient who is asymptomatic or has minimal signs and symptoms (Ross, 2005a, 2005b).

The primary question concerning subclinical thyroid disease is whether early intervention is beneficial and patients should be screened. The only disease state that has been directly related to subclinical thyroid disease is overt hypothyroidism. Individuals with subclinical hypothyroidism have a higher incidence of progression to overt hypothyroidism than the general population. Annually, 3% to 5% of patients identified with subclinical hypothyroidism will progress to overt hypothyroidism with sTSH levels over 10.0 mIU/L (Toft and Beckett, 2005). The majority of these represent early CAT (Hashimoto's thyroiditis). Currently, no consensus exists among national organizations as to whether these patients should start therapy during this phase of their disease. Treating those with symptoms seems appropriate, but there is no evidence to support the premise that early treatment alters the disease course or associated comorbidities (hyperlipidemia, hypertension, CAD) (Helfand, 2004).

Studies demonstrate a two to three times higher incidence of atrial fibrillation in patients with subclinical hyperthyroidism compared to individuals with normal sTSH levels (Ross, 2005b). The Framingham data suggest some individuals with subclinical hyperthyroidism are at increased risk of paroxysmal atrial fibrillation (Oiknine and Mooradian, 2006). However, no data support early intervention. Osteoporosis is associated with overt hyperthyroidism, and some speculate that treating subclinical hyperthyroidism may prevent or delay this process. The American Association of Clinical Endocrinologists (AACE, 2002) recommends treatment of subclinical hyperthyroidism caused by nodular thyroid disease.

Anatomic Diseases

Anatomic diseases of the thyroid gland include a number of primary and secondary disorders (Box 35-5). The list includes goiter, nodules, primary neoplasia, metastatic neoplasia (rare), and familial disorders.

Goiter

Goiter is the most common anatomic disease, and the major cause of goiter worldwide is iodine deficiency. When simple goiter occurs in areas of adequate iodine intake, there appears to be a strong genetic component to the disease. In the United States, goiter is usually associated with CAT

Box 35-5 Anatomic Diseases of Thyroid

Goiter: Simple, toxic, iodine deficiency
Nodule: Adenoma, incidental, toxic
Cyst: Simple, complex
Malignancy
Primary: Papillary/follicular, medullary, lymphoma
Metastatic: Lymphoma, breast, pulmonary, other
Familial: Multiple endocrine neoplasia type IIA (MEN-IIA)
      Familial medullary carcinoma of thyroid (FMCT)

(Hashimoto's thyroiditis) as the disease progresses to a hypothyroid state. Goiter is the result of both hypertrophy and hyperplasia of the thyroid gland. In the case of iodine deficiency, this is caused by excess thyrotropin production, leading to glandular growth and colloid production.

In Graves' disease, stimulation of the thyroid by TSH-RS Abs causes excess production of T$_4$ and T$_3$, in turn resulting in uncontrolled production of colloid to store the excess production of thyroid hormone. In fact, goiter is the most common clinical finding in Graves' disease after thyrotoxicosis, occurring in almost 100% of patients (Chiovato et al., 2001). Goiter is one of the five hallmarks of Graves' disease. Goiter, associated with hypothyroidism, will often improve once euthyroid doses of thyroxine have been achieved, although it may take 6 months to 1 year. If the goiter does not involute with thyroxine replacement, excision may be required. Besides goiter, the other four hallmarks of Graves' disease are thyrotoxicosis, ophthalmopathy, local myxedema, and acropachy (clubbing of fingers and toes).

Nodules and Cysts

Thyroid nodules come in a variety of sizes and types. The incidence of malignancy in nodules less than 1.0 cm, which are found incidentally during nonthyroid-related diagnostic procedures (e.g., head and neck ultrasonography), is less than 0.5%. Current recommendations for evaluation of incidentalomas include a sTSH and FT$_4$ and careful palpation of the thyroid gland (Cooper et al., 2009). If tests and palpation are normal, only annual follow-up with palpation by the physician is recommended. As long as growth remains minimal, and there are no ultrasonographic hallmarks of malignancy on the initial scan, these nodules can be monitored clinically. Exceptions might include patients with a family history of thyroid cancer, personal history of head and neck radiation, primary malignancy in another part of the body, or rapid growth.

A palpable thyroid mass requires evaluation. If the sTSH is within normal range, and a local endocrinologist experienced in FNA is available, referral without imaging is appropriate. If the patient has a suppressed sTSH, however, the nodule may be functioning autonomously. Before any intervention (surgical or FNA), a radioisotope ^{123}I scan is indicated. If the lesion is "hot," suppression is the course of action. If "cold," this could represent a cystic, mixed, or solid mass requiring further evaluation by FNA (first choice) or surgical exploration (Fig. 35-2).

Benign nodules do not require therapeutic intervention. If the nodule is large, a trial of thyroxine to decrease its size is

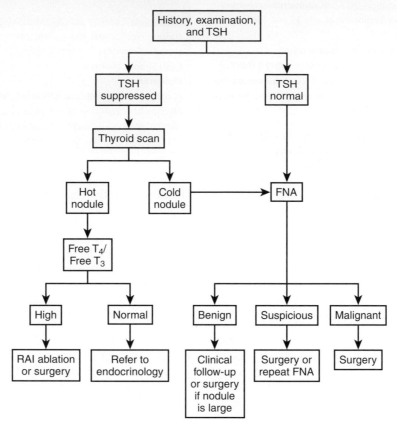

Figure 35-2 Algorithm for clinical evaluation of thyroid nodule.

appropriate but generally ineffective. If the nodule's size is causing symptoms (tracheal compression or pain), excision is the treatment of choice.

Malignancy

Malignancy of the thyroid, both primary and secondary, is rare, accounting for less than 2% of all cancers, and generally, tumors are not aggressive. *Papillary carcinoma* is the most common, accounting for approximately 80% of primary thyroid malignancies. Follicular carcinoma, which arises from the same cell type as papillary carcinoma, accounts for about 5% of thyroid neoplasia. Undifferentiated and anaplastic carcinoma makes up less than 10% of all thyroid malignancies and medullary carcinoma of the thyroid about 5% (Baloch and Livolsi, 2005). The most common cancers that metastasize to the thyroid are breast, lung, and kidney. Primary lymphoid cancer occurs in the thyroid, but its incidence is unknown since it cannot be distinguished from lymphoma that originates elsewhere in the body. Treatment of thyroid cancers is generally surgical with ^{131}I therapy after near-total thyroidectomy. As with cancer elsewhere in the body, primary treatment will depend on tissue diagnosis and clinical evaluation.

Two familial thyroid malignancies are multiple endocrine neoplasia type IIA (MEN-IIA) and familial medullary thyroid carcinoma (FMTC). MEN-IIA is an autosomal dominant disorder that can cause "C" cell hyperplasia and hyperparathyroidism. Diagnosis is often serendipitously found during evaluation for hypercalcemia or renal calculi.

Nodules less than 1.0 cm usually do not require FNA, but any solitary nodule occurring before 14 years of age is an exception, with greater than 50% incidence of malignancy.

Long-Term Follow-up of Thyroid Disorders

For patients receiving long-term thyroid therapy for hypothyroidism, monitoring is through sTSH unless there is hypothalamic-pituitary disease. It takes 2 to 4 weeks after initiating treatment (or changing dose) before clinically significant change occurs in sTSH level. In most patients, checking sTSH once monthly is sufficient until steady state is reached. After the patient is stabilized, sTSH can be checked annually unless the patient develops new symptoms or dosing changes.

Patients with benign nodules should be followed annually with careful palpation of the thyroid gland. Unless there is a change in size, no additional testing is required. Ultrasound of the thyroid is not recommended for follow-up of nodules less than 1.0 cm. Repeat ultrasound is required in patients with an enlarging nodule, evidence of a new thyroid mass, or who complain of pain or pressure. Unless the patient is experiencing symptoms of hyperthyroid or hypothyroid, repeat testing of sTSH or FT_4 is not indicated.

Sick Euthyroid Syndrome (Thyroid Hormone Adaptation Syndrome)

Thyroid function can be suppressed during severe illness and may not represent abnormal thyroid function. Serious illness has been shown to affect laboratory tests of thyroid function (sTSH, T_4, thyroglobulin), but there is no clear evidence this reflects a disease state (Chopra, 1997). Because these changes appear to have no direct adverse effect on the patient's overall clinical state, this condition is labeled "sick euthyroid syndrome." In broad terms, sick euthyroid syndrome is more of academic interest than clinical. Administration of T_4 to a seriously ill individual does not improve outcome for most patients, although evidence suggests that high doses of T_3 immediately after cardiac surgery may be beneficial (Wiersinga, 2005). The physician should remember the rare patient whose thyroid disease is uncovered by serious illness. If a seriously ill patient is not responding as expected (e.g., difficulty in weaning from ventilator support), checking thyroid function may be appropriate, although any interpretation of results should be reviewed by a clinician experienced in interpreting thyroid tests in seriously ill patients before intervention. Patients with preexisting thyroid dysfunction will continue to require thyroid therapy during a severe illness. However, individuals who were euthyroid at presentation generally do not require or improve with thyroid replacement therapy.

Drugs Affecting Thyroid Function and Testing

Key Points

- Therapeutic drugs have a variety of effects on thyroid function, including delayed or suppressed synthesis.
- Therapeutic drugs may block the effect of thyroid hormone at the cellular level.
- Phenothiazines, dopamine, phenytoin, and glucocorticoids block release of TSH from the pituitary.
- Amiodarone can cause both hyperthyroidism and hypothyroidism. In the United States, because of generally adequate dietary iodine, amiodarone causes a hypothyroid state.

Many common drugs can affect thyroid function, bioavailability of thyroid hormone, and laboratory testing. Drugs that affect thyroid function fall into several categories; some inhibit synthesis of T_4, some block secretion of T_4, some block TSH release, some affect extrathyroidal conversion of T_4 to T_3, and some influence thyroxine at the tissue/cellular level. PTU and methimazole (MMI) inhibit thyroid hormone synthesis by interfering with thyroid peroxidase. PTU has the added advantage of inhibiting extrathyroidal conversion of T_4 to T_3. Neither PTU nor MMI inhibits T_4 release (secretion) from the thyroid gland.

Amiodarone, lithium, and cytokines can affect synthesis and secretion. In the absence of iodine, amiodarone can precipitate both hyperthyroid and hypothyroid events. In the United States, where dietary iodine is plentiful, patients taking amiodarone tend to develop hypothyroidism from fibrosis of the thyroid gland. The incidence is approximately 20% (Harjai and Licata 1997; Roti and Vagenakis, 2005). Patients taking these drugs, especially amiodarone, should be screened regularly with sTSH for developing thyroid dysfunction. Dopamine, glucocorticoids, and phenytoin inhibit release of TSH from the anterior pituitary. Salicylates and other NSAIDs, furosemide, heparin, and enoxaparin compete for binding sites on thyroid hormone transport proteins. Use of these drugs in acute thyroid disease can potentially exacerbate thyrotoxic symptoms by releasing thyroid hormone into the peripheral circulation. TSH and FT_4 should be monitored in regular users of these medications (Table 35-2).

Phenytoin, phenobarbital, carbamazepine, and rifampin stimulate hepatic enzymatic activity, thus shortening thyroid hormone clearance times and increasing conversion of T_4 to T_3. Serum TSH levels should be monitored routinely, until stable, when these medications are added or deleted from a patient's regimen. Sucralfate, cholestyramine, calcium carbonate, aluminum hydroxide, soy products, and ferrous sulfate inhibit absorption of exogenous L-thyroxine from the gut. Again, oral L-thyroxine should be taken on an empty stomach.

Beta blockers exert their effect on thyroid hormones at the cellular level, and benzodiazepines block T_3 uptake at the cellular level (Wartofsky, 2005; Tiegens and Leinung, 1995; Hedley et al., 1989). Calcium channel–blocking agents inhibit uptake of thyroid hormone by hepatic and muscle cells (Table 35-3).

Thyroid Disease in Pregnancy

Pregnancy can exacerbate an already-existing thyroid disorder, thus requiring extra vigilance by the family physician. Careful monitoring and proactive clinical intervention are key. The majority of women with hypothyroidism, who are euthyroid on stable doses of thyroid replacement, will require increased doses of thyroxine replacement during their pregnancy. Being aware of this need and prepared to make dosage adjustments in a timely manner is important. Consulting an endocrinologist to help with the care of these patients is advised (Shankar et al., 2001).

Silent (postpartum) thyroiditis during pregnancy is essentially a benign, short-term disease and requires only symptomatic treatment. Occasional checks of sTSH and FT_4 levels are justified to monitor recovery.

Table 35-2 Drugs that Affect Thyroid Function at Glandular Level

Drug	Inhibits T_4 Synthesis	Blocks T_4 Secretion	Blocks TSH Release
Iodine	Yes	—	—
Propylthiouracil	Yes	—	—
Methimazole	Yes	—	—
Antipsychotic	—	—	Yes
Amiodarone	Yes	Yes	—
Lithium	Yes	Yes	—
Phenytoin	—	—	Yes
Dopamine	—	—	Yes
Glucocorticoid	—	—	Yes
Cytokines	Yes	Yes	—

T_4, Thyroxine; *TSH*, thyroid-stimulating hormone (thyrotropin).

Table 35-3 Drugs that Affect Thyroid Function at the Peripheral Level

Drugs	Compete for Protein Binding	Inhibit Deiodi-nation of T_4 to T_3	Inhibit Action at Tissue Level	Inhibit Uptake of T_3 at Tissue Level	Affect Thyroid Hormone Clearance Time	Inhibit GI Absorption	Adverse Effect on Lab Tests
Phenytoin	—	—	—	—	Yes	—	—
Phenobarbital	—	—	—	—	Yes	—	—
Carbamazepine	—	—	—	—	Yes	—	—
Rifampin	—	—	—	—	Yes	—	—
Salicylates	Yes	—	—	—	—	—	Yes
NSAID	Yes	—	—	—	—	—	Yes
Furosemide	Yes	—	—	—	—	—	Yes
Heparin	Yes	—	—	—	—	—	Yes
Enoxaparin	Yes	—	—	—	—	—	Yes
Sucralfate	—	—	—	—	—	Yes	—
Ca carbonate	—	—	—	—	—	Yes	—
Al hydroxide	—	—	—	—	—	Yes	—
Soy	—	—	—	—	—	Yes	—
Ferrous sulfate	—	—	—	—	—	Yes	—
PTU	—	—	Yes	—	—	—	Yes
Dexamethasone	—	Yes	—	—	—	—	Yes
Beta blocker	—	Yes	Yes	—	—	—	Yes
Benzodiazepine	—	—	—	Yes	—	—	—
CCB	—	—	—	Yes	—	—	—
Amiodarone	—	Yes	—	—	—	—	—
Contrast agent	—	Yes	—	—	—	—	—

GI, Gastrointestinal; *NSAID*, nonsteroidal anti-inflammatory drug; *Al*, aluminum; *Ca*, calcium, *PTU*, propylthiouracil; *CCB*, calcium channel blocker.

For the rare pregnant patient who requires suppression of T_4 synthesis, judicious use of antithyroid drugs (PTU and MMI) is generally considered safe. There is some concern that MMI may cross the placental barrier more readily than PTU, but this has not proved to be a concern in the clinical setting. It is important, however, to remember that prolonged suppression of the thyroid, or suppression late in pregnancy, can result in a transient depression of neonatal thyroid function and may induce goiters in the neonate. PTU and MMI can be found in breast milk. This has not been of concern as long as the dose is kept low. PTU (maximum, 150 mg/day) and MMI (maximum, 20 mg/day) caused no problems with a nursing child (Glinoer, 2005). Both PTU and MMI are category D pregnancy risk; the American Academy of Pediatrics reports no sign or symptom in infants of adverse effects on lactation and supports use of drugs during breastfeeding. In the United States, PTU has generally been the antithyroid drug of choice in pregnant and nursing women, although in June 2009 the FDA issued a MedWatch warning for PTU concerning reports of hepatotoxicity, which may change this pattern.

Screening for Thyroid Disease

Screening for asymptomatic thyroid disease is controversial, although screening in specific populations may be beneficial. Women over age 50 have the highest incidence of spontaneous hypothyroidism compared with all males and mixed younger populations, approaching 5% per year. Thus, screening has a good chance of finding disease early. However, the evidence supporting benefit from early intervention is weak and probably does not justify cost. Patients who present with paroxysmal atrial fibrillation should be routinely screened for hyperthyroidism, although the incidence of positive findings is low (AACE, 2002).

One area where screening is advantageous is patients with newly diagnosed dementia. This is especially true if the clinical course is atypical or accelerated. Both hypothyroidism (myxedema) and hyperthyroidism (apathetic thyrotoxicosis) can present with dementia-like symptoms, and in these patients, timely intervention can completely reverse the signs and symptoms of dementia or depression caused by thyroid dysfunction. If screening is undertaken, the test of choice is sTSH. When coupled with FT_4, the vast majority of clinically significant hyperthyroidism and hypothyroidism can be diagnosed. If symptoms are present, or there are overt signs of disease, the initial testing should include sTSH, FT_4, and FT_3. Thyroid panels providing T_4, T_3, T_7, FT_4 index, and T_3 uptake are no longer advocated (AAFP, 2009; Helfand, 2004; Ladenson et al., 2000).

KEY TREATMENT

Thyrotoxicosis is treated initially with beta blockers and antithyroid medication to control symptoms and stop synthesis/release of thyroid hormone into the peripheral circulation (Oiknine et al., 2006; Trivalle et al., 1996) (SOR: A).

Hypothyroid (TSH >10 mIU/L) replacement T_4 dose is approximately 1.6 µg/kg/day (Oiknine et al., 2006) (SOR: A).

With the exception of thyroid antibody–positive subclinical hypothyroidism, prophylactic treatment has not shown positive effect on lipids or CAD risk (Helfand, 2004) (SOR: A).

Subclinical hyperthyroidism should be treated when caused by nodular thyroid disease (ACCE, 2002) (SOR: B).

Adrenal Glands

The adrenal glands are located at the superomedial aspects of the kidneys. The glands consist of two endocrine tissues of different embryologic origin: the primarily steroid-producing adrenocortical tissue in the cortex and the catecholamine-producing chromaffin cells in the medulla. The adrenal cortex consists of three zones that vary in both morphologic features and hormones produced. The outer *zona glomerulosa* is the unique source of the mineralocorticoid aldosterone. The intermediate *zona fasciculata* and the inner *zona reticularis* produce the glucocorticoids cortisol and corticosterone and the androgens dehydroepiandrosterone (DHEA) and DHEA sulfate. The chromaffin cells in the adrenal medulla mainly secrete the catecholamines epinephrine and norepinephrine (Williams and Dluhy, 2008) (Box 35-6).

Mineralocorticoids are major regulators of extracellular fluid volume and potassium metabolism. Volume is regulated through a direct effect on the collecting duct of the kidney, where aldosterone causes an increase in sodium retention and in potassium excretion. The release of aldosterone is regulated by the renin-angiotensin system, plasma potassium levels, and adrenocorticotropic hormone (ACTH). The renin-angiotensin system maintains the circulating blood volume constant by regulating aldosterone secretion. Aldosterone-induced sodium retention occurs in volume deficiency states, but the aldosterone-dependent sodium retention is reduced when volume is ample. An increase in plasma potassium or a decrease in plasma sodium stimulates aldosterone release. ACTH stimulates mineralocorticoid output, but this effect on aldosterone secretion is transient.

Box 35-6 Adrenal Gland Anatomy and Steroids

Cortex

Zona glomerulosa
- Aldosterone

Zona fasciculata

Zona reticularis
- Glucocorticoids
- Cortisol
- Corticosterone
- Dehydroepiandrostenedione (DHEA)
- DHEA sulfate (DHEA-S)

Medulla
- Epinephrine
- Norepinephrine
- Dopamine

The release of *cortisol*, the main glucocorticoid in humans, is pulsatile and is directly stimulated by ACTH or its precursors, such as pro-opiomelanocortin. The release of ACTH from the anterior pituitary is regulated by corticotropin-releasing hormone (CRH) produced by the hypothalamus. High cortisol levels inhibit the biosynthesis and secretion of CRH and ACTH through a negative-feedback mechanism. Cortisol release follows a circadian rhythm, with its highest level in the morning, and is sensitive to light, sleep, stress and disease. The glucocorticoid effects are multisystemic. They stimulate proteolysis and gluconeogenesis, inhibit muscle protein synthesis, and increase fatty acid mobilization. Gluconeogenesis results in the increase of blood glucose concentrations. At high levels, glucocorticoids are catabolic and result in loss of lean body mass. Glucocorticoids modulate the immune response through their anti-inflammatory effects, and modulate perception and emotion in the CNS.

The production of the adrenal androgens is controlled by ACTH, not by gonadotropins. Among the adrenal androgens, DHEA is the most abundant circulating hormone in the body and is readily conjugated to its sulfate ester DHEA-S. The adrenal androgens are converted into androstenedione and subsequently into potent androgens (testosterone) or estrogens (estradiol) in the peripheral tissues. The adrenal secretion of DHEA and DHEA-S increases in children at age 6 to 8 years and peaks at 20 to 30 years. However, the production of DHEA-S by the adrenal glands is reduced by 70% to 95% during the aging process; at age 70, serum DHEA-S levels are at approximately 20% of their peak values and continue to decrease with age. Adrenal androgens have minimal effects in males whose sexual characteristics are predominantly determined by gonadal steroids (testosterone). In females, adrenal-derived testosterone is important in maintaining pubic and axillary hair. Adrenal androgen hypersecretion in adult males causes no clinical signs but in females manifests with signs of hirsutism and masculinization.

The adrenal medulla secretes epinephrine, norepinephrine, and dopamine. Most catecholamine output in the adrenal vein is epinephrine; norepinephrine also enters the circulation from noradrenergic nerve endings. In emergency situations, secretion of adrenal catecholamines is increased to prepare the individual for stress ("fight or flight" response). Hypoglycemia and certain drugs are also potent stimuli to catecholamine secretion.

Disorders of Cortical Hypofunction

Primary Adrenal Insufficiency

Key Points

- Primary adrenal insufficiency is defined as the failure of the adrenal cortex to produce glucocorticoids and mineralocorticoids.
- The most frequent cause of primary adrenal insufficiency is autoimmune. In the developing world, however, tuberculosis remains the most common cause.
- Symptoms are usually insidious, including fatigue, orthostatic hypotension, weight loss, and hyperpigmentation.
- Acute adrenal insufficiency should be considered in critically ill patients with unexplained hypotension.
- A baseline cortisol and ACTH level followed by an ACTH stimulation test can establish diagnosis.
- Detection of adrenal cortex antibodies or 21-hydroxylase autoantibodies supports the diagnosis of autoimmune adrenalitis. Abdominal CT may be helpful if other causes are suspected.

Primary adrenal insufficiency (AI) is defined as the failure of the adrenal cortex to produce adequate amounts of glucocorticoids and mineralocorticoids. Primary AI can result from processes that damage the adrenal glands or from drugs (ketoconazole, etomidate) that block the synthesis of cortisol. All causes of primary AI involve the adrenal cortex as a whole and result in a deficiency of cortisol and aldosterone (plus adrenal androgen), although the severity of the deficiencies may vary. An exception is the *syndrome of isolated glucocorticoid deficiency*. The reported prevalence of primary AI (Addison's disease) in developed countries is 39 to 60 per 1 million population. In adult patients, mean age at diagnosis is 40 years (range, 17-72).

The most frequent cause of primary AI in developed countries is *autoimmune adrenalitis*. However, in the developing world, tuberculosis remains the most common cause of adrenal failure. Autoimmune adrenalitis is sometimes accompanied by other autoimmune endocrine deficiencies (autoimmune polyglandular syndromes, APS). The adult form (type II, Schmidt's syndrome) of polyglandular syndrome consists mainly of AI, autoimmune thyroid disease, and insulin-dependent (type 1) diabetes mellitus. Several infectious processes associated with acquired immunodeficiency syndrome (AIDS) such as cytomegalovirus (CMV), *Mycobacterium tuberculosis, Cryptococcus neoformans, Mycobacterium avium intracellulare, Histoplasma capsulatum,* and Kaposi's sarcoma, may damage the adrenal gland and lead to insufficiency. In young males, adrenoleukodystrophy (or the less severe adrenomyeloneuropathy), an X-linked recessive disorder of metabolism of long-chain fatty acids, can cause spastic paralysis and adrenal insufficiency. AI can precede neurologic symptoms and should prompt the clinician to perform careful neurologic examination in young males with primary AI. Other causes are listed in Box 35-7.

Box 35-7 Causes of Primary Adrenal Insufficiency

Autoimmune
Isolated adrenal insufficiency (Addison's disease)
Polyglandular autoimmune syndrome types I and II

Infectious
Tuberculosis
Fungal
 Histoplasmosis
 Paracoccidioidomycosis
HIV/AIDS
Cytomegalovirus
Syphilis
African trypanosomiasis

Vascular
Bilateral adrenal hemorrhage
Sepsis (Waterhouse-Friderichsen syndrome)
Coagulopathy
Thrombosis, embolism
Infarction

Infiltrative
Metastatic carcinoma (most often lung, breast, stomach, colon)
Lymphoma
Sarcoidosis
Amyloidosis
Hemochromatosis

Congenital
Congenital adrenal hyperplasia
 21α-Hydroxylase deficiency
 11β-Hydroxylase deficiency
 3β-ol-Dehydrogenase deficiency
 20,22-Desmolase deficiency
 Familial adrenocorticotropic hormone resistance syndromes
 Familial glucocorticoid deficiency
 Adrenoleukodystrophy
 Adrenomyeloneuropathy
Adrenal hypoplasia

Iatrogenic
Bilateral adrenalectomy
Anticoagulation therapy
Drugs
 Adrenolytic: mitotane, aminoglutethimide, metyrapone, trilostane
 Other: ketoconazole, rifampin, etomidate, phenytoin, barbiturates, megestrol acetate

---

Chronic (Primary) Adrenal Insufficiency

Most of the symptoms are nonspecific and occur insidiously. Chronic AI manifestations include weakness, chronic fatigue, anorexia, unintentional weight loss, listlessness, joint pain, and orthostatic hypotension. Some patients may initially present with GI symptoms (abdominal pain, nausea, vomiting, diarrhea), whereas others may present with symptoms that can be attributed to depression or anorexia nervosa. In contrast to secondary AI, primary AI is often associated with lack of aldosterone as well as cortisol. Thus, signs of mineralocorticoid deficiency (salt craving, postural hypotension, electrolyte abnormalities) are usually indicative of primary AI. The most specific sign of primary AI is *hyperpigmentation* of the skin and mucosal surfaces, which results from the melanocyte-stimulating activity of β-lipotropin derived from the same precursor as ACTH. Patients with autoimmune adrenalitis present with vitiligo, Hashimoto's thyroiditis (70% in APS-II), type 1 diabetes, and pernicious anemia. Thinning or loss of pubic and axillary hair may occur in women as a result of lack of androgen production by the adrenal cortex. Both systolic and diastolic blood pressure (BP) are usually reduced (systolic BP <110 mm Hg).

Acute (Primary) Adrenal Insufficiency

In critically ill patients, it is crucial to consider the possibility of adrenal insufficiency. AI should be suspected in the presence of unexplained catecholamine-resistant hypotension, especially if the patient has pallor, hyperpigmentation, vitiligo, scanty axillary and pubic hair, hyponatremia, or hyperkalemia. Furthermore, AI due to adrenal hemorrhage and adrenal vein thrombosis should be considered in a severely ill patient with abdominal pain or rigidity, vomiting, confusion, and arterial hypotension. In acutely ill patients, plasma cortisol level greater than 25 g/dL rules out adrenal insufficiency, but a level in the normal range does not; further testing may be required.

Laboratory Evaluation

Patients with adrenal insufficiency present with hyponatremia (frequent), hyperkalemia, acidosis, mild elevation of plasma creatinine concentrations, hypoglycemia, hypercalcemia (rare), mild normocytic anemia, lymphocytosis, and mild eosinophilia. In addition, hormone levels are useful in diagnosis. A random measurement of serum cortisol level is usually inadequate to assess adrenal function because of the pulsatile and diurnal variation of cortisol secretion. However, a morning cortisol level (8-9 AM) of 3 μg/dL or less indicates primary AI and obviates the need for further tests; a level of 19 μg/dL or greater rules AI out; patients with levels of 3 to 19 μg/dL need further testing. If primary AI is suspected, basal ACTH and cortisol levels should be measured, followed by a short ACTH stimulation test. For testing, synthetic ACTH (cosyntropin) is given IV or IM at 250 μg and serum cortisol is measured 60 minutes after injection. A normal response to this test (cortisol 20 μg/dL or higher) excludes primary AI. In patients with severe secondary AI, plasma cortisol increases little or not at all after the administration of cosyntropin because of adrenocortical atrophy.

Detection of adrenocortical antibodies or 21-hydroxylase autoantibodies supports the diagnosis of autoimmune adrenalitis. Antibodies against other endocrine glands are common in patients with autoimmune AI, and evaluation might be warranted. However, the incidence of antiadrenal antibodies in serum from patients with normal adrenal function who have other autoimmune endocrine diseases is low (2%), with the exception of those with hypoparathyroidism (16%). Abdominal CT scan may be helpful if infection, hemorrhage, infiltration, or neoplastic disease is suspected.

Treatment

In chronic AI, any underlying cause, such as infection or malignancy, should be treated. Glucocorticoid replacement is usually required for symptomatic patients and is given in two or three daily doses with half to two thirds of the daily dose given in the morning to mimic the physiologic daily pattern of cortisol secretion. Hydrocortisone (15-25 mg/day) or cortisone acetate (25-37.5 mg/day) is preferred because of its mineralocorticoid action and shorter biologic half-life, which prevents unfavorably high nighttime glucocorticoid activity. The goal is to use the smallest dose that relieves the patient's symptoms to prevent side effects from steroid use, such as weight gain and osteoporosis. Because a reliable marker of glucocorticoid action is lacking, clinical judgment and careful assessment of clinical signs and symptoms guide treatment.

In patients with primary AI, mineralocorticoid replacement is necessary and is attained by fludrocortisone, in a single daily dose of 0.05 to 0.2 mg, as a substitute for aldosterone. The dose can be adjusted based on measurements of BP, serum sodium and potassium, and renin activity (aiming at concentrations within the middle or upper-normal range). All patients should carry a card or wear a medical alert bracelet or necklace with information on current treatment and recommendations in emergency situations. Patients should be advised to double or triple the dose of hydrocortisone temporarily when they have a febrile illness or injury. In addition, they should be given ampules of glucocorticoid for self-injection or glucocorticoid suppositories to be used in case of vomiting.

Secondary and Tertiary Adrenal Insufficiency

Key Points

- Secondary adrenal insufficiency results from ACTH deficiency and is often seen in panhypopituitarism or after chronic glucocorticoid excess.
- Lack of production of CRH from the hypothalamus results in tertiary adrenal insufficiency.
- In secondary adrenal insufficiency, mineralocorticoid production is maintained by the renin-angiotensin system. Thus, hyperkalemia is absent while hyponatremia may result from loss of glucocorticoid effect on free-water clearance.
- Low ACTH and cortisol levels suggest secondary or tertiary adrenal insufficiency.

Secondary adrenal insufficiency is defined as a deficiency of ACTH. Isolated ACTH deficiency is rare and may be congenital or caused by lymphocytic hypophysitis. Secondary AI more often occurs in the setting of panhypopituitarism from underlying causes such as pituitary or metastatic tumors, craniopharyngioma, infections (TB, histoplasmosis), infiltrative disease (sarcoidosis), head trauma, or postpartum pituitary necrosis (Sheehan's syndrome). Chronic glucocorticoid excess, either exogenous (glucocorticoid treatment for more than 4 weeks) or endogenous (Cushing's syndrome), causes secondary AI by prolonged suppression of CRH production. Tertiary adrenal insufficiency results from the lack of CRH production from the hypothalamus.

Clinical Presentation

Signs and symptoms are similar to those of primary AI, but electrolyte and fluid abnormalities and hypotensive symptoms are absent because the mineralocorticoid production is still maintained by the renin-angiotensin system. Hyperpigmentation is not seen. Menstrual dysfunction, headache and visual symptoms, hypothyroidism, and diabetes insipidus may be present as a result of panhypopituitarism (see Pituitary Disorders).

Laboratory Evaluation

Plasma cortisol and ACTH levels should be checked initially. Low ACTH (<5 pg/mL) and cortisol levels suggest secondary or tertiary adrenal insufficiency, and pituitary CT or MRI is indicated. The cosyntropin stimulation test may be helpful in identifying adrenal insufficiency. With an abnormal result, ACTH level may determine primary (high ACTH) versus secondary (normal or low ACTH) disease. However, in secondary AI the ACTH-stimulation test might not be abnormal because sufficient ACTH might be present to prevent adrenal gland atrophy. In these patients, CRH stimulation test can assess ACTH response. Secondary AI shows little or no increase in the ACTH or cortisol level throughout the test, but in tertiary AI the ACTH increases in an exaggerated fashion and remains elevated longer. The insulin tolerance test and the metyrapone test are also available (but less often used) to assess the integrity of the hypothalamic-pituitary-adrenal (HPA) axis by its response to hypoglycemia or the inhibited cortisol synthesis, respectively.

Treatment

As described in primary AI, treatment of underlying disorders and glucocorticoid replacement are necessary in secondary and tertiary AI, but not mineralocorticoid replacement.

Isolated Aldosterone Deficiency

See the discussion online at www.expertconsult.com.

Disorders of Cortical Hyperfunction: Hypercortisolism

Cushing's Syndrome

Key Points

- Cushing's syndrome results from chronic exposure to excessive levels of glucocorticoids.
- Cushing's syndrome may be ACTH dependent (pituitary or ectopic tumors) or ACTH independent (exogenous glucocorticoids).
- Reddish purple striae, plethora, proximal muscle weakness, easy bruising, and unexplained osteoporosis are discriminatory symptoms.
- CT or MRI of the adrenals may differentiate between the various types of ACTH-independent Cushing's syndrome.

Cushing's syndrome is a group of signs and symptoms that result from prolonged and inappropriately high exposure of tissue to glucocorticoids. Excess cortisol production is the hallmark of endogenous Cushing's syndrome and may result from excess ACTH secretion from the pituitary (Cushing's disease) or from ectopic tumors secreting ACTH or CRH. ACTH-independent adrenal production of cortisol is caused by adrenocortical tumors or hyperplasias. However, the most common cause of Cushing's syndrome is *iatrogenic* from exogenous glucocorticoid administration. Certain psychiatric disorders (anxiety, depression), poorly controlled diabetes, and alcoholism can be associated with mild hypercortisolism and may produce results suggestive of Cushing's syndrome (Nieman et al., 2009).

Clinical Presentation

Although Cushing's syndrome might be easy to diagnose when full blown, the diagnosis can be challenging in mild cases. The spectrum of clinical presentation is broad. Some discriminatory symptoms include reddish purple striae, plethora, proximal muscle weakness, bruising without any obvious trauma, and unexplained osteoporosis. More often, patients present with features caused by cortisol excess, such as obesity, depression, diabetes, hypertension, or menstrual irregularity. Dorsocervical fat pad (buffalo hump), facial and supraclavicular fullness, thin skin, peripheral edema, hirsutism or female balding, and poor skin healing are typically seen in Cushing's syndrome. Children usually have slow growth, abnormal genital virilization, short stature, and pseudoprecocious or delayed puberty.

Laboratory Evaluation

Before the diagnosis of Cushing's syndrome is considered, exogenous intake of glucocorticoids should be excluded. According to the 2008 Endocrine Society Clinical Practice Guidelines, tests to consider for diagnosis include urine free cortisol (UFC), late-night salivary cortisol, 1-mg overnight dexamethasone suppression test (DST), or the longer, low-dose DST (2 mg/day for 48 hours). UFC and salivary cortisol should be obtained at least twice. The diagnosis of Cushing's syndrome is made if two tests are unequivocally abnormal. The diagnostic accuracy of other tests previously used, such as random cortisol levels, is too low to recommend them for testing (Fig. 35-3).

The UFC provides an integrated assessment of cortisol secretion over 24 hours and measures the cortisol not bound to cortisol-binding globulin (CBG). Unlike serum cortisol, which measures both free and CBG-bound cortisol, UFC is not affected by conditions and medications that alter CBG. A 24-hour urine cortisol secretion or an overnight urine sample (10 PM to 8 AM) can be ordered in conjunction with urine creatinine to ensure accuracy of the results. UFC reflects renal filtration, and values are significantly lower in moderate to severe renal impairment. A patient can be assumed to have Cushing's syndrome if basal urinary cortisol secretion is more than three times the upper limit of normal and one other test is abnormal. However, UFC may be normal in patients with mild Cushing's syndrome, in whom salivary cortisol may be more useful.

Late-night salivary cortisol is usually measured at bedtime or between 11 PM and 12 AM as the loss of circadian rhythm, with absence of a late-night cortisol nadir, is a consistent biochemical abnormality with Cushing's syndrome. The active free cortisol in the blood is in equilibrium with cortisol in the saliva, and the concentration of salivary cortisol does not appear to be affected by the rate of saliva production. Overall in adults, the accuracy of the test is similar to that of UFC.

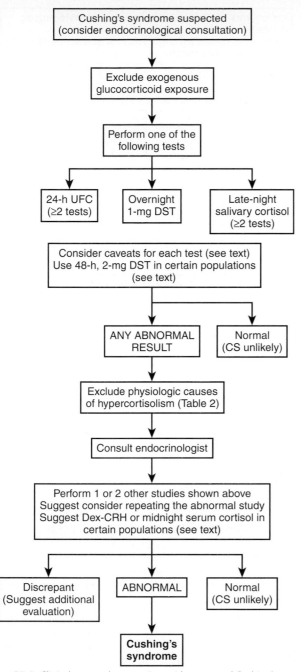

Figure 35-3 Clinical approach to a patient with suspected Cushing's syndrome. *(Courtesy The Endocrine Society.)*

may be helpful in conditions with overactivation of the HPA axis but without true Cushing's syndrome, such as in certain psychiatric disorders, obesity, and alcoholism. Dexamethasone is given in doses of 0.5 mg every 6 hours for 48 hours, beginning at 9 AM on day 1, at 6-hour intervals (at 9 AM, 3 PM, 9 PM, and 3 AM). Serum cortisol is measured at 9 AM, 6 hours after the last dose of dexamethasone (Funder et al., 2008).

Additional testing is recommended for patients with initial abnormal or discordant results, such as the dexamethasone-CRH stimulation test or the midnight serum cortisol test. The dexamethasone-CRH stimulation test has been developed to improve the sensitivity of the LDDST. Dexamethasone at 2 mg/day over 48 hours is followed by administration of CRH (1 μg/kg IV) 2 hours after the last dose of dexamethasone. Cortisol is measured 15 minutes later. ACTH and cortisol should increase after administration of CRH in patients with Cushing's disease.

After hypersecretion of cortisol is confirmed, the next step is to determine if the Cushing's syndrome is ACTH dependent or independent. This is accomplished through measurement of the late-afternoon ACTH level, which is normally low. Cushing's syndrome is ACTH *dependent* if plasma ACTH is greater than 10 pg/mL and ACTH *independent* if ACTH is less than 5 pg/mL. For an intermediate ACTH level, further testing with the CRH stimulation test is performed. A rise in cortisol by 20% or in ACTH of at least 50% over baseline after administration of CRH is considered evidence for an ACTH-dependent lesion. In these patients, high-dose dexamethasone suppression test (HDDST), combined with cranial MRI studies, may help in localizing the site of ACTH overproduction. HDDST (2 mg dexamethasone every 6 hours for 2 days) provides close to 100% specificity if the criterion used is suppression of urinary free cortisol by more than 90% and can differentiate Cushing's disease from ectopic ACTH production. If workup results are still equivocal, or suggestive of ectopic ACTH production, inferior petrosal sampling is performed, obtaining ACTH samples from the periphery and petrosal sinuses simultaneously. A petrosal sinus/peripheral ACTH ratio of 2:1 is diagnostic of a pituitary source and can be further used to localize the side of ACTH production from the pituitary gland.

For patients with ACTH-independent lesions, abdominal CT or MRI may localize the site of the lesion.

Treatment

The treatment of Cushing's syndrome depends on the cause. For endogenous disease, surgical resection of the causative tumor is indicated. The treatment of choice for Cushing's disease is transsphenoidal hypophysectomy. Other treatments include various forms of radiation therapy and pharmacologic inhibition of ACTH secretion.

Patients with adrenal adenomas are treated with unilateral adrenalectomy and have excellent prognosis. These patients require glucocorticoid therapy both during and after surgery until the residual adrenal gland recovers. For patients with biopsy-proven adrenal carcinoma that is not amenable to surgery, mitotane is the treatment of choice. For ectopic ACTH syndrome, ideal treatment is the excision of identified benign tumors. However, for ectopic tumors that are unidentified or unresectable, medications that block steroidogenesis, such as ketoconazole, metyrapone, and aminoglutethimide, may be useful.

Various protocols have been used for the DST but most often, 1 mg of dexamethasone is given between 11 PM and 12 AM and cortisol measured between 8 and 9 AM the following morning. In patients with endogenous Cushing's syndrome, a low dose of dexamethasone fails to suppress ACTH and cortisol secretion. A normal response is a serum cortisol of 5 μg/dL or less. To enhance DST sensitivity, experts advocate requiring a lower cutoff for suppression of the serum cortisol to 1.8 μg/dL or less to achieve sensitivity rates greater than 95%.

Some endocrinologists prefer to use the 48-hour, 2-mg/day, low-dose DST (LDDST) as an initial test because of its improved specificity compared with the 1-mg test. LDDST

Aldosteronism

Key Points

- In primary aldosteronism, secretion of aldosterone is inappropriately high and, when the result of an adrenal adenoma, it is relatively autonomous from renin-angiotensin secretion.

- Secondary aldosteronism is generally related to hypertension, and the aldosterone secretion is driven by high plasma renin.

- Patients present with hypokalemia and hypertension that may be resistant to treatment.

- The plasma aldosterone/renin ratio is the most reliable test for screening for primary aldosteronism.

- A plasma aldosterone/renin ratio of 20 or greater and plasma aldosterone higher than 15 ng/dL support the diagnosis of primary hyperaldosteronism.

Primary aldosteronism (PA) was first described by Jerome Conn in 1955 as a syndrome (Conn's syndrome) characterized by hypertension and hypokalemia caused by an adrenal aldosterone-producing adenoma. The secretion of aldosterone from the adrenal zona glomerulosa is regulated mainly by the renin-angiotensin system (RAS) and by potassium anions. PA is now recognized to be the most common form of secondary hypertension. In PA the secretion of aldosterone is inappropriately high, relatively autonomous from the RAS, and nonsuppressible by volume expansion or sodium loading. In secondary aldosteronism associated with hypertension, the aldosterone secretion is driven by high plasma renin and is suppressed by volume expansion (Funder et al., 2008; Young, 2007).

Primary aldosteronism is typically caused by an aldosterone-producing adenoma (APA, 35% of cases), by unilateral or bilateral idiopathic adrenal hyperplasia (IHA) (2% and 60%, respectively), by an adrenal carcinoma (rare), or in rare cases, familial hyperaldosteronism (FH), either type I (glucocorticoid-remediable aldosteronism [GRA]) or type II (familial occurrence of APA or IHA, or both). There are two types of aldosteronomas: a corticotrophin-responsive (and renin-unresponsive) type and a renin-responsive type. PA had been previously described in less than 1% of patients with hypertension. However, recent studies estimate the prevalence of PA is 5% to 13% among hypertensive patients.

Clinical Presentation

Few symptoms are specific to the syndrome. Patients present with moderate to severe hypertension that may be resistant to usual pharmacologic treatments. Hypokalemia is usually present, and serum sodium concentration tends to be high-normal or slightly above the upper limit of normal. Patients with marked hypokalemia may have muscle weakness and cramping, headaches, palpitations, polydipsia, polyuria, or nocturia. However, hypokalemia might be absent; thus any patient with hypertension could be a candidate for this disorder. Patients with PA may be at higher risk than other patients with hypertension for target-organ damage of the heart and kidney. A significantly higher rate of cardiovascular events (stroke, atrial fibrillation, myocardial infarction) has been noted in patients with APA or IHA when compared with patients matched for age, gender, and hypertension. Patients with APA have more severe hypertension, more frequent hypokalemia, higher plasma and

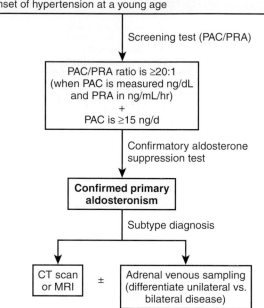

Figure 35-4 Indications for screening for primary aldosteronism and flow chart for clinical assessment.

urinary levels of aldosterone, and are younger (<50 years) than those with IHA.

Hypokalemia, when present, strongly suggests associated mineralocorticoid excess. However, most patients with primary PA have baseline blood levels of potassium in the normal range. Therefore, hypokalemia should not be the criterion used to make the diagnosis of PA. Screening for PA should be considered in patients with: hypertension and hypokalemia, treatment-resistant hypertension (three antihypertensive drugs and poor control), severe hypertension (≥160 mm Hg systolic or ≥100 diastolic), hypertension and an incidental adrenal mass, and onset of hypertension at a young age (Fig. 35-4). When an evaluation for secondary hypertension is performed, the diagnosis of PA should also be considered. In patients with suspected PA, the screening can be accomplished by measuring a morning ambulatory paired random plasma aldosterone concentration (PAC) and plasma renin activity or concentration (PRA or PRC). This test can be performed while the patient is taking antihypertensive medications (except for spironolactone, eplerenone, and high-dose amiloride) and without posture stimulation. The aldosterone/renin ratio (ARR) is currently the most reliable means of PA screening. A test is considered positive when the PAC/PRA ratio is 20:1 or greater (when PAC is measured in ng/dL and PRA in ng/mL/hr) and the PAC is higher than 15 ng/dL. All positive results should be followed by a confirmatory aldosterone suppression test to verify autonomous aldosterone production before treatment is initiated.

Aldosterone suppression testing can be performed with oral sodium chloride and measurement of urinary aldosterone or with IV sodium chloride loading and measurement of PAC. On the third day of the high-sodium diet, a 24-hour urine specimen is collected for measurement of aldosterone, sodium, and creatinine. Hypertension and hypokalemia should be controlled before the administration of the sodium load. Urinary aldosterone excretion greater than 12 μg/24 hr, when there is adequate sodium repletion (24-hour urinary sodium excretion ≥200 mmol), is consistent with autonomous aldosterone secretion. The IV saline infusion will suppress PAC to less than 5 ng/dL in normal subjects, but not to less than 10 ng/dL in patients with PA.

If the diagnosis of PA is confirmed, lateralization of the source of the excessive aldosterone secretion is critical to guide further management. All patients with PA should undergo an adrenal CT scan as the initial study in subtype testing and to exclude large masses that may represent adrenocortical carcinoma. MRI has no advantage over CT in subtype evaluation of PA. In patients with PA, adrenal venous sampling is the reference standard test to differentiate unilateral from bilateral disease. This is important because unilateral adrenalectomy in patients with APA or primary adrenal hyperplasia results in normalization of hypokalemia and improvement of hypertension in all patients and cure of hypertension in 30% to 60%. Glucocorticoid-remediable aldosteronism is an autosomal dominant disease and may be diagnosed by genetic testing.

Treatment

The treatment approach depends on the cause of PA. Unilateral laparoscopic adrenalectomy is an excellent treatment option for patients with APA or unilateral hyperplasia. BP control improves in almost 100% of these patients postoperatively, and the average long-term cure rates of hypertension after unilateral adrenalectomy for APA range from 30% to 72%. A potassium supplement and/or a mineralocorticoid receptor antagonist should be given preoperatively to correct the hypokalemia but should be discontinued postoperatively.

Medical management is recommended for patients with APA who do not undergo surgery and for these with IHA or GRA. Spironolactone has been the drug of choice for PA and is titrated to achieve BP control and normokalemia without the aid of oral potassium supplement. Eplerenone is a competitive and selective aldosterone receptor antagonist and may be used as an alternative agent. Compared with spironolactone, eplerenone has less antiandrogenic and progestational actions but is more expensive. In patients intolerant to aldosterone receptor antagonists, amiloride may be an alternative treatment that can reduce BP and normalize potassium levels, but it does not protect against the negative effects of aldosterone excess. Patients with IHA may be resistant to drug therapy because of hypervolemia and may require a second antihypertensive agent such as a thiazide diuretic in combination with the aldosterone receptor antagonist.

Disorders of Hyperfunction: Adrenal Medulla

Pheochromocytoma

Key Points

- Pheochromocytomas are catecholamine-secreting neuroendocrine tumors that originate in the adrenal medulla (85% of cases) or in any sympathetic ganglion (paragangliomas).
- Hypertension, tachycardia, pallor, palpitations, diaphoresis, and anxiety are common.

- Paroxysmal hypertension often occurs, even in normotensive persons, and may result in hypertensive emergencies.
- Plasma and urine catecholamines and metanephrines are measured to diagnose pheochromocytoma.
- CT, MRI, and ^{123}I-MIBG may be helpful for tumor localization.

Pheochromocytomas are catecholamine-secreting neuroendocrine tumors arising from chromaffin cells of neural crest origin. About 80% to 85% of pheochromocytomas originate in the adrenal medulla, and 15% to 20% are extra-adrenal (paragangliomas). Pheochromocytomas are rare tumors, with an incidence of 1 to 2 per 100,000 adults per year. Sporadic forms of pheochromocytoma are usually diagnosed in individuals age 40 to 50 years, whereas hereditary forms are diagnosed earlier, most often before age 40. The traditional "rule of 10" for pheochromocytomas (10% bilateral, 10% extra-adrenal, 10% familial, 10% malignant) is now challenged by advances in diagnosis and genetics. Hereditary pheochromocytomas occur in MEN-II, von Hippel–Lindau syndrome, neurofibromatosis type 1, and familial paragangliomas. Pheochromocytoma is rare in children but, when found, are often extra-adrenal, multifocal, and associated with hereditary syndromes (Lenders et al., 2005).

Clinical Presentation

Paroxysmal signs and symptoms caused by the episodic secretion of catecholamines provide clues to the diagnosis of pheochromocytoma. The presentation can vary greatly, and therefore the pheochromocytoma is often referred to as the "great mimic." Anesthesia and tumor manipulation are the most well-known stimuli to elicit a catecholaminergic crisis. Hypertension, tachycardia, pallor, palpitations, diaphoresis, headache, and feelings of panic or anxiety are common. The hypertension is often paroxysmal and may occur in patients with hypertension or in normotensive persons. The hypertensive episodes can be severe, resulting in hypertensive emergencies. Persons with paragangliomas may have normal BP or hypotension. Orthostatic hypotension (a result of hypovolemia), fever, nausea, flushing, leukocytosis, and polycythemia are less common findings. Metabolic abnormalities may be present and include hyperglycemia, lactic acidosis, and weight loss.

Laboratory Evaluation

All patients with suspected pheochromocytoma should undergo biochemical testing. Traditional tests include measurements of urinary and plasma catecholamines, urinary metanephrines (normetanephrine and metanephrine), and urinary vanillylmandelic acid (VMA). Measurement of plasma-fractionated metanephrines (normetanephrine and metanephrine) is a newer test. Plasma and urine metanephrine measurements are the most sensitive tests for diagnosis but do not always indicate a pheochromocytoma. Many physiologic stimuli (e.g., stress), drugs (e..g, phenoxybenzamine, tricyclic antidepressants), and clinical conditions (e.g., hyperthyroidism, heart failure, stroke) may cause an increase in circulating catecholamines and metabolites and lead to false-positive results. The use of clonidine or glucagon to suppress catecholamine release from the sympathoadrenal system provides a dynamic pharmacologic test to distinguish increased catecholamine release due to sympathetic activation from increased release due to a pheochromocytoma.

If there is biochemical evidence for pheochromocytoma, tumor localization by CT scan of the entire abdomen (and pelvis), with and without contrast, should be performed. MRI with gadolinium has similar diagnostic sensitivity (90%-100%) and specificity (70%-80%) and is usually the preferred modality, especially for extra-adrenal lesions. Iiodine-123 metaiodobenzylguanidine (^{123}I-MIBG) isotope scanning has increased specificity (95%-100%) over CT and MRI and is more appropriate for patients with extra-adrenal, metastatic, multifocal, or recurrent disease.

Treatment

Preoperatively, phenoxybenzamine, prazosin, doxazosin, or urapidil can be used for the blockade of alpha adrenoceptors. Phenoxybenzamine is often preferred because it blocks alpha adrenoceptors noncompetitively. Alternative drugs for preoperative management are labetalol or calcium channel blockers, either alone or in combination with α-adrenergic receptor blockers. Treatment must be initiated 10 to 14 days preoperatively and is titrated until mild orthostasis (systolic BP should not fall below 90 mm Hg in standing position) is present. Blockade of beta adrenoceptors should never be initiated before blockade of alpha adrenoceptors. Laparoscopic removal of intra- and extra-adrenal pheochromocytomas is the preferred surgical approach. All patients should be followed up every year for at least 10 years after surgery. BP and catecholamines should be monitored indefinitely in patients with extra-adrenal or familial pheochromocytoma to detect possible recurrence. For malignant disease, radical surgical removal is recommended, but survival remains poor (~50%). Treatment with ^{131}I-MIBG or combination chemotherapy has shown disappointing results.

Mixed Disorder: Congenital Adrenal Hyperplasia

See the discussion online at www.expertconsult.com.

KEY TREATMENT

In primary adrenal insufficiency, long-term glucocorticoid and mineralocorticoid replacement is necessary. Baseline steroid dose should be increased twofold to threefold during febrile illness or injury (Arlt and Allolio, 2003; Oelkers, 1996; Salvatori, 2005) (SOR: A).

Therapeutic intervention for secondary and tertiary adrenal insufficiency requires treatment of underlying disorders. Glucocorticoid replacement is necessary (Arlt and Allolio, 2003; Oelkers, 1996; Salvatori, 2005) (SOR: A).

Oral fludrocortisone (0.05-0.20 mg daily) is the treatment of choice for aldosterone deficiency. In hyporeninemic hypoaldosteronism, furosemide with reduced salt intake can ameliorate acidosis and hyperkalemia (Arlt Allolio, 2003; Oelkers, 1996) (SOR: A).

Surgical resection is usually the treatment of choice for Cushing's disease and ACTH-independent Cushing's syndrome (Nieman et al., 2009) (SOR: A).

Treatment of aldosteronism is directed at the underlying cause. Aldosterone antagonists such as spironolactone are effective therapy (Funder et al., 2008) (SOR: A).

Laparoscopic removal of intra- and extra-adrenal pheochromocytomas after alpha-adrenoceptor blockade is the preferred treatment (Lenders et al., 2005) (SOR: A).

Treatment of congenital adrenal hyperplasia with glucocorticoids may result in amelioration of symptoms (New, 2004) (SOR: A).

Ovarian and Testicular Disorders

Sexual development in both males and females is driven by the hypothalamic-pituitary axis. The normal process is the result of pulsatile release of GnRH from the hypothalamus, which stimulates the pituitary to release FSH and LH (GHRH and GH also play a role). Release of FSH and LH activates the ovary and testis to produce estrogen and testosterone and is responsible for stimulation of gametogenesis. This process is assisted by conversion of adrenal androgens from the adrenal cortex into androstenedione and subsequently into potent androgens (testosterone) or estrogens (estradiol) in the peripheral tissues (see Adrenal Glands). Errors can occur along this complex pathway, resulting in early sexual development (precocity), delayed sexual development (delayed menarche), errors of translation (male feminization syndrome), early loss of reproductive function (premature menopause), and inappropriate response to stimuli (polycystic ovary syndrome).

Normal Sexual Development

Sexual differentiation in humans is controlled by genetics (presence of Y chromosome determines development of testis and absence determines development of ovary with additional X chromosome), environment (e.g., nutrition), and hormones (MacLaughlin and Donahoe, 2004). Congenital conditions associated with aberrations of chromosomal, gonadal, or anatomic sexual development are called "disorders of sex development (DSD)" (Houk et al., 2006). In the postgonadal phase, hormones control external genitalia differentiation and secondary sexual development. Puberty refers to a physiologic transition phase (>4 years) between childhood and adulthood during which there is pubertal growth spurt and development of secondary sexual characteristics. Puberty is preceded by adrenarche (6-7 years in females and 7-8 years in males), marked by increasing amounts of adrenal androgens (DHEA, DHEA-S, and androstenedione). The growth spurt (striking increase in growth velocity during puberty) is a complex hormonal phenomenon in which GH, thyroid hormones, and sex steroids play a major role. Gonadarche (secretion of gonadal sex steroids) follows adrenarche and is initiated by activation of the GnRH pulse generator in the hypothalamus. These GnRH pulses result in increased gonadotropin secretion and subsequent production of sex hormones by the gonads.

Sexual maturation in females starts with breast development (thelarche) at a mean age of 11 years, followed by pubic hair development and menses (menarche). In males it starts with scrotal corrugation and testicular enlargement at a mean age of 11.5 years, followed by growth of the penis and pubic hair.

In males, release of LH stimulates testicular Leydig cells to produce testosterone. FSH, in conjunction with testosterone, stimulates spermatogenesis. In females, FSH stimulates development of primary ovarian follicles and increases production of estrogen from ovarian granulosa cells. LH in females stimulates ovarian theca cells to produce androgens and the corpus luteum to synthesize progesterone. LH induces ovulation through the midcycle surge.

Estradiol production in males increases the bone age, bone mineral density, and rate of epiphyseal fusion. In females it stimulates the development of breasts, labia, vagina, and uterus and proliferation of endometrium. In addition, estradiol enhances development of, and increase in, the ducts of the breast and body fat. Estrogen in low levels enhances linear growth, and high levels increase the rate of fusion of epiphyses. Testosterone is responsible for the increase in muscle mass, sebaceous glands, and voice changes seen in pubertal males and is a linear growth accelerator. In females, testosterone accelerates linear growth and stimulates pubic and axillary hair development. Progesterone in females is responsible for development of a secretory endometrium and plays a role in breast development. Linear growth and pubic hair development in both males and females are caused by androgens from the adrenal gland. Figures 35-5 and 35-6 show normal pubertal developmental stages of Marshall and Tanner.

Abnormal Puberty

Key Points

- Evaluation should begin if signs of puberty develop in girls younger than 8 years or boys younger than 9 years.

- Diagnoses of true puberty and pseudopuberty should be differentiated.
- Evaluation includes a comprehensive history and physical examination, growth chart, and wrist radiograph.
- If true puberty is suspected, consider cranial CT or MRI to rule out CNS lesions.

Evaluation of suspected abnormal puberty begins with obtaining a detailed history, including growth and development (timing of physical and developmental milestones), medical conditions, dietary history, social history, ethnicity, and family history. Physical examination should be thorough, including current weight and a focus on development of secondary sexual characteristics and genitalia. A detailed growth chart from birth to present day should be obtained. A radiograph of the left wrist is needed to estimate bone age (Blondell et al., 1999).

Precocious Puberty

Precocious puberty (early puberty) may be defined as the appearance of secondary sexual maturation at an early age. The age of onset of puberty before age 8 years in girls and

Tanner stage	Breasts*	Standard	Pubic hair*	Standard	Growth	Other
1	Prepubertal, elevation of papilla only	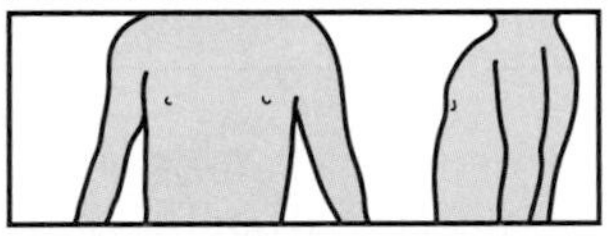	Prepubertal, villus hair only	—	Basal; about 5.0 to 6.0 cm (2.0 to 2.4 in) per year	Adrenarche Ovarian growth
2	Breast bud appears under enlarged areola (11.2 years)	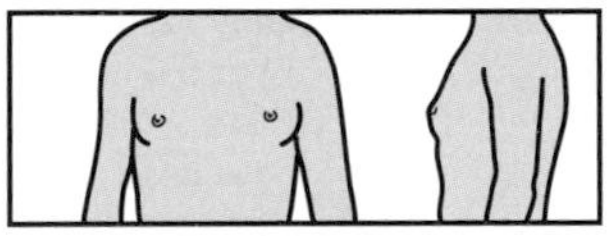	Sparse growth of slightly pigmented hair along the labia (11.9 years)	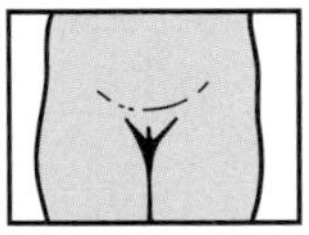	Accelerated: about 7.0 to 8.0 cm (2.8 to 3.2 in) per year	Clitoral enlargement Labia pigmentation Uterus enlargement
3	Breast tissue beyond areola without contour separation (12.4 years)	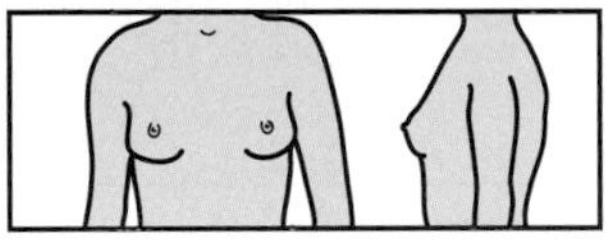	Hair is coarser, curled and pigmented; spreads across the pubes (12.7 years)	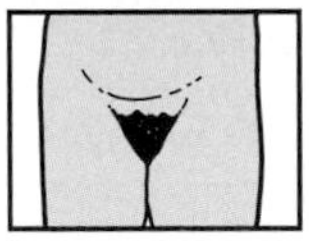	Peak velocity: about 8.0 cm (3.2 in) per year (12.5 years)	Axillary hair (13.1 years) Acne (13.2 years)
4	Projection of areola and papilla forms a secondary mound (13.1 years)	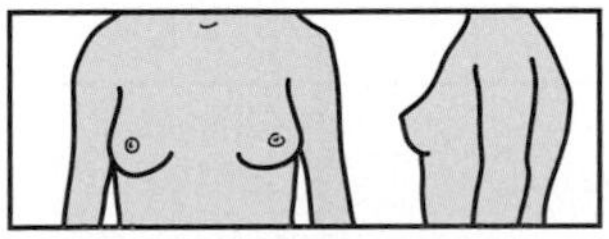	Adult-type hair but no spread to medial thigh (13.4 years)	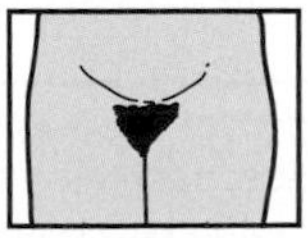	Deceleration: <7.0 cm (2.8 in) per year	Menarch (13.3 years) Regular menses (13.9 years)
5	Adult breast contour with projection of papilla only (14.5 years)	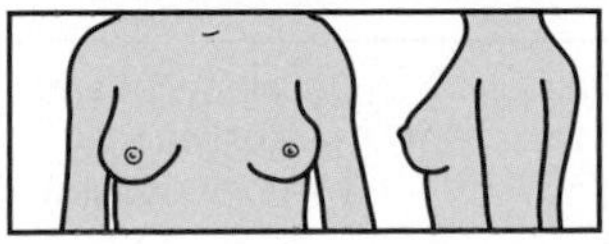	Adult-type hair with spread to medial thigh but not up linea alba (14.6 years)	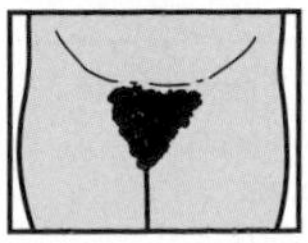	Cessation at about 16 years	Adult genitalia

*The Tanner stages of puberty in girls are based on breast size and shape and pubic hair distribution. Mean age of milestone attainment is shown in parentheses for the reference population of Marshall and Tanner. Actual age at milestone attainment may vary among individuals and among different study populations.

Figure 35-5 Pubertal milestones for girls. (*From Blondell Rd, Foster MB, Dave KC. Disorders of puberty. Am Fam Physician 1999;60:209, 223.*)

9 years in boys is considered precocious puberty. The Lawson Wilkins Pediatric Endocrine Society guidelines recommend that breast development or pubic hair in white girls before age 7 and black girls before age 6 should be evaluated for precocious puberty. Boys of all races should be evaluated for precocious puberty with signs of secondary sexual development at age 9 or younger (Kaplowitz and Oberfield, 1999). These guidelines are under some debate as setting perhaps too early an age for defining precocity. Some child endocrinologists believe that defining precocity as only those children with sexual development younger than 7 years will lead to missing some conditions that may respond to early intervention; they prefer the formerly used age of less than 8 years in girls to trigger investigation (Carel and Léger, 2008; Midyett et al., 2003; Traggiai and Stanhope, 2003). Children with developmental disabilities have a higher incidence of precocity (Siddiqui et al., 1999). However, most patients (>75%) investigated for precocious puberty will have benign diagnoses that are considered normal variations and do not require treatment (Kaplowitz, 2004).

Precocious puberty is classified as *central* (GnRH dependent) or *peripheral* (non–GnRH dependent). The peripheral group includes autonomous gonadal activation, gonadal tumors with production of sex steroids, adrenal disorders, and exposure to exogenous agents with properties of sex steroids. Precocious puberty may be differentiated into *progressive* (one stage to next in 3-6 months) or *nonprogressive* (no progression of pubertal signs over time). Other terminology is based on the pubertal signs in relation to the individual's gender. *Isosexual* refers to precocity in the same gender (e.g., feminization of a female). *Heterosexual* (or contrasexual) would be precocious puberty resulting in virilization of a female.

Benign variants of precocious pubertal development (incomplete precocious puberty or variations in pubertal development) include nonprogressive precocious puberty, isolated precocious thelarche, isolated precocious pubarche, isolated menarche, and adolescent (male) gynecomastia. *Isolated thelarche* (unilateral or bilateral breast development) without progression of other signs of puberty generally resolves spontaneously, especially in girls younger than 2 years, and requires no treatment. *Isolated precocious pubarche* (pubic hair development) as a result of early adrenarche is usually self-limited. Evaluation beyond a complete history, physical examination, and bone-age determination would include ACTH stimulation test to rule out late-onset congenital adrenal hyperplasia. *Gynecomastia* in adolescent males is common and presents more of a social than a physical problem. Careful explanation with reassurance for the child and parent that this is a self-limited condition is the best approach.

Tanner stage	Standard	Genitalia*	Pubic hair*	Growth	Other
1	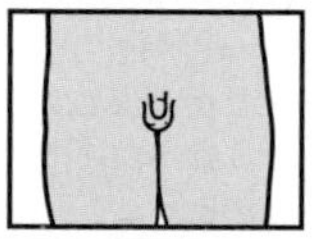	Prepubertal testes: <2.5 cm (1.0 in)	Prepubertal, villus hair only	Basal: about 5.0 to 6.0 cm (2.0 to 2.4 in) per year	Adrenarche
2	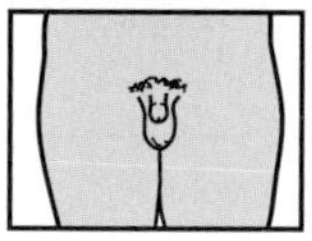	Thinning and reddening of scrotum (11.9 years) Testes: 2.5 to 3.2 cm (1.0 to 1.28 in)	Sparse growth of slightly pigmented hair at base of penis (12.3 years)	Basal: about 5.0 to 6.0 cm (2.0 to 2.4 in) per year	Decrease in total body fat
3	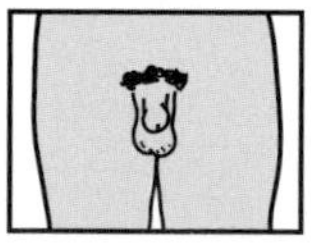	Growth of penis, especially length (13.2 years) Testes: 3.3 to 4.0 cm (1.32 to 1.6 in)	Thicker, curlier hair spreads to the mons pubis (13.9 years)	Accelerated: about 7.0 to 8.0 cm (2.8 to 3.2 in) per year	Gynecomastia (13.2 years) Voice break (13.5 years) Muscle mass increase
4	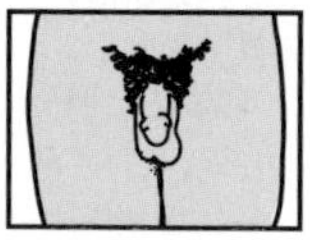	Growth of penis and glands, darkening of scrotum (14.3 years) Testes: 4.1 to 4.5 cm (1.64 to 1.8 in)	Adult-type hair but no spread to medial thigh (14.7 years)	Peak velocity: about 10.0 cm (4.0 in) per year (13.8 years)	Axillary hair (14.0 years) Voice change (14.1 years) Acne (14.3 years)
5	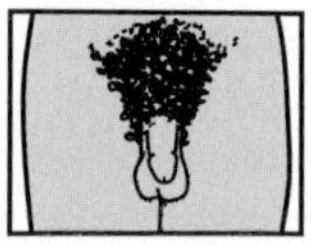	Adult genitalia (15.1 years) Testes: >4.5 cm (1.8 in)	Adult-type hair with spread to medial thighs but not up linea alba (15.3 years)	Deceleration and cessation (about 17 years)	Facial hair (14.9 years) Muscle mass continues to increase after Stage 5

*The Tanner stages of puberty in boys are based on the development of the genitalia and pubic hair distribution. Mean age of milestone attainment is shown in parentheses for the reference population of Marshall and Tanner. Actual age at milestone attainment may vary among individuals and among different study populations.

Figure 35-6 Pubertal milestones for boys. *(From Blondell Rd, Foster MB, Dave KC. Disorders of puberty. Am Fam Physician 1999;60:209, 223.)*

Accidental precocity occasionally results from unusual dietary habits or inappropriate use of medications (estrogen creams). A careful review for these habits early in the evaluation is helpful.

Central (GnRH-Dependent) Precocious Puberty

Central (or true) precocious puberty is caused by early activation of hypothalamic GnRH secretion. Most patients have no identifiable cause, and the precocity is labeled "idiopathic." Initial evaluation begins with history, examination, growth chart, and wrist radiographs. Morning testosterone levels are useful in boys, and GnRH-agonist stimulation tests are helpful in females to identify a central etiology. Various CNS lesions are known to cause central isosexual precocity, so cranial CT or MRI is indicated to rule out these pathologies. An underlying CNS disorder is not unusual in boys presenting with precocious puberty. Treatment is focused on managing the underlying cause. GnRH analogues that reversibly inhibit gonadotropin secretion can be used to prevent secondary sexual development and early epiphyseal fusion that occurs in children who are very young at the onset of puberty, especially when it progresses rapidly (Carel et al., 2004). Optimal age to discontinue therapy is 11 years. When therapy is discontinued, puberty commences normally. There is a slowly progressive form of central isosexual precocity in which no height is lost. These patients may be considered for a nontherapeutic approach with careful observation (Palmert et al., 1999) (Table 35-4).

In many studies the most common causes of precocity are benign and need no treatment. Detailed evaluation with hormonal studies and imaging may be reserved for patients with severe symptoms and signs (de Vries and Phillip, 2005; Kaplowitz, 2004, 2005).

Delayed Puberty

Key Points

- Lack of thelarche (breast development) by age 12 years in girls or lack of testicular enlargement by age 14 years in boys indicates delayed puberty.
- Constitutional delay is characterized by delayed but spontaneous onset of puberty, whereas organic delay is caused by gonadal, pituitary, or central dysfunction.

Delayed puberty in girls is defined as lack of thelarche by age 12 years or duration between thelarche and menarche longer than 5 years. In boys, delayed puberty is defined as no testicular enlargement by age 14 years with more than 5 years between initial and complete development of the genitalia. Delayed puberty in both males and females is classified as *constitutional* (idiopathic) or *organic* (gonadal, pituitary, or central cause). A retrospective study of 232 male and female patients with delayed puberty revealed that the majority (53%) had constitutional delay of growth and maturation, with much higher incidence in males (63%) than females (30%). The remaining 47% of the total 232 patients had mixed etiologies; 19% had functional hypogonadotropic hypogonadism, 12% permanent hypogonadotropic hypogonadism, 13% permanent hypergonadotropic hypogonadism, and no clear etiology for the remaining 3% (Sedlmeyer and Palmert, 2002).

Constitutional delay is characterized by physiologic delay but subsequent spontaneous onset of puberty and is a diagnosis of exclusion. The cause is a delay in GnRH pulse generation, with low levels of gonadotropins. Height and weight in these children tend to be below the fifth percentile, but most catch up during adolescence, reaching normal adult height and weight. Family history may reveal similar delays of puberty in one or both parents, which can be reassuring for the child and parent. Values for FSH, LH, DHEA-S, prolactin, testosterone, and estradiol levels will be consistent with prepubertal values until onset of puberty and normal sexual maturation.

The two common causes of delayed puberty from organic etiologies are pituitary dysfunction or hypogonadotropic hypogonadism. Panhypopituitarism in children may present as delayed puberty, but in conjunction with growth failure, secondary hypothyroidism, and adrenal insufficiency. Differentiation of organic forms of delay from constitutional delay may be difficult to establish in certain patients, requiring a series of observations and testing (no single study or imaging technique will differentiate these). *Hypogonadotropic* hypogonadism presents with low levels of FSH and LH as a result of defective GnRH pulsation. Causes include anorexia nervosa, excessive weight loss, extreme exercise (cross country runners), tumors, head trauma, infiltrative processes, infection, and radiation. *Hypergonadotropic* hypogonadism is usually caused by gonadal failure and presents with high levels of gonadotropins and low levels of sex steroids.

Evaluation of delayed puberty, as with all evaluations for abnormal sexual development, begins with a detailed history focusing on growth patterns, presence of any secondary sexual development, diet, exercise habits, congenital abnormalities, neurologic symptoms, and family history. Physical examination includes a thorough search for early signs of sexual maturation using Tanner staging. Measurement of arm span in relation to height is helpful in growth assessment. Arm span that exceeds height more than 5 cm is consistent with adult configuration. When present in children, this may mean delayed epiphyseal closure due to hypogonadism. Wrist radiography is useful to determine bone age. Initial laboratory screening should include complete blood cell count (CBC), erythrocyte sedimentation rate (ESR), and liver function tests (LFTs). Serum FSH, LH, estradiol, and testosterone levels can distinguish between primary and secondary hypogonadism. In primary hypogonadism (ovarian and testicular failure), serum gonadotropin levels will be elevated. In patients with constitutional delay of puberty and congenital GnRH deficiency, serum gonadotropin levels will be low. Prolactin, TSH, adrenal androgens, and karyotype (to rule out Turner's, Klinefelter's, and Noonan's syndromes) should be evaluated if the clinical presentation warrants.

Therapy for delayed puberty is targeted at the underlying disorder, if identified. If the cause is unknown, observation with reassurance and psychosocial support and reevaluation after 4 to 6 months is an option. Hormonal therapy with estrogen (girls older than 12 years) or testosterone (boys older than 14 years) is another option. Short-term use of exogenous hormones does not appear to have long-term sequelae, except for the potential effect on skeletal maturation, which might result in failure to achieve potential adult

Table 35-4 Precocious Puberty: Types, Causes, and Treatment

Etiology	Symptoms	Tests/Treatment
Central Precocity*		
Idiopathic	Secondary sexual characters development	GnRH analogues Discontinue at 11 years.
CNS lesions (including congenital defects): hamartomas, tumors, infection, trauma, radiation, after androgen exposure, craniopharyngioma, others	History of trauma Medical history Headache, visual changes possible	FSH, LH, prolactin, sex steroids, TSH MRI of brain Treatment per pathology
Primary hypothyroidism	Signs of hypothyroidism without increase in growth velocity	Thyroid profile Treatment with thyroxine
Incomplete Isosexual Precocity		
Females: Isolated precocious thelarche	Breast enlargement without other secondary sexual changes	Most cases are benign.
Females: Isolated precocious adrenarche	Pubic hair development, adult odor, acne	DHEA may be increased. Adrenal steroid hormones and sex hormones: normal ACTH stimulation test to exclude CAH Usually benign; no treatment needed
Females: Isolated precocious menarche	Menarche precedes breast development or appearance of pubic hair.	Normal bone age Ultrasound: normal pelvis with prepubertal uterus Usually benign; check for abuse and ovarian and genital pathology.
Females: Estrogen-secreting tumors of ovary or adrenals Ovarian cysts	Abdominal symptoms Signs of precocious puberty	CT or MRI in addition to hormonal tests Treat as per pathology
Females/males: McCune-Albright syndrome	Autonomous hyperfunction of gonads; rapid development of precocity Café au lait spots, fibrous dysplasia	Ultrasound/CT of abdomen: large ovarian masses LFTs, DHEA sulfate, TSH, phosphate, cortisol
Males: Gonadotropin-secreting tumors; excessive androgen production Testicular or adrenal tumors Virilizing CAH Premature Leydig's and germinal cell maturation	Excessive virilization Enlargement of testis (unilateral)	CT/MRI of abdomen Ultrasound Hormonal tests Treat per pathology. Surgery may be indicated.
Males/females: Iatrogenic	History of using sex steroids and related products	Stop causative agent.
Contrasexual Precocity (Isolated Virilization)		
Isolated precocious adrenarche.		
Females: Virilizing CAH; androgen-secreting ovarian or adrenal neoplasm; Cushing's syndrome; glucocorticoid resistance; arrhenoblastoma	Prepubertal masculinization	Tests for CAH Cortisol Testosterone MRI of abdomen and pelvis Treat per pathology.
Males: Estrogen-secreting tumor, chorionepithelioma; increased extraglandular aromatization of adrenal steroids causing increased extraglandular estrogen production and unusual CAH variations	Prepubertal feminization in boys is rare.	Tests for CAH Cortisol and estrogen levels Testosterone MRI of abdomen and pelvis Treat per pathology.
Iatrogenic	History of using sex steroids and related products	Stop causative agent.
Nonprogressive precocious puberty	Stabilization of precocity Normal bone age	Normal bone age Ultrasound: normal pelvis with prepubertal uterus

Modified from Carel JC, Léger J. Precocious puberty. N Engl J Med 2008;358(22):2366-2377.
*True precocious puberty: gonadotropin dependent.
CNS, Central nervous system; *GnRH*, gonadotropin-releasing hormone; *FSH*, follicle-stimulating hormone; *LH*, luteinizing hormone; *TSH*, thyroid-stimulating hormone; *MRI*, magnetic resonance imaging; *DHEA*, dehydroepiandrosterone; *ACTH*, adrenocorticotropic hormone; *LFTs*, liver function tests; *CT*, computed tomography; *CAH*, congenital adrenal hyperplasia.

height. In females taking estrogen replacement therapy, progestins should be added to the regimen after breakthrough bleeding occurs or after 1 year of therapy.

Problems of the Testicle and Other Male Endocrine Issues

Male Hypogonadism

Male hypogonadism is defined as "inadequate gonadal function" manifested by deficiency in gametogenesis or secretion of gonadal hormones. Primary hypogonadism is caused by dysfunction in the testes from either chromosomal or acquired disorders (Box 35-8). Secondary hypogonadism is caused by an abnormality of the hypothalamic-pituitary axis. Males may present with infertility, decreased testicular size, changes in libido, impotency, gynecomastia, delayed puberty, or a combination of these (Swerdloff and Wang, 2004).

Diagnosis

Clinical diagnosis again begins with history, including information about sexual developmental milestones, current symptoms, ambiguous genitalia at birth, cryptorchidism, behavioral abnormalities, anosmia, surgeries, sexually transmitted diseases (STDs), and medications. History should include the presence of acute and chronic medical conditions and neurologic symptoms. Physical examination is directed toward sexual characteristics, body habitus, gynecomastia, and signs of hypogonadism. Testis should be measured for length and width with an orchidometer. Consistency of the testes should be noted and a scrotal examination done for the presence of varicocele. A nonpalpable prostate may imply testosterone deficiency. A low morning (8-10 AM) serum testosterone level confirms hypogonadism. Serum LH and FSH levels are elevated in primary hypogonadism and are normal to low in secondary hypogonadism. Semen analysis will assess the capability of spermatogenesis. An increase in sex hormone–binding globulin (SHBG) may imply hyperthyroidism, severe androgen deficiency, liver disease, or estrogen excess. A low level of SHBG may indicate hypothyroidism, polycystic ovary syndrome (PCOS), obesity, or acromegaly. Prolactin level should be measured to identify a prolactinoma, followed by CT or MRI, if elevated. Other studies, such as bone mineral density (BMD), pituitary imaging, genetic studies, and in some cases testicular biopsy, may be indicated.

Klinefelter's syndrome is the most common genetic cause of male infertility. It is caused by a chromosomal aberration, most often 47,XXY. Phenotypic males can present with small firm testicles, infertility, tall height, long legs, gynecomastia, and varying symptoms of androgen deficiency and undervirilization. Treatment is replacement of testosterone to prevent the sequelae of androgen deficiency.

Kallmann syndrome is an inherited disorder (see Pituitary Disorders). The most common form is isolated gonadotropin deficiency caused by defective GnRH secretion from the hypothalamus. Patients with Kallmann syndrome usually come to medical attention because of delayed puberty or incomplete sexual development. Anosmia or hyposmia is present in 80% of patients (remember the coffee grounds everyone carried around in medical school?) and establishes the diagnosis of Kallmann syndrome in those with isolated gonadotropin deficiency. Treatment is aimed at virilization by the administration of testosterone.

Cryptorchidism

See online text for discussion.

Box 35-8 Causes of Hypogonadotropic Hypogonadism (HH)

Congenital

Isolated gonadotropin deficiency

Idiopathic HH

Kallmann's syndrome

Non-X-linked

Partial HH (fertile eunuch syndrome)

Associated with CNS disorders

Prader-Willi syndrome

Laurence-Moon-Biedl syndrome

Möbius' syndrome

Lowe's syndrome

Noonan's syndrome

LEOPARD syndrome

X-linked ichthyosis

Genetic defects

    GnRH receptor gene mutations

    FGFR1

    GPR54

    Adrenal hypoplasia, congenital

Multiple pituitary hormone deficiency

Acquired

Organic lesions

Tumors

    Craniopharyngiomas

    Pituitary adenomas (e.g., prolactinoma, nonfunctioning tumor)

    Meningioma

Pituitary apoplexy

Infiltrative disorders

    Sarcoidosis, hemochromatosis

    Histiocytosis X

    Head trauma

    Leydig cell tumors, choriocarcinoma

    CNS radiation therapy

Systemic disorders affecting HPT axis

Critical illness, including burns

Extreme exercise

Malnutrition (anorexia nervosa)

Morbid obesity

Anabolic steroid abuse

Glucocorticoid excess (endogenous: Cushing's syndrome; exogenous)

Narcotics

From Allan CA, McLachlan RI. Androgen deficiency disorders. In DeGroot LJ, Jameson, JL (eds). Endocrinology, 5th ed, vol 3. Philadelphia, Elsevier-Saunders, 2006. *CNS*, Central nervous system; *GnRH*, gonadotropin-releasing hormone: *HPT*, hypothalamic-pituitary-testicular.

Table 35-5 Common Diagnoses in Men Evaluated for Infertility

Diagnostic Category	Incidence (%)
Idiopathic infertility	50-60
Primary testicular failure (chromosomal disorders including Klinefelter's syndrome, Y-chromosome microdeletions, undescended testis, irradiation, orchitis, drugs)	10-20
Genital tract obstruction (congenital absence of vas, vasectomy, epididymal obstruction)	5
Coital disorders	<1
Hypogonadotropic hypogonadism (pituitary adenomas, panhypopituitarism, idiopathic hypogonadotropic hypogonadism, hyperprolactinemia)	3-4
Varicocele[*]	15-35
Other (sperm autoimmunity, drugs, toxins, systemic illness)	5

From Griffin JE, Wilson JD. Disorders of the testes and the male reproductive tract. In Larsen PR et al (eds). Williams' Textbook of Endocrinology, 10th ed. Philadelphia, Elsevier-Saunders, 2003.

Male Infertility

Infertility is defined as failure to achieve pregnancy after 1 year of unprotected intercourse. A specific cause can be identified in approximately 80% of couples, one third of which are female factors alone, one third male factors alone, and one third a combination of both. Unexplained infertility, in which no specific cause can be identified, occurs in approximately 20% of infertile couples. The initial step in evaluation of the male is a thorough medical history, focusing on general health, erectile function, STD history, medications, surgical history, previous successful pregnancy, contraception use, drug or alcohol use, and family history of genetic disease. The first and often only test needed in evaluating male factors is semen analysis. If two consecutive analyses indicate oligospermia or azoospermia, ordering blood tests for testosterone, LH, FSH, and prolactin levels is warranted. *Varicocele* is the most common cause of male infertility (Griffin and Wilson, 2003)(Table 35-5).

Management consists of treating underlying infection with appropriate antibiotics, varicocelectomy, appropriate counseling about environmental factors, and referral to an infertility specialist for more extensive therapy (Frey and Patel, 2004).

Gynecomastia

Key Point

- Although breast cancer is an uncommon cause of breast enlargement in men, this diagnosis must be ruled out because the prognosis is worse for men diagnosed with breast cancer than for women.

Gynecomastia refers to a benign enlargement of the male breast resulting from proliferation of breast glandular tissue. When the male breast is enlarged from adipose tissue, it is called *lipomastia* or *pseudogynecomastia* and is not caused by proliferation of breast tissue. Gynecomastia can be unilateral or bilateral, or it can be asymmetric. Any palpable breast tissue in men is abnormal except for three physiologic situations: transient gynecomastia of the newborn (caused by maternal or placental estrogens), pubertal gynecomastia (observed in 40%-70% of adolescent boys, resolving by age 18), and gynecomastia that occasionally occurs in older adult men (resulting from changes in estrogen and androgen metabolism). Gynecomastia can also be iatrogenic as a result of some medications.

Gynecomastia occurs as concentric, palpable glandular tissue beneath the areola that is not fixed to underlying structures. Prevalence is highest in men 50 to 80 years old and generally presents as bilateral. The cause of pathologic gynecomastia is a relative or absolute increase in circulating estrogen compared with androgen. Careful history (including drugs, legal and illegal) and physical examination can usually rule out Klinefelter's syndrome, androgen insensitivity syndrome, and testicular tumors (Griffin and Wilson, 1995) (Table 35-6).

Breast cancer is very uncommon in men but does occur, and generally the prognosis is much worse for men than for women diagnosed with breast cancer. Typically, breast cancer will present as a painless, central breast lump that may advance to pain, bloody discharge, and skin ulceration. Diagnosis is confirmed by biopsy (Wise et al., 2005).

Treatment of nonphysiologic gynecomastia involves removal of the offending drug or correction of the underlying condition, either of which usually results in regression of the glandular breast tissue. If the gynecomastia persists, a trial of antiestrogen therapy may be considered. Gynecomastia present for more than 1 year will undergo fibrosis and usually will not respond to medications. Surgical correction is required for alleviation of symptoms.

Problems of the Ovary and Other Female Endocrine Issues

Menopause and Hormone Replacement Therapy

See the discussion online at www.expertconsult.com. (Table 35-7).

Amenorrhea

Key Points

- Amenorrhea is categorized as primary or secondary, although this distinction may be misleading in certain patients.
- Primary amenorrhea can be caused by obstruction of the outflow tract, androgen insensitivity, gonadal dysgenesis, hyperprolactinemia, and dysfunction of the hypothalamus, pituitary, or thyroid.
- Pregnancy is the most common cause of secondary amenorrhea.

Primary Amenorrhea

Menses is a normal, physiologic function in a sexually mature female. Amenorrhea is the absence of menses in a sexually mature female. Amenorrhea is divided into two large categories, primary and secondary, depending on whether the female has ever had menarche, with attendant menstrual flow. *Primary* amenorrhea is defined as failure of menarche

Table 35-6 Causes of Pathologic Gynecomastia

Estradiol Excess

Estradiol Secretion

Adrenal tumors
Sporadic testicular tumors (sex cord, Sertoli, germ, Leydig cells)
Testicular tumors associated with familial syndromes (Peutz-Jeghers, Carney complex)

Exogenous Estrogens or Estrogenic Substances

Drug therapy with estrogens
Estrogen creams and lotions
Embalming fluid exposure
Delousing powder
Hair oil
Marijuana
Estrogen analogues: digitoxin

Elevated Estrogen Precursors: Aromatizable Androgens

Human chorionic gonadotropin (hCG) excess (eutopic or ectopic)

Exogenous hormones

Testosterone enanthate
Testosterone propionate
Anabolic steroids
hCG administration

Testosterone Deficiency

Anorchia
Hypogonadotropic syndromes
Drugs or exogenous substances
Ketoconazole
Heroin
Methadone
Alcohol

Estradiol/Testosterone Imbalance

Hypergonadotropic syndromes
Hypogonadotropic hypogonadism syndromes
Primary gonadal diseases
Drugs

Regulatory Hormone Excess

Hyperthyroidism
Acromegaly
Prolactin excess
Hypothyroidism
Pituitary tumor

Drug therapy with:
Catecholamine antagonists or depleters
Domperidone
Haloperidol
Methyldopa
Metoclopramide
Phenothiazines
Reserpine
Sulpiride
Tricyclic antidepressants
Administration of growth hormone
Cushing's syndrome

Other Causes

Local Trauma

Hip spica cast
Chest injury
Herpes zoster of chest wall
Post thoracotomy
Spinal cord injury
Primary breast tumor

Uncertain Causes

Other Chronic Illnesses

Renal failure
Pulmonary tuberculosis
HIV
Diabetes mellitus
Leprosy
Refeeding gynecomastia
Persistent pubertal macromastia
Idiopathic

Drugs associated with gynecomastia with uncertain mechanisms:

Cytotoxic drug-induced hypogonadism from:

Busulfan
Nitrosourea
Vincristine
Combination chemotherapy
Steroid synthesis inhibitory drugs
Androgen resistance
Complete testicular feminization
Partial: Reifenstein, Lubs, Rosewater, and Dreyfus syndromes
Androgen antagonistic drugs
Bicalutamide
Cimetidine
Cyproterone acetate
Flutamide
Spironolactone
Blockers of 5α-reductase
Finasteride
Tumor-related: hCG-producing tumors (testis, lung, gastrointestinal tract, etc.)
Hypogonadotropic syndromes
Isolated gonadotropin deficiency, particularly fertile eunuch syndrome
Panhypopituitarism
Systemic illnesses
Renal disease
Severe liver disease

Amiodarone
Amphetamines
Auranofin
Beta blockers
Calcium channel blockers
Captopril
Cyclosporin
Diazepam
Diethylpropion

Continued

Table 35-6 Causes of Pathologic Gynecomastia—cont'd

Enalapril	Narcotic analgesics
Ethionamide	Nitrates
Etretinate	Omeprazole
Griseofulvin	Penicillamine
Heparin	Phenytoin
Indinavir	Quinidine
Isoniazid	Sulindac
Methotrexate	Theophylline
Metronidazole	Thiacetazone
	Vitamin E

From Santen RJ. Gynecomastia. In DeGroot LJ, Jameson, JL (eds). Endocrinology, 5th ed, vol 3. Philadelphia, Elsevier-Saunders, 2006.

Table 35-7 Menopausal Symptoms* and Treatment

Symptoms	Pre (%)	Peri (%)	Post (%)	Treatment
Vasomotor symptoms	14-51	35-50	30-80	ET/EPT (SOR A)
Vaginal dryness and painful intercourse	4-22	7-39	17-30	ET/EPT Vaginal ET preferred (SOR A)
Mood symptoms	8-37	11-21	8-38	ET may be beneficial (SOR A).
Urinary symptoms	10-36	17-39	15-36	Vaginal estrogens (SOR B)
Sleep disturbances	16-42	39-47	35-60	Sleep hygiene; other agents

Modified from http://consensus.nih.gov/2005/2005MenopausalSymptomsSOS025html.htm.
*Incidence of *premenopausal*, *perimenopausal*, and *post*menopausal symptoms.
ET, Estrogen therapy; *EPT*, cyclic combined estrogen-progestogen therapy; *SOR*, strength of recommendation.

by age 16 in a female with apparently normal sexual development or in a female age 14 who does not demonstrate evidence of developing secondary sexual characteristics. *Secondary* amenorrhea is failure of menstruation after normal menses are established, with the caveat that at least 3 months have passed with apparently normal menses or 9 months have passed in a woman with oligomenorrhea.

Menstruation is a complex process with many interacting and co-dependent processes that must occur in specific chronologic order. Dysfunction of any organ or system involved with these processes has the potential to disrupt the menstrual cycle and cause amenorrhea. The organs and systems involved in the menstrual cycle are CNS (influenced by environment, stress), hypothalamus (through GnRH), anterior pituitary (FSH, LH), thyroid gland, adrenals, ovary (estrogen, progesterone), and uterus. Secondary amenorrhea is more common than primary amenorrhea, with the most common cause being pregnancy. The distinction between etiologies of primary and secondary amenorrhea may be misleading, as in the woman with PCOS who presents with primary amenorrhea, or the woman with partial gonadal dysgenesis who has rudimentary ovarian development and may initially ovulate, thus presenting with secondary amenorrhea (Box 35-9).

The more common causes of primary amenorrhea fall into congenital or anatomic abnormalities. Congenital absence of the uterus and vagina, known as müllerian agenesis or Mayer-Rokitansky-Küster-Hauser (MRKH) syndrome, is a significant cause of amenorrhea. Other congenital causes of primary amenorrhea include chromosomal abnormalities, prenatal adrenal hyperplasia, and female virilization syndrome. An anatomic cause of primary amenorrhea, usually discovered at menarche, is imperforate hymen.

To evaluate a patient with primary amenorrhea, after a thorough clinical history, the physical examination must focus on development of secondary sexual characteristics (breast development, pubic/axillary hair). Pregnancy as a cause of primary amenorrhea is less common than in secondary amenorrhea, although it should be excluded before any testing or imaging is initiated. Laboratory testing includes FSH, LH, TSH, and prolactin. If FSH is normal or reduced, this may mean the patient has chronic anovulation, functional hypothalamic amenorrhea, or PCOS. Increased FSH with breast development is likely secondary to ovarian failure. Increased FSH without secondary sexual characteristics may be caused by congenital agenesis of the ovaries. In the patient without a uterus, serum testosterone level and karyotype should be determined. In the presence of a uterus and normal secondary sexual characteristics, serum TSH levels should be evaluated (Sybert and McCauley, 2004) (Box 35-10).

Secondary Amenorrhea

Pregnancy is the most common cause of secondary amenorrhea and must always be ruled out at the initial clinical visit. Structural changes may cause amenorrhea, such as adhesions

Box 35-9 Causes of Amenorrhea*

Hyperprolactinemia

    Prolactin-secreting tumor

    Centrally acting medications, including dopamine antagonists

Pituitary disease

    Non–prolactin-secreting pituitary tumor

    Generalized pituitary insufficiency, including previous pituitary surgery

Hypothalamic amenorrhea

    Nutrition/exercise disorders

    Idiopathic hypogonadotropic hypogonadism

From Illingworth P. Amenorrhea, anovulation, and dysfunctional uterine bleeding. In DeGroot LJ, Jameson, JL (eds). Endocrinology, 5th ed, vol 3. Philadelphia, Elsevier-Saunders, 2006.
*Resulting from disorders of the hypothalamus and pituitary.

Box 35-10 Causes of Primary Ovarian Failure

Iatrogenic

Surgery

Chemotherapy

Radiotherapy

Environmental

Smoking

Viral infections

Autoimmune

Association with other autoimmune disease

Abnormal karyotypes

46,XY

45,XO

Genetic disorders with normal karyotype

Fragile X permutations

Galactosemia

Carbohydrate-deficient glycoprotein syndrome type 1 (CDG-1)

Inhibin α-gene mutations

Follicle-stimulating hormone (FSH) receptor gene mutations

From Peter Illingworth. Amenorrhea, anovulation, and dysfunctional uterine bleeding. In DeGroot LJ, Jameson, JL (eds). Endocrinology, 5th ed, vol 3. Philadelphia, Elsevier-Saunders, 2006.

after instrumentation (Asherman's syndrome) or infection in the form of TB or endometritis. Patients with PCOS present with irregular or absent menses, hirsutism, acne, subfertility secondary to a hyperandrogenic state, or a combination. Adrenal or ovarian tumors, hyperthecosis, and late-onset or mild congenital adrenal hyperplasia may also result in secondary amenorrhea and hyperandrogenism. Hypergonadotropic hypogonadism (premature ovarian failure), hypogonadotropic hypogonadism, thyroid disease, menopause, extreme exercise, anorexia nervosa, bulimia, and hyperprolactinemia are all potential causes of secondary amenorrhea.

A thorough history and physical examination will provide the diagnosis, with laboratory studies and imaging serving as collaborative evidence. Particular attention should be paid to menstrual history, diet, exercise, medications, pubertal development, hirsutism, acne, galactorrhea, and other medical conditions. Initial laboratory evaluation includes pregnancy test and TSH and prolactin levels. If these are normal, and there are no signs of hyperandrogenism (e.g., hirsutism, acne, voice change), proceed with progesterone challenge by using medroxyprogesterone (Provera), 10 to 20 mg daily for 5 to 10 days. In the presence of a uterus, the progesterone withdrawal test will induce withdrawal bleeding within 10 days in a woman with adequate estrogen production. If there is no withdrawal bleed, consider repeating the test with progesterone in oil (100-200 mg IM) or with norethindrone or micronized progesterone. If this test is also negative, a 21-day course of conjugated estrogen (1.25 mg/day) or a cycle of combined oral contraceptives (OCs) should provide adequate stimulation of the endometrium to support a withdrawal bleed. If all these measures fail to result in menstrual flow, additional tests may be ordered, beginning with FSH and, if there are clinical signs of hyperandrogenism, DHEA-S and testosterone levels. Elevated FSH indicates ovarian failure (including gonadal dysgenesis and secondary ovarian failure or menopause); normal or low values indicate hypogonadotropic hypogonadism or uterine abnormality (Asherman's syndrome). Proceed with a workup for PCOS (discussed later), late-onset congenital adrenal hyperplasia, or Cushing's syndrome if there are features consistent with these illnesses. Features of hyperandrogenemia or substantially increased serum testosterone levels should prompt appropriate studies to rule out a neoplastic source of

androgen. Figure 35-7 is a diagnostic algorithm for evaluating a patient with primary and secondary amenorrhea. Hirsutism can be subjective.

Management of amenorrhea depends on establishing a diagnosis, specific treatment directed to the underlying cause, restoration of ovulatory cycles, and treating infertility, if desired. Also, appropriate treatment is provided for hypoestrogenemia and hyperandrogenemia (medical and surgical).

Turner's Syndrome

See the discussion online at www.expertconsult.com.

Female Infertility

Infertility is defined as failure of conception after 1 year of unprotected intercourse. From 15% to 20% of all couples are infertile. In women, fertility peaks between ages 20 and 24. After this, there is progressive decline in fertility until about age 32, followed by a steep decline after 40. Causes of infertility in couples tend to be one-third male factors, one-third female factors, and one-third combination. Female causes of infertility include ovarian dysfunction (40%), tubal factors (20%), cervical factors (infection, stenosis), uterine factors (infection, fibroids), and other (endometriosis, adhesions). The course of investigation for infertility should be based on a couple's wishes for fertility, their age, duration of infertility, and unique features in the history and physical examination.

Evaluation of the male partner is an integral part of the infertility workup and should coincide with the female partner's evaluation. Comprehensive history and physical examination of the female partner should include menstrual

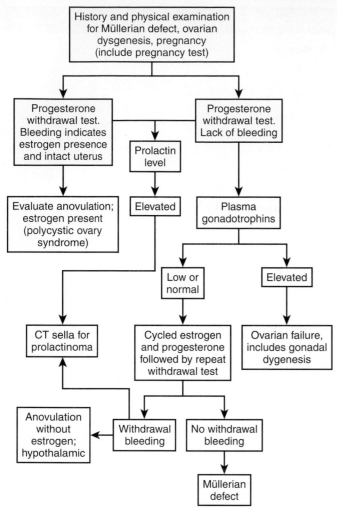

Figure 35-7 Diagnostic algorithm for evaluating a patient with primary and secondary amenorrhea. *(Modified from Carr BR. Disorders of the ovaries and female reproductive tract. In Wilson JD, Foster DW [eds]. Williams' Textbook of Endocrinology, 8th ed. Philadelphia, Saunders, 1992.)*

Table 35-8 Tests for evaluating Female Infertility

Female Infertility	Common Tests
Ovulatory factors	Basal body temperature or urinary LH test (ovulatory predictor test); serum progesterone (during luteal phase); transvaginal ultrasound; TSH, FSH, prolactin, and androgens
Cervical factors	Cervical mucus evaluation; postcoital test (not sensitive)
Uterine factors	Ultrasound, hysterosalpingography, hysteroscopy, sonohysterography (for submucosal myomas and endometrial polyps), magnetic resonance imaging
Tubal factors	Hysterosalpingography; laparoscopy and chromotubation; fluoroscopic/hysteroscopic tubal cannulation
Peritoneal factors	Ultrasound, laparoscopy

Modified from: Brassard M, AinMelk Y, Baillargeon JP. Basic infertility including polycystic ovary syndrome. Med Clin North Am 2008;92:1163-1192.

history, prior obstetric history, secondary sexual characteristics, recent and remote history of STDs, pelvic inflammatory disease (PID), pelvic surgeries or instrumentation, hirsutism, weight changes (up and down), medications, and comorbidities. Personal and family history should include use of drugs (including alcohol, tobacco, caffeine), physical activity, douching, frequency and timing of sexual intercourse, and family history of infertility or genetic disorders. Initial laboratory testing for the female partner includes a CBC, urinalysis, STD screen, confirmation of rubella and varicella immunity, and Papanicolaou smear. Ovulation should be verified by urinary ovulation prediction kits that detect the LH surge, determination of the mid–luteal phase serum progesterone level (7 days before anticipated menses), or both. Assessment of fallopian tube patency is by hysterosalpingography (first choice) or laparoscopy (if history strongly suggests prior tubal damage). Women over age 35 should have serum FSH checked on day 3 of their menstrual cycle. A value higher than 12 IU/L is associated with poor ovarian response, and referral to a reproductive endocrinologist should be considered. Postcoital tests, endometrial biopsies, and basal body temperature records

are no longer recommended as routine studies in the initial evaluation (Brassard et al., 2008; Practice Committee, 2004) (Table 35-8).

Treatment should be directed toward the underlying cause. For tubal disease, surgery and in vitro fertilization are options. Endometriosis can be managed with conservative surgery based on the degree of disease or can be circumvented through intrauterine insemination or in vitro fertilization. Ovulatory dysfunction is treated based on the underlying cause: bromocriptine for prolactinoma, metformin or clomiphene citrate for PCOS, human menopausal gonadotropin for hypogonadotropic hypogonadism, clomiphene citrate plus glucocorticoids for adrenal hyperplasia with elevated levels of androgens, and antibiotics for infection. The family physician should strongly consider early referral to a reproductive specialist if the patient or couple have complex medical histories or advanced reproductive age.

Galactorrhea and Hirsutism

See the discussions online at www.expertconsult.com.

Polycystic Ovary Syndrome

Polycystic ovary syndrome is the clinical condition seen most frequently with androgen excess. Women with PCOS present with complaints of abnormal menses, infertility, hirsutism, acne, and obesity, all of which are related to excess androgen. PCOS is the single most common endocrine abnormality of women of reproductive age and affects 6% to 8% of women worldwide. The definition of PCOS is constantly being revised. The Task Force on the Phenotype of the Polycystic Ovary Syndrome from the Androgen Excess and PCOS Society (AE-PCOS Society) defines PCOS by the presence of hyperandrogenism (clinical and/or biochemical), ovarian dysfunction (oligo-anovulation and/or polycystic ovaries),

Box 35-11 Causes of Androgen Excess in Women

I. Adrenal hyperandrogenism
   A. Premature adrenarche
   B. Functional adrenal hyperandrogenism
   C. Congenital adrenal hyperplasia
   D. Cushing's syndrome
   E. Hyperprolactinemia and acromegaly
   F. Abnormal cortisol action/metabolism
   G. Adrenal neoplasms
II. Gonadal hyperandrogenism
   A. Ovarian hyperandrogenism
      1. Functional ovarian hyperandrogenism/polycystic ovary syndrome
      2. Adrenal virilizing disorders and rests
      3. Ovarian steroidogenic blocks
      4. Syndromes of extreme insulin resistance
      5. Ovarian neoplasms
   B. True hermaphroditism
   C. Pregnancy-related hyperandrogenism
III. Peripheral androgen overproduction
   A. Obesity
   B. Idiopathic

From Ehrmann DA, Barnes RB, Rosenfield RL. Hyperandrogenism, hirsutism, and the polycystic ovary syndrome. In DeGroot LJ, Jameson, JL (eds). Endocrinology, 5th ed, vol 3. Philadelphia, Elsevier-Saunders, 2006.

Table 35-9 Signs and Symptoms in Relation to Presence of Polycystic Ovary Syndrome (PCOS)

Symptoms/Signs	Patients with PCOS (% and % range)
Hirsutism and unwanted hair growth	78.4
Acne	36
Alopecia	36.5
Hyperandrogenemia,	70
Hirsutism	72
Persistent acne	20-40
Normal androgen levels	20-40
Overt menstrual dysfunction	75-85
Oligomenorrhea	79.11
Polycystic ovaries	75-90
LH/FSH ratio	40
Insulin resistance	50-70
Type 2 diabetes	26.7
Dyslipidemia	70
Oligoanovulation	40
Obesity	50
Hyperprolactinemia	<1

Modified from Azziz R, Carmina E, Dewailly D, et al. Task Force on the Phenotype of the Polycystic Ovary Syndrome of the Androgen Excess and PCOS Society. The Androgen Excess and PCOS Society criteria for the polycystic ovary syndrome: the complete task force report. Fertil Steril 2009;91:456-488.

and the exclusion of related disorders (Azziz et al., 2009) (Box 35-11).

Typical presentation of PCOS includes hirsutism, menstrual dysfunction, obesity, insulin resistance, acanthosis nigricans, decreased fertility, and polycystic appearance to the ovaries. The onset of symptoms is usually around menarche, but it may occur after puberty as a result of weight gain or other environmental factors. Differential diagnosis includes idiopathic hirsutism, ovarian hyperthecosis, ovarian tumor, adrenal tumor, nonclassic adrenal hyperplasia, Cushing's syndrome, glucocorticoid resistance, and androgen-producing neoplasms.

A patient with PCOS is at higher risk for infertility, dysfunctional bleeding, obesity, endometrial hyperplasia, endometrial carcinoma, type 2 diabetes mellitus, dyslipidemia, hypertension, obstructive sleep apnea, and possibly cardiovascular disease with familial tendency (increased risk for mother and daughter) (Azziz et al., 2009; Ehrmann, 2005) (Table 35-9).

The diagnosis of PCOS is made with evidence of hyperandrogenism (clinical or biochemical), presence of ovarian dysfunction (clinical or anatomical), and excluding other conditions producing hyperandrogenism and ovarian dysfunction. Initial laboratory testing should include the determination of serum free testosterone, androstenedione, DHEA-S, and 17-hydroxyprogesterone. Other studies include prolactin, TSH, fasting glucose/insulin, and serum lipid profile. Obtaining circulating levels of LH and FSH does not contribute significantly to the diagnosis of PCOS, so these laboratory tests are not indicated with initial evaluation. Pelvic or transvaginal ultrasound should be performed to identify the ovaries and determine their size and shape and the presence of cysts;

typical PCOS ovaries have increased volume and contain 10 to 12 subcapsular follicular cysts 2 to 9 mm in diameter.

Treatment of hirsutism and acne in PCOS focuses on decreasing androgen levels, production, and effects. Metformin is used extensively to reduce insulin resistance and hyperinsulinemia related to hormonal changes and ovulation (Nestler, 2008). To decrease risk of endometrial hyperplasia and carcinoma, cyclic progestin or a combination OC should be considered to inhibit endometrial proliferation.

In the long-term management of PCOS, steps should be taken to reduce cardiovascular complications, diabetes, obesity, and psychosocial morbidities (Fig. 35-8). Screening for glucose-intolerance with a 75-g 2-hour FTT and determination of serum lipid levels (total cholesterol, LDL, HDL, triglycerides) should be carried out. Lifestyle management changes include weight loss, exercise, and use of metformin and thiazolidinediones for patients with abnormal GTT results. In addition, clinicians should consider cardiovascular risk reduction, psychosocial issues, management of subfertility and hirsutism, and other lifetime management with insulin sensitizers and protection of the endometrium with hormonal manipulations.

KEY TREATMENT

Common causes of precocity are benign and require no treatment. Careful nontherapeutic observation may be considered (Carel et al., 2004) (SOR: A).

Treatment of precocity with GnRH analogues, which reversibly inhibit gonadotropin secretion, can be used to prevent secondary sexual development and early epiphyseal fusion (Carel et al., 2004) (SOR: A).

Hormonal therapy with hCG or GnRH can be used to increase the likelihood of testicular descent (Henna, 2004) (SOR: A).

Inguinal orchiopexy is a well-established procedure for palpable undescended testicle and is generally considered the standard of care for cryptorchidism in the United States (Engeler, 2000; Kollin, 2007; Ritzèn, 2008) (SOR: A).

Present clinical practice suggests treating menopausal symptoms on an individual basis; predominantly with lifestyle therapies, risk modification, screening strategies, and nonhormonal therapies (Barton and Loprinzi, 2004; Brewer et al., 2003; Krebs et al., 2004; MacGregor et al., 2005) (SOR: C).

SSRIs, clonidine, and gabapentin are recommended for treatment of menopausal symptoms (Barton and Loprinzi, 2004; Brewer et al., 2003; Krebs et al., 2004; MacGregor et al., 2005) (SOR: C).

Tibolone is effective in controlling menopausal symptoms and reduces risk of fracture and breast cancer, but with an increased risk of stroke (Cummings et al., 2008) (SOR: A).

Patients with polycystic ovary syndrome require cardiovascular risk reduction, psychosocial counseling, management of subfertility and hirsutism, and possible insulin sensitizers and protection of endometrium with hormonal manipulations (Azziz, 2003; Azziz et al., 2009; Ehrmann, 2005; Nestler, 2008) (SOR: A).

Newer selective estrogen receptor modulators (SERMs) are being used to treat depressed libido in women, which minimizes risk to the endometrium while preserving benefits to breast and bone (MacGregor et al., 2005) (SOR: A).

Diagnosis of secondary amenorrhea can be facilitated with a progesterone challenge (Sheeler et al., 2007) (SOR: B).

Disturbances in Calcium and Phosphate

Calcium homeostasis is a delicate balance among a number of organ systems and functions. These include kidneys, thyroid, parathyroid, bone, adrenal glands, gastrointestinal tract, nutrition, infectious disease, and medication. Malfunction in any of these modalities can result in hypercalcemia or hypocalcemia with the potential for serious morbidity and mortality. Total body calcium is balanced between plasma and the bony skeleton in a state of dynamic equilibrium. Approximately 1% of total calcium is in circulation, and the remaining 99% is stored in bone. In plasma, circulating calcium is approximately 40% protein (albumin) bound; 45% exists in an ionized state (Ca^{++}); and about 15% is found as various salts (calcium citrate, calcium lactate, calcium phosphate, calcium sulfate). Bony calcium exists in an active state with constant deposition and resorption under the influence of parathyroid hormone (PTH, parathormone), calcitonin, osteoclastic and osteoblastic activity, and neoplastic disease.

The primary factor driving increases in circulating calcium is PTH, which increases bone resorption and converts vitamin D_3 (cholecalciferol) into 1,25-dihydroxycholecalciferol, the active form of vitamin D_3. Cholecalciferol is primarily formed in the skin from solar irradiation, and some evidence suggests that ultraviolet (UV) radiation exposure of tanning beds can raise vitamin D_3 (Tangpricha et al., 2004). Dietary sources are also important and can be obtained from fortified milk, fruit juices, fish oil, and other sources. The active form of vitamin D_3 is required to facilitate calcium absorption from the gut. Calcium homeostasis is further maintained by circulating levels of ionized calcium and calcitonin's negative effect on osteoclastic bone resorption (Hall, 2011). Figure 35-9 shows the pathway for conversion of vitamin D_3 into its active form and vitamin D's role in controlling plasma calcium concentration.

Normal levels of total circulating calcium, with normal albumin levels, range between 8.5 and 10.5 mg/dL ($\approx$ 2.4 mmol/L). Ionized levels, which are not albumin dependent, will range between 1.17 and 1.33 mmol/L ($\approx$ 4.7 mg/dL) (Bringhurst and Leder, 2006).

Hypercalcemia

Causes of hypercalcemia are generally divided into two types; primary and secondary. Primary causes are excessive parathormone secretion, and secondary causes include disease processes that directly affect bone metabolism and calcium excretion. The most common cause of primary hyperparathyroidism (PHPT) is a solitary parathyroid adenoma, accounting for approximately 80% of cases. Multiple adenomas are found in 2% to 4% of cases. The second most common cause of PHPT (15%) is parathyroid hyperplasia of multiple (usually ≥4) parathyroid glands. The etiologies for these include a mix of congenital and familial diseases (MEN-I, MEN-IIA). Less than 1% of PHPT is caused by primary parathyroid malignancy (Silverberg and Bilezikian, 2006) (Box 35-12).

Primary hyperparathyroidism does not present with classic symptoms. Symptoms may be as nonspecific as generalized weakness in the proximal muscles, fatigue, headache, weight loss, and constipation or as profound as renal failure, hypovolemic shock, and death (usually in patients with malignancy, although sometimes previously undiagnosed). Patients rarely present with signs and symptoms immediately suggesting hypercalcemia. PHPT is usually uncovered through routine nonspecific screening laboratory tests, during evaluation for nephrolithiasis, or occasionally in a patient with accelerated osteoporosis and pathologic fracture.

There is a classic "quadrad" of symptoms associated with hypercalcemia that, although seen in many disease processes, may be helpful in a patient with hypercalcemia, irrespective of etiology. The mnemonic taught to medical students is "bones, stones, moans, and abdominal groans," representing the four symptoms of the classic quadrad: bone pain, renal calculi, psychiatric disorder, and nausea and vomiting (Silverberg and Bilezikian, 2006).

The primary dysfunction in PHPT is an excess of circulating parathormone. However, with bony metastases, PTH levels will be appropriately suppressed in the presence of elevated serum calcium levels caused by osteolytic metastases. When the cause of hypercalcemia is malignancy, the patient usually has a history; an exception is unsuspected multiple myeloma, which may present with chronic low back pain and elevated serum calcium. Calcium levels in malignancy are typically higher (>14 mg/dL) than those found with parathyroid adenomas (<13 mg/dL), although this is not always the case (Table 35-10).

Thiazide diuretics, lithium, and calcium carbonate are common medications seen in primary care that, if not properly

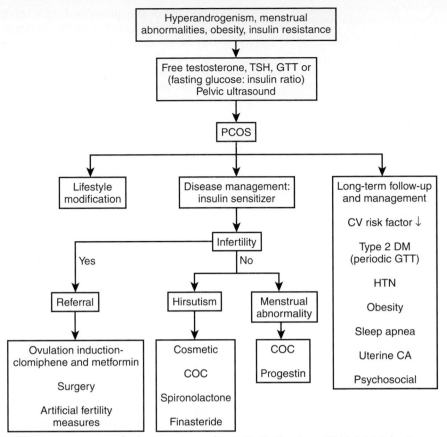

Figure 35-8 Therapeutic algorithm for management of polycystic ovary syndrome. *(Modified from Samraj GPN, Kuritzky L. Polycystic ovary syndrome: comprehensive management in primary care. Comp Ther 2002;28:208-221q.)*

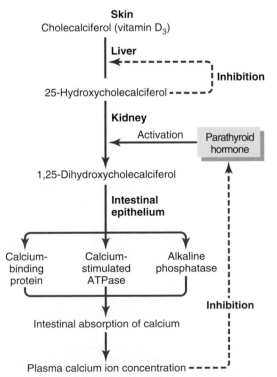

Figure 35-9 Pathway for conversion of vitamin D_3 into its active form (1,25-dihydroxycholecalciferol) and the role vitamin D plays in control of plasma calcium concentration. *(From Hall JE. Parathyroid hormone, calcitonin, calcium and phosphate metabolism, vitamin D, bone, and teeth. In Guyton AC, Hall JE [eds]. Textbook of Medical Physiology, 12th ed. Philadelphia, Saunders-Elsevier, 2011.)*

Box 35-12 Differential Diagnosis of Hypercalcemia

Primary hyperparathyroidism
Parathyroid carcinoma
Hypercalcemia of malignancy
Nonparathyroid endocrine causes
    Thyrotoxicosis
    Pheochromocytoma
    Addison's disease
    Islet cell tumors
Drug-related hypercalcemia
    Vitamin D
    Vitamin A
    Thiazide diuretics
    Lithium
    Estrogen and antiestrogens
Familial hypocalciuric hypercalcemia
Miscellaneous
Immobilization
Milk-alkali syndrome
Parenteral nutrition

From Silverberg SJ, Bilezikian JP. Primary hyperparathyroidism. In DeGroot LJ, Jameson JL (eds). Endocrinology, 5th ed, vol 2. Philadelphia, Elsevier-Saunders, 2006.

Table 35-10 Biochemical Profile in Primary Hyperparathyroidism

	Patients (mean +/- SEM)	Normal Range
Serum calcium	10.7 ±mg/dL	8.2-10.2 mg/dL
Serum phosphorus	2.8 ±0.1 mg/dL	2.5-4.5 mg/dL
Total alkaline phosphatase	114 ±5 IU/L	<100 IU/L
Serum magnesium	2.0 ±0.1 mg/dL	1.8-2.4 mg/dL
PTH (IRMA)	119 ±7 pg/mL	10-65 pg/mL
25(OH) vitamin D	19 ±1 ng/mL	9-52 ng/mL
1,25(OH)$_2$ vitamin D	54 ±2 pg/mL	15-60 pg/mL
Urinary calcium	240 ±11 mg/g creatinine	
Urine DPD	17.6 ± nmol/L/ mmol/L creatinine	<14.6 nmol/L/mmol/ L creatinine
Urine PYD	46.8 ±2.7 nmol/L/ mmol/L creatinine	<51.8 nmol/L/mmol/ L creatinine

From Silverberg SJ, Bilezikian JP. Primary hyperparathyroidism. In DeGroot LJ, Jameson JL (eds). Endocrinology, 5th ed, vol 2. Philadelphia, Elsevier-Saunders, 2006.

monitored and prescribed, can result in hypercalcemia. It is also important to inquire about nonprescription (OTC) medications because excess vitamin D (intoxication) can be a cause. If a patient is taking any of these substances and is asymptomatic, with serum calcium level less than 14 mg/dL, the approach is to discontinue the medication and repeat the calcium level in a week. If the serum calcium is stable or declining, continue to monitor until it returns to normal.

Occasionally, adrenal insufficiency and hyperthyroidism are uncovered in the evaluation of a patient with an elevated serum calcium level.

Patients who have symptoms consistent with hypercalcemia or serum calcium levels in excess of 13.5 mg/dL may require more aggressive treatment. These patients will almost always be volume depleted as a result of hypercalciuria with resultant polyuria. Treatment is aimed initially at aggressive rehydration. Isotonic saline at 2 to 4 L/day until calcium level returns to normal is appropriate. Furosemide (loop diuretic) can be used with fluid replacement in older patients and those with renal or cardiac disorders to prevent fluid overload. Careful fluid management must be maintained to prevent inadvertent fluid overload or depletion (Table 35-11). Other treatments include IV bisphosphonate, calcitonin, and gallium nitrate or plicamycin (Table 35-12).

If the patient is determined to have a parathyroid adenoma, the only currently available option for cure is parathyroidectomy. For asymptomatic patients, patients who have failed surgery, and those who do not meet surgical criteria, medical treatment includes moderate calcium intake,

Table 35-11 Summary of Most Generally Useful Medical Therapies for Hypercalcemia

Treatment	Onset of Action	Duration of Action	Advantages	Disadvantages
Rehydration	Hours	During treatment	Rapid action Rehydration invariably needed	None
Forced saline diuresis (with or without loop diuretics)	Hours	During treatment	Rapid action	Modest calcium-lowering effect Potential for volume overload Electrolyte disturbance Transient efficacy Inconvenient for patients
Calcitonin	Hours	1-2 days	Rapid onset of action	Modest calcium-lowering effect Tachyphylaxis develops in a few days
Bisphosphonates				
Etidronate	1-3 days	5-7 days	First-generation bisphosphonate Well tolerated	3-day infusion protocol Less effective than other bisphosphonates
Pamidronate	1-2 days	Weeks to months	Second-generation bisphosphonate Normalizes calcium levels in many patients	Fever Occasional hypocalcemia, hypophosphatemia, and hypomagnesemia
Zoledronate	1-2 days	Weeks to months	Third-generation bisphosphonate More potent than second-generation bisphosphonates Normalizes calcium levels in 90% of patients Can be given in 30 min	Fever Hypophosphatemia Hypocalcemia Renal toxicity occasional

From Finkelstein JS, Potts JT. Medical management of hypercalcemia. In DeGroot LJ, Jameson JL (eds). Endocrinology, 5th ed, vol 2. Philadelphia, Elsevier-Saunders, 2006.

Table 35-12 Summary of Therapies for Hypercalcemia Useful in Special Circumstances

Treatment	Onset of Action	Duration of Action	Advantages	Disadvantages
Gallium nitrate	5 days	7-10 days	May normalize calcium in patients resistant to bisphosphonates	Must be infused continuously over 5 days Occasional nephrotoxicity or hypophosphatemia
Glucocorticoids	Days	Days to weeks	Oral administration	Effective in granulomatous disorders and certain types of malignancies, especially hematologic
Dialysis	Hours	During use and for 24-48 hours afterward	Rapid onset of action Useful in patients with renal failure and heart failure Useful to treat life-threatening hypercalcemia	Complex procedure Reserved for extreme or special circumstances
Oral phosphate	24 hours	During use	Minimal toxicity if serum phosphate low Oral administration	Modest calcium-lowering effect Diarrhea

From Finkelstein JS, Potts JT. Medical management of hypercalcemia. In DeGroot LJ, Jameson JL (eds). Endocrinology, 5th ed, vol 2. Philadelphia, Elsevier-Saunders, 2006.

estrogen replacement (when applicable), bisphosphonates, and selective estrogen receptor modulators (SERMs).

For the patient with PHPT not caused by malignancy, determining if there is one adenoma or multiple functioning adenomas and the location(s) is important in minimizing both duration and extent of surgery. It is possible to determine preoperatively which parathyroid gland(s) may be the source of the PTH utilizing ultrasound, CT, or MRI. If none of these provides definitive results, technetium-labeled (Tc-99m) sestamibi nuclear scan may localize the adenoma (Silverberg and Bilezikian, 2006).

Hypocalcemia

Hypocalcemia has a number of primary and secondary causes. Primary causes involve some defect in PTH availability, including (1) lack of production (surgical removal of parathyroid gland or hypoparathyroidism from autoimmune disease), (2) impaired secretion (with profound hypomagnesemia), and (3) end-organ resistance. With the first two, there is a deficit in circulating PTH, but with the third, PTH is elevated, in contrast to a low serum calcium and hyperphosphatemia. An example of end-organ resistance is Albright's syndrome. Secondary causes include severe vitamin D deficiency, "hungry bone syndrome" with chondrosarcoma, and HIV/AIDS (Box 35-13).

Signs and symptoms are generally lacking in the outpatient setting. The primary clinical findings are caused by neuromuscular irritability. If hypocalcemia is suspected, although negative responses do not rule out hypocalcemia, two physical tests may assist in the diagnosis: Chvostek sign (tapping the facial nerve across the cheek with contraction of the facial muscle) and Trousseau's sign (carpal spasm via BP cuff). Deep tendon reflexes may be hyperactive, and the patient may appear anxious, confused, demented, or psychotic. The signs and symptoms of hypocalcemia are related to the level of ionized calcium rather than total calcium, as well as the rapidity of decline (Levine, 2006). Alkalosis,

either primary or compensatory, can cause a shift in ionized calcium to a bound state, thus exacerbating a borderline hypocalcemia situation.

Cardiac changes caused by hypocalcemia include prolongation of the QT interval, resulting in life-threatening dysrhythmia and cardiac dysfunction. Generalized seizures are also possible. The cardiac dysfunction is generally reversible with normalization of the ionized calcium levels. In acute and severe cases, IV calcium is the treatment of choice. Concurrent management of hyperphosphatemia, alkalosis, and hypomagnesemia is required. Long-term management is with oral calcium and vitamin D. Although use of thiazide diuretics is contraindicated in patients with hypercalcemia, they can be used with hypocalcemia and may have a beneficial effect. On the other hand, loop diuretics must be used cautiously because they increase renal excretion of calcium and may exacerbate the problem.

Pseudohypoparathyroidism is a rare phenomenon representative of several congenital endocrinologic disorders in which tissue resistance to PTH is present. The classic form of this disorder is *Albright's hereditary osteodystrophy* (AHO). The AHO patient has short stature, mental retardation, brachydactyly, and PTH resistance (elevated PTH levels). Another form of AHO does not involve PTH dysfunction, called pseudo-pseudohypoparathyroidism. Although the clinical course of these diseases may vary and in some cases is protracted, AHO usually is associated with a shortened life expectancy. Treatment is primarily supportive (Levine, 2006).

Hyperphosphatemia

The most common cause of hyperphosphatemia, and most familiar to primary care physicians, is impaired renal function. It is also a characteristic of all forms of hypoparathyroidism, from the loss of inhibitory effect of PTH on phosphate reabsorption at the proximal renal tubule (Levine, 2006). High-phosphate formula provided to infants can result in hypocalcemia and tetany (Box 35-14).

Box 35-13 Causes of Functional Hypoparathyroidism

A. Surgery
B. Toxic agents
   1. High-dose radiation (rarely)
   2. Asparaginase
   3. Ethiofos
C. Infiltrative processes
   1. Iron deposition
   2. Copper deposition
   3. Tumor or granuloma
D. Defective secretion of PTH
   1. Magnesium deficiency
   2. Magnesium excess
   3. Activating mutation of calcium-sensing receptor gene (MIM 145980)
   4. Antibodies that activate the calcium-sensing receptor
   5. Burn injury and upregulation of calcium-sensing receptor
   6. Alcohol
   7. Maternal hypercalcemia
   8. Neonatal hypocalcemia
E. Autoimmune destruction of parathyroid glands
   1. Autoimmune hypoparathyroidism
   2. Autoimmune polyglandular syndrome, type 1 (APECED, MIM 240300)
F. Idiopathic hypoparathyroidism
   1. Autosomal recessive (MIM 241400)
   2. X-linked (MIM 307700)

G. Embryologic defects in parathyroid gland development
   1. DiGeorge syndrome (del 22q or TBX1 Mutation); DGS1; MIM 188400
   2. DiGeorge syndrome (del 10p) DGS2; MIM 601362
   3. Velocardiofacial syndrome (del 22q); MIM 192430
   a. Kenny-Caffey/Sanjad-Sakati syndromes (TCBE, MIM 244460)
H. Defective synthesis of parathyroid hormone; MIM 168450
   1. Autosomal dominant mutation in prepro-PTH gene
   2. Autosomal recessive mutation in prepro-PTH gene
I. Metabolic defects and mitochondrial neuromyopathies
   1. Kearn-Sayre syndrome
   2. Person's syndrome
   3. tRNA *leu* mutations
J. Resistance to parathyroid hormone
   1. Pseudohypoparathyroidism type 1a (MIM 103580)
   2. Pseudohypoparathyroidism type 1b
   3. Pseudohypoparathyroidism type 1c
   4. Pseudohypoparathyroidism type 2

From Levine MA. Hypoparathyroidism and pseudohypoparathyroidism. In DeGroot LJ, Jameson JL (eds). Endocrinology, 5th ed, vol 2. Philadelphia, Elsevier-Saunders, 2006.

PTH, Parathyroid hormone (parathormone).

Hypophosphatemia

Dietary causes of hypophosphatemia are virtually non-existent, although excessive use of oral phosphate binders (aluminum and magnesium hydroxide antacids) can result in binding of phosphate in the intestine, thus preventing absorption. Generally, when use of oral antacids is excluded, the most common cause of hypophosphatemia is elevated levels of serum calcium caused by increased PTH or malignancy (Silverberg and Bilezikian, 2006). Hypophosphatemia in association with hypocalcemia is usually caused by renal wasting or is seen in severe illness. One form of infant hypophosphatemic rickets is transmitted as an autosomal dominant trait (Box 35-15).

Osteoporosis and Osteomalacia

See the discussion online at www.expertconsult.com.

Box 35-14 Causes of Hyperphosphatemia

Impaired renal phosphate excretion

Renal insufficiency
Tumoral calcinosis
Hypoparathyroidism, pseudohypoparathyroidism
Acromegaly
Etidronate
Heparin

Increased extracellular phosphate

Rapid administration of phosphate (IV, oral, rectal)
Rapid cellular catabolism or lysis
   Catabolic states
   Tissue injury
      Hyperthermia
      Crush injuries
      Fulminant hepatitis
   Cellular lysis
      Hemolytic anemia
      Rhabdomyolysis
      Cytotoxic therapy
   Transcellular shifts of phosphate
      Metabolic acidosis
      Respiratory acidosis

From Bringhurst FR, Leder BZ. Regulation of calcium and phosphate homeostasis. In DeGroot LJ, Jameson JL (eds). Endocrinology, 5th ed, vol 2. Philadelphia, Elsevier-Saunders, 2006.

Box 35-15 Causes of Hypophosphatemia

Impaired intestinal phosphate reabsorption

Selective binding of dietary phosphate
  Aluminum-containing antacids

Impaired renal tubular phosphate reabsorption

Renal tubular disorders

Fanconi syndrome(s), other renal tubular disorders
Cystinosis
Wilson's disease
Inactivating NA/P$_1$2 mutations
Dent's disease
Hypophosphatemia in idiopathic hypercalciuria

Elevated PTH or PTHrP

Primary hyperparathyroidism
PTHrP-dependent hypercalcemia (malignancy)
Secondary hyperparathyroidism
  Vitamin D deficiency resistance
  Calcium starvation or malabsorption
  Bartter's syndrome
  Autosomal recessive renal hypomagnesemia/hypercalciuria

Humoral phosphate-wasting syndromes

X-linked hypophosphatemic rickets
Autosomal dominant hypophosphatemic rickets
Tumor-induced osteomalacia
McCune-Albright syndrome

Other systemic disorders

Glucosuria
Hyperaldosteronism
Magnesium or potassium depletion
Amyloidosis
Renal transplantation
Rewarming, induced hyperthermia

Drugs and Toxins

Ethanol	Glucocorticoids
Ifosfamide	Rapamycin
Acetazolamide	Estrogens
Cisplatin	Foscarnet
Toluene	Suramin
Heavy metals	Pamidronate

Accelerated phosphate redistribution into cells or bone

Acute intracellular shifts

Insulin therapy (for hyperglycemia, diabetic ketoacidosis
Intravenous glucose, fructose, glycerol (in NPO patients)
Catecholamines (epinephrine, albuterol, terbutaline, dopamine)
Acute respiratory alkalosis (salicylate intoxication, acute gout)
Gram-negative sepsis, toxic shock syndrome, thyrotoxic periodic paralysis
Recovery from acidosis, starvation, hypothermia

Rapid formation of new cells

Leukemic blast crisis
Bone marrow, stem cell therapy
Erythropoietin, GM-CSF therapy
Treatment of pernicious anemia
Status post–partial hepatectomy

Accelerated net bone formation

Postparathyroidectomy
Treatment of vitamin D deficiency
Early phase of bisphosphonate therapy
Osteoblastic metastases

Bringhurst FR, Leder BZ. Regulation of Calcium and Phosphate Homeostasis. In DeGroot LJ, Jameson JL (eds). Endocrinology, 5th ed, vol 2. Philadelphia, Elsevier-Saunders, 2006.

PTH, Parathyroid hormone; *GM-CSF,* granulocyte macrophage-colony-stimulating factor.

References

The complete reference list is available online at www.expertconsult.com.

Web Resources

www.ncbi.nlm.nih.gov/sites/entrez
  PubMed is a general reference source that provides search access based on subject, author, journal, etc.
www.endo-society.org/guidelines
  Direct access to current and past treatment guidelines for most endocrine-related diseases.
www.hormone.org/Resources/Patient_Guides
  Ready resource for current recommendations for physicians and the public for endocrine disorders.
www.jama.ama-assn.org
  Reference site sponsored by the American Medical Association with access to current and past *JAMA* publications, by author, subject, etc.

www.aafp.org/online/en/home/clinical.html
  American Academy of Family Physicians maintains a website that can be accessed by members (more selection) and nonmembers with information on recommendations for clinical screening and treatment.
www.acponline.org/clinical_information/guidelines/
  American College of Physicians maintains this website for general information as well as specific information on disease screening.
www.aace.com/pub/guidelines/
  American Association of Clinical Endocrinologists.

36 CHAPTER

Obesity

Gregory J. Anderson and Donald D. Hensrud

Chapter contents

Overview

Key Points

- Body mass index (BMI) determines the classification of obesity for clinical use.
- Waist circumference reflects the distribution of adipose tissue and helps determine obesity risk.
- Central obesity, reflected by a high waist measurement, is associated with more complications.

Obesity has been a rapidly developing health concern in the United States. The ongoing Behavioral Risk Factor Surveillance System (BRFSS) and National Health and Nutrition Examination Survey (NHANES) provide a longitudinal view of changes in the obesity problem. BRFSS data are from a state-based telephone survey, and NHANES data are based on measurements of a representative sample of the U.S. population. The self-reporting design of BRFSS tends to underestimate weight, but ongoing studies can be examined for trends. NHANES reported that the prevalence of U.S. adults in the overweight category (BMI ≥25 kg/m²) increased from 46% to 61% between the late 1970s and 1990s

(Zimmerman, 2002). As of 1999–2000, 64.5% of adults were overweight and 30.5% were obese (BMI ≥30 kg/m²) (Flegal et al., 2002). Prevalence estimates from the Centers for Disease Control and Prevention (CDC) for 2007–2008 found that 32.2% of men and 35.5% of women were obese. In addition, surveys from 1976–1980 and 2003–2006 found that obesity increased from 5.0% to 12.4% among children age 2 to 5 years; from 6.5% to 17.0% for ages 6 to 11 years; and 5.0% to 17.6% for ages 12 to 19 years. Changes in obesity prevalence have affected all U.S. regions (Fig. 36-1).

The problem of obesity is not limited to the United States. Globally, *overnutrition* has now surpassed undernutrition as a public health concern. An estimated 8.5% of the world population is overweight versus 5.8% underweight (Zimmerman, 2002). Although obesity prevalence estimates vary among countries, the World Health Organization (WHO) has projected that 2.3 billion adults will be overweight and 700,000 million obese by 2015.

Improved treatment of comorbidities has made assessing obesity's impact on mortality more difficult, but estimates of the excess mortality associated with obesity in the United States range from 100,000 to 300,000 deaths each year. Persons in the overweight category have 20% to 40% increased mortality, and obese persons have a twofold to threefold increase in mortality (Adams et al., 2006).

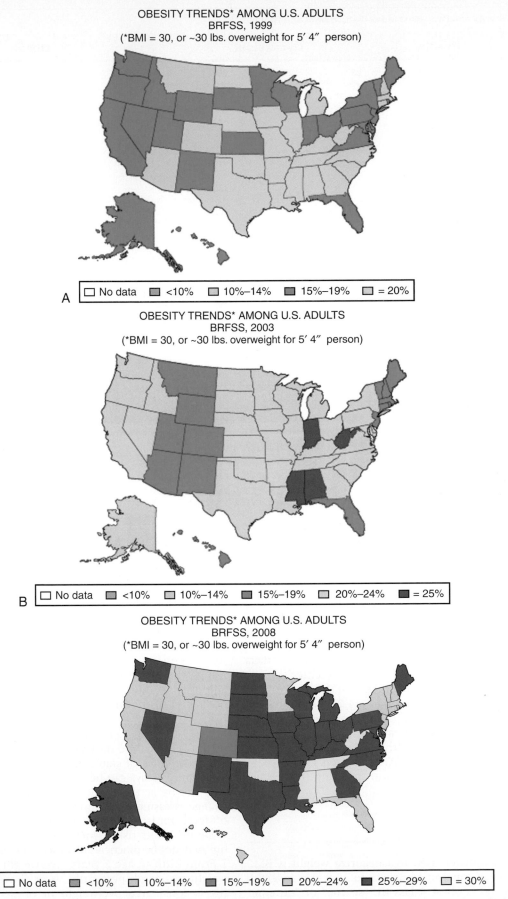

Figure 36-1 U.S. maps reflecting changes in obesity prevalence estimates over time. *(Courtesy Centers for Disease Control and Prevention. Behavioral Risk Factor Surveillance System.)*

Table 36-1 Obesity and Body Mass Index (BMI): Height and Weight

	Healthy		Overweight			Obese			
BMI (kg/m²)	18.5	24.9	25	27	29.9	30	35	40	45
Height					Weight (lb)				
4'10"	89	119	120	129	143	144	167	191	215
4'11"	92	123	124	134	147	148	173	198	223
5'0"	95	127	128	138	153	154	179	205	230
5'1"	98	131	132	143	158	159	185	211	238
5'2"	101	136	137	148	163	164	191	218	246
5'3"	104	140	141	152	168	169	197	226	254
5'4"	108	145	146	157	174	175	204	233	262
5'5"	111	149	150	162	179	180	210	240	270
5'6"	115	154	155	167	185	186	217	247	278
5'7"	118	158	159	172	190	191	223	255	287
5'8"	122	163	164	177	196	197	230	263	296
5'9"	125	168	169	183	202	203	237	270	304
5'10"	129	173	174	188	208	209	244	278	313
5'11"	133	178	179	193	214	215	251	286	322
6'0"	136	183	184	199	220	221	258	294	331
6'1"	140	188	189	204	226	227	265	303	340
6'2"	144	193	194	210	232	233	272	311	350
6'3"	148	199	200	216	239	240	280	319	359
6'4"	152	204	205	221	245	246	287	328	369

The increased prevalence of obesity has many other health ramifications. An increase in body mass index (BMI) is a risk factor for short-term disability in the workplace. Overweight and obese individuals have odds ratios of 1.26 and 1.76, respectively, compared to normal-weight workers (Arena et al., 2006). Obesity increases "presenteeism," or the reduced productivity in workers still on the job. Workers with BMI over 35 kg/m² experienced a 4.2% health-related drop in productivity (Gates et al., 2008). Evidence indicates that the 37% increase in obesity rates (BRFSS) between 1998 and 2006 is a significant factor driving health care costs. The medical consequences of obesity have been estimated to account for 9.1% of annual medical spending (Finkelstein et al., 2009).

Assessment

The primary parameter used to categorize weight is BMI: 18.5 and 24.9 is normal in adults; 25 to 29.9 is overweight; and 30 or greater is obese. Class III, "severe," or "extreme" obesity is 40 and higher. Calculated from height and weight

and expressed in kg/m², BMI is a readily available tool in the assessment of obesity (Table 36-1). Because it correlates with total body fat and with the complications of obesity better than body weight, BMI is a recommended parameter to assess obesity, but an imperfect tool to measure adiposity. A high value may reflect greater lean body mass rather than adiposity in muscular individuals. In addition, BMI does not reflect distribution of body fat, a factor that influences risk.

Body fat percentage is a more precise assessment of adiposity but is difficult to measure accurately in the office setting. The techniques of skin fold measurements and bioelectric impedance assays can be used, but skin fold measurements may not be accurate, and both measures generally do not change assessment or treatment goals for most patients. Cutoff levels for body fat percentage selected by WHO are used to stratify health risks associated with overweight and obesity but may not be practical in clinical practice.

From birth to age 2 years, overweight is assessed by the weight-for-length percentile; at or above the 95th percentile is considered overweight or obese. For the pediatric population age 2 to 19 years, percentile ranks based on

Table 36-2 Classification of Obesity Based on BMI and Waist Circumference

	BMI* (kg/m²)	Obesity Class	Disease Risk	
			Low Waist Cir	High Waist Cir†
Underweight	<18.5	—	—	—
Normal	18.5-24.9	—	—	—
Overweight	25.0-29.9	—	Increased	High
Obesity	30.0-34.9	I	High	Very high
	35.0-39.9	II	Very high	Very high
Extreme obesity	≥40	III	Extremely high	Extremely high

From National Heart, Lung, and Blood Institute, National Institutes of Health. The Practical Guide to the Identification, Evaluation, and Treatment of Overweight and Obesity in Adults (NIH). Pub No 00-4084. NIH, Bethesda, Md, 2000.
*Body mass index can be calculated as wt (kg)/ht² (m), or wt (lb) × 703/ht² (in).
†High waist circumference is defined as >40 inches in men and >35 inches in women.

the 2000 CDC growth charts for the United States are used to define overweight and obesity. The CDC defines overweight between ages 2 and 19 years as a BMI between the 85th and 95th percentiles for age and sex. A child or adolescent with BMI at or above the 95th percentile is considered obese.

The *distribution* of body fat also affects health risks. *Central obesity,* also referred to as visceral, abdominal, or android obesity, is associated with a greater risk of complications, including the metabolic syndrome, as discussed later. Waist-to-hip ratio has been used to assess central obesity, but gender-specific waist circumference, taken at the level of the iliac crest, has proved to be a better assessment of the distribution of body fat. Health risks increase above a waist circumference of 35 inches in women and 40 inches in men, and as a continuous variable with increasing waist circumference, but these cutoffs facilitate a simple classification of risk in a continuous variable. Magnetic resonance imaging (MRI) and computed tomography (CT) of the abdomen have also been used to assess visceral deposition of fat in research settings, but cost and lack of easy accessibility make them impractical for clinical use. Table 36-2 lists the classification of obesity based on BMI and waist circumference.

Demographics

Key Points

- Men are more likely than women to have central obesity.
- African Americans, Hispanics, and Native Americans are at greater risk of obesity than whites.
- Obesity is inversely related to education and socioeconomic status.
- Obesity is more prevalent in rural than urban areas.

Table 36-3 Obesity Prevalence (BRFSS Surveys, 2006–2008)

	White, non-Hispanic	Black, non-Hispanic	Hispanic
Men	25.4%	31.69%	27.8%
Women	21.8%	39.2%	29.4%
Both	23.7%	35.7%	28.7%

Data from Behavior Risk Factor Surveillance System. Differences in prevalence of obesity among black, white, and Hispanic adults—United States, 2006–2008. http://www.cdc.gov/mmwr/preview/mmwrhtml/mm5827a2.htm..

Obesity is a concern within virtually all demographic groups (Table 36-3). The high prevalence of obesity is seen in both genders, most ethnic groups, and at all ages. Within those groups, the impact is not uniform.

Gender Differences

Men are more likely than women to be overweight, whereas women are more likely to be obese. Men, however, are more likely to have central obesity, associated with greater health risks.

Race and Ethnic Origin

African Americans, Hispanics, and Native Americans are at greater risk for obesity. Blacks have a 51% higher prevalence of obesity and Hispanics a 21% higher prevalence than whites (Pan et al., 2009). Asians are at lower risk as an ethnic group. However, health risks of overweight and obesity may appear at a lower weight in Asians, and thus a lower cutoff for overweight has been proposed for Asians (BMI >23 kg/m²). Gender differences are seen within ethnic groups. The prevalence of obesity is greater among African American women than among African American men, whereas these differences are not as evident among non-Hispanic whites. Immigrants have an increased incidence of obesity, starting about 10 years after arrival in the United States (Goel et al., 2004).

Socioeconomic Status

The increase in the prevalence of obesity worldwide reflects, in part, economic development. The prevalence ranges from approximately 2% in the least developed countries to over 30% in the most developed countries. In developed countries, however, lower socioeconomic status is associated with an increased risk. Proposed reasons for this observed difference include reduced access to medical care, healthy foods, and exercise facilities among lower socioeconomic groups. Furthermore, foods that are more energy dense (through the addition of added sugar) are less costly than nutrient-dense foods (Thompson et al., 2009).

Education Level

Education level is inversely related to the risk of obesity, which may partly explain the decreased risk with increased socioeconomic status in developed countries. Access to health care, greater awareness of healthy lifestyle habits, and more access to recreational facilities are potential factors in this association.

Rural and Urban Differences

Analysis of BRFSS data shows that the prevalence of obesity is greater in rural than urban areas. Factors that reduce physical activity may play a role, ranging from less access to exercise facilities to lack of sidewalks. Reduced availability of healthy food choices is also thought to contribute. As in other settings, African Americans and Native Americans in rural areas have the highest prevalence of obesity. Although Asians in urban environments have a low prevalence of obesity, the prevalence among Asians in rural settings approaches that of other ethnic groups (Jackson et al., 2005).

Age

The incidence of overweight increases steadily after age 20 until the seventh decade of life. At that point, it levels off and begins a gradual decline. Even within the low-risk age ranges of 18 to 29 and older than 70 years, the prevalence of overweight has increased according to BRFSS. The increased prevalence of overweight is especially alarming in the pediatric population, in whom the most dramatic increase has been in the severely obese, similar to the adult population. More than 30% of children and adolescents are overweight or obese. Older children are more likely to be in a higher weight category.

Determinants of Obesity

Key Points

- Obesity results from the interaction of genetic makeup, environment, and lifestyle.
- Genetic factors are estimated to account for 30% to 40% of the variability in adult weight.
- Genetic influence is polygenic.
- Specific metabolic or endocrine disorders account for less than 1% of the obese population.

When reduced to basics, obesity results from calorie consumption in excess of expenditure. What complicates this simple principle is the role of genetics, lifestyle, and environmental factors. Throughout human evolution there has been a survival advantage to storing energy as fat. The conveniences of modern life have led to a decrease in energy expenditure. At the same time, greater access to energy-dense food, along with other factors, has increased energy consumption. These changes, in the relatively recent past, negate the survival advantage of fat storage for most segments of the population.

Genetics vs. Lifestyle

The relative contribution of genes versus lifestyle and environment in the development of obesity has not been precisely delineated. A child's risk of adulthood obesity is three times greater if one parent is obese and 10 times greater if both are obese. Indeed, for children younger than 3 years, parental weight is a greater determinant of risk of obesity than the child's own weight (Whitaker et al., 1997). However, the influence of parental weight does not reflect only genetic predisposition, because family members also share the same environment. A correlation in adult weight between identical twins is seen, even when they have been raised apart. Among adoptees, weight correlates with the weight of their biologic parents, but the correlation is not as strong as in twin studies. In summary, genetic makeup plays a permissive role, with adult weight being determined by interaction with the environment. Overall, genetic factors are estimated to be responsible for 30% to 40% of the variability in adult weight.

Genetic Factors

Most of the genetic influence on obesity is polygenic. More than 250 genes and chromosomal regions are associated with phenotypic obesity (Larsen et al., 2003). In some cases, the genes code specifically for visceral as opposed to subcutaneous obesity. Although specific genetic factors to explain common obesity have not been identified, several single-gene defects cause obesity in animals, with some correlates in humans.

Single-gene mutations related to obesity often involve leptin and melanocortin. *Leptin* is a protein produced in adipose tissue that provides negative feedback to appetite control centers. Obesity may reflect lack of hormone production or a lack of leptin receptors. There are leptin-deficient animal models, and rarely, this deficiency has been identified in humans. In leptin-deficient people, weight loss results when leptin is replaced. Leptin supplementation in non–leptin-deficient obese subjects does not result in weight loss (Bray, 2002).

Rare defects in *melanocortin* receptors in the adrenals have also been associated with obesity. Most often, a person must be homozygous for the abnormal gene for the trait to be expressed. A defect in the melanocortin-4 receptor is the most common single-gene mutation associated with severe obesity but still accounts for only about 5% of this population. Other single-gene mutations have been found in animal models as well as humans, but all are extremely rare. Recently identified genes include the FTO (fat mass and obesity-associated) gene. Each of these genes seems to be associated with a modest increase in weight.

There are a number of congenital syndromes in which obesity is part of the phenotype. The best known, *Prader-Willi syndrome*, results from a defect in the long arm of chromosome 15 and causes poor muscle tone in the newborn period, with hyperphagia, hypogonadism, behavioral problems, and developmental delay noted later. As with other medical causes of childhood obesity, linear growth is poor while growth in weight is excessive. Although the exact mechanisms by which the genetic abnormalities lead to obesity are unclear, patients with Prader-Willi syndrome have elevated levels of *ghrelin*, a peptide produced in the stomach and duodenum that stimulates eating.

Modulation of Appetite

Many hormonal factors are involved in appetite, as well as in the absorption, storage, and use of calories. Factors providing input to the brain include leptin levels, vagal afferent activity, and fluctuation in plasma glucose levels. Neuropeptides and monoamine neurotransmitters are also involved in appetite control. Some weight loss medications exert their influence through modulation of neurotransmitter levels, which may affect appetite or satiety.

Influences on Central Obesity

Central obesity suggests increased visceral fat deposits, likely caused by increased production of peptides and other metabolic messengers. Hormonal influences most likely play a role in the distribution of fat. Central obesity is believed to result partly from increased androgenic effects, which is why men have a greater tendency for central obesity. Central obesity is also associated with hyperandrogenic states in women, such as polycystic ovary syndrome (PCOS). The increase in visceral deposition of fat that can occur after menopause in women may be related to a decrease in growth hormone and estrogen production (see Chapter 35).

Lifestyle Influences

Key Points

- Increased caloric intake is related in part to "portion distortion," linked to eating away from home.
- Smoking cessation is associated with weight gain of 4 to 5 kg (on average).
- Many antidepressants, neuroleptics, and anticonvulsants are associated with weight gain.
- Decreased overall physical activity (not just "exercise") is a major factor associated with the increasing prevalence of overweight and obesity.

As mentioned, obesity develops when caloric intake exceeds caloric expenditure against a background of genetic influences. The chief determinants of energy imbalance are lifestyle factors. Individual total energy requirements depend on the *basal metabolic rate* (BMR), thermic effect of food, and energy needed for the day's physical activities. The chief determinant of BMR is the amount of lean body mass, which can be difficult to increase. Some data indicate that the *thermic effect* of food (amount of energy needed to absorb, digest, and assimilate nutrients) is lower in obese persons than in lean subjects, but this difference is quite small. Physical activity (exercise and activity throughout the day) is the most variable component of energy expenditure. The major reasons for weight gain are therefore excessive calorie intake and decreased overall physical activity.

Caloric Intake

Over the past 40 years, the tendency in the U.S. population has been to consume more calories needed; per-capita consumption of calories increased from 2220 kcal in 1970 to 2680 kcal in 1997 (Putnam, 2000). Some of this increase is related to increased portion size; a normal portion in 1970 is much less than a normal portion in 2010. This "portion distortion" has been linked to people eating more away from home. The typically larger restaurant portion size has been adopted as the in-home standard as well (Foreyt and Poston, 2002).

Energy density also plays a role. Satiety helps determine food intake and is largely determined by the volume and weight of food consumed. Foods that are high in caloric content for a given volume lead to excessive calorie intake. This includes fat and highly processed foods such as sugar and other refined carbohydrates that are high in energy density. Per-capita consumption of sugar has greatly increased at the same time as the increasing prevalence of obesity.

The frequency of meals may play a small role. Eating smaller meals more frequently is associated with less overweight. Large meals are associated with more insulin release. This might be a mechanism whereby meal size influences weight gain.

Activity Changes

Decreased energy expenditure may play a greater role in the development of obesity than increased caloric intake. In the United States a progressive decrease in energy expenditure has coincided with the increase in calorie consumption (Foreyt and Poston, 2002). The amount of exercise has not changed much over the past few decades, so most of the decrease in physical activity energy expenditure has occurred in daily physical activities, not exercise.

Smoking Cessation

Often cited by smokers as a reason to continue smoking, stopping cigarette smoking does lead to weight gain. The average weight gain is 4 to 5 kg (~9-11 lb) over months (Flegal et al., 1995). Typically, the person gains 1 to 2 kg (~2-4 lb) in the first few weeks after cessation (Bray, 2002). Approximately 10% of people gain 10 kg (22 lb) or more.

Medications

A number of medications are associated with weight gain, including antidepressants, antipsychotics, anticonvulsants, and hypoglycemic agents. Tricyclic antidepressants, monoamine oxidase inhibitors, and mirtazapine are the antidepressants most likely to cause weight gain. Of the more common selective serotonin reuptake inhibitors (SSRIs), paroxetine is most likely to be associated with weight gain, although individual effects vary. Many neuroleptics can lead to weight gain. Phenothiazines and haloperidol, as well as some newer agents such as clozapine and olanzapine, tend to increase weight. Among anticonvulsants, valproic acid and gabapentin have been most closely tied to weight gain. Lamotrigine is thought to be weight neutral, whereas topiramate may actually promote weight loss. Insulin, as well as oral hypoglycemics that increase production or release of insulin, promote weight gain. It should be noted that metformin, which increases insulin sensitivity, is associated with modest weight loss and may ameliorate the weight gain from other hypoglycemics. Chronic systemic steroid use can cause a cushingoid type of obesity.

Endocrine and Metabolic Factors

Specific identifiable endocrine or metabolic disorders known to cause obesity account for less than 1% of the obese population, contrary to what is commonly believed (see also Chapter 34).

Hypothyroidism

Although rarely found in children, hypothyroidism is associated with slow statural growth and developmental delay. More common among adults and more often seen in women, hypothyroidism is a relatively rare cause of obesity. If undiagnosed, it is typically accompanied by other symptoms of thyroid deficiency, such as cold intolerance, decreased energy, obstipation, and increased thinning of the scalp.

Neuroendocrine Factors

The rarely seen neuroendocrine causes for obesity result from injury to the ventromedial hypothalamus, the result of tumor, trauma, or surgery to the posterior fossa. Other symptoms indicative of endocrine and neurologic abnormalities are seen along with hyperphagia and subsequent obesity (Bray, 2002).

Cushing's Syndrome

This endocrine disorder is associated with central obesity and "buffalo hump" along with axillary striae, glucose intolerance and hypertension. In children with Cushing's syndrome, linear growth is restricted.

Polycystic Ovary Syndrome

More than 50% of women affected by this relatively common disorder are obese. Some controversy surrounds whether PCOS is a cause or consequence of obesity, although most evidence points to the latter. Other common features include menstrual irregularities, hirsutism, and elevated testosterone and luteinizing hormone blood levels. Insulin resistance is a consistent finding, even in the absence of obesity. This resistance is thought to be associated with other findings in PCOS, although exact mechanisms are unclear.

Growth Hormone Deficiency

Although growth in height is impaired in growth hormone deficiency, there is also an increase in truncal obesity. This corrects with replacement of growth hormone.

Medical Complications

Key Points

- Obesity is more closely related to elevated triglycerides and low HDL cholesterol than elevated total and LDL cholesterol.
- Weight loss is the most effective lifestyle change to lower blood pressure.
- Up to 80% of cases of type 2 diabetes mellitus are attributable to overweight and obesity.
- Obesity plays a role in 14% of cancer deaths in men and 20% in women.

Based on observational studies, obesity is a risk factor for a number of chronic medical conditions. In conjunction with other risk factors, obesity can greatly impact the chances of developing many diseases. In general, the increased risk for morbidity and mortality begins in the overweight range and correlates more strongly with BMI over 30 kg/m^2 (Flegal et al., 2004). The risk of specific conditions associated with obesity, such as diabetes and hypertension, varies with gender and ethnic origin.

Hypertension

Obesity has long been recognized as a risk factor for hypertension and appears to be associated with the increasing incidence of hypertension seen with aging. The obesity-related increase in blood pressure (BP) is associated with an increase in vascular resistance as well as sodium resorption. The increased vascular tone may reflect increased sympathetic tone because of insulin resistance and the resultant increase in insulin levels. In the Nurses' Health Study (NHS), for BMI at age 18 and again at midlife, the relative risk of hypertension in women gaining 5 to 9.9 kg (11-22 lb) in that time was 1.7, and in those with weight gain over 25 kg (55 lb) was 5.2 (Huang et al., 1998). Controlling overweight would reduce the incidence of hypertension in whites by an estimated 48% and in African Americans by 28% (Bray, 2003). Weight loss is the most effective lifestyle change to decrease blood pressure. For every 1-kg loss in weight, there is an average decrease of 0.6 mm Hg in systolic and 0.34 mm Hg in diastolic BP (Stevens et al., 1993). In the National Heart, Lung, and Blood Institute (NHLBI) obesity guidelines, weight loss is recommended to lower elevated BP in overweight and obese persons.

> **KEY TREATMENT**
>
> Modest weight loss can reduce morbidity of obesity-related disease (Shepherd, 2003) (SOR: A).

Dyslipidemia

Obesity is associated with elevated triglyceride (TG) levels, reduced high-density lipoprotein cholesterol (HDL-C), and an increase in the more atherogenic, small, dense LDL particles. Despite common belief, obesity causes only a small mean elevation in total and low-density lipoprotein cholesterol (LDL-C) values. There is strong evidence that weight loss through lifestyle measures will reduce TG and increase HDL-C levels. This weight loss is generally accompanied by a decrease in total cholesterol and LDL-C, in part because the same lifestyle changes in diet that decrease weight also decrease LDL-C. The favorable effect on lipids from aerobic exercise is most noticeable when accompanied by weight loss. NHLBI recommends weight loss to reduce elevated total cholesterol, LDL-C, and TG levels and to raise HDL-C in overweight/obese persons.

Type 2 Diabetes Mellitus

According to BRFSS, the prevalence of type 2 diabetes mellitus (T2DM) increased from 4.9% in 1990 to 7.9% in 2000 (Mokdad et al., 2003). This change has been clearly linked to the increase in obesity. The risk of T2DM is lowest below a BMI of 22 to 23 kg/m^2. At a BMI of 31, the risk for women in the NHS was 40-fold greater than in women with a BMI less than 22 (Colditz et al., 1995). For men in the Health Professionals Follow-up Study, the risk of T2DM above a BMI of 35 kg/m^2 was increased 60-fold. Up to 80% of cases of T2DM can be attributed to overweight and obesity. There appears to be a time delay of about 10 years between the development of overweight and onset of the diabetes (Bray, 2003). As weight increases, insulin resistance and compensatory insulin secretion also increase. At some point, the body's ability to secrete insulin does not meet requirements, and blood glucose rises. Weight loss is recommended to lower elevated glucose levels in overweight and obese persons with T2DM.

Metabolic Syndrome

The metabolic syndrome brings together a number of the comorbidities associated with obesity. The definition used by the National Cholesterol Education Program (NCEP) Adult Treatment Panel III requires the presence of three of the following five disorders: (1) BP elevation of at least 130/85 mm Hg, (2) serum TG level higher than 150 mg/dL, (3) HDL-C level less than 50 mg/dL in women and 40 mg/dL in men, (4) fasting blood glucose level at least 110 mg%, and (5) waist circumference more than 35 inches in women and 40 inches in men. WHO and American Association of Clinical Endocrinologists (AACE) criteria are similar but add increased urinary albumin excretion and require the presence of impaired glucose tolerance or T2DM. The waist circumference indicates abdominal or visceral obesity. It is not clear whether visceral obesity is a factor in the development of the metabolic syndrome or if it is simply a marker for the disorder. An estimated 40% of the U.S. population over age 65 meet the criteria for the metabolic syndrome. Although other factors may be involved in the pathogenesis, a common thread linking these disorders is insulin resistance. The presence of the metabolic syndrome increases the risk of T2DM, hypertension, coronary artery disease (CAD), and cerebrovascular disease.

Heart Disease

The presence of obesity in the absence of other risk factors may lead to cardiomyopathy and congestive heart failure (CHF) as the workload of the heart increases. Beyond the direct impact on cardiac function, obesity may be an independent risk factor for CAD. Obesity is associated with a number of well-established risk factors for CAD, and most of the increased risk associated with obesity is caused by these factors. The NHS indicated that for women with BMI more than 29 kg/m^2, CAD risk increases 3.3-fold compared with women with BMI less than 21 kg/m^2 (Manson et al., 1995). The Finnish Heart Study found that for each increase in weight of approximately 1 kg, the risk of mortality from CAD was increased by 1% to 1.5% (Jousilahti et al., 1996). The NHS and the Health Professionals Follow-up Study showed a significant increased risk of CAD among participants who gained more than 10 kg after age 20. A 4% increased risk of atrial fibrillation has been found for each 1-unit increase in BMI. Left atrial enlargement is a predictor of atrial fibrillation and has been associated with increased BMI (Zalesin et al., 2008).

Cancer

Although not all studies have found a positive correlation between specific cancers and obesity, it is thought to be associated with many and perhaps most cancers. Obesity may be the largest avoidable cause of cancer for nonsmokers. A 16-year prospective study of over 900,000 people found a 52% increase in cancer mortality in men and a 62% increase in women who were severely obese (Calle et al., 2003). Cancers of many different primary sites were associated with obesity, with increased mortality risk from cancer of the esophagus, colon, kidney, gallbladder, and pancreas, as well as multiple myeloma and non-Hodgkin's lymphoma. There was a significant trend toward increased risk of prostate, gastric, ovarian, and endometrial cancers. The relative risk for obese subjects who had never smoked was even greater than for smokers. It was estimated that overweight and obesity played a role in 14% of cancer deaths in men and 20% in women.

The mechanisms accounting for the increased risk of cancers vary with the primary site. One proposed mechanism for endometrial and breast cancer is an increase in circulating estrogen levels. Central obesity in particular has been associated with breast cancer. Increasing evidence shows an association between obesity and prostate cancer, with the increased risk likely related to changes in testosterone as well as leptin, insulin-like growth factor 1, and interleukin-6 levels.

The World Cancer Research Fund and American Institute for Cancer Research (2007) state that maintenance of a healthy weight throughout life may be one of the most important ways to protect against cancer. Adults should maintain BMI between 21 and 23.

Obstructive Sleep Apnea

Although obstructive sleep apnea (OSA) is not always associated with obesity, excessive weight is a major risk factor. About 70% of OSA patients are obese. Among obese persons, the incidence of OSA is approximately 40% (Poulain et al., 2006). The increased risk may be related to increased neck circumference and pharyngeal fat deposits. Often unrecognized, OSA has significance beyond daytime somnolence and the spousal impact of disruptive snoring and has been associated with systemic effects as well, such as pulmonary hypertension, right-sided CHF, and erectile dysfunction. Weight loss may benefit the OSA patient. Conversely, a patient with mild OSA who has a 10% increase in body weight then has a sixfold increased risk of progressing to moderate or severe sleep apnea (Caples et al., 2005).

Pulmonary Disease

Obesity can have an impact on overall lung function. It increases the work of breathing through a decrease in chest wall compliance as well as a reduction in respiratory muscle strength. Obesity increases pressure on the diaphragm, reducing residual lung volume (reduced FEV$_1$, FVC, TLC, and FRC). The result can be a mild restrictive pattern, although typically only in the severely obese population (Poulain et al., 2006). Asthma is exacerbated with increased weight, and obesity-hypoventilation syndrome (hypercapnic respiratory failure and cor pulmonale) is associated with marked degrees of obesity.

Fatty Liver Disease

Fatty liver disease is the most common reason for elevated serum liver enzymes and affects an estimated 20% of the U.S. population (Angelico et al., 2005). First described in obese diabetic females, fatty liver disease is widely recognized as a complication of obesity and is associated with the features of the metabolic syndrome. The spectrum of fatty liver disease ranges from nonalcoholic fatty liver disease (NAFLD) to nonalcoholic steatohepatitis (NASH). Fibrosis and cirrhosis can develop in NASH, which has been linked to insulin resistance, as with metabolic syndrome (Choudhury and Sanyal, 2004). The increased insulin level likely causes fatty acid flux from adipose tissue to be deposited in the liver. Inflammatory cytokine release triggered by hyperinsulinemia contributes to the steatohepatitis and fibrosis.

Orthopedic Disorders

Overweight children have an increased risk of slipped femoral capital epiphysis, genu valga, pes planus, and scoliosis (Speiser et al., 2005). In adults, an association between obesity and degenerative joint disease (DJD), particularly of the knee, is related in part to mechanical factors resulting in increased compressive forces on the knee. Obesity-related cytokine production has been associated with a chronic inflammatory state promoting osteoarthritis. Obesity is associated with knee weakness and balance problems, increasing the risk of falls. Functional impairment from obesity in elderly persons has been linked to these factors (Messier, 2008).

Gallbladder Disease

Obesity, along with hyperinsulinemia and the metabolic syndrome, are risk factors for gallbladder disease, apparently related to changes in cholesterol metabolism. Cholesterol production increases with weight gain, and cholesterol is excreted into bile. The increased cholesterol relative to bile acids can lead to the formation of stones. Cholesterol flux during weight loss increases risk of symptomatic gallbladder disease, which increases with the rapidity of weight loss (Bray, 2003).

Psychological Impact

Self-awareness of overweight and the associated psychological impact can be seen in children as young as 5 years old. The social repercussions of overweight can result in poor self-esteem. This may result in poor body image, especially in young women. Eating disorders, particularly binge eating, can complicate the management of obesity. In adults, obesity is associated with depression in women, although not in men (Carpenter et al., 2000).

Complications in Childhood and Adolescence

In addition to childhood overweight being a risk factor for adult obesity, medical complications of excessive weight occur in the pediatric population. These range from a slipped femoral capital epiphysis to self-esteem issues. Adult diseases (T2DM, NAFLD, OSA) are being increasingly identified in the pediatric population.

Management and Interventions

Key Points

- An initial goal of a 5% to 10% reduction in weight is reasonable.
- A process-oriented target (lifestyle) may be more beneficial for some than a target weight.
- A weight reduction rate of 1 to 2 pounds weekly is achievable if intake is reduced by 500 to 1000 kcal daily.
- Caloric restriction alone is not as effective as combining it with an exercise program.
- A low-energy-dense diet composed of generous quantities of vegetables and fruits promotes health and facilitates weight management.

Although long-term treatment of obesity has generally had disappointing results, some individuals have lost and maintained significant amounts of weight. Weight loss programs have typically shown modest benefit, with variable results depending on the method, but most weight is eventually regained in 4 to 5 years. An exception is bariatric surgery, although its use is restricted to a small subset of the extremely obese population. Primary prevention strategies using many interventions at the individual and population levels are needed to limit the growing epidemic of obesity. Early intervention should start in childhood, and because excessive weight gain can occur at any age, strategies should be continued through adulthood. Family physicians should calculate BMI for all patients at least yearly to monitor for a developing weight disorder, with further screening for comorbidities if overweight is found.

Childhood Overweight and Obesity

Key Points

- Childhood obesity rarely is associated with a primary medical disorder.
- When present in childhood obesity, underlying disorders are almost always associated with statural growth reduction.
- The risk of adult obesity increases with the age of the obese child.
- Intervention can be more effective in children than in adults and should involve the entire family.

Only a small proportion of obese children participate in a medically supervised program. Although many studies of obesity management in the pediatric population have had methodologic limitations, efforts to make lifestyle behavioral changes in physical activity and diet have been found to be of benefit (Oude et al., 2009). Family therapy, school-based programs, and in particular involvement of parents are also beneficial (Hill et al., 2002). Interventions for children may be more effective than those for adults.

The approach of treatment in childhood is primarily related to the lifestyle issues of proper diet and exercise. The goals of treatment should be a reduction in BMI to less than the 95th percentile for age and prevention or reversal of comorbidities. Parental involvement is a key component in childhood weight management. However, parents may not recognize the problem of overweight and obesity in their children, particularly in their sons (Jeffery et al., 2005). Poor parental recognition of their own obesity is also noted. In addition, health care providers may overlook obesity at well-child visits (Cook et al., 2005). Therefore, health care providers may need to educate themselves and their patients about the appropriate recognition and treatment of obesity. Individual and family counseling may be indicated in patients with more severe obesity.

During well-child visits, BMI should be calculated and risk factors for obesity noted. These include parental obesity, maternal smoking during pregnancy, a predilection for sedentary activities, and poor dietary habits. When followed through early childhood, BMI typically will decrease until a period known as *adiposity rebound* occurs between ages 5 and 7 years. An early adiposity rebound noted on BMI for age charts increases the risk of adult obesity. The physician should discuss with all parents the importance of developing healthy eating habits early in life, as well as limiting sedentary activities such as television and computer games. Encouraging parents to model this lifestyle is beneficial.

In children, underlying hormonal factors leading to obesity also tend to lead to short stature. The association of short stature with excess weight gain should therefore prompt an investigation into a possible underlying endocrine disorder (Brown et al., 2002). In contrast, childhood obesity related to exogenous factors is associated with an increased rate of statural growth. This increased growth in height is associated with increased bone age and early puberty.

An adolescent who has been identified as overweight should be screened for comorbidities. The Expert Committee on Clinical Guidelines for Overweight in Adolescent Preventive Services recommends a lipid panel and fasting blood glucose for adolescents with a BMI over the 85th percentile if there is a family history of lipid disorders or early-onset cardiovascular disease (Brown et al., 2002).

A staged treatment approach is recommended depending on the child's age and degree of obesity (Barlow, 2007). For the child between the 85th and 95th percentile for BMI, diet and exercise continue to be key components of treatment. The approach should involve modest calorie restriction while increasing energy expenditure. Overly restrictive diets have the potential of interfering with growth rate, bone mineralization, and menstruation. At a BMI over the 95th percentile, a more structured and aggressive approach may be appropriate, perhaps with referral to a subspecialist.

In an infant, breastfeeding should be encouraged up to the age of 1 year. Restriction or elimination of sweetened beverages such as soft drinks and sports drinks can greatly reduce calorie consumption in children who consume large amounts. The American Academy of Pediatrics (AAP) recommends that sweetened beverages and fruit juice be limited to 4 to 6 ounces daily for children age 1 to 6 years and 8 to 12 ounces for children and adolescents age 7 to 18 years. Replacing sugar-sweetened beverages with milk not only reduces calorie intake but also provides calcium needed for adequate mineralization of bone. All children older than 2 years should be receiving low-fat dairy products such as skim or 1% milk rather than whole milk, which has higher saturated-fat content. Increasing consumption of foods low in energy density but high in nutritional density, such as

vegetables and fruits, can reduce calorie intake and improve nutritional status. In general, food should not be used as a reward, and children should not be required to clean their plate at every meal; rather, they should be taught to choose an appropriate portion size when selecting food. Health-supporting foods should be available through school cafeterias and vending machines.

A sedentary lifestyle is a risk factor for obesity among children and, therefore, there is good reason to promote a physically active lifestyle as a key component in the prevention and treatment of obesity. AAP recommends that sedentary activities (e.g., TV, computer) be limited to no more than 2 hours daily. Rather than requiring specific physical activities, limiting time spent in sedentary activities allows children or teenagers to explore options and find activities they enjoy and are more likely to maintain. School districts should be encouraged to include and fund physical education programs, and community exercise facilities should be readily available to children.

Because of the potential problems of restrictive dieting in children, parents should work with their children through lifestyle changes to maintain a stable weight while height increases, which will result in a decreasing BMI. However, particularly if complications of obesity have developed, a more aggressive approach might be indicated. Nutritional adequacy, growth, and maturation should be closely monitored during more restrictive diets, and referral to a registered dietitian can be beneficial.

Medication use is rarely indicated in children. Sibutramine is approved for use in those older than 16 years and orlistat in those over 12. Both medications are associated with potential side effects. In obese adolescents, sibutramine with behavioral approaches resulted in greater improvement in BMI than with placebo, but almost half the active-treatment group experienced elevated BP or heart rate, necessitating a reduction or discontinuation of the medication (Berkowitz et al., 2003). Bariatric surgery in children and adolescents is also controversial. Although good data are lacking, guidelines are available for both pharmacotherapy and bariatric surgery in children and adolescents (Apovian et al., 2005; August et al., 2008).

Management in Adults

The benefits of screening for obesity have been examined by a number of organizations. The U.S. Preventive Services Task Force (USPSTF, 2003) recommends screening adults for obesity. The amount of information needed to make the diagnosis and establish the most effective approach is modest and can be handled in the context of a typical office visit. The initial approach can be framed through three questions (Hensrud, 2004): (1) what is the patient's BMI? (2) what is the waist circumference? and (3) what comorbidities are present? Determining comorbidities may involve obtaining fasting blood glucose, thyroid-stimulating hormone (TSH), aspartate transaminase (AST) or alanine transaminase (ALT), and lipid profile, as well as BP and history information suggesting associated disorders (e.g., OSA, DJD). Having identified overweight or obesity as a medical concern, it is important to help patients become aware of the medical implications and to engage them in management. Box 36-1 lists areas to discuss with the patient that will affect management (Hensrud, 2002).

Box 36-1 Assessment Areas of Medical History in Obese Patient Evaluation

Readiness/motivation to undertake weight loss

Reasons/expectations for weight loss

Available support

Previous methods of weight loss and results (including why results were not successful)

Potential barriers to weight loss and maintenance (time, finances, established habits)

High school graduation weight, minimum and maximum adult weight

Periods of increased weight gain (e.g., pregnancy, smoking cessation, stressful life periods)

Current (and past) diet

Triggers to eating

Current (and past) exercise/activity

Factors the patient believes are responsible for weight

Binge eating, purging, laxative or diuretic use

Family history of obesity

Medications

(From Hensrud DD. Obesity. In Rakel RE, Bope (eds). Conn's Current Therapy. Philadelphia, Saunders, 2002.)

Many patients are unaware that their weight is excessive or, if aware, do not fully understand the health consequences. Given the negative societal connotations of obesity, patients may not be receptive to addressing weight issues. When obesity is approached nonjudgmentally from the perspective of health risk, patients may be more accepting of the need to change and more willing to partner with the physician in addressing the problem. Readiness to change should be assessed, and addressing barriers to success is key in weight loss and maintenance. Barriers may include emotional factors (stress, depression) or time constraints that limit exercise. A support system can be helpful for someone attempting weight loss, including a spouse or a program incorporating group support (e.g., Weight Watchers).

Preventing or reversing obesity involves finding ways to balance energy intake and energy expenditure better. To obtain the best results, people should change both sides of the energy equation—that is, raise their energy expenditure by increasing physical activity and lower their energy intake by decreasing calories consumed. Physical activity and exercise appear to be more important than diet in preventing both initial weight gain and regaining weight after weight loss. Dietary restriction appears to be more important than physical activity in promoting weight loss.

Physical activity should be increased in daily activities as well as exercise. Aerobic exercise is the most efficient way to burn calories by directly increasing energy expenditure. However, increasing physical activity during the daily routine can result in large energy expenditure. Exercise programs that incorporate resistance training may slightly increase lean body mass, possibly increasing resting energy expenditure. Dietary treatment in the absence of an exercise program produces weight loss but not as much as combining both. In addition, weight loss solely through caloric restriction without an exercise program may result in greater loss of lean body mass.

Although all weight loss programs should involve a combination of caloric restriction and increased physical activity, certain patients may be candidates for adjunctive weight loss medications or, in some situations, bariatric surgery. If the patient has BMI of 27 kg/m² or greater and an obesity-related comorbidity (e.g., T2DM, OSA), sibutramine or orlistat may be indicated as an adjunctive measure. If BMI is 30 or greater, medications may be used even without a comorbid condition, although at Mayo Clinic, we usually prescribe these medications only if the patient also has a comorbid condition. Bariatric surgery can be considered for a patient with BMI of 40 or greater with associated complications or with BMI of 35 or greater if medical complications are present. Table 36-4 outlines the treatment options available based on BMI and comorbid conditions.

Setting Goals

Discussing expectations for weight loss is important as the process begins. If a target goal is too difficult, the patient may quit in frustration. Studies show that a 5% to 10% body weight reduction is achievable through lifestyle approaches, and that this amount of weight loss will benefit health. If this goal is achieved and weight is still above the desired weight, a lower target can be set. Randomized trials demonstrate that weekly weight loss of 1 to 2 lb can be achieved with a daily calorie deficit of 500 to 1000 kcal (because 1 lb of fat contains 3500 kcal). Setting a target weight may not always be the most effective approach. For some patients, a *process*-oriented target (lifestyle) rather than an *outcome*-oriented target (weight) is more effective in the long run in terms of improving health. People who have made lifestyle changes by reducing caloric and saturated-fat intake and improving cardiovascular fitness have improved their health by reducing the risk of obesity-related complications, even if they have not reached a specific weight goal. Using the process-oriented target approach may be less frustrating to some patients, allowing them to sustain their lifestyle changes more effectively, which will have greater impact on their health.

Process and other goals should be specific, measurable, achievable, realistic, and trackable (SMART). For example, instead of setting a goal of just exercising more, a starting SMART goal is exercising by walking 20 minutes 3 days per week. Progress is logged and the goal gradually and regularly increased as fitness improves. A SMART dietary goal would be to eat 1 more piece of fruit and 1 more serving of vegetables daily, monitoring progress through diet records.

Patients should be counseled about the need to maintain indefinitely the lifestyle changes found to be effective. Because the specific type of lifestyle change may vary among patients, individual management is necessary. The NHLBI (2000) recommends that the initial goal of weight loss therapy should be 10% of baseline weight.

Diet

Many different and sometimes physiologically impossible weight reduction diets exist. Patients can access information on weight loss diet plans through books, Internet sites, magazines, and organizations such as Weight Watchers, although few data exist on their effectiveness. One study comparing the

Table 36-4 NHLB/NHI Guidelines for Treatment of Obesity

Treatment	BMI Category*				
	25-26.9	27-29.9	30-34.9	35-39.9	≥40
Diet, physical activity, and behavior therapy[†]	w/co	w/co	+	+	+
Pharmacotherapy[‡]	—	w/co	+	+	+
Surgery	—	—	w/co	w/co	w/co

From National Heart, Lung, and Blood Institute, National Institutes of Health. The Practical Guide to the Identification, Evaluation, and Treatment of Overweight and Obesity in Adults (NIH). Pub No 00-4084. NIH, Bethesda, Md, 2000.

w/co, With comorbidities; +, use of treatment regardless of comorbidities.

*Prevention of weight gain with lifestyle therapy is indicated in any patient with BMI ≥25, even without comorbidities, whereas weight loss is not necessarily recommended for those with BMI of 25-29.9 or a high waist circumference, unless they have two or more comorbidities.

[†]Combined therapy with a low-calorie diet (LCD), increased physical activity, and behavior therapy provides the most successful intervention for weight loss and weight maintenance.

[‡]Consider pharmacotherapy only if a patient has not lost 1 pound per week after 6 months of combined lifestyle therapy.

effectiveness of four popular diets (Ornish, Weight Watchers, Atkins, Zone) showed little difference in results (Dansinger et al., 2005). Although differing in nutritional composition, the diets were equally effective. Results were modest, with average weight loss ranging from 2.1 to 3.3 kg at 1 year. There was a significant attrition rate noted in each program. Adherence to the respective diet was associated with greater weight loss. Thus, one dietary program appears to be no better than another, and adherence is important regardless of the dietary approach. Individualization of dietary therapy may enhance adherence.

Low-carbohydrate diets have been popular in recent years. The rationale involves lowering the insulin levels through reducing carbohydrate intake and blood glucose levels. Reducing the anabolic effect of insulin is the proposed mechanism by which people lose weight. Decreased appetite from ketosis, resulting from carbohydrate restriction, and satiety from fat are other possible mechanisms. A recent study evaluated four diets with varying compositions of carbohydrate (35%-65%), fat (20% or 40%), and protein (15% or 25%) (Sacks et al., 2009). After 2 years, weight loss was not statistically significantly different among diets. Regardless of the calorie source, total calorie intake must be reduced below energy expenditure for weight loss to occur. Difficulty adhering to any diet over time, including low-carbohydrate diets, limits effectiveness; in clinical trials of at least 1 year, almost 40% of subjects randomized to a low-carbohydrate diet dropped out, only slightly lower than those randomized to a calorie-controlled diet. Elimination or restriction of fruits and vegetables on some low-carbohydrate diets may have health consequences as well.

Very-low-calorie diets (VLCDs) restrict calories to 400 to 800 kcal/day. Usually, this consists of a high-protein drink. VLCDs may produce a more rapid initial weight loss than other diets, but results are similar over time. Close medical monitoring during a VLCD program is needed (Kazaks and Stern, 2003).

Most often, a low-calorie diet (LCD) is recommended. Reducing daily caloric intake by 500 to 1000 kcal/day can result in weight loss of 1 to 2 lb per week. Women should consider initially consuming 1000 to 1200 kcal/day, with men consuming 1200 to 1600 kcal/day (NHLBI, 2000). This type of diet plan modestly restricts saturated fats and refined carbohydrates (e.g., sugar) as part of overall caloric restriction. Dietary recommendations should be individualized within certain parameters. For example, a dietary program may be relatively low or high in the proportion of carbohydrates and fats while lowering overall calorie intake. Regardless of diet composition, the types of carbohydrates and fats should be health supporting. Whole-grain carbohydrates such as whole-wheat bread or pasta, brown rice, and oatmeal are preferred over refined carbohydrates such as sugar and white flour. Unsaturated fats such as olive oil, canola oil, and other vegetable oils are preferred over saturated and *trans* fats, which include many cuts of meat, full-fat dairy products, margarine, and other foods that contain partially hydrogenated vegetable fats.

There are many strategies to lower overall caloric intake, such as counting calories and monitoring number of servings of certain food groups. *Portion control* is generally an important part of dietary recommendations to reduce calorie intake; dining at restaurants can be especially challenging. Eating breakfast is associated with better weight management, along with keeping diet records. Substituting low-calorie foods for higher calorie versions can be useful. Meal replacements are another strategy to consider and have been shown to be as effective as conventional dietary recommendations on weight loss (Heymsfeld et al., 2003).

The *energy density* of foods is a potentially important part of reducing calorie intake. Grapes, for example, are less energy-dense than raisins. Because people tend to eat until they feel full, consuming less energy-dense foods will in itself reduce caloric consumption. A reasonable approach is to recommend a diet high in fruits and vegetables, along with moderate amounts of whole grains, unsaturated fats, and lean sources of protein, including low-fat dairy products. This reduction in calories can be achieved by choosing foods that are less energy-dense and by reducing portion size of high energy-dense foods. Because fats and sugar are more energy-dense, the overall volume of food consumed may be closer to the individual's former eating habits. A dietician can help the patient make the proper choices; further resources are available from the American Dietetic Association and other groups to help with education and practical implementation. A major determinant of long-term success is the ability of the person to adhere to the diet. If the program departs too much from former eating patterns, the diet may not be sustainable over time, and any weight loss may be temporary.

KEY TREATMENT

Average weight loss on low-calorie diets is 8% at 3 to 12 months. Very-low-calorie diets may increase weight loss, but results at 1 year are similar to low-calorie diets (Shepherd, 2003) (SOR: A).

Physical Activity and Exercise

Physical activity is a key component of a healthy lifestyle for reasons ranging from stress reduction to decreased risk of cardiovascular disease. It is also an important component of preventing and treating obesity. Everyone should include physical activity in their daily routine whenever possible (e.g., walk over lunch hour, using stairs) as well as a more formal exercise program. An advantage of exercise is that more calories can be expended in a given period. The choice of exercise depends on individual interests and should be scheduled into the day as a priority. For those who have been sedentary, gradually starting an exercise is advisable. In general, the goal should be 30 minutes of moderately vigorous physical activity most days of the week. To promote weight loss, a goal of 60 minutes may be more appropriate and, to maintain weight loss, even up to 90 minutes a day may be necessary. A popular program promoting physical activity encourages people to walk 10,000 steps each day or at least an initial increase of 2000 steps over baseline. A simple pedometer allows people to follow their progress. As noted earlier, children's sedentary activities (e.g., TV/computer time) can be limited to 2 hours daily or less. A similar attempt to limit sedentary activities during adult off-work hours may also be helpful (Table 36-5) (Hu et al., 2003).

Behavioral Approaches

Behaviorally based approaches have been found to improve the results of weight loss programs. In general, the longer the program, the longer the weight loss is maintained. A variety of approaches have been used, without a clear advantage to a specific modality, including self-monitoring with diet and activity records or rewarding specific behaviors such as exercise or diet changes. Identifying and avoiding environmental or social triggers for excessive eating can also help. Group support may be helpful for some people. Because emotions often play a role in eating, stress and depression should be addressed before undertaking weight loss or as part of a behavioral weight loss program.

Medications

Various medications have been used in the treatment of obesity. At one time, these included amphetamines, exogenous thyroid hormone to induce a hyperthyroid state, fenfluramine, dexfenfluramine, and phenylpropanolamine, none of which should be used currently. Appetite suppressants work through their effects on neurotransmitters. Increased levels

Table 36-5 Examples of Moderate Amounts of Physical Activity*

Energy expended in common physical activities: number of minutes to burn 150 kcal

Common Chores (min)	Sporting Activities (min)	
Washing and waxing car (45-60)	Playing volleyball (45-60)	Less vigorous, more time†
Washing windows or floors (45-60)	Playing touch football (45)	
Gardening (30-45)	Walking 1.25 miles (35; 20 min/mile)	
Wheeling self in wheelchair (30-40)	Basketball (shooting baskets) (30)	↑
Pushing stroller 1.5 miles (30)	Bicycling 5 miles (30)	
Raking leaves (30)	Dancing fast (social) (30)	
Walking 2 miles (30; 15 min/mile)	Water aerobics (30)	
Shoveling snow (15)	Swimming laps (20)	↓
Stairwalking (15)	Basketball (playing a game) (15-20)	More vigorous, less time
	Jumping rope (15)	
	Running 1.5 miles (15; 15 min/mile)	

*A moderate amount of physical activity is roughly equivalent to physical activity that uses approximately 150 calories per day or 1000 calories per week.
†Some activities can be performed at various intensities; the suggested durations correspond to expected intensity of effort.
From National Heart, Lung, and Blood Institute, National Institutes of Health. The Practical Guide to the Identification, Evaluation, and Treatment of Overweight and Obesity in Adults (NIH). Pub No 00-4084. NIH, Bethesda, Md, 2000.

of norepinephrine and serotonin in neurologic synapses through increased release or inhibition of neurotransmitter reuptake produce this effect. Fenfluramine and dexfenfluramine, both of which promote serotonin release, were taken off the market in 1997 after they were found to be associated with damage to heart valves. These two drugs have also been associated with pulmonary hypertension. Prolonged elevation of serotonin levels is thought to increase pulmonary vasoconstriction.

Sibutramine, a nonselective inhibitor of serotonin, norepinephrine, and dopamine reuptake, produces a feeling of satiety rather than a decrease in appetite. Until recently, sibutramine was one of the most commonly used medications for weight loss. In October 2010 sibutramine was withdrawn from the market when postmarketing data showed an increased risk of heart attack and stroke in patients with heart disease.

Orlistat inhibits gastric and pancreatic lipase, thereby reducing digestion and absorption of fats. After 1 year, subjects taking orlistat lost 2.9 kg more than those taking placebo (Rucker et al., 2007). Side effects, primarily gastrointestinal and related to fat malabsorption, occur in about 20%

of subjects but only last up to 1 week in half the patients affected. During the second year of treatment, prevalence of side effects is no greater than with placebo. Because absorption of fat-soluble vitamins may be decreased, patients taking orlistat should also take a daily multivitamin. Orlistat is not absorbed, making systemic side effects unlikely. The recommended dose is 120 mg three times daily with meals that contain fat. If patients choose high-calorie but low-fat foods, little benefit will be seen. Orlistat is available over the counter in a reduced dose of 60 mg. Whether this is effective for long-term weight loss has not been established.

Fluoxetine has shown mixed but generally unimpressive results because any initial weight loss is often regained, and side effects include nervousness, tremor, fatigue, hypersomnia, insomnia, and diarrhea. Snow and colleagues (2005) reported a 3.6-kg weight loss at 6 months with *phentermine* and a 3.0-kg loss with *diethylpropion* over placebo. *Metformin* increases peripheral insulin sensitivity and therefore insulin levels can drop. When used in glucose-intolerant patients, metformin has been associated with a decreased risk of diabetes and modest weight loss of a few pounds.

Follow-up visits after starting pharmacotherapy assess response and monitor for adverse effects. A suggested schedule includes visits at 2 to 4 weeks, then monthly for 3 months, and then every 3 months for the first year (ICSI, 2005). The weight loss seen with medication use in conjunction with diet and exercise occurs primarily in the first 6 months. If a patient has not lost 2 kg in the first 4 weeks, the drug may be ineffective for that patient and might be stopped. When the medication is effective, its continuation can help maintain weight loss, although some people do regain weight despite maintenance therapy.

Complementary and Alternative Medicine

Complementary and alternative medicine (CAM) treatments are attractive to patients with various medical concerns. The perceived safety of natural products and their availability without the expense of seeing a physician have contributed to this interest.

Ephedrine, often in combination with caffeine, has been marketed in purified form or in herbal products as *ma huang*. *Guarana* and *gotu kola* are herbal sources of caffeine. A small study showed a significantly greater loss of weight with the combination of ma huang and guarana (4.0 ±3.4 kg, vs. 0.8 ±2.4 kg in placebo group) (Boozer et al., 2001). Ephedrine, the most potent isomer in *ephedra*, increases thermogenesis in adipose tissue through the stimulation of beta receptors. Side effects reflect the increased sympathetic activity and typically include insomnia, tachyarrhythmias, headache, and elevated BP. Because of its association with more serious side effects (stroke, tachyarrhythmias, seizures, death), ephedra was removed from the market in 2004. *Bitter orange* has also been used for weight loss and contains the sympathomimetic alkaloids of Synephrine and octopamine. An action similar to that of ephedrine has been suggested, and because little evidence supports use of bitter orange, this supplement is not recommended (Heber, 2003).

Caffeine can increase sympathetic nervous system activity and is thought to increase weight reduction through an increase in metabolic rate and fat oxidation. *Green tea* contains, along with caffeine, catechins. These antioxidants have been thought to have sympathetic activity, increasing thermogenesis and aiding in weight loss. Any effect attributable to catechins is difficult to assess because of the presence of caffeine.

Conjugated linoleic acid (CLA) was not found to be effective for weight loss, although it may have a slight effect on body composition. Animal studies show an increase in insulin resistance that suggests safety concerns, although limited human studies have not shown adverse effects. *Hydroxycitric acid*, found in *Garcinia cambogia* (Brindall berry), was also found to be ineffective for weight loss. Increased *dietary fiber*, particularly water-soluble fiber, has been associated with modest weight reduction benefits. *Chitosan*, a nonabsorbable carbohydrate derived from the exoskeletons of crustaceans, has been purported to have fat-blocking effects through binding with dietary fats, but human studies have found no benefit (Heber, 2003).

Surgery

Weight loss surgery has been found to be effective in carefully selected patients (Maggard et al., 2005). In the United States, approximately 220,000 bariatric surgeries were performed in 2008. As noted earlier, candidates for bariatric surgery should have a BMI of more than 35 kg/m^2 and obesity-related complications. Before considering surgery, patients should have a strong attempt to achieve weight loss through conservative means, including diet, exercise, and behavioral modification. For the patient considering surgery, it is important to work with a team experienced in the different aspects of bariatric surgery and weight loss, including a psychologist or psychiatrist, registered dietitian, physician nutrition specialist (if available), and experienced surgeon. Patients should be well informed of the life-changing nature of the surgery, as well as potential complications.

Bariatric Procedures

The complications and degree of weight loss differ depending on the surgical approach. Current procedures are classified as being malabsorptive or restrictive, or a combination, in their mechanism of reducing calorie absorption (Box 36-2). The first surgical procedure to be widely used was the *jejunoileal bypass*, a malabsorptive approach in which most of the small bowel is bypassed by connecting the proximal with the distal small bowel. Side effects, including steatorrhea, electrolyte imbalance, and hepatic and renal injury, led to this approach being abandoned.

Current *malabsorptive* procedures include biliopancreatic diversion with or without duodenal switch. The *duodenal switch* refers to the portion of the small intestine that is transected. The *biliopancreatic diversion* is similar to the jejunoileal bypass in that much of the small intestine is bypassed. However, the bypassed small intestine continues to supply bile and pancreatic enzymes, preventing some of the most severe complications of the jejunoileal bypass. Nutrient deficiencies are still much more common than with restrictive procedures. Both types of biliopancreatic diversion include a limited partial gastrectomy, with the pylorus being maintained in the duodenal switch.

In general, *restrictive* procedures tend to result in less dramatic weight loss than malabsorptive procedures. The

Box 36-2 Types of Bariatric Surgical Procedures

Malabsorptive
Jejunoileal bypass
Biliopancreatic diversion

Restrictive
Vertical-banded gastroplasty
Gastric banding

Malabsorptive and Restrictive
Roux-en-Y gastric bypass

Roux-en-Y gastric bypass, by far the most widely used procedure, works predominantly by restricting caloric intake, but it may also have a component of malabsorption, depending on the length of the bypassed intestine (Fig. 36-2). Most of the stomach is transected with this procedure. The small intestine is also transected, and the distal limb is attached to the stomach remnant. The bypassed stomach is attached to the remaining intact intestine through the proximal limb of the transected small intestine. The *vertical-banded gastroplasty* is also a restrictive procedure, but weight loss is less than with the Roux-en-Y gastric bypass. Restrictive procedures cause more vomiting but overall have fewer side effects related to persistent diarrhea and malabsorption of nutrients than malabsorptive procedures. Malabsorptive procedures may be more appropriate when a greater degree of weight loss is desired, but the patient should be aware of the increased side effects.

The adjustable *gastric band* is a purely restrictive procedure, usually placed laparoscopically, and its use is increasing. A band is placed around the upper portion of the stomach (Fig. 36-3). Part of the stomach is sutured over the band to help keep it in place. This band contains fluid that can be infused through a port just under the skin. By infusing fluid in the port, the band can be tightened or loosened. Adjustments in the fluid are often necessary as people lose weight because the band may loosen.

One of the side effects with the Roux-en-Y gastric bypass is *dumping syndrome,* which occurs when high-osmolality foods such as ice cream or soda are consumed and presented immediately to the small bowel through the remnant stomach. Symptoms include cramping, diarrhea, malaise, and sweating, and therefore this can be a deterrent to consuming these generally high-calorie foods. However, because the anatomy is intact with the gastric band, dumping syndrome does not occur. In fact, liquid foods such as ice cream and soda may slide more easily through the band, and therefore greater behavioral changes are required to decrease consumption of these foods with a gastric band compared to the Roux-en-Y gastric bypass. This is one reason why weight loss is not as great with the band compared to the bypass.

Perioperative risks increase with bariatric procedures because of the patient population and type of surgery, but overall mortality is under 1%. All currently used procedures can be performed laparoscopically, which is more technically difficult but associated with faster recovery.

During the immediate postoperative period, it can be anticipated that pharmacotherapy for weight-related conditions will quickly be reduced. Insulin dosing will usually need to

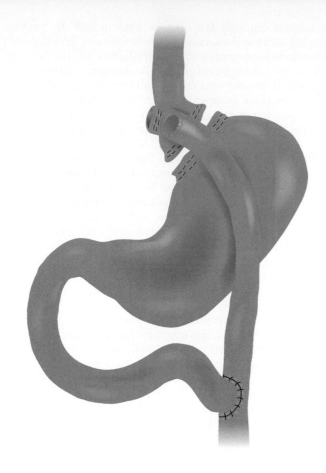

Figure 36-2 Roux-en-Y gastric bypass for obesity. *(Redrawn from and courtesy Mayo Clinic © 2000.)*

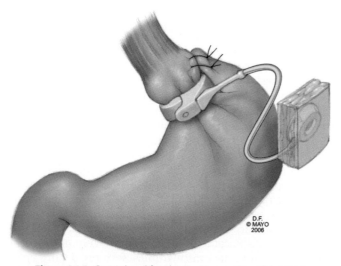

Figure 36-3 Gastric band for obesity. *(Courtesy Mayo Clinic © 2006.)*

be decreased immediately. Patients taking oral hypoglycemics preoperatively may be better controlled on a sliding scale of short-acting insulin in planning for a decreased postoperative need for medications. Similarly, antihypertensive and other medications may need to be reevaluated. Immediate-release agents may be better suited to the patient after a malabsorptive procedure than sustained-release types, because altered gastrointestinal absorption can be anticipated.

Long-term management of surgical patients requires supplementation with vitamins and minerals. Vitamin B_{12} deficiency is common. Clinical practice at Mayo Clinic is to treat all bariatric surgery patients with 2 multivitamins (starting with chewable form), daily calcium supplementation (carbonate or citrate), vitamin D (1000-2000 U daily), and 1 mL (1000 μg/mL) of subcutaneous cyanocobalamin (vitamin B_{12}) monthly. Ferritin levels should be monitored and iron deficiency treated, as necessary. The altered ability to absorb medications will persist, and serum drug concentrations may need to be performed more frequently.

The Swedish Obese Subjects (SOS) study reported on extremely obese patients treated by bariatric surgery or conventional nonsurgical approaches over 10 years (Sjostrom et al., 2004). Peak weight loss occurred at 6 months in the control group (1% of baseline weight) and at 1 year in the surgical groups. At 1 year, weight loss was 38% for gastric bypass, 27% for vertical-banded gastroplasty, and 21% for those undergoing gastric banding. By 10 years, percentage weight loss from baseline fell to 25%, 16%, and 13%, respectively, for the three procedures, compared with 1.6% weight gain in the control group. Improvement in hypertension, T2DM, and dyslipidemia was greater in the surgical group than the control group at 2 and 10 years. Improvement in hypercholesterolemia did not differ between the groups. Reduction in the incidence of T2DM and hypertriglyceridemia was greater in the surgical patients than the control group at 2 and 10 years. The incidence of hypertension and hypercholesterolemia did not differ between the groups.

KEY TREATMENT

Diet and exercise together with behavioral modification can improve short-term outcomes, though long-term effectiveness is lacking (Shepherd, 2003) (SOR: A).

Both sibutramine and orlistat may achieve modest additional weight loss when added to diet and physical activity in patients who are appropriate candidates for pharmacotherapy (Rucker et al., 2007) (SOR: A).

Gastric bypass is more effective than vertical-banded gastroplasty for weight loss and is associated with fewer revisions but more side effects (Everson et al., 2004) (SOR: A).

Summary

The epidemic of obesity has major implications for health care now and in the future. Family physicians are in a unique position to affect this epidemic through primary as well as secondary prevention. This strategy should start in childhood but must also continue as a lifelong process. Over a lifetime, gradual restriction in caloric intake and continued participation in physical activity are necessary to maintain weight and health. Weight management should be addressed with patients and therapy tailored to the individual. Community endeavors to reduce calorie intake and increase physical activity should be supported. These efforts should be viewed as public health priorities.

References

The complete reference list is available online at www.expertconsult.com.

Web Resources

www.icsi.org
  Institute for Clinical Systems Improvement; evidence-based guidelines on prevention and management of obesity.
www.cdc.gov/obesity
  Compilation of current statistics and overview of obesity.
www.cdc.gov/obesity/causes/economics.html

www.cdc.gov/obesity/data/index.html
  Centers for Disease Control and Prevention.
www.who.int/mediacentre/factsheets/fs311/en/index.html-world
www.ahrq.gov/clinic/3rduspstf/obesity/obesrr.htm
www.ahrq.gov/clinic/uspstf/uspsobes.htm
  U.S. Preventive Services Task Force; screening for obesity in adults.

Nutrition and Family Medicine

Mary Barth Noel, Margaret Thompson, William C. Wadland, and Jodi Summers Holtrop

Overview

The goal of improving the health of the U.S. population through approaches such as physical activity and nutrition has come to the forefront of medical concerns. The efforts of public service and health care professionals in promoting nutrition's potential to improve health is beginning to result in constructive action. The public health approach to improving diet through education is part of the focus on preventing chronic diseases in an aging population. The clinical medicine approach to nutrition is using nutritional therapies as part of disease management. This chapter discusses both approaches.

Current Dietary Guidance

The latest version of the public health dietary guidance program was introduced in 2010. This is in connection with the MyPyramid food guidance system (www.MyPyramid.gov). The MyPyramid recommendations are based on the following:
- *Variety:* Eat foods from all food groups and subgroups.
- *Proportionality:* Eat more of some foods (e.g., fruits, vegetables, whole grains, fat-free or low-fat milk products) and less of others (e.g., foods high in saturated or *trans* fats, added sugars, cholesterol, salt, alcohol).
- *Moderation:* Choose forms of foods that limit the intake of saturated or *trans* fats, added sugars, cholesterol, salt, and alcohol.
- *Activity:* Be physically active every day.

The new food pyramid has an interactive interface, allowing for customization of the food plan as well as key concepts into a visual image (see Web Resources). Although there is general agreement, many argue that the recommendations are vague and that food amounts and groupings are inappropriate. The major addition in this version of the food guidance system has been *physical activity,* which seems to be critical in the considerations of diet and the balancing of energy needs with intake. The overarching concepts of the 2010 Dietary Guidelines (www.dietaryguidelines.gov) explain the educational framework for the MyPyramid, as follows:
- Maintain calorie balance over time to achieve and sustain a healthy weight.
- Focus on consuming nutrient-dense foods and beverages.

There are more than 23 key recommendations in the latest Dietary Guidelines for the general population and six additional key recommendations for specific populations. The Key Recommendations of the latest version of the Dietary Guidelines are as follows:
- Balance calories to manage weight
  - Prevent and/or reduce overweight and obesity through eating and physical activity
  - Control total calorie intake to manage body weight
  - Increase physical activity and reduce time spent in sedentary behaviors
  - Maintain appropriate calorie balance during each stage of life

- Foods and food components to reduce
  - Reduce daily sodium to less than 2300 milligrams per day
  - Consume less than 10% of calories from saturated fats per day
  - Consume less than 300 milligrams from dietary cholesterol per day
  - Keep trans fatty acid consumption low as possible
  - Reduce calories from solid fats and added sugars
  - Limit consumption of foods that contain refined grains
  - If alcohol is consumed, it should be consumed in moderation
- Foods and nutrients to increase
  - Increase vegetable and fruit intake
  - Eat a variety of vegetables
  - Consume at least half of all grains as whole grains
  - Increase intake of fat-free or low-fat milk and milk products
  - Choose a variety of protein foods
  - Increase the amount and variety of seafood consumed by choosing seafood in place of some meat and poultry
  - Replace protein foods that are higher in solid fats with choices that are lower in solid fats and calories
  - Use oils to replace solid fats when possible
  - Choose foods that provide more potassium, dietary fiber, calcium, and vitamin D, which are nutrients of concern in American diets.

There are additional recommendations for women capable of becoming pregnant, women who are pregnant or breastfeeding, and individuals ages 50 years and older.

The specifics are many, and the latest dietary guidelines might be as confusing as previous guidelines. They are a combination of food- and nutrient-based recommendations, the latter of which is often difficult to explain. Both the professional community and general public recognize the important role of proper nutrition in maintaining health, but neither always heeds current evidence. This chapter highlights the current evidence for supporting nutritional approaches to common medical and health concerns. The recent changes in recommendations recognize that the whole diet seems to be more of a concern than specific nutrients.

Nutrition Assessment

A nutrition assessment is the process of determining an individual's nutritional status or whether adequate amounts of required nutrients are available to and absorbed by the body. Every patient in a family medicine practice deserves some level of nutrition assessment. This assessment can be a brief screen, when the patient is relatively healthy, or more in-depth, if the patient appears to have nutritional inadequacy or risk factors for malnutrition. The depth of the assessment is based on the patient and the presenting situation. Those who may require a more in-depth evaluation include patients who are grossly overweight or underweight, patients with a chronic or severe acute illness, growing infants and children, patients in poverty or otherwise unable to obtain a variety of foods, most frail older adults, and patients who maintain nontraditional diets, such as recent immigrants or fad dieters.

History

As with any other health assessment, the patient history is the first step in determining nutritional status. In a reasonably healthy adult or child, this history may be a brief screen, including determining changes in weight and appetite, eating habits such as the number of meals daily and the variety of foods consumed, and symptoms of underlying chronic or debilitating illness. Information about the ability to perform activities of daily living (ADLs), including shopping and cooking, is important when interviewing older adults or the infirm population.

Patients with chronic illness deserve a more thorough history assessment, as do patients with symptoms or signs potentially related to poor nutrition (Table 37-1). Physicians should review gastrointestinal (GI) symptoms and elicit information about supplemental vitamins or other nutritional products, alcohol and illicit drugs, appetite suppressants or stimulants, glucocorticoids, and laxatives. In at-risk patients or those with clinical evidence of poor nutrition, clinicians should consider the presence of conditions that may increase nutritional requirements. Physicians should also investigate the patient's ability to obtain, ingest, digest, metabolize, and absorb nutrients; consider whether a treatment or medication will require modification of the diet; and use information obtained in the history to plan for that change.

Conditions that May Increase Nutritional Requirements

Any condition that increases the metabolic rate of the patient is likely to increase nutritional requirements (Box 37-1).

Ability to Obtain Food

Patients in poverty and who cannot or do not receive financial assistance are at risk for poor nutrition because of an inability to obtain enough food or a variety of foods. Those who lack transportation or have other shopping access issues, such as language barriers or distance from a store, may also not be able to acquire sufficient food. Patients who rely on others to provide or prepare foods, or both, may have inadequate dietary intake. Many patients, because of poor mobility and declining health, gradually lose the ability to perform ADLs, such as shopping, cooking, and cleaning, so the history should contain specific questions directed at these activities. Individuals with substance abuse problems or poor mental health may lack the initiative or ability to acquire healthy foods.

Ability to Ingest Nutrients

Various conditions may contribute to a patient's inability or lack of desire to eat (see Box 37-1).

Digestion

A number of processes can affect the normal digestive process. Any factor that interferes with the secretion of acid or enzymes into the stomach or small intestine may impair digestion. For example, patients with partial gastrectomy or even vagotomy for peptic ulcer disease may have maldigestion and nutritional deficiencies. Similarly, patients with chronic pancreatitis may lack certain digestive enzymes and thus cannot absorb all nutrients.

Table 37-1 Summary of Major Nutrients

Nutrient	Major Dietary Sources	Major Functions	Signs of Deficiency	Usual Causes of Deficiency	Effects of Excess	Normal Laboratory Value
Protein (Pro) (supplies 4 kcal/g)	Fish, chicken, beef, other animals; lentils, seeds, legumes, dried beans; dairy products; eggs, nuts	Building materials (AAs) for growth, maintenance, repair of all cells; regulates fluid balance between blood and cells; provides energy; essential AAs are threonine, tryptophan, histidine, lysine, leucine, isoleucine, methionine, valine, phenylalanine	Kwashiorkor (protein malnutrition); decreased immune response; edema; stunted growth and development; poor musculature; marasmus (protein-energy malnutrition)	Poor intake of protein, especially high-quality protein; too few calories so that protein is used for energy; malabsorption; genetic diseases of protein, AAs (e.g., PKU)	Reduced calcium retention; weight gain, obesity	Albumin, 3.5-5.0 g/dL; BUN 9-20 mg/dL; creatinine, 0.31.3 mg/dL; prealbumin 10-40 mg/dL; total protein, 6.0-8.0 g/dL
Carbohydrates (CHO) (supplies 4 kcal/g)	Cereal grains, dried peas and beans, bread, pasta, vegetables, fruits, dairy products, sugar, jellies, other sweets	Provides energy for body processes and physical activity; aids in use of fat and spares protein; provides energy; many vitamins and most fibers are CHO	Growth retardation; weight loss	Poor intake; malabsorption; genetic diseases of CHO (e.g., glycogen storage disease)	Weight gain, obesity; increased blood triglyceride levels	None
Fat (supplies 9 kcal/g)	Saturated fats: meats, dairy fats (e.g., ice cream, sour cream, butter), bacon, sausages Unsaturated fats: avocado, oils (e.g., corn, safflower, vegetable) Monounsaturated fats: olive oil, canola oil	Supplies concentrated source of energy; carries fat-soluble vitamins; supplies essential fatty acids (e.g., linoleic, linolenic, arachidonic acids); membrane structures; transport processes of cells	Flaky, scaly skin; poor growth; hair loss; impaired wound healing and immune functioning	Poor intake; malabsorption, extreme diets or supplementary feedings for long periods (e.g., IV lines, TPN without fats)	Increased blood cholesterol and/or triglyceride levels; weight gain, obesity	Total cholesterol, <200 to >140 mg/dL; HDL >45 mg/dL; LDL <100-130 mg/dL
Water	Water, beverages, fruits; almost all foods contain some water	Provides substrate for most of body's reactions; helps move materials to and waste from cells; helps control body temperature; lubricates joints in body	Dehydration, death	Poor intake; medications; diarrhea; vomiting; high temperatures	Excess retention of fluid related to imbalance of minerals; overconsumption rare but can result in death	Dehydration: increased albumin, BUN Fluid overload: decreased albumin, BUN

Vitamins

Water-Soluble Vitamins

Nutrient	Major Dietary Sources	Major Functions	Signs of Deficiency	Usual Causes of Deficiency	Effects of Excess	Normal Laboratory Value
Vitamin B$_1$ (thiamin)	Lean pork, wheat germ, whole/fortified cereals, legumes, bread products	Assists in use of CHO and fat for energy; promotes growth, appetite, and muscle tone; promotes normal functioning of nervous system; coenzyme in metabolism of CHO branched-chain AAs	Beriberi; changes in nerves; excessive water retention; loss of appetite; depression; muscle tenderness; high-output cardiac failure; polyneuritis	Poor intake; malabsorption; hemodialysis	None reported	Thiamine pyrophosphate (TPP); stimulation >20% (index >.2% indicates deficiency)
Vitamin B$_2$ (riboflavin)	Dairy products, liver and other organ meats, meat, fish, dark green vegetables, fortified grain products	Functions as part of energy release; essential for growth; part of flavin coenzymes required in cellular oxidation	Cheilosis; photophobia, angular stomatitis, magenta tongue, glossitis, seborrhea, corneal vascularization	Poor intake; malabsorption	None reported	Flavin adenine dinucleotide (FAD); stimulation >40% (index >1.4% indicates deficiency)

Nutrient	Major Dietary Sources	Major Functions	Signs of Deficiency	Usual Causes of Deficiency	Effects of Excess	Normal Laboratory Value
Vitamin B$_6$ comprises six compounds: pyridoxal, pyridoxine, pyridoxamine, and three 5'-phosphates: pyridoxal (PLP), pyridoxine (PNP), and pyridoxamine (PMP)	Liver, pork, poultry, whole/fortified grain products, bananas, legumes, lentils, fortified soy-based meat substitutes, nuts	Cofactor for many enzymes in metabolism of protein and AAs; functions in hemoglobin synthesis	Anemia; irritability; convulsions (in infants); skin lesions; smooth red tongue (glossitis); peripheral neuropathies; impaired all-mediated immunity	Poor intake; malabsorption; aging (increased need), medications	Sensory neuropathy marked by changes in gait and peripheral sensation	—
Vitamin B$_{12}$* (cobalamin)	Liver, beef, poultry, fish, eggs, brewer's yeast, (not present in plant foods) Oral initial dose: 1000-2000 μg per 1-2 weeks Maintenance: 1000 μg daily for life IM initial dose: 100-1000 μg daily or every other day for 1-2 weeks Maintenance: 100-1000 μg every 1-3 months	Maintenance of nervous tissue and blood formation; nucleic acid synthesis; recycling of tetrahydrofolate	Megaloblastic anemia (pernicious anemia); permanent damage to nervous system; peripheral neuropathy; weight loss; glossitis	Deficiency of hydrochloric acid in stomach (as occurs with aging); strict vegetarians; high intakes of folate can mask deficiency of vitamin B$_{12}$	None reported	Schilling test: 8% of radioactivity per 24-hour urine[†]
Vitamin C (ascorbic acid))	Citrus fruits and juices, tomatoes, potatoes, cabbage, broccoli, strawberries, spinach	Cofactor for reactions requiring reduced copper or iron metalloenzymes; protective antioxidant	Scurvy; easy bruising; slow wound healing; degeneration of skin, teeth, gums, blood vessels	Smokers have increased need, poor intake	GI disturbances; kidney stones; excess iron absorption	Plasma or leukocyte vitamin C measured by chromatography; plasma vitamin C, 0.50-1.40 mg/dL (30-80 μmol/L)
Folate (folic acid, folacin, pteroylpoly-glutamates)	Dark-green leafy vegetables, whole grains, legumes, nuts, organ meats, orange juice, fortified cereal products	Assists in red blood cell maturation; cofactor for synthesis of purine and pyrimidine; coenzyme in metabolism of nucleic acids and AAs	Megaloblastic anemia; general weakness; depression; polyneuropathy; GI upsets; poor growth; maternal deficiency linked to neural tube defects in fetus (400 μg/day recommended prepregnancy)	Poor intake; malabsorption	Masks deficiency of vitamin B$_{12}$	Red blood cell folate, 4-20 ng/mL
Niacin (includes nicotinic acid amide, nicotinic acid, nicotinamide)	Liver, meat, bran/fortified cereal products, fish, poultry, whole/fortified grains, peanuts, tuna	Part of coenzymes for oxidation-reduction reactions; active in release of energy and biosynthesis of fatty acids	Pellagra; pigmented dermatitis; dementia; diarrhea; inflammation of mucous membranes; weakness; tremors	Poor intake; malabsorption; consumption of processed grains that have niacin removed; hemodialysis	Flushing, burning, tingling around face, neck, hands; liver damage; gastrointestinal distress	—

Continued

Table 37-1 Summary of Major Nutrients—cont'd

Nutrient	Major Dietary Sources	Major Functions	Signs of Deficiency	Usual Causes of Deficiency	Effects of Excess	Normal Laboratory Value
Pantothenic acid	Liver, egg yolks, meat, mushrooms, whole grains, brewer's yeast, broccoli, skim milk, sweet potatoes, avocados	Component of coenzyme A; functions in release of energy from CHO, Pro, and fat; coenzyme in fatty acid metabolism	Fatigue; malaise; insomnia; burning paresthesias; depression, weakness (rare)	Poor intake; malabsorption; incomplete PEN or TPN formulas	Unknown	—
Biotin	Nuts, soy, eggs, nonfat milk, sweet potatoes	Coenzyme for carboxylation reactions; plays a role in CHO and fat metabolism; coenzyme in synthesis of fat, glycogen, and AAs	Dermatitis; neuritis; appetite loss; nausea; glossitis; insomnia; thin hair; depression hypercholesterolemia (few known cases)	Incomplete PEN or TPN formulas	Unknown	—
Fat-Soluble Vitamins						
Vitamin A (includes provitamin A such as retinols, carotenoids)	Liver, dairy products, fish; turkey (carotene); carrots, dark-green leafy vegetables, sweet potatoes, cantaloupe, apricots, broccoli, tomatoes	Maintenance of skin and mucous membranes; component in visual process; particular adaptation to darkness; immune function	Night blindness; xerophthalmia, keratomalacia; Bitot's spots; follicular hyperkeratosis; reduced immunity; poor growth	Poor intake; malabsorption with steatorrhea; liver disease	Loss of appetite; headache; vomiting; blurred vision with eventual eye damage; liver toxicity; teratogen in fetal growth	Serum retinol and retinol ester vitamin A, 30-80 µg/dL (1.0-2.8 µmol/L
Vitamin D (also called calciferol) uptake; glucocorticoid	Fortified dairy products,‡ fish, eggs; sunlight (15min/day for 3-4 days/wk)	Mineralization of bones and teeth; intestinal regulation of calcium and phosphorus	Rickets (children); osteomalacia (adults); costochondral beading; muscle weakness and twitching; low serum calcium	Poor sunlight exposure; poor intake; with aging, poor uptake glucocorticoid therapy may need additional vitamin D	Poor growth; weight loss; poor appetite; calcium deposits in soft tissues	25-hydroxy-vitamin D test, costochondral
Vitamin E (also called α-tocopherol)	Nuts, fats, polyunsaturated vegetable oils, margarine, seeds, whole grains	Antioxidant; prevents peroxidation of polyunsaturated lipids; free radical scavenger	Hemolytic anemia of newborn; increased fragility of red blood cells; nerve and muscle disturbances in severe malabsorption	Lipid malabsorption	Interferes with vitamin K (risk of bleeding, especially in trauma); hemorrhagic toxicity; monitor patients taking anticoagulants and vitamin E supplements	Serum tocopherol measured by chromatography, 0.5-1.8 mg/dL (12-42 µmol/L)
Vitamin K	Dark-green leafy vegetables, liver, vegetable oils, margarines, cabbage family	Synthesis of prothrombin and clotting factors II, VII, IX, and X	Bleeding (especially in newborns); ecchymosis; epistaxis; prolonged clotting time	Bacteria destroyed in gut that produce vitamin K; liver disease; lipid malabsorption	Unknown; monitor patients taking anticoagulants with vitamin K intake	Prothrombin time (PT) to assess vitamin K indirectly
Minerals						
Calcium	Dairy products, fish with small bones, dark-green leafy vegetables (mustard greens, kale); corn tortillas, calcium-set tofu	Structure of bones and teeth; nerve transmission; muscle contraction; essential role in blood clotting	Stunted growth; bone loss; rickets; osteomalacia; osteoporosis; tetany; possibly hypertension	Poor intake; poor consumption of vitamin D, poor sunlight exposure; lack of physical activity; high phosphorus intake	Decreased absorption of other minerals; kidney stones; hypercalcemia; milk-alkali syndrome; renal insufficiency	8.5-10.5 g/dL

Nutrient	Major Dietary Sources	Major Functions	Signs of Deficiency	Usual Causes of Deficiency	Effects of Excess	Normal Laboratory Value
Chloride	Table salt, seafood, meat	Acid-base balance; constituent of gastric juice; major anion of extracellular fluid	Rare; mental apathy, muscle cramps, usually seen with sodium depletion	Rare in United States (has occurred in babies whose formula did not have chloride)	None reported	96-106 mEq/L
Chromium	Fish, cheese, meat, poultry, whole-grain cereals, beer	Insulin cofactor; glucose and energy metabolism	Insulin resistance; glucose intolerance	Unknown	None reported	—
Cobalt	Organ and muscle meats, dairy products	Constituent of vitamin B_{12}	Only as vitamin B_{12} deficiency; pernicious anemia	Those associated with vitamin B_{12}	None reported	—
Copper	Liver, shellfish, nuts, whole grains, cereals, legumes, cocoa products	Absorption and use of iron; enzyme cofactor; in myelin nerve sheath	Anemia; kinky hair; neutropenia; disturbance of bone formation	Usually genetic	Wilson's disease (genetic); iron deficiency anemia; chronic renal failure	—
Fluoride	Fluoridated drinking water, fluoridated dental products, seafood	Structure of bone and teeth enamel; reduces dental caries	Dental caries	Nonfluoridated water or dental products	Mottled teeth; enamel and skeletal fluorosis	—
Iodine	Iodized salt; seafood, saltwater fish	Constituent of thyroid hormone	Goiter; cretinism	Lack of iodine in food or in soil where food grown	Rare; goiter may be caused by excess iodine; elevated TSH	—
Iron	Liver, lean meats, legumes, egg yolk, fortified cereals and breads	Constituent of hemoglobin; involved in oxygen and electron transport	Microcytic hypochromic anemia; fatigue; decreased immune response	Poor intake; blood loss	Liver and pancreas damage; large dose at one time: shock, death; GI distress	Serum iron, 50-150 µg/dL
Magnesium	Bran cereals, nuts, legumes, green leafy vegetables, meat	Part of protein synthesis; helps muscles contract and helps nerve impulse transmission	Rare; behavioral disturbances, tremor, spasms, neuromuscular irritability	Rare	Rare; diarrhea; fatigue; nervous system disturbances (usually from pharmacologic agents, not food sources)	1.5-2.5 mEq/dL
Manganese	Nuts, legumes, whole-grain cereals	Involved in formation of bone and enzymes in AAs, cholesterol, and CHO metabolism	Rare; dermatitis; weight loss	Rare	Rare; inhaled manganese linked to CNS disorders, neurotoxicity	—
Molybdenum	Whole-grain cereals, legumes, nuts	Oxidation-reduction reactions; enzyme helps in catabolism of sulfur AAs; metabolism of purine, pyrimidines	None	None	Unknown	—
Phosphorus	Dairy products, eggs, meat, whole-grain cereals, soda	Structure of bone and teeth; component of phospholipids; helps regulate acid-base balance; energy metabolism	Rare; demineralization of bone; weakness; poor growth; paresthesias of hands and feet	Rare in United States	May cause deficiency of calcium, skeletal porosity; interference with calcium absorption	2.5-4.5 mg/dL

Continued

Table 37-1 Summary of Major Nutrients—cont'd

Nutrient	Major Dietary Sources	Major Functions	Signs of Deficiency	Usual Causes of Deficiency	Effects of Excess	Normal Laboratory Value
Potassium	Fruits (particularly bananas, citrus juices), dairy products, potatoes, vegetables	Major component of intracellular fluid; regulates acid-base and water balance; maintains heart/nerve function	Muscle weakness; rapid, irregular heart rate; paralysis, death	Medications (e.g., diuretics), especially with poor intake	Electrolyte imbalance; muscle weakness; disturbed heart function; death	3.5-5.0 mEq/dL
Selenium	Organ meat, seafood, plants from selenium-containing soil	Antioxidant; constituent of glutathione oxidase	Rare; cardiac myopathy; muscle tenderness	Rare	Rare; hair and nail brittleness and loss	—
Sodium	Table salt, processed foods, in most foods except fruits	Maintains water balance; influences muscle contraction and nerve irritability	Rare; muscle cramps and reduced appetite	Rare; restricted diet with excessive medication	In some people, retention of fluids and hypertension	135-145 mEq/dL
Sulfur	Protein foods (e.g., meat, dairy, legumes)	Constituent of coenzyme A, AAs, hair, cartilage	No dietary deficiency with adequate protein	Rare	Rare	—
Zinc	Meat, seafood, dark meat of poultry, whole grains, legumes	Component of enzymes and proteins; involved in regulation of gene expression	Growth failure; impaired wound healing, taste changes, decreased immune response	Poor consumption of protein foods; phytate consumption inhibits absorption	Fever, nausea, vomiting, diarrhea; reduction in copper	115 ±12 ng/dL

Modified from Noel, Thompson. Nutrition and obesity. In Paulman PM, Susman J, Harrison J, et al (eds). Family Medicine Clerkship Guide. St. Louis, Mosby-Elsevier, 2005, Chapter 49.
*Dosages from Lederle FA. Oral cobalamin for pernicious anemia: medicine's best kept secret? JAMA 1991;265:94-95.
†From Mahan LK, Escott-Stump S. Krause's Food and Nutrition Therapy, 11th ed, Philadelphia, Saunders, 2003, pp.1208-1219.
‡Not all dairy products are fortified.
AAs, Amino acids; *BUN,* blood urea nitrogen; *CNS,* central nervous system; *GI,* gastrointestinal; *HDL,* high-density lipoprotein; *LDL,* low-density lipoprotein; *PEN,* peripheral enteral nutrition; *PKU,* phenylketonuria; *TPN,* total parenteral nutrition; *TSH,* thyroid-stimulating hormone.

Box 37-1 Select Conditions that Increase Nutrient Requirements

Pregnancy
Lactation
Healing wounds, including skin ulcers
Surgery
Trauma
Burns
Chronic lung disease
Cancer
Acquired immunodeficiency syndrome
Infection
Inflammatory diseases
Hyperthyroidism

Absorption

Patients may demonstrate poor absorption of nutrients for a variety of reasons, including loss of absorptive surface area in the intestinal tract from surgery, Crohn's disease, infectious processes, or other inflammatory conditions, such as celiac disease (National Digestive Diseases Information Clearinghouse [NDDIC], 2005) (Table 37-2). Incomplete digestion and processing of fats, carbohydrates, proteins, and vitamins can also lead to decreased absorption of those nutrients. Table 37-3 lists various nutrients and their sites of metabolism and absorption.

Metabolism and Excretion

Many chronic diseases result in poor metabolism of foods, which leads to poor availability of calories and other nutrients. Additionally, any condition that results in excessive losses of nutrients through the intestinal tract or kidneys may also result in malnutrition. Certain foods, such as nonabsorbable fat substitutes, cause excessive loss of fat-soluble vitamins, with steatorrhea caused by the fat not being absorbed (Table 37-4).

Dietary History

It is important to obtain information about the patient's usual and recent diet as part of the history. The dietary history refers to a patient's usual pattern of food intake and any factors that may influence food choices and availability.

Table 37-2 Celiac Disease: Grains with and without Gluten

Grains or Flours Allowed		Grains or Flours with Gluten: Not Allowed
Rice	Millet	Wheat (e.g., durum, semolina, kamut, spelt)
Soy	Buckwheat	
Potato	Arrowroot	Rye
Tapioca	Amaranth	Barley
Beans	Tef	Triticale
Garfava	Wild grass seeds (Montina)	Oats (most likely because of contamination)
Sorghum		
Quinoa	Nut flours	

Table 37-3 Nutrients and Sites of Metabolism/Absorption

Nutrient	Site of Absorption
Macronutrients	
Amino acids	Throughout small intestine (more rapid proximally)
Sugars	Throughout small intestine
Fats	
Fatty acids	Throughout small intestine (mostly proximal)
Bile acids	Ileum
Short-chain fatty acids	Colon
Minerals	
Calcium	Duodenum, jejunum
Iron	Duodenum
Magnesium	Small intestine
Vitamins	
Folic acid	Proximal small intestine
Vitamin B$_{12}$	Ileum
Fat-soluble (A, D, E, K)	Small intestine

Table 37-4 Conditions Affecting Metabolism and Excretion

Type of Impairment	Possible Contributing Condition
Impaired dietary intake	AIDS
	Anorexia nervosa
	Cancer
	Depression
	Dental problems
	Hyperemesis gravidarum
	Poverty
	Stroke
	Substance abuse
Maldigestion	Cholestasis
	Enzyme deficiencies
	Intestinal bacterial stasis
	Pancreatitis or insufficiency
	Radiation enteritis
	Short bowel syndrome
Malabsorption	AIDS
	Celiac disease
	Intestinal lymphoma
	Radiation enteritis
Impaired metabolism	AIDS
	Cancer
	Chronic disease (liver, kidney)
	Corticosteroid use
Increased excretion of nutrients	Diarrhea (zinc, magnesium)
	Glucosuria
	Inflammatory bowel disease
	Protein-losing enteropathy
	Gastrointestinal bleeding (iron)
Increased requirements	Burns
	Trauma
	Surgery
	Chronic infection
	Inflammation
	Chronic lung disease
	Hyperthyroidism
	Sepsis

Modified from Newton JM, Halsted CH. Clinical and functional assessment of adults. In Shils ME, Olson JA, Shike M, Ross AC (eds). Modern Nutrition in Health and Disease, 9th ed. Lippincott–Williams & Wilkins, 1999, Chapter 55.
AIDS, Acquired immunodeficiency syndrome.

Screening questions include number of daily meals and examples of food consumed. A more thorough evaluation delves into cultural or religious food practices, personal preferences, and use of the food pyramid as a tool to help patients identify food groups from which they may be consuming too few or too many servings.

A specific part of the dietary history is a *nutrient intake* analysis. This history relies on a food diary kept by the patient for a specific period, usually 3 to 7 days, including times, food and beverages consumed, and activity. Clinicians also use *dietary recall* as a method to assess nutrient intake. With this tool, patients report foods and beverages consumed over the past 24 to 48 hours. This retrospective analysis has less validity than the prospective food diary because people typically are unable to remember the details of their past eating habits accurately (Hammond, 2004).

Physical Examination

Key Points

- Significant weight loss— 5% in 1 month, 7.5% in 3 months, or 10% in 6 months, from usual weight— indicates the need for further evaluation to determine the cause.
- Albumin and transferrin can be artificially low when C-reactive protein level (inflammation) is high. Prealbumin is a more accurate marker of nutritional status with systemic inflammation.

A systematic physical examination is important in evaluating nutritional status. General inspection may immediately reveal obvious overweight or underweight. Anthropometry, or physical measurements of an individual that are compared with reference standards, plays a role as well. These parameters include height, weight, skin fold thickness, head circumference (especially in infants and children), and waist and hip circumferences. These measurements are most helpful when taken at several intervals over time.

Height and Weight

It is useful to measure height and weight to assess nutrition. Patients tend to overestimate their height and underestimate their weight. In considering weight alone in adults, the *usual body weight* is a more useful parameter than ideal body weight obtained from published tables. In children, body weight is more useful than height in estimating body fat and also provides information about recent nutrient intake (Hammond, 2004). Changes in weight over time from the usual body weight may reflect a change in nutritional status. However, it is important to remember that acutely, weight loss or gain may signify a change in fluid status rather than in nutritional well-being. In an obese individual or older adult, loss of lean body mass indicating malnutrition may be masked by the presence of excess body fat.

Significant weight loss is defined as a 5% loss in 1 month, a 7.5% loss in 3 months, or a 10% loss in 6 months. A severe weight loss is defined as any loss higher than those percentages in the same interval. The following method is also used to assess nutritional status as a function of weight loss (Hammond, 2004):

- Weight within 85% to 90% of usual body weight—*mild* malnutrition.
- Weight within 75% to 84% of usual body weight—*moderate* malnutrition.
- Weight less than 74% of usual body weight—*severe* malnutrition.

Both height and weight are needed to calculate the body mass index (BMI), which is highly correlated with independent measures of body fat in adults (Balcombe et al., 2001; Keys et al., 1972). The formula for calculating BMI is weight (kg)/[height (m)]^2. Table 37-5 lists parameters for overweight, obesity, and underweight according to the BMI (see Web Resources for BMI calculator).

It is important to note the limitations of the BMI as a nutritional assessment tool. It may overestimate body fat in trained athletes, and it may underestimate body fat in older patients and in those who have lost lean body mass because

Table 37-5 Weight Categories according to Body Mass Index (BMI)

Category	BMI (kg/m²)
Underweight	<18.5
Normal	18.5-24.9
Overweight	25-29.9
Obese	≥30

From National Heart, Lung, and Blood Institute (NHLBI). Clinical guidelines on the identification, evaluation, and treatment of overweight and obesity in adults, BMI calculator. http://www.nhlbisupport.com/bmi/bmicalc.htm.

of nutritional deficiency. There are no clear guidelines on the use of the BMI in pregnancy (National Heart, Lung, and Blood Institute [NHLBI], 2000).

Body Composition

Assessment of body composition reveals the relative amount of body fat and lean body mass. One common method for assessing subcutaneous fat is the measurement of *skin fold thickness*. Several areas of the body have demonstrated good correlation with body fat, including the triceps, biceps, subscapular tissue, and tissue above the iliac crest. Measurements are taken with calipers and compared with standardized tables to determine the percentage of body fat. This type of assessment can be limited by the accuracy of the measuring technique. Changes in skin fold thickness take place over 3 to 4 weeks, so this measurement is not a useful gauge for determining acute changes in nutritional status.

Circumference measurements are useful in assessing nutritional status. The waist circumference correlates with abdominal fat content. Increased waist circumference has been associated with cardiovascular disease risk factors (Dalton et al., 2003). The correct method for waist circumference is to measure the distance around the smallest area below the rib cage and above the umbilicus. Waist measurements of more than 40 inches in men and 35 inches in women are independent risk factors for disease (NHLBI, 2005). The waist circumference has less predictive value in patients shorter than 5 feet tall and in those with BMI greater than 35.

General Physical Examination

Certain findings on physical examination may alert the physician to the potential for malnutrition. These include temporal wasting, decreased muscle mass in general, proximal muscle weakness, and certain skin changes, such as scaling, poor wound healing, and bruising. Tissues in the body that undergo rapid cell turnover, such as mucous membranes, skin, and hair, may be the first to show signs of nutritional insufficiency (see Table 37-1).

Laboratory Evaluation

Physiologic changes related to adequacy of nutrition occur slowly; the first signs of a change in nutritional status usually appear at the cellular level. These changes may be detected by a variety of laboratory tests. Single laboratory tests may have value in screening for nutritional problems, whereas a series of values is important for assessing ongoing nutritional problems and treatment.

Assessment of Protein Status

One traditional method of determining nutritional status is to measure the *nitrogen balance*, calculated by comparing protein gain with protein loss. In healthy adults the nitrogen balance is zero; that is, the amount of nitrogen consumed should equal the amount of nitrogen excreted. Calculation of the nitrogen balance gives an indication of short-term changes in protein status. Approximately 16% of protein mass in the body is made up of nitrogen. In calculating nitrogen balance, the clinician can determine protein intake in the diet and then measure nitrogen output in urine and feces. The nitrogen balance is negative when protein-calorie intake is insufficient; it is positive in growing children and pregnant women. The following formula is used for calculating nitrogen balance:

$$\text{Nitrogen balance} = \text{Nitrogen intake}(g/24 \text{ hr})$$
$$- (\text{Urinary nitrogen } [g/24 \text{ hr}] + 2 g/24 \text{ hr})$$

where the 2 g/24 hr accounts for nitrogen losses from GI epithelium, skin, hair loss, and sweat. The total urine nitrogen can be determined by dividing the 24-hour urinary urea nitrogen by 0.85. In patients with extensive diarrhea or other losses of nitrogen (e.g., through pancreatic fistula), other methods must be used to calculate nitrogen losses, such as by the use of pyrochemiluminescence.

There are limitations in calculating nitrogen balance. It is difficult to assess the amount of protein intake in a person eating by mouth because of the need to measure portions and amounts consumed accurately. Determination of the nitrogen balance is more accurate for patients receiving defined formulas of enteral or parenteral nutrition.

Measuring Visceral Protein: Albumin

The protein contained in visceral organs constitutes about 10% of total body protein, whereas the protein in plasma and extravascular body fluids makes up about 3% of total protein. *Albumin* is a plasma protein produced by the liver that can be used as an indicator of visceral protein balance. The measurement of serum albumin reflects changes in the protein status over a longer time than the nitrogen balance, in part because albumin has a serum half-life of 2 to 3 weeks.

Using serum albumin as a marker for protein nutrition status also has limitations. Albumin is a negative acute-phase reactant and tends to decrease in concentration under conditions of inflammation. Because of its long half-life, this change may be misleading. In protein-calorie starvation, albumin levels tend to decrease, but in total-calorie deprivation, albumin levels may remain more stable (Hammond, 2004). Finally, there is a large extravascular albumin pool, which tends to equilibrate by entering the vascular system when plasma concentration of albumin decreases.

Transferrin

Transferrin is another plasma protein that reflects overall protein balance. Like albumin, transferrin is a negative acute-phase reactant, but because of its shorter half-life (8 days), it may be somewhat more accurate than albumin as a tool for assessing nutritional status. Transferrin has limitations, however, in that its concentration is related to the patient's overall iron status. Also, as with albumin, serum concentration of transferrin does not change rapidly with changes in protein-calorie intake.

Other Plasma Proteins

Several other plasma proteins have been proposed as good markers for protein energy status. The level of transthyretin (TTY), also known as *prealbumin,* has been shown to correlate with visceral protein status, but it is an acute-phase reactant and is also affected by zinc concentrations. Retinol-binding protein (RBP) has a short serum half-life (12 hours) and correlates with protein energy status in some patients with malnutrition, but it also is a negative acute-phase reactant and has limitations for the assessment of nutritional status.

It is possible to circumvent the problems raised by inflammation in interpreting the plasma levels of the proteins mentioned. *C-reactive protein* (CRP) level provides an indication of the amount of inflammation present at a given time. Some clinicians may ascribe more usefulness to levels of albumin, transferrin, transthyretin, and RBP when the CRP level is low.

Urinary Creatinine and Creatinine/Height Ratio

The urinary creatinine level reflects the amount of ongoing muscle metabolism. The amount of creatinine excreted in the urine is proportional to the muscle mass of an individual. Using a mathematical formula, it is possible to derive an expected amount of creatinine excretion over 24 hours based on a person's height. This formula is limited in the case of a tall, thin, or short muscular subject. The amount of urinary creatinine also varies depending on the diet; diets high in meat will result in increased urinary creatinine excretion.

Vitamin and Mineral Assays

In general, protein-calorie malnutrition is associated with low levels of vitamin A, zinc, and magnesium. Fat-soluble vitamins may be deficient in conditions of malabsorption of fat. Folic acid and iron are not well absorbed in celiac disease.

Hematologic Tests

Changes in red blood cell production may result from insufficient levels of iron, vitamin B_1, folic acid, and other vitamins. It is important to note that determining the complete blood count (CBC) is important in assessing nutritional status. Patients with poor nutritional status may also demonstrate weak immune status. T-cell–mediated responses are more severely affected by nutritional inadequacy than B-cell functions, such as immunoglobulin function. Evaluating the total lymphocyte count can be helpful in assessing T cells. Using skin testing for energy is one method of testing T-cell immune competence.

Nutrition in the Life Cycle

Pregnancy and Lactation

Pregnancy has long been recognized as a time of increased nutritional needs. Recommendations vary but one constant remains: with adequate caloric intake comes a greater likelihood of ingesting adequate nutrients. Weight checks are a standard part of all prenatal visits. In recent years, concern has focused on the woman's health status after the pregnancy. As Table 37-6 demonstrates, in older pregnant women or biologically immature women (those who become pregnant within 5 years of starting to menstruate), the caloric intake and weight gain are specific to the particular health needs of the woman during as well as after the pregnancy. The usual weight retained with each pregnancy by women in the United States is 10 pounds (McGanity et al., 1999). This retained weight may have a significant influence on future chronic disease development for women.

Table 37-6 Pregnancy Outcomes Linked to Weight Gain

Increased Risk of LBW Infant	Best Outcomes		Increased Risk of Gestational Diabetes*
Biologically immature or too thin (BMI <18.5 kg/m²)	BMI 18.5-24.9 kg/m²	BMI 25-29.9 kg/m²	BMI ≥30 kg/m² or older than 35 years
Recommended Weight Gain			
Approximately 28-40 pounds (1.1 lb/wk)	25-30lb (0.7 lb/wk) Not nursing: 0.8 lb/wk Nursing: 0.9 lb/wk Twins: 1.4 lb/wk	15-25 lb	11-20 lb

Data from Institutes of Medicine (IOM). Report on weight gain during pregnancy: reexamining the guidelines, 2009.
*Increased risk of LBW infant or infant too large.
LBW, Low-birth-weight; *BMI*, body mass index.

Table 37-7 Intake of Nutrients in Maternal Diet and Effect on Amount of Breast Milk

Intake Causes No Increase in Amount of Breast Milk	Intake Causes Some Increase	Intake Causes Significant Increase
Calories Fluid Protein Calcium Phosphorus Magnesium Sodium Potassium Folate Vitamin C Iron*	Fatty acid content Selenium Iodine Water-soluble vitamins (excluding folate and C) Fat-soluble vitamins	Vitamin D Vitamin B₆ Iodine Selenium

*Although supplementation is needed because of increased needs of infant (IOM. Nutrition during Lactation, 1991.)

It is now known that the nutritional needs for pregnancy begin before conception. The state of nutrition 60 to 90 days before conception influences pregnancy outcomes. The major nutrient changes from conception through the first trimester are increases in folic acid, iron, and calories. The overall nutritional needs throughout the pregnancy are as follows:

1. Adequate calories for development of the fetus, placenta, and lactation after delivery (with adequate calories increasing the opportunity for adequate nutrients)
2. Adequate protein
3. Adequate iron
4. Adequate folic acid, vitamin C (especially critical if the woman is a smoker, because there is a much higher need in smokers), and vitamin B_{12}
5. Adequate calcium and iodine

Community-based programs such as Women, Infants, and Children (WIC) can be a resource for helping women in need. It has been demonstrated that infants of women who participate in these programs have higher birth weights than those who were not in the programs and who are in the same social, economic, or other problematic circumstances.

Many of the nutritional issues in *lactation* are influenced by the nutritional status of the pregnant woman. The nutritional stores of the newly delivered woman are an important source of supplies for her and the infant. Certain nutrients are stable regardless of the maternal diet (Table 37-7). Studies of lactation have found that after about 6 months of breastfeeding, maternal weight decreases by about 10 pounds without any changes in the composition or production of breast milk (Barbosa et al., 1997). This may be important when considering that the average weight retained with each pregnancy is about 10 pounds.

Infancy and Childhood

An excellent summary of the nutrients and development needs for food in this age group has been recently published (Fig. 37-1). This figure provides guidance about major nutrient needs and how the infant and child can meet these needs. These evidence-based guidelines were developed by a panel of pediatricians, nutritionists, and the U.S Department of Agriculture (USDA) after comprehensive review of the literature.

It is important to help parents understand that the introduction of new foods takes time. Researchers found that it takes at least eight different attempts of introducing a new food before a child will show true acceptance or rejection (Birch et al., 1991; Satter, 2000). Parents must understand that their role is to provide a healthy range and variety of foods in a pleasant eating environment, whereas the child's role is to consume the food in the amounts that he or she needs and wants. This foundation of good food habits will carry through to the adolescent stage, in which independence and finding ways of expressing this independence are achieved not only in social functioning but also in food and health habits.

Adolescence

Adolescents gain independence by taking a greater role in food choices and amounts eaten. It is frustrating for parents who worked to establish standards to see the young person seek independence, even with foods consumed. This is a stage in life that demands high caloric intake, because growth needs are second only to those in infancy—more kilocalories per kilogram are needed than in any other life stage. This high caloric consumption is favorable to nutritional status because with high calories comes the increased likelihood of taking in more nutrients. Parents must remain hopeful that good health habits will guide the teenager. There may be concern over peer pressure leading to "strange" or different food habits, such as disordered eating, sports nutrition, and vegetarian diets, which many teens attempt. Such exploration is often a natural part of expressing independence. These food patterns can be healthy, such as improving food habits with vegetarianism or sports nutrition. The family physician needs to determine when the teen's exploration could become harmful. Nutrition assessment is appropriate in this life stage in regard to determining whether a nutritional problem is present.

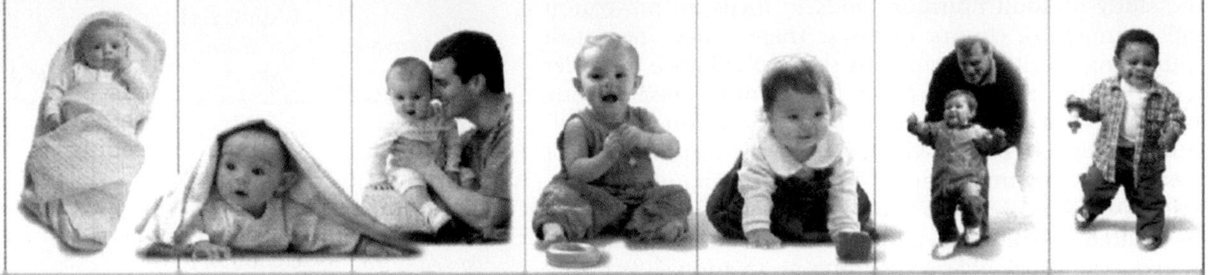

Development stage	Newborn	Head up	Supported sitter	Independent sitter	Crawler	Beginning to walk	Independent toddler
Physical skills	• Needs head support	• More skillful head control with support emerging	• Sits with help or support • On tummy, pushes up on arms with straight elbows	• Sits independently • Can pick up and hold small object in hand • Leans toward food or spoon	• Learns to crawl • May pull self to stand	• Pulls self to stand • Stands alone • Takes early steps	• Walks well alone • Runs
Eating skills	• Baby establishes a suck-swallow-breathe pattern during breast or bottle feeding	• Breastfeeds or bottle feeds • Tongue moves forward and back to suck	• May push food out of mouth with tongue, which gradually decreases with age • Moves pureed food forward and backward in mouth with tongue to swallow • Recognizes spoon and holds mouth open as spoon approaches	• Learns to keep thick purees in mouth • Pulls head downward and presses upper lip to draw food from spoon • Tries to rake foods toward self into fist • Can transfer food from one hand to the other • Can drink from a cup held by feeder	• Learns to move tongue from side to side to transfer food around mouth and push food to the side of the mouth so food can be mashed • Begins to use jaw and tongue to mash food • Plays with spoon at mealtime, may bring it to mouth, but does not use it for self-feeding yet • Can feed self finger foods • Holds cup independently • Holds small foods between thumb and first finger	• Feeds self easily with fingers • Can drink from a straw • Can hold cup with two hands and take swallows • More skillful at chewing • Dips spoon in food rather than scooping • Demands to spoon-feed self • Bites through a variety of textures	• Chews and swallows firmer foods skillfully • Learns to use a fork for spearing • Uses spoon with less spilling • Can hold cup in one hand and set it down skillfully
Baby's hunger and fullness cues	• Cries or fusses to show hunger • Gazes at caregiver, opens mouth during feeding indicating desire to continue • Spits out nipple or falls asleep when full • Stops sucking when full	• Cries or fusses to show hunger • Smiles, gazes at caregiver, or coos during feeding to indicate desire to continue • Spits out nipple or falls asleep when full • Stops sucking when full	• Moves head forward to reach spoon or food when hungry • May swipe the food toward the mouth when hungry • Turns head away from spoon when full • May be distracted or notice surroundings more when full	• Reaches for spoon or food when hungry • Points to food when hungry • Slows down in eating when full • Clenches mouth shut or pushes food away when full	• Reaches for food when hungry • Points to food when hungry • Shows excitement when food is presented when hungry • Pushes food away when full • Slows down in eating when full	• Expresses desire for specific foods with words or sounds • Shakes head to say "no more" when full	• Combines phrases with gestures, such as "want that" and pointing • Can lead parent to refrigerator and point to a desired food or drink • Uses words like "all done" and "get down" • Plays with food or throws food when full
Appropriate foods and textures	• Breastmilk or infant formula	• Breastmilk or infant formula	• Breastmilk or infant formula • Infant cereals • Thin pureed foods	• Breastmilk or infant formula • Infant cereals • Thin pureed baby foods • Thicker pureed baby foods • Soft mashed foods without lumps • 100% juice	• Breastmilk or infant formula • 100% juice • Infant cereals • Pureed foods • Ground or soft mashed foods with tiny soft noticeable lumps • Foods with soft texture • Crunchy foods that dissolve (such as baby biscuits or crackers) • Increase variety of flavors offered	• Breastmilk, infant formula or whole milk • 100% juice • Coarsely chopped foods, including foods with noticeable pieces • Foods with soft to moderate texture • Toddler foods • Bite-sized pieces of foods • Bites through a variety of textures	• Whole milk • 100% juice • Coarsely chopped foods • Toddler foods • Bite-sized pieces of foods • Becomes efficient at eating foods of varying textures and taking controlled bites of soft solids, hard solids or crunchy foods by 2 years

© 2003 Gerber Products Company

Figure 37-1 Summary of physical and eating skills, hunger and fullness cues, and appropriate food textures for infants and children. *(From Butte N, Cobb K, Dwyer J, et al. The Start Healthy feeding guidelines for infants and toddlers. J Am Diet Assoc 2004;104:455-467.)*

Adulthood

The study of adult nutrition tends to focus on prevention and treatment of chronic diseases. There is new interest in optimizing nutrition during this stage to enhance the older adult's quality of life. The public has demonstrated a strong interest in this process with the use of nutrition and nutritional products as an alternative medicine source. Some of these developments, such as antioxidant vitamins, plant-based estrogens, and other functional foods, have not had the desired outcomes (i.e., longer life, enhanced functional status). The *Dietary Reference Intakes* (National Academy of Sciences, 2005) has addressed this concept of enhanced nutrient intakes through supplements and other products by introducing a new category called *tolerable upper intake levels* (see Terminology). Many values in this category of nutrient levels are still being researched.

The research on caloric restriction as a means for decreasing the problems of aging is still at an animal model level. Studies concerning the risks of obesity and the positive effects of physical activity have the most promise to helping to understand the effects of overnutrition and caloric restriction on human longevity.

Osteoporosis

With the possibility of a 20% bone mass loss in the 5 to 7 years following menopause, the best treatment for osteoporosis (reduction in amount of bone mass) is the prevention of bone loss. The following three steps are recognized as most helpful for women (80% of osteoporosis population):
1. Balanced diet rich in calcium and vitamin D (Table 37-8; see also Table 37-1)
2. Weight-bearing exercise, such as walking
3. Healthy lifestyle, with no smoking or excessive alcohol intake

Peak bone development occurs throughout adolescence, with smaller bone gain during the 20s and less calcium needed at this age. Bone loss starts with menopause for women, which increases the need for calcium and vitamin D to prevent bone loss. High dietary intake of calcium does not seem to present any risk; previous concern about kidney stone formation with increased calcium intake appears to be unfounded (Curhan et al., 1997). Side effects of high calcium supplement intake include constipation and dyspepsia, and calcium supplementation with more than 2000 mg/day of vitamin D may lead to soft tissue calcification.

Cancer Prevention through Nutrition

Caloric Restriction

In animal studies, caloric restriction has shown promise in increasing the life span of the animals studied, but human studies have not been as encouraging. This may be an extremely difficult area to investigate because there is no clear understanding of where in the human life span caloric restriction would be the most beneficial. In humans the balance between starvation and overnutrition seems to be more difficult to determine. People with a BMI less than 18 kg/m2 seem to have a higher mortality rate, but those who are obese (BMI >30) also probably do less well. Currently, there is insufficient evidence to recommend caloric restriction as a means

Table 37-8 Supplement or Food Sources of Calcium and Vitamin D

Supplement or Food	Elemental Calcium/ Tablet	Calcium Compound	Vitamin D (IU)*
Supplement			
Caltrate 600	600 mg	Carbonate	0
Caltrate 600 + D	600 mg	Carbonate	200
Tums	600 mg	Carbonate	0
Citracal	400 mg	Citrate	0
Calcium Gummy Bears (2)	200 mg	Phosphate	200
Viactiv	500 mg	Carbonate	100
Food (1 cup)			
Milk (skim)	300 mg		100
Juice fortified with calcium	300 mg		0
Tofu prepared by calcium precipitation	260 mg		0

*Adequate intake of vitamin D in cholecalciferol (1 μg cholecalciferol = 40 IU vitamin D): 31-50 years old, 5 μg/day; 51-70 years old, 10 μg/day; older than 70 years of age, 15 μg/day.

of treatment or prevention of cancer, although evidence does suggest that a high BMI (>30) may be a cancer-promoting factor. Physical activity to balance the energy intake is probably the best preventive measure against cancer at this time.

Vitamin Supplementation

Epidemiologic studies note that populations who consume diets high in vitamins and minerals have a lower incidence of cancer. Three studies, the Alpha-Tocopherol Beta-Carotene Cancer Prevention Study Group (1994), β-Carotene and Retinol Efficacy Trial (CARET; Omenn et al., 1996), and Physicians' Health Study (PHS; Hennekens et al., 1996), investigated smokers and asbestos workers to see whether provitamin A and beta carotene supplementation would decrease the incidence of cancer. Those who received supplementation developed cancers earlier than those who did not, and the studies were suspended. The question of whether supplementation with antioxidant vitamins prevents cancer has not been answered, because several other antioxidant vitamins have not been studied. Supplementation has lost its support as a positive intervention, particularly in men who smoke. Foods rich in the antioxidant vitamins (beta carotene, vitamins C and E) and minerals (potassium) are recommended rather than supplements until the problems of dietary supplement research can be solved.

Therefore, the dietary elements that seem to be the most favorable, according to epidemiologic studies, are as follows:
More fruits, vegetables, whole-grain products, and calcium-containing foods
Less saturated fats, particularly those found in red meats

Box 37-2 Different Nutrient Needs in Aging

Decreased Need

Calories

Vitamin A

Increased Need

Fluid needs

Protein (slightly increased)

Vitamin D

Calcium

Vitamin B_{12}

Vitamin B_6 (pyridoxine)

Aging

The only difference in the nutritional needs of older adults was long thought to be the decrease in caloric needs, about a 2% to 5% decrease with each decade of life. The smaller decrease in caloric need (2%) is for those who exercise and the higher decrease (5%) is for those who do not exercise. Decrease in caloric need is complicated by the well-established phenomenon that weight gain tapers as humans age. Peak weights for men are at around 55 years, with weight loss after that age (slowly, because rapid weight loss has significant risks in the older adult). Peak weights for women are at around 65 years with decreases after that age. Rapid weight loss can identify critical problems; one of the first signs of dementia is often unintended weight loss. Additional changes in nutrient needs occur mainly because of the physiologic changes of aging (Box 37-2). The Tufts University USDA Human Nutrition Center on Aging has developed a food pyramid based on the different nutrient needs that are critical to older adults (Russell et al., 1999).

Because psychosocial components are so important in determining nutritional status in older adults, reliable nutrition assessment includes consideration of these elements for evaluation (Fig. 37-2). Functional status and mental status influence nutrition and well-being.

Diet in Prevention and Management of Major Disease

Vascular and Related Conditions

Key Points

- Dietary improvements for the general population as well as for patients with cardiovascular disease, including low saturated fats, increased omega-3 fatty acids of nuts and fish, and nutrient-rich foods, seem to improve disease risk.
- Dietary supplements have not reduced the risk of cardiovascular disease in the general population or in patients with cardiovascular disease.
- Foods seem to be better than supplements in disease prevention.

Hypertension

The report of the Seventh Joint National Committee on Prevention, Detection, Evaluation and Treatment of Hypertension (JNC-7) has identified patients with systolic blood pressure (SBP) of 130 to 139 mm Hg and diastolic blood pressure (DBP) of 85 to 89 mm Hg as having *prehypertension* (Chobanian et al., 2003). Persons with prehypertension and stage I hypertension (SBP 140-159; DBP 90-99) are candidates for lifestyle and diet modification. Persons with stage I hypertension with complicating conditions such as diabetes or cardiovascular disease or stage II hypertension (SBP 160-179; DBP 100-109) and stage III hypertension (SBP ≥180; DBP ≥110) not only should receive recommendations for dietary and lifestyle modification, but also are candidates for appropriate pharmacotherapy, with diuretics as the mainstay of treatment.

Several lifestyle modifications are recommended for prehypertension and all treatment categories (stages I-III), regardless of whether medications are indicated for ideal control (Dosh, 2002). Aerobic exercise (45-60 minutes at least 3 days/wk and preferably daily); a low-salt, low-fat, high-fruit, high-vegetable diet; limited alcohol consumption (<3 drinks/day); and modest weight loss (3%-9% of total body weight) have been shown to result in modest blood pressure reductions. There is insufficient evidence that these measures alone reduce morbidity and mortality rates in persons with hypertension.

A Cochrane review of 58 clinical trials found that sodium restriction led to significant reductions in systolic and diastolic blood pressures, with a greater effect in blacks than in whites (Jurgens and Graudal, 2004). SBP decreased by an average of 4.2 mm Hg and DBP by 2.0 mm Hg in white patients. Trials in black patients indicated that SBP decreased by an average of 6.4 mm Hg and DBP by 2.0 mm Hg. Based on these trials, JNC-7 recommended that patients with hypertension limit daily sodium intake to about 2 to 4 g daily (Chobanian et al., 2003). This recommendation may be suitable for prehypertension and early stage I hypertension, but not for stages II and III hypertension alone. Isolated systolic hypertension, which is more common in older adults, is also more responsive to sodium restriction. Reducing sodium intake (<2-4 g/day) does lead to a slightly lower average BP, especially in black Americans. No evidence has shown that reducing sodium intake decreases morbidity or mortality or that modest sodium restriction is harmful (Smucny and FPIN, 2004).

A combination diet known as DASH (*d*ietary *a*pproach to *s*top *h*ypertension) is low in saturated fat, high in fruits and vegetables (8-10 servings, or 4-5 cups/day), and high in low-fat dairy products. DASH resulted in significant reductions in systolic (>11 mm Hg) and diastolic (>5 mm Hg) BP in persons with stage I hypertension (Appel et al., 1997; Svetkey et al., 1999). With the addition of sodium restriction (<2 g daily), further BP reductions have been observed (He and MacGregor, 2004; NIH, 1992). The DASH diet, or a similar combination, with modest sodium restriction should be considered as first-line treatment for prehypertension and early stage I hypertension.

Other dietary considerations for hypertension, but with weaker evidence than sodium restriction, include increasing fiber and maintaining potassium intake; these recommendations are based on observational studies comparing

NESTLÉ NUTRITION SERVICES

Updated Version

Nestlé

Mini Nutritional Assessment
MNA®

Last name:	First name:	Sex:	Date:

Age:	Weight, kg:	Height, cm:	I.D. Number:

Complete the screen by filling in the boxes with the appropriate numbers.
Add the numbers for the screen. If score is 11 or less, continue with the assessment to gain a Malnutrition Indicator Score.

Screening

A Has food intake declined over the past 3 months due to loss of appetite, digestive problems, chewing or swallowing difficulties?
0 = severe loss of appetite
1 = moderate loss of appetite
2 = no loss of appetite □

B Weight loss during last months
0 = weight loss greater than 3 kg (6.6 lbs)
1 = does not know
2 = weight loss between 1 and 3 kg (2.2 and 6.6 lbs)
3 = no weight loss □

C Mobility
0 = bed or chair bound
1 = able to get out of bed/chair but does not go out
2 = goes out □

D Has suffered psychological stress or acute disease in the past 3 months
0 = yes   2 = no □

E Neuropsychological problems
0 = severe dementia or depression
1 = mild dementia
2 = no psychological problems □

F Body Mass Index (BMI) (weight in kg)/(height in m)^2
0 = BMI less than 19
1 = BMI 19 to less than 21
2 = BMI 21 to less than 23
3 = BMI 23 or greater □

Screening score (subtotal max. 14 points) □ □

12 points or greater — Normal – not at risk – no need to complete assessment

11 points or below — Possible malnutrition – continue assessment

Assessment

G Lives independently (not in a nursing home or hospital)
0 = no   1 = yes □

H Takes more than 3 prescription drugs per day
0 = yes   1 = no □

I Pressure sores or skin ulcers
0 = yes   1 = no □

J How many full meals does the patient eat daily?
0 = 1 meal
1 = 2 meals
2 = 3 meals □

K Selected consumption markers for protein intake
• At least one serving of dairy products (milk, cheese, yogurt) per day?   yes □ no □
• Two or more serving of legumes or eggs per week?   yes □ no □
• Meat, fish or poultry every day   yes □ no □
0.0 = if 0 or 1 yes
0.5 = if 2 yes
1.0 = if 3 yes □.□

L Consumes two or more servings of fruits or vegetables per day?
0 = no   1 = yes □

M How much fluid (water, juice, coffee, tea, milk…) is consumed per day?
0.0 = less than 3 cups
0.5 = 3 to 5 cups
1.0 = more than 5 cups □.□

N Mode of feeding
0 = unable to eat without assistance
1 = self-fed with some difficulty
2 = self-fed without any problem □

O Self view of nutritional status
0 = view self as being malnourished
1 = is uncertain of nutritional state
2 = views self as having no nutritional problem □

P In comparison with other people of the same age, how do they consider their health status?
0.0 = not as good
0.5 = does not know
1.0 = as good
2.0 = better □.□

Q Mid-arm circumference (MAC) in cm
0.0 = MAC less than 21
0.5 = MAC 21 to 22
1.0 = MAC 22 or greater □.□

R Calf circumference (CC) in cm
0 = CC less than 31   1 = CC 31 or greater □

Assessment (max. 16 points) □ □.□

Screening score □ □

Total Assessment (max. 30 points) □ □.□

Malnutrition Indicator Score

17 to 23.5 points — at risk of malnutrition □

Less than 17 points — malnourished □

06.98 USA

® Société des Produits Nestlé S.A., Vevey, Switzerland, Trademark Owners

Figure 37-2 Mini Nutritional Assessment (MNA). *(From Vellas B, Garry PJ, Guigoz V [eds]. Mini Nutritional Assessment [MNA]: Research and Practice in the Elderly, vol 1. Nestlé Nutrition Workshop Series. Basel, S Karger, 1999, p 158.)*

vegetarians with nonvegetarians and differences in systolic and diastolic BP (Berkow and Barnard, 2005). Vegetarian diets are generally high in fruits, vegetables, legumes, and nuts. They have a relatively low total fat and high potassium, magnesium, and fiber content. No evidence shows that potassium or magnesium supplementation has beneficial effects in hypertension, except when there is wasting of these elements because of diuretic use (Beyer et al., 2006).

Hyperlipidemia

Diet is the mainstay of therapy for mild and moderate hyperlipidemia. Patients with high low-density lipoprotein (LDL) levels (>160 mg/dL) and those with borderline high LDL cholesterol (130-160 mg/dL), but with two risk factors for coronary heart disease, should be considered for dietary modification. The National Cholesterol Education Program (NCEP) has recommended a diet for therapeutic lifestyle changes that includes less than 200 mg of cholesterol daily and less than 7% saturated fat, 25% to 35% total fat, 50% to 60% carbohydrates, and 15% protein of total calories (Expert Panel, 2001; Henley, 2002). Although diet will reduce the cholesterol level, there is no clear evidence that diet low in saturated fat or cholesterol will reduce cardiovascular morbidity and mortality. The Irish Heart Foundation focused on limiting saturated fat intake and encourages the use of eggs in a balanced, healthy diet (Gray and Griffin, 2009). Dietary therapy should be offered in conjunction with weight reduction and exercise, all of which also reduce triglyceride levels, increase high-density lipoprotein (HDL) levels, reduce BP, and improve glucose tolerance.

Increased consumption of fruits and vegetables is associated with a lower incidence of vascular disease events in observational studies (Clinical Evidence, 2001). The Ornish program, which combines a high-vegetable and very-low-fat diet with stress reduction and prescribed exercises, has shown reversal of coronary vascular disease on pre- and postangiographic studies (Ornish et al., 1998; Pischke et al., 2008). Many patients found long-term maintenance difficult because of the strict dietary modification required.

In an attempt to increase the effectiveness of diet in reducing serum cholesterol, NCEP has recommended the use of functional foods high in components that reduce cholesterol, such as viscous fibers, soy protein, plant sterols, and nuts (Expert Panel, 2001).

Dietary fiber intake, independent of fat intake, has been shown to have an inverse association with myocardial infarction (MI) (Rimm et al., 1996). During a 6-year follow-up of 734 cases of MI, patients in the highest quartile of dietary fiber had the lowest incidence of MI. A 10-g increase in total dietary fiber corresponded to a relative risk reduction (RR) of 0.81 in MI. A multicenter, population-based cohort study of 2909 healthy black and white adults followed for 10 years showed inverse linear associations with increasing fiber diets with reductions in weight gain, insulin levels, LDL levels, and BP (Ludwig et al., 1999). Fiber consumption predicted these coronary vascular disease risk factors more strongly than total-fat or saturated-fat consumption. Similar associations, especially with higher oral fiber intake, have been reported in women (Wolk et al., 1999) and elderly patients (Mozaffarian et al., 2003).

No evidence shows that treating isolated high triglyceride (TG) levels in the absence of other risk factors prevents coronary events. Weight reduction, restricting alcohol use, and increased exercise are the important interventions in lowering TGs. Although carbohydrate intake may influence blood TGs in some individuals, the practicality of the glycemic index of foods has not shown improvement in risk factors for heart disease (Kelly et al., 2004). Coincident lowering of TG levels while treating other dyslipidemias (e.g., high LDL, low HDL) can contribute to decreasing coronary events (Cucuzzella et al., 2004).

Secondary Prevention of Cardiovascular and Cerebrovascular Disease

A systematic review graded the evidence of dietary recommendations for the prevention of further events in patients with existing cardiovascular disease (Hooper et al., 2004a). The recommendation is ranked grade 1 (evidence from RCTs, systematic reviews of RCTs) and level A evidence of the effect of the intervention on morbidity and mortality rates (SOR A, 1).

Recommend an increase in omega-3 fats to all patients with established coronary disease. Reduced saturated fat results in decreased recurrent coronary events. Recommend the Mediterranean diet to all patients after MI (Hooper et al., 2004b). The Mediterranean diet is a combination of increased omega-3 fats, fruits, vegetables, and fresh foods, together with a reduction in saturated fats and processed foods. In a prospective cohort of 1302 Greek men and women with CAD followed for 3.78 years, a 27% reduction in all-cause mortality and 31% reduction in cardiovascular disease–specific mortality were seen in those with the highest adherence to the Mediterranean diet (Trichopoulou et al., 2005) (see Web Resources, American Heart Association). There is no clear systematic evidence for dietary protection in patients with cerebrovascular disease. Multicomponent programs focusing on diet, exercise, and stress management can have additive benefit to patients with CHD (Daubenmier et al., 2007).

Dietary Supplements and Vascular Diseases

Is folate supplementation indicated with coronary artery disease (CAD)? Evidence is insufficient to recommend the routine use of folate supplementation to treat CAD (Albert et al., 2008). High levels of serum homocysteine are associated with increased risk for CAD in case-control studies. Folate supplementation decreases the level of serum homocysteine (Gill, 2004). The American Heart Association and American College of Cardiology do not recommend the routine use of high-dose folic acid or vitamin B supplements for primary or secondary prevention of cardiovascular events. The Canadian Task Force on Preventive Health Care has not recommended screening for homocystinemia but has recommended meeting the daily allowances for folate (400 µg), vitamin B_1 (2.4 µg), and vitamin B_6 (1.7 µg) (Booth and Wang, 2000).

Do vitamin C supplements reduce cardiovascular disease mortality (Aukerman, 2004; Bloom et al., 2002; Riccioni et al., 2007; Sesso et al., 2008)? There is insufficient evidence to recommend vitamin supplements for prevention of cardiovascular disease (USPSTF, 2003).

Does vitamin E supplementation have a benefit in reducing cardiovascular disease? The Heart Outcomes Prevention Evaluation (HOPE) followed 3994 patients with vascular disease or diabetes over age 55 for 5 to 7 years (Lonn et al., 2005). Patients received 400 IU of vitamin E or matching placebo. Vitamin E supplementation had no long-term benefit to prevent major cardiovascular events and may increase the risk of heart failure. Vitamin E supplementation, in a variety of doses, does not decrease the incidence of cardiovascular or all-cause mortality. There is no evidence that vitamin C decreases mortality in patients at CAD risk (Aukerman, 2004; Bloom et al., 2002).

Vitamin D deficiency and low blood levels of D have been associated with heart disease and hypertension, especially in regions with low sunlight and in individuals with dark skin pigmentation. Whether supplementation of vitamin D would reduce high BP or heart disease is unclear; research is ongoing.

The dietary supplement of omega-3 fatty acids for the prevention and treatment of cardiovascular disease has received widespread interest. It is unclear whether omega-3 fatty acid intake alters mortality, cardiovascular events, or cancers in those at risk or in the general public (Cochrane review; Hooper et al., 2004b). Further studies are being conducted.

KEY TREATMENT

Sodium restriction significantly reduces systolic and diastolic blood pressure, with a greater effect in blacks than whites (Jurgens and Graudal, 2004) (SOR: A).

The DASH diet significantly reduces systolic (>11 mm Hg) and diastolic (>5 mm Hg) BP in persons with stage I hypertension (Appel et al., 1997; Svetkey et al., 1999) (SOR: A).

Diabetes Mellitus

Diet is one of the cornerstones of management of types 1 and 2 diabetes mellitus. The American Diabetes Association (ADA, 2006) has published a comprehensive guide to the management of diabetes, including recommendations for *medical nutrition therapy* (MNT). Some goals for all diabetic patients include controlling weight, blood lipids, and BP and keeping blood sugar levels in the normal range or at a level that avoids acute complications of diabetes. Diabetic patients should consume a diet that is appropriate for their particular needs, with consideration of coexisting medical conditions, cultural patterns, tastes, and levels of physical activity.

Type 1

Some specific goals of MNT in type 1 diabetes are to provide adequate nutrition to allow normal growth in children and to provide food intake that, when combined with insulin therapy, results in stable and safe blood glucose levels.

The ADA recommends the terms *sugar, starch,* and *fiber* to refer to the different types of carbohydrate. Traditionally, dietitians have paid great attention to carbohydrates in the diet in patients with diabetes. Many diabetic diets affirm the role of the *glycemic index,* which is the amount that the blood glucose level increases in 2 to 3 hours after consuming different foods. Some believed that the different glycemic responses from different types of carbohydrate influenced diabetic outcomes, but studies have shown that the glycemic response in type 1 and type 2 diabetes is related to the total amount of carbohydrate consumed and does not depend on the type of carbohydrate (Franz et al., 2002). Most patients have a limited ability to maintain a diet containing only foods with a low glycemic index. No definitive evidence exists on the value of low-glycemic index diets. Thus, it is probably not practical or realistic to educate type 1 diabetic patients about the roles of various carbohydrates in maintaining the glycemic index.

Fiber

Patients with type 1 diabetes should be educated about the healthy benefits of fiber in the diet. Although early studies showed some benefit for blood glucose levels with a high-fiber diet, these results have not been supported by larger trials (Franz et al., 2002).

Sweeteners

Many diabetics and health care providers operate under the misconception that plain sucrose as a sweetener results in hyperglycemia and should be avoided. However, studies have not shown this to be true, and patients do not need to restrict sucrose intake, but rather should monitor the total carbohydrate load in the diet. Some recommend replacing sucrose with fructose in the diet because fructose has a lower glycemic index. There is some concern that fructose adversely affects lipids, however, so this substitution is probably not beneficial. All appear to be safe.

Diabetic patients should consume carbohydrates through fruits, whole grains, vegetables, and low-fat milk. The total amount of carbohydrate in a meal is important; it is not necessary to consume particular foods based on the glycemic index. Sucrose and sucrose-containing foods do not need to be avoided by diabetic patients, but should be counted as part of the total carbohydrate load in the diet. The four FDA-approved nonnutritive sweeteners—aspartame, saccharin, acesulfame, and sucralose—are generally safe when consumed in recommended amounts established by the U.S. Food and Drug Administration (ADA, 2002).

Because the postprandial glycemic response is strongly related to the premeal insulin dose, patients should learn how to adjust insulin doses based on the total carbohydrate content of the meal. The usual calculation of carbohydrate (CHO) to insulin starts at 15 g CHO for each unit of regular insulin (see Web Resources for additional information on foods and portion sizes). Adjustments are then made for the individual patient based on how closely this works to help maintain blood glucose levels.

Protein

Some patients with hyperglycemia need extra protein in the diet—0.8 g protein/kg body weight in adults (National Academy of Sciences, 2004). Most adults consume at least 50% more protein than required, so modifying the amount of protein in the diet is usually not necessary for diabetic patients. Dietary intake of the usual amount of protein does not appear to affect the development of nephropathy. However, there are no long-term studies to evaluate the nephropathic effect of consuming more than 20% of calories from protein.

Dietary Fat

Patients with diabetes should attempt to limit the amount of saturated fat and cholesterol in the diet. No studies have demonstrated that modifying fat in the diet of diabetic patients modifies serum lipid levels any differently than such changes in the nondiabetic population. Interestingly, some metabolic studies show that low–saturated fat (10% of energy level), high-carbohydrate diets actually increase postprandial glucose, insulin, and TG levels compared with diets consisting of high proportions of monounsaturated fats. However, high–monounsaturated fat diets have not been shown to improve hemoglobin A_{1c} (HbA_{1c}) levels, and instructing patients to increase consumption of a particular type of fat may result in undesirable weight gain.

Diabetic patients should lower the amount of fat in their diet by replacing high-fat foods with those containing lower amounts of fat, and they should avoid saturated fats. Although FDA-approved fat substitutes are safe, when included as fat replacers in the diet, these substances have not resulted in significant weight loss over time and can cause diarrhea when overconsumed.

Diabetic patients should obtain less than 10% of their daily calories from saturated fats. Some patients (e.g., those with elevated LDL levels) may benefit by lowering their total daily saturated fat intake to less than 7% of total calories. Dietary cholesterol intake should be less than 300 mg/day in diabetic patients, and patients with elevated LDL levels may benefit by lowering daily cholesterol consumption to less than 200 mg (ADA, 2002).

Micronutrients

Although diabetes puts body tissues under increased oxidative stress, there is no evidence that increasing dietary consumption of antioxidants improves health outcomes in diabetic patients. Deficiencies of the minerals potassium, chromium, magnesium, and zinc may exacerbate glucose intolerance. Supplementation with these minerals has not been of benefit, except in the case of potassium and magnesium, for which serum levels can easily demonstrate correctable deficiencies.

KEY TREATMENT

Diet as a whole should be considered in the balanced food intake (with energy expenditure and basal metabolic rate) for determining medication needs of diabetic patient. Diet should be individualized to the patient's unique needs (ADA, 2008) (SOR: A).

Monitoring carbohydrate intake, despite the form of carbohydrate, is a crucial component in dietary management of type 1 diabetes (ADA, 2008) (SOR: A).

Nonnutritive sweeteners are safe when used at established intake levels (FDA, 2008) (SOR: A).

Diabetic patients should limit saturated fat intake to less than 7% of daily energy intake (ADA, 2008) (SOR: A).

Type 2 Diabetes Mellitus

Prevention

Obesity and overweight are important risk factors for developing type 2 diabetes mellitus. Lifestyle modifications, including diet, have been shown to reduce the risk of developing type 2. Diets that result in long-term weight loss of 5% to 7%, along with exercise of moderate intensity for at least 150 minutes per week (30 minutes for 5 days per week), reduce the incidence of type 2 diabetes (Knowles et al., 2002).

Treatment

Obesity tends to increase insulin resistance, so weight loss is an important tool in the prevention and management of type 2 diabetes (see Chapter 36). Dietary recommendations for type 2 patients are similar to those for type 1 patients. It is important to emphasize the importance of other lifestyle changes, such as increasing activity by these patients.

In patients with insulin resistance, reduced calorie intake and modest weight loss can improve insulin resistance and blood glucose levels in the short term. Structured programs for making lifestyle modifications (e.g., increased physical activity, <30% of calories from fat, regular participant contact) can result in weight loss of 5% to 7% (ADA, 2002).

Metabolic Syndrome

The metabolic syndrome consists of components that are all susceptible to dietary management (NCEP Expert Panel, 2001). Because many patients with the metabolic syndrome are overweight or obese, a focus on modest weight loss with dietary modification and increased activity is important.

The dietary recommendations for patients with the metabolic syndrome should be similar to those for patients with diabetes. Additionally, these patients should lower sodium intake, as with hypertension. The Diabetes Prevention Program was a study that evaluated the effect of intensive lifestyle changes; it focused on diet and exercise versus the use of standard lifestyle changes with or without metformin (placebo group) in the prevention of metabolic syndrome in over 3000 patients with impaired fasting glucose levels (Orchard et al., 2005). Patients were evaluated over a 3-year period. At the end of 3 years, significantly more patients in the group receiving standard lifestyle change recommendations and medication had developed the metabolic syndrome than patients with intensive lifestyle modification alone. In the study, intensive lifestyle changes were also associated with a decrease in the prevalence of the metabolic syndrome in patients who met criteria for the syndrome at baseline.

KEY TREATMENT

Lifestyle changes (increased activity, weight loss, smoking cessation, decreased saturated fat and increased fiber intake, moderation in alcohol intake) are the only treatment shown to affect all components of the metabolic syndrome and should be implemented in all patients (Finnish Medical Society, 2007) (SOR: A).

Nutrition Decisions in the Hospitalized Patient

Patients who are hospitalized require appropriate nutritional support to heal wounds and recover from illness. Up to 40% of hospitalized patients have some degree of malnutrition (Coates et al., 1993). Clinical studies have shown that length of stay and hospital costs are higher in patients at risk for poor nutrition than patients who are not at risk (Chima et al., 1997). The Joint Commission (formerly Joint Commission on Accreditation of Healthcare Organizations, JCAHO) requires a nutritional screen to be completed on each patient within 24 hours of admission. Often, patients with chronic illness are nutritionally depleted before hospitalization, and trauma and surgery increase nutritional demands significantly. Patients may rapidly fall behind in caloric and nutrient intake, particularly older adults.

Subjective Global Assessment

A useful instrument for assessing nutritional status in the hospitalized patient is the subjective global assessment (SGA) (Brugler et al., 2005). The SGA incorporates five features of the history and four components of the physical examination findings, enabling the physician to make a rapid determination of a patient's nutritional status (Fig. 37-3). The history components are weight loss, food intake, presence of significant GI symptoms, functional status or energy level, and metabolic demand of the underlying disease state. The physical components are depletion of subcutaneous fat, muscle wasting in the quadriceps and deltoid muscles, edema, and ascites. Each component is evaluated as category A (patient well nourished), B (mildly malnourished), or C (severely malnourished).

Weight loss is one of the most important components of the assessment. Generally, if the patient loses at least 5% of body weight over 2 weeks, the ranking in that category is B; a 10% loss puts the patient in category C.

After completing the assessment, the clinician makes a global judgment about the overall status. This is not a numeric assessment, but rather is based on the clinician's sense of the overall nutritional picture, mainly through evidence of weight loss, poor intake, muscle wasting, and loss of subcutaneous fat. This instrument has been validated with

SUBJECTIVE GLOBAL ASSESSMENT SCORING SHEET

Patient name: ____________ Patient ID: ____________ Date: ____________

Part 1: Medical history — SGA Score: A | B | C

1. **Weight change**
   - A. Overall change in past 6 months: ________ kgs.
   - B. Percent change: ________ Gain < 5% loss; ________ 5–10% loss; ________ > 10% loss
   - C. Change in past 2 weeks: ________ Increase; ________ No change; ________ Decrease
2. **Dietary intake**
   - A. Overall change: ________ No change; ________ Change
   - B. Duration: ________ Weeks
   - C. Type of change: ________ Suboptimal solid diet; ________ Full liquid diet; ________ Hypocaloric liquid; ________ Starvation
3. **Gastrointestinal symptoms (persisting for >2 weeks)**
   ____ None ____ Nausea ____ Vomiting ____ Diarrhea ____ Anorexia
4. **Functional impairment (nutritionally related)**
   - A. Overall impairment: ________ None; ________ Moderate; ________ Severe
   - B. Change in past 2 weeks: ________ Improved; ________ No change; ________ Regressed

Part 2: Physical examination

SGA Score

5. **Evidence of:**	Normal	Mild	Moderate	Severe
Loss of subcutaneous fat				
Muscle wasting				
Edema				
Ascites (hemo only)				

Part 3: SGA rating (check one)

A. ☐ Well-nourished B. ☐ Mildly-moderately malnourished C. ☐ Severely malnourished

Figure 37-3 Subjective global assessment (SGA). *(From Kalantar-Zadeh K, Kleiner M, Dunne E, et al. Total iron-binding capacity-estimated transferring correlates with nutritional subjective global assessment in hemodialysis patients. Am J Kidney Dis 1998;31:263-272; and Brugler L, Stankovic AK, Schlefer M, Bernstein L. A simplified nutrition screen for hospitalized patients using readily available laboratory and patient information. Nutrition 2005;21:650-658.)*

trained clinicians (Baker et al., 1982a, 1982b; Detsky et al., 1984) but not with untrained physicians.

Other assessment tools have been proposed and may eventually be validated (Brugler et al., 2005). Most of these take into account the same key factors: risk for malnutrition based on preexisting conditions, oral intake, need to heal wounds, and biochemical or hematologic parameters, such as serum albumin level and total lymphocyte count. The family physician can find most of these data readily and obtain a reasonable assessment of nutritional status.

Deterioration of Nutritional Status and Need for Support

Caloric Requirements

Even previously healthy patients may lose nutritional ground rapidly once they are hospitalized. Surgery and the stress of disease increase caloric requirements. The amount of these increases can be calculated using one of a number of predictive equations for determining *resting metabolic rate* (RMR) in kilocalories per day (kcal/day), which is the largest component of overall calorie expenditure. One frequently used model is the *Harris-Benedict equation* (1919), as follows:
For men:

$$RMR = 66.47 + (13.75 \times Weight\ [kg]) + (5.0 \times Height\ [cm]) - (6.75 \times Age\ [yr])$$

For women:

$$RMR = 665.09 + (9.56 \times Weight\ [kg]) + (1.84 \times Height\ [cm]) - (4.67 \times Age\ [yr])$$

Frankenfield and colleagues (2005) compared validation studies on several equations and found that the *Mifflin–St. Jeor equation* performed best in terms of predicting RMR compared with calorimetry. Although all the equations are less accurate for obese subjects, the following Mifflin–St. Jeor equation is least affected by obesity.
For men:

$$RMR = (9.99 \times Weight\ [kg]) + (6.25 \times Height\ [cm]) - (4.92 \times Age\ [yr]) + 5$$

For women:

$$RMR = (9.99 \times Weight\ [kg]) + (6.25 \times Height\ [cm]) - (4.92 \times Age\ [yr]) - 161$$

(See Web Resources for resting metabolic rate/basal metabolic rate and resting energy energy/basal energy expenditure calculators.)

These predictive equations do have weaknesses. They have not been validated in all subsets of the population, such as the elderly and nonwhite ethnic groups. Chronic illness can affect the relationship between RMR and body size, with loss of lean body mass in chronic illness.

These equations predict the *resting* metabolic rate, and caloric requirements increase beyond this figure, based on the patient's illness and other metabolic demands. The *resting energy expenditure* (REE) is 1.2 to 1.3 multiplied by the RMR. This figure is further altered by the level of stress. An example is to multiply REE by 1.1

by the number of degrees (Celsius) above normal in a patient with fever. Other multiples are 1.2 for mild stress, 1.4 for moderate stress, and 1.6 for severe stress. It is important to remember that all these calculations only *estimate* caloric requirements and should be considered as a starting point in nutrition repletion rather than the goal (Table 37-9).

Macronutrient Requirements

Hospitalized patients, and especially surgery and trauma patients, often suffer from *protein-calorie malnutrition* (PCM). It is important that patients in the hospital receive adequate calories to meet energy needs and adequate protein to maintain cellular integrity. Caloric requirement can be estimated by a formula, as noted earlier. Protein should make up 1.5 to 2 g/kg/day of that caloric requirement. Specific amino acids (e.g., glutamine, arginine) may be especially important in catabolic states (e.g., cancer, burns). These amino acids are therefore called *conditionally essential* amino acids. Carbohydrates make up about 70% of the total caloric requirement and lipids about 30%.

When to Start Nutritional Supplementation

There is a general trend to delay nutritional supplementation in hospitalized patients in the belief that oral intake will improve imminently, but this may exacerbate the existing malnutrition. The decision to initiate supplemental feeding (over what the patient willingly consumes at meals) must be individualized according to the patient's overall health and likely clinical outcome.

Calorie counts can be obtained for patients receiving oral nutrition. If the patient is falling short on caloric or protein intake, oral supplements are appropriate, given one to three times daily. The commercially available, canned oral supplements provide about 250 kcal and 9 g of protein per can.

For a variety of reasons, hospitalized patients are often unable to consume the calories and protein required to maintain nutrition. At some point, a patient may require enteral or parenteral nutrition. The American Society for Enteral and Parenteral Nutrition has published evidence-based guidelines for assessment and management of supplemental

Table 37-9 Estimated Caloric Need (kcal/kg)

Weight Goal	Level of Activity or Severity of Illness		
	Low kcal/kg	Moderate kcal/kg	High kcal/kg
Lose weight	15	20	25
Maintain weight	20	25	30
Gain weight	25	30	35

Examples: A 165-pound woman (height 5'2"; BMI 30.2) needs to lose weight but does not want to do any physical activity (low activity, lose weight); 165 lb = 75 kg, 75 × 15 = 1125 kcal estimated. A 200-pound man (height 6'4"; BMI 24.3) is hospitalized with sepsis and needs to maintain his weight (moderate activity, maintain weight); 200 lb = 91 kg, 91 × 25 = 2275 kcal estimated.

nutrition in patients with various disease states and surgical procedures (Albina et al., 2002; also available through the National Guideline Clearinghouse, www.guideline.gov). Depending on the disease state, these guidelines recommend that hospitalized patients begin *specialized nutrition support* (SNS) (enteral or parenteral feeding) when it is anticipated that patients will not otherwise be able to meet their nutritional needs for 7 to 10 days.

Enteral Nutrition

Most experts agree that when SNS is required, enteral feeding is the most appropriate method as long as the GI tract is competent (ADA, 2006; SORT A). This is partly because enteral feeding can supply complex nutrients such as fiber and intact proteins that parenteral nutrition cannot supply. Also, evidence indicates that enteral feeding has beneficial effects on the GI mucosa. Some cells lining the GI tract rely on luminal nutrients to flourish, and enteral feeding maintains the absorptive capacity of the epithelial cells. Enteral feeding also stimulates the immune function of the gut. Enteral feeding is usually safer and less expensive than parenteral feeding.

Delivery Methods

Nasogastric feeding is the least invasive form of enteral feeding and is appropriate when there is no gastric outlet obstruction, delayed gastric emptying, or elevated risk for aspiration. If a patient does not tolerate gastric feeding, has one of the previous contraindications, or requires prolonged nutritional supplementation, as is often the case with head and neck cancers, a *postpyloric feeding method* such as duodenal or jejunal tube placement is appropriate. Jejunal tubes are preferred to duodenal tubes because the latter still pose a reasonably high risk for aspiration.

Formulas

One type of tube-feeding formula is blenderized food, which can be any type of food that can be successfully liquefied. There are also nutritionally complete commercial formulas that are sterile, easy to use, and appropriate for patients with normal digestive and absorptive function. Elemental formulas contain predigested, chemically formulated nutrients in low-molecular-weight form and may be useful in patients with a stressed GI tract that cannot digest and absorb nutrients in a more complex form. Specialized modular formulas are available for specific disease states, such as a formula appropriate for a patient with chronic kidney or lung disease.

Complications

Clinicians should be aware of the potential complications of enteral feeding, such as aspiration (especially with gastric feeding), gut perforation, and functional problems, such as gastric distention, nausea, vomiting, and diarrhea. Serum electrolyte and glucose level abnormalities are common in patients receiving enteral nutrition, and monitoring of these parameters is important.

Parenteral Nutrition

Most hospitals now use multidisciplinary teams to help plan and implement parenteral nutrition when it is deemed appropriate. *Peripheral* parenteral nutrition (PPN), using a peripheral vein, is appropriate for short-term administration of nutrients (7-10 days) when the GI tract is not functional. *Total* parenteral nutrition (TPN) is administered through a more central vein and is used longer term (>10 days). TPN may be used to administer higher concentrations of glucose and protein than PPN, as well as for infusion of lipids.

Complications

The complications of PPN and TPN include phlebitis and other local reactions to infusion, maintenance of venous access, infection, air embolism, and refeeding syndrome. The *refeeding syndrome* is more common with TPN and may result in sudden death, more often affecting severely malnourished patients as they transition suddenly from deriving energy from stored fat to obtaining energy from infused glucose. This can cause a sudden depletion of phosphate stores, resulting in cardiac dysfunction. Patients who have lost more than 30% of their body weight should undergo gradual repletion of nutrients, with a slow increase in the rate of TPN over several days.

EVIDENCE-BASED SUMMARY

- To determine total daily calorie needs, multiply the basal metabolic rate (BMR) by the appropriate activity factor:
  Sedentary (little or no exercise; mild stress): BMR × 1.2
  Light activity (light exercise, sports 1-3 days/wk; moderate stress): BMR × 1.4
  Moderately active (moderate exercise, sports 3-5 days/wk; severe stress): BMR × 1.6
  Very active (hard exercise, sports 6-7 days/wk): BMR × 1.725
  Extra active (very hard exercise, sports + physical job or cross-training): BMR × 1.9
- To determine the BMR or basal energy expenditure (BEE), use the on-line calculator (http://www.calculator.org/bmr.html).
- Whenever possible, nutritional supplementation should be through the enteral route rather than parenteral.

Behavioral Modifications to Improve Diet and Lifestyle

Diet and lifestyle can be improved to promote good health through changes in behavior.

Patient Counseling on Dietary Changes

The family physician advising the patient about improving diet and lifestyle must specify the behaviors needed (rather than outcomes), help build the patient's behavioral change skills, address factors impeding change, and have an interactive discussion.

Specify Behaviors, Not Just Outcomes

Many chronic conditions have dietary implications, and dietary change is required for the condition to improve. For example, obesity involves calorie reduction; diabetes involves changes in food types eaten, portions, and spacing of eating episodes; and hypertension often involves sodium restriction. Thus, it is important to focus on the behavior necessary (e.g., reducing intake of simple carbohydrates) to reach the outcome (improved HbA$_{1c}$ levels). Often, dietary advice involves the patient being told to do the outcome, such as "lose some weight" or "improve A1c." Although important goals, these should not be confused with what *action* a patient can take. A patient cannot stand still and lose weight but can only change eating patterns and increase physical activity (behaviors). In communicating with patients, it is important to state not only the desired outcome and why (e.g., "It is important to get your hemoglobin A1c below 7% so that you can reduce the chance that you will have complications from your diabetes, such as loss of vision or amputation"), but also to discuss how the patient might accomplish that outcome (e.g., "Eating a healthy diet and increasing physical activity can improve A1c. Which of these would you like to talk about today?").

Build Skills for Behavior Change

A second common problem with diet counseling is that the focus is often on the patient acquiring knowledge rather than learning the skills for change. Patients who are critically ill need specific instructions on dietary restrictions for their condition. However, most patients who need diet counseling (e.g., those with hypertension, obesity, type 2 diabetes) need to know how to change their habits more than specific details of "dieting dos and don'ts." Too much information also overwhelms most patients, who begin to feel helpless to make all these changes correctly. Instead, encourage patients to consider how they will make the diet changes needed. Use a stepwise approach; start with small goals in short time increments and build to long-term goals so that patients may gain confidence in their ability to be successful with a new diet plan. Research shows that patients are best able to change behavior when the following elements are incorporated into the plan:

- *Readiness to change.* Patients are in different places with regard to their readiness to change (see Chapter 7). Some are ready to make a change immediately, some are reluctant and cannot decide, and others have tried repeatedly and failed. The family physician's goal is to move the patient to the next logical step (Prochaska et al., 1992).
- *Goal setting and tracking.* Proper goal setting and knowing the patient's current state can facilitate successful change by encouraging confidence in the ability to change. Start off with a small, attainable goal and build over time (Locke et al., 1981; Strecher et al., 1995).
- *Relapse prevention.* Patients who have an active plan for avoiding temptation and returning to past behaviors are much more successful than patients who have not planned coping strategies to use during tempting situations (Larimer et al., 1999; Marlatt and George, 1990).
- *Support.* Consider how people and environments can support the patient making changes.

These strategies collectively affect self-efficacy and perception of the patient's ability to make successful change in a specific area (Bandura, 1977, 2004).

Consider Factors Impeding Change

Many behavioral theories describe why patients act appropriately or not in regard to healthy behaviors, but in the daily practice of medicine, it is useful to break this into a simple and workable system. *Motivational interviewing* shows great promise as a technique for encouraging behavior change discussions with patients regarding diet improvement (Burke et al., 2003; Thorpe, 2003; vanWormer and Boucher, 2004). Physicians should consider two main factors affecting patient motivation for changing a behavior: importance and confidence. *Importance* is the priority the patient places on the behavior change in question. "How important is it that I make this change?" *Confidence* is the patient's perception that he or she can actually execute the change. Both are needed. When discussing dietary change with patients, it is important both to engage the patient in considering his or her level of importance and confidence relating to the behavior or task in question and to encourage the patient to consider how the importance and confidence are preventing progress toward a goal, as well as what specific barrier to change (Miller and Rollnick, 2002; Rollnick, 1996).

Factors that influence importance include the following:
- The expected benefit of the change and the value of that benefit
- Competing priorities
- How others view the behavior, and how much the patient values their views
- Cues in the environment
- Perception of connection to a healthy outcome (how severe, how likely)
- Quality of available information

Factors that influence confidence are as follows:
- Success of options for change (does anything work?)
- Past experiences with change
- Barriers
- Support from others
- Resources and skills needed
- Supportive environment(e.g., foods available, social situation)

Have an Interactive Discussion

It is important to communicate dietary information in a way tailored to each patient by considering each patient's specific circumstances, readiness to change, and motivation. Patients often tire of a canned lecture. Consider the patient an expert on him/herself, and ask open-ended inquiring questions, then incorporate the patient's response into a plan. In general, try to focus on encouraging your patient in the process of change rather than the emphasis on specific foods or details of diet instructions that they can read or learn about on their own.

Office Changes

To assist patients with dietary change, it is helpful to have a system in place to accomplish the following (at the least): identify dietary risks, assess readiness to change, and assist with change and referral to programs. Although not thoroughly tested for dietary interventions, many family physicians find that the "five As" construct—assess, advise, agree, assist, and arrange—adapted from tobacco cessation interventions in clinical care, is a workable framework to use for health behavior clinical interventions (Whitlock et al., 2002). Practices that incorporate a systematic process, with specified roles for clinical staff members to be involved in the five As, have the greatest success with helping patients meet their health behavior change goals. For example, receptionists can provide patients as they are waiting with a short dietary assessment; medical assistants can ask dietary assessment questions and cue the physician with a brochure or notation on the record; clinicians can advise patients to choose healthy foods and explain the importance to their health; and other practice team members can create referral mechanisms to community programs. Practice support tools may include flow sheets, chart cues, readily available patient education information, program referral forms and information, and mechanisms for tracking and obtaining feedback about the system.

Current research is investigating the patient-centered medical home (Backer, 2007; Berenson et al., 2008; Lewis, 2008; Nutting et al., 2009; Reid et al. , 2009; Rosenthal, 2008; http://www.pcpcc.net/node/14). One component of the medical home is a physician-directed team approach to care that may include practice support in the form of nurses, health educators, dietitians, and other health professionals who directly or indirectly work with primary care practices (see Chapter 2). As such approaches emerge, there is greater opportunity to assist the patient with dietary needs in this team care model.

Community Resources

Physicians at a primary care or family medical practice may not have the time or necessary training to guide patients regarding dietary change. Most communities have resources for patient referral, including diet counseling (dietitian), commercial programs (e.g., Weight Watchers), hospital programs, health plans (on-line, telephone education resources; case management for disease-specific diet concerns), and Internet sites. The most common referral is to a dietitian for dietary counseling. Many patients report frustration after a visit with the dietitian for the reasons outlined earlier: too much information that is too difficult to change too fast, as well as a lack of follow-up with the physician on the necessary changes. For this reason, it is important to consider how a program will help the patient learn the necessary information about nutrition and diet changes and how to make these behavior changes. Other considerations regarding community programs include cost, availability, and user needs.

Summary

- Dietary changes are difficult to make and thus need to be small, stepwise changes that patients can sustain.
- Dietary change instructions need to be straightforward, direct, and understandable.
- The patient needs to feel "ownership" of the dietary changes and must be able and agree to make the changes.
- The behavior changes need to be reviewed and must continue to be supported by the physician so that the patient is motivated to continue.
- Practice redesign may provide opportunities for other health professionals to work with physicians to support dietary and other behavioral needs of patients.

Future in Nutrition

Genomics and Diet: The Future

Consider the following hypothetical case:

A woman in her early 60s is seen by a nutritional genomic counselor because she has had difficulty controlling her significantly elevated low-density lipoprotein (LDL) cholesterol level with diet and exercise. Several different statins were tried without effect.

Her diet history reveals total fat intake less than 30%, polyunsaturated fatty acid (PUFA) intake near 5%, and monounsaturated fat intake as 17% of total energy intake. Her diet suggests appropriate fat intake, but her genome includes a polymorphism in the APOA1 gene. This polymorphism results in a low high-density lipoprotein (HDL) level when PUFA intake is low. She will need to increase her PUFA intake to improve her HDL as a protective effect against heart disease. She has a hepatic lipase gene that raises HDL when her fat intake is less than 30% of total energy. Her 3-hydroxy-3-methylglutaryl–CoA reductase gene has a variant that explains her poor response to statins in lower lipid levels. Lifestyle changes and keeping her PUFA intake relatively elevated with a diet low in animal fat are specific options for prevention of cardiovascular disease based on her genotype (Debusk et al., 2005).

This scenario may become a reality in the future. The emerging field of nutritional genomics may improve treatment options and preventive measures so that they are tailored to the specific genetic makeup and needs of the individual. A central theme in a comprehensive review of studies on genomics and nutrition is the importance of the family history "as a tool for chronic disease prevention and health promotion" (Khoury and Mensah, 2005). In 2004 the U.S. Surgeon General launched a campaign urging all citizens to know their family history and to discuss it with health care providers using an online family history collection tool (USDHHS, 2004). The presence of a disease in a family member, especially a first-degree relative, increases individual risk. Although "old-fashioned," family history remains the least expensive and "best genomic tool" compared with other tests (Khoury and Mensah, 2005). Family physicians who often see a number of family members at once are in a perfect position to construct the best family histories that may predict individual risks for diseases.

Diet-related diseases that will benefit from nutritional genomics research and applications are chronic diseases such as cardiovascular diseases, cancers, diabetes, neurologic disorders, obesity, osteoporosis, and inflammatory disorders (Debusk et al., 2005). These conditions result when homeostasis is disrupted by bioactive dietary components affecting the genotype and environmental factors influencing cellular changes, leading to altered protein and metabolite expression and, eventually, altered physiologic function.

The approach that "one diet fits everyone" for prevention and for treatment may be obsolete with the onset of nutritional genomics. Presently, standardized diet programs tested with experimentally designed population-based studies with significant long-term outcomes are the best approaches that clinicians can offer patients. Nutritional genomics has considerable potential for diet-related diseases in the future. Family physicians are well suited to assist individual patients who may have a diet-related disease or who are at risk for these diseases because of family history. Family physicians should prepare themselves to become more sophisticated with genomic medicine and nutrition as research advances.

Terminology

The following list of definitions is taken from *Dietary Reference Intakes* (National Academy of Sciences, 2004).

Recommended daily allowance (RDA): Average daily nutrient intake level sufficient to meet the nutrient requirements of nearly all those (97% to 98%) in a life stage and gender group. It is intended to be used for assessing the diets of healthy subjects, not for assessing or planning diets for groups.

Estimated energy requirement (EER): Dietary energy intake that is predicted to allow for a level of physical activity consistent with normal health and development and for the deposition of tissues at a rate consistent with growth.

Acceptable macronutrient distribution range (AMDR): Range of macronutrient intakes for a particular energy source associated with reduced risk of chronic disease while providing adequate intakes of essential nutrients.

Tolerable upper intake levels (TULs): Highest average daily nutrient intake likely to pose no risks of adverse health effects to almost all those in a life stage and gender group.

Adequate intake (AI): Recommended average daily nutrient level based on observed or experimentally determined estimates of average nutrient intakes by a group of healthy subjects. It is used when an RDA cannot be determined and may be used to plan and evaluate diets of individual subjects or groups.

Estimated average requirement (EAR): Nutrient intake value estimated to meet the requirement defined by a specific indicator of adequacy in 50% of those in a life stage and gender group, expressed as a daily value over time (for most nutrients, at least 1 week). It includes an adjustment for bioavailability, is intended to be used as one factor in assessing the adequacy of intake of groups or individual subjects, and should not be used as an intake goal for just one person.

PEARLS AND PITFALLS

PEARLS

- Changing one's diet is hard, and the outcome is often unpredictable. Small changes can often be maintained and are influential in improving health. Before any changes, assessment of the current diet and nutritional status is imperative.
- Extreme changes, whether medically prescribed or self-prescribed, often lack supporting evidence, and moderate changes might work for the biologic improvements desired.
- The interaction between diet and genetics (nutrient needs) is still being researched. Although genetic differences exist in humans' nutrient needs, their extent is not currently well understood.
- Behavioral changes for improving dietary intake involve a series of conversations over time, not just handing out a diet sheet.

PITFALLS

- A nutrient being beneficial for humans does not mean that more of that nutrient will be even better. An example of this is iron; an adequate amount is important, and too much iron is dangerous. The tolerable upper intake levels recognize this dangerous pitfall (National Academy of Sciences, 2004).
- Assumptions about nutritional status are problematic. Often, men assume that if they exercise, it does not matter what they eat. Women often assume that if their weight is within normal limits (or even lower), their diet or exercise patterns, or both, are healthy. These gender assumptions will misdirect the physician about the nutritional status of their patients.
- Health through nutrition is influenced throughout the life cycle. A single short period of eating well or eating poorly will not profoundly affect a person's health status. However, poor food and nutrient intake at certain periods in the life cycle, such as at conception and in older adults, may set a new or different course for that life stage.

Conclusion

Nutrition is a foundation for human health. In the future, as more is understood about genetics, nutritional needs will become more tailored to individual diverse needs. In the review of a person's nutritional status, the clinician should consider food and supplements, as well as how these balance with exercise, diseases, and other environmental factors (e.g., smoking). Overweight, normal-weight, and underweight people are not necessarily well nourished, and weight may not be an indicator of healthy eating. *Biologic balance* involves energy balance (between what is needed or eaten and what is used) and nutrient balance; too few nutrients can cause malnutrition and even chronic diseases, and too many nutrients may be toxic or may even cause chronic disease.

References

The complete reference list is available online at www.expertconsult.com.

Web Resources

www.diabetes.org/home.jsp
American Diabetes Association.

www.eatright.org/
American Dietetic Association public information site.

www.aafp.org/afp/20000301/1409.html
American Association of Family Physicians; a "stages of change" approach for helping patients change behavior.

www.americanheart.org/presenter.jhtml?identifier=4644
Mediterranean Diet from American Heart Association.

www.calculator.org/bmr.html
For calculating basal metabolic rate for adults.

www.uri.edu/research//cprc/transtheoretical.htm
Cancer Prevention Research Center; summary of transtheoretical model.

www.cdc.gov/nccdphp/dnpa/bmi/calc-bmi.htm
Body mass index (BMI) calculator from Centers for Disease Control and Prevention.

www-users.med.cornell.edu/~spon/picu/calc/beecalc.htm
Basal energy expenditure (Harris-Benedict equation) calculator from Cornell University, Weill Medical College.

http:diabetes.niddk.nih.gov/dm/pubs/eating_ez/
National Institutes of Health; information diabetes and diet for the public.

http://motivationalinterview.org
Mid-Atlantic Addiction Technology Transfer Center; information on motivational interviewing.

www.genome.gov
Genomics information from National Human Genome Research Institute, National Institutes of Health.

www.nlm.nih.gov/medlineplus
National Library of Medicine, National Institutes of Health (MedlinePlus); reliable health information on nutrition, diet, and dietary supplements.

www.nlm.nih.gov/medlineplus/druginfo/natural/patient-vitamind.html
Ongoing research into vitamin D and cardiovascular disease (MedlinePlus).

www.nutrition.org/cgi/content/full/129/3/751.
Modified food guide pyramid for people over 70 years of age.

www.nutrition.gov
Portal for all government websites on nutrition information; available through U.S. Department of Agriculture (USDA), National Agricultural Library.

www.MyPyramid.gov
Current Food Pyramid called "Steps to a Healthier You" (USDA).

www.dietaryguidelines.gov

www.healthfinder.gov/prevention

CHAPTER 38

Gastroenterology

Joel J. Heidelbaugh

Chapter contents

He who does not mind his belly will hardly mind anything else.

Samuel Johnson (1763)

Thought depends absolutely on the stomach, but in spite of that, those who have the best stomachs are not the best thinkers.

Voltaire (1770)

Epidemiology and Social Impact of Gastrointestinal Disease

Although diseases of other organ systems (e.g., cardiovascular disease) may appear to be more dramatic illnesses with higher rates of morbidity and mortality, the overall impact of gastrointestinal (GI) disorders is often underestimated from both a biopsychosocial and a resource standpoint. Typically, diseases of the GI tract are misdiagnosed, mistreated, misunderstood, or missed altogether, ultimately leading to substantial psychological morbidity and tremendous direct and indirect expense. Digestive diseases cost an estimated $91 billion annually in U.S. health care costs, lost days from work, and premature deaths. More than 70 million Americans are diagnosed each year with disorders of the digestive tract, including gastroesophageal reflux disease, peptic ulcer disease, inflammatory bowel disease, GI cancers, motility disorders, hepatitis, cirrhosis, and food-borne illness (Foundation, 2009).

This chapter serves as an overview of common GI diseases and disorders encountered in family medicine practices, encompassing both adult and pediatric populations. The most recent evidence-based diagnostic and therapeutic guidelines and reviews are highlighted, and radiographs, endoscopy photos, and video segments are integrated where applicable.

Approach to the Patient with Gastrointestinal Complaints

Psychosocial Factors of Gastrointestinal Disease

Locke's review in *Sleisenger and Fordtran's Gastrointestinal and Liver Disease* (8th edition) provides an excellent framework of the biopsychosocial approach to the patient with GI complaints. In caring for patients with both acute and chronic GI disorders, family physicians should obtain a patient-centered, nondirected history, using open-ended questions that enable patients to tell the history in their words. Medical and social histories should be integrated so that symptomatic complaints are described in the context of the psychosocial events surrounding the presenting illness, including the setting of symptom onset and exacerbation. Throughout the encounter, the provider's questions should communicate a sincere willingness to address both biologic and psychologic aspects of the illness. Evaluation and treatment of GI symptoms depend on a strong physician-patient therapeutic relationship, allowing the family physician to elicit, evaluate, and communicate the role of potential psychosocial factors in the disease state. Patient reassurance, acknowledgment of patient adaptations to chronic illness, reinforcement of healthy behaviors, and the consideration of psychopharmacologic medication are paramount (Locke, 2006).

The failure to find a specific structural etiology for a patient's GI symptoms is usually the rule rather than the exception in the ambulatory care setting. Because functional GI disorders may represent an "illness without an evident disease," some providers do not regard these as legitimate, especially within the biopsychosocial model of disease. This phenomenon often leads physicians (and patients to coerce physicians) to pursue unnecessary, costly, and invasive diagnostic tests to find the etiology of a patient's symptoms, rather than focusing directly on symptom management and potential psychological comorbidities. Family physicians must establish clear boundaries with their patients to prevent unnecessary workups and, when indicated, should consider a referral to a mental health professional skilled in the care of patients with functional GI conditions, to assist in symptom management (Locke, 2006).

The Abdominal Examination

For descriptive purposes of location, the abdomen has been divided into four quadrants, constructed by an imaginary vertical line from the tip of the xyphoid process to the pubic symphysis and an imaginary horizontal line bridging the anterior superior iliac crests, referred to as the right upper (RUQ), right lower (RLQ), left upper (LUQ), and left lower (LLQ) quadrants (Bickley, 2008). The abdomen can be further divided into the epigastric, umbilical, hypogastric or suprapubic, and right and left flank regions. Knowledge of anatomic structures that lie in each of these quadrants and regions is imperative for the clinician to form an accurate differential diagnosis in relation to a patient's presenting symptoms (Box 38-1).

Clinicians should remember that a comprehensive physical examination, not just abdominal, should be performed in patients presenting with digestive complaints. The clinician should ensure patient comfort and modesty because the abdominal examination (and pelvic, if indicated) may cause significant pain, anxiety, and embarrassment to the patient. Infants, young children, and pregnant women may require additional care during the abdominal examination. A thorough explanation of examination techniques and findings is necessary to minimize patient anxiety.

The anorectal examination is an important component of the abdominal examination that may often be omitted. Although uncomfortable and embarrassing to the patient, it should not be neglected and should be approached with a calm, gentle attitude on the part of the clinician. The examiner should comment on both external and internal components of the anorectal examination, specifically anal sphincter tone; presence or absence of hemorrhoids, fissures, fistulas, or masses; prostatic abnormality in the male patient; and consistency of the stool. Anoscopy should be considered as an adjunct to the anorectal examination when indicated, allowing for direct visualization of the internal anorectal canal. In female patients, the pelvic examination may provide additional information in the diagnosis of abdominal symptoms, as it is often challenging to differentiate between GI and genitourinary complaints.

Common Pediatric Gastrointestinal Disorders

Infantile Regurgitation

In the infant with recurrent vomiting, a thorough history and physical examination are often sufficient to establish a diagnosis of uncomplicated gastroesophageal reflux disease (GERD), labeling the infant as "the happy spitter." Diagnostic evaluation is indicated if there are signs of poor weight gain, GI obstruction, excessive crying and irritability, disturbed sleep, or feeding or respiratory problems suggesting suspected asthma or recurrent pneumonia. In the infant with uncomplicated GERD, parental education, reassurance, and anticipatory guidance are recommended; no specific intervention is necessary because the process is usually self-limited. Thickened formula and a trial of a hypoallergenic formula are the best treatment options. A trial of time-limited acid-suppression therapy, usually with histamine-2 receptor antagonists (H_2RAs), is useful in determining if GERD is causing vomiting and regurgitation. If symptoms worsen or do not improve by 18 to 24 months of age, reevaluation for complications of GERD is recommended, including an upper GI series (barium swallow study) and consultation with a pediatric gastroenterologist. In otherwise normal children who have recurrent vomiting or regurgitation after age 2 years, management options include an upper GI series, upper endoscopy with biopsy, and antisecretory therapy (Rudolph, 2001).

Diarrhea and Dehydration

Diarrhea is exceedingly common in pediatric and adult populations worldwide. Dehydration and electrolyte (e.g., sodium, potassium, bicarbonate) losses associated with severe diarrhea account for significant morbidity and may lead to mortality in cases of acute gastroenteritis, especially in countries with poor access to adequate healthcare. Rotavirus infection is the most common cause of diarrhea in U.S. infants and children, especially in winter months and temperate climates; Norwalk-like virus is the most common agent in adults (King et al., 2003).

A thorough history should be the first step in evaluating the patient who presents with a significant diarrheal illness, including the following (Guerrant et al., 2001):

- When and how the illness began (abrupt or gradual onset and duration of symptoms)
- Stool characteristics (watery, bloody, mucous, purulent, greasy)
- Frequency of bowel movements and relative quantity of stool produced
- Presence of dysenteric symptoms (fever, tenesmus, blood/pus in stool)
- Symptoms of volume depletion (increased thirst, tachycardia, orthostasis, decreased urine output, lethargy, decreased skin turgor, decreased tear production)
- Associated symptoms and their frequency and intensity (nausea, vomiting, abdominal pain, cramps, headache, myalgias, altered sensorium)

Box 38-1 Differential Diagnosis for Abdominal Pain Based on Location

Left upper quadrant

Cardiac: Angina pectoris, myocardial infarction

Dermatologic: Herpes zoster

Gastric: Peptic ulcer disease, gastritis, pyloric stenosis, hiatal hernia

Intestinal: High fecal impaction, perforated colon, diverticulitis

Pancreatic: Pancreatitis, neoplasm, stone in pancreatic duct or ampulla

Pulmonary: Pneumonia, empyema, pulmonary infarction

Renal: Calculi, pyelonephritis, neoplasm

Splenic: Splenomegaly, rupture, abscess, splenic infarction

Trauma

Vascular: Dissecting or ruptured aortic aneurysm

Right upper quadrant

Biliary: Calculi, infection, inflammation, neoplasm

Cardiac: Myocardial ischemia or infarction (particularly involving the inferior wall), pericarditis

Dermatologic: Herpes zoster

Fitz-Hugh-Curtis syndrome (perihepatitis)

Gastric: peptic ulcer disease, pyloric stenosis, neoplasm, alcoholic gastritis, hiatal hernia

Hepatic: Hepatitis, abscess, hepatic congestion, neoplasm, trauma

Pancreatic: Pancreatitis, neoplasm, stone in pancreatic duct or ampulla

Pulmonary: Pneumonia, pulmonary infarction, right-sided pleurisy

Renal: calculi, infection, inflammation, neoplasm, rupture of kidney

Intestinal: retrocecal appendicitis, intestinal obstruction, high fecal impaction, diverticulitis

Trauma

Left lower quadrant

Intestinal: Diverticulitis, intestinal obstruction, perforated ulcer, inflammatory bowel disease, perforated descending colon, inguinal hernia, neoplasm, appendicitis

Psoas abscess

Renal: Renal or ureteral calculi, pyelonephritis, neoplasm

Reproductive: Ectopic pregnancy, ovarian cyst, torsion of ovarian cyst, salpingitis, tuboovarian abscess, mittelschmerz, endometriosis, seminal vesiculitis

Trauma

Vascular: Dissecting, ruptured, or leaking aortic aneurysm

Right lower quadrant

Cholecystitis

Intestinal: Acute appendicitis, regional enteritis, incarcerated hernia, cecal diverticulitis, intestinal obstruction, perforated ulcer, perforated cecum, Meckel's diverticulitis

Psoas abscess

Reproductive: Ectopic pregnancy, ovarian cyst, torsion of ovarian cyst, salpingitis, tuboovarian abscess, mittelschmerz, endometriosis, seminal vesiculitis

Renal: Renal or ureteral calculi, pyelonephritis, neoplasm

Trauma

Vascular: Dissecting, ruptured, or leaking aortic aneurysm

Other regions

Epigastric

Biliary: Cholecystitis, cholangitis

Cardiac: Angina, myocardial infarction, pericarditis

Duodenal: Peptic ulcer disease, duodenitis

Gastric: Peptic ulcer disease, gastric outlet obstruction, gastric ulcer

Hepatitic: Hepatitis, abscess

Intestinal: High small bowel obstruction, early appendicitis

Pancreatitis

Pulmonary: Pneumonia, pleurisy, pneumothorax

Subphrenic abscess

Vascular: Dissecting, ruptured, or leaking aortic aneurysm, mesenteric ischemia

Periumbilical

Intestinal: Small bowel obstruction or gangrene, early appendicitis

Vascular: Mesenteric thrombosis, dissecting, ruptured, or leaking aortic aneurysm

Suprapubic

Genitourinary: Cystitis, rupture of urinary bladder

Intestinal: Colonic obstruction or gangrene, diverticulitis, appendicitis

Reproductive: Ectopic pregnancy, mittelschmerz, torsion of ovarian cyst, pelvic inflammatory disease, salpingitis, endometriosis, rupture of endometrioma

Diffuse

Genitourinary: Urinary tract infection, pelvic inflammatory disease

Intestinal: Diverticulitis, early appendicitis, gastroenteritis, inflammatory bowel disease, intestinal obstruction, irritable bowel syndrome, mesenteric adenitis, insufficiency, or infarction

Metabolic: Toxins, lead poisoning, uremia, drug overdose, diabetic ketoacidosis, heavy metal poisoning

Pancreatitis

Peritonitis

Pneumonia (rare)

Sickle cell crisis

Trauma

Other: Acute intermittent porphyria, tabes dorsalis, periarteritis nodosa, Henoch-Schönlein purpura, adrenal insufficiency

Vascular: Aortic aneurysm

Modified from Differential diagnosis. In Ferri FF. Ferri's Clinical Advisor 2010. Philadelphia, Saunders-Elsevier, 2010.

In addition, all patients should be asked about potential epidemiologic risk factors for diarrheal diseases, including the following:

- Travel to an underdeveloped area
- Daycare center attendance or employment
- Consumption of unsafe foods (e.g., raw meats, eggs, or shellfish; unpasteurized milk or juices) or swimming in or drinking untreated fresh surface water from a lake or stream
- Visiting a farm or petting zoo or having contact with reptiles or with pets with diarrhea
- Knowledge of other ill persons (e.g., in a dormitory, office, or social function)
- Recent or regular medications (e.g., antibiotics, antacids, antimotility agents)
- Underlying medical conditions predisposing to infectious diarrhea (AIDS, immunosuppressive medications, prior gastrectomy, extremes of age)

- Receptive anal intercourse or oral-anal sexual contact
- Occupation as a food-handler or caregiver

In the majority of patients with acute gastroenteritis, the "gold standard" stool cultures and ova and parasite testing are seldom required, because the disease is most often viral in etiology and self-limited. In more severe cases with dehydration, metabolic derangement, longer duration, bloody stools (dysentery) and mucus in the stool, or known or suspected transmission of a pathogen, these tests are often required to identify the pathogen and to direct appropriate antimicrobial therapy (Table 38-1). Viral cultures are rarely performed and are unnecessary, except in rare cases and immunocompromised patients. Although fecal leukocytes and lactoferrin often suggest an inflammatory etiology of diarrhea, there is no consensus regarding the routine use of these tests in the initial testing of patients with either community-acquired or nosocomial diarrhea. Hospitalized patients with diarrhea, especially those with abdominal pain, should be tested for Clostridium difficile toxin (Guerrant et al., 2001). Oral metronidazole and oral vancomycin have been shown to be equally effective in the treatment of C. difficile–associated diarrhea (CDAD). Vancomycin is significantly more expensive and may select for colonization with vancomycin-resistant enterococci (VRE), and thus metronidazole should be recommended as first-line therapy.

Nonpathogenic causes of diarrhea should be considered when a viral etiology is unlikely and a diagnostic evaluation has not identified a pathogen. Differential diagnosis includes irritable bowel syndrome, inflammatory or ischemic bowel disease, laxative abuse, partial bowel obstruction, rectosigmoid abscess, Whipple's disease, pernicious anemia, diabetes mellitus, malabsorption syndromes (e.g. celiac disease), small bowel diverticulosis, and scleroderma in primarily adult patients, and an appropriate workup should be considered.

KEY TREATMENT

Oral metronidazole and vancomycin are equally effective in the treatment of *Clostridium difficile*–associated diarrhea (Guerrant et al., 2001) (SOR: A).

In cases of traveler's diarrhea, (e.g. enterotoxigenic *Escherichia coli, Shigella, Salmonella,* or *Campylobacter*), prompt treatment with a fluoroquinolone or, in children, trimethoprim-sulfamethoxazole (TMP-SMX) has been shown to reduce the duration of the illness from 3 to 5 days to less than 1 to 2 days (Guerrant et al., 2001) (SOR: A).

Appendicitis

A diagnosis of appendicitis should be considered in any pediatric patient presenting with acute abdominal pain. Acute appendicitis often presents with a constellation of signs and symptoms, including fever, anorexia, nausea, vomiting, tenesmus, migratory RLQ abdominal pain, abdominal

---

Table 38-1 Common Pathogens and Recommended Therapy for Acute Diarrhea

Pathogen	Therapy (Adult Doses)
Campylobacter jejuni	Azithromycin, 500 mg qd for 3 days *or* Ciprofloxacin,* 500 mg bid for 7 days
Clostridium difficile	Metronidazole, 500 mg tid, or 250 mg qid, for 10 14 days *or* Vancomycin, 125 mg qid for 10-14 days
Entamoeba histolytica	Metronidazole, 500-750 mg tid for 10 days *or* Tinidazole, 2 g qd for 3 days *followed by* Paromomycin, 500 mg orally tid for 7 days *or* Iodoquinol, 650 mg tid for 20 days
Escherichia coli 0157:H7	No treatment with antimicrobials or antimotility drugs
E. coli (toxigenic)	Azithromycin, 1 g in 1 dose *or* Rifaximin, 200 mg tid for 3 days *or* Levofloxacin,* 500 mg for 1 dose
Giardia lamblia	Tinidazole, 2 g in 1 dose *or* Nitazoxanide, 500 mg bid for 3 days *or* Metronidazole, 500-750 mg tid for 5 days
Salmonella spp. (non-*typhi*)†	Ciprofloxacin, 500 mg bid for 5-7 days *or* Azithromycin, 1 g for 1 day, then 500 mg qd for 6 days
Shigella spp.	Ciprofloxacin, 500 mg bid for 5-7 days *or* Levofloxacin, 500 mg qd for 3 days *or* TMP-SMX-DS, 1 tablet bid for 3 days *or* Azithromycin, 500 mg for 1 dose, then 250 mg qd for 4 days
Staphylococcus aureus (food poisoning)	No treatment with antimicrobials or antimotility drugs
Vibrio cholerae	Ciprofloxacin, 1 g in 1 dose, plus aggressive fluid hydration
Vibrio parahaemolyticus	No treatment with antimicrobials or antimotility drugs
Yersinia enterocolitica	No treatment unless severe; if severe: Doxycycline, 100 mg IV bid, *and* Tobramycin or gentamicin, 5 mg/kg/day qd, *or* TMP-SMX and fluoroquinolones as alternatives

Modified from Gilbert DN, Moellering RC, Eliopoulos GM, et al. The Sanford Guide to Antimicrobial Therapy, 39th ed. Vermont, Antimicrobial Therapy, 2009.
*Avoid fluoroquinolones in pediatric patients and pregnant women.
†Antimicrobial therapy not indicated in asymptomatic patients or those with mild illness. Treatment advised in patients less than 1 year old or greater than 50 years old, if immunocompromised, or if patient has a vascular graft or prosthetic joints.
TMP-SMX, Trimethoprim-sulfamethoxazole; *DS,* double strength; *IV,* intravenously; *qd,* once daily; *bid,* twice daily; *tid,* three times daily; *qid,* four times daily.

tenderness and guarding, and signs of peritoneal irritation. Classically, hours after onset, the pain migrates to *McBurney's point*, defined as the point two-thirds the distance from the umbilicus along a straight line toward the anterosuperior iliac spine of the pelvis. *Rovsing's sign* (referred tenderness from LLQ to RLQ during palpation), *psoas sign* (pain elicited by extending hip posteriorly with patient lying prone), and *obturator sign* (pain elicited by abducting right hip with patient lying supine) are often conducted but are of little diagnostic value. No sign or combination of signs has accurately predicted acute appendicitis in children (Cincinnati Children's Hospital [CCH], 2002).

While none has proved adequately predictive of acute appendicitis in the pediatric population, laboratory studies are typically performed in the emergency department because other diagnoses may need to be excluded. A series of studies discovered an elevated white blood cell (WBC) count in 87% to 92% of patients with acute appendicitis, although 8% to 13% of patients with appendicitis had a normal WBC count (CCH, 2002). The abdominal examination is particularly unreliable in women of reproductive age, so pelvic exam, urinalysis, and urine pregnancy test represent a reasonable clinical strategy to exclude genitourinary pathology.

Diagnostic imaging is not routinely recommended in patients with a high or a low probability of appendicitis, because it can alter management strategies and has not proved cost-effective; imaging is most helpful when the clinical assessment is equivocal. Controversy exists over the superiority of ultrasound versus computed tomography (CT) in accurately diagnosing appendicitis, and both tests have a positive predictive value approaching 100%. Although ultrasound may be advantageous in thin patients, CT is preferred in the evaluation of a more obese child (Halter et al., 2004). Typical radiographic findings in the evaluation of acute appendicitis include appendicoliths (Fig. 38-1), dilation of the appendix with adjacent hazy fat (Fig. 38-2), and periappendiceal abscesses (Fig. 38-3). If the abdominal CT does not show evidence of acute appendicitis, the patient may either be admitted for observation or discharged at the discretion of the examiner and parents, with instructions for follow-up if symptoms worsen. Expert opinion states that if there is high suspicion of appendicitis on the basis of history, physical examination, and laboratory studies, the patient should go directly to the operating room for an exploratory laparotomy to evaluate the appendix, without an imaging study.

Common Adult Gastrointestinal Disorders

Esophagus

Barrett's Esophagus and Esophageal Adenocarcinoma

Barrett's esophagus is a premalignant condition related to chronic GERD. The hallmark is a change in the mucosal lining of the distal esophagus from the normal squamous epithelium to columnar-appearing mucosa resembling that of the stomach and small intestines, referred to as *intestinal metaplasia* (Fig. 38-4). The estimated risk of progression to adenocarcinoma of the esophagus with Barrett's esophagus is approximately 0.5% per year, whereas without Barrett's esophagus the risk is 0.07%, prompting development of clinical practice guidelines for surveillance endoscopy.

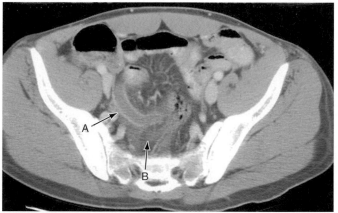

Figure 38-2 Appendicitis. Dilated thickened appendix *(A)*, with adjacent hazy fat *(B)*. *(Courtesy Dr. Perry Pernicano.)*

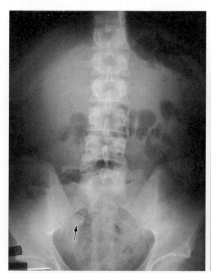
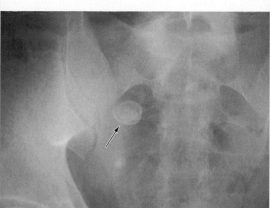
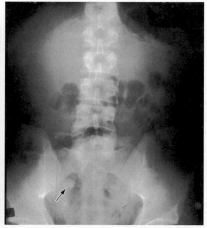

Figure 38-1 Appendicolith. *(Courtesy Dr. Perry Pernicano, Clinical Assistant Professor, Department of Radiology, University of Michigan Medical School, Ann Arbor.)*

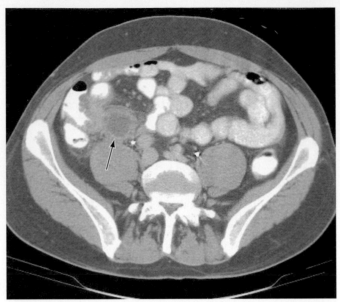

Figure 38-3 Periappendiceal abscess *(arrow)*. *(Courtesy Dr. Perry Pernicano.)*

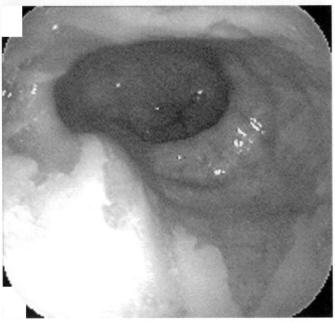

Figure 38-4 Barrett's esophagus. *(Courtesy Dr. Erik-Jan Wamsteker.)*

Adenocarcinoma of the esophagus has had the fastest-rising incidence of any cancer in the United States and Western Europe over the last two decades. Family and other primary care physicians who see the vast majority of patients with GERD in its nonerosive and more complicated forms are charged with the task of suspecting and appropriately referring patients with Barrett's esophagus for EGD. Although risk factors for Barrett's esophagus and adenocarcinoma are not evidence-based, there is suggestive evidence that male gender, white race, older age, dysplasia, smoking, and obesity place patients at a higher risk (Sampliner, 2002).

Currently, no evidence-based guidelines exist for the assessment and surveillance of patients with Barrett's esophagus; routine screening will not be cost-effective unless criteria can be identified to select patients at high risk. Recommendations from the American Society for Gastrointestinal Endoscopy

(ASGE) state that screening esophagogastroduodenoscopy (EGD) for Barrett's esophagus should be considered in select patients with chronic, long-standing GERD. After a negative screening examination, further screening endoscopy is not indicated. For patients with established Barrett's esophagus of any length and with no dysplasia, after two consecutive examinations within 1 year, an acceptable interval for additional surveillance is every 3 years. Surveillance in patients with low-grade dysplasia is recommended, although the optimal interval and biopsy protocol have not been established. A follow-up EGD at 6 months should be performed, and if low-grade dysplasia is confirmed, surveillance at 12 months and yearly thereafter as long as dysplasia persists is advised (Hirota et al., 2006).

Stomach and Duodenum

Dyspepsia

Dyspepsia ("bad digestion") accounts for approximately 5% of all visits to family practitioners and is the most common reason for referral to a gastroenterologist in the United States, accounting for 20% to 40% of consultations (Jones and Lacy, 2004). The term *dyspepsia* refers to episodic or recurrent pain or discomfort arising from the proximal GI tract related to meals and is associated with heartburn, reflux, regurgitation, indigestion, bloating, early satiety, and weight loss. The lack of a standardized definition affects accurate prevalence data, given the challenge of clearly defining dyspepsia as either *functional* or *nonulcer dyspepsia* (~60% of cases), or that caused by structural or biochemical disease (40%) (Dickerson and King, 2004). Regardless of cause, dyspepsia has a profoundly negative impact on patients' health-related quality of life (HRQOL) and results in significant economic burden.

Nonulcer dyspepsia (NUD) is defined in patients who have undergone either formal radiographic or endoscopic evaluation and who do not have an organic lesion (e.g., ulcer, tumor) to explain their symptoms. Potential etiologies for NUD include gastric acid hypersecretion, gastroduodenal dysmotility, visceral hypersensitivity, emotional stress, and psychological factors. As with other functional GI disorders, the potential for underlying psychosocial and lifestyle factors must be addressed. There is no current recommendation on the role of prokinetics, cytoprotectives, or antidepressants in the management of functional dyspepsia; similarly, no clear evidence supports specific diet and lifestyle modifications or psychosocial interventions.

Peptic Ulcer Disease

Key Points

- A noninvasive *H. pylori* "test and treat" strategy is as effective as endoscopy in the initial management of patients under age 45 with uncomplicated dyspepsia.
- Eradication of *H. pylori* infection in patients with a duodenal or gastric ulcer reduces symptom recurrence.
- Ulcer prophylaxis with an H₂RA or PPI should be considered in patients at high risk for NSAID-associated PUD, including those with a history of PUD, elderly patients, and patients taking corticosteroids or anticoagulants.

Peptic ulcer disease (PUD) is the most common cause of *upper gastrointestinal bleeding* (UGIB) and a leading cause of dyspepsia (Box 38-2), with a cumulative lifetime prevalence of 8% to 14% (Fig. 38-5). Although up to 70% of patients with gastric and duodenal ulcers are 25 to 64 years old, the peak prevalence of complicated ulcer disease requiring hospitalization is age 65 to 74 (Saad and Scheiman, 2004).

Numerous options exist for the management of uninvestigated dyspepsia in primary care (Fig. 38-6). Given the high cost and often limited access to endoscopy testing, not all patients with uninvestigated dyspepsia should undergo an invasive investigation of their symptoms. The presence of "alarm symptoms" for PUD raises concern for a gastric malignancy. The American Gastroenterological Association (AGA, 2005) endorses prompt endoscopic evaluation in any patient over age 45 with new-onset dyspepsia.

The most common complications of PUD include UGIB, perforation, penetration, and gastric outlet obstruction. An upper GI hemorrhage can occur in up to 15% of patients with PUD and is most common in patients older than 60, with mortality as high as 10%. Perforation occurs in approximately 7% of patients with PUD, again classically in elderly patients receiving long-term nonsteroidal anti-inflammatory drugs (NSAIDs). Perforation can be confirmed on plain abdominal radiography; barium contrast studies and upper endoscopy are contraindicated with suspected perforation, and urgent surgical consultation is mandatory. Mortality may be as high as 30% to 50% in patients with perforation, particularly in elderly and debilitated patients. Penetration occurs when the ulcer crater erodes through and into adjacent organs, including the small bowel, pancreas, liver, and biliary tree. Often subtle, it typically presents as acute pancreatitis. Gastric outlet obstruction occurs in 1% to 3% of PUD patients, resulting from acute inflammation or mechanical obstruction caused by scarring at the gastroduodenal junction (Saad and Scheiman, 2004).

Approaches to confirm a diagnosis of PUD include double-contrast barium esophagography (upper GI series) and upper endoscopy. Although the upper GI series has accuracy of 80% to 90%, upper endoscopy is the preferred diagnostic modality, with multiple studies showing consistent diagnostic superiority in identifying gastric and duodenal ulcers. Despite a higher procedural cost and a slightly increased risk in procedure-related complications (bleeding, perforation, oversedation), upper endoscopy should be the initial diagnostic study performed in suspected PUD. Most importantly, upper endoscopy provides the distinct advantage of permitting biopsies and brushings to identify underlying pathology.

Fecal-oral infection with the bacterium *Helicobacter pylori* is a major risk factor for the development of PUD. Its prevalence and association with PUD is higher in populations who have a lower standard of living than in the United States, especially in Africa and Central America, although this may be declining. Approximately 90% of patients worldwide with duodenal ulcers are infected with the *H. pylori* pathogen, whereas 30% to 40% of U.S. ulcer patients are infected (Chey and Wong, 2007). The strongest evidence to support the role of *H. pylori* as an etiology of PUD is the elimination of ulcer recurrence when the infection has been successfully eradicated.

The evidence-based standard of care dictates that patients with dyspepsia and no alarm symptoms should be tested

---

Box 38-2 Causes of Dyspepsia

Common*

GERD (with and without esophagitis)
Functional (nonulcer dyspepsia)
Peptic ulcer disease

Less common†

Alcohol consumption
Biliary colic
Celiac sprue
Gastrointestinal malignancy
Gastroparesis
Infection (viral, bacterial, spirochetal, parasitic)
Inflammatory and infiltrative processes (esophagus, stomach, small bowel)
Intestinal ischemia
Lactose intolerance
Medications (primarily aspirin and NSAIDs)
Pancreatitis
Pregnancy
Other systemic and metabolic disorders

*In order of relative frequency.
†Alphabetical order.
Modified from Saad R, Scheiman JM. Diagnosis and management of peptic ulcer disease. Clin Fam Pract 2004;6:569-587.
GERD, Gastroesophageal reflux disease; NSAIDs, nonsteroidal anti-inflammatory drugs.

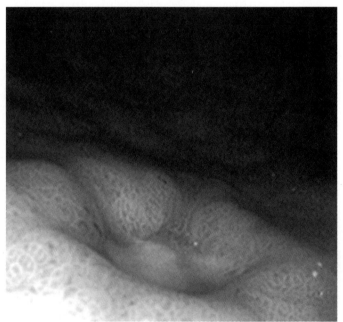

Figure 38-5 Gastric ulcer. *(Courtesy Dr. Erik-Jan Wamsteker.)*

for *H. pylori* infection and then given eradication therapy if positive, ("test and treat") (Chey and Wong, 2007). *H. pylori*–positive or *H. pylori*–negative patients who do not undergo endoscopy initially should do so if their symptoms persist. The effectiveness of this approach depends on the prevalence of *H. pylori* infection in patients with ulcers in the

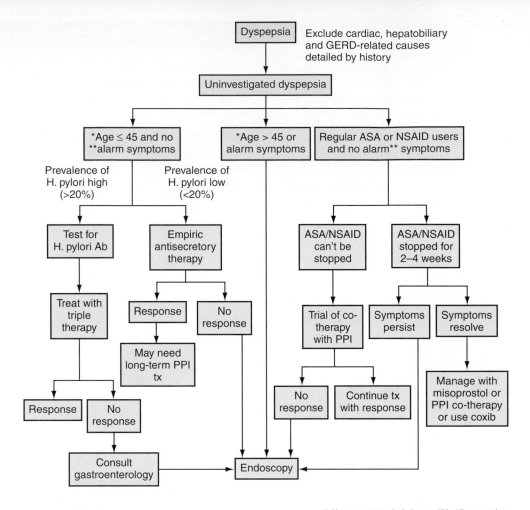

GERD: gastroesophageal reflux disease
ASA: aspirin
NSAIDs nonsteroidal anti-inflammatory drugs
PPI: proton pump inhibitor
H. pylori: Helicobacter pylori

* Age cutoff is controversial.
Risk of pathology increases
slightly with age but older age
(50–55) cutoff in many guidelines

** Alarm symptoms include rectal bleeding or melena,
weight loss, anorexia, early satiety, persistent vomiting,
anemia. The presence of an abdominal mass,
lymphadenopathy, dysphagia, odynophagia, family
history of upper GI cancer, personal history of peptic
ulcer, prior gastric surgery or malignancy should
eliminate consideration of noninvasive approaches.

Figure 38-6 Evaluation of uninvestigated dyspepsia. *(Modified from Saad R, Scheiman JM. Diagnosis and management of peptic ulcer disease. Clin Fam Pract 2004;6:569-587.)*

community; as in some geographic areas, prevalence may be too low to make this approach effective.

Nonendoscopic testing for *H. pylori* includes a quantitative assay for serum immunoglobulin G (IgG) antibodies, the radiolabeled urea breath test, and the stool antigen test. The median sensitivity and specificity for serologic IgG tests are 92% and 83%, respectively (SIGN, 2003). Some patients may have persistently positive IgG antibodies for months to years after eradication therapy, yielding a false-positive result during that period if retested. In comparative studies, urea breath tests are more accurate than serologic tests. The stool antigen test is recommended as the preferred initial noninvasive diagnostic test. The urea breath test is the recommended standard to determine if H. pylori has been successfully eradicated (Chey and Wong, 2007).

Several medication regimens have been developed for the treatment of confirmed *H. pylori* infection, based on data from randomized controlled trials (RCTs), meta-analyses, and systematic reviews (Table 38-2). The best evidence-based recommendation for *H. pylori* eradication is for 14-day triple therapy with the use of a proton pump inhibitor (PPI), clarithromycin, and either amoxicillin or metronidazole,

yielding eradication rates from 70% to 85%. The most common salvage regimen in patients with persistent *H. pylori* is bismuth quadruple therapy. Recent data suggest that 10-day therapy with a PPI, levofloxacin, and amoxicillin is more effective and better tolerated than bismuth quadruple therapy for persistent *H. pylori* infection (Chey and Wong, 2007).

Another major etiology of PUD is the increasing and widespread use of both NSAIDs and aspirin. The use and overuse of these medications is the most common cause of PUD in *H. pylori*–negative patients, and up to 60% of unexplained cases of PUD are attributed to unrecognized NSAID use. In a meta-analysis of observational studies of GI bleeding risk from various NSAIDs, a fourfold increased risk associated with NSAID-use persisted throughout therapy and fell to baseline within 2 months of discontinuation of the drug (Hernandez-Diaz and Rodriguez, 2000). Although both *H. pylori* and aspirin/NSAIDs are involved in the overwhelming majority of PUD cases, other factors contribute to the remaining 1% to 5% (Box 38-3).

Independent risk factors that augment the impact of *H. pylori* and NSAID-related PUD risk and may promote ulcer complications include advancing age; history of PUD

Table 38-2 First-Line Regimens for Helicobacter pylori Eradication

Regimen	Duration (days)	Eradication Rates (%)	Comments
Standard-dose PPI bid (esomeprazole, qd); clarithromycin, 500 mg, *or* amoxicillin, 1000 mg	10-14	70-85	Consider in non-penicillin-allergic patients who have not previously received a macrolide.
Standard-dose PPI bid; clarithromycin, 500 mg, *or* metronidazole, 500 mg	10-14	70-85	Consider in penicillin-allergic patients who have not previously received a macrolide or are unable to tolerate bismuth quadruple therapy.
Bismuth subsalicylate, 525 mg qid; metronidazole, 250 mg qid; tetracycline, 500 mg qid; ranitidine, 150 mg bid; *or* standard-dose PPI qd-bid	10-14	75-90	Consider in penicillin-allergic patients.
PPI + amoxicillin, 1 g bid, *followed by:*	5	>90	Requires validation in North America.
PPI + clarithromycin 500 mg, tinidazole 500 mg bid	5		

Modified from Chey WD, Wong BC. American College of Gastroenterology guideline on the management of *Helicobacter pylori* infection. Am J Gastroenterol 2007;102:1808-1825. *PPI*, Proton pump inhibitor.

Box 38-3 Etiology of Peptic Ulcer Disease

Major causes

Helicobacter pylori infection

Nonsteroidal anti-inflammatory drugs (NSAIDs)

Aspirin

Minor causes

Duodenal obstruction from annular pancreas

Use of topically injurious drugs (potassium chloride, nitrogen-containing bisphosphonates)

Immunosuppressants (e.g., mycophenolate)

Helicobacter heilmannii infection

Mucosal infection (herpes simplex 1, cytomegalovirus, tuberculosis, syphilis)

Systemic processes (systemic mastocytosis, Crohn's disease, lymphoma, carcinomas)

Radiation involving duodenum

Use of cocaine or "crack" cocaine

Zollinger-Ellison syndrome

From Heidelbaugh JJ. Peptic ulcer disease. In Rakel RE (ed). Essential Family Medicine, 3rd ed. Philadelphia, Saunders-Elsevier, 2006.

---

or complicated ulcer disease with perforation, penetration, or gastric outlet obstruction; use of multiple NSAIDs (including concomitant use of low-dose aspirin and an NSAID); and concurrent warfarin or corticosteroid use. Evidence suggests that smoking may increase the risk of PUD and ulcer complications by impairing gastric mucosal healing. Alcohol use may increase the risk of ulcer complications in NSAID users, but its overall effect in those patients without concomitant liver disease has not been clearly defined. Currently, no solid evidence implicates dietary factors in the development of PUD.

Use of NSAIDs and aspirin is frequently associated with symptoms of dyspepsia, even in the absence of PUD. Empiric antisecretory therapy with PPIs is an attractive strategy that involves subjecting only those patients to upper endoscopy who fail to respond to a 4-week course of pharmacotherapy. The rationale for this approach is that most patients with dyspepsia do not have *H. pylori* infection or PUD (most typically have GERD), and their response to antisecretory therapy eliminates the need for further, expensive and invasive diagnostic testing (Saad and Scheiman, 2004).

KEY TREATMENT

The most efficacious therapy for *H. pylori* eradication consists of 14-day triple therapy with a PPI, clarithromycin, and amoxicillin or metronidazole, yielding eradication rates of 70% to 85% (Chey and Wong, 2007) (SOR: A).

Gastroesophageal Reflux Disease

Key Points

- The PPIs provide the most rapid symptomatic relief and healing of esophagitis in the highest percentage of patients.
- Although less effective than PPIs, H$_2$RAs given in divided doses may be effective in some patients with less severe symptoms of GERD; continuous therapy to control symptoms and prevent complications is appropriate.
- Chronic acid suppression has been associated with malabsorption of iron, vitamin B$_{12}$, and calcium; small bowel bacterial overgrowth; increased risk of hip fracture; and community-acquired pneumonia.

A complex, chronic, and relapsing condition, GERD carries a risk of significant morbidity and resultant complications. Population-based studies revealed that 40% of U.S. adults experience heartburn at least once a month; age- and gender-adjusted prevalence of weekly heartburn or acid regurgitation approaches 20% (Heartburn, 1998; Locke 1997). Most patients with GERD self-treat with over-the-counter (OTC) medications and do not seek medical attention for their symptoms.

Most patients with GERD evaluated in primary care practices have *nonerosive reflux disease* (NERD), although some will progress to *erosive esophagitis* (Fig. 38-7), and even fewer to more severe disease resulting in esophageal strictures, Barrett's esophagus, and adenocarcinoma of the esophagus (DeVault and Castell, 2005). Patients with NERD are prone to develop atypical or extraesophageal manifestations of disease (Box 38-4). Because of a small risk of disease progression, however, they generally do not require long-term surveillance despite persistent reflux symptoms. Symptom relapse rates in patients with NERD are similar to those in patients with erosive esophagitis, and although many will require continuous pharmacotherapy to control their symptoms, almost all continue to exhibit no definable erosive esophagitis on upper endoscopy (Fass, 2002).

Upper endoscopy is considered the gold standard in assessing esophageal complications of GERD (e.g., erosive esophagitis, Barrett's esophagus) but lacks an appreciable sensitivity and specificity for identifying pathologic reflux. Double-contrast barium radiography has limited usefulness in making an accurate diagnosis of GERD but may be useful in defining the presence of anatomic abnormalities, such as pyloric stenosis, malrotation, and annular pancreas in the vomiting infant, as well as hiatal hernia and esophageal strictures in children and adults.

The goals of GERD treatment are to relieve symptoms, heal erosive esophagitis if present, manage and prevent complications, and avoid recurrence and progression of disease using acid-suppressive medications. Initial empiric pharmacotherapy should consist of either an H_2RA or a PPI, without the need for immediate diagnostic testing in the vast majority of cases. Expert opinion supports either step-up or step-down therapy for the initial treatment of patients with GERD (Inadomi, 2002). In patients who incompletely respond to H_2RAs, PPIs taken once daily 30 minutes before the first meal of the day are preferred over continuing H_2RA therapy because of greater efficacy and faster symptom control with PPIs. An inadequate response to a 4- or 8-week trial of standard-dose PPI may indicate the need for longer treatment, more severe disease, or an incorrect diagnosis (Fig. 38-8). Additional benefit may be obtained by extending treatment for another 4 to 8 weeks with the same or a double dose of PPI (Medical Advisory Panel, 2003).

Diagnostic testing is recommended in patients with GERD who have an inadequate response to PPI therapy, need continuous chronic therapy to control frequent GERD symptoms, have chronic symptoms (>5 years) and are at risk for Barrett's esophagus, have atypical or extraesophageal manifestations suggesting complicated disease, or have alarm symptoms suggesting cancer (Box 38-5).

Lifestyle modifications should be recommended as adjunctive therapy in all patients with GERD (Box 38-6). Evidence is lacking to support the use of nonpharmacologic measures as the sole initial or long-term therapy for GERD, but expert opinion considers these to be of some potential benefit and no proven harm, although not sufficiently effective in treatment.

The basic tenets of antireflux surgery include reduction of the hiatal hernia, repair of the diaphragmatic hiatus, strengthening of the gastroesophageal junction–posterior diaphragm attachment, and strengthening of the antireflux barrier by adding a gastric wrap around the gastroesophageal junction (Nissen/Toupet fundoplication). In controlled studies comparing antireflux surgery to H_2RAs and PPIs, surgery has shown marginal superiority as measured by heartburn relief,

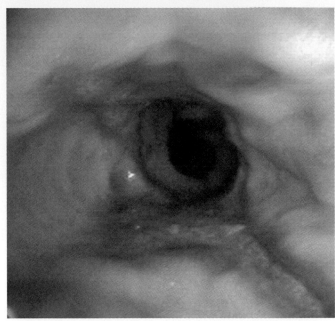

Figure 38-7 Esophagitis. *(Courtesy Dr. Erik-Jan Wamsteker.)*

Box 38-4 Atypical or Extraesophageal Manifestations of GERD
Aspiration
Asthma
Chronic cough
Dental enamel loss
Globus sensation
Noncardiac chest pain
Recurrent laryngitis
Recurrent sore throat
Subglottic stenosis
Modified from Heidelbaugh JJ, Nostrant TT. Medical and surgical management of gastroesophageal reflux disease. Clin Fam Pract 2004;6:547-568.

esophagitis healing, and improved quality of life in patients with erosive esophagitis. Long-term follow-up trials found that over half of patients resumed taking antireflux medications 3 to 5 years after surgery, most likely as a result of poor patient selection and surgical breakdown (Heidelbaugh and Nostrant, 2004).

KEY TREATMENT

Acid suppression with PPIs (proton pump inhibitors) is the mainstay of therapy for esophagitis (DeVault and Castell, 2005) (SOR: A). Lifestyle modifications should be recommended as an adjunctive therapy in patients with GERD (DeVault and Castell, 2005) (SOR: B).

Upper Gastrointestinal Bleeding

Key Points

- Comorbid risk factors for GI bleeding severity, including advanced age, shock, congestive heart failure, ischemic heart disease, and stigmata of recent hemorrhage, accurately predict the likelihood of death or rebleeding.

DIAGNOSIS AND TREATMENT OF GERD

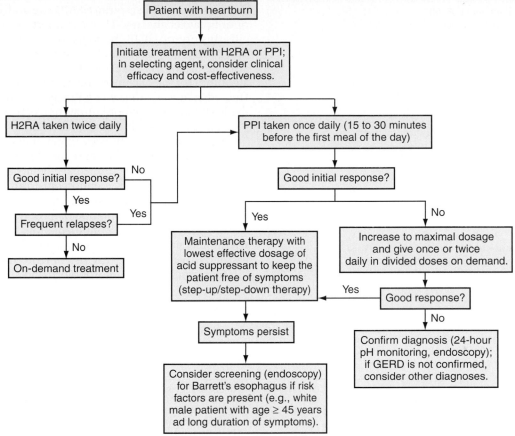

Figure 38-8 Algorithm for the diagnosis and treatment of gastroesophageal reflux disease. *(Modified from Heidelbaugh JJ, Nostrant TT. Medical and surgical management of gastroesophageal reflux disease. Clin Fam Pract 2004;6:547-568.)*

Box 38-5 Alarm symptoms of GERD Suggesting Complicated Disease

Black or bloody stools
Choking
Chronic coughing
Dysphagia
Early satiety
Hematemesis
Hoarseness
Iron deficiency anemia
Odynophagia
Weight loss

Modified from Heidelbaugh JJ, Nostrant TT. Medical and surgical management of gastroesophageal reflux disease. Clin Fam Pract 2004;6:547-568.

Box 38-6 Suggested Lifestyle Modifications in GERD Management

Avoid acidic foods (citrus and tomato-based products), alcohol, caffeinated beverages, chocolate, onions, garlic, salt, and peppermint.
Avoid large meals.
Avoid medications that may potentiate GERD symptoms (calcium channel blockers, β-agonists, α-agonists, theophylline, nitrates, sedatives)
Avoid recumbency 3 to 4 hours after meals.
Avoid tight clothing around the waist
Decrease dietary intake of fat.
Elevating head of bed 4 to 8 inches (10-20 cm).
Losing weight
Smoking cessation
*Dietary fibers and physical exercise may be protective

Modified from DeVault KR, Castell DO. Updated guidelines for the diagnosis and treatment of gastroesophageal reflux disease. The Practice Parameters Committee of the American College of Gastroenterology. Am J Gastroenterol 1999;94:1434-1442; and Nilsson M, Johnsen R, Ye W, et al. Lifestyle related risk factors in the aetiology of gastro-oesophageal reflux. Gut 2004;53:1730-1735.

- UGIB is confirmed by upper endoscopy, permitting direct visualization of the cause and location of the bleeding and allowing an attempt at immediate hemostasis.

Significant UGIB is defined as bleeding that results in hemodynamic instability and a decrease in the hemoglobin (Hb) and hematocrit (Hct). Although most patients with UGIB resolve spontaneously, those with an acute UGIB requiring hemostasis often present with a recent history of hematemesis (vomiting fresh blood) or "coffee grounds" emesis (black, partially digested blood). UGIB has an incidence of 40 to 150 episodes per 100,000 persons annually in the United States, with mortality of 6% to 10% (Oh and Pisegna, 2004). Box 38-7 lists the most common causes of UGIB.

Box 38-7 Common Causes of Upper Gastrointestinal Bleeding

Arteriovenous malformations (AVMs)

Bleeding from the nose or pharynx

Dieulafoy's lesion (ruptured mucosal artery)

Erosive esophagitis (severe)

Esophageal rupture (Boerhaave's syndrome)

Helicobacter pylori infection

Hemobilia

Hemoptysis

Mallory-Weiss tears (esophagogastric mucosal tears)

Neoplasm (carcinoma, lymphoma, leiomyoma, leiomyosarcoma, polyps)

Nonsteroidal anti-inflammatory drugs (NSAIDs)

Ulcers (gastric, duodenal)

Vascular-enteric fistulas, usually from aortic aneurysm or graft

Varices (esophageal, gastric, duodenal)

Modified from Oh DS, Pisegna JR. Pharmacologic treatment of upper gastrointestinal bleeding. Curr Treat Options Gastroenterol 2003;6:157-162.

It is important to characterize patients with risk factors for the development of UGIB to identify potential preventive measures, including aspirin/NSAID use and anticoagulation or antiplatelet therapy. *H. pylori* infection, erosive esophagitis, history of UGIB, perioperative period, intensive care unit (ICU) admission, and Zollinger-Ellison syndrome are also significant risk factors for UGIB. Figure 38-9 outlines an algorithm for the diagnosis and management of acute UGIB. Hemodynamically unstable patients should be admitted to the ICU, have a large-bore intravenous (IV) and nasogastric tube placed, and should not be fed orally.

Confirmation of UGIB is by upper endoscopy, permitting direct visualization of the cause and location of the bleeding and an attempt at immediate hemostasis. During the diagnostic evaluation, the endoscopist can treat the source of UGIB by using electrocautery, injection of 0.9% saline or 100% ethanol, or a combination of these techniques. Alternative methods include laser photoablation, band ligation, and sclerotherapy and balloon tamponade for esophageal and gastric variceal bleeding. The risk of rebleeding after therapy can be predicted by the morphology and size of the ulcer at

ALGORITHM FOR ACUTE UPPER GI BLEEDING

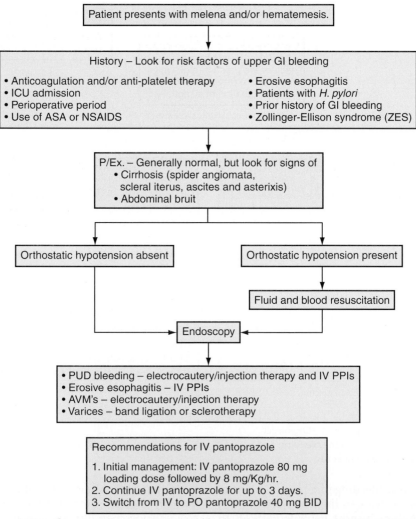

Figure 38-9 Algorithm for the evaluation of acute upper gastrointestinal (GI) bleeding. *ASA,* Acetylsalicylic acid; *AVM,* arteriovenous malformation; *NSAIDs,* nonsteroidal anti-inflammatory drugs; *PPI,* proton pump inhibitor; *PUD,* peptic ulcer disease. *(Modified from Oh DS, Pisegna JR. Management of upper gastrointestinal bleeding. Clin Fam Pract 2004;6:631-645.)*

upper endoscopy. Most cases of rebleeding occur within the first 72 hours after hospital admission; patients at increased risk for upper GI rebleeding should have ICU monitoring during their admission (Oh and Pisegna, 2004). The use of PPIs in reducing the risk of UGI rebleeding was demonstrated in a landmark study with IV omeprazole, showing the clinical efficacy of acid reduction therapy in preventing the complications of PUD rebleeding (Lau et al., 2000).

Gastroparesis

Clinical symptoms suggesting gastroparesis, or impaired and delayed gastric emptying, include nausea, vomiting, and postprandial abdominal fullness. Most often, gastroparesis is related to poorly controlled diabetes mellitus, autonomic neuropathies, postsurgical conditions (e.g., vagotomy, Billroth pyloroplasty), and anorexia nervosa. Vomiting needs to be differentiated from regurgitation, rumination, and even bulimia; the duration, frequency, and severity of symptoms together should be described along with any associated symptoms.

Gastric-emptying scintigraphy of a radiolabeled solid meal is the most accepted method to test for gastroparesis. Conventionally, the test is performed for 2 hours after ingestion of a radiolabeled meal; however, performing the test for up to 4 hours may increase the yield in detecting delayed gastric emptying in symptomatic patients. Breath testing can be used to measure gastric emptying using the nonradioactive isotope carbon 13 (^{13}C) (Parkman et al., 2004).

Primary treatment of gastroparesis includes dietary manipulation and administration of antiemetic and prokinetic agents. Dietary recommendations include eating more frequent and smaller meals and replacing solid food with liquids, such as soups. Foods consumed should be low in both fat and fiber content. Common antiemetic agents include prochlorperazine, trimethobenzamide, and promethazine. Currently used prokinetic agents include metoclopramide and erythromycin, administered orally or intravenously. Domperidone, a dopamine (D_2) receptor antagonist, is not approved in the United States for treatment of gastroparesis but is available in Canada, Mexico, and Europe (Parkman et al., 2004). Endoscopic injection of botulinum toxin into the pyloric sphincter can aid in relaxing pyloric sphincter resistance, allowing more food to empty from the stomach. No placebo-controlled trials have yet been reported for this therapy, and long-term control of gastroparesis should not be expected from using botulinum toxin.

Gallbladder

Cholelithiasis and Cholecystitis

Gallstones are exceedingly common among women and men of all ages, affecting approximately 20% of Americans during their lifetime. Population-based studies reveal a prevalence of gallbladder disease in women age 20 to 55 of 5% to 20%, increasing to 25% to 30% after age 50. By age 75, an estimated 35% of women and 20% of men will develop either symptomatic or asymptomatic gallstones (Attili et al., 1995). The prevalence for men is approximately one-third to one-half that for women in any given age group. The traditional clinical picture of a patient likely to have gallstones is

an obese woman over 40 years of age (The four F's: female, "fat", 40, and fertile). Prevalence is also increased in patients with cystic fibrosis with pancreatic insufficiency, diabetes mellitus, or family history of biliary colic; pregnancy; rapid weight loss; Native American Pima Indian or Scandinavian descent; patients taking estrogens, progestins, or ceftriaxone; and those requiring total parenteral nutrition (TPN).

The Rome Group for the Epidemiology and Prevention of Cholelithiasis (GREPCO, 1984) found that the overall cumulative probability of developing biliary colic over time was 11.9% at 2 years, 16.5% at 4 years, and 25.8% at 10 years, with a cumulative probability of 3% of developing complications at 10 years. The incidence of the development of biliary complications as the presenting complaint of gallstone disease is rare, ranging from zero to 5.5%. Based on these data, evidence from well-designed cohort and case-control studies summarized by GREPCO favors expectant treatment of asymptomatic gallstones.

In the approach to the patient with symptomatic gallstones, clinicians should effectively rule out other potential causes of RUQ and epigastric abdominal pain, distinguishing biliary from nonbiliary etiologies as the primary source of disease (see Table 38-1). A gallstone blocking the cystic duct or common bile duct (CBD; *choledocholithiasis*) results in acute biliary colic, which can evolve into acute suppurative cholecystitis or cholangitis. The onset of pain from biliary colic is rarely related to meals or the type of food consumed, contrary to popular opinion. Many patients with postprandial abdominal pain believe that they have gallbladder disease, but many of them suffer from dyspepsia or GERD. One meta-analysis found that heartburn, flatulence, regurgitation, and fatty food intolerance were not associated with gallstones, but that epigastric pain, nausea, and vomiting were associated with a higher odds ratio of having gallstones (Kragg et al., 1995).

In cases of acute cholecystitis, laboratory tests frequently lack adequate predictive value in making an accurate diagnosis. A complete blood count (CBC) usually reveals a moderate leukocytosis, often with a "bandemia" in cases of ascending cholangitis. Serum amylase and lipase values are usually normal but may be elevated if there is associated pancreatitis. Serum alkaline phosphatase (ALP), liver transaminases, and bilirubin levels are rarely elevated except when CBD stones are causing obstruction. Patients with choledocholithiasis often present similar to those with cholelithiasis, although they may also have obstructive jaundice, cholangitis, and pancreatitis.

The evaluation of gallstones using abdominal ultrasound is currently the best screening modality, with sensitivity and specificity above 90%. When calculi, gallbladder wall thickening, and gallbladder sludge are found, the diagnosis of acute cholecystitis is almost certain, yet the presence of stones by itself does not ensure the diagnosis of acute cholecystitis. Only 10% to 15% of gallstones are visible on plain radiographs (Fig. 38-10). A CT scan of the upper abdomen is more sensitive than conventional radiography but may miss a significant amount of cholesterol gallstones and biliary sludge readily seen on US (Fig. 38-11). Biliary scintigraphy (HIDA scan) uses technetium 99m (^{99m}Tc)–labeled derivatives of excreted bile acids to determine CBD obstruction. Endoscopic retrograde cholangiopancreatography (ERCP) with stent placement and/or sphincterotomy is useful

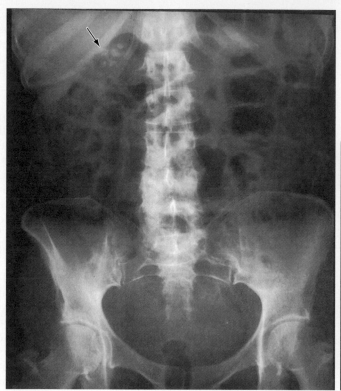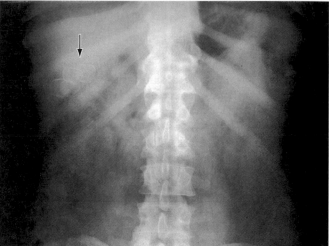

Figure 38-10 Radiographs of gallstones. *(Courtesy Dr. Perry Pernicano.)*

in identifying and treating CBD stones, but is invasive, expensive, and often fraught with complications, including iatrogenic pancreatitis (Fig. 38-12).

Endoscopic ultrasound is a widely used, noninvasive method with excellent sensitivity and specificity for detecting and evaluating CBD stones. Magnetic resonance cholangiopancreatography (MRCP) is another noninvasive modality for identifying gallstones and CBD stones, but it often has lower sensitivity and specificity than ultrasound and is more costly (Browning and Sreenarasimhaiah, 2006). The natural history of CBD stones suggests that 70% will pass safely into the duodenum and will not require ERCP for stone extraction.

Most surgeons advocate expectant management in patients with asymptomatic gallstones. Nonsurgical treatments include pain relief with narcotic analgesics, excluding morphine and its derivatives (which may precipitate sphincter of Oddi spasm and worsen symptoms) extracorporeal shockwave lithotripsy, and gallstone dissolution using oral bile acid therapy and contact solvents such as MTBE). Numerous RCTs have confirmed the adoption of laparoscopic cholecystectomy as the gold standard for the treatment of gallstone disease over the open procedure (Glasgow and Mulvihill, 2006).

Liver

Hepatitis

Hepatitis is defined as acute inflammation of hepatic parenchyma. In the United States the most common types of hepatitis are secondary to viral etiologies and are labeled as hepatitis A, B, and C. Table 38-3 outlines the various

serologic markers for viral hepatitis. Viral hepatitis is less frequently attributed to Epstein-Barr virus, toxoplasmosis, and cytomegalovirus. Additional causes of hepatitis include bacterial and fungal sources, autoimmune and metabolic disorders, toxic poisoning, and various hepatotoxic medications (e.g., isoniazid, acetaminophen) and alternative supplements. Acetaminophen overdose should be considered in acute nonviral hepatitis and treated immediately with n-acetylcysteine to avoid permanent hepatic damage and death. Patients presenting with acute hepatitis often exhibit low-grade fever, fatigue, lethargy, anorexia, RUQ pain, nausea, vomiting, diarrhea, arthralgias and myalgias, and in severe cases, dark urine and jaundice.

Serum bilirubin, transaminases, and ALP levels can be greatly elevated in all forms of acute hepatitis, but the specific values have poor prognostic value. Alarm symptoms of severe hepatic parenchymal destruction include mental status changes (hepatic encephalopathy), asterixis, ascites, and prolongation of prothrombin time (PT). These patients may require hospitalization, with attention toward improving nutritional status and specialist referral for liver transplantation evaluation. Most cases of acute hepatitis resolve without complications, so most patients can be managed as an outpatient, although they must take proper contact isolation precautions and allow for a slow return to usual activity. A patient's symptomatic improvement usually precedes the resolution of liver function serologies.

Viral Hepatitis

Hepatitis A is endemic worldwide, with 10% of U.S. children seropositive and up to 100% of preschool children seropositive in areas where sanitation and socioeconomic status is

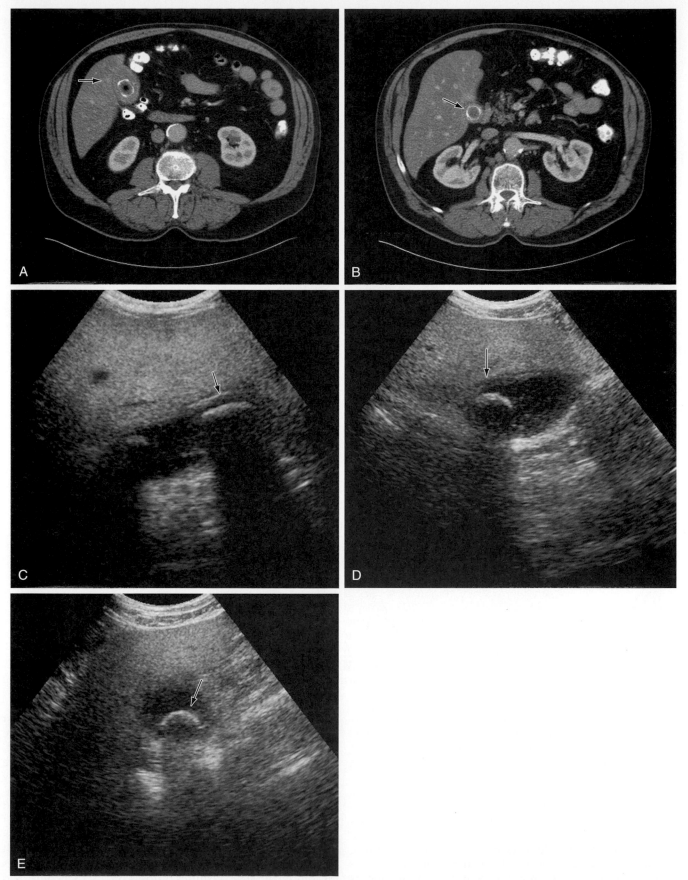

Figure 38-11 CT scans **(A, B)** and ultrasound **(C-E)** of gallstones *(arrows)*. *(Courtesy Dr. Perry Pernicano.)*

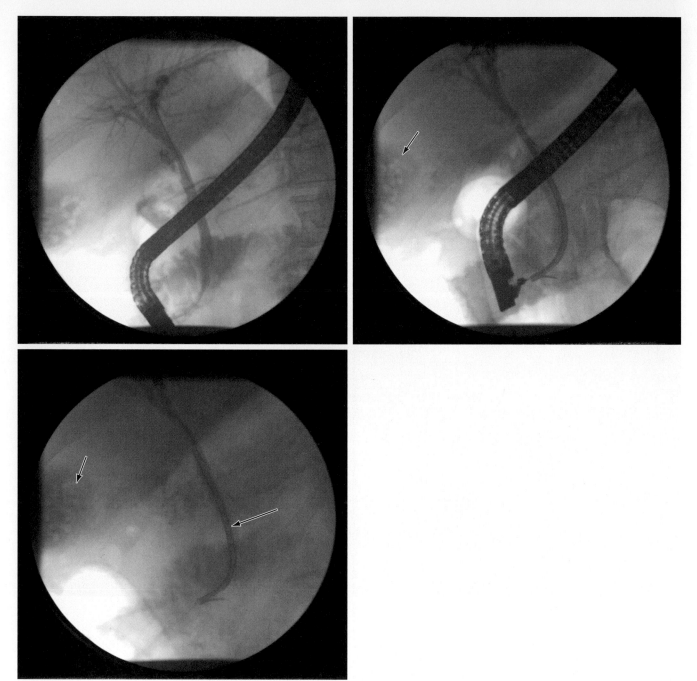

Figure 38-12 Endoscopic retrograde cholangiopancreatography (ERCP) with stent placement to identify and treat gallstones *(arrows)*. *(Courtesy Dr. Perry Pernicano.)*

poor in less developed countries (Marsano, 2003). The virus has received sporadic national attention in the United States from outbreaks in restaurants from undercooked meat and vegetable sources. Spread through the fecal-oral route, severe hepatitis can be seen after an incubation period of 2 to 6 weeks, but the vast majority of patients recover completely within this time frame and without permanent hepatic damage. Once a patient contracts hepatitis A, immunity follows with the appearance of anti-HAV IgG antibodies, and there is no chronic carrier state. If exposed to hepatitis A during a known incubation period, the patient should be passively immunized with immune globulin. Vaccination is recommended in high-risk populations and before travel to endemic areas (CDC, 1999).

Despite the availability of a highly effective vaccine against *hepatitis B*, approximately 2 billion people worldwide are infected, 350 million with chronic active infection accounting for 600,000 attributable deaths annually worldwide (WHO, 2009). Hepatitis B is spread via blood and body fluid contact through heterosexual and homosexual relations, by sharing of needles by infected drug abusers, and by accidental needle sticks in the medical setting. In areas of high disease prevalence (e.g., Southeast Asia, China), transmission is primarily from mother to child during childbirth or in early childhood. The vaccination for hepatitis B uses recombinant DNA, requires 3 doses on a set schedule, and confers immunity in the majority of recipients. In a child born to a mother positive for hepatitis B surface antigen

Table 38-3 Viral Hepatitis Serologic Tests and definitions

Test	Description
Hepatitis A virus (HAV)	
Anti-HAV IgM	Immunoglobulin M (IgM) antibody to hepatitis antigen. Antibody of IgM class signifies recent acute infection. This develops at onset of symptoms and resolves in less than 1 year.
Anti-HAV IgG	Immunoglobulin G (IgG) antibody to hepatitis A antigen. With negative anti-HAV IgM, this indicates past HAV infection, and that patient is immune. It appears 1 to 2 weeks after IgM antibody.
Hepatitis B virus (HBV)	
HBsAg	Hepatitis B surface antigen is earliest indicator of acute infection. It can be present for several months before symptoms and may remain detectable for up to 6 months. Persistence after 6 months may indicate a chronic carrier state.
Anti-HBs	Antibody to hepatitis B surface antigen is indicator of clinical recovery and subsequent immunity. It appears 1 to 2 months after HBsAg disappears, and it may be present for life.
HBcAg	No clinical significance, not readily available.
Anti-HBc IgG	Antibody to hepatitis B core antigen is early indicator of acute infection. It is also a lifelong marker that represents past exposure. It may precede the detection of HBsAg. This persists for years but does not necessarily confer immunity.
IgM Anti-HBc	Early indicator of acute active infection; usually short-lived (3-6 wk). Persistence of e antigen suggests progression to chronic carrier state.
HBe g	Active infection is present, and patient is highly contagious.
Anti-HBe	Seroconversion from antigen to antibody is prognostic for resolution of infection and, in a carrier, means very low infectivity.
IgM anti-HBc	IgM fraction of antibody to hepatitis B core antigen is test of choice to rule out acute HBV infection. IgM fraction disappears in first few months.
Hepatitis C Anti-HCV	An antibody to HCV that appears 3 to 12 months after exposure.
Hepatitis D Anti-HDV	This antibody to HDV may appear late and may be short-lived.
Hepatitis E (non-A, non-B)	No markers detectable, epidemiology parallels that of hepatitis B.

Modified from: Rodney WM. Gastrointestinal disorders. In Rakel RE (ed). Textbook of Family Medicine, 6th ed. Philadelphia, Saunders, 2002.

(HBsAg), in addition to the vaccine, hepatitis B hyperimmune globulin should be administered during the first 12 hours of life. Patients with chronic infection can develop cirrhosis and end-stage liver disease. Antiviral treatments for hepatitis B are indicated for patients with moderate to severe disease activity diagnosed on liver biopsy. Current therapies include interferon and more recently, lamivudine and adefovir (Marsano, 2003).

Hepatitis C affects more than 300 million people worldwide and 4 million people in the United States. At least six genotypes and 100 subtypes have been identified (Bukh, 2000). The diagnosis is established with serum testing for HCV RNA antibodies; although an antibody is induced, it is not protective against disease contraction and progression. Transmission occurs via blood or body fluid contamination through IV and intranasal drug use, blood transfusions, and in health care workers (e.g., needle stick or skin disruption with contaminated instrument). Data on sexual transmission and though tattooing have been inconsistent. Co-infection with human immunodeficiency virus (HIV) increases the risk of transmission sexually, as well as vertically mother to child. In patients with chronic hepatitis C, alcohol use rapidly accelerates liver damage and cirrhosis. Many experts believe lifelong abstinence from alcohol and IV and intranasal drugs should be immediate on diagnosis and enforced before initiating antiviral therapies.

Therapy with pegylated interferon and ribavirin has been shown to achieve sustained viral eradication in almost 50% of patients with hepatitis C (Shehab, 2004). Patients should be monitored for side effects of antiviral treatment, which may require dose adjustments or discontinuation of therapy. Duration and success of therapy depend on viral genotype and possible downward adjustments in therapeutic doses. Sustained virologic response ranges from 42% in genotype 1 to 80% in genotypes 2 and 3 (Marsano, 2003).

Hepatitis D virus (delta hepatitis) is usually only seen in IV drug users and in former carriers of hepatitis B as a co-infection. *Hepatitis E* is an enteric virus only rarely identified in the United States, characterized by an acute self-limited illness without a chronic carrier state.

Cirrhosis

Cirrhosis and chronic liver failure rank as the 12th leading cause of death in the United States, accounting for 27,555 deaths (9.2 per 100,000 population) in 2006, with a slight male predominance (NCHS, 2009). The vast majority of cirrhosis-related morbidity and mortality is secondary to excessive alcohol consumption, hepatitis B and C, and obesity (nonalcoholic fatty liver disease [NAFLD]), and is theoretically preventable. The term *cirrhosis* refers to a progressive diffuse, fibrosing, and nodular condition that disrupts the entire normal architecture of the liver. Portal hypertension ensues with multiple long-term complications. Approximately 40% of patients are asymptomatic, with cirrhosis often discovered during a routine examination, including laboratory and radiographic studies (Figs. 38-13 and 38-14), or often at autopsy. Mortality rates in patients with alcoholic liver disease are considerably higher than in those with other forms of cirrhosis.

The major complications of cirrhosis that affect HRQOL and survival include ascites formation, spontaneous bacterial peritonitis, hepatorenal syndrome, encephalopathy, and GI bleeding secondary to portal hypertension and varices. Another serious complication of cirrhosis is the development of hepatocellular carcinoma, for which screening protocols with ultrasound and serum alpha-fetoprotein testing are cost-effective (Marrero, 2005). All patients with ascites

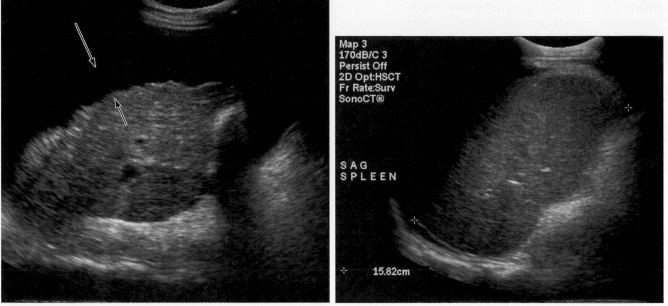

Figure 38-13 Cirrhosis. Ultrasound shows lobulated shrunken liver with ascites and splenomegaly. *(Courtesy Dr. Perry Pernicano.)*

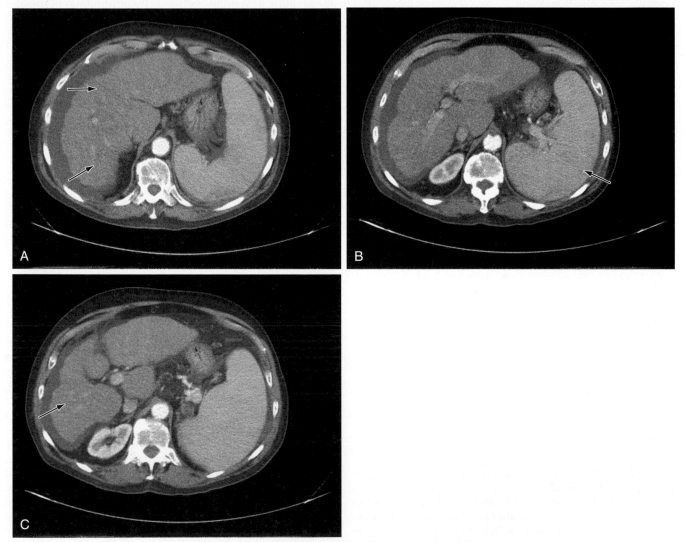

Figure 38-14 Cirrhosis. CT scans show **A,** lobulated contour of liver; **B,** splenomegaly; and **C,** ascites. *(Courtesy Dr. Perry Pernicano.)*

should be evaluated for liver transplantation because of poor 5-year survival (30%-40%) (Gines et al., 2004) (Fig. 38-15).

Pancreas

Acute Pancreatitis

Acute pancreatitis continues to cause significant morbidity and mortality despite dramatic advances in the understanding of its pathophysiology and its critical care management. Some studies suggest a high rate of undiagnosed pancreatitis, with approximately 40% of acute cases recognized only at autopsy. Thus, it is imperative for primary and emergency care physicians to make the diagnosis of pancreatitis within the first 48 hours of admission (AGA, 2007). In severe acute pancreatitis, parenchymal and fat necrosis ensues, as well as profound multisystem organ failure, infection, and life-threatening hemodynamic instability.

The causes of acute pancreatitis are diverse and demonstrate changing trends over time and variation by geography. Gallstones, biliary sludge, and microlithiasis are recognized as the proximate cause in more than half of reported cases. Ethyl alcohol ingestion is the second most common reported cause of acute pancreatitis, about 30% of cases, although it is unclear whether alcohol is a toxin or an exacerbating factor in individuals who have compromised pancreatic function. The remaining causes of acute pancreatitis account for less than 15% of total cases, including hypertriglyceridemia, trauma, medications, ERCP, neoplasms, perforated PUD, viral infection, and idiopathic causes.

Serum markers of acute pancreatitis have high sensitivity and specificity but no role in predicting the severity or course of disease. The most common enzymes assayed, amylase and lipase, are released at approximately the same time after the initial insult to the pancreas but are cleared from the bloodstream at different rates. Therefore, relying on total serum amylase alone to make an accurate diagnosis of acute pancreatitis is error-prone, because it is cleared almost

totally from the blood within 48 to 72 hours. The sensitivity of pancreatic amylase for the diagnosis of acute pancreatitis decreases to less than 30% between the second and fourth day after onset of the acute episode. By contrast, an elevated serum lipase level can be detected up to 14 days after the acute event and has sensitivity greater than 90% for acute pancreatitis (Orbuch, 2004).

Early prognostic factors that can be measured and indicate severity of disease include the Acute Physiology and Chronic Health Evaluation II (APACHE-II) score. The overall success at prediction of mortality from acute pancreatitis at hospital admission remains at 40%, and even at 48 hours it is no better than 80% when all diagnostic strategies of morbidity and mortality prediction are compared (Papachristou, 2004). The most important factor in the management of patients with acute pancreatitis is maintaining appropriate intravascular volume status (AGA, 2007). Many predictors of pancreatitis severity are directly related to "third spacing" of fluids and include hemoconcentration and rising creatinine level. The hematocrit may be high as a result of hypovolemia secondary to third spacing of fluids. Volume resuscitation during the first 24 hours is important because this may minimize or even prevent pancreatic necrosis (Mayerle et al., 2004).

If the bilirubin, liver transaminases, and ALP increase, a CBD stone may exist (Fig. 38-16). Similar laboratory abnormalities with a less acute presentation may occur in patients with chronic pancreatitis when bile duct stricture occurs. This possibility should be further explored with abdominal US and possibly ERCP, which can be both diagnostic and therapeutic. ERCP is especially useful in the setting of biliary pancreatitis with associated cholangitis or severe pancreatitis within 72 hours of presentation (AGA, 2007). Leukocytosis (>20,000 WBCs/mL) suggests a more severe disease (Ranson et al., 1974). Since respiratory distress syndrome may ensue, chest radiographs and arterial blood gases should be considered. In severe cases, renal failure may appear despite adequate fluid intake, and thus urine output should be closely monitored.

Contrast-enhanced computed tomography (CECT) is the most extensively studied modality for the confirmation of

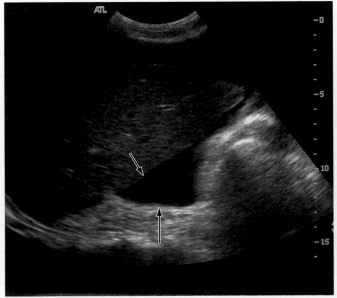
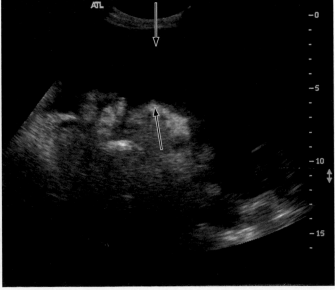

Figure 38-15 Ascites *(arrows). (Courtesy Dr. Perry Pernicano.)*

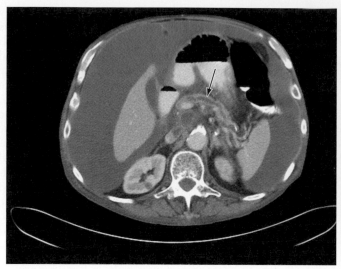
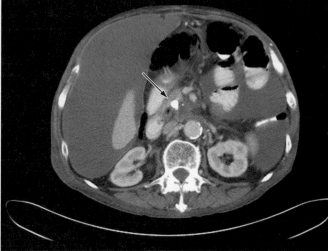

Figure 38-16 CT scans of dilated pancreatic duct secondary to stone pancreatitis. *(Courtesy Dr. Perry Pernicano.)*

acute pancreatitis and provides the highest level of sensitivity and specificity of current imaging technologies (Fig. 38-17) (Papachristou and Whitcomb, 2004). Sensitivities using ultrasound for the diagnosis of acute pancreatitis range between 62% and 95% and probably reflect the failure to visualize the organ in as many as 30% of cases. When the pancreas is visualized in the setting of acute disease, tissue abnormalities are detected in 90% of those studied. The milder the disease presentation, the less likely it is that abnormalities will manifest that are detectable on CT examination. Magnetic resonance imaging (MRI) and MRCP have specific yet limited roles in diagnosing acute pancreatitis.

Medical therapy of acute pancreatitis is primarily supportive, with the major objective being hemodynamic stabilization. Nutritional support should be provided in those patients likely to remain "nothing by mouth" (NPO) for more than 7 days. Nasojejunal tube feeding, using an elemental or semielemental formula, is preferred over TPN (AGA, 2007). Pain management in the hospital setting is best achieved using morphine derivatives. Infrequently, patient-controlled anesthesia may be used for severe abdominal pain, and alternative diagnoses and complications should be considered.

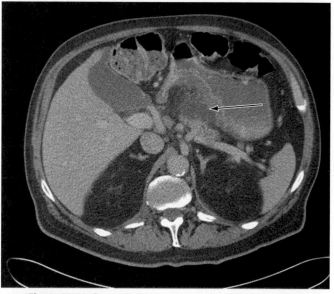

Figure 38-17 Pancreatitis (CT scan). *(Courtesy of Dr. Perry Pernicano.)*

Chronic Pancreatitis

Permanent pathologic damage to the pancreas results in chronic pancreatitis. In addition to exocrine deficiency (with malabsorption, diabetes, or both), a chronic pain syndrome may evolve and become a management challenge. Many patients suffer from substance abuse and other behavioral problems that require time, patience, compassion, and skill to resolve. Patients who continue to consume alcohol are more likely to have recurrent attacks. Carefully selected patients may benefit from therapeutic ERCP or pancreatic surgery, with some pain relief. Exocrine deficiency may be treated with pancreatic enzyme supplementation with each meal (Apte et al., 1999).

Chronic pancreatitis indicates some degree of progressive and permanent damage to the pancreas, usually visualized as calcifications on radiographs and CT (Figs. 38-18 and 38-19). This damage often leads to diabetes and pancreatic

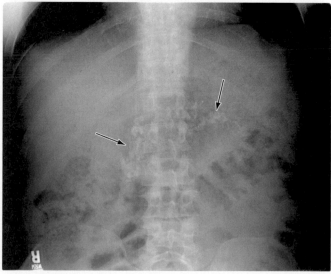

Figure 38-18 Chronic pancreatitis with calcifications. *(Courtesy Dr. Perry Pernicano.)*

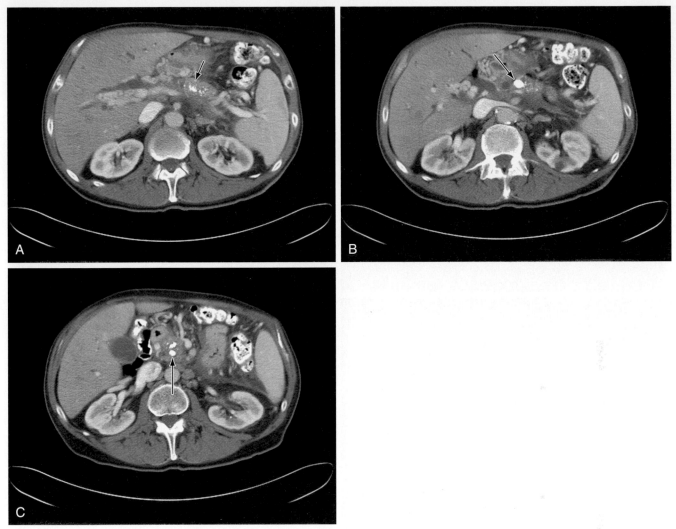

Figure 38-19 Pancreatic calcifications. *(Courtesy of Dr. Perry Pernicano.)*

insufficiency, resulting in malabsorption with chronic diarrhea. Patients with chronic pancreatitis present with repeated attacks of abdominal pain and are often admitted for acute or chronic exacerbations. Potential complications include pseudocyst (Fig. 38-20) and abscess formation, fistula formation between pseudocysts and the gut, persistent pancreatic ascites caused by a disrupted pancreatic duct system, communication with the peritoneal cavity, mesenteric venous thrombosis, and arterial pseudoaneurysm (Apte et al., 1999).

Pancreatic Cancer

More than 37,000 people in the United States were diagnosed with pancreatic cancer in 2008, and more than 34,000 died from their disease (Cancer Facts, 2008). The major risk factors are advancing age and a history of tobacco and alcohol use; the diagnosis is rarely made early in the disease course because of vague presenting symptoms of nonspecific abdominal pain, weight loss, cachexia, and painless obstructive jaundice. Approximately 85% of patients present with locally advanced or metastatic disease, with median survival of 3 to 12 months. For these patients, conventional treatments include palliative surgery. Radiation and chemotherapy

have not substantially impacted survival. Endoscopic ultrasound and high-resolution CT allow for better preoperative selection for patients likely to benefit from exploration for resection (Fig. 38-21).

Lower Gastrointestinal Tract

Inflammatory Bowel Disease

Key Points

- Steroids are effective for inducing but not maintaining remission in IBD.
- The 5-ASA medications are effective in ulcerative colitis for therapy induction and maintenance therapy but largely are ineffective for Crohn's disease.

Inflammatory bowel disease (IBD) is a chronic condition that often requires long-term maintenance therapy for the majority of the half-million Americans affected. The two major categories include ulcerative colitis (UC) and Crohn's disease; a more recent and less common third category of *microscopic colitis* has also been identified. The incidence of

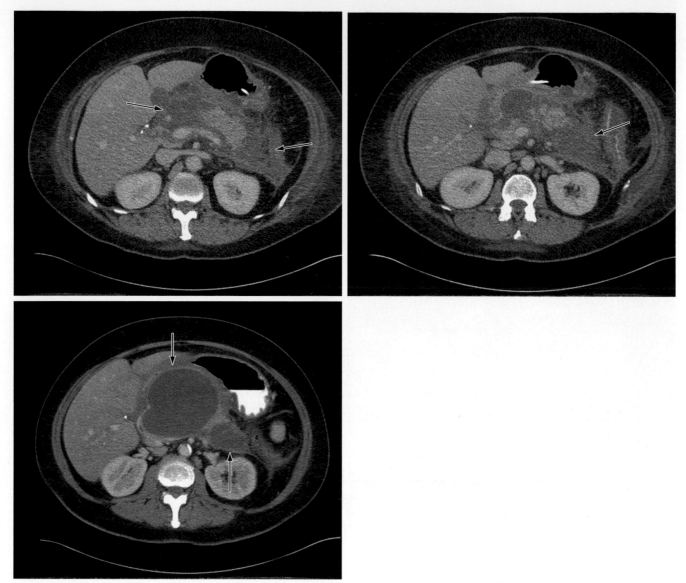

Figure 38-20 CT scans showing severe pancreatitis evolving into pseudocysts *(arrows)* over 2 months. *(Courtesy Dr. Perry Pernicano.)*

UC and Crohn's disease is 1.5 to 8 new cases per 100,000 U.S. population per year, more often in Caucasians and with no specific gender predominance, although some suggest a male predominance in Crohn's disease and a female predominance in UC. Most patients are diagnosed with IBD between ages 15 and 25, with a second peak between 55 and 65 years. The incidence of microscopic colitis is most likely underestimated because it is not well known; estimated incidence ranges from 4.3 to 9.2 per 100,000 in Western European and Icelandic population studies (Loftus, 2003).

Genetic factors play an important role in the development of IBD. First-degree relatives of patients with either form of IBD have been shown to have an almost 10% lifetime risk of developing disease and often present with a similar disease type and course as the affected family member (Higgins and Zimmerman, 2004).

Ulcerative colitis involves the mucosal layer of the sigmoid colon and rectum in the vast majority of cases, causing proctitis and proctosigmoiditis (Fig. 38-22). When there is proximal spread, it tends to be continuous and symmetric, causing intestinal mucosal inflammation with edema and friability that is visualized from the rectum proximally. Pancolitis is caused by inflammatory exudates producing a backwash ileitis by way of a patent ileocecal valve, and can cause small bowel involvement.

Crohn's disease differs from UC in that it may involve any part of the GI tract from the mouth to the anus, including the gallbladder and biliary tree, and involves the entire thickness of the bowel wall. It is most often found in the immunologically rich terminal ileum, and Crohn's disease involves the rectum in less than 50% of cases. In contrast to UC, the mucosal abnormalities are discontinuous ("skip lesions"), asymmetric, and patchy, which account for obstruction, abscesses, and perianal fistulas and those to other organs and skin. Recurrent disease flares and healing can result in significant muscular hypertrophy and fibrosis of the intestinal wall, leading to small bowel strictures, upstream dilation of intestine and increased fistula formation, and eventual bowel obstruction and the imminent need for surgical intervention (Higgins and Zimmerman, 2004).

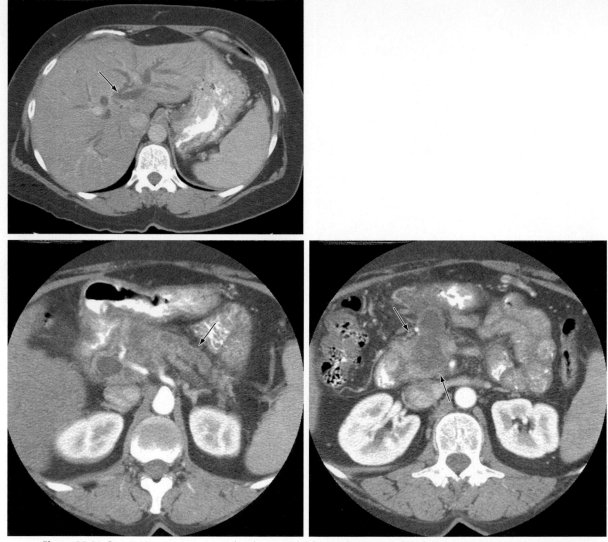

Figure 38-21 Pancreatic cancer, pancreatic head mass, with biliary and pancreatic ductal dilation. *(Courtesy Dr. Perry Pernicano.)*

Most patients with UC present with mild to moderate diarrhea without constitutional symptoms. Typically, the more severe the illness, the greater is the number of bowel movements, and the more likely that constitutional symptoms such as fever, fatigue, dehydration, and weight loss will also occur. UC can be intermittent with flare-ups, and remission can occur without therapy. A minority of patients with UC present with severe or fulminant panniculitis, ranging from an acute abdomen to toxic megacolon. Frequent urgent and bloody diarrhea usually suggests rectal disease and is most consistent with UC.

In patients with mild Crohn's disease, abdominal pain may be vague, the diarrhea intermittent, and weight loss absent. Postprandial crampy pain can suggest transient small bowel obstruction from inflamed or fibrotic, narrowed small bowel segments. Colonic involvement with Crohn's disease may present similar to UC, with predominantly bloody diarrhea. Rectal involvement produces more urgent and frequent small, bloody stools as a result of an inflamed, nondistensible rectum. Mucus in the stool is nonspecific and is found in both IBD and irritable bowel syndrome (IBS) (Higgins and Zimmerman, 2004).

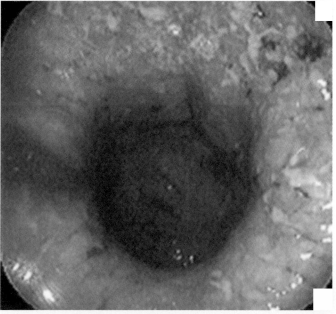

Figure 38-22 Severe colitis. *(Courtesy Dr. Erik-Jan Wamsteker.)*

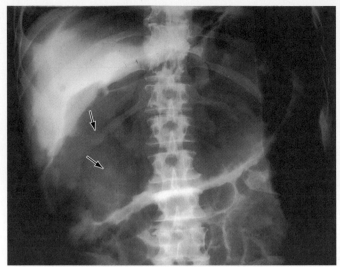

Figure 38-23 Ulcerative colitis, pseudopolyps. *(Courtesy Dr. Perry Pernicano.)*

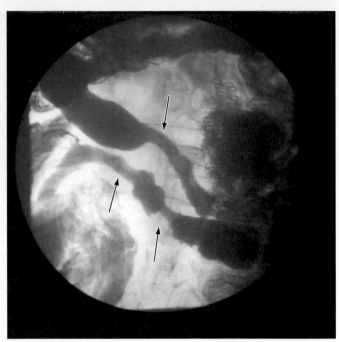

Figure 38-24 Crohn's disease. *(Courtesy Dr. Perry Pernicano.)*

Extraintestinal manifestations may be the presenting symptoms of UC or Crohn's disease. Uveitis, iritis, or episcleritis often flare concomitantly with intestinal symptoms. Large-joint pain and sacroiliitis may be a form of enteropathic arthritis. Common skin manifestations include erythema nodosum, perianal fistulas, and pyoderma gangrenosum. IBS is much more prevalent than IBD, and thus a major pitfall in the diagnosis of IBD is the mislabeling of patients with IBS.

The finding of confluent erythematous rectal inflammation is most consistent with UC and infectious colitis. Pseudopolyp formations indicate chronic inflammatory colitis (Fig. 38-23), while solitary aphthous ulcers, "rake-like" lesions, strictures, and rectal sparing are consistent with Crohn's disease. Colonoscopic evaluation should include ileal intubation and biopsies of both normal and abnormal mucosa. Anal or perianal lesions, including sinus tracts, rectovaginal fistulas, and abscesses, is consistent with Crohn's disease but not with UC. The mucosa in a patient with Crohn's disease may appear cobblestoned or nodular. Loss of haustra, distortion of normal architecture, or both may be found (Figs. 38-24 and 38-25).

Pharmacologic treatment of IBD is aimed at inducing remission and maintaining a symptom-free life, often after consultation with a gastroenterologist. Treatment of active flares with systemic steroids has been the mainstay of remission induction therapy, producing remission rates up to 70% in Crohn's disease versus 30% with placebo; similar results have been shown in the remission of UC. Budesonide, a nonsystemic steroid used in an enema formulation, has been effective for induction of remission in Crohn's disease and distal UC flares. Mild flares of UC are usually treated with 5-aminosalicylic acid (5-ASA) derivatives such as sulfasalazine, although RCTs have shown 5-ASA only marginally superior to placebo at controlling flare-ups of Crohn's disease. 5-ASA products are thought to be inferior to budesonide and systemic steroids for remission induction in Crohn's disease and generally are not used (Higgins and Zimmerman, 2004).

Azathioprine and its metabolite, 6-mercaptopurine, are slow-acting compounds proved effective for inducing remission in Crohn's disease. They often are added to systemic steroids to help induce and maintain remission and to ease steroid tapering. Methotrexate is also effective for remission induction in Crohn's disease. Close monitoring of CBC and serum transaminases is recommended, with monthly testing on initiation and with dosage changes. Pregnancy and exposure to live-virus vaccines should be avoided. Infliximab, an anti–tumor necrosis factor alpha antibody, is remarkably effective in treating approximately 60% of steroid-resistant patients with Crohn's disease. Infliximab has significant side effect risks, including infusion reactions, and rarely, worsening of heart failure, activation of latent tuberculosis, serum sickness, and invasive fungal infections (Feagan, 2003).

KEY TREATMENT

Systemic steroid therapy is effective in the treatment of active flare-ups of Crohn's disease and ulcerative colitis (Hanauer and Baert, 1994) (SOR: A).

Budesonide is effective for remission induction in Crohn's disease and distal ulcerative colitis flares (Kuhbacher and Fölsch, 2007) (SOR: A).

Irritable Bowel Syndrome

Key Points

- Irritable bowel syndrome likely represents the clinical expression of multiple potential pathophysiologic factors, including a genetic predisposition to the disease, disturbed CNS pain processing, visceral hypersensitivity, mucosal inflammation, abnormal colonic motility, and emotional stress.
- Anxiety disorders, somatoform disorders, and history of physical or sexual abuse have been identified in 42% to 61% of patients with IBS referred to gastroenterologists.

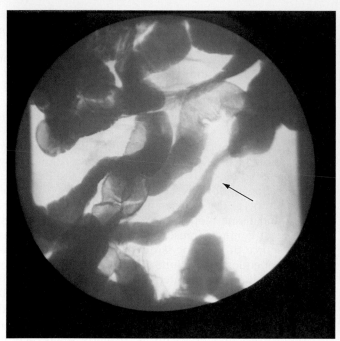
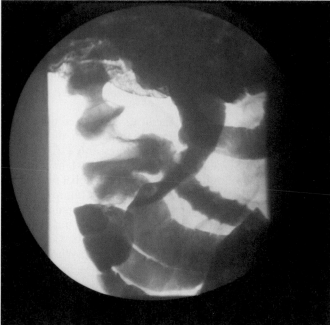

Figure 38-25 Crohn's disease. *(Courtesy Dr. Perry Pernicano.)*

Irritable bowel syndrome (IBS) is one of the most common conditions encountered in family practices, with a prevalence ranging from 1% to 20% worldwide and approximately 7% in the United States. IBS is characterized by abdominal pain, bloating, and disturbed defecation in the absence of known structural or biochemical abnormality. It typically appears in the late 20s, although it may present in teenagers and in patients as old as age 45; patients over 45 with suspected IBS should be evaluated for organic disease. IBS is responsible for over $20 billion in direct and indirect expenditures annually in the United States, and patients with IBS consume 50% more health care resources than matched controls without IBS (ACG, 2009).

Irritable bowel syndrome likely represents the clinical expression of multiple potential pathophysiologic factors, including a genetic predisposition to the disease, disturbed central nervous system (CNS) pain processing, visceral hypersensitivity, mucosal inflammation, abnormal colonic motility, and emotional stress. Given the degree of variation of IBS symptoms in affected patients, it is likely that the etiology of IBS is a heterogeneous combination of these factors, as well as other undetermined mechanisms. Psychosocial stressors likely exacerbate symptoms in patients with functional GI disorders. Anxiety disorders, somatoform disorders, and a history of physical and/or sexual abuse have been identified in 42 to 61% of patients with IBS who have been referred to gastroenterologists (Miller et al., 2001).

The physical examination in patients with IBS is often non-specific, and may demonstrate a normal abdomen examination, a diffusely tender abdomen, or a focally tender abdomen. Multiple diagnostic screening tests have been recommended including a CBC, erythrocyte sedimentation rate (ESR), serum chemistries, thyroid function tests, stool cultures including ova and parasites, fecal occult blood test, colonoscopy, and hydrogen breath testing, specifically to rule out other causes of disease (ACG, 2009). Despite these

Box 38-8 Diagnosis of Irritable Bowel Syndrome: Rome III Criteria

Symptoms of recurrent abdominal pain or discomfort and a marked change in bowel habit for at least 6 months, with symptoms experienced on at least 3 days of at least 3 months.
Two or more of the following must apply:
   Pain is relieved by a bowel movement.
   Onset of pain is related to a change in frequency of stool.
   Onset of pain is related to a change in the appearance of stool.

Modified from Longstreth GF, Thompson WG, Chey WD, et.al. Functional bowel disorders. Gastroenterology 2006;130:1480-1491.

recommendations, diagnostic testing should depend on the pretest probability of organic disease.

The differential diagnosis of IBS includes IBD, lactose intolerance, acute gastroenteritis, celiac disease, small intestinal bacterial overgrowth, colorectal cancer, and motility-altering metabolic disturbances (e.g., from hypo/hyperthyroidism. Currently, the Rome III criteria are the most widely accepted symptomatic classification of IBS (Box 38-8) (Longstreth et al., 2006).

There is no single evidence-based, consistently successful therapeutic approach for patients with IBS. Because it is largely a chronic condition, the goals of therapy should focus on patient reassurance, education about the natural course of the syndrome, and global symptomatic improvement, rather than on disease cure. This is best achieved through a well-developed physician-patient relationship with a clear delineation of realistic goals and expectations.

Newer treatments of IBS include tegaserod (Zelnorm), a 5-HT4 receptor agonist, shown to be more effective than placebo in relieving global symptoms in women with constipation-predominant IBS. Alosetron (Lotronex), a 5-HT3 antagonist, is indicated for women with diarrhea-predominant IBS and also is more effective than placebo in RCTs. Reports of ischemic colitis have limited the use of alosetron to physicians participating in the manufacturer's risk management program. Treatment of diarrhea-predominant IBS can be achieved with loperamide, although no effect over placebo for global IBS symptoms has been reported (Brandt et al., 2002).

To date, all other classes of medications used in the management of IBS have more limited impact on the global symptoms of IBS. The tricyclic antidepressants (TCAs) and selective serotonin reuptake inhibitors (SSRIs) have been shown to reduce abdominal pain, although global symptom reduction and HRQOL did not significantly improve compared with placebo. Treatment of constipation-predominant IBS can be achieved with fiber-bulking agents, but has not improved global IBS symptoms over placebo. Cognitive-behavioral therapy (CBT), interpersonal psychotherapy, group therapy, biofeedback, and hypnosis have been shown to improve individual aspects of diarrhea-predominant IBS, but these have also not been shown to improve global IBS symptoms (see Key Treatment). Complementary and alternative medicine (CAM) techniques include acupuncture, enteric-coated peppermint oil, probiotic therapy, and Chinese herbal medicine. CAM therapies are becoming increasingly popular in the treatment of GI disorders and have shown some limited symptomatic improvement in select patients with IBS (ACG, 2009).

KEY TREATMENT

Cognitive-behavioral therapy for IBS (efficacy defined as >50% reduction of symptoms) showed significant benefit with a mean number needed to treat (NTT) versus controls of approximately two (2 patients NTT for 1 to benefit) (meta-analysis of 17 studies; Lackner et al., 2004) (SOR: A).

Gut-directed hypnotherapy (GDH) can have long-lasting effects; of 204 patients with resistant IBS symptoms, 81% of initial responders had benefit 5 years after completion of treatment (Gonsalkorale et al., 2003) (SOR: B).

Fiber bulking agents can help treat constipation-predominant IBS (Mertz, 2003) (SOR: B).

Enteric-coated peppermint oil (0.2-0.4 mL [200-400 mg] three times daily in adults) reduced pain and spasm of IBS (Ford et al., 2008; Merat et al., 2009) (SOR: B).

Tricyclic antidepressants should be considered in the treatment of pain-predominant IBS (Mertz, 2003) (SOR: B).

Tegaserod is more effective than placebo at relieving global IBS symptoms in female patients who have constipation-predominant IBS (ACG, 2009) (SOR: A).

Alosetron is more effective than placebo at relieving global IBS symptoms in female patients who have diarrhea-predominant IBS (ACG, 2009) (SOR: A).

Lower Gastrointestinal Bleeding

Lower GI bleeding (LGIB) is defined as bleeding arising from a source distal to the ligament of Treitz, with the resultant potential for rapid hemodynamic instability. Physical signs of hemodynamic compromise include orthostatic hypotension, fatigue, pallor, palpitations, chest pain, dyspnea, tachypnea, and tachycardia. Hemodynamic stabilization through large-bore IV fluid resuscitation should be initiated immediately if acute LGIB is suspected, and blood transfusion may be necessary. Laboratory testing should include CBC, comprehensive panel, coagulation profile, iron studies including transferrin saturation, and reticulocyte count (before transfusion), and blood type and crossmatch. Clotting disorders and anticoagulant use, including daily aspirin or NSAIDs, should be identified during history taking. Figures 38-26 and 38-27 provide a detailed algorithm for the workup of LGIB.

The American Society for Gastrointestinal Endoscopy Standards of Practice Committee recommends colonoscopy as the preferred modality for the evaluation and treatment of LGIB, allowing for direct visualization of the source of bleeding in over 70% of cases, as well as therapeutic intervention and tissue biopsy. Table 38-4 lists the frequency of the most common causes of LGIB. When no obvious colonic source of bleeding is discovered on lower endoscopy, upper endoscopy is done to evaluate potential causes of rapid, significant UGIB interpreted as LGIB. If there is still no identifiable source of bleeding, examination of the small intestine using enteroclysis or capsule endoscopy should be considered. Intubation of the terminal ileum at the time of colonoscopy may be useful, particularly when there is blood throughout the colon; fresh blood emanating from the ileum indicates small intestinal bleeding (Eisen et al., 2001).

The combination of an overall higher diagnostic yield and a lower rate of complications makes colonoscopy the preferred choice over angiography as the initial test in most patients with suspected GI bleeding. Colonoscopy may be performed urgently or electively, depending on the patient's hemodynamic status and risk-stratification criteria. Comorbid risk factors for GI bleeding severity, including advanced age, presence or absence of shock, congestive heart failure (CHF), ischemic heart disease, and stigmata of recent hemorrhage, accurately predict the likelihood of death or rebleeding (Rockall et al., 1996). In patients with LGIB who are hemodynamically stable, a clean-out preparation (e.g., GoLytely) should be used before colonoscopy to increase visibility and diagnostic yield. In patients with hematochezia and hemodynamic compromise, consideration should be given to a rapidly bleeding upper GI source, the patient should be kept NPO, and a nasogastric tube should be placed. A bloody aspirate or one without blood or bile, a history of NSAID use or previous PUD, or a patient with massive bleeding may prompt performance of upper endoscopy before evaluation of the colon (Eisen et al., 2001).

The ^{99m}Tc pertechnetate–labeled red blood cell (RBC) scan is a safe and noninvasive alternative to angiography. Slower rates of bleeding may be detected with this technique, but it is not as accurate in identifying the exact location of a bleeding site. When arteriography is used in association with a ^{99m}Tc-tagged RBC blush, the sensitivity of the arteriogram is increased to 61 to 72% (Zuckerman et al., 2000). A retrospective study using these scans showed that an "immediate blush" (positive scan) had 60% predictive value for an associated positive angiogram, and a "delayed blush" correlated with 93% predictive value for a negative angiogram.

Preoperative localization of the origin of LGIB is the standard practice, except in life-threatening cases of massive GI hemorrhage that necessitate emergency surgical

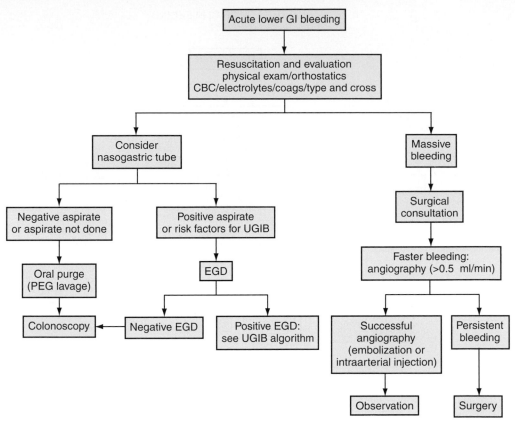

Figure 38-26 Algorithm for the management of acute lower gastrointestinal bleeding (part 1). *CBC,* Complete blood count; *UGIB,* upper gastrointestinal bleeding; *PEG,* percutaneous endoscopic gastrostomy; *EGD,* esophagogastroduodenoscopy. *(Modified from Eisen GM, Dominitz JA, Faigel DO, et al; American Society for Gastrointestinal Endoscopy, Standards of Practice Committee. An annotated algorithmic approach to acute lower gastrointestinal bleeding. Gastrointest Endosc 2001; 53:859-863.)*

exploration. Directed segmental resection is advised when the bleeding site is identified preoperatively, as seen in adenocarcinoma of the colon or diverticular disease limited to the left colon with persistent or recurrent bleeding. The removal of identified colonic lesions does not always result in effective treatment of the underlying source of bleeding. In these cases, arteriography can be used intraoperatively as an adjunct to localize a source of bleeding, facilitate segmental resection of the bowel, and prevent "blind hemicolectomy" (Manning-Dimmitt et al., 2005). A transfusion requirement of greater than 4 units of packed RBCs in 24 hours and recurrent diverticular bleeding (seen in up to 30% of patients) are common indications for surgical intervention. Other factors, such as comorbidities and individual surgical practices, play a significant role in this decision (Eisen et al., 2001).

In patients with chronic intermittent rectal bleeding, upper endoscopy is the preferred test for evaluation, with sensitivity and specificity of 92% and 100%, respectively. A barium-contrast upper GI series with small bowel follow-through (SBFT) may be considered if there is a relative contraindication to endoscopy (e.g., anticoagulation therapy, high risk for complications with conscious sedation, endoscopist unavailable). This test has sensitivity and specificity of 54% and 91% in the detection of upper GI lesions located above the ligament of Treitz (Zuckerman et al., 2000). Transcatheter embolization is an alternative when vasopressin is unsuccessful or contraindicated, but carries a risk of

acute abdominal pain and intestinal infarction (Eisen et al., 2001).

Small intestinal sources of GI bleeding account for less than 10% of all cases. When upper and lower endoscopy have failed to determine the suspected cause of bleeding, the physician should consider *push enteroscopy* (extension of upper endoscopy that allows visualization of up to 160 cm of small bowel distal to ligament of Treitz), although this procedure is limited by its inability to visualize the entire small bowel and thus carries a low diagnostic yield. The barium-contrast upper GI series with SBFT carries a very low sensitivity of zero to 5.6%. *Enteroclysis* (endoscopic placement of radiopaque contrast directly into proximal small bowel) also has low sensitivity, but has a shorter procedure time and can be used in the unconscious or uncooperative patient. Enteroclysis combined with push enteroscopy has higher diagnostic sensitivity than either method alone. Arteriography can be used in challenging cases to evaluate bleeding not identified by endoscopy. It is particularly helpful in the evaluation of older patients in whom arteriovenous malformations (AVMs) or neoplasms are suspected, because both of these lesions are associated with characteristic vascular patterns that can be identified on arteriogram. Capsule endoscopy is being studied as another modality for identifying small bowel bleeding and neoplastic pathology, but is limited in that biopsy samples cannot be obtained. Enhanced helical CT scanning is being explored as an alternative means of evaluating GI bleeding. Laparotomy with intraoperative

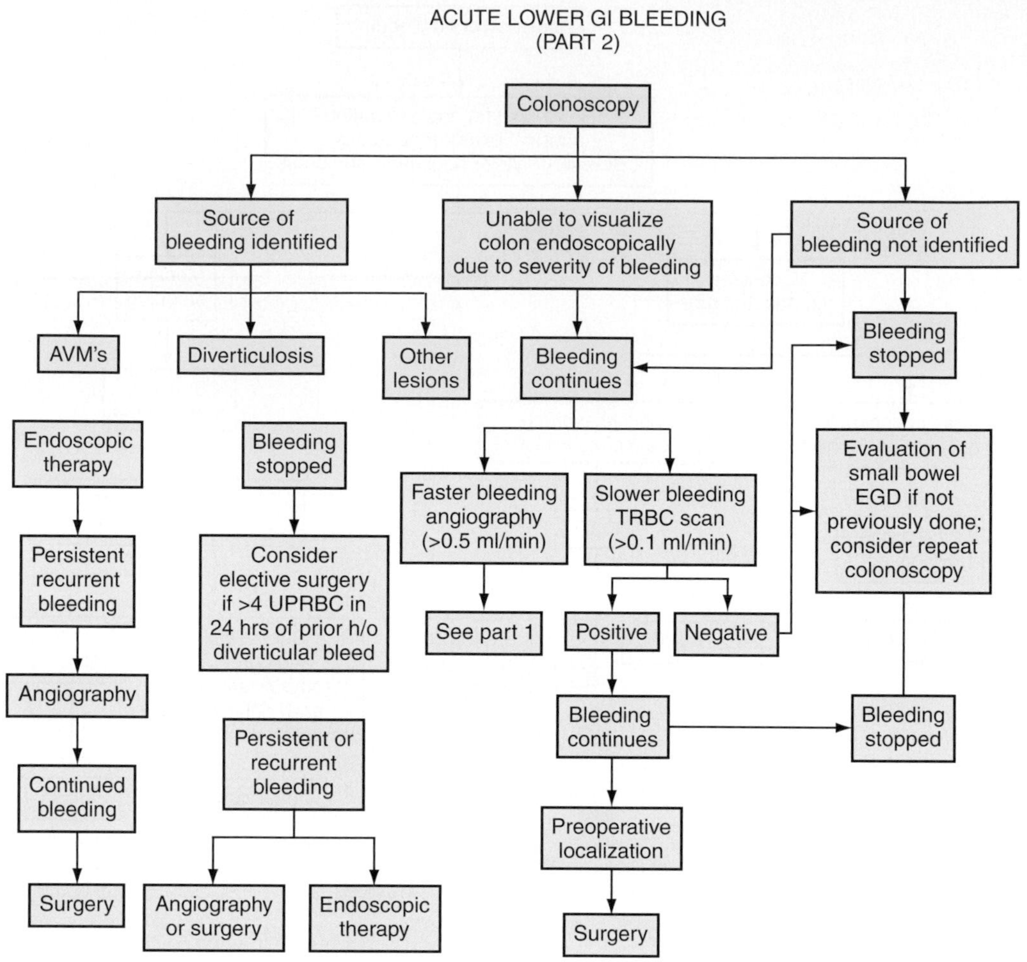

ACUTE LOWER GI BLEEDING
(PART 2)

Figure 38-27 Algorithm for the management of acute lower gastrointestinal bleeding (part 2). *AVM,* Arteriovenous malformation; *UPRBC,* units of packed red blood cells; *TRBC,* tagged (radiolabeled) red blood cell. *(Modified from Eisen GM, Dominitz JA, Faigel DO, et al; American Society for Gastrointestinal Endoscopy, Standards of Practice Committee. An annotated algorithmic approach to acute lower gastrointestinal bleeding. Gastrointest Endosc 2001;53:859-863.)*

enteroscopy should be considered a "last resort" in the diagnostic evaluation of nonemergent cases of GI bleeding because it is associated with higher rates of morbidity and mortality (Zuckerman et al., 2000).

KEY TREATMENT

Colonoscopy is the preferred modality used in the treatment of lower GI bleeding (Zuccaro, 1998) (SOR: A).

Diverticular Disease

Diverticulosis refers to the presence of diverticula, or herniations of the intestinal mucosa and submucosa, most often in the sigmoid colon (Figs. 38-28 and 38-29). More than one half of patients over age 50 have incidental colonic diverticula. *Diverticulitis* is the most common complication of diverticulosis, occurring in up to 20% of patients, and results from a microperforation of a diverticulum from inspissated fecal material that often becomes a phlegmon, or a pericolic or intra-abdominal abscess.

The initial assessment of the patient with suspected diverticulitis should include a thorough history and physical examination, including abdominal, rectal, and pelvic examinations.

The majority of patients will have LLQ pain (93%-100%), fever (57%-100%), and leukocytosis (69%-83%). Other associated features include nausea, vomiting, constipation, diarrhea, dysuria, and urinary frequency. The differential diagnosis includes IBS, IBD, colon cancer, ischemic colitis, bowel obstruction, and gynecologic and urologic disorders (ASCRS, 2000). Initial evaluation of the patient with abdominal pain and suspected diverticulitis includes CBC, urinalysis, and flat and upright abdominal radiographs.

The American Society of Colon and Rectal Surgeons Standards Task Force for the treatment of diverticulitis state that if the patient's clinical picture clearly suggests acute diverticulitis, the diagnosis can be made on the basis of clinical criteria alone (ASCRS, 2000). The need for additional tests in the patient with suspected diverticulitis is determined by the severity of the presenting signs and symptoms and diagnostic confidence. When the diagnosis of diverticulitis is in question, other tests may include water-soluble contrast enema, abdominal CT, or ultrasonography.

Criteria for the diagnosis of diverticulitis on water-soluble contrast enema include the presence of diverticula (Figs. 38-30 and 38-31), mass effect, intramural mass, sinus tract, and extravasation of contrast. Ultrasound may reveal bowel wall thickening, abscess, and rigid hyperechogenicity of the colon caused by inflammation and may be helpful in female

Table 38-4 Causes of Massive Acute Rectal Bleeding

Cause	Frequency (%)
Upper GI Tract	
Peptic ulcer disease	40-79
Gastritis, duodenitis	5-30
Esophageal varices	6-21
Mallory-Weiss tear	3-15
Esophagitis	2-8
Gastric cancer	2-3
Dieulafoy's lesion	<1
Gastric arteriovenous malformations	<1
Portal gastropathy	<1
Lower GI tract	
Small Bowel	
Angiodysplasia	70-80
Jejunoileal diverticula	<1
Meckel's diverticulum	<1
Neoplasms/lymphomas (benign and malignant)	<1
Enteritis, Crohn's disease	<1
Aortoduodenal fistula in patient with synthetic vascular graft	<1
Large Bowel	
Diverticular disease	17-40
Arteriovenous malformations	2-30
Colitis	9-21
Colonic neoplasms, postpolypectomy bleeding	11-14
Anorectal causes (hemorrhoids, rectal varices, fissures)	4-10
Colonic tuberculosis	<1

Modified from Manning-Dimmitt LL, Dimmitt SG, Wilson GR. Diagnosis of gastrointestinal bleeding in adults. Am Fam Physician 2005;71:1339-1346.

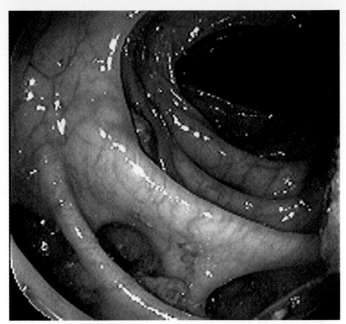

Figure 38-28 Diverticulosis. *(Courtesy Dr. Erik-Jan Wamsteker.)*

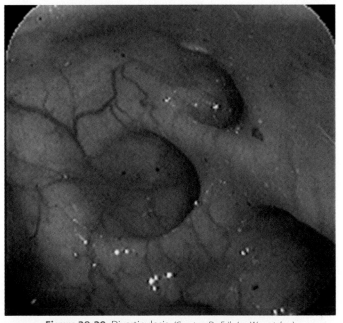

Figure 38-29 Diverticulosis. *(Courtesy Dr. Erik-Jan Wamsteker.)*

patients to exclude pelvic or gynecologic pathology. CT with oral and IV contrast is increasingly used as the initial imaging test for patients with suspected diverticulitis, particularly if disease of moderate severity or abscess is anticipated. Endoscopy is usually avoided in the setting of acute diverticulitis because of the risk of perforating the inflamed colon, either with the instrument itself or by insufflation of air. When the diagnosis of acute colonic diverticulitis is uncertain, limited flexible sigmoidoscopy with minimum insufflation of air may be performed to exclude other diagnoses.

Conservative medical management of uncomplicated diverticulitis without associated abscess, fistula, obstruction, or perforation includes bowel rest and IV fluoroquinolones or extended-spectrum penicillins. If the patient does not improve after several days, an abscess should be suspected and diagnostic imaging considered. Conservative treatment results in resolution in 70% to 100% of cases (ASCRS, 2000). After recovery from an initial episode of diverticulitis, when the inflammation has subsided, the patient should be reevaluated. Appropriate examinations include a combination of flexible sigmoidoscopy and single-contrast or double-contrast barium enema or colonoscopy. Eventual resumption of a high-fiber diet is recommended after acute inflammation resolves; long-term fiber supplementation after the first

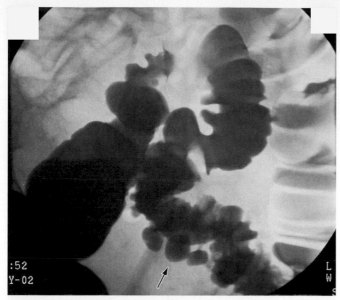

Figure 38-30 Sigmoid diverticula. *(Courtesy Dr. Perry Pernicano.)*

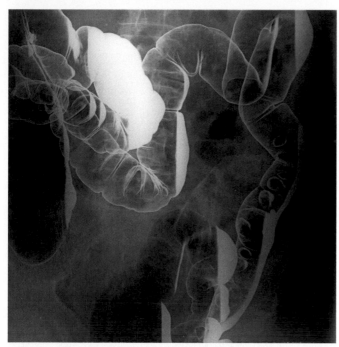

Figure 38-31 Diverticula. *(Courtesy Dr. Perry Pernicano.)*

episode of diverticulitis has been shown to prevent recurrence in more than 70% of patients followed up for more than 5 years.

The decision of whether to proceed with inpatient or outpatient treatment of diverticulitis depends on the clinical judgment of the physician, the severity of the disease process, and likelihood that the patient's condition will respond to outpatient therapy. Patients who are able to tolerate a diet, who do not have systemic symptoms, and who do not have significant peritoneal signs may be treated on an outpatient basis with TMP-SMX or a fluoroquinolone plus metronidazole (Gilbert et al., 2009).

Primary resection and anastomosis without a protective stoma has become the surgical treatment of choice for

uncomplicated diverticulitis and may also be performed for patients with localized pericolic or pelvic abscess. A single-stage procedure is associated with decreased hospital stay and has lower mortality and morbidity compared with two-stage and three-stage procedures. The most common two-stage operation is Hartmann's procedure, which carries a mortality range of 2.6% to 36.8% (ASCRS, 2000). Surgical treatment of diverticulitis, in both acute and chronic settings, has been successfully accomplished by laparoscopic and laparoscopic-assisted means.

Treatment of the patient with multiple attacks of diverticulitis or recurrent diverticulitis is individualized to minimize the morbidity and mortality of intervention. Factors considered when deciding whether to proceed with resection include patient's age; number, severity, and interval of attacks; rapidity and degree of response to medical therapy; and persistence of symptoms after an acute attack. The risk of recurrent symptoms after an attack of diverticulitis ranges from 7% to 45%. With each episode, the patient is less likely to respond to medical therapy (70% respond to medical therapy after first attack vs. 6% after third). Thus, after two attacks of uncomplicated diverticulitis, resection is usually recommended (ASCRS, 2000).

> ### KEY TREATMENT
>
> Patients who can tolerate a diet and do not have systemic symptoms or significant peritoneal signs may be treated as outpatients with TMP-SMX or a fluoroquinolone plus metronidazole (Gilbert et al., 2009) (SOR: B).
> Surgery may be necessary in some patients both in uncomplicated and complicated diverticulitis and should be individualized (Stollman and Raskin, 2004) (SOR: B).

Celiac Disease

Key Points

- Tests to consider in testing for celiac disease include transglutaminase IgA, antiendomysial antibody, antigliadin antibody, and the genetic test HLA DQ2/DQ8.
- A negative HLA DQ2/DQ8 test is most helpful in ruling out celiac disease. A positive test does not rule it in but is associated with an increased risk.
- Consider an elimination/challenge diet for 2 weeks. If symptoms improve, a rechallenge with gluten-containing foods will cause a recurrence of symptoms.
- The antibody tests (TTG IgA, antiendomysial, antigliadin) can become negative after elimination of gluten protein and may be false negative.

Adult presentation of celiac disease is characterized by weight loss, diarrhea, fatigue, and anemia. Children frequently present with failure to thrive, vomiting, diarrhea, muscle wasting, signs of hypoproteinemia including possible ascites, and general irritability. Common comorbidities include type 1 diabetes mellitus, cerebral calcifications, Sjögren's syndrome, and thyroid disease. Celiac disease should be considered in cases of unexplained folic acid, iron or B_{12} deficiency, reduced serum albumin, osteoporosis, and osteomalacia.

Other presentations may include infertility or recurrent miscarriage. Splenic atrophy commonly occurs in celiac sprue, and pneumococcal immunization should be administered in these patients.

Immunoglobulin A (IgA) antiendomysial antibodies are currently the most accurate serologic test for diagnosing celiac sprue with a sensitivity of 97% to 100% and specificity of 98% to 99%. Antigliadin antibodies are also usually quantified. Enzyme tissue transglutaminase, the antigen for antiendomysial antibodies, has a sensitivity of 95% and specificity of 94% in diagnosing celiac disease (AGA, 2006). HLA testing can now be done to evaluate persons at risk for celiac disease. About 95% of celiac patients are positive for HLA-DQ2 and 5% for HLA-DQ8. The majority of people who test positive for HLA-DQ2/DQ8 are at risk, but only 2% to 3% actually develop celiac disease. Celiac disease is rarely seen with a negative test, and thus this test is most useful when negative. A positive test does not make the diagnosis. A CBC, comprehensive biochemical profile including serum albumin concentration, transferrin saturation, serum or RBC folate, vitamin B_{12}, and liver function tests should also be obtained on diagnosis. Deficiencies of iron, folic acid, calcium, and vitamins B_{12} and D frequently often correct after initiating a gluten-free diet, without the need for vitamin supplementation.

The diagnostic standard for celiac disease is a small intestinal biopsy using endoscopy, although this is usually not necessary to establish an accurate diagnosis. Characteristic changes include damage to the normal villous morphology with decreased villous height/crypt depth, decreased epithelial surface cell height, and increased lymphocytic infiltration of the intestinal mucosa. The accepted AGA diagnostic criteria state that small intestinal mucosa should be abnormal while patients continue on a gluten diet. A repeat biopsy should be taken 4 to 6 months after induction of treatment, and if there has been no improvement in the small intestinal mucosal morphology, the original diagnosis should be questioned. Many gastroenterologists do not obtain a subsequent biopsy specimen, and the cost-effectiveness of this approach has not been demonstrated. A gluten challenge is recommended if there is any doubt concerning the correct diagnosis (AGA, 2006).

The AGA guidelines state that the cornerstone of treatment of celiac disease and its resultant complications is gluten-free diet therapy under a nutritionist's guidance. Patients should completely omit wheat, rye, barley, beer, and breakfast cereals from their diet. It is important to explain the disease process and toxicity of gluten-containing foods to the patient, including the potential for the reversal of current celiac-related problems, including anemia, depression, and infertility. Gluten-free breads, pasta, and other products are commercially available and should be recommended as substitutes. Patients with celiac disease usually experience rapid symptomatic improvement within weeks of the exclusion of dietary gluten, providing additional diagnostic confirmation. Monitoring of antiendomysial or tissue transglutaminase antibody (TTG IgA) titers, which usually normalize with the institution of a gluten-free diet, may prove useful to check dietary compliance, but have neither become standard practice nor been cost-effective. Life-threatening hypokalemia or hypomagnesemia rarely occurs and should be appropriately corrected. Expert panels suggest that yearly weight, CBC, ferritin, folate, calcium, and ALP levels should be obtained for disease monitoring. Oral corticosteroids may be used in unresponsive patients, but only when other causes of small intestinal villous atrophy have been excluded (AGA, 2006).

Dermatitis herpetiformis is a common extraintestinal manifestation of gluten-sensitive enteropathy, characterized by a pruritic, blistering, and vesicular rash. The diagnosis is made with immunofluorescent staining of granular IgA after skin biopsy. Treatment involves oral dapsone and a gluten-free diet, and with sufficient symptom relapse after 6 months, dapsone can be withdrawn and the gluten-free diet continued indefinitely. Osteopenia and osteoporosis, as well as bone pain, pseudofractures, and orthopedic deformities, are common features of celiac disease. Osteoporosis carries a significant fracture risk, and thus dual-energy x-ray absorptiometry (DEXA) screening of patients with celiac disease is recommended yearly. If osteoporosis is discovered, measures include strict adherence to a gluten-free diet, calcium supplementation of up to 1500 mg/day, bisphosphonate or calcitonin therapy, or consideration of hormone replacement therapy in postmenopausal women. Smoking cessation should be encouraged and an exercise regimen advised in all patients. Ulcerative jejunitis is a serious complication of celiac disease that carries a high mortality risk after intestinal hemorrhage, perforation, or obstruction in patients with a history of significant malnutrition. Diagnosis can be challenging, and small intestine radiography often is not helpful. If small intestinal ulceration or lymphoma is suspected, enteroscopy may be used to obtain biopsy specimens for histologic assessment. Surgical resection of the ulcer, especially if localized to one part of the intestine, can be curative. Again, a strict gluten-free diet should be initiated, and treatment with steroids has shown significant benefit. If a diagnosis of enteropathy-associated T-cell lymphoma is made, the patient should be referred to an oncologist for appropriate chemotherapy.

Overall mortality risks are higher in patients with celiac disease, attributed to malignant intestinal lymphoma and adenocarcinoma. One study found a fivefold increased risk of developing malignancy in patients with celiac disease, with a relative risk of 40 for developing non-Hodgkin's lymphoma. These risks decreased to the level of the normal population after patients maintained a gluten-free diet for 5 years (AGA, 2006).

Colorectal Cancer

Key Points

- Average-risk individuals should begin colorectal cancer screening at age 50, and at age 45 in African Americans.

Colorectal cancer (CRC) is the third leading cause of cancer mortality in the United States, accounting for an estimated 9% of all cancer deaths in 2009. Risk factors include increasing age, a family history of CRC, obesity, sedentary lifestyle, a diet high in red meat and low in vegetables, and excessive alcohol and/or tobacco use. Diets high in fiber, fruits, vegetables, and calcium may be protective, but data are inconclusive. African Americans have a 50% higher likelihood of dying from CRC than Caucasians, because they may have more proximal distribution of colonic adenomas and carcinomas than the general population, and these may be missed more often on suboptimal screening (ACS, 2009).

Approximately 75% of CRCs are diagnosed in individuals who have no risk factors other than advanced age; 90% of patients are older than 50. Other risk factors include prior or family history of CRC or adenomatous polyps, chronic IBD, and genetic syndromes. Several case-control and cohort studies found an inverse association between physical activity and risk in men and women of all ages and in various racial and ethnic groups in diverse geographic areas worldwide. The long-term use of aspirin may be associated with a decreased risk of CRC, yet the risk/benefit profile for chemoprevention cannot justify broad recommendations for its use in the general population (Nease, 2004).

Up to 30% of CRCs are believed to arise secondary to a genetic predisposition. Approximately 20% of cases occur among patients who have a history of CRC in a first-degree relative. About 6% are attributable to identifiable, inherited genetic mutations known as *hereditary colorectal cancer syndromes*, including familial adenomatous polyposis (FAP) and hereditary nonpolyposis colorectal cancer (HNPCC). Although these syndromes are relatively uncommon, they confer a lifetime risk of CRC ranging from 80% to 100%.

Currently accepted methods for screening of CRC include the digital rectal examination (DRE), fecal immunochemical test (FIT), double-contrast barium enema (DCBE), flexible sigmoidoscopy, and colonoscopy. According to the AGA, "the relative virtues of each screening test can be debated, but the best test is that one that gets done" (Burt et al., 2004). Screening should begin by classifying a patient's level of risk based on personal, family, and medical history, which together determine the approach to screening in that person. Box 38-9 details current CRC screening recommendations.

The DRE is a simple, inexpensive, and minimally invasive test that can be routinely performed in the office during yearly health maintenance examinations. It allows for palpation of the internal anal canal and examination of the prostate. Along with DRE, FIT should be performed to assess for occult blood. The DRE itself has a very low diagnostic yield, identifying less than 10% of colorectal tumors. Sensitivity of DCBE varies widely, ranging from 50% to 80% for polyps less than 1 cm, 70% to 90% for polyps greater than 1 cm, and 55% to 85% for Dukes stage A and B colon cancers (Winawer et al., 1997). In a comparison study with colonoscopy, sensitivity of barium enema for neoplasia was significantly lower (32% for polyps ≤5 mm, 53% for polyps 0.6-10 mm, 48% for polyps >1 cm) (Winawer et al., 2000). Any suspected lesions identified by DCBE need to be confirmed, biopsied, and removed by colonoscopy. Rarely, the classic "apple core" hallmark sign of a colonic mass may be visualized on DCBE (Fig. 38-32).

Flexible sigmoidoscopy is an efficient screening tool for individuals at an average risk for CRC, allowing for direct visualization and biopsy of the colonic mucosa in the rectosigmoid, descending, and distal transverse colon. To date, no RCTs or case-control studies have shown that screening with this method decreases CRC mortality for tumors within the reach of the standard 60-cm scope. The limitation of this method is that advanced lesions may be missed in the ascending and proximal transverse colon in individuals who

---

Box 38-9 Current Colorectal Cancer (CRC) Screening Recommendations

Preferred Screening Tests

Cancer prevention tests should be offered first. The preferred CRC prevention test is colonoscopy every 10 years, beginning at age 50. Screening should begin at age 45 years in African Americans.

Cancer detection test should be offered to patients who decline colonoscopy or another cancer prevention test. The preferred cancer detection test is annual FIT for blood.

Alternative CRC Prevention Tests

Flexible sigmoidoscopy every 5 to 10 years.

CT colonography every 5 years.

Alternative Cancer Detection Tests

Annual Hemoccult Sensa.

Fecal DNA testing every 3 years.

Positive Family History but HNPCC Evaluation Not Indicated

Single first-degree relative with CRC or advanced adenoma diagnosed at age 60 years or older.

> *Recommended screening:* Same as average risk.

Single first-degree with CRC or advanced adenoma diagnosed before age 60 years, or two first-degree relatives with CRC or advanced adenomas:

> *Recommended screening:* Colonoscopy every 5 years beginning at age 40 years or 10 years younger than age at diagnosis of the youngest affected relative

Familial Adenomatous Polyposis

Patients with classic FAP (>100 adenomas) should be advised to pursue genetic counseling and genetic testing, if they have siblings or children who could potentially benefit from this testing.

Patients with known FAP or who are at risk of FAP based on family history (and genetic testing has not been performed) should undergo annual flexible sigmoidoscopy or colonoscopy, as appropriate, until colectomy is deemed by physician and patient to be the best treatment.

Patients with retained rectum after subtotal colectomy should undergo flexible sigmoidoscopy every 6 to 12 months.

Patients with classic FAP, in whom genetic testing is negative, should undergo genetic testing for bi-allelic MYH mutations. Patients with 10 to 100 adenomas can be considered for genetic testing for attenuated FAP and if negative, MYH-associated polyposis.

Hereditary Nonpolyposis CRC

Patients who meet the Bethesda criteria should undergo microsatellite instability testing of their tumor or a family member's tumor, and/or tumor immunohistochemical staining for mismatch repair proteins.

Patients with positive tests can be offered genetic testing. Those with positive genetic testing, or those at risk when genetic testing is unsuccessful in an affected proband, should undergo colonoscopy every 2 years beginning at age 20 to 25 years, until age 40 years, then annually thereafter.

Modified from Rex DK, Johnson DA, Anderson JC, et al. American College of Gastroenterology guidelines for colorectal cancer screening 2008. Am J Gastroenterol 2009;104:739-750.

CT, Computed tomography, *FAP,* familial adenomatous polyposis; *FIT,* fecal immunochemical test; *HNPCC,* hereditary nonpolyposis colorectal cancer.

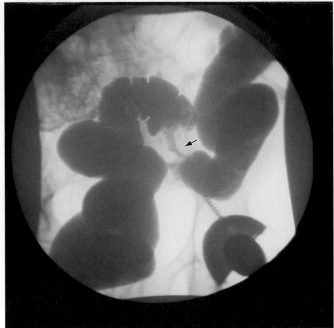
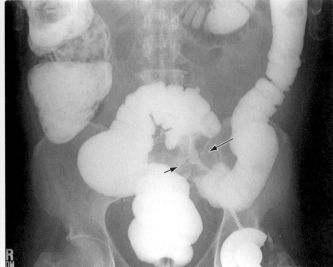

Figure 38-32 "Apple core" lesion in colon cancer. *(Courtesy Dr. Perry Pernicano.)*

do not have distal polyps. Although advocated as being more convenient than colonoscopy, because it is generally done in the office without the need for conscious sedation, only an estimated 30% of eligible patients undergo screening with flexible sigmoidoscopy (Nease et al., 2004). If polyps are identified during flexible sigmoidoscopy, a full colonoscopy is required to visualize the remaining colonic segments and to remove any remaining identified polyps.

Colonoscopy provides the most complete visualization of the entire colon and is the gold standard test for CRC screening. Since greater than half of all individuals who have advanced proximal adenomas may not have distal polyps, many investigators advocate the use of colonoscopy as the primary modality for CRC screening. The removal of precancerous adenomas decreases CRC incidence by as much as 76% to 90% compared with no screening methodology (Figs. 38-33 and 38-34). One study using colonoscopy as a screening tool in U.S. military veterans discovered advanced villous adenomas in 10.5% of subjects (Fig. 38-35). Colonoscopy carries a higher risk of adverse events attributed to therapeutic interventions such as biopsy and polyp removal, compared to FIT, DCBE, and flexible sigmoidoscopy, specifically bowel perforation and postpolypectomy hemorrhage.

Newer modalities for CRC screening are being developed. Virtual colonoscopy, or CT colonography, uses thin-section helical CT scans to generate high-resolution two-dimensional images that are reconstructed into three-dimensional images of the colon to evaluate for the presence of polyps. Direct comparison of CT colonography to colonoscopy in asymptomatic adults has shown sensitivity and specificity for polyp detection comparable to that of colonoscopy for polyps larger than 6 mm. CT colonography may be viewed as a more acceptable approach for CRC screening because it is less invasive and requires less time, without the potential adverse risks of sedation or bowel perforation. Most patients prefer conventional colonoscopy, reporting more pain, more

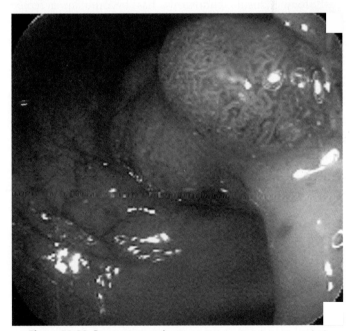

Figure 38-33 Precancerous adenomas. *(Courtesy Dr. Erik-Jan Wamsteker.)*

discomfort, and less respect from staff with CT colonography. As with conventional colonoscopy, CT colonography is limited by quality of the bowel preparation, procedural cost, lack of insurance coverage, variable physician training, and procedural time.

Capsule endoscopy is another emerging technology in the detection of CRC. The patient fasts overnight, ingests a disposable capsule, and begins water intake 2 hours after the capsule is ingested; the capsule is usually expelled within 48 hours of ingestion. The recorded information from the capsule is then downloaded and reviewed for abnormal

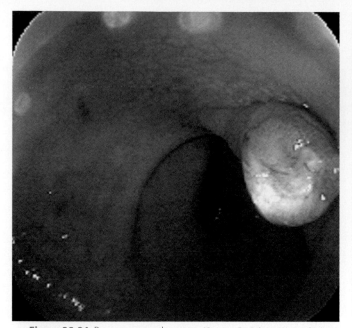

Figure 38-34 Precancerous adenomas. *(Courtesy Dr. Erik-Jan Wamsteker.)*

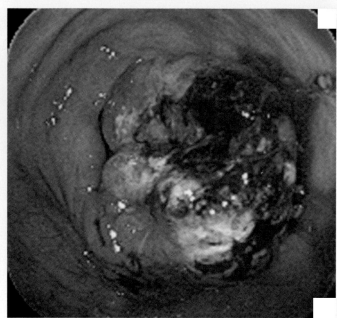

Figure 38-35 Advanced villous adenomas. *(Courtesy Dr. Erik-Jan Wamsteker.)*

pathology. Capsule endoscopy has become an accepted method for screening the small intestine for obscure GI bleeding. For colonic imaging, however, its use has been limited because of the larger colonic diameter, residual stool, and limited battery life of the capsule.

KEY TREATMENT

The removal of precancerous adenomas can significantly decrease colorectal cancer incidence by as much as 76% to 90% (Winawer et al., 1993) (SOR: A).

References

The complete reference list is available online at www.expertconsult.com.

Web Resources

www.gastro.org
  American Gastroenterological Association site contains useful practice parameters and position statements.
www.acg.gi.org
  American College of Gastroenterology site contains useful practice parameters and position statements.
www.guidelines.gov
  National Guideline Clearinghouse provides evidence-based practice guidelines.

www.nlm.nih.gov
  National Library of Medicine provides a thorough overview of disease processes.
http://daveproject.org
  Digital Atlas of Video Education contains real-time endoscopic footage of various gastrointestinal disorders.
www.aafp.org
  American Association of Family Physicians; topic-specific search of *American Family Physician* articles provides a concise overview of various diseases.

Hematology

Alan K. David

Overview

Key Point

- Iron deficiency anemia is more prevalent in children, women, and older adults.

Family physicians develop communication styles and relationships with patients and families that facilitate the physician's ability to define and prioritize patient problems, develop diagnostic and treatment plans for more common problems, and coordinate patients' care of less common problems with the rest of the health care system. Recognizing this primary function, the family physician needs to know how to diagnose a variety of conditions, understand their pathophysiology, know when and how to treat more common disorders, and know how to diagnose and refer more unusual disorders. This chapter organizes the subject of hematology by cellular, elemental, and functional categories; delineates the pathophysiology of hematologic disorders; and discusses the recognition, diagnostic criteria, and treatment of disorders more likely to be seen in family medicine.

Hematology is the study of the cellular elements of the blood—their origins, functions, and disorders. The frequency with which these disorders are discovered and treated in primary care varies with the population being served. The National Ambulatory Medical Care Survey of the 15 to 20 major diagnostic clusters seen in primary care practice by age group mentions only "anemia" in the cluster table of visits made by patients age 75 years and older (Woodwell and Cherry, 2004). In the National Health and Nutrition Examination Survey (NHANES 1999–2000), the prevalence of *iron deficiency anemia* was 7% in 1- to 2-year-old and 12% in 12- to 49-year-old females, versus 3% to 5% in 12- to 60-year-old males (NCHS, 2005a). This remains largely unchanged. In a practice largely populated by younger African American patients, predominantly women of child-bearing age, the prevalence of sickle cell anemia and iron deficiency anemia would be greater than in more heterogeneous populations. Disorders of white blood cells, such as neutropenia and leukemia, are encountered infrequently in most primary care practices. Nonetheless, understanding the presentation of uncommon disorders and their pathophysiology, diagnostic criteria, and treatment principles is imperative for a competent family physician.

Hematopoiesis: Regulation of Cellular Elements of Blood

Key Points

- Stem cells have self-renewal capability and differentiate into red blood cells, granulocytes, monocytes, lymphocytes, and platelets.
- Red cell production is controlled by erythropoietin and white cell production by granulocyte colony-stimulating factor.

Blood cell production normally takes place in the bone marrow, and all the circulating cellular elements of the blood arise from the level of a pluripotent hematopoietic stem cell (Fig. 39-1). Hematopoietic stem cells have two important properties, extensive self-renewal and ability to differentiate and mature into red blood cells, granulocytes

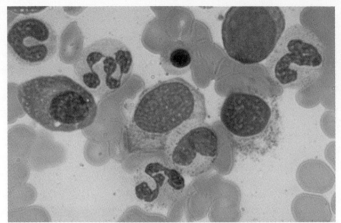

Figure 39-1 Common cellular elements seen in bone marrow aspirate, including plasma cell, polymorphonuclear neutrophil and band, eosinophil, and nucleated red blood cell. *(From the American Society of Hematology Image Bank image #505. Copyright 1996 American Society of Hematology, used with permission.)*

Table 39-1 Cellular Elements of the Blood (Adult)

Red Blood Cells (RBCs)	Men	Women
Hematocrit (%)	46.0 ±4.0	40.0 ±4.0
Hemoglobin (g/dL)	15.7 ±1.7	13.8 ±1.5
RBC count (×106/µL)	5.3 ±0.7	4.6 ±0.5
Reticulocytes (%)	1.6 ±0.5	1.4 ±0.5
Mean corpuscular volume (fl)	88.0 ±8.0	
Mean cell hemoglobin (pg/RBC)	30.4 ±2.8	
Mean cell hemoglobin concentration (g/dL of RBC)	34.4 ±1.1	
Red cell volume distribution width (RDW) (%)	13.1 ±1.4	
Platelets (/µL)	150,000-300,000	

White Blood Cells	Range (/µL)	Range (%)
All white blood cells	4300-10,000	100
Total neutrophils	2000-7000	20-70
Segmented neutrophils	1500-6000	15-60
Band neutrophils	500-1000	5-10
Lymphocytes	1500-4000	15-40
Monocytes	100-900	1-9
Eosinophils	100-700	1-7
Basophils	0-150	0-1.5

(neutrophils, eosinophils, basophils), monocytes, platelets, and lymphocytes (T cells, B cells, and NK cells). Little is known about the molecular mechanisms that control self-renewal, but this ability of stem cells is critical to the success of treatments such as bone marrow transplantation. More is known about the factors that control hematopoietic differentiation and maturation.

Hematopoietic stem cells are rare in number, estimated at approximately 1 in 1 × 10^6 bone marrow cells, or 0.05% of all marrow cells. The fact that they exist at all is best defined by their ability to support bone marrow regrowth after stem cell transplantation or marrow recovery after severe marrow suppression from chemotherapy or radiation. Two major lineages arise from the pluripotent hematopoietic stem cell: the common *myeloid* progenitor cell and the common *lymphoid* progenitor cell. Lymphopoiesis then proceeds to the differentiation of T cells, B cells, natural killer (NK) cells, and some dendritic cells. The common myeloid progenitor gives rise to red cells, granulocytes of all types, monocytes and macrophages (and some dendritic cells), and platelets.

The regulation of the terminal stages of hematopoietic differentiation and maturation is under the control of a variety of hormones and cytokines. Red cell production is under the control of erythropoietin (EPO), a glycoprotein hormone secreted by the kidney in response to hypoxia or anemia. Neutrophil production is under the control of granulocyte colony-stimulating factor (G-CSF). Eosinophil production is under the control of interleukin-5 (IL-5). Monocyte and macrophage production is under the control of macrophage colony-stimulating factor (M-CSF) and, to a lesser extent, granulocyte-macrophage colony-stimulating factor (GM-CSF). Platelet production is under the control of thrombopoietin (TPO), produced in the liver. TPO also stimulates proliferation and release of hematopoietic stem cells. Of these various growth factors, EPO and G-CSF have important uses clinically; TPO is under clinical development. The number of cellular elements in the blood is tightly controlled by these regulatory hormones. Table 39-1 shows the normal ranges for the various cellular elements of the blood in adults.

Disorders of Red Blood Cells

Key Points

- The RBC mass reflects the oxygen-carrying capacity of the body.
- Oxygen supply depends on RBC mass, lung function, circulatory system, supply of EPO, and bone marrow.

The major role of the red blood cell (RBC, erythrocyte) is to transport oxygen from the lungs to the tissues and organs in the body. This is accomplished by the reversible binding of oxygen to the heme moiety of the hemoglobin molecule. Hemoglobin (Hb) is the most prominent RBC protein. The functional ability of the Hb molecule is determined by primary amino acid structure, pH (Bohr effect), temperature, and intracellular concentration of 2,3-biphosphoglycerate (2,3-BPG). Abnormalities of Hb function most frequently result from mutations (amino acid substitutions) in one or more of the globin genes. These mutations, such as the mutation that causes sickle cell disease, can alter the stability of the Hb molecule or its oxygen-binding properties. Many of these mutations result in tissue hypoxia because the instability of the molecule results in the early death of the RBC in circulation (hemolysis). Other Hb mutations can affect oxygen binding and release or can produce free-globin chains that may bind to the inner RBC membrane, resulting in membrane instability (Heinz bodies). Hemoglobin is also recognized as the major "sink" of nitric oxide (NO) in the blood. This has important implications for the control of vascular tone in the microcirculation.

Under normal conditions, regulation of erythropoiesis can be viewed as a positive control loop. Red cell production is regulated by EPO. Production of EPO occurs primarily in the kidney, although a small amount is produced by the liver; this is a holdover from fetal life, when the liver was the major source of EPO production. EPO stimulates RBC production by binding to specific receptors on the surface of erythroid progenitor cells in the marrow. This activates a number of cell division steps that results in approximately 16 to 32 mature RBCs for each progenitor cell stimulated. These new RBCs leave the bone marrow and circulate for about 120 days as mature cells. The circulating red blood cells make up the RBC mass.

The RBC mass represents the oxygen-carrying capacity of the body. As RBCs traverse the circulation, the cells provide oxygen for all metabolic functions. In the kidney, oxygen availability is sensed by specialized peritubular capillary lining cells. The sensing mechanism is mediated by hypoxia-inducible factor 1α (HIF-1α). The adequacy of the oxygen supply depends not only on RBC mass, but also on normal lung function, a normal circulatory system that allows RBCs to be delivered effectively to all parts of the body, an adequate supply of EPO to stimulate RBC production, and a normally functioning bone marrow. Abnormalities in any of these factors can affect RBC production and result in anemia (too few RBCs) or erythrocytosis (too many RBCs).

Anemia

Key Points

- Anemia is a reduced RBC mass, resulting in decreased oxygen-carrying capacity of the blood (>2 SD from mean for age, gender, and race).
- Patients with unrecognized anemia often present with symptoms of fatigue, loss of stamina, shortness of breath, and tachycardia (with exercise).
- Acute blood loss or anemia is almost always caused by hemorrhage or hemolysis.
- Loss of 30% of blood volume results in postural symptoms; loss of 40% blood volume produces signs of shock.
- Bone marrow responsiveness to anemia is best evaluated by reticulocyte index and marrow production index.
- Anemias can be best understood by classifying them into three types: hypoproliferative anemia, maturation disorders, and hemolytic-hemorrhagic anemia.
- Anemia of chronic disease is a hypoproliferative anemia now referred to as the anemia of inflammation (AI).

- Serum ferritin is normal or increased in AI and low in true iron deficiency
- Treatment of folate deficiency with alcoholic neuropathy without confirming vitamin B_{12} deficiency may result in a progressively worsening neuropathy.
- Values below lower limits of normal for age/gender indicate only 25% likelihood that the person is *not* anemic.
- If creatinine is greater than 2 mg/dL and no other cause for anemia can be found, the anemia probably results from renal inefficiency.
- Bilirubin gallstones occur in 40% to 60% of sickle cell disease patients.
- The absence of free haptoglobin is diagnostic of hemolytic anemia.
- Sickle cell disease is a form of hemolytic anemia; thrombosis is more common in children, whereas hemorrhage occurs more often in adults with sickle cell disease.
- Coombs test is the diagnostic choice for autoimmune hemolytic anemia.

Definition

Anemia is best defined as a reduced RBC mass resulting in decreased oxygen-carrying capacity of the blood. Table 39-1 lists normal values for hemoglobin and hematocrit (Hct); values below the lower limits of normal for age and gender indicate only 25% likelihood that the person is not anemic. Previous Hb and Hct values for a given patient are useful comparisons when interpreting currently determined levels. Both pregnant women and long-distance athletes may have increases in plasma volume so that the Hct or the Hb value, or both, fall artificially below normal ranges. They still have a normal oxygen-carrying capacity with a normal RBC mass and should not be considered anemic. Conversely, a dehydrated patient admitted to the hospital may have Hb or Hct that appears normal because of plasma volume contraction. Correction of their volume-depleted state will allow appropriate determination of their true RBC oxygen-carrying capacity. When Hct or Hb is abnormal, further investigation is indicated, whether or not the subject appears clinically well.

Prevalence

Mean hemoglobin concentration for all U.S. males older than 1 year is 14.67 g/dL, and for females older than 1 year, 13.19 g/dL (NHANES-III; NCHS, 2005b). These values vary by ethnic group; non-Hispanic white males had mean Hb of 14.05 g/dL, versus 13.87 g/dL for Mexican Americans and 13.14 g/dL for African Americans. Hb values for African American men and women are 1 g/dL lower than their white counterparts. The median Hb concentration was the same for both genders in all race and ethnic groups younger than 9 years. Mean Hb level tends to peak at 15.4 g/dL between ages 20 and 29 years and decreases to 14.36 g/dL by age 70. Anemia is defined as Hb level more than 2 standard deviations (SD) from the mean for age and race for the entire population.

The most prevalent cause of anemia in the United States is iron deficiency. Table 39-2 categorizes the prevalence of iron deficiency and iron deficiency anemia (NHANES-III,

Table 39-2 Prevalence of Iron Deficiency and Iron Deficiency Anemia—United States

Age Group (yr)	Deficiency		Anemia	
	1988–1994	1999–2000	1988–1994	1999–2000
Both genders				
1-2	9%	7%	3%	2%*
3-5	3%	5%		
6-11	2%	4%		
Males				
12-15	1%*	5%†		
16-69	1%†	2%†		
≥70	4%	3%*		
Females				
12-49	11%	12%	4%	3%
12-15	9%	9%	2% (12-19)	2% (12-19)
16-19	11%	16%		
20-49	11%	12%	5%	
50-69	5%	9%	2%	3%*
≥70	7%	6%	2%	1%
Ethnic or racial group				
White	8%	10%		
Black	15%	19%		
Mexican American	19%	22%		

Modified from CDC. Iron deficiency—United States, 1999–2000. MMWR 2002;51:897-879; NCHS. NHANES, 1999–2000, 2005. http://www.cdc.gov/nchs/about/major/nhanes/nhanes99_00.htm; NCHS. NHANES-III, 1988–1994, 2005. http://www.cdc.gov/nchs/nhanes.htm.
*Unreliable comparison data.
†*p* ≥0.05 for survey comparisons.

1988–1994, 1999–2000; NCHS, 2005a, 2005b). The prevalence of iron deficiency is 9% and of iron deficiency anemia 3%, in both genders age 1 to 2 years. The prevalence for children age 3 to 5 years is 3% for iron deficiency and less than 1% for iron deficiency anemia; those 6 to 11 years old have a 2% prevalence of iron deficiency and less than 1% for iron deficiency anemia. The prevalence of iron deficiency in the nonblack population is 1% lower than the prevalence in all races combined. Women have a much higher prevalence; those age 12 to 15 have 9% prevalence of iron deficiency and 2% for iron deficiency anemia; those age 16 to 19 have 11% and 3% prevalence; women 20 to 49 years, 11% and 5%; and those 50 to 69 years, 5% and 2%, respectively. In women over age 70, prevalence of iron deficiency rises to 7% and iron deficiency anemia to 2%. Males in general have less than a 1% prevalence of iron deficiency or iron deficiency anemia until age 50, when the prevalence of iron deficiency rises to 2%. In those older than 70, prevalence of iron deficiency is 4% and iron deficiency anemia 2%.

In a comparative study (Netherlands, Japan, Poland, United States) of diagnostic encounters, blood disorders comprised 1% of all encounters, and iron deficiency was the 27th most frequent diagnosis seen in all four countries (Okkes et al., 2002). Anemia is the most frequent hematologic disorder seen in family medicine and occurs often enough that knowledge of RBC function, classification of RBC disorders, evaluation of laboratory data, and treatment of common anemias constitute an important part of the knowledge base of the competent family physician.

Clinical Features

Anemia is most often recognized by abnormal screening laboratory test results. Much less frequently, patients will present to their family physician with previously unrecognized anemia, complaining of fatigue, loss of stamina, shortness of breath, and rapid heart rate (particularly with physical exercise). In younger patients, if the anemia comes on gradually, several compensatory mechanisms help maintain tissue oxygenation. These include peripheral vasodilation, increased cardiac output, a change in the oxygen-hemoglobin dissociation curve that facilitates oxygen unloading in the tissues, and shunting of blood away from circulation-rich organs (e.g., gut, skin, kidney) to critical organs (e.g., heart, brain).

Physicians must recognize that the signs and symptoms of anemia will be determined in part by the acuteness of onset. Acute anemia is almost always caused by blood loss or hemolysis. If blood loss is mild, enhanced oxygen delivery is achieved through changes in the oxyhemoglobin dissociation curve and in hemodynamics. With acute blood loss, however, the changes in blood volume dominate the clinical picture, and Hct and Hb levels do not reflect the volume of blood lost for at least 48 hours. Signs of vascular instability appear with acute blood losses of 10% to 15% of the total blood volume. In such patients, management issues are related not to the anemia, but to hypotension and decreased organ perfusion. When more than 30% of the blood volume is lost suddenly, patients are unable to compensate with the usual mechanisms of vascular contraction and changes in regional or organ blood flow. The patient prefers to remain lying flat and will show postural hypotension and tachycardia if placed in an upright position. If the volume of blood loss is more than 40% (>2 L in average-sized adult), signs of shock are prominent, including confusion, air hunger, sweating, hypotension, and tachycardia. These patients have significant deficits in vital organ perfusion and require immediate volume replacement.

For the family physician, certain disorders are associated more often with anemia. These include chronic inflammatory states (e.g., infection, rheumatoid arthritis, cancer) associated with mild to moderate anemia, whereas lymphoproliferative disorders (e.g., chronic lymphocytic leukemia, other B-cell neoplasms) may be associated with immune-mediated hemolysis.

Laboratory Evaluation

Key laboratory tests in the office evaluation of the anemic patient include complete blood count (CBC), reticulocyte count, and iron studies (Box 39-1). The laboratory evaluation of anemia is designed primarily to determine effective response of the bone marrow to the anemia stimulus and to detect any disturbance in iron metabolism; this information allows physiologic classification of the most common anemias. The evaluation of the marrow's response to anemia is best approximated through corrected reticulocyte count (Fig. 39-2), which provides information about the number of newly released RBCs in circulation. Normally, a newly released RBC can be seen as a reticulocyte for about 24 hours. The reticulum of a reticulocyte is made up of residual ribosomal ribonucleic acid (RNA); the cell is somewhat larger and appears bluer than mature RBCs on a Wright-Giemsa–stained peripheral blood smear.

First, however, the raw reticulocyte percentage must be corrected if it is to reflect the marrow production index. The first correction of the reticulocyte count is for dilution, as shown by the following equation for determining reticulocyte index (RI):

$$RI = \text{Reticulocyte count (\%)} \times (\text{Patient's Hb or Hct}) / (\text{Normal Hb or Hct})$$

Box 39-1 Laboratory Tests in Office Evaluation of Anemia

1. Complete blood count (hemoglobin, hematocrit, red cell indices [MCV, MCH, MCHC], white cell count, and differential, platelet count)
2. Reticulocyte count (appropriately corrected)
3. Studies of iron status, including serum iron level, total iron-binding capacity (from which transferrin saturation [%] is calculated), and serum ferritin level

MCV, Mean corpuscular volume; *MCH*, mean cell hemoglobin; *MCHC*, mean cell hemoglobin concentration.

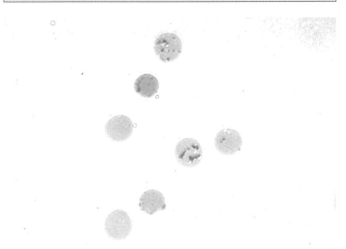

Figure 39-2 An increased number of reticulocytes are seen on a peripheral blood smear stained for reticulocytes. *(From the American Society of Hematology Image Bank image #1333. Copyright 1996 American Society of Hematology, used with permission.)*

The normal reticulocyte count is 1% to 2% and the normal RI is 1.0. This correction is not necessary if the laboratory reports reticulocyte count as an absolute number, normally about 40,000 to 50,000 cells/μL.

A further correction of the reticulocyte count is necessary if there is evidence from the peripheral blood smear that reticulocytes are being released prematurely from the bone marrow (shift cells or shift reticulocytes). Under these circumstances, reticulocytes live longer than the usual 24 hours in circulation, and thus the uncorrected reticulocyte count will overestimate the rate of new cell production. The second correction is shown by the equation for determining the marrow production index: MPI = RI/2. The normal MPI value is 1.0. The RI is divided by a factor of 2 to account for the prolonged reticulocyte life span in the circulation.

For example, if the reticulocyte count is 15% and Hct is 15%, there is evidence of shift reticulocytes on the peripheral smear. The MPI can be calculated as follows:

$$MPI = ([15\% \times 15\%]/45)2 = 2.5$$

Also critical to understanding the pathophysiology of most anemias is to characterize the availability of iron for hemoglobin synthesis. This is done by measuring the serum iron level, total iron-binding capacity (TIBC), and serum ferritin level. Transferrin saturation percent is the proportion of iron binding sites occupied by iron atoms, reflecting the amount of iron immediately available for Hb synthesis, and is very labile. Serum ferritin is an indirect reflection of the body's total iron stores and is more stable. These values provide information about the two most common forms of anemia seen in the hospital or in the family physician's office—iron deficiency anemia and the anemia of chronic inflammation.

Physiologic Classification

The physiologic classification of anemia is based on response of the bone marrow. The three major categories are hypoproliferative anemia, maturation disorders (ineffective erythropoiesis), and hemolytic-hemorrhagic anemia (Box 39-2).

Hypoproliferative Anemia

In hypoproliferative anemias the response of the bone marrow is impaired by one of three general mechanisms. The first is *marrow damage,* which results from an injury to the bone marrow and makes it impossible for the marrow to respond to adequate EPO stimulation. Aplastic anemia is a classic example, but chemotherapy-induced marrow aplasia is more common (Box 39-3). The physiologic hallmark of marrow damage is a low RPI (<2 at Hb >10 g/dL; <2.5 at Hb of 7-10 g/dL). EPO is typically elevated, with evidence of premature release of reticulocytes from the bone marrow (shift reticulocytes, including nucleated RBCs in some cases). Despite EPO stimulation, however, the bone marrow is unable to proliferate. Bone marrow examination may reveal an empty or hypocellular marrow or one replaced by tumor cells or fibrosis. Treating these patients with recombinant human EPO is rarely useful.

A second mechanism of hypoproliferation is *inflammation,* which is the most common form of anemia seen in hospitalized patients. Often referred to as the "anemia of chronic disease" (ACD), it has more recently been termed the *anemia of inflammation* (AI) (Weiss and Goodnough, 2005). The anemia associated with inflammatory states is complex and involves altered iron homeostasis as well as decreased EPO production and an impaired response of erythroid progenitor cells in the marrow to EPO. Inflammation comes in many forms in addition to acute and chronic infection. Also

associated with changes consistent with AI is tissue damage, as caused by necrosis, surgery, myocardial infarction, and other tissue injury.

The major effect of AI is on iron metabolism. With inflammation, iron absorption from the gut is blocked, as is iron release to transferrin from reticuloendothelial stores. The net effect is a decrease in the serum iron level and in transferrin saturation. This results in an inadequate supply of iron to the erythroid marrow for hemoglobin synthesis. Over time, the clinical picture (e.g., microcytic, hypochromic RBCs) may come to resemble true iron deficiency anemia, despite the fact that iron stores in the body are normal or increased. The mediator of these alterations in iron metabolism is *hepcidin,* a small molecule made in the liver that is critical to iron homeostasis and that is upregulated in the presence of inflammation. Hepcidin interferes with the cellular iron export protein *ferroportin*. The ferroportin pathway is the mechanism by which iron absorbed from the diet is shunted through the gut and reticuloendothelial cells and released to circulating transferrin. Iron regulatory proteins (IRP-1 and IRP-2) also play a role in balancing iron storage as well as circulating iron. Although there are many similarities to iron deficiency, providing iron in this setting is generally ineffective. Recombinant human EPO (epoetin) may stimulate RBC production, but the approach to treatment is primarily to identify and reverse, if possible, the inflammatory trigger.

In addition to changes in iron homeostasis, inflammation results in the release of proinflammatory cytokines such as IL-1, tumor necrosis factor alpha (TNF-α) and interferon γ (IFN-γ). These cytokines have many effects on erythropoiesis, such as decreasing EPO production and blunting the response of erythroid progenitors in the marrow to EPO. All these changes result in marrow hypoproliferation and an inadequate marrow response to anemia.

The third major category of hypoproliferative anemia is that associated with *inadequate EPO production,* which results in understimulation of the marrow. Typically, this is seen in patients with chronic renal insufficiency whose diseased kidney cannot produce EPO despite often profound anemia. The advent of successful renal replacement therapy (peritoneal or hemodialysis) has resulted in an increasingly large population of severely and chronically anemic patients. For these patients, epoetin therapy has been lifesaving in terms of quality of life and overall health.

Box 39-2 Classification of Anemias

Hypoproliferative anemias

Aplastic anemia
Anemia of inflammation
Chronic renal insufficiency
Hypothyroidism
Mild iron deficiency

Maturation disorders

Megaloblastic anemias
Myelodysplasia
Severe iron deficiency
Thalassemia syndromes

Hemolytic-Hemorrhagic anemia

Autoimmune hemolysis
Drug- or chemical-induced hemolysis
Acute or chronic blood loss
Sickle cell anemia

Box 39-3 Mechanisms of Marrow Damage

Aplasia

Drug-induced (immunologic)
Gold
Benzene
Autoimmune (idiopathic aplastic anemia)
Chemotherapy
Congenital anemia (Fanconi's, Blackfan-Diamond)

Marrow replacement

Metastatic malignancy
Leukemia
Fibrosis

In the family physician's office, the question often is how much anemia can be ascribed to mild or moderate renal insufficiency. There is no easy answer, but generally, if the creatinine level is higher than 2 mg/dL with no other obvious or reversible cause for the anemia (blood loss, hemolysis after appropriate testing), it is reasonable to ascribe the anemia to renal insufficiency.

Another pathologic process resulting in inadequate EPO stimulation is *hypometabolism*, particularly hypothyroidism. The anemia may reflect a reduced need for oxygen-carrying capacity because of the reduced metabolic load resulting from the thyroid hormone deficiency.

Mild iron deficiency anemia also is associated with a hypoproliferative marrow response. Iron deficiency, with mild to moderate anemia, impairs the erythroid marrow response. If the anemia is mild, circulating RBCs are normocytic or slightly microcytic, and the red cell distribution width (RDW) index is normal (Fig. 39-3). The serum iron is usually low, transferrin saturation less than 15%, and serum ferritin less than 15 ng/mL.

Table 39-3 compares anemia of inflammation and classic iron deficiency anemia. The major difference is the serum ferritin level, which is typically normal or increased with AI and characteristically low with true iron deficiency. Making this distinction is important because the mechanisms that lead to inflammation or iron deficiency are generally distinct, as is the approach to treatment.

Maturation Disorders

Maturation disorders are characterized by adequate EPO stimulation and erythroid marrow hyperplasia, but in the absence of a sufficiently increased reticulocyte production index. Under these conditions, premature cell death (apoptosis) takes place in the marrow, and a mismatch occurs between degree of erythroid hyperplasia on bone marrow aspiration or biopsy and the reticulocyte (effective) production index. Consequently, RBC production in such patients is considered ineffective and can involve nuclear or cytoplasmic maturation defects.

Nuclear maturation defects result in a megaloblastic bone marrow and are typical in patients with severe folate or vitamin B_{12} deficiency. The RBCs are macrocytic, and the reticulocyte production index is normal or slightly above normal (Fig. 39-4). Examining the bone marrow of patients with vitamin B_{12} or folate deficiency reveals increased erythroid marrow precursors and loosening of nuclear chromatin, as well as more cells with nuclear degeneration (karyorrhexis and karyolysis). These are the features of apoptosis.

Because of the degree of RBC destruction in the bone marrow, serum bilirubin may be elevated and haptoglobin decreased. It is important to distinguish between vitamin B_{12} and folate deficiency because the pathogenesis is different and the treatment must be specific. Patients who present with folate deficiency and alcoholic neuropathy pose a particularly difficult diagnostic challenge; the neuropathy of vitamin B_{12} deficiency should not be treated inappropriately with folic acid, because the anemia may be partly corrected with folic acid, but the neuropathy associated with vitamin B_{12} deficiency will progress. This is rarely seen at present. The neurologic symptoms may precede the anemia, so it is important to screen older adults with unexplained memory loss for vitamin B_{12} deficiency.

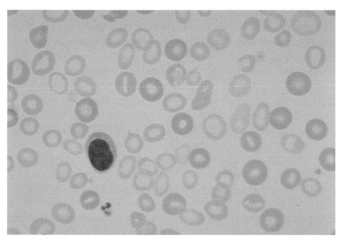

Figure 39-3 Hypochromic, microcytic red blood cells, with anisocytosis. *(From the American Society of Hematology Image Bank image #1214. Copyright 1996 American Society of Hematology, used with permission.)*

Table 39-3 Comparison of Anemia of Inflammation and Iron Deficiency Anemia

Iron Deficiency	Anemia of Inflammation
Low serum iron level	Low serum iron level
Elevated TIBC	TIBC normal or reduced
Transferrin saturation low (<15%)	Transferrin saturation low (15%-20%)
Serum ferritin level low (<15 ng/mL)	Serum ferritin level normal or elevated
Microcytic, hypochromic RBCs	Normocytic to microcytic RBCs
RBC protoporphyrin level elevated	RBC protoporphyrin level elevated

TIBC, Total iron-binding capacity; *RBCs,* red blood cells.

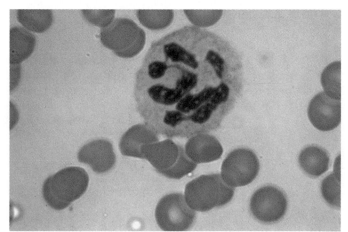

Figure 39-4 Megaloblastic changes of macrocytosis and hypersegmented neutrophils. *(From the American Society of Hematology Image Bank image #2611. Copyright 1996 American Society of Hematology, used with permission.)*

The diagnosis of these disorders is relatively straightforward and can be made with laboratory testing for serum vitamin B_{12} and folate levels. RBC levels of folate may also be useful, particularly in a folate-deficient patient receiving diet therapy or an undernourished alcoholic patient being fed. Alcohol inhibits the entry of folic acid, decreasing serum folic acid levels. Thus, folic acid deficiency may result from both dietary insufficiency and inhibition of folic acid release in patients with chronic alcohol intake. Folic acid deficiency has greatly decreased since 1998, when most grains began to be fortified with folic acid in the United States.

Treatment of vitamin B_{12} or folic acid deficiency is simply replacement with the appropriate vitamin. In patients who appear with severe megaloblastic anemia and who need treatment immediately, it is prudent to obtain blood samples, both whole blood and serum, for later diagnostic tests and then to treat the patient with both vitamins. This ensures that the anemia and central nervous system (CNS) manifestations of potential vitamin B_{12} deficiency are adequately treated.

The *Schilling test* is useful to specify the defect leading to B_{12} deficiency. This involves a small, oral dose of radiolabeled vitamin B_{12} along with a large, parenteral flushing dose of B_{12}. The B_{12} absorbed from the diet is excreted in the urine because there are no transport binding sites in the circulation. This first stage of the absorption test indicates if the patient can absorb vitamin B_{12}. The second stage is similar to the first, except the oral dose of B_{12} is given with intrinsic factor (IF). Theoretically, the addition of IF should correct the absorption defect associated with pernicious anemia. If the absorption defect is caused by disease of the terminal ileum, both stages of the Schilling test will be positive. A host of surrogate markers for pernicious anemia include measurement of IF or anti–parietal cell antibodies. However, these markers are positive in an increasing percentage of patients as they grow older, and consequently cannot be considered definitive for the diagnosis.

Another cause of a macrocytic anemia associated with ineffective erythropoiesis is *myelodysplasia.* The myelodysplastic syndromes are primary bone marrow neoplasms, and the macrocytosis does not respond to vitamin replacement therapy. This is now an increasingly frequent diagnosis, particularly because it is a more common diagnosis in older adults and the population is aging.

Transient megaloblastic and macrocytic anemia may be seen with certain types of anticancer drugs that interfere directly with DNA synthesis and cell division. Common drugs in this category include hydroxyurea and thymidine inhibitors. Family physicians also see patients with mild anemia and macrocytosis who have a history of excessive alcoholic intake, with or without a mild to moderate degree of liver disease. The macrocytosis in these cases has two probable causes: spurious macrocytosis caused by lipid loading of the RBC membrane, and macrocytosis caused by intermittent folate deficiency associated with bouts of high alcohol consumption in the absence of other caloric intake.

Iron Deficiency

In addition to nuclear maturation defects that result in macrocytic anemia, cytoplasmic maturation defects such as severe iron deficiency occur. Extreme iron deficiency and

severe anemia may result in a pattern of ineffective RBC production. With mild anemia, iron deficiency limits erythroid proliferation, and the anemia appears to be hypoproliferative. However, as anemia becomes more profound and EPO stimulation of the marrow increases, the marrow becomes more ineffective in appearance. In either case, laboratory test results indicating low serum iron, low transferrin saturation, and extremely low ferritin are diagnostic.

Once the diagnosis of iron deficiency is definitive, the family physician needs to consider the cause. Women in their childbearing years typically have marginal iron stores, and even being an occasional blood donor may result in mild anemia, with iron deficiency. The case is different in an adult male or postmenopausal woman. Unless there is a clear explanation, gastrointestinal (GI) blood loss should be the prime suspect and must carefully be ruled out.

Treatment of iron deficiency is not always straightforward. The goal is to remedy the hemoglobin deficit and replace iron stores. Many oral iron preparations are available, but ferrous sulfate and ferrous gluconate are most often used and inexpensive. The best regimen is to give 3 iron tablets daily; this provides about 150 mg of elemental iron daily. If the patient is compliant and absorption normal, reticulocytosis will occur in a week and Hb level will increase at least 1 g/dL within 2 weeks. Microcytosis may take up to 4 months to resolve. The iron is best taken on an empty stomach because certain foods interfere with iron absorption. However, 15% to 20% of patients will have significant gastric upset with oral iron and may not be compliant. If poor absorption or noncompliance is of concern, parenteral iron may be given. Several preparations are available, including iron sucrose and iron gluconate intravenously (IV) at 125 to 250 mg/day, and have a good safety profile compared with iron dextran. In treating iron deficiency, the target for therapy is not just to correct the anemia, but also to provide some degree of iron stores, so it is recommended that iron treatment be continued for 2 to 3 months after a normal Hb level is reached.

Various preparations of ferrous salts are equally tolerated and effective for the treatment of iron deficiency anemia. Controlled-release (CR) iron formulations cause fewer GI side effects than non-CR salt preparations, but discontinuation rates are similar. Ferrous salts are the treatment of choice for iron deficiency anemia (McDiarmid and Johnson, 2002).

Hemochromatosis in hereditary form has a homozygous incidence of 0.44% and a 10% heterozygous incidence, all in populations of white European descent. Elevated transferrin saturation levels (>45%-50%) and elevated ferritin levels (>300 mg/L) are markers of increased iron stores that may indicate the need for further evaluation.

Thalassemia

Severe cytoplasmic maturation defects are usually inherited and are characteristic of the thalassemic syndromes or defects in heme synthesis. The inherited thalassemias represent a large number of mutations in the globin genes themselves or in the regulation of globin gene expression. When either the alpha or the beta globin chains are produced in unequal amounts, the excess chains aggregate and the erythroid precursor cells die, leading to ineffective erythropoiesis. β-Thalassemia produces decreased numbers of beta chains and α-thalassemia decreased alpha chains. Homozygous β-thalassemia is one of the most severe forms of human anemia; more than 200 million people worldwide carry the β-thalassemia gene. Because of the large number of mutations that can result in thalassemia, most patients who have the clinical phenotype of homozygous thalassemia are compound heterozygotes. Homozygous α-thalassemia is not seen in adults because it results in hydrops fetalis in the newborn. β-Thalassemia trait and α-thalassemia trait, however, are common but are usually associated with only mild anemia.

With increasing numbers of immigrants from Southeast Asia, there are more people with a complex thalassemia syndrome, known as *hemoglobin Constant Spring*, who might be seen in practice. Obtaining a definitive diagnosis is important so as not to prescribe iron or other therapies inappropriately.

Hemolytic-Hemorrhagic Anemia

Hemolytic-hemorrhagic anemia (HHA) is diagnosed in patients with persistent anemia or decreasing Hb and Hct levels despite what appears to be an adequate bone marrow erythropoietic response. For patients with chronic hemolytic disease, this means a marrow production index of 3. In patients with hemorrhagic disease, this level of production may not be reached quickly because of the ongoing iron loss, and production indices about 2 to 2.5 times normal are more common. In the latter case, however, blood loss dominates the clinical picture unless the loss is internal.

In a discussion of the hemolytic anemias, which can be complex to diagnose, it is helpful to consider the pathophysiology of disease and how to categorize the hemolytic process. One should first consider whether the hemolysis appears to be intravascular or extravascular.

Intravascular Hemolysis

Intravascular hemolysis is associated with the rupture of erythrocytes and dispersion of their contents into the plasma. This results in free hemoglobin in the plasma and, if sufficient RBC destruction takes place, there is Hb spillover into the urine (hemoglobinuria). The primary Hb-binding protein in the plasma is haptoglobin, but in the presence of intravascular hemolysis, free haptoglobin becomes undetectable. This is a useful test only if the results are negative because ineffective RBC production, associated with substantial destruction of RBCs in the bone marrow (or even primarily extravascular hemolysis), will result in the release of sufficient Hb to reduce circulating haptoglobin levels.

Intravascular hemolysis can be life threatening if acute and can have several causes. For example, RBC membrane damage and intravascular hemolysis can result from burns or exposure to certain toxins that target the RBC membrane, such as *Clostridium perfringens*. Hypotonic lysis is rarely seen but could occur because of the IV infusion of free water. Immune-mediated lysis of RBCs can occur when mismatched transfusions are given. With ABO incompatibility, the operative mechanism is immunoglobulin M (IgM) antibodies that fix complement to the RBC surface and cause rapid lysis.

Mechanical fragmentation is probably the most common form of intravascular hemolysis seen in North America and is associated with microvascular diseases such as thrombotic thrombocytopenic purpura, *hemolytic uremic syndrome* (HUS; Fig. 39-5), defective mechanical heart valves, and disseminated intravascular coagulation. Acute attacks of malaria

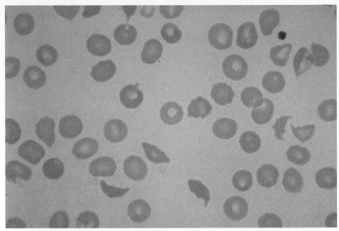

Figure 39-5 Schistocytes and helmet cells characteristic of a hemolytic process (hemolytic uremic syndrome). *(From the American Society of Hematology Image Bank image #4678. Copyright 1996 American Society of Hematology, used with permission.)*

are also associated with intravascular hemolysis. *Paroxysmal nocturnal hemoglobinuria* (PNH) is an unusual form of intravascular hemolysis caused by an acquired X-linked defect in the hematopoietic stem cell. Patients with PNH have varying degrees of hemolysis throughout the day, and in crisis, this can be severe.

An inherited condition that predisposes patients to intravascular hemolysis is the Mediterranean form of *glucose-6-phosphate dehydrogenase* (G6PD) *deficiency*. G6PD deficiency is the most common inborn error of RBC metabolism worldwide, affecting almost 0.5 billion people. Because it is an X-linked genetic disorder, it is most severe in men. G6PD protects RBCs from oxidative stressors such as superoxide anions and hydrogen peroxide. Oxidative products in RBCs are normally neutralized by reduced glutathione, which is generated by glutathione reductase. This pathway is part of the hexose monophosphate shunt pathway and requires G6PD for proper functioning. The Mediterranean abnormality of G6PD deficiency is associated with moderate chronic hemolysis, but this may become overwhelming and even fatal when the RBCs are exposed to oxidative stress. Any oxidative stress in these patients may have severe clinical consequences that could require transfusion or exchange transfusion as part of therapy.

The more common variety of G6PD deficiency in North America is G6PD^{A-}, which affects approximately 10% of the African American population. G6PD^{A-} is an enzyme with reduced stability and catalytic activity that become more prominent as the red cell ages. In these people, hemolytic events typically involve older RBCs and are therefore benign and relatively self-limited. The accumulation of oxidized glutathione reacts with hemoglobin and causes precipitation of Hb into Heinz bodies, resulting in hemolytic disease. The hemolytic process can be enhanced by infection, surgical stress, diabetic acidosis, and certain medications, such as the antimalarials primaquine and quinacrine.

Extravascular Hemolysis

Contrasted with intravascular hemolysis is the destruction of RBCs that occurs primarily in the reticuloendothelial system (RES), so-called extravascular hemolysis. The primary site of destruction is outside the vascular compartment, in the liver, spleen, and bone marrow. A form of extravascular hemolysis is the ineffective RBC production seen with nuclear or severe cytoplasmic maturation defects. More common sites for extravascular destruction are the liver and particularly the spleen. Again, it is useful to determine whether the hemolysis is congenital or acquired. Congenital forms include inherited hemoglobinopathies (thalassemias, sickle cell disease), inherited membrane defects (hereditary spherocytosis or elliptocytosis), and enzyme defects. Defective RBC metabolism usually causes hemolysis by creating unstable Hb or by failing to generate adequate adenosine triphosphatase (ATP) to maintain RBC membrane plasticity, as occurs in pyruvate kinase deficiency; this autosomal recessive disorder is the most common enzyme deficiency of the glycolytic pathway. Most patients with pyruvate kinase deficiency have a mild anemia and generally do not require transfusions.

Sickle Cell Anemia

Sickle cell anemia is an inherited autosomal condition in which glutamic acid in the sixth position on the β-globin chain is replaced by a valine (Glu6Val). This results in hemoglobin SS in the homozygous state. Sickle cell trait, or hemoglobin AS, is found in 8% to 10% of African Americans in the United States, and sickle cell anemia occurs in about 1 in 400, or about 70,000 individuals. The gene for HbS is prevalent in sub-Saharan Africa. Persons of Mediterranean descent from India or Saudi Arabia have varying but somewhat lower percentages of the carrier state for HbSS. Sickle cell anemia occurs worldwide but predominates in Mediterranean, Saudi Arabian, and Indian populations. This distribution appears to be associated with independent mutations in these regions. People with hemoglobin AS or SS are somewhat protected against malaria because their erythrocytes are resistant to invasion by malarial parasites. If the parasite infects the cell, the rate of sickling increases, causing the cell with the parasite to be removed from the circulation more rapidly.

The pathophysiology of the sickling process is related to the oxygenation of the molecule. When deoxygenated, HbSS tends to polymerize into long, tubelike fibrils. This results in an elongated, rigid cell subject to trapping in the microcirculation, resulting in vaso-occlusive crisis. Hypoxemia, acidosis, dehydration of the RBC, hyperosmolality of the renal medulla, and viral infections can play a role in triggering or accentuating the sickling process. Sickled RBCs are also more adhesive to endothelial cells, activate endothelial cells, and contribute to the interaction between neutrophils and activated endothelium in the microvasculature. When the conditions that cause sickling are corrected, the sickle cell may return to a more normal shape and function. However, some sickled RBCs are irreversibly changed, indicating that the membrane cytoskeleton has been damaged. Irreversibly sickled cells are generally removed in the sinusoidal RES networks, but approximately one-third may be hemolyzed intravascularly. Some degree of anemia has a protective effect in vaso-occlusive crises by helping reduce blood viscosity and deoxygenation, thereby reducing the likelihood of polymerization.

During vaso-occlusive crises, the microvascular capillaries, capillary bed, and veins become occluded. Contributing to this locally are low pH, prolonged capillary transit time, and infection. Increased numbers of sickled RBCs occlude the vessels, which leads to painful ischemia, infarction, and reduced organ function over time. Areas particularly affected include the portal circulation, in which oxygen tension is low; the kidney, in which the renal medulla is hyperosmolar and dehydrates RBCs, increasing mean corpuscular hemoglobin concentration (MCHC); the lungs; and the brain. It is not clear why some patients have severe, frequent episodes and others do not. *Avascular necrosis* of the bone marrow is usually the cause of severe pain.

Clinical Diagnosis

A patient with sickle cell disease usually has chronic hemolysis that results in a moderate anemia, intermittent jaundice, and a marrow with a thinned, bony cortex. Vaso-occlusive episodes and the appearance of Howell-Jolly bodies occur by the time the patient becomes an adult. The presence of Howell-Jolly bodies indicates that the patient has undergone an autoinfarction of the spleen.

The diagnosis of sickle cell disease is easily made by finding sickled cells on the peripheral smear, preparing a sickle cell sample, and carrying out a screening hemoglobin electrophoresis, which will confirm the Hb type. For a sickle cell preparation, blood is mixed with 2% sodium metabisulfite, which produces sickling. The proportion of sickled cells is measured initially and then 1 hour later to make the diagnosis. The "gold standard" diagnosis is Hb electrophoresis, which shows the relative amounts of Hb forms.

Patients with long-standing sickle cell anemia may have pain syndromes related to bone marrow vaso-occlusive crises and aseptic necrosis of the femoral head. Bilirubin gallbladder stones occur in 40% to 60% of patients. Hepatic and cardiac complications may also develop. Other associated problems include vascular occlusion in the pulmonary bed, leading to acute chest syndrome. Breakdown of the skin over bony prominences in the lower extremities is common and may lead to chronic, poorly healing ulcers. Papillary necrosis of the kidney may occur and, with age, renal function may decline. In the eye, conditions such as hemorrhage and neovascularization may occur. Patients with sickle cell anemia are particularly susceptible to *Salmonella* infections because of decreased complement activation, and asplenic patients are also subject to an increased likelihood of infection from encapsulated organisms such as *Pneumococcus*. Patients with sickle cell anemia should be given Pneumovax vaccine to prevent streptococcal pneumonia and sepsis. *Haemophilus influenzae* infection is responsible for a high percentage of pneumonia cases in sickle cell anemia patients.

Neurologically, patients with sickle cell anemia are subject to cerebrovascular accident (CVA, stroke). Particularly disturbing, children with severe sickle cell anemia will have evidence of multiple small strokes on magnetic resonance imaging (MRI) or computed tomography (CT) of the head by age 10 years. This has been associated with learning impairments in affected children. Aggressive transfusion protocols have been tested to reduce the incidence of this complication, with some success. Thrombosis is more common in children, whereas hemorrhage is more common in adults, possibly because of the occlusion of small vessels in hypoxic situations. Also, sickled cells show increased attraction to the endothelium, causing proliferation of the endothelial intimal surface, which can contribute to vascular occlusion. There is a high rate of recurrent stroke within 3 years of the initial event. Parvovirus infection can also cause pure RBC aplasia in these patients and lead to a devastating exacerbation of the anemia.

Treatment

Patients with sickle cell anemia should have Hb and Hct maintained at moderately low level to protect against vaso-occlusive complications related to viscosity. Patients with a painful crisis should be put on bed rest, hydrated vigorously, and given oral analgesics. Nonsteroidal anti-inflammatory drugs (NSAIDs), antihistamines, and benzodiazepines may also be helpful. Mild alkalinization of the blood is recommended. Oxygen should be given by nasal cannula or mask to keep the hemoglobin well oxygenated. Parenteral narcotics are rarely necessary, especially if the patient is given large volumes of fluid, oxygen, and oral morphine (or similar preparation) for pain control. Avascular necrosis of the bone marrow causes severe pain, and the patient may require intravenous (IV) narcotics and hydration for pain control.

Treatment with drugs that increase the proportion of fetal hemoglobin (HbF) show promise. Mixed polymers of HbF and HbS do not have the same propensity to sickle as SS tetramers. Azacitidine (5-AZA) increases the proportion of HbF but has significant toxicity. Hydroxyurea increases HbF level, which often results in fewer painful episodes, hospital admissions, and transfusions. The goal is to raise HbF level, if possible, to 20% to 30% of the total hemoglobin. Mortality can be reduced by as much as 40%. Unfortunately, not all patients respond to these types of interventions. Because both are antitumor drugs, azacitidine and hydroxyurea have significant toxicity, such as tumor induction. Gene therapies are being investigated but are not yet successful. In severe situations, allogenic (sibling) bone marrow transplantation has been tried, resulting in an 86% event-free survival at 5 years after transplant (Bhetia and Walters, 2008).

Patients undergoing surgery with general anesthesia are at increased risk of hypoxemia, sickling, and sickle cell crisis. They should be transfused before surgery with packed RBCs to bring the HbA level to 50% or higher. This decreases the likelihood of sickle cell episodes.

Pregnancy increases the risk of vaso-occlusive crisis for the mother. There is a high incidence of fetal loss among women who have sickle cell anemia. Vaso-occlusive episodes in the placenta may result in lower-birth-weight infants or fetal death.

Sickle Cell Trait

Patients with sickle cell trait are heterozygous for the sickle gene and have a much lower likelihood of sickling than those who are homozygous. Most heterozygotes are asymptomatic throughout life. Patients with sickle cell trait, however, may develop complications if put into an extremely hypoxic environment such as high altitude, suffer heat stroke and dehydration, or acquire pulmonary infections.

Acquired Forms of Hemolysis

The acquired forms of reticuloendothelial or extravascular hemolysis are dominated by patients with acquired immune-mediated hemolytic disease. Patients with *autoimmune hemolytic anemia* (AHA) can present with severe anemia; this is usually associated with another disease such as a collagen vascular disease (e.g., rheumatoid arthritis, severe systemic lupus erythematosus) or drugs, or it is idiopathic. AHA is uncommon but can be dramatic on presentation. About 50% of patients have no associated disease. The Coombs antiglobulin test, performed directly and indirectly determines the presence of antibody coating the patient's RBCs or free antibody in the plasma capable of binding to RBCs in AHA diagnosis. The autoantibodies may fix complement or may target the red cell for phagocytosis by the RES.

Therapy of AHA depends on the severity and causative mechanism. If the AHA is drug-induced, it is often sufficient to stop the drug and wait for the antibodies to clear, although this may take some time. Drug-induced hemolytic disease is uncommon and requires a specialized laboratory to make a precise diagnosis. AHA associated with collagen vascular diseases, lymphomas, or Hodgkin's disease may be controlled with treatment of the primary underlying condition. The mainstay of treatment of AHA is high-dose corticosteroid therapy, at least 1 mg/kg of prednisone daily; refractory cases may require up to 2 mg/kg/day. Patients who do not respond to steroid therapy may be candidates for splenectomy, because the spleen is the primary site of removal of antibody-coated RBCs. Other drugs used as second- and third-line therapies for their immunosuppressive effects include cyclophosphamide, chlorambucil, and intravenous immune globulin (IVIG).

A final mechanism of acquired extravascular hemolysis is *hypersplenism.* Typically, patients with hypersplenism have an enlarged spleen because of infiltrative disease of the spleen, or they have splenomegaly as a result of portal hypertension. Under these circumstances, the RBCs are trapped for an unusually long period in the splenic circulation. Splenectomy may be beneficial.

Polycythemia

Polycythemia (or *erythrocytosis*) is the overproduction of red blood cells (erythrocytes). The mechanism of action resulting in polycythemia may be primary or secondary. *Primary* polycythemia indicates that the disorder arises at the level of the hematopoietic stem cells (see later), whereas *secondary* polycythemia represents the overproduction of RBCs caused by the increased stimulation of the bone marrow by EPO.

Polycythemia is typically identified initially in the laboratory by Hb and Hct values that are substantially above normal, requiring an explanation. Hb values of 18 to 20 g/dL lie in a range in which it is unclear whether the elevated Hb is caused by increased RBC production or a decreased plasma volume. In the latter case, the elevated Hb and Hct levels are caused by a contraction of the plasma volume and not by an increase in the RBC mass, so-called spurious polycythemia (pseudopolycythemia), or Gaisbock's syndrome, and may not warrant therapeutic intervention. Typically, Hb level above 20 g/dL is unequivocally associated with increased RBC mass.

In the evaluation of patients with polycythemia or suspected polycythemia, it is important to first establish that the RBC mass has increased. This is achieved through direct measurement of the red cell mass using isotope dilution techniques, and the test can be performed at most large hospitals. Once that issue has been resolved, and assuming that there is evidence of RBC overproduction, it is important to determine whether the polycythemia is primary or secondary by measuring the circulating EPO level. If elevated, causes of the increased EPO production to consider include heart or chronic pulmonary disease, in which there is desaturation of Hb as it leaves the lungs, or less common causes such as renal cysts, hepatic or cerebellar tumors, uterine leiomyoma, or impaired Hb function caused by heavy smoking, which results in elevated levels of carboxyhemoglobin, which is essentially inert as an oxygen transporter. Severe obstructive sleep apnea may cause enough desaturation to raise EPO levels, resulting in secondary polycythemia. Athletes using EPO, androgens, or blood doping may also present with secondary polycythemia.

Certain forms of polycythemia are inherited. These can be associated with mutations in the Hb molecule that increase Hb's affinity for oxygen, making it more difficult to offload oxygen within the tissues. These are referred to as "high-affinity mutants," and more than 20 have been identified. It is important to identify the various possibilities because different causative factors have different long-term consequences.

Primary polycythemia, or *polycythemia vera* (PV), is a disorder of the hematopoietic stem cell. It is acquired typically in midlife and thereafter and, when full-blown, is associated with an increase in the platelet count, white cell count, splenomegaly, and severe itching following hot showers or baths. Pruritus can be disabling and presumably results from degranulation of skin basophils. Unlike secondary forms of erythrocytosis, EPO level is in the normal or low-normal range.

Treatment of PV strives to reduce the RBC mass to normal. Because PV is usually associated with an increase in total blood volume, the goal of phlebotomy therapy should be Hb and Hct levels in the normal range. Eventually, repeated phlebotomies induce iron deficiency, which is a reasonable end point. For patients with more aggressive disease (e.g., a growing spleen, increasing white cell and platelet counts), hydroxyurea therapy is effective. The goal is to maintain blood counts as close to normal as possible, or at least in an acceptable range.

Myeloproliferative Disorders

Polycythemia vera is one of a group of conditions referred to as the myeloproliferative disorders. These include essential thrombocytosis (ET) and agnogenic myeloid metaplasia with myelofibrosis (AMM/MF), also known as idiopathic myelofibrosis. All these disorders are characterized by the overproduction of one or more cell types. In PV the clinical picture is dominated by the increased production of RBCs. In ET the clinical picture is dominated by increased numbers of platelets, which may reach values as high as $2 \times 10^6/\mu L$. With AMM/MF the clinical picture is dominated by various cytopenias associated with marrow fibrosis and splenomegaly. Splenomegaly, in this case, likely represents extramedullary hematopoiesis.

Many features of these diseases overlap. In PV, the spent phase may resemble myelofibrosis. Some patients with ET will eventually manifest an increased RBC mass. The occasional overlapping and thus confusing nature of these disorders has been partially explained by the recent demonstration of a very high frequency of a point mutation in a signaling molecule on the EPO signaling pathway (Kralovics et al., 2005). In several reports, almost two thirds to three quarters of patients with PV had this mutation in *JAK2*, with lower frequencies seen in patients with ET and AMM/MF. The mutation results in a constitutively activated pathway and the overproduction of bone marrow cellular elements.

It can be anticipated that this will become a useful molecular test in the differential diagnosis of these disorders and will almost certainly become a target for drug development.

In ET the peripheral smear reveals increased numbers of platelets of various sizes. Platelet counts may be high, in excess of 1 or $2 \times 10^6/\mu L$. There may be an associated leukocytosis, and Hb level is typically normal. The decision to treat such patients is not always easy. Generally, patients with platelet count approaching $1 \times 10^6/\mu L$ are treated, even with no associated symptoms or signs. Asymptomatic young women with ET require special consideration; watchful waiting is probably sufficient, although hydroxyurea plus aspirin is the most effective approach for patients who require treatment.

Patients with AMM/MF tend to run an indolent course. Usually, over time, the spleen continues to enlarge, and peripheral RBC destruction increases. There also may be varying degrees of thrombocytopenia caused by impaired bone marrow production and increased splenic sequestration. In all the myeloproliferative disorders, platelet function may be abnormal. Treatment of AMM/MF is largely symptomatic. The anemia can be treated with transfusions, or epoetin therapy can be attempted, although no good clinical trials support these approaches. In advanced cases of myeloid metaplasia, the spleen may grow to such a size that it may require removal to stabilize peripheral blood counts. Proper management of all the myeloproliferative disorders is associated with extended survival.

KEY TREATMENT

Different preparations of iron salts are equally well tolerated and effective in the treatment of iron deficiency anemia. Controlled-release iron preparations have fewer GI side effects but similar discontinuation rates, so they are no more effective (McDiarmid and Johnson, 2002) (SOR: A).

Pneumovax vaccine should be given to patients with sickle cell disease because they tend to undergo auto splenectomy (Nabel, 2009) (SOR: B).

Treatment of a sickle cell crisis consists of rest, hydration, and oral analgesics, such as NSAIDs, antihistamines, and oral morphine (Nabel, 2009) (SOR: B).

In severe cases of sickle cell, allogenic (sibling) bone marrow transplantation results in an 86% event-free survival at 5 years (Bhetia and Walters, 2008) (SOR: B).

High-dose corticosteroid therapy is the treatment of choice for autoimmune hemolytic anemia (Nabel, 2009) (SOR: B).

White Blood Cells

Key Points

- Leukocytosis is WBC count 2 SD above the mean, generally higher than 11,000/μL.
- Only 10% of all neutrophils are found in the peripheral blood, where they survive only 6 to 10 hours.
- Neutrophilia is caused by inflammation, stress, or steroid therapy.
- Infection is probable when band neutrophils are more than 20% of the total WBC count and Döhle bodies and toxic granulations are seen.
- The risk of severe infection does not usually occur unless the absolute neutrophil count is less than 500/μL.

The white blood cells (WBCs, leukocytes) are made up of neutrophils, lymphocytes, eosinophils, basophils, monocytes, and plasma cells, although plasma cells are rarely found in the circulation. Most are produced in the bone marrow and some primarily in lymphoid tissue. The normal WBC count ranges from approximately 4300 to 10,000 cells/µL with some variation, depending on the laboratory reference control samples. An abnormal WBC count can be defined as more than 2 SD from the mean of 7000 cells/µL.

Leukocytosis is defined as a WBC count 2 SD higher than the mean, generally greater than 11,000 cells/µL. WBCs are composed of two types of cells with different functions. *Phagocytic cells*, consisting of neutrophils, eosinophils, monocytes, and macrophages, are primarily responsible for the ingestion and killing of microorganisms. *Lymphocytes* are responsible for cellular-mediated immunity and humoral immunity expressed through the production of antibodies. Table 39-4 lists normal WBC values and ranges. White cells produce cytokines (interleukins and growth factors), vasoactive substances, and enzymes, which allow them to interact and formulate immune responses. This section focuses primarily on phagocytic cells and their disorders; lymphocytes and lymphocytic disorders are discussed in a later section. When a patient has an increasing number or severity of bacterial or fungal infections, or both, abnormalities of phagocytic cells should be suspected. Conversely, when any phagocytic cell line is increased, such as neutrophils or eosinophils, an infectious process should be suspected.

Types of White Blood Cells

See online text for discussion of granulocytes, eosinophils, and monocytes/macrophages.

Disorders of Neutrophils

Neutrophilia

Neutrophilia is defined as a WBC count higher than 10,000 cells/µL plus an absolute neutrophil count more than 2 SD above the mean, or higher than 7000 cells/µL. The *absolute neutrophil count* (ANC) can be calculated by multiplying the total WBC count by the percentage of polymorphonuclear neutrophil (PMN) leukocytes and bands (PMNs + bands)

Table 39-4 Normal White Blood Cell (WBC) Counts in Peripheral Blood

WBC Type	Range (cells/µL)	Range (%)
All white cells	4300-10,000	100
Total neutrophils	2000-7000	20-70
Segmented neutrophils	1500-6000	15-60
Band neutrophils	500-1000	5-10
Lymphocytes	1500-4000	15-40
Monocytes	100-900	1-9
Eosinophils	100-700	1-7
Basophils	0-150	0-1.5

in the WBC differential. There are two major categories of neutrophilia, primary and secondary. *Primary* neutrophilia is related to defects in the production or maturation of neutrophil precursors in the bone marrow, associated with conditions such as chronic myelogenous leukemia (CML) and PV. Rare genetic forms of neutrophilia include the type associated with Down syndrome infants, who may express intermittent leukemoid reactions. In the presence of an enlarged spleen, myelocytic precursors in the peripheral blood, increased levels of basophils and eosinophils, and a low leukocyte alkaline phosphatase (LAP) level, the diagnosis of CML is highly probable. Unless neutrophilia is caused by a myeloproliferative syndrome, treatment is usually not indicated.

Secondary neutrophilia is caused primarily by three major mechanisms: inflammation (or infection), stress, and steroid therapy. *Inflammation* can result from active inflammation or infection; cigarette smoking; burns, surgery, or trauma; and vaccination or snakebite. *Stress* may be caused by pregnancy and spontaneous or cesarean delivery; chronic anxiety state, panic disorders, posttraumatic stress disorder, and depression; vigorous exercise; splenectomy; and sickle cell disease.

The physician must consider the history and physical examination to determine the appropriate diagnosis for the cause of neutrophilia. *Severe* neutrophilia (30,000-50,000 cells/µL and higher) is called a *leukemoid reaction* and is related to severe infections such as sepsis, hemorrhagic shock, and major tissue injury, but must be distinguished from acute or chronic leukemia. Infections and chronic inflammation may change the characteristics of neutrophils in the peripheral circulation. Increasing numbers of young cells, such as bands and metamyelocytes, the presence of Döhle bodies (residual endoplasmic reticulum), and toxic granulations are indicators of infectious and inflammatory causes of neutrophilia. Recognition allows the probable cause to be appropriately treated, particularly because treatment of chronic inflammation, infection, and stress is different.

A pseudoleukocytosis occasionally occurs, usually related to clumping of platelets in a blood sample, which alters the electronic determinations of WBC and platelet counts. Platelet clumping may be related to inadequate anticoagulation of the blood sample or the presence of abnormal proteins in a patient's blood, leading to platelet clumping. Cold, insoluble plasma proteins, known as cryoglobulins, may also cause increased WBC and platelet counts, particularly when the patient's temperature is 30° C (86° F) or lower.

The highest specificity for the presence of infection occurs when more than 20% of the total WBC count is made up of band neutrophils. The highest sensitivity for infection is the presence of Döhle bodies, toxic granulations, and cytoplasmic vacuoles when the peripheral smear is examined. The most accurate predictor of the presence of acute inflammation is a total WBC count higher than 10,500 cells/µL (Neutrophilia, 2009).

Neutropenia

Neutropenia is defined as ANC less than 1800 cells/µL, approximately 2 SD below the mean, and includes both mature PMN and band forms. Some ethnic populations, such as those of African descent or Yemenite Jews, may have a lower total WBC count and ANC that can be normal at 1000 neutrophils/µL. The primary concern with neutropenia is the risk of infection. Severe infection does not usually occur unless ANC is less than 500 cells/μL (Table 39-5). When severe neutropenia occurs, patients are at risk for serious infection from breaks in cutaneous or mucosal barriers in areas such as the GI tract or oropharynx. If they are taking corticosteroids, the risk of infection in the presence of neutropenia is greatly enhanced because of the steroidal effect on immune responsiveness.

As with RBC disorders, neutropenia can be classified as production disorders, maturation disorders, and increased destruction disorders (Box 39-4). Production disorders may be congenital or caused by genetic abnormalities, such as cyclic neutropenia, characterized by recurrent mouth infec-

Table 39-5 Relation of Absolute Neutrophil Count (ANC) to Risk of Infection

ANC (cells/μL)	Risk/Management
>1500	None.
1000-1500	No significant risk of infection; fever can be managed on outpatient basis
500-1000	Some risk of infection; fever can occasionally be managed on outpatient basis.
<500	Significant risk of infection; fever should always be managed on inpatient basis with parenteral antibiotics; clinical signs of infection present.
<200	Very significant risk of infection; fever should always be managed on inpatient basis with parenteral antibiotics; clinical signs of infection may be late phenomena.

From Neutrophilia. http://www.uptodate.com. November 2009.

Box 39-4 Classification of Neutropenia

Production disorders

Congenital neutropenia
Cyclic neutropenia
Chédiak-Higashi syndrome
Cancer drugs (cyclophosphamide, methotrexate, azathioprine)

Maturation disorders

Vitamin B_{12}, folate deficiencies
Myelodysplastic syndromes
Viral infections

Disorders of Increased destruction

Immune induction agents
Postinfection disorders (HBV, EBV, HIV/AIDS, bacteria)

Autoimmune disorders

Felty's syndrome
Systemic lupus erythematosus
Acute respiratory disease
Hypersplenism
Rheumatoid arthritis
Transfusion reaction

---

tions and 21-day fluctuations in the neutrophil count. *Congenital neutropenia,* also known as infantile genetic agranulocytosis, is a chromosomal abnormality possibly related to a G-CSF receptor defect. *Chédiak-Higashi syndrome* is an autosomal recessive chromosomal abnormality characterized by recurrent infections, partial albinism, and lymphoproliferative features caused by defective neutrophil migration and bactericidal properties. Cancer chemotherapeutic agents (e.g., cyclophosphamide, methotrexate, azathioprine) also directly suppress neutrophil production, in a dose-dependent manner.

Maturation disorders include vitamin B_{12} and folic acid deficiencies, myelodysplastic syndromes, and viral infections. Disorders of increased neutrophil destruction include those caused by antibodies to neutrophils induced by drugs such as antibiotics, antithyroid medications, and sulfa-containing compounds. Infections caused by hepatitis B, Epstein-Barr virus (EBV), human immunodeficiency virus (HIV), rickettsiae, and parasites may induce the production of antibodies that adversely effect the sequestration and destruction of neutrophils.

Autoimmune causes of neutropenia may also have an associated thrombocytopenia and hemolytic anemia. *Felty's syndrome* is the combination of rheumatoid arthritis, splenomegaly, and neutropenia, which is caused by antineutrophil antibodies. Similar antibodies can also be found in systemic lupus erythematous and Sjögren's syndrome. Antineutrophil antibodies can occasionally be found in hyperthyroidism and Wegener's granulomatosis as well. Antibodies to G-CSF also play a role in some of these autoimmune disorders. Isoimmune neonatal neutropenia is a disorder in infants secondary to transplacental transfer of IgG antibodies that react with neutrophilic antigens. These antigens are inherited from the father of the infant, and the disease process is similar to that of Rh-hemolytic disease of the newborn. This disorder resolves spontaneously, but occasionally the administration of G-CSF is necessary.

Treatment

Treatment of neutropenia depends on its cause and relative severity. Chronic neutropenia will necessitate a careful family history, a chronology of the types and severity of infections, and recurrent findings, such as oral ulcers, cellulitis, and sepsis. A medication history is extremely important in determining the cause of recent-onset neutropenia. Bone marrow aspiration is indicated if a production deficit is suspected or if there is any question of a myelodysplastic or malignant cause. If a viral infection is suspected, serologic testing for infectious mononucleosis, hepatitis, HIV, EBV, and parvovirus may be indicated. When an autoimmune disorder is implicated, testing for antinuclear antibodies and rheumatoid factor is necessary. When neutropenia is found, a direct review of the peripheral blood smear using Wright-Giemsa stain not only confirms the relative absence or decreased number of neutrophils, but also can provide clues if there are toxic granulations, Döhle bodies, or changes seen in the maturation of the available neutrophils. If anemia or thrombocytopenia (or both) is found along with neutropenia, bone marrow aspiration and biopsy should be performed to determine the cause of this deficit in bone marrow production.

The Infectious Disease Society of America (IDSA; www.idsociety.org) and the American Society of Clinical

Oncology (www.asco.org) have developed evidence-based guidelines for the treatment of neutropenia associated with acute febrile episodes and those associated with cancer chemotherapy. These websites are kept current for use in clinical practice. Box 39-5 provides guidelines for the management of febrile neutropenia.

Mild neutropenia in the absence of a recurrent or protracted infection is most likely benign and can be observed. The history of a recent viral infection or new medication is often associated with mild neutropenia. The patient should be examined carefully and ANC monitored until it returns to normal. Once the neutropenia resolves, CBC should be determined whenever a fever occurs. If the neutropenia continues for 8 weeks or longer, a bone marrow aspiration and biopsy may help determine the cause and prognosis.

In patients with *moderate to severe neutropenia* with recurrent infection, a more vigorous approach should be undertaken to determine the cause. Bone marrow aspiration and biopsy, appropriate serologic tests, and blood cultures are necessary. Determination of antinuclear antibodies, complement levels, and antineutrophil antibodies and serologic studies for entities such as HIV infection are needed. An acute episode of febrile neutropenia requires a careful history and examination for potential sites of infection; blood and body fluid samples should be tested, and immediate implementation of IV antibiotic therapy is required. If indicated, antibiotics should be adjusted after 3 days, depending on culture results. Low-risk patients and patients responding quickly may be switched to oral antibiotic therapy. If the patient is severely

ill and is not responding, treatment with antifungal agents and G-CSF should be considered.

Chronic neutropenia in Felty's syndrome may respond to splenectomy and regular doses of methotrexate. The long-term use of corticosteroids, gamma globulin injections, and splenectomy are generally not indicated in patients who have chronic neutropenia. Long-term antibiotics have no proven benefit in preventing infections in patients with chronic or recurrent neutropenia. Patients with fever and ANC higher than 1000 cells/μL can generally be managed on an outpatient basis with oral antibiotics.

The use of myeloid growth factors (G-CSF, GM-CSF) may be helpful for some neutropenic patients. These recombinant-manufactured products can correct neutropenia and reduce infectious morbidity, particularly in patients subject to recurrent infections, such as those with severe congenital neutropenia, cyclic neutropenia, HIV infection, and long-term bone marrow suppression from cancer chemotherapy. In controlled studies in patients with severe chronic neutropenia or HIV disease with low CD4+ cell count and ANC less than 1000/μL, administration of G-CSF reduced the incidence of infection by 30% to 40% (Jadersten et al., 2005). G-CSF is now recommended to be given in the first cycle of chemotherapy, when the incidence of febrile neutropenia is likely to be higher than 20%. Patients receiving G-CSF may have more intensive chemotherapy and better survival but a greater risk of leukemia (Dale, 2009). Patients older than 55 with neutropenia or with acute myeloid leukemia may benefit from the administration of CSFs after completion of induction therapy. These agents can be started 24 to 72 hours after chemotherapy and are continued until ANC reaches or exceeds 1000/μL.

Disorders of Neutrophil Function

Some patients have normal numbers of neutrophils but have recurrent, severe, or unusual infections and therefore have a neutrophil function disorder. Defects in function include neutrophil adherence, chemotaxis, degranulation, and metabolic problems. The evaluation is complex but involves family history, complete examination of peripheral smear, and determination of immunoglobulin and complement levels. Neutrophil function can be evaluated by the nitroblue tetrazolium (NBT) test and other assays. Chronic granulomatous disease and severe G6PD deficiency may be found in this evaluation. Referral to a specialist is usually necessary to investigate disorders of neutrophil function adequately.

Eosinophilia

Eosinophilia is an absolute eosinophil count greater than 700 cells/μL, with primary and secondary causes. Secondary eosinophilia may result from immunodeficiency, neoplasms, collagen vascular disease, and dermatologic disorders. When seen in a family medicine setting, allergic disorders and infections caused by parasites are more likely causes of eosinophilia. The primary form of eosinophilia is often called *hypereosinophilic syndrome* (HES). Characteristics of HES are an eosinophil count higher than 1500 cells/μL, longer than 6 months in duration, and evidence that eosinophils have infiltrated into tissues. Studies have shown that this may be a mutation in chromosome 4 that results in the linkage of

---

Box 39-5 Guidelines for Management and Prevention of Febrile Neutropenia

Management

Take careful history and conduct thorough physical examination of the patient.

Examine patient carefully for portal for bacterial or fungal infections.

Culture blood and other appropriate body fluids.

Start antibiotics immediately.

Treat with monotherapy (e.g., ceftazidime or imipenem) or duotherapy (e.g., aminoglycoside such as gentamicin, with β-lactam drug effective against *Pseudomonas*, such as piperacillin).

Add vancomycin if there is a significant risk of gram-positive sepsis.

Adjust antibiotic therapy after 3 days, depending on the results of cultures and the patient's clinical status.

Switch low-risk patients to oral therapy.

Continue broad-spectrum therapy for severely ill patients.

Consider antifungal treatments.

Consider colony-stimulating factors as an adjunct to antibiotics for febrile neutropenia in severely ill, high-risk patients.

Prevention

Primary prophylaxis with granulocyte colony-stimulating factor (G-CSF) reduces the incidence of febrile neutropenia by about 50% when risk of febrile neutropenia is about 40%.

Use G-CSF or granulocyte-macrophage colony-stimulating factor (GM-CSF) as a preventive strategy for patients who have had their cancer treatment reduced or experience a delay in treatment because of an episode of febrile neutropenia or a prolonged period of neutropenia.

Consider reducing the intensity of chemotherapy.

the *RHCE* and *PDGFRd* genes. Clinical features are a rash, fever, cough, dyspnea, peripheral neuropathy, diarrhea, and development of congestive heart failure, with valvular abnormalities and mural thrombi. The blood smear reveals many eosinophils with vacuoles and decreased numbers of granules. The total WBC count may range from 10,000 to 30,000 WBCs/μL, of which 30% to 70% are eosinophils. Care should be taken to eliminate severe allergic reactions, eosinophilic leukemias, and invasive parasitic infections before this diagnosis is firmly established. If there are cardiopulmonary problems, initial therapy with prednisone at high doses, followed by lower doses for up to 3 months or longer, is often successful. If this not helpful, hydroxyurea can be used to lower the WBC count to below 10,000 cells/μL.

Monocyte and Macrophage Disorders

These disorders are histiocytic syndromes in which macrophages and dendritic cells are abnormal, such as acute monocytic leukemia, monocytic sarcoma, nonmalignant disorders such as histiocytosis syndromes, and Hand-Schüller-Christian and Letterer-Siwe disease. Most of these are rare and infrequently seen in family medicine. Lysosomal storage diseases are enzymatic disorders that are usually congenital, such as lipid and polysaccharide storage diseases.

KEY TREATMENT

Patients with severe neutropenia and fever empirically need IV antibiotics started in an inpatient setting (e.g., cefepime, 2 g every 8 hours) (IDSA, 2008) (SOR: C).

In patients with severe chronic neutropenia or HIV disease with low CD4+ count and absolute neutrophil count less than 1000 cells/μL, G-CSF reduced the rate of infection by 30% to 40% (Jadersten et al., 2005) (SOR: A).

Platelets

Key Points

- Petechiae and bleeding do not usually occur until the platelet count is below 20,000 cells/μL.
- Platelet dysfunction should be considered in a patient with clinical evidence of hemorrhage and platelet count above 100,000 cells/μL.
- Primary marrow-related thrombocytosis is more likely to cause thrombosis.
- Aspirin irreversibly inactivates cyclooxygenase in platelets, whereas nonsteroidal anti-inflammatory drugs do not.

Platelet Origins

Platelets are produced by megakaryocytes, which develop from the same stem cells as leukocytes and red cells in the bone marrow. Production of megakaryocytes is under the control of thrombopoietin. Megakaryocytes are large cells with abundant cytoplasm that undergo division of the nucleus without concomitant cell division (endomitosis). As the cell matures, it develops a vacuolated blue-gray appearance with strands. Beads of the strands pinch off to become

platelets. The youngest platelets are the largest, as reflected in the mean platelet volume (MPV), which is an automatically determined parameter in the CBC. Smaller platelets are older, have less activity, and are less effective. Platelets live approximately 8½ to 10 days in the circulation, with a half-life of 4 days.

Although there is no reserve pool of platelets in the bone marrow, the marrow can increase its production of platelets sevenfold to eightfold above normal in response to stress (Fig. 39-6). From 30% to 40% of the platelet pool is in the spleen. Platelets freely move between the spleen and the circulation. (See further discussion online.)

Platelet Functions

The primary role of the platelet is to maintain the integrity of the endothelial lining of small vessels. This process is not completely understood but most likely indicates that platelets are constantly being recruited to repair submicroscopic rents between endothelial lining cells in small arterioles and venules. Thus, when the platelet count falls below a certain level, petechiae begin to appear, particularly in the dependent portions of the body such as the ankles and lower legs. Minor trauma may induce unusual bruising at these sites. (See discussion at www.expertconsult.com.)

Platelet Disorders

Disorders of platelets can be classified into three major categories: thrombocytopenia, thrombocytosis, and platelet function disorders.

Thrombocytopenia

Thrombocytopenia is a platelet count below the lower normal limit of 150,000 cells/μL and has two major causes, reduced platelet production and accelerated platelet removal. Bleeding does not generally occur until the platelet count falls below 20,000 cells/μL or the patient is an older adult, has coexistent diseases such as liver dysfunction or a connective tissue disorder, or is taking a drug that impairs platelet function.

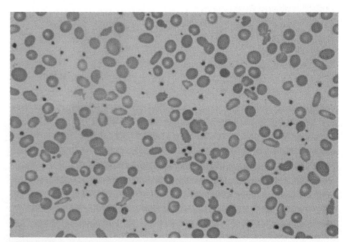

Figure 39-6 Increased number of platelets seen on a peripheral blood smear. *(From the American Society of Hematology Image Bank image #2695. Copyright 1996 American Society of Hematology, used with permission.)*

Clinical signs of thrombocytopenia include the appearance of *petechiae,* small spots of pinpoint (millimeters) bleeding in the skin and subcutaneous tissue in which red blood cells leak from small capillaries or venules. Petechiae occur most frequently at sites in the lower extremities, around the mouth, or where there is constrictive clothing causing pressure on small vessels. Mucosal bleeding, recurrent nosebleeds, small bruises, and excessive menstrual bleeding are likely to be associated with von Willebrand's disease or discrete platelet disorders. If the clinical picture involves deep tissue bleeding into muscles or joints, a clotting factor disorder such as hemophilia is more likely.

Aspirin plays a key role in impairing platelet function and is used prophylactically in small doses to prevent coronary insufficiency syndromes and strokes. The investigation and treatment of thrombocytopenia are significantly affected by whether it is a solitary phenomenon or is associated with other cytopenias. Confirmation of a low platelet count should be done by repeating the CBC, because low platelet numbers can result from clumping caused by inappropriate anticoagulation of the blood sample or cold agglutinins. MPV can provide additional diagnostic information; low values suggest poor production and very old platelets, and high values suggest rapid production of new platelets. Bone marrow aspiration with biopsy may be important in the diagnosis of thrombocytopenia when the cause is unclear, because it may indicate aplasia, hypoplasia, drug toxicity, or bone marrow infiltration with leukemic cells or fibrosis.

Box 39-6 divides the causes of thrombocytopenia into production defects and accelerated platelet removal mechanisms. Platelets may not be produced in adequate numbers or may have dysfunctional characteristics if the marrow has been damaged by radiation or chemotherapeutic drugs or has been infiltrated by cancer or fibrous tissue. Drugs such as gold, sulfa products, thiazides, and ethanol can inhibit platelet production, and certain infections (e.g., HIV, rubella) or vaccines may cause deficits in production. Drug etiologies are more frequently related to drugs started within the previous 1 to 2 months. Deficiencies of vitamins (e.g., B_{12}, folic acid) may render the development of platelets ineffective.

Box 39-6 Classification of Thrombocytopenic Disorders

Platelet production defect

Pancytopenia, aplasia: Radiation, cancer drugs

Marrow infiltration: Fibrosis, cancer

Impaired platelet production: Infections (rubella, HIV) drugs; gold, sulfa compounds, alcohol

Impaired platelet development: Folate, vitamin B_{12} deficiencies, alcohol

Accelerated platelet removal

Immune destruction: Autoantibodies—idiopathic thrombocytopenic purpura, systemic lupus erythematosus; infections (HIV, sepsis, mononucleosis); drugs

Nonimmune destruction: Disseminated intravascular coagulation, vasculitis, thrombotic thrombocytopenic purpura, HELLP syndrome*

Hypersplenism: Various causes

*Hemolysis (microangiopathic), elevated liver enzymes, and low platelets.

The most common phenomenon in accelerated platelet removal is *immune destruction.* Antibodies produced by the body may facilitate the enhanced removal of platelets from the circulation. Diseases involving immune platelet destruction include idiopathic thrombocytopenic purpura, systemic lupus erythematosus (SLE), drug-induced thrombocytopenia, infectious mononucleosis, HIV/AIDS, malaria, and even posttransfusion purpura. Diseases involving no immunologic mechanism, but in which platelets are removed from the circulation more rapidly than normal, include disseminated intravascular coagulation (DIC), preeclampsia, vasculitis, thrombotic thrombocytopenic purpura, and gram-negative septicemia. Also, a significantly enlarged spleen represents an increased platelet pool, thus lowering the platelet count.

Removal of drugs that could be causing production problems and replacement of vitamins (B_{12} and folic acid) are probably the easiest remedies to address platelet production defects. Recombinant thrombopoietin is in development, but has not yet been approved for clinical use. Platelet counts greater than 50,000 cells/μL are generally safe for interventional procedures, except major surgery or epidural anesthesia. Childbirth and tooth extractions may occur safely with stable platelet levels (30,000-50,000) and no evidence of bleeding.

Accelerated Platelet Removal Caused by Immune Destruction

Idiopathic Thrombocytopenic Purpura

Formerly seen most often in young women, idiopathic thrombocytopenic purpura (ITP) is now seen more often in HIV-positive men. Associated illnesses or causes may include infectious mononucleosis, Graves' disease, thyroiditis, and other viral illnesses. ITP has an insidious onset, with the only physical finding being petechiae in the lower extremities. There may be some gingival bleeding with brushing or flossing of the teeth; splenomegaly is uncommon. ITP is characterized as an autoimmune disorder in which IgG antibodies are formed against the patient's own platelets. These antibodies attach to platelets, causing them to be identified as abnormal. The platelets are then removed by the RES, most often in the spleen. The bone marrow responds to the rapid destruction of platelets by increasing production, resulting in functionally large platelets, which accounts for the low incidence of bleeding in this disorder. The laboratory evaluation reveals a higher-than-normal MPV and the presence of few platelets on a peripheral blood smear (Bain, 2005); however, the platelets present are large and well granulated. If schistocytes or helmet cells are seen, this suggests a mechanical hemolytic process as well. The bone marrow reveals a plethora of megakaryocytes, whereas other test results for autoimmune diseases should be negative. Other, similar presentations might include a falsely low platelet count resulting from the anticoagulant used in the blood sampling (e.g., pseudothrombocytopenia caused by clumping), cold agglutinins, gestational thrombocytopenia, and myelodysplastic syndrome.

Treatment of ITP varies with the degree of bleeding, whether the patient is pregnant, CNS involvement, and to some extent, the patient's age. The goal is to prevent serious bleeding. The American Society of Hematology has made the following evidence-based recommendations for the management of ITP (George et al., 1996):

1. Patients with platelet counts above 50,000 cells/μL do not require treatment routinely.
2. Treatment is indicated in patients with platelet counts of 20,000 to 30,000 and in patients with platelets below 50,000 with significant mucosal bleeding or risk factors for bleeding.
3. Patients with platelets below 20,000 need not be hospitalized if they are asymptomatic or if they have only mild purpura.

Patients in the second category who have mucosal bleeding with a platelet count between 20,000 and 30,000 cells/μL are often treated with prednisone, 60 to 100 mg/day, to reduce the amount of antiplatelet antibodies produced by lymphocytes in the marrow and spleen. When the platelet count rises after 2 to 3 weeks of therapy, the prednisone can be tapered over another 3 to 4 weeks. Long-term complete response occurs in probably 15% to 20% of patients. If the platelet counts remain below 30,000 after 6 to 8 weeks of therapy, or if the platelet count begins to fall after the steroids have been tapered, splenectomy should be considered. If splenectomy is planned, steroid therapy should be resumed to boost the platelet count to a more acceptable level. The lymphoid system in the spleen can respond best to immunizations, such as pneumococcal, *Haemophilus influenzae*, or meningococcal vaccine, which should be administered 1 to 2 weeks before surgery. If steroids do not raise the platelet level to an acceptable presurgical level, IVIG at 0.4 to 1.0 mg/kg may also be administered before surgery but will take 1 to 3 days to increase platelet counts to safe levels. CNS bleeding is a medical emergency in which hospitalization, large doses of prednisone, and IVIG are used as concomitant therapeutic measures.

Patients who go into remission and later relapse or fail to respond to these measures are considered to have refractory ITP. If the platelet count is above 30,000, the best course of action is to consider it an incomplete response and manage the patient conservatively, without further therapy. If therapy is indicated in these refractory cases, the physician can consider agents such as azathioprine or cyclophosphamide, plus prednisone. Referral of these patients to a hematologist is often necessary.

Other Disorders Caused by Immune Destruction

Immune-mediated thrombocytopenia may occur in patients with SLE or lymphoma; treatment is similar to that of ITP in other patients. If the ITP is associated with a hemolytic anemia, the clinical picture is that of Evans' syndrome. Treatment is similar to that for ITP without autoimmune hemolytic anemia. Patients with aggressively treated HIV may develop antibodies to the platelet GP-IIb/IIIa, causing thrombocytopenia; if platelet count is below 10,000, prednisone or splenectomy (or both) can be used. Patients treated with GP-IIb/IIIa antagonists may develop thrombocytopenia. Removal of the antagonist is usually effective. For platelet counts less than 10,000, one platelet transfusion is usually effective in restoring platelets to safe levels.

Approximately 5% of all pregnant women have a platelet count as low as 70,000 cells/μL. If the platelet count drops lower, preeclampsia should be ruled out before making a diagnosis of ITP. Splenectomy carries significant risks of miscarriage, which can be reduced by administering corticosteroids or IVIG.

Multiparous women receiving a blood or platelet transfusion may have posttransfusion thrombocytopenia at a level of 10,000 cells/μL or lower. This is apparently the result of having previously been sensitized to blood and platelet antigens that induced an antibody not only to the foreign platelets in the transfusion, but also to endogenous platelets. This occurs 2 to 10 days after the transfusion and may last for as long as 4 weeks. Platelet transfusions are not effective. Therapeutic use of IVIG and sometimes high doses of corticosteroids are more likely to be effective.

Specific drugs can elicit immune-mediated platelet destruction that mimics ITP, including cocaine, gold, heparin, quinidine, and platelet glycoprotein antagonists (e.g., abciximab [ReoPro]). Removal of the offending drug is usually sufficient, along with time to allow the situation to resolve. A few cases of thrombocytopenia have occurred in patients taking a combination of naproxen and acetaminophen; their metabolism caused an immune reaction involving normal platelets, leading to their enhanced destruction.

Nonimmunologic-Enhanced Destruction of Platelets

A common theme in nonimmune platelet destruction is blood vessel wall injury, resulting in thrombin and platelet activation, with ensuing consumption of platelets and a reduction in the platelet count. Heparin-induced thrombocytopenia may result from heparin flushes used in settings where large, vascular access lines are needed.

Thrombotic Thrombocytopenic Purpura and Hemolytic Uremic Syndrome

One of the more serious entities in this category is thrombotic thrombocytopenic purpura (TTP) and the adult hemolytic uremic syndrome (HUS). These disorders may be stimulated by similar agents or factors, but their pathophysiology differ. In both, damage to the endothelium of small vessels triggers platelet deposition in small arterioles and capillaries, resulting in a thrombotic microangiopathy. TTP is characterized by five major clinical features: (1) microangiopathic hemolytic anemia with a high lactate dehydrogenase (LDH) level, (2) severe thrombocytopenia, (3) fever, (4) CNS symptoms and signs, and (5) renal compromise.

The physician should suspect TTP or HUS in the patient with thrombocytopenia and microangiopathic hemolytic anemia alone, with no other apparent cause. The blood smear in both disorders will show reduced platelets, helmet cells, and schistocytes, indicative of the microangiopathic hemolytic process. If assayed, bone marrow will reveal increased numbers of megakaryocytes. Renal disease will be more severe in HUS, whereas CNS symptoms may be more prominent in TTP. Not all patients have all five features on presentation. Differentiation must be made from other disorders such as Evans' syndrome, SLE, and leukemia. Hemolysis, leukocytosis, and a negative direct Coombs test are hallmarks of TTP and HUS. The absence of abnormal coagulation results essentially eliminates DIC. Causes of these syndromes may range from pregnancy to bone marrow transplantation, drugs, cancer, and in children, infection with *Escherichia coli* O157:H7. Treatment of this *E. coli* infection with antibiotics does not help and may make the disease worse. Various drugs may also cause TTP and HUS, such as cancer chemotherapeutic drugs, immunosuppressive agents such as cyclosporine, antiplatelet drugs such as ticlopidine, oral contraceptives, and quinine.

A number of theories exist concerning the cause of these syndromes. Damage to the endothelial surface of small arteries may stimulate extensive platelet aggregation, thereby plugging up small vessels. Some investigators have found that there are abnormally large von Willebrand factor multimers in the circulation, suggesting that there is a deficiency in the enzyme (ADAMTS-13) that cleaves this blood-clotting factor. These large proteins then bind to platelets and cause plugging of small arterioles and capillaries.

A large, randomized clinical trial in Canada found that plasma exchange transfusions at 1.5 to 2 times the total body plasma volume were significantly more effective than simple plasma transfusions (Rock et al., 1991). This therapy must use a higher volume during the first 3 days and a lower volume over the next 4 to 5 days, for a minimum of 7 days. Other therapies, such as aspirin and steroids, have not been studied in randomized clinical trials. Splenectomy has been used occasionally, but only by experts seeing larger numbers of cases than normally seen in a family medicine setting.

HELLP Syndrome

The HELLP syndrome—*h*emolysis (microangiopathic), *ele*vated *l*iver enzymes, and *l*ow *p*latelets (≤100,000/μL)—can occur in pregnant women between the 23rd and 39th weeks of gestation. This is a form of preeclampsia in which the patients are extremely ill. Treatment is delivery of the infant. The lowest platelet counts occur several days after delivery, although in some cases, thrombocytopenia does not present until after delivery. If a clinical picture of TTP emerges, plasma exchange should be strongly considered.

Thrombocytosis

Thrombocytosis can be a primary marrow-related disorder or secondary/reactive to a surgical or medical condition and is defined as a platelet count greater than 500,000/uL. Primary marrow related thrombocytosis may occur in the face of a chronic myeloproliferative or myelodysplastic disorder such as polycythemia vera (PV), primary myelofibrosis (MF), chronic myelogenous leukemia (CML) and essential thrombocythemia (ET). ET can be diagnosed by eliminating secondary causes and the other myeloproliferative disorders. (See earlier section: Myeloproliferative Disorders).

Secondary or reactive thrombocytosis can occur in the setting of infection, post surgical conditions with and without infection, cancer, postsplenectomy, acute blood loss or iron deficiency. Other situations, such as celiac disease, amyloidosis, rheumatoid arthritis, or rebound after alcohol- or drug-induced thrombocytopenia, can lead to thrombocytosis as well. Symptoms are more likely to be associated with primary rather than secondary thrombocytosis and include headache, lightheadedness, chest pain, visual disturbance, fingertip or toe paresthesia, and bleeding or thrombosis. Platelet morphology is also helpful. In most reactive thrombocytoses, the increased platelets on the peripheral blood smear are typically small and relatively uniform in size. In contrast, increased platelets of patients with myeloproliferative disorders may vary in size, including macrothrombocytes, misshapen platelets, and large patches of bluish-staining

material that may represent megakaryocyte cytoplasmic fragments. Patients with iron deficiency and increased platelets will have low serum ferritin levels, and splenectomized patients will have Howell-Jolly bodies in their RBCs and target cells on peripheral blood smears. C-reactive protein (CRP) should be elevated in inflammatory states and normal in primary marrow-induced thrombocytosis disorders. Diagnostic criteria for ET require platelet counts greater than 600,000. Patients with a primary marrow thrombocytosis have a mutation in *JAK2*.

Secondary thrombocytosis rarely causes thrombosis, and treatment is directed at the underlying disorder (e.g., infection, anemia). In primary marrow-related thrombocytosis, thrombosis is more likely. If thrombosis has occurred and the platelet count is greater than 800,000, prompt platelet apheresis is recommended. Chronically, the platelet count can be reduced with platelet-lowering agents (e.g., aspirin, hydroxyurea) with a goal of keeping the level below 400,000. Vasomotor symptoms may be controlled by low-dose aspirin (81 mg/day).

Platelet Function Disorders

Impaired platelet function may be acquired or inherited. Certain drugs are designed to interfere with platelet function and have proved useful in preventing recurrent strokes or other cardiovascular events, such as transient ischemic attacks (TIAs), in patients with established vascular disease. Particularly useful are drugs such as aspirin and nonsteroidal anti-inflammatory drugs (NSAIDs). An important distinction between aspirin and NSAIDs is that aspirin irreversibly inactivates cyclooxygenase in platelets, and aspirin-treated platelets will not normally contribute to clot formation. In contrast, NSAIDs reversibly interfere with platelet function. Clopidogrel inhibits platelet aggregation and selectively inhibits the binding of adenosine diphosphate (ADP) to its platelet receptor and the subsequent ADP-mediated activation of the GP-IIb/IIIa complex. Even more effectively than aspirin, clopidogrel reduces myocardial infarction, TIA, unstable angina, and other adverse events in patients with established arteriosclerotic cardiovascular disease.

Inherited disorders of platelet function are uncommon, although Glanzmann thrombasthenia may be seen most often. This congenital disorder has identified mutations in the GP-IIb/IIIa complex. ADP-induced platelet aggregation is abnormal, as is platelet contribution to clot retraction. Abnormalities involving impaired granular release or relative absence of granules characterize Bernard-Soulier and Wiskott-Aldrich syndromes; these rare disorders are also associated with thrombocytopenia. Von Willebrand's disease is an example of impaired platelet adhesion and aggregation caused by the deficiency of the von Willebrand factor, which significantly affects platelet function.

Unusual causes of acquired platelet dysfunction include liver disease and chronic renal failure. The role of the platelet function lesion in uremia or chronic liver disease is unclear, although the bleeding time may be prolonged in both disorders. The correction of the anemia with epoetin therapy in patients with end-stage renal disease appears to lessen the bleeding tendency in these patients.

Acquired platelet dysfunction can occur in myeloproliferative disease, uremia, liver disease, dysproteinemia, and drug-induced conditions. Some drugs that affect platelet function include aspirin, NSAIDs, alcohol, dextrans, semi-synthetic penicillins, heroin, and GP-IIb/IIIa antagonists. Platelet dysfunction usually requires hematologic consultation and special laboratory testing to determine the cause.

KEY TREATMENT

Treatment starts with high-dose corticosteroids in ITP patients with platelet count less than 20,000/μL and mucosal bleeding (Cines and McMillan, 2003) (SOR: B).

Splenectomy is indicated in ITP patients in whom steroids fail to sustain platelet counts greater than 30,000/μL (Nabel, 2009) (SOR: C).

Patients should receive pneumococcal, *H. influenzae*, and meningococcal vaccines 1 to 2 weeks before splenectomy (Nabel, 2009) (SOR: C).

Patients with TTP are best treated with plasma exchange transfusions (Rock et al., 1991) (SOR: A).

Patients with chronic thrombocytosis can be treated with a platelet-lowering agent such as aspirin or hydroxyurea (Harrison et al., 2005) (SOR: A).

Lymphoid System

Key Points

- B lymphocytes produce immunoglobulins; T lymphocytes function as helper, suppressor, or cytotoxic cells; NK lymphocytes function as natural killer cells.

- Suspect malignancy for lymph node enlargement that is one sided, in the neck or mandibular region, in older patients with no evidence of infection.

- Biopsy reveals malignancy in 17% of patients with persistent lymph node enlargement from strictly primary care practices.

The lymphoid system is made up of the primary and secondary tissues or organs. The primary lymphoid system consists of the bone marrow and thymus and generates B and T lymphocytes. The secondary lymphoid system consists of the lymph nodes, spleen, tonsils, and special lymphocytic tissue in the GI and respiratory tracts. Lymphocytes reside in these tissues; B and T cells may be segregated but can interact. T cells are more localized between follicles and B cells more within follicles. Macrophages, histiocytes, dendritic cells, and endothelial cells form the supporting structures of lymphoid organs and facilitate interactions that allow lymphocytes to generate appropriate cellular and humoral immune responses. T cells make up 60% to 80% of the normal lymphocyte population, B cells 10% to 20%, and natural killer (NK) cells 5% to 10%. NK cells are related to T cells in that they both arise from thymic precursors.

Functions of Lymphocytes

See discussion online at www.expertconsult.com.

Lymphocyte Disorders

Lymphocytosis

The presentation of lymphocytosis varies somewhat with age. In those older than 12 years, the upper limit of normal is 4000 cells/μL. Neonates and young children may have normal absolute lymphocyte counts up to 8000 cells/μL. The absolute lymphocyte count can be calculated by multiplying the WBC count by the percentage of lymphocytes in the differential. When an absolute lymphocytosis is encountered, the peripheral smear should be examined for atypical lymphocytes, granular lymphocytes, blastocytes (blasts), smudge cells, and other abnormalities of morphology and diversity.

Lymphocytosis can be classified as primary (malignant) or secondary (reactive). *Primary* lymphocytosis is defined in the context of an acute or chronic lymphoproliferative disorder, often caused by dysregulation of lymphocyte development and production. Leukemias (chronic lymphocytic, acute lymphocytic, hairy cell), lymphoma, and B-cell lymphocytosis are examples of primary or malignant lymphocytosis. *Secondary* lymphocytosis is defined as a lymphocytosis in a patient who does not have a known hematologic disorder and in whom the lymphocyte count is expected to return to normal in less than 2 months after cessation of the inciting condition. *Reactive* lymphocytosis can sometimes be mistaken for a primary or malignant lymphocytosis when examining the peripheral blood smear, particularly in infectious mononucleosis with a marked increase in larger, atypical, or transformed lymphocytes. Other causes of secondary lymphocytosis may generate small lymphocytes, as in pertussis. Viral infections are the most prevalent cause of secondary lymphocytosis, including Epstein-Barr, cytomegalovirus, herpes simplex, varicella, rubella, HIV, adenovirus, and hepatitis. Occasionally, toxoplasmosis and pertussis in children can cause a lymphocytosis that is extremely high, up to levels of 50,000 to 70,000 cells/μL. Some forms of extreme stress can cause an increase in lymphocytes, such as cardiovascular collapse, septic shock, status epilepticus, surgery, or major hypersensitivity or allergic disorders. *Chronic* lymphocytosis may be seen in patients with cancer, sarcoidosis, and certain autoimmune disorders, as well as in cigarette smokers.

Lymphocytopenia

When a paucity of lymphocytes occurs, because most lymphocytes are T cells, it is preponderantly a reduction in the T-cell count. Lymphocytopenia is defined as a total lymphocyte count of 1000 cells/μL or lower. Inherited causes of lymphocytopenia include severe combined immunodeficiency, ataxia-telangiectasia, Wiskott-Aldrich syndrome, and idiopathic CD4+ T-cell lymphocytopenia. Acquired causes of decreased lymphocyte counts include mostly viral infections, such as HIV, hepatitis, influenza, or respiratory syncytial virus (RSV), and unusual bacterial infections, such as typhoid fever or tuberculosis. Miscellaneous causes include aplastic anemia, autoimmune diseases, Hodgkin's disease, sarcoidosis, chronic alcohol ingestion, immunosuppressive agents, particularly corticosteroids, and radiation.

Lymphadenopathy

Enlarged lymph nodes, single or multiple, are a common problem seen by family physicians in ambulatory practice. Nodes may be enlarged as a reactive phenomenon to infection, inflammation, malignancy, or systemic generalized disease (Box 39-7). Most enlarged lymph nodes seen in younger patients are benign. Table 39-6 summarizes the four major determinants of significant lymphadenopathy:

Box 39-7 Causes of Lymphadenopathy

Infections

Bacterial: Streptococci, staphylococci, cat-scratch fever, mycobacteria, tularemia

Viral: Infectious mononucleosis, adenovirus, HIV, herpes simplex

Chlamydial: *Chlamydia trachomatis*

Mycotic: Sporotrichosis, histoplasmosis

Protozoal: Toxoplasmosis

Rickettsial: Rocky Mountain spotted fever, typhus

Malignancies

Hodgkin's lymphoma, acute and chronic leukemias, lymphoma

Metastatic tumors and sarcoma

Immune system

Drug reactions

Insect stings

Connective tissue diseases

Serum sickness

Miscellaneous

Sarcoidosis, amyloidosis

Chronic granulomatous disease

Histiocytic disorders

Necrotizing lymphadenitis

Table 39-6 Lymphadenopathy: Clinical Signs and Implications

Considerations	Significance
Age of patient (yr)	
<30	80% lymphadenopathy benign, most often infectious
>50	40% benign probability
Location of node enlargement	
Cervical nodes, axillary nodes, epitrochlear nodes, bilateral hilar adenopathy	Benign, infectious
Generalized; unilateral, jugular, or mandibular areas; supraclavicular, scalene nodes; Virchow's node; thoracic, retroperitoneal; unilateral hilar adenopathy	Malignant
Characteristics of node enlargement	
Soft, mobile, tender	Benign
Rubbery, matted, nontender	Lymphoma
Hard, fixed	Chronic lymphocytic leukemia (CLL), metastatic
Clinical setting of patient*	
Older adult, smoker	Malignant
College student	Infectious with pharyngitis and fever

*In which solitary, nontender, enlarged cervical node occurs.

age of patient, location of adenopathy, character of lymph node, and clinical settings in which enlarged lymph nodes can occur. For example, a relatively soft, small (<1 cm), movable node may be found in the submandibular or anterior cervical region in as many as 50% to 60% of those younger than 50 years. Inguinal nodes up to 1 to 2 cm may be found in normal healthy adults. Patients younger than 50 are much more likely to have lymphadenopathy from a benign or infectious process than patients older than 50, in whom only 40% of the causes of lymphadenopathy are of a benign or infectious nature.

Enlarged lymph nodes in the anteroposterior cervical regions or the occipital area in younger persons are generally benign, but this also depends on the character of the node and the clinical setting in which this enlargement occurs. If two distinct but separate lymph node groups are enlarged, a hematologic malignancy is more likely, such as chronic lymphocytic leukemia or lymphoma. Infectious processes such as infectious mononucleosis, viral hepatitis, secondary syphilis, histoplasmosis, toxoplasmosis, or cytomegalovirus infection are more probable when generalized lymphadenopathy is found. If one-sided lymph node enlargements without obvious infectious cause are discovered in the neck or mandibular region, and in older patients in the anterior scalene node region, malignancy deserves much greater consideration.

Virchow's node is an enlarged left supraclavicular node usually infiltrated with a metastatic tumor from below the diaphragm, especially of GI origin. An enlarged right supraclavicular node is more likely associated with a tumor of thoracic origin. A matted node that is enlarged could be caused by a local phenomenon such as an infection, bite, or trauma to the arm, but it may also represent a melanoma, lymphoma, or metastatic breast cancer in a young woman. Bilateral hilar adenopathy and enlargement of nodes in the femoral triangle are more likely to be seen with systemic disease, generalized infection, or occasionally lymphoma.

The character of the node, overall size, and relation to other lymph node groups help determine whether biopsy is indicated. When there is thoracic adenopathy, unilateral hilar adenopathy, or mediastinal adenopathy, particularly in older adults, lung cancer, sarcoidosis, or lymphoma must be strongly considered, depending on the clinical setting. Mediastinal adenopathy in young persons, however, may be associated with sarcoidosis or infectious mononucleosis. Enlarged nodes found in the abdomen or retroperitoneal space are more likely to be malignant and are characteristic of lymphomas or germ cell tumors in men.

Nodes that are enlarged, well circumscribed, rubbery, firm, mobile, and not particularly tender are more likely to be reactive lymph nodes related to infection. Some may also be painful, particularly if the rate of the growth has been rapid, caused by inflammation. Lymph nodes that are hard, nontender, nonmovable, and fixed to the underlying tissues are more likely to be infiltrated with metastatic tumor from a regionally proximate cancer.

The clinical setting is important. An older adult who smokes and has an enlarged supraclavicular or cervical lymph node may be more likely to have a cancer in the mouth, head and neck, or lung than a younger person with enlarged cervical lymph nodes accompanied by a fever and sore throat, indicative of infectious mononucleosis.

Auxiliary and supraclavicular nodes may increase in size in women with silicone breast implants. Patients with acquired immunodeficiency syndrome (AIDS) may have generalized lymphadenopathy indicative of a severe systemic infection or lymphoma. Associated symptoms such as fatigue and intermittent fevers are common.

When an enlarged lymph node or lymph node group that does not have striking hallmarks of malignancy is seen, and there are no other symptoms, it is appropriate to watch and observe the patient over several weeks. Nodes that do not become smaller or revert to a more benign appearance should be biopsied. In primary care practices, referral yielded a 17% prevalence of malignancy (Chau et al., 2003). Nodes that are difficult for the pathologist to read as reactive and lymph nodes diagnosed with follicular hyperplasia may have an occult lymphoma, and a second opinion might be beneficial. For a patient with repeated lymph node enlargements that have no clearly infectious cause, serologic studies for infections and repeat lymph node biopsies are indicated to establish a diagnosis. Most lymph node enlargements found by the family physician are benign and resolve within a short time. Those that do not resolve require further investigation and ultimately biopsy if no cause can be found.

Classification of Hematopoietic and Lymphoid Tissue Tumors

The World Health Organization (WHO) updated its classification of blood and lymphoid tissue tumors in 2008 by utilizing more molecular characteristics or markers instead of primarily morphologic changes seen in malignant cells. It includes genetic, morphologic, immunophenotypic, and clinical characteristics to formulate a diagnosis. Tumors of heme and lymphoid cells are divided into three main cell types: (1) myeloid cell neoplasms, originating in leukocytes and RBCs found in the marrow; (2) lymphoid neoplasms, from B-cell and T-cell lymphocyte precursors and mature forms; and (3) dendritic/histiocytic neoplasms, derived from precursors to dendritic cells or tissue microphages (Box 39-8).

Box 39-8 WHO Classification of Hematologic and Lymphoid Neoplasms

Myeloid Neoplasms

Acute myeloid leukemia (AML)

Myelodysplastic syndromes

Myeloproliferative disorders

  Chronic myelogenous leukemia (CML)

  Chronic neutrophilia leukemia

  Polycythemia vera (PV)

Essential thrombocytopenia (ET)

  Chronic eosinophilic leukemia

  Mastocytosis

Myelodysplastic/myeloproliferative syndromes

  Myelomonocytic leukemia: chronic/juvenile

  Atypical CML

Dendritic/Histiocytic Neoplasms

Tumors from precursors to dendritic cells

Tumors from tissue microphages

Lymphoid Neoplasms

Precursor lymphoid neoplasms (precursor B or T cell)

  Leukemia/lymphomas

Mature B-cell neoplasms

  Chronic lymphocytic leukemia

  Follicular lymphoma

  Diffuse large B-cell lymphoma

  Plasma cell myeloma

  Harry cell leukemia

Hodgkin's lymphoma (HL)

  Nodular lymphocyte-predominant HL

  Classic HL

Mature T-cell or NK-cell neoplasms

  Anaplastic large-cell lymphoma

  Adult T-cell lymphoma/leukemia

Leukemia

See the discussions of acute leukemia (myeloid, lymphoblastic), chronic leukemia (myelogenous, lymphocytic), and lymphomas (Hodgkin's, non-Hodgkin's) online at www.expertconsult.com.

References

The complete reference list is available online at www.expertconsult.com.

Web Resources

www.IDsociety.org *and* www.asco.org
Infectious Disease Society of America and American Society of Clinical Oncology have developed guidelines for the treatment of neutropenia in patients with acute febrile episodes and those receiving chemotherapy.

www.wadsworth.org/chemheme/heme/microscope/celllist.htm
Pictures of normal and abnormal blood cells and specific hematologic disease states.

www.bloodthevitalconnection.org/blood-basics/other-resources.aspx
Patient information resource for hematologic disease; updated by American Society of Hematology (ASH).

www.cancer.gov/cancertopics/pdq/cancerdatabase
National Cancer Institute (NCI) provides information on clinical trials, references for staging hematologic cancers, and patient handouts.

CHAPTER 40

Urinary Tract Disorders

Charles Carter, James Stallworth, and Robert Holleman

Urogenital health care concerns account for 4.4% of all ambulatory patient visits in the United States, more than half with primary care physicians (Schappert and Rechtsteiner, 2008). Disease in the urogenital system can be categorized as anatomic, functional, infectious, and neoplastic disorders. Although there is inevitable overlap between these categories, as in benign prostatic hyperplasia (neoplastic) causing outflow obstruction and incontinence (functional), this framework is useful for characterizing urinary tract abnormalities.

Evaluation of the Urinary Tract

The urinary system includes the kidneys, ureters, bladder, and urethra; a system history most often focuses on *voiding*, its primary function. Other issues may include *sexual function* or areas of overlap with other systems (e.g., abdominal pain). Patients often present with, or are found to have, common concerns specific to the urinary tract (see later discussion). A thorough drug history is critical because many common medications have urologic side effects (Thomas et al., 2003) (see **eTable 40-1** online).

Physical Examination

Physical examination is limited with urinary tract disorders, but special techniques are available. Many physical findings are helpful, if present, although their absence does not imply normalcy. For example, a renal bruit may indicate arterial stenosis, but its absence does not rule out the condition. Variations in examiner skill and patient factors also limit the accuracy and reliability of physical findings.

The kidneys are retroperitoneal organs and are difficult to palpate, except in very thin persons and children. The right kidney sits more inferiorly than the left because of the liver. The ureters are nonpalpable but, as with the kidneys, may radiate pain to the flank area. The bladder is typically nonpalpable unless distended with at least 150 mL of urine, and percussion is preferred over palpation for diagnosing distention (Gerber and Brendler, 2007). In women an enlarged bladder may also be noted on bimanual examination.

Pelvic examination is useful for diagnosing *cystocele* in women. Two fingers can be placed in the introitus and opened to visualize the vaginal cavity. The patient then performs the Valsalva maneuver. The anterior wall dipping down into the vaginal cavity may signify a cystocele. More subtle cystoceles can be detected by placing a lubricated cotton swab in the urethral meatus and having the patient perform the Valsalva maneuver. If the swab moves upward (anteriorly), it may indicate movement of the bladder neck with straining.

Examination of the external genitalia in men may reveal penile lesions, regional adenopathy, or disorders of the scrotum and testicles. Uncircumcised men should have the foreskin retracted to rule out phimosis and visualize the glans. Careful palpation of the testicular complex is needed to detect and differentiate masses and anatomic abnormalities. Digital rectal examination (DRE) can estimate prostate size and detect masses or inflammation. It is usually performed with the patient leaning forward on the examination table with his elbows bent. Prostate tenderness, warmth, or a boggy consistency suggests prostatitis. Prostate enlargement consistent with benign prostatic hyperplasia is typical in older men. Masses or asymmetry may indicate a tumor.

Laboratory Tests

Key Points

- Routine screening urinalysis is not recommended, even in pediatric prevention.
- Evaluate for sexually transmitted infections in patients with UTI symptoms, positive leukocyte esterase, and negative urine cultures.
- Do not use urine from a catheter bag for culture.
- Microalbuminuria screening is routine in diabetes care.

Urinalysis

Urinalysis is the most common office laboratory test, with dipstick urinalysis most often used (Cherry et al., 2007). Urinalysis is inexpensive, noninvasive, easily carried out, and could indicate a number of urinary and systemic conditions. Performing urinalysis in otherwise healthy people as a preventive health service is commonplace. However, screening is not recommended in asymptomatic adults for many of the conditions that urinalysis can identify (e.g., asymptomatic bacteriuria, bladder cancer; see later). Routine urinalysis lacks evidence of benefit, and guidelines recommend against routine urinalysis as part of adult or child preventive care, suggesting it only be done if clinically indicated (Grenz et al., 2009a, 2009b; Stephens and Wilder, 2003). The American Academy of Pediatrics also no longer recommends urinalysis as part of routine pediatric prevention (AAP, 2007).

Although urinalysis can detect occult disease, most positive results will not yield this outcome; more patients would incur unnecessary or potentially dangerous medical evaluations than would benefit. Thus, the potential value is elusive while there is the possibility of harm. It is important, however, not to confuse broad population screening recommendations with those specific to certain patients or problems. For example, microalbuminuria screening is routine in diabetes care (ADA, 2009).

Physicians should be aware that there is a good chance of false-positive and false-negative results with dipstick tests. Thus, abnormal results are not necessarily indicative of disease and may need confirmatory testing (Gerber and Brendler, 2007; Simerville et al., 2005).

Specimen Preparation

A midstream clean-catch specimen is the recommended standard for urinalysis. Uncircumcised men should retract the foreskin before urinating. Urine should be examined immediately, if possible, and should be refrigerated if it will not be examined in 1 to 2 hours.

Inspection

Normal urine color varies from clear (dilute) to yellow to deep golden and cloudy. Many substances can cause urine color to appear abnormal (Table 40-1). Cloudy urine may be caused by infection *(pyuria)*, but the most common cause is *phosphaturia*, in which phosphate crystals precipitate in alkaline urine. Microscopic analysis can differentiate these two entities. A strong or foul-smelling sample does not necessarily indicate infection. Urine odor may change because of dietary intake (e.g., asparagus), medications, illness, or concentration. Fecal odor suggests gastrointestinal-vesical fistula.

Dipstick Urinalysis

Specific Gravity

Urine specific gravity ranges from 1.001 to 1.035. It reflects the urine concentration and is a marker of hydration status. However, conditions affecting renal functions, such as chronic kidney disease and syndrome of inappropriate antidiuretic hormone secretion (SIADH), alter specific gravity and its relation to hydration. The glomerular filtrate has a specific gravity of 1.010, and urine with this fixed specific gravity may indicate renal dysfunction.

pH

Average urinary pH is usually acidic, ranging from 5.5 to 6.5. It reflects the serum pH except in patients with *renal tubular acidosis* (RTA) (Simerville et al., 2005). These patients have

Table 40-1 Factors Affecting Urine Color

Color	Causative Factor
Colorless	Very dilute urine; overhydration
Cloudy, milky	Phosphaturia; pyuria; chyluria
Red	Hematuria; hemoglobinuria, myoglobinuria; anthocyanin in beets and blackberries; chronic lead and mercury poisoning; phenolphthalein (in bowel evacuants); phenothiazines (e.g., prochlorperazine [Compazine]); rifampin
Orange	Dehydration; phenazopyridine (Pyridium); sulfasalazine (Azulfidine)
Green-blue	Biliverdin; indicanuria (tryptophan indole metabolites); amitriptyline (Elavil); indigo carmine; methylene blue; phenols (e.g., IV cimetidine [Tagamet]; IV promethazine [Phenergan]); resorcinol; triamterene (Dyrenium)
Brown	Urobilinogen; porphyria; aloe, fava beans, rhubarb; chloroquine, primaquine; furazolidone (Furoxone); metronidazole (Flagyl); nitrofurantoin (Furadantin)
Brown-black	Alkaptonuria (homogentisic acid); hemorrhage; melanin; tyrosinosis (hydroxyphenylpyruvic acid); cascara, senna (laxatives); methocarbamol (Robaxin); methyldopa (Aldomet); sorbitol

From Hanno PM, Wein AJ. A Clinical Manual of Urology. Norwalk, Conn, Appleton-Century-Crofts, 1987, p 67.

alkaline urine because the kidneys cannot acidify urine. Type 1 RTA will always have alkaline urine, whereas urine in type 2 RTA may become acidic as the acidosis worsens. Urine infected with urease-producing organisms such as *Proteus* species becomes alkaline.

Blood

Dipstick urinalysis has a sensitivity of 91% to 100% and a specificity of 65% to 99% for microscopic hematuria (Grossfeld et al., 2001a). Myoglobin and hemoglobin can cause a false-positive dipstick reaction. Thus, heme-positive urine specimens require microscopic examination.

Glucose

Glucose in the urine *(glycosuria)* occurs when the glucose concentration of the glomerular filtrate exceeds the proximal tubule's ability to resorb it. The dipstick only reacts to glucose. A finding in uncontrolled diabetes mellitus, glycosuria occurs when the serum glucose level exceeds 180 mg/dL.

Ketones

Urinary ketone bodies are a main feature of diabetic ketoacidosis. They may also be found in starvation states and pregnancy. Dipsticks detect acetoacetic acid. False-positive results may occur with very concentrated or acidic urine.

Leukocyte Esterase

Leukocyte esterase is a substance produced by neutrophils that signifies possible pyuria. It is sensitive (72%-97%), but not very specific (41%-86%) for urinary tract infection (UTI). Urine contamination by vaginal cells is the most common reason for false-positive results. Patients with typical UTI symptoms, positive leukocyte esterase, and negative urine cultures should be evaluated for sexually transmitted infections (STIs) (Graham and Galloway, 2001).

Nitrite

The finding of nitrites in the urine is 92% to 100% specific for a UTI (Simerville et al., 2005). However, many patients with UTIs will not be nitrite positive (i.e., low sensitivity). Gram-negative coliform organisms convert urinary nitrates to nitrite, but not *Staphylococcus saprophyticus* or enterococci. The test loses accuracy with lower bacterial colony counts. The reagent is air sensitive, so a dipstick may yield false-positive results if strips in the container are not tightly sealed (Gallagher et al., 1990).

Protein

Urine dipsticks are very sensitive and specific for albuminuria. The reagent color change roughly corresponds to the protein concentration in the sample (Table 40-2). Very dilute, alkaline, or nonalbumin proteinuria may cause false-negative results. Microalbuminuria screening usually requires a separate dipstick designed specifically for this purpose. A urine protein electrophoresis is needed to evaluate nonalbumin proteinuria, such as globulinuria or Bence Jones protein.

Urobilinogen

Urobilinogen is a breakdown product of conjugated bilirubin. There is normally a small amount present, but elevations indicate possible hemolysis or liver disease. Conjugated bilirubinuria is abnormal and signifies hepatic disease or biliary

obstruction. Unconjugated bilirubin is not filtered by the glomerulus.

Urine Microscopy

To prepare a urine sample for microscopic analysis, centrifuge 10 mL of urine for 5 minutes at 2000 rpm. After centrifugation, pour off the supernatant and resuspend the remaining sample (0.5-1.0 mL). Place a drop of this sample on the slide and focus up to high power. Samples showing probable skin or vaginal contamination should be retested or a catheterized specimen obtained (Grossfeld et al., 2001a). Sediment counts should be estimated as the average number of elements viewed per high-power field (hpf).

Red Blood Cells

Urine specific gravity may affect findings, because red cells may lyse at values lower than 1.007 (Vaughan and Wyker, 1971). Normal-appearing red blood cells (RBCs) suggest a lesion in the urinary tract, whereas dysmorphic RBCs are probably of glomerular origin (Fig. 40-1). Red cell casts are typically found at the edges of the glass coverslip and are highly suspicious for renal parenchymal disease.

White Blood Cells

Normal urine samples may show some white blood cells (WBCs) on high-power examination (Fig. 40-2). For women, fewer than 5 WBCs/hpf is normal, and for men fewer than 2 WBCs/hpf is normal (Simerville et al., 2005). Values in excess of these limits constitute microscopic pyuria. Purulent, cloudy urine with WBCs too numerous to count describes gross pyuria.

White cells are inflammatory markers, so infection cannot be confirmed by their presence or ruled out by their absence. Common causes of sterile pyuria include STIs, kidney stones, prostatitis, and urinary tract neoplasms. In children, pyuria may occur during a febrile illness, even if a UTI is not present (Graham and Galloway, 2001).

Casts

RBC casts signify a nephritic or vasculitic process. WBC casts are often considered pathognomonic for pyelonephritis, but may be found in other types of nephritis. Granular and waxy casts signify renal parenchymal disease. Hyaline casts may

Table 40-2 Dipstick Protein Findings

Dipstick Color	Estimated Corresponding Protein Level (mg/dL)
Yellow	Negative (no protein)
Yellow-green	Trace (10-20)
Green	1+ (30)
Dark green	2+ (100)
Green-blue	3+ (300)
Blue	4+ (>1000)

From Simerville JA, Maxted WC, Pahira JJ. Urinalysis: a comprehensive review. Am Fam Physician 2005;71:1153-1162.

be normal in concentrated specimens or a marker of renal infection or disease.

Crystals

Various crystal morphologies may be seen in urine samples (Fig. 40-3).

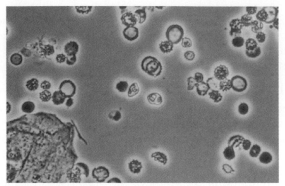

Figure 40-1 Urinalysis: dysmorphic red blood cells. *(From Gerber GS, Brendler CB. Evaluation of the urologic patient. In Wein AJ [ed]. Campbell-Walsh Urology, 9th ed, vol 1. Philadelphia, Saunders-Elsevier, 2007, p 106.)*

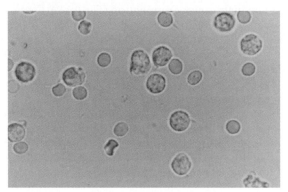

Figure 40-2 Urinalysis: white blood cells. *(From Gerber GS, Brendler CB. Evaluation of the urologic patient. In Wein AJ [ed]. Campbell-Walsh Urology, 9th ed, vol 1. Philadelphia, Saunders-Elsevier, 2007, p 107.)*

Crystals

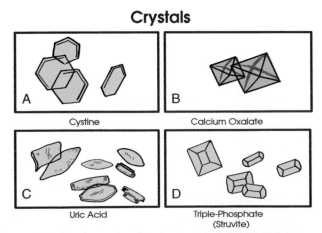

Cystine

Calcium Oxalate

Uric Acid

Triple-Phosphate (Struvite)

Figure 40-3 Crystal types found in urine samples. **A,** Cystine. **B,** Calcium oxalate. **C,** Uric acid stones are found in acidic urine. **D,** Triple-phosphate crystals are found in alkaline specimens. *(From Gerber GS, Brendler CB. Evaluation of the urologic patient. In Wein AJ [ed]. Campbell-Walsh Urology, 9th ed, vol 1. Philadelphia, Saunders-Elsevier, 2007, p 108.)*

Urinary Epithelial (Urothelial) Cells

Transitional epithelial cells are normally found in microscopic specimens. They are uniform in shape and have a large, central nucleus. In contrast, squamous cells have irregular borders and a small nucleus. Squamous cells indicate skin contamination.

Bacteria

Bacteria may signify bacteruria, although in women vaginal contamination is also likely. A urine Gram stain is also helpful for identifying bacterial characteristics in urine samples in which infection is suspected.

Fungi

Yeast seen in urine specimens most likely indicates contamination from the skin or vagina. However, it may signify systemic *Candida* infection if found in a catheterized specimen (Graham and Galloway, 2001).

Trichomonads

These motile organisms signify a common STI and may be seen in urine samples. Treatment with metronidazole (2 g as a single dose or 500 mg twice daily for 7 days) is effective. Patients should be evaluated for other STIs.

Urine Culture

Urine culture is the "gold standard" test for diagnosing UTIs. Many sources have emphasized the midstream clean-catch technique as necessary for preventing contamination, although the value of this practice is uncertain (Lifshitz and Kramer, 2000). Bladder aspiration and catheterization are invasive sampling techniques. Urine from a catheter bag should not be used for culture, because bacterial contamination is typical.

More than one bacterial isolate on culture suggests contamination. Controversy exists regarding the threshold colony counts that define bacteriuria consistent with infection. Although more than 10^5 colony-forming units per milliliter (CFU/mL) is a well-known cutoff, lower values are meaningful in certain patients. In patients with typical UTI symptoms, counts as low as 10^2 CFU/mL signify infection if *Escherichia coli* or other enterobacteriaceae are isolated. A cutoff of 10^3 CFU/mL is appropriate in men with symptoms (Graham and Galloway, 2001).

Other Diagnostic Tests

Postvoid Residual Measurement

Postvoid residual measurement assesses the volume of urine in the bladder after voiding and can be performed in the office. One method is to have the patient void and then measure any residual urine by catheterization. Less than 50 mL of residual urine is normal, and 200 mL or greater is abnormal (Nitti and Blaivas, 2007). Portable ultrasound units can also estimate postvoid residual urine. *Urodynamics* refers to a battery of tests examining micturition, which may include postvoid residual measurement as well as various tests of bladder and sphincter pressures.

Endoscopy

Urinary endoscopy (cystoscopy) provides visual diagnosis and the opportunity for intervention. Rigid or flexible endoscopic procedures are available. Common interventional techniques include stone retrieval, stent placement, tumor biopsy and resection, and laser treatment. Risks include infection, bleeding, urethral damage, and bladder perforation.

Imaging Studies

Key Points

- Ultrasound studies are ideal for evaluating renal parenchymal disease and testicular disorders.
- Computed tomography is a better choice for evaluating solid renal masses, renal infections, perirenal masses, and renal calculi.

Intravenous Urography

The standard method of upper urinary tract imaging is intravenous urography (IVU), also known as intravenous pyelography (IVP). It is widely available, has a low cost, and can detect upper tract urothelial tumors and renal calculi. However, it cannot distinguish solid from cystic masses. Thus, ultrasound studies are often required to evaluate abnormal findings. Ultrasound and IVU are limited in their ability to detect small renal masses, particularly those smaller than 3 cm. Further, IVU is only 52% to 59% sensitive for detecting renal calculi (Grossfeld et al., 2001b). IVU also requires administering radiographic contrast.

Ultrasound

Ultrasound has many applications for evaluating urinary tract disease. It is the method of choice for imaging renal cysts and the renal parenchyma as part of a renal disease workup. Ultrasound is also the test of choice for evaluating scrotal and testicular disorders. It can usually differentiate masses such as hydrocele, inguinal hernia, and varicocele. Furthermore, regular and color Doppler ultrasound are essential parts of evaluating acute scrotal pathology, such as epididymitis, orchitis, and testicular torsion.

Ultrasound is almost 100% sensitive for testicular tumors (Dogra et al., 2003). However, it does not provide tissue diagnosis. Rather, ultrasonography helps define the nature of the suspected lesion, differentiating it from the many other conditions that might mimic an intratesticular tumor.

Computed Tomography

Computed tomography (CT) is a better choice for evaluating solid renal masses, perirenal masses, and renal infections (Grossfeld et al., 2001b). CT is the test of choice for renal calculi (Lindbloom and Meadows, 2001). Other uses include CT angiography, trauma imaging, and cancer staging.

Other Techniques

Magnetic resonance imaging (MRI) is an option comparable with CT for detecting renal masses. MR urography is also available. MRI studies are more expensive than CT, however, and availability varies (Brehmer, 2002). Thus, this modality is often used when CT examination is equivocal or contraindicated. MRI is used for staging prostate cancers (Harisinghani et al., 2003).

Voiding cystourethrography (VCUG) uses contrast imaging of the bladder and urethra during urination. Contrast material is delivered via catheter, and the images are obtained while the patient voids. It is most often used to diagnose suspected vesicoureteral reflux. Nuclear medicine studies may also be used to examine possible vesicoureteral reflux, as well as renal function or suspected testicular torsion.

Common Urinary Tract Concerns

Key Points

- Dysuria most often indicates UTI, vaginitis, or STI.
- Gross hematuria requires aggressive evaluation.
- Urine microscopy is required to diagnose hematuria. In adults, risk factors for malignancy should be assessed; isolated hematuria is most common in children.
- Hematuria of renal origin often has dysmorphic red cells. Hematuria of bladder origin should show normal red cells.
- Nocturia is common in both genders and increases the risk of falling in older adults.
- The urine protein/creatinine (Upr/UCr) ratio correlates well with a 24-hour urine and is much easier to obtain.
- Proteinuria in children is most often orthostatic.

Dysuria

Urinary burning or pain most often represents UTI or vaginitis. It is common in middle-aged and/or sexually active women. In men, it is more likely to occur as they grow older (Bremnor and Sadovsky, 2002). Both voiding history and sexual history are essential. Questions regarding vaginal symptoms are important in women. Also, use of medications and personal hygiene products should be reviewed.

Dysuria significantly increases the chance that a patient has a UTI. However, there are many potential causes of dysuria (Box 40-1), and empiric treatment based on this symptom alone leads to unnecessary antibiotic use. Incorporating other symptoms increases the likelihood that a UTI is the

---

Box 40-1 Differential Diagnosis of Dysuria

Calculi

Meatal stenosis

Medications

Neoplasm—bladder, benign prostate hyperplasia, prostate, penile, vulvovaginal

Prostatitis

Sexually transmitted infection—*Chlamydia,* gonorrhea, herpes simplex virus, *Mycoplasma, Trichomonas*

Somatization

Trauma—foreign body, mechanical, masturbation, postcoital

Urethral syndrome

Urethritis—infectious, irritant, chemical, spondyloarthropathy

Urinary tract infection—cystitis, pyelonephritis, prostatitis

Vaginitis—allergic, atrophic, bacterial vaginosis, candidiasis, chemical

Modified from Seller RH. Urethral discharge and dysuria. In Differential Diagnosis of Common Complaints, 3rd ed. Philadelphia, Saunders, 1996; and Brenmor JD, Sadovsky R. Evaluation of dysuria in adults. Am Fam Physician 2002;65:1589-1596.

cause (see Urinary Tract Infection) (Bent et al., 2002; McIsaac et al., 2002).

Flank Pain

Flank pain may be a presenting complaint indicating urinary tract disorder. It is typically not relieved by position changes and is colicky in nature. Nausea and vomiting may coincide. Obstruction (e.g., kidney stones) and inflammation (e.g., pyelonephritis) are the two most common causes. The location may help localize the underlying cause (Fig. 40-4). Tumors are less likely, because they are usually only symptomatic if they distend the renal capsule or obstruct the ureter.

Urinary Frequency

As a complaint, urinary frequency implies a deviation from a patient's normal urination pattern. Thus, it may either be truly abnormal or simply more than the patient's custom (but still normal). It may exist alone or in concert with other symptoms. For example, UTI often causes urinary frequency, urgency, and dysuria.

Adults typically urinate five to six times a day (Gerber and Brendler, 2007). Frequency usually represents an increased number of episodes with small volumes of urine as opposed to increased urine volumes, such as in polyuria. These factors help narrow the differential diagnosis (Box 40-2).

Hematuria

Hematuria is often an incidental finding on urinalysis, and evaluation depends on whether it is gross or microscopic and whether it occurs in adults, children, or adolescents. Most patients with hematuria do not have significant pathology, but this depends on the type of hematuria and underlying risk factors. One prospective study found that 61% of patients with hematuria had no finding after evaluation (Khadra et al., 2000).

Gross hematuria is blood in the urine visible to the patient or physician. Microscopic hematuria is the more

common entity. Various cutoff points exist; for adults, the American Urological Association (AUA) Best Practice Policy has defined *microscopic* hematuria as 3 or more (RBCs/hpf (Grossfeld et al., 2001a). In children, clear consensus is lacking, although more than 5 RBCs/hpf found in at least two weekly urine samples is considered abnormal (Dodge et al., 1976; Vehaskari et al., 1979). The reasons for the different definitions may reflect a lower evaluation threshold in adults because of the larger spectrum of potential causes.

Dipstick urinalysis alone is insufficient for diagnosing hematuria, because certain substances (e.g., myoglobin) and test characteristics (e.g., specificity) can cause false-positive results. Thus, microscopic analysis is necessary and inherent in the definition.

Hematuria in Adults

Gross Hematuria

Gross hematuria is a common presenting symptom for patients with bladder or renal cancer (Yun et al., 2004). The sensitivity of gross hematuria for bladder cancer is 83%, and the positive predictive value (PPV) is 22% (Buntinx and Wauters, 1997). However, the studies generating these values were of low quality and based on referral populations. No studies are available on the likelihood that family medicine patients with this finding will have serious pathology. Pending this research, the approach to gross hematuria should remain aggressive (Khadra et al., 2000).

Confirmation of blood in the urine with dipstick and microscopy is needed in cases of red-tinted urine, because certain substances can discolor the urine (see Table 40-1). However, visible clots are unlikely to have a mimic. History should focus on signs and symptoms of infection, trauma, as well as risk factors for urinary tract malignancy (see Bladder Cancer). Physical examination should assess the external

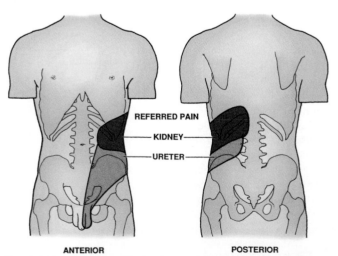

Figure 40-4 Localization of flank pain. *(From Anderson JK, Kabalin JN, Cadeddu. Surgical anatomy of the retroperitoneum, adrenals, kidneys, and ureters. In Wein AJ [ed]. Campbell-Walsh Urology, 9th ed, vol 1. Philadelphia, Saunders-Elsevier, 2007, p 37.)*

Box 40-2 Differential Diagnosis of Urinary Frequency
Anxiety
Bladder calculus
Bladder outlet obstruction
Chemical irritation
Cystitis
Diabetes insipidus
Diabetes mellitus
Detrusor instability
Diuretics
Excessive fluid intake
External genital lesion
Habit
Pelvic mass
Pregnancy
Somatization
Upper motor neuron lesion
Urethritis
Urinary tract infection
Vaginitis
From Hanno PM. Interstitial cystitis and related disorders. In Walsh PC (ed). Campbell's Urology, 8th ed, vol 2. Philadelphia, Saunders, 2002, p 661.

genitalia and include a pelvic examination in women and a prostate examination in men. Urology consultation is appropriate, except when an obviously benign (e.g., menses) or treatable cause is found. Even when a treatable cause is identified (e.g., renal calculi), close follow-up with repeat urinalysis is needed because gross hematuria is frequently a harbinger of serious urinary tract pathology (Khadra et al., 2000).

Microscopic Hematuria

Asymptomatic hematuria potentially signals serious urinary tract disease, although there are many causes, often benign. Hematuria may occur in 9% to 18% of normal subjects (Grossfeld et al., 2001a). Most studies evaluating and defining this problem were not performed in typical family medicine populations or are of lower quality, or both. No prospective studies demonstrate an improved outcome from routine screening. For the general population, finding asymptomatic microscopic hematuria carries a predictive value of only 0.5% (Brehmer, 2002). Thus, benefit from routine microhematuria screening is unlikely (Kryszczuk et al., 2004).

Because routine screening is unhelpful, family physicians encountering microhematuria should consider patient risk characteristics and systematic laboratory testing and imaging (Fig. 40-5). The first step in approaching asymptomatic microscopic hematuria is to verify it is a consistent finding. Patients should have repeat urinalysis, and if two separate follow-up samples are normal, no further evaluation is needed. Transient hematuria is not unusual, and serious urinary tract pathology is unlikely in patients younger than 40 years. Furthermore, history or examination may reveal a benign cause—menses, sexual activity, vigorous exercise, viral illness, or trauma. If repeat examination is normal after these considerations, no further examination is needed. A caveat would be the patient at risk for bladder cancer, because intermittent hematuria can precede this finding, and more extensive follow-up may be warranted (Grossfeld et al., 2001b). Family physicians should be cautious not to misattribute certain causes as benign. For example, warfarin (Coumadin) may cause hematuria if the patient is excessively anticoagulated, but it should not cause hematuria within its goal international normalized ratio (INR) range. Hematuria in this setting is often a sign of urologic disease (Culclasure et al., 1994).

If hematuria is consistently found, the next step is to risk-stratify the patient based on history, physical, and baseline laboratory findings. Initial laboratory testing should include urinalysis, urine culture (if indicated), and serum creatinine level. If UTI is present, a repeat examination 6 weeks after treatment is appropriate. High-risk patients are those at increased risk for urologic malignancy—older than 40 years, tobacco history, analgesic abuse, pelvic irradiation, occupational exposures (see Bladder Cancer), prior urologic disease, irritative voiding symptoms, history of UTIs, and cyclophosphamide use (Grossfeld et al., 2001b). These patients should undergo a more thorough evaluation for the cause of their hematuria, whereas lower-risk patients can have a more limited testing battery (Grossfeld et al., 2001a). Hematuria of renal origin may be associated with microscopic red cell casts or dysmorphic RBCs. Other findings may include proteinuria, elevated serum creatinine, or a physical finding such as

hypertension or edema. These patients need evaluation for renal disease, including urine protein quantification. Some patients will have risk factors and findings for both renal and urologic disease or may already have a history of chronic kidney disease (CKD), so simultaneous evaluations for both causes may be necessary.

Patients whose initial evaluation does not suggest primary renal disease should undergo urologic evaluation based on their risk category. This includes upper urinary tract imaging, urine cytology, and cystoscopy. There are no prospective outcome data on the impact of imaging on asymptomatic microscopic hematuria. Thus, patient-oriented recommendations are unavailable, and family physicians should consider the advantages and disadvantages of the different techniques (see earlier Imaging Studies) when deciding on the appropriate method. IVU is widely available and less costly, and has a low chance of missing pathology when appropriate follow-up studies are used. CT is a good choice for a broad range of urinary tract disorders. Non-contrast-enhanced scans can be performed initially. If these show calculi in a low-risk patient, no further imaging is needed. Contrast studies can follow in all other cases (Grossfeld et al., 2001b). CT is the modality of choice when other techniques fail to reveal a cause (Lang et al., 2002). Deciding between IVU and CT is challenging because the lower cost of IVU may be offset by the eventual need for CT (McDonald et al., 2006). Radiation exposure must be considered as well. Kidney, ureter, and bladder (KUB) studies with ultrasound or MRI are alternatives for patients unable to receive radiographic contrast. However, in the case of CKD patients, the risk of nephrogenic systemic sclerosis from gadolinium contrast may also limit use of MRI.

Cystoscopy is necessary to rule out bladder cancer confidently because no imaging study is adequate for evaluation. Urine cytology is often performed with cystoscopy and has a sensitivity of 40% to 76% for bladder cancer. A positive finding is diagnostic, but a negative finding does not rule out disease. Thus, in high-risk patients, cytology is used adjunctively and in follow-up. Cystoscopy is optional in low-risk patients because it is unlikely to yield a definitive finding. These patients should undergo urine cytology. Furthermore, if they develop any high-risk characteristics, they should undergo cystoscopy (Grossfeld et al., 2001b). Urine tumor markers are available but not yet validated for routine use (Cohen and Brown, 2003).

A cause for hematuria is often not found even after a complete evaluation. Isolated hematuria is *asymptomatic microscopic hematuria* with a normal urologic evaluation and no signs of systemic disease or microscopic evidence of intrinsic renal disease (the definition slightly differs for children). The prognosis is good, although some studies indicate a high proportion of renal abnormalities (e.g., IgA nephropathy). Thus, surveillance for signs of renal disease is appropriate (Grossfeld et al., 2001b). Also, up to 3% of patients with initially negative workups are later found to have a urinary tract malignancy. High-risk patients should have periodic follow-up with focused history, blood pressure, urinalysis, and urine cytology for up to 3 years. This regimen can also be considered for low-risk patients (see Fig. 40-5). Evaluation and treatment of *symptomatic microscopic hematuria* is directed at the condition. However, family physicians should consider the underlying risk of urinary tract abnormalities when deciding

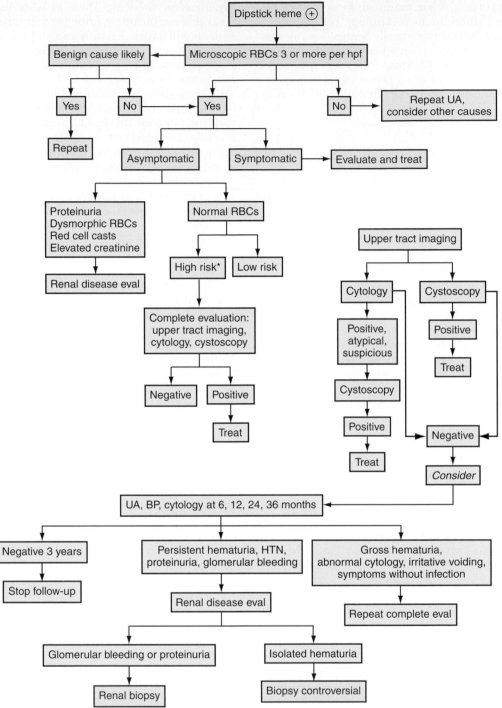

Figure 40-5 Evaluation and follow-up of asymptomatic microscopic hematuria. *BP,* Blood pressure; *HTN,* hypertension; *RBCs,* red blood cells; *UA,* urinalysis.

on follow-up. For example, a patient with a symptomatic kidney stone may have microhematuria. Although this provides the most likely explanation for the bleeding, if the patient has a background risk for malignancy (e.g., smoking) or renal disease, repeat urinalysis is needed to ensure resolution.

Hematuria in Children and Adolescents

Hematuria is a relatively common finding in children, with an estimated prevalence of 0.5% to 2% of asymptomatic school-age children (Dodge et al., 1976). Those with hematuria and proteinuria, particularly when associated with hypertension, edema, or urinary casts, need aggressive evaluation for underlying glomerular disease or uropathy. The vast majority of children with hematuria, however, present with isolated hematuria. This is typically detected on a random urine sample obtained in the context of a routine physical examination but may also present as asymptomatic gross hematuria. In children, the term *isolated* refers to the complete absence of symptoms, significant past medical or family history, physical examination findings, or other abnormalities on urinalysis. This distinction often separates those children with benign processes from those with underlying pathology.

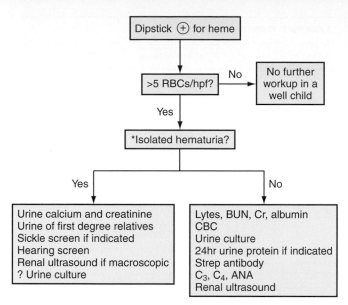

* Negative history, normal physical exam, and absence of symptoms, HTN, pyuria, proteinuria, or cellular casts

Figure 40-6 Approach to the child with hematuria. *ANA*, Antinuclear antibody; *BUN*, blood urea nitrogen; *CBC*, complete blood cell count; *Cr*, creatinine; *RBCs/hpf*, red blood cells per high-power field.

Once the diagnosis of hematuria has been confirmed and a complete history obtained and physical examination performed, a staged evaluation should ensue (Fig. 40-6). Significant underlying renal or urologic disease is highly unlikely in children with isolated microscopic hematuria (Bergstein et al., 2005). A more thorough evaluation is indicated for asymptomatic macroscopic hematuria.

The most common glomerular diseases associated with isolated hematuria are subclinical postinfectious glomerulonephritis, IgA nephropathy, and Alport's syndrome. In the absence of proteinuria or more advanced disease, there is no treatment given for these conditions. Yearly follow-up with blood pressure and urinalysis is indicated for all forms of persistent hematuria.

Hypercalciuria may or may not be associated with pain. The exact mechanism by which hypercalciuria causes hematuria is unproven but probably secondary to crystalluria (Stapleton, 1994). Hypercalciuria is generally defined by a urinary calcium excretion higher than 4 mg/kg/day or a random urine calcium/creatinine ratio higher than 0.2. Higher excretion rates are expected in infants and toddlers. Patients with documented hypercalciuria should undergo a renal ultrasound to rule out nephrocalcinosis or significant stone disease. The treatment is to increase fluid intake and restrict dietary sodium (<3 g/day) while maintaining the recommended daily allowance of calcium (Srivastava and Alon, 2005). This dietary intervention may lower the urine calcium concentration and ultimately result in resolution of the hematuria. A thiazide diuretic should be considered if there is evidence of nephrocalcinosis or nephrolithiasis.

Lower Urinary Tract Symptoms

Lower urinary tract symptoms (LUTS) are the symptoms traditionally associated with *benign prostatic hyperplasia* (BPH). Many subcategories of LUTS exist, but the two most

---

Box 40-3 Lower Urinary Tract Symptoms

Voiding

Hesitancy
Poor urinary flow
Straining
Incomplete bladder emptying
Terminal or postmicturition dribbling
Prolonged urination

Storage

Urinary frequency
Nocturia
Urgency
Urge incontinence

Modified from Thorpe A, Neal D. Benign prostatic hyperplasia. Lancet 2003;361:1359-1367.

---

prominent are storage and voiding symptoms (Box 40-3). *Voiding* symptoms imply obstruction, but physical obstruction may not be responsible. In men with BPH, for example, detrusor overactivity, neurologic disorders, or age-related smooth muscle dysfunction may be the cause. Thus, LUTS should shift attention toward a larger symptom complex with many potential causes. This is particularly important when dealing with urinary tract disorders such as BPH, incontinence, and overactive bladder.

Nocturia

Nocturia describes waking at night to urinate. It is more common in older adults, but no population data define a normal range for any group; therefore the complaint implies a deviation from a perceived norm. Furthermore, the primary complaint often centers on the sleep disturbance rather than on urination. It may represent frequent nocturnal urination or excessive nocturnal urine production (nocturnal polyuria). Although often thought of as a prostatic symptom, it is common in both men and women. The many secondary causes in addition to local causes include prostatic hyperplasia and bladder dysfunction (Box 40-4). In patients with prominent lower urinary tract symptoms, the problem is compounded by urination difficulty. Furthermore, studies in older adults indicate that nocturia/LUTS increases risk of falling (Parsons, et al., 2009). Age-related variations in arginine vasopressin secretion may play a role in nocturnal polyuria (Weiss and Blaivas, 2000).

Treatment centers on the underlying cause, and a voiding diary may aid clinical decisions. Prostate hyperplasia or bladder dysfunction often receives first attention. Treating BPH may help, although BPH often does not result in true physical obstruction, and epidemiologic data have indicated that nocturia is common in men without prostatic obstruction. Thus, family physicians should consider the contribution of nocturnal polyuria. For example, patients with chronic heart failure and leg edema may benefit from fluid restriction and napping with leg elevation during the day. Treating obstructive sleep apnea helps alleviate the increased urine production resulting from increased atrial natriuretic peptide production. Behavioral

Box 40-4 Causes of Nocturia

Alcohol consumption
Anxiety
Benign prostatic hyperplasia
Bladder outlet obstruction
Caffeine
Calculi
Chronic heart failure
Cystitis
Detrusor instability
Diabetes insipidus
Diabetes mellitus
Diuretics
Dysfunctional voiding
Edema
Excessive nighttime fluid consumption
Myeloneuropathy
Nephrotic syndrome
Neurogenic bladder
Obstructive sleep apnea
Overactive bladder syndrome
Sleep disorders
Somatization
Stroke
Urologic cancer

From Weiss JP, Blaivas JG. Nocturia. J Urol 2000;163:5-12.

Table 40-3 Proteinuria Values

Test	Protein Value
Dipstick	≥1+ if urine specific gravity ≤1.015 *or* ≥2+ if urine specific gravity >1.015
UPr/UCr[*]	Children >0.5 (age 6 mo to 2 yr) >0.25 (>2 yr) Adults: >0.2
24-hour urine assay	Children >4 mg/m^2/hr >100 mg/m^2/day Adults 30-300 mg/24 hr—microalbuminuria >300 mg/24 hr—albuminuria >3.5 g/24 hr—nephritic-range proteinuria

[*]Urine protein/creatinine ratio.

interventions include avoiding excess nighttime alcohol or fluid intake and afternoon napping. Adjusting diuretic doses so they are given earlier in the evening should negate medication effects during sleep (Weiss and Blaivas, 2000).

Proteinuria

The kidneys normally excrete a small amount of protein daily, usually glycoproteins. Only very small amounts of globulins, light-chain proteins, or albumin are released. Functional proteinuria may result from physiologic changes in glomerular filtration, as occurs with exercise (Venkat, 2004). However, consistent albuminuria implies glomerular or tubular dysfunction.

The urine dipstick is the most convenient measurement, but a more accurate test is the Upr/UCr ratio, obtained by dividing the random urine sample protein level by the urine creatinine level (both in mg/dL). This ratio has proven correlation with 24-hour excretion rates (Ginsberg et al., 1983). Thus, random urine samples are the best way to identify and follow proteinuria, and 24-hour collections are usually not needed (Levey et al., 2003) (Table 40-3). However, results from those with low or high levels of muscle mass may not correlate as well with 24-hour measurements (Venkat, 2004).

Proteinuria in Adults

Proteinuria is a marker of kidney disease in adults and may actually contribute to renal impairment. Patients with diabetes should be periodically tested for microalbuminuria. Others at risk for kidney disease, such as patients with hypertension, should also be tested.

Adults with proteinuria need their UPr/Ucr determined. Those with values outside the normal range should undergo an evaluation for CKD (see later). Patients with dipstick proteinuria but normal-range UPr/UCr values should be rechecked at periodic follow-up (Fig. 40-7).

Proteinuria in Children and Adolescents

Most proteinuria in children is transient when followed up with weekly urine sample testing. Persistent proteinuria found in at least two of three weekly urine samples warrants further evaluation to identify those children who may have chronic renal disease.

Proteinuria in children may be classified as functional, isolated, or symptomatic. *Functional* proteinuria may occur with fever or exercise. *Isolated* proteinuria is defined by the absence of abnormal history, physical examination findings, symptoms, or other urinary abnormalities. The most common cause of this form is *benign orthostatic proteinuria,* defined by normal protein excretion overnight or in the supine position. The initial evaluation for isolated proteinuria involves obtaining a first-morning urine sample for protein and creatinine as well as a formal urinalysis for microscopy review (Hogg et al., 2000). The absence of morning proteinuria, as evidenced by normal UPr/UCr, supports the diagnosis of benign orthostatic proteinuria. A more accurate assessment is a split 24-hour urine collection for protein. Benign orthostatic proteinuria may be transient or fixed and in either case has an excellent prognosis (Springberg et al., 1982). In contrast, *nonorthostatic* isolated proteinuria with a duration of 1 year or longer may represent significant renal pathology (Trachtman et al., 1994). Thus, these patients need yearly or twice-yearly clinical follow-up with assessment of blood pressure, renal function, serum albumin, urine microscopy, and urine protein.

Pathologic proteinuria, whether isolated or symptomatic, occurs in the setting of a variety of glomerular and tubulointerstitial diseases (Box 40-5). Some children may present with the *nephrotic syndrome* (proteinuria, hypoalbuminemia, edema). Depending on the degree of proteinuria and the results of the initial laboratory evaluation, a renal biopsy may be indicated (Fig. 40-8).

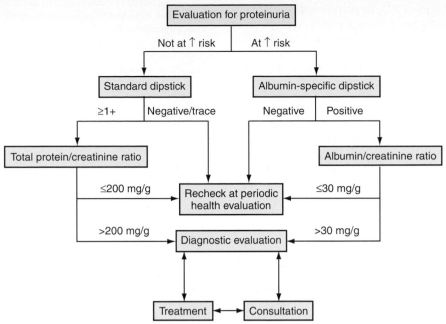

Figure 40-7 Approach to proteinuria in adults. *(Modified from Levey AS, Coresh J, Balk E, et al. National Kidney Foundation practice guidelines for chronic kidney disease: evaluation, classification, and stratification. Ann Intern Med 2003;139:137-147, E148-E149. Redrawn from National Kidney Foundation/Kidney Disease Quality Initiative. See Web Resources.)*

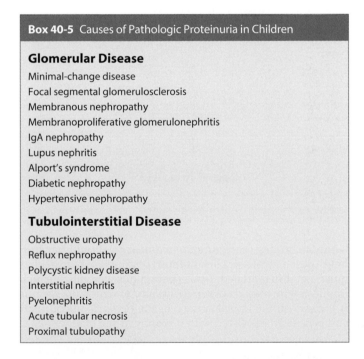

Box 40-5 Causes of Pathologic Proteinuria in Children

Glomerular Disease

Minimal-change disease
Focal segmental glomerulosclerosis
Membranous nephropathy
Membranoproliferative glomerulonephritis
IgA nephropathy
Lupus nephritis
Alport's syndrome
Diabetic nephropathy
Hypertensive nephropathy

Tubulointerstitial Disease

Obstructive uropathy
Reflux nephropathy
Polycystic kidney disease
Interstitial nephritis
Pyelonephritis
Acute tubular necrosis
Proximal tubulopathy

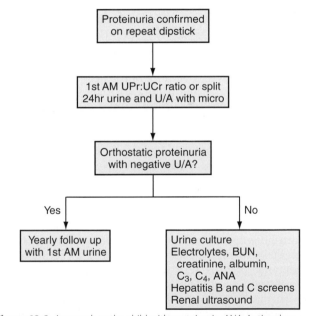

Figure 40-8 Approach to the child with proteinuria. *ANA,* Antinuclear antibody; *BUN,* blood urea nitrogen; *U/A,* urinalysis; *UPr:UCr,* urine protein/ urine creatinine.

Anatomic Disorders

Key Points

- Prenatally identified hydronephrosis may be caused by underlying urinary tract obstruction. These infants need close follow-up with ultrasound in the first week of life.
- Hydroceles in infants often resolve by age 2 years. Hydroceles in adults may have a secondary cause.
- Reassure patients with Peyronie's disease that it is usually self-limited.

- Testicular torsion is a medical emergency. Torsion of the appendix testis is less severe and can be managed with supportive care.
- Undescended testes increase the risk for testicular cancer in the undescended as well as contralateral testicle.

Anatomic urinary tract disorders involve various congenital and acquired abnormalities, most notably of the external genitalia. Testicular disorders are seen more often than abnormalities of the penis, particularly undescended testes. Anatomic derangements of the bladder, ureter, and kidney are often only discovered incidentally or during an evaluation for UTIs, voiding problems, CKD, or pain possibly related to the urinary tract. For example, posterior urethral valves cause vesicoureteral reflux and may contribute to recurrent UTIs (see Urinary Tract Infections in Children).

Scrotal masses are frequently encountered in family medicine. Anatomic causes of scrotal masses are not limited to the urinary tract, and neoplastic and infectious causes are also in the differential diagnosis (Table 40-4). Scrotal or testicular pain, the so-called acute scrotum, implies a more urgent or emergent cause (e.g., testicular torsion). Because the history and physical examination may not be adequate to differentiate certain conditions (e.g., epididymo-orchitis from testicular torsion), adjunctive imaging such as ultrasound is often used.

Fetal Hydronephrosis

With the pervasive use of fetal ultrasound, hydronephrosis is more often diagnosed prenatally. A dilated renal collecting system is often the only indication of a number of congenital uropathies (Ismaili et al., 2004). Two processes cause hydronephrosis, reverse urine flow (vesicoureteral reflux, VUR) and impaired forward urine flow (obstruction). VUR occurs as an isolated entity or can be associated with a more complicated uropathy, such as bladder outlet obstruction with VUR. Obstructive uropathy may occur at different sites along the urinary tract, most often the ureteropelvic junction (UPJ).

Infants with fetal hydronephrosis need an ultrasound in the first week of life. If normal, a repeat ultrasound should be done in 2 to 4 weeks because of the possibility of a false-negative study in the low urine flow state characteristic of the newborn (Becker and Avner, 1995). Once the diagnosis is confirmed, evaluation includes a urinalysis, urine culture, basic metabolic panel (if bilateral), and a VCUG. If the VCUG is normal, a furosemide renogram is needed to determine the presence and degree of obstruction.

Hydrocele

Hydroceles are fluid accumulations in the tunica vaginalis and can be *primary*, resulting from a failure of the processus vaginalis to close during development, or secondary to epididymitis, orchitis, testicular torsion, trauma, or tumors (Brenner and Ojo, 2004). Hydroceles typically transilluminate, whereas inguinal hernias do not. In young children, management is supportive, with the hydrocele often resolving by age 2 years. Hydroceles presenting beyond 2 years or those associated with inguinal hernias require surgical consultation. Also, some hydroceles are communicating; that is, fluid can pass from the peritoneal cavity into the hydrocele. These may change in size with activity or during the day and need surgical evaluation (Schneck and Bellinger, 2007). Hydroceles arising de novo in adults often have a secondary cause and require evaluation (Dogra et al., 2003).

Hypospadias

Hypospadias, in which the urethra opens on the underside of the penis, is infrequently seen (Fig. 40-9). However, it is important that hypospadias is recognized early, preferably at the initial newborn examination. It can occur with or

Table 40-4 Selected Differential Diagnosis of Scrotal Masses with Physical Findings

Abnormality	Physical Finding
Epididymitis, orchitis	Tender mass
Hydrocele	Transilluminates
Inguinal hernia	Does not transilluminate
Testicular torsion	Pain and loss of cremasteric reflex
Torsion of the appendix testis	Blue dot sign
Trauma	Tender scrotum, edema, trauma history
Tumor	Solid mass
Spermatocele	Nontender cystic mass
Varicocele	Bag of worms appearance

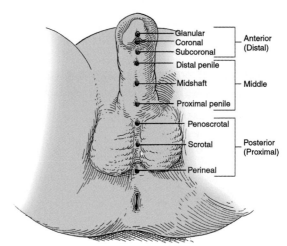

Figure 40-9 Hypospadias. *(From Borer JG, Retik AB. Hypospadias. In Wein AJ [ed]. Campbell-Walsh Urology, 9th ed, vol IV, Philadelphia, Elsevier, 2007.)*

without chordee (curvature). Circumcision should be withheld and a urology consultation obtained. Hypospadias must be differentiated from ambiguous genitalia, which implies an intersex disorder. *Epispadias*, in which the meatus is located on the dorsal surface of the penis, is uncommon and is usually associated with extrophy of the bladder.

Labial Adhesions

Labial adhesions may be seen in young girls and may be partial or complete (fusion) and asymptomatic. However, labial adhesions can be associated with difficult or abnormal urination and may contribute to the development of UTIs. It is important to perform an external genital examination in the female with her first UTI (Fig. 40-10). Retrospective data and case series support topical estrogen cream to the affected areas, with gentle traction until the adhesions have separated (Bacon, 2002). In a recent study, however, labial separation occurred more quickly and with less recurrence in patients treated with betamethasone than in those treated with estrogen cream (Mayoglou et al., 2009).

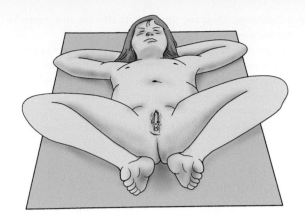

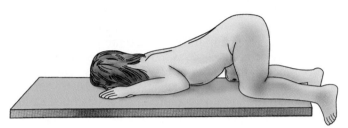

Figure 40-10 Techniques for pediatric female genital examination. *(From Canning DA, Nguyen MT. Evaluation of the pediatric urologic patient. In Wein AJ [ed]. Campbell-Walsh Urology, 9th ed, vol 1. Philadelphia, Saunders, 2007.)*

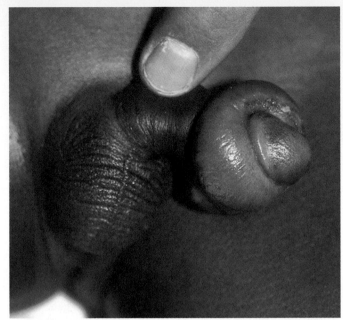

Figure 40-11 Paraphimosis. *(From Kleigman R, et al. Nelson Textbook of Pediatrics, ed 18. Philadelphia, Saunders-Elsevier, 2007, p 2256.)*

Peyronie's Disease

Peyronie's disease is characterized by formation of fibrosis in the tunica albuginea, with resulting penile deformity and pain. Symptoms include painful erection, physical penile deformity (often curvature), palpable penile plaque (fibrosis), and erectile dysfunction. Pain is typically transient, and most cases do not result in a deformity so severe that it impairs intercourse. Sexual history, counseling, and partner involvement are important, because Peyronie's disease can be disruptive to a relationship. Most patients do not require any treatment beyond reassurance and counseling. Nonsurgical treatments are available (e.g., colchicine, intralesional verapamil), but supporting evidence is limited, and urologic consultation should be considered before exploring treatment. Steroid injection is best avoided. Surgery is an option in severe cases (Lewis and Munarriz, 2007).

Phimosis and Paraphimosis

Phimosis (inability to retract foreskin over glans) and paraphimosis (inability to return retracted foreskin over glans) are possible complications seen in the uncircumcised male (Fig. 40-11). About 50% of boys typically are able to retract their foreskin by 1 year of age and 80% by age 3 (Anderson and Anderson, 1999). Topical estrogen therapy has been reported as successful, but no randomized trials support its use (Yanagisawa et al., 2000). However, low-potency topical corticosteroid therapy combined with daily prepuce retraction appears effective for phimosis (Zampieri et al., 2005).

Because vascular engorgement leads to necrosis of the glans, acute paraphimosis needs urgent medical attention. A dorsal slit procedure may be required if other reduction techniques are unsuccessful. Ice packs and plastic wrap may reduce the edema enough to allow manual reduction (Choe, 2000). Circumcision is generally indicated after the reduction and edema resolution. Methods of reduction included manual, osmotic, puncture and aspiration (Little and White, 2004).

Spermatoceles

Spermatoceles (epididymal cysts) are painless cysts filled with sperm and can be palpated distinct from the testis. They transilluminate, are generally of no consequence, and do not affect fertility.

Testicular Disorders

Testicular Torsion

Although occasionally seen in the newborn male, testicular torsion is an acquired condition seen during puberty and is an emergency. It usually presents with abrupt onset of severe scrotal pain, at times waking the patient up in the early morning. Associated signs and symptoms include fever, nausea, vomiting, and abdominal pain. Intermittent testicular torsion has been described. On physical examination, the testis may lie in a more horizontal position, caused by a lack of normal attachment to the tunica vaginalis ("bell clapper" deformity), and demonstrate a loss of the cremasteric reflex. The diagnosis of testicular torsion can be made by physical examination or with the assistance of color Doppler ultrasound; however, physical examination is unreliable for ruling torsion in or out (Schmitz and Safranek, 2009). Timeliness of the diagnosis is critical, because testicular viability declines to 0% if detorsion occurs 24 hours after the onset of symptoms (Brenner and Ojo, 2004). Testicular torsion can occur in systemic illnesses, such as Henoch-Schönlein purpura, or can mimic the symptoms of other conditions, such as appendicitis or nephrolithiasis.

Torsion of the appendix testis presents similar to testicular torsion, although the symptoms are not as severe. The classic patient is a boy age 7 to 12 years. Palpation of the testis is normal except for a small, tender, palpable mass located on the superior or inferior pole. The cremasteric reflex is intact. The "blue dot" sign may be present and represents the compromised appendix testis as viewed through the scrotum. Diagnosis is generally made clinically and treatment is supportive, including analgesia and scrotal elevation. It is not unusual for the pain to last 5 to 10 days, but chronic pain may occur and warrants urology consultation.

Undescended Testis

Undescended testis (testes) occurs in 2.7% to 5.9% of full-term male infants, decreasing to 1.2% to 1.8% by age 1 year (Pillai and Bassner, 1998); the incidence is higher in premature infants. An undescended testis must be differentiated from a *retractile* testis, which may occur as the cremasteric reflex is developed. As opposed to an undescended testis, a retractile testis can be manually coaxed into the scrotum. In general, the patient with truly undescended testes needs urology evaluation. Failure to respond to human chorionic gonadotropin (hCG) is an indication for orchiopexy, especially if the testes have not descended by the first birthday. This should be accomplished before the child is 6 years old. The testicular examination should be taught to orchiopexy patients because of the slightly increased risk of cancer in either testicle (Altman, 1967).

Varicoceles

A varicocele is a collection of dilated and tortuous veins surrounding the spermatic cord. It is most often asymptomatic and left-sided. Varicoceles arise in adolescence and are estimated to occur in 10% to 15% of the male population (Schneck and Bellinger, 2007). Evidence that varicoceles cause infertility is limited, but they are found in 12% of men presenting with infertility and in mature adolescents with varicoceles, 26% had abnormal semen analyses (Brenner and Ojo, 2004; Biyani et al., 2009). The "bag of worms" appearance on scrotal examination is the hallmark of this diagnosis. Inferior vena cava obstruction should be considered if the varicocele is right sided, of acute onset, or occurs in a prepubertal boy.

Functional Disorders

Key Points

- Patients with proteinuria and elevated Upr/UCr should be evaluated for chronic kidney disease. The serum creatinine level may not correlate with glomerular filtration rate; GFR estimates are adequate to diagnose kidney disease; 24-hour urine testing is usually not needed.
- Patients with chronic kidney disease need systemic management.
- Enuresis typically resolves with age. A bed-wetting alarm is effective if treatment is needed.
- Erectile dysfunction has many causes and may be a marker of vascular disease.
- Pelvic floor muscle exercises are first-line treatment for stress and mixed urinary incontinence.

- Anticholinergic drugs and trospium are effective treatments for urge incontinence.
- Anticholinergic drugs for an overactive bladder may not have clinically significant benefits and often cause dry mouth.
- Men with recurrent kidney stones and idiopathic hypercalciuria should be on a low-sodium, low-protein diet. Low-calcium diets do not reduce stone formation.
- Non-contrast-enhanced CT is the test of choice for diagnosing kidney stones.

Chronic Kidney Disease

Renal disease is a significant public health burden, with almost 20 million persons in the United States having chronic kidney disease (Coresh et al., 2003). In 2002 the National Kidney Foundation issued guidelines on the evaluation and management of CKD. The centerpiece of this new approach is defining CKD as kidney damage or decreased kidney function for 3 months or longer (Levey et al., 2003).

Proteinuria is a clinical sign of kidney disease. Patients with proteinuria should be approached as described earlier. Patients with abnormal urinary protein values (e.g., UPr/UCr) or other markers of kidney damage should be assessed for CKD (Johnson et al., 2004). The primary measure of kidney function is the glomerular filtration rate (GFR), and the stages of CKD are based on GFR (calculated by Cockcroft-Gault or MDRD equation) (Table 40-5). The modification of diet in renal disease (MDRD) equation performs as well or better than measured creatinine clearance (Levey et al., 1999). However, physicians should be aware that the values obtained by the equations may differ slightly, and the

Table 40-5 Stages of Chronic Kidney Disease

Stage	Defining Features	GFR[†] (mL/min/1.73 m²)
1	Kidney damage,* normal GFR	≥90
2	Kidney damage, mild decrease in GFR	60-89
3	Moderate decrease in GFR	30-59
4	Severe decrease in GFR	15-29
5	Kidney failure	<15

*Pathologic renal abnormalities; markers of damage: abnormal blood, urine, or imaging studies.
Calculators for office use are available from National Kidney Disease Education Program (NKDEP). http://www.nkdep.nih.gov/professionals/gfr_calculators/index.htm.
[†]Glomerular filtration rate (GFR) equations
Cockcroft-Gault equation:

$$C_{Cr}(mL/min) = \frac{([140 - Age] \times Weight)/72 \times S_{Cr})}{(\times 0.85, if\ female)}$$

Abbreviated MDRD:

$$GFR(mL/min/1.73m^2) = \frac{1.86 \times (S_{Cr})^{1.154} \times (Age)}{(0.742[if\ female] \times 1.210[if\ black])}$$

C_{Cr}, Creatinine clearance; *MDRD*, modification of diet in renal disease study equation; S_{Cr}, serum creatinine level (mg/dL).
From Johnson CA, Levey AS, Coresh J, et al. Clinical practice guidelines for chronic kidney disease in adults. Part II. Glomerular filtration rate, proteinuria, and other markers. Am Fam Physician 2004;70:1091-1097.

Cockcroft-Gault equation is the primary measure used when validating recommended medication dosing adjustments for creatinine clearance. Slightly elevated (or even "normal range") serum creatinine levels may correlate with impaired GFR, depending on factors such as age or race (Table 40-6). Thus, the serum creatinine level alone is an inadequate clinical marker for a patient's risk for, or the presence of, renal impairment (Levey et al., 2003).

Workup of persons identified as having CKD (by GFR) includes a complete urinalysis, renal ultrasound, and determination of the serum creatinine and serum electrolyte levels and albumin/creatinine ratio. Patients should also be assessed for background risk factors that may worsen their disease. Particular emphasis should be placed on the most common problems—diabetes, hypertension, and tobacco use. Patients with class 1 CKD have evidence of renal disease (e.g., diabetes, proteinuria) but a normal GFR. Patients with type 2 diabetes and nephropathy clearly benefit from treatment with an angiotensin-converting enzyme (ACE) inhibitor or an angiotensin receptor blocker (ARB). Furthermore, blood pressure control is critical for preventing nephropathy progression. The evidence is stronger for ARBs for preventing end-stage failure in patients with advanced nephropathy (Shlipak, 2009).

Management of patients with stage 1 or 2 CKD focuses on risk factors and preventing disease progression. Particular attention should be directed toward controlling diabetes and hypertension, if present. CKD has numerous complications requiring regular assessment. In stage 3 CKD, family physicians should assess for anemia, neuropathy, nutrition, and disorders of bone metabolism. Patients with a GFR less than 30 should be referred to a nephrologist. Stage 4 patients should be proactively prepared for dialysis or transplantation. Patients in stage 5 should be monitored for uremia and dialysis initiated at that point (Levey et al., 2003).

Chronic Nonbacterial Prostatitis

The term *prostatitis* means prostate inflammation but often also implies infection (infectious causes are discussed later). However, prostatitis encompasses many different clinical entities (Table 40-7). Chronic nonbacterial prostatitis, also

Table 40-6 Serum Creatinine Levels and Chronic Kidney Disease*

| Age (yr) | Serum Creatinine (mg/dL) MDRD Study Equation | | | | Cockcroft-Gault Equation | |
| | European American | | African American | | | |
	Men	Women	Men	Women	Men	Women
30	1.47	1.13	1.73	1.34	1.83	1.56
40	1.39	1.08	1.65	1.27	1.67	1.42
50	1.34	1.03	1.58	1.22	1.50	1.28
60	1.30	1.00	1.53	1.18	1.33	1.13
70	1.26	0.97	1.49	1.15	1.17	0.99
80	1.23	0.95	1.46	1.12	1.00	0.85

Modified from Levey AS, Coresh J, Balk E, et al. National Kidney Foundation practice guidelines for chronic kidney disease: evaluation, classification, and stratification. Ann Intern Med 2003;139:137-147, E148-E149.
*These values correspond to a GFR of 60 mL/min/1.73 m^2.
MDRD, Modification of diet in renal disease.

Table 40-7 NIH and NIDDK Classification System for Prostatitis

Category	Name	Defining Characteristics
I	Acute bacterial prostatitis	Acute prostate infection
II	Chronic bacterial prostatitis	Recurrent prostate infection
IIIa	Chronic nonbacterial prostatitis—inflammatory chronic pelvic pain syndrome	No infection; white cells evident in semen, prostatic secretions, or postprostate massage voided urine
IIIb	Chronic nonbacterial prostatitis—noninflammatory chronic pelvic pain syndrome	No infection; no white cells in semen, prostatic secretions, or postprostate massage voided urine
IV	Asymptomatic inflammatory prostatitis	No subjective symptoms; white cells in prostatic secretions or prostate tissue

From McNaughton-Collins M, Joyce GF, Wise M, Pontari MA. Prostatitis. In Litwin MS, Saigal CS (eds). Urologic Diseases in America. US Department of Health and Human Services, Public Health Service, National Institutes of Health (NIH), National Institute of Diabetes and Digestive and Kidney Diseases (NIDDK). Washington, DC, US Government Printing Office, 2007; NIH Pub No 07-5512, p 13.

known as *chronic pelvic pain syndrome,* is poorly understood and better classified as a *functional* urinary tract disorder. Patients with chronic nonbacterial prostatitis can experience genital, ejaculatory, perineal, back, pelvic, or rectal pain; irritative voiding symptoms; and sexual dysfunction. Unlike those with category II prostatitis, however, patients with nonbacterial prostatitis do not experience recurrent UTIs (Stevermer and Easley, 2000). Physical examination may be normal or reveal a tender prostate.

Chronic nonbacterial prostatitis negatively affects quality of life and is associated with depression, anxiety, and somatization (McNaughton-Collins, 2003). A potentially helpful clinical tool is the validate National Institutes of Health (NIH) Chronic Prostatitis Symptom Index, which can help define a patient's symptoms (McNaughton-Collins et al., 2007). Treatment is problematic because the underlying pathogenesis is uncertain and the evidence base poor. Alpha-adrenergic blockers reduce pain and improve quality of life (Erickson et al., 2008). There is not enough evidence to recommend routine antibiotic use (McNaughton-Collins et al., 2001). Patients with NIH category IIIa prostatitis can receive a trial of a fluoroquinolone antibiotic for 2 to 4 weeks or a prolonged course (4-6 weeks total) if they benefit. However, antibiotics in categories IIIb and IV prostatitis appear ineffective (Erickson et al., 2008; Wagenlehner and Naber, 2003). Allopurinol, 5α-reductase inhibitors, anti-inflammatory drugs, biofeedback, pentosan (Elmiron), prostate massage, thermotherapy and sitz baths are alternatives of uncertain effectiveness (McNaughton-Collins and Wilt, 2002). As in other somatic syndromes, patients benefit from a supportive physician relationship focused on quality of life rather than cure.

Enuresis

Nocturnal Enuresis

Enuresis is a common childhood complaint. Distinguishing *primary* enuresis (children who have never achieved a satisfactory period of nighttime dryness) from *secondary* enuresis (return of nighttime wetting after 6 months of nighttime dryness) is important; secondary enuresis indicates possible dysfunctional voiding or other pathologic condition. A child needs to be 5 years old to be considered enuretic, and children younger than 7 years may not exhibit the commitment necessary for treatment to be effective (Kiddoo, 2007). It is more common in boys and has a genetic tendency. The exact cause is unknown. Family background, life stressors, and psychological problems have not shown a causal relationship (Theidke, 2003). Enuresis typically resolves with age, although 1% of adults may have an average of two wet nights per week.

History should focus on birth and development, family history, voiding and defecation history, signs of abnormal voiding, and parental response to the problem. A voiding diary may be helpful (Theidke, 2003). Evaluation with a urinalysis and an age-appropriate neurologic examination, including gait and anal reflex (wink), as well as close examination of the lumbosacral area, is mandatory to determine the need for further evaluation in the patient with primary nocturnal enuresis. If the history, physical exam, and urinalysis are normal, usually no further workup is indicated.

Interventions found to be beneficial for managing nocturnal enuresis include dry-bed training with positive reinforcement, decreasing fluids at night, medications such as desmopressin and tricyclics, and conditioning therapy with nighttime bed-wetting alarms. Waking children age 4 to 5 years after 1.5 to 2 hours of sleep ("lifting") may help reduce the number of wet nights (vanDommelen et al., 2009) A bed-wetting alarm is the most effective treatment for nocturnal enuresis (Glazener et al., 2005b). Desmopressin is effective, but the effects are temporary, with a high relapse rate once discontinued (Glazener and Evans, 2002; Kiddoo, 2007). Tricyclic medications have proved efficacious for nocturnal enuresis, but side effects such as anorexia, drowsiness, and cardiac arrhythmias limit their use. A limited study found that reboxetine, a nonadrenaline reuptake inhibitor without apparent cardiac toxicity, successfully treated enuresis, especially in conjunction with desmopressin (Neveus, 2006). Because most children will be dry by 7 years old, reassurance may be most appropriate until that point (Kiddoo, 2007).

Dysfunctional Voiding

Dysfunctional voiding, a term used to describe impairments of micturition, encompasses a wide array of symptoms and can lead to significant morbidity. The typical patient is a school-age girl who may be enuretic or have recurrent UTIs. Parents will often give a history that the child "holds her urine" or demonstrates urgency with infrequent voiding. *Vincent's curtsy* is a well-known posture assumed by these girls to help alleviate the pressure of a full bladder, which can result in a non-neurogenic neurogenic bladder. The dysfunctional voiding scoring system (DVSS) is a validated tool instrument that can be used to diagnose and evaluate children with dysfunctional voiding (Farhat et al., 2000). Urodynamic studies, cystoscopy, and imaging studies are available in the workup of voiding dysfunction, if indicated by the history and physical examination. Treatment is designed to improve bladder tone by placing the patient on a timed voiding schedule.

Erectile Disorders

Erectile Dysfunction

Erectile dysfunction (ED) refers to "the inability to attain and/or maintain penile erection sufficient for satisfactory sexual performance" (NIH Consensus Development Panel on Impotence, 1993). Sexual function declines with age, and normal erectile function depends on a number of body systems—cardiovascular, endocrine, muscular, nervous, psychological (Lue, 2000). Disorders in any of these can lead to ED, although many factors often are involved.

As many as 30 million men have ED (Fink et al., 2003, 2002). Risk factors include diabetes, cardiovascular diseases (e.g., hypertension, coronary heart disease, hyperlipidemia), lifestyle (e.g., alcohol, obesity, smoking), depression, neurologic disease or damage, pelvic or vascular surgery, and medications, and other endocrine and urologic disorders (Fink et al., 2002. Medications such as antidepressants and antihypertensives are often implicated, and medications play a role in as many as 25% of cases (McVary, 2007) (see eTable 40-1). As many as two thirds of men with cardiovascular

---

Box 40-6 Erectile Dysfunction Treatment Options

Alprostadil[*][†]
    Intracavernosal (Caverject, Edex)[*]
    Intraurethral (Muse)[*]
    Topical
Apomorphine (sublingual)[*]
Cognitive-behavioral therapy
Ginseng
Phosphodiesterase (type 5) inhibitors
    Sildenafil (Viagra)[*]
    Tadalafil (Cialis)[*]
    Vardenafil (Levitra)[*]
Yohimbine (Yocon, Yohimex, generic)
Papaverine[‡] (alone or mixed with phentolamine or phentolamine and alprostadil)
Penile prosthesis surgery
Psychosexual counseling
Therapeutic lifestyle changes—smoking cessation, weight loss, limited alcohol consumption
Vacuum device[*]

Modified from Tharyan P, Gopalakrishanan G. Erectile dysfunction. Clin Evid 2009;05:1803.
[*]These treatments have good evidence of benefit.
[†]Harms may limit use. Alprostadil may cause penile pain.
[‡]Harms may limit use. Papaverine injections may alter liver function and cause penile bruising or fibrosis.

---

disease experience ED before the onset of cardiac symptoms (Billups, 2005), suggesting clinical risk assessment in men presenting with ED.

Assessment should include a general health history, with particular focus on risk factors and psychosocial issues, such as substance use, libido, and partner relationship. Clinical survey tools such as the sexual health inventory for men (SHIM) can aid in diagnosis and treatment (Cappelleri and Rosen, 2005). Surgical and medication history is essential. The examination should focus on genitourinary, endocrine, and vascular function. Laboratory work includes urinalysis, blood count, and assessment of renal function and glucose, lipid, and serum testosterone levels. Hyperprolactinemia may cause ED, although this occurs in fewer than 2% of cases (Mikhail, 2005). Thus, determination of prolactin levels, along with free testosterone and luteinizing hormone (LH) levels, should be reserved for patients with signs or findings consistent with hypogonadism (e.g., low serum testosterone level) (Lue, 2000).

Alprostadil (intracavernosal, intraurethral), apomorphine, and phosphodiesterase type 5 (PDE-5) inhibitors are effective ED treatments (Box 40-6). Potentially beneficial alternative therapies include yohimbine and Korean red ginseng, with yohimbine having the stronger evidence base (Tharyan and Gopalakrishanan, 2009). Attention to lifestyle issues is important. For example, weight loss may improve sexual function in obese patients (Esposito et al., 2004). Discontinuing potentially causative medicines is an option, although risks and benefits of this choice and its effect on other conditions must be considered. The advent of oral treatment with PDE-5 inhibitors has made these medications the drugs of first choice (Table 40-8). Cardiovascular disease is a concern with PDE-5 inhibitors because these patients may be taking nitrates or may experience cardiac symptoms from sexual exertion. The medicine itself does not cause ischemia. Furthermore, no increase in cardiovascular events or death was found in randomized trials (Fink et al., 2002). Patients with antidepressant-induced ED, primarily from selective serotonin reuptake inhibitors (SSRIs), may benefit from the addition of a PDE-5 inhibitor, a switch to a different antidepressant (e.g., bupropion), or a drug holiday (Rudkin et al., 2004; Sturpe et al., 2002). PDE-5 inhibitors may also be beneficial in patients with ED from diabetes or spinal cord injury.

One unintended consequence of widely publicized ED treatments is the negative emotions when these treatments fail, which they often do (Fink et al., 2002; Tomlinson and Wright, 2004). Psychosexual counseling and cognitive-behavioral may be beneficial, although evidence is limited for these interventions (Tharyan and Gopalakrishanan, 2009).

Premature Ejaculation

Although various definitions exist, premature ejaculation is "ejaculation that occurs sooner than desired, either before or shortly after penetration, causing distress to either one or both partners" (AUA, 2004). Sexual history, psychological history, and differentiation from ED are essential. Treatment should be tailored to the individual patient. Psychological interventions are options for willing patients. Although no medicines are U.S. Food and Drug Administration (FDA) approved for this problem, exploiting side effects of SSRIs and topical anesthetics is an option.

Incontinence

Urinary incontinence is defined by the involuntary loss of urine. Many systems for classifying incontinence exist, but the most widely accepted divides the problem into stress, urge, and mixed incontinence (Abrams et al., 2010). *Stress* incontinence is the loss of urine with effort, exertion, or the Valsalva maneuver (e.g., coughing). *Urge* incontinence is urine leakage preceded by an urge to void. *Mixed* incontinence describes patients with symptoms from both categories. *Functional* incontinence can be used to describe patients who have incontinence with clear functional causes and who do not fit the previous categories (e.g., spinal cord injury, bedridden patient).

Urinary incontinence negatively affects quality of life through social isolation, depression, sexual dysfunction, and impaired activities of daily living (SIGN, 2004). Women are more likely to experience incontinence at a younger age than men. Risk increases with age, increased weight, depression, hysterectomy, smoking, and childbirth (Melville et al., 2005, Onwude, 2009). Causes for men are not well defined but include prostate procedures. Women are less likely than men to seek medical advice for this problem (SIGN, 2004). In community-dwelling elderly persons the rates may approach 35%, up to 60% in those at long-term care facilities (Griebling, 2009).

Evaluation should address bowel and bladder history, symptom characteristics, surgical history, and medication review. A voiding diary may be helpful in characterizing the

Table 40-8 Oral Phosphodiesterase (PDE-5) Inhibitors for Erectile Dysfunction

Drug	Doses, Duration	Dosing	Side Effects, Precautions, Drug Contraindications
Sildenafil (Viagra)	25, 50, 100 mg 4 hr	50 mg (25 mg if >65 yr); 100 mg/24 hr; take 0.5-4 hr before intercourse.	Common—headache, flushing, dyspepsia, nasal congestion, abnormal vision; serious—priapism Caution if sexual activity or exertion risky because of existing cardiovascular disease; caution with potent CYP3A4 inhibitors; caution in renal, hepatic impairment; caution in older adults (>65 yr); caution with α-blockers.* Nitrates
Tadalafil (Cialis)	2.5, 5, 10, 20 mg Up to 36 hr	Daily use: 2.5 mg, may increase to 5 mg PRN use: 10 mg, 1 dose/24 hr; take before intercourse.	Common—headache, dyspepsia, back pain, myalgia, nasal congestion; serious—priapism Caution if sexual activity, exertion risky because of existing cardiovascular disease; caution with alcohol; caution in renal, hepatic impairment; caution in left ventricular (LV) outflow obstruction; caution with potent CYP3 inhibitors; caution in older adults (>65 yr); caution with α-blockers.* Nitrates
Vardenafil (Levitra)	2.5, 5, 10, and 20 mg 4-5 hr	10 mg (5 mg if >65 yr); 1 dose/24 hr; take1 hour before intercourse.	Common—headache, flushing, dyspepsia, rhinitis; serious—priapism Caution in hepatic impairment; caution if sexual activity, exertion risky because of existing cardiovascular disease; caution in LV outflow obstruction; caution with potent CYP3A4 inhibitors; caution in older adults (>65 yr). α-Blockers, nitrates Avoid in patients with prolonged QT taking class IA or III antiarrhythmics.

From Physicians' Desk Reference, 64th ed. Montvale, NJ, Thompson, 2010. www.pdr.net.

*PDE-5 inhibitors should be used with caution in patients taking alpha-adrenergic blockers. This is no longer a contraindication based on labeling, but a number of precautions are based on potential for additive vasodilation in concomitant use:
1. Patients should be on α-blocker therapy and stable before starting PDE-5 inhibitor.
2. Patients who already have hemodynamic instability on α-blockers are at increased risk of additive vasodilatory effects.
3. Use the lowest recommended dose to start.
4. If starting α-blocker in a patient on a PDE-5 inhibitor, use the lowest dose of α-blocker.
5. Other medications or volume status may also contribute to vasodilation and should be considered.

type of incontinence and possible overlap with syndromes such as overactive bladder. Genitourinary and neurologic examinations as well as urinalysis should be performed. A postvoid residual urine measurement is useful for men with obstructive symptoms or patients with voiding difficulty (SIGN, 2004). Urodynamic studies are of uncertain benefit. No studies have shown that these tests improve outcomes or predict who will succeed with surgical treatment (Glazener and Lapitan, 2002; Lemack, 2004). Urodynamics may be helpful if the cause of incontinence is uncertain (Lopez et al., 2002). Children who are thought to be incontinent—that is, those who cannot be categorized as simply enuretic or dysfunctional voiders—need more extensive evaluation.

Incontinence treatment should focus on improving quality of life. Stress and urge incontinence may be treated differently, depending on the underlying cause. Physical therapies, medications, alternative treatments, and surgery are options. Pelvic floor exercises are effective and a reasonable first choice for stress and mixed symptoms. It is unknown whether these are effective for urge symptoms (Hay-Smith et al., 2001). Bladder training is effective for urge incontinence (Teunissen et al., 2004). Other options include biofeedback and electrical stimulation (Onwude, 2009). Evidence does not currently support acupuncture treatment (SIGN, 2004).

Medications include alpha agonists, anticholinergics, estrogen, serotonin and norepinephrine reuptake inhibitors,

and tricyclic antidepressants (TCAs). Oral estrogen replacement therapy should not be used because of the underlying cardiac and cancer risk, as well as the finding that it worsens incontinence (Hendrix et al., 2005). Topical vaginal estrogen appears effective; however, data on long-term use and effects after treatment cessation are limited or lacking. Thus, short-term use is likely most prudent at present (Cody et al., 2009).

For stress incontinence, some evidence has shown that α-agonists are more effective than placebo, but the only available form in the United States is pseudoephedrine and side effects limit its use. TCAs are an option, but no randomized controlled trials (RCTs) have evaluated this use (SIGN, 2004). Duloxetine (Cymbalta) improves stress incontinence compared to placebo, but long-term data are lacking (Guay, 2005, Onwude 2009). Anticholinergic drugs such as oxybutynin, tolterodine, solifenacin, and darifenacin are effective for urge incontinence (Table 40-9). Trospium, a quaternary ammonium compound, is also effective (Athanasopoulos and Perimenis, 2009). Preventing incontinence would be ideal. Methods such as pelvic muscle exercises are often recommended for women after childbirth, although evidence on effectiveness is insufficient at present (Hay-Smith et al., 2002). Episiotomy does not appear to reduce urinary incontinency in women (Hartmann et al., 2005).

Table 40-9 Medications for Urinary Incontinence

Medication	Dosage
Stress Incontinence	
Duloxetine (Cymbalta)*	40 mg twice daily
Pseudoephedrine	30, 60 mg every 4-6 hr 120 mg SR daily
Estrogen*	Topical
Urge Incontinence/Overactive Bladder	
Tolterodine (Detrol, Detrol LA)	1, 2 mg twice daily 2, 4 mg daily (LA)
Trospium (Sanctura, Sanctura XR)	20 mg twice daily 60 mg daily (XR)
Solifenacin (Vesicare)	5, 10 mg daily
Darifenacin (Enablex)	7.5, 15 mg daily
Oxybutynin (Ditropan, Ditropan XL)	5 mg twice daily 5, 10 mg daily (XL)
Oxybutynin transdermal (Oxytrol)	3.9 mg transdermal patch twice weekly
Oxybutynin transdermal gel (Gelnique)	100 mg/g topical daily
Imipramine (Tofranil)*	10, 25, 50 mg at bedtime; max dose 150 mg

Modified from Athanasopoulos A, Perimenis P. Pharmacotherapy of urinary incontinence. Int Urogynecol J Pelvic Floor Dysfunct. 2009;20:475-482; and Physicians' Desk Reference, 64th ed. Montvale, NJ, Thompson, 2010. www.pdr.net.
*Non–FDA-approved use.
SR, Sustained release.

Interstitial Cystitis

Interstitial cystitis is a chronic, noninfectious bladder disorder predominantly diagnosed in women. Symptoms mimic those of a UTI (urgency, frequency) with the addition of chronic pelvic pain, dyspareunia, or both and varying with bladder filling. Although not associated with cellular change, epithelial inflammation and prolonged symptoms can lead to epithelial damage (Kahn et al., 2005). Two forms are identified: "classic" interstitial cystitis, demonstrating inflammatory bladder wall changes identifiable on cystoscopy, and *painful bladder syndrome,* defined by the symptoms of interstitial cystitis in the absence of any objective cystoscopic findings (Marinkovic et al., 2009).

The main impact of interstitial cystitis is on quality of life. Patients often express somatization and depression or anxiety; as with other somatic pain syndromes, its pathogenesis is unclear. Differential diagnosis includes other somatic syndromes such as fibromyalgia, irritable bowel, and chronic pelvic pain, as well as UTI, overactive bladder, uterine fibroids, and endometriosis. Interstitial cystitis should be considered in any patient presenting frequently with UTI symptoms. There may also be association with autoimmune disorders.

Pentosan polysulfate sodium (Elmiron), 100 mg three times daily, is the only FDA-approved medication for interstitial cystitis. Adjunctive medications include antihistamines, TCAs, gabapentin, anticholinergics, prednisone, and cyclosporine (Marinkovic et al., 2009). Urologic consultation should be considered. Physical therapy, counseling, and bladder training may help (Kahn et al., 2005). Many dietary avoidance recommendations have focused on acidic, high-potassium foods and drinks with acid, caffeine, or alcohol. However, prospective data on dietary interventions are lacking, so such restrictions should be individualized to each patient.

Overactive Bladder

Overactive bladder describes a clinical syndrome characterized by lower urinary tract voiding dysfunction. The International Continence Society has defined overactive bladder as "urgency, with or without urge incontinence, usually with frequency and nocturia" (Wein and Rovner, 2002). The lack of specificity inherent in this definition creates potential for overlap with other urinary tract symptom complexes (e.g., LUTS) and diseases. The pathogenesis is uncertain, and urinary tract abnormalities that could cause symptoms should be ruled out. The primary dysfunction revolves around improper detrusor muscle activity and functional reductions in bladder volume. However, the definition does not exclude patients with the symptoms who do not have objective bladder hypercontractility. Furthermore, voluntary control of bladder contraction may be impaired so that the urge to void cannot be controlled (Herbison et al., 2003).

Neurologic conditions may contribute. For example, patients with multiple sclerosis, stroke, or diabetic neuropathy might manifest overactive bladder. This might be better described as *neurogenic detrusor overactivity,* whereas patients without cause or contributor might be described as having *idiopathic* detrusor overactivity (Herbison et al., 2003). Thus, overactive bladder is best viewed as a descriptive, symptom-driven complex rather than a disease.

Overactive bladder affects approximately 16% of adults, with equal gender distribution. However, women are more likely to experience urge incontinence as a feature (Stewart et al., 2003). Patients may plan their days around issues such as restroom access or avoiding social settings because of incontinence. Patients may be reluctant to discuss these symptoms because of embarrassment, so family physicians may not detect the true impact of these symptoms without specific inquiry.

Many pharmacotherapy options are available for overactive bladder (see Table 40-9). Bladder retraining is another option. There are no systematic reviews comparing these treatments, although incontinence data have suggested that physical therapies are a reasonable option. There are no important differences in effectiveness among medications. Systematic review of anticholinergic medications versus placebo shows statistically significant effectiveness. However, the clinical significance is uncertain, with the exception of side effects, and long-term treatment effects are unknown (Herbison et al., 2003). Anticholinergic treatment will likely result in one less leakage or voiding episode every 48 hours, but one third of patients experience dry mouth (Hay-Smith et al., 2005b).

Renal Calculi

Adults

Approximately 5% to 12% of adults will have a kidney stone, and the chance of a recurrent stone is 50% (Parmar, 2004; Teichman, 2004). Whites have the highest risk, particularly men. Family history increases the risk threefold and is present in 55% of recurrent stone formers (Teichman, 2004).

A classic history suggesting renal calculi is the abrupt onset of unilateral flank pain. It often radiates into the groin and may be accompanied by nausea and vomiting. Patients with kidney stones typically have great difficulty finding a comfortable position. On examination, there may be costovertebral angle or lower abdominal pain, and hematuria occurs in 90% of patients (Teichman, 2004). Patients may experience UTI symptoms such as dysuria, frequency, and urgency as the stone passes from the ureter into the bladder. However, patients with fever, microscopic signs of infection, or signs of systemic sepsis may have superimposed UTI. Complete obstruction and hydronephrosis can result in renal failure.

Helical non-contrast-enhanced CT is the test of choice for diagnosing renal calculi (Lindbloom and Meadows, 2001). Renal ultrasound and IV urography may be helpful for radiopaque stones and pregnant women (ultrasound only) (Sheafor et al., 2000). Stones larger than 5 mm found in the proximal ureter on more than one imaging study will probably need urology consultation and intervention (Grossfeld et al., 2001b). Stones smaller than 5 mm will likely pass without intervention (Teichman, 2004).

Treatment initially focuses on analgesia and relieving nausea and vomiting. Pain results from ureteral obstruction and renal capsular distention and/or hydronephrosis. Pain can be effectively managed with narcotic analgesics or nonsteroidal anti-inflammatory drugs (NSAIDs; ketorolac, indomethacin). Ketorolac (Toradol) is more effective than meperidine (Demerol) and probably as effective as narcotics (Larkin et al., 1999; Teichman, 2004). Alpha blockers such as terazosin or tamsulosin appear to increase the likelihood of a stone passing (DasGupta et al., 2009).

Two thirds of stones pass spontaneously. Stones that have not passed within 4 weeks are unlikely to pass (Teichman, 2004). Urine straining is important because a captured stone can be analyzed for content. Repeat imaging is needed when stone passage has not occurred or is uncertain.

It is debatable whether all patients should receive an evaluation for metabolic disorders after a first kidney stone. A reasonable workup includes an electrolyte panel, urinalysis, blood urea nitrogen (BUN), creatinine, calcium, parathyroid hormone (if calcium elevated), and stone analysis, if possible. Calcium oxalate is found in 60% to 80% of stones (Parmar, 2004). Patients with recurrent stones need a more extensive evaluation, including urine culture and a 24-hour urine study to determine calcium, oxalate, uric acid, citrate, phosphate, sodium, and creatinine levels (Teichman, 2004).

Proper hydration is essential in preventing stones. Patients should aim for urine output of 2 to 3 L/day (Parmar, 2004). Cost-effectiveness data suggest that dietary intervention is appropriate for first episodes (Lotan et al., 2004). Patients with recurrent stones need dietary intervention, a metabolic evaluation, and potassium citrate measurement. Hypercalciuria is an indication for prophylaxis with thiazide diuretics, which effectively reduce recurrence of calcium oxalate stones. Evidence is less clear for other treatments, such as citrate (Pearle et al., 1999). Men with recurrent stones and idiopathic hypercalciuria will have fewer stones on a low-sodium, low-protein diet than men on a low-calcium diet (NNT = 5.5 for 5 years). Low-calcium diets do not reduce stone formation (Borghi et al., 2002).

Patients with uric acid stones respond to urinary alkalinization with potassium citrate (Teichman, 2004).

Children

Although usually considered an adult problem, children are not immune to urolithiasis. Older children present with typical symptoms, and younger children may have signs mimicking those of colic. About 15% of children presenting to the emergency department who were ultimately diagnosed with urolithiasis by CT did not have hematuria (Persaud et al., 2009). Metabolic disorders are often the cause of pediatric stones, most often hypercalciuria (Peitrow et al., 2002).

The mainstay of treatment is a high fluid intake. Urinary alkalinization inhibits cystine and uric acid stones. For calcium-based stones, a diet low in sodium and oxalate and high in potassium is recommended. Excess intake of vitamins D and C is discouraged. Thiazide diuretics are also a treatment option. Gated and ungated shock wave lithotripsy has been successful treatment in children, with minimal morbidity (Shouman et al., 2009).

KEY TREATMENT

Use ACE inhibitors and angiotensin receptor blockers for nephropathy prevention in diabetes (Shlipak, 2009) (SOR: A).

Antibiotics are ineffective for chronic nonbacterial prostatitis (category IIIb, IV) (Erickson et al., 2008) (SOR: A).

Enuresis alarm helps manage nocturnal enuresis (Kiddoo, 2007) (SOR: A).

Pelvic floor muscle exercises are used for stress incontinence (Onwude, 2009) (SOR: B).

Duloxetine is effective for stress incontinence (Onwude, 2009) (SOR: A).

Anticholinergics (oxybutynin, tolterodine, solifenacin, darifenacin) and trospium are effective for urge incontinence (Athanasopoulos and Perimenis, 2009) (SOR: A).

PDE-5 inhibitors (sildenafil, tadalafil, vardenafil) are used for erectile dysfunction (Tharyan and Gopalakrishanan, 2009) (SOR: A).

Infectious Disorders

Key Points

- *Neisseria gonorrhoeae* and *Chlamydia trachomatis* cause most cases of urethritis and typically coexist.
- Identifying and treating asymptomatic bacteriuria are only important in pregnant women.
- Evaluate for urethritis, prostatitis, or both in men with UTI symptoms.
- Women with dysuria and frequency without vaginal symptoms have a 90% chance of UTI.
- Both antibiotic prophylaxis and cranberry juice prevent recurrent UTI.
- The ideal evaluation of children with UTIs is controversial.

Balanitis

Balanitis refers to inflammation of the glans penis (Fig. 40-12). It may occur as a local infectious process, as part of a urethritis syndrome (e.g., Reiter's syndrome), or as a skin disease (e.g., lichen sclerosis). In uncircumcised men, yeast balanitis may result from poor hygiene. Consideration should be given to dermatologic conditions and immunodeficiency in circumcised men.

Epididymitis

Epididymitis (epididymo-orchitis) often presents with testicular pain or swelling. It is usually unilateral, with a palpable, tender epididymis and possibly hydrocele. Risk factors include STI, insertive anal intercourse, invasive urinary tract procedures, and anatomic urinary tract disorders. Anatomic abnormalities are the most likely explanation in children. Epididymitis may occur as an STI in men during insertive anal intercourse or in men older than 35 who have undergone invasive procedures (e.g., cystoscopy). The differential diagnosis includes trauma, infarction, testicular cancer, and testicular torsion. Testicular cancer can be misdiagnosed as epididymitis. Thus, family physicians should emphasize close follow-up.

Chlamydia trachomatis and *Neisseria gonorrhoeae* cause most cases in men younger than 35 and usually coexist with asymptomatic urethritis (CDC, 2006). Other causative organisms include gram-negative enteric bacteria. Fungi and tuberculosis are other possible infectious causes.

Treatment includes antibiotics, analgesia, and scrotal elevation. In patients in whom gonorrhea or chlamydia is the likely cause, ceftriaxone (single dose, 250 mg IM) and doxycycline (100 mg twice daily for 10 days) is the treatment of choice. In patients who are allergic to these, or likely to have an enteric organism as the cause, 10 days of treatment with ofloxacin or levofloxacin is appropriate (CDC, 2006; del Rio, 2007).

Prostatitis

Prostatitis is a fairly common urinary tract disorder in men (Krieger et al., 2003) (see Table 40-7). Categories I (acute) and II (chronic) prostatitis are treated as infectious disorders.

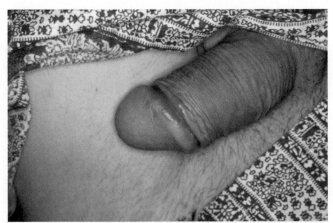

Figure 40-12 Circinate balanitis in a patient diagnosed with Reiter's syndrome (arthritis, conjunctivitis, urethritis). *(From the CDC Public Health Image Library image 5806. Courtesy Susan Lindsley and Dr. M. Rein.)*

The four-glass method for diagnosing and localizing prostatitis is often recommended but has not been prospectively validated (Stevermer and Easley, 2000).

Acute Bacterial Prostatitis

Acute bacterial prostatitis should be suspected in men presenting with symptoms of UTI. Age and immunodeficiency contribute to men having UTIs, so prostatitis is more likely in otherwise healthy men with these symptoms (Lipsky, 1999). Patients may have UTI symptoms (e.g., dysuria, frequency, urgency) and typically systemic symptoms of acute illness, such as fever, chills, and myalgias. Local discomfort in the form of pelvic or back pain is also typical. Examination reveals a tender, boggy prostate. Most experts have recommended against prostate massage in acute prostatitis because it would be very uncomfortable and theoretically could disseminate the infection (Benway and Moon, 2008; Wagenlehner and Naber, 2003).

Urine culture is typically positive for the causative organism. Treatment is empiric pending the results. Depending on the degree of illness, patients may need an IV broad-spectrum penicillin or third-generation cephalosporin, possibly with an aminoglycoside, or a fluoroquinolone (Wagenlehner and Naber, 2003). Less severe cases can be managed with oral antibiotics. Options include fluoroquinolones and trimethoprim-sulfamethoxazole (TMP-SMX) (Lipsky, 1999). An alternative when STI is likely is intramuscular (IM) ceftriaxone followed by oral doxycycline. Antibiotic therapy is typically 10 to 14 days, although some recommend 4 weeks because of concerns about antibiotics poorly penetrating prostatic tissue. Obstructive uropathy may result from prostatic enlargement; thus, assessment for this clinically or with postvoid residual assessment should be considered (Benway and Moon, 2008).

Chronic Bacterial Prostatitis

Chronic bacterial prostatitis may manifest with irritative voiding symptoms, prostatitic obstruction, or recurrent UTIs (Lipsky, 1999). Patients may have microscopic pyuria but negative cultures. Other symptoms include hemospermia, penile discharge, and systemic symptoms.

Longer courses of antibiotics are generally considered standard practice. Options include TMP-SMX and fluoroquinolones for 4 to 6 weeks (Lipsky, 1999). Alpha-adrenergic blockers have limited evidence of benefit when added to antimicrobials for category II prostatitis (Erickson et al., 2008). Patients with recurrent symptoms may need longer antibiotic courses, urologic consultation, or reconsideration of their diagnosis.

Sexually Transmitted Infections

Chancroid

Chancroid is caused by infection with *Haemophilus ducreyi*. A clinical syndrome of painful genital ulcers and adenopathy (patient does not have syphilis; ulcers are herpes negative) allows for presumptive diagnosis (Fig. 40-13). Many treatment options exist (Table 40-10).

Gonorrhea and Nongonococcal Urethritis

Urethritis may present as a urethral discharge or simply dysuria. Family physicians should suspect urethritis in patients with symptoms of UTI, pyuria, presence of leukocyte esterase, and negative urine culture. *N. gonorrhoeae* and *C. trachomatis* are the most important causative organisms. Gonococcal urethritis is typically symptomatic. Chlamydia causes most cases of nongonococcal urethritis (CDC, 2006). Various treatment options exist (see Table 40-10). Fluoroquinolones are no longer recommended as a treatment option due to resistance rates (del Rio et al., 2007). Patients with gonorrhea who are not ruled out for chlamydia should be treated for it because co-infection is common (CDC, 2006).

Herpes Genitalis

Herpes simplex virus type 2 (HSV-2) causes most genital herpes infections, although HSV-1 causes 50% of first cases (CDC, 2006). An estimated 20% of those older than 12 years have it, and infection is often asymptomatic (USPSTF, 2005). Symptoms, if present, may present as multiple,

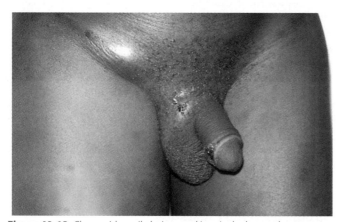

Figure 40-13 Chancroid: penile lesions and inguinal adenopathy. *(From the CDC Public Health Image Library image 4419. Courtesy Pledger.)*

small, painful ulcers or vesicles (Fig. 40-14). Causative virus is prognostically important, so confirmatory testing is recommended. Polymerase chain reaction testing is sensitive, whereas a Tzanck test is not (CDC, 2006). Serologic tests for herpes IgG are available but do not differentiate acute from remote infection. The U.S. Preventive Services Task Force (USPSTF, 2005) recommends against routine screening for HSV in asymptomatic adults because there is no evidence that this decreases disease transmission or reduces morbidity. Antiviral medications can treat acute outbreaks and be used as prophylaxis to prevent recurrent outbreaks.

Human Papillomavirus

Human papillomavirus (HPV) may cause symptomatic genital warts, although most patients do not manifest them. HPV types 6 and 11 cause most visible warts (CDC, 2006). Certain HPV types are associated with genital squamous neoplasia. Patients with penile plaques suspicious for warts can be examined by placing an acetic acid solution on the plaque and looking for an acetowhite change. Untreated warts will regress, remain stable, or spread. Symptomatic relief is the main treatment goal. Treatment options include podofilox 0.5%, imiquimod (1%, 5%), topical interferon, cryotherapy, office-based chemical treatments (acetic acid), or surgery (Buck, 2007; CDC, 2006,).

Syphilis

Primary *Treponema pallidum* infection manifests as a painless genital ulcer known as a *chancre* (Fig. 40-15). Diagnosis is typically confirmed with a combination of nontreponemal screening tests (rapid plasma reagin [RPR], Venereal Disease Research Laboratories [VDRL]) and a treponema-specific test (fluorescent treponemal antibody absorption [FTA-ABS]). *T. pallidum* is difficult to culture, so darkfield microscopy or fluorescent antibody testing of a tissue specimen provides definitive diagnosis. Primary syphilis is treated with a single dose of penicillin, 2.4 million units IM in adults and 50,000 to 2.4 million U/kg IM in children) (CDC, 2006).

Table 40-10 Treatment for Selected Sexually Transmitted Infections (STIs)

STI	Medication	Dose	Route*	Duration
Chancroid	Azithromycin	1000 mg	PO	Single dose
	Ceftriaxone	250 mg	IM	Single dose
	Ciprofloxacin	500 mg	PO	Twice daily for 3 days
	Erythromycin base	500 mg	PO	Three times daily for 7 days
Chlamydia	Azithromycin	1000 mg	PO	Single dose
	Doxycycline	100 mg	PO	Twice daily 7 days
Gonorrhea	Cefixime	400 mg	PO	Single dose
	Ceftriaxone	125 mg	IM	Single dose
Syphilis, primary	Penicillin	2.4 million U	IM	Single dose

*PO, Oral; IM, Intramuscular.

Doxycycline and tetracycline are alternatives for penicillin-allergic patients.

Urinary Tract Infections

Urinary tract infections are the most common urologic issue encountered by family physicians and one of the most common diagnoses overall (Stange et al., 1998). Most are uncomplicated lower UTIs, such as cystitis.

Asymptomatic Bacteriuria

Approximately 5% of reproductive-age women have asymptomatic bacteriuria (Bent et al., 2002). It is also common in older adults. This is important for understanding the community risk of UTI when evaluating a patient with UTI symptoms. However, although asymptomatic bacteriuria may conceptually place a patient at risk for UTI, identification and treatment do not appear to affect morbidity or mortality (Gartlehner et al., 2004; Lin and Fajardo, 2008). Thus, bacteriuria screening is not recommended (USPSTF, 2008a).

In contrast, pregnant women do benefit from screening. Testing with urine culture should be done in all pregnant women at 12 to 16 weeks of gestation (USPSTF, 2008a). Urine culture is the best method, because dipstick testing and microscopy are not accurate enough tests to predict this condition.

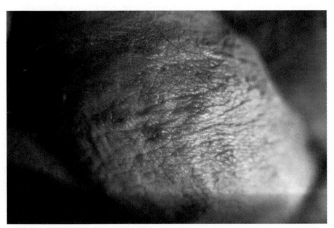

Figure 40-14 Crusted lesions of genital herpes on penile shaft. *(From CDC Public Health Image Library image 6480. Courtesy Susan Lindsley.)*

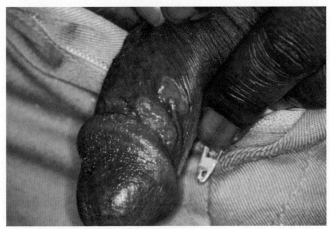

Figure 40-15 Chancre of primary syphilis. *(From CDC Public Health Image Library image 6803. Courtesy Dr. M. Rein.)*

Uncomplicated Cystitis

Most UTIs manifest as acute uncomplicated bacterial cystitis, and women experience most of these episodes. *Escherichia coli* causes up to 90% of cases, with the rest probably caused by *Staphylococcus saprophyticus*. Other causative organisms include *Proteus mirabilis*, enterococci, and *Klebsiella* (Fihn, 2003). To have "uncomplicated cystitis," women must have no underlying urinary tract abnormalities or immune compromise (Bent et al., 2002).

Dysuria, frequency, and urgency are the classic clinical triad. The condition most commonly mimicking UTI is vaginitis. Other conditions have been described (see Dysuria). Patients may also experience back or flank pain and suprapubic abdominal pain. Dipstick urinalysis may show leukocyte esterase or nitrite or may be heme positive. Microscopic analysis should assess for pyuria, hematuria, and bacteriuria. The gold standard for diagnosis is urine culture.

Women presenting with at least one UTI symptom have a 50% chance of having a UTI. The combination of dysuria and frequency without vaginal symptoms increases the chance to 90% (likelihood ratio, 24.6). Four symptoms significantly increase the chance of UTI—dysuria, frequency, hematuria, and back pain (Bent et al., 2002). Nitrite-positive or leukocyte esterase–positive dipsticks are the most accurate tests, but cannot rule out a UTI.

Antibiotics are the mainstay of treatment, usually for 3 days (Table 40-11). A shorter duration is as effective as longer therapy for most women, including older adult women (Lutters and Vogt, 2002; Milo et al., 2005). In the southeastern and southwestern United States, there is growing *E. coli* resistance to TMP-SMX, leading some to recommend that this should no longer be first-line treatment for UTI. However, many women treated with TMP-SMX who have a resistant organism on culture achieve clinical cure (Fihn, 2003). Compared with quinolones' propensity for resistance, TMP-SMX is still a reasonable first choice for many patients, and family physicians should base treatment choices on documented local resistance patterns. If resistance to TMP-SMX exceeds 20%, an alternative treatment should be employed (Nicolle, 2008).

Complicated Infection

Complicated UTIs are characterized by signs and symptoms of upper tract (i.e., renal) involvement or by factors that predispose to upper tract involvement. UTIs with signs of renal or systemic involvement are also called *pyelonephritis*. Most cases of pyelonephritis are caused by ascending bacterial infection from the bladder (Ramakrishnan and Scheid, 2005).

Symptoms include fever, flank pain, nausea, vomiting, and costovertebral angle tenderness. Findings such as pyuria are typical, and urine culture is usually positive. White cell casts may be present on urine microscopy. Hospitalized patients with UTIs are best managed based on culture results. *E. coli* is the typical pathogen for uncomplicated outpatient UTIs and pyelonephritis. *E. coli* is still the most common isolate in hospitalized patients, but now to a lesser extent, as

Table 40-11 Treatment Options for Acute Uncomplicated UTIs

Medication	Dose	Regimen	Duration
Trimethoprim/ sulfamethoxazole (Bactrim DS, Cotrim DS, Septra DS)	160/800 mg	Twice daily	3 days
Trimethoprim (Primsol)	100 mg	Twice daily	3 days
Nitrofurantoin macrocrystals (Macrodantin)	50 or 100 mg	4 times daily	7 days
Nitrofurantoin monohydrate macrocrystals (Macrobid)	100 mg	Twice daily	7 days
Ciprofloxacin (Cipro)	250 mg	Twice daily	3 days
Gatifloxacin (Tequin)	400 mg	Daily	1 single dose or 3 days
Lomefloxacin (Maxaquin)	400 mg	Twice daily	3 day
Levofloxacin (Levaquin)	250 mg	Once daily	3 days
Norfloxacin (Noroxin)	400 mg	Twice daily	3 day
Fosfomycin (Monurol)	3 g	Single dose	Single dose

From Fihn SD. Acute uncomplicated urinary tract infection in women. N Engl J Med 2003;349:259-266.
UTIs, Urinary tract infections; *DS*, double strength.

Table 40-12 Antibiotics for Uncomplicated UTI Prophylaxis

Drug	Pediatric Dose	Adult Dose*
Amoxicillin	10 mg/kg, once daily	N/A
TMP-SMX	2 mg/kg, once daily based on TMP	Single strength (80/400 mg), half-tablet at night or three times weekly
Trimethoprim	N/A	100 mg nightly
Nitrofurantoin	1-2mg/kg, once daily	50 or 100 mg nightly
Norfloxacin	N/A	200 mg nightly

Postcoital prophylaxis options: TMP-SMX, nitrofurantoin, fluoroquinolones.
TMP-SMX, Trimethoprim-sulfamethoxazole; *N/A*, not applicable.

Enterococcus, Pseudomonas, and *Staphylococcus* species become more likely (Graham and Galloway, 2001; Scholes et al., 2005). Blood cultures do not necessarily change management (Ramakrishnan and Scheid, 2005). Imaging, such as renal ultrasonography, is sometimes recommended, but it also does not necessarily change management and thus can be employed at clinical discretion (Nicolle, 2008).

Outpatients can be managed with an oral fluoroquinolone. Hospitalized patients should receive a fluoroquinolone, an aminoglycoside with or without ampicillin, or an extended-spectrum cephalosporin with or without an aminoglycoside. Patients with cultures showing gram-positive cocci should receive ampicillin-sulbactam with or without an aminoglycoside (Warren et al., 1999). Treatment for 7 to 14 days is usually adequate. Resistant bacteria and renal calculi are the most common causes of treatment failure (Ramakrishnan and Scheid, 2005).

Recurrent Infections

Recurrent UTI can be defined as three episodes in 1 year or two episodes in 6 months (Sen, 2008). Self-diagnosis has an 84% PPV in women with recurrent UTIs (Bent et al., 2002). Cultures are helpful in guiding antibiotic choice (Table 40-12). Prophylactic antibiotics are effective for the subset of women with recurrent symptomatic UTI, although choice of patient and duration is uncertain. Because sexual activity

is associated with developing UTIs, many physicians recommend that women void immediately after intercourse. However, the poor-quality study examining this practice found no significant effect (Beisel et al., 2002). Thus, no evidence supports recommending this practice to patients. In contrast, postcoital antibiotic prophylaxis reduces the incidence of cystitis (Sen, 2008). Furthermore, it may be as effective as continuous prophylaxis at reducing recurrence, because women in one RCT comparing these methods showed no difference in UTI rates (Albert et al., 2004). In postmenopausal women, topical estrogen is often proposed, but this too lacks good supporting evidence (Sen, 2008).

Cranberry juice has potential as a preventive treatment for recurrent UTI. Its effect is likely caused by chemicals that inhibit bacterial adherence to uroepithelial cells rather than urinary acidification (Raz et al., 2004). RCTs support its use in community-dwelling women. Ingesting pure cranberry juice, from 200 mL daily to 250 mL three times daily, or taking cranberry concentrate tablets (1:30) resulted in a 12% to 20% absolute reduction in symptomatic UTIs (NNT = 58). The type of juice is likely a factor, although type and amount have yet to be well defined (Jepson and Craig, 2008; Sen, 2008).

Urinary Tract Infections in Children

An estimated 3% to 8% of girls and 1% to 2% of boys will have a UTI (Foxman, 2002; Hellstrom et al., 1991). *Pyelonephritis* is a clinical diagnosis and is the most common documented serious bacterial infection in febrile infants. *Cystitis* is common in school-age children and adolescents and, as a general rule, is not a condition of infants or pre–toilet-trained toddlers. Risk factors for UTI range from constipation and dysfunctional voiding to congenital uropathies. Presenting symptoms vary with age and site of infection and may be nonspecific in younger children. Pyelonephritis in infants, for example, may present with fever, irritability, vomiting, diarrhea, poor feeding, or failure to thrive. School-age children and adolescents may present with fever, vomiting and flank pain. Symptoms of cystitis are more common after age 2 years and may include dysuria, frequency, urgency, and low-grade fever (<38.3° C).

As with adults, the gold standard test in children is an appropriately obtained urine culture. In neonates and young infants, a suprapubic aspiration is the ideal collection method. Catheterization is otherwise preferred until the child is old enough to collect a midstream clean-catch specimen. Bag urine collections are unreliable and increase the number of ambiguous cultures (Schroeder et al., 2005). Many elements of the urinalysis have been viewed as tools for aiding diagnosis of UTI. Inadequate sensitivity and specificity continue to support use of urine culture (AAP, 1999). Furthermore, no RCTs have evaluated clinical empiric treatment versus awaiting culture results (Larcombe, 2004). However, pyuria (>5 WBCs/hpf) and a positive Gram stain are helpful in making the decision to initiate early antibiotic therapy, pending culture results.

Treatment remains somewhat controversial, particularly the choice between parenteral and oral antibiotics in the setting of pyelonephritis. For children with pyelonephritis, therapeutic goals include treating or preventing systemic complications of bacteremia, preventing renal sequelae, and ameliorating acute symptoms. Historically, parenteral antibiotics have been the preferred option, particularly in younger children with pyelonephritis. This remains true for infants younger than 4 weeks, who should be hospitalized and receive parenteral therapy. This is also true for older infants and children assessed at high risk because of a septic appearance, vomiting or inability to take oral fluids and medications, dehydration, or concerns regarding compliance. Choice of parenteral antibiotic includes ampicillin in combination with gentamicin or cefotaxime for neonates and third-generation cephalosporin alone for older children. In these cases, transition to oral therapy follows once culture results and sensitivities are known and signs of systemic infection have resolved. Follow-up urine cultures to test for cure are unnecessary in patients with good clinical response (AAP, 1999). Prolonged parenteral therapy is indicated for septic infants. For children 1 month and older not assessed as high risk, it now appears that oral antibiotics are equally effective not only regarding course of illness but also in preventing renal scarring (Montini et al., 2007). Options for initial oral therapy would include amoxicillin–clavulanic acid, TMP-SMX (>2 months), and cephalosporins. Because of the increasing incidence of UTI with ampicillin-resistant *E. coli*, amoxicillin is no longer the preferred initial choice. The recommended length of therapy is typically 7 to 10 days for an uncomplicated UTI (i.e., cystitis) and 10 to 14 days for pyelonephritis (Larcombe, 2007).

The most appropriate evaluation after first UTI is controversial (Layton, 2003). Traditionally, children have undergone a complete evaluation for underlying urologic abnormalities that would increase the risk of further infections and renal scarring. This includes renal ultrasound and VCUG. In 309 children younger than 24 months with their first febrile UTI, ultrasound was of limited value because it did not change management, and other tests may be obviated by routine cultures for children with a febrile illness after a prior UTI (Hoberman et al., 2003). However, 29% of 390 children under age 5 years with a first-time febrile UTI had abnormal renal ultrasound findings (Huang et al., 2008).

The most common uropathy associated with pediatric UTI is *vesicoureteral reflux* (VUR), occurring in 30% to 40% of cases. Reflux is diagnosed by VCUG and graded on a scale of 1 to 5, with grade 5 being the most severe. The degree of VUR is directly proportional to the incidence of renal scarring. In addition to the standard fluoroscopic VCUG, radionuclide cystography may be performed. This test has the advantage of less radiation exposure but is lacking in anatomic detail

and is most often used for follow-up studies. The traditional approach to the patient with VUR has been prophylactic antibiotics, with surgical intervention reserved for complicated patients with breakthrough UTIs and evidence of renal injury (see Table 40-12). "Deflux" is a newer, less invasive procedure performed using cystoscopy and is proving to be highly effective in the treatment of reflux. However, the management of VUR is a rapidly evolving field and remains controversial. Evidence supporting prolonged antibiotic prophylaxis is weak because of a lack of properly designed RCTs (Williams et al., 2005). Also, evidence that surgical repair reduces negative outcomes in children with normal renal function is weak or absent (Larcombe, 2007). The Randomized Intervention for Children with Vesicoureteral Reflux (RIVUR) is a multicenter, randomized, double-blind prospective study currently in progress in the United States designed to assess the efficacy of prophylactic antibiotics in the treatment of grade 1 to 4 VUR in children age 2 months to 6 years. If emerging evidence supports withholding antibiotic prophylaxis, the need for routine VCUG will be obviated. Renal scintigraphy (dimercaptosuccinic acid [DMSA] scan) has been recommended to help diagnose pyelonephritis. This is also controversial because false-negative results could lead to undertreating children with pyelonephritis. DMSA scanning has shown promise in predicting higher grades of reflux in older infants and children (Lee et al., 2009), but this has not been true in neonates (Siomou et al., 2009). DMSA scans are not recommended routinely in children with UTI (AAP, 1999). The prudent course with evaluation is to await more evidence-based management guidelines, which appear to be forthcoming.

The ultimate goal in the approach to patients with UTI is to prevent morbidity. Renal scarring may ultimately manifest as hypertension, proteinuria, or both. The incidence of renal scarring in patients with UTI is increased in children younger than 3 years, presence of VUR proportional to grade of reflux, recurrent UTI, and delayed or inadequate therapy.

KEY TREATMENT

Continuous or postcoital antibiotics are equally effective for recurrent UTI (Sen, 2008) (SOR: A).

Ceftriaxone and cefixime are used for gonorrhea (CDC, 2006) (SOR: C).

Fluoroquinolones should not be used to treat gonorrhea (CDC, 2006; del Rio, 2007) (SOR: C).

Treat for chlamydia and gonorrhea if treating urethritis presumptively (CDC, 2006) (SOR: C).

Neoplastic Disorders

Key Points

- Benign prostatic hyperplasia affects most men by age 80 years. Lower urinary tract symptoms vary and may not correlate with prostate size. Other factors such as detrusor dysfunction contribute to LUTS.
- Alpha-adrenergic antagonists and 5α-reductase inhibitors are effective for BPH and LUTS.
- Smoking is the top risk factor for bladder cancer, and hematuria is the most common presenting sign.

- Prostate cancer is the most common cancer in men and second most common cause of male cancer death.
- There is no PSA value that is both sensitive and specific for prostate cancer.
- When ordering a PSA test, family physicians should discuss the risk, benefits, and uncertainties with patients and make a shared decision about whether to screen.
- The value of testicular self-examination is unknown.

Benign Neoplasia: Benign Prostatic Hyperplasia

Benign prostatic hyperplasia is a common problem for men. More than 50% of men older than 60 years have BPH, and this reaches 80% by 80 years of age (Dull et al., 2002; Thorpe and Neal, 2003). The exact pathogenesis of BPH is uncertain, but it is characterized by epithelial and stromal cell proliferation in the periurethral prostate tissue.

The LUTS syndrome (see earlier) overlaps with BPH because up to 30% of men have lower urinary tract symptoms (Thorpe and Neal, 2003). The symptoms defining LUTS were once thought to be solely indicative of BPH. However, LUTS may arise from other disorders (e.g., detrusor dysfunction), and there is a lack of symptomatic correlation with prostate size. However, outflow obstruction from an enlarged prostate may contribute to the development of detrusor dysfunction and urinary retention, referred to as LUTS-BPH.

Diagnosis focuses on patient history, rectal examination, and impact on quality of life. Symptoms can vary over time, even without treatment; however, the course is typically progressive, and 1% to 2% of men with BPH experience acute urinary retention annually (Webber, 2006).Various measures exist for measuring symptom severity. The most widely used and well validated is the International Prostate Symptom Score. This scoring system can discriminate the severity of symptoms and treatment response. However, it does not correlate with anatomic findings or objective measures of urinary flow (Barry and O'Leary, 1995). Prostate-specific antigen (PSA) values may increase with prostate hyperplasia, but the overlap with prostate cancer makes this of limited use in managing BPH (Barry, 2001).

Medical therapies have overtaken surgical as the most common treatments. Alpha-adrenergic blocking drugs improve urinary symptoms in BPH (Wilt et al., 2008). Alpha-adrenergic antagonists block adrenoreceptors in the prostate and bladder neck (Table 40-13). They may also induce prostate epithelial apoptosis (Thorpe and Neal, 2003). Side effects, particularly blood pressure effects, are important, because these drugs will most often be used in older adults (Schulman, 2003). The α-blocker tamsulosin has recently been implicated in association with serious postoperative ocular complications in patients undergoing cataract surgery (Bell et al., 2009).

Prostate tissue is androgen responsive throughout life. 5α-Reductase inhibitors inhibit the conversion of testosterone to dihydrotestosterone, leading to glandular atrophy and reduced prostate volume (20%-30%) (Thorpe and Neal, 2003). It takes many months for these medicines to become effective. Sexual side effects are the most prominent. These drugs also reduce PSA by up to 50%. Based on the Prostate Cancer Prevention Trial, family physicians should discuss potential benefits and harms of 5α-reductase inhibitors (see Prostate Cancer) when using these medications for BPH and LUTS (Kramer et al., 2009). Prostate enlargement can progress

Table 40-13 Pharmacotherapy for Benign Prostatic Hyperplasia

Drug	Dosage	Adverse Effects
Alpha-Adrenergic Blockers		
Alfuzosin (Uroxatral)	10 mg daily	Cardiovascular: dizziness, postural hypotension, syncope Sexual: ejaculatory dysfunction Systemic: asthenia, drowsiness, fatigue, headache
Doxazosin (Cardura, generic)	1-8 mg daily	
Terazosin (Hytrin, generic)	1-10 mg at bedtime	
Tamsulosin (Flomax)* †	0.4 mg daily	
5α-Reductase Inhibitors		
Dutasteride (Avodart)	0.5 mg daily	Sexual: impotence, decreased libido, ejaculatory dysfunction
Finasteride (Proscar)	5 mg daily	

From Schulman CC: Lower urinary tract symptoms/benign prostatic hyperplasia: Minimizing morbidity caused by treatment. Urology 2003;62:24-33; Schwinn DA, Price DT, Narayan P: α₁-Adrenoreceptor subtype selectivity and lower urinary tract symptoms. Mayo Clin Proc 2004;79:1423-1434; and Thorpe A, Neal D: Benign prostatic hyperplasia. Lancet 2003;361:1359-1367.
*Alpha-1 adrenoreceptor selective.
†Associated with postoperative complications from cataract surgery.

enough to obstruct the bladder outlet completely, leading to acute urinary retention. If this occurs, catheterization is warranted. The addition of an α-blocker may aid in voiding once the catheter is removed (Thorpe and Neal, 2003). A randomized, double-blind trial of doxazosin and finasteride over 4 years showed that combining these two medications significantly slowed symptomatic progression and reduced the risk of urinary retention and invasive treatment. Treatment was safe, and the effect of combined treatment on symptom scores was greater than the effect of either agent alone (McConnell et al., 2003). In addition to prescription medicines, a number of alternative therapies are available. Saw palmetto extract *(Serenoa repens)* is one of the most studied herbal medicines (Buck, 2004). Earlier studies found it is as effective as tamsulosin or finasteride for BPH. Other herbal medicines include β-sitosterols (promising), pygeum (African plum, *Prunus africanus*), and rye grass pollen (cernilton), with efficacy of the latter two uncertain (Webber, 2006).

Malignant Neoplasias

With the exception of prostate cancer, urologic malignancy is relatively uncommon in the general population. After prostate cancer, which is the most common cancer diagnosed in men, the next most common cancers are bladder and renal cell cancers (American Cancer Society, 2009). Testicular cancer is relatively common in young men compared with other cancers in that age group.

Bladder Cancer

Bladder cancer occurs in approximately 38.4 per 100,000 men and 9.8 per 100,000 women. Its incidence in white men is twofold higher than in black men (ACS, 2009). The incidence increases with age, with 80% of new cases occurring in patients older than 60 (National Cancer Institute, 2009a).

Cigarette smoking is the most prominent risk factor, increasing the risk fourfold to sevenfold. Aminobiphenyl is a cigarette carcinogen linked to bladder cancer. Smoking cessation decreases risk, although it still remains twofold higher 10 years after cessation. Other risk factors include exposure to the aromatic amines used in the dye and rubber industry, benzidine production, dry cleaning, garment manufacturing, and rope and twine manufacturing, as well as exposure to gases and soot from coal. Medical risks include cyclophosphamide, radiation, and prolonged exposure to foreign bodies (e.g., catheter). Finally, aristolochic acid, found in certain weight loss supplements and traditional Chinese herbal compounds containing *Aristolochia fangchi*, may increase risk. Banned in many western countries, this is still available in the United States (NCI, 2009a).

Hematuria is the most common sign of bladder cancer (NCI, 2009a), and diagnosis is most often made by direct bladder visualization (cystoscopy) and biopsy. Positive urine cytology is essentially diagnostic, although false-negative results limit the usefulness of this approach alone. No imaging test can reliably detect bladder cancers.

The USPSTF (2004a) recommends against routine screening of asymptomatic persons for bladder cancer. The prevalence of bladder cancer is low, and most patients with hematuria do not have bladder tumors. Most positive screening tests yield false-positive results, prompting unnecessary evaluation.

Penile Cancers

Penile cancers are rare; with 1250 new U.S. cases in 2010 (ACS, 2010). Penile cancers are most often squamous cell, and there may be a connection to HPV infection. As expected from this cell type, lesions may appear as a superficial plaque or ulcer. Biopsy or consultation is appropriate in the evaluation of a suspicious penile lesion.

Prostate Cancer

Prostate cancer is the most common cancer diagnosed in men and is the second most common cause of cancer death in men after lung cancer. The gap between the annual numbers of diagnoses (217,730) and deaths (32,050) is wide (ACS, 2010). Major risk factors include age, African American race, and family history. Most cases occur in men older than 65. African Americans have a 60% higher incidence compared with whites and experience a disproportionate share of prostate cancer deaths (Harris and Lohr, 2002).

Dietary factors may play a role, including the proandrogenic effects of dietary fat, carcinogenic compounds in grilled meats, and antioxidants in vegetables (Nelson et al., 2003). Dietary antioxidants such as lycopene show epidemiologic links (mostly related to tomato consumption) supporting a preventive effect, with possible mechanisms including androgen inhibition (Wertz et al., 2004). However, an RCT using vitamin E and selenium, alone or in combination, failed to show any preventive effect. Given these results and prior disappointing results of other antioxidant trials, clinicians should not recommend supplements for prostate cancer prevention (Lippman et al., 2009).

Prostate cancer is most often indolent, with symptoms typically arising later in the disease course. Physical examination is most often unrevealing. A firm nodule on DRE may indicate a tumor. However, DRE accuracy depends on the performing physician and is imprecise. An abnormal DRE predicts prostate cancer in 18% to 28% of cases (Schwartz et al., 2005). Further, up to 25% of biopsy-detected cancers after an abnormal DRE occur on the side opposite the palpated nodule (McNaughton-Collins et al., 1997).

Tumors are most often diagnosed after biopsy for an abnormal screening result. The Gleason score grades cellular differentiation of the two most common patterns seen in a biopsy specimen. Scores range from 2 to 10, with higher scores indicating a more poorly differentiated tumor (Schwartz, 2005). The risk of prostate cancer death is higher with poorly differentiated cancer. Men with low Gleason scores (2 to 4) have a low risk of death, whereas those with higher scores (8 to 10) had a high probability of dying from prostate cancer within 10 years (Albertson et al., 2005).

Treatment options for prostate cancer include watchful waiting, brachytherapy, external beam radiation, radical prostatectomy, androgen ablation, and combinations of these options. High-grade tumors receive aggressive treatment, but the ideal treatment for intermediate-grade tumors (Gleason score of 5 to 7) is controversial. Low-grade tumors are candidates for watchful waiting. Treatment for localized disease, regardless of method, carries the risk of persistent negative effects on quality of life, such as sexual, urinary, and bowel dysfunction (Smith et al., 2009). An RCT of prostatectomy versus watchful waiting for low-grade tumors in Scandinavian men found little difference in outcomes during early follow-up, but at 10 years, the prostatectomy group had a lower risk of metastasis or progression and a slightly lower overall mortality (Bill-Axelson et al., 2005; Holmberg et al., 2002).

Prostate-specific antigen is a glycoprotein produced by prostatic epithelial cells. Its level increases with prostate adenocarcinoma, hyperplasia, inflammation, procedures, ejaculation, and massage. However, clinical DRE should not affect the PSA level (Barry, 2001). The most widely accepted upper limit of normal for total PSA is 4.0 ng/mL. The Prostate Cancer Prevention Trial, using a biopsy standard, indicated that as PSA levels increase, sensitivity declines and specificity increases, and at no point is there a good balance between the two. Thus, cancer appears ubiquitous—men with normal-range PSA levels may have prostate cancer; 15% of men with a PSA less than 4.0 ng/mL have cancer, 15% of which are high-grade tumors (Thompson et al., 2004). Furthermore, although some studies have concluded that a lower abnormal PSA cutoff level would detect more cancer (Punglia et al., 2003), these findings indicate that more men would have unnecessary biopsies. Thus, PSA testing suffers from both a high false-positive rate and false negatives as (Harvey et al., 2009).

It is unknown whether PSA screening reduces all-cause mortality. Two large, randomized screening trials, the Prostate, Lung, Colorectal, and Ovary (PLCO) trial, and the European Randomized Study of Screening for Prostate Cancer (ERSPC), were initiated to evaluate the impact of screening on mortality. The ERSPC study did show a 20% reduction in prostate cancer death; 1410 men would need to be screened and 48 prostate cancer cases treated to prevent one death in 10 years. Overdiagnosis of clinically insignificant prostate cancer was a problem (Schroder et al., 2009). In contrast, interim reports from the ongoing PLCO trial found no differences in prostate cancer mortality between the test and control groups (Andriole et al., 2009).

Should screening prove beneficial, African American men and patients with first-degree family histories (age <65) may be most likely to benefit, beginning at age 45 years (ACS, 2009b). Although older men have a higher risk, competing causes of death and the low chance of progression make screening men with less than 10 years in remaining life expectancy of little benefit (Fisher, 2002; Ilic et al., 2006).

Preventing prostate cancer with prophylactic measures can be considered (Unger et al., 2005). The Prostate Cancer Prevention Trial showed that finasteride significantly reduced cancer compared with placebo in an RCT (absolute risk reduction, 6% at 7 years). However, patients taking finasteride had an increased risk of high-grade cancer (Thompson et al., 2003). The American Society for Clinical Oncology and American Urological Association joint guideline recommends clinicians consider discussing the risks and benefits of 5α-reductase inhibitors for men with PSA values less than 3.0 who either undergo regular PSA screening or are planning to do so. The impact on PSA values and how PSA screening is interpreted must also be considered (Kramer et al., 2009).

Because PSA testing will detect cancers early, patients may live longer with the disease but not actually live longer lives (lead-time bias). Also, some patients treated for PSA-detected cancer may not have aggressive tumors. Treating them may artificially elevate treatment success and survival rates (length-time bias). Thus, mortality rate reductions may reflect the success of screening, misattribution of cause of death, research bias, improved treatments, or changing disease patterns. The most significant challenge remains that there is no way to differentiate patients with aggressive disease from those with clinically unimportant disease using current screening tools. Until this is resolved, controversy surrounding prostate cancer screening is likely to persist.

Despite any clear evidence showing that screening saves lives, over half of U.S. men are regularly screened with PSA testing (Thompson et al., 2005). PSA testing is a well-known test, with men possibly believing that being screened is beneficial and responsible behavior (Chapple et al., 2002). Furthermore, the PSA test has accuracy problems, which makes reassuring patients with normal-range results difficult. The controversies surrounding screening are reflected in the disparate prostate cancer screening guidelines (Box 40-7). However, one consistency emerges—family physicians should engage in an informed-consent discussion with their patients before screening. The risks, benefits, and limitations should be discussed so that patients are fully informed and can incorporate their personal preferences into the screening decision. Thus, although screening remains debatable, it appears inappropriate to order PSA testing routinely without this type of discussion.

As with any screening method, false-positive test results have potential for physical and psychological harm. Prostate biopsy carries procedural risks as well as the risk of discovering and treating a cancer that would not be significant in the patient's lifetime.

Box 40-7 Prostate Cancer Screening Recommendations

U.S. Preventive Services Task Force (USPSTF)
Evidence insufficient for recommendation in men younger than 75 years.
Recommend against PSA screening in men 75 and older.

American Cancer Society
Routine screening should not occur without an informed consent discussion.
Asymptomatic men with a life expectancy greater than 10 years should have the opportunity to make an informed decision on screening. Men with an average risk should have this at age 50; African-Americans or men with a first-degree relative with prostate cancer at age 45; and men with multiple affected relatives at age 40.
Men with less than a 10 year life expectancy should not be offered screening.
If screening is chosen, then PSA with or without DRE is the method. For men who choose screening:

○ PSA < 2.5 ng/mL may be screened every 2 years.
○ PSA > 2.5 ng/mL should be screened every year.
○ PSA > 4.0 ng/mL should be referred for biopsy. Consider individual risk for prostate cancer in men with PSA between 2.5 and 4.0 ng/mL.

Does not support routine testing.
Offer PSA testing and DRE annually beginning at age 50 years for men with at least 10-year remaining life expectancy as part of risk/benefit discussion; African Americans, and those with family history in one or more first-degree relatives diagnosed at an early age, should begin at 45 years.

American Academy of Family Physicians
Recommends against screening men 75 and older.

American Urological Association
Offer DRE and PSA testing to asymptomatic men 40 years or older with remaining life expectancy more than 10 years.

Modified from American Academy of Family Physicians. Recommendations for clinical preventive services; American Cancer Society guideline for early detection of cancer; American Urological Association. Prostate-specific antigen: best practice statement: 2009 update; US Preventive Services Task Force. Screening for prostate cancer: recommendation statement. Ann Intern Med 2008;149:185-191.
DRE, Digital rectal examination; *PSA*, prostate-specific antigen.

Renal Cancers

Renal cancers are twice as common in men as in women; more than 57,000 cases are diagnosed annually in men (ACS, 2010). Risk factors are less well understood than for other urologic cancers. Heavy tobacco use (>20 packs/year) is a risk factor in men, and severe obesity is a risk in both genders. Risks from occupational or medication exposure are less certain (Dhote et al., 2004).

Diagnosis of renal cancer is often incidental to an imaging study (e.g., ultrasound) obtained for another reason. Hematuria is also a clinical sign that may lead to the diagnosis. Although renal cell cancers are curable if localized (88%-100%), overall survival rates (40%-60% at 5 years) are not as encouraging as in other urologic cancers (Dhote et al., 2004; NCI, 2009d).

Testicular Cancer

Approximately 8400 men were diagnosed with testicular cancer in 2010 (ACS, 2010). It is unusual in that it occurs mostly in young men (15-35 years) and is the most common cancer in this group. Orchiopexy in children with cryptorchidism does not necessarily prevent cancer, so these patients should be followed closely (NCI, 2009e).

Most testicular tumors are initially discovered by patients. Typical presentations include painless testicular lumps or scrotal pain, edema, or hardness. Symptoms can mimic those of epididymitis, and tumor should be in the differential of this condition (Kinkade, 1999). Ultrasound is the initial study of choice for suspected testicular masses. Most tumors are germ cell neoplasms. Thus, serum tumor markers (β-hCG, lactate dehydrogenase, alpha-fetoprotein) are important in the diagnosis, prognosis, and monitoring aspects of care. However, normal values do not rule out cancer in patients with a mass, and they are not appropriate as screening tools, so they should not be used to decide whether a confirmed mass is cancerous (Kinkade, 1999). Patients are typically followed for many years for treatment failure or recurrence, and family physicians play an important role in ensuring that patients participate adequately with follow-up.

Testicular self-examination or clinical examination might detect cancer at an earlier stage but is highly unlikely to have a significant impact on testicular cancer mortality, with survival rates already so high. Thus, USPSTF (2004b) does not recommend testicular cancer screening in the general population.

Wilms' Tumor

Wilms' tumor presents in childhood as an abdominal mass. It is a rare cancer, with approximately 500 cases annually. Wilms' tumor has good cure potential, with survival rates greater than 90% at 4 years (NCI, 2009f).

KEY TREATMENT

Use of 5α-reductase inhibitors is effective for benign prostatic hyperplasia (BPH) (Kramer et al., 2009; Thorpe and Neal, 2003) (SOR: A).
Alpha-adrenergic blockers are also used to treat BPH (Wilt et al., 2000) (SOR: A).
5α-Reductase inhibitors are used for prostate cancer prevention (SOR: B).
Surgical treatments may be needed for BPH (SOR: A).

References

The complete reference list is available online at www.expertconsult.com.

Web Resources

www.aafp.org/online/en/home/clinical/exam/p-t.html.
American Academy of Family Physicians; recommendations for clinical preventive services.
www.cancer.org/docroot/PED/content/PED
American Cancer Society; guidelines for early cancer detection.
www.cdc.gov/STD/treatment/default.htm
Centers for Disease Control and Prevention; guidelines for treating sexually transmitted infections.
http://phil.cdc.gov/phil
CDC Public Health Image Library.
http://nkdep.nih.gov/professionals/index.htm
National Kidney Disease Education Program site on chronic kidney disease with guidelines and GFR calculators for adults and children.
www.cpcn.org/ipss.pdf
International Prostate Symptom Score.

www.cancer.gov/
National Cancer Institute main site, with information on various cancers and treatment.
www.auanet.org/
American Urological Association; guidelines and patient education resources.
http://www2.niddk.nih.gov/NR/rdonlyres/93B6388F-B429-4603-9C3C-6765BDEB49A1/0/NIHCPSIEnglish.pdf
National Institutes of Health Chronic Prostatitis Symptom Index.
www.kidney.org/professionals/kdoqi/guidelines_ckd/p9_approach.htm.
National Kidney Foundation/Kidney Disease Quality Initiative; clinical practice guidelines for chronic kidney disease: evaluation, classification, and stratification.

Ophthalmology

Earl R. Crouch, Jr., Eric R. Crouch, and Thomas R. Grant, Jr.

Patients present to the family physician with a limited set of symptoms, often with subtle differences to indicate mild or serious ocular conditions. To decide when to treat patients and when to refer them to an ophthalmologist, the family physician must possess a complete appreciation of these subtle differences. Knowledge of the basic anatomy of the eye is essential in determining these diagnostic differences (Fig. 41-1).

Red Eye

The family physician frequently encounters patients who complain of a "red eye." Usually, the condition causing the red eye is a simple disorder, such as conjunctivitis or subconjunctival hemorrhage. These conditions improve spontaneously or are readily treated. A red eye, however, may be a symptom of a more serious disorder, such as herpetic dendritic ulcer, iritis, acute angle-closure glaucoma, ophthalmia neonatorum, or congenital glaucoma. These conditions must be clearly distinguished from the much more common conjunctivitis and subconjunctival hemorrhage because *immediate referral* to the ophthalmologist is paramount. To evaluate the red eye, the family physician needs to have available a penlight, magnifying glasses, visual acuity chart, fluorescein dye, anesthetic drops, and tonometer.

Evaluation

Symptoms and Signs

Patients who complain of a red eye generally can tell the physician whether the eye irritation occurred rapidly or progressed slowly. This information is important because a small foreign body, such as a grain of sand, lodged in the conjunctival sac produces a rapid hyperemia, whereas a viral or allergic conjunctivitis, or an iritis, generally produces a slowly progressive redness. Ocular pain is an important symptom (Table 41-1). Irritation of the superficial layer of the cornea, as caused by a small foreign body, is accompanied by a superficial "grain of sand" sensation in the eye. Deeper inflammatory processes, such as iritis or iridocyclitis, or a deeper penetrating foreign body in the cornea, present with more severe, dull pain in the eye.

Abnormal light sensitivity (photophobia) is a third danger symptom that must be elicited by the family physician. Photophobia occurs with corneal inflammation, iritis, and angle-closure glaucoma. Patients who have conjunctivitis usually do not have abnormal light sensitivity (Box 41-1).

Patients who complain of a red eye often complain of discharge from the eye (Table 41-2). If they do not complain of eye discharge spontaneously, the physician must inquire about the presence, type, and quantity of discharge. Purulent (creamy white or yellow watery) discharge suggests a bacterial cause. A serous or clear discharge suggests a viral cause. Scanty, white, stringy exudate occurs most often with allergic conjunctivitis. The absence of discharge indicates an unusual cause for red eye, such as iridocyclitis, ultraviolet (UV) light keratitis (snow blindness), or acute angle-closure glaucoma. A complaint of diminished visual acuity is a serious danger sign and must be elicited in the history.

Physical Examination

It is important to examine both eyes because many patients with conjunctivitis in one eye have clear signs of early conjunctivitis in the other. The type of infection must be closely

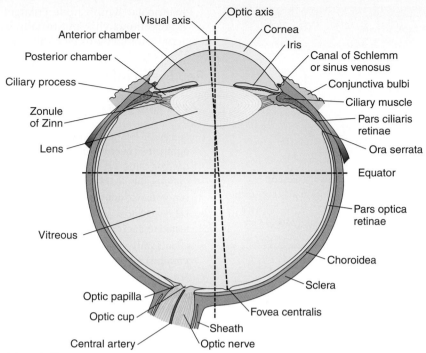

Figure 41-1 Anatomy of the right eyeball. *(From Scheie HG, Albert DM. Textbook of Ophthalmology, 9th ed. Philadelphia, Saunders, 1977.)*

Table 41-1 Red Eye: Differential Diagnosis

Parameter	Conjunctivitis, Bacterial	Iritis	Keratitis	Acute Glaucoma
Vision	Normal	Blurred	Blurred	Marked blurring
Pain	None	Moderately severe; intermittent stabbing	Sharp, severe	Severe; sometimes nausea/vomiting
Photophobia	None	Moderate	Moderate	Moderate
Discharge	Usually significant with crusting of lashes	None	None to mild	None
Conjunctival injection	Diffuse	Circumcorneal	Circumcorneal	Diffuse
Appearance of cornea	Clear	Clear	Cloudy	Cloudy
Pupil size	Normal	Constricted	Normal	Dilated
Intraocular pressure*	Normal	Normal or low	Normal	Elevated

From American Academy of Ophthalmology. The Red Eye. AAO Professional Information Committee, San Francisco, 1986.
Caution: Do not measure IOP with discharge present.

inspected; *conjunctival* infection is characterized by individually visible vessels in the conjunctiva branching from the sclera toward the cornea, whereas *ciliary* infection appears as a red ring surrounding the cornea in which individual vessels are not clearly visible. The significance of ciliary infection is that the deep ciliary vessels are involved, indicating a much more serious inflammatory condition of the eye, such as a deep corneal infection, iritis, or iridocyclitis. Inspect the palpebral conjunctiva carefully with magnification to determine whether lymphoid hyperplasia (cobblestone appearance) exists. The type and quantity of discharge are assessed by pulling down the lower lid. The appearance of the punctum should be examined to determine whether pus is coming out

of the tear duct. Palpation of the tear sac on the upper portion of the nose (lacrimal crest) demonstrates tenderness in cases of acute dacryocystitis.

Carefully examine the cornea. Normally, the cornea is perfectly transparent. Excessive fluid within the stroma of the cornea results in partial opacification that can be observed by direct illumination with a penlight. A diffuse corneal haze can occur with congenital glaucoma and angle-closure glaucoma. After inspection with a penlight under magnification, perform corneal staining with fluorescein using sterile filter paper strips. The stained part of the strip is moistened with water and touched to the conjunctiva away from the cornea. With blinking, the fluorescein

Box 41-1 Approach to Patient Presenting with Red Eye (No History of Trauma)

1. Check for the following symptoms or signs.
   a. Reduced vision
   b. Pain
   c. Photophobia
   d. Corneal staining
   e. Corneal edema
   f. Unequal pupils
   g. Elevated intraocular pressure
2. Refer to ophthalmologist if any of these signals are present.
3. If none of the above is present, the diagnosis is probably conjunctivitis.
4. The triad of a red eye, pain, and loss of vision should *always* alert the examiner to a potentially blinding condition.

Table 41-2 Conjunctivitis Clues

Finding	Cause
Purulent discharge	Bacterial
Serous or clear discharge	Viral
Stringy, white discharge	Allergic
Preauricular lymph node enlargement	Viral

spreads over the cornea. A UV light source enhances fluorescence. Areas of bright-green staining denote absent or diseased epithelium. Corneal staining readily demonstrates a corneal abrasion and helps identify corneal foreign bodies and infectious epithelial defects, such as herpetic dendritic keratitis (Fig. 41-2).

Examine the pupils carefully for size and shape. In most people the pupils are of equal size; a small percentage have congenital variation in the size of the pupils (anisocoria). These patients are often aware that their pupils are unequal. In patients with previously equal pupils, inequality of the pupil may indicate iritis, typically with the affected pupil partially constricted. In acute angle-closure glaucoma the pupil is usually partially dilated and may not be round. Unequal pupil size is an important sign of significant ocular trauma or third nerve palsies.

Estimate the anterior chamber depth by side illumination with a penlight. If the anterior chamber is normal or deep, the entire surface of the iris is well illuminated. When the anterior chamber is shallow, the iris on the more distant side of the pupil is in shadow. A shallow anterior chamber in a red eye may indicate acute angle-closure glaucoma or ocular trauma. The anterior chamber appears deep in patients with congenital glaucoma.

If the red eye does not have an obvious infection, measure the *intraocular pressure* (IOP) with a tonometer. IOP is normal in most patients with red eye, except for those with acute angle-closure glaucoma. With iritis and traumatic, perforating ocular injuries, IOP is generally low. Sterilize the tonometer before and after application to a red eye, preferably by heat sterilization.

Preauricular lymph node enlargement is a frequent sign of viral conjunctivitis and usually is not present with acute bacterial conjunctivitis (see Table 41-2).

Red Eye in Infants

Key Points

- Red eye in infants requires special attention to differentiate ophthalmia neonatorum, congenital glaucoma, conjunctivitis, and dacryocystitis.
- Cultures should be obtained in neonates with symptoms suggestive of ophthalmia neonatorum.
- Febrile children with acute dacryocystitis should have cultures tested to direct management.
- Infants with symptoms of congenital glaucoma should be promptly referred to an ophthalmologist.
- For chronic dacryocystitis, the best age for surgical intervention is 6 to 12 months.
- Infants with a dacryocystocele require prompt ophthalmologist referral and systemic antibiotics.

Several conditions occur specifically during the first year of life. They include ophthalmia neonatorum, acute and chronic dacryocystitis, bacterial conjunctivitis, and congenital glaucoma.

Ophthalmia Neonatorum

Ophthalmia neonatorum is an infection or inflammation of the conjunctiva that occurs during the first 4 weeks of life. Possible causes include chemical conjunctivitis, *Neisseria gonorrhoeae*, and chlamydial infection. The increased incidence of venereal disease and shortcomings in silver nitrate prophylaxis are significant factors in the constantly evolving clinical picture. Ophthalmia neonatorum frequently is a manifestation of a systemic infection, requiring determination of the exact cause in all but the most transient cases. Table 41-3 outlines the management of the various types of ophthalmia neonatorum. At present, erythromycin is the medication of choice. Povidone-iodine ophthalmic solution (0.5%) is less toxic, inexpensive, and effective, but is not generally used because of confusion over povidone solution versus povidone soap.

Silver nitrate has been replaced by erythromycin, so the incidence of chemical conjunctivitis has decreased significantly. Before the neonatal prophylaxis, gonorrhea was a common cause of ophthalmia neonatorum. Half of patients with *gonococcal* conjunctivitis develop corneal clouding, a major cause of blindness. Gonococcal conjunctivitis still occurs, despite erythromycin prophylaxis. Frequently, the infant with gonococcal conjunctivitis presents with swollen lids, purulent exudates, beefy-red conjunctiva, and conjunctival edema. The gonococcal organism can rapidly penetrate the intact corneal epithelium and produce corneal perforation if recognition and treatment are delayed. When gonococcal conjunctivitis is suspected, referral to an ophthalmologist is critical. Patients may also have systemic involvement, with associated central nervous system (CNS) signs. Both parents should be examined for venereal disease and treated, if necessary.

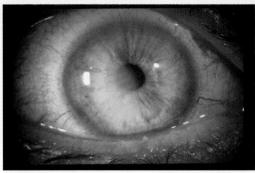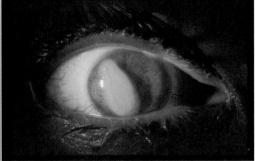

Figure 41-2 Corneal abrasion. The patient had a fingernail injury caused by the daughter *(left)*. Characteristic fluorescein staining is displayed in the adjacent photomicrograph *(right)*.

Table 41-3 Management of Ophthalmia Neonatorum

Disease	Diagnosis	Treatment
Gonococcal conjunctivitis	Gram-negative intracellular diplococci *plus* Growth on chocolate agar or Thayer-Martin agar *plus* Fermentation glucose negative and maltose negative	Ceftriaxone, 125 mg IM single dose *plus* one of the following: Oral tetracycline, 500 mg qid Oral doxycycline, 100 mg bid Oral erythromycin, 500 mg qid Ophthalmology consultation
Other bacterial conjunctivitis	Gram stain *plus* Growth on blood agar or chocolate agar	Gram positive: erythromycin ointment qid, or fluoroquinolone qid, for 2 wk Gram negative: gentamicin, tobramycin, or fluoroquinolone, qid for 2 wk
Chlamydial conjunctivitis	Giemsa stain— basophilic intracytoplasmic inclusion bodies *plus* Chlamydial culture	Tetracycline, 500 mg qid for 3-4 wk Erythromycin, 250-500 mg for 3 wk Doxycycline, 100 mg bid for 2 wk Azithromycin, 1 g (one dose)

IM, Intramuscularly; *bid,* twice daily; *qid,* four times daily.

A recommended regimen for ophthalmia neonatorum prophylaxis is a single application of silver nitrate 1% aqueous solution, erythromycin 0.5% ophthalmic ointment, or tetracycline 1% ophthalmic ointment (CDC, 2002b).

Chlamydial Infection

Chlamydial infections are a leading cause of ophthalmia neonatorum. There is a high incidence of this type of infection because of the frequent exposure to the newborn during delivery and the lack of effective prophylaxis. The onset of infection can occur at any time. The typical picture is a mild unilateral or bilateral mucopurulent conjunctivitis with moderate lid edema, chemosis, and conjunctival injection. Systemic involvement may include rhinitis, vaginitis, and otitis media.

Treatment is with tetracycline ointment or erythromycin four times daily for 4 weeks. In addition, both parents should be treated with oral tetracycline or azithromycin. Alternative treatments include oral erythromycin or doxycycline for 3 weeks. Systemic tetracycline should be avoided in breastfeeding women with this infection.

Conjunctival cultures are indicated in all cases of suspected infectious neonatal conjunctivitis (CDC, 2002).

Bacterial Conjunctivitis

The most common gram-positive bacteria that are causative agents of conjunctivitis include *Staphylococcus aureus*, *Streptococcus pneumoniae*, and group A and B streptococci (Fig. 41-3). Gram-negative organisms include *Haemophilus influenzae*, *Escherichia coli*, and *Pseudomonas aeruginosa*. Bacterial conjunctivitis can occur at any age from the first day of life. Chemosis (edema of bulbar conjunctiva), purulent discharge, lid edema, and injection are common signs. Associated systemic septicemia can occur, especially with *Pseudomonas* infection. Cultures should be prepared on blood and chocolate agar.

A topical fluoroquinolone often provides effective treatment for severe cases before culture results (Leibowitz, 1991). Gram-negative organisms are best treated with tobramycin or a topical fluoroquinolone. Systemic antibiotics are recommended when there is evidence of systemic disease. Physicians should use caution with gentamicin, neomycin, and sulfacetamide eye medications, because these drugs may cause a toxic chemical conjunctivitis and complicate management. Patients with mild conjunctivitis generally respond to erythromycin or bacitracin ointment.

Acute Dacryocystitis

Neonates may present with acute dacryocystitis, an inflammation of the lacrimal sac (Fig. 41-4). Pain, tearing, redness, and discharge usually occur. If the child is febrile, culture testing and Gram staining should be done. *S. pneumoniae* and *S. aureus* are the most common pathogens. Systemic antibiotics are indicated for the acute stage. The ophthalmologist should be consulted immediately, because irrigation and probing may be necessary to establish drainage as quickly as possible. Severe cases may progress to a dacryocystocele, sepsis, meningitis, or even death, especially in young infants.

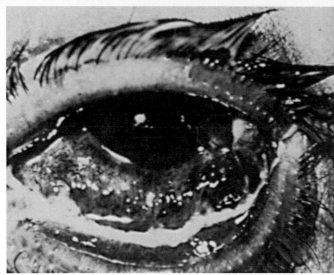

Figure 41-3 Purulent conjunctivitis may indicate infection with *Staphylococcus, Haemophilus influenzae, Streptococcus,* or *Pseudomonas. (From American Academy of Ophthalmology. The Red Eye. San Francisco, AAO Professional Information Committee, 1986 [AAO. The Red Eye].)*

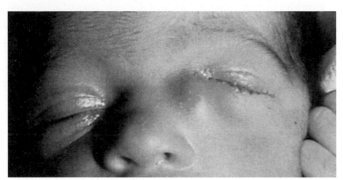

Figure 41-4 Acute dacryocystitis in a neonate with fever and malaise. Lacrimal sac massage and systemic antibiotics relieved the acute infection.

Chronic Dacryocystitis and Nasolacrimal Duct Obstruction

Infants with chronic dacryocystitis usually present to the physician with a chronic history of tearing and crusting with a chronic yellow discharge. Topical antibiotics, such as a fluoroquinolone four times daily, should be used. The mother should be taught to compress or massage the lacrimal sac four to six times daily. Approximately 80% of these inflammations resolve spontaneously by age 6 to 12 months. If treatment is not successful or if dacryocystitis persists, the patient should be referred and the nasolacrimal duct system irrigated between 6 and 10 months of age. Before age 14 months, a single probing is curative in about 90% of cases.

Congenital Glaucoma

Congenital glaucoma is a potentially blinding condition with an incidence of 1 per 10,000 births. It is often confused with chronic dacryocystitis. About two thirds of these cases are bilateral. These patients, similar to those with dacryocystitis, present with excessive tearing. The infants usually are light sensitive (photophobic) and frequently bury their head in a pillow or blanket. These infants often have intense

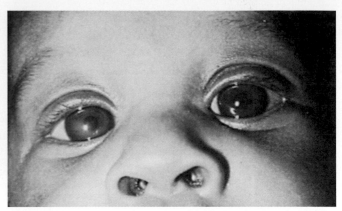

Figure 41-5 Congenital glaucoma in a 2-month-old infant who presented with a cloudy cornea involving the right eye. Intraocular pressure was elevated. The diagnosis was congenital glaucoma.

blinking or lid spasm (blepharospasm). An enlarged cornea or corneal clouding can be detected clinically and measured with a plastic ruler (normal, ≤12 mm) (Fig. 41-5). Corneal edema is the result of elevated IOP, which causes breaks in the inner corneal layers (Descemet's membrane) and intrusion of anterior chamber fluid into the corneal stroma. Increased IOP causes significant optic nerve damage, which can lead to blindness. Whenever glaucoma is suspected, immediate consultation is indicated. Surgical treatment of congenital glaucoma is successful in approximately 90% of cases. These patients must be followed by an ophthalmologist for life as a precaution against recurrent IOP elevation and amblyopia.

KEY TREATMENT

Newborns should be prophylactically treated with erythromycin 0.5% or tetracycline 1% ophthalmic ointment to reduce the risk of ophthalmia neonatorum (CDC, 2002) (SOR: A).

Ciprofloxacin 0.3% ophthalmic solution is effective empiric treatment of bacterial conjunctivitis (Leibowitz, 1991) (SOR: A).

A broad-spectrum antibiotic for 5 to 7 days is generally effective for most cases of bacterial conjunctivitis (American Academy of Ophthalmology [AAO], 2008) (SOR: A).

Children with nasolacrimal duct obstruction may undergo nasolacrimal duct surgery between 6 and 12 months of age, or sooner if clinically indicated (Katowitz et al., 1987) (SOR: C).

Children with congenital glaucoma should be promptly referred to a pediatric ophthalmologist or glaucoma specialist (AAO, 2008) (SOR: A).

Red Eye in Adults and Older Children

Key Points

- Red eye in adults and older children requires careful evaluation to differentiate the various causes of inflammation.
- Purulent conjunctival discharge warrants culturing and broad-spectrum antibiotics.
- Allergic conjunctivitis generally responds well to topical treatment; symptoms may manifest or worsen on initiation of systemic antihistamines.

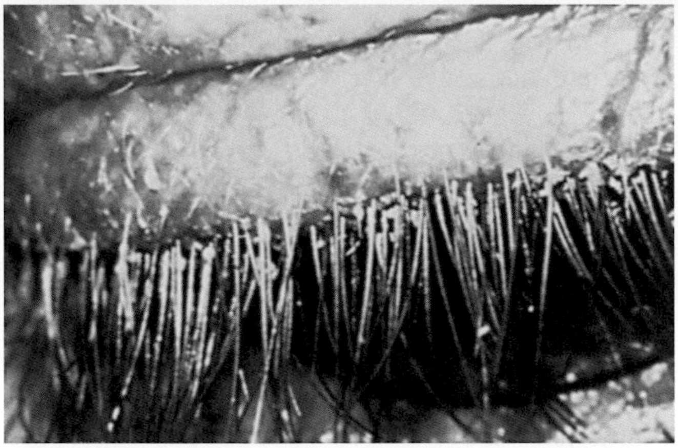

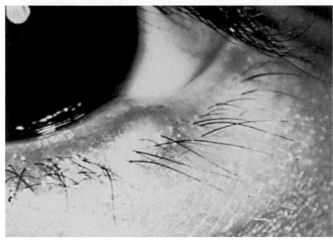

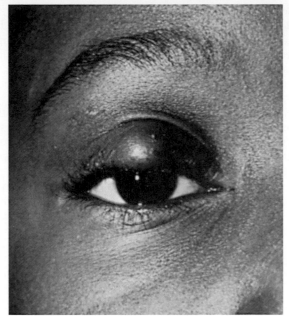

Figure 41-6 Seborrheic blepharitis is characterized by greasy, dandruff-like scales on the lashes. *(From AAO. The Red Eye.)*

Figure 41-8 Chalazion of right upper eyelid in 10-year-old girl. *(From AAO. The Red Eye.)*

Figure 41-7 Acute hordeolum, or stye. The swollen, tender, red eyelid includes an acute, boil-like lesion. Treatment includes warm compresses and topical antibiotics. *(From AAO. The Red Eye.)*

- Orbital cellulitis requires prompt computed tomography and systemic antibiotics. Cultures should be obtained from the nasopharynx, conjunctiva, and blood.
- Iritis is characterized by pain, photophobia, miosis, and circumciliary injection and generally occurs after blunt trauma.
- A red eye in a contact lens wearer requires prompt evaluation for a corneal ulcer.
- Acute angle-closure glaucoma is an ocular emergency and requires immediate treatment by an ophthalmologist.

Blepharitis

Blepharitis is a chronic lid inflammation that involves abnormalities of the glands surrounding the eyelashes. The two most common types are chronic staphylococcal infections of the lid and seborrheic blepharitis (Fig. 41-6). *Staphylococcal blepharitis* is the most common inflammation of the external eye. It is frequently asymptomatic initially, but as the disease progresses, the patient complains of foreign body sensation, matting of the lashes, and burning. Lid crusting, discharge, redness, and loss of lashes are observed. *Seborrheic blepharitis* is associated with seborrhea of the scalp, lashes, eyebrows, and ears, characterized by greasy, dandruff-like scales on the lashes. Blepharitis is not associated with skin ulcerations.

Treatment of both these conditions is long and laborious. Lid hygiene is recommended for both conditions. Topical antibiotics are prescribed for staphylococcal blepharitis. Both conditions are recurrent and require repeated therapy.

Stye

A stye is the most common localized infection of one of the glands of the eyelid margin (Fig. 41-7). It is an acute boil-like lesion, and the patient usually has a swollen, tender, red eyelid. There may be a moderate amount of conjunctival injection. Treatment includes warm compresses for 15 minutes four times per day and topical antibiotics. Systemic antibiotics are usually not indicated unless there is a preseptal cellulitis component. Generally, the stye drains spontaneously within several days. If resolution does not occur within 2 weeks, the patient should be referred.

Chalazion

A chalazion is a chronic swelling of the eyelids not associated with conjunctivitis (Fig. 41-8). The chalazion, a granulomatous inflammatory reaction, may persist for weeks or even months. Chalazia are generally not amenable to oral or topical antibiotics, unless the lesion is secondarily infected. Chalazia are usually rubbery, cystic, and nontender on palpation. When the upper lid is involved, vision may be temporarily blurred. If the chalazion persists for more than 4 to 6 weeks, it may require incision and curettage. Recurrent chalazia may be caused by an underlying sebaceous carcinoma, so the lesion should be biopsied and sent for pathologic testing.

Bacterial Conjunctivitis

All common bacteria may cause acute conjunctivitis. Presently, *S. pneumoniae, H. influenzae, S. aureus,* and *P. aeruginosa* are the most common pathogens. The most frequent causes of hyperacute conjunctivitis are *N. gonorrhoeae* and *N. meningitidis*. Risk factors for bacterial conjunctivitis include contact lens wear, exposure to infectious persons, compromised immune systems, nasolacrimal duct obstruction, and sinusitis. In the presence of a severe purulent discharge, culture of the conjunctiva is mandatory (see Fig. 41-3). Subconjunctival hemorrhage may occur with bacterial conjunctivitis and is especially common with *H. influenzae* conjunctivitis.

Treatment of conjunctivitis is with a topical antibiotic, such as erythromycin or bacitracin. Tobramycin ophthalmic ointment may be used for many gram-positive and gram-negative conjunctivitis cases. Ciprofloxacin and ofloxacin also provide effective broad coverage of most types of conjunctivitis. Gonococcal and *Haemophilus* conjunctivitis require systemic and topical therapy. If the conjunctivitis does not improve within 2 to 3 days or the worsening symptoms develop, the patient should be referred to an ophthalmologist.

Ciprofloxacin and ofloxacin provide effective broad coverage of most causative organisms. Newer fluoroquinolones such as gatifloxacin and moxifloxacin provide more potent coverage and better penetration for gram-positive organisms than earlier types of fluoroquinolones. Topical steroids or antibiotic-steroid combinations for conjunctivitis or other causes of red eye should not be used unless the patient is under the care of an ophthalmologist.

Topical corticosteroids have four potentially serious ocular side effects and are contraindicated for conjunctivitis, as follows:

1. Steroids can facilitate penetration of an undetected corneal herpetic infection to the deeper corneal layers and cause corneal perforation.
2. Prolonged local use of the corticosteroids (usually >2 weeks) can cause chronic open-angle glaucoma.
3. Prolonged use of topical corticosteroids can cause cataracts.
4. Topical corticosteroids are capable of potentiating the development of fungal corneal ulcers.

In general, topical steroids should be reserved for patients under the care of an ophthalmologist.

KEY TREATMENT

Cultures of the conjunctiva are indicated in all cases of suspected infectious neonatal conjunctivitis (AAO, 2003) (SOR: A).

Viral Conjunctivitis

Viral conjunctivitis, in contrast to bacterial conjunctivitis, has a less prominent discharge that is usually watery. The condition is highly contagious, and handwashing is important to avoid infection. When infected, hospital personnel, daycare workers, and institutional personnel should avoid contact with others. Palpable preauricular lymph nodes frequently are present with viral conjunctivitis and represent an important sign that can differentiate it from bacterial conjunctivitis. An associated upper respiratory infection may occur. In advanced cases, true photophobia and blurred vision caused by corneal involvement may be present and require consultation. However, most viral conjunctivitis is self-limiting, and no specific treatment is indicated. Topical

steroids are contraindicated. Most viral infections resolve within 10 to 14 days, and specific serologic diagnosis is not necessary. If the conjunctivitis persists or there is any pain or change in vision, the patient should be referred.

Allergic Conjunctivitis

Allergic conjunctivitis is frequently found in pediatric patients and adults. It is usually seasonal, most often the spring and fall. Although often associated with allergic rhinitis, allergic conjunctivitis may occur without systemic symptoms. There is an increase in itching, redness, and swelling, which is variable from day to day. Seasonal allergic conjunctivitis is related to tree and grass pollens, each of which has a distinct season and severity. The condition may be asymmetric. Chronic allergic conjunctivitis is most often related to various indoor allergens, including dust mites, animal dander, molds, and cockroaches. Cats are especially irritating to the eye for the allergic patient.

Treatment for allergic conjunctivitis involves avoidance procedures for outdoor allergens, keeping windows closed at night during allergy season, and eye protection (even sunglasses can reduce exposure to allergens). Washing the face after coming indoors, washing the hair when showering, and keeping the patient's hands away from the eyes can reduce allergen exposure. Bed linens should be washed weekly. Occasionally, allergy testing and allergy shots may be necessary in severe recalcitrant cases.

Symptomatic treatment of allergic conjunctivitis includes cool compresses, artificial tears, and over-the-counter (OTC) antihistamines. Topical antihistamine-decongestant combinations include naphazoline hydrochloride/antazoline phosphate (Vasocon-A) and naphazoline hydrochloride/pheniramine maleate (Naphcon-A), which are reasonably safe and effective. However, rebound vasodilation can occur and cause chronic hyperemia and conjunctival injection.

Cromolyn sodium 4% and olopatadine hydrochloride (Patanol) are effective mast cell stabilizers. Ketorolac tromethamine (Acular), azelastine hydrochloride (Optivar), and lodoxamide tromethamine (Alomide) are also reasonable options for managing allergic conjunctivitis. Systemic allergy medications may cause allergic conjunctivitis to manifest because of reduced tear film production.

Subconjunctival Hemorrhage

A patient may present with a bright-red eye, normal vision, and no pain. Usually, no obvious cause exists, but in some patients there is a history of coughing, sneezing, or straining before the hemorrhage is present. The patient should be reassured that it is nothing more than hemorrhage of the conjunctiva. There is no therapy, except reassurance that the blood will clear within 2 to 3 weeks. Hematologic blood coagulation studies are usually of limited value in patients with subconjunctival hemorrhages unless there is a history of recurrence. Additionally, it is unusual for a hemorrhage to involve the relatively avascular sclera. If trauma is suspected, the patient should be referred to an ophthalmologist to rule out more serious injuries, such as perforation, contusion, or occult rupture of the globe. Subconjunctival hemorrhage may indicate that the patient is a battered child or adult, and other signs of bodily trauma should be investigated.

Corneal Herpetic Infections

Herpetic infections of the eye can produce conjunctivitis, corneal inflammation (keratitis), and uveitis (inflamed iris, ciliary body, and choroid). The herpes simplex virus (HSV) is the most common cause of corneal opacification in temperate-zone countries. The human is the only natural host for this DNA virus. Approximately 90% of the population has systemic antibodies to HSV. The incubation period of HSV infection is 2 to 12 days. HSV type 1 (HSV-1) is the most common cause of ocular infection, but transmission of HSV-2 also can occur. Although classically HSV-1 is the oral type and HSV-2 is the genital type, current epidemiologic studies indicate that either type may be the source of corneal infection, and therefore cultures and viral titers are often sent for both types.

Primary Herpes Simplex Infection

Primary ocular infection in a nonimmune subject usually presents as conjunctivitis with a clear watery discharge, skin vesicles on the lids, and preauricular nodes. Associated vesicles and ulcers on the oral mucosa and skin are common. Corneal involvement also may occur with single or multiple dendrites. If dendrites are present, the patient should be referred for treatment. Particular attention should be given to inspecting the nose for possible lesions. A lesion at the tip of the nose indicates involvement of the cornea through the nasociliary branch of cranial nerve V. Treatment generally involves trifluridine 1% (Viroptic) drops five times daily for 10 to 14 days. If other regions are involved, oral acyclovir is added to trifluridine, as in eyelid or corneal involvement. These patients should be managed by an ophthalmologist.

Recurrent Corneal Herpetic Infections

At the time of the primary herpetic infection, the virus gains access to the CNS, where it resides in a latent state in the trigeminal and other ganglia. Recurrent attacks occur when the latent state is reversed. The virus travels via the sensory nerves to target tissues, one of which is the eye. Recurrent corneal involvement also includes the development of single or multiple dendritic ulcers. After a brief period, the plaque of epithelial cells desquamates to form a linear branching ulcer (dendrite). When a corneal dendrite is detected by corneal staining with fluorescein, the patient should be referred.

Preseptal Cellulitis

Preseptal cellulitis involves the eyelid and periorbital soft tissues and is characterized by acute eyelid erythema and edema. The infection usually occurs in the setting of an upper respiratory tract infection, external ocular infection, or trauma to the eyelids. Patients may have a mild fever and tend to complain of epiphora, conjunctivitis, and localized tenderness. However, the signs of orbital cellulitis are generally absent, unless a preseptal cellulitis evolves into an orbital cellulitis. Treatment is initiated empirically in most cases with cefuroxime, ceftriaxone, or nafcillin.

Orbital Cellulitis

Orbital cellulitis, most frequently caused by an extension of infection from the ethmoid sinus, can occur in adults and children (Fig. 41-9). It is the most common cause of

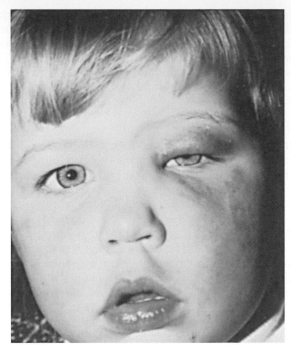

Figure 41-9 Orbital cellulites in 3-year-old patient. *(From AAO. The Red Eye.)*

exophthalmos in children. It may be difficult to differentiate a periorbital or anterior lid cellulitis from a true posterior orbital cellulitis. With a true orbital cellulitis, the child or adult has pain on movement of the eye, conjunctival edema, and limited extraocular movements. The most common causative organisms are *S. aureus*, *Streptococcus*, and *H. influenzae*. Cultures should be obtained from the nasopharynx, conjunctiva, and blood.

Immediate hospitalization and ophthalmic consultation are necessary. Emergent computed tomography (CT) should be performed to rule out orbital cellulitis. If orbital cellulitis is diagnosed, immediate hospitalization with intravenous (IV) antibiotics and ophthalmologic consultation should be undertaken. Appropriate systemic antibiotic treatment depends on the causative organism. Cavernous sinus thrombosis, meningitis, and blindness are serious complications of orbital cellulitis.

Iritis

Iritis is an inflammatory process of the anterior chamber, often associated with blunt trauma or infection. Redness, pain, and photophobia occur with iritis. No discharge is seen, and the pupil is constricted. Circumcorneal (ciliary) injection may occur. IOP is normal or low. Initial treatment may include dilation with homatropine and loteprednol etabonate (Lotemax) for patient comfort, with immediate referral to an ophthalmologist. Consultation should be obtained for all such patients as soon as possible.

Corneal Ulcers

The most common causes of corneal ulcers include gram-positive organisms, such as staphylococci and streptococci; and gram-negative organisms, such as *Pseudomonas aeruginosa* and Enterobacteriaceae. Less common gram-negative organisms include *Bacteroides.* Risk factors for corneal ulcers include patients with corneal erosions, persistent epithelial defects, impaired immunologic mechanisms, contact lenses, chronic topical or systemic steroid use, diabetes, and alcoholism. Corneal ulcers require consultation with an ophthalmologist for appropriate culture and antibiotic therapy.

Angle-Closure Glaucoma

Acute elevations in IOP can occur when the outflow of aqueous humor is suddenly blocked. The condition is more common in Asians but may occur in any patient. An acute angle-closure attack may follow an episode of emotional or physical stress, dilation of the pupil in dim lighting, or rarely, after instillation of dilating eyedrops. A patient having an acute attack usually has severe ocular pain, redness, blurred vision, rainbow-colored halos around lights, and sometimes nausea and vomiting. On examination, the eye is usually red, pupil mid-dilated and poorly reactive, and IOP greatly elevated. Generally, only one eye is affected at a time. Corneal clouding or corneal edema may be present in advanced cases.

An acute episode of angle-closure glaucoma is an ocular emergency and requires immediate treatment to lower IOP by medical treatment. Once IOP is under control, yttrium-argon-garnet (YAG) or argon laser peripheral iridectomy is performed.

Ocular Trauma and Other Emergencies

Key Points

- Chemical burns require immediate evaluation and treatment to stabilize the ocular surface.
- Central retinal artery occlusion requires immediate intervention to return oxygenation to the retina. Patients should be thoroughly evaluated to determine the source of the retinal artery occlusion.
- Hyphema should be carefully managed with bed rest, shielding the injured eye, and appropriate pharmacologic or surgical treatment to minimize potential complications. Patients with hyphema and angle recession require lifelong evaluation for possible glaucoma.
- Ocular foreign bodies of the surface can be conservatively managed with removal of the foreign material and appropriate antibiotic ointment. Care should always be taken to rule out an occult ruptured globe.
- The early signs of a retinal detachment include an increase in floaters or flashing lights. Retinal detachments warrant careful evaluation and prompt intervention.

Emergencies

True emergencies can be classified as those for which therapy should be instituted within minutes. Two true emergencies in the eye are chemical burns of the cornea and central retinal artery occlusion.

Chemical Burns

Most acids produce the extent of their damage immediately on contact—the more concentrated the acid, the more severe the immediate effect. Alkali burns are more devastating to the eye because they continue to cause damage long after the initial chemical contact. Corneal melting can lead to perforation, and severe chronic glaucoma can occur as a later complication. Burns of the eye by acids or alkalis are true ocular emergencies. An alkaline substance, such as lye, can cause permanent and irreversible blindness.

The immediate treatment of chemical burns must be continual irrigation of the eyes, with up to 1000 mL of normal saline (NS) or lactated Ringer's (LR) solution. If these solutions are not available, water from a shower, spigot, bathtub, or drinking fountain is appropriate. The conjunctival pH should be assessed after irrigation and again 30 minutes later to confirm stabilization of the ocular surface; pH value should be 7.5 to 8. If the pH remains abnormal, irrigation should be repeated until the pH is normal. Patients are managed with aggressive antibiotic ointment therapy and lubrication following a chemical burn. After the initial ocular irrigation, ophthalmologic consultation must be immediate.

KEY TREATMENT

Chemical burns of the ocular surface should be washed with at least 1 liter of fluid and tested until the pH returns to normal. An ophthalmologist should evaluate the affected eye within 24 hours after treatment (AAO, 2007) (SOR: C).

Central Retinal Artery Occlusion

With an incidence of about 1 in 10,000 people, central retinal artery occlusion is generally not the result of trauma. Risk factors include atrial fibrillation, mitral valve disease, atherosclerosis, a hypercoagulable state, and hypertension. Additionally, prolonged intraorbital swelling can cause occlusion of the central retinal artery. Such situations occur particularly in patients who are having surgery in the face-down position. The characteristic fundus appearance with central retinal artery occlusion is narrow arterioles and a pale optic disc. In addition, there is diffuse retinal whitening. A cherry-red spot occurs only several hours after the initial retinal artery occlusion (Fig. 41-10).

Treatment of central retinal artery occlusion must be immediate, including breathing into a small paper bag to help increase the patient's carbon dioxide level. Emergency paracentesis is a rapid method to decompress the eye and may actually provide immediate restoration of vision. However, most physicians are reluctant to perform paracentesis on a patient within a few minutes. Ocular massage is another means of decompressing the eye. Some centers have hyperbaric oxygen available, which may also be helpful in restoring retinal perfusion for some patients. Treatment should be instituted within 90 minutes if any realistic hope of possible visual recovery can be expected. Patients with central retinal artery occlusion should be thoroughly evaluated for cardiac and carotid disease.

Urgent Situations

Urgent situations include those for which therapy should be instituted within minutes or a few hours. They include penetrating injuries of the globe, acute angle-closure glaucoma,

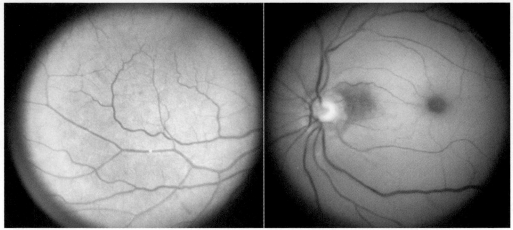

Figure 41-10 Central retinal artery occlusion of left eye with Hollenhorst plaque in right eye. Patient has a characteristic cherry-red spot involving the macula of left eye *(left)*. Hollenhorst plaque with a retinal arcade in right eye suggests bilateral carotid disease and cardiovascular disease *(right)*.

papillary block, orbital cellulitis, corneal ulcer, corneal foreign body, gonococcal conjunctivitis, ophthalmia neonatorum, and acute iritis. In addition, trauma with retinal tears, vitreous hemorrhage, retinal detachment, and hyphemas constitute urgent situations.

Ocular Foreign Body and Other Eye Injuries

The most common eye injury encountered in family practice is a foreign body in the eye. The most common causes of a foreign body in the conjunctival sac or one embedded in the cornea are particles blown in by the wind, occupational or work-related injuries, and metallic foreign bodies that may fly into the eye, such as after a person hits a metal object with a hammer. It is important to evaluate the location of the foreign body and, in the case of corneal foreign bodies, the depth of penetration. Symptoms may be helpful; superficial foreign bodies in the cornea generally present with the complaint of a dust particle in the eye. Foreign bodies that have penetrated deeper into the corneal stroma produce a dull, aching pain perceived in or behind the eye.

On examination, it is important to look carefully at the inflammatory response of the eye. A purely localized conjunctival inflammation pattern is generally associated with superficial foreign bodies. Ciliary injection is a warning sign that a deep penetration may have taken place, and an ophthalmologic consultation should be sought immediately. Examine the eye after the instillation of ophthalmic local anesthetic to avoid blepharospasm and evasive eye movements. Inspect the cornea with a penlight or ophthalmoscope in a darkened room. Use of the slit on the ophthalmoscope can help visualize irregularities in the corneal surface. Staining with fluorescein demonstrates abrasions and helps identify otherwise transparent foreign bodies.

The family physician may elect to remove a foreign body in the conjunctival sac by irrigation with a sterile solution or after eversion of the upper lid with a moistened cotton swab. In the case of superficial corneal foreign bodies, a physician may attempt to remove it with a moist sterile swab, but embedded foreign bodies should be referred to an ophthalmologist.

Corneal Abrasions

Corneal abrasions are often caused by foreign bodies underneath the upper lid or inadvertent injury from a finger or small object. Evert the lid and examine for conjunctival foreign bodies. To evert the lid, the patient is seated and asked to look downward. The upper lid is grasped by its central lashes and pulled downward and slightly outward. The examiner then depresses the upper lid with a cotton applicator proximal to the upper tarsus margin. Gentle pressure is maintained until the upper lid is flipped into the everted position. Frequently, the foreign body is observed and can be removed with a cotton applicator or forceps. Corneal abrasions generally can be treated with an antibiotic ointment. Small abrasions often do not require patching. Large corneal abrasions may require pressure patching or bandage contact lens.

If the conjunctival or corneal foreign body is not easily removed with a cotton applicator, the family physician should obtain ophthalmologic consultation. If the abrasion is not healed within 24 hours, an ophthalmic consultation should be obtained. Corneal abrasions should also be carefully inspected for other ocular injury. Any irregularity of the pupil in the presence of a corneal abrasion could signify an underlying occult penetrating injury. In such cases, the patient should be immediately directed to an ophthalmologist for further evaluation.

Contact Lens Overwear

Patients suffering from contact lens overwear syndrome have worn their lenses longer than usual and typically awaken during the early-morning hours with severe pain and tearing. In response to prolonged wear, the cornea becomes swollen and develops epithelial defects. Patients need reassurance that the condition is usually not serious, even though the pain is severe. However, occasional contact lens–induced corneal abrasions, especially those associated with soft lenses, can rapidly progress to severe corneal infection. Patients should be seen the next day and referred if they have not improved. Contact lens wear may be resumed only after the corneal epithelium is well healed.

Metallic Foreign Bodies

Metallic foreign bodies, if allowed to stay in the eye for a number of hours, frequently leave a "rust ring" that is clearly visible after removal of the foreign body. Rust rings irritate the cornea and result in long-lasting inflammatory changes in the eye. Follow-up should be daily, with staining of the cornea to demonstrate the expected rapid healing. If healing does not take place over 24 to 48 hours, suspect an infection in the corneal stroma and obtain consultation. Topical antibiotic ointments are used after removal of foreign bodies in an attempt to prevent this complication.

Corneal and Scleral Lacerations

Corneal and scleral lacerations fall within the realm of the ophthalmologist and should be referred immediately after a shield is placed over the eye. Frequently, signs of corneal and scleral lacerations include unequal pupils, decreased IOP, iris prolapse, and hyphema, and a corneal laceration often also involves the lens. It is important to consider posterior injuries to the globe, including retinal detachment, retinal tear, and vitreous hemorrhage (Fig. 41-11). Patients can often be managed as outpatients with oral antibiotics. Intravitreal antibiotics may be given at ruptured-globe repair. Some patients are hospitalized for IV antibiotics, although current intravitreal penetration of many antibiotics is often comparable. Corneoscleral lacerations should be principally repaired at the presenting institution when possible with available ophthalmology services. Hospital transfers delay wound closure or risk wound extension or prolapse of intraocular contents.

Blunt Eye Injuries

Blunt eye injuries are common and may result from relatively trivial injuries or high-velocity impact projectiles. An exact history of the trauma must be obtained to assess the velocity involved, which in turn may indicate the extent of ocular damage. Inquiry must be made to determine whether visual acuity changes occurred immediately after the injury. Flashing lights are often seen at the instant of injury and indicate irritation of the retina, because any message to the brain from the retina is perceived as light. Persistent blurred vision is indicative of a more serious injury. It may indicate blood in the anterior chamber that is suspended in the aqueous humor. Free-floating blood in the anterior chamber is generally not appreciated by direct ophthalmoscopy. A slit-lamp examination is necessary to observe the suspended red blood cells in the anterior chamber.

Black Eye (Eyelid Contusion)

A black eye may be serious or relatively minor. If accompanied by severe pain, bleeding, or constant blurred vision, more serious eye trauma must be considered. In such patients, orbital CT scan and ophthalmologic consultation may be necessary to rule out a ruptured globe.

Red Eye

Almost all ocular trauma cases include bleeding or dilation of blood vessels on the surface of the eye (subconjunctival hemorrhage). This may be observed with any degree of eye

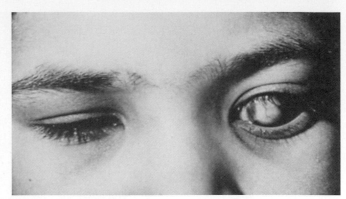

Figure 41-11 Corneal leukoma in 6-year-old boy. Diagnosis was ocular trauma and penetrating corneal laceration.

injury. For example, a subconjunctival hemorrhage may be spontaneous and often indicates minor injury. In the presence of other findings, a subconjunctival hemorrhage suggests more serious injury, particularly if a concomitant hyphema or vitreous hemorrhage is present.

Pupillary Change

Blunt trauma to the eye may result in lacerations of the sphincter muscle of the pupil. These are manifested by traumatic mydriasis. Unlike the unequal pupils seen with congenital anisocoria, traumatic mydriasis is characterized by recent onset of unequal pupils and by the irregularity of the dilated pupil. Although traumatic mydriasis by itself is not harmful, it suggests severe blunt trauma and is an indication for a careful assessment of other ocular structures, including the vitreous and retinal periphery.

Traumatic Hyphema

Blunt trauma to the eye may cause injury to the iris, angle structures, and other intraocular structures. Hemorrhage into the anterior chamber, or *hyphema,* is most often found in children. The agent producing the hyphema is usually a projectile that strikes the exposed portion of the eye. A great variety of missiles and objects may be responsible, including balls, rocks, projectile toys, air gun, paint balls, bungee cords, and the human fist. With the increase of child abuse, fists and belts have started to play a prominent role. Boys are involved in 75% of cases.

Rarely, spontaneous hyphemas occur and may be confused with traumatic hyphemas. *Spontaneous* hyphemas are secondary to neovascularization, ocular neoplasms (retinoblastoma), and vascular anomalies (juvenile xanthogranuloma). Vascular tufts that exist at the pupillary border have been implicated in spontaneous hyphema. A *traumatic* hyphema may be graded by measuring the height of the layered hyphema in the anterior chamber in millimeters. A hyphema is an ocular emergency and should be referred immediately.

Cataract, choroidal rupture, vitreous hemorrhage, angle recession glaucoma, and retinal detachment are often associated with traumatic hyphema and compromise the final visual acuity prognosis. It is important to recognize that the prognosis for visual recovery from traumatic hyphema is directly related to three factors: (1) amount of associated damage to other ocular structures (e.g., choroidal rupture or macular scarring), (2) presence or absence of secondary hemorrhage, and (3) presence or absence of complications of glaucoma, corneal blood staining, or optic atrophy. With treatment, most hyphema patients have a good visual outcome. (See the discussion of hyphema grading and complications, as well as treatment and prognosis, online at www.expertconsult.com.)

KEY TREATMENT

Hyphemas are generally well managed with bed rest, shielding of the injured eye, and medical control of the hyphema and intraocular pressure (Crouch et al., 2009) (SOR: A).

If IOP remains elevated or hyphema occupies more than 50% of the anterior chamber, surgical evacuation of the clot may be required to lower IOP, preserve corneal clarity, and reduce optic atrophy (Sheppard et al., 2009) (SOR: A).

Nonaccidental Inflicted Neurotrauma (Formerly "Shaken Baby Syndrome")

The true incidence of nonaccidental inflicted neurotrauma is unknown because of the difficulty collecting statistical data. An estimated 1300 children in the United States experience fatal head trauma from child abuse annually (JAMA, 2003). The findings of nonaccidental inflicted neurotrauma involve repetitive, violent, unrestrained, acceleration-deceleration, head and neck movements. Neurotrauma can occur without blunt head trauma. Cases primarily occur in children under 3 years old, usually during the first year of life. Typically, patients present with fracture and intracranial or intraocular hemorrhages; not all findings are required to establish the diagnosis. An ophthalmologic consult should be obtained for all patients with suspected nonaccidental inflicted neurotrauma, with carefully documented retinal drawings or preferably fundus photography. Approximately 20% of cases are fatal within the first few days of presentation. Traumatic *retinoschisis*, if present, is highly specific for nonaccidental inflicted neurotrauma, particularly if the child is younger than 5 years.

Retinal Detachment

An increase in previous floaters or the onset of new floaters may occur in a retinal detachment. Traumatic detachment of the retina can be observed after blunt eye injury, especially in older adults. Retinal detachment may also occur spontaneously, especially in patients with high myopia. The patient may complain of reduced overall brightness in the involved eye or may have continuous light flashes, indicating retinal traction. After eye trauma, it is imperative to inspect not only the central portions of the retina, but the peripheral portions as well. This examination should be performed in a darkened room after instillation of a short-acting mydriatic agent. Any questionable findings should be referred to an ophthalmologist immediately.

Other serious injuries are traumatic tears of the iris, subluxation or dislocation of the lens that occasionally displaces into the anterior chamber, and blowout fracture of the orbit, with impaired upward eye movement caused by entrapment of the inferior rectus muscle. These injuries are usually readily identified.

Pediatric Ophthalmology

Key Points

- Children should be screened at birth, birth to 3 months, 3 to 6 months, 6 to 12 months, 3 years, 5 years, and then every 1 to 2 years.
- Amblyopia and strabismus are distinct but may be associated. Children can have amblyopia without having strabismus. All children with amblyopia or strabismus should be referred to a pediatric ophthalmologist.
- Cataracts are an important cause of amblyopia in children and require prompt intervention.
- Pediatric cataracts may be a sign of a metabolic disorder, TORCH infection (*toxoplasmosis, other agents, rubella, cytomegalovirus, herpes simplex*), or chromosomal abnormality.
- Leukocoria warrants further investigation; significant causes include cataracts, *Toxocara canis* infection, retinal disease, and retinoblastoma.

Evaluation of Vision within First 4 Months of Life

Parents may report that their baby does not appear to look at them. This statement requires the physician to document a history of prematurity, fetal distress, anoxia, or birth trauma carefully. A failure to reach developmental milestones may indicate neurologic abnormalities. A history of seizure disorder, cerebral palsy, or chromosomal abnormalities helps identify potentially serious causes. In this case, visual acuity or the child's ability to fixate must be assessed. Normal newborns follow faces. By age 2 or 3 months, infants normally follow light and high-contrast objects. Assessment of vision can be achieved by using an optokinetic nystagmus drum. Oculomotor disturbances may be the underlying cause of the child's apparent visual inattention. Bilateral cranial nerve III palsy, congenital fibrosis syndrome, or partial cranial nerve III palsy may give this impression as well.

Searching or roving eye movements are a form of profound nystagmus, with little foveal perception. Nystagmus is an important sign of decreased vision, indicating visual acuity often in the range of 20/200. The onset is usually at birth or shortly thereafter. The nystagmus can be a jerk or pendular nystagmus. The direction should be characterized as horizontal, vertical, or rotary.

Abnormalities of the anterior portion of the eye can cause profound visual loss and are easily visible with a +10 magnification. They include corneal opacities (leucoma) caused by congenital glaucoma, *Peter's anomaly* (abnormal cornea and lens), and *leukocoria* (white pupil) related to congenital cataracts, inflammatory disease, or retinal disease.

Evaluation of the posterior aspect of the eye, including examination of the red reflexes, may indicate an early retinal detachment or retinoblastoma. Optic nerve abnormalities may be associated with midline CNS defects, such as an absent septum pellucidum, agenesis of the corpus callosum, or hypopituitarism. Optic nerve abnormalities such as optic nerve hypoplasia are associated with nystagmus. CT or magnetic resonance imaging (MRI) can identify these abnormalities. Electroretinography (ERG) may be helpful for determining the cause of decreased visual acuity. An abnormal ERG is seen with Leber's congenital amaurosis, congenital achromatopsia, and congenital stationary night blindness. Visual-evoked potential testing may be necessary to determine whether vision is intact.

Some infants who have a completely normal eye examination but demonstrate poor fixation may actually have a delay in maturation of the visual system. Normally, the initial visual system development matures by 4 to 6 months of age. Visual-evoked potential acuities are about 20/400 during the first few days of life and improve to about 20/40 by 6 months of age. In some patients, visual-evoked responses and clinically assessed visual function may be abnormal, only to improve between 4 and 12 months of age. Although incompletely defined, in delayed visual maturation the vision is decreased, but the ocular examination appears normal, including brisk pupillary response to light. Typically, there is no nystagmus, and ERG is normal.

Vision Screening and Ocular Examination

Appropriate vision screening is one of the most important factors in pediatric eye care. Because focused visual stimuli are critical to normal development, early detection and correction of visual problems reduce serious vision impairment or blindness. The American Academy of Ophthalmology (AAO), American Academy of Pediatrics (AAP), and American Association of Pediatric Ophthalmology and Strabismus (AAPOS) strongly support the goal of early detection and treatment of eye problems in children. In particular, vision screening is needed to detect four major conditions: strabismus, amblyopia, ocular disease, and refractive errors. Family physicians are ideal vision screeners because of their ability to detect abnormalities at an early age. Essential components of vision screening are age, testing format, testing procedures, efficacy, and referral criteria. On a practical level, vision screening must be cost-effective and time-efficient. The testing devices must be readily available and relatively easy to use. High sensitivity is essential to keep overreferrals and underreferrals to a minimum.

Four Stages of Screening

The AAO and AAPOS recommend that children be examined for eye problems in the following four stages (Table 41-4):

1. In the newborn nursery, physicians should examine all infants. Ophthalmologists should be consulted to examine patients at high risk for conditions such as retinopathy of prematurity (ROP), cataracts, congenital defects, and other ocular pathology.
2. At 6 months
3. At 3 years
4. At 5 years and older

The AAO statement recommends that family physicians establish a close working relationship with a local ophthalmologist who is familiar with children's eye problems. The collaboration can help clarify questions about vision screening and the need for referral. (See online content for specific information on different stages of vision screening.)

Also, special groups may need additional vision screening. The following children should also be screened, even if they are not due to be examined by their age: all children

Table 41-4 Recommended Vision Screening by Family Physicians

Age	Examination	Referral Criteria
Newborn	Penlight examination of cornea Rule out nystagmus Red reflexes	Any ocular pathology Nystagmus Abnormal red reflexes or white reflex
6 months	Fixation to light and small toys Penlight examination Corneal light reflex test, cover test Red reflexes	Object to occlusion Nystagmus; any ocular pathology Strabismus Abnormal red reflexes or white reflex
3 years	Visual acuity: Snellen letters, tumbling E, or HOTV wall chart Corneal light reflex test, cover test Fundus examination	Acuity of 20/40 or less in one or both eyes Strabismus Any ocular pathology
≥5 years	Visual acuity: Snellen letter, tumbling E, or HOTV (see online text) Corneal light reflex test, cover test Fundus examination	Acuity of 20/30 or less in one or both eyes Strabismus Any ocular pathology

at high risk of having vision disorders, including those who are mentally retarded or who have trisomy 21 or cerebral palsy; and all children who show signs or symptoms of visual problems, experience school failure, or have reading difficulties or other learning problems (e.g., dyslexia). It is important to note that children with learning disabilities such as dyslexia have the same incidence of ocular abnormalities (strabismus, refractive error) as children without such disabilities. Dyslexia involves interpretation by cortical processing centers and does not generally indicate any ocular pathology. Eye defects do not cause letter, number, or word reversal.

Testing Visual Acuity

Several diagnostic tests are used to detect strabismus, amblyopia, ocular disease, and refractive errors. These include visual acuity and fixation preference tests, corneal light reflex test, cover test, simultaneous red reflexes test, fundus examination, stereoscopic tests, and photorefractive techniques.

The best way to screen for possible visual loss caused by amblyopia is to measure the visual acuity or fixation preference of each eye separately. The covered eye should be firmly occluded during the assessment to avoid any peeking. When there is no apparent sign of amblyopia, the only clue to poor vision may be the child's objection to having the better eye occluded. Additionally, the child may demonstrate a fixation preference of the better-seeing eye, with an inability to fixate on distance objects in the amblyopic eye. Both are common signs of amblyopia that may be caused by a refractive error, media opacities, retinal or optic nerve abnormality, or cortical processing problem.

Equipment required for testing children older than 42 months consists of standard wall charts containing Snellen letters, Snellen numbers, tumbling Es, and HOTV monitors, as well as some means of occluding the nontested eye, ideally, occluder patches (Opticlude, Coverlet).

Stereoscopic and Photorefractive Tests

The visual acuity test is the most widely used vision screening test, but use of this test alone will underrefer many patients with amblyopia and undiagnosed strabismus. Stereoscopic tests such as the random dot E stereogram are relatively inexpensive, fairly accurate, and easy to use. Stereopsis tests are complementary and offer additional information regarding a patient's visual health.

The use of photorefractive apparatus is relatively new. Reproducible results of photography of the red reflex can screen the nonverbal infant or child. The sensitivity is high (95%) for refractive error in the range of 1.00 to 2.00 diopters. A problem with this technique is that cycloplegia is usually required to prevent obtaining false-positive results, especially for myopia. In addition, two photographs are needed to avoid missing an astigmatic refractive error. The technology offers great promise, but it must be cost-effective. As newer, more rapid and accurate vision tests are developed, these may be incorporated into the screening process.

Strabismus and Amblyopia

Strabismus and amblyopia are two of the most common visual problems affecting children. Strabismus occurs in 4% and amblyopia in 4% of the population. Half of all amblyopia patients have a concomitant strabismus. Conversely, half of all amblyopia patients will have no demonstrable strabismus.

Movements of the eyes horizontally and vertically are controlled by the six muscles attached to the sclera of each eye. Movement of both eyes in unison allows vision of singular images. Through a blending process called *fusion,* the brain combines the two images into a single, three-dimensional image. As long as the eye muscles are able to work together, the brain can process incoming visual information. When the eye muscles are not coordinated, one eye deviates inward, outward, or upward, and the other eye remains straight. When this occurs, the brain receives a different image from each eye and cannot combine the two disparate images into a single image frame.

Misalignment of the eye muscles results in strabismus. In addition to a breakdown or absence of fusion, the causes of strabismus may include refractive errors, anatomic anomalies, and abnormal tonic innervation. Adults with acquired strabismus frequently develop double vision, but children with strabismus quickly learn to ignore or suppress the image seen by the deviated eye. As a result of suppression, the straight eye takes over most of the work of seeing, and the crossed eye develops reduced central vision because of lack of use. There are various types of strabismus and may be horizontal, vertical, or rotational (cyclotorsional). (See online text for additional information on specific types of strabismus.)

Loss of vision in a relatively normal eye is called *amblyopia.* The phrase "lazy eye" should not be used in diagnosing patients because it can be confused with amblyopia and strabismus. As mentioned earlier, these two distinct clinical entities

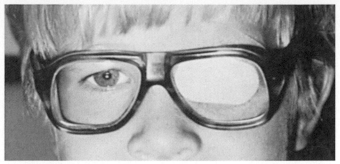

Figure 41-12 Amblyopia. This 5-year-old patient also required patching of the better-seeing eye to improve vision in the amblyopic eye.

are associated with each other in only 50% of cases. In children younger than 4 years, amblyopia is the most frequent cause of unilateral vision loss (Fig. 41-12). The condition is usually unilateral, although bilateral high myopia, hyperopia, or astigmatism may occur. Unless treatment begins early, loss of vision in the affected eye may be permanent. Amblyopia is usually treatable if detected at age 3 to 4 years but is generally considered irreversible after 13 years; however, treating amblyopia in patients older than 13 years has had some success. The earlier treatment begins, the better the prognosis for the patient. The primary treatment of amblyopia includes the use of patches, glasses, or both. The better eye is occluded, and underlying conditions such as cataracts or refractive errors are treated.

Testing for Strabismus

The corneal light reflex test, cover test, red reflex, and extraocular rotations are four basic tests for strabismus. To perform the corneal light test, project a penlight onto the cornea of both eyes simultaneously while the child looks straight ahead. Compare the placement of the two corneal reflections. When the eyes are straight, the light appears at the same point on each cornea. If a muscle deviation is present, the reflected light appears slightly off center in one eye. Figure 41-13 illustrates the placement of corneal reflections as they would appear for each direction of deviation. In part *A,* note that the light is centered on the cornea of the left eye but is displaced laterally, or outward, on the right cornea, indicating that the right eye is turned inward, or is *esotropic.* In *B,* note that the light is centered again on the left cornea but is displaced medially, or inward, on the right cornea, demonstrating an outward-turning, *exotropia* of the right eye. In part *C* the light indicates that the right eye is turned upward, or is *hypertropic,* and the left eye is straight.

The cover test is performed by having the child look straight ahead at an object 20 feet away (Fig. 41-14). An eye chart is usually used to test children older than 3 years. For younger children, it is helpful to use a colorful, moving object or toy. As the child looks at the target, cover the child's right eye and look for movement of the uncovered eye. If the left eye moves to pick up fixation, it was deviated before placing the cover over the right eye. Repeat the procedure for the left eye, and watch for any movement in the uncovered right eye. If the eye moves inward to pick up fixation, the eye is exotropic. If the eye moves outward to pick up fixation, the eye is esotropic.

The third test involves simultaneous examination of the pupillary red reflexes. This is a useful test to assess ocular

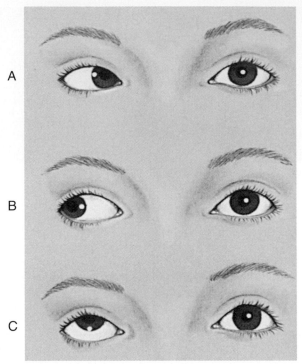

Figure 41-13 Strabismus of right esotropia **(A),** right exotropia **(B),** and right hypertropia **(C).** *(From American Academy of Ophthalmology. The Child's Eye: Strabismus and Amblyopia. American Academy of Ophthalmology, Professional Information Committee, San Francisco, 1982 [AAO. The Child's Eye].)*

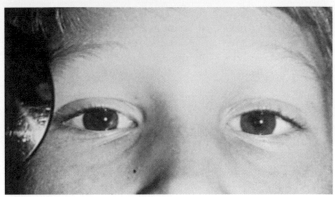

Figure 41-14 Cover-uncover test. Evaluate the unoccluded eye for strabismus. *(From AAO. The Child's Eye.)*

alignment and rule out abnormal ocular media, such as cataracts. The test should be performed in a darkened room with the examiner approximately 18 to 24 inches from the patient. Both red reflexes should be simultaneously assessed and compared using the direct ophthalmoscope. If an abnormality exists in the ocular media, the red reflex will be asymmetric or a white reflex may be present. An abnormal reflex may also signify a high refractive error or a small strabismus. The red reflexes should be equal and symmetric. Ophthalmoscopy also permits direct visualization of the fundus and optic disc. The fourth test checks the extraocular movements in the cardinal positions of gaze (Fig. 41-15). The results of these tests provide a good basis for determining whether there is any misalignment present. This is an important screening for all family physicians to learn, because early intervention can help improve the overall visual and binocular status of the patient.

Table 41-5 lists several forms of strabismus. For congenital esotropia, surgery is the primary treatment for this condition and is performed between 6 and 12 months of age (Fig. 41-16). Esotropia may also be related to refractive error and managed with spectacle correction (Figs. 41-17 and 41-18). Large deviations of exotropia and hypertropia are also managed surgically (Figs. 41-19 to 41-23). (See online text for further discussion.)

Pseudostrabismus

A common misconception is that children with cross-eye (esotropia) outgrow the condition, but this is generally not the case. This belief stems from confusion between true strabismus and what is known as pseudostrabismus, or false strabismus.

A child with pseudostrabismus has broad folds of skin that partially cover the top of each eye and a flat nasal bridge that creates the illusion of crossed eyes. As the child ages and the skin fold becomes less apparent, the condition becomes less noticeable. When a child's eyes are truly crossed, it is always a serious condition and requires the care of an ophthalmologist.

Other Causes of Strabismus

Acute strabismus may be brought on by a viral upper respiratory tract infection, which can cause acute cranial nerve VI palsy. With the advent of antibiotics, middle ear infections with associated petrositis and cranial nerve VI palsies are relatively uncommon. Sudden-onset strabismus may also indicate underlying neurologic disease. Another cause is spasm of the near reflex. A hallmark of spasm of convergence is a constricted pupil. Paralytic or mechanical causes of strabismus occur with trauma and Duane's syndrome. In addition, neurologic trauma accounts for paralysis to cranial nerves III, IV, and VI (Fig. 41-24).

The proper corrective treatment for strabismus includes nonsurgical treatment, such as patching and glasses, and surgical treatment, when indicated. Eye muscle surgery is performed when nonsurgical methods cannot correct the misalignment, as well as with worsening misalignment, no effect on the deviation or stereopsis, or progressive loss of fusion. Four aspects of strabismus surgery should also be stressed, as follows:

1. The surgery is safe and effective.
2. The eyeball is never removed from the orbit to perform the surgery.
3. More than one procedure may be required to establish alignment.
4. Both eyes may require surgery to correct the strabismus.

The goals when treating strabismus include the ability to provide and maintain equal vision in both eyes, enable the eye to work together rather than independently, and improve depth perception, whenever possible.

KEY TREATMENT

Surgical and nonsurgical treatment of strabismus is beneficial to appropriate visual development, reduction of amblyopia, and rehabilitation of sensorimotor function or depth perception (AAO, 2007) (SOR: A).

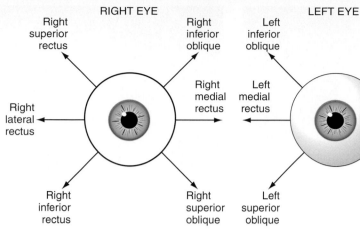

RIGHT EYE

Right superior rectus

Right inferior oblique

Right medial rectus

Right lateral rectus

Right inferior rectus

Right superior oblique

LEFT EYE

Left inferior oblique

Left superior rectus

Left medial rectus

Left lateral rectus

Left superior oblique

Left inferior rectus

Figure 41-15 Ocular muscle movement in cardinal fields of gaze.

Table 41-5 Classification of Strabismus

Type	Cases (%)	Age of Onset
Congenital or infantile esotropia	20	Birth to 6 mo
Accommodative esotropia	45-50	6 mo to 7 yr (usually 2 yr)
Nonaccommodative (acquired) esotropia	10	Variable, depending on cause
Exotropia	20	Variable (usually during infancy to 4 yr)
Hypertropia	<5	Variable, depending on cause

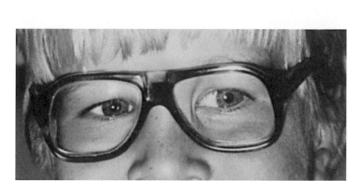

Figure 41-17 Accommodative esotropia and anisometropic amblyopia in 5-year-old patient who has unequal refractive errors between the two eyes as well as accommodative esotropia.

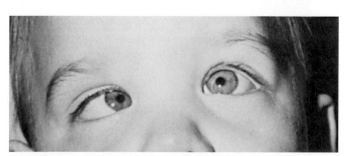

Figure 41-16 Clinical esotropia in 12-month-old infant. With the right eye fixing, there is a left esotropia.

Refractive Errors and Color Vision

Some eyes are either too long or too short and need help focusing light onto the retina. If an eye is too long, the light rays focus in front of the retina and the image is blurred; the person can move things closer to see better or can wear glasses. This condition is called nearsightedness *(myopia)*. With farsightedness *(hyperopia)*, the light focuses behind the retina because the eye is too short and causes a blurred image. Both conditions are corrected by glasses or contact lenses. *Astigmatism*, another common error in the eye's focusing abilities, is caused by unequal curvature of the front surface of the cornea. Corrective glasses are necessary if it

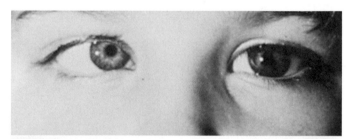

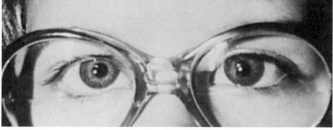

Figure 41-18 Accommodative esotropia in 3-year-old patient uncorrected *(top)* and corrected by hyperopic (farsighted) glasses *(bottom)*. *(From AAO. The Child's Eye.)*

causes blurred vision or discomfort. Unless there is a marked amount of myopia (nearsightedness), hyperopia (farsightedness), or astigmatism, or a significant refractive difference between the eyes, eyeglasses can adequately compensate for these problems. Refractive errors requiring eyeglasses affect almost 20% of the pediatric population before full growth is attained.

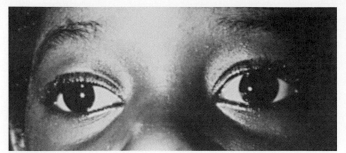

Figure 41-19 Exotropia in 8-year-old patient with right exotropia.

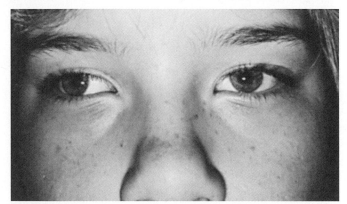

Figure 41-20 Positive angle kappa, which appears similar to exotropia, in 8-year-old patient. Actually, this patient has retinopathy of prematurity, with bilateral dragged maculas.

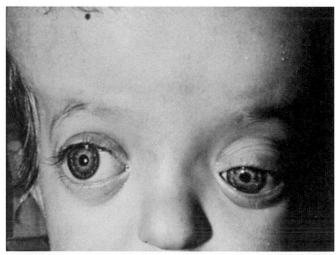

Figure 41-21 Patient with diagnosis of Crouzon's syndrome presented with proptosis, amblyopia, and left exotropia.

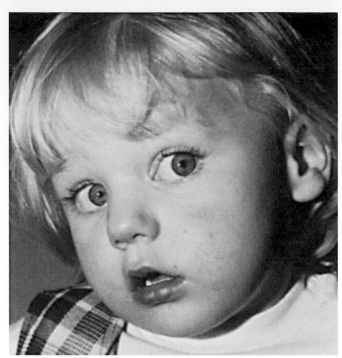

Figure 41-22 Positive head tilt in 4-year-old child could indicate a vertical deviation, especially superior oblique palsy. *(From AAO. The Child's Eye.)*

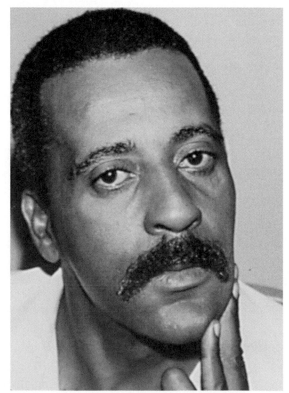

Figure 41-23 Ocular torticollis in 34-year-old patient. Note the abnormal head tilt.

Color vision defects rarely result in significant visual difficulties. About 8% of white males have some red-green color deficiency, whereas less than 1% of females are affected. In isolation, this defect rarely results in any real drawback to normal function, especially during childhood. Although the identification of such defects can be helpful in a classroom situation, emphasis should not be placed on these minor abnormalities at this age. Color vision testing is not required unless a retinal dystrophy or optic nerve disease is suspected, the family history is positive, or the family specifically requests it.

Headaches

Headache is one of the most common conditions of humans, and children seem to complain less about headaches than adults. Most headaches are not serious and frequently are caused by tension. Many people believe incorrectly that eye

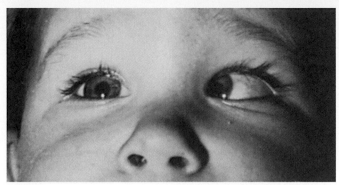

Figure 41-24 Chief presenting complaint of underaction of the left lateral rectus muscle and left esotropia after upper respiratory infection in 14-month-old patient, who actually had cranial nerve VI palsy related to the viral syndrome.

strain and the need for glasses are common causes of headaches, although this is certainly possible. Headaches caused by eye disease are usually felt in the eye or in the brow on the same side as the involved eye. Frequently, these headaches are associated with some other symptom, such as blurred vision, halos around lights, or extreme sensitivity to light. Most headaches are related to stress.

Learning Disabilities and the Eye

Although reading may be easier and faster when sight is clear, visual problems generally do not cause learning disabilities, and eye defects are not responsible for reversal of letters. In the past, reading problems were blamed on the eyes, although children with a learning disability have no greater incidence of eye problems than the rest of the population. Other issues, such as dyslexia, attention-deficit hyperactivity disorder, social issues, or family problems are often found to be contributing to a child's poor attention in class or learning difficulties.

It is important that a thorough medical eye examination be performed. The presence or absence of visual defects can be diagnosed and corrected. Once vision is corrected, no other examinations or therapies involving the eyes diminish a learning disability. Meta-analysis shows that children with learning disabilities do not benefit from visual training, muscle exercises, perceptual training, or hand-eye coordination exercises (AAO/AAP/AAPOS Policy Statement, 2009). It may be difficult to diagnose a learning disability definitively before a child is 6 to 7 years old. However, once a diagnosis is made, educational assistance is needed promptly.

Pediatric Cataracts

Approximately 40% of acquired pediatric cataracts are secondary to trauma, and as many as approximately one third of pediatric cataracts are inherited. The basic approach to the patient with pediatric cataracts is to determine whether the cataract is an isolated finding, part of a systemic abnormality, or associated with ocular disease. When several members of the same family are affected by congenital cataracts, a hereditary origin may be assumed. Autosomal dominant hereditary patterns are the most frequent mode of transmission.

X-linked cataracts are rare and occur primarily with the oculocerebrorenal syndrome. Congenital or infantile cataracts have been described in association with a large number of congenital anomalies. (See online content for additional information on pediatric cataract differential.)

History and Ocular Examination

In patients with pediatric cataracts, the physician should determine the age when the cataract or decreased vision occurred. A detailed history of maternal intrauterine infections should include rubella, toxoplasmosis, herpes simplex, cytomegalovirus, and varicella. Drug and medication use during pregnancy and birth trauma should be ruled out.

A complete ocular examination should be performed, including visual acuity assessment using fixation and following responses. Infants with complete bilateral congenital cataracts usually demonstrate decreased visual interest and may have delayed development. Nystagmus results from early visual deprivation and is an ominous sign of poor vision. Ocular fixation and following movements may be decreased or absent. In some cases, strabismus is a presenting sign, especially in children with monocular cataracts.

Glaucoma and other ocular disorders must be ruled out. Examination of the red reflexes by retinoscopy can reveal even minute lens opacities. Direct ophthalmoscopy or retinoscopy through the child's nondilated pupil is helpful for estimating potential vision in an eye harboring a cataract. Any central opacity or surrounding cortical distortion larger than 3 mm can be visually significant. Generally, the more posterior lens opacity carries more visual significance. The presence of retinal detachment, retinoblastoma, or other ocular pathologies that preclude good visual outcome must be ruled out by indirect ophthalmoscopy or ultrasonography.

Most *anterior polar cataracts* are small, less than 1 to 2 mm, and are usually not progressive. Surgery is seldom required for small, anterior polar cataracts, and the visual prognosis is excellent. If the cataracts increase in size, visual acuity may be compromised and may require surgical intervention.

Nuclear cataracts are typically congenital, dense axial opacities 3 mm or larger. Nuclear cataracts are frequently associated with microphthalmos and are inherited as autosomal dominant traits. Visual results are generally only fair, even if surgery is done early, and poor if done late. Aphakic glaucoma has a much higher incidence in these patients. *Rubella cataracts* may occur as a manifestation of the classic rubella syndrome—the triad of cardiac defects, hearing impairment, and cataracts.

Partial Lens Opacities

The evaluation of partial lens opacities is related to the location of the cataract. *Anterior cataracts* include anterior lenticonus, polar cataracts, persistent pupillary membrane opacities, and those occurring with anterior segment dysgenesis. *Posterior cataracts* include posterior polar, posterior lenticonus, persistent hyperplastic primary vitreous, and posterior subcapsular lens opacities. Posterior subcapsular cataracts are typically associated with corticosteroid use, atopic dermatitis, or inflammatory diseases and are generally bilateral.

Traumatic and Posterior Lenticonus

Traumatic cataract, the most common cause of unilateral cataract in children, is caused by penetrating or blunt trauma. Posterior lenticonus cataracts are the second most common cause of unilateral acquired cataract in children. *Posterior lenticonus* is a circumscribed oval or round bulge in the infant's or child's posterior lens capsule and cortex, restricted generally to a 2 × 7–mm axial diameter. The bulge increases progressively, and cataractous changes occur in the cortex surrounding the posterior lenticonus. Generally, there is a reduced red reflex initially with posterior lenticonus, and cataractous changes occur in the surrounding cortex. In 21 patients with posterior lenticonus, only two had bilateral posterior lenticonus. The interval between the "oil droplet" posterior lenticonus and cataract development is variable. The eyes are normal in size, and visual results are good with surgery. Posterior lenticonus cataracts occur as early as 3 months of age or as late as 15 years. If the vision becomes worse than 20/70, the cataract should be removed by specialized instrumentation, followed by contact lens fitting or an intraocular lens.

Complete Lens Opacities

Workup for complete cataracts includes systemic evaluation, ocular ultrasonography, metabolic evaluation, serum chemistry, and chromosomal analysis. Congenital cataract causes include intrauterine infection, metabolic disorders, chromosomal anomalies, and systemic syndromes. Workup for congenital cataracts includes urinalysis for reducing substances and amino acids. Serum chemistry for calcium, phosphorus, glucose, and blood urea nitrogen (BUN) levels and TORCH (*t*oxoplasmosis, *o*ther agents, *r*ubella, *c*ytomegalovirus, *h*erpes simplex) titers should be obtained. When warranted, genetic and pediatric consultations should be requested. Radiologic imaging, including CT or MRI, may be needed.

Surgical Issues

Prompt clearing of the visual axis with immediate optical correction offers the best chance for visual recovery in pediatric patients with unilateral or bilateral cataracts. The surgical procedure recommended depends on the patient's age, risk of amblyopia and expected ocular growth, and reactivity to surgery. In patients younger than 6 months to 2 years old, the best option is to clear the visual axis and have it remain clear throughout the critical period of vision development with a lensectomy-vitrectomy procedure and 6-mm posterior capsulectomy with anterior vitrectomy. This procedure eliminates reopacification of the posterior capsule, which occurs in more than 90% of pediatric patients younger than 2 years. In children older than 2 years, lensectomy with vitrectomy and a 4-mm posterior capsulectomy are performed. Most of these children can be fitted with contact lenses, although an intraocular lens is indicated for some traumatic cataract patients. Traumatic unilateral cataracts present the least controversial situation in which intraocular lenses are considered in young children. Advances in intraocular lenses and surgical techniques have afforded significant improvements in pediatric cataract management.

The prognosis for children with monocular and binocular congenital and pediatric cataracts has improved markedly. Ongoing clinical studies will determine the best indications and procedures for use in pediatric cataract patients.

KEY TREATMENT

The decision for cataract surgery with intraocular lens implantation depends on the degree of vision loss and potential for amblyopia. Among newborns and infants with cataracts, visually significant cataracts should be removed and corrected with intraocular lens, aphakic contact lens, or aphakic spectacles (AAPOS, 2007) (SOR: C).

The decision for cataract surgery with intraocular lens implantation in older children depends on the degree of vision loss, comorbidities, and systemic disease (AAPOS, 2007) (SOR: C).

Retinoblastoma

Retinoblastoma is the second most common primary intraocular malignancy in all age groups (melanoma is most common in adults) and is the most common intraocular malignancy of childhood. Its incidence is approximately 1 in every 14,000 births. Generally, there are 250 to 300 new cases in the United States annually.

The tumor occurs bilaterally in as many as 40% of cases. It is generally diagnosed between 14 and 18 months of age, and more than 90% of the tumors are diagnosed by the age of 3 years. Familial retinoblastoma accounts for 6% of patients, but 15% of unilateral cases are carriers for the retinoblastoma gene. The remaining 94% of cases are sporadic. Germinal mutations account for 25% of retinoblastoma cases and somatic mutations for 75%. Most bilateral cases are caused by germinal mutations. The disease is inherited through an autosomal recessive tumor suppressor gene; thus the phenotype appears similar to that of autosomal dominant inheritance with incomplete penetrance. It is difficult, if not impossible, to differentiate the genetic mutations clinically and to determine which tumors will be passed on to offspring. There are occasional rare cases of retinoblastoma related to chromosomal abnormalities (partial deletion of long arm of chromosome 13). It has also been associated with trisomy 21.

The diagnosis of retinoblastoma is made by the patient presenting with a white pupil (leukocoria) in 61% of cases, strabismus in 22% of cases, and sometimes with a retinal detachment, red painful eye, or spontaneous hyphema (Fig. 41-25). Generally, patients with small retinoblastomas have problems with vision or strabismus. More advanced lesions present with leukocoria and occasionally secondary glaucoma. The advanced lesions may metastasize to the orbit and produce proptosis through the orbital spread. In addition, patients with retinoblastoma may have systemic metastases to the CNS, skull bones, lymph nodes, and other organs.

The treatment of retinoblastoma is generally enucleation for patients with advanced retinoblastoma involving more than 50% of the eye. If the second eye is involved, treatment depends on the size of tumor and whether there is extraocular extension. External beam irradiation treatment may be performed on the second eye or bilaterally, when necessary. Photocoagulation and cryotherapy are equally effective for small retinoblastomas confined to the retinal periphery. Newer modalities are incorporating chemoreduction and radioactive plaque therapy for localized retinoblastoma and possible vision preservation. Systemic chemotherapy may be indicated after enucleation for advanced unilateral or bilateral cases.

KEY TREATMENT

Patients with retinoblastoma should receive long-term follow-up for evaluation of associated systemic cancers (Children's Oncology Group, 2006) (SOR: C).
Surgery for retinoblastoma requires specialist services and should be referred to supraregional centers when possible (National Collaborating Centre for Cancer, 2005) (SOR: C)

Adult Ophthalmology

Key Points

- Refractive errors in adults may be corrected with glasses or contact lens or more recent advanced techniques in refractive surgery. Risks and benefits associated with each option vary considerably.

- Patients with an acquired unilateral ptosis should be evaluated for Horner's syndrome, myasthenia gravis, and cranial nerve III palsy.

- Patients with recurrent anterior uveitis should be evaluated for ankylosing spondylitis, inflammatory bowel disease, sarcoidosis, juvenile rheumatoid arthritis, Reiter's syndrome, herpetic keratitis, and Lyme disease. Patients should be seen by an ophthalmologist for further evaluation.

- Common causes of posterior uveitis include toxoplasmosis, sarcoidosis, cytomegalovirus, Epstein-Barr virus, Behçet's disease, and *Bartonella* infection.

- Ocular medications, particularly antiglaucoma medications, are well known for having a variety of systemic side effects. Medications such as β-blockers may have implications for patients with heart or lung disease.

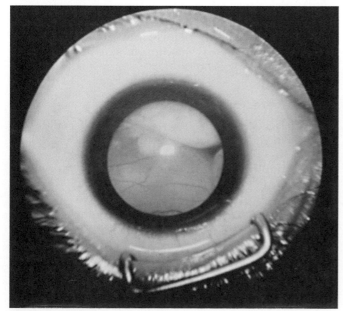

Figure 41-25 Total retinal detachment and advanced retinoblastoma in 23-month-old infant who presented with leukokoria (white reflex).

Correction of Refractive Errors

Contact Lenses

A major use of contact lenses is to correct myopia, aphakia, and astigmatism. It is critical to have a well-motivated patient who will wear contacts successfully. The many types of contact lenses mainly fall into four groups: (1) daily-wear hard lenses, (2) daily-wear soft lenses, (3) rigid, gas-permeable lenses, and (4) extended-wear soft lenses. Hard lenses have generally been constructed of polymethyl methacrylate. The material absorbs less fluid than soft contact lenses. Soft contacts may become 80% or more hydrated. New materials for hard and soft lenses continue to be developed. Complications of contact lenses, particularly extended-wear contacts, include infection, ocular allergies, follicular conjunctivitis, contact lens opacification, corneal edema, and corneal vascularization. Therefore, patients wearing contacts and complaining of red eyes require urgent evaluation.

Refractive Surgery

The latest treatment option for myopia, hyperopia, and astigmatism is laser refractive surgery with the excimer laser. Photorefractive keratectomy (PRK) and laser-assisted in situ keratomileusis (LASIK) use the excimer laser to remove corneal tissue to flatten the cornea or make it steeper. In the PRK procedure, the laser cuts through the surface cornea. Myopia of −1.00 to −10.00 diopters can be successfully corrected with PRK. This procedure does not involve a corneal flap, unlike LASIK, and has good visual recovery response. However, it is more painful than LASIK. The LASIK procedure is performed under a corneal flap. A 6-mm zone is cut with a microkeratome and the laser treatment directed to the exposed stromal tissue. LASIK is the preferred procedure for more than 6 to 8 diopters of myopia; its benefits are greater accuracy with the laser, reduced postoperative complications, quicker recovery of vision, and predictable healing. Some studies have suggested that LASIK has a slightly higher retreatment rate.

Hyperopia and astigmatism can now also be corrected with laser refractive surgery. The LASIK procedure is the preferred treatment for these conditions; PRK and LASIK are widely available. In the past several years, refractive surgery for myopia, hyperopia, and astigmatism has been considered instead of contact lenses or glasses. Recently, conductive keratoplasty has been advanced for treating presbyopia. However, there may be a compromise in balancing distance and near-vision postoperatively. Potential surgical complications include infections, epithelial ingrowth, halos, and loss of contrast sensitivity. In a patient with moderate cataracts, cataract surgery is more advisable than refractive surgery, because the patient will often have only a few years of vision correction before needing cataract surgery.

Decisions regarding refractive surgery procedures should be based on surgeon expertise, patient refraction, and available equipment. The patient should be informed about the possible options. For patients who are not candidates for laser refractive surgery, other surgical methods can correct refractive error. For example, implantable collamer lenses (ICLs) are particularly useful for high myopic patients, are generally well tolerated, and have a lower incidence of postoperative symptoms (e.g., halos).

Ocular Medications

Ocular medications may have significant systemic side effects, such as many of the glaucoma medications. Glaucoma medications can generally be classified into β-blockers, prostaglandins and prostamides, carbonic anhydrase inhibitors, α-blockers, and older medications, such as epinephrine and pilocarpine.

Systemic absorption of beta-adrenergic blockers, such as timolol (Timoptic), may exacerbate asthma. β-Blockers may also cause problems with breathing, bradycardia, and hypotension. These medications are contraindicated in patients with heart block, congestive heart failure, asthma, or obstructive lung disease.

Carbonic anhydrase inhibitors, such as methazolamide (Neptazane), lower IOP and decrease aqueous production. Carbonic anhydrase inhibitors, such as acetazolamide (Diamox), cause increased urination, decreased appetite, headache, nausea, malaise, and kidney stones. Additionally, these medications lower the serum potassium level, particularly in patients taking diuretics. Potassium supplements should be prescribed to prevent hypokalemia.

Alpha-adrenergic agonists, such as brimonidine tartrate (Alphagan), can lower blood pressure as well as intraocular pressure. Side effects include dry mouth and fatigue. Additionally, brimonidine can cross the blood-brain barrier and produce somnolence. Apraclonidine (Iopidine) induces allergy in 20% to 25% of patients and is found to be ineffective in about 25% of all patients.

A newer class of glaucoma medications includes the prostaglandins and prostamides. These medications, such as latanoprost (Xalatan), travoprost (Travatan), and unoprostone isopropyl (Rescula), are associated with increased eyelash growth and increased pigmentation of the iris, conjunctiva, and eyelids. Additionally, these medications can induce conjunctival hyperemia and can increase the risk of postoperative retinal edema.

Other ocular medications include antibiotics, anti-inflammatory agents, and steroids. Patients are occasionally given an antibiotic-steroid combination, such as tobramycin-dexamethasone (TobraDex), that may increase IOP, cause cataracts, or potentiate fungal ulcers. Steroid glaucoma is a form of open-angle glaucoma. If the condition is undetected and the patient continues to refill the medication, damage may occur to the optic nerve, including glaucomatous optic atrophy. Generally, IOP is lowered once the steroids have been discontinued. However, it may take several months for IOP to return to a normal level. Vision loss that occurs during this period may be permanent. Because of the relative frequency of steroid glaucoma, cataract, and exacerbations of viral infections, topical corticosteroids should be avoided for minor ocular inflammations. Generally, ocular conditions that warrant the use of topical steroids also warrant consultation with an ophthalmologist.

Ophthalmic Conditions in Older Adults

The most important causes of central and peripheral visual impairment in older adults include glaucoma, cataract, diabetic retinopathy, and macular degeneration. Most of these conditions can be controlled or, as in the case of cataracts, vision can be restored to a significant level to improve the

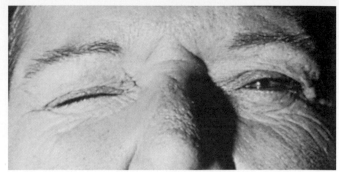

Figure 41-26 Blepharospasm in 68-year-old woman with a history of uncontrollable lid spasm resulted in her being unable to drive.

quality of life. Glaucoma and macular degeneration progression may be slowed with proper treatment. Regular eye examinations for older adults can detect early signs of ocular abnormalities and ensure that proper treatment is initiated. Generally, adults older than 40 years should have a complete examination at least every 3 years. After age 65, the examination should be at 1- to 2-year intervals.

Diseases of the Eyelid

Entropion is a turning in of the eyelid margin so that there is a rubbing of eyelashes or cilia, with resultant ocular irritation. An *ectropion* is a turning out of the eyelid margin so that the eye builds up excessive tears and becomes inflamed. Both conditions are more common in the older adult population. Entropion and ectropion can cause symptoms of irritation and corneal changes.

Basal cell carcinoma is much more common in older adults. It occurs more often on the lower lid. Generally, basal cell carcinomas have pearly edges and a central depression that becomes ulcerated.

Dermatochalasis, or baggy eyelids, may interfere with vision, covering part of the eye. This condition is caused by atrophy of the eyelid skin and elasticity changes. Dermatochalasis causes no permanent damage to vision.

Blepharospasm is a chronic spasm of the eyelid in older adults (Fig. 41-26). It may interfere with reading and driving. Botulinum toxin (Botox) injection in small doses is presently the treatment of choice.

Herpes Zoster and Herpes Simplex

Herpes zoster occurs more frequently in the older adult population. When the skin lesions involve the eyelids and tip of the nose, the ophthalmologist should be consulted for evaluation. Corneal dendrites and ulcers can occur with herpes zoster virus and HSV infection (Fig. 41-27). HSV infection is more frequently associated with uveitis. Herpes simplex infection responds to trifluridine (Viroptic) eyedrops, whereas HSV infection requires topical steroids.

Ptosis

Ptosis can occur in a number of forms, including congenital ptosis, pseudoptosis, and acquired ptosis (Fig. 41-28). Congenital ptosis can occur as a unilateral or bilateral ptosis. A Marcus Gunn, jaw-winking ptosis results from a misdirected

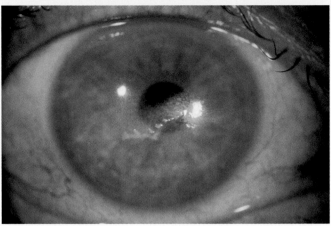

Figure 41-27 Herpes zoster keratitis. Photomicrograph shows pseudodentrites.

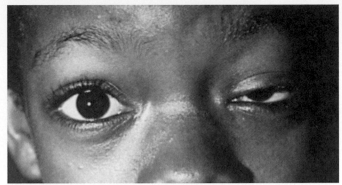

Figure 41-29 Ptosis of left upper lid in 8-year-old patient who had ocular myasthenia and subsequently developed ptosis of right upper lid and exotropia.

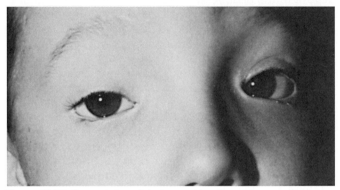

Figure 41-28 Congenital ptosis in 4-year-old patient with congenital bilateral ptosis.

cranial nerve III. Acquired forms of ptosis include *myogenic* forms, such as myasthenia gravis and progressive external ophthalmoplegia, and *neurogenic* forms, such as Horner syndrome and cranial nerve III palsy (Fig. 41-29). *Pseudoptosis* is caused by conditions giving the appearance of a ptosis. It is particularly common with microphthalmia (small eye, or phthisis bulbi). Pseudoptosis may also be secondary to hypotropia.

Congenital ptosis generally is corrected with bilateral fascia lata brow suspension or a levator resection in patients with good levator function. Treatment of adult forms of ptosis includes correction with a tarsoconjunctival resection, strengthening of the levator aponeurosis, and levator resection.

Myasthenia Gravis

Myasthenia gravis is an autoimmune disease. It can occur at any age and is more common in women. There are some genetic associations, but usually it is sporadic. In myasthenia gravis, acetylcholine receptor antibodies decrease postsynaptic receptor activity at the neuromuscular junction. The muscle cannot receive the message propagated by the action potential. The clinical effect is muscle weakness, which may be variable, chronic, localized, or diffuse. The immunologic component (B and T cells produced in thymus) plays a role. About 75% of patients have thymic abnormalities, and 10% have thymomas.

Common ocular findings include unilateral or bilateral ptosis, which is usually asymmetric lid fasciculations, and lid retraction. Patients with myasthenia gravis frequently have eye muscle deviations with double vision. Systemic manifestations include involvement of the jaw and neck, inability to hold the body erect because of weakness of the spinal muscles, and limb weakness. In addition, symptoms may include choking on food and shortness of breath, which is considered a *myasthenic crisis*. Speech difficulties may also occur. A neurologist usually prescribes treatment for myasthenic patients. The prognosis is generally good in patients who present with ocular abnormalities initially.

Strabismus in Adults

Adult strabismus results in both visual and psychosocial disabilities. Adults with strabismus may not be offered appropriate surgical treatment because of misconceptions regarding surgical and nonsurgical correction. Successful strabismus surgery can relieve diplopia and visual confusion, restore or establish depth perception, expand the visual field, eliminate an abnormal head posture, and improve psychosocial function and employability.

Adults with strabismus should be referred to an ophthalmologist who specializes in surgical and nonsurgical correction of adults. Patients should understand the management of strabismus, if possible, and can be educated regarding the relative risks and benefits of surgery.

KEY TREATMENT

The surgical and nonsurgical treatment of strabismus in adults results in improved binocular visual function, visual rehabilitation of sensorimotor system, and improved psychosocial benefits (AAO, 2007) (SOR: A).

Dry Eye (Keratitis Sicca)

Tears, because of their lubricating and bacteriostatic properties, are essential for maintaining a healthy cornea and conjunctiva. A deficiency in tear production may result in a dry eye, also known as keratitis sicca. *Keratoconjunctivitis sicca* is an acquired disorder seen frequently during the fifth decade of life that occurs more often in women. Initial symptoms include a foreign body sensation, dryness, and burning, which often worsens as this condition progresses. Paradoxical tearing from reflex stimulation of the lacrimal gland occurs. Symptoms usually exceed the signs of this common condition. Examination reveals a lack of corneal and conjunctival luster, with punctate erosions. With a decrease in aqueous tears, there is an attempt to compensate by an increase in mucin production, leading sometimes to a stringy, ropelike discharge.

Some cases of keratoconjunctivitis sicca are related to an autoimmune cause, particularly those patients with dryness of other mucous membranes. It also often occurs with rheumatoid arthritis, systemic lupus erythematosus, and Sjögren's syndrome. Initial treatment includes lubrication with artificial tears and ointments to supplement or replace the tear film deficit. In moderate or severe cases, an ophthalmologist may need to occlude the eyelid punctum surgically and perform a tarsorrhaphy to protect the corneal surface. Moisture chambers may also be prescribed. Topical antibiotics are required only if secondary infection occurs. Cyclosporine 0.05% (Restasis) is also useful in addressing inflammatory components of tear film insufficiency, when other treatments are insufficient.

Exposure keratitis is a condition symptomatically similar to dry eyes that is caused by incomplete eyelid closure during blinking or with sleep. It may result from Bell's palsy, scarred or malpositioned eyelids, or thyroid exophthalmos. Management involves the use of ophthalmic lubricating solutions and ointments. Mechanical measures designed to assist normal eyelid closure may be necessary, including frequent manual massage of the lids during the day to assist closure, forceful blinking exercises to elicit Bell's reflex, and taping the lids shut at night. Merely patching the eye should be avoided because of an increased risk of corneal abrasion if the lids do not cover the eye underneath the patch.

Thyroid Eye Disease (Thyroid Orbitopathy)

Hyperthyroidism may induce an orbitopathy in some patients. In such cases, there is diffuse hyperplasia of the thyroid and infiltrative ophthalmopathy. Thyroid eye disease is seen in association with thyroid dysfunction, although thyroid function test results may be normal. With thyroid orbitopathy, the extraocular muscle becomes infiltrated; this may occur even when the disease appears to be under good systemic control. The precise extraocular mechanism is unknown and the genetic predisposition uncertain.

Graves' ophthalmopathy occurs in approximately 95% of patients with Graves' thyroid disease, but is only rarely seen with Hashimoto's thyroid disease. The diagnosis of *euthyroid* Graves' ophthalmopathy is primarily a clinical diagnosis, confirmed with orbital CT imaging. Clinical characteristics include hypotropia, esotropia, or a combination of vertical and horizontal strabismus. Many patients are euthyroid at diagnosis, but there may be a history of previous thyroid dysfunction. Thyroid myopathy is a common cause of acquired vertical deviation in adults but relatively uncommon in children. Werner has classified eye involvement in Graves' disease by the NO-SPECS mnemonic: *n*o signs of symptoms, *o*nly signs of lid retraction or gaze palsy with or without lid lag or proptosis, *s*igns and symptoms of soft tissue involvement, *p*roptosis, *e*xtraocular muscle involvement, *c*orneal involvement with corneal drying, and *s*ight loss with optic nerve involvement.

The total muscle volume of the extraocular muscles increases as the disease worsens. The volume can be computed by averaging serial CT sections. Indications for treatment of thyroid ophthalmopathy include diplopia, abnormal head position, a large horizontal or vertical strabismus, and loss of vision. Generally, the preferred treatment is orbital decompression if loss of vision is threatened. Nonsurgical management of the patient includes prisms to alleviate the diplopia in primary position. Eye muscle surgery can be performed with adjustable sutures.

Ocular Changes with Aging

Arcus senilis, or corneal arcus, is a hazy, white or yellow arc or deposit in the peripheral cornea. It has many causes and is more common in older adults. The deposit is composed of cholesterol and other lipids and does not generally indicate an underlying systemic abnormality. It does not interfere with vision or eye function. In white patients, this finding may indicate lipid abnormalities and an increased propensity for cardiovascular disease. No such clear correlation has been identified in African Americans, who are much more likely to have an arcus. The pupil becomes miotic and does not respond well to dilation or darkness. The vitreous body detaches from the retina, resulting in the perception of flashing lights secondary to retinal traction. The retinal pigment epithelium atrophies, making the choroidal vessels more visible. The lens becomes progressively stiffer with age. Symptoms begin in the mid-40s, with increasing difficulty in near-vision focusing. By age 60, most patients have had a major reduction in accommodative amplitudes. The universal stiffening of the lens with age causes the well-known symptoms of presbyopia, requiring the use of reading glasses.

Cataracts

A cataract is a condition that affects a large percentage of the population. As a result, cataract surgery is the most common U.S. surgery performed. Currently, cataracts affect approximately 40 million people in the United States. Generally, the normal aging and cataractous changes in the lens are related to its metabolic activity. *Acquired cataracts* may be caused by penetrating trauma, irradiation, heat, or blunt trauma. Metabolic cataracts occur particularly in association with diabetes. Changes in the blood glucose concentration may alter the refractive power of the lens. With hyperglycemia, glucose byproducts enter the lens, causing it to swell and inducing a myopic shift. *Nuclear sclerosis cataract* is the most common cause of lens opacity seen by the ophthalmologist; an increased central density makes lens power stronger. As a result, frequent changes in the eyeglass prescription are necessary to correct the changing lens power. This type of cataract develops slowly, and surgery may not be necessary for several years.

The decision for cataract surgery with intraocular lens implantation depends on the degree of vision loss and the daily requirements of the patient. In patients with cataracts, indications for surgery include the patient's preference and needs, functional disability by Snellen visual acuity test and visual field testing, and concomitant ocular problems.

Cataract surgery involves removal of the cataractous lens and insertion of an intraocular lens. Generally, the procedure is performed under local anesthesia, although the patient may have general anesthesia. Modern cataract surgery primarily entails removing the lens through an extracapsular technique, which can be done en bloc or through a small corneal incision with phacoemulsification. In children, cataracts are generally soft and often require aspiration equipment.

Phacoemulsification is a technique that uses ultrasonic energy to break up the lens material so that it may be withdrawn through a small needle. Unfortunately, phacoemulsification has been confused with laser treatment for cataract removal. It is important to emphasize to patients that the laser is not used to remove the cataractous lens. Part of the confusion lies in the fact that secondary cataracts or opacification of the posterior capsule can be eliminated using the YAG laser. With the YAG laser there is photodisruption of the capsule, which creates an opening and provides good visual acuity. Cataract removal is one of the most successful operations performed. Generally, adult patients are treated with intraocular lenses after cataract removal. If the patient has bilateral aphakia, contact lenses or cataract spectacles may be worn. However, moderate visual distortion occurs with aphakic spectacles, as well as restriction of peripheral vision. Routine preoperative testing does not improve clinical outcomes for healthy patients undergoing cataract surgery.

Uveitis

A red painful eye with photophobia and increased tearing often occurs with the presentation of anterior uveitis. In addition, the patient may have decreased vision. *Vascular injection,* a circumcorneal injection involving the deep vessels of the sclera, is one of the primary signs of anterior uveitis. Generally, uveitis patients are moderately light sensitive. In addition, the inflammatory process may hinder aqueous production and reduce intraocular pressure.

Patients suspected of an *anterior uveitis* should be referred to an ophthalmologist for consultation and treatment. The most common cause of anterior uveitis is idiopathic; other common causes include ankylosing spondylitis, inflammatory bowel disease, sarcoidosis, juvenile rheumatoid arthritis, Reiter's syndrome (urethritis, polyarteritis, and ocular inflammation), herpetic keratitis, and Lyme disease.

Patients with *posterior uveitis* usually present with a reduction in vision and vitreous floaters. They may have clinical signs of retinal vasculitis, retinal ischemia, optic nerve edema, and exudative retinal detachment. On careful inspection, cells may be visible floating in the vitreous. Common causes of posterior uveitis are toxoplasmosis, sarcoidosis, cytomegalovirus, Epstein-Barr virus, Behçet's disease, and *Bartonella* infection. *Toxoplasmosis* accounts for up to 30% of cases and may destroy the macula or other important visual structures. Characteristically, there is an exudation in the retina caused by an inflammatory process. *Toxocara canis* may also present as uveitis.

Diseases of the Retina and Optic Nerve

Key Points

- Glaucoma is a leading cause of blindness and is managed medically and surgically.
- Choroidal melanoma is the most common intraocular malignancy.
- Posterior vitreous detachment is a common cause of vitreous floaters but may present similar to retinal detachment.
- Age-related maculopathy represents a significant cause of central vision loss in older adults.
- Some patients with macular degeneration may benefit from advances in therapeutic laser treatments.
- Vitamin supplements have been shown to be beneficial for some patients with macular degeneration.
- Routine funduscopy should be performed to evaluate for hypertensive retinopathy and diabetic retinopathy.
- Diabetic retinopathy is the most common cause of blindness in Americans age 20 to 74.
- Giant cell arteritis generally occurs in patients 55 and older, with headache, scalp tenderness, jaw claudication, malaise, fatigue, and amaurosis fugax.
- Carotid artery disease is an important cause of transient ischemic attacks; 50% of patients with TIA involving carotid artery disease have a major stroke within 1 month of first attack.
- About 75% of women and 34% of men with optic neuritis will develop multiple sclerosis within 15 years.

Retinal diseases account for 10% to 15% of blindness. Common retinal diseases include macular degeneration, diabetic retinopathy, retinal detachment, and retinal vascular disease. Sudden loss of vision can have various causes; four common causes are retinal detachment, temporal arteritis, ischemic optic neuropathy, and optic neuritis (Table 41-6).

Vitreous Floaters

The vitreous gel degenerates during middle age and forms microscopic strands within the eye. An increase in previous floaters, acute flashing lights, or the appearance of a veil or curtain over a patient's vision may signify a retinal detachment. Posterior vitreous detachment is a common cause of vitreous floaters. The sudden onset of vitreous floaters can be alarming for the patient. Generally, they are simply the result of the normal aging process. Vitreous floaters may interfere with clear vision, particularly reading. Although generally benign, posterior vitreous detachments can create retinal hemorrhages and are associated with retinal tears and detachments.

Melanoma

Choroidal melanoma, a pigmented elevated mass in the choroid, is the most common intraocular malignancy. As the tumor spreads, it may produce a retinal detachment. In addition, retinal pigment epithelial alterations can occur in the form of *drusen* or *lipofuscin* (Fig. 41-30). The differential diagnosis of choroidal melanoma includes choroidal nevus, retinal detachment, and metastatic tumor to the choroid. All patients with intraocular tumors should have an extensive physical examination and laboratory testing to exclude metastatic spread of the neoplasm. Many ocular melanomas have already metastasized at diagnosis. Treatment modalities generally

Table 41-6 Systematic Approach to Patient Presenting with Rapid or Sudden Loss of Vision

Presentation	Symptoms	Signs	Treatment
Painful Acute narrow, angle-closure glaucoma	Pain, tearing, headache	Shallow anterior chamber	**Refer immediately.**
	Halos around light with intermittent blurring of vision	Sudden rise of intraocular pressure	If no ophthalmologist available, begin oral glycerin (1 mL/kg), intramuscular acetazolamide (500 mg), and topical pilocarpine (1%-4%) every 15 min.
	Nausea, vomiting	Circumcorneal injection Cornea edematous and cloudy	
Painless Central retinal artery occlusion	Sudden unilateral visual loss (may be preceded by transient blurring)	Cherry-red spot in macula	Digital ocular massage
		Narrowed arteries Pale optic nerve head Edematous retina	Elevation of blood CO_2 level through rebreathing into paper bag or breathing 95% O_2 and 5% CO_2 (carbogen) if available
Painless Cranial (giant cell) arteritis	Sudden unilateral visual loss preceded by vague migrating joint pains Low-grade fever, depressed appetite No localized pain in eyeball but scalp pain; severe, boring headaches	Enlarged and painful temporal artery Increased erythrocyte sedimentation rate is key to diagnosis.	**Refer immediately.** Definitive treatment is high doses of systemic corticosteroids. Involvement of other eye in relatively short time; therefore, immediate referral is imperative.
Retinal detachment	Usually rapid loss of vision but *may vary* Frequently preceded by flashing lights and floaters; more common in patients with myopia; after cataract extraction; after blunt trauma	Retinal elevation on ophthalmoscopic examination	Refer to ophthalmologist promptly.

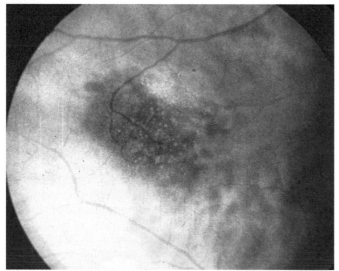

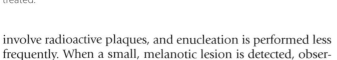

Figure 41-30 Choroidal melanoma. Increased pigmentation involves the choroid, with characteristic lipofuscin overlying the lesion, which is slightly elevated with bowing of the overlying vessels. This melanoma was locally treated.

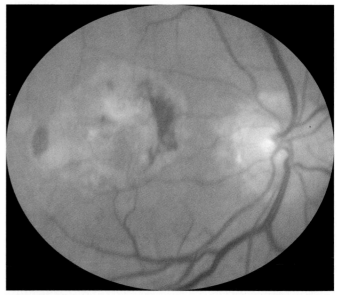

Figure 41-31 Age-related maculopathy in 73 year–old woman who demonstrated evidence of geographic atrophy with her macular degeneration.

involve radioactive plaques, and enucleation is performed less frequently. When a small, melanotic lesion is detected, observation is indicated in older adults with slow-growing lesions.

Macular Degeneration

Age-related macular degeneration (ARMD) is the most common form of breakdown in the macular area, accounting for 70% of all cases. *Age-related maculopathy*, formerly called "macular degeneration," leads to loss of fine or central vision but not side vision. Laser treatment is of benefit in select

patients. Macular degeneration begins with nonexudative changes (Fig. 41-31). However, many people with macular degeneration have an abnormal vascularization that is not always amenable to laser therapy (Fig. 41-32). The condition occurs in the other eye within 1 year in 10% of cases. Another form of macular degeneration is *exudative macular degeneration*, which accounts for 10% of cases.

Normally, the macula is protected by thin tissue that separates it from the fine blood vessels that nourish the posterior aspect of the eye. When these blood vessels break or leak, scar

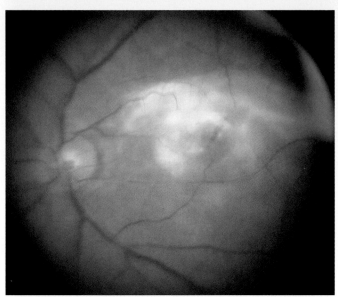

Figure 41-32 Age-related maculopathy with choroidal neovascularization. Abnormal blood vessels have formed in the area of macular degeneration and require further studies to determine whether laser treatment is indicated.

tissue may form, often leading to abnormal growth of new blood vessels (neovascularization). These new vessels are particularly fragile, and leakage and bleeding may occur. If macular degeneration involves both eyes, near activities become difficult. If an individual loses central vision related to macular degeneration, generally the peripheral vision is unaffected.

An ophthalmologist can confirm the diagnosis of macular degeneration; assessment includes color vision testing, ophthalmoscopy, and fluorescein angiography, when indicated. Examination reveals an accumulation of membranous debris on the posterior aspect of the retinal pigment epithelium, presence of drusen, and atrophy of the retinal pigment epithelium. In addition, there may be detachment of the retinal pigment epithelium and choroidal neovascularization.

There is no cure for patients with ARMD. Ophthalmic laser surgery may be beneficial in reducing the spread of the exudative macular degeneration, but it is successful only in the early stages. Laser therapy and anti-VEGF (vascular endothelial growth factor) medications have been helpful in treating membranes and neovascularization. Advanced cases of macular degeneration have been treated with macular translocation with some success. At present, use of multivitamins with beta-carotene and vitamin E may delay progression for many patients with ARMD. However, beta-carotene supplements in smokers have been associated with an increase in lung cancer. Vitamin supplements have no impact on cataract formation.

KEY TREATMENT

Patients with intermediate age-related macular degeneration had a 25% reduction in the progression of ARMD with the following vitamin and mineral supplements: vitamin C (500 mg), vitamin E (400 IU), beta-carotene (15 mg [25,000 IU]), zinc oxide (80 mg), and cupric oxide (2 mg) (AREDS Research Group, 2001) (SOR: A). Management options for macular degeneration include observation, antioxidant vitamin and mineral supplements, intravitreal injection of anti-VEGF agents, PDT, and laser photocoagulation surgery (AAO Preferred Practice Patterns, 2008) (SOR: A).

Hypertensive Retinopathy

Routine ophthalmoscopy in hypertensive patients affords the physician a direct view of the arterioles and helps assess the long-term duration and severity of the hypertension as well as evidence of accelerated or malignant hypertension. In the vascular system, arterioles serve as the resistance vessels, and the overall cross section of the arteriolar bed determines peripheral resistance. With the fundus examination, the physician can directly observe the degree of spasm in arterioles and the effects of long-term hypertension on the arteriolar wall. Severe hypertensive retinopathy can lead to profound vision loss, although usually the patient is completely asymptomatic.

The normal arteriolar wall is transparent, and the visible image is of the blood column as it passes through the arteriolar lumen. An additional anatomic consideration is that at the point of crossing of the arteriole and venule, the vasculature shares a common adventitial layer. Therefore, when arteriolar thickening occurs, the venule is compressed, resulting in arteriolar-venous (A-V) nicking. It is practical to divide the changes in the fundus seen in hypertension into two scales, a hypertensive scale and an arteriole-sclerotic scale (see online text, Hypertensive Retinopathy Grading).

Diabetic Retinopathy

Diabetic retinopathy is the most common cause of blindness in Americans 20 to 74 years old. Diabetic patients are at 25 times greater risk of becoming blind from diabetic retinopathy than nondiabetic persons of becoming blind from all other causes. Diabetic retinopathy is more common in women, but men appear to develop a more complicated and severe proliferative retinopathy. Findings have shown that in type 1 diabetes mellitus, it is unusual to detect diabetic retinopathy before 5 years after onset of disease. After 15 years from diagnosis, most patients with type 1 diabetes have some diabetic retinopathy, with incidence of proliferative disease greater than 40%. In type 2 diabetes, with onset after age 30, diabetic retinopathy is often detectable at the initial diagnosis. Diabetic patients requiring insulin have a higher incidence of diabetic retinopathy and proliferative disease.

The precise pathogenesis of diabetic retinopathy remains unclear, but the target tissue is the retinal capillary. Localized ischemia has been shown to increase levels of vascular endothelial growth factor (VEGF) and result in a corresponding area of vascular proliferation. The vascular complications evolve through states defined by ophthalmoscopic findings.

The first stage is called *nonproliferative* or "background" retinopathy (Fig. 41-33). Capillaries leak and later become occluded. The retinal findings include aneurysms, hard exudates, intraretinal hemorrhages, and macular edema. In the nonproliferative stage, patients will only experience visual loss if there is macular involvement. Visual loss from macular edema is present in 5% to 20% of diabetic patients, depending on the type and duration of disease. With progression, patients will develop *preproliferative* diabetic retinopathy. This stage frequently progresses to proliferative diabetic retinopathy. The most readily recognized abnormality of preproliferative retinopathy is the cotton-wool spot, a white opacity with feathery edges indicative of localized retinal infarct of the nerve fiber layer.

Proliferative diabetic retinopathy (PDR) is responsible for most serious vision loss in patient with diabetes. As a result of continued retinal ischemia, new blood vessels form in the area of the optic disc or elsewhere on the retinal surface (Fig. 41-34). Without laser photocoagulation, these vessels typically progress to retinal detachment and form vascularization within the vitreous cavity. Neovascularization results in vitreous hemorrhage and retinal traction. Once fibrous proliferation has detached the retina, surgical repair can be challenging. Prophylactic laser photocoagulation is the best way to avoid this complication for diabetic patients with proliferative diabetic retinopathy.

Screening Recommendations.

Screening eye examinations for patients with type 2 diabetes reduce the chance of vision loss (FPIN, 2004) (SOR A, 1). Type 1 diabetic patients should have their first eye examination 5 years after onset.

Type 2 diabetic patients should have their first eye examination at diagnosis.

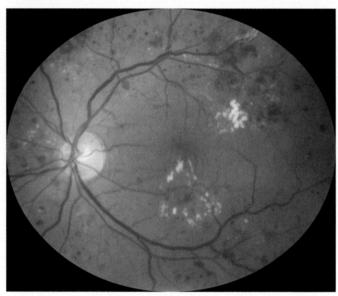

Figure 41-33 Nonproliferative diabetic retinopathy of left eye. There is extensive nonproliferative disease with macroaneurysms, hemorrhages, and exudates. Although there is no neovascularization, this patient is at risk of developing proliferative disease.

Diabetic patients should have a baseline eye examination before becoming pregnant or early in the first trimester. On initiation of ophthalmic screening, all diabetic patients should have annual dilated fundus examinations by an ophthalmologist, or sooner if poor diabetic control or visual symptoms develop (AAO, 2007) (SOR A, 1).

Retinal Detachment

Retinal detachment is separation of the retina from its blood supply. It usually follows a tear or hole in the retina. Retinal tears may be caused by trauma or retinal disease, but the cause of most tears is unclear. When the retina is detached, vision is lost from the involved area of the retina. If the macula detaches, irreversible loss of vision may occur unless the detachment is treated within 24 hours. Anatomic reattachment of the retina is successful in up to 90% of cases.

Giant Cell Arteritis (Temporal Arteritis)

Temporal arteritis is a systemic autoimmune disorder. Pathologically, there is a granulomatous inflammation of large and medium-sized arteries. It generally occurs in patients older than 55 years, with no gender predilection. Involvement may occur in any organ system. Ocular involvement is generally associated with inflammation of the posterior ciliary arteries. General symptoms include amaurosis fugax, headaches, scalp tenderness, jaw claudication, occasional ear pain or arthralgias, pain and tenderness on one or both temples, malaise, and intermittent fevers. Ocular symptoms include loss of vision, diplopia, pain, red eye, and ocularischemic syndrome. The workup of patients suspected to have giant cell arteritis includes a careful history of nonvisual symptoms, examination, and laboratory studies to include erythrocyte sedimentation rate (ESR), C-reactive protein, and complete blood count with differential. Using the Westergren method, the value for a normal ESR is 30 mm/hr for a 60-year-old man; for women, top of normal range is age plus 10 divided by 2, so 35 mm/hr is the upper range of normal for a 60-year-old woman. The differential diagnosis of sudden vision loss also includes emboli, central retinal artery occlusion, and retinal detachment.

The visual loss of giant cell arteritis is caused by an ischemic process in the optic nerve. Central retinal artery occlusion

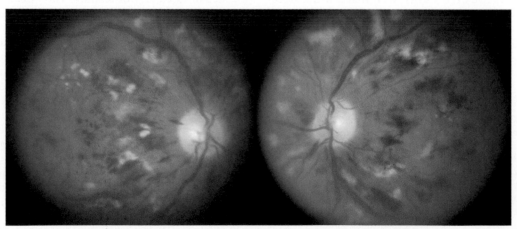

Figure 41-34 Proliferative diabetic retinopathy. Patient has severe disease, with diffuse retinal hemorrhages in all quadrants and evidence of neovascularization, and requires urgent panretinal photocoagulation. There is evidence of neovascularization of the optic disc in the left eye.

may also occur with giant cell arteritis. It is important to diagnose giant cell arteritis as early as possible. Without corticosteroid treatment, patients often develop permanent vision loss bilaterally. When one eye is involved with giant cell arteritis, the second eye loses vision in 65% of untreated patients. Generally, involvement of the second eye occurs with 10 days of onset. When the diagnosis is suspected on the basis of clinical symptoms and signs, temporal artery biopsy is necessary to confirm the diagnosis. The ESR is often greatly elevated, although it may be normal for age. If there is any doubt regarding the diagnosis, a temporal artery biopsy is warranted.

Once the diagnosis is established, steroid therapy should be instituted immediately. Up to 100 mg of prednisone (1.0-1.5 mg/kg/day) should be given orally if giant cell arteritis is suspected. Some physicians recommend IV steroids. Patients often require treatment for several months pending a positive biopsy or strong suspicion of giant cell arteritis. Steroids should not be delayed because of the temporal artery biopsy. Biopsy results will remain positive for up to 1 week after beginning steroid therapy. The patient can be monitored by symptoms occurring after institution of treatment and by ESR. Because of the severe systemic effects of giant cell arteritis, the patient should be followed closely.

> ### KEY TREATMENT
>
> Giant cell arteritis should be promptly treated with oral or intravenous steroids before obtaining a temporal artery biopsy; treatment should not be delayed for laboratory confirmation (Turbin et al., 1999) (SOR: A).

Glaucoma

Glaucoma is responsible for at least 10% of people with blindness in the United States. Glaucoma is four times more common in African Americans, who are also eight times more likely to develop blindness from glaucoma. Glaucoma appears to increase with age in the United States and decreases with age in Japan. Diabetic patients also have an increased risk for developing glaucoma.

The most common form of glaucoma in the United States is primary *open-angle glaucoma*, which accounts for about two thirds of all cases. In Asia the most common form of glaucoma is *angle-closure glaucoma*. Open-angle glaucoma tends to be genetically based, with multifactorial inheritance or as an autosomal recessive trait, with a high prevalence of carriers. Glaucoma is bilateral and occurs predominantly after age 50, although incidence is significant during the 30s and 40s, and it may even occur during the teenage years. Glaucoma is more severe in the African American population. Current incidence of glaucoma is 2% in the United States. The family physician can measure intraocular pressure using tonometry to detect elevated IOP. Tonometry can be performed with a Schiøtz tonometer, Perkins applanation tonometer, Tono-Pen XL tonometer, or Goldmann applanation tonometer held horizontally. This test should be performed at least every 3 years, beginning at age 35 years.

The damage to vision caused by glaucoma is irreversible. If the glaucoma can be detected early, it can usually be controlled and is curable by medial treatment, laser surgery, trabeculectomy, or some other filtering procedure. It is important to emphasize that glaucoma may occur at any age. Causes include congenital glaucoma, chronic open-angle glaucoma, narrow-angle glaucoma, or other forms of glaucoma, including pigmentary glaucoma.

One of the most common forms of secondary glaucoma is *steroid glaucoma*, which occurs in a substantial number of patients who use corticosteroid eyedrops or ointment for several weeks or longer. This condition also may occur with oral or systemic corticosteroid use, although it is rare. Steroid glaucoma is a form of open-angle glaucoma and, like primary open-angle glaucoma, can be effectively treated if detected early. If IOP is not lowered in time, there may be permanent damage to the optic nerve. Treatment for this type of glaucoma is discontinuation of corticosteroids and initiation of topical glaucoma medications. The IOP elevation is reversible once the steroids have been discontinued, but it may take 2 to 3 months or longer for pressure to return to a normal level. Any visual loss that occurs during this period may be permanent. There is no reliably safe dose of topical steroids that can ensure the prevention of steroid glaucoma. Even topical medications that consist of a combination of steroids and antibiotics or other type of medication can increase IOP. Because of the relative frequency of steroid glaucoma, as well as other ocular complications resulting from steroid use (e.g., cataract, exacerbation of viral infections), topical steroids should not be used for minor ocular inflammations, except in special circumstances.

Secondary glaucoma also may be caused by ocular trauma, intraocular inflammations, intraocular tumors, and carotid vascular disease. Regardless of cause, any patient suspected of having secondary glaucoma should be referred to an ophthalmologist as soon as possible for further evaluation and therapy. Management depends on the cause of the disease and character of the IOP elevation. Some medications can also result in glaucoma and include a warning related to developing angle-closure glaucoma. Additionally, topiramate (Topamax) is associated with an idiosyncratic acute glaucoma caused by uveal effusions.

With increased IOP, damage to the optic nerve and visual field abnormalities can occur. Almost all elevated pressures are caused by an obstruction to the outflow of aqueous humor. *Aqueous humor*, formed inside the eye in the ciliary body, circulates around the lens and through the pupil into the anterior portion of the eye. The aqueous humor exits through the anterior angle structures (trabecular meshwork and Schlemm's canal) (Fig. 41-35). About 10% of glaucoma cases occur in the setting of normal IOP, suggesting that these eyes are particularly susceptible to pressure changes. Glaucoma management involves more than controlling IOP. Possible sources of damage to the optic nerve involve mechanical factors affecting the optic nerve, decreased optic nerve perfusion, and blockage of axoplasmic flow in the lamina cribrosa. Carotid artery stenosis can also cause problems because of decreased perfusion to the optic nerve. Occasionally, elevations result from impeded outflow caused by elevated venous pressure, such as in patients with Sturge-Weber syndrome.

The most serious consequence of elevated IOP is damage to the optic nerve (Fig. 41-36). As IOP rises, retinal nerve

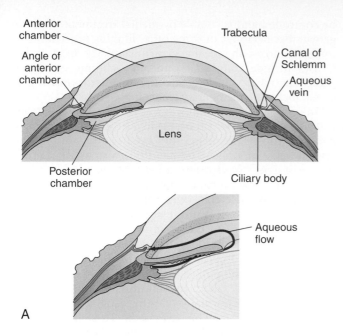

Anterior chamber

Angle of anterior chamber

Trabecula

Canal of Schlemm

Aqueous vein

Lens

Posterior chamber

Ciliary body

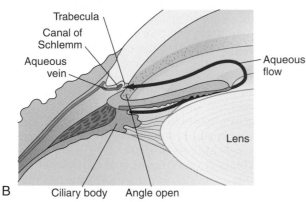

Aqueous flow

A

Trabecula

Canal of Schlemm

Aqueous vein

Aqueous flow

Lens

B   Ciliary body   Angle open

Figure 41-35 A, Flow of aqueous from the ciliary body, leaving the eye through the trabecula and canal of Schlemm via a normal, open, wide angle. **B,** Chronic open-angle glaucoma. *(From Scheie HG, Albert DM. Textbook of Ophthalmology, 9th ed. Philadelphia, Saunders, 1977.)*

fibers are destroyed at the optic nerve head, resulting in permanent visual loss. Peripheral vision is usually affected first, followed by progressive visual loss involving the entire visual field (Fig. 41-37).

KEY TREATMENT

Long-term monitoring is essential for successful management of glaucoma (AAO, 2000) (SOR: A).

For chronic open-angle glaucoma, initial treatment is topical medications (AAO, 2000) (SOR: C).

For uncontrolled chronic open-angle glaucoma, surgical treatment should be considered (AAO, 2000) (SOR: C).

For acute angle- closure glaucoma, medical treatment and surgery (laser or incision) should be implemented as soon as medically possible (Saw et al., 1993) (SOR: A).

Anterior Ischemic Optic Neuropathy

The clinical characteristics of ischemic optic neuropathy include age at onset generally older than 60 years, painless vision loss, and afferent pupillary defect (Marcus Gunn pupil). These patients also usually have a visual field abnormality. Examination of the optic disc reveals edema in almost all cases. Pathology appears to be related to a diseased ciliary circulation. It is generally difficult to determine whether the disc edema will result in a mild peripheral (side) visual field defect and good visual acuity, or reduced central acuity and a significant visual field defect. Giant cell arteritis must be ruled out in these patients. A general physical examination and associated blood work are indicated. No treatment prevents the progression of ischemic optic neuropathy, including steroids and anticoagulants.

Transient Ischemic Attacks in Carotid Artery Disease

Transient ischemic attacks are neurologic deficits lasting less than 24 hours and are reversible. The most common ophthalmologic TIA is *amaurosis fugax*, which is a fleeting monocular blindness caused by an embolic event. There is a sudden graying or reduction of vision, often moving from the peripheral vision to the center to cover the entire visual field within a few seconds. After 1 to 5 minutes, the central vision

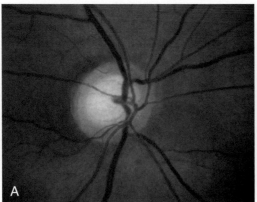
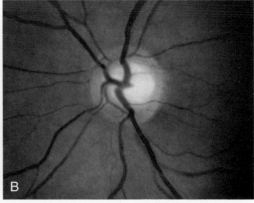

Figure 41-36 Bilateral glaucoma in 60-year-old man. Patient also had history of diabetes mellitus. The glaucoma is characterized by prominent optic nerve cupping. **A,** Enlarged optic nerve cup, right eye. **B,** Enlarged optic nerve cup, left eye. Note thinning of optic nerve rim.

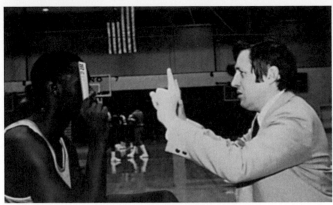

Figure 41-37 Testing peripheral fields by confrontation. *(From American Academy of Ophthalmology. The Athlete's Eye. San Francisco, AAO Professional Information Committee, 1986.)*

begins to return first. Other causes of TIAs include chronic disc edema (in which vision loss lasts seconds, not minutes), chronic papilledema with bilateral blackouts based on optic nerve disease (often also lasting a few seconds and caused by postural changes), and basilar artery insufficiency. TIAs related to basilar artery insufficiency are usually bilateral blackouts lasting seconds or minutes, often with changes in the posterior circulation.

The most important mechanisms involving carotid TIAs with stroke are embolization from the carotid artery or its branches, reduced perfusion caused by carotid stenosis or occlusion, or a combination of the two. In most patients (up to 90%), the site of the obstruction is the carotid sinus. Hollenhorst plaques are bright-yellow cholesterol emboli that may occlude the retinal arterioles (see Fig. 41-10). Fibrin platelet emboli can occur near retinal arterioles and produce visual symptoms. A cholesterol or fibrin platelet embolus is indicative of ulcerative disease in the carotid arteries and is associated with a high incidence of ischemic heart disease, peripheral vascular disease, stroke, and aortic abdominal aneurysm. A rarer form of carotid TIA is related to valvular heart disease, particularly with a prolapsed mitral valve or cardiac arrhythmia. Approximately 30% to 50% of patients with TIAs and carotid artery disease have a major stroke within 1 month of the first attack.

Optic Neuritis

Optic neuritis is localized inflammation of the optic nerve sheath, resulting in reduced neuronal transmission and decreased visual acuity. Generally, there is a loss of color vision and red desaturation noticed by the patients. The symptoms generally worsen during the first few days and progressively improve over several weeks. In children, optic neuritis has various causes, typically associated with viral infections. In young adults, optic neuritis has a high association with multiple sclerosis (MS). Approximately 75% of women and 34% of men with optic neuritis will develop MS within 15 years of the onset of optic neuritis. Patients should undergo MR neuroimaging to investigate for plaque formations. They should be questioned regarding constitutional symptoms of fatigue, weakness, difficulty moving or seeing after strenuous activity, and previous attacks.

Intravenous methylprednisolone (1 g/day for 3 days) followed by oral prednisone (1 mg/kg/day for 11 days) reduced the rate of MS development for 2 years (Optic Neuritis Study Group). Patients at high risk had a 44% reduction in the rate of developing MS when treated with interferon (Controlled High Risk Avonex Multiple Sclerosis Trial, CHAMPS). Newer treatments with interferon beta-1a (Avonex) and interferon beta-1b (Betaseron, Copaxone) have shown significant improvement in quality of life for patients and reduction in relapses. The Optic Neuritis Treatment Trial recommendations included giving patients with optic neuritis IV methylprednisolone (1 g/day) for 3 days, followed by 11 days of oral prednisone (1 mg/kg/day) (Beck et al., 1993). The dose is generally modified for children with 1 mg/kg/day whether using IV or oral steroids. Patients who receive oral rather than IV steroids for the first 3 days generally have more relapsing of their symptoms. Additionally, although corticosteroids hasten visual recovery, administration of steroids does not affect the overall visual acuity. The main benefit is delay of onset of multiple sclerosis.

References

The complete reference list is available online at www.expertconsult.com.

Web Resources

www.aao.org
American Academy of Ophthalmology; includes education, practice guidelines, practice management tips, and news.

www.aapos.org
American Association of Pediatric Ophthalmology and Strabismus; focuses on research and training in pediatric ophthalmology and the advanced care of adults with strabismus.

www.ascrs.org
American Society of Cataract and Refractive Surgeons; provides clinical and practice management information to members.

www.asotonline.org/ots.html
American Society of Ocular Trauma Ocular Trauma Score; estimates whether an eye trauma patient will obtain a specific visual range by 6 months after surgery.

www.aafp.org/afp/2007/1215/p1815.html
American Family Physician; differential diagnosis of the swollen red eyelid.

www.aao.org/practice_mgmt/eyesmart/snapshot_2009_results.cfm
AAO 2009 survey of eye injuries in the United States.

www.aapos.org/faq_bucket/cellulitis
AAPOS guidelines; diagnosis and treatment of preseptal and orbital cellulitis.

www.aapos.org/client_data/files/37_policyvisionscreeningforinfantsand children.pdf
AAPOS Vision Screening Guidelines for Children.

www.aapos.org/faq_bucket/thyroid_eye_disorders
AAPOS site that focuses on thyroid eye disease.

www.childrenseyefoundation.org/
Children's Eye Foundation; programs to help parents and physicians prevent vision loss and eye disease, especially related to amblyopia and strabismus.

www.eyecareamerica.org/
EyeCare America website, Foundation of American Academy of Ophthalmology; includes information on cataracts, glaucoma, diabetic neuropathy, macular degeneration, and how patients can gain access to no-cost care.

www.preventblindness.org/
Prevent Blindness America; volunteer eye health and safety organization to prevent blindness and preserve sight through vision screening and research.

www.aao.org/eyecare/conditions/uveitis/index.cfm
Uveitis diagnosis, treatment, and potential causes.

www.nei.nih.gov/health/glaucoma/glaucoma_facts.asp
Government site that includes many facts about glaucoma.

www.nlm.nih.gov/medlineplus/maculardegeneration.html
Macular degeneration reference for patients.

www.nei.nih.gov/health/maculardegen/nei_wysk_amd.PDF
Age-related macular degeneration handout for patients.

http://public.pedig.jaeb.org/Publications.aspx
Pediatric Eye Disease Investigator Group; list of current publications on amblyopia and strabismus.

http://pediatrics.aappublications.org/cgi/content/extract/100/6/1021
American Academy of Pediatrics Perinatal Guidelines.

https://secure3.aao.org/pdf/0240407.pdf
American Academy of Pediatrics (AAP) red reflex policy statement.

http://emedicine.medscape.com/article/1217083-overview
Summary of optic neuritis treatment.

http://telemedicine.orbis.org/learning/bins/login.asp?cid=740
Orbis Cyber-Sight Telemedicine Learning of Ophthalmology.

http://pediatrics.aappublications.org/cgi/content/extract/100/6/1021
AAP perinatal guidelines.

http://one.aao.org/CE/PracticeGuidelines/PPP_Content.aspx?cid=9d96 50fb-39a3-439c-9225-5fbb013cf472
AAO Preferred Practice Patterns for managing conjunctivitis.

http://one.aao.org/CE/PracticeGuidelines/ClinicalStatements_Content. aspx?cid=31b2cc0f-cf5e-4005-889e-d291a7ef8674
AAO guidelines for appropriate referral of persons with possible eye diseases or injury.

http://one.aao.org/CE/PracticeGuidelines/PPP_Content.aspx?cid=a6a3 402d-3fc6-44a4-9a52-46b74d37b830
Thorough discussion of primary angle closure, including AAOS guidelines for care.

CHAPTER 42

Neurology

Curtis Gingrich and William E. Carroll

Family physicians regularly encounter and manage a range of neurologic conditions. Many are fairly common in certain age groups, such as febrile seizures in children and Alzheimer's dementia in older adults. Other conditions, such as dysautonomia, are less common but present first to the primary care physician. This chapter discusses the neurologic disorders that family physicians are most likely to encounter, with guidelines for assessment and management.

Neurologic Examination

The neurologic examination begins with information obtained from the neurologic history, which is similar to a general medical history. The chief complaint is determined by asking open-ended questions. Analysis of the chief complaint should include the following:

Date of onset
Character and severity
Location and extension
Time relationship (acute, subacute, or chronic)
Associated complaints
Aggravating and alleviating factors
Previous treatment and effects

The sequence of the events and their progression is helpful in localizing the lesion and developing a differential diagnosis. A brief neurologic review of systems should include questions about headaches, visual changes, weakness, sensory changes, gait disturbances, and bowel and bladder function. The past medical history, social history, and family history are reviewed as well.

Much of the initial neurologic examination, including cranial nerve testing, carotid artery auscultation, and reflex and sensory assessment, can be conducted with the patient seated in a chair, on the bed, or on the examination table. Superficial reflexes, tests for meningeal irritability, and rectal examination are performed with the patient lying down. Gait, strength, and coordination can subsequently be evaluated with the patient standing. Traditionally, the neurologic examination is divided into five major areas: mental status, cranial nerves, motor system, sensory system, and reflexes.

Mental Status Examination

The mental status examination assesses appearance and behavior (including level of consciousness), speech and language, mood, thoughts and perceptions, and cognition. Speech abnormalities can interfere with the initial history. Abnormalities of speech include hearing deficits, aphasia (problems with understanding, thought, and word finding), and dysarthria (problems with articulation). *Aphasia* results from damage to the dominant hemisphere. *Wernicke's* aphasia refers to poor comprehension, with fluent but often meaningless speech. In *Broca's* aphasia, comprehension is preserved, but speech is nonfluent. Repetition, naming, reading, and writing are impaired in Wernicke's and Broca's aphasia. With *conductive* aphasia, there is a loss of repetition but preserved comprehension. Reading comprehension is thus relatively preserved, but reading aloud and writing are impaired. *Dysarthria* refers to difficulties with the production of speech caused by injury to the vocal cords, larynx, palate, tongue, or facial muscles. It is also seen with extrapyramidal or cerebellar lesions. Cognitive function is often assessed by tools such as the Mini–Mental State Examination, a simple, quick screening test for cognitive function. Errors in copying several simple drawings can be indicative of organic brain damage, particularly in those with dementia or parietal lobe damage.

Cranial Nerve Examination

The cranial nerve examination usually evaluates all cranial nerves, with the exception of CN I. CN I testing is generally reserved for patients with complaints of loss of smell or a closed-head injury. Smell can be decreased or lost in degenerative diseases, such as Parkinson's or Alzheimer's disease.

Cranial Nerve II (Optic Nerve)

The principal function of the optic nerve is vision. Testing of the optic nerve includes assessment of visual acuity and visual fields, funduscopic examination, and pupillary light reflex. Visual acuity is assessed in each eye individually. Visual fields are evaluated by confrontation. When performing the funduscopic examination, look for papilledema, hemorrhages, cholesterol emboli, and atrophy. Atrophy is characterized by a small, pale disc. Pupillary function assesses CNs II and III as well as sympathetic activity. The direct and consensual responses require CNs II and III to work correctly. If CN II is damaged, an afferent pupillary defect is often present. If the optic nerve is damaged, the light reflex is sluggish.

Cranial Nerves III (Oculomotor), IV (Trochlear), and VI (Abducens)

The principal functions of these nerves include ocular rotation, lid elevation (III), and pupillary constriction. CN III innervates the medial, inferior, and superior rectus muscles; the inferior oblique, which allows inward and upward gaze; and the levator palpebrae superioris muscle, which raises the upper eyelid. It also innervates the pupillary constrictor muscle. CN IV innervates the superior oblique muscle, which causes the eye to look inward and down. CN VI innervates the lateral rectus muscle.

To test ocular rotation, the patient should first be examined by looking straight ahead, to note any imbalances between the eyes. Next, ocular rotation of each eye is tested separately. First, abduction is tested with the patient following the examiner's finger horizontally; this tests the lateral rectus muscle. The patient then looks laterally and upward, to test the superior rectus, and downward, to test the inferior rectus. Adduction of the eye tests the medial rectus muscle. With the eye adducted, the patient looks up, to test the inferior oblique, and downward, to test the superior oblique.

The pupils should be observed for symmetry. Most unequal pupils (anisocoria) are congenital and not clinically significant. The light reflex, direct and consensual, is checked by shining a bright light directly into the pupil. The response to light should be brisk.

Cranial Nerve V (Trigeminal)

The principal functions of the trigeminal nerve include control of the muscles of mastication and sensation in the face, anterior half of the scalp, and mucous membranes of the mouth, nose, and sinuses. The nerve also mediates the afferent arc of the corneal reflex. The three sensory divisions are ophthalmic, maxillary, and mandibular. Each division is tested by light touch, pinprick, and temperature. The motor division of CN V can be assessed by palpating the jaw as the patient bites down. CN V is the afferent limb of the corneal reflex, and CN VII is the efferent limb. This reflex is tested by lightly touching the cornea with a wisp of cotton; the reflex, integrated through the pons, results in brisk, bilateral eye closure.

Cranial Nerve VII (Facial)

The principal functions of the facial nerve are control of the muscles of facial expression and provision of taste for the anterior two thirds of the tongue. It also innervates the lacrimal, sublingual, and submaxillary glands. To test the facial nerve, the patient is asked to smile, close the eyes tightly, and wrinkle the forehead. Taste is tested on each side separately using bitter and sweet substances.

Cranial Nerve VIII (Vestibulocochlear Nerve)

The principal functions of the vestibulocochlear nerve are hearing and vestibular function. Hearing is tested one ear at a time. Testing of hearing can be done by comparing each side with a finger rub, watch tick, or vibration of a tuning fork. The Rinne test compares bone conduction with air conduction on both sides. A tuning fork is placed on the mastoid process to assess bone conduction and then in front of the ear to assess air conduction. Air conduction should be louder than bone conduction. The Weber test evaluates middle ear conduction. A vibrating tuning fork is placed on the forehead. With normal hearing, there should be equal sound in both ears. Sound lateralized to one side indicates a conductive loss on that side or a neural loss on the opposite side. Vestibular function is not routinely tested.

Cranial Nerve IX (Glossopharyngeal)

The principal function of CN IX is to supply sensation to the pharynx and tonsillar fossa and taste to the posterior one third of the tongue. Clinical testing is done by eliciting a gag reflex. It should be done on both sides of the pharynx.

Cranial Nerve X (Vagus)

The principal functions of the vagus nerve are motor control to the pharynx, palate, and larynx and parasympathetic innervation of the thoracic and abdominal viscera. Motor control is tested by observing for symmetric elevation of the palate. The uvula should not deviate. Vocal cord paralysis can present with hoarseness or dysphonia and can occur with injury to the recurrent laryngeal branch.

Cranial Nerve XI (Spinal Accessory)

The principal functions of this nerve are to allow turning of the head and assist in shrugging of the shoulders. It innervates the sternocleidomastoid and upper trapezius. Strength is tested by shrugging the shoulders and turning the head to both sides against resistance.

Cranial Nerve XII (Hypoglossal)

The principal function of the hypoglossal nerve is innervation of intrinsic muscles of the tongue. To test this nerve, ask the patient to protrude the tongue. It should be midline.

If not, it protrudes to the paretic side. Also, observe for atrophy or fasciculations of the tongue.

Motor Examination

The motor examination includes assessment of body position, strength, tone, involuntary movements, coordination, and gait. Strength is graded as follows:

5—Normal.
4—Weak but can overcome gravity plus some additional resistance.
3—Can overcome gravity but not additional resistance.
2—Can move joint but cannot overcome the force of gravity.
1—Muscle contracts, but with little or no joint movement.
0—No muscle contraction.

Muscle tone is tested by passively flexing and extending the arm or wrist. Abnormal responses include spasticity, rigidity and flaccidity. *Spasticity* refers to increased muscle resistance when the muscle is passively stretched. This is seen with lesions to the cortical spinal tract. *Rigidity* or *cogwheeling* is observed with extrapyramidal lesions and Parkinson's disease. *Flaccid* refers to the absence of muscle tone.

Muscular weakness can result from upper motor neuron (UMN) lesions, lower motor neuron (LMN) lesions, muscle disease, neuromuscular junction disorders, or functional weakness. UMN disease is characterized by increased tone and reflexes, whereas LMN disease presents with wasting, fasciculations, decreased tone, and absent reflexes. With neuromuscular junction disorders, the patient complains of fatigable weakness but has normal or decreased tone and normal reflexes. A patient with functional weakness has normal tone, normal reflexes without wasting, and erratic power. The motor examination also includes observation for any abnormal movements, including tremors, choreiform movements, myoclonus, and dystonia.

Gait should be examined, even if assistance is needed. Assessment includes stride length, arm swing, posture, and turning, starting and stopping. Watch for specific gait abnormalities, such as *hemiplegia,* which is seen with unilateral UMN damage; *spasticity,* in which both legs have UMN lesions; *steppage,* in which there is footdrop; *waddling,* caused by weakness of the trunk and pelvic girdle; and *parkinsonism,* characterized by a stooped posture, short steps, and flexed arms with decreased arm swing.

Balance is maintained by the cerebellum, proprioceptive system, basal ganglia, and vestibular system. The Romberg sign is tested with the patient standing with feet together and then with eyes closed. If the patient falls with eyes closed, the test is considered positive. A positive test indicates proprioceptive loss, which can be from a peripheral cause or a posterior column lesion. The Romberg test can be positive with cerebellar or vestibular disease. Postural stability can be checked by gently pushing the patient while the feet are together.

Coordination can be tested with simple tests. For the finger-to-nose test, ask the patient to extend the arm, touch the tip of the nose, and then touch the examiner's index finger. This is repeated after the examiner has moved the index finger several times. The heel-knee-shin test is performed by asking the supine patient to slide one heel smoothly down the opposite leg from knee to shin. Two other tests of coordination are finger tapping and rapidly alternating hand movements. Injury to the cerebellar hemisphere impairs smooth coordination of limb movements on the same side of the body. With cerebellar lesions, these tests will be inaccurate, will have increased amplitude, and will be initiated more slowly.

Sensory Examination

The sensory examination requires an alert and cooperative patient. Sensory testing includes light touch, pinprick, proprioception, and vibration. Start by testing for light touch using a wisp of cotton or tissue on the major dermatomes of the extremities and trunk. Observe for dermatomal losses or a distal-to-proximal gradient. The same areas are then tested for superficial pain with a pin. Temperature is mediated by the same pathway as pain, so any deficits of pain sensation should have a corresponding deficit in temperature sensation. Vibration is tested by placing a 128-cycles/sec tuning fork on the bony prominences of the extremities and asking the patient to identify when it stops vibrating. Comparisons are made side to side. If there is a question of myelopathy, a vibration level may be noted as the tuning fork is moved up the spinous processes. Position is best tested using the great toe and distal phalanx of the thumb or another finger. The digit is grasped on the sides and moved up and down. Even a very slight movement of a finger should be detected. Proprioception, vibration, and light touch are functions of the dorsal column, and pain, temperature, crude touch, and pressure are functions of the spinothalamic tract.

Stereognosis, graphesthesia, and touch localization are integrated cortical sensations and are difficult to test if primary sensations are impaired. To test *stereognosis,* several small familiar objects are placed in the patient's hand and the patient is asked to identify them. To test *graphesthesia,* the examiner writes numbers on the patient's palm and asks the patient to identify them.

Reflexes

The reflex examination includes the deep tendon reflexes (DTRs) and the pathologic reflexes. In testing the deep tendon reflexes, it is important to look for symmetry. DTRs are graded using the following scale:

0—Absent
1—Present but diminished
2—Normal
3—Normal, but brisker than average
4—Increased and pathologic, with one or more beats of clonus

The DTRs assist with localization of a lesion because these reflexes are integrated at different levels of the spinal cord. DTRs help in distinguishing whether a lesion is a UMN lesion with pathologic hyperreflexia or possibly an LMN lesion with hyporeflexia. Table 42-1 summarizes the most important reflexes and their nerve root innervations.

The Babinski sign, or extensor toe sign, is tested by stroking the sole of the foot with a sharp object. A normal response is toe flexion. A pathologic response is extension of the great toe and flaring of the other toes. A positive response is always abnormal in patients older than 3 years and is a sign of pyramidal tract disorder.

Table 42-1 Nerve Root Innervations and Main Reflexes

Root	Movement	Reflex
C5	Shoulder abduction, elbow flexion	Biceps
C6	Elbow flexion	Supinator
C7	Finger extension, elbow extension	Triceps
C8	Finger flexors	Finger
T1	Small muscles of hand	None
L1, L2	Hip flexion	None
L3, L4	Knee extension	Knee
L5	Extension of great toe	None
S1	Hip extension, knee flexion, plantar flexion	Ankle

C, Cervical; T, thoracic; L, lumbar, S, sacral.

Neurologic Conditions

Headaches

Key Points

- More than 90% of men and women will have at least one headache each year.
- If there is a history typical of a particular primary headache with a normal examination, neuroimaging and electroencephalography are not necessary.
- Prophylactic treatment of migraine headaches is recommended when they occur with increasing frequency and there appears to be a potential overuse of acute therapies.
- Giant cell or temporal arteritis is a serious headache to consider in older adults and can be associated with blindness.

Headaches are a common problem encountered by family physicians. More than 90% of men and women will have at least one headache each year, and as many as 4.5 million Americans will experience recurrent headaches. The International Headache Society established a system for the classification of headaches to assist in diagnosis and treatment with a standard of care for family physicians. Migraine with aura, migraine without aura, tension, and cluster headaches constitute most primary headaches. Secondary headaches are symptoms of organic disease (Sarchielli, 2004). The initial evaluation of a patient with headache requires a complete history and physical examination with the following information:

- Age at onset
- Location, frequency, and duration
- Intensity and character
- Associated symptoms
- Triggering and ameliorating factors
- Medications
- Associated physical and neurologic symptoms
- Impact on work and family
- Psychological symptoms
- History of head trauma
- Previous imaging results
- Family history

Features of the history that should warn of an ominous cause for headache include the following:
Sudden onset of first headache
Worst headache ever
Late onset of new headache (after age 50 years)
Headache associated with fever, rash, or stiff neck
Progressively worsening headache
Headache associated with neurologic signs and symptoms other than aura
Headache associated with mental status changes
Headache associated with papilledema
Headache with exertion, sexual activity, coughing, or sneezing

The physical examination of a patient first presenting for evaluation of headache should include vital signs, cardiac examination, cervical spine examination, including nuchal rigidity, and ophthalmologic examination, including the optic fundi, pupils, and visual fields. The neurologic examination should include an assessment of cognitive function, motor function, reflexes, plantar response, cranial nerves, coordination, and gait.

If there is a history typical of a particular primary headache with a normal examination, neuroimaging and electroencephalography (EEG) are not necessary. A lumbar puncture, after neuroimaging, is recommended only if there is suspicion of subarachnoid hemorrhage, infection, or idiopathic intracranial hypertension (pseudotumor cerebri). Routine EEG is not indicated but may be useful in evaluating patients with associated mental status or consciousness changes, a history of head injury, or a history of syncope.

Migraine

Migraine headaches include migraine without aura, migraine with aura, and other migrainous disorders. Women suffer from migraines three times as often as men, and 90% of migraine sufferers have a positive family history. Migraines can begin in childhood, and as many as 4% to 10% of school-age children have migraines. The International Headache Society has developed diagnostic criteria for these types of headaches (Sarchielli, 2004). To establish a diagnosis of *migraine without aura*, there must have been at least five attacks fulfilling the following criteria:

1. Headache attacks lasting 4 to 72 hours
2. Headache with at least two of the following characteristics:
   a. Unilateral location
   b. Pulsating quality
   c. Moderate or severe intensity (inhibits or prohibits daily activities or causes avoidance of routine)
   d. Aggravated by physical activity such as walking or climbing
3. During the headache, at least one of the following occurs:
   a. Nausea and vomiting
   b. Photophobia and phonophobia

Migraine with aura has comparable diagnostic criteria but includes an aura. *Auras* can be a visual, sensory, motor, or speech aura. Visual changes include parallel zigzag lines and are often associated with scotomatous defects. Sensory deficits can involve an ipsilateral arm or paraorbital numbness or tingling. The tongue may be involved in some patients. The sensation has a marching characteristic. Motor deficits can be similar to sensory in that the deficits spread from one area to another. Speech problems may manifest as a mild dysphasia.

Other migraine types include basilar-type migraine, retinal migraine, status migrainosus, and migrainous infarction. *Basilar-type migraine* aura symptoms are referable to the brainstem or bilateral hemispheres, including dysarthria, vertigo, tinnitus, diplopia, and bilateral paresthesias. Reversible monocular, positive or negative visual disturbances associated with migraine are characteristic of *retinal migraine*. A diagnosis of *status migrainosus* requires an ongoing migraine of at least 72 hours in duration. Neuroimaging evidence of a cerebral infarct associated with a migraine is indicative of *migrainous infarction*.

Treatment

Migraine headache management includes acute analgesia, pharmacologic prophylaxis, and nonpharmacologic management. Factors to consider before starting prophylactic medications include frequency, severity, and lack of response or contraindications to analgesic medications. Nonpharmacologic management includes identification and avoidance of triggering factors, stress management, regular sleep and exercise, and physical therapy. Factors that can aggravate or trigger migraines include alcohol, oral contraceptives, hormonal replacement, caffeine or caffeine withdrawal, stress, changes in weather, strong scents, foods (nitrates, dairy products, chocolate, aged cheese), and fasting or missing meals.

The goal of pharmacologic treatment is to reduce the patient's disability and maintain an acceptable quality of life. The choice of abortive drug therapy depends on the severity of the patient's symptoms. A plan can be developed with the patient to use some medications for mild to moderate attacks and other medications for more severe attacks. For mild attacks, combination medicines, such as aspirin, acetaminophen, and caffeine (Excedrin or generic equivalent) are effective. For more severe headaches, the triptans are the drugs of choice (the triptans are not indicated for basilar migraines or hemiplegic migraines) (Polizzotto, 2002).

Dihydroergotamine (DHE) and other ergotamine compounds are useful. Aqueous lidocaine applied intranasally is another option. Briefly, 0.5 mL of a 4% aqueous solution of lidocaine is slowly dripped into one nostril with the patient supine, head hyperextended 45 degrees, and rotated 30 degrees toward the side affected by the headache (Maizels et al., 1996). Antiemetics, such as metoclopramide or chlorpromazine, can be used in conjunction with most abortive medications (Table 42-2).

Prophylactic treatment of migraine is recommended when headaches occur with increasing frequency and the patient may be overusing acute therapies. The daily use of symptomatic medications, including acetaminophen and nonsteroidal anti-inflammatory drugs (NSAIDs), can cause liver and kidney injury. Also, regular use of certain medications (e.g., propoxyphene, butalbital, ergotamines, triptans) can result in habituation or rebound headaches. Preventive treatment is also recommended for patients who have

Table 42-2 Symptomatic Migraine Medications

Drug Name	Dose Range	Adverse Effects
Acetaminophen, 325 mg; isometheptene, 65 mg; and dichloralphenazone, 100 mg (Midrin)	2 capsules at onset, then qh for 3 hr	Liver toxicity, dizziness
Lidocaine 4% aqueous solution for nasal spray (Xylocaine)	0.5 mL to nostrils, repeat after 2 min	None known
Ergotamine, 1 mg with caffeine, 100-mg oral tablets (Cafergot)	2 tablets, then 1 every 30 min four times	Nausea, vasoconstriction, fetal harm
Ergotamine, 2 mg with caffeine, 100-mg suppository (Cafergot)	1 rectally, up to 2 per attack	
Parenteral agents		
Dihydroergotamine, 1 mg/mL (D.H.E. 45)	0.5-1 mg IM, SC, or IV qh for 3 hr (2 hr for IV)	Nausea, vasoconstriction
Dihydroergotamine, 0.5 mg/mL (Migranal)	0.5 mg spray in each nostril, repeat in 15 min	
Ketorolac (Toradol)	15-30 mg IM or IV q6h	Gastrointestinal upset, renal toxicity
Selective Serotonin (5-HT) Agonists		
Sumatriptan (Imitrex)		
Autoinjector	6 mg qh 12 mg/day	Chest and neck discomfort
Nasal spray	5 or 20 mg q2h 40 mg/day	
Tablet	50 mg q2h 300 mg/day	
Naratriptan (Amerge)	2.5 mg q4h 5 mg/day	
Rizatriptan (Maxalt)	5 or 10 mg q2h 30 mg/day	
Zolmitriptan (Zomig)	2.5 or 5 mg q2h 10 mg/day	
Eletriptan (Relpax)	20 or 40 mg q2h 80 mg/day	
Frovatriptan (Frova)	2.5 mg q2h 7.5 mg/day	
Almotriptan (Axert)	6.25 or 12.5 mg q2h 25 mg/day	

qh, Every hour; *q2h*, every 2 hours; *IM*, intramuscularly; *SC*, subcutaneously; *IV*, intravenously; *5-HT*, 5-hydroxytryptamine.

Table 42-3 Preventive Antimigraine Therapy

Type of Drug	Dose Range	Adverse Effects
Beta-Adrenergic Blockers		
Propranolol (Inderal)	40-240 mg/day	Bronchospasm, bradycardia, hypotension, fatigue, depression
Timolol (Blocadren)	10-30 mg/day	Bronchospasm, bradycardia, hypotension, fatigue, depression
Calcium Channel Blockers		
Verapamil (Calan)	240-480 mg/day	Hypotension, constipation, edema
Tricyclic Antidepressants		
Amitriptyline (Elavil)	10-150 mg/day	Sedation, dry mouth, weight gain, tremor, cardiac arrhythmias, difficulty voiding
Nortriptyline (Pamelor)	10-150 mg/day	Sedation, dry mouth, weight gain, tremor, cardiac arrhythmias, difficulty voiding
Anticonvulsants		
Divalproex sodium (Depakote)	250-1000 mg/day	Nausea, fatigue, weigh gain, hair loss, tremor, liver toxicity, fetal harm
Gabapentin (Neurontin)	100-3600 mg/day	Fatigue
Topiramate (Topamax)	25-200 mg/day	Fatigue, paresthesias, weight loss, memory loss, nephrolithiasis
Cyproheptadine	4-16 mg/day	Drowsiness, dizziness, constipation, urinary retention

frequent attacks, often four or more, throughout the month or when headaches are so severe that acute treatment is no longer completely effective. The overall goal of preventive treatment is to reduce the frequency and severity of migraine attacks. Prophylactic agents include beta-adrenergic blockers, calcium channel blockers, selective serotonin reuptake inhibitors (SSRIs), tricyclic antidepressants (TCAs), and anticonvulsant medications (Table 42-3). Beta blockers such as propranolol have proven efficacy in this role (Polizzotto, 2002).

Tension-Type Headaches

Tension-type headaches can be episodic or chronic. There is a slight female preponderance, and the prevalence may be directly related to socioeconomic status. Chronic tension headaches can sometimes develop in migraine patients and are frequently associated with overuse of analgesics. The International Headache Society has further subdivided tension-type headaches into those with and without *pericranial tenderness* (Sarchielli, 2004). Headaches can be classified by cause, such as temporomandibular joint dysfunction, psychosocial stress, and analgesic overuse. Tension-type headaches require a comprehensive assessment to determine whether any comorbid conditions exacerbate the headache. The diagnostic criteria for episodic tension-type headaches include at least 10 previous headache episodes fulfilling the following criteria:

1. Headaches lasting for 30 minutes to 7 days, with at least two of the following pain characteristics:
    a. Pressing or tightening (nonpulsating) quality
    b. Mild or moderate intensity
    c. Bilateral location
    d. No aggravation by walking, climbing stairs, or similar routine physical activity
2. Both of the following:
    a. No nausea or vomiting
    b. Photophobia and phonophobia—both absent, or only one present

Frequently, the initial symptoms of a tension headache are described as a bandlike, squeezing, or tight pressure sensation. It is generally diffuse, often concentrated in the occipital region or in the temples. This can also be associated with depression or anxiety and aggravated by stress. No neurologic abnormalities should be noted in the history or physical examination.

A chronic tension headache requires that the pain be present for 15 days/month for more than 3 months. The other criteria are the same as those for episodic tension-type headaches.

The treatment for tension-type headaches is generally difficult. There is always the concern of analgesic abuse. Amitriptyline is frequently a reasonable drug choice, 10 to 100 mg daily. Muscle relaxants can be helpful as a short-term intervention when the pain extends into the shoulder trapezius muscles. In addition to therapeutic options, it is beneficial to use relaxation therapy, physical therapy, and stress management programs. Improvement of posture, stretching exercises, and even traction can be beneficial. On occasion, relief can be obtained with injections or occipital nerve blocks.

Medications can be used for abortive treatment and can include NSAIDs and analgesics with caffeine. The choice of medication depends on the severity and frequency of the headaches. Care needs to be used when prescribing butalbital-containing compounds, because their addiction potential is high. In addition, there is always the problem of analgesic overuse, which could lead to the development of chronic daily headaches.

Cluster Headaches

Cluster headaches are less common than migraines, and almost 80% of patients are male. Cluster headaches present with unilateral pain. Attacks may last 15 to 180 minutes and can occur every other day, up to eight times daily. The cycle may last for 4 to 12 weeks. These headaches frequently are triggered by alcohol, with some nausea. They tend to occur at a similar time during the day or night. The pain is frequently in the orbital or periorbital region. It is an extremely sharp, continuous, incapacitating pain.

The criteria for diagnosis include at least five attacks with the following elements:

1. Severe unilateral orbital or supraorbital pain lasting 15 to 180 minutes
2. Headache associated with at least one of the following ipsilateral signs in addition to the headache:
   a. Conjunctival infection
   b. Lacrimation
   c. Nasal congestion
   d. Miosis, ptosis
   e. Eye edema
   f. Forehead and facial sweating
   g. Sense of restlessness or agitation
3. Frequency from every other day to eight times a day

Cluster headaches are unusual in that they may come at certain intervals throughout the year. Headaches may last for a few weeks and then disappear, or can become chronic and persist throughout the year.

Medications for the treatment of cluster headaches include some of the same drugs used for abortive treatment for migraines: DHE, ergotamines, intranasal 4% aqueous lidocaine solution, and triptans. The nasal and injectable forms have a more rapid onset of action than the oral preparations. Cluster headaches are also unusual in that they may respond to oxygen. Inhaled 100% oxygen can relieve an attack within 10 to 15 minutes.

For headaches that are intense, do not respond to abortive treatment, or require excessive use of abortive treatment, prophylaxis is recommended. Divalproex (Depakote) can be used for the treatment of the chronic cluster headache. Doses range up to 1000 mg/day in divided doses. A pulse dose of steroids can also be effective, as can verapamil.

Medication Overuse Headaches

Headache sufferers can begin to experience daily or almost daily headaches when medication doses are excessive or too frequent. Rebound can occur with opioids, acetaminophen, aspirin, analgesic-codeine or analgesic-barbiturate combinations, NSAIDs, ergotamines, and triptans. Characteristics of rebound headaches include a diffuse, bilateral, almost daily headache, often aggravated by mild physical or mental exertion. The headache is frequently present on waking and can be associated with restlessness, nausea, forgetfulness, and depression. Tolerance develops to abortive medications, and there is decreased responsiveness to preventive medications.

Treatment of rebound headaches can be difficult. The causative medications must be identified, and there may be some psychological as well as physical dependence. The key to treatment is to discontinue the overused medication and thus break the cycle. Stopping the medication may result in withdrawal symptoms and an initial period of increased headaches, with subsequent improvement. Patients may need to be hospitalized to stop the medication. Specific limits need to be set for the use of analgesics, ergotamines, and triptans to reduce the likelihood of rebound headaches.

Miscellaneous Headaches

Episodic and chronic *paroxysmal hemicrania* is an unusual headache that tends to occur in women. The attacks are short, and the pain is similar to that of a cluster headache.

These headaches respond to indomethacin, with a maximum of 150 mg/day in divided doses.

Posttraumatic headaches can follow a head injury, with presentation similar to migraine headache. No clear correlation appears to exist between intensity of the head trauma and development of headache. These headaches may be associated with dizziness and impaired concentration. Treatment is difficult, but many of the migraine compounds are effective.

Trigeminal neuralgia is described as a piercing, sudden, severe pain that can last for seconds to minutes in the area of the cheek or jaw and can be aggravated by chewing or talking. Treatment options include carbamazepine, oxcarbazepine, baclofen, and gabapentin. Surgical intervention is an option when medical treatment fails.

Headaches in Older Adults

A serious headache that presents in the older adult population is *giant cell arteritis,* or temporal arteritis. The pain can be bitemporal or unilateral, moderate to severe in intensity, and is diffuse, not always throbbing, and persists throughout the day and often worsens at night. This headache is often associated with systemic complaints (e.g., weight loss, joint tenderness) and can be aggravated with jaw movement. It is important to treat giant cell arteritis because it can be associated with blindness. The Westergren erythrocyte sedimentation rate (ESR) is frequently elevated. If temporal arteritis is suspected, a diagnostic temporal artery biopsy is performed. It is important not to delay treatment while waiting for the biopsy. Steroid treatment can be initiated up to 2 weeks before the biopsy without compromising the results. The patient with headache of giant cell arteritis requires high doses of prednisone, usually for several months or longer.

Ophthalmic zoster is another type of head pain in the older adult. The pain is described as a burning, constant, piercing, shocklike pain. It follows the distribution of the trigeminal nerve. This is a difficult headache to treat, but it responds well to anticonvulsants, particularly carbamazepine and gabapentin.

Glaucoma can cause a migrainelike headache, with severe pain around the affected eye.

Stroke (Cerebrovascular Accident)

Key Points

- Strokes usually occur without warning, and less than 20% of CVAs are preceded by a warning TIA.
- Stroke risk factors include hypertension, smoking, atrial fibrillation, internal carotid artery stenosis, and diabetes.
- The time-related cellular death in areas of hypoperfusion requires reperfusing the ischemic penumbra.
- Both dipyridamole (plus aspirin) and clopidogrel are reasonable first-line antiplatelet agents for secondary stroke prevention.
- During the first day after an ischemic stroke, most patients with elevated blood pressure should not be treated unless systolic is consistently higher than 220 or diastolic is consistently higher than 120 mm Hg.

Cerebrovascular accident (CVA, stroke) is the third leading cause of death in the United States and the leading cause of significant disability in adults. About 750,000 new cases of stroke occur each year. Despite a decline in ischemic stroke rate (which accounts for most strokes), the absolute number of strokes in the United States continues to rise. This continued annual increase is the result of an increase in the mean age of the population. Current projections predict 1 million strokes each year in the United States by 2050. The mortality rate for CVA is about 15%, and only slightly less than one third of patients who suffer a stroke regain normal cerebral function. Furthermore, the recurrence rate for patients who survive a stroke is about 10% per year. Thus, CVA remains a major public health problem in the United States (Benavente and Hart, 1999; Hart and Benavente, 1999).

Stroke is generally defined as the rapid onset of a neurologic deficit involving a certain vascular territory that lasts longer than 24 hours. A *transient ischemic attack* (TIA) is similarly characterized by the rapid onset of a neurologic deficit, but it generally lasts for less than 24 hours, and usually for only minutes. CVAs may be of ischemic or hemorrhagic origin, whereas TIAs are generally ischemic events. Statistically, most patients have ischemic rather than hemorrhagic strokes. About two thirds of ischemic strokes are caused by thrombosis, and slightly less than one third are caused by embolus. *Ischemic* strokes result from many causes, including intracranial atherosclerosis, cervical carotid artery stenosis, and occlusive disease of the small, penetrating arteries, leading to lacunar infarcts. *Hemorrhagic* strokes are generally related to intracranial or subarachnoid hemorrhage, with intracranial hemorrhages being more common. No specific cause is identified in as many as 30% of patients with stroke; patients with cryptogenic CVA are often younger.

Strokes usually occur without warning, and less than 20% are preceded by a warning TIA. Patients with a previous TIA or CVA have a 4.5% to 6.6% annual risk for subsequent stroke. The risk for CVA after a retinal TIA (amaurosis fugax) is much lower than that after a hemispheric TIA.

Risk Factors

Hypertension

Patients with a systolic blood pressure (SBP) higher than 160 mm Hg or a diastolic blood pressure (DBP) higher than 95 mm Hg have a fourfold increased risk of stroke compared with the general population. Decreasing DBP by as little as 5 mm Hg reduces the relative risk of CVAs by 43%, and a decrease of 10 mm Hg results in a 50% relative risk reduction. Treatment of older adults with isolated SBP elevations higher than 160 mm Hg reduces their risk of stroke and is usually well tolerated if approached carefully.

Smoking

Cigarette smoking is an independent risk factor for CVA. The risk of stroke is almost twice as high for smokers, and the relative risk of subarachnoid hemorrhage is almost three times as high as for the general population.

Atrial Fibrillation

Clinical trials continue to demonstrate the benefits of warfarin for primary and secondary stroke prevention among high-risk patients with nonvalvular atrial fibrillation. The CVA risk in patients with atrial fibrillation is reduced by about two thirds when they are treated with warfarin

adjusted to achieve a target international normalized ratio (INR) of 2 or 3.

Hypercholesterolemia

The role of cholesterol reduction in stroke prevention is not clear. Large observational studies have failed to implicate increased cholesterol as an independent risk factor for CVA. Statins are effective for the primary prevention of ischemic stroke for patients with a history of occlusive arterial disease, coronary artery disease (CAD), or diabetes, without a history of cerebrovascular disease. Statins reduce the risk of ischemic stroke in hypertensive patients with multiple cardiovascular risk factors and nonfasting cholesterol levels lower than 250 mg/dL, reduce CVA risk for patients with CAD or equivalent (e.g., diabetes, peripheral artery disease), and prevent recurrent ischemic stroke in CAD patients (Busch et al., 2004). Statins have also been shown to reduce the incidence of CVA and TIA in patients without preexisting CAD (Amarenco et al., 2006).

Carotid Artery Stenosis

Patients with internal carotid artery stenosis of less than 75% have an annual risk of stroke of approximately 1.3%. In contrast, patients with internal carotid stenosis greater than 75% have annual TIA risk of 7.2% and annual CVA risk of 3.3%. Patients with asymptomatic carotid stenosis have a relatively low rate of ipsilateral stroke, probably about 2% per year (Norris et al., 1991). Select patients with asymptomatic carotid stenosis may benefit from carotid endarterectomy. The Asymptomatic Carotid Atherosclerosis Study (ACAS) showed a benefit from endarterectomy in patients with a stenosis more than 60%, although the overall benefit was relatively small (Young et al., 1996). A low perioperative complication rate is crucial if endarterectomy is to offer asymptomatic patients a beneficial option. Carotid angioplasty and stenting are emerging as viable alternatives to carotid endarterectomy but are limited to patients at high risk for endarterectomy. When used with an embolus protection device, the safety and efficacy of carotid stenting has been established and its noninferiority compared with endarterectomy has been demonstrated. When medical management is elected, it should include control of hypertension, smoking cessation, education regarding the symptoms of TIA, efforts to identify and treat existing CAD, antiplatelet therapy, statin therapy, and serial carotid ultrasound studies to monitor the progression of carotid stenosis.

The management of symptomatic carotid artery stenosis—that is, cervical carotid stenosis associated with ipsilateral focal ischemic events—is less controversial. Clinical trials consistently demonstrate the benefits of carotid endarterectomy for patients with high-grade (70%) cervical carotid stenosis who are symptomatic. Conversely, symptomatic patients with mild (<50%) carotid stenosis do not benefit from surgery. Patients with moderate stenosis obtain a moderate benefit from surgery. These patients may be appropriately treated with surgery or medical therapy, depending on the clinical judgment of the treating physicians. Physicians should remember that women have a lower incidence of subsequent stroke than men with similar degrees of carotid stenosis. Women also have higher rates of perioperative complications than men.

Diabetes

Diabetic patients who suffer stroke tend to be younger and have a higher incidence of intracerebral bleeding. There is no evidence that controlling the hyperglycemia decreases the incidence of stroke.

Acute Intervention

When oxygen deprivation occurs, neuronal cellular death occurs within minutes. Thus, in nonperfused areas of the brain, necrosis results in minutes. These areas of necrosis are typically surrounded by areas of decreased blood flow. This diminished blood flow may be barely enough to keep the neurons in these areas alive. Such areas of hypoperfusion are electrically silent and are referred to as the *ischemic penumbra*. If timely reperfusion of the ischemic penumbra occurs, these neurons can recover. However, failure to reperfuse the ischemic penumbra promptly results in time-related neuronal cell death and transformation of an area of hypoperfusion into an area of frank infarction. Resuscitation of the ischemic penumbra is therefore a primary goal of acute stroke management. Because of the time-related cellular death that occurs in areas of hypoperfusion, interventions aimed at reperfusing the ischemic penumbra must be instituted expeditiously if maximal benefit is to be realized.

Many agents and interventions have been under investigation for the treatment of acute stroke. Although therapeutic options for acute stroke management are expanding, *tissue plasminogen activator* (t-PA) is currently the only specific medication validated for this purpose by clinical trials and labeled for this use by the U.S. Food and Drug Administration (FDA). The National Institute of Neurologic Disorders and Stroke recommends t-PA for acute intervention in select stroke patients (NINDS, 1995). The t-PA trials showed substantial improvement in long-term functional outcome for patients treated with t-PA within 3 hours of ischemic stroke onset, compared with the placebo group (NINDS, 1997). For every 100 patients given t-PA, 12 more experienced complete neurologic recovery than those receiving placebo. However, there was an approximately 6% increase in intracerebral hemorrhage in t-PA recipients, not all of which are symptomatic. This risk of intracerebral hemorrhage increased significantly if computed tomography (CT) demonstrated early infarction changes. More recently, the European Cooperative Acute Stroke Study III has demonstrated that the time window for administration of t-PA can be safely and effectively extended to 4.5 hours in select patients. Those older than 80, those with a history of stroke and diabetes, those taking oral anticoagulants, and those with NIH Stroke Scale greater than 25 are excluded from this extended timeframe.

The administration of t-PA for the treatment of acute stroke requires strict adherence to established eligibility criteria, emergency CT capability with experienced interpretation, and 24-hour intensive care unit monitoring (Box 42-1). The limit from stroke onset to treatment with t-PA must be respected, whether the patient meets criteria for the 3-hour time window or the 4.5 hour time window. If a patient wakes from sleep with a neurologic deficit, the stroke must be assumed to have had its onset at the time sleep commenced. If the exact time of stroke onset is in question, t-PA should not be given. Patients and their families should understand that although treatment of acute ischemic stroke with t-PA

Box 42-1 Criteria for t-PA Use in Patients with Thromboembolic Stroke

Considering t-PA as Treatment Option

Age ≥18 years

Noncontrast CT without evidence of hemorrhage

Time since onset of symptoms clearly <3 hours (4.5 hours for select patients) before t-PA administration would begin

Excluding t-PA as Treatment Option

Historical and Clinical Findings

Clinical presentation suggests subarachnoid hemorrhage, even if CT is normal:

- Sudden, severe headache, often with loss of consciousness at onset
- Vomiting common

Active internal bleeding, increased risk of bleeding, or known bleeding diathesis, including:

- Recent use of warfarin with prolonged INR
- Use of heparin within 48 hours with prolonged aPTT
- Platelet count < 100,000 cells/mm^3
- History of intracranial hemorrhage
- Known arteriovenous malformation or aneurysm
- GI or GU bleeding in past 21 days
- Arterial puncture in past 7 days at noncompressible site

Recent lumbar puncture

Stroke, intracranial surgery, or head trauma in previous 3 months

Major surgery or serious trauma in preceding 14 days

Persistent systolic blood pressure > 185 or diastolic > 110 mm Hg

Seizure at stroke onset

Rapidly improving neurologic signs

Isolated, mild neurologic deficits

Acute myocardial infarction (MI)

Post-MI pericarditis

Blood glucose < 50 mg/dL or > 400 mg/dL

Patient pregnant or lactating

CT Findings

Evidence of intracranial hemorrhage

Hypodensity or effacement of the sulci in one third of the region of the middle cerebral artery

t-PA, Tissue plasminogen activator (alteplase [Activase]); *aPTT*, activated partial thromboplastin time; *CT*, computed tomography; *INR*, international normalized ratio; *GI*, gastrointestinal; *GU*, genitourinary.

---

is potentially beneficial, there is an approximately 1 in 15 chance of suffering a serious cerebral hemorrhage, even if t-PA is used in accordance with strict guidelines. They should also understand that although patients with severe ischemic strokes have the most to gain from t-PA, they also have a higher risk of t-PA–associated intracerebral hemorrhage. Finally, the CT must not demonstrate intracranial bleeding if t-PA is to be given, and some experts recommend withholding t-PA if the CT demonstrates evidence of early infarction.

In some referral centers, intra-arterial thrombolysis is also a treatment option. Such intervention extends the treatment window to 6 hours, principally because of the lower dose of t-PA administered and the ability to deliver the agent directly into the clot. Additionally, mechanical removal of intra-arterial thrombus is also a treatment option, using a corkscrew-like mechanism (Merci device) or a suction mechanism (Penumbra device) to extract the clot and thereby reestablish blood flow to the ischemic penumbra.

Pharmacologic Therapy

Published studies to date overwhelmingly support the ability of *aspirin* to reduce stroke incidence and death in patients who present with TIA or CVA. Aspirin and other agents that affect platelet function are frequently used for long-term secondary stroke prevention. It therefore seems reasonable, after hemorrhage has been excluded by CT, to begin aspirin therapy in the setting of acute stroke, provided the patient does not have a contraindication to aspirin therapy. Aspirin doses between 50 and 1300 mg/day have been shown to be effective for stroke prevention. In the absence of convincing evidence favoring a specific dosage, most clinicians prescribe 81 or 325 mg/day. The FDA recommends that aspirin doses of 50 to 325 mg/day be used for stroke prevention.

*Clopidogrel (*Plavix) inhibits platelet function by irreversibly binding to adenosine diphosphate receptors. Compared with aspirin, clopidogrel significantly decreases the constellation of CVA, myocardial infarction (MI), and vascular death and has a toxicity comparable with that of aspirin. Thrombotic thrombocytopenic purpura (TTP) has been reported after the initiation of clopidogrel, often within the first 2 weeks of therapy (Bennett et al., 2000).

Dipyridamole (Persantine) was widely used in combination with aspirin in the early 1980s for the prevention of stroke until critical analysis cast doubt on its efficacy. A European study found high-dose sustained-release dipyridamole plus aspirin to be superior to aspirin alone for the prevention of stroke (Diener et al., 1996). The side effects of this therapy included headache and required discontinuation in approximately 6% of patients.

Selection of the appropriate antiplatelet agent for stroke prevention can become complicated, especially for patients with comorbid cardiovascular disease. Both extended-release dipyridamole plus aspirin (Aggrenox) and clopidogrel (Plavix) are reasonable first line antiplatelet agents for secondary stroke prevention, shown to be more effective than aspirin alone. Randomized controlled trials (RCTs) have shown no additional benefit of the combination of clopidogrel and aspirin, which only increase the risk of hemorrhage.

The use of *heparin* therapy for the prevention of recurrent TIA or stroke progression is limited. Progression of CVA is common, occurring in 15% to 20% of carotid-distribution strokes and 35% to 40% of vertebrobasilar CVAs. Even in patients with angiographically minimal or absent cerebral artery occlusion, clinical worsening of neurologic findings frequently occurs. Furthermore, heparin has not been shown in adequate clinical trials to improve clinical outcome among patients with stroke. The International Stroke Trial (IST, 1997) reported that patients receiving subcutaneous heparin had fewer recurrent ischemic strokes, but this improvement was offset by an increase in hemorrhagic strokes. There was no net benefit. Trials with heparinoids have also failed to demonstrate a clear benefit and have shown an increased risk of non–central nervous system (non-CNS) bleeding. Studies have also failed to demonstrate a clear benefit for low-molecular-weight (LMW) heparin.

Box 42-2 Cardiac Conditions Substantially Associated with Embolism

Atrial fibrillation
Mitral stenosis
Mechanical cardiac valves
Recent myocardial infarction
Left ventricular thrombus, especially if mobile and protruding
Atrial myxoma
Infective endocarditis
Dilated cardiomyopathy
Marantic (nonbacterial thrombotic) endocarditis

Currently, *warfarin* (Coumadin) cannot be recommended as initial therapy for most patients with stroke of primarily cerebrovascular origin. In two large-scale RCTs of warfarin compared with aspirin in the prevention of recurrent stroke (SPIRIT, WARSS), warfarin was not superior to aspirin for patients without cardioembolic disease or operable carotid stenosis (Sacco et al., 2006). Furthermore, the hemorrhagic risk with warfarin was higher than with aspirin. In contrast to ischemic stroke, there is good evidence that warfarin is beneficial for patients with several major cardiac disorders predisposing them to embolic stroke. Box 42-2 summarizes cardiac conditions that are substantially associated with cardioembolic stroke and often warrant prophylactic therapy with warfarin. Other cardiac conditions, such as mitral valve prolapse with or without myxomatous changes, severe mitral annular calcification, and calcific aortic stenosis, have a low or uncertain risk of embolism, and warfarin therapy is generally reserved for secondary prevention.

Management of Acute Stroke

Initial Management in Emergency Department

Patients suspected of having suffered an acute stroke should be stabilized in accordance with usual emergency management, which focuses initially on basic cardiopulmonary resuscitation (CPR) and support. All patients should have a thorough but timely physical examination, looking especially for head and neck trauma and cardiovascular abnormalities, followed by neurologic evaluation, including assessment of mental status, cranial nerve function, cerebellar function, and motor and sensory function, using the NIH Stroke Scale. Initial laboratory studies should generally include determination of a complete blood count (CBC) with differential and platelet count, prothrombin time and partial thromboplastin time (PT/PTT), electrolyte, blood urea nitrogen (BUN), creatinine, and glucose levels, oxygen saturation by pulse oximetry, and a metabolic panel. Depending on the clinical history, some patients should have studies for possible altered coagulation or connective tissue diseases. A CT scan of the head should be obtained expeditiously to evaluate for hemorrhage. Most patients should have additional studies, including electrocardiography (ECG), chest radiography, echocardiography, and carotid duplex ultrasonography. Consultation with neurology, speech therapy, physical therapy, occupational therapy, and social services should be considered (Box 42-3).

Box 42-3 Initial Treatment Considerations for Stroke Patients

Provide Initial Care.

Stabilize the patient, secure the airway, and provide adequate oxygenation.

Assess level of consciousness, language, visual fields, eye movements, and pupillary movements.

Obtain history and perform physical examination.

Perform CT of head without contrast.

Obtain CBC with platelets and differential, electrolytes, creatinine, BUN, glucose, PT/PTT, and oxygen saturation.

Consider Toxicology Screen.

Consider special coagulation studies such as antiphospholipid antibodies, factor V Leiden assay, protein C and protein S, antithrombin III, ANA, fibrinogen, RPR, homocysteine, serum protein electrophoresis, prothrombin gene 20210.

Consider Acute Intervention with T-PA.

Consider the Following with Admission Orders:

Transesophageal echocardiography

Carotid duplex ultrasonography

Telemetry

Supplemental oxygen and appropriate oxygen saturation monitoring

Antiplatelet therapy

Fluid restriction if infarct is large, to reduce cerebral edema

Close monitoring of intake and output

Regular determinations of blood glucose levels to avoid hyperglycemia

NPO until there is certainty about the gag reflex pending swallowing evaluation

Elevate head of bed 20 to 30 degrees to reduce cerebral edema.

Bed rest for first 24 hours with fall precautions, then advance as appropriate.

Vital signs and neurologic checks every 2 hours × 4, then every 4 hours for 24 hr

Prophylaxis for DVT while immobile

Speech therapy consultation to evaluate swallowing

Neurology, physical therapy, occupational therapy, nutrition, and social services consultations

ANA, Antinuclear antibodies; *BUN,* blood urea nitrogen; *CBC,* complete blood count; *CT,* computed tomography; *DVT,* deep vein thrombosis; *NPO,* nothing by mouth; *PT/PTT,* prothrombin time/partial thromboplastin time; *RPR,* rapid plasma reagin; *t-PA,* tissue plasminogen activator.

Box 42-4 Antihypertensive Agents for Patients with Acute Stroke

Labetalol (Normodyne)

    10 mg intravenously (IV) over 1 to 2 minutes; may repeat or double dosage every 10 to 20 minutes until blood pressure controlled or maximum dose of 300 mg has been reached.

    100 mg orally twice daily

Nicardipine (Cardene)

    5 mg/hr IV, titrated upward as necessary, typically to a maximum of 15 mg/hr

Sodium nitroprusside (Nipride)

    0.3 µg/kg/min IV, titrated upward as necessary, typically to a maximum of 10 µg/kg/min

---

When antihypertensive agents are used shortly after CVA, one with rapid action and predictable response, such as nicardipine (Cardene), labetalol (Normodyne), or sodium nitroprusside, should be chosen (Box 42-4). Nicardipine is currently considered first-line treatment in this setting. Labetalol is preferable to sodium nitroprusside because of nitroprusside's ability to cause cerebral vasodilation, which can worsen cerebral edema in some patients. Sublingual calcium channel antagonists should be avoided because of their ability to cause precipitous BP declines, which could significantly reduce cerebral blood flow and result in further ischemic damage.

Cerebral Edema

Cerebral edema usually peaks within 2 to 4 days after a stroke. It is seldom a problem during the first 24 hours, except in cases of large cerebellar CVAs. Steroids are not used to treat cerebral edema related to thromboembolic strokes. Steroids are generally ineffective and may exacerbate hyperglycemia and raise BP. Cerebral edema related to thromboembolic stroke is first treated by raising the head of the bed 20 to 30 degrees. Hyperventilation can work rapidly to reduce *intracranial pressure* (ICP) but has only a transient effect. Mannitol can be given to lower ICP at 0.25 to 0.5 g/kg intravenously (IV) over 30 minutes, but its use is controversial because of possible pooling in the area of ischemia and potential worsening of edema. Mannitol can rapidly lower ICP and can be repeated every 6 hours. The maximum dose of mannitol is 2 g/kg IV. Hypertonic saline has also been used to reduce cerebral edema in this context. Hemicraniectomy with durotomy is performed for malignant MCA-distribution infarct in select cases and has been shown to improve survival and functional outcome.

Other Management Issues

Hypoxia should be avoided. Any circumstance that is likely to impair oxygen delivery to the ischemic penumbra needs to be avoided. Patients with acute stroke should therefore have their oxygen saturation monitored, and supplemental oxygen provided if desaturation occurs.

The use of subcutaneous heparin for the prevention of *deep venous thrombosis* (DVT) in nonhemorrhagic stroke patients has been well accepted. Heparin should be dosed based on weight. LMW heparin is a reasonable alternative in this setting. Intermittent pneumatic compression stockings are the best prophylactic alternative for patients unable to receive

Elevated Blood Pressure

During the first day after an ischemic stroke, elevated blood pressure (BP) should not be treated unless systolic is consistently higher than 220 mm Hg or diastolic is consistently higher than 120 mm Hg. There are exceptions to this recommendation. Patients who have received t-PA should have BP maintained below 185/110 mm Hg, and patients with MI, heart failure, aortic dissection, or renal failure should have more aggressive BP control. Areas of cerebral ischemia lose their normal autoregulatory capacity, and tissue perfusion becomes directly linked to mean arterial pressure. When cerebral ischemia occurs, BP elevations are often transient and spontaneous declines common. Overzealous BP treatment can therefore convert an area of ischemia that retains the potential for recovery into an area of frank infarction with no potential for recovery.

anticoagulants. Patients able to ambulate 50 feet daily are at low risk for venous thromboembolism.

Fever is seen quite often after an acute stroke. Regardless of cause, fever should be reduced, because ischemic cerebral insults accompanied by even mild elevations in body temperature have been associated with less favorable outcomes in both experimental models and clinical studies.

Hyperglycemia can be harmful for the ischemic penumbra because it permits anaerobic metabolism, which results in local generation of lactic acidosis. Serum glucose levels should generally be maintained below 150 mg/dL. Nevertheless, it should be recognized that controlling blood glucose has not been shown to improve stroke outcome in humans.

Patients who suffer a *seizure* after a stroke have a higher mortality. Some believe that such patients should receive anticonvulsant therapy indefinitely, whereas others note that a trial off medication after several years without seizure activity seems reasonable.

Delirium

Key Points

- A confused older adult patient should generally be assumed to have delirium until proved otherwise.
- Delirium is a transient, global disorder of cognition and consciousness; changes in consciousness typically develop quickly and fluctuate during the day.
- Underlying dementia is a significant risk factor for delirium.
- The history, physical examination, and test results usually suggest a cause for delirium.
- Delirium is best managed by correction of the causative disturbances.

Delirium is a common problem encountered in patients seen by family physicians, especially in the hospital or skilled nursing facility. Delirium is characterized by a change in cognition and attention that develops rapidly, usually over hours to days, and fluctuates throughout the day. It may present as *hyperactive delirium,* with agitation, disorientation, and delusions; *hypoactive delirium,* demonstrated by the lethargic patient who is difficult to arouse and engage in conversation; or a mixed-type delirium with features of both. Hypoactive delirium is the most common encountered form of delirium, which may explain why it goes unrecognized in up to 70% of patients experiencing delirium (Gillis et al., 2006). Because of this, any confused older adult patient should generally be assumed to have delirium until proved otherwise. Delirium is a serious condition that has long-term ramifications, including increased hospital length of stay, increased mortality, failure to return to baseline cognitive and functional status, and increased need for prolonged, skilled nursing facility care. Box 42-5 summarizes risk factors for the development of delirium. Two thirds of delirium cases occur in patients with underlying dementia, placing these patients at significant risk when being treated for other health problems (Cole, 2004).

The mainstay of treatment for delirium is to identify and correct the underlying cause. This cause can usually be determined through a thorough history, physical examination, and evaluation of selected laboratory tests. Box 42-6

Box 42-5 Risk Factors for Development of Delirium

Age >65 years
Chronic kidney disease
Dehydration
Dependence with activities of daily living
Hearing impairment
Infection
Malnutrition
Multiple comorbid conditions
Polypharmacy
Underlying dementia
Vision impairment

Box 42-6 Common Causes of delirium

Dehydration
Electrolyte abnormalities
Infection
Myocardial infarction
Heart failure
Neurologic disorder (stroke, seizure)
Hypoxia
Medications (anticholinergics, antihistamines, antidepressants, benzodiazepines, narcotics)
Intoxication
Environmental changes (change in location or caregiver, overstimulation)
Pain
Sleep deprivation
Surgery
Urinary catheter
Urinary retention
Fecal impaction

---

summarizes some of the common causes that should be considered. Special attention should focus on recently started medications. Although almost any medication can precipitate delirium, analgesics, antiarrhythmics, antidepressants, Parkinson's medications, and anticholinergic medications such as antihistamines, benzodiazepines, β-blockers, calcium channel blockers, steroids, diuretics, clonidine, and digoxin are common culprits. A targeted laboratory evaluation should be undertaken, including a CBC, determination of electrolytes, BUN, creatinine, glucose, calcium, magnesium, phosphate, and liver function tests (LFTs). Oxygenation should be assessed by oximetry or arterial blood gases (ABGs). ECG should be considered, especially for patients with angina, dyspnea, or a cardiac history. A chest x-ray film and urinalysis to evaluate for occult infection, especially in older-adult patients, should also be considered.

If this evaluation does not elicit a likely cause for a patient's delirium, further testing may be necessary. Additional laboratory studies to consider include thyroid function tests, human immunodeficiency virus (HIV) testing, rapid plasma reagin (RPR) test, drug levels, toxicology screening, serum ammonia level, and serum vitamin B$_{12}$ level. Lumbar puncture is usually reserved for patients with fever and signs suggesting meningitis. Neuroimaging may be indicated for patients with new neurologic signs or a history of head trauma. EEG may be helpful in the evaluation of patients with a suspected seizure disorder or to differentiate delirium from a functional psychiatric disorder.

Delirium can be treated with both nonpharmacologic and pharmacologic measures. Environmental modifications should be instituted early, before pharmacologic intervention or mechanical restraint is considered. A supportive and familiar environment should be created for the patient. Family members should be encouraged to remain nearby as much as possible. The staff should visit the patient frequently or move the patient to be near them. The room should be well illuminated, with a large, easily read clock and calendar. The family should bring familiar items from home to be placed in the patient's room. Whenever possible, normal sleep hygiene patterns should be maintained with minimal interruptions during the night hours.

Pharmacologic management of delirium should be considered when the previous treatments have failed to control agitation and should involve the use of antipsychotic medications. Among the antipsychotic agents, haloperidol (Haldol) at 1 to 2 mg orally every 4 hours as needed, or 0.25 to 0.5 mg orally every 4 hours for elderly patients, is recommended (American Psychiatric Association, 1999). Other antipsychotic medications, such as risperidone (Risperdal), 0.5 to 1 mg orally daily, and olanzapine (Zyprexa), 2.5 to 5 mg orally daily, may also be used; as yet, no RCTs have established the safety and effectiveness of one antipsychotic medication over another for the management of delirium symptoms (Seitz et al., 2007). Risperidone and olanzapine do not work as quickly as haloperidol, often require slow titration, and can be associated with significant orthostasis. More recent studies have also demonstrated a potentially elevated risk of mortality in older adults with dementia who were treated with atypical antipsychotics (Schneider et al., 2005). Therefore, these risks must be considered when initiating pharmacologic treatment for delirium. Further recommendations for initiating antipsychotics for the treatment of delirium include using the lowest possible doses, frequent reassessments to limit the duration of antipsychotic use, and a baseline ECG to rule out susceptibility to an arrhythmia from a prolonged QT interval (Seitz et al., 2007). Lorazepam (Ativan), a benzodiazepine, has also been used for the treatment of agitation associated with delirium, although a Cochrane review concluded that benzodiazepines cannot be recommended for the treatment of non-alcohol-related delirium (Lonergan et al., 2009). Physical restraints should be a last resort, reserved for the protection of patients who do not adequately respond to environmental and pharmacologic interventions.

Dementia

Key Points

- Dementia is a gradual, progressive impairment of memory and other cognitive functions that is severe enough to impact work, social activities, and relationships.
- Dementia can be divided into four categories: Alzheimer's disease (60% of cases), dementia with Lewy bodies (15%), vascular dementia (15%), and all other causes (10%).

- Comprehensive, longitudinal, well-coordinated care delivered by the family physician for both the patient and the caregiver is the cornerstone of effective management of patients with dementia.
- The cholinesterase inhibitors are effective in slowing the progression of cognitive and functional decline and may be used in conjunction with memantine (NMDA receptor antagonist) to treat moderate to severe dementia.

Dementia is characterized by the development of an acquired impairment in memory associated with impairment in one or more cognitive domains, including executive function, language (expressive or receptive), *praxis* (learned motor sequences), or *gnosis* (ability to recognize objects, faces, or other sensory information). The impairments are severe enough to interfere with work, social activities or relationships (American Psychiatric Association, 1994). The course is usually one of gradual, progressive decline and causes impairment in the ability to perform activities of daily living (ADLs). The incidence of dementia increases with age. By 75 years, 10% to 15% of people have dementia, increasing to 35% to 50% for those over 85.

Classification and Pathophysiology

Dementia is usually divided into four main categories. Dementia of Alzheimer's type accounts for approximately 60% of cases; dementia with Lewy bodies, 15%; and vascular dementia, 15%. The remaining category includes multiple other forms, including mixed dementias that exhibit components of both Alzheimer's and vascular dementia and dementias resulting from CNS trauma, Parkinson's disease, Pick's disease, Creutzfeldt-Jakob disease, and Huntington's disease.

Alzheimer's disease patients have brains that demonstrate atrophy with ventricular and sulcal enlargement. They reveal evidence of neuronal loss as well as the presence of amyloid plaques and neurofibrillary tangles. Amyloid plaques are composed of misfolded β-amyloid that initiates a pathogenic cascade resulting in neurotoxicity and nerve cell death.

Dementia with Lewy bodies is similar to Alzheimer's disease, but visual hallucinations and motor symptoms similar to parkinsonism develop early in the course of the disease. Histologically, Lewy bodies are present, cytoplasmic inclusions found in the temporal, parietal, and paralimbic regions of the brain.

Vascular dementia is usually subdivided into multi-infarct dementia and subcortical vascular dementia. *Multi-infarct dementia* should be suspected when focal, asymmetric neurologic abnormalities accompany dementia. Neuroimaging may show multiple strokes. *Subcortical vascular dementia* should be suspected if the patient manifests significant problems with gait early in the course of the dementia. The CT or magnetic resonance imaging (MRI) scan is usually normal in these patients, except for increased signal in the deep white matter, a nonspecific sign.

Evaluation

The diagnosis of dementia is still made clinically, so evaluation of a patient with suspected dementia begins with a complete history and physical examination. The history should include questions regarding the time frame surrounding symptom progression. The relation to any recent vascular events such as stroke should be noted. Risk factors for vascular disease (hypertension, diabetes, hyperlipidemia, atrial fibrillation, smoking history) should be reviewed. Changes in the ability to perform ADLs should also be addressed. The patient's ability to perform dressing, eating, ambulating, toileting, and bathing tasks should be recorded as independent, requiring assistance, or dependent. The physical examination should include a thorough neurologic examination for signs of underlying vascular disease and stoke. Cognitive testing should be done, ideally with the Mini–Mental State Examination, which allows for quantification of cognitive impairment over time (Table 42-4). A score less than 24 is considered abnormal, but because of educational bias, highly educated patients may have inflated scores and those with limited education artificially low scores (Tombaugh, 1992).

When considering which tests to perform as part of the evaluation of a patient with dementia, physicians have traditionally been taught to search for reversible causes of dementia. It is now recognized that reversible dementia rarely occurs (Sloane, 1998). Current recommendations for laboratory testing generally recommend that all patients be evaluated with a CBC, thyroid-stimulating hormone (TSH), serum calcium, electrolytes, and fasting glucose, as well as a serum B_{12} level. Selective testing based on the presenting medical history, physical examination, and cognitive testing may include a red blood cell (RBC) folate level, RPR for syphilis screening, and HIV antibodies. Testing for

homocysteine levels and genetic testing for apolipoprotein E gene is not recommended (Feldman, 2008). Although neuroimaging is not recommended for all patients in the workup of dementia, selective use of CT or MRI is recommended for patients with suspected tumor, subdural hematoma, or normal-pressure hydrocephalus (NPH) (Feldman et al., 2008).

Management

Comprehensive, longitudinal, well-coordinated care delivered by the family physician for both the patient and the caregiver is the cornerstone of effective management of patients with dementia. Patients should be seen regularly in the office, and the physician should be readily available by telephone. The family should maintain frequent contact with the patient and physician. The family physician should update vaccinations, monitor visual acuity and hearing, and address other appropriate health issues. Families should be counseled regarding behavioral and environmental modifications that may be helpful, including reducing hazards in the home for falls and injuries. A discussion regarding the timing of cessation of driving should be undertaken early in the course of treatment. Decisions regarding advanced directives and planning for the later stages of the disease should begin early in the process as well. The patient should legally designate a durable power of attorney for health care. The discussion of the placement of feeding tubes should begin before difficulties with feeding develop. Families should be aware that feeding tubes do not prolong life, are associated with discomfort and medical complications, and are generally not recommended for patients in the final stages of a dementing illness (Li, 2002). The role of palliative care and hospice care should also be discussed early in the course of the illness, when the patient has the opportunity to participate in the decision-making process.

Pharmacotherapy

The cholinesterase inhibitors donepezil (Aricept), galantamine (Razadyne), and rivastigmine (Exelon) have received FDA approval for the treatment of patients with Alzheimer's disease. Tacrine (Cognex), which is associated with elevated liver transaminase levels in about 30% of patients, is rarely used. The cholinesterase inhibitors act by blocking acetylcholinesterase breakdown of acetylcholine, believed to increase acetylcholine in affected areas of the brain. All these agents show comparable response rates, and choice is therefore individualized according to patient and caregiver needs as well as the drug's side effect profile. Pharmacologic effectiveness is measured by a slowing of the decline in cognitive and global functioning over 6 to 12 months. The cholinesterase inhibitors are generally well tolerated, although side effects include nausea, vomiting, diarrhea, dyspepsia, anorexia, weight loss, bradycardia, and agitation. When these medicines are discontinued, the patient may experience a rapid decline in global functioning.

Another medication, memantine (Namenda), an N-methyl-D-aspartate (NMDA) receptor antagonist, has been FDA approved for the treatment of moderate to severe dementia as monotherapy or in combination with a cholinesterase inhibitor (Reisberg, 2003). Memantine appears to have fewer

Table 42-4 Mini–Mental Status Examination

Max Score*	Task
5	Orientation: Year, season, date, day, and month.
5	Orientation: State, county, town, building, and floor (as applicable)
3	Registration: Name three objects. Record the number of trials required to learn.
5	Attention and calculation: Serial 7 subtraction: Subtract from 100 by 7 (stop after 5 answers) or Spell the word "world" backward (score number of correct letters in correct location).
3	Recall: Recall the three objects registered above.
2	Language: Name two objects (pencil and watch).
1	Repeat "No ifs, ands, or buts."
3	Follow a three-step command.
1	Read and obey: "Close your eyes" written in print large enough for patient to see clearly.
1	Write a sentence.
1	Copy a picture of intersecting pentagons.

Modified from Folstein MF, Folstein SE, McHugh PR. Mini–Mental State: a practical method for grading the cognitive state of patients for the clinician. J Psychiatr Res 1975;12:189.
*Total possible score: 30.

side effects than the cholinesterase inhibitors, although dizziness, insomnia, and hallucination may be seen. Alternative agents such as *Ginkgo biloba*, nicotine, vitamin C, and vitamin E could be beneficial in the treatment of Alzheimer's disease. At present, however, no other prescribed medication, supplement, or herbal preparation can be recommended for the cognitive or functional manifestations of dementia (Hogan et al., 2008).

Seizures

Key Points

- Febrile seizures usually occur between age 3 months and 5 years and represent the most common convulsive disorder of young children (2%-5%).
- Risk factors for a first febrile seizure include family history, developmental delays, high fever, and child care attendance.

One in 11 Americans who lives to the age of 80 years experiences at least one seizure. About 1% of the U.S. population have epilepsy or recurrent unprovoked seizures. Treatment of patients with epilepsy reduces the risk of recurrent seizures while optimizing quality of life. This requires minimizing the adverse effects of antiepileptic medications and maximizing the patient's ability to engage in normal activities and responsibilities (Scheuer and Pedley, 1990).

Seizures are a manifestation of disturbed neurologic function and therefore often associated with acute neurologic disorders such as meningitis. In some patients the seizures are self-limited and resolve when an acute neurologic disturbance resolves. In others the seizures persist and result in a diagnosis of epilepsy. Some patients who appear medically and neurologically normal after appropriate evaluation may experience a single seizure and the cause never determined. Such patients do not have epilepsy.

Seizures are typically classified as partial or generalized. *Partial*, or *focal*, seizures arise in a portion of one cerebral hemisphere and are accompanied by focal EEG abnormalities, whereas *generalized* seizures appear to involve simultaneously all or large parts of both cerebral hemispheres from their onset. Partial seizures are subclassified according to whether consciousness is preserved (simple partial seizures) or impaired (complex partial seizures). Generalized seizures are subclassified by their associated patterns of convulsive movements (Box 42-7).

It is not always possible to classify accurately a seizure based exclusively on clinical observations. A seizure with generalized convulsive activity may have a focal onset with rapid generalization. Such a seizure would best be classified as a partial seizure with secondary generalization, rather than as a generalized tonic-clonic seizure. Accurate classification of such a seizure could not be accomplished, however, without EEG. Also, not every paroxysmal event that appears to be a seizure is a seizure. Movement disorders, psychological disorders, and sleep disorders can produce activity that is similar to seizure activity. Thus, accurate seizure diagnosis often requires both clinical observation and corroborative EEG. Because EEG is usually done in the absence of seizures, certain steps should be taken to increase its diagnostic yield. Both sleep and sleep deprivation increase the likelihood of recording epileptiform abnormalities by EEG. Obtaining multiple recordings can also increase the diagnostic yield. In some cases, accurate diagnosis can be accomplished only with continuous video and EEG monitoring. A small number of patients with seizure disorders have normal interictal EEG recordings, despite efforts made to record epileptiform abnormalities.

Febrile Seizures

Febrile seizures are seizures without a definite cause that are associated with fever. Febrile seizures, by definition, do not include seizures occurring in patients with an intracranial infection, such as meningitis or encephalitis, toxic encephalopathy, or any other neurologic illness. The definition also excludes seizures associated with fever that occur in patients who have a history of a previous nonfebrile seizure. Febrile seizures usually occur in children between the ages of 3 months and 5 years and represent the most common convulsive disorder of young children, affecting 2% to 5% of U.S. children. The most common age of onset is in the second year of life, and boys are affected slightly more often than girls (Freeman and Vining, 1995; Hirtz, 1997).

Risk factors for a first febrile seizure include a family history of febrile seizures, developmental delays, very high fever, and child care attendance. Approximately one third of children who experience a first febrile seizure will experience at least one more. The younger the child when the first febrile seizure occurs, the more likely the child is to have another febrile seizure. Most recurrences occur within 1 year. A family history of febrile seizures also increases the likelihood of recurrence. Fortunately, less than 5% of children who experience a febrile seizure develop epilepsy.

Febrile seizures can be of any type, but are most often tonic-clonic. Febrile seizures are usually shorter than 6 minutes, and fewer than 8% last longer than 15 minutes. Most children therefore do not come to the attention of the family physician until after the seizure is over. Although it is commonly believed that the rate of fever increase is an important factor in the development of febrile seizures, no data support this as being more important than fever severity.

Box 42-7 Seizure Classification

Partial Seizures

Simple (consciousness is preserved)

Complex (consciousness is impaired)

Secondarily generalized

    Simple partial seizures evolving to generalized tonic-clonic

    Complex partial seizures evolving to generalized tonic-clonic

    Simple partial seizures evolving to complex partial, then to generalized tonic-clonic

Generalized Seizures

Tonic-clonic

Absence

Atypical absence

Myoclonic

Tonic

Atonic

The evaluation of a child who has had a febrile seizure should begin with a careful history and physical examination. The history should include symptoms of infection, medication use, toxic ingestions, developmental and health problems, prenatal/birth and family history, and detailed description of the seizure by witnesses. The physical examination should pay particular attention to signs of severe illness, including petechiae, meningismus, tense or bulging fontanelle, Kernig's and Brudzinski's signs, and signs of neurologic abnormality, including decreased alertness or cognition and deficits of motor strength or tone. Even in children with a previous history of febrile seizures, a seizure associated with fever may be a sign of an intracranial infection. If intracranial infection is suspected, a *lumbar puncture* (LP) should be performed. Otherwise, LP is not necessary. Children older than 18 months who have meningitis or encephalitis usually demonstrate typical clinical signs and symptoms. Many of these children lack histories, symptoms, or signs suggesting meningitis and thus do not require LP. However, children younger than 12 to 18 months may lack the typical clinical signs and symptoms of intracranial infection and are more likely to require LP. If a child is already taking antibiotics and experiences a seizure associated with fever, partially treated meningitis should be considered. The presence of a source of infection, such as otitis media, does not exclude the possibility of meningitis. Other features in the history that should also raise suspicion of meningitis in children with seizures and fever include evaluation for illness by a physician within the past 48 hours, a seizure that occurs in the office or emergency department (ED), or a focal seizure.

Most children with febrile seizures do not require routine laboratory testing. The only laboratory studies needed are those that will assist in evaluating the source of the child's fever. Radiography of the skull, neuroimaging studies such as CT and MRI, and EEG are not usually indicated. Children who are diagnosed with a febrile seizure should be observed in the ED or physician's office for several hours. These children may then be sent home, provided (1) they demonstrate satisfactory clinical improvement and are alert, (2) their fever has been appropriately evaluated and treated, and (3) close outpatient follow-up is possible. If there is any question about intracranial infection, if a child does not demonstrate expected clinical improvement during observation, or if follow-up cannot be ensured, hospital admission is recommended.

One of the most important components of outpatient management of children with febrile seizures is education of the parents. Seizures are frightening events for most parents. They should be reassured that febrile seizures do not result in brain damage and that the risk of epilepsy is very low. Slightly more than one in six children, however, experience another seizure within 24 hours, and about one in three experiences another febrile seizure at some point. If another seizure occurs, parents should be advised to place the child on his or her side or face down on the abdomen. Contrary to common belief, they should not attempt to place anything between the child's teeth during a seizure. The parents should carefully observe the child, and if the seizure does not spontaneously resolve after 10 minutes, they should call 9-1-1. Parents may have concerns about routine vaccinations for children with a history of febrile seizures. The diphtheria and tetanus toxoids and pertussis (DTP) and measles, mumps, and rubella (MMR) vaccinations are most likely to produce fever associated with seizure. If a febrile seizure is going to occur after vaccination, it is most likely to occur within 48 hours of the DTP vaccination or within 10 days of the MMR vaccination.

Initial Diagnostic Evaluation of a First Seizure in Adults

A careful history and physical examination, along with routine blood work, can detect many medical problems that may be associated with seizures. Such problems include infection, electrolyte and glucose abnormalities, impaired hepatic or renal function, and cardiopulmonary disease. Most patients with new-onset seizures should have a CBC with platelet count and differential, toxicology screen, thyroid function testing, PT/PTT, determination of serum transaminase, electrolyte, calcium, magnesium, phosphorus, BUN, creatinine, glucose, ABGs, or pulse oximetry. If cardiopulmonary disease is suspected, ECG and chest radiograph should be obtained. Meningitis or encephalitis suspected clinically indicates LP, which is otherwise not necessary. Patients usually recover rapidly after a first seizure, and their clinical progress can be gauged after several hours of observation. Hospitalization is not usually necessary after a first seizure unless an underlying illness is suspected or there are concerns about the patient's clinical progress, inadequate social support or observation, or patient's ability or motivation to complete outpatient follow-up.

Patients with new-onset seizures should be scheduled for appropriate EEG and neuroimaging studies. MRI and CT are important complements to EEG because of their ability to identify structural abnormalities that may be related to the development of seizures. MRI is preferable to CT because of its superior ability to identify cortical architectural abnormalities, visualize the temporal lobes, detect gliomas, and identify cavernous malformations. CT, however, is appropriate in the emergency setting because it is readily available and can detect hemorrhages acutely. If the patient is seen in the office shortly after a first seizure, neuroimaging does not need to be performed immediately unless the history and physical examination suggest focal brain injury or marked cognitive impairment. In contrast to MRI and CT, positron emission tomography (PET) and single-photon emission CT (SPECT) can provide functional views of the brain. These studies can identify areas of relative hypoperfusion or hypometabolism that appear to be structurally normal but might play an important role in the development of partial seizures. Although such studies can be useful, especially for patients with conditions such as localization-related epilepsy, they are not routinely obtained or widely available.

Pharmacologic Therapy

Whether antiepileptic drug therapy should be initiated after a first seizure remains a topic of debate. The data regarding the likelihood of recurrent seizures after a first seizure are wanting or questionable, and estimates of the rate of recurrence after a single unprovoked seizure range widely. Certain findings and characteristics do seem to increase the likelihood of recurrence after a first seizure, including EEG abnormalities, previous neurologic injury, partial seizures, and a family history of seizures. Also, it is not known whether antiepileptic pharmacologic therapy following a single seizure alters the subsequent risk of epilepsy. Because of these uncertainties and because antiepileptic pharmacologic therapy is associated with a significant incidence of adverse effects, often exceeding the risk of recurrent seizures, many family physicians elect not to prescribe antiepileptic medications for most patients after a single seizure.

Although many agents are available for the treatment of seizures, carbamazepine (Tegretol), phenytoin (Dilantin), phenobarbital, and divalproex (Depakote) have been traditional first-line therapies for most patients with epilepsy. Increasing availability of newer agents to treat seizures has often resulted in more favorable side effect profiles. Phenobarbital is the oldest agent but has certain disadvantages. Its adverse effects include irritability, decreased cognition, and hyperactivity or lethargy. The degree of sedation and cognitive effects produced at therapeutic dosages are frequently significant enough that many family physicians do not prescribe phenobarbital as a first-line agent. The recommended dosage for common antiepileptics and adverse effects are summarized in Table 42-5. Most patients with epilepsy can achieve remission with the use of a single medication. Because the addition of another antiepileptic agent is usually associated with an increase in adverse drug effects, patients not controlled with one agent should be given a trial of a different agent rather than combining agents early in the course of treatment. Treatment with more than one agent is usually attempted only after a number of trials of monotherapy have failed.

Family physicians should exercise caution when measuring levels of antiepileptic drugs. Therapeutic ranges for most antiepileptics are only guidelines for treatment. Some patients achieve therapeutic remission without significant side effects with drug concentrations ordinarily toxic. Other patients develop intolerable side effects with subtherapeutic serum levels. Serum levels of most antiepileptic drugs should generally be determined when remission of seizures is achieved or the patient develops significant side effects. Drug concentrations can also provide evidence of compliance. More frequent serum testing is necessary for patients taking more than one agent, pregnant women, older adults, patients with hepatic or renal dysfunction, and patients taking medications for other medical problems. Box 42-8 lists drugs used to treat other medical conditions that can lower the seizure threshold. Nevertheless, serum levels should not be the primary basis for decisions regarding antiepileptic drug dosing. Seizure control and the development of adverse effects related to drug therapy are more important than serum levels alone.

Status Epilepticus

Status epilepticus is generally defined as more than 30 minutes of unconsciousness and continuous or intermittent, generalized seizure activity. However, because most seizures last 2 minutes or less, any seizure longer than 5 minutes may progress to status epilepticus. Patients with recurrent seizures without recovery to wakefulness should also be considered to be in status epilepticus. Status epilepticus can be alarming to observe, even for experienced clinicians. A systematic approach to patients in status epilepticus can facilitate

optimal patient care during such an episode. The first step in the management of patients with status epilepticus is to support vital functions. The airway should be protected. Although the patient should be intubated if necessary, this usually requires neuromuscular blockade, and bag and mask ventilation is often preferable. The patient's vital signs should be closely monitored, including continuous oximetry and ECG. Supplemental oxygen at a rate of about 4 L/min is recommended. Intravenous access should be secured for the administration of parenteral medications and blood drawn for a CBC, toxicology screen, and determination of electrolyte, glucose, calcium, magnesium, and anticonvulsant drug levels. The patient should receive thiamine, 100 mg IV, followed by 50 mL of D50W.

If the patient continues to seize, parenteral agents may be given, including lorazepam, 0.1 mg/kg IV at 2 mg/min, or diazepam, 0.2 mg/kg (max 10 mg) at a maximum rate of 5 mg/min. These agents have a relatively rapid onset and short duration of action. Simultaneous loading with phenytoin is therefore recommended. Phenytoin is loaded at 20 mg/kg IV at a rate of less than 50 mg/min through a line infusing glucose-free saline, to avoid precipitation of phenytoin in the line. Fosphenytoin (Cerebyx) is the prodrug of phenytoin and has a more favorable safety profile compared with phenytoin, can be given at a faster rate (150 mg/min), and converts to phenytoin after first-pass metabolism, but it is more costly than phenytoin. Blood pressure and cardiac rhythm must be closely observed because of the ability of phenytoin to precipitate hypotension and heart block. If these side effects appear, they often resolve when the rate of administration is decreased. If seizures continue despite these measures, phenobarbital may be administered parenterally. As a last resort, barbiturate coma or general anesthesia can be instituted. Propofol (Diprivan) and midazolam (Versed) administered as continuous IV drips are often used in neurocritical care settings to induce coma for status epilepticus.

Central Nervous System Infection and Inflammation

Key Points

- Bacterial meningitis is a neurologic emergency.
- Acute bacterial meningitis has a high morbidity and mortality.
- Antibiotic therapy should be started as soon as possible after meningitis is considered likely, usually by CSF analysis.
- Knowing the most prevalent organisms that cause bacterial meningitis in different age groups is important in guiding therapy.
- Gram stain of CSF is recommended for all patients with suspected bacterial meningitis.
- Adjunctive dexamethasone therapy for infants, children, and adults who have already received antibiotics is not recommended.

Bacterial Meningitis

Acute bacterial meningitis has a high morbidity and mortality rate, even under the best circumstances. For this reason, prompt recognition of the clinical syndrome, performance of appropriate testing to confirm the diagnosis, and initiation of appropriate therapy are essential.

Table 42-5 Common Antiepileptic Agents

Agent	Usual Dosage	Adverse Effects
Carbamazepine (Tegretol)	Start: 3 mg/kg/day (adults), 5 mg/kg/day (children) Maintenance: 5-20 mg/kg/day (adults), 20-40 mg/kg/day (children) Usually divided qid	Drowsiness or agitation, diplopia and blurred vision, disequilibrium, benign leukopenia, hepatic failure, rare SIADH, rare aplastic anemia
Phenytoin (Dilantin)	Start: 4-6 mg/kg/day (adults), 3-10 mg/kg/day (children) Maintenance: same Usually divided tid	Dose related: nausea and vomiting, nystagmus, ataxia Not dose related: gingival hyperplasia, hirsutism, acne, coarsening of features, hepatic failure, osteomalacia
Divalproex (Depakote)	Start: 10-15 mg/kg/day Maintenance: 15-30 mg/kg/day Usually divided bid-qid	Transient GI side effects Toxic effects: tremor, thrombocytopenia Side effects: weight increase, alopecia, hepatotoxicity (controversial whether LFTs detect in time to avoid), pancreatitis
Phenobarbital	Starting and maintenance: 1-3 mg/kg/day (adults) and -5 mg/kg/day (children) Usually given in single or divided doses	Lethargy, sedation, decreased cognition, decreased attention, hyperactivity, depression
Levetiracetam (Keppra)	Start: 1000 mg/kg/day (adults), 20 mg/kg/day (children) Maintenance: max 3000 mg/day (adults), 60 mg/kg/day (children) Usually divided bid	Depression, hostility, aggressive behavior, psychosis, somnolence, headache, URI symptoms, infection, fatigue, irritability
Oxcarbazepine (Trileptal)	Start: 600 mg/day (adults), 16 mg/kg/day (children) Maintenance: max 2400 mg/day (adults), 60 mg/kg/day (children) Usually divided bid	Hyponatremia, hypersensitivity reaction, leukopenia, thrombocytopenia, angioedema, Stevens-Johnson syndrome, dizziness, somnolence, diplopia, headache, nausea, ataxia
Lamotrigine (Lamictal)	Start: dosing varies with concomitant anti-epileptics Maintenance: max 400 mg/day Usually divided bid	Rash, Stevens-Johnson syndrome, angioedema, neutropenia, pancreatitis, dizziness, headache, ataxia, nausea, somnolence
Tiagabine (Gabitril)	Start: 4 mg/day (adults/children >12 yr) Maintenance: max 56 mg/day Usually divided bid-qid	CNS depression, seizures, weakness, rash, dizziness, asthenia, somnolence, nausea, diarrhea, tremor, confusion, impaired concentration
Gabapentin (Neurontin)	Start: 300 mg/day (adults), 10 mg/kg/day (children) Maintenance: up to 3600 mg/day (adults), 50 mg/kg/day (children) Usually divided tid	Leukopenia, depression, dizziness, somnolence, ataxia, fatigue, peripheral edema, weight gain, tremor, diarrhea
Pregabalin (Lyrica)	Start: 150 mg/day (adults) Maintenance: up to 300 mg/day Usually divided bid-tid	Thrombocytopenia, hypersensitivity reaction, angioedema, dizziness, somnolence, ataxia, peripheral edema, weight gain
Lacosamide (Vimpat)	Start: 100 mg/day (adults) Maintenance: up to 400 mg/day Usually divided bid	Syncope, atrial fibrillation (rare), dizziness, headache, diplopia, vomiting, fatigue, ataxia
Rufinamide (Banzel)	Start: (Lennox-Gastaut) 10 mg/kg/day (children) Maintenance: 45 mg/kg/day Usually divided bid	Suicidality, seizures, QT shortening, hypersensitivity reaction, leucopenia, somnolence, vomiting, headache, dizziness, nausea
Vigabatrin (Sabril)	Start: (infantile spasms) 50 mg/kg/day (children) Maintenance: up to 150 mg/kg/day Usually divided bid	(Restricted in U.S.) permanent vision loss, anemia, neuropathy, headache, dizziness, fatigue, somnolence, weight gain

LFTs, Liver function tests; *SIADH,* syndrome of inappropriate secretion of antidiuretic hormone; *URI,* upper respiratory infection; *CNS,* central nervous system; *bid,* twice daily; *tid,* three times daily; *qid,* four times daily.

Most adult patients (85%) present with the classic triad of fever, headache, and neck stiffness (Roos et al., 1997). Other symptoms include nausea and vomiting (35%), seizures (30%), cranial nerve palsies, and other focal neurologic signs (10%-20%). Meningismus (50%) may be subtle or marked, as with Kernig's sign (resistance to knee extension after flexion of hip and knees by examiner) or Brudzinski's sign (involuntary flexion of knees in supine patient in response to rapid neck flexion by examiner) (Tunkel and Scheld, 1997). Other symptoms include nuchal rigidity, lethargy, photophobia, confusion, sweats, and rigors. Papilledema occurs in less than 1% of patients during the early phases of the disease. When papilledema is present early, an alternative diagnosis such as a brain abscess or mass lesion should be sought.

Box 42-8 Drugs that Can Lower Seizure Threshold

Theophylline
Isoniazid
Tricyclic antidepressants
Penicillin
Phenothiazines
Diphenhydramine
Pseudoephedrine
Cocaine
Amphetamines
Alcohol (withdrawal)
Benzodiazepines
Barbiturates (including phenobarbital)

Table 42-6 Common Pathogens of Bacterial Meningitis Based on Age

Age	Pathogens
0-1 mo	Group B streptococcus, *Listeria monocytogenes, Escherichia coli, Streptococcus pneumoniae*
1-3 mo	Group B streptococcus, *E. coli, L. monocytogenes, S. pneumoniae, Neisseria meningitidis, Haemophilus influenza*
3 mo-18 yr	*H. influenzae, N. meningitidis, S. pneumoniae*
18-50 yr	*H. influenzae, N. meningitidis, S. pneumoniae*
>50 yr	*S. pneumoniae, L. monocytogenes, gram-negative bacilli*

Not all patients present with the classic signs and symptoms. Neonates may present with poor feeding or weak sucking response, irritability, vomiting, temperature instability (hyperthermia or hypothermia), diarrhea, and apnea. Nuchal rigidity and meningismus are not reliable signs in children younger than 1 year (Prober, 1996). A bulging fontanelle may occur late in the disease, and seizures occur in 40% of neonates. A maculopapular rash that later becomes petechial and purpuric on the extremities should suggest meningococcal meningitis. Older-adult patients may have a more insidious presentation, with variable meningeal signs, change in mental status, lethargy, obtundation, and no fever.

The host is an important determinant of susceptibility to meningitis. Obvious risk factors include a history of recent open trauma, surgery (especially neurosurgery), and burns. Closed-head trauma can cause cerebrospinal fluid (CSF) leaks, which have been associated with pneumococcal meningitis. Common predisposing factors include otitis media (most common), sinusitis, mastoiditis, alcoholism, perinatal exposure, and nonimmunized, immunocompromised, or asplenic status (Swartz, 1997).

Knowing the most prevalent organisms that cause bacterial meningitis in the various age groups is important in guiding empiric therapeutic choices (Table 42-6). The three most common pathogens for community-acquired bacterial meningitis are *Haemophilus influenzae, Neisseria meningitidis,* and *Streptococcus pneumoniae,* accounting for about 80% of cases in the United States. Until the development of the *H. influenzae* type b (Hib) vaccine in the early 1990s, this was the most common bacterial meningitis, occurring in almost 50% of cases. As a result, *S. pneumoniae* and *N. meningitidis* have become relatively more common, especially in the pediatric population. *Escherichia coli* has been superseded by group B streptococci as the most common cause in infants during the first months of life. Other common pathogens include *Listeria monocytogenes, Klebsiella pneumoniae, Staphylococcus aureus* and *S. epidermidis,* other gram-negative bacilli, and other streptococci.

Initial Management

The Infectious Disease Society of America (IDSA) practice guidelines call for prompt blood cultures and lumbar puncture for most patients with suspected acute bacterial meningitis (Tunkel et al., 2004). Nevertheless, emergency LP may not be successful or prudent because of overriding

Table 42-7 Criteria for Adult Patients with Suspected Bacterial Meningitis Recommended for CT before LP

Criterion	Comment
Immunocompromised state	HIV infection or AIDS, receiving immunosuppressive therapy, or after transplantation
History of CNS disease	Mass lesion, stroke, or focal infection
New-onset seizure	Within 1 week of presentation; some authorities would not perform LP on patients with prolonged seizures or would delay LP for 30 minutes in patients with short, convulsive seizures.
Papilledema	Presence of venous pulsations suggests absence of increased intracranial pressure.
Abnormal level of consciousness	—
Focal neurologic deficit	Includes dilated nonreactive pupil, abnormalities of ocular motility, abnormal visual fields, gaze palsy, arm or leg drift.

From Tunkel AR, Barry J, Hartman SL, et al. Practice guidelines for the management of bacterial meningitis. Clin Infect Dis 2004;39:1267.
CT, Computed tomography; *LP,* lumbar puncture; *HIV,* human immunodeficiency virus; *AIDS,* acquired immunodeficiency syndrome; *CNS,* central nervous system.

concerns about a CNS mass lesion or other cause of increased ICP, necessitating CT before LP. In these patients, blood samples should be drawn and appropriate antibiotic and adjunctive therapy provided before LP or CT (Table 42-7).

The LP is the foundation of the diagnosis of bacterial meningitis. In adults, opening pressure is typically 200 to 500 mm H_2O, although lower values may be observed in infants and children. Table 42-8 illustrates typical CSF findings. Gram stain is recommended for all patients, because it permits rapid organism identification in 60% to 90% of patients with community-acquired bacterial meningitis, with a specificity of more than 97% (Tunkel et al., 2004). Other rapid diagnostic tests, such as latex agglutination, and limulus lysate assay have not shown clinical usefulness in diagnosis

Table 42-8 Typical Cerebrospinal Fluid Findings in Bacterial and Viral Meningitides

Parameter	Bacterial Meningitis	Viral Meningitis
Opening pressure (mm H$_2$O)	>180	Often normal or significantly elevated
Leukocyte count (cells/mm^3)	1000-10,000 Median: 1195 Range: 100-20,000	<300 Median: 100 Range: 100-1000
Neutrophils (%)	>80	<20
Glucose (mg/dL)	<40	>40
Protein (mg/dL)	100-500	Often normal
Gram stain (% positive)	60-90	Negative
Culture (% positive)	70-85	50

Table 42-9 Antimicrobial Therapy in Adult Patients with Presumptive Pathogen Identification by Positive Gram Stain

Microorganism	Recommended Therapy	Alternative Therapies
Streptococcus pneumoniae	Vancomycin *plus* third-generation cephalosporin* †	Meropenem (C), fluoroquinolone‡ (B)
Neisseria meningitidis	Third-generation cephalosporin*	Penicillin G, ampicillin, chloramphenicol, fluoroquinolone, aztreonam
Listeria monocytogenes	Ampicillin§ *or* penicillin G§	TMP-SMP, meropenem (B)
Streptococcus agalactiae	Ampicillin§ *or* penicillin G§	Third-generation cephalosporin*(B)
Haemophilus influenzae	Third-generation cephalosporin*	Chloramphenicol, cefepime meropenem, fluoroquinolone
Escherichia coli	Third-generation cephalosporin*	Cefepime, meropenem, aztreonam, fluoroquinolone, TMP-SMP

Modified from Tunkel AR, Barry J, Hartman SL, et al: Practice guidelines for the management of bacterial meningitis. Clin Infect Dis 39,1267, 2004.
Note: All recommendations are (A) unless otherwise indicated. In children, ampicillin is added to the standard therapeutic regimen of cefotaxime or ceftriaxone plus vancomycin when *L. monocytogenes* is considered and to an aminoglycoside if a gram-negative enteric pathogen is of concern.
*Ceftriaxone or cefotaxime.
†Some experts would add rifampin if dexamethasone is also given (B).
‡Gatifloxacin or moxifloxacin.
§Addition of an aminoglycoside should be considered.
TMP-SMP, trimethoprim-sulfamethoxazole.

or management of bacterial meningitis. Polymerase chain reaction (PCR) assay to amplify DNA may be helpful, particularly for patients with negative Gram stains. The serum C-reactive protein (CRP) concentration may be particularly helpful for patients with findings consistent with meningitis, but for whom the Gram stain is negative and withholding antibiotics is being contemplated, because a normal CRP has a high negative predictive value (Tunkel et al., 2004).

Additional laboratory studies include CBC, platelet count, PT, PTT, ABGs, and determination of electrolyte, protein, glucose, BUN, and creatinine levels. Further laboratory workup and imaging studies (chest film, sinus series, skull films) may be indicated, depending on the clinical setting.

Bacterial meningitis is a neurologic emergency. Accordingly, antibiotic therapy should be started as soon as possible after the diagnosis is considered likely, usually once the diagnosis has been established by CSF analysis. Antibiotic therapy is generally targeted by the results of the Gram stain (Table 42-9), or may be chosen empirically based on age and predisposing conditions (Table 42-10). Table 42-11 outlines recommendations for specific antimicrobial therapy based on isolates and susceptibility, and Table 42-12 recommends doses.

Role of Corticosteroids

The theoretic goal of using corticosteroids in bacterial meningitis is to minimize meningeal inflammation, thereby decreasing the severity and incidence of brain injury. However, IDSA recommends adjunctive dexamethasone therapy in certain patients based on age.

Neonates

There are currently insufficient data to make recommendations involving newborns (Tunkel et al., 2004).

Infants and Children

Available evidence supports the use of adjunctive dexamethasone in infants and children with *H. influenzae* type b meningitis initiated 10 to 20 minutes before (or at least concomitant with) the first doses of antibiotic at a dose of 0.15 mg/kg every 6 hours for 2 to 4 days. However, adjunctive dexamethasone should not be given to infants and children who have already received antimicrobial therapy, because it is unlikely to improve patient outcome (Tunkel et al., 2004). Adjunctive dexamethasone in infants and children with pneumococcal meningitis is controversial. On the use of steroids for pneumococcal meningitis, the Committee on Infectious Diseases of the American Academy of Pediatrics stated, "For infants and children 6 weeks of age and older, adjunctive therapy with dexamethasone may be considered after weighing the potential benefits and possible risks. Experts vary in recommending the use of corticosteroids in pneumococcal meningitis; data are not sufficient to demonstrate clear benefit in children" (AAP, 2003). Also, data support adjunctive corticosteroids in children from high-income countries, but show no beneficial effect for children in low-income countries (Cochrane review; van de Beek et al., 2007).

Adults

Adjunctive dexamethasone, 0.15 mg/kg every 6 hours for 2 to 4 days, with the first dose administered 10 to 20 minutes before (or at least concomitant with) the first dose of antibiotic, should be initiated in all adult

Table 42-10 Empiric Antimicrobial Therapy for Purulent Meningitis Based on Patient Age and Specific Predisposing Condition (A)

Predisposing Factor	Common Bacterial Pathogens	Antimicrobial Therapy
Age		
<1 mo	*Streptococcus agalactiae, Escherichia coli, Listeria monocytogenes, Klebsiella* spp.	Ampicillin *plus* cefotaxime or ampicillin *plus* an aminoglycoside
1-23 mo	*Streptococcus pneumoniae, Neisseria meningitidis, S. agalactiae, Haemophilus influenzae, E. coli*	Vancomycin *plus* third-generation cephalosporin* †
2-50 yr	*N. meningitidis, S. pneumoniae*	Vancomycin *plus* third-generation cephalosporin* †
>50 yr	*S. pneumoniae, N. meningitidis, L. monocytogenes,* aerobic gram-negative bacilli	Vancomycin *plus* ampicillin *plus* third-generation cephalosporin* †
Head Trauma		
Basilar skull fracture	*S. pneumoniae, H. influenzae,* group A ß-hemolytic streptococci	Vancomycin *plus* third-generation cephalosporin*
Penetrating trauma	*Staphylococcus aureus,* coagulase-negative staphylococci (especially *Staphylococcus epidermidis*), aerobic gram-negative bacilli (including *Pseudomonas aeruginosa*)	Vancomycin *plus* cefepime, vancomycin *plus* ceftazidime, *or* vancomycin *plus* meropenem
Postneurosurgery	Aerobic gram-negative bacilli (including *P. aeruginosa*), *S. aureus,* coagulase-negative staphylococci (especially *S. epidermidis*)	Vancomycin *plus* cefepime, vancomycin *plus* ceftazidime, or vancomycin *plus* meropenem
Cerebrospinal fluid shunt	Coagulase-negative staphylococci (especially *S. epidermidis*), *S. aureus,* aerobic gram-negative bacilli (including *P. aeruginosa*), *Propionibacterium acnes*	Vancomycin *plus* cefepime, ‡ vancomycin *plus* ceftazidime, ‡ *or* vancomycin plus meropenem ‡

Modified from Tunkel AR, Barry J, Hartman SL, et al: Practice guidelines for the management of bacterial meningitis. Clin Infect Dis 2004;39,1267.
*Ceftriaxone or cefotaxime.
†Some experts would add rifampin if dexamethasone is also given.
‡In infants and children, vancomycin alone is reasonable unless Gram stain reveals gram-negative bacilli.

Table 42-11 Specific Antimicrobial Therapy in Bacterial Meningitis Based on Isolated Pathogen and Susceptibility Testing

Microorganism, Susceptibility	Standard Therapy	Alternative Therapies
Streptococcus pneumoniae		
Penicillin MIC		
<0.1 µg/mL	Penicillin G *or* ampicillin	Third-generation cephalosporin,* chloramphenicol
0.1-1.0 µg/mL†	Third-generation cephalosporin*	Cefepime (B), meropenem (B)
≥2.0 µg/mL	Vancomycin *plus* third-generation cephalosporin* ‡	Fluoroquinolone§ (B)
Cefotaxime or ceftriaxone MIC ≥1.0 µg/mL	Vancomycin *plus* third-generation cephalosporin* ‡	Fluoroquinolone§ (B)
Neisseria meningitidis		
Penicillin MIC		
<0.1 µg/mL	Penicillin G *or* ampicillin	Third-generation cephalosporin,* chloramphenicol
0.1-1.0 µg/mL	Third-generation cephalosporin*	Chloramphenicol, fluoroquinolone, meropenem
Listeria monocytogenes	Ampicillin or penicillin G¶	Trimethoprim-sulfamethoxazole, Meropenem (B)
Streptococcus agalactiae	Ampicillin or penicillin G¶	Third-generation cephalosporin* (B)
Escherichia coli and other Enterobacteriaceae**	Third-generation cephalosporin	Aztreonam, fluoroquinolone, meropenem, TMP-SMX, ampicillin

Table 42-11 Specific Antimicrobial Therapy in Bacterial Meningitis Based on Isolated Pathogen and Susceptibility Testing— *cont'd*

Microorganism, Susceptibility	Standard Therapy	Alternative Therapies
*Pseudomonas aeruginosa***	Cefepime¶ or ceftazidime¶	Aztreonam,¶ ciprofloxacin,¶ meropenem¶
Haemophilus influenza		
β-Lactamase negative	Ampicillin	Third-generation cephalosporin,* cefepime, chloramphenicol, fluoroquinolone
β-Lactamase positive	Third-generation cephalosporin	Cefepime, chloramphenicol, fluoroquinolone
Staphylococcus aureus		
Methicillin susceptible	Nafcillin or oxacillin	Vancomycin, meropenem (B)
Methicillin resistant	Vancomycin¶¶	Trimethoprim-sulfamethoxazole, Linezolid (B)
Staphylococcus epidermidis	Vancomycin¶¶	Linezolid (B)
Enterococcus spp.		
Ampicillin susceptible	Ampicillin plus gentamicin	—
Ampicillin resistant	Vancomycin plus gentamicin	—
Ampicillin and vancomycin resistant	Linezolid (B)	

—Modified from Tunkel AR, Barry J, Hartman SL, et al. Practice guidelines for the management of bacterial meningitis. Clin Infect Dis 2004;39:1267.
Note: All recommendations are (A), unless otherwise indicated.
TMP-SMX, Trimethoprim-sulfamethoxazole; *MIC,* minimum inhibitory concentration.
*Ceftriaxone or cefotaxime.
†Ceftriaxone/cefotaxime-susceptible isolates.
‡Consider addition of rifampin if the MIC of ceftriaxone is >2 μg/mL.
§Gatifloxacin or moxifloxacin.
¶Addition of an aminoglycoside should be considered.
¶¶Consider addition of rifampin.
**Choice of a specific antimicrobial agent must be guided by in vitro susceptibility test results.

patients with suspected or proven pneumococcal meningitis. Although data are insufficient to make this recommendation for other bacterial pathogens, many experts would initiate dexamethasone in all adults because the cause of meningitis is not always ascertained at the initial evaluation. As in children, dexamethasone should not be given to adult patients who have already received antibiotics (Tunkel et al., 2004).

Dexamethasone should only be continued if the CSF stain reveals gram-positive diplococci, or if the blood or CSF cultures are positive for *S. pneumoniae.*

Antimicrobial Therapy

Prompt and accurate treatment of meningitis is essential to increase survival and reduce morbidity. Treatment recommendations for a known pathogen of community-acquired bacterial meningitis and for selected clinical settings are listed in Tables 42-13 and 42-14. Duration of therapy is based more on tradition than on clinical evidence and varies, depending on the pathogen. Repeat LP for CSF analysis of response to therapy is not necessary for most patients who demonstrate clinical improvement within 24 to 48 hours. Patients who do not demonstrate significant clinical improvement and show high resistance on culture and sensitivity, as well as neonates with meningitis caused by gram-negative bacilli, should undergo repeat LP (Tunkel et al., 2004).

Prophylaxis and Prevention

Prophylaxis is indicated for any close contacts of persons with documented meningococcal meningitis or *H. influenzae* type b meningitis. For meningococcal meningitis, adults should receive 600 mg of rifampin orally twice daily for 2 days; children older than 1 month should receive 10 mg/kg every 12 hours orally for 2 days (5 mg/kg every 12 hours if younger than 1 month). Rifampin is not recommended for pregnant women, and the reliability of oral contraceptives may be affected by rifampin therapy. An alternative for children is ceftriaxone intramuscularly as a single dose, 125 mg for those 15 years and younger and 250 mg for those older than 15 years. Ciprofloxacin, 500 mg orally as a single dose, is another alternative to rifampin in nonpregnant, nonlactating adults (ACIP, 1997; CDC, 2000; Pickering, 2003).

Prevention of nasopharyngeal carriage in patients treated for meningitis is achieved by starting prophylaxis doses (same as earlier) before discharge. Prevention is also achieved by immunoprophylaxis. The Hib vaccine is now part of the primary vaccination series for children and has been immensely successful at almost eliminating *H. influenzae* meningitis. A vaccine for meningococcal disease is now a part of the standard immunization regiment for all children between the ages of 11 and 12 years. It should also be administered to children between the ages of 13-18 years and all previously unvaccinated freshmen living in a dormitory setting (Advisory Committee of Immunization Practices, 2009).

Table 42-12 Recommended Dosages of Antimicrobial Therapy in Patients with Bacterial Meningitis (A)

| Antimicrobial Agent | Total Daily Dose (Dosing Interval in hr) | | Infants and Children | Adults |
| | Neonates (Age in days) | | | |
	0-7*	8-28*		
Amikacin	15-20 mg/kg (12)	30 mg/kg (8)	20-30 mg/kg (8)	15 mg/kg (8)
Ampicillin	150 mg/kg (8)	200 mg/kg (6-8)	300 mg/kg (6)	12 g (4)
Aztreonam	—	—	—	6-8 g (6-8)
Cefepime	—	—	150 mg/kg (8)	6 g (8)
Cefotaxime	100-150 mg/kg (8-12)	150-200 mg/kg (6-8)	225-300 mg/kg (6-8)	8-12g (4-6)
Ceftazidime	100-150 mg/kg (8-12)	150 mg/kg (8)	150 mg/kg (8)	6 g (8)
Ceftriaxone	—	—	80-100 mg/kg (12-24)	4 g (12-24)
Chloramphenicol	25 mg/kg (24)	50 mg/kg (12-24)	75-100 mg/kg (6)	4-6 g (6)‡
Ciprofloxacin	—	—	—	800-1200 mg (8-12)
Gatifloxacin	—	—	—	400 mg (24)§
Gentamicin†	5 mg/kg (12)	7.5 mg/kg (8)	7.5 mg/kg (8)	5 mg/kg (8)
Meropenem	—	—	120 mg/kg (8)	6 g (8)
Moxifloxacin	—	—	—	400 mg (24)§
Nafcillin	75 mg/kg (8-12)	100-150 mg/kg (6-8)	200 mg/kg (6)	9-12 g (4)
Oxacillin	75 mg/kg (8-12)	150-200 mg/kg (6-8)	200 mg/kg (6)	9-12 g (4)
Penicillin G	0.15 mU/kg (8-12)	0.2 mU/kg (6-8)	0.3 mU/kg (4-6)	24 mU (4)
Rifampin	—	10-20 mg/kg (12)	10-20mg/kg (12-24)¶	600mg (24)
Tobramycin†	5 mg/kg (12)	7.5 mg/kg (8)	7.5 mg/kg (8)	5mg/kg (8)
TMP-SMX§	—	—	10-20mg/kg (6-12)	10-20mg/kg (6-12)
Vancomycin**	20-30 mg/kg (8-12)	30-45 mg/kg (6-8)	60 mg/kg (6)	30-45 mg/kg (8-12)

Modified from Tunkel AR, Barry J, Hartman SL, et al. Practice guidelines for the management of bacterial meningitis. Clin Infect Dis 2004;39:1267.

*Smaller doses and longer intervals of administration may be advisable for very-low-birth-weight neonates (<2000 g).

†Need to monitor peak and trough serum concentrations.

‡Higher dose recommended for patients with pneumococcal meningitis.

§No data on optimal dosage needed in patients with bacterial meningitis.

¶Maximum daily dose of 600 mg.

**Maintain serum trough concentrations of 15-20 μg/mL.

¶¶Dosage based on trimethoprim component.

TMP-SMX, Trimethoprim-sulfamethoxazole.

The heptavalent pneumococcal conjugate vaccine (PCV-7) is recommended for all children as part of the Advisory Committee of Immunization Practices immunization schedule (ACIP, 2009).

KEY TREATMENT

Evidence supports the use of adjunctive dexamethasone in infants and children with *Haemophilus influenzae* type b meningitis (IDSA; Tunkel et al., 2004) (SOR: A).

Adjunctive dexamethasone is recommended for adult patients with suspected or proven pneumococcal meningitis (IDSA; Tunkel et al., 2004) (SOR: A).

Recurrent Meningitis

Recurrent meningitis can have both infectious and noninfectious causes. A CSF leak accounts for approximately 75% of cases of recurrent meningitis. Clinically, it presents more like aseptic meningitis. A careful history may detect a drug exposure, structural lesion, or associated systemic disorder. To be truly recurrent, the CSF must confirm pleocytosis. Between episodes, the CSF must also be documented to return to normal. The interval between recurrences can be months to years. Unless the source is bacterial, the course of recurrent meningitis is usually self-limited, and spontaneous recovery is generally the rule. Optimal treatment is aimed at the underlying cause.

Table 42-13 Specific Antibiotic Treatments for Known Pathogens

Pathogen	Primary Therapy	Alternative*
Group B streptococcus	Penicillin G *or* ampicillin	Vancomycin *or* third-generation cephalosporin[†]
Streptococcus pneumoniae (MIC <0.1)	Third-generation cephalosporin[†]	Meropenem penicillin
S. pneumoniae (MIC >0.1)	Vancomycin *plus* third-generation cephalosporin*	Substitute rifampin for vancomycin; *or* meropenem; *or* vancomycin as monotherapy if highly allergic to other alternatives
Haemophilus influenzae (ß-lactamase negative)	Ampicillin	Third-generation cephalosporin[†] *or* chloramphenicol *or* aztreonam
H. influenzae (ß-lactamase positive)	Third-generation cephalosporin[†]	Chloramphenicol *or* aztreonam *or* fluoroquinolones[‡]
Listeria monocytogenes	Ampicillin *plus* gentamicin	TMP-SMX
Neisseria meningitidis	Penicillin G *or* ampicillin	Third-generation cephalosporin[†]
Enterobacteriaceae	Third-generation cephalosporin[†] *plus* aminoglycoside	TMP-SMX *or* aztreonam *or* fluoroquinolones or antipseudomonal penicillin[§] (or ampicillin) *plus* aminoglycoside
Pseudomonas aeruginosa	Ceftazidime *plus* aminoglycoside	Aminoglycoside *plus* aztreonam *or* aminoglycoside *plus* antipseudomonal penicillin[§]
Staphylococcus aureus (methicillin sensitive)	Antistaphylococcal penicillin[¶] ± rifampin	Vancomycin *plus* rifampin *or* TMP-SMX *plus* rifampin
S. aureus (methicillin resistant)	Vancomycin *plus* rifampin	
Staphylococcus epidermidis	Vancomycin *plus* rifampin	

*If patient is highly allergic or intolerant of primary therapy.
[†]Ceftriaxone or cefotaxime.
[‡]Ciprofloxacin or levofloxacin.
[§]Piperacillin, mezlocillin, or ticarcillin.
[¶]Nafcillin, oxacillin, or methicillin.
MIC, Minimum inhibitory concentration; *TMP-SMX,* trimethoprim-sulfamethoxazole.

Table 42-14 Common Pathogens of Bacterial Meningitis and Empiric Treatment Based on Age

Age	Common Pathogens	Treatment*	Duration (days)
0-1 mo	Group B streptococcus *Listeria monocytogenes* *Escherichia coli* *Streptococcus pneumoniae*	Ampicillin *plus* third-generation cephalosporin[†] *or* ampicillin *plus* aminoglycoside	14-21 14-21 21 10-14
1-3 mo	Group B streptococcus, *E. coli, L. monocytogenes* *S. pneumoniae* *Neisseria meningitidis, Haemophilus influenzae*	Ampicillin *plus* third-generation cephalosporin[†]	14-21 10-14 7-10
3 mo-18 yr	*H. influenzae, N. meningitidis* *S. pneumoniae*	Third-generation cephalosporin[†] *or* meropenem *or* chloramphenicol	7-10 10-14
18-50 yr	*H. influenzae, N. meningitidis* *S. pneumoniae*	Third-generation cephalosporin[†] *or* meropenem *or* ampicillin *plus* chloramphenicol	7-10 10-14
>50 yr	*S. pneumoniae* *L. monocytogenes* Gram-negative bacilli (other than *H. influenzae*)	Ampicillin *plus* third-generation cephalosporin[†] *or* ampicillin *plus* fluoroquinolone[‡] *or* meropenem	10-14 14-21 21

*Add vancomycin in areas where there is greater than 2% incidence of highly drug-resistant *S. pneumoniae.*
[†]Ceftriaxone or cefotaxime.
[‡]Ciprofloxacin or levofloxacin.

Chronic Meningitis

There are no pathognomonic features of chronic meningitis. The classic symptoms, if present, may be extremely subtle and variable. There may be unusual symptoms such as psychoses, movement disorders, and parkinsonian syndrome. The average duration of symptoms is 17 to 43 months, during which symptoms may fluctuate or remain static. CSF that shows a mildly decreased glucose level in the setting of mononuclear pleocytosis should always raise the suspicion of chronic meningitis. The causes are numerous, and attention should be paid to a history of previous systemic diseases, specific infections that could involve the meninges, possible exposures, geographic risk factors, immunologic compromise, and concurrent extraneural involvement (Boxes 42-9 and 42-10).

Viral Meningitis

Viral meningitis is actually a subset of aseptic meningitis. *Aseptic meningitis* antedates the modern science of virology and signifies an infection of the subarachnoid space and meninges with no obvious bacterial cause. *Encephalitis* occurs when there is inflammation of brain tissue. *Viral meningitis* presents with similar signs and symptoms as bacterial meningitis, but with less severity. A history of a preceding viral respiratory infection is common. Obtaining LP for CSF evaluation is the only method for determining the difference. There are numerous causes of viral meningitis (Box 42-11). Outbreaks are often seasonal.

Treatment is mainly supportive, with the exception of herpesvirus (herpes simplex virus [HSV]) and HIV, for which specific antiviral therapy is available. Data regarding herpes meningitis treatment are limited, and both high-dose acyclovir (60 mg/kg/day) and lower-dose therapies have been advocated (Kohlhoff et al., 2004). For HIV and acquired immunodeficiency syndrome (AIDS)–dementia complex (ADC), many antiviral combinations have been suggested. The factors to be considered when choosing a combination therapy for ADC include toxicity, the many potential drug interactions, CNS penetration, and resistance. Because the treatments for HIV and its complications are often changing, consultation with an infectious disease specialist should be considered.

With the exception of HSV encephalitis and ADC, the prognosis is generally very good for other viral meningitides. Children seem to recover within 1 to 2 weeks, whereas adults may take several months.

Brain Abscess

Brain abscess, a rare disease in the United States, can occur in single or multiple sites. It usually arises from a secondary focus outside the CNS. Examples may include upper or lower respiratory infection, intracardiac infection, penetration skull trauma, local osteomyelitis, any source of bacteremia, or no source (20%). Risk factors include IV drug use, HIV infection, and any other immunocompromised state. Common pathogens include streptococci, staphylococci, enteric gram-negative organisms, and anaerobes.

Clinically, brain abscess usually has a more aggressive onset of symptoms than bacterial meningitis. Symptoms usually present as typical meningeal irritation, along with

---

Box 42-9 Causes of Chronic Meningitis

Bacterial

Tuberculosis
Brucellosis
Nocardiosis
Syphilis
Lyme disease
Actinomycosis
Listeriosis
Subacute bacterial endocarditis
Tularemia
Leptospirosis
Meningococcal infection

Fungal

Cryptococcosis
Coccidioidomycosis
Histoplasmosis
Blastomycosis
Candida
Aspergillus
Zygomycetes
Sporothrix

Viral

Retroviruses
Herpesvirus
Enteroviruses
Lymphocytic choriomeningitis
Mumps

Parasitic

Cysticercosis
Schistosomiasis
Trichinosis
Paragonimiasis
Echinococcosis
Toxoplasmosis
Visceral larva migrans

Noninfectious

Neoplasm
Vasculitis
Chemical meningitis
Collagen vascular disease
Behçet's disease
Sarcoidosis
Systemic lupus erythematosus
Fabry's disease
Foreign body in central nervous system
Vogt-Koyanagi-Harada syndrome

Other

Parameningeal focus
Chronic lymphocytic meningitis

Box 42-10 Laboratory Evaluation for Chronic Meningitis

Blood

Complete blood count, differential

Chemistries, erythrocyte sedimentation rate, antinuclear antibodies

Human immunodeficiency virus (HIV) serology

Rapid plasma reagin (RPR)

Consider angiotensin-converting enzyme (ACE), antineutrophilic cytoplasmic antibodies, specific serologies, blood smears

Cerebrospinal Fluid

Cell count with differential, protein, glucose

Cytology

Venereal Disease Research Laboratories (VDRL)

Cultures (TB, fungal, bacterial, viral)

Stain (Gram, acid-fast, India ink)

Cryptococcal antigen

Oligoclonal bands, IgG index

Consider ACE; polymerase chain reaction (PCR; viruses, mycobacteria, *T. whippelii*); *Histoplasma* antigen, immunocytochemistry (*T. whippelii* and other selected agents); paired antibodies for *B. burgdorferi*, *Brucella*, *Histoplasma*, *Coccidioides*, other fungal agents; neoplastic markers

Neuroimaging

Brain MRI with contrast

Consider CT, spinal MRI, angiography

Cultures

Blood (parasites, fungi, viruses, rare bacteria)

Urine (mycobacteria, viruses, fungi)

Sputum (mycobacteria, fungi)

Consider gastric washings, stool, bone marrow, liver (mycobacteria, fungi)

Ancillary

Chest radiography

Electrocardiography

Select testing (e.g., mammography, chest/abdominal CT)

Biopsy

Extraneural sites (bone marrow, lymph node, peripheral nerve, liver, lung, skin, small bowel)

Leptomeningeal/brain (with or without special stains)

CT, Computed tomography; *MRI*, magnetic resonance imaging; *IgG*, immunoglobulin G; *TB*, tuberculosis.

Modified from Coyle PK. Overview of acute and chronic meningitis. Neurol Clin 1999;17:691.

Box 42-11 Causes of Viral Meningitis

Enteroviruses
   Echovirus
   Poliovirus
   Coxsackieviruses A and B
Herpesviruses
   Herpes simplex virus (HSV) types 1 and 2
   Varicella-zoster virus (VZV)
Lymphocytic choriomeningitis
Flaviviruses (St. Louis encephalitis)
Morbillivirus (measles)
Bunyaviruses (LaCrosse)
Epstein-Barr virus (EBV)
Adenoviruses
Cytomegalovirus (CMV)
Mumps
Hepatitis B virus (HBV)
Human immunodeficiency virus (HIV)

in 5% to 10% of patients. Morbidity is significant and includes the risk of epilepsy (10%-70%), focal neurologic sequelae (25%), and cognitive impairment (15%). Overall mortality is 5% to 10%.

Dizziness

Key Points

- Dizziness is a risk factor for falls and functional decline in older adults.
- Characterizing the type of dizziness can narrow the differential diagnosis.
- Benign paroxysmal positional vertigo patients complain of episodic vertigo without aural symptoms.

Dizziness is a common problem encountered by the family physician. It is a typical complaint of elderly patients and has a broad differential diagnosis. Fortunately, dizziness is usually benign and self-limited. Nevertheless, it is a risk factor for falls and functional decline in the geriatric population and, in a small subset of patients, can signal a life-threatening condition.

Evaluation

The evaluation of dizziness is often frustrating for both patients and physicians. This frustration arises from the vast differential diagnosis, the potential for multiple etiologies, and the lack of a dependable method of diagnosing the more serious causes of dizziness. The initial step in the evaluation of a patient with dizziness is a thorough history. First, the physician should clarify the category of dizziness reported by the patient. Dizziness can be categorized as *vertigo*, which is the sensation of spinning or motion; *presyncopal lightheadedness*, which is a sensation of impending faint; *disequilibrium*, a sensation of unsteadiness; or dizziness that cannot be adequately quantified, reported by patients as a feeling of lightheadedness or floating sensation. Categorizing the type of dizziness can

mental status changes that progress to stupor or coma, seizures, and focal neurologic findings. Laboratory studies are not impressive. Caution should be exercised before performing LP because brain edema is often present. Once past the initial cerebritis stage, CT or MRI of the brain often identifies the abscess. A search for a secondary cause is important. A radionuclide-labeled leukocyte scan may be needed to differentiate a brain tumor from infection. Aspiration or biopsy of the area in question usually confers a definitive diagnosis.

Treatment is directed toward the cause and lasts for 4 to 6 weeks. Drainage of the abscess is achieved by CT-guided needle aspiration or craniotomy. Recurrence can be expected

Table 42-15 Types of Dizziness

Category	Differential Diagnosis
Vertigo (sensation of spinning)	Inner ear, vestibular, brainstem and cerebellar abnormalities, sinusitis, drug toxicity, panic disorder, cervical spine disease
Presyncopal lightheadedness	Cerebral hypoperfusion, venous pooling in extremities, low blood volume, cardiac abnormalities (arrhythmia, cardiac insufficiency),vasovagal phenomenon
Disequilibrium (unsteadiness more prominent when standing)	Broad differential—any disturbance of the neurosensory system
Other (vague descriptions of lightheadedness without presyncope, or a floating sensation)	Broad differential, but many times associated with psychological disorders

Box 42-12 Medications associated with dizziness

Alcohol
Alpha blockers
Anticholinergic
    Antihistamines
    Tricyclic antidepressants
    Meclizine
Anticonvulsants
Beta blockers
Caffeine
Calcium channel blockers
Cough and cold medication
Diuretics
Muscle relaxants
Nonsteroidal medications
Psychotropic medicines
Vasodilating agents

limit the differential diagnosis (Table 42-15). Many patients, however, will be unable to limit their dizziness symptoms to one specific category. Classically, the category of vertigo was further defined as peripheral or central vertigo based on symptoms and signs, including nystagmus. This is not clinically useful, especially in the older-adult population, because many of these findings are seen in normal patients as well.

After categorizing the type of dizziness experienced by the patient, the physician should next determine the temporal pattern of the symptoms. *Continuous* dizziness is typically produced by a stroke. *Episodic* dizziness lasting a few seconds to a minute and associated with head movement is usually a sign of benign positional vertigo. Meniere's disease tends to cause dizziness lasting hours to days. Finally, the history should focus on the onset of the symptoms, alleviating or aggravating factors, and a review of the patient's medications (Box 42-12).

The physical examination should include orthostatic blood pressure and pulse determinations; examination of ears, nose, and throat for signs of infection; cardiovascular examination for murmurs and arrhythmias, with auscultation for carotid bruits; and neurologic examination, including evaluation of cranial nerves, hearing and vision screening, observation of gait, cerebellar testing, and neuromuscular assessment of extremities. A Dix-Hallpike maneuver should be tested if the differential diagnosis includes benign positional vertigo, because a positive test confirms this diagnosis. Screening audiometry should be considered to rule out Meniere's disease and acoustic neuroma, if warranted by the type of dizziness described by the history.

Laboratory and imaging studies should be ordered based on history and physical examination findings. Laboratory tests frequently include CBC, electrolytes, BUN, creatinine, glucose, serum calcium, LFTs, and TSH. If neuroimaging is indicated, MRI is the preferred modality because of its superior ability to evaluate the posterior fossa and brainstem. In some patients, carotid Doppler evaluation, cardiac event monitoring, or echocardiography may be necessary. Subspecialty consultation should be considered before proceeding with further, extensive testing.

Conditions Associated with Dizziness

Benign Positional Vertigo

Benign positional vertigo is believed to be caused by a dislodged otolith from the semicircular canal. Symptoms include episodic vertigo without aural symptoms. Nausea and vomiting may also be present secondary to the vertigo. Common histories include vertigo precipitated by rolling over in bed or bending over to tie shoes. The diagnosis can usually be made by the history and eliciting a positive Dix-Hallpike maneuver. Patients can be expected to have gradual resolution of their symptoms over 4 to 6 weeks with supportive therapy. The canalith repositioning (Epley) maneuver provides short-term resolution of the vertiginous symptoms (Cochrane review; Pinder, 2004).

Postural Dizziness

Nonvertiginous postural dizziness suggests postural hypotension. *Orthostatic hypotension* is usually defined as a 20 mm Hg drop in systolic BP or 10 mm Hg drop in diastolic BP 2 minutes after moving from a recumbent to standing position. Older-adult patients, however, can develop postural dizziness without apparent postural hypotension. In some cases, no BP decline occurs, although enough blood pools in the older adult's lower extremities to impair cerebral perfusion. When postural dizziness without postural hypotension is suspected, an evaluation of the cardiovascular system should be considered. If significant cardiovascular pathology, such as congestive heart failure, is not identified, a therapeutic trial of support stockings and optimized hydration can be contemplated.

Labyrinthitis, Vestibular Abnormalities, and Meniere's Disease

A comprehensive review of these topics is beyond the scope of this chapter but should be considered when evaluating any patient with dizziness. Patients with the abrupt onset of a single episode of vertigo that gradually resolves over several days often have *labyrinthitis* or *vestibular neuronitis,* usually distinguished clinically by the presence or absence of hearing changes. Patients with labyrinthitis usually experience hearing changes, whereas those with vestibular neuronitis do not. A viral infection is the usual cause in younger patients while infarction becomes more likely in the older adult. Older-adult patients may recover more slowly and experience feelings of imbalance for several months. Treatment during the symptomatic period may include vestibular rehab exercises and pharmacologic agents such as meclizine, promethazine, or low-dose benzodiazepine (e.g., lorazepam). *Meniere's disease* should be suspected when an older adult reports recurrent episodes of vertigo, tinnitus, gradual development of low-frequency hearing loss, and in some cases ear fullness before onset of vertigo.

Dizziness of Cervical Origin

Cervical spine problems, especially osteoarthritic changes, can cause dizziness that may be vertiginous in nature and of vascular or proprioceptive origin. In cases of vascular origin, flow through one of the vertebral arteries is temporarily disrupted by an osteoarthritic spur that compresses the vessel when the patient turns the head or looks up. In cases of proprioceptive origin, overstimulation of the proprioceptive receptors in the facet joints produces the sensation of dizziness. Either of these conditions can cause a "drop attack." These patients should avoid the position that precipitates the symptoms and, in some cases, cervical collars or cervical traction may be helpful.

Vertebrobasilar Transient Ischemic Attacks and Stroke

The TIAs that produce vertigo of abrupt onset lasting minutes to hours are a manifestation of ischemia in the distribution of the vertebrobasilar arteries, not the carotid arteries. Unfortunately, the TIA diagnosis can be difficult to make because vertigo may be the only symptom reported, and more definitive neurologic symptoms suggestive of a vertebrobasilar event may be absent, such as blurred vision, visual field deficits, diplopia, dysarthria, and unilateral motor or sensory changes. When a patient presents with symptoms of a vertebrobasilar TIA, the physician should consider causes such as cardioembolic disease, polycythemia, and subclavian steal syndrome. A significant BP difference in the arms and symptoms with arm abduction may signal subclavian steal syndrome, which may be corrected surgically. If the cause of these symptoms is related to vertebrobasilar vascular disease, treatment is usually medical with aspirin or other antiplatelet agents.

Vertigo is also a component of several well-recognized *vertebrobasilar stroke syndromes* (Table 42-16). *Lacunar strokes,* particularly those affecting the cerebellum, are also an important cause of dizziness. The dizziness associated with lacunar strokes is often reported as a sense of disequilibrium that is difficult to explain clinically. Such patients often report a sense of imbalance when standing that started when they were not feeling well and persists even after they return to their otherwise usual state of health. Neuroimaging is rarely helpful. CT lacks the necessary resolution to identify many of these strokes, and MRI, which may demonstrate lacunar disease, rarely identifies the lesion responsible for the patient's symptoms. Aggressive efforts to control blood pressure are advised for patients believed to have experienced lacunar strokes.

Table 42-16 Vertebrobasilar Stroke Syndromes

Anatomy	Symptoms
Occlusion of vertebral artery	Lateral medullary syndrome: vertigo, nausea, ipsilateral facial numbness, Horner's syndrome, contralateral body loss of pain and temperature sensation, tendency to fall to affected side
Occlusion of anterior inferior cerebellar artery: affects labyrinth, pontomedullary region, and inferolateral cerebellum	Lateral pontomedullary syndrome: severe vertigo, nausea, vomiting, unilateral hearing loss, tinnitus, facial paralysis, asymmetric cerebellar testing
Cerebellar infarction	Severe vomiting, vertigo, and ataxia; brainstem signs may be absent, making differentiation from labyrinthitis difficult or impossible.

Peripheral Neuropathies

Key Points

- In developed countries, diabetes and alcoholism are the most common causes of peripheral neuropathy in adults.
- Polyneuropathies are often inflammatory and caused by HIV infection, Lyme disease, and leprosy; no cause can be found in up to 20% of cases.
- There is no specific laboratory study or serum marker for the diagnosis of peripheral neuropathy.
- Electromyography and nerve conduction studies are most useful for evaluation of peripheral neuropathy and should be considered early.
- Mononeuropathies are usually caused by entrapment, compression, or other physical injury to a specific nerve.
- Carpal tunnel syndrome is a common mononeuropathy caused by decreased tunnel size (Colles' fracture, rheumatoid arthritis), enlargement of median nerve (diabetes, amyloidosis), or increased volume of other structures (tenosynovitis, gout).
- Common symptoms of CTS include numbness and paresthesias in the median nerve sensory distribution, pain at rest (especially at night), weakness in the thumb, and thenar atrophy.

The incidence of peripheral neuropathy is not known, but it is a common feature of many systemic diseases. In developed countries, diabetes and alcoholism are the most common causes of peripheral neuropathy in adults (Poncelet, 1998). Worldwide, leprosy is the primary treatable cause of peripheral neuropathy, and HIV is one of the fastest-growing causes (Sabin et al., 1993).

Peripheral neuropathies are frequently overlooked. The evaluation can be time-consuming and costly without a systematic approach based on a careful history, clinical evaluation, and select studies. Despite a thoughtful approach, however, no cause can be found in up to 20% of cases (Dyck et al., 1981; McLeod et al., 1984). The goal in treating peripheral neuropathy should be to identify the treatable cause or underlying medical condition, such as diabetes, alcohol, drugs, or nutritional disorder. Hereditary neuropathies are uncommon but underdiagnosed; thus a careful family history (e.g., long-standing distal neuropathy) should not be neglected.

Anatomy

The peripheral nervous system (PNS) consists of cranial nerves III to XII, spinal roots (dorsal and ventral), spinal nerves, dorsal root ganglia, and most autonomic ganglia and roots. Because the motor neuron cell bodies are located in the spinal cord or CNS, diseases affecting these are considered separately. Peripheral nerves consist of different types of fiber bundles called *axons.* Large and medium-sized axons are normally myelinated and carry information about proprioception, vibration, and light touch. Small axons, consisting of myelinated and unmyelinated types, are responsible for light touch, pain, and temperature, as well as autonomic information. These small, unmyelinated fibers of the autonomic PNS travel within most peripheral nerves and convey poorly defined visceral sensations and monitor autonomic functions. Most peripheral nerves carry incoming sensory information (afferent fibers) and outgoing motor and autonomic messages (efferent fibers).

Clinical Pathophysiology

Sensory Changes

Large-fiber and small-fiber neuropathies can often be distinguished clinically by whether they affect proprioception and vibration or pain and temperature. Because processes that affect small fibers cause pain and sensory changes, symptoms may include reduced sensitivity to stimuli (hypoesthesia) or burning and tingling sensations (dysesthesias and paresthesias, respectively). There may also be impaired pain or temperature sensation and autonomic dysfunction. When large fibers are damaged, vibratory sense and proprioception are affected. This can lead to unsteady gait, complaints of coolness in the extremities, or *allodynia,* in which non-noxious stimuli such as light touch are perceived as pain. In polyneuropathies, pain and sensation are commonly affected in a stocking-glove distribution.

Motor Changes

Symptoms are usually most pronounced distally. This is especially true with polyneuropathies, in which symptoms of stumbling, clumsiness, and weakness are most common because of the effects on the intrinsic muscles. Motor symptoms can range from mild weakness to complete paralysis. Diminished DTRs may be one of the early signs of motor dysfunction. Denervation of muscles causes eventual atrophy. An example is the "sharp shin" sign, whereby atrophy of the tibialis anterior muscle gives a prominent appearance to the tibia. As the intrinsic muscles deteriorate, the wasting gives the hands and feet a skeletal appearance. In long-standing neuropathies, trophic changes such as high-arched feet (pes cavus), hammertoes, kyphoscoliosis, and hair loss with or without ulcerations can be seen. Cramps, fasciculations, and restless legs may also be present.

Autonomic Changes

Autonomic changes are especially common with diabetes. The skin may become smooth, cold, and shiny. It may be unusually dry and devoid of perspiration. Orthostatic hypotension is one of the most common autonomic symptoms associated with neuropathy from systemic disease. The genitourinary and gastrointestinal systems are also often affected.

Classification

Peripheral neuropathies are often categorized in terms of the anatomy affected, pathophysiologic process, temporal development, and functional outcome.

Anatomic Classification

The major anatomic patterns of peripheral nerve disease can be distinguished by the clinical presentation—mononeuropathy, multiple mononeuropathy, and polyneuropathy. *Mononeuropathies* occur when there is damage to a single peripheral nerve or root. This is seen with local entrapment from causes such as trauma (acute or chronic), tumor infiltration, or infarction. *Multiple mononeuropathies* (mononeuropathy multiplex) occur when several nerves are individually affected by a disease process. Involvement is usually asymmetric and noncontiguous. These mononeuropathies are much less common than other peripheral neuropathies and are more difficult to recognize and treat. Multiple mononeuropathies are usually seen with systemic diseases such as vasculitis, diabetes, and rheumatoid arthritis. *Polyneuropathies* occur in a symmetric, diffuse, bilateral pattern and produce a characteristic stocking-glove pattern of sensory changes. However, most polyneuropathies affect both sensory and motor nerves. Some can affect peripheral autonomic nerves. Many common peripheral neuropathies fall into this category.

Pathophysiologic Classification

Based on the primary site of involvement, peripheral neuropathies can be classified as neuronopathies, axonal neuropathies, and myelinopathies. Electrodiagnostic studies can help define this in a clinical setting. *Neuronopathies* result from damage to the sensory cell bodies in the dorsal root ganglia or motor neuron cell bodies in the spinal cord. Their location in the CNS usually results in a degenerative process that produces incomplete recovery. Diseases that specifically affect the motor neuron cell bodies in the CNS are usually not categorized as peripheral neuropathies. *Axonal neuropathies* occur when damage occurs at the level of the axon. When the axon is disrupted (e.g., by trauma), the axon and distal myelin sheath may degenerate distal to the site of injury (wallerian degeneration). In toxic or metabolic injuries, when the distal axon is injured and myelin degeneration spreads proximally, it is known as "dying back" neuropathy. With the dying back process, the longer nerves tend to be affected earlier and more severely. *Myelinopathies* (demyelinating neuropathies) result from a process affecting primarily the myelin sheath. They can result from acute conditions such as Guillain-Barré syndrome (GBS), chronic inflammatory demyelinating polyradiculoneuropathies (CIDPs), and certain hereditary neuropathies.

Temporal Classification

Acute peripheral neuropathies develop over a few days. When motor signs are predominant, GBS should be suspected first. Vasculitic or toxic processes can also present acutely. A subacute presentation may be seen in toxic, inflammatory, infiltrative, or carcinomatous processes that develop over weeks. A chronic-onset neuropathy may develop gradually and progress over months to years, as is the case in metabolic or hereditary neuropathies. Peripheral neuropathies may also have a relapsing course (Box 42-13).

Box 42-13 Neuropathies Classified by Temporal Presentation

Acute Onset (within days)

GBS
Vasculitis
Porphyria
Diphtheria
Thallium toxicity
Ischemia
Penetrating trauma
Rheumatoid arthritis
Diabetic plexopathy or cranial neuropathy
Acute nerve compression
Polyarteritis nodosa
Burns
Iatrogenic (e.g., improper injection techniques)

Subacute Onset (weeks to months)

Most toxins
Most drugs
Nutritional deficiencies
Abnormal metabolic state
Diabetic plexopathy
Neoplasms
Uremia

Chronic Course (months to years)

CIDP
Alcohol
Diabetes
Hereditary neuropathies

Relapsing

GBS
HIV
Porphyria
Refsum's disease
CIDP

GBS, Guillain-Barré syndrome; *CIDP*, chronic inflammatory demyelinating polyradiculoneuropathy; *HIV*, human immunodeficiency virus.

Box 42-14 Small-Fiber Neuropathies

Diabetes	HIV/AIDS
Leprosy	Amyloidosis
Hereditary	Alcoholism

HIV/AIDS, Human immunodeficiency virus/acquired immunodeficiency syndrome. Modified from Poncelet AN. An algorithm for the evaluation of peripheral neuropathy. Am Fam Physician 1998;57:755.

Electromyography (EMG) and nerve conduction studies (NCS) are probably the most useful laboratory studies for the evaluation of peripheral neuropathy and should be considered early. They can confirm the presence of peripheral neuropathy and provide information about the type of fibers involved (sensory, motor, or both) and whether the problem is symmetric, asymmetric, or multifocal. EMG can define entrapment neuropathies and differentiate these from more proximal radicular compression. It can also help differentiate muscle wasting caused by neuropathic or myopathic disorders from simple disuse atrophy. NCS can help define pathophysiology (axonal loss vs. demyelination). EMG and NCS are useful but have limitations and should complement the history and examination. EMG is usually not as helpful in diseases that cause a diffuse small-fiber peripheral neuropathy, in which only pinprick and temperature sensation are affected (Box 42-14). In fact, the electromyogram may be normal. EMG needles also mildly inflame the muscles into which they are inserted. Thus, if a muscle biopsy is anticipated, that muscle should not be tested with EMG (Corse and Kuncl, 1999). NCS are most diagnostic with diseases affecting large, fast fibers and thus may be normal in patients with small-fiber neuropathies. Evaluation of small, proximal sensory nerves is not reliably done using EMG or NCS.

Nerve biopsy is helpful only in specific cases and is usually a last step in the workup. This includes patients with suspected amyloidosis, vasculitis, leprosy, leukodystrophies, sarcoidosis, or demyelinating disorders. Because the sural nerve, a sensory nerve, is generally used, disease affecting only motor nerves may be missed. Possible complications include permanent numbness or dysesthesia in the distribution of the excised nerve (typically lateral heel and ankle), infection, and poor wound healing.

In the evaluation of neuropathies, a carefully performed history that identifies key features of the presentation correlated with the findings of electrodiagnostic studies is the critical first step in developing a reasonable diagnosis. Questions include the following:

- Is the pattern of involvement focal or multifocal (Box 42-15)?
- Is the pattern symmetric (Boxes 42-16 and 42-17)?
- Did symptoms evolve acutely, subacutely, or chronically? Was there a predilection for the upper extremities (Box 42-18)?
- Were the extremities affected in a distal versus a proximal distribution (see Boxes 42-16 and 42-17)?
- Are the symptoms sensory, motor, or both (Box 42-19; see also Boxes 42-16 and 42-17)?
- Is there autonomic or cranial nerve involvement (Boxes 42-20 and 42-21)?

Laboratory Evaluation

There is no specific laboratory study or serum marker for the diagnosis of peripheral neuropathy. Information from the history and physical examination may direct specific laboratory tests (e.g., testing for specific toxins, infections, or inflammatory disorders). If the cause of neuropathy is not obvious, some screening laboratory studies should be considered: ESR, CBC, LFTs, and determination of fasting blood glucose, glycosylated hemoglobin, BUN, creatinine, serum vitamin B_{12}, and TSH levels. Additional studies may be warranted, depending on the initial workup, such as chest radiograph to rule out sarcoidosis, pulmonary function tests for GBS, or ECG for processes that affect cardiac conduction. An LP for CSF showing an elevated protein level with normal white blood cells (WBCs) may indicate an acquired inflammatory neuropathy (GBS or CIDP).

Box 42-15 Neuropathies by Pattern of Involvement

Focal	Multifocal
Common entrapment neuropathies:	Diabetes mellitus
Endocrine	Vasculitis
Myxedema	Polyarteritis nodosa
Acromegaly	Churg-Strauss syndrome
Hypothyroidism	Giant cell arteritis
Diabetes	Wegener's granulomatosis
Infection/inflammation	Rheumatoid arthritis
Septic arthritis	Sjögren's syndrome
Lyme disease	Systemic lupus erythematosus
Tuberculosis	HIV (e.g., cytomegalovirus)
Histoplasmosis	Leprosy
Sarcoidosis	Sarcoidosis
Rheumatoid arthritis	Cryoglobulinemia
Amyloidosis	Multifocal variant of CIDP
Tumors	
Ganglion	
Neurofibroma	
Lipoma	
Hemangioma	
Congenital: Anatomic anomalies of muscles, bones, vessels	
Trauma	
Fractures	
Hematoma	
Hemorrhage from anticoagulation	
Pregnancy	
Hemodialysis	
Idiopathic	
Occupational	
Repetitive stress	
Neoplastic infiltration or compression	
Leprosy	
Ischemic lesions	
Diabetes mellitus	
Vasculitis	

CIDP, Chronic inflammatory demyelinating polyneuroradiculopathy; *HIV*, human immunodeficiency virus.

Box 42-16 Distal Symmetric Sensorimotor Polyneuropathies

Nutritional diseases	Medications and toxins
B-complex deficiencies	(see Box 42-22)
Vitamin E deficiency	Infectious
Folate deficiency	Human immunodeficiency virus
Whipple's disease	Lyme disease
Postgastrectomy syndrome	Hypophosphatemia
Alcoholism	Metabolic
Gastric resection for obesity	Uremia
Endocrine diseases	Porphyria
Diabetes mellitus	Gout
Hypothyroidism	Critical illness polyneuropathy
Acromegaly	Amyloidosis
Neoplastic	Metal neuropathy
Multiple myeloma	Thallium
Lymphoma	Gold
Carcinoma	Arsenic
Paraneoplastic	Mercury
Connective tissue disease	Inherited metabolic disease
Rheumatoid arthritis	Refsum's disease
Cryoglobulinemia	Adrenoleukodystrophy
Polyarteritis nodosa	Hereditary neuropathies
Systemic lupus erythematosus	
Scleroderma	
Sarcoidosis	
Churg-Strauss vasculitis	

Modified from Poncelet AN: An algorithm for the evaluation of peripheral neuropathy. Am Fam Physician 1998;57:755.

Box 42-17 Distal Symmetric Motor Polyneuropathies

Lead neuropathy	Porphyria
Diphtheria	Acute arsenic polyneuropathy
Guillain-Barré syndrome	Osteoclastic myeloma
Hereditary neuropathies	Human immunodeficiency virus
Diabetes mellitus	Waldenström's macroglobulinemia
Lymphoma	Chronic inflammatory demyelinating polyradiculoneuropathy
Lyme disease	
Vincristine toxicity	Monoclonal gammopathy of undetermined significance
Hypothyroidism	Motor neuropathy with multifocal conduction block

Modified from Poncelet AN. An algorithm for the evaluation of peripheral neuropathy. Am Fam Physician 1998; 57:4755.

- What did the EMG and NCS show? Were other significant laboratory studies done?

Taking this approach to peripheral neuropathies will prove to be more efficient and fruitful than less ordered approaches, despite the often elusive nature of these diagnoses.

Mononeuropathies

Mononeuropathies are usually caused by entrapment, compression, or other physical injury to a specific nerve. Peripheral nerves most at risk are those that occupy spaces with confining borders. Electrodiagnostic studies are useful in confirming the diagnosis and quantifying the degree of injury. Treatment is generally conservative, involving protection of the affected nerve from further injury by the use of activity avoidance or modification, ergonomic workplace correction, and bracing. Local (by injection) or systemic anti-inflammatory treatment is often helpful. Surgical intervention is usually reserved for patients who fail conservative therapy, have evidence of progressive weakness and atrophy, or have a significant focal conduction block on electrodiagnostic examination.

Brachial Plexus Neuropathy

Brachial plexus neuropathy (plexopathy) can result from blunt or penetrating trauma. The typical injury is directed into the axilla or violently increases the angle between the shoulder and head. In the latter case, *stingers* or *burners*, which frequently occur in football players, result in temporary

Box 42-18 Neuropathies with Predilection for the Upper Limbs

Diabetes
Porphyria
Hereditary neuropathies
Hereditary amyloid neuropathy type II (causes carpal tunnel syndrome from amyloid deposits)
Guillain-Barré syndrome
Myeloma
Lead neuropathy
Vitamin B_{12} deficiency

Modified from Poncelet AN. An algorithm for the evaluation of peripheral neuropathy. Am Fam Physician 1998;57:4755.

Box 42-19 Predominantly Sensory Neuropathies and Neuronopathies

Idiopathic sensory neuropathy	Carcinoma
Paraneoplastic	Lymphoma
Pyridoxine toxicity	Paraproteinemias
Sjögren's syndrome	Crohn's disease
Primary biliary sclerosis	Hereditary neuropathies
Vitamin E deficiency	Friedreich's ataxia
Medications	Chronic gluten enteropathy
Cisplatin	Nonsystemic vasculitic neuropathy
Metronidazole	Styrene-induced peripheral neuropathy
Misonidazole	
Thalidomide	

Modified from Poncelet AN. An algorithm for the evaluation of peripheral neuropathy. Am Fam Physician 1998;57:755.

Box 42-20 Neuropathies with Autonomic Symptoms

Diabetic neuropathy	Human immunodeficiency virus
Amyloidosis	Porphyria
Thiamine deficiency	Thallium, mercury, arsenic toxicity
Alcoholic neuropathy	Dysautonomia (Riley-Day)
Guillain-Barré syndrome	Lymphoma
Vincristine toxicity	Paraneoplastic neuropathy

Modified from Poncelet AN. An algorithm for the evaluation of peripheral neuropathy. Am Fam Physician 1998;57:755.

Box 42-21 Neuropathies with Cranial Nerve Involvement

Primary
Bell's palsy
Trigeminal neuralgia

Secondary
Diabetes mellitus
Diphtheria
Lyme disease
Sarcoidosis with cranial invasion
Guillain-Barré syndrome
Human immunodeficiency virus

paresthesias and diffuse weakness in the upper extremity. Recurrent stretch injuries to the brachial plexus can result in permanent weakness and atrophy. Also, apical lung tumors with direct extension or compression can cause pain in the upper extremity and hand numbness. Radiation therapy also can result in brachial plexopathies. *Idiopathic brachial plexopathy* (Parsonage-Turner syndrome) often occurs abruptly without any clear precipitating factor, although it can develop after an infection, injection, surgery, or childbirth. It typically begins with an aching sensation in the neck or shoulder and progresses over days to produce weakness, sensory loss, and diminished reflexes. Patients with brachial plexopathy often have considerable pain. Recovery is usually spontaneous but can take weeks to months. Some residual weakness may be present in a few patients.

Median Neuropathy (Carpal Tunnel Syndrome)

Carpal tunnel syndrome (CTS) is one of the most common mononeuropathies. It typically occurs within the confines of the carpal tunnel in the wrist. The median nerve can also be entrapped in the forearm as a pronator or interosseous syndrome. The entrapment can be caused by anything that causes a decrease in the size of the carpal tunnel (e.g., Colles' fracture, rheumatoid arthritis, congenital carpal tunnel stenosis), enlargement of the median nerve (e.g., diabetes, amyloidosis, thyroid disease, neuroma), or an increase in the volume of other structures within the carpal tunnel (e.g., tenosynovitis, ganglion, gout, urate deposits, lipoma, hematoma, fluid retention in pregnancy).

Other risk factors include any tasks that require repeated or sustained stress over the base of the palm. Low-frequency vibration exposure is another well-recognized risk factor for CTS. Repetitive wrist and hand movements such as knitting, typing, painting, woodworking, and weightlifting are also implicated as high-risk factors.

Common symptoms include numbness and paresthesias in the sensory distribution of the median nerve (palmar surface of thumb, index finger, and middle finger; radial side of ring finger; radial two thirds of palm). The patient may also have pain at rest (especially at night), weakness in the thumb, and thenar atrophy. Signs include a positive Tinel's sign at the wrist (tingling in median nerve distribution on percussion over ventral wrist), positive Phalen's sign (similar findings within 45 seconds after placing patient's wrist in maximal flexion), pain or paresthesias in a median distribution with thumb pressure over the median nerve for up to 30 seconds, and thenar atrophy. CTS can present with many variations, including proximal pain in the arm and shoulder, and with normal EMG.

Ulnar Neuropathy

The most common place to have ulnar nerve injury is at the elbow, where the nerve is anatomically most exposed and vulnerable as it traverses superficially in the ulnar groove. Pressure at the elbow such as with prolonged elbow weight bearing, coma, intoxication, or anesthesia can account for this problem.

Cubital tunnel syndrome occurs when the nerve is compressed as it runs beneath the aponeurosis of the flexor carpi ulnaris just distal to the medial epicondyle (cubital tunnel). Activities that involve repetitive or sustained elbow flexion, such as baseball pitching, can injure and stretch the nerve. This results in hypermobility of the ulnar nerve and allows recurrent subluxation over the medial epicondyle. Common symptoms include paresthesias or pain in the ring and small fingers and dorsoulnar aspect of the hand and forearm. There may be generalized loss of grip or fine motor control in the hand because of impairment of the intrinsic muscles. Symptoms may improve with elbow extension. Recurrent subluxation of the ulnar nerve at the elbow, especially in young throwing athletes, often requires surgical intervention.

Ulnar neuropathy distal to the elbow usually presents as *ulnar tunnel syndrome* when the nerve is compressed within Guyon's canal in the wrist. Prolonged pressure over the hypothenar eminence, as occurs with cycling, is a common cause, as are similar causes listed for CTS. Dysesthesias may or may not be present in the ulnar regions. Depending on where the specific entrapment occurs, all the intrinsic hand muscles may be weak, or hypothenar function may be selectively preserved.

Radial Neuropathy

Radial nerve injuries are much less common than other upper extremity neuropathies. Proximally, the radial nerve is most vulnerable in the axilla, where it can be injured by hyperabduction of the arm, which puts traction on the nerve. This is the case with "Saturday night palsy," when an intoxicated person sleeps with an arm draped over a chair. A similar circumstance occurs when the nerve is compressed against the humerus at the spiral groove. It is also seen with improper fit or use of crutches. Other sources of compression that can injure the radial nerve along its course include lipoma, fibroma, and new or previous (from callus) humerus fracture.

The radial nerve is predominantly a motor nerve, so symptoms depend on the level of injury. If the compression is proximal enough, there will be sensory loss over the dorsum of the hand, along with weakened triceps (elbow extension) and brachioradialis (elbow extension and supination) motor function. The most obvious finding in radial palsy is wristdrop and drop finger (digital extensor paralysis).

In *posterior interosseous syndrome* (radial tunnel syndrome) the compression is more distal; the purely motor branch of the radial nerve, the posterior interosseous nerve, is entrapped at the supinator muscle, causing only weakness in the finger extensors without affecting wrist extension.

Lumbosacral Neuropathy

Compared with the brachial plexus, the lumbosacral plexus is less susceptible to trauma. Injury caused by trauma or compression from surgery, pregnancy, childbirth, tumors, or aortic aneurysm can occur. Diabetes can also cause multiple mononeuropathy of the plexus (see later).

Meralgia Paresthetica

Compression of the lateral femoral cutaneous nerve as it passes over the anterior superior iliac spine at the lateral end of the inguinal canal is common. It is seen in those who have diabetes, are obese, or wear their pants too tight. Patients experience numbness, paresthesias, and pain over the anterolateral aspect of the thigh, without weakness.

Femoral Neuropathy

Any blunt or penetrating trauma, surgery or angiography in the groin, prolonged lithotomy position, or hyperextension during dance or gymnastics can injure the femoral nerve. A tumor or inguinal hernia involving the plexus can also compress the nerve. The femoral nerve supplies the quadriceps muscles for knee extension and provides sensory information from the anterior medial thigh and medial leg. Dysfunction in this nerve can result in pain in the groin that radiates to the thigh, buckling of the knee caused by quadriceps weakness, and sensory loss over its area of distribution. Weakness in the hip flexors indicates a more proximal lesion in the lumbar plexus or roots. Diabetic lumbosacral plexopathy should also be distinguished from femoral neuropathies. With the former, patients are older than 50 years, with diabetes, and develop acute severe pain in the thigh that progresses over days to weakness in the femoral nerve distribution. Sensory symptoms are mild. EMG helps distinguish these different conditions.

Sciatic Neuropathy

The sciatic nerve arises from the sacral portion of the plexus. It leaves the pelvis through the sciatic notch and divides into the tibial and peroneal nerves at the popliteal fossa. The sciatic nerve provides sensation to the perineum, posterior thigh, lateral calf, and foot. It innervates the thigh extensors, hamstrings, and all the muscles of the lower leg and foot. Pain, weakness, and sensory changes caused by injury of the sciatic nerve or one of its two branches can be caused by trauma from gunshots, hip fracture or dislocation, compression from surgery or prolonged sitting on a hard edge, tumor, endometriosis, lipoma, aneurysm of the gluteal artery, or improper intramuscular injection into the gluteus. Symptoms of sciatic nerve compression can mimic L5-S1 radiculopathy. Again, EMG is helpful in these clinical situations.

Peroneal Neuropathy

The common peroneal nerve is most often compressed as it passes close to the fibular head. Such compression occurs from prolonged leg crossing, squatting, or kneeling, improperly fitted cast or stockings, or prolonged pressure in an intoxicated or comatose patient. Symptoms of peroneal palsy consist of sensory loss over the lateral calf and dorsum of the foot and a weakness of ankle dorsiflexion (footdrop) and foot eversion without pain. If a clear history of trauma or compression cannot be elicited, imaging of the posterior fossa is necessary to rule out a mass lesion. Patients with a more permanent injury to the peroneal nerve may need an ankle-foot orthotic device to provide ankle stability and prevent plantar flexion contractures.

Tibial Neuropathy (Tarsal Tunnel Syndrome)

The tarsal tunnel is located at the inferoposterior margin of the medial malleolus. Its boundaries include the bones of the ankle and fibrous flexor retinaculum. The posterior tibial nerve and three flexor tendons of the foot and vessels lie within this tunnel. Compression can occur within the tunnel from tenosynovitis, enlarged veins, and fracture or dislocation of the ankle. Prolonged standing or walking may lead to vascular stasis and engorgement within the tunnel. A horse jockey is in one of the few occupations associated with this syndrome. The primary symptom of tarsal tunnel syndrome is painful, burning paresthesias in the sole of the foot that are worse after a day of activity and may extend into the night. The symptoms can be reproduced or exacerbated by gentle percussion over the tarsal tunnel (Tinel's sign). The patient may also have weakness in the intrinsic muscles of the foot, making it difficult to push off during walking. Definitive treatment is surgical decompression involving release of the retinaculum.

Interdigital Neuropathy

A common cause of foot pain, entrapment of an interdigital nerve is often caused by a Morton's neuroma or benign swelling of the nerve. Tenderness is appreciated in the web space between the metatarsal heads. Any space can be affected, but the second and third web spaces are most often involved. Running, ballet dancing, and wearing tight shoes or high heels are all risk factors. Modifying risk factors, local corticosteroid injection, and surgical release are treatment options.

Polyneuropathies

Inflammatory Neuropathies

With inflammatory neuropathies, an inflammatory process is directed against the peripheral nerve; the most common causes follow. Treatment is usually directed toward the causative agent.

Human Immunodeficiency Virus

Several opportunistic infections of the PNS may result from HIV infection. The HIV itself, cytomegalovirus, and herpes zoster are most common. Painful sensorimotor polyneuropathies or demyelinating polyradiculoneuropathies occur during the early and late stages of HIV disease. Symptomatic relief of neuropathic pain may be achieved with antidepressants (e.g., amitriptyline) or anticonvulsants (e.g., carbamazepine).

Lyme Disease

The early stages of disseminated Lyme disease have resulted in Bell's palsy or an inflammation of CN VII (facial nerve) in approximately 11% of Lyme disease patients (Wilkinson, 1998). In the later stages of Lyme disease, a neuropathy mimicking CIDP can occur.

Leprosy

Although uncommon in the United States, leprosy is the most common worldwide treatable cause of neuropathy. Symptoms of neuropathy can occur before the systemic manifestations of disease are present. As leprosy progresses, with its characteristic skin lesions, the risk for peripheral nerve injury increases. Sensory loss of some degree is expected. Treatment is directed toward the disease itself.

Acute Inflammatory Demyelinating Polyradiculoneuropathy

Guillain-Barré syndrome, or acute inflammatory demyelinating polyradiculoneuropathy, is a rapidly progressive paralytic syndrome affecting persons of all ages. GBS seems to occur through an immune-mediated process. Many cases follow a mild gastrointestinal or upper respiratory viral illness by 1 to 3 weeks. Other risk factors include pregnancy, influenza immunization, the postoperative period, and HIV infection. A particularly strong link between *Campylobacter jejuni* infection and GBS has been suggested in up to 20% of cases (Dyck et al., 1993).

The traditional description of a rapid progression of ascending symmetric weakness starting in the lower extremities and moving to the upper extremities is often useful, *but variations are quite common.* Indeed, early development of proximal weakness is frequently seen, and involvement of upper extremities before lower extremities is not rare. In general, the presentation is one of rapid progression of an ascending symmetric weakness, usually starting in the lower extremities and moving to the upper extremities. Patients may initially complain of pain and paresthesias in the back and proximal limbs. The progressive weakness that involves the legs as well as the upper extremities, trunk, intercostals, head, and neck muscles may take several days to 4 weeks and often results in paralysis. There may be mild sensory impairment in the extremities, early loss of DTRs, and bilateral facial nerve palsy in up to 40% of patients. Nerve conduction studies demonstrate demyelination, and the CSF may show an increased protein level, with normal cell counts.

The differential diagnosis of a rapid-onset polyradiculoneuropathy includes botulism, diphtheria, hypophosphatemia, acute intermittent porphyria, poliomyelitis, Lyme disease, poisoning from contaminated shellfish (e.g., tetrodotoxin), and toxic neuropathies (e.g., arsenic, mercury, thallium).

Because of the rapidly progressive nature of GBS, patients should be monitored in the hospital for signs of respiratory failure and autonomic instability (arrhythmias, hypotension, hypertension, and hyperpyrexia in two thirds of patients). Treatment usually consists of plasmapheresis or intravenous human immune globulin (IVIG). There is no role for steroids in the acute treatment of GBS. In most patients, recovery is complete or nearly complete, although it may take a few weeks to 18 months. About 10% of cases result in severe permanent disability. Even under the best circumstances, 3% to 5% of patients do not survive.

Chronic Inflammatory Demyelinating Polyradiculoneuropathy

CIDP is an acquired motor and sensory neuropathy of unknown cause. As with GBS, an immune-mediated pathogenesis is suspected. Unlike GBS, CIDP usually occurs in the absence of a preceding illness. Unusual exceptions include HIV infection, dysproteinemias, and lupus erythematosus. CIDP is predominantly a motor polyneuropathy affecting those of all ages, with a progressive or relapsing course. Weakness can be proximal or distal but usually develops in the legs over at least 2 months, distinguishing CIDP from GBS. Sensory changes include numbness or paresthesias but can be variable. DTRs are decreased or absent. Electrodiagnostic and CSF findings are similar to those found in GBS. Treatment includes prednisone, along with plasmapheresis or IVIG. CIDP should be distinguished from other acquired and hereditary neuropathies.

Metabolic Neuropathies

Diabetic Neuropathy

Diabetes is the cause of the most common polyneuropathy seen by family physicians, occurring in up to 50% of all diabetic patients. Its incidence usually rises with disease progression. Diabetic peripheral neuropathy has a widely variable presentation but usually is seen as a symmetric polyneuropathy, with predominant sensory signs and mild motor signs. Patients experience burning dysesthesias and pain in the soles of the feet. Impaired position sense leading to ataxia and arthropathy (Charcot's joints) implies the involvement of large, myelinated, sensory fibers. Patients with diabetic neuropathy experience bilateral symptoms that include burning pain in the back and thigh with proximal muscle weakness, decreased patellar DTRs, and normal sensory function. This is thought to be caused by microvascular ischemia of the proximal motor trunks. Diabetes is also associated with autonomic neuropathies. Symptoms may include postural hypotension, gastroparesis, intestinal dysmotility, atonic bladder, impotence, and loss of pain fibers in the cardiac sympathetic system, permitting silent MI.

Uremic Neuropathy

Patients with chronic renal disease develop a symmetric sensorimotor neuropathy involving the upper and lower extremities. They complain mostly of burning paresthesias. Uremic neuropathy is thought to be secondary to a toxic effect on the peripheral nerves. Because many chronic renal patients also have diabetes, it is often difficult to isolate a single cause. However, patients with true uremic neuropathy who have undergone renal transplantation can have dramatic improvement of symptoms (Rees, 1995).

Nutritional Neuropathies

Most nutritional neuropathies involve one of the B-complex vitamins. Patients at risk for these neuropathies usually have chronic alcoholism, malabsorption syndrome, eating disorder, or unusual diet (food faddist). It presents as a symmetric polyneuropathy with burning in the feet. Weakness, atrophy, and hypoactive reflexes may also occur.

Alcoholic neuropathy is caused from inadequate intake and poor absorption. Treatment with multivitamin supplementation is usually adequate but may take time to be effective. Thiamine (vitamin B_1) deficiency, or beriberi, is seen most often with chronic alcoholism. It may present as a distal polyneuropathy or as a more serious Wernicke-Korsakoff encephalopathy, with mental status changes. In the latter case, intramuscular thiamine (100 mg/day) is preferred initially over oral administration. Pyridoxine (vitamin B_6) deficiency can be associated with the use of dapsone or isoniazid, which interfere with vitamin B_6 metabolism. Prevention requires supplementation with 50 mg of pyridoxine three times daily. Prolonged intake of pyridoxine of more than 2 g/day has also been associated with sensory neuropathy (Rostami, 1995). Vitamin B_{12} deficiency may present only with vague paresthesias. Determining the serum vitamin B_{12} level is the best way to assess a patient when this problem is suspected, because abnormal RBC indices may not be apparent until irreversible neurologic symptoms have already occurred.

Hereditary Neuropathies

The hereditary neuropathies are often missed by family physicians and even by those close to the affected patient. These indolent, slowly progressive polyneuropathies may present with motor, autonomic, and less often, sensory symptoms.

Box 42-22 Neuropathies Caused by Drugs and Toxins

Drugs

Axonal
Amitriptyline
Chloroquine
Cimetidine
Colchicine
Dapsone
Didanosine
Disulfiram
Ethambutol
Hydralazine
Interferon alfa
Isoniazid
Lithium
Metronidazole
Nitrous oxide
Nitrofurantoin
Paclitaxel
Phenytoin
Pyridoxine
Procainamide
Vincristine

Demyelinating
Amiodarone
Colchicine
Gold

Neuronopathy
Cisplatin
Pyridoxine
Thalidomide

Toxins

Industrial
Organophosphates
Lead, arsenic, mercury
Thallium, methyl bromide
Plastics, synthetic fabrics
Carbon monoxide
Ethylene oxide

Euphoriants
Glue
Solvents

These include pes cavus, absent tendon reflexes, a high-stepping or slapping gait, footdrop, slowly progressive wasting and weakness of peroneal muscles, foot ulcers, joint arthropathy, and absence of sweating. Without a specific treatment for these neuropathies, efforts are focused on management of physical disabilities, education, genetic counseling, and reassurance. Hereditary neuropathies and CIDP can both have a familial pattern, the important difference being that CIDP is treatable.

Toxic Neuropathies

Toxic neuropathies occur from repeated exposure to drugs, industrial toxins, or heavy metals (Box 42-22). Presentation depends on the exact exposure and what part of the nerve is affected. It may present as a progressive, symmetric, ascending polyneuropathy, as in many occupational exposures, or with vague sensory changes similar to those of nutritional neuropathies. Lead intoxication creates a motor neuropathy starting in the upper limbs, affecting the radial nerve and causing wristdrop. Many of these neuropathies slowly improve once the offending agent is removed; however, this is not always the case. A careful medical and occupation history is important. Treatment is directed accordingly.

Dysproteinemic Neuropathies

Dysproteinemias such as cryoglobulinemia, myeloma, amyloidosis, lymphoma, monoclonal gammopathies, and some leukemias are associated with peripheral neuropathy. In patients with idiopathic peripheral neuropathies, a *monoclonal gammopathy* can be identified in up to 10% (Kissel and Mendell, 1996). Plasma exchange is useful as a treatment option for some of the dysproteinemic neuropathies.

Carcinomatous Neuropathies

Carcinomatous neuropathies may result from direct compression by a solid tumor or local infiltration of nerves. The most common association is lung carcinoma. Some chemotherapeutic agents, such as vincristine and cisplatin, have neurotoxic side effects. The most common presentation is that of a distal sensorimotor polyneuropathy. In up to 16% of patients with lung carcinoma and 4% of those with breast carcinomas, peripheral neuropathy preceded the actual signs of the disease.

Cranial Neuropathies

Key Points

- Bell's palsy is an acute unilateral paralysis of the facial nerve and involves the forehead muscles.
- Trigeminal neuralgia is usually a unilateral severe lancinating pain lasting a few seconds, triggered by innocuous stimuli (light touch to face, toothbrushing).
- Trigeminal neuralgia is rarely seen in patients less than 40 years of age.

Many conditions or infections may affect the cranial nerves and cause a peripheral neuropathy. Two common problems encountered by family physicians are idiopathic acute peripheral facial paralysis (Bell's palsy) and trigeminal neuralgia (tic douloureux).

Idiopathic Acute Peripheral Facial Paralysis

Bell's palsy is an acute, unilateral paralysis of the facial nerve of unknown etiology but possibly linked to an antecedent herpes infection (Adour, 1975). Bell's palsy is likely the most common isolated cranial neuropathy (23 per 100,000) seen by family physicians (Hauser, 1971). Symptoms tend to develop over hours to days and may be associated with recent upper respiratory infection. Symptoms include partial or complete paralysis of the ipsilateral facial muscles, forehead involvement, otalgia, phonophobia, and cephalgia. If the forehead muscles are spared, one must consider a central etiology to the symptoms. Bilateral findings of Bell's palsy should prompt consideration of GBS, sarcoidosis, disseminated Lyme disease, or diabetes.

Most patients with Bell's palsy will recover with only supportive therapy within a few days to a few months. This makes aggressive treatment controversial. A recent meta-analysis showed that high-dose corticosteroids (>450 mg total dose) were associated with greater benefit and decreased risk of unsatisfactory recovery, whereas antiviral agents showed no benefit alone but may have additional benefit when used with corticosteroids (de Almeida et al., 2009). A typical corticosteroid regimen may include oral prednisone, 60 mg/day for 7 days, then tapering by 10 mg/day, with or without valacyclovir, 500 mg orally three times daily for 7 days.

KEY TREATMENT

High-dose corticosteroids (>450 mg total dose) help reduce the risk of unsatisfactory recovery from Bell's palsy (de Almeida et al., 2009) (SOR: A).

Trigeminal Neuralgia

Trigeminal neuralgia (tic douloureux) usually involves the second and third (maxillary and mandibular) divisions of the trigeminal nerve, causing pain of the innervated structures (lips, gums, teeth). It is almost always unilateral, with the pain sudden, sharp, and severe, lasting a few seconds at a time. This cycle of pain can occur hundreds of times a day. It may be described as lancinating, ice pick like, or an electric shock and characteristically is precipitated by innocuous stimuli such as light touch to the face or toothbrushing. It is rarely seen in patients younger than 40. Pain that is longer in duration, bilateral, or described as more aching or pressure like is usually not related to trigeminal neuralgia and should cause the physician to search for another cause. Other conditions that should be considered include multiple sclerosis, acoustic neurinoma, aneurysm, meningioma, trigeminal neuroma, and early herpes zoster or postherpetic neuralgia. Herpes zoster should be suspected in patients younger than 40 who present with pain following the upper division of the trigeminal nerve (forehead and eye). Neuroimaging with MRI scanning of the brain is recommended to exclude these causes from idiopathic disease.

A common initial pharmacologic treatment for idiopathic trigeminal neuralgia is carbamazepine (Tegretol), up to 800 mg/day, or oxcarbazepine (Trileptal), up to 1200 mg/day. Usually, these medications are started at relatively low doses (100-200 mg once or twice daily) and increased at 7- to 10-day intervals until adequate symptom control is achieved. Patients should be educated that these medicines will only work when taken on a consistent basis and not as an analgesic medication. Other medications that have been used but are not FDA approved include gabapentin (Neurontin), amitriptyline, and baclofen. Toxicities from these medications, including allergic reactions, bone marrow suppression, and liver toxicity, may develop and thus require close monitoring. Patients with refractory symptoms or who do not tolerate pharmacologic treatment should be considered for neurosurgical evaluation.

Parkinson's Disease

Key Points

- The hallmark clinical features of Parkinson's disease include resting tremor, rigidity and bradykinesia of asymmetric onset.
- Symptoms such as hallucinations, gait abnormalities, paralysis of upward gaze, early dementia, early postural instability, early autonomic dysfunction, involuntary movements other than a tremor and a failure to respond to levodopa suggest a parkinsonism-plus syndrome and require further evaluation.
- Drug therapy for Parkinson's disease should be initiated when the symptoms are significant enough to cause functional impairment.

Parkinson's disease is the second most common progressive neurodegenerative disorder in the United States after Alzheimer's disease. Parkinson's affects about 1% of the population over age 60 and 4% to 5% of those older than 85. The disease is uncommon before age 40, and incidence is higher in men than women. A genetic predisposition to Parkinson's disease may be present; up to 15% of patients will have a first- or second-degree relative with Parkinson's disease. At present, no clear environmental links to Parkinson's disease have been identified. The disease is caused by a disruption of dopaminergic neurotransmission in the basal ganglia and the development of eosinophilic intracytoplasmic inclusions (Lewy bodies) in the residual dopaminergic neurons.

Symptoms and Signs

The hallmark clinical features of Parkinson's disease include tremor, rigidity, and bradykinesia, usually of asymmetric onset. Tremor is the presenting symptom in up to 70% of patients, and in fact, an asymmetric rest tremor is virtually pathognomonic of Parkinson's disease. Many patients present to the family physician complaining of a tremor and the concern they may have Parkinson's disease. Most will have *essential tremor,* which can be differentiated from the tremor of Parkinson's disease in that essential tremor is usually symmetric and exacerbated by action, whereas the tremor of Parkinson's disease is usually at rest and asymmetric.

Rigidity is often associated with *cogwheeling,* a ratchety quality during passive movement of the limb. *Bradykinesia* refers to the slowness of movements, which usually begins in an asymmetric fashion, described by the patient as "weakness" of an extremity, although no abnormalities are noted with strength testing. Other clinical features associated with Parkinson's disease include micrographia, paucity of facial expression (masked facies), narrow shuffling gait, and postural instability (late finding). Behavioral and cognitive symptoms are frequently seen in patients with Parkinson's disease as well.

Differential Diagnosis

Up to 20% of patients initially diagnosed with Parkinson's disease ultimately have an alternative diagnosis. The term *parkinsonism-plus syndrome* is used for patients who have similar symptoms but also have additional abnormalities or do not respond to the usual medications. Symptoms that suggest a parkinsonism-plus syndrome include hallucinations, gait abnormalities, paralysis of upward gaze, early dementia, early postural instability, early autonomic dysfunction, involuntary movements other than tremor, and a failure to respond to levodopa (Italian Neurological Society, 2003). Conditions that frequently may be confused with Parkinson's disease include progressive supranuclear palsy, dementia with Lewy bodies, multiple-system atrophy, vascular parkinsonism, and drug-induced parkinsonism.

Progressive supranuclear palsy (PSP) may initially be mistaken for Parkinson's disease. Patients have ophthalmoparesis of vertical gaze, primarily downward gaze. Early loss of postural reflexes, predominantly axial rigidity, pseudobulbar palsy, and frontal lobe signs are other characteristics of PSP. Response to dopaminergic medications is minimal.

Dementia with Lewy bodies has motor symptoms similar to those of Parkinson's disease, and there may be a response to levodopa. Rigidity is usually more prominent than bradykinesia or tremor. Additionally, there is early cognitive impairment and hallucinations early in the disease course.

Multisystem atrophy includes a number of diseases, and it is not clear if they represent distinct diseases or a single, pathologic continuum. This group includes olivopontocerebellar atrophy, striatonigral degeneration, and Shy-Drager syndrome.

Symptoms are related to autonomic nervous system dysfunction and include orthostatic hypotension, cerebellar dysfunction, bladder dysfunction, and a poor levodopa response.

Vascular parkinsonism may be associated with multiple vascular lesions in the basal ganglia. There is usually a stepwise progression to the disease. Tremor at rest is not a common finding, and the bradykinesia and rigidity tend to be more significant in the legs. The gait is often broad based. Associated symptoms include dementia, spasticity, and weakness. MRI studies show multi-infarct changes, and the response to levodopa is poor.

A final category of Parkinson-like conditions is *drug-induced parkinsonism.* It is important to identify this cause because it is usually reversible. Drug-induced parkinsonism accounted for 20% of cases of parkinsonism-plus conditions in a population-based study (Bower et al., 1999). Medications that can cause these symptoms include neuroleptics, atypical neuroleptics, antiemetic medications (e.g., metoclopramide, prochlorperazine), amiodarone, valproic acid, and lithium. Medicines that block the synthesis of dopamine, such as methyldopa (Aldomet), or deplete dopamine (e.g., reserpine), can also induce parkinsonism (Nutt and Wooten, 2005).

Diagnostic Evaluation

An extensive diagnostic evaluation is not necessary when the history and physical examination reveal classic findings of Parkinson's disease. Imaging of the brain with CT or MRI may be performed if the diagnosis is in question and to rule out other conditions such as NPH or vascular parkinsonism. Consultation with a neurologist may be helpful, especially if the diagnosis is in question or a parkinsonism-plus diagnosis is likely.

Treatment

Currently, diagnosis of Parkinson's disease does not relegate a patient to pharmacologic treatment. Drug therapy should be initiated when the symptoms are significant enough to cause functional impairment (Rao et al., 2006). Current therapies do not appear to slow the progression of the disease and no studies have clearly demonstrated a best initial treatment for this condition (Schreck et al., 2003). Table 42-17 summarizes the pharmacologic agents available to treat Parkinson's disease.

Pharmacotherapy

Levodopa, a precursor of dopamine, is the most frequently prescribed agent for the treatment of symptomatic Parkinson's disease and is particularly effective at controlling bradykinesia and rigidity (Miyasaki et al., 2002). Alone, levodopa is absorbed but is peripherally metabolized to dopamine by dopa-decarboxylase enzymes. This peripheral conversion limits the overall effectiveness of levodopa and increases the side effects, including nausea, vomiting, and hypotension. To remedy this, levodopa is combined with carbidopa, which prevents this peripheral conversion. Dopa-decarboxylase is saturated with 70 to 100 mg of carbidopa. Thus the usual starting dose of carbidopa-levodopa is 25 mg/100 mg three times daily (Rao et al., 2006).

Dopamine agonists directly stimulate dopamine receptors, thus bypassing the presynaptic synthesis of dopamine. These medications cause less dyskinesia and fewer fluctuations

Table 42-17 Medications for Parkinson's Disease

Generic Name	Recommended Dosage	Side Effects/Comments
Anticholinergics		
Trihexyphenidyl (Artane)	1 mg tid; increase to 2 mg tid	Effective for tremor. Side effects include impaired memory, blurred vision, and urinary retention.
Benztropine (Cogentin)	0.5 mg at bedtime; increase by 0.5 mg up to max 1 mg bid.	Same as for trihexyphenidyl.
Carbidopa-Levodopa Combinations		
Immediate release (Sinemet)	25 mg/100 mg initially ½ tablet tid; increase by ½ tablet every 4-7 days.	"Gold standard" of therapy. Long-term therapy may result in motor fluctuations, dyskinesias, confusion, and hallucinations.
Controlled release (Sinemet-CR)	1 tablet bid	Same as for immediate release.
Carbidopa-levodopa plus entacapone (Stalevo)	1 tablet tid	Same as for other carbidopa-levodopa preparations, plus diarrhea.
Catechol-*O*-Methyltransferase (COMT) Inhibitors		
Tolcapone (Tasmar)	100 mg or 200 mg tid	Adjunct to levodopa to prevent motor fluctuations. Monitor liver functions.
Entacapone (Comtan)	200 mg with each dose of carbidopa-levodopa, up to 8 times daily	Same as for tolcapone.
Dopamine Agonists		
Bromocriptine (Parlodel)	1.25 mg with meals bid; increase by 2.5 mg every 2-4 weeks to max 15 mg/day.	Effective in monotherapy or as adjunct to levodopa.
Pramipexole (Mirapex)	0.125 mg tid, max 1.5 mg tid	Side effects include excessive daytime somnolence, hypotension, confusion, and hallucinations.
Ropinirole (ReQuip)	25 mg tid; increase weekly by 0.25 mg tid to 3 mg tid. Max dose 8 mg tid	Same as for pramipexole.
Monoamine Oxidase Type B (MAO-B) Inhibitors		
Selegiline (Eldepryl)	5 mg at breakfast and lunch	Avoid use with SSRIs, TCAs, and meperidine. Side effects include nausea, dizziness, hallucinations, abdominal pain, and vivid dreams.
Rasagiline (Azilect)	0.5 mg/day to 1 mg/day	Side effects include extrapyramidal symptoms, dyskinesia, hallucinations, hypotension, and depression.
N-Methyl-D-Aspartate (NMDA) Antagonist (Receptor Inhibitor)		
Amantadine (Symmetrel)	100 mg twice daily	May be used as monotherapy. Side effects include dizziness, confusion, livedo reticularis, and hallucinations.

bid, Twice daily; *tid*, three times daily; *SSRIs*, selective serotonin reuptake inhibitors; *TCAs*, tricyclic antidepressants.

than levodopa. They can be used alone or in conjunction with levodopa. Currently, bromocriptine (Parlodel), pramipexole (Mirapex), and ropinirole (ReQuip) are medications in this class available for the treatment of Parkinson's disease. Apomorphine (Apokyn) is also available as a subcutaneous injection for the treatment of sudden, resistant "off" periods (Goetz et al., 2005). It has significant adverse effects and should only be used by individuals experienced with its use. Dopamine agonists should not be used in patients with dementia because of the high likelihood of producing hallucinations (Nutt and Wooten, 2005).

Monoamine oxidase type B (MAO-B) *inhibitors* were initially thought to provide a neuroprotective effect to patients with Parkinson's disease. This has not been supported in the literature. Agents available in the United States in this class include selegiline (Eldepryl), orally disintegrating selegiline (Zelapar), and rasagiline (Azilect). A meta-analysis of 17 trials comparing MAO-B inhibitors with placebo or levodopa revealed MAOIs reduce disability, incidence of motor fluctuations, and need for levodopa (Ives et al., 2004).

Anticholinergic medications primarily work on the muscarinic acetylcholine receptors. These medications have low effectiveness and a high incidence of side effects which limit their overall usefulness to patients younger than 70 years and with preserved cognitive function.

Degradation of levodopa in the periphery is known to be associated with motor fluctuations and dyskinesia in Parkinson's disease. The enzyme catechol-O-methyltransferase (COMT) is responsible for part of this degradation. *COMT inhibitors* prolong the dopamine response. Two medications in this category are tolcapone (Tasmar) and entacapone (Comtan). These medications reduced "off" time, reduced total levodopa dose, and improved motor symptoms in patients with advanced Parkinson's disease and motor complications (Cochrane review; Deane et al., 2004). As such, COMT inhibitors are usually reserved for more advanced cases.

Among *NMDA antagonists* (NMDA receptor inhibitors), amantadine (Symmetrel), originally developed as an antiviral agent, is useful for tremor, rigidity, and bradykinesia associated with Parkinson's disease, although few studies demonstrate its clear efficacy. Amantadine may also have a dopamine agonist effect as well as an anticholinergic effect. Side effects include dizziness, insomnia, nausea, and vomiting.

Surgical Treatment

Surgical treatments are options to be considered when tremor, motor fluctuations, and dyskinesia are not adequately controlled with medications alone. Techniques that offer potential benefit include unilateral pallidotomy and deep brain stimulation of the globus pallidus interna or subthalamic nucleus (Goetz et al., 2005). Patients with symptoms not controlled medically should be referred to specialized centers with surgeons experienced in performing these procedures.

Treatment of Nonmotor Symptoms

Patients with Parkinson's disease frequently develop other comorbid conditions such as depression or dementia. In the case of depression, an SSRI can be used. Up to 40% of patients develop dementia (Aarsland et al., 2003). In these patients the cholinesterase inhibitors can be effective. Parkinson's disease is a progressive illness, so it is important for the family physician to discuss advanced directives, establishment of power of attorney for health care decisions, and the patient's wishes surrounding the use of artificial nutrition. Living wills and other legal documents should be prepared and appropriate discussions documented. Common symptoms such as constipation, sleep disturbance, and orthostatic hypotension should be aggressively treated.

> **KEY TREATMENT**
>
> Levodopa, dopamine agonists, and MAO-B inhibitors, alone or in combination, are effective in treating the symptoms of Parkinson's disease (Rao et al., 2006) (SOR: A).
> Usual starting dose of carbidopa-levodopa is 25 mg/100 mg three times daily (Rao et al., 2006) (SOR: A).
> Surgical therapies (unilateral pallidotomy, deep brain stimulation) are effective when medical therapy fails to control Parkinson symptoms (Goetz et al., 2005) (SOR: B).

Multiple Sclerosis

Key Points

- The diagnosis of multiple sclerosis requires evidence of demyelinating disseminated disease.
- Optic neuritis, nystagmus from internuclear ophthalmoplegia, and Lhermitte's sign are highly suggestive of MS.
- The currently most widely accepted diagnostic criteria for MS are the McDonald criteria, established by an international panel in 2001 and revised in 2005.

Multiple sclerosis (MS) is a recurrent, chronic, demyelinating, autoimmune disorder that affects the central nervous system. The mean age of onset for MS is 29 to 33 years, although the range is 15 to 50 years, which makes this the most common cause of neurologic disability in young adults.

Diagnosis

The diagnosis of MS is based on clinical signs and symptoms combined with diagnostic testing, which may include MRI, CSF analysis, and visual-evoked potentials (VEPs). Definitive diagnosis of MS requires evidence of demyelinating disease disseminated over time and space (McDonald et al., 2001). That is, clinical symptoms should last at least 24 hours and should be separated by at least 30 days, and should affect two different areas of the CNS: the brain, spinal cord, or optic nerves. The clinical symptoms vary, depending on which part of the CNS is involved. Three symptoms are highly suggestive of MS: optic neuritis, nystagmus resulting from internuclear ophthalmoplegia, and Lhermitte's sign, which is an electrical sensation extending down the back and legs with flexion of the neck. The International Panel of the Diagnosis of Multiple Sclerosis developed criteria for the diagnosis of MS (McDonald et al., 2001), revised in 2005 and summarized in Table 42-18 (Polman et al., 2005). It is important to remember that alternative diagnoses should be considered and excluded. These would include CNS vasculitis, paraneoplastic syndromes, sarcoidosis, leukodystrophies, CNS tumors, infections, CNS lymphoma, and nutritional deficiencies, such as B_{12} deficiency.

The precise relationship between clinical symptoms and MR findings are not well understood. Thus, MRI alone is not useful in predicting the clinical course of MS. T2-weighted MR images best define the size of white matter lesions, and gadolinium can reveal the disruption of the blood-brain barrier associated with an active MS lesion. In general, MR findings consistent with MS must include at least three of these findings: (1) one gadolinium-enhancing lesion or nine T2 hyperintense lesions if gadolinium-enhancing lesions are not present; (2) at least one infratentorial lesion; (3) at least one juxtacortical lesion; and (4) at least three periventricular lesions. These lesions should be at least 3 mm in cross section (Barkof et al., 1997; Tintore et al., 2000). Spinal cord lesions can be substituted for one of the brain lesions as long as it reveals little or no swelling of the spinal cord, is unequivocally hyperintense if detected with T2-weighted MR images, at least 3 mm in size but less than two vertebral segments in length, and occupies only part of the cross section of the spinal cord (Polman et al., 2005).

Table 42-18 Criteria for Multiple Sclerosis (MS)

Clinical Presentation	Additional Data Needed
Two or more attacks (relapses); two or more objective clinical lesions	None; clinical evidence will suffice (additional evidence desirable but must be consistent with MS)
Two or more attacks; one objective clinical lesion	Dissemination in space, demonstrated by MRI *or* Positive CSF and two or more MRI lesions consistent with MS *or* further clinical attack involving different site
One attack; two or more objective clinical lesions	Dissemination in time, demonstrated by MRI *or* second clinical attack
One attack; one objective clinical lesion (monosymptomatic presentation)	Dissemination in space by demonstrated by MRI *or* Positive CSF and two or more MRI lesions consistent with MS *and* Dissemination in time demonstrated by MRI *or* Second clinical attack
Insidious neurologic progression suggestive of MS (primary progressive MS)	Positive CSF *and* Dissemination in space demonstrated by MRI evidence of nine or more T2 brain lesions *or* Two or more spinal cord lesions *or* Four to eight brain and one spinal cord lesion *or* Positive VEP with four to eight MRI lesions *or* Positive VEP with less than four brain lesions and one spinal cord lesion *and* Dissemination in time demonstrated by MRI *or* Continued progression for 1 year

Modified from McDonald WI, Compston A, Edan G, et al. Recommended diagnostic criteria for multiple sclerosis: Guidelines from the International Panel on the diagnosis of multiple sclerosis. Ann Neurol 200;150:121.
MRI, Magnetic resonance imaging; *CSF,* cerebrospinal fluid; *VEP,* visual-evoked potential.

The CSF analysis of patients with MS generally demonstrates a normal opening pressure, cell count, glucose level, protein level, and culture. The most clinically useful CSF abnormality is the presence of oligoclonal immunoglobulin G (IgG) bands resulting from intrathecal IgG synthesis, which can be found in up to 90% of patients with MS (Freedman et al., 2005). IgG bands are not specific to MS and are also seen in sarcoidosis, AIDS, and subacute sclerosis panencephalitis. The value of CSF analysis is mainly limited to MS patients with only a few lesions on MRI, or to make the diagnosis of primary progressive MS, as discussed later. Visual-evoked responses may also provide supporting evidence for MS, particularly in situations with few abnormalities on MRI. Other VEP analysis offers little in establishing a diagnosis of MS (Gronseth and Ashman, 2000).

Clinical Course

Four subtypes of MS are currently described—relapsing remitting, secondary-progressive, primary progressive, and progressive-relapsing. *Relapsing-remitting* MS accounts for about 85% of the initial diagnosis of MS patients and is characterized by acute attacks followed by full recovery. The interval between relapses can be variable and is characterized by a lack of disease progression. *Secondary-progressive* MS is characterized by a pattern that is initially relapsing-remitting but then evolves into a pattern of progressive neurologic decline. MRI demonstrates more extensive lesions, and approximately 50% of patients initially diagnosed with relapsing-remitting MS will develop secondary-progressive disease. *Primary-progressive* MS, characterized by a gradual disease progression from the initial onset, accounts for approximately 10% of MS diagnoses and has limited treatment options. *Progressive-relapsing* MS demonstrates a pattern of steady progression from the time of onset that may be punctuated by clearly defined relapses. The patients may or may not fully recover from these acute relapses.

Treatment

The treatment of MS can be divided into disease-modifying therapies, medications for acute relapses, and symptomatic management. Although there is no definitive cure, disease-modifying therapies may reduce the frequency of relapses, slow the rate of progression, and reduce the acute inflammatory response. Symptomatic therapy can improve the control of many of the functional disabilities and thus improve quality of life.

Disease-Modifying Therapies

It is generally held that disease-modifying therapy should be initiated immediately on the diagnosis of MS (Coyle and Hartung, 2002). Disease-modifying therapy has been shown to be more effective in preventing new lesion formation than repairing old lesions. These therapies include interferon beta-1b (Betaseron), interferon beta-1a (Avonex, Rebif), and glatiramer acetate (Copaxone). The beta interferons are immunomodulating medications that also have antiviral activities. They have been shown to reduce relapses in patients with the relapsing-remitting form of MS. Betaseron is given as an alternating-day subcutaneous (SC) injection, Rebif is a three-times-weekly SC injection, and Avonex is administered as a weekly intramuscular injection. All have similar side effects, including injection site reactions, influenza-like symptoms, and worsening of preexisting depression. Bone marrow suppression and transient elevation of liver enzymes may also occur.

Glatiramer (Copaxone) is a synthetic polypeptide consisting of four amino acids. It is thought to lead to the induction of antigen-specific suppressor T cells. It is administered as a daily SC injection and has been shown to reduce relapses by approximately 30% (Comi et al., 2001). Side effects include postinjection reactions and occasionally a reaction involving flushing, chest pain, anxiety, and dyspnea. The reaction is self-limited and does not require discontinuation of the medication.

Two other disease-modifying drugs for MS are mitoxantrone and natalizumab. Mitoxantrone is a synthetic anthracenedione given by IV infusion once every 3 months. It has been shown to reduce MS relapses by 67% (Hartung et al., 2002). Mitoxantrone is blue and can lead to transient bluish discoloration of the sclera and urine. It also can cause cardiotoxicity, and as a chemotherapeutic agent, should only be prescribed for worsening cases of MS not responding to first-line agents. Also, only experienced health care professionals should prescribe mitoxantrone.

Natalizumab is a monoclonal antibody that blocks α_4-integrin. This molecule is involved in moving circulating leukocytes into the brain in response to inflammation. It is administered as a 1-hour infusion every 4 weeks. Natalizumab has been shown to reduce clinical relapses, slow the progression of disability, and reduce the development of new brain lesions (Polman et al., 2006). Complications that limit its use include a hypersensitivity reaction up to an hour after infusion. Natalizumab has also been associated with progressive multifocal leukoencephalopathy, a destructive brain infection caused by JC virus. Therefore the distribution and use of natalizumab is closely monitored, and it can be administered only by registered physicians.

Medications for Acute Relapses

Glucocorticoids are still widely used for the treatment of acute exacerbations of MS. The principal effects of corticosteroids appear to be related to their anti-inflammatory and antiedema effects. It is recommended as standard therapy for any patient with an acute attack of MS (Goodin et al., 2002). Treatment normally consists of 3 to 5 days of a 1-g/day IV infusion of methylprednisolone. Oral prednisone taper may or may not be used after infusion.

Symptomatic Management

Medications used for symptomatic management depend on the specific symptoms encountered by the patient. MS patients frequently develop spasticity, which can be treated with baclofen, tizanidine, or benzodiazepines. Physical therapy can also help with spasticity. Bladder dysfunction can also occur in patients with MS. New bladder symptoms should be evaluated with a urine culture to rule out infection. A postvoid residual should also be obtained, as well as urodynamic testing to determine whether the problem is overflow incontinence from urinary retention or urge incontinence from detrusor instability. In the presence of urge incontinence, the anticholinergics oxybutynin (Ditropan) and tolterodine (Detrol) may be useful. If the problem is urinary retention and overflow incontinence, patients will usually need to be treated with intermittent self-catheterization. Patient may also experience depression, constipation, and sexual dysfunction. The usual evaluation and treatment options should be considered for patients who experience these problems.

KEY TREATMENT

Beta interferons have been shown to reduce the number of relapse in patients with the relapsing remitting form of MS (Coyle and Hartung, 2002) (SOR: A).

Glucocorticoids are recommended as standard therapy for any patient with an acute attack of MS (Goodin et al., 2002) (SOR: A).

Disease-modifying therapy should begin at diagnosis of MS (Coyle and Hartung, 2002) (SOR: B).

References

The complete reference list is available online at www.expertconsult.com.

Web Resources

http://neuromuscular.wustl.edu/
   Washington University Neuromuscular Disease Center; comprehensive resource for disorders affecting peripheral nerve, muscle, and neuromuscular junction.
www.cdc.gov/vaccines/recs/schedules/child-schedule.htm
   Centers for Disease Control and Prevention recommended immunization schedule.
www.aan.com
   American Academy of Neurology practice parameters and neurologic news.

www.wemove.org/
WE MOVE; resource for both patients and practitioners concerning movement disorders.
www.strokecenter.org/trials/
   Internet Stroke Center–Stroke Trials; updated resource for ongoing and completed trials related to stroke.

43 CHAPTER

Medical Human Sexuality

Wendy S. Biggs

Overview

Sexuality is a fundamental aspect of human self-concept and a complex biopsychosocial process. Physiologic aspects of sexuality are interpreted within the patient's cultural and social context. Family physicians and primary care providers are well situated to offer patients basic information regarding human sexual health issues and to evaluate and treat most common sexual problems; however, they seldom ask patients about sexual functioning. This chapter describes the basic principles of evaluation of female and male sexual dysfunction and clinical management of common disorders.

Sexual Self-Concept

Humans possess a gender identity and a sexual orientation. *Gender,* in many Western cultures, is synonymous with their chromosomal or genital phenotype (male or female sex). *Gender identity,* however, is a more comprehensive internal self-perception of being male or female, masculine or feminine. Many cultures, including Native American and African groups, do not regard gender as being determined by sex characteristics, and these cultures may provide an accepted role for persons in whom these aspects are not congruent. *Sexual orientation* may be defined as the attraction individuals feel toward sexual partners of their own or the other gender. Sexual orientation is self-defined, and individuals may describe themselves at different points in their lifetime as exclusively attracted to their own gender (homosexuality) or the opposite gender (heterosexuality), or somewhere between these two (bisexuality).

Models of Human Sexual Response

Masters and Johnson first described the physiology of "human sexual response cycle" in 1966. Based on the physical components of sexual functioning, they described four phases of the sexual response cycle: excitement, plateau, orgasm, and resolution (Fig. 43-1). Helen Singer Kaplan subsequently described a more subjective, psychologically oriented sexual responsiveness model with three phases: desire, excitement, and orgasm. Recently, however, nonlinear alternative models have been suggested, especially for women's sexual response (Basson and Schultz, 2007) (Fig. 43-2). In certain settings, men may have similar nonlinear sexual responses. Response phases establish a framework to discuss sexual dysfunction.

Initial Evaluation of Sexual Problems

Many patients would benefit from detection and treatment of sexual problems; however, many clinicians do not ask, and patients may not volunteer the information. In the Global Study of Sexual Attitudes and Behaviors, which surveyed more than 27,000 adults age 40 to 80 in 29 countries, 49% of women and 43% of men reported experiencing at least one sexual problem; fewer than 20% had sought medical assistance for sexual issues (Moreira et al., 2005). Health care providers should proactively and routinely address sexual health.

The sexual health interview may be approached with a screening or abbreviated method, followed by in-depth questioning, if necessary (Nusbaum and Hamilton, 2002) (Box 43-1). The answers on the detailed sexual history then direct the physical examination and appropriate laboratory testing. A physician may open the sexual history questioning with an *inclusion* technique: "Sexual health is important to overall health, therefore, I ask all my patients about it. I'm going to ask you a few questions on sexual matters now."

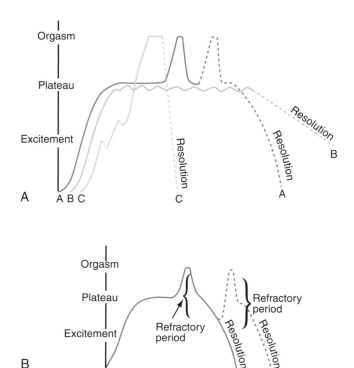

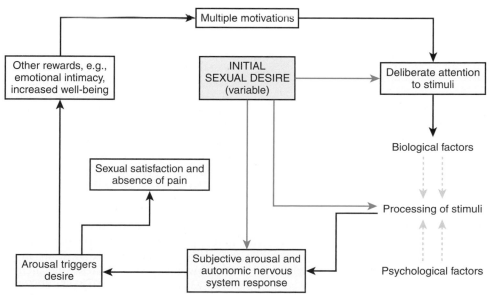

Figure 43-1 Female **(A)** and male **(B)** sexual response cycles. Desire precedes both cycles in this model. The phases illustrated are excitement, plateau, and orgasm. The length of the plateau phase is variable. Women may have a brief plateau followed by orgasm (cycle *C*) or a long plateau with no orgasm (cycle *B*). Women may have multiple orgasms before resolution, although many do not (cycle *A*). For men with premature ejaculation, the plateau phase is brief. After ejaculation, men enter a refractory period lasting minutes to hours during which they are unable to ejaculate.

The clinician can use normalization or universalization techniques. In *normalization* the clinician introduces emotionally laden or difficult subjects by implying these experiences are quite prevalent: "Many people have been sexually abused or molested as children. Did you have any experiences like that when you were young?" *Universalization* phrases questions as if everyone has done everything, making an affirmative answer easier for sensitive questions. For example, patients may be asked "How often do you masturbate?" instead of "Do you masturbate?" The clinician should also reassure the patient about physician-patient confidentiality.

Jack Annon in 1976 proposed the PLISSIT model to approach sexual concerns: Permission, Limited Information, Specific Suggestions, and Intensive Treatment (Box 43-2). The clinician can alternatively use the ALLOW acronym: Ask, Legitimize, Limitations, Open up, and Work together (Hatzichristou et al., 2004), as discussed next.

Ask. Questions regarding sexual functioning should be asked in a matter-of-fact yet sensitive manner. Physicians should avoid terms that make assumptions regarding patients' sexual behaviors. When inquiring about past or recent sexual encounters, the clinician may inquire "with men, women, or both?" Using the term "partner" instead of "husband" or "boyfriend" or "wife" or "girlfriend" may allow patients to discuss their sexual orientation openly. Slang words should be redefined in medical terminology so that the clinician and patient may communicate clearly.

Legitimize. By acknowledging the clinical relevance of sexual dysfunction, the clinician legitimizes the patient's sexual problem. Opening questions also can be linked to the patient's medical problems: "Many people with hypertension and heart disease notice a change in sexual functioning. Have you noticed any change?"

Limitations. The patient's knowledge may have limitations, and patient education may address the patient's perceived sexual dysfunction. For example, an older man with longer time between erections may not know the refractory period normally increases with age. Patient education and

Figure 43-2 Circular model of female sexual response showing cycle of overlapping phases. *(From Basson R, Schultz WW. Sexual sequelae of general medical disorders. Lancet 2007;369:409-424.*)

reassurance may eliminate his perceived "sexual dysfunction." Physicians should recognize their own limitations and, if necessary, refer a patient to the appropriate specialist for further evaluation and treatment of a sexual dysfunction.

Open up, for further discussion and evaluation. A detailed sexual history may be needed to evaluate fully a patient's

---

Box 43-1 Questions for a Detailed Sexual History

Are you currently sexually active? Have you ever been sexually active?

Are your sexual partners men, women, or both?

How many sexual partners have you had in the past month? Past 6 months? Lifetime?

How satisfied are you with your (and/or your partner's) sexual functioning?

Has there been any change in your (or your partner's) sexual desire or the frequency of sexual activity?

Do you have, or have you ever had, any risk factors for HIV (blood transfusion, needle stick injuries, IV drug use, STIs, partners who placed you at risk)?

Have you ever had any sexually related diseases?

Have you ever been tested for HIV? Would you like to be?

What do you do to protect yourself from contracting HIV?

What method do you use for contraception?

Are you trying to become pregnant (or father a child)?

Do you participate in oral sex? Anal sex?

Do you or your partner(s) use any particular devices or substances to enhance your sexual pleasure?

Do you ever have pain with intercourse?

Women: Do you have any difficulty achieving orgasm?

Men: Do you have any difficulty obtaining and maintaining an erection? Difficulty with ejaculation?

Do you have any questions or concerns about your sexual functioning?

Is there anything about your (or your partner's) sexual activity (as individuals or as a couple) that you would like to change?

From Nusbaum MRH, Hamilton CD. The proactive sexual health history. Am Fam Physician 2002;66:1705-1712.

HIV, Human immunodeficiency virus; *STIs*, sexually transmitted infections; *IV*, intravenous.

Box 43-2 PLISSIT Model for Approaching Sexual Problems

Permission

  For physician to discuss sex with the patient.

  For the patient to discuss concerns now or in the future.

  To continue sexual behaviors not potentially harmful.

Limited **I**nformation

  Clarify misinformation.

  Dispel myths.

  Provide factual information in a limited manner.

Specific **S**uggestions

  Provide specific suggestion directly related to the particular problem.

Intensive **T**reatment

  Provide highly individualized therapy for more complex issues.

Modified from Annon JS. The Behavioral Treatment of Sexual Problems. Honolulu, Enabling System, 1974-1975.

---

sexual concern (see Box 43-1). If the time constraints limit the current visit, the physician should offer the patient a future follow-up visit.

Work together, to develop a treatment plan. In some cases, simply following the previous four steps may be therapeutic. Many clinical cases can be managed with brief education or limited advice, such as discussing normal physiologic sexual changes with aging or recommending books or products (e.g., water-based lubricant for vaginal dryness). When a referral has been made, scheduled follow-up supports the patient during the process and helps address administrative or adherence issues. Counseling may be extremely important, and the physician should research local resources. The American Association of Sex Educators, Counselors, and Therapists (AASECT) may be contacted for referral information (http://www.aasect.org).

Female Sexual Dysfunction

Key Points

- Low sex drive is the most common sexual problem reported by women. A woman distressed by her low sexual drive has hypoactive sexual drive disorder.
- The cyclic model of sexual functioning postulates that arousal may be the initial trigger for a woman's sexual encounter, not desire.
- Ovarian androgens may play an important role in female sexual drive. Androgen levels in premenopausal women should be measured at the peak on days 8 to 10 of a 28-day menstrual cycle.
- Women may believe they have primary inhibited orgasm disorder because, unlike many men, they do not reach orgasm solely with vaginal intercourse.
- In most cases of orgasmic dysfunction, no specific physical examination or laboratory testing is necessary.
- Vaginismus is an involuntary, usually painful, spastic contraction of the pelvic musculature surrounding the outer third of the vagina and is complete, partial, or situational.

The linear model of sexual functioning classifies female sexual dysfunction as disorders of sexual interest/desire, arousal, orgasm, or pain. The cross-sectional, population-based PRESIDE study (Prevalence and Correlates of Female Sexual Disorders and Determinants of Treatment Seeking) estimated the prevalence of any female sexual problems was 44.2%, with "personal distress" reported by 22.8% of participants (Hatzichristou et al., 2004). Sexual dysfunction associated with personal distress became a disorder defined in the American Psychiatric Association's *Diagnostic and Statistical Manual of Mental Disorders,* 4th edition, text revision (DSM-IV-TR).

Hypoactive Sexual Desire Disorder

For women, low sexual drive is the most frequently reported sexual problem. Four in 10 women state they have low sexual drive. The lack of sexual desire may not be distressing for all women, with "distress" prevalence ranging in studies from 23% to 61% (Lindau et al., 2007; Shifren et al., 2008). Hypoactive sexual desire disorder (HSDD) may be *general* (a general lack of sexual desire), *situational* (previously present sexual desire is now absent), *acquired* (beginning after a period of normal sexual function), or *lifelong* (persistent no or low sexual desire). The cyclic model of sexual functioning postulates that arousal, not desire, may be the initial trigger for a woman's sexual encounter. Recently, therefore, experts suggest defining HSDD as a recurrent, consistent lack of ability to experience any desire or arousal (Basson et al., 2004). A brief questionnaire can be helpful to screen patients for HSDD (see **eTable 43-1** online).

Female sexual desire is a complex interaction among biologic, psychological, social, interpersonal, and environmental components. Ovarian function, especially ovarian androgens, may play an important role. In women age 20 to 49, HSDD is almost threefold more likely in surgical postmenopausal women than premenopausal women. However, no significant difference in HSDD exists between naturally or surgical postmenopausal women over age 50 (Leiblum et al., 2006). Medical illnesses, such as thyroid disease, chronic pain conditions, urinary incontinence, and depression/anxiety, may negatively impact sexual desire. Medications can affect sexual drive, especially selective serotonin reuptake inhibitor (SSRI) antidepressants, antihypertensives, antipsychotics, and narcotics. Fear of pregnancy or sexually transmitted infection and discord or communication difficulty in a couple's relationship may diminish sexual desire. The clinician must explore all aspects of the biopsychosocial model when evaluating a woman with hypoactive sexual desire.

Evaluation for HSDD includes a thorough history and physical examination to detect any gynecologic, neurologic, cardiovascular, or endocrine disorders. Laboratory testing should include thyroid function, fasting glucose, lipid profile, and liver function. If a hormonal problem is suspected, prolactin, total and free testosterone, sex hormone–binding globulin (SHBG), dihydroepiandrosterone (DHEA), and estrogen levels may be drawn. Androgen levels in premenopausal women should be measured at the peak on days 8 to 10 of a 28-day menstrual cycle.

Treatment

The U.S. Food and Drug Administration (FDA) has not approved any medication specifically for treatment of HSDD. Estrogen therapy improves vaginal dryness but does not affect sexual desire. The manufacturer of oral esterified estrogen and methyltestosterone discontinued distribution in the United States in March 2009. Although the transdermal testosterone patch is approved in Europe (Intrinsa), in 2004 the FDA did not approve it because of concerns regarding relatively low effectiveness, large placebo response, masculinizing side effects, and possible long-term consequences (cardiovascular and breast cancer when given with estrogen). Further Phase III clinical trials are ongoing. A randomized controlled trial (RCT) of sildenafil in postmenopausal women with SSRI-associated sexual dysfunction demonstrated a significant improvement in delayed orgasm and arousal (lubrication), but no improvement in desire (Nurnberg, 2008).

In small studies, bupropion improves HSDD in premenopausal women and women taking SSRIs, but large-study data are lacking (Segraves et al., 2004). Given the lack of allopathic treatment for HSDD, many women turn to complementary and alternative therapies (CAM). DHEA, an adrenocorticosteroid the body converts to testosterone, was found to improve sexual interest, thoughts, and fantasies in women with adrenal insufficiency, but studies are conflicting for women without adrenal insufficiency (Arlt et al., 1999). Limited data exist for *Ginkgo biloba*, damiana leaf, ginseng, and other proprietary herbal blends that are marketed to improve HSDD (Simon, 2009). For psychological interventions for HSDD, cognitive-behavioral therapy appears most beneficial (Basson et al., 2004).

Female Sexual Arousal Disorder

The DSM-IV-TR defines female sexual arousal disorder as the inability to attain or maintain a genital lubrication-swelling response during sexual activity. The American Foundation for Urologic Disease recommended division of this diagnosis into subjective, genital, and combined subtypes. It also urged recognition of "persistent" sexual arousal disorder characterized by "spontaneous, intrusive, and unwanted genital arousal . . . unrelieved by one or more orgasms" (Basson et al., 2003).

With the exception of persistent sexual arousal disorder, evaluation should include assessment for hypoactive sexual desire disorder. Neurologic and vascular causes should be considered when adequate genital vasocongestion and swelling do not occur but subjective arousal and lubrication are intact.

Treatment is based on the suspected cause of the sexual arousal disorder. Supplemental water-soluble lubrication may be needed. Off-label use of PDE-5 inhibitors (e.g., sildenafil) may be helpful in restoring the vascular response (Kaplan et al., 1999). The FDA-approved Eros Clitoral Therapy Device uses a silicon cup to apply a vacuum to increase blood flow to the clitoris and surrounding tissue. The device appears effective in women without detectable disease and after radiation treatment for cervical cancer (Munarriz et al., 2003, Schroder et al., 2005), although sample sizes have been small. Herbal supplements and botanical genital massage oil showed some effect in small studies (Ito et al., 2001, Ferguson et al., 2003). Partner issues and situational factors may need to be addressed.

Female Orgasmic Disorder

Orgasmic dysfunction, the inability to reach orgasm when desired, may be *primary*, with the patient never having experienced orgasm, or *secondary*, with the dysfunction manifesting after previous satisfactory orgasmic functioning. Some women may believe they have primary inhibited-orgasm disorder because, unlike many men, they do not reach orgasm solely with vaginal intercourse. Portrayals of female orgasm in novels and films are often overstated or misleading. A basic description of physical orgasm (i.e., pleasurable sensation in genital area and contractions of vagina, followed by a feeling of physical and psychological relaxation) may facilitate discussion of orgasm. Many women prefer simultaneous vaginal and clitoral stimulation, oral-genital sex, or clitoral stimulation alone to have an orgasm and do not have an orgasmic disorder.

In both primary and secondary orgasmic dysfunction, it is important to ask about past or current experiences of violence, victimization, and abuse. Social factors also affect a woman's experience of orgasm. Women taught negative messages regarding sexuality or with strict religious or cultural prohibitions on sexual attraction and thoughts may experience orgasmic difficulty, even if the specified conditions for sexual behavior (e.g., marriage) have been fulfilled. Women who were born later in the 20th century are more likely to experience orgasm than those born earlier, likely reflecting social changes. Secondary inhibited orgasm can be caused by other medical illnesses and contributing contextual factors.

The clinical history in secondary inhibited orgasm should focus on the patient's perception of this dysfunction: time and circumstances of onset, possible causes, effect on relationship(s), and treatment goals. Physiologic functioning during sexual stimulation, including adequacy of lubrication and ability to sustain states of high arousal, should be explored. Contributing factors such as fatigue, depression, postpartum physical and social changes, preoccupation with other life issues, substance abuse, and other medical illnesses should be considered. Contextual and relationship issues, including lack of tenderness or interest in non-intercourse stimulation by the partner, early ejaculation, problems regarding contraceptive responsibility, lack of privacy, relationship conflicts, and the possibility of abuse, should be discussed. In most cases of orgasmic dysfunction, no specific physical examination or laboratory testing is necessary. As with other sexual dysfunctions, neurologic, gynecologic, or other examination may be suggested by the clinical history.

Treatment of orgasmic dysfunction usually involves increasing knowledge and sexual options for the patient and partner. Masturbation (self-pleasuring) may provide information about sexual responsiveness and preferred stimulations, which can then be transferred to sexual situations with the partner. Partner education regarding clitoral stimulation and adequate pre-intercourse lovemaking (foreplay) can change the focus from intercourse to mutual pleasuring, spontaneity, and sexual satisfaction. Referral for more in-depth therapy is indicated if the evaluation reveals significant relationship dysfunction, past abuse, or other severe medical or psychosocial complications.

Sexual Pain Disorders

Vaginismus

Vaginismus is an involuntary, usually painful, spastic contraction of the pelvic musculature surrounding the outer third of the vagina. It is classified as *complete* (e.g., precluding intercourse, tampon insertion, or other vaginal penetration), *partial* (resulting in dyspareunia or difficulty with other forms of vaginal penetration, including speculum examination), or *situational* (e.g., occurring when intercourse is anticipated). Vaginismus is often idiopathic. Many cases, however, may follow pelvic trauma, such as painful intercourse, sexual assault, rough gynecologic examination, complicated episiotomy, vaginal infections, pelvic inflammatory disease, or pelvic surgery. Childhood or adolescent sexual abuse may also lead to vaginismus during adulthood. Regardless of the cause of vaginismus (traumatic, psychological, or idiopathic), once a pattern of pain and anticipation of pain has been established, it will likely recur unless treatment is provided.

Diagnosis is usually made by history. Patients report pain and difficulty with, or inability to engage in, vaginal intercourse or digital vaginal stimulation; using tampons or vaginal contraceptives; or having a pelvic examination.

Patients may demonstrate visible contraction of the pelvic floor musculature with anticipated speculum examination. Physical examination may detect pertinent anatomic abnormalities, such as vaginal septa.

Few studies exist on vaginismus. Uncontrolled reports suggest that sex therapy may be helpful (McGuire and Hawton, 2005). Vaginismus is not under the patient's conscious control. Therapy must be directed at restoring conscious control under conditions that respect the patient's autonomy and maintain the patient's safety from further trauma. If the patient expresses fear or anxiety, pelvic examination may be deferred, and in severe cases, sedation may be necessary. Any physical abnormalities detected on pelvic examination, such as infections, should first be treated. After this, the patient may begin self-treatment with size-graded plastic or silicone vaginal dilators, gradually teaching her vagina to remain relaxed and receive nonpainful, self-controlled penetration (see Web Resources). Specialized physical therapists teach patients to use biofeedback to relax the pelvic floor musculature; this can be more effective than treatment with dilators and is often preferred by patients. Treatment of posttraumatic stress disorder and other sequelae of past trauma may be crucial. Referral to a sex therapist is often helpful.

KEY TREATMENT

Cognitive-behavioral therapy appears beneficial for hypoactive sexual desire disorder (Basson et al., 2004) (SOR: B).
Treatment of orgasmic dysfunction usually involves increasing knowledge and sexual options for the patient and partner (SOR: C).
Sex therapy and vaginal dilators of increasing size may help treat vaginismus (SOR: C).

Dyspareunia

Dyspareunia refers to pain experienced immediately before, during, or after intercourse. Diagnosis of dyspareunia is made by history and physical examination. Useful questions include the onset, duration, and circumstances in which this problem occurred, the location of the pain (e.g., superficial, deep, unilateral, bilateral), and whether it is specific to a particular partner or practice. Physical exam may reveal perineal trauma or vaginal infection, vaginal mucosal atrophy, or other anatomic factors (e.g., vaginal septa, partial vaginismus). Emotional factors may contribute, such as ambivalence or distaste regarding the sexual relationship, as well as the sequelae of childhood abuse. Inadequate lubrication, relationship difficulties, poor sexual technique or a rough or abusive partner can cause dyspareunia.

Treatment of physiologic dyspareunia caused by atrophic vaginitis may require vaginal estrogen. Vaginal infections must be diagnosed and treated. For poor lubrication, supplemental water-based lubrication may be sufficient. Deep dyspareunia is often caused by overvigorous penetration or excess cervical pressure and may respond to brief educational interventions. Many people do not realize that penises and vaginas vary in length, and the vagina may not stretch to accommodate full penile engulfment. Changing position to allow the woman to control the amount of cervical pressure may ameliorate the dyspareunia. Referral for sex therapy for the couple may prove helpful. In some cases, the patient may be able to bring about change in the sexual relationship with sufficient information and assertiveness. If dyspareunia is the result of deliberate carelessness or abuse by the partner, ending the relationship is usually the only reasonable option.

Male Sexual Dysfunction

Key Points

- The prevalence of erectile dysfunction increases with age.
- Vascular risk factors (e.g. diabetes, smoking, sedentary lifestyle, and being overweight) increase the risk for ED.
- Behavioral techniques for premature ejaculation are important for sustained success without pharmacologic treatment.

Erectile Dysfunction

Historically, male sexual dysfunction was described as "impotence"; however, the term *erectile dysfunction* (ED) is now preferred. The National Institutes of Health (NIH) Consensus Development Conference (1992) defined ED as "the inability for a male to achieve an erect penis as part of the overall multifaceted process of male sexual function." ED becomes "male erectile disorder" defined by the DSM-IV-TR when "marked distress or interpersonal difficulty" accompanies it, and is not better accounted for by another mental health disorder (other than a sexual dysfunction), and not exclusively caused by the direct physiologic effects of a substance (e.g., drug of abuse, medication) or a general medical condition.

Both sympathetic and parasympathetic nerves regulate blood flow into the corpus cavernosum of the penis. Stimulation of the parasympathetic nerves causes release of nitric oxide (NO) from the noradrenergic, noncholinergic nerves and endothelial cells. NO increases the intracellular levels of cyclic guanosine monophosphate (cGMP) in the cavernosal smooth muscle, which relaxes the cavernosal tissues. With the resultant rapid blood flow into the corporal bodies of the penis, the small emissary veins that cross the tunica albuginea are occluded, and blood is trapped inside the corpus cavernosum, leading to an erection. The level of cGMP is also affected by prostaglandins. Phosphodiesterase-5 (PDE-5) is the main cGMP-catalyzing enzyme in human smooth muscle. PDE-5 inhibitors (sildenafil, tadalafil, vardenafil) increase cGMP levels and facilitate and maintain penile erection. The intact functioning of four body systems—vascular, neurologic, endocrine, and usually psychological—is necessary for a man to experience a penile erection.

Erectile dysfunction can occur at any age, but prevalence increases with age; 2% for ages 40 to 49, 6% for 50 to 59, 17% for 60 to 69, and 39% for 70 or older (Inman et al., 2009). Medical conditions associated with peripheral vascular disease, such as diabetes, coronary artery disease, stroke, and hypertension, increase the prevalence of ED. In men younger than 60, smoking, sedentary lifestyle, and being overweight increased the risk for ED (Bacon et al., 2003).

Evaluation

Clinicians should carefully evaluate the patient's complaint of ED, because some men consider premature ejaculation as "erectile dysfunction." After obtaining the pertinent history, the clinician should carefully review the patient's past medical history. Because penile erection depends on intact vasculature, the medical history is similar to one assessing cardiovascular risk factors: "What is bad for the heart is bad for the penis." Several common classes of medicines can cause sexual dysfunctions (Box 43-3). The social history should include the patient's smoking, alcohol, and marijuana use, and the patient's important social and sexual relationships. The physician should also assess psychological factors such as depression and anxiety.

Physical examination focuses on signs related to the vascular, neurologic, and endocrine systems. Peripheral pulses should be palpated and carotids auscultated for bruits. The thyroid should be examined for enlargement or nodular disease. A thorough genitourinary examination should be performed. The clinician can assess perineal enervation with anal sphincter tone, perianal sensation, and the bulbocavernosus reflex. The penile shaft may show Peyronie's disease (fibrous plaques of corpus cavernosa affecting erectile function or causing pain with erection). The prostate should be evaluated. Testicular atrophy may indicate low testosterone levels. If secondary sexual characteristics are lacking or the patient has other signs of hypogonadism, further endocrine evaluation should be undertaken.

Few laboratory tests are necessary. Vascular risk factors should be assessed with fasting glucose and lipid profile. Blood urea nitrogen (BUN) and creatinine, serum transaminases (AST, ALT), thyroid-stimulating hormone (TSH), and prostate-specific antigen (PSA) levels should be considered. If the patient is young, is deficient in secondary sexual characteristics, or has other signs of hypogonadism, testosterone level should be determined. A low testosterone level, however, cannot be considered a definitive cause of ED. Many

---

Box 43-3 Medications Affecting Sexual Function

Antihypertensives
    Beta blockers (atenolol, metoprolol, bisoprolol, propranolol)
    Thiazide diuretics (hydrochlorothiazide, chlorthalidone)
    Sympatholytics (clonidine, methyldopa)
    Calcium channel blockers (nifedipine, amlodipine)
    ACE inhibitors (enalapril, lisinopril)
Antipsychotics
Antidepressants (TCAs, SSRIs)
Anxiolytics/tranquilizers
Antiandrogens
    5α-Reductase inhibitors
    Gonadotropin-releasing hormone agonists
    Ketoconazole
    Spironolactone
    H_2 blockers (cimetidine)
HIV medications
Fibrates (gemfibrozil, fenofibrate)
Statins
Digoxin
Cytotoxic agents (methotrexate)

ACE, Angiotensin-converting enzyme; *TCAs*, tricyclic antidepressants; *SSRIs*, selective serotonin reuptake inhibitors; *HIV*, human immunodeficiency virus.

men with very low levels of circulating testosterone have normal libido and erectile function. Testosterone is highly protein-bound to SHGB, with only about 2% circulating as free testosterone; therefore, total testosterone levels may not reflect the bioavailable testosterone. The prevalence of abnormally low serum testosterone levels, even among men with ED, is only about 7%. Controversy surrounds testosterone supplementation for ED treatment.

Treatment

Phosphodiesterase-5 inhibitors are first-line therapy for ED and are effective in most cases, including antidepressant-induced ED and diabetes related (Rudkin et al., 2004; Vardi and Nini, 2007). In 1998, sildenafil (Viagra) was the first PDE-5 inhibitor to become FDA approved, followed by vardenafil (Levitra) and tadalafil (Cialis) in 2003. The medications differ in absorption, potential effective time interval, and some side effects (Table 43-1). Evidence is insufficient to support one inhibitor over another (McVay, 2007). These medications have similar side effects, caused by their vasodilatory action. All PDE-5 inhibitors can cause increased vasodilation with nitrates and should not be used concomitantly; fatalities have been reported. Use with alpha-adrenergic blocker

medications should also be avoided due to risk of significant hypotension. Human immunodeficiency virus (HIV) protease inhibitors significantly increase the half-life of PDE-5 inhibitors by interfering with hepatic metabolism. PDE-5 medications have several dosages available to facilitate titration upward to an effective dose or dose reduction for age and hepatic or renal impairment.

Prostaglandin E_1 (PGE$_1$; alprostadil) is second-line treatment for men who have a contraindication for or have failed PDE-5 inhibitors. Intraurethral alprostadil (MUSE—*medicated urethral system for erection*) is a pellet of synthetic PGE$_1$ that is absorbed across the urethral mucosa and increases corpus cavernosum blood flow. Treatment has been effective in 50% of men with ED from radical prostectomy after sildenafil failed (Jaffe et al., 2004). Intracavernous self-injection of alprostadil (Caverject, Edex) is another alternative, especially for patients with mild to moderate vascular disease not responsive to PDE-5 inhibitors. Complications, although relatively uncommon, include ecchymosis, hematoma, and painful erection. Although priapism occurs in less than 1% of users, patients should be warned to seek prompt medical attention if an erection lasts longer than 4 hours. Injection can also cause minor bleeding, so condom use is advised if blood-borne infection risk is present. Long-term

Table 43-1 Phosphodiesterase-5 (PDE5) Inhibitors

Parameter	Sildenafil (Viagra)	Vardenafil (Levitra)	Tadalafil (Cialis)
Dosages	25, 50, 100 mg	2.5, 5, 10, 20 mg	2.5 mg (taken daily), 5 mg, 10 mg (as needed dosing)
Absorption	Decreased if taken with high-fat foods	Decreased if taken with high-fat foods	Unchanged with food; decreased if taken with antacids
Onset of action	30-60 minutes	30-120 minutes	16-30 minutes
Length of effect	3-5 hours	4-5 hours	24-72 hours
Side effects	Headache, flushing, nasal congestion, dyspepsia, abnormal color vision	Headache, flushing, dyspepsia, nasal congestion, abnormal color vision	Headache, flushing, nasal congestion, dyspepsia; back pain, myalgia 12-24 hr after dose; color vision changes very rare
Metabolism	Hepatic	Hepatic	Hepatic
Drug interactions	Strong CYP3A4 inhibitors (e.g., ritonavir, indinavir, ketoconazole, itraconazole), moderate CYP3A4 (e.g., erythromycin), nonspecific	Strong CYP3A4 inhibitors (e.g., ritonavir, indinavir, ketoconazole, itraconazole) increase plasma levels; potential hypotension with nitrates and alpha-adrenergic blockers	Strong CYP3A4 inhibitors (e.g., ritonavir, indinavir, ketoconazole, itraconazole) increase plasma levels; potential hypotension with nitrates and alpha-adrenergic blockers
Dose reduction	CYP450 inhibitor (cimetidine) causes significant increase in plasma levels; potential hypotension with nitrates and alpha-adrenergic blockers	Patients older than 65 years; hepatic impairment; no adjustment for moderate to severe renal impairment (CrCl <30 mL/min)	No dosage adjustment for age; not recommended in patients with severe hepatic impairment Daily use: no adjustment for moderate to severe renal impairment (CrCl >30 mL/min); not recommended for CrCl <30 mL/min As-needed use: reduce dose for CrCl <50 mL/min
Additional information	Patients older than 65 years; hepatic impairment; severe renal impairment (CrCl < 30 mL/min)	May prolong QT interval	Nitrates given no sooner than 48 hr after dose; substantial consumption of alcohol (e.g., 6 oz of 80-proof vodka) increases orthostatic hypotension; no blood pressure drop with tamsulosin (selective alpha-adrenergic blocker)

Data from Lexi-Comp, 2009.
CrCl, Creatinine clearance

use can result in fibrosis of the corpus cavernosum, and administration more frequently than three times weekly is not recommended.

Vacuum constriction devices (VCDs) can be used by men with ED from any cause. The penis is inserted into a tube in which a vacuum is applied, filling the corpus cavernosum with blood. A soft, constricting ring is placed at the base of the penis to prevent venous drainage from the corpus. Side effects include penile pain and numbness, bruising, and trapped ejaculation. Anticoagulant therapy is a relative contraindication (Lue et al., 2004).

Apomorphine is a centrally acting dopamine agonist with affinity for dopamine receptors in the brain that are believed to be involved in sexual functioning. Apomorphine effectively treats ED, although it appears less effective than PDE-5 inhibitors (Eardley et al., 2004; Perimenis et al., 2004). Significant dose-related side effects include nausea, dizziness, severe sweating, and drowsiness. At present, sublingual apomorphine has been approved for use in Europe. In the United States, a subcutaneous form is approved only for treatment of Parkinson's disease.

Yohimbine antagonizes α_2-adrenergic receptors. In one systematic review, yohimbine improved self-reported sexual function and penile rigidity compared with placebo (Ernst and Pittler, 1998). It has not been clinically researched for ED in the last decade. Yohimbine has significant adverse effects, including elevation of blood pressure and heart rate, increased motor activity, nervousness, irritability, and tremor.

Testosterone supplementation may or may not improve erectile function in hypogonadal men. One study found that previously unresponsive hypogonadal men using testosterone supplementation responded to sildenafil or apomorphine (Foresta et al., 2004). Other research showed that hypogonadal men who received testosterone supplementation and normalized their testosterone level had only short-term improvement in erectile function (Mulhall et al., 2004). Topical testosterone gel (AndroGel, Testim) is the most common form of supplementation and provides relatively steady serum testosterone levels. Transdermal patches can be applied on the upper body (Androderm) or scrotum (Testoderm), but skin irritation may occur in up to 15% of men. Intramuscular injection of testosterone enanthate or testosterone cypionate every 10 to 21 days may provide adequate supplementation but often causes significant peaks and troughs in testosterone levels.

Patients with ED primarily (or exclusively) of psychological origin may benefit from individual psychotherapy or pharmacologic therapy. Focused group therapy demonstrates greater efficacy than no therapy for ED (Melnik et al., 2007). Men who are experiencing sexual dysfunction often develop the "spectator effect"; fear of recurrent failure or difficulty focuses attention on self-performance rather than pleasuring and enjoyment, further decreasing arousal. Similarly, "performance anxiety" increases sympathetic tone, which physiologically impedes erectile function. Relationship conflicts, contraception or fertility concerns, and religious or moral conflicts regarding sexual activity can affect erectile function. Depression, anxiety, adjustment disorders, substance abuse, and other psychiatric symptoms should be evaluated and treated or referred. Survivors of physical or sexual abuse may require long-term treatment and support with a therapist experienced in this area.

> ## KEY TREATMENT
>
> Phosphodiesterase-5 inhibitors (sildenafil, tadalafil, vardenafil) are first-line therapy for erectile dysfunction (ED) (Rudkin et al., 2004; Vardi and Nini, 2007) (SOR: A).
>
> Prostaglandin E$_1$, intraurethral or injected into the corpus cavernosum, is second-line treatment of ED (Jaffe et al., 2004) (SOR: A).
>
> Vacuum constriction devices may help ED of any cause (Lue et al., 2004) (SOR: B).
>
> Focused group therapy improves erectile function better than no therapy (Melnik et al., 2007) (SOR: A).
>
> Off-label use of SSRI antidepressants improves premature ejaculation by prolonging the preorgasmic plateau (Arafa and Shamioul, 2007) (SOR: A).

Premature (Rapid) Ejaculation

Premature ejaculation refers to the occurrence of male ejaculation, usually with orgasm, before desired by the individual, his partner, or both. Premature ejaculation is also referred to as *rapid ejaculation* or *difficulty with ejaculatory control.*

Evaluation of premature ejaculation is by history. Onset, circumstances, and meaning (personal and relationship) of the dysfunction should be explored, as well as pertinent past sexual experiences. For example, young men whose first sexual experiences were rushed may later have difficulty establishing ejaculatory control in more relaxed contexts. Men having intercourse infrequently are more likely to ejaculate rapidly. The clinician should determine whether a patient can delay his ejaculation while masturbating. In addition, information regarding the patient's level of sexual knowledge and his partner's expectations may be significant.

Behavioral techniques, such as the squeeze technique, stop and start, masturbation training, and non-intercourse-based pleasuring may be used to treat premature ejaculation. In the "squeeze technique," firm (squeezing) pressure for 3 to 5 seconds on the ventral surface of the penis at the frenulum or base, followed by quick release, will temporarily relieve the need to ejaculate. "Stop and start" refers to the man learning to stop or reduce penile stimulation when ejaculation is approaching (but not imminent) and resume when arousal has partially dissipated. Masturbation training aimed at increasing ejaculatory control may also be useful. Changing the focus of the relationship from achieving partner orgasm with intercourse to mutual pleasuring often results in an improved sexual relationship, regardless of immediate success in delaying ejaculation.

The SSRI antidepressants can cause prolongation of the preorgasmic plateau and thus may delay ejaculation. Using SSRIs for premature ejaculation is currently an off-label use, although research is ongoing. In a single-blinded prospective study of paroxetine, fluoxetine, and escitalopram, 100% of men complaining of premature ejaculation experienced an improvement in their symptoms, with no difference detected between the three treatment groups (Arafa and Shamioul, 2007). Dapoxetine is a short-acting SSRI that can be taken as needed, instead of daily as with other SSRIs, but is not yet approved by the FDA for use in the United States. Phase III randomized, double-blind, placebo-controlled trials show dapoxetine, 30 and 60 mg as needed, achieved statistically significant improvements in perceived control over ejaculation (Hellstrom, 2009). PDE-5 inhibitors added to SSRIs may further improve premature ejaculation. Sildenafil with paroxetine or fluoxetine and tadalafil with fluoxetine have been shown to improve premature ejaculation better than the SSRI alone (Husseini and Yarmohammadi, 2007; Mattos et al., 2008; Salonia et al., 2002). Several studies show various formulations of topical treatments that reduce the sensory stimuli to the penis (e.g., topical eutectic mixture of lidocaine-prilocaine spray) appear to increase ejaculatory latency time compared to baseline or placebo (Morales et al., 2007). However, unless behavioral means of delaying ejaculation are also used, success is often not sustained following discontinuation of medication. In patients without underlying relationship difficulties, prognosis for premature ejaculation is excellent.

Male Orgasmic Disorder

Men who can sustain a full erection for a reasonable duration of sexual activity will usually be able to reach orgasm. When this is not the case, a more complete evaluation should be undertaken, evaluating the central and peripheral nervous systems, use of medications and substances, and relationship issues. SSRI antidepressants are well known to interfere with orgasm. Alcohol use can cause difficulty with sustaining arousal or with orgasm. Many contextual and partner issues discussed with regard to female patients also apply to men.

Dyspareunia

Although dyspareunia is a gender-neutral term, men experience dyspareunia much less often with vaginal-penile intercourse than women. Dyspareunia in men is often caused by concurrent medical illness, such as Peyronie's disease or neuropathy, although relationship dynamics and poor sexual technique may also cause sexual discomfort. Anal dyspareunia can occur with the anally receptive or insertive partner and is usually caused by insufficient lubrication or spasm of the anal musculature. Evaluation consists of the history and physical examination. As with most sexual dysfunctions, onset, context, patient perceptions regarding possible causes, and impact on the relationship(s) are important. Physical examination may reveal evidence of neuropathy, urethritis, epididymitis, Peyronie's disease, prostatitis, anal fissures, hemorrhoids, or other pertinent findings. Treatment of dyspareunia involves correction of underlying physical pathology, counseling regarding sexual technique, and referral of complicated cases to a urologist or sex therapist, as indicated.

Sexual Orientation Spectrum

Key Points

- Sexual orientation may be a continuous spectrum from exclusive homosexuality to exclusive heterosexuality.
- Some people who have been sexually active with members of their own gender identify themselves as heterosexual.
- Lesbians are less likely to obtain health maintenance services, such as mammography or Pap smears.
- Any intact organ in a transgendered individual should be screened according to current guidelines.

Sexual orientation is a social construct. Customs regarding which sexual acts are acceptable, with whom, and under what circumstances, have varied in different cultures and eras. In the *Sexual Behavior in the Human Male* in 1948, Kinsey and colleagues hypothesized sexual orientation might be a continuous spectrum, from exclusive heterosexuality through exclusive homosexuality, and might vary across the life span in different people. Researchers have attempted to measure the prevalence of homosexuality and bisexuality in populations, with varying success and controversy. Some people who have been sexually active with members of their own gender identify themselves as heterosexual. In one study, although only 2.8% of male respondents and 1.4% of female respondents self-identified as gay, lesbian, or bisexual, 10.9% of men and 4.3% of women ages 40 to 49 years reported having had at least one same-gender sexual experience since puberty (Laumann, 1994). Because many gay, lesbian, and bisexual patients do not share information regarding sexual orientation and past sexual behavior with their physicians, most physicians likely overestimate the number of exclusively heterosexual patients in their clinical practices.

Clinical Considerations in the Care of Lesbian, Gay, and Bisexual Patients

All patients have the same medical needs and expectations, regardless of sexual orientation, such as accurate diagnosis and treatment and respectful communication. However, several issues are especially important to remember for the medical care of gay, lesbian, and bisexual patients.

Lesbians are less likely to obtain health maintenance services, including clinical breast examination, mammography, and cervical cancer screening than heterosexual women, perhaps because of an underinsured or uninsured status. Patients in same-gender couples are often not eligible for spousal health insurance benefits and may be less likely than their heterosexual counterparts to be adequately insured. Many lesbians mistakenly believe they do not need Papanicolaou smears. However, women self-identified as lesbian may have been a victim of childhood sexual abuse, had a remote history of consensual male sexual contact, or they are bisexual. Nulliparous lesbians are at a high risk for cancers of the breast, endometrium, and ovary. Female-to-female transmission of sexually transmitted diseases (STDs, including HIV infection) is much less efficient than male-to-female transmission; however, genital-oral sex and fomites such as sex toys can transmit gonorrhea and *Trichomonas,* respectively.

Gay men sometimes report difficulty in obtaining adequate health care caused by providers' bias and fear of discrimination. Any male patient who presents for treatment of urethritis should be asked about participation in oral-genital sex or receptive anal intercourse, because some treatment regimens for urethral gonorrhea and chlamydia are not effective against pharyngeal and anal infections. A careful exposure history should be taken, even if the patient self-identifies as heterosexual, because some heterosexual-identified men may have same-gender sexual experiences.

Spectrum of Gender Identity and Expression

People may seek medical assistance in changing their physical sex to be congruent with their internal self-perception. *Transsexuals* usually desire full hormonal transition and sex reassignment surgery. *Cross-dressers* (previously referred to as "transvestites") are persons who at times may dress as the other gender to be publicly perceived as such or for sexual pleasure. A *transgendered* individual is one who seeks to take on the social role of the other gender, either full- or part-time, often with the assistance of hormone therapy, but does not desire genital surgery. *Intersex* (transsexual) is a different medical concept and refers to persons born with ambiguous genitalia or for whom phenotypic and chromosomal sex do not match (e.g., 5α-reductase deficiency). Some persons do not perceive themselves as being fully male or fully female and seek to create new gender identities, similar to those found in many indigenous cultures. Reliable population prevalence estimates for transgendered and transsexual people are difficult to obtain and vary among cultures. In Belgium, overall prevalence was 1:12,900 for male-to-female (MTF) and 1:33,800 for female-to-male (FTM) transsexuals (DeCuypere et al., 2007). People who identify as transgendered or who cross-dress, however, are likely to be more numerous than individuals seeking sexual reassignment surgery.

Transgender Health Care

Cross-dressers and transgendered persons often encounter difficulty in obtaining adequate medical services. In one study, 26% of respondents reported being denied medical care because they were transgender (Kenagy, 2005). Transgendered persons also suffer "hate crime" victimization, with more than half the transgendered people in one study reporting some form of harassment or violence within their lifetime, and a quarter experiencing a violent incident (Lombardi et al., 2001).

Transgendered people receiving hormones can present an unusual blend of gender-associated physical characteristics and may be reluctant to reveal their treatments. MTF sex reassignment surgery is currently technically advanced, with postoperative MTF individuals often not identified as such, even on cursory gynecologic examination. FTM surgery is less sophisticated, and results are more variable. Patients may obtain medical services without revealing their preoperative history.

Transgender patients need routine health promotion and preventive services. Any intact organ should be screened according to current guidelines (e.g., a woman with a prostate gland needs prostate cancer screening counseling). Similarly, screening mammography guidelines do not distinguish between natal women and transsexual women, although specific guidelines have been proposed. FTM reconstructive chest surgery does not remove all the glandular tissue, as with a mastectomy; thus FTM men who retain the axillary tail should at minimum continue self-examination. A transsexual, transgendered, or cross-dressed patient should be asked how he or she would like to be addressed. If a legal name change has not been finalized, cross-referenced filing of the medical chart under both names may be needed.

The initiation of hormone therapy for modification of visible sex characteristics and sex reassignment surgery are life-changing medical interventions that should only be undertaken for patients who have completed an appropriate mental health evaluation and are in supportive mental health care. For clinical gender transition, a multidisciplinary team approach is ideal, such as in a comprehensive program (e.g., University of Michigan's Comprehensive Gender Services Program; www.med.umich.edu/transgender/) or concurrent care from a mental health professional with experience in this area, a primary care physician knowledgeable about hormone supplementation and general transgender medical care, and urology, gynecology, and plastic surgery specialists. The World Professional Association for Transgender Health (formerly the Harry Benjamin International Gender Dysphoria Association) has resource links for patients (www.wpath.org).

Sexuality Issues at Specific Times of Life

Adolescence

Key Points

- Almost half of high school students report having experienced sexual intercourse.
- Adolescents perceive less health, social, and emotional risks with oral sex than vaginal intercourse.
- Adolescents report increased condom use over the last decade.
- About 8% of adolescents report being forced to have sexual intercourse they did not want.
- Nonheterosexual adolescents are more likely to engage in high-risk behaviors and are at risk for harassment and violence.

Physical, social, and sexual maturation can be a source of both pride and confusion or anxiety for teenagers. Peers, television, and the Internet provide information about sex, although often inaccurate, misleading, and inappropriate. School-based education regarding health and development, including sexuality, is often limited. Although shyness, reticence, and embarrassment are common, most adolescents (77% in one survey) would like their health care provider to ask them directly about their sexual knowledge and experience (Rosenthal et al., 1999). Family physicians can use routine outpatient visits for school, camp, or preemployment physical examination to offer medical information as it relates to the teenager's current concerns.

Masturbation

Masturbation is a normal and healthy sexual activity at all ages and may serve as an appropriate substitute for partnered sexual behavior during adolescence. Adolescent boys usually learn about masturbation from their peers and demonstrate an increase in masturbation activity at age 13 to 15 years. Although some begin masturbation at preschool ages, girls tend to learn to masturbate at a later age, usually through self-discovery. Both boys and girls learn early in life that a social stigma is associated with masturbation and that it is not a topic for public discussion. Family physicians can reassure adolescents regarding the normal nature of masturbation behavior.

Partnered Sexual Activity

Human sexual behavior is an instinctive drive. Sexual urges often awaken or intensify at puberty. In premodern society, puberty marked adulthood and subsequent reproduction.

In modern Western society, full adulthood is delayed through the adolescent years. As the teenager undergoes sexual physical development, biologic urges for physical intimacy and reproduction may affect sexual behavior. Although many adolescents delay their sexual debut for a variety of reasons, the modern assumption that *all* teenagers will be willing or able to delay participation in intercourse and other sexual behaviors until age 18, marriage, or some other milestone is at odds with the experience of human history.

The Centers for Disease Control and Prevention (CDC) conducts the Youth Risk Behavior Surveillance (YRBS) surveys every 2 years. In 2007, 14,041 questionnaires were completed in 157 high schools nationally, with an overall response rate of 68%. Nationwide, almost half (48%) of all students reported having experienced sexual intercourse, with the prevalence by state ranging from 36% to 60%. Although 14% of teenagers reported experience with four or more sexual partners, prevalence varied by gender and ethnic/racial background. Significantly more African American boys (38%) reported four or more sexual partners than Hispanic (23%) and white (12%) boys. Similarly, 18% of African American girls compared to 11% of both Hispanic and white girls reported four or more sexual partners (degree of reporting bias is unknown). Psychosocially, adolescents frequently practice *serial monogamy;* they begin an exclusive relationship that over time may involve sexual behavior, then end that relationship and initiate another. Serial monogamy is the lifestyle practiced by most American adults, although the length of the sequential relationships often increases; a 17-year-old may experience two steady relationships during a single year, whereas a 40-year-old is more likely to have been married twice during the preceding 20 years.

Family physicians should remain mindful that teenagers may practice sexual acts other than intercourse. Some teens maintain sexual relationships involving mutual genital touching and masturbation (also referred to as "outercourse") for months or years before beginning intercourse. In one study, a significantly greater number of ninth-grade students had engaged in oral sex than in vaginal sex (19.6% vs. 13.5%), and more participants intended to have oral sex than vaginal sex during the next 6 months (31.5% vs. 26.3%). These adolescents also perceived less health, social, and emotional risks with oral sex than vaginal intercourse (Halpern-Felscher et al., 2005). The Kaiser Family Foundation Survey (2000) of sexually active teenagers 15 to 17 years old found that 26% believed that one cannot become infected with HIV by having unprotected oral sex, and 15% did not know whether or not one could become infected. Risks involved in oral-genital or anal sexual acts, such as oral transmission of gonorrhea or HIV infection with unprotected anal intercourse, should be discussed frankly with adolescents.

Encouragingly, over the last 10 years, more adolescents report condom use with their last vaginal intercourse. The 1997 YRBS survey reported 57% of teens used condoms with their last vaginal intercourse, versus 62% in 2007. The prevalence of condom use, however, appears to diminish over time; 69% of sexually active ninth-grade students reported condom use with sexual intercourse, decreasing to 62% and 54% of 11th graders and 12th graders, respectively. After 5 years, sexual activity among teenagers who had taken "virginity pledges did not differ from non-pledgers, but did decrease the likelihood of taking precautions during sexual activity" (Rosenbaum, 2009). Family physicians should remind sexually active adolescents to use a condom with each oral, genital, or anal intercourse to minimize HIV and other sexually transmitted infection (STI) risk.

Contextual Issues

Family physicians should not assume that adolescent sexual experiences are consensual or desired, even when the teenager denies having been sexually assaulted or raped. Both young women and men should be asked about unwanted sexual contact. In the YRBS 2007, 7.8% of youth reported having been forced to have sexual intercourse they did not want (11.3% female, 4.5% male). Many teenagers who have had coercive sexual experiences do not identify these as rape or abuse. Asking a neutrally worded question (e.g., "Have you ever done anything sexual when you really didn't want to?") may open the door to further dialogue regarding exploitive or traumatic sex.

For adolescent patients, drug and alcohol use is a significant risk factor for unprotected sexual activity. In the 2007 YRBS, 23% of teenagers reported alcohol or drug use immediately before they last had sexual intercourse. Long-acting contraception is often the best option for young women who are at risk for pregnancy because of substance use. Referral for treatment of addiction should be considered for adolescents who combine drinking with driving or sex and who are unable to discontinue this risk behavior without assistance.

Sexual Orientation

While in the process of discovering their adult identity, many adolescents have questions regarding sexual orientation, gender identity, or gender role. Concurrent heterosexual and homosexual feelings and attractions are common; a single or small number of same-sex sexual encounters are not necessarily predictive of a gay, lesbian, or bisexual identity as an adult. Predominantly homosexual attractions during adolescence, however, are unlikely to change with time. By maintaining an opening questioning style, such as asking, "When you think of people to whom you are sexually or romantically attracted, are they men, women, both, neither, or are you not sure yet?", the health care provider gives the adolescent permission to express their sexual orientation freely.

In an environment critical of their emerging sexual orientation, nonheterosexual adolescents may experience profound isolation and fear of discovery, which interfere with achieving the developmental tasks related to self-esteem, identity, and intimacy. Censure, alienation, and abandonment by the family of origin represent a particularly devastating consequence for many gay and lesbian teenagers. Nonheterosexual adolescents are more likely to have had sexual intercourse, to have had three or more sexual partners, and to have experienced sexual intercourse against their will, putting them at increased risk of STDs, including HIV infection. Nonheterosexual teenagers are more likely than heterosexual peers to start using tobacco, alcohol, and illegal drugs at an earlier age. They are also at higher risk of dropping out of school, becoming homeless, and turning to prostitution or drug trafficking for survival (Garafolo et al., 1998). They are often subjected to harassment and violence; 45% of gay men and 20% of lesbians surveyed were victims of verbal and physical assaults in secondary school, specifically because of their sexual orientation (Kreiss and Patterson, 1997).

Teenagers seeking family-planning or obstetric services are not necessarily heterosexual; bisexual and lesbian respondents are two to seven times more likely to become pregnant than their heterosexual peers (Saewyc et al., 2008). Although for American adults, no differences in suicide rates are detectable between heterosexual and homosexual cohorts, gay, lesbian, bisexual, and "not sure" high school students were three times more likely to report a suicide attempt than their heterosexual peers (Garafolo et al., 1998). Primary care providers who care for adolescents, especially gay, lesbian, or bisexual youth, should be alert to the possibility of depression and suicide. For support, clinicians can suggest they contact the Gay, Lesbian, Bisexual, and Transgender National Youth Talkline at 800-246-PRIDE or the Trevor Helpline (866-488-7386; 866-4UTREVOR), a 24-hour suicide prevention hotline that focuses on the needs of gay youth.

Older Adults

Key Points

- Although the likelihood of being sexually active declines with age, many older adults remain sexually active.
- Approximately half of sexually active older adults report at least one sexual problem, and two-thirds have at least two.
- The likelihood of being sexually active correlates with good health.
- Although testosterone levels decline with age, androgen supplementation is recommended only in hypogonadal men.

Although the likelihood of being sexually active declines steadily with age, many older adults remain sexually active; 84% of men and 62% of women age 57 to 64 and 67% of men and 40% of women age 65 to 74 report being sexually active in the previous 12 months, with two thirds of both genders in each cohort sexually active more than two to three times a month. For those age 75 to -85, only 39% of men and 17% of women reported sexual activity within 12 months (those sexually active still had >2-3/mo) (Lindau et al., 2007). Several factors impact the decline in sexual activity. As men and women age, physiologic changes in sexual functioning occur. During arousal, older men experience less scrotal vasoconstriction and testicular elevation, erection may be delayed or insufficient, and orgasm may be of shorter duration with less ejaculatory fluid. Women may have decreased labial engorgement and less vaginal lubrication during arousal and fewer and weaker uterine contractions during orgasm. Regardless of these physical changes, many older adults continue to have active sexual lives.

In one large U.S. study, approximately half of sexually active older adults reported at least one sexual problem, with almost two-thirds having at least two bothersome sexual problems. Sexual problems most often reported by women were lack of interest (43%), difficulty with lubrication (39%), inability to climax (34%), finding sex not pleasurable (23%), and pain (17%). Among men, the most common sexual problems were difficulty in achieving or maintaining an erection (37%), lack of interest in sex (28%), climaxing too quickly (28%), anxiety about performance (27%), and inability to climax (20%). The likelihood of being sexually active is associated with good health. Men and women who reported good to excellent health were 80% and 70%, respectively, more likely to be sexually active than men and women with "poor" or "fair" health status (Lindau et al., 2007). Many common health conditions, such as arthritis or back pain, can inhibit sexual activity. Vascular disease and its risk factors, including coronary artery disease, stroke, diabetes, hypertension, hyperlipidemia, and smoking, correlated with ED in the Global Study of Sexual Attitudes and Behaviors (GSSAB). Women with diabetes are also less likely to be sexually active than women without diabetes (Laumann et al., 2005). Pudendal nerve disruption following hysterectomy and bladder, rectal, or prostate surgery may cause sexual dysfunction. Since they take more medications, older adults may be particularly susceptible to iatrogenic sexual dysfunction, because many common medications affect sexual functioning, especially antihypertensives and antidepressants (see Table 43-1).

At all ages, women are less likely to be sexually active than men. For example, 50% of women age 60 to 69 reported that a healthy sexual life was at least "moderately important" to them; however, only 30% reported continued regular participation in sexual intercourse (Ponholzer et al., 2005). Women may be more likely not to have a spouse or intimate partner because of their greater longevity. In those age 75 to 85, men are almost twice as likely as women to have an intimate partner (78% vs. 40%). In addition, women are frequently younger than their male partners. Partner health may be an issue; 64% of women reported the male partner's physical health as the reason for sexual inactivity longer than 3 months (Lindau et al., 2007). Data from the 2005 Vermont Civil Unions suggest a similar age discrepancy among same-sex partners; for women and men age 40 to 44, more than 25% and about 50%, respectively, had a partner more than 5 years older (see Web Resources). Lack of privacy may be problematic for elderly adults, who may live with family members or in long-term care settings.

Decline in sex steroid production is a factor in sexual dysfunction for both women and men. Postmenopausal estrogen deficiency is responsible for loss of vaginal lubrication and elasticity. The Women's Health Initiative (WHI) raised concerns regarding deleterious effects of systemic estrogen replacement (Rossouw et al., 2002). Clinicians should counsel women desiring long-term oral estrogen supplementation to diminish vaginal atrophy symptoms regarding the increased risk of coronary artery disease, thrombotic disease, and breast cancer. Vaginal estrogen supplementation may be helpful to decrease vaginal mucosal atrophy with much less systemic absorption. Using creams, pessaries, or a vaginal ring to apply estrogen vaginally relieves the symptoms of vaginal atrophy, although some creams may cause adverse effects such as uterine bleeding, breast pain, and perineal pain (Suckling et al., 2006). Women who remain sexually active may avoid significant vaginal atrophy through continued stimulation of the epithelium and vascular supply.

Androgen deficiency in adult males (ADAM), often called "male menopause" or "andropause," is controversial. Testosterone levels do decline with age, eventually by 50% from midlife to old age, and predictable physiologic changes occur. One large, double-blind RCT demonstrated that supplementing older men with low-normal circulating testosterone levels with 80 mg of oral testosterone undecenoate twice daily for 6 months increased lean body mass and decreased fat mass, but it did not improve functional mobility or muscle strength. There also was no demonstrable beneficial effect on cognition or quality-of-life measures (Emmelot-Vonk et al., 2008). Androgen supplementation does have risks, such as altering cholesterol metabolism; thus it currently is not recommended unless the man has hypogonadism (Bhasin et al., 2006).

In one global study in men 40 to 80 years old who visited a primary care physician, almost half (49%) had ED (Mulhall et al., 2008). Despite the increasing prevalence of sexual difficulties in aging persons, the GSSAB reported only 9% of both men and women had been asked about sexual health by their physician during the preceding 3 years. Only 18% of the men and women in that study population sought medical assistance for their sexual problems (Moreira et al., 2005). The increased acceptance and availability of PDE-5 inhibitors may have improved physician-patient discussions over the last few years. In a recent study, 38% of men and 22% of women reported having discussed sex with a physician since age 50 (Lindau et al., 2007). Clinicians can improve their older-adult care by inquiring about sexual health and illness during the course of routine geriatric health care. Normal physical changes can be explained. ED and other sexual problems can often be treated effectively, thus assisting elderly patients in maintaining healthy sexual lives.

Conclusion

Sexuality is a core aspect of personal identity. Knowledge regarding human sexual behavior in health and illness across the life span will enable family physicians to provide appropriate care to patients who are experiencing sexual difficulties. Many sexual problems can be treated by family physicians and other primary health care providers without assistance. Referral to a certified sex therapist should be pursued for more complicated cases. Family physicians should maintain awareness of the health care needs of persons with same-gender sexual experience or orientation. Transgendered persons may have the health care needs of their former and present gender. Sexual health issues are pertinent for adolescent and older-adult well-health care. Family physicians should routinely include questions regarding sexual behavior, relationships, and personal identity during the clinical interview of all patients, to help maintain their optimum health.

EVIDENCE-BASED SUMMARY

- Estrogen creams, pessaries, tablets, and estradiol vaginal ring appear equally effective for the symptoms of vaginal atrophy. Women seem to favor the estradiol-releasing vaginal ring for ease of use, comfort of product, and overall satisfaction (SOR: A).
- In men with antidepressant-induced erectile dysfunction, addition of sildenafil is an effective strategy (SOR: A).
- PDE-5 inhibitors are a valuable treatment option for ED in men with diabetes (SOR: A).
- Group psychotherapy may improve erectile function, both compared to no treatment or sildenafil alone (SOR: A).

References

The complete reference list is available online at www.expertconsult.com.

Web Resources

www.aasect.org
American Association of Sex Educators, Counselors, and Therapists; can help locate local resources for sexual counseling.
www.cdc.gov/HealthyYouth/yrbs/pdf/yrbss07_mmwr.pdf
Center for Disease Control and Prevention Youth Risk Behavior Surveillance Survey; data on adolescent high-risk behaviors.
www.endo-society.org/guidelines/Current-Clinical-Practice-Guidelines.cfm
Endocrine Society Treatment Guideline; testosterone therapy in adult men with androgen deficiency syndromes.
www.med.umich.edu/transgender/
University of Michigan Comprehensive Gender Services Program; health care services for individuals who are transgendered and in need of gender-related care, including endocrinologic, surgical, mental, and general health care services.

http://wpath.org
World Professional Association for Transgender Health; multidisciplinary group whose mission is to promote evidence-based care, education, research, advocacy, public policy, and respect in transgender health.
www.vaginismus.com
Site to order plastic dilators for vaginismus treatment.
www.soulsourceenterprises.com
Site to order silicone dilators.
http://healthvermont.gov/research/stats/2005/i04fp.htm
Data from the 2005 Vermont Civil Unions.

CHAPTER **44**

Clinical Genetics (Genomics)

W. Gregory Feero, Philip Zazove, and Nancy G. Stevens

Overview

Key Points

- Discoveries related to common conditions such as diabetes, heart disease, and cancer are rapidly changing the role of genetics in health care.
- Primary care providers should know the limits of their own knowledge in genetics and should become familiar with supportive resources and seek out expert consult when in doubt.

We stand at a remarkable time in history regarding our understanding of how variations in the human genome contribute to health and disease. At least some of this progress can be attributed to the technologies developed to complete the Human Genome Project. The tools of genomics and molecular biology have begun to unlock the fundamental underpinnings of previously enigmatic conditions, shedding light on the fundamental nature of the human species.

The most exciting developments since 2005 are related to the genetics of common disease, a mainstay of primary care medicine. For the first time, geneticists have been able to use a very powerful technique known as *genome-wide association study* (GWAS) to identify human genome variations associated with common disease risk. Hundreds of risk markers known as *single nucleotide polymorphisms* (SNPs) have been reliably associated with the presence of a long list of common conditions. Although each individual marker confers only a small risk of disease (which greatly limits their use in the clinic to predict risk in individual patients), each has helped to better define disease pathogenesis (Kraft and Hunter, 2009; Manolio et al., 2008). With the advent of low-cost whole-genome sequencing, discoveries related to disease risk, prognosis, and treatment relevant to primary care should accelerate (Feero et al., 2010). Most chapters in a family medicine textbook will eventually include the relevant information to the specific topic derived from genetics and genomics.

We are at an early stage in the discovery process, and our embryonic understanding of the human genome is *not* easily yielding improvements in clinical care. This perspective is often lost in the media hype and attention given to the latest genetic discovery. The lack of a rapid translation from a new discovery to a proven clinical application (e.g., genetic test, targeted therapy) frustrates clinicians and patients alike and can lead to unrealistic and potentially harmful expectations. Clinicians should recognize where the application of knowledge from genetic discovery is of proven benefit, and where it is not. Perhaps most importantly, physicians should recognize that a substantial and rapidly expanding number of genomic applications fall into a gray area of unexplored benefit. It is incumbent on providers to seek additional information from a reputable source when in doubt.

Genetics vs. Genomics

The terms genetics and genomics are often used interchangeably in the literature, and this chapter is no exception. However, *genetics* is best viewed as the study of *single genes*, what they do, and how mutations in these genes cause disease. It is a snapshot of a specific situation, and environmental and behavioral factors often play a subordinate role. A prototypical genetic condition, cystic fibrosis, is usually caused by a deletion mutation ΔF508 in the *CFTR* gene. *Genomics* is the broader study of "the functions and interactions of all the genes in the genome," including how those genes interact with environmental and behavioral factors (Guttmacher and Collins, 2002). When considering genomics, it is important to recognize that environmental factors may be much more important in determining phenotype than genetic mutations. Common, so-called complex conditions, such as diabetes, cancer, and heart disease, are best considered from the perspective of genomics.

Genetics and Evidence-Based Medicine

As a discipline, *clinical genetics* developed in an environment that focused on the diagnosis and treatment of rare, or at least uncommon, disease. Often, large numbers of patients were not available for clinical trials, and in many cases the severity of the conditions made randomized placebo-controlled trials (RCTs) untenable. This contrasts with *evidence-based medicine* (EBM), which primarily deals with common conditions and values large, prospective RCTs, as well as the societal consequences of individual medical choices. As genomic discoveries increasingly impact health care for common conditions, new applications should be evaluated through a lens of *evidence of benefit.* Established groups that follow EBM precepts, such as the U.S. Preventive Services Task Force (USPSTF, 2009), have addressed screening and testing for hereditary breast and ovarian cancer syndrome and hemochromatosis. The U.S. Centers for Disease Control and Prevention (CDC) has established newer groups such as the Evaluation of Genetic Applications in Practice and Prevention (EGAPP, 2009) specifically to review the evidence supporting genetic and genomic applications intended for health care use. Modeled after USPSTF, EGAPP has begun to produce evidence reviews and recommendations (Table 44-1). Considerable growing pains will occur as EBM and genomic medicine intersect.

Family History: Best Guide to Genetic Components of Disease

Key Points

- Family history is the best general tool for assessing a patient's risk for heritable conditions.
- Numerous guidelines relevant to primary care providers incorporate family history information.
- Evidence-based reviews have found that family history obtained from patients is generally accurate.
- Patient-completed web-based tools offer a convenient way to gather family history information.

Family history is arguably the single best tool for recognizing genetic components of disease in the primary care setting. In the context of single-gene disorders, family history has proved valuable for generations of clinicians and plays a major role in making a diagnosis and identifying at-risk individuals. Family physicians should be familiar with common patterns of inheritance of single-gene disorders, including X-linked recessive, X-linked dominant, autosomal dominant, autosomal recessive, and multifactorial/complex (Table 44-2). Classically, the three-generation genetic history

Table 44-1 Select Evidence-Based Recommendations for Genetic/Genomic Applications

Condition	Clinical Scenario	Recommendation	Organization
Breast cancer	Screening	Recommend referral of women with family history consistent with increased risk for hereditary breast and ovarian cancer syndrome for genetic counseling.	USPSTF, 2005
	Screening	Recommend against using *BRCA1* and *BRCA2* testing as screening tool in average-risk populations.	USPSTF, 2005
	Treatment	Insufficient evidence to recommend for or against routine use of expression profiles to guide care in specific populations of women with breast cancer.	EGAPP, 2008
Colorectal cancer	Screening	Insufficient evidence to determine if fecal DNA testing is effective means to screen for colorectal cancer.	USPSTF, 2006
	Case finding	Recommend offering counseling and tumor sample testing for Lynch syndrome to all patients with newly diagnosed colorectal cancer, to reduce morbidity and mortality in relatives.	EGAPP, 2009
	Pharmaco-genetic testing	Insufficient evidence to recommend for or against *UGT1A1* testing for patients with metastatic colorectal cancer.	EGAPP, 2009
Hemo-chromatosis	Screening	Recommend against screening for hemochromatosis in asymptomatic individuals.	USPSTF, 2008
Hyperlipidemia	Screening	Recommend earlier screening for hyperlipidemia in patients with family history of premature cardiovascular disease.	USPSTF, 2008
Depression	Pharmaco-genetic testing	Insufficient evidence, and recommend against routine use of CYP450 testing before prescribing SSRIs in adults with depression.	EGAPP, 2007

From the U.S. Preventive Services Task Force (USPSTF) and CDC Evaluation of Genomic Applications in Practice and Prevention (EGAPP) Working Group relevant to primary care.
USPSTF. http://www.ahrq.gov/CLINIC/uspstf/uspstopics.htm.
EGAPP. http://www.egappreviews.org/workingrp/recommendations.htm.
SSRIs, Selective serotonin reuptake inhibitors.

known as a *pedigree* or *genogram* has been taught as the "gold standard" of family history collection. Certainly, once a potential genetic issue has been identified, a family physician should be comfortable in collecting and accurately representing a complete family history. However, taking a complete family history can be time-consuming, and on a practical level, it is not always possible to collect in the context of a brief office visit. It is perfectly reasonable to gather, review, and update family history longitudinally.

Common diseases such as type 2 diabetes, coronary artery disease, and cancer also cluster in families. Family history captures both hereditary and environmental risks and is an important component of many validated risk algorithms for these and other conditions. Recent attention has focused on the systematic collection of family history as a screening tool in primary care settings. Family history information supplied by patients is generally fairly accurate for a wide range of conditions. However, few well-designed trials have examined health outcomes associated with use of family history as a screening tool (NIH Consensus Development Program, 2009).

Given competing demands on family physicians' time and resources, what genetic family history is the most important to capture? A national collaboration of primary care and genetics professionals has developed mnemonics to help clinicians think genetically as they provide patient care (Burke et al., 2001). FamilyGENES highlights "red flags" that signal a genetic concern, as follows (Whelan et al., 2004):

- *Family* history—multiple affected siblings or individuals in multiple generations
- Groups of congenital anomalies
- *Extreme* (or *e*xceptional) presentation of common conditions
- *N*eurodevelopmental delay or degeneration
- *E*xtreme or exceptional pathology
- *S*urprising laboratory values

SCREEN (for familial disease) uses the following set of family history questions to uncover genetic implications:

- *S*ome *C*oncerns: Do you have any (some) concerns about diseases or conditions that seem to run in the family?

- *R*eproduction: Have there been any problems with pregnancy, infertility, or birth defects in your family?
- *E*arly disease, death, or disability: "Have any members of your family died or become sick at an early age?
- *E*thnicity: How would you describe your ethnicity? *or* Where were your grandparents born?
- *N*ongenetic: Are there any other risk factors or nonmedical conditions that run in your family?

Electronic health record (EHR) systems seldom offer efficient and complete ways to collect and represent family history information. National efforts are underway to address this deficiency. Patient-completed paper and electronic tools provide another way to obtain a detailed genetic history. The U.S. Surgeon General's Family History Initiative (2005) includes a web-based tool that can be completed by patients, stored on their local computer, and shared with relatives and their health care providers in pedigree or table format (My Family Health Portrait; https://familyhistory.hhs.gov/). This free, easy-to-use tool is an excellent way for patients with Internet access to record family history and is time-saving for the clinician. The family history collected by the tool is now stored using emerging data standards that allow the data to be shared with EHR and personal health record systems. Alternatively, a number of organizations have created paper family history tools for patients and providers that are available on the Internet.

Genetic Testing

Key Points

- Knowledge of the indications for and limitations of genetic testing is relevant to common clinical situations in family medicine.
- The context of testing and its limitations are important for proper interpretation.
- Pretest and post-test counseling are currently recommended for genetic testing, although the need for such counseling in all testing situations is controversial.

Table 44-2 Patterns of Inheritance Often Encountered in Primary Care

Pattern of Inheritance	Characteristics Of Family History	Example Conditions
X-linked recessive	Males affected more than females, maternal inheritance, 50% risk of female carrier sons affected	X-linked color blindness X-linked muscular dystrophy
X-linked dominant	Males and females may be affected, males more severe, daughters of affected males affected, male and female transmission	Fragile-X syndrome
Autosomal dominant	Affected individuals usually in every generation, 50% probability of affected individuals having affected offspring, M = F	Huntington's disease Hyperkalemic periodic paralysis Lynch syndrome Marfan's syndrome
Autosomal recessive	Often multiple affected individuals in same generation, skipped generations, 25% risk of affected child for carriers, M = F	α_1-Antitrypsin deficiency Cystic fibrosis Sickle cell disease Most inborn errors of metabolism
Multifactorial	Clustering of cases in families, risk to first-degree relatives high; consequences of shared environment might be evident.	Coronary artery disease Types 1 and 2 diabetes Many cancers

- Genetic testing results can have implications for the family, and providers generally have a duty to warn potentially affected members.
- Family physicians should be involved in ordering, interpreting, and managing the consequences of genetic testing with health implications.

Identifying what constitutes a genetic or genomic test can be challenging. Traditionally, a genetic test measures changes in the sequence of deoxyribonucleic acid (DNA), but a "genetic test" can also be a measure of a protein or metabolite (Table 44-3). From this perspective, a fasting lipid panel could be considered a genetic test. Also, a genetic test does not always need to be relevant to other family members, as when an individual's cancer cells are tested for mutations that affect prognosis and therapy. In some cases a family physician's most important role is simply to reassure low-risk individuals that they do not need genetic testing.

The indications for genetic testing include confirming a diagnosis, identifying disease risk, and guiding therapeutic interventions. A genetic test can be done using many types of specimens, although testing for mutations in DNA is often done on DNA extracted from whole blood, saliva, or a cheek swab. Some tests look for only specific mutations, whereas others scan for all mutations in a specific DNA region. Testing costs can range from $100 to thousands of dollars, depending on the complexity and patent status of the test. Often, testing an affected family member first is the preferred strategy. Without knowing the mutation present in a family, an asymptomatic patient's negative test result may not be informative, because the particular test done may not include the mutation affecting that family.

Family physicians should be aware that genetic testing may have implications for the extended family as well as the patient. For example, studies with Huntington's patients have shown that genetic test results, whether positive or negative, have significant implications for patients and their families. This includes depression, lifestyle behavior changes, and relationship changes among family members. Those testing negative may have survivor's guilt or may be treated as being outside the family. Patients can benefit from counseling about implications before undergoing genetic testing that is both highly predictive and associated with profound health consequences (Martin and Wilikofsky, 2004). For genetic tests that are less predictive or are associated with conditions with less profound health consequences, the benefits of formal genetic counseling are less clear-cut.

Obtaining and interpreting molecular tests for DNA mutations often has unique considerations. First, it is important to order the correct test for the patient's condition; this is not always obvious, particularly when multiple tests are available. Second, the presence of a mutation in an asymptomatic individual only rarely predicts disease onset, course, or severity. This is particularly true for the multitude of recently discovered SNP markers associated with risk for common complex conditions. Third, absence of a known causal mutation in a gene may not mean that an individual is at no or low risk of disease. For example, in families meeting the clinical criteria for hereditary breast and ovarian cancer syndrome, testing for mutations in the *BRCA1* or *BRCA2* occasionally fails to detect a mutation in affected members. The absence of detectable mutations in affected individuals means that the test is essentially uninformative, and the risk to asymptomatic family members needs to be estimated from the clinical scenario and is not that of the average population (GeneTests, 2009). Because of the complex factors involved, genetic tests are frequently ordered by physicians with particular expertise regarding the condition for which testing is being considered. Currently, there are insufficient genetics professionals in all U.S. areas to handle the counseling associated with genetic tests. As a result, primary care physicians will most likely be providing more genetic counseling and testing in the future. The next section provides a more in-depth look at settings in which different types of genetic testing are relevant to primary care.

Examples of Genetic Testing

Preconception and Prenatal Screening

Genetic screening or testing can occur either before conception or during the pregnancy. When possible, screening or testing before a pregnancy is ideal, because this provides the broadest range of choices if increased risk of a genetic defect is detected. Preimplantation genetic testing is available for

Table 44-3 Types of Genetic/Genomic Testing

Test	Example Methods	Clinical Scenarios	Example Conditions
Chromosomal analysis	Fluorescent in situ hybridization, karyotype, array comparative genomic hybridization	Pediatrics, prenatal testing	Down syndrome, unexplained mental retardation
DNA analysis	Allele-specific oligonucleotide hybridization, sequencing, fluorescent PCR assays, DNA microarrays	Adult, pediatric, prenatal testing, pharmacogenetic testing	Hereditary breast and ovarian cancer syndrome, Huntington's disease, cystic fibrosis, warfarin pharmacogenomics
Biochemical tests	Various	Adult, pediatric, prenatal	Hyperlipidemia, phenylketonuria, quadruple screen
Expression profiling	cDNA measurement on microarrays, quantitative PCR	Adult, pediatric	Breast cancer, melanoma, colorectal cancer

PCR, Polymerase chain reaction; *cDNA,* complementary (copy) deoxyribonucleic acid.

an increasing number of conditions but is costly and not accessible to many individuals. Most genetic evaluations occur after the pregnancy is established. The ability to detect genetic defects has grown rapidly over the past decade. Many ethical issues exist in both the preconception and the prenatal screening or testing environment, including the course of action if the fetus is found to have an incurable, life-altering condition. Common indications for prenatal testing are advanced maternal age, previous child with a chromosomal abnormality, family history of abnormality or single-gene disorder, family history of neural tube defect or other structural abnormality, abnormalities identified in pregnancy (e.g., on ultrasound), parental consanguinity, recurrent miscarriages, previous unexplained stillbirth, parental ancestral origin, and use of certain medications. The American College of Obstetricians and Gynecologists (ACOG) and the American College of Medical Geneticists (ACMG) have developed guidelines for recommended tests (Solomon and Feero, 2008). However, these guidelines are often based on consensus or expert opinion and do not always agree.

High-resolution ultrasound and quadruple serum panel are screening tests for congenital anomalies associated with a variety of genetic conditions. More invasive testing, such as chorionic villus sampling (CVS) and amniocentesis, may provide more accurate diagnosis, but at the cost of higher risk of complications. Recent guidelines suggest that amniocentesis be offered to all pregnant women to aid in the detection of Down syndrome (ACOG, 2007). The family physician should evaluate the risks and benefits of all forms of prenatal genetic screening or testing, discuss them with the patient and her partner, and make referrals to health care providers with genetics expertise as appropriate.

Pharmacogenetics

Pharmacogenetics is the study of genetically determined variations in response to medication. This can include variations in how a drug is metabolized as well as how drugs interact with intended as well as unintended targets in the body. Pharmacogenetic testing can be useful in ensuring accurate drug dosing, avoiding adverse side effects, and selecting drugs. The U.S. Food and Drug Administration (FDA) mandates that many drugs reference pharmacogenetic testing in their labeling. Although family physicians should be aware that such labeling exists, the evidence of benefit of testing for these variations is not uniform across drugs. Currently, several pharmacogenetic tests are routinely used to guide treatment of oncology and infectious disease patients. Pharmacogenetic testing is likely relevant to some of the family physician's patients (Table 44-4). This number will grow as more pharmacogenetic tests become available.

Recent promising applications of pharmacogenomics measure variations relevant to drug responsiveness in cancer. Often, cancer drugs are toxic and expensive, so more individually targeted therapy (personalized medicine) based on the mutations present in a patient's tumor prove valuable over time. Examples include testing breast cancer tumors for overexpression of *HER2* receptor to guide use of targeted therapies. Such testing is becoming a part of routine oncologic care. More recently, the American Society of Clinical Oncology (ASCO) has developed guidelines for testing for *KRAS* oncogene mutations to guide colorectal cancer treatment

(Allegra et al., 2009). More clinical applications of pharmacogenetic testing relevant to cancer care are in the pipeline for clinical release.

Direct-to-Consumer Testing

Since the completion of the Human Genome Project in 2003, more companies now offer direct-to-consumer (DTC) genetic testing. The public profile of DTC testing increased dramatically over the last several years with the advent of inexpensive, genome-wide scans for SNPs. Tests that measure millions of genetic variations simultaneously can be obtained with a saliva sample and a few hundred dollars. The majority of these markers are probably of little significance to the tested individual's health, and patients may both overestimate and underestimate their personal risk of disease based on the results of such testing. The other types of tests offered can be grouped into "medical" and "nonmedical" categories. Medical tests include highly validated DNA testing for specific mutations in classic single-gene mendelian disorders, pharmacogenetic testing, and paternity testing. Nonmedical testing ranges from determining one's ethnic and geographic origins or athletic prowess to ear wax type. DTC testing can offer advantages of anonymity for testing as well as easy access to genetic tests that might be difficult to obtain through routine health care channels. The consumer pays for most DTC genetic testing.

Clinicians should recognize that "buyer beware" applies to DTC genetic testing. National regulatory oversight ensuring the analytic and clinical validity of these tests is inadequate, although some states (California, New York) have enacted laws to increase scrutiny of consumer-oriented tests. Even

Table 44-4 Pharmacogenetic Testing

Drug	Gene	Notes
Abacavir	HLA-B*5701	HIV-1 patients
Aminoglycosides	A1555G	Not routinely
Antifolate chemotherapy	MTHFR	Not routinely
Azathioprine	TPMT	Not routinely
Beta blockers	CYP2D6	Not routinely
Irinotecan	UGT1A1	Not routinely
Opioids	CYP2D6	Not routinely
Oral contraceptives	FVL, prothrombin G20210A, others	Family and personal history of VT can be used
SSRIs	CYP450	EGAPP recommended against, 2007.
Carbamazepine	HLA-B*1502	For Asian-Americans
Warfarin	CYP2C9 and VKORC1	Algorithms may work as well/better.

HIV-1, Human immunodeficiency virus type 1; *EGAPP*, Evaluation of Genomic Applications in Practice and Prevention; *SSRIs*, selective serotonin reuptake inhibitors; *VT*, venous thrombosis.

with accurate testing, there is no assurance that the result will be clinically useful to the individual. This is particularly problematic when a trained health professional is not available to help individuals appropriately select and interpret genetic testing. Companies now offer phone-based genetic counseling services independent of any testing services. Phone counseling has been shown to be effective for a variety of genetic conditions, and it remains to be seen how this type of counseling service might affect the movement to increasing DTC access to genetic tests. Ideally, a trained health professional should be involved in ordering and interpreting any genetic or genomic testing with health implications.

Ethical, Legal, and Social Issues

Key Points

- Clinicians should consider potential ELSIs when discussing genetic testing with patients.
- GINA provides national protections against health insurance and employment discrimination based on genetic information. HIPAA provides insurance portability and privacy protections. Some states have more comprehensive statutes to prevent genetic discrimination.
- Case law suggests that family members have a right to know whether genetic information affects their personal health, and that health care providers have a duty to warn family members of health risks.
- Minors incapable of providing informed consent should not be tested for conditions not immediately relevant to their health or not treatable in childhood.

Significant potential ethical, legal, and social issues (ELSIs) are associated with the use of genomic technologies in health care, and funding for research regarding ELSIs was part of the Human Genome Project from the outset. ELSIs include concerns regarding potential for discrimination or stigmatization based on one's genome, the right to know or not know one's genetic status in family settings, potential adverse effects of genetic testing on reproductive decision making, and discomfort with genetic testing of conditions for which treatment in childhood is not recommended or is not available.

Many patients are concerned that genetic information could be used as a tool for discrimination by health insurers and employers. In 2008 the Genetic Information Nondiscrimination Act (GINA) became U.S. law and provides national protection against use of genetic and family history information as a basis for discrimination by health insurers or employers (Hudson, 2008). However, the law does not prevent use of genetic information by life, long term care, or disability insurers. Some states have laws providing for more stringent protections than those afforded by GINA, and physicians should be aware of the protections their states provide (National Conference of State Legislatures, 2008).

Family physicians must remember that a genetic diagnosis affecting a patient has implications for the entire family. Before genetic testing, they should discuss the need to inform family members of abnormal results that might affect them. When a patient does not want family members to know that they have a genetic disease, the Health Insurance Portability and Accountability Act (HIPAA) has clarified and strengthened the patient's right to privacy of medical information. When knowledge of the patient's condition would not change health outcomes for the relative, the physician has no duty to warn. If the information can affect other family members' health, this presents a quandary. Some courts have ruled that physicians are liable for failure to inform other family members. Physician assistance in informing family members can also help the patient (Offit et al., 2004).

Several national groups of genetics professionals have developed consensus guidelines against genetic testing in *minors,* unless there is a potential immediate benefit to the child's health. Experience in adult-onset conditions has revealed that many people choose not to know if they are at risk for a genetically determined condition. Knowing about the risk of developing an adult illness in childhood, when no treatment or intervention is available, may present unnecessary intrusion into normal child and family development. Consequently, rather than test minors, it is often advisable to wait until adulthood so that a fully informed decision can be made about testing.

Reproductive decision making can be complex. It is important to remember that the quadruple screen or high-resolution ultrasound during pregnancy is genetic testing. Before patients undergo preconception or prenatal screening or testing, family physicians need to discuss the patient's expectations about results and subsequent pregnancy planning. Counseling before fetal testing should include detailed information about risks, benefits to parents and infants, probability of abnormal result, and implications of possible results, including inconclusive results or those indicating alternate paternity. Reproductive counseling has followed a nondirective model, in which the health professional avoids biasing the woman's or the couple's decision-making process.

Genetics in Primary Care Practice: Disease Illustrations

Key Points

- Health care providers should recognize when genetic factors contribute meaningfully to risk assessment, diagnosis, or disease management for rare conditions as well as common multifactorial conditions.
- Staying current with advances in diagnosis and treatment of genetic conditions challenges both genetic specialists and family physicians.
- Family physicians should identify and utilize credible and current information resources to support their care of patients with heritable conditions because proper diagnosis and management can be lifesaving.

Table 44-5 lists examples of multifactorial, single-gene, and chromosomal disorders seen in family medicine, including genetic information about each disease (Acheson and Wiesner, 2004; Christiansen et al., 2005; Gaston et al., 1986). In aggregate, single-gene and chromosomal disorders are relatively common. Physicians should remain alert for

Table 44-5 Multifactorial, Single-Gene, and Chromosomal Disorders Seen in Family Medicine

Condition	Inheritance Pattern	Genes Involved*
Single-gene diseases		
Early-onset Alzheimer's disease	Autosomal dominant	APP, PSEN1, PSEN2
Breast cancer	Autosomal dominant with incomplete penetrance	BRCA1, BRCA2
Colon cancer (Lynch syndrome)	Autosomal dominant with incomplete penetrance	MLH1, MSH2, MSH6, and PMS2
Cystic fibrosis	Autosomal recessive	CFTR
Hemachromatosis, adult	Autosomal recessive	HFE
Marfan's syndrome	Autosomal dominant	FBN1, TGFBR2
Sickle cell disease	Autosomal recessive	HBB
Tay-Sachs disease	Autosomal recessive	HEXA
β-Thalassemia	Autosomal recessive	HBB
Familial hypercholesterolemia	Various	LDLR, ApoB, PCSK9, LDLRAP1
Chromosomal diseases		
Down syndrome	Sporadic	Trisomy 21
Fragile X syndrome	X-linked dominant with incomplete penetrance	FMR1, with >200 CGG repeats
Turner' syndrome	Sporadic	XO karyotype
XXY Males (Klinefelter's syndrome)	Sporadic	XXY karyotype
Multifactorial diseases		
Alzheimer's disease	Multifactorial	APOE E4, multiple SNPs
Asthma	Multifactorial	Multiple SNPs
Coronary artery disease	Multifactorial	Multiple SNPs
Depression	Multifactorial	Multiple SNPs
Diabetes type 2	Multifactorial	Multiple SNPs
Diabetes, type I	Multifactorial	HLA variants and multiple SNPs
Venous thromboembolism	Multifactorial/autosomal dominant	Factor V Leiden FVL, proteins C and S, prothrombin G20210A, antithrombin III

Data from Gene Tests (www.genetests.org); Online Mendelian Inheritance in Man (http://www.ncbi.nlm.nih.gov/omim/); and NHGRI GWAS catalog (http://www.genome.gov/26525384).
*Most common mode of inheritance for each condition listed; for many common multifactorial conditions, there are rare instances of mutations in single genes causing a similar disease.
SNPs, Single nucleotide polymorphisms.

single-gene diseases when seeing patients, which can include causes of cancers, anemia, liver disease, developmental delay, and deep vein thrombosis. Making a correct genetic diagnosis can lead to lifesaving interventions for affected patients and their families.

Much research is needed regarding the genetics of multifactorial disorders, and predispositional genetic testing for such conditions using newer markers (e.g., disease-associated SNPs) is not currently recommended. A few examples illustrate what can currently be done with genetics and genomics in primary care.

Hereditary Breast and Ovarian Cancer

A family history of premenopausal breast cancer in a first-degree relative doubles personal breast cancer risk. These women may benefit from earlier screening and should be counseled about the benefits of early detection. An autosomal dominant pattern of inheritance is seen in a much smaller number of families, perhaps 5% of women with breast cancer, known as hereditary breast and ovarian cancer (HBOC) syndrome. Current USPSTF guidelines suggest that physicians should recognize individuals from such families because they may benefit from counseling about HBOC and testing for mutations in the *BRCA1* and *BRCA2* genes. The USPSTF recommends against using *BRCA* and mutation testing as a screening tool in the absence of a suggestive personal or family history. Numerous *BRCA* mutations have been found, and their prevalence in the general population is about 1 in 800, but up to 1 in 40 in people of Ashkenazi Jewish descent. Pretest and post-test counseling is very important for HBOC. The presence of many rare mutations and mutations of unknown clinical significance in the population can make interpretation of testing complicated, and involvement of a clinician with specialized knowledge is advisable.

Women with *BRCA* mutations may have up to an 80% lifetime risk of breast cancer and a 40% risk of ovarian cancer depending on the mutation. The risk of other cancers is also greater, although less so. It is important to recognize that males with a *BRCA* mutation develop breast cancer at much higher rates than the general population. In fact, a diagnosis of male breast cancer should lead to a careful review of family history. Personal risk depends on the specific gene variant involved and other risk factors. Aggressive strategies aimed at early detection (e.g., breast MRI) are frequently recommended, but evidence of comparative effectiveness is lacking. Interventions such as bilateral mastectomy and oophorectomy have an enormous impact on women's lives, but evidence suggests these surgeries may confer up to a 90% reduction in cancer risk (NCCN, 2008).

Evidence regarding prophylaxis with tamoxifen or related agents is equivocal and may be related to the specific causal mutation. Although routinely offered to individuals with *BRCA* mutations, little evidence supports the use of annual CA-125 and transvaginal ultrasound to screen for ovarian cancer. Options for prevention and treatment are increasing over time, and more targeted and less invasive options may become available.

KEY TREATMENT

Women with a family history suggestive of hereditary breast and ovarian cancer (HBOC) syndrome should be offered genetic counseling (USPSTF, 2005) (SOR: A).

Enhanced breast cancer screening with annual mammograms and breast magnetic resonance imaging (MRI) starting at age 25, or 10 years earlier than the age of earliest diagnosis in the family, are recommended for individuals with *BRCA* mutations (NCCN, 2008; Saslow et al., 2007) (SOR: C).

Prophylactic mastectomy and oophorectomy dramatically reduce the risk of breast and ovarian cancer in HBOC patients (NCCN, 2008) (SOR: B).

Hereditary Colorectal Cancer

About 10% of the general population has a first-degree relative with colorectal cancer (CRC); this history increases personal lifetime risk for CRC to 9% to 16%. Many guidelines recommend early screening for these individuals—by age 40, or 10 years earlier than the age at diagnosis of a family member. Early detection and removal of adenomatous polyps have made determining family history more difficult. Patients should be asked about removal of polyps in relatives, and those who have adenomatous polyps should be encouraged to tell their families.

A family history that contains many relatives with CRC, adenomatous polyps, or endometrial cancer, especially in more than one generation or with early-onset (age <50) suggests an autosomal dominant pattern of inheritance. Two relatively common, autosomal dominant, hereditary colorectal cancer syndromes account for about 3% to 5% of all CRC cases. *Lynch syndrome,* or *hereditary nonpolyposis colon cancer syndrome* (HNPCC), occurs in about 1 in 200 to 800 families and is underdiagnosed in primary care settings. Lynch syndrome is caused by mutations in mismatched repair genes and confers an approximately 80% lifetime risk of CRC. Often these cancers are right-sided and occur at an earlier age than sporadic CRC. Women with HNPCC have an increased risk for endometrial cancer; the incidence of other gastrointestinal and central nervous system cancers is also increased, but to a lesser degree. Evidence-based guidelines suggest that CRC screening with colonoscopy should begin in the 20s for affected individuals. Screening for endometrial cancer is also recommended, but there is less evidence of benefit. Evidence indicates that the disease burden could be reduced by screening tissue samples from all new CRC cases for molecular findings suggestive of Lynch syndrome. Family members of individuals testing positive then could be offered testing and enhanced surveillance if positive (EGAPP Working Group, 2009).

Familial adenomatous polyposis (FAP) is seen in about 1 in 8000 families, and affected individuals have a 100% lifetime risk of CRC. Management usually involves early screening (age 10-12) with sigmoidoscopy and early colectomy. Chemoprophylaxis with nonsteroidal anti-inflammatory drugs (NSAIDs) may also be of benefit.

Family physicians should recognize both FAP and HNPCC and ensure that genetic evaluation is offered to these families. If a specific mutation is identified, early screening of family members can be stopped for those testing negative. In the absence of a known mutation, all family members should be screened at an early age and the screening repeated at shorter intervals.

KEY TREATMENT

Individuals with a single first-degree relative (parent, sibling, child) affected by colon cancer should be offered screening at 40 years of age, or 10 years before the age at diagnosis of the affected relative (NCCN, 2009) (SOR: B).

All colon cancer tumor samples should be tested for changes suggestive of Lynch syndrome (HNPCC), to reduce morbidity and mortality in family members (EGAPP Working Group, 2009) (SOR: A).

Accelerated screening for colon cancer is recommended for individuals with Lynch syndrome (NCCN, 2009) (SOR: A).

Colon cancer screening beginning in the second decade of life and early colectomy are recommended to reduce risk of colorectal cancer for individuals with familial adenomatous polyposis syndrome (NCCN, 2009) (SOR: A).

Cystic Fibrosis

Cystic fibrosis (CF) is a relatively common autosomal recessive condition that causes progressive lung disease and exocrine pancreatic insufficiency. CF affects approximately 1 in 3200 U.S. Caucasians but is less common in other population groups. CF results from inheriting two mutated copies of the *CTFR* gene, which is known to play a role in regulating chloride transport across epithelial membranes. More than 1000 *CFTR* mutations have been described, but the ΔF508 mutation accounts for the great majority of classic CF cases.

The diagnosis of CF in symptomatic individuals can be made by the chloride sweat test, transepithelial nasal potential difference measurement, or genetic testing for *CFTR* mutations. Once almost universally fatal in adolescence or early adulthood, improved management has resulted in more CF patients surviving well into adulthood. Patient management in specialized CF centers is common, although it is unclear to what extent management by a specialized center is associated with improved patient outcomes. Lung transplantation has been used as a "cure" for the pulmonary complications of CF.

All women should be offered CF carrier screening as part of prenatal or preconception care to determine risk, so that reproductive planning is an option (ACOG, 2005). It is important to recognize that the common panels offered for prenatal CF screening contain tests for a variety of CF mutations but perform less well in certain ethnic groups. This lowered sensitivity results in residual risk of having an infant with CF despite a negative screening test in certain population groups.

Several U.S. states include CF in their newborn screening programs, and some evidence suggests that screening is associated with improved outcomes (Grosse et al., 2006; Southern et al., 2009). Newborn screening for CF illustrates some important dilemmas. As a result of this screening, we now know that many patients with nonclassic *CFTR* mutations have only mild disease, such as congenital absence of the vas deferens or chronic sinus infections. Does diagnosis before the onset of symptoms improve outcomes for these individuals? What about the risks of informing parents of a serious disease in their apparently normal newborn—will it change parenting and child development? The answers to these questions are under investigation, but they are important factors to consider when assessing risks and benefits of early CF detection.

KEY TREATMENT

Newborn screening for cystic fibrosis occurs in some U.S. states and is associated with improved outcomes (Grosse et al., 2006; Southern et al., 2009) (SOR: B).

It is reasonable to offer CF carrier screening to women in the preconception or prenatal setting, regardless of race or ethnicity (ACOG, 2005) (SOR: C).

Consensus guidelines suggest sweat chloride testing or genetic testing for *CFTR* mutations for CF diagnosis in symptomatic individuals (GeneReviews, 2008) (SOR: C).

References

The complete reference list is available online at www.expertconsult.com.

Web Resources

http://ghr.nlm.nih.gov/
Excellent and up-to-date basic resource for genetics and health, including glossary.

http://genetests.org
National Library of Medicine; detailed information on many genetic diseases, a genetics services searchable database, a list of laboratories performing specific genetic tests, and illustrated glossary linked to text.

www.ncbi.nlm.nih.gov/omim
National Library of Medicine Online Mendelian Inheritance in Man; compendium of information on most genetic diseases, but may have more information than most nongeneticists need.

www.genome.gov/Health
National Human Genome Research Institute; useful resources for patients and patient care, including links to family history tools and guidelines, the Genetics and Rare Disease website (genetics help desk), National Cancer Institute's cancer PDQ, and genetic professional locators.

www.egappreviews.org/
Evaluation of Genomic Applications in Practice and Prevention; evidence-based guidelines for genomic applications.

www.nchpeg.org/
National Coalition of Health Professional Education in Genetics, dedicated to educating health professionals about genetics and genomics.

http://genes-r-us.uthscsa.edu/
National Newborn Screening and Genetics Resource Center; extensive information related to newborn screening, including links to the ACT sheets and general genetics resources.

www.cdc.gov/genomics
Centers for Disease Control and Prevention Office of Public Health Genomics; extensive information on public health aspects of genetics and genomics, including family history; provides links to other CDC resources related to genomics.

Crisis Intervention, Trauma, and Intimate Partner Violence

Robert E. Feinstein and Abby Snavely

Family medicine physicians are frequently asked to assist a patient who is in a crisis, whether a life-threatening illness, intimate partner violence, suicide attempt, job loss, loss of insurance, depression, panic attack, or bipolar episode. In this emotional state of crisis, the patient feels panicked, helpless, and overwhelmed and cannot perform basic activities involving work, family relations, and even daily living. Urgent safety concerns surround patients with acute medical conditions, as well as those with suicidal ideation and victims of violence. Many family physicians feel unprepared to offer patients practical help during a general office visit.

The *crisis intervention approach* provides both a theory and a treatment model that can be readily applied to patients in crisis or to victims of intimate partner violence. This chapter describes the general principles of crisis intervention theory and treatment, as well as crisis evaluation and treatment of *intimate partner violence,* which is a pervasive and often underrecognized public health problem.

Development of Crisis Intervention, Trauma, and Disaster Theory

Historical Considerations

Key Points

- Crises can be effectively treated. Three core principles of crisis treatment are (1) the expectation that the patient will recover, (2) the provision of immediate treatment, and (3) the encouragement of the patient to return to normal daily functioning as soon as possible. A crisis typically last 6 weeks and can resolve spontaneously. Crisis resolution depends on the severity of the crisis, personal reaction, support system, and effects on the community.

- A crisis is a brief psychological upheaval, precipitated by a stressor, resulting in an inability to cope, adapt, or function in daily life.

- A crisis may resolve with improved functioning, a return to baseline, or may be stabilized at a lower level of functioning.

Thomas Salmon (1917), a British military physician during World War I, was asked to evaluate severe "shell shock" (traumatic neurosis), which was producing psychological paralysis in Allied soldiers. In this first medical description of the psychological effects of war, Salmon noted that French soldiers suffered fewer psychological casualties than British soldiers. Three factors seemed to account for the French advantage: (1) French soldiers were told that they could expect to recover from their psychological traumas; (2) soldiers received immediate psychological treatment, close to the battlefront; and (3) soldiers were returned to battle as quickly as possible. These principles became the cornerstone of modern crisis theory and disaster management strategies. Patients entering crisis treatment can expect to be treated immediately, in their natural environments, with an expectation that they will recover from the crisis or disaster. Efforts should be made to return patients to their normal life and community as soon as possible.

Eric Lindemann (1944) applied and expanded Salmon's theories. He studied the acute grief reactions of persons who lost family members in the Coconut Grove fire in Boston, which claimed 500 lives. Lindemann discovered that normal people surviving such a horrific experience would develop an emotional crisis of pain, confusion, anxiety, and temporary difficulty in daily functioning. Also, he discovered that the psychological trauma caused by the crisis had little relation to preexisting psychopathology, and that only a small group of the victims declined to a lower level of functioning. Generally, the outcome of the crisis was most closely related to the severity of the stressor, personal reaction to the trauma, effect of trauma on the person's family and friends, and degree of community disruption. Lindemann found that most crisis survivors recovered spontaneously within 6 weeks.

Erik Erikson (1959), a sociologist, introduced the idea of a life cycle composed of developmental stages and developmental crises. His eight stages were seen as normative processes during which age-specific psychological tasks, transitions, and crises were routinely encountered. A difficulty or inability to negotiate a stage successfully affects the ability to progress to the next stage. For example, an adolescent seeks an adult identity and redefines social roles that emphasize peer relationships and increasing autonomy from parents. Those who do not successfully traverse adolescence develop a childlike dependence on parental figures and often have difficulty developing a career, getting married, or developing autonomous social relations.

Other crisis practitioners have expanded Erikson's basic concept of eight developmental crises to include other crises such as leaving home for the first time, the midlife crisis, and parents' experience of the "empty nest syndrome." For many patients, a transition from one life phase to the next, such as marriage, divorce, retirement, or an illness, may bring the potential for a new developmental crisis.

Gerald Caplan (1961, 1964) synthesized many of these earlier ideas into modern crisis theory and treatment. He defined the crisis state as a brief, personal, psychological upheaval precipitated by a stressor, or "hazard." A precipitant produces emotional turmoil so that the person is temporarily unable to cope, adapt, or function in daily activities. Caplan demonstrated that a crisis implies the potential for danger and an opportunity for growth. Although subscribing to Lindemann's theories of acute precipitants, Caplan believed that a person's preexisting psychiatric condition could influence the development, evolution, and resolution of a crisis. A crisis may be based on the failure of a person's individual coping style and ability to adapt. Caplan confirmed that most acute crises resolve in about 6 weeks, with four possible outcomes: improved functioning, functioning restored to precrisis levels, incompletely restored functioning with a susceptibility to the development of future crises, or a severely impaired but stable level of lower functioning. He corroborated Lindemann's findings that some people cope with a crisis by spontaneously and flexibly developing new coping or problem-solving styles. Caplan developed a crisis treatment focus on development of better coping mechanisms and adaptations to life's traumas.

Current Understanding of Crisis

Key Points

- Approximately 13% of the U.S. population has reported a lifetime exposure to natural or human-generated disaster.
- Posttraumatic stress disorder in the United States has an estimated lifetime prevalence of 8%, with women twice as likely as men to be affected.

The current understanding of "crisis" has been used as one of several core strategies in the management and treatment of trauma. The frequency of traumatic experiences is defined by the type of events called "traumatic." For example, early studies limited traumatic events to wars, natural disasters, and plane crashes, whereas more recent epidemiologic studies include intimate partner violence, car accidents, crime, or foreclosures. Estimates of lifetime trauma exposure vary with the definition of a "traumatic event," so community studies of exposure to lifetime trauma also varies (25%-90%). According to the American Psychiatric Association's *Diagnostic and Statistical Manual of Mental Disorders*, 4th edition, text revision (DSM IV-TR), the lifetime rate of posttraumatic stress disorder (PTSD) ranges between 1% and 14%.

Natural disasters such as earthquakes, tsunamis, hurricanes, tornadoes, and volcanic eruptions can traumatize individuals, devastate whole communities, and disturb an entire population in a large geographic area. Man-made disasters, such as 9-11 (2001), Oklahoma City (1995), suicide bombings, plane crashes, and environmental accidents, are all byproducts of the 21st century and, unfortunately, have become a part of modern life.

The prevalence of exposure to mass trauma is difficult to estimate. In one study, 13% of the U.S. population reported a lifetime exposure to natural or human-generated disaster (Burkle, 1996). The U.S. National Comorbidity Survey estimated that 18.9% of men and 15.2% of women reported a lifetime experience of a natural disaster (Kessler et al., 1995). These are merely exposure rates to trauma. Fortunately, most victims recover from traumatic exposure over time, without long-term sequelae. However, some will go on to develop *posttraumatic stress disorder* (PTSD). According to the National Center for Posttraumatic Stress Disorder, the estimated lifetime prevalence of PTSD among adult Americans is approximately 8%, with women twice as likely as men to be affected at some time during their life (Stein et al., 2003). Women who are victims of intimate partner violence are almost four times more likely than nonabused women to develop PTSD (Campbell, 2002).

The most common traumatic events include witnessing an injury, murder, fire, flood, or natural disaster; life-threatening accident; and combat exposure. According to the World Health Organization (WHO), 1.2 million people are killed in motor vehicle crashes and 50 million injured annually (Mayou et al., 1993). Well-known man-made disasters include the U.S. atomic bombings of Hiroshima and Nagasaki (WWII, 1945), the Chernobyl nuclear power plant accident in Russia (1986), the domestic terrorist bombing of Murrah federal building in Oklahoma City (1995), and foreign terrorist destruction of the World Trade Center in New York (2001). In addition, violence and trauma in American society continues with shootings in schools, community centers, and businesses.

Intimate Partner Violence

Key Points

- The American Association of Family Physicians estimates that one third of patients cared for by family physicians are affected by family violence.

- Children are adversely affected by intimate partner violence and may need a referral to child-focused treatment.
- Family violence leads to 39,000 physician visits and 73,000 hospitalizations annually.

Intimate partner violence (IPV) is a specific type of crisis requiring some special consideration; we use this term throughout this chapter to account for diverse populations and types of abuse. The Family Violence Prevention Fund (FVPF, 2004) defines intimate partner violence as "a pattern of assaultive and coercive behaviors that may include inflicted physical injury, psychological abuse, sexual assault, progressive social isolation, stalking, deprivation, intimidation, and threats. These behaviors are perpetrated by someone who is, was, or wishes to be involved in an intimate or dating relationship with an adult or adolescent, and are aimed at establishing control by one partner over the other."

Worldwide, at least 10% to 50% of women have been physically or sexually abused in their lifetime (WHO, 2001). Annually, 2 to 4 million women and 835,000 men are assaulted by intimate partners in the United States (National Institute of Justice). Lifetime prevalence of physical or sexual abuse by an intimate partner of U.S. women is 20% to 30%, and for men, 7.5% (FVPF, 2004). From 22% to 46% of gays and lesbians have been victims of physical IPV (AAFP, 2000). Between 2000 and 4000 U.S. women die from these injuries each year. Up to one in six pregnant women is abused during pregnancy (AAFP, 2000). One study showed that IPV increased health care costs in affected women by 92% (Ramsay et al., 2009). Family violence leads to 39,000 physician visits and 73,000 hospitalizations annually (Kass-Bartelmes and Rutherford, 2004).

A common and costly problem, IPV is receiving increased attention. Several professional organizations and other groups have made policy statements and recommendations; some mandate screening. The majority of IVP research is about violence committed by men against women, although recent epidemiologic studies show that IPV remains a significant problem in male homosexual relationships and occurs in all types of relationships (FVPF, 2004). The previous statistics on IPV are even more striking when considering that IPV is almost universally underreported (Watts and Zimmerman, 2002). Many studies assess only physical violence, not accounting for the psychological, economic, and emotional abuse that may exist alone or with other forms of violence.

Health Effects

Intimate partner violence leads to significant morbidity and mortality and contributes to high health care costs. Victims of IPV experience similar problems as patients with general crisis or trauma (Box 45-1). Abused U.S. women show increased rates of poor general health, digestive problems, abdominal pain, urinary and vaginal infections, pelvic pain, sexual dysfunction, headache, and chronic pain (Campbell, 2002). In particular, these women suffer from gynecologic, central nervous system (CNS), and stress-related problems at an increased rate of 50% to 70% (Wathen and MacMillan, 2003). The largest difference between sexually abused and non–sexually abused women is in gynecologic complaints. In addition to direct harm caused by trauma, perinatal complications include low birth weight, antepartum

---

Box 45-1 Common Symptoms Associated with a Crisis or Trauma

Physical

General

Insomnia

Tremors

Profuse sweating

Chills

Loss of or increased sexual drive

Increased substance use or abuse

Gastrointestinal

Nausea

Vomiting

Upset stomach

Loss of or increased appetite

Cardiac

Racing heart/ palpitations

Chest discomfort

Neurologic

Headaches

Dizziness

Numbness, tingling

Acute or chronic pain

Thoughts

Recurring traumatic dreams or nightmares

Difficulty with memory, attention, concentration

Difficulty in making decisions

Obsessions or compulsions related to the trauma

Reconstructing events of crisis to master the trauma

Questioning spiritual or religious beliefs

Psychosis (extreme)

Suicidal ideation

Homicidal ideation

Feelings

Numbness, irritability, restlessness

Anhedonia

Fear, anxiety when reminded of traumatic event

Feeling sad, blue, depressed

Emotional outbursts and angry feelings

Hopelessness, helplessness

Behaviors

Overprotection of self and family

Easily startled

Isolation from others

Avoidance of activities associated with the event

Avoidance of places and people that trigger memories

Keeping busy to avoid thinking

Increase in conflict with family members

Agitation

Drug seeking

Suicidal behaviors

Acting out, violent behaviors

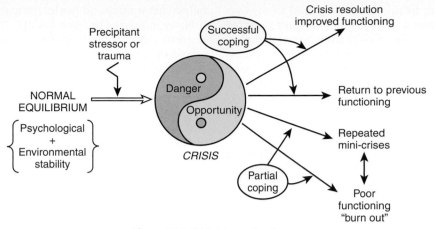

Figure 45-1 Crisis intervention theory.

hemorrhage, labor complications, preeclampsia, and mental health problems in the mother (Cherniak et al., 2005).

Children

Children are also adversely affected by exposure to IPV. Between 3.3 and 10 million children are exposed to IPV each year in the United States (Edelson, 1999). Exposure may be directly witnessing physical abuse, emotional abuse, or the sequelae of such abuse without viewing the violent acts. As a result of IVP, children may experience significant physical and behavioral symptoms acutely and throughout life, including somatic complaints, violence, substance abuse, and psychiatric illness (e.g., anxiety, depression, PTSD) (FVPF, 2009). When IPV is detected, the physician should decide if the children should be referred to child-focused mental health services. Furthermore, up to 60% of children exposed to IPV are themselves directly abused (Edelson, 1999). Physicians who detect IPV should be alert for child abuse and aware of mandatory reporting laws (see later Documentation and Reporting of IPV).

Evaluating the Crisis or Disaster

Key Points

A comprehensive evaluation of a crisis, trauma, or disaster includes assessment of the following:
- The normal equilibrium state
- The precipitant stressor or trauma
- The personal interpretation or meaning of the events
- The crisis state
- Preexisting personality or psychiatric conditions
- Selective past history
- System of social supports
- Effects on local society or community resources
- Special considerations for IPV (see later Key Points for IPV Approach).

Figure 45-1 presents an overview of a modern crisis intervention theory that is useful for the treatment of a crisis, IPV, or trauma.

Normal Equilibrium State and Stressors

Under normal circumstances, a person has a sense of internal psychological equilibrium and environmental support that generally permits activities of daily living (ADLs), working, and experiencing pleasure. A delicate balance among the person's internal wishes and fears, skills and capacities, and values and ideals determines psychological equilibrium. *Environmental equilibrium* refers to a stable balance among basic needs for food, water, shelter, physical comfort, and the integrity of community and social supports for job, family, religion, and society.

A patient in crisis enters an emotional storm after a stressor disturbs the normal equilibrium. Environmental precipitants typically seen in a family physician's office include IPV, sickness, and the stress of coping with death, divorce, marital separation, job loss, a financial crisis, and so forth. *Disasters* are acute environmental crises during which all concerned are focused on basic survival, acute medical care, and provisions of basic human needs. *Psychological stressors* may be related to events such as witnessing a trauma, surviving a disaster, loss of self-esteem, loss of love, a disturbing dream, sexual dysfunction, or sudden overwhelming fear, panic, or rage. *Developmental crises* such as latency, puberty, adolescence, marriage, birth of a child, midlife crisis, chronic medical illness, and retirement are common factors precipitating a crisis or may be comorbid factors.

Hobson and associates (1998) revised the Holmes and Rahe (1967) social readjustment scale. This newer scale lists 51 external life stressors that precipitate significant stress in most people. The top 20 items in this scale were in five separate domains: death and dying, health care issues, stress related to crime and criminal justice system, financial and economic issues, and family stresses. This scale includes events that range in severity from the most stressful being death of a spouse (rated as 1), divorce (7), experiencing domestic violence or sexual abuse (11), and surviving a disaster (16). It also includes events that many would consider positive yet stressful, such as getting married (32), experiencing a large monetary gain (42), and retirement (rated as 49). This list of stressors represents the most common precipitants causing a crisis. It is these types of stressors, and the internally disturbing feelings attached to the event, that produce emotional turmoil and a transient inability to adapt during the early stages of a crisis.

Most patients seeking treatment are surprised to discover that a major, unrecognized life stressor may have occurred on the same day or several days before the onset of the crisis. Less often, the stressor occurred sometime in the previous 6 weeks. Generally, events that occurred more than 6 weeks earlier are not acute stressors. Instead, these important past events may represent a previous crisis that was incompletely resolved and may be linked to the current crisis, as illustrated in Case Study 1.

Case Study 1

Melinda is a 42-year-old woman who presented to the office with insomnia, fear of public places, increased alcohol use, and irritability. Assisted by her physician's questions, Melinda realized that her symptoms had begun approximately 5 weeks ago, when she read about a violent local robbery in the newspaper. Since then, she felt anxious in public, coped by doing errands early in the morning, and began avoiding social interactions. Recently, she found it difficult to tolerate sex with her husband and unexpectedly felt emotionally distant from him. She began drinking alcohol so she could fall asleep and manage her anxiety. Her husband felt that she was "overreacting" to the robbery and expressed his concern about her escalating alcohol use. Nightmares returned of her experience in Hurricane Andrew 10 years earlier. She and a boyfriend stayed behind to protect their home, which was destroyed, and she witnessed a looter assaulting her friend. The couple broke up shortly thereafter, and she developed PTSD. A therapist helped Melinda move past the trauma and recover. She had been without symptoms for years.

Interpretation or Meaning of the Stressor

Whether a crisis is precipitated by an external life event or an internal psychological thought or feeling, each person interprets or adds meaning to the acute precipitant. For some people, like Melinda in Case Study 1, a local violent crime precipitated a major emotional crisis and a recurrence of her PTSD symptoms.

When listening for the precipitant of a crisis, it is important to understand the meaning of even minor stressors in the context of a patient's life. The robbery in Melinda's community had a personalized meaning to her that reawakened old wounds and PTSD symptoms, fueling a major emotional crisis. The following sequence of events, filtered through the lens of Melinda's select past personal experiences, created this current crisis. On learning of a local robbery, Melinda perceived a threat to her home and safety. This precipitant inundated her with traumatic memories of the hurricane and its aftereffects, which destroyed her home and her relationship. She felt anxious, insecure, and emotionally numb, and she was newly avoiding crowded places. The turmoil of her earlier relationship was being reenacted in her current marriage. Her nightmares interrupted her sleep, and she began using alcohol to fall asleep and quell her anxiety. Her alcohol abuse contributed to insomnia and feelings of numbness and intensified her anxiety. The violent robbery and her internal reactions and interpretation culminated in an acute crisis with recurrent PTSD symptoms, alcohol abuse, and marital discord.

Melinda presented to her physician unable to articulate her problem fully. As they discussed her symptoms and situation, Melinda realized that her current reaction was rooted in the seemingly unrelated events from her past. Her physician

helped her understand her interpretation of the local violent robbery in light of her past trauma. The patient realized that the reemergence of her PTSD symptoms was triggered by perceived threats to her current security. She could now better understand her reactions to her husband and acknowledge the pain and loss she suffered in the hurricane. Additionally, she recognized that her alcohol abuse was part of a maladaptive coping style. Based on her physician's input, Melinda was able to discontinue her alcohol use, felt more secure, and began efforts to reconnect with her husband.

Crisis State

The crisis state can be defined as a brief psychological upheaval, precipitated by a stressor, that produces an intense state of inner turmoil or disorganization that overwhelms a person's ability to cope and adapt. As with Melinda, the crisis state can be experienced as panic, disbelief, fear, confusion, sudden awareness of vulnerability, initial elation at having survived, or beginning of a grief reaction. For some, the crisis state may be denied or experienced as psychological numbing.

Often, patients in a crisis or suffering from a trauma present to their family physician with a confusing array of physical complaints. Patients like Melinda, who seek help while in an acute crisis, are typically impaired in some aspect of their daily interpersonal, work, social, or family life. Patients may have obvious psychological symptoms, unconscious psychological distress and pain associated with substance abuse, or physical symptoms. Four clusters of symptoms are typically experienced by patients during a crisis or secondary to a trauma (Box 45-1).

Case Study 2

Seth, an accountant and father of two, presented to his family physician at the urging of his wife. He complained of fatigue, difficulty concentrating, and anhedonia. His symptoms began the day of his son's 8th birthday party. He recalled inexplicably feeling a sense of dread and was near tears that day, despite having a good relationship with his son and looking forward to the party. His physician discovered that Seth's mother had died from a heart attack when Seth was 8 years old. Seth and his mother had been close; he remembered that she called him her "perfect little angel." After her death, Seth's family coped by telling him that he was too young to understand. His family avoided all conversations about his mother. He never fully mourned her. He maintained his attachment to his mother by his ambitious achievements and his perfectionism. His son's 8th birthday party reawakened Seth's unresolved maternal grief, sadness, and new symptoms of depression.

Typically, a patient in crisis such as Seth cannot explain what is upsetting him, although he is certainly aware that something is wrong. Seth's family physician asked, "Why now, at this point in time, are you depressed and feeling in crisis?" When asked, Seth felt distressed and confused. As he began to talk about his son and the birthday party, he realized that he was the same age as his son when his own mother died. He began to cry with the unresolved grief and the pride he imagined that she would have for him and her grandson.

Frequently, people in the crisis do not seek help by themselves and instead are brought in by concerned family members, lovers, friends, or perhaps the police or an ambulance. In these cases, it may take hours for the "Why now?" causes to be identified. Patients typically are not able to identify the specific cause of their crisis. Physician questioning and asking patients to retell their experience is typically how the "Why now?" of the crisis emerges. "Why now?" questioning is the first step in treating a crisis.

Acute Crisis Resolution and Adaptation to the Crisis (Within 6 Weeks)

For many patients, the acute nature of the crisis is often resolved within 6 weeks as the patient learns to cope or adapt to the acute stress. The DSM-IV-TR (APA, 2000) has classified the initial 1-month period of a crisis marked by impaired functioning as an "acute stress disorder." DSM IV-TR specifies that the acute symptom picture must last more than 2 days and no more than 4 weeks and must cause significant distress or impairment in social or occupational functioning. The result of the acute stages of the crisis is one of four possible outcomes specified in Figure 45-1. Successful coping and adaptation to a crisis can lead to crisis resolution that ultimately promotes growth and can even lead to improved functioning. For most patients, however, crisis resolution means a return to a previous level of baseline functioning. Still other patients only partially resolve the crisis and instead "seal over" and deny the significance of their feelings or recent events, setting the stage for a future crisis. Those with the worst prognosis typically have poor adaptation skills and, at best, stabilize at a lower level of daily functioning. For example, a patient who swallowed many pills after being left by her boyfriend may in retrospect deny any suicidal intent and instead say, "I just had a headache." This patient has sealed over her crisis. Denial of her suicidal intent and anger with her boyfriend will probably lead to poor adaptation and latent weakness, called a *missed* or *unresolved crisis*. The patient may continue to use unsuccessful coping strategies, such as drinking or repeated suicide gestures, as a way to deal with her feelings. Unresolved crises predispose the patient to future episodes that may be caused by even less stressful precipitants. For example, this same patient may once again become suicidal after a minor argument with a male friend. Fortunately, future crises can afford new opportunities to rework past unresolved crisis, with better adaptation and coping.

Sequelae of Crisis, Trauma, or Disaster (6 Weeks to Lifetime)

Although many patients completely recover from a crisis within 4 to 6 weeks, others may suffer with the sequelae of trauma or a crisis. The prognosis generally depends on three groups of factors: pretraumatic, traumatic, and posttraumatic risk factors (Ursano et al., 1995). *Pretraumatic* factors may include prior psychiatric illness, genetics, typical coping styles, gender, and culture. *Traumatic* risk factors relate to the type of trauma, severity and duration of the trauma, and seriousness of a physical injury. *Posttraumatic* risk factors involve coping styles, resources available for repair, individual or community response, capacity for problem solving, and adaptation. In general, recovery is more likely if the crisis is not too severe and is short in duration. If the crisis is prolonged or totally devastating to the fabric of a community (as with a hurricane or earthquake), the resources available for repair and the coping strategies used are the best predictors of outcome.

When dealing with a patient who has been in a crisis or suffered a trauma, it is important for the family physician to assess for associated trauma-related conditions. This assessment begins with attention to physical illness or psychosomatic complaints, then focuses on basic health care needs (food, warmth, shelter, clean drinking water, good sanitation). From a psychiatric standpoint, the family physician must remember that it is normal to have symptoms of trauma after a crisis event. Most patients' symptoms will wane gradually or resolve spontaneously and may not require psychological treatment. At 1 year, however, 30% to 40% of those exposed to a disaster will show lingering evidence of psychiatric morbidity (Raphael, 1986). For example, 1 year after being involved in a car crash, about 25% of patients will show signs of a psychiatric disorder, and 11% will go on to develop PTSD (Mayou et al., 1993). Table 45-1 summarizes the spectrum of psychiatric disorders that can occur in the wake of a crisis or trauma.

Previous Psychiatric Illness or Personality Disorder

For many people, there is little correlation between a previous psychiatric illness or personality disorder and their capacity to cope or adapt to an acute crisis or trauma. A person with schizophrenia may be just as capable of handling an acute crisis as others who do not have psychiatric disorders. How well a person handles an acute crisis or trauma depends primarily on the variables discussed earlier, including the precipitant, the meaning of the events, the crisis situation itself, the patient's coping skills and styles, and the effectiveness of the patient's support network.

However, there are many cases in which a preexisting psychiatric disorder or an unresolved trauma or crisis may influence the development of a new crisis. Consider the case of a mentally retarded boy who becomes severely violent because his mother ran out of his favorite breakfast cereal. This change would be a minor stressor for most people, but for this boy, disruption of his daily breakfast food and routine are perceived as catastrophic. His low IQ and lack of verbal skills, related to his mental retardation, predispose him to a crisis involving violence because he lacks the ability to consider other options. Patients with severe psychiatric illness or personality disorders, those with trauma-related disorders (see Table 45-1), and those who have rigid coping styles or poor adaptation skills all are at greater risk for future crisis.

Selective Past History

For an acute crisis, the patient's past history is relevant only as it can help explain and resolve the current crisis. Many patients, wanting to avoid the pain of the current crisis, may unconsciously lead the family physician "down the garden path" to chronic problems, avoiding the pain of the current issues. To avoid the past history trap, the physician must try to understand the dynamics of the current crisis and then look for similar events in the patient's past that can be used to understand more about the current situation. For example, a selective past history of suicide attempts and the circumstances surrounding those attempts may provide valuable clues to understanding a current suicidal crisis. This selective history can assist in developing an understanding of the "Why now?" of the current suicide attempt.

Table 45-1 Psychiatric Disorders Related to Trauma or Crisis

Diagnosis	Diagnostic Criteria* and Symptom Picture	Onset/Duration
Adjustment disorder	Emotional, behavioral symptoms in response to identifiable stressor(s) Distress in excess of what would be expected from exposure to stressor Symptoms create marked distress or impairment in social or occupational functioning Does not represent bereavement	Begins within 3 mo of onset of stressor Symptoms usually resolve within 6 mo of termination of stressor.
Acute stress disorder	Exposure to traumatic event that involved actual or threatened death or threat of serious injury to self or others Response to threat—intense fear, helplessness, or horror Marked avoidance of stimuli associated with the trauma (including thoughts, places, conversations) Dissociative symptoms (e.g., numbing, detachment, feeling dazed, depersonalization, derealization, dissociative amnesia) Trauma reexperienced through flashbacks, distressing recollections, dreams, sense of reliving, or psychological-physiologic reactions when exposed to cues that represent the trauma Symptoms of increased arousal, exaggerated startle response, hypervigilance, motor restlessness, or anxiety Clinically significant impairment in social or occupational functioning Not merely an exaggeration of existing psychiatric condition	Lasts minimum of 2 days and maximum of 4 wk†
PTSD	Same as for acute stress disorder, with three possible time courses: acute, chronic, or delayed	Acute: 1-3 mo Chronic: >3 mo Delayed: >6 mo
Major depressive disorder	Must have depressed mood or loss of interest or pleasure In addition to above, 5 of following 9 symptoms present for at least 2 weeks: depressed mood most of day, anhedonia, weight loss or gain, insomnia or hypersomnia, agitation or motor retardation, fatigue, feelings of worthlessness or excessive guilt, poor or decreased concentration, and recurrent thoughts of suicide or death Symptoms represent change from previous functioning Causes distress or social or occupational impairment	Onset common 6-12 mo after crisis or disaster Symptoms present for most of day, nearly every day, for 2 wk
Substance use or abuse	Numbing substances (e.g., alcohol, heroin, marijuana) and sedative-hypnotic abuse usually preferred	Most common 6-12 mo after crisis
Dissociative disorders	Dissociative amnesia, dissociative fugue, dissociative identity disorder (formerly multiple personality disorder), depersonalization disorder Disturbance consists of one or more episodes of inability to recall important personal information, usually of traumatic nature	Sequelae of enduring chronic trauma, abuse, or neglect
Generalized anxiety disorder	Persistent symptoms of excessive anxiety or worry for at least 6 mo Also associated with restlessness, being easily fatigued, poor concentration, irritability, and sleep disturbances Free-floating anxiety unrelated to specific person(s) or situation	Any time after trauma
Panic disorder (with or without agoraphobia)	Recurrent, unexpected panic attacks, defined as episodic periods of intense anxiety, often with physical symptoms (e.g., palpitations, tremors, chest discomfort) Symptoms develop abruptly, increase in intensity over 10 min Persistent concerns about having additional attacks Anxiety, worry about implications or consequences of attack (e.g., heart attack, losing control)	Any time after trauma
Specific phobia, social phobia (social anxiety disorder)	Specific phobias: excessive or unreasonable fear of specific objects or situations (e.g., animals, heights, needles), which provokes immediate anxiety response Patient avoids feared situation or object. Social phobias: fear of social or performance situations in which patient fears possible excessive scrutiny by others Patient constantly worried about acting in humiliating or embarrassing way.	Any time after trauma

Modified from American Psychiatric Association. Diagnostic and Statistical Manual of Mental Disorders, 4th ed, text revision. Washington, DC, APA, 2000.
*DSM-IV-TR abridged criteria, 2000.
†More than 4 weeks; see criteria for posttraumatic stress disorder (PTSD).

Continued

Table 45-1 Psychiatric Disorders Related to Trauma or Crisis—cont'd

Diagnosis	Diagnostic Criteria* and Symptom Picture	Onset/Duration
Brief psychosis	Presence of one or more: hallucinations, delusions, disorganized speech, and disorganized or catatonic behavior Eventual full return to premorbid level of functioning	At least 1 day to <1 mo
Somatization disorder	Unexplained physical symptoms (e.g., pain, gastrointestinal, sexual, neurologic) Symptoms begin before age 30 and occur over several years. Symptoms are not intentionally produced or feigned.	Any time after trauma
Conversion disorder	One or more symptoms affecting motor or sensory function suggest neurologic or general medical condition. Initiation or exacerbation of symptoms often is preceded by conflicts or stressors. Symptoms are not intentionally produced or feigned.	Any time after trauma

Additional events from the past history that might be helpful in understanding a suicide attempt include deaths, separations, severe medical illnesses, and a history of depression, alcoholism, or family suicide. Selective past history that could be relevant for understanding an acute violent crisis might be the timing and circumstances of past episodes of violence, childhood experiences of abuse or neglect, previous hospitalizations for violence, prior incarcerations, past legal problems, and past neurologic or medical illness.

When dealing with trauma victims, it is important to ask about past trauma, previous successful coping styles or adaptations, and cultural and religious beliefs, because this information can help promote recovery. The less severe the current traumatic event, the more critical are predisaster variables, such as neuroticism or history of a psychiatric illness.

Social Systems

Everyone lives within a network of social interaction, social support, and community and national resources. Most of our daily social interactions are with family, friends, and work colleagues. These daily social interactions are made possible by the community supports that enable a person to obtain clean water, adequate sanitation, housing, food, clothing, work, education, finances, and medical care. Community structures are generally made possible because of the support of the country or nation. National resources support the entire infrastructure of the civilization, from roads to a monetary system to constitutional protections. In general, stable social systems at different levels tend to provide the greatest buffers against crises or disasters of all types. A patient's social system can be represented by an ecological map (see Case Study 3 and review Figure 45-3).

Often, a patient goes into a crisis because the immediate social environment is threatened or disrupted by such issues as divorce, a dysfunctional family, drug abuse, unemployment, or an eviction notice. Relative damage to a local support network can have profoundly varied effects on a patient. For example, the death of a spouse produces a more severe crisis if the deceased was also the sole financial provider. Even a minor disturbance in a small or dysfunctional support network can produce a major crisis. For example, an elderly woman who is housebound and without family, friends, or a telephone can experience a major crisis when her home health aide misses a scheduled visit.

When assessing the local support network of a patient, a family physician should consider whether the patient's network is interested, available, and competent to help. Some networks are helpful and should be included, whereas other networks may be harmful to the patient. This determination may be especially complicated in IPV cases where a marital separation is necessary but results in the woman needing to face financial stresses, loss of her home, and the loss of her social network. When a patient is in a crisis, the family physician can help the patient choose and mobilize the most helpful people in the patient's immediate support network and exclude others. Such helpful mobilizations may include calling in a specific family member, speaking to a supportive boss, helping the patient retain an attorney, establishing health care, or obtaining Medicaid.

In general, social disruptions at the local level of support (e.g., job loss) are less damaging than community level disruptions (e.g., tsunami). National disruptions such as wars or earthquakes in poor countries cause a devastation from which many never recover. Disasters are long-lasting when the needed resources remain greater than the available resources. During a disaster, the social structure of a society can be damaged to such an extent that the existence and functioning of the entire community or nation are threatened (Eranen and Liebkind, 1993). This is the experience of Hurricane Katrina in 2005 and the earthquake in Haiti in 2010. Disasters of this magnitude require local, state, national, and even international support if there is to be a chance of restoring the social integrity of the community to the predisaster level of functioning.

Crisis Intervention Treatment in the Office Setting

Basic Approach

Key Points

- Develop a timeline of events starting with the "Why now?" and work from the initial presentation backward in time.
- Focus on acute risk assessment, including risk of suicide, violence, and acute medical conditions.

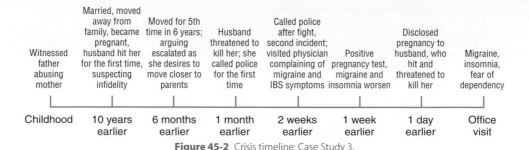

Figure 45-2 Crisis timeline: Case Study 3.

- Develop an eco-map or support network map, beginning with a three-generational genogram and other psychosocial supports.
- Select a single problem or symptom to begin crisis treatment.
- Build a wheel-and-spoke treatment plan with the single problem or symptom in the center and biopsychosociocultural factors as spokes.
- Treat the problem or symptoms by fostering the use of adaptive coping skills.
- Use a crisis resolution strategy.
- Use psychiatric medication, as needed, for symptom relief.

The focus of a crisis assessment involves the evaluation of the precipitants of the crisis or trauma, personal meaning of the events, crisis state itself, selective past history, support network, and current psychiatric illness, if relevant. These assessments are subsequently used to help formulate the causes of the crisis, so that if necessary, specific crisis intervention treatment and problem-solving approaches can be implemented.

A tailored crisis intervention treatment is typically one to five sessions, offered on a voluntary basis. The treatment is specifically geared toward helping the patient survive and cope with the acute biopsychosocial or cultural effects from the crisis. The time required for each session depends on the complexity of the case and the practitioner's skill. A family physician can begin the crisis assessment and treatment by exploring the "Why now?" or acute precipitant of the crisis. This inquiry can be followed by detective-style questioning designed to uncover the specific chronology and sequence of events, feelings, thoughts, and behaviors that led to the development of the acute crisis. Patients seeking help should be encouraged to tell the details of their traumatic experiences.

Helping the patient to describe the stressors and evolution of the acute problem may offer clues to problem-solving approaches to crisis resolution. Crises or disasters involving the lack of food, clothing, shelter, poor sanitation, or inadequate medical care should be given first priority. Crises involving violence, suicide, or a life-threatening medical illness have secondary priority and should become the focus of the crisis treatment. Crises in everyday life can be treated according to the patient's preferences.

Crisis treatment focuses on the dynamic interplay of events from the most recent precipitants and days, the previous 6 weeks, and selective elements from the patient's past history. Important tools and approaches that can guide a crisis formulation and treatment are the timeline, ecologic (eco) map/support network tool, wheel-and-spoke formulation, symptom-oriented treatment, and assessment and development of more adaptive coping styles. All these components can be used for the development of a general crisis resolution strategy.

Timeline

A timeline is a pictorial representation of the immediate, recent, and selective events from the past history contributing to the current crisis. A family physician can build a timeline while interviewing the patient. The physician asks the patient to discuss the immediate events and precipitants of the crisis on the day of the office visit or events from the past week. Together, the physician and the patient reconstruct the history by working backward over the previous 6 weeks. Finally, the physician tries to elicit the selective past history that may relate to the current crisis. Use of the timeline is illustrated in Case Study 3 (Fig. 45-2).

Developing a timeline with a patient helps both physician and patient focus on recent events and begins the process of formulating treatment. As illustrated in Figure 45-2, for

Case Study 3

Denise is a 30-year-old woman living with her husband and 10-year-old son. She presented to her family physician complaining of severe migraines and insomnia over the past week after having a positive home pregnancy test. She feared that having another child would make her permanently dependent on her husband. The couple met while she was a college student living with her parents. They married within weeks and moved frequently because of his jobs. She lost weight with each move and was eventually diagnosed with irritable bowel syndrome (IBS). He managed their finances and believed that women should not work outside the home. She was so afraid of him that she quickly abandoned her secret plans to become a teacher. When she was 7 months pregnant, her husband saw her talking with a male neighbor and accused her of infidelity. He then hit her for the first time.

Denise witnessed her alcoholic father physically abusing her mother throughout her childhood. Her father favored her brothers and spared them any abuse, while verbally and emotionally abusing her and her mother. When Denise left home, she and her mother remained close allies and maintained a lifelong bond. Denise's relationship with her father continued to be strained.

Since moving to the area 6 months ago, Denise and her husband argued daily about finances and her desire to move closer to her parents. One month ago, he threatened to kill her and their child. She had called the police twice in the past month, but she never pressed charges. In the past 6 months she had visited her physician 10 times, with various complaints (headaches, IBS, emotional symptoms). Ultimately, her physical injuries alerted the physician to abuse. He had asked about domestic violence during past visits, but she disclosed nothing. When she told her husband of the pregnancy, he became enraged, blamed her for getting pregnant, and hit her in the face and belly while threatening to kill her. During her appointment the next day, she was tearful and scared. Her physician asked her again if she was safe and when she said "no," they were able to discuss the beatings.

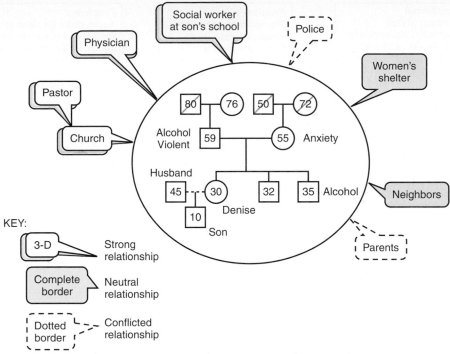

Figure 45-3 Eco-map (ecologic support network): Case Study 3.

Denise, her crisis was both becoming pregnant and being assaulted and threatened by her husband. During the office visit, her physician helped her build her timeline. Denise was able to recognize how her migraines and IBS were related to her growing anger at her husband for controlling and isolating her. The timeline highlighted the pattern of her husband's escalating abuse and how this endangered her and her pregnancy. This awareness enabled her to accept her physician's help. They developed a safety plan to move her and her child into a shelter for battered pregnant women.

Ecological Map

An ecological map (eco-map) is a pictorial representation of the patient's entire support network. Included in this eco-map are a genogram and the immediate support network. This map should include the patient's current family, the family of origin for three generations, and all the people and community resources in the patient's immediate living environment (e.g., family, neighbors, law enforcement, physician, church, social services agencies). An eco-map can be used by a family physician to help decide who can help the patient, who needs to be excluded, or what social, religious, legal, or economic resources need to be mobilized to assist the patient in crisis.

Using Case Study 3, Denise's eco-map is illustrated in Figure 45-3. Her physician, church, social worker from her son's school, a local shelter, and neighbors might be called on to assist her during this crisis. Her parents and the local police could also be important for her immediate safety. The decisions about which support elements to use should be negotiated with the patient. Denise and her physician decided that the safety plan would utilize church members to get her child to her at the local women's shelter. While there, she began talks with her parents about moving in with them.

Selecting the Problem or Symptom

Because most crises present with a number of problems and symptoms simultaneously, it is important to select the starting point of the treatment. Immediate survival and safety issues are almost always first priority. Preventing IPV, homicide, suicide risk, or acute medical emergency, or providing for food or shelter, must supersede all other concerns as was the case for Denise. Less severe problems or symptoms can be handled according to the patient's preferences.

Wheel-and-Spoke Formulation of the Crisis

The wheel-and-spoke format is a useful tool to help develop a formulation that specifies the causes of the crisis and can assist in the development of an effective, prioritized treatment plan. The acute crisis should be pictured as the center of a wheel. The spokes of the wheel are the problems or symptoms that are likely causing or contributing to the crisis. The physician can establish a numbered priority list for problem solving. For each problem listed, the family physician recommends a specific evaluation, test, or treatment approach designed to ameliorate the crisis. An application of the wheel-and-spoke diagram for Denise's case is illustrated in Figure 45-4.

Problem-Focused or Symptom-Oriented Treatment

Once the physician has formulated the case using the timeline and eco-map and developed a wheel-and-spoke treatment plan, the problem-focused or symptom-oriented crisis treatment can begin. A family practitioner may use educational, psychotherapeutic, or supportive approaches with or without medications. The cornerstone approaches to crisis treatment are fostering coping skills and adaptive problem

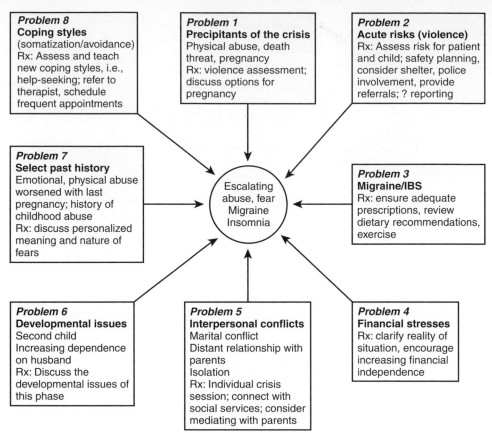

Problem 8
Coping styles
(somatization/avoidance)
Rx: Assess and teach
new coping styles, i.e.,
help-seeking; refer to
therapist, schedule
frequent appointments

Problem 1
Precipitants of the crisis
Physical abuse, death
threat, pregnancy
Rx: violence assessment;
discuss options for
pregnancy

Problem 2
Acute risks (violence)
Rx: Assess risk for patient
and child; safety planning,
consider shelter, police
involvement, provide
referrals; ? reporting

Problem 7
Select past history
Emotional, physical abuse
worsened with last
pregnancy; history of
childhood abuse
Rx: discuss personalized
meaning and nature of
fears

Escalating
abuse, fear
Migraine
Insomnia

Problem 3
Migraine/IBS
Rx: ensure adequate
prescriptions, review
dietary recommendations,
exercise

Problem 6
Developmental issues
Second child
Increasing dependence
on husband
Rx: Discuss the
developmental issues of
this phase

Problem 5
Interpersonal conflicts
Marital conflict
Distant relationship with
parents
Isolation
Rx: Individual crisis
session; connect with
social services; consider
mediating with parents

Problem 4
Financial stresses
Rx: clarify reality of
situation, encourage
increasing financial
independence

Figure 45-4 Wheel-and-spoke crisis formulation and treatment plan: Case Study 3.

solving, using a crisis resolution strategy. Medications may be necessary for symptom relief or as part of the treatment approach to a major psychiatric illness. In IPV cases, safety planning is of paramount importance (see Box 45-3).

Coping Skills and Adaptive Problem Solving

Fortunately, most people will find new ways to handle or cope with a crisis. Coping styles are the unique ways that patients deal with stress. For example, some cope with a stressful crisis by analyzing it, asking others for help, or gathering additional information. Some coping styles work better in certain situations than others. Box 45-2 lists some typical adaptive coping styles that can be suggested to patients, as well as pathologic coping styles that should be avoided whenever possible. Crisis resolution can be promoted by evaluating a patient's coping style and, when necessary, suggesting an alternative or more adaptive coping style. These new skills facilitate a patient's adaptation to the stressful life circumstances. In general, those who can flexibly use many coping styles are the most successful at crisis resolution and problem solving. Often, patients in crisis rely too heavily on one coping style, which may not be the most adaptive for a particular situation. Those patients who lack the capacity to develop new, more adaptive coping styles may become dysfunctional when confronted with a crisis.

To illustrate coping styles and new coping skills, review Case Study 3. Denise copes with threats of violence, isolation, and being controlled by her husband by keeping quiet and submitting to her husband's demands. This is patterned

after the relationship with her father. After her physician discussed her somatic and avoidant coping style, he suggested that she could use his help and talk openly and directly about her safety concerns and needs. Denise's use of a new help-seeking and informational style enabled her to develop a safety plan, prepare to leave her home, and utilize church members to help get her child to a local shelter for battered women. She also was able to tell her parents about her fears and ask for their support and help.

Crisis Resolution Strategy

In addition to teaching coping styles and coping skills, a family physician can also provide a patient with general strategies for crisis resolution and provide specific strategies that are necessary in the special case of IPV. A crisis resolution strategy, based on the crisis principles, is composed of 18 steps (Box 45-3). The family physician may need to walk through some or all of these steps with the patient first before encouraging the patient to attempt some steps as a self-help strategy for the future.

Intimate Partner Violence Approach

Key Points

- Universal screening for IPV is controversial but recommended by several professional organizations.
- Screening and referral of IPV patients are often the primary interventions in family medicine settings.

Box 45-2 Coping Styles

Adaptive coping styles

Intuitive: Using imagination, feelings, and perceptions to solve a problem

Logical, rational: Carefully reasoned, logical, deductive style

Trial and error: Trying a random solution; if it fails, modifying it and trying again

Help seeking: Gathering information, then proceeding

Wait and see: Allowing time or circumstance to determine the outcome

Action oriented: Taking action to rectify the problem immediately

Contemplative: Quietly thinking over the problem before acting

Spiritual: Asking for God's direction

Emotional: Using emotions such as tears, anger, or fear to help solve problem

Controlling: Controlling people or oneself to gain power to solve problem

Manipulative: Using various manipulative styles to resolve crisis

Pathologic coping styles

Deceptive, antisocial: Use of dishonesty, lying, cheating, or stealing to resolve crisis

Suicidal: Using threat of suicide or suicide attempts to coerce someone or to solve problem

Violent: Using threat or actual violence to establish control and solve problem

Avoidance, denial: Failure to confront or acknowledge problems

Somatization: Displaying physical symptoms as a method of expressing emotions

Impulsive: Unpredictable or impulsive responses without anticipation of possible outcomes

Random, chaotic: Nonproductive and extreme form of trial and error and impulsive style; often seen in prolonged psychotic states

- Evidence shows the efficacy of legal interventions and batterer's treatment.
- Safety and safety planning are critical, regardless of stage of abuse.

General Recommendations

Intimate partner violence can be a sensitive issue, and it may be difficult for physicians to inquire about IPV and for patients to disclose it. Physicians should use direct and nonjudgmental language, conduct the interview in private, maintain confidentiality, and when needed, use professional interpreters who do not know the patient (FVPF, 2004). However, confidentiality may not be absolute, because threats of violence and suicide risk must be disclosed to reporting authorities or others. Effective interventions are often based on empowerment of the abused person, allowing her to define her own goals, explore her own solutions, and arrive at her own understanding of the situation (Ramsay et al., 2009). An analysis of provider-patient communications in emergency departments demonstrated that disclosure of IPV is facilitated by open-ended questions, responding to psychosocial cues, and asking at least one follow-up question (Rhodes et al., 2007). However, disclosure of IPV is not the only goal of inquiry. Well-conducted interviews may help a victim, even if she does not disclose the abuse (Rhodes and Levinson, 2003).

Screening

Universal screening for IPV in primary care settings is controversial. Multiple major medical organizations recommend universal screening, including the American Association of Family Physicians (AAFP), despite the US Preventive Services Task Force (USPSTF) finding that there is "insufficient evidence to recommend for or against routine screening of women for IPV." Proponents believe that screening is widely acceptable to patients, and that the availability of reliable screeners, the opportunity for intervention in identified victims, and the high prevalence and costs of IPV are good reasons for universal screening (MacMillan et al., 2009). Evidence overall is equivocal for the efficacy of advocacy interventions (Cochrane review; Ramsay, 2009).

Although evidence does not support universal screening, many physicians may still want to screen their patients. When using routine screening, begin with framing questions: "As violence is a major factor in people's lives, I have begun to inquire about this with every patient"; or, "I am concerned that some of your symptoms may be a result of someone hurting you." This should be followed with direct questions that focus on behavior: "Has someone physically harmed you: hit, slapped, kicked, or thrown something at you? Threatened you? Forced you to have sex when you did not want to? Do you feel controlled or isolated by your partner?" Several empirically validated screening tools focus on physical abuse by an intimate partner. The SAFE questions screen for nonphysical aspects of abuse provides a logical framework for interventions: The physician can inquire about stress and safety in patient's relationships (S), if the patient feels afraid or abused (A), awareness and support of friends and family (F), and emergency plans (E) (Neufeld, 1996).

Treatment of Intimate Batterers

An abusing partner may also present to the family physician's office and directly or indirectly disclose the violence. These perpetrators may portray themselves as the victim, may ask the physician for referrals to couples counseling or anger management, or present their situation as one of mutual conflict (Rhodes and Levinson, 2003). When domestic abuse is disclosed by the perpetrator, the physician should conduct a violence risk assessment. The physician may have a duty to warn or protect the threatened person, depending on state laws. As is clinically helpful, the physician may alternatively want to educate the patient regarding the effects of violence on the family or ask the patient to be responsible for his actions and seek treatment. Unfortunately, batterer's treatment only produces a marginal overall effect on recidivism rates (Babcock et al., 2004).

Optimal legal interventions for IPV are similarly unclear. Based on early studies, arrest has been shown to have variable outcomes on recidivism rates, despite widespread popularity. Orders of protection are another option for legal intervention, but also leading to mixed results. In one study, permanent protective orders lasting 12 months led to a significant decrease in reports of physical violence, whereas temporary orders actually led to an increase in psychological abuse (Wathen and MacMillan, 2003). Because of the lack of clearly efficacious interventions for intimate batterers, a prudent clinician will need to use his best judgment based on a thorough safety assessment and in accordance with local and state laws.

Box 45-3 Crisis Resolution Strategy

Assess safety. If a patient is in acute danger due to violence, suicide risk, or acute medical problems, more help may be required. Contact medical providers, law enforcement, or other resources as indicated.

In cases of intimate partner violence (IPV), use specific strategies for assessment, safety planning, and documentation (see Box 45-4).

1. Teach the patient to recognize the early warning signs of a crisis, which typically includes anxiety or depressive symptoms, occasional panic symptoms, feelings of being overwhelmed, sense of urgency, vigilance, confusion, disorganization, intrusive thoughts, flashbacks, nightmares, self-defeating actions, and suicidal or homicidal feelings.

2. Set the patient's expectations for recovery.

3. Inform the patient that after an acute event, most acute life crises take approximately 6 weeks to subside, stabilize, or resolve.

4. Normalize the patient's symptoms. Patients need to know that, after an acute crisis or trauma, somatic and psychiatric symptoms, and atypical daily routines (e.g., not going to work), are common and are part of normal, healthy coping.

5. It is important for patients to know that if problems and symptoms do not resolve after 6 weeks, they should obtain further evaluation and treatment, as necessary.

6. If desired, the patient can talk over the crisis with the family physician or a trusted friend. It is often best if these friends or family members are not directly involved in the crisis. For prevention or early intervention for the next crisis, the physician can assist the patient in developing a list of contacts of available friends, other physicians or specialists, and available community resources.

7. If a patient is overwhelmed with emotion, is coping poorly, or has a dysfunctional daily routine (beyond typical posttraumatic reaction), the patient may benefit by sharing painful feelings or discussing recurrent or intrusive thoughts, which may provide some immediate relief.

8. Identify the specific symptoms, problems, and area of the patient's functioning that is most affected by the crisis (e.g., work, home, interpersonal, economic).

9. Identify the specific precipitants, other stressors, and symptoms (e.g., insomnia) that are currently contributing to the crisis. This can be done by helping the patient develop a timeline (see Fig. 45-2).

10. Evaluate the support system by use of an ecological map (see Fig. 45-3). Using this support network tool, patients can be assisted in discovering who can help and who might exacerbate the situation.

11. Select the problem(s) or symptom(s) to treat first. This can be the most difficult part, because it requires an understanding or formulation of the causes of the crisis to prioritize what problem or symptom to treat first.

12. Use a wheel-and-spoke format to develop the treatment plan for a core crisis and prioritize the order of problems or symptoms that need to be treated (see Fig. 45-4).

13. Teach the patient to understand his or her current coping style and why and how it may not be working. Introduce other, more adaptive coping styles (see Box 45-2).

14. Obtain additional information from others who may be able to assist with crisis resolution. This should only be done once the crisis has been formulated and the focus of the treatment chosen.

15. Make a specific plan for crisis resolution based on additional information, newly discovered feelings, a crisis formulation, and treatment focus. This plan should involve the use of novel coping styles, a specific sequence of actions, and psychopharmacology, as clinically appropriate (see Box 45-4).

16. The patient should implement the plan. Initially, it may be less overwhelming to resolve one cause of the crisis at a time, instead of trying to handle many problems simultaneously.

17. Assess the results. Has the problem been resolved? If yes, go to step 1 and tackle a new symptom or problem. If not, go to step 18.

18. If the initial plan has not helped, try again, obtain additional help, or consult with a psychiatrist or other professional.

Couples

If the victim and the violent partner are both patients of the same family physician, this will present unique challenges. An American Medical Association consensus statement advises that this dual relationship is not a conflict of interest, but that each patient should be handled independently (Ferris et al., 1997). Confidentiality must be maintained unless the victim has given consent. Couples counseling is generally contraindicated, especially when violence is ongoing. Family physicians may have neither the time nor the training to address this complex situation; couples who are safe and desire counseling should generally be referred to appropriate mental health professionals.

Safety Planning

Safety planning is a key intervention for victims of IPV. Planning between the physician and patient helps to send the message that IPV is serious. The patient needs to hear that IVP will typically continue without an intervention, and that IVP can be life threatening and may require immediate action. This message can help reduce the patient's sense of isolation and despair, and is especially helpful for patients who are not yet ready to make or implement a safety plan on their own. Safety planning is important regardless of whether a victim is in the midst of a violent incident, planning to leave, or living apart from her abuser. Safety planning should include gathering all essential documents, setting aside required finances, developing packing lists, developing child care plans, having a list of emergency numbers, and having shelter contact information (Box 45-4).

Documentation and Reporting

Documentation of cases of known or suspected IPV should include the patient's report, the physician's assessment and examination, interventions, and follow-up plans. Photographic evidence, body maps, and a clear discussion of the relationships between abuse and medical problems may also be prudent (FVPF, 2004). These practices may serve as both medicolegal necessity and advocacy measure for patients who may take legal action against the perpetrator.

A physician should have a basic understanding of local reporting laws. Mandatory reporting of intimate partner violence varies from state to state and may depend on type of injury, if a weapon was used and which type, if rape occurred, or other criminal conduct occurred. Cases that involve child abuse must also be reported. When children have not been directly abused, state laws vary as to what is a reportable IPV offense. Physicians have discretion in these cases and may be required to do a careful assessment of imminent risk and

---

Box 45-4 Intimate Partner Violence (IPV) Safety Planning

During a violent incident

Know where to go.

Know how to get there.

Have keys and a packed bag ready.

Move to a room with an exit.

Avoid bathroom, kitchen, and other areas with access to dangerous items that could be used as weapons.

Train children to call police/911.

Use judgment and stay safe.

Alert police and/or trusted friend or family once safe.

Planning to leave

Pack and keep hidden or with a friend:

1. Copies of important documents: legal documents, birth certificates, school and medical records, insurance information, financial records (deeds, mortgages)
2. Money and bank account numbers
3. Keys to house, car, safety deposit box
4. Personal items for self and children (e.g., medications, clothing)
5. List of important contact information. Cell phone use is risky because it may reveal details about your location and people with you.

Living apart from abuser

Neighbors, friends, and someone at work should know about the situation, including how and when to call the police.

Inform school and child care providers if a partner is not allowed to pick up the children.

Consider additional safeguards at the residence, including extra locks or alarm systems.

Consider seeking a protection (restraining) order.

---

benefits of reporting. In IPV cases that do not require mandatory reporting and do not involve children, the physician should be prepared to help victims make decisions about their use of the legal system.

KEY TREATMENT

Patients in IPV situations should be treated individually, not as a couple, and children should be referred to child focus treatments as needed (SOR: C).

Safety planning is recommended if IPV is detected (AMA; Ferris et al., 1997) (SOR: B).

Referrals and resource information should be provided for every patient (AMA; Ferris et al., 1997) (SOR: B).

Other Trauma Treatments

Patients in an acute crisis or with disaster-related trauma may or may not require treatment. Crisis treatment is often necessary if the patient is suicidal or at risk for violence, has an acute medical emergency, or has a major psychiatric disorder (psychosis, PTSD, bipolar disorder, depression, overwhelming anxiety). All treatment is best when it is offered voluntarily or upon patient request.

Psychological treatment of trauma should be offered immediately, with the patient allowed to pursue treatment

voluntarily. Treatment should be vigorously pursued and possibly mandated if a major, life-threatening psychiatric illness appears acutely (APA, 2004; NICE, 2005).

No acute psychiatric treatment is often the best course of action if symptoms and non-life-threatening problems are resolving and if social and occupational functioning have remained intact over the first 6 weeks. Evidence indicates that mandatory crisis intervention in non-life-threatening circumstances, often called *critical incident stress management* (CISM), or "debriefing" (Mitchell et al., 1983), is not helpful (Rose et al., 2004). Patients who have experienced a mass trauma or disaster may benefit from "psychological first aid" (Bisson et al., 2007). This approach fosters safety, calmness, self and community efficacy, social connectedness, and optimism. The best personnel to deliver this treatment remains controversial (clinician responder or emergency responder with community leader?) (Watson, 2007).

Exposure-based cognitive-behavioral therapy (CBT) is recommended for patients with PTSD (Bradley et al., 2005). CBT includes reexposure to past trauma through imagined, in vivo, directed therapeutic, written, verbal, or taped narrative. In addition, psychoeducation, breathing and relaxation training, and homework are often included (APA, 2004; Benedek et al., 2009; NICE, 2005).

KEY TREATMENT

Crisis intervention and psychotherapeutic techniques are a first-line approach for a crisis or mass trauma (Bradley et al., 2005; NICE, 2005) (SOR: A).

Exposure-based CBT is recommended for patients with PTSD (Bradley et al., 2005) (SOR: A).

Psychoeducation, breathing and relaxation training, and homework can be helpful for PTSD (APA, 2004; Benedek et al., 2009; NICE, 2005) (SOR: B).

Psychological intervention is helpful after mass trauma or disaster if offered on a voluntary basis (Bisson, 2007) (SOR: B).

Mandatory critical incident stress management (CISM, debriefing) is not helpful (Rose et al., 2004) (SOR: C).

Medications for Symptoms of Psychiatric Disorders

Although psychotherapeutic techniques are a first-line approach for a crisis or mass trauma (Bradley et al., 2005; NICE, 2005), use of medications for treatment of specific symptoms or psychiatric disorders can also be helpful. In general, pharmacology targeting symptom reduction parallels the pharmacology of the treatment for the major psychiatric disorders. For example, if a patient has an isolated sleep disturbance, use of the newer hypnotics is warranted. Similarly, for depressive or psychotic symptoms, antidepressants or antipsychotics can be used. This symptom-oriented approach has not been well studied.

During the acute crisis or immediate posttraumatic state, insomnia or other sleep disturbances may greatly affect coping. Use of a nonbenzodiazepine such as zolpidem, zaleplon, or eszopiclone can be considered as first-line pharmacologic treatment for acute sleep disturbances. The use of benzodiazepines for sleep or anxiety in the acute postcrisis state is questionable, with little support for efficacy and concerns that benzodiazepines may inhibit effective coping. Benzodiazepines also carry the risk of dependence and addiction. Although data are sparse regarding the effectiveness, trazodone is also often used clinically for chronic sleep difficulties because it carries no risk of dependence.

Thus far, no known interventions have prevented PTSD. For the primary treatment of PTSD, medications include selective serotonin reuptake inhibitors (SSRIs), prazosin, propranolol, and antiepileptics. PTSD symptoms, including reexperiencing the trauma, avoidance, numbing, and hyperarousal, are effectively treated with SSRIs, including sertraline, paroxetine, venlafaxine, and fluoxetine (APA, 2004; Benedek et al., 2009; Stein et al., 2006).

A distinction between non-combat-related and combat-related PSTD is warranted when considering pharmacologic therapy (Benedek et al., 2009). Non-combat-related PTSD includes civilian trauma, childhood or adult sexual assault, IPV, interpersonal trauma, or trauma caused by a motor vehicle crash. For non-combat-related PTSD, sertraline, paroxetine, fluoxetine, and venlafaxine are effective in short-term trials. These SSRIs either can be a primary form of treatment, if the patient does not want exposure-based CBT, or can be combined with CBT; no evidence yet shows that combined treatment is superior to SSRI or CBT alone. The efficacy of the antidepressant mirtazapine and the anticonvulsants topiramate and tiagabine is equivocal but reportedly somewhat beneficial (Benedek et al., 2009). No efficacy for beta blockers or bupropion has been established.

The results for pharmacologic treatment of combat-related trauma are less convincing. It seems that younger veterans with PTSD from more recent wars are responsive to the same SSRIs and SNRIs as non-combat-related patients. However, older veterans from previous wars do not appear to respond to sertraline or fluoxetine. Thus the common SSRIs may be only somewhat effective for this group (Benedek et al., 2009). For PTSD nightmares in both groups, prazosin (3-15 mg/night) has been used with some success.

Although SSRIs are the first-line choice for the pharmacotherapy of PTSD, not all patients will have a full treatment response. Adjunctive treatment with risperidone and olanzapine may be helpful. Augmentation with a mood stabilizer such as divalproex or lithium may be considered, but evidence for success is limited. Buspirone or benzodiazepines may also be used, but only sparingly and adjunctively, to decrease anxiety or panic attacks. These medications are not recommended as monotherapy.

KEY TREATMENT

Acutely, nonbenzodiazepine sleeping medications may be used as first-line treatment for insomnia (Bradley et al., 2005; NICE, 2005) (SOR: B).

PTSD is often effectively treated with SSRIs, including sertraline, paroxetine, venlafaxine, and fluoxetine, though this effect may be less in older veterans (APA, 2004; Benedek et al., 2009; Stein et al., 2006) (SOR: A).

The antidepressant mirtazapine and the anticonvulsants topiramate and tiagabine may be beneficial in PTSD therapy (Benedek et al., 2009) (SOR: B).

For PTSD nightmares, prazosin may be effective (SOR: B).

Risperidone and olanzapine may be effective augmentation to SSRIs for persistent PTSD symptoms (Benedek et al, 2009) (SOR: B).

Conclusion

Family physicians are routinely faced with a variety of acute crises, patient-reported traumas, intimate partner violence, and disaster situations that require a specialized knowledge to understand patient complaints and to successfully develop management and intervention strategies. The goal of crisis intervention and disaster management is to evaluate the precipitants of the crisis, understand the personal meaning of the events, deal with the crisis state itself, and use the selective past history to comprehend the current situation better. It is also important to mobilize the support network and, if relevant, diagnose and treat any comorbid psychiatric illnesses. A crisis evaluation strategy using a timeline, eco-map, and wheel-and-spoke formulation can be used to help implement a specific problem-solving approach. Crisis treatment includes problem or symptom-oriented therapy, use of adaptive coping styles, 18-step crisis intervention approach, and medications when indicated. Cases involving intimate partner violence require particular attention to violence risk, safety planning, and documentation. All these interventions can be helpful when seeking a resolution of the crisis.

References

The complete reference list is available online at www.expertconsult.com.

Web Resources

www.suicidepreventionlifeline.org/
National Suicide Prevention Lifeline, (800) 273-TALK; free, confidential, 24-hour/day access to crisis counselors, with services for Spanish speakers, veterans, and TTY users.

http://ndvh.org/
National Domestic Violence Hotline, (800) 799-SAFE; education, resources, and 24/7 anonymous and confidential help for victims or others calling on their behalf.

www.endabuse.org/
Information about family violence education, prevention, and advocacy, including an action center for health care providers.

www.safe4all.org/
Stop Abuse for Everyone (SAFE) offers resources and information concentrating on battered straight men; gay, lesbian, bisexual, and transgender (GLBT) victims, teenagers, and elderly victims.

http://endabuse.org/userfiles/file/HealthCare/MandReport2007FINAL MMS.pdf/
State reporting requirements.

CHAPTER 46

Difficult Patients: Personality Disorders and Somatoform Complaints

Robert E. Feinstein and Frank Verloin deGruy III

The chapters in Part Two of this book generally are devoted to topics in family medicine practice that can be understood and managed as discrete clinical problems. Although several problems might coexist in a patient, this is the usual way the family physician approaches health problems. In this chapter, however, we follow our conviction that the clinical encounter is the ground on which *all* problems in family medicine are addressed. An effective clinical encounter, at its best, develops as an extended, trusting partnership between patient and physician. However, disturbances or difficulties in the encounter can ruin even the best therapeutic plan. In this chapter we use the term *difficult patients* to refer to two patient groups: those with personality traits (styles) or personality disorders and those with unexplained physical symptoms or somatoform disorders.

Our treatment of "personality styles" follows a spectrum or dimensional approach. In the mildest form, *personality traits* are present in normal, healthy patients, and under certain circumstances are assets. Although sometimes unpleasant, these are not necessarily pathologic. At the other end of the spectrum are features of personality that are so extreme as to constitute full-blown disorders: Axis II of the DSM-IV-TR contains a set of *personality disorders* that are real, difficult, and disabling and that often present in primary care settings.

Our treatment of patients with "unexplained physical symptoms," as with personality styles, also follows this spectrum or dimensional approach. In it mildest form, unexplained physical complaints will present in generally normal, healthy patients. These benign physical complaints are often accompanied by psychological issues just as often as psychological symptoms are accompanied by physical complaints. Features of psychological problems just as psychological symptoms always accompany physical problems (Kroenke et al., 1994). Moreover, symptoms of both a physical and a psychological nature frequently appear in patients—indeed, in all people—without obvious explanation. Mild physical symptoms such as "butterflies" in the epigastrium just before a public speech may disappear as mysteriously as they appear and are of no consequence. At the other end of the spectrum are increasingly severe, persistent, or disabling, unexplained physical symptoms that eventually cross a threshold and become a disorder in their own right. The *somatoform disorders* are this family of full-blown diagnostic conditions, characterized by disabling physical symptoms with no physical explanation.

This chapter discusses difficult patients at all points on the personality and somatic continuum, from normal to disordered, to patients with comorbid conditions. Success in managing these difficult patients depends more often on the physician's reaction to the patient's personality traits or somatic complaints (and resulting interventions) than on assignment of a specific diagnosis. These problems do not exist in the patient, but rather in the transactions between patient and physician. Here the physician's task is not simply to discover and describe patient problems, but also to create a relationship with the patient that is therapeutic rather than problematic. Our approach here is to address difficult clinical encounters in terms of patients' personality style and somatic presentation and the responses elicited in physicians. Interventions based on the physician's responses and an understanding of the patient's issues offer a convenient and parsimonious framework for constructive management strategies.

Personality Style vs. Personality Disorder

A personality style is the lifelong habitual way that a person thinks, feels, and behaves. Styles are determined by genetics and are often called *temperament*. Temperamental aspects, such as the ability to filter external stimuli or shyness, are often observable at birth. Other personality traits are determined by upbringing from early parent-child interactions, such as *mentalization*, which is the ability to empathize with another's emotions or perspective and utilize this to read the intentions of others. Each personality has unique, enduring, and slowly evolving characteristics, including the organization of perception, a set of core beliefs, thinking style, fantasy life, hierarchy of emotional needs, value system, ideals, characteristic ways of relating to self and others, and adaptation to external reality.

The distinction between personality style and a personality disorder is a matter of degree. Personality styles tend to be relatively stable over a lifetime but can be modified by psychotherapy or needs to adapt to the environment. Personality disorders are also stable, but are more difficult to modify, if at all, and then by long-term or special forms of psychotherapy or by life events. Personality styles that become rigid, extreme, maladaptive, or damaging to self or others, or that lead to social or occupational impairment, are called "personality disorders." Although everyone is unique, there seems to be a set of personality styles and disorders that are commonly encountered. Some personality disorders can be recognized in the movies (schizotypal personality disorder, Robert DeNiro in *Taxi Driver*; narcissistic personality disorder, Tom Cruise in *Top Gun*; dependent-borderline personality disorder, Bill Murray in *What About Bob?*).

Classification

Personality Disorders

Inflexible and maladaptive personality disorders cause distress or social or occupational impairment. A patient with a personality disorder typically has problems in at least two of these areas: cognition, affectivity, interpersonal functioning, and impulse control. Pervasive manifestations occur across a range of situations. A *personality disorder* is stable and of long duration, typically begins in adolescence or early adulthood, and is diagnosed in adulthood.

The two primary classification approaches to personality disorders are categorical and dimensional. The *categorical* approach, currently represented in DSM-IV-TR, describes people as having clusters of associated traits, symptoms, or behaviors that form discrete "prototypes," or categories of personality. The *dimensional* approach, likely the wave of the future, assesses multiple traits or dimensions of a personality that are present, absent, or have varying degrees of intensity; measurable dimensions of personality might include novelty seeking, harm avoidance, reward dependence, cooperativeness, and self-directedness. Categorical approaches have the advantage of colorfully describing and differentiating distinct groups of different personality types. This classification convention remains popular with family physicians because it follows the concept of disease categories within general medicine. The *Diagnostic and Statistical Manual of Mental Disorders*, fourth edition, text revision (DSM-IV-TR), uses a categorical personality disorder classification as part of a multiaxial system that encourages physicians to consider personality variables in every patient (American Psychiatric Association [APA], 2000).

The preliminary diagnosis of a personality disorder begins by identifying the appropriate cluster or dimension, because it is easiest to recognize the broad traits of a cluster diagnosis first. The three clusters of personality disorders are *cluster A*, odd and eccentric; *cluster B*, dramatic, emotional, or erratic; and *cluster C*, anxious or fearful. These clusters or dimensions are subdivided into specific personality subtypes with general characteristics (Box 46-1). Because personalities are complicated, it is not unusual for a patient to meet the criteria for two cluster diagnoses and more than one specific personality disorder diagnosis.

Unexplained Physical Symptoms vs. Somatoform Disorders

Physical symptoms appear and disappear on a regular basis in normal people. Less than 3% of these symptoms result in a visit to a physician (Banks et al., 1975), but more than half the visits to primary care physicians are for symptoms. Even symptoms severe enough to trigger a visit are usually self-limited; about three-quarters improve or disappear in 2 weeks, and over half of those remaining have improved or disappeared at 3 months (Kroenke and Jackson, 1998). Most patients do not remember having a symptom that they reported 1 year earlier (Simon and Guerje, 1999). From this cohort of symptomatic patients, a substantial number have symptoms sufficiently persistent, severe, or numerous to justify a diagnostic workup, which usually reveals a medical problem that the family physician manages in the usual

Box 46-1 Personality Disorder Clusters*

Cluster A (Odd, Eccentric)

1. **Paranoid**

Expects exploitation, harm; questions loyalty, fidelity; bears grudges; easily slighted

2. **Schizoid**

Loner; aloof; indifferent to praise or criticism; social anxiety; constricted affect

3. **Schizotypal**

Odd, eccentric; social anxiety; magical thinking; suspicious, paranoid ideation

Cluster B (Dramatic, Emotional)

1. **Antisocial**

Cruelty; problems with authority, unlawful behaviors, exploits others, dishonesty, irresponsibility

2. **Histrionic**

Overly emotional; seductive, sexual attention seeking; shallow, superficial

3. **Borderline**

Unstable intense relationships; self-destructive, suicidal; impulsive; affect instability; identity disturbances

4. **Narcissistic**

Grandiose; inflated self-importance; entitled; exploits others; lacks empathy; needs admiration; hypersensitive to criticism

Self-Defeating†

Suffers; self-sacrificing; defeats others; self-destructive; cannot enjoy; easily hurt

Cluster C (Anxious, Fearful)

1. **Dependent**

Indecisive; lacks initiative; submissive; helpless; dependent; fears abandonment

2. **Obsessive-compulsive**

Perfectionism; inflexibility; preoccupation with details; wishes to control others; stingy; overconscientiousness; excessive morality or ethics

3. **Avoidant**

Easily hurt; timid, fearful; social discomfort; avoids interpersonal interactions

From American Psychiatric Association. Diagnostic and Statistical Manual of Mental Disorders, 4th ed, text revision. Washington, DC, APA, 2000.

*DSM-IV-TR abridged criteria, 2000.

†From APA. Diagnostic and Statistical Manual of Mental Disorders, 3rd ed revised. Washington, DC, APA, 1986.

way, as described throughout this text. In about one third of patients, however, the symptoms are causing impairment and no physical explanation can be found; alternatively the symptom is out of proportion to the supposed explanatory finding; these patients are *somatic*. At the more severe end of the continuum, somatic symptoms cluster into discrete diagnostic categories: the somatoform disorders, including somatization disorder, conversion disorder, somatoform pain disorder, hypochondriasis, factitious disorder, malingering, and body dysmorphic disorder. Primary care physicians tend not to pursue diagnoses to the level of these categories, because it is a time-consuming process not yet shown to improve patient outcomes. However, these categories have promising implications for managing the difficult

clinical relationship, particularly in the context of personality types and disorders.

About 15% of primary care encounters are experienced by physicians as "difficult," as determined by the self-administered DDPRQ (Hahn et al., 1996). Patients classified as difficult are not distinguished by the usual demographic categories (age, gender, race, social status) but rather by the presence of somatoform complaints; other DSM Axis I conditions, particularly depression and anxiety disorders; and unique personality styles, up to and including DSM Axis II personality disorders. There is extensive overlap among these symptom clusters, particularly at the less severe end of the spectrum.

Unexplained physical symptoms are often benign and transitory, and only 3% of patients with these symptoms see a physician. Somatic complaints are described by patients within all domains of the traditional review of symptoms. Somatoform disorders are a group of severe psychiatric conditions that present with physical symptoms that suggest a medical condition but that cannot be adequately explained by a medical condition. Patients can have both a medical condition and unexplained physical symptoms that meet criteria for a somatoform condition. Box 46-2 describes somatoform disorders (DSM-IV-TR classification). Social or occupational impairment in these patients exceeds what would be expected based on physical complaints.

Comorbidity of Personality and Somatoform Disorders

Personality and somatoform disorders have significant comorbidity, and clinical management of these disorders frequently overlaps. According to the DSM IV-TR, 1% to 5% of primary care patients meet the criteria for somatization disorder (APA, 2000). Prevalence rates for personality disorders are reported to be 4% to 13% in the general population and up to 24% of patients in primary care settings (Gross et al., 2002; Moran et al., 2000).

A meta-analysis of 18 studies demonstrated that significant comorbidity exists between somatization disorder and five personality disorders (Bornstein and Gold, 2008). The most robust comorbidity is between somatization disorders and antisocial, borderline, and histrionic personality disorders, with less robust but significant comorbidity with avoidant and dependent personality disorders. Exploring the connections between these two groups of disorders offers some insight into the intrapsychic and interpersonal dynamics of both groups. One clinically relevant factor common to both groups is that the early family relationships of these difficult patients were both rejecting and tenuous. This may have led both groups to an anxious or insecure attachment style. This translates into the persistent care-seeking style so recognizable by physicians, in both somatic patients and in patients with a personality disorder. Both groups may display clinging, dependent, manipulative, and ambivalent attachment styles, often seen in those with borderline, histrionic, antisocial, and dependent personality disorders.

Significant comorbidity also exists between other somatoform disorders and other personality disorders. For example, patients with hypochondriasis and body dysmorphic disorders are obsessed with fear of illness and fear of a body defect, respectively. Patients with both of these also display

Box 46-2 Somatoform Disorders

Hypochondriasis

Fears or ideas that one has a serious disease, which persist despite a negative medical workup and causes social or occupational dysfunction that lasts at least 6 months. Hypochondriasis is clinically similar to *obsessive-compulsive disorder*. Hypochondriac ruminations are common in patients with *obsessive-compulsive personality disorder*.

Somatization Disorder

Consists of four pain symptoms, two gastrointestinal symptoms, one sexual symptom, and one pseudoneurologic symptom; symptoms are not fully explained by known medical conditions. Somatization disorder develops over years and causes significant social and occupational dysfunction. Patients with somatization disorder or a subthreshold disorder show a significant comorbidity with *antisocial, borderline, histrionic, dependent,* and *avoidant personality disorders*.

Conversion Disorder

One or more symptoms or deficits affecting voluntary motor or sensory function; symptoms may include paralysis, somnambulism, pseudoseizure, psychogenic blindness, and mutism. Symptoms can also mimic other neurologic or medical disorders. No clear physical cause is found. Psychological conflict is important in symptom development and is unconscious. Social and occupational dysfunction is typical. Patients with *histrionic personality disorder* often present with conversion symptoms.

Pain Disorder

Symptom is pain, and no medical cause is obvious. Psychological factors are important and unconscious. The pain causes social or occupational dysfunction and may be acute (<6 months) or chronic (>6 months).

Body Dysmorphic Disorder

Preoccupation and excessive concern with an imagined body defect, presenting with social or occupational dysfunction.

Factitious Disorder

Intentional production or feigning of physical signs or psychological symptoms, motivated by a desire to assume the sick role, with no other secondary gain in evidence. Factitious disorder is often comorbid with *antisocial personality disorder*.

Malingering

Intentional production or feigning of physical or psychological illness, motivated by secondary gain (e.g., monetary [disability], avoid the military, procure drugs). Malingering is often comorbid with *antisocial personality disorder*.

compulsive requests for medical care. Clinically, these disorders have overlapping features with obsessive-compulsive disorder (OCD) and may be variants of OCD. Interestingly, all three of these disorders can be managed similarly and are somewhat responsive to treatment with antidepressants. Conversion disorders also have a long-standing connection to hysteria and more recently to Briquet's syndrome (somatization disorder) and can be understood and managed similarly to the histrionic personality disorder. Also, reports of somatic symptoms in patients with factitious and malingering disorder may represent a form of antisocial personality disorder. All three of these disorders have in common a conscious desire to lie and mislead others for secondary gain.

Management

Management of the physician-patient relationship requires special skills when dealing with a difficult patient. The following five-step process is useful for family physicians:

1. Understand the patient's core beliefs, fears, and irrational thoughts.
2. Identify the patient's defense mechanisms and coping style, and use confrontation, clarification, and interpretation to modify these.
3. Recognize recurrent patient behaviors and how these will likely affect patient adherence and use of medical services.
4. Learn to use the physician's own reactions to the patient to help identify the diagnosis and management strategy.
5. Recognize that specific interventions are helpful for different types of patients.

To create therapeutic relationships with patients who might otherwise be experienced as difficult, the clinician must first understand patients' core beliefs, thoughts, and fears; then understand their defenses and coping styles; and finally, understand the health-related behaviors that follow from these beliefs and styles. This understanding helps physicians utilize the reactions such behaviors evoke in them, thereby leading to alternative responses and potential interventions. Tables 46-1 and 46-2 outline this process using DSM-IV-TR classification.

Patient Core Beliefs, Irrational Thoughts, and Fears

Understanding core beliefs has therapeutic implications. The family physician can use simple principles of *cognitive-behavioral therapy* (CBT) to facilitate the management of these patients. The theory of CBT is that patients have core beliefs, a worldview, and personality/somatic-specific fears that can be identified and modified by bringing them to conscious awareness (Beck and Freeman, 1990; Greenberger and Padesky, 1995).

Core beliefs and fears are deeply held, intense, and idiosyncratic in quality. When stress occurs against the background of a core belief, a reinforcing feedback sequence ensues. The core belief is acted on by the stressor, which leads to irrational fears, negative moods or emotions that lead to maladaptive physical symptoms or behaviors, which in turn confirm or amplify the core belief or fear. Core beliefs and fears are readily activated during a visit to the physician, when a patient has symptoms, feels sick, or is vulnerable. For example, a patient with hypochondriasis may fear she has a serious illness. She may have a core belief and fear that she is dying. She may believe that the physician knows she is severely ill but will not tell her. The physician, however, by understanding the patient's core beliefs and associated fears, can prevent unnecessary worry. The physician can empathize with the patient; discuss the patient's core beliefs and fears of an illness; help the patient recognized the distorted, irrational, or illogical thoughts; and ultimately, interpret the patient's defenses and suggest alternative ways for coping.

The CBT sequence of stress, acting on core beliefs and irrational fears, and subsequent development of symptoms or maladaptive behaviors is described for difficult patients in Table 46-1. Adherence to medical recommendations and use

Table 46-1 Schema for Managing Difficult Patients

DSM-IV-TR	Patient Core Beliefs	Patient Fears	Defenses	Coping Styles	Patient Health Behaviors
Paranoid	Others are adversaries and are to blame; I am being examined; They are out to get me; I can't trust anyone.	Exploitation; slights; betrayal; humiliation; physical intrusions from medical procedures.	*Projection:* ascribe one's impulses to others. *Projective identification:* project one's impulse plus control of others as way to control one's own impulses. *Denial:* refusal to admit painful realities. *Splitting:* self and others seen as all good or all bad.	Guarded and protective of their autonomy, often with arrogant belief in their own superiority.	Wariness, suspicion, mistrust, jealousy, self-sufficiency, counterattacking, anger, and violence.
Schizoid	I need space; I need to be alone; people are replaceable or unimportant.	Emotional contact; warmth; intimacy; caring; intrusions or violation of privacy.	*Isolation of affect:* thoughts stored without emotion. *Intellectualization:* replace feelings with facts. Denial, splitting (see above). *Regression:* revert to childlike thoughts, feelings, or behaviors.	Inner world is defended and/or insulated from others.	Withdrawal; seeking isolation and privacy.
Schizotypal	Idiosyncratic, magical, or eccentric beliefs (I know what they're thinking/feeling); premonitions.	Emotional contact; intimacy; warmth, caring; violation of privacy.	*Schizoid fantasy:* retreat to idiosyncratic fantasy when faced with painful experience. *Undoing:* symbolic magical action designed to reverse or cancel unacceptable thoughts, feelings, or actions. Regression, denial, splitting (see above).	Chaotic, idiosyncratic, disorganized.	Withdrawal; odd, autistic, or magical behaviors and movements; seeks isolation and privacy.
Antisocial	People are there to be used and exploited; I come before all others.	Boredom; loss of prestige, power, or esteem.	*Acting out:* expression in action or behavior rather than in words or emotions. Splitting (see above).	Seeks autonomy, freedom; seeks advantage or secondary gain.	Lies, deceit, and manipulation; violence; seeks secondary gain.
Histrionic	I need to impress, be admired/loved; I need to be taken care of, or helped; emotions rule.	Loss of love, admiration, attention, or dependent care.	*Sexualization:* functions or objects changed into sexual symbols to avoid anxieties. Regression, acting out, splitting (see above). *Dissociation:* disruption of perceptions or sensations, consciousness, memory, or personal identity. *Somatization:* physical symptoms caused by mental processes. *Repression:* involuntary forgetting of painful memories, feelings, experiences.	Self-centered, emotion driven, flirtatious, flighty.	Dramatics, exhibitionism, expressiveness, impressionistic.
Borderline	I am very bad or very good. Who am I? I can't be alone.	Separations, loss; emotional abandonment; not being loved and cared for; fluctuating self-esteem.	Splitting, projection, projective identification, dissociation, regression, acting out (see above). *Omnipotence:* seeing self or others as all-powerful. *Idealization/devaluation:* vacillates between seeing self or others as ideal, then deprecating self or others. Minipsychotic experiences.	Hostile dependency; chaotic lifestyle; threatening, intimidating, or seeking intimacy, dependency, or pseudoautonomy.	Impulsive behaviors, suicidal actions, cutting, anger/violence, panic, anxiety, poor reality, stormy relationships.

Continued

Table 46-1 Schema for Managing Difficult Patients—cont'd

DSM-IV-TR	Patient Core Beliefs	Patient Fears	Defenses	Coping Styles	Patient Health Behaviors
Narcissistic	I am special; I am important; I come first; The world should revolve around me.	Loss of prestige, image, beauty, power, or esteem.	Splitting, projection, projective identification, acting out, denial, regression (see above).	Superiority and arrogance, self-aggrandizing, self-centered, self-protecting, demeaning, demanding, critical.	Self-aggrandizement; inflated/deflated self-view; entitled; devalue/idealize; viciousness; envy; competitive.
Avoidant	I must avoid harm or be cautious, as I may get rejected, exposed, or be humiliated.	Rejection; embarrassment in social situations; humiliation; exposure of inadequacies.	*Inhibition:* restriction of thoughts, feelings, behaviors to avoid shame, exposure of inadequacies, rejection, humiliation. *Phobias:* fears of objects, people, situations; avoided to prevent anxiety. Avoidance, withdrawal, regression, somatization (see above).	Withdraw or escape, avoiding criticism.	Avoidance, withdrawal, social timidity, caution, fear/anxiety.
Dependent	I am helpless without others; I can't make a decision; I need constant reassurance and care.	Fears separation, independence; making decisions; and anger.	*Dependent:* yearning for care, clinging, needing direction. *Passive-aggressive:* superficial compliance and passivity disguising stubbornness and anger. *Reaction formation:* unacceptable impulses expressed as the opposite. Regression, splitting (see above).	Passive, dependent, helpless.	Unusually submissive; clinging, indecisive, childlike, needing to be taken care of.
Obsessive-compulsive disorder (OCD)	People should do better; try harder; I must be perfect; make no errors or mistakes; details, rule.	Disorder, mistakes, imperfection; fears feelings, especially rage/anger, anxiety, self-doubt, dependency.	Isolation of affect, intellectualization, reaction formation, undoing, dependent, phobias, repression (see above). *Controlling:* efforts to regulate objects or others to avoid anxiety. *Displacement:* transfer of one's feelings from one person on to another. *Inhibition:* restricting thoughts, feelings, or behaviors for fear that unacceptable impulses will create anxiety or damage.	Inflexible, constricted, governed by details and rules, safety, or security concerns.	Perfectionism, driven orderliness; logical, obsessions and/or compulsions; controlling, critical; stubbornness, stinginess; workaholic; rational.
Self-defeating	I must suffer and sacrifice; I am a martyr; I should be punished.	Loss of love; fears pleasure; fears recovery.	*Ambivalence:* coexistence of opposite feelings. Displacement, denial, projective identification, reaction formation, passive-aggressive, splitting (see above).	Self-defeating, self-destructive.	Feels worse with good news; self-defeating, self-destructive.
Hypochondriasis (shares many features with both OCD and OCPD)	I am afraid that I have a horrible disease [based on symptom misinterpretation]. The doctor could be wrong or may have missed something. I must be absolutely certain that I am well. I must worry. I need to obsess and use compulsions.	Fears of a catastrophic illness; fears uncertainty; unconscious emotional fears.	Denial; avoiding awareness of painful experience; anger elicited when denial of emotions is suggested. *Externalization:* attributing internal state to external explanations. Hypochondriasis dominant; exaggerating or overemphasizing illness; somatization (less common); psychic or emotional experience converted to somatic symptoms; regression (returning to earlier developmental levels of functioning).	Highly anxious coping style.	Dependent: clinging is attached to their fears; demanding excessive health testing; doubting test results and physician assertions; seeks authoritarian, paternalistic doctors who give them answers.

Disorder	Belief	Fears	Defenses	Coping style	Behavior
Somatoform disorders (may be comorbid with antisocial, borderline, histrionic, avoidant, or dependent personality traits, sometimes disorders)	I will always have pain (or neurologic symptoms, or sexual symptoms).	Fears labeling their emotions; unable to see psychosocial stress as part of the explanation for physical symptoms; unconscious emotional fears.	Somatization dominates; psychic experience converted to somatic or physical symptoms; sexualization (expression of trauma as sexual); denial; externalization; attributing internal state to external explanations; regression.	Low anxious coping style. Anxiety converted to physical symptoms; do not recognize their own anxiety (but others do).	Entitled demander; attached to physical symptoms; expecting or demanding medical treatment for symptoms; dissatisfied with care or rejecting of help.
Conversion disorder/pain disorder (often associated with histrionic personality traits disorder)	I have a neurological disorder. I am powerless (and/or impaired).	Frightened by pain, which appears as varied neurologic symptoms; unconscious fears of anger or sexual wishes.	Repression, dissociation, sexualization (pseudoseizures), externalization.	Repressive coping style. Failure to recognize being upset or have difficulty recognizing their own emotional responses.	Requesting or demanding relief, analgesics, or surgery; assuming role of invalid.
Body dysmorphic disorder (shares many features with both OCD and OCPD)	Fear that a body part is deformed, defective, or ugly (nose, thinning hair, acne, scars, swelling, facial asymmetry); other defective body parts.	Tormenting distress, worry, shame, or embarrassment and fear about a specific body defect.	*Distortion:* reshaping external reality to internal needs. Hypochondrias; denial, dissociation, sexualization (see above).	Highly anxious coping style.	Demanding or pressuring physician to "fix the defect" (often surgically).
Factitious disorder (may be comorbid or part of antisocial personality disorder)	I will fake or feign physical or psychological symptoms to be taken care of as if I am sick child.	Fears reexperiencing painful, frightening, or traumatic early life experiences. Fears being discovered as fraudulent, abandoned, accused (See Dependent and Antisocial personality disorders).	*Acting out:* consciously feigning physical or psychological symptoms. Denial, splitting (see above).	Manipulative coping style. Seeks the patient sick role.	Outward concern while consciously misleading physician in pursuit of close medical relationship as substitute for desired, caring parent–child bond; defensive hostility when confronted that symptoms or history has been manufactured to obtain treatment or assume the sick role.
Malingering (may be comorbid or part of antisocial personality traits or disorder)	I will fake or feign physical or psychological symptoms to gain specific nonmedical benefits (e.g., money, disability payments, drugs, free food, shelter, avoiding police).	Fears true manipulative intention will be discovered (See Antisocial and Narcissistic personality disorders).	*Acting out:* consciously feigning physical or psychological symptoms. Denial, splitting (see above).	Manipulative coping style. Deceitful; seeks secondary gain.	Lies; uses conscious deceit and manipulation to mislead for secondary gain. Symptoms or history manufactured for a specific gain.

OCPD, Obsessive-compulsive personality disorder.

Table 46-2 Difficult Patients: Adherence, Utilization, Physician Reactions, and Interventions (DSM-IV-TR)

Adherence	Utilization	Physician Reactions	Interventions
Paranoid Personality Disorder			
Difficult when requested by physician since patient is suspicious of need for compliance. Problematic, but may be easier when patient is seeking relief from symptoms.	Limited utilization; or as a condition for medical service utilization, the patient may seek detailed explanations or reasons for diagnostic testing or needs for other services.	Fearful; sense of danger; mistrust; feeling accused, blamed, or threatened.	1. Empathize with patient's fear of being hurt; acknowledge complaints without arguing or ignoring. 2. Openly and honestly explain medical illness. 3. Correct reality distortions and unreasonable patient expectations. 4. Gently question irrational thoughts, and suggest more rational thoughts. 5. Do not confront delusions. 6. If patient refuses care out of mistrust, rather than insisting, ask if you can disagree about need for the test or the specific medical care. 7. Interpret projection (blame) and other defenses. 8. Foster more adaptive coping styles.
Schizoid Personality Disorder			
May be difficult. Will need reinforcement and monitoring. May need outreach services.	Underutilization Outreach, if not too frequent, may help foster appropriate use of medical services.	Detached or removed; wish to involve patient with others; to break through the isolation.	1. Empathize with patient's need for privacy and contact. 2. Accept patient's unsociability. 3. Reduce patient's isolation as tolerated. 4. Neutrally impart medical information. 5. Do not demand involvement or permit total withdrawal. 6. Correct reality distortions and unreasonable patient expectations. 7. Question irrational thoughts; suggest more rational ones. 8. Interpret isolation and other defenses. 9. Foster more adaptive coping styles.
Schizotypal Personality Disorder			
May be difficult. May need outreach, visiting nurse, community resources, or case management.	Underutilization May need outreach to gain reasonable and appropriate utilization of medical services.	Detached; removed; "weird and alone"; wish to involve patient in additional medical care; or to break through the isolation.	1. Empathize with patient's idiosyncratic style, magical thinking, and perceptions without directly confronting. 2. Recognize the need for privacy and contact. 3. Accept patient's unsociability; reduce patient's isolation, as tolerated. 4. Neutrally impart information. 5. Do not demand involvement or permit total withdrawal. 6. Correct reality distortions and unreasonable patient expectations. 7. Question irrational thoughts; suggest more rational ones. 8. Interpret regression and other defenses. 9. Foster more adaptive coping styles.
Antisocial Personality Disorder			
May be resistant, problematic, and intolerant of the need for ongoing compliance.	May misuse medical resources for secondary gain.	Used, exploited or deceived; anger, and wish to uncover lies, punish, or imprison.	1. Empathize with patient's fear of exploitation and low self-esteem. 2. Determine if you are being used for secondary gain. Should you suspect dishonesty, verify symptoms and illness progression with others. 3. Do not moralize. Explain that deception results in the physician giving the patient poor care. 4. Correct reality distortions and unreasonable patient expectations. 5. Question irrational thoughts; suggest more rational ones. 6. Interpret defenses. 7. Foster more adaptive coping styles.

Table 46-2 Difficult Patients: Adherence, Utilization, Physician Reactions, and Interventions (DSM-IV-TR)—cont'd

Adherence	Utilization	Physician Reactions	Interventions
Histrionic Personality Disorder			
Often dependent on others or inconsistent.	May misuse or overuse medical resources to gain attention from the physician or staff.	Flattered, captivated, seduced or aroused; flooded by emotions; depleted; wish to rescue.	1. Empathize with patient's fear of losing love or care. 2. Interact in a friendly way, not too reserved or too warm. 3. Discuss patient's fears; reassure when possible. 4. Use logic to counteract an emotional style of thinking. 5. Set limits if the patient regresses. 6. Correct reality distortions and unreasonable patient expectations. 7. Question irrational thoughts; suggest more rational ones. 8. Interpret sexualization, regression, and other specific defenses. 9. Foster more adaptive coping styles.
Borderline Personality Disorder			
Inconsistent, because adherence is easily influenced by emotional storms, interpersonal conflicts, and chaotic lifestyles.	Misuse or high use for maladaptive behaviors, such as suicidal or disruptive behaviors.	Feeling manipulated, angry, impotent, depleted, self-doubting; wish to rescue or get rid of the patient; guilty.	1. Empathize with patient's fear of abandonment and separation, and plan for absences by arranging coverage. 2. Express a wish to help and satisfy reasonable needs. 3. Ask the patient to monitor impulsive behaviors with a diary or log. 4. Set firm limits and do not punish. 5. Correct reality distortions and unreasonable patient expectations. 6. Question irrational thoughts; suggest more rational ones. 7. Interpret splitting and other defenses. 8. Negotiate emergency procedures in advance. If suicidal, patient must go to emergency room, if not safe. If patient refuses emergency help when you offer, tell patient in advance that this therapeutic breach may end the relationship. 9. Foster more adaptive coping styles.
Narcissistic Personality Disorder			
Can be problematic. Intolerant of need for ongoing compliance requirements.	Entitled to use, or may abuse medical services when needed.	Devalue/overvalue; inferior/superior; fearful of patient's criticism or anger; wish to retaliate, devalue, or get rid of the patient.	1. Empathize with patient's vulnerability and low self-esteem. 2. Do not mistake patient's superior attitude for *real* confidence, and do not confront entitlement. 3. When devalued or attacked, acknowledge patient's hurt, your mistakes, and express your continued wish to help. 4. If devaluing continues, offer referral as option, not as punishment. 5. Correct reality distortions and unreasonable patient expectations. 6. Question irrational thoughts; suggest more rational ones. 7. Interpret splitting and other defenses. 8. Foster more adaptive coping styles.
Avoidant Personality Disorder			
Diverted or delayed by avoidant behavior. Guided by a wish to avoid disapproval of medical staff.	Seeks medical services to secure approval or avoid criticism, not necessarily seeking health benefits.	Frustrated because patient often cannot articulate fears; annoyed at patient's weakness.	1. Empathize with patient's social fears, shame, shyness, and fears of revealing inadequacies, rejection, embarrassment, humiliation, and anger. 2. Help patient describe in detail the feared situation(s). 3. Encourage and support the need for the patient to gradually face their fears and tendency to avoid; if this seems overwhelming, choose smaller fears to confront or refer. 4. If frustrated or unclear about nature of the fears, ask for detailed descriptions of the problem. 5. Gently elicit irrational thoughts, and suggest more rational thoughts. 6. Correct reality distortions. 7. Interpret avoidance, phobias, and other defenses. 8. Foster more adaptive coping styles.

Continued

Table 46-2 Difficult Patients: Adherence, Utilization, Physician Reactions, and Interventions (DSM-IV-TR)—cont'd

Adherence	Utilization	Physician Reactions	Interventions
Dependent Personality Disorder			
Dependent on others for medical supervision and easily overwhelmed by demands of self-monitoring compliance.	Underuse when left to self, but may overuse service when physician or medical staff becomes the source of needed gratification.	Depleted; annoyed at patient's dependence/neediness; may deny patient's reasonable needs.	1. Empathize with patient's need for care. 2. Frustrate total dependence. 3. Be careful to avoid telling patient what to do. 4. Encourage independent thinking and action. 5. Realize that what patient says he wants (caretaking) is not necessarily what he needs. 6. Ask patient what is so frightening about independence. 7. Do not abandon or threaten termination, because some dependent patients need regular physician contact for life. 8. Correct reality distortions and unreasonable patient expectations. 9. Gently elicit irrational thoughts, and suggest more rational thoughts. 10. Interpret regression and other specific defenses. 11. Foster more adaptive coping styles.
Obsessive-Compulsive Personality Disorder			
Rigid and inflexibly follows the rules; disrupted or anxious if unexpected changes are required.	Conflicted about utilization. Fears of uncertainty may drive increased use, whereas fears of loss of control may decrease use.	In a battle of control with negative reactions to patient stinginess, need for details, order, and stubbornness; distanced from feelings; bored with details.	1. Empathize with patient's logical, detailed, unemotional style of thinking. 2. If obsessive thoughts are interfering with medical care, ask about patient's feelings. 3. Do not struggle with patient about control or critical judgments. 4. Avoid abandoning patient. 5. Correct reality distortions and unreasonable patient expectations. 6. Elicit irrational thoughts; suggest more rational thoughts. 7. Interpret specific defenses. 8. Foster more adaptive coping styles.
Self-Defeating Personality Disorder*			
Dependent on others; may be "help seeking," then "help rejecting."	Underutilization; because patient feels undeserving of services, or believes they will not help. Overutilization, when patient perceives being treated badly.	Wish to rescue; fantasies that patient will suffer/die; defeated; self-blame; self-doubt, or hopelessness, helplessness.	1. Empathize with patient's suffering. Acknowledge and appreciate the difficulty associated with illness and treatment. 2. Emphasize that recovery may be a slow, steady process. 3. Patient's need for recovery can be presented as necessary to benefit others. 4. Inquire about obviously self-destructive or self-defeating behaviors. 5. Do not abandon patient. 6. Correct reality distortions and unreasonable patient expectations. 7. Elicit irrational thoughts, and suggest more rational ones. 8. Interpret specific defenses. 9. Foster more adaptive coping styles.
Hypochondriasis			
"Doctor shopping" Adhere to medical testing, but have difficulty adhering to recommendations for psychosocial evaluation or treatment.	High utilization. Repetitive physician visits, or avoidance of doctors because the situation is hopeless.	Frustrated, angry, and annoyed with patient's needs, demands, and help-rejecting behaviors. Wants patient to stop complaining. Wants to end the doctor-patient relationship.	1. Empathize/understand involuntary nature of symptoms. 2. Use parallel diagnostic inquiry. (Suggest from start that symptoms have biopsycho-sociocultural components.) Workup proceeds simultaneously in all domains. 3. Use emotion-focused interviewing **Kroenke's algorithm*** Is the symptom medically explained? Acutely serious? Seriously persistent or bothersome? What are patient's specific concerns or expectations? What else is the patient worried about? Anything else helpful? Does patient have depression, anxiety disorder, or abuse history? Has the patient been tried on antidepressants? Does patient have history of chronic somatization? 4. Reassure the patient that the disorder is not lethal. 5. Do not abandon the patient. 6. Correct reality distortions and unreasonable patient expectations. 7. Elicit irrational thoughts, and suggest more rational ones. 8. Interpret specific defenses.

Table 46-2 Difficult Patients: Adherence, Utilization, Physician Reactions, and Interventions (DSM-IV-TR)—cont'd

Adherence	Utilization	Physician Reactions	Interventions
Hypochondriasis—cont'd			
			9. Foster more adaptive coping styles. 10. Provide additional treatment. Encourage regular office visits. With physical complaint, do a focused physical exam. Refer for consultation rather than hospitalization. Goal is preservation and restoration of function, not elimination of symptoms.
Somatization Disorder			
"Doctor shopping" Adhere to requests for medical testing, but highly resistant to psychosocial exploration, evaluation, or treatment.	Up to 9× the health care expenditures of typical primary care patients. Utilization increases depending on number of symptoms. Doctor seeking until patients can find a physician who believes them or will do what they seek.	With more somatic complaints, perceives patient as more difficult. Frustrated, puzzled with inability to explain or diagnose problem. Wants patient to stop complaining.	1. Empathize/understand involuntary nature of symptoms. 2. Screen for reasonable medical condition that could explain symptoms. 3. Use parallel diagnostic inquiry. (Suggest from start that symptoms have biopsycho-sociocultural components.) Workup proceeds simultaneously in all domains. 4. Use emotion-focused interviewing (see above). 5. Do not abandon the patient. 6. Correct reality distortions and unreasonable patient expectations. 7. Elicit irrational thoughts and suggest more rational ones. 8. Interpret specific defenses. 9. Foster more adaptive coping styles.
Conversion Disorder			
Adhere to medical recommendation. May accept psychosocial explanations.	Doctor seeking until patients can find one who believes them or will do what they seek.	Puzzled initially. Often feel helpless to address psychosocial or emotion conflict.	1. Empathize/understand involuntary nature of "symptoms. 2. Perform thorough neurologic and medical evaluation. 2. Make a timely diagnosis. 3. Give therapeutic reassurance that symptoms are not caused by a medical or neurologic condition but are secondary to underlying psychological conflict. 4. Combined medical model approach and psychological modalities best address physical needs and invite patient to engage in treatment without feeling humiliated (combined, if appropriate, with progressive physical therapy to promote sense of mastery and control). 5. Treat any comorbid psychiatric disorder. 6. Work through patient's defenses and help to develop more mature and adaptive defense mechanisms to prevent future conversion episodes. 7. Foster more adaptive coping styles.
Body Dysmorphic Disorder			
Initially avoid medical care. Once disorder is acknowledged by patient, can be intensely medical seeking to correct the defect.	Avoid doctors initially, but then may overuse medical care, seeking variety of surgical and medical treatments.	Puzzled by patient's complaints of body defect that is not readily visible or apparent. Frustrated that reassurance does not work.	1. Empathize; understand involuntary nature of symptoms. 2. *Stepped care* attempts to provide most effective but least intrusive treatments appropriate to a person's needs. Step 1: awareness and recognition Step 2: recognition and assessment *Treatment options:* exposure response; CBT or SSRI; or combined treatment. 3. NICE guidelines: SSRI or clomipramine, CBT (including exposure response prevention [ERP]), or combination of SSRI or clomipramine and CBT (including ERP); consider care coordination, augmentation strategies, admission, social care. 4. Do not abandon or threaten termination. 5. Correct unreasonable patients expectations. 6. Gently elicit irrational thoughts and suggest more rational thoughts. 7. Interprets specific defenses. 8. Foster more adaptive coping styles.

Continued

Table 46-2 Difficult Patients: Adherence, Utilization, Physician Reactions, and Interventions (DSM-IV-TR)—cont'd

Adherence	Utilization	Physician Reactions	Interventions
Factitious Disorder			
Patients will only adhere to medical recommendations when these support the patient's goal of assuming the sick role.	Extremely high use of inpatient medical hospitalization and occasionally psychiatric hospitalizations. Willing to undergo mutilating procedures.	Initial wish to help, then anger/rejection of patient's complaints. Wish to expose, retaliate, punish, or terminate care.	1. Empathize/explore with patient's history of trauma and painful early life experiences. 2. Clarify that you are being used to help patient seek dependent care. 3. Do not moralize. Explain that seeking care in a medical setting is fraught with iatrogenic injury. 4. Explain that there are other, more adaptive ways of receiving care, such as seeking psychiatric help. 5. Set limits on medical care; correct reality distortions. 6. Question irrational thoughts; suggest more rational ones. 7. Interpret defenses and maladaptive coping style. 8. Foster more adaptive coping styles.
Malingering			
Only adhere to medical recommendations when these support patient's secondary goal.	Exploit both inpatient but more often outpatient settings when needed. Symptoms abate or disappear as goals are obtained.	Initial wish to help, then anger/rejection of patient's complaints. Wish to expose, retaliate, punish, or terminate care.	1. Empathize with fear of being discovered in lying and exploiting other. 2. Determine the secondary gain that patient seeks. If dishonesty suspected, verify symptoms and illness progression with others. 3. Do not moralize. Direct patient to use of other, appropriate resources. 4. Correct reality distortions and unreasonable patient expectations. 5. Question irrational thoughts; suggest more rational ones. 6. Interpret defenses and maladaptive coping style. 7. Foster more adaptive coping styles.

CBT, Cognitive-behavioral therapy; *SSRI*, selective serotonin reuptake inhibitor.
*From American Psychiatric Association: Diagnostic and Statistical Manual of Mental Disorders, 3rd ed revised. Washington, DC, APA, 1986.

of medical services are somewhat predictable based on the particular personality or somatoform disorder.

Defenses and Coping Styles

Patients with severe unexplained somatic symptoms tend to use denial, externalization, and somatization, converting psychosocial distress and problematic interpersonal relationships into unexplained physical complaints. Patients with severe unexplained somatic symptoms tend to use high/low anxious coping or manipulative coping styles (see Table 46-1).

A family physician can attempt to relieve a core problem or a symptom interfering with medical care by fostering the patient's awareness of his or her problems. It is important to appreciate the unconscious psychological processes known as *defense mechanisms*. These psychological processes (e.g., denial, projection) are used to resolve internal conflicts, manage moods, mediate external dangers, and facilitate adaptations to reality. *Coping styles*, on the other hand, are typically behavioral patterns and methods of coping with the external environment.

By understanding the constellation of defenses and coping styles used by difficult patients, the physician may be able to modify the pathologic defense or coping style that is interfering with the patient-physician alliance and the delivery of medical care. A physician can use clarification, confrontation, and interpretation (see Table 46-1). For example, a borderline patient may feel hurt and abandoned by the physician's vacation and accuse the physician of not caring. This patient may use a defense mechanism called *devaluation* (physician

is deprecated as uncaring) and a coping style of manipulation (threatens suicide). With this understanding, the physician can begin to help the patient by not taking the patient's efforts to devalue or manipulate personally. The physician can respond to the patient by empathizing with the patient's fears of abandonment. The physician may clarify that the patient has a distorted belief, and that the vacation is being incorrectly experienced as a personal abandonment of the patient. The physician may further clarify that the vacation does not communicate anything about the physician's future ability or wish to care for the patient. The patient can be reassured of the physician's return, future realistic medical availability, specific limits of availability, and medical coverage by another physician. In a preventive effort to allay a crisis and help a borderline patient manage separation fears, the physician (before the vacation) could suggest a new coping style of having the patient schedule a meeting with a medical colleague who will provide coverage while the physician is away. Often, it is helpful to anticipate issues that may arise for the patient and suggest specific problem solving and coping.

Patient Behaviors, Adherence, and Use of Medical Services

Difficult patients often display characteristic behaviors that affect their adherence to medical recommendations and use of medical services. Understanding these behaviors can also help physicians manage their expectations of these difficult patients and improve the chances for effective interventions that might improve medical adherence and health outcomes. In general, patients with cluster A personality disorders (paranoid, schizoid, and schizotypal) tend not to adhere to medical recommendations and underuse medical services. They may require outreach to involve them in their own medical care. Cluster B patients (antisocial, histrionic, borderline, narcissistic, and self-defeating) tend to have variable adherence to medical recommendations and may misuse, overuse, or underuse medical care. Cluster C patients (dependent, obsessive-compulsive, avoidant) tend to adhere to medical recommendations because of fear of the consequences of nonadherence. They are ambivalent users of the medical system and tend to use medical services appropriately when others are involved in their care.

Patients with somatic symptoms tend to overuse medical services and are reluctant to adhere to medical recommendations, even while seeking care from several providers. Somatic patients usually seek relief of physical symptoms through medical, not psychological, interventions. Patients with hypochondriasis or body dysmorphic disorder often initially avoid physicians out of fear or shame that they will be viewed as "crazy." Once they become patients, however, somatic patients also tend to pressure physicians to order many diagnostic tests and perform multiple procedures. They also tend not to adhere to medical recommendations.

Physician Reactions to Difficult Patients

Although DSM-IV-TR is a useful aid for making a diagnosis, family physicians often recognize a patient with a personality trait or unexplained physical complaint by their own reaction to the patient. Physicians working with difficult patients seem to have specific and characteristic reactions to these patients that need to be recognized, understood, and used for the patient's benefit. Patient-generated feelings provoked in the physician are created through the interpersonal interaction between patient and physician. These reactions to a patient should alert the physician to a possible diagnosis of a difficult patient. Typical physician reactions to patients that are provoked by the patient are also called *patient-generated countertransferences*. These include intense feelings, uncharacteristic fantasies, or atypical behaviors by the physician.

Intense Affects

Intense physician feelings elicited through patient interactions may include hate, fury, or frustration toward a patient (Groves, 1978; Strous et al., 2006). Alternatively, the physician may have strong feelings of love, sexual arousal, or wanting to rescue the patient or provide exceptionally good medical care. These may alternate with other wishes to avoid the patient, terminate the relationship, or transfer the patient to a colleague. In extreme cases, intense feelings aroused in a physician can become a focal point for leading the physician into boundary violations with a patient. These are extremely damaging to both parties and violate the tenets of professional behavior.

Fantasies

Physicians may recognize that they are interacting with a difficult patient by their own fantasies. These might include excessive worrying about a patient after normal work hours, dreams of discovering or being unable to discover a medical cause for complex somatic complaints, dreaming about a patient, or experiencing exaggerated or intrusive, angry, sexual, or curious fantasies about the patient during personal time.

Atypical Behaviors

A physician may notice behaviors with certain patients that are atypical for their usual customary medical practice. These unusual physician behaviors should trigger self-examination by the physician and consideration that the patient may have a personality or somatoform disorder. Frequently, difficult patients are capable of arousing unconscious reactions that lead to new and unusual physician behaviors.

Common atypical physician behaviors may include ordering tests to placate a patient, asking for more than the usual number of consults on a patient whose case does not seem medically complicated, suggesting increasingly aggressive diagnostic testing or procedures when the yield of these tests is likely to be low, repeatedly extending the time spent with a particular patient or family, lowering the customary fee, offering free treatment, or developing a personal (not professional) relationship with a patient. Common physician reactions associated with difficult patients are reviewed in Table 46-2.

Physicians can use the scope of patient-generated countertransferences (their feelings, fantasies, and atypical medical behaviors) as a valuable diagnostic aid, because difficult patients tend to provoke the same feelings in most physicians who deal with them. For example, a patient with a borderline personality disorder often leaves many physicians exhausted and worried about the patient's suicidal threats. A patient with multiple somatic complaints may leave physicians feeling frustrated that they cannot alleviate the patient's pain symptoms or suffering. Physicians who learn to recognize feelings provoked by patients will find it easier to identify the subtype of difficult patients according to the feelings elicited. More importantly, physicians who can recognize their unusual reactions will be better able to tolerate them and avoid acting out their feelings with a patient. This will improve the physician-patient relationship, medical decision making, and ultimately patient care (Feinstein et al., 1999).

General Management Principles for Difficult Patients

Attend to the physician-patient relationship.
Focus the interview on manageable goals within the time frame available.
Use psychotherapeutic techniques when interviewing the patient.
Attend to the patient's emotional needs.
Modify the patient's surroundings.
Improve the patient's capacity to test reality.
Empathize with the patient's worldview.
Accept the patient's limitations and strengths.
Manage unreasonable patient expectations, and set limits.
Question illogical feelings, thoughts, or behaviors.
Discuss and interpret defenses and coping style.
Prescribe medications as needed.
Use specific interventions and suggest better coping styles for each type of difficult patient.

Attending to a Problematic Alliance

To establish a good working alliance based on trust, acceptance, and confidence, the family physician should begin each patient encounter by listening, asking open-ended questions, and continually striving for empathy. The alliance is also fostered by the physician's own self-awareness, ability to acknowledge mistakes, and efforts to adapt to the patient's wishes or needs that will foster improved health. Problems often occur in developing an alliance with a patient who has a personality or somatoform disorder. If tension develops in the alliance, the physician should first ask what the patient thinks of the current problem. If the patient expresses the problem clearly, the physician should join with the patient in solving the problem to deliver effective medical care. If the problem is the physician-patient relationship, nondefensive reflective listening, clarifications, admitting mistakes, and expressing new efforts to improve the situation are often helpful. If the physician believes that there is a different problem affecting the alliance, the physician may say, "I believe that there is a different problem [identify the problem, e.g., psychosocial distress, problem drinking] that is affecting my ability to help you get well and offer you the best medical care available. We need to think about this problem and come up with some solutions."

Choosing a Focus for the Interview

When delivering medical care with a difficult patient, it is important to be consistent, reliable, and predictable to avoid future problems. Difficult patients typically experience an inability to verbalize or prioritize their most important medical or psychosocial concerns. For these patients, it is particularly important to strive for a mutually agreed focus for short-term and long-term treatment goals. It is often helpful to use a process called *informed shared decision making*, in which the physician takes time with the patient to discuss and negotiate the acute focus of medical care, long-term medical goals, strategies to achieve these goals, and specific timelines for accomplishing the prioritized medical plan (Feinstein et al., 1999).

Using Basic Psychotherapy Techniques

As is often the case, a general medical approach may not be sufficient to help a difficult patient. After a brief period of immersion in the patient's complaints, the family physician can respond with empathic responses, initially acknowledging the patient's fears and symptoms (see Table 46-1). If this is not helpful, the physician can use general psychotherapeutic techniques, such as confrontations, clarifications, or interpretations, directed toward the current problem interfering with medical care.

A *confrontation* is an observation by the physician offered to a patient for examination. It is usually a comment that draws attention to contradictions in the patient's beliefs, thoughts, feelings, or behaviors. For example, one might say to an anxious-somatic patient who denies that psychosocial factors might be contributing to her symptomatology, that her physical complaints may be caused by medical, psychological, or social stresses, and that her high levels of anxiety could be making her physical symptoms worse.

A *clarification* adds new information or perspective or elucidates misunderstandings, miscommunications, or other information that seems vague or confusing. The need for repeated clarifications occurs regularly with difficult patients. It is important to use clarifications before suggesting a new plan to correct the problem.

Interpretations are integrating comments that link confrontations and clarifications with the patient's current problem that is interfering with medical care. Interpretations can be made about the immediate medical situation and may address the patient's core beliefs, irrational thoughts, fears, maladaptive symptoms or behaviors, defense mechanisms, or coping style. Interpretations can also be directed at a difficulty in the physician-patient interaction, problems with the patient coping with the disease, problems in the patient's life circumstances, or patient refusal of a necessary medical workup or treatment. For example, an interpretation to a somatic patient who is refusing to acknowledge any psychosocial contribution to her symptoms might be the following:

I think you want relief from your physical symptoms. However, your refusal to consider that any of your psychosocial stress is contributing to your pain makes relief from your physical symptoms less likely [confrontation]. You then get annoyed with me and more depressed, which leads you to have new physical symptoms, and then you feel hopeless [clarification]. Instead of accepting my help to look broadly at all factors causing your pain, you blame me for not making you better. Your physical symptoms become an excuse for why you have difficulty managing your life [interpretation].

Such interpretations take practice but can powerfully restore a realistic and helpful physician-patient relationship.

Attending to Patient's Emotional Needs

Difficult patients are often exquisitely sensitive and distressed by internal emotional states, desires, and physical complaints. At a basic level, this often means listening empathically and carefully before attempting an intervention. It may be important initially to attend to physical or psychological pain. The most helpful initial intervention for some patients may be pain medication, to address physical complaints, or psychiatric medication, to address the patient's anxious, depressed, or agitated moods.

Modifying Patient's Surroundings

Difficult patients will often show fewer symptoms and a dramatic improvement in their acute emotional, physical, and behavioral functioning when the physician recruits additional support from the environment. This may mean bringing in a helpful spouse, friend, or other personal support into the patient's medical care. Other approaches to improving the patient's external environment may include allowing the nurse or office staff to spend more time with the patient and adding social services, self-help support groups, or psychiatric care. In extreme situations, using the psychiatric or medical emergency services can be helpful interventions. Some patients with personality disorders need to be managed with the help of the police.

Improving the Capacity to Test Reality

Difficult patients often have distorted views of realty. Stressed patients with cluster A and B personality disorders may transiently hear voices, hallucinate, have brief episodes of delusional thinking, or have other severe distortions in perception of reality (e.g., paranoia). This can occur with paranoid, schizotypal, and borderline personality disorders. If psychotic disturbances in reality are present, assess and treat these first before providing the requested medical care. Mobilizing external supports, using medications, or placing the patient in a safe and calm environment is often sufficient.

A stressed or somatic patient can also present with a tenuous or disturbed relationship to reality. Some hypochondriac patients appear delusional in their belief that they have a serious medical condition, even when medical testing contradicts this. Patients with body dysmorphic disorder are certain that a part of their body is defective, even when no visual evidence confirms this. Difficult patients may have a disturbance in the sense of reality, such as *derealization* (watching own life as if it were a movie), *depersonalization* (not feeling a part of one's own life), dramatic distortions of what has been said, transient misperceptions of real events (interpreted according to core beliefs or irrational thoughts), or misunderstanding the physician or patient role. Such reality distortions are not usually dangerous but can lead to severe problems in the physician-patient relationship if they are not recognized and addressed. Verbal techniques include uncovering and clarifying the patient's irrational thoughts or core beliefs and using confrontation, clarification, and interpretation to improve the patient's reality testing.

Empathizing with Patient's Worldview

All psychological interventions depend on the patient feeling understood by the physician. Listening and reflecting back the problems identified by the patient while empathizing with the patient's worldview can be extremely helpful in management. For example, an avoidant patient may refuse a prostate examination while having complaints of urinary hesitation and dribbling. The physician could say:

> *I understand your wish to avoid dealing with this problem. The testing—a blood test, the prostate-specific antigen (PSA) test, and a rectal examination—take only a few minutes and are not terribly uncomfortable. I am not trying to criticize you. I just think it is in your interest to get these examinations. Could we do this today? Then we can plan a way to relieve your symptoms.*

A patient may be certain there is a medical cause of pain. Empathy can be shown by performing a detailed physical exam; often the physical touch allows the patient to feel that the physician is taking him seriously.

Accepting Patient's Limitations and Strengths

Difficult patients are often rigid in their approach to the world and limited in their capacity for social and occupational functioning. They do not seek or make changes quickly. However, because they often seem reasonable at first impression, there can be a temptation to try to change the patient's belief. This typically leads to frustration for all concerned. It is more effective to accept the patient's beliefs and limited functioning, focus on the patient's strengths, and address how other issues or circumstances can be modified to help the patient cope.

Managing Unreasonable Expectations and Setting Reasonable Limits

Difficult patients often have unreasonable expectations. They may expect an unrealistic cure, never-ending diagnostic testing, constant availability of the medical team, special treatment, an unwarranted disability diagnosis, excessive pain medication, or many consultations. The physician must set limits on a patient's unreasonable expectations. Effective limit setting involves exploring why the patient believes that her particular expectation can or should be met. This involves a reasonable physician response about what can or cannot be done. Ultimately, limit setting is about agreeing to a reasonable approximation of the patient's request and tactfully saying "no" to requests that are not appropriate.

Questioning Illogical Feelings, Thoughts, and Behaviors

Patients often have irrational thoughts about their illness and the care that they will receive. They may also misunderstand the physician's efforts to communicate. For example, a patient may think that nothing can be done to ameliorate his physical complaints, or that a prescribed medication may make him sick; another may think that magnetic resonance imaging (MRI) will cure her, or that MRI may give her cancer. These types of irrational thoughts should be explored and the reality clarified. If done tactfully, this usually reduces anxiety in most patients. If a patient is frankly delusional, it is not useful to confront a patient's fixed belief. It is better to accept the patient's viewpoint while asking the patient's permission to have a different viewpoint.

Discussing Defense Mechanisms and Coping Styles

Patients may benefit from discussing their maladaptive defenses and coping styles and exploring ways of effectively dealing with their situation. For example, an obsessive-compulsive patient has a high cholesterol level and is calling the physician's office for more details about other laboratory tests. The results of the lipid profile are given to the patient, who now wants to know whether a lifestyle change or a statin medication would work better. With the recommendation for an initial lifestyle plan of more exercise and nutritional counseling, the patient becomes concerned about how to pay for this. Repeated efforts to help the patient with additional information are not making the patient feel any better. In fact, more information just raises more requests for additional information. The patient is asked to come for another visit. At this visit, the physician might say, "I can continue to give you more information, but it seems that anxiety is driving your questions. What are you worried about?" In essence, this says, "Your coping style of seeking information and details is not helping you. If you can recognize your anxiety about this subject, you may feel calmer." Review Table 46-1 for specific defenses and coping styles. Interpreting defenses or modifying a coping style requires the ability to recognize these and then to implement the preparatory confrontations and clarifications before making an interpretation and subsequently suggesting new ways to cope with the situation.

Prescribing Medication

Prescribing medication for patients with personality disorders is similar to prescribing for the major psychiatric disorders. Low-dose, typical or newer antipsychotics can be tried if the patient has psychotic symptoms, such as ideas of reference or severe paranoid ideation. A full dose of the newer antidepressants—selective serotonin reuptake inhibitors (SSRIs) or selective noradrenergic reuptake inhibitors (SNRIs)—is often recommended if the patient has depressive symptoms. Patients with an unstable mood who may be irritable or impulsive may be treated with full doses of a newer antidepressant, a monoamine oxidase inhibitor (MAOI), lithium, an anticonvulsant, or other mood stabilizer. An anxious patient can be treated with benzodiazepines, as needed. If the anxiety is persistent or chronic, the patient can be treated with low-dose and full-dose antidepressants (SSRI, SNRI) or MAOIs. The use of medication for patients with personality disorder can be very important for acute and long-term management.

The psychopharmacology of personality disorders can also be steered in the categorical direction toward specific personality disorders. There is evidence for the effectiveness of pharmacotherapy for patients with borderline personality disorder (Soloff, 2000, 2009; Nose et al., 2006). Affective instability and anger are treated with SSRIs and mood stabilizers, not antipsychotics, and impulsivity and aggressions are best treated with antipsychotics. Some studies of schizotypal personality disorder also indicate the effectiveness of antipsychotics (Markovitz, 2004; Soloff, 2009). The pharmacotherapy used for other personality disorders is variable.

Another approach to the pharmacology of personality disorders is to treat target symptoms. Using this approach with patients with borderline personality disorder has also been studied (Nose et al., 2006; Ypriitham, 2004). Borderline patients have three main symptom clusters: *cognitive-perceptual symptoms* (e.g., suspiciousness, referential thinking, paranoid ideation, hallucinations), *affective dysregulation* (e.g., irritability, unstable moods, anger or temper outbursts, hypomania, depression), *and impulse control symptoms* (e.g., suicide attempts, cutting, binge eating, substance abuse, reckless spending, gambling, promiscuity). Table 46-3 lists medications that have been used with some efficacy in treating symptoms associated with borderline personality disorder.

KEY TREATMENT

Mood symptoms can be treated with an SSRI, mood stabilizer, or antipsychotic medication (Nose et al., 2006; Soloff, 2009) (SOR: B).
Somatic symptoms can be treated with pain medications or SSRIs (SOR: B).
Psychotic symptoms can be treated with low doses of typical or atypical antipsychotic medications (SOR: B).
Irritability or impulsive behaviors can be treated with an SSRI, low-dose antipsychotic, or mood stabilizer (Markovitz, 2004; Soloff, 2009)† (SOR: B).
Drugs used for other personality disorders have trended toward SOR B and C and have variable effectiveness.

Table 46-3 Medication Dosages for Symptom Clusters in Personality Disorders*

Mood Symptoms, Anger	Psychotic Symptoms	Irritability, Impulsivity, Aggression
SSRIs Fluoxetine, 20-80 Sertraline, 100-200 Venlafaxine, 75-225	**Atypical Antipsychotic** Olanzapine, 2.5-10 Risperidone, 1-4 Aripiprazole 2.5-15 Clozapine, 75-460	**SSRIs** Fluoxetine, 20-80 Sertraline, 100-200 Venlafaxine, 75-400
Other Antidepressants Amitriptyline, 100-300 Amoxapine, 200-250	**Typical Antipsychotics** Haloperidol, 1-4 Perphenazine, 12-16	**Low-Dose Antipsychotic** See Psychotic Symptoms.
Antipsychotic for Anger See Psychotic Symptoms.	Trifluoperazine, 2-6 Thiothixene, 2-40 Loxapine, 13.5-14.5	**Mood Stabilizers** Divalproex, 1000-2000 Carbamazepine, 800-1200
Mood Stabilizers Divalproex, 1000-2000 Omega-3 fatty acid, 1000	Chlorpromazine, 105-120	Lamotrigine, 25-200 Lithium, 1000-2000 **Anxiety†** Alprazolam, 1-7 Clonazepam, 0.25-4

*All doses are daily doses in milligrams.
†Use with caution if anger, impulsivity, or substance abuse is present.
SSRIs, Selective serotonin reuptake inhibitors.

Strategic Principles for Working with Somatic Patients

Key Points

- Trying to explain somatic symptoms through a medical workup is the usual approach, although this is not always effective.
- Parallel diagnostic inquiry can help the physician maintain a therapeutic relationship with somatizing patients, even when physical explanations for symptoms cannot be found.
- Positive diagnostic features of somatization (chronicity, number of symptoms, patient defensiveness, provider suspicion, psychosocial evidence, medication history) help the clinician judge the likelihood that symptoms are somatoform.
- Emotion-focused interviewing may prove to be a useful technique for diagnosing specific subsets of somatizing behavior.
- The somatoform module of the PRIME-MD, or its self-administered counterpart, the PHQ-15, is the best diagnostic instruments for the clinician to use for formal diagnosis of somatization in primary care.

Parallel Diagnostic Inquiry

Although most clinicians regard patients with somatization as difficult, effective and rewarding approaches exist for recognizing and managing these patients. We first present a general approach to the diagnostic strategy with somatic patients, then describe a more specific diagnostic algorithm that has proved useful in managing patients with somatization.

In the course of a normal clinical encounter, a clinician (1) hears a complaint, (2) asks questions to elicit related symptoms and to understand the context of the symptoms more fully, and (3) performs the appropriate physical and laboratory examination. In other words, the clinician attempts to *explain* the symptoms. This universal clinical process is appropriate for many presenting complaints but has at least three important limitations. First, some symptoms are not easily explained; at some point, explanatory efforts can be seen as increasingly futile and irrelevant. Second, poor interrater reliability exists between explainers; on close inspection, symptom explanations do not meet scientific standards. Third, in some patients the sheer number of symptoms overwhelms the capacities of a symptom-by-symptom diagnostic approach. In other words, at some point it does not make sense to try to continue explaining symptoms or to pursue diagnostic workups. Even the most compulsive, biologically oriented physician knows when a diagnostic pursuit is pointless.

Before reaching this point, the physician needs a different mode of diagnostic pursuit. For example, a patient presents with several days of intermittent, heavy chest pain. The physician might test for angina pectoris, then for other cardiac causes, then for gastroesophageal reflux disease (GERD), while looking for pleuritic explanations and perhaps ruling out costochondritis. If all these tests are negative, the physician might initiate an exploration of psychological or psychosocial factors that could be responsible. After an exhaustive focus on various physical explanations for this pain, the patient might question the physician's competency. With no explanation for the chest pain, the patient also may think the physician is saying, in effect, "It must all be in your head."

It is not good practice to complete a physical workup for a symptom with no explanation. By that time, the physician could have elaborated a set of psychosocial connections to the symptoms. By pursuing a strategy of *parallel diagnostic inquiry*, the physician can avoid this trap. This process begins by explaining that all symptoms, illnesses, and diseases are produced, sustained, and amplified by interacting physical and psychosocial factors. Symptoms can be explained as having a physical cause with psychosocial factors that are secondarily important, and vice versa. Many symptoms, diseases, and illnesses with biomedical or psychosocial etiology produce symptoms and problems in both domains. Therefore the physician should inquire into both domains concurrently, in parallel. Thus, while eliciting the characteristics of the chest pain and arranging for an electrocardiogram, the physician should also ask about stressors, depression, and panic. The physician can incorporate both physical and psychosocial inquiry into a comprehensive understanding of the presenting problem and of the patient. If the workup for angina pectoris, valvular disease, pericarditis, pleuritis, GERD, and costochondritis is negative, the physician is already far down the road with the psychosocial inquiry. The point is never to communicate directly or give the impression that the "real" workup has failed, leaving a psychosocial explanation. Rather than viewing psychosocial explanations simply as the only ones left after a failed biomedical workup, the physician should remember that positive diagnostic features are also associated with somatization spectrum disorders. The physician should consider the following issues as suggestive of, but not definitive for, somatization:

Chronicity. Most symptoms are quick to improve or disappear. The longer a symptom persists, particularly after diagnostic efforts, the greater the likelihood that it is a somatic complaint.

Number of symptoms. Somatization disorder, abridged somatization disorder, and multisomatoform disorder are all defined by the presence of numerous unexplained symptoms; the more explained symptoms, the more unexplained symptoms. Therefore, patients with many symptoms should be provisionally regarded as having a somatoform component to the illness.

Provider suspicion. An experienced physician's initial judgment about an explanation eventually being found has about 90% accuracy.

Patient defensiveness. Fierce denials or anger by the patient when exploring psychosocial dimensions suggests somatization.

Psychosocial evidence. Major current stressors, a family history of illness behavior, violence or abuse, or comorbid depression or anxiety are all associated with somatization. Moreover, these factors have management implications.

Medication history. Look for polypharmacy, multiple drug reactions or "allergies," multiple drug failures, and prior use of psychotropic drugs and controlled substances.

For the family practitioner, the finer points of diagnostic classification of somatic manifestations do not generally contain corresponding management differences. Thus, the physician would manage a patient with somatization disorder similar to one with multisomatoform disorder, or even somatoform pain disorder. There may be exceptions. However, using videotaped case studies and clinical trials, Davanloo (1990, 2001) proposed four main patterns of somatization: striated muscle tension, smooth muscle tension, cognitive-perceptual disruption, and conversion. These patterns can be elicited with a simple interviewing technique known as *emotion-focused interviewing* (Abbass, 2005). This technique involves examining the emotional system by actively exploring emotionally charged situations and observing the response. This allows classification into a somatization category for specific short-term psychotherapy. Psychiatrists have developed credible research efforts aimed at classifying somatic patients into more refined, therapeutically meaningful categories, which are beyond the scope of this chapter.

Although there is no formal evidence that active case finding (testing for disease in patients whose presenting complaint does not suggest it) for somatization is beneficial, there is a place for confirmatory testing in suspected cases, and perhaps for diagnostic testing in high-risk situations. A number of diagnostic instruments are available, but the emerging "gold standard" in primary care, both for research and clinical purposes, is the somatoform module of the PRIME-MD (Spitzer et al., 1994) or its self-administered derivative, the PHQ-15 (Kroenke et al., 2002). This instrument can make the diagnosis of multisomatoform disorder in a few minutes and can track the severity of the symptoms.

Management Algorithm for Somatization

Kroenke's algorithm can lead to a medical explanation, an antidepressant-responsive condition, or presumptive evidence of chronic somatization. Primary care clinicians can use the following guidelines when dealing with patients who present with symptoms (Kroenke, 2002):

- In the patient with chronic somatization, the physician should follow the guidelines offered in Smith's consultation letter (see next section).
- Many somatic patients have sustained serious abuse. The physician should inquire about abuse, and in most cases offer a referral to a skilled mental health professional.

- Antidepressants may be effective against some forms of somatization. Further study is needed.
- Cognitive-behavioral therapy, group psychotherapy, and short-term dynamic psychotherapy are effective for somatic patients. If available, such therapy should be offered.
- St. John's wort has been shown to be effective against somatoform disorders.
- Massage therapy may be effective for somatic pain syndromes.

When dealing with potential somatization, the clinician can never become complacent and assume without further inquiry that any given symptom is somatoform. If the symptom is not medically explained, a focused history and physical examination are warranted, and if there are physical abnormalities, additional laboratory work may be indicated. Some symptoms suggest conditions that require immediate attention, such as dyspnea, crushing chest pain, syncope, severe abdominal pain, and sudden severe headache. Because many symptoms resolve spontaneously, however, the physician is often justified in deferring an extensive workup until nonthreatening symptoms have time to resolve. Follow-up is preferable to workup; if symptoms persist at follow-up, the physician is justified in beginning a focused diagnostic workup.

What are the patient's specific concerns or expectations? For the one third of patients whose symptoms are neither acutely serious nor readily explainable, two patient questions are in order:

1. "Is there anything else you are worried about?" This question elicits unexpressed concerns. Patients can be concerned that their symptoms might mean something serious, or they can be concerned about a particular disease such as cancer. They might be concerned about the prognosis of the symptom, wondering whether it is advisable to take a planned vacation, or whether they are likely to miss work. They might be concerned about whether further testing is ahead.
2. "Is there anything else you have thought might be helpful?" This question is designed to elicit additional expectations. Some patients present for symptom relief, others for an explanation. Some patients want further diagnostic tests, and others expect a referral to a specialist or a mental health professional. This question helps the clinician address expectations that might not have been voiced during the discussion of specific symptoms.

The physician should ask himself or herself three additional questions:

1. Does the patient have a depressive or anxiety disorder? Most patients with somatic symptoms meet criteria for a mental diagnosis. If such a diagnosis is present, prescribing an antidepressant or other treatment known to be effective is appropriate. In addition to the benefit to the patient's overall health, it can specifically improve the symptom severity.
2. Does the patient have a syndrome known to respond to antidepressants? There is some evidence that syndromes such as fibromyalgia, irritable bowel syndrome, premenstrual syndrome, chronic pain disorders, and chronic headaches, or even recurrent migraine headaches respond to antidepressants (O'Malley et al., 1999). Thus, a trial of antidepressants is warranted in these patients.

3. Does the patient have a history of chronic somatization? The physician can answer this question affirmatively only after working through the previous questions and determining that the patient has had a number of unexplained complaints over time, or at least had a single unexplained symptom that has persisted for a long time. At this point, a number of management recommendations apply.

Consultation Letter

It has been shown that writing a consultation letter to assist other physicians or health care providers improves the health of patients with somatization disorder (Smith et al., 1986), abridged somatization disorder (Smith et al., 1995), and multisomatoform disorder (Dickinson et al., 2003) and also reduces costs. The recommendations in the consultation letter improve outcomes for somatic patients, as well as making these patients seem less burdensome and difficult for clinicians. The consultation letter should include the following:

- Notification of physician or other health care provider that the patient meets criteria for somatization.
- Reassuring information about the nonlethal prognosis of somatization.
- Encouragement to schedule the patient for regular, brief visits, rather than waiting for the patient to develop a new symptom or schedule an urgent visit.
- Recommendation to follow all complaints with a focused physical examination and generally to pursue workups only if physical findings are present.
- To avoid hospitalization, surgery, and subspecialty referral, if possible.
- To view the symptoms as part of an unconscious process, and to avoid telling the patient, "It's all in your head."

Pharmacotherapy and Psychotherapy for Somatoform Disorders

In a review of 34 randomized clinical trials of treatments for somatoform disorders, two thirds involved somatization disorder or one of its less severe variants (Kroenke, 2007). CBT was effective in 11 of these 13 studies. Antidepressants were effective in four of five pharmacotherapy trials. The consultation letter was effective in 8 of 16 studies. Effective treatments for conversion disorder and pain disorder have not yet been demonstrated.

Short-term group therapy has been shown in at least two trials to have modest effectiveness for somatizing patients (Kashner et al., 1995; Lidbeck, 1997). These interventions may be difficult to offer in the primary care setting, unless the physician has access to mental health professionals trained in these techniques.

Other treatments have also proved effective. Short-term dynamic psychotherapy has been studied extensively for a variety of somatizing syndromes and appears to be effective in reducing symptom severity and reducing costs. Access to this therapy depends on the availability of a skilled psychotherapist. St. John's wort has been shown to be unambiguously effective for somatizing patients in two randomized, double-blind, placebo-controlled trials (Muller et al., 2004; Volz et al., 2002). Massage therapy should be mentioned as a potential therapy for the somatic patient

KEY TREATMENT

Cognitive-behavioral therapy is effective in the treatment of somatoform disorder (Kroenke, 2007) (SOR: A).

Antidepressants are effective in treatment of somatoform disorders (Kroenke, 2007) (SOR: A).

Short-term group therapy has modest effectiveness for somatizing patients (Kashner et al., 1995; Lidbeck, 1997) (SOR: A).

Short-term dynamic psychotherapy may be effective in reducing symptom severity in somatizing syndromes (Abbass et al., 2004) (SOR: B).

St. John's wort is effective in somatizing patients (Muller et al., 2004; Volz et al., 2002) (SOR: B).

Massage therapy is effective against somatoform back pain and other pain syndromes (Cherkin et al., 2001; Owens and Ehrenreich, 1991) (SOR: B).

with musculoskeletal symptoms; it has been shown effective against somatoform back pain and other pain syndromes.

Interventions for Specific Personality Disorders

To utilize specific interventions for each subtype of personality disorders is the art of medicine. A basic specific approach is outlined for each disorder in Tables 46-1 and 46-2. This schema includes choosing the correct DSM-IV-TR cluster; identifying the specific personality diagnosis; understanding the patient's core beliefs, irrational thoughts, specific fears, main defense mechanisms, and coping style; and recognizing common physician reactions to each personality disorder. Using this knowledge, interventions are then tailored for each disorder (see Table 46-2). This conceptual framework allows the formulation of helpful interventions for the primary care management of specific personality disorders.

Paranoid Personality Disorder

When interacting with a paranoid patient, the physician typically reacts with fear, mistrust, and a sense of danger. The physician may also feel blamed or accused. The patients may have a similar fear of being hurt, exploited, or invaded. Patients often react to suggestions for medical care with mistrust, excessive fault finding, sensitivity to criticism, or hypervigilance. They may collect small insults as proof of the world's injustices. When invasive medical procedures are performed, the paranoid patient may react with full-blown panic and anxiety; many paranoid patients unconsciously experience a body invasion as a homosexual assault. Patients with paranoid personality disorder rely most heavily on projection as their main defense. Using projection, they accuse the physician of hurts that reflect their own aggressive style of hurting others.

A physician working with the paranoid patient needs to empathize with the patient's mistrust and hypersensitivity. The physician should avoid arguing or attempting to reason the patient out of the paranoid worldview. It is extremely important to use confrontations and clarifications to help correct the patient's distorted perceptions about his medical care. Unfortunately, direct confrontation of a delusion or hallucinations (the most troubling deficits in reality testing) often has the paradoxical effect of making these patients more suspicious of the physician.

Acknowledging that the patient's suspicion has an emotional reality can be helpful. Rather than confronting mistrust or suspicions directly, the physician can acknowledge responsibility for any actions that the patient might have perceived as mistakes. For example, the physician could say, "I did not appreciate how it might hurt you when I ordered that lab test." It may also help to express understanding and concern for the patient's rights. If there is a medical need for special testing of which the patient is suspicious, acknowledge the patient's fears, and describe openly and honestly the details of the procedures, potential for pain, and likely risks and benefits. If the patient still refuses to comply, do not use direct persuasion. Ask the patient, "Is it all right with you if we have different opinions?" With the patient's consent to hearing a different opinion, openly discuss the medical necessity of the testing without trying to resolve the problem. At future office visits, attempt new and ongoing discussions of the patient's fears of complying with the request for specialized testing. It may take months for the paranoid patient to trust enough to consent to the appropriate treatment. Counterprojective statements by the physician can diffuse the projections and distortions directed at the physician. The physician can use counterprojective remarks to help the patient access her feelings while focusing angry or suspicious feelings away from the physician toward others who are not present. For example, a physician harassed by an angry, suspicious, or blaming patient could use a counterprojective statement such as, "You felt angry and hurt when the lab technician drew your blood. You must be fearful of the results of these tests."

Schizoid and Schizotypal Personality

Physicians typically feel uninvolved or detached or have a desire to break through the aloofness of schizoid and schizotypal patients. *Schizoid* patients may give the physician the impression that the patient is a loner. A common physician reaction to *schizotypal* patients is a feeling that the patient is alone and "weird or strange." Superficially, patients with either diagnosis fear personal contact, emotional involvement, and invasion of their privacy. At the deepest level, they long for emotional contact that is not overwhelming. They may react to suggestions for medical care with avoidance, withdrawal, apparent emotional detachment, or denial of the medical problem. Schizotypal patients function at a psychotic level, with impaired reality testing manifested by magical, odd, or psychotic modes of thinking. Schizotypal patients use regression to schizoid fantasy and, to a lesser extent, denial as their main defenses. They appear increasingly idiosyncratic and withdrawn when stressed. Schizotypal personality disorder appears to be a significant risk factor for the future development of schizophrenia, although most patients do not go on to develop overt schizophrenia.

Schizoid patients do not appear psychotic or idiosyncratic in their behavior. They are disinterested in intimate contacts with others, appear detached and unemotional, and wish to be left alone. Infrequently, the schizoid personality will also be associated with the future development of schizophrenia. When stressed by a medical problem, schizoid patients will use isolation and intellectualization to hide their emotions. If necessary, they will regress to childlike functioning or use psychotic denial of their illness as their main defenses.

Patients with schizotypal and schizoid personalities tend to experience their physician as intruding into their privacy, which may drive them away from the physician. They are relieved when the physician is not present and prefer fewer medical appointments and contacts. It is generally helpful to accept their lack of sociability at a level that does not demand involvement or permit total withdrawal. Neutral or unemotional expressions of medical information are most likely to be heard and used.

Antisocial Personality Disorder, Malingering, and Factitious Disorders

Common physician reactions to a patient with antisocial personality disorder are feelings of being used, exploited, or deceived. This can lead to physician anger and wishes to be free of the patient, uncover lies, and punish or imprison the patient. These patients fear that they will become vulnerable, lose respect or admiration from others, and become easy prey to manipulation when they become ill. They expect to be exploited, demeaned, or humiliated. Like the narcissistic patient, they often have low self-esteem, excessive self-love, compensatory feelings of superiority, grandiosity, recklessness, emotional shallowness, and show a lack of concern for others. They often react to medical care with entitled demands for special treatment. When caught in dishonesty, they may angrily attack or devalue the physician. They may resort to other psychopathic manipulations of deception, lying, cheating, or stealing. In fact, their friendly, facile, slick, superficial charm, and intelligent appearance is often beguiling for the physician. They can lose reality testing when stressed by the potential of getting caught in their deceptive practices. This is typically manifested by impulsive actions that reveal severely impaired or sometimes psychotic judgments. When receiving medical care for a legitimate illness, they typically function at the same level and often appear to have the same characteristic issues as the narcissistic personality disorder (Kernberg, 1992). They can often be managed similarly (see Narcissistic Personality Disorder).

To intervene with an antisocial patient, the family physician needs to be alert and anticipate that the patient may be requesting unnecessary medical care or even malingering or presenting a factitious disorder This patient may be seeking the secondary gain of illegal benefits or money, excuses for work absenteeism, or avoidance of legal problems, or just seeking caretaking. It is important not to collude with the patient's plans for secondary gain inadvertently. For example, if the physician thinks that a patient's request for disability is fraudulent or unwarranted, the patient should not be referred for additional evaluations. If deception is suspected, the physician can ask for verification of symptoms from other reliable sources. There is often dishonesty in a patient's communication in the form of withholding important information, partial truths, or outright lying, cheating, or stealing. If this occurs, avoid the common reaction of moralizing. Instead, grant the patient the reality that he has the ability to fool all the physicians if he wants. The patient can be told that the result of deception is that the physician may make poorly informed medical decisions. This will ultimately result in the patient receiving inadequate or poor medical care. The physician can explore with the patient why he needs to act self-destructively. Patients may need to be reminded that the physician's role is to help with medical problems and not to pass judgment or help the patient obtain unfair medical benefits.

Histrionic Personality Disorder; Conversion or Somatic Symptoms

Patients with histrionic personality disorder have an emotionally expressive style, seek excessive attention, are often dramatic, and may present with a conversion disorder. Physicians may feel flattered, captivated, seduced, or sexually aroused by these patients. Alternatively, the physician may feel overwhelmed by the patient's exaggerated or excessive emotions, embarrassed by the sexual overtures, depleted, or confounded by unexplained physical symptoms, such as pseudoseizures, paralysis, and mutism. These patients may unconsciously use their symptoms to elicit attention or support from the physician (Bornstein and Gold, 2008). They may also use their sexuality to recruit others to satisfy their needs to be taken care of or romantically pursued. They fear that they are not desired and will lose the care or admiration of others.

There are two different levels of functioning with the histrionic personality disorder. Kernberg (1984, 1992) describes a neurotically functioning "hysteric" who shows intact reality testing, defenses centered on repression, and stable and mature relations with others. The female hysteric has a flirtatious, clinging, childlike dependence in intimate relationships but can function at mature levels in social and work situations. Male hysterics have similar psychological conflicts, but may appear as "macho" or "effeminate" (Kernberg, 1992). The hysteric of either sex often reacts to medical care with regression to a childlike, sexualized, dependent, and clinging position. They seek to gratify their wishes for dependent care by seducing or flattering others. Outside the office, they usually function well.

By contrast, the "histrionic patient" (Kernberg, 1984, 1992) can display transient losses of reality testing, defenses centered on splitting, and chaotic sexualized relations with others and a range of unexplained physical or somatic complaints. The histrionic patient is self-centered and self-indulgent, with a pervasive childlike dependence that extends from intimate relationships into all aspects of social and occupational functioning. Female histrionics typically act flirtatiously but may become indignant when a man shows sexual interest. Male histrionics also show the self-centered and dependent pattern, but may also have hypochondrical and antisocial features. Histrionics of both genders may seek medical care because of unexplained medical symptoms. They may react to medical care with regression but, unlike the hysteric, use defenses centered on "splitting"; they may see the physician as "all good or all bad" and can be extremely devaluing. They may appear severely self-centered, attention seeking, diffusely sexual, hypochondrical, somatic, and exploitative. All this may be coupled with an exhausting dependency on the physician.

In working with hysterics and histrionic patients, a physician needs to be friendly, not overly warm or reserved. Hysterics and histrionics often are helped when the physician uses parallel inquiry when they present with somatic complaints. Hysterics also may benefit from some gratification of their dependent wishes and a free discussion of their fears and emotions. They can often be reassured by an educational and informational approach to their medical illness and are capable of expressing gratitude to the physician. In contrast, the intense dependency of histrionics is often made worse by gratifying the patient's needs. Offering excessive emotional care may make them greedy or demanding for satisfaction of their needs. Histrionics benefit from firm, kind limit setting (especially to their sexual overtures), with neutral acknowledgment and gratification of their reasonable needs. They may be further helped by focusing on their distortions in reality perception and through interpretation of their splitting mechanisms.

Borderline Personality Disorder; Somatization Symptoms or Disorder

Borderline patients, many of whom also have somatization disorders, frequently become dependent on their physicians in an extremely demanding, clinging, helpless, or self-destructive manner. Physicians may feel manipulated, angry, depleted, exhausted, or self-doubting. They may want to end the patient relationship or rescue the patient from herself, or they can be drawn into a cycle of extensive medical testing to try and explain many somatic complaints. These patients fear separation or abandonment and may react to potential losses with panic, emotional instability, anger, or impulsive (suicidal or self-destructive) actions. They may seek care and utilize defenses, which appears as a somatization disorder. These somatic symptoms and borderline personality structure often represent the sequelae of childhood abuse, sexual abuse, or other trauma (Kernberg, 1975; Sansone et al., 2001).

Use of parallel inquiry to uncover a history of trauma is often most helpful for the patient complaining of multiple somatic complaints. Borderline patients often react to medical care with an aggressive or dependent clinging to their physician and other caretakers. They may angrily devalue the physician who does not adequately explain their symptoms and may make entitled demands for special treatment when they become worried or frustrated. They tend to relate to others as "all good or all bad," which significantly contributes to their poor life functioning.

Typically, reality testing is intact. However, under stress, borderline patients may temporarily lose reality testing and manifest severe distortions in perceptions or sense of reality. They may misunderstand the physician's intentions or instructions. They may also experience episodes of derealization, depersonalization, or brief psychotic episodes. Borderline patients have *identity diffusion*, extreme fluctuations in self-perception from the grandiose to an excessively harsh underestimation of their abilities. They also have stormy and chaotic relationships with others. They rely heavily on splitting, projective identification, projection, and devaluing.

Office management of borderline patients involves an empathic understanding of their fears. These fears revolve around the threat to their security or fears of separation or abandonment and, secondarily, sensitivity to rejection, or fears of humiliation. They require firm limit setting (e.g., what physician can realistically offer). Attempts to satisfy these patients' intense needs often result in an exhausted or angry physician. This can be avoided by setting realistic limits while offering the patient different ideas or options for medical care, and suggestions of more adaptive behaviors. Initial interventions should attempt to establish reality testing or correct reality distortions. If reality testing is intact, the most helpful interventions can be aimed at attending to medical care while decreasing the pathologic splitting defenses by using confrontation, clarification, and interpretations of the problematic situation.

The primary treatment for borderline personality disorder is psychotherapy complemented by symptom-targeted pharmacotherapy. Certain types of psychotherapy and medications are effective in the treatment of borderline patients. Most will need extended psychotherapy to attain and maintain lasting improvement in their personality, interpersonal problems, and overall functioning. Pharmacotherapy often has an important adjunctive role, especially for diminution of symptoms such as affective instability, impulsivity, psychotic-like symptoms, and self-destructive behavior (APA, 2001; Soloff, 2008).

Narcissistic Personality Disorder

The family physician's reactions to the narcissistic patient are often difficult to manage. The superior, entitled, self-loving, arrogant attitude of these patients can be intimidating. They may elicit feelings of being devalued and inferior. The physician may have concerns about the patient's anger and criticism. Alternatively, the lack of empathy and interpersonal exploitation of these patients can readily provoke the physician to anger, a wish to retaliate with harsh criticism, or a desire to end the patient-physician relationship.

The core fears of narcissistic patients are the result of a fragile self-esteem and their need for constant approval and praise from others. They fear loss of admiration, potency, and power, and fear being exploited when vulnerable. Any perceived insult to their "grandiose self" (Kernberg, 1984, 1992) makes them feel rejected, deflated, and criticized and frequently results in feelings of rage, shame, or humiliation.

The narcissistic patient has generally intact reality testing, yet can undergo severe reality distortions when he perceives slights, rejection, or competition from others with talent. Those narcissistic patients who have paranoid and antisocial features (Kernberg, 1992) have a worse prognosis. They often have a fragile identity that can swing from the grandiose to the worthless. They rely heavily on splitting mechanisms to regulate their self-esteem. They portray themselves as grandiose and superior. This helps defend against feelings of extreme inadequacy and vulnerability. They can devalue, viciously attack, or degrade those around them when they act in a self-important way. Alternatively, as splitting operates, they may idealize or be envious of others who are, for the moment, seen as more powerful or successful. In this position, their self-esteem plummets, as evidenced by their sense of worthlessness and their reports of deprecating and degrading self-attacks.

Office management of the narcissistic patient, as well as many antisocial patients, requires that the physician not mistake the patient's superior and entitled manner for genuine confidence. When being verbally devaluing, it may help the physician to view the demeaning or verbally attacking patient as a wounded child having a "temper tantrum." This may prevent the physician from retaliating, by demeaning the patient, which only escalates a maladaptive interaction. Intervening in the face of a devaluing attack involves acknowledging that the patient feels hurt and that the patient also has a right to her opinions. If this patient can discuss these hurt feelings with a nonjudgmental and empathic physician, the problems generally resolve and a good physician-patient alliance can be restored. If this is not possible, offer the patient the right to seek another expert for consultation. This offer needs to be made without malice, defensiveness, or apology. This may help the patient calm down and reconsider his position.

In a long-term relationship with a narcissistic patient, the current splitting can be interpreted. This can be done by reminding patients that they previously praised the skill and abilities of the physician. Patients can be asked why they are now so critical and angry. When this is effective, it will allow patients to discuss their perception of insults to their self-esteem.

Avoidant Personality Disorder and Somatization Disorder

Patients with avoidant personality disorder suffer with feelings of inadequacy and fear of criticism. They have low self-esteem and believe that they are inept and inadequate. They believe that others are critical and disapproving until proved otherwise. Although avoidant patients crave human relationships and affection, their fear of being criticized, rejected, embarrassed, or hurt causes them to initially avoid social situations or meeting new people. Their shyness and avoidance protect them from their fears of being rejected or humiliated. In medical encounters, they often can seek psychosocial help through somatic complaints. This somatic approach of physical complaints can conceal psychological issues and makes them feel safer than revealing unconscious or unexpressed emotions. They prefer not to divulge personal aspects of themselves because this may leave them vulnerable. Their timidity, hypersensitivity, and cautiousness can generate feelings of frustration or annoyance in the physician. Patients with avoidant personality disorder typically use defense mechanisms based on repression, including inhibition, phobia, and isolation.

Managing avoidant patients is more effective when the physician utilizes both parallel inquiry and emotion-focused interviewing. It is most helpful when the physician can recognize and empathize with the patient's social fears, including the fear of the physician. Patients may minimize symptoms or delay seeking help because of fear of the physician or the feeling that they are unworthy or unimportant. Some avoidant patients do the reverse; they can only ask for emotional help through somatic symptoms. The physician should help the patient understand her symptoms and any specific fears revolving around the diagnostic or therapeutic plan. Irrational fears and thoughts can be gently corrected and alternative interpretations offered. Patients should be encouraged, with appropriate support, to face their somatic and other fears as the best way of mastering them. If the physician feels frustration or annoyance, it is often helpful to encourage the patient to describe what he is finding most difficult in the medical care or proposed medical plan.

Dependent Personality Disorder and Somatization Disorder

Patients with dependent personality disorder may be characterized by an exaggerated need for care or a need for direction from another person, or both. Dependent patients may present initially with a physical illness. These initial medical complaints, which often elicit and exaggerated caretaking response from physicians and may introduce into the medical relationship a tendency to return to the physician with increasing somatic complaints (Bornstein and Gold, 2008). Dependent patients often feel helpless and inadequate in making even minor decisions, such as what to do next medically, what to wear, or whom to befriend. They have a core belief that they cannot function alone, are completely incapable of taking care of themselves, and must have someone else provide care and make decisions. Their major fear is of independence.

Although both borderline patients and dependent patients are extremely dependent on others, they react very differently to the threat of losing a significant other. The borderline patient becomes angry or enraged, whereas the dependent patient becomes submissive and obsequious. Dependent personality disorder patients use defenses that include regression, passive-aggression, and reaction formation.

Patients with dependent personality disorder are submissive and clinging with their caretakers because of fear of losing them. The dependence of these patients can make physicians feel annoyed, drained, or depleted. Physicians may tend to deny reasonable needs of the excessively dependent patient. The secondary gains that dependent personality patients receive from an illness also create extra challenges for the physician. Use of parallel diagnostic inquiry and emotion-focused interviewing is helpful. The physician must understand and empathize with the patient's need for being taken care of while encouraging and fostering independent thinking and action by the patient. Because these patients often use medication, alcohol, food, and other means to satisfy their dependency needs, the physician must exercise caution in how these are used in the therapeutic plan. Unreasonable expectations for being taken care of should be gently discouraged by the physician.

Obsessive-Compulsive Personality Disorder, Hypochondriasis, and Body Dysmorphic Disorders

Patients with obsessive-compulsive personality disorder (OCPD) are preoccupied with details, order, and control. Although their labels are similar, these patients differ in substantial ways from patients with obsessive-compulsive disorder (OCD). OCD patients have recurrent disturbing thoughts or obsessions that create marked subjective distress. Patients with hypochondriasis are obsessed about fear of an illness triggered by somatic sensations. Patients with body dysmorphic syndrome obsess about a bodily defect, such as a malformed nose, which is not readily apparent to an observer. OCD patients may be driven to ritualistic or compulsive behaviors, such as handwashing or checking rituals. Patients with hypochondriasis and body dysmorphic syndromes are often compulsively "doctor shopping." These behaviors help them manage, control, and distract them from intense anxiety.

The core adaptive traits of patients with OCPD are orderliness, attention to detail, and an emphasis on rational thinking and logic. These traits are lifelong patterns that many patients use adaptively in their professional life. Patients with OCPD often view these traits as a personal strength. However, often their attention to detail leads them to perfectionist beliefs, worry, or ruminations that they must not make mistakes or be imperfect. They can interpret rules, regulations, and values rigidly and stubbornly. Patients with OCPD often ruminate and are prone to interpret minor physical changes as worrisome somatic complaints (McGuire and Shore, 2001).

Because they are uncomfortable with feelings and emotions, patients with somatic presentations may be unconsciously motivated to seek reassurance from their physician. They may fear disorderliness and dirt. The compulsive, critical, controlling, self-righteous side of their personalities often creates difficulty in relationships with co-workers, friends, and family. They can be stingy, orderly, and obstinate. Physicians, who often have obsessive-compulsive traits themselves, may feel irritated and competitive with these patients about who controls the diagnostic workup or treatment plan.

Patients with OCPD use defense mechanisms such as intellectualization, isolation, displacement, doing/undoing, and reaction formation. Using reaction formation, they may behave in a superficially deferential or obsequious manner to repress from themselves and hide from others their critical and self-righteous feelings. These defenses are used against their anger and dependency needs, which are often consciously denied. Illness often represents a dangerous threat to the sense of self-control in OCPD patients. A past illness can lead to a future somatic presentation. The physician should understand and empathize with this loss of self-control while helping the patient regain some control in the management of the problem. Struggle or conflict with the patient over control of medical care should be avoided. Reality distortions, including excessive perfectionism, idealization of logic, and avoidance of feeling, can be gently elicited, explored, and worked through with the patient.

Self-Defeating Personality Disorder

Self-defeating patients are often depressed, suffering, and self-sacrificing. They repeatedly make bad choices that lead to failure or pain. This diagnostic category was eliminated from DSM-IV-TR because of a gender bias (female) and an inability to reach a general agreement for the diagnostic features. However, it is included in this chapter because patients who are self-defeating are frequently seen and present difficult clinical problems for many physicians that still need to be addressed. A common physician reaction to self-defeating patients is an urge to rescue them from their own self-destructiveness. Trying too vigorously to help these patients often results in a worsening of their hypochondriasis or somatic complaints. This often leaves the physician frustrated, angry, defeated, self-doubting, self-blaming, or hopeless; alternatively, the physician may fantasize about the patient suffering or dying. Self-defeating patients are excessively dependent on love,

support, and acceptance from others. They cannot directly express their anger and may be harshly self-judgmental. They fear recovery, which to them means losing love and care. Improvement of their medical condition often leads to the development of new complaints that have no somatic basis.

Mildly self-defeating patients can make the physician feel mildly guilty that the physician is causing pain or suffering or not helping enough. The patient and the physician both suffer. However, these patients ultimately can be helped and can express genuine gratitude toward the physician. The patients with a severe self-defeating personality disorder may passive-aggressively reject the help of their physicians and make the physician feel helpless and responsible for the patients' severe suffering or self-destructiveness.

Physicians can manage self-defeating patients by empathizing with the patient's realistic medical suffering, symptoms, or complaints from the illness. It should not be suggested that the patient's symptoms are psychological or that they will improve or be cured quickly. These optimistic predictions by the physician may paradoxically increase the patient's symptoms, complaints, telephone calls, and office visits. Potential recovery can be presented as a likely but distant reality. If patients cannot permit or admit relief of the symptoms, they can be asked to speak less about their symptoms for the benefit of other family members.

Conclusion

Difficult patients contribute significantly to physician dissatisfaction with medical practice. The result is often poor quality of medical care for this difficult but all too common patient population. Special diagnostic, management, and intervention strategies exist for working with patients who have personality disorders or somatic complaints in the family medicine setting. The schema combines DSM-IV-TR diagnosis and cognitive-behavioral and psychodynamic viewpoints involving the patient's core beliefs and irrational thoughts, fears, defenses and coping style, behaviors, adherence to medical treatment, and use of medical services. Common physician reactions, general strategies, and specific physician interventions are also addressed, to maintain a working physician-patient relationship that permits the delivery of needed medical care.

References

The complete reference list is available online at www.expertconsult.com.

Web Resources

www.ncbi.nlm.nih.gov/pubmedhealth/PMH0001935
    National Center for Biotechnology Information
    Reviews of the major personality disorders and treatments

www.nmha.org/go/information/get-info/personality-disorders
    Mental Health America
    Consumer information about personality disorders

www.nice.org.uk/search/guidancesearchresults.jsp?keywords=Personailty+Disorders&newSearch=true&searchType=Guidance
    National Institute for Health and Clinical Excellence (NICE)
    Practice guidelines for personality disorders

www.guideline.gov/search/search.aspx?term=personality+disorders
    National Guideline Clearinghouse
    Practice guidelines for borderline and antisocial personality disorders

www.nlm.nih.gov
    National Institute of Mental Health on Somatization and Personality Disorders

www.psych.org
    American Psychiatric Association
    Information on somatic and personality disorders

Anxiety and Depression

Brian Rothberg and Christopher D. Schneck

Overview

Key Points

- Depression and anxiety increase medical morbidity and mortality.
- Mood disorders comprise unipolar and bipolar disorder.
- Anxiety disorders comprise eight disorders, of which generalized anxiety disorder and panic disorder are frequently encountered in primary care settings.
- Treatment of depression and anxiety improves overall health outcomes.
- The majority of mood and anxiety disorders are treated in primary care settings.

Major depression and anxiety disorders are the two most common psychiatric illnesses in the United States and are particularly prevalent in primary care settings. Despite the relative availability of specialty psychiatric care in the United States, most patients with depression or anxiety disorder continue to receive their treatment from primary care physicians. Moreover, patients with both medical illness and comorbid mood or anxiety disorder frequently have poorer outcomes, experience more prolonged and difficult treatment, and have greater morbidity and mortality than patients without psychiatric illness (Katon, 2003). Conversely, treating underlying depressive and anxiety disorders not only improves the emotional well-being of patients, but also improves overall health outcomes and lowers health care costs. Given their frequency, severity, prevalence, morbidity, and mortality, depression and anxiety disorders remain important illnesses for primary care physicians to identify and treat.

The broader categories of mood and anxiety disorders comprise a large number of specific illnesses. *Mood disorders* include major depression (also called unipolar depression), bipolar disorder (which includes bipolar I and bipolar II disorder), cyclothymia, and dysthymia. The category of *anxiety disorders* includes generalized anxiety disorder (GAD), panic disorder with and without agoraphobia, agoraphobia without a history of panic disorder, specific phobia (e.g., fear of heights), social phobia (social anxiety disorder), obsessive-compulsive disorder (OCD), posttraumatic stress disorder (PTSD), and acute stress disorder. Describing the specific symptoms, epidemiology, assessment, and treatment of each illness is beyond the scope of this chapter; rather, we examine the illnesses that primary care physicians are most likely to encounter in clinical settings, and provide the most common strategies used in assessment, diagnosis, and treatment.

Epidemiology

Key Points

- Major depression and anxiety disorders are the two most common psychiatric illnesses in the United States.
- The economic burden of anxiety and depressive disorders is substantial in terms of workdays lost, disability, health care expenditures, and mortality.

- Anxiety and depression are chronic illnesses that typically run a waxing/waning course.
- Prevalence rates for anxiety disorders appear to decline with advancing age, except for GAD, which may increase in geriatric populations.
- Depression is often a highly recurrent illness; each episode of depression increases the likelihood of future episodes.

Prevalence estimates of mental disorders in the United States continue to find that anxiety and mood disorders are the two most common mental disorders in the general population. Lifetime prevalence for anxiety disorders is estimated at 16.6% to 28.8% (Conway et al., 2006; Kessler et al., 2005a) and for major depression is 14.9% to 16.2% (Kessler et al., 2003). Recent 12-month prevalence rates show a similar stratification, with anxiety disorders most common (18.1%), followed by mood disorders (9.5%). Lifetime prevalence rates of panic disorder and GAD are 4.7% and 5.7%, respectively (Kessler et al., 2005a). Anxiety disorders make up approximately 2% of all office visits to physicians in the United States, but almost 50% occur in primary care settings. In comparison, approximately 40% of patients presenting with anxiety disorders are seen by psychiatrists (Harman et al., 2002).

Major depression remains a common disorder and is associated with substantial symptom severity and role impairment (Kessler et al., 2003). One-year prevalence rates for major depression are approximately 6% in the general population, followed by dysthymia (1.8%) and bipolar disorders (1%-2%). Rates in primary care settings remain substantially higher, with prevalence of 10% or greater (Spitzer et al., 1994), although many of these patients suffer from depressions that are unrecognized by their primary care physician (Schultheis et al., 1999).

Costs

Both anxiety and depressive disorders account for substantial health care costs and thus constitute a major public health and economic concern. Despite an increasing treatment rate of depression in the United States between 1990 and 2000, estimated costs from depression failed to decline and were calculated to be $83.1 billion in 2000, of which $26.1 billion were for direct medical costs, $5.4 billion for suicide mortality costs, and $51.5 billion for work-related costs (Greenberg et al., 2003). Similarly, estimates from the 1990s placed the annual economic burden of anxiety disorders at $63.1 billion (in 1998 dollars), of which nonpsychiatric direct medical costs accounted for 54% of the total, and direct psychiatric care accounted for 31% (Greenberg et al., 1999). Not surprisingly, patients with anxiety disorders are much more likely to see their primary care physicians or utilize emergency services. Patients with pure GAD (i.e., no comorbid medical illnesses), for example, were 1.6 times more likely to have seen a primary care physician four or more times in the past year than those without GAD or depression (Wittchen et al., 2002). Patients with panic disorder were almost twice as likely as controls to have visited an emergency room in the previous 6 months (Roy-Byrne et al., 1999).

Disease Course

Both anxiety and depressive disorders tend to run a chronic course, with waxing and waning symptomatology. Illness severity typically worsens the longer the illness remains untreated. The age of onset for anxiety disorders varies greatly, depending on the specific condition. Specific phobias and separation anxiety, for example, often begin in childhood (median age of onset, 7 years), while panic disorder (median age, 21) and GAD (median age, 31) are typically seen in early to mid-adulthood (Kessler et al., 2005b). In elderly persons (>65 years) the prevalence of all anxiety disorders appears to decline, except for GAD, which is maintained at 4% prevalence and may increase over time (Krasucki et al., 1998). GAD is often a recurring illness in which patients may experience periods of residual symptoms and occasional interepisode remissions (Angst et al., 2009). More than one third of patients with panic disorder have full remission with treatment, but about 20% have an unremitting and chronic course despite treatment (Katschnig and Amering, 1998).

The onset of major depression can occur at any age, although the median age of onset is 30 (Kessler et al., 2005b). Depression is a highly recurrent illness, and each episode increases the likelihood of future episodes. Patients with a single episode have a 50% lifetime chance of recurrence, whereas those with three or more episodes have an almost 100% chance of recurrence without treatment (Eaton et al., 2008). Untreated depressive episodes can last 6 months or longer (Kessler et al., 2003).The Sequenced Treatment Alternatives to Relieve Depression (STAR*D) study found that a substantial number of patients receiving first-line treatment may require 8 weeks or more of treatment to achieve response or remission (Trivedi et al., 2006). Although most patients will recover from their depressive episode and return to normal functioning with treatment, approximately 15% of patients will continue to have an unremitting course, with worsening psychosocial functioning and higher risk for suicide (Eaton et al., 2008).

Neurobiology and Genetics

The neurobiology of both depressive and anxiety disorders is complex and incompletely understood. In contrast to illnesses such as Parkinson's or Huntington's disease, no single area of brain pathology or anatomic lesion has been implicated in the development of anxiety or depression; rather, these illnesses appear to be mediated by dysregulation of complex interactions between neural circuits (Nestler et al., 2002). In depression, most lines of investigation have involved dysregulation of the hypothalamic-pituitary axis (HPA) and hippocampus, along with investigations of neural circuitry mediating mood, reward, sleep, appetite, motivation, and cognition. In particular, hyperactivity of the HPA axis in some depressed patients has been found to lead to hippocampal volume reduction, likely by reduction of brain-derived neurotrophic factor (BDNF) and changes in the mechanisms that mediate BDNF expression. However, whether reduced hippocampal volume is a partial cause or merely a result of depression is currently unclear, and it is not seen in all patients diagnosed with depression. Although epidemiologic studies show that depression appears highly heritable, with some studies showing that 40 to 50% of the risk may be genetic, no one gene appears implicated, and depression likely is the phenotypic expression of multiple genetic vulnerabilities, coupled with environmental stresses (physical/emotional trauma, viral illness), physical factors (e.g., preexisting or comorbid medical illnesses such as hypothyroidism or stroke), and random processes during brain development (Nestler et al., 2002).

Neurobiologic research in anxiety disorders has focused on elucidating the neural networks involved in the *fear response*, but despite advances in neuroimaging, the exact mechanism of each anxiety disorder has yet to be completely understood. Strategies to understand the neuroanatomic underpinnings of panic disorder have focused on translational research, using conditioned fear in animals as a model for panic attacks in humans. Panic disorder patients may have an especially sensitive fear mechanism involving the central nucleus of the amygdala, the hippocampus, thalamus, hypothalamus, periaqueductal gray region, locus ceruleus, and other brainstem sites (Gorman et al., 2000). Other areas of focus in anxiety disorders have involved investigations into alterations of interoceptive processing of the anterior insula (Mathew et al., 2008). Both the insula and the anterior cingulate cortex (ACC) are thought to be the regions of the brain that form a representation of the visceral state of the body. A heightened sensitivity of this region may underlie the misinterpretation of bodily signals in panic disorder.

Genetic epidemiologic studies have clearly documented that anxiety disorders aggregate in families and that this familial link primarily results from genetic factors (Smoller and Faraone, 2008). First-degree relatives of probands with the major anxiety disorders (panic disorder, social anxiety disorder, specific phobias, OCD) have a fourfold to sixfold increased risk of the index disorders compared to relatives of unaffected probands (Hettema et al., 2001). Genetic studies of GAD suggest that a common genetic susceptibility may apply to "clusters" of anxiety disorders and other comorbid disorders (Norrholm and Ressler, 2009). An overlap of genes may play a role in the development of multiple psychiatric conditions, including anxiety and depression.

Anxiety, Major Depression, and Medical Illnesses

Key Points

- Anxiety disorders and major depression often coexist.
- The more severe the anxiety disorder, the greater is the likelihood of major depression.
- Medical illnesses are associated with higher prevalence of anxiety and depression, and vice versa.
- Medically ill patients with comorbid anxiety or depressive disorders adapt more poorly to physical symptoms, complicating disease management.

Interaction of Depression and Anxiety

Major depression and anxiety are often found together, and each illness complicates the course and outcome of the other. Studies have consistently shown that anxiety disorders are the most frequently occurring comorbid disorder with major depression, with 50% to 60% of major depressed patients with both illnesses (Zimmerman et al., 2002). Anxiety can lead to depression in almost 60% of patients, whereas depression leads to anxiety in only 15% of patients (Mineka et al., 1998). Not surprisingly, the more severe anxiety

disorders are more likely to lead to subsequent depression; that is, panic disorder, agoraphobia, OCD, PTSD and GAD more frequently lead to depression compared to either social phobia or simple phobia. In addition, patients with both illnesses often have increased severity of symptoms, increased frequency of episodes (either mood or anxiety episodes), poorer response to treatment, higher suicide rates, a more chronic course, and overall poorer prognosis.

Treatment is complicated by the fewer studies on coexisting depression and anxiety, providing clinicians with a smaller evidence-base for treatment decisions. Patients with comorbid major depressive disorders are half as likely subsequently to recover from panic disorder with agoraphobia or GAD, and comorbid major depression almost doubles the likelihood of recurrence of panic disorder with agoraphobia (Bruce et al., 2005). In addition, children and adolescents with anxiety disorders are at eight times the risk of additional depression (Angold et al., 1999). Practitioners must therefore be aggressive in screening for anxiety disorders in patients reporting depressive symptoms, as well as screening for depression in patients reporting anxiety symptoms.

Interaction of Depression, Anxiety, and Medical Illness

A complex and reciprocal relationship exists between medical illnesses and comorbid anxiety and depressive disorders. Medical illnesses are associated with higher prevalence rates of anxiety and depression, and anxiety and depression are associated with higher rates of comorbid medical illnesses. Studies of patients with diabetes, cancer, stroke, myocardial infarction, HIV-related illness, and Parkinson's disease have higher rates of depression compared to patients without such illnesses (Katon, 2003a). Common medical disorders seen in primary care settings have high comorbidity with anxiety disorders as well. Cardiovascular disease is associated with a 1.5 times greater risk of both GAD and panic disorder (Goodwin et al., 2008). Patients with back pain or arthritis are almost twice as likely to have panic attacks or GAD (McWilliams et al., 2004), whereas patients with asthma (pediatric or adult) may have a 30% increased likelihood of anxiety disorders (Katon et al., 2004). The prevalence of anxiety and depression in patients with diabetes is more than double that in the general population (Collins et al., 2009). Almost 100% of patients with irritable bowel syndrome will have major depression, GAD, or panic disorder (Lydiard et al., 1993).

Medical illnesses are associated with a higher risk for mood and anxiety disorders, so the presence of these disorders places patients at higher risk for multiple medical conditions. Patients with GAD or panic disorder are almost six times more likely to have a cardiac disorder, three times more likely to have a gastrointestinal (GI) disorder, twice as likely to have respiratory difficulties, and twice as likely to have migraine headaches compared to patients without anxiety disorders (Harter et al., 2003). Depression may be a predictor for the subsequent development of medical illness. Several studies found an association between history of major depression and subsequent development of type II diabetes (Eaton et al., 1996; Kawakami et al., 1999) and coronary artery disease (Rugulies, 2002).

Management of patients with comorbid medical illness and anxiety or depression is complex. Such patients have higher rates of unexplained symptoms than patients without these disorders, even after adjusting for the severity of medical illness (Katon and Walker, 1998). An increasing body of literature suggests that patients with medical illness and comorbid depression/anxiety adapt more poorly to chronic symptoms, such as fatigue or pain, and tend to focus on both symptoms of their physical illnesses and physical symptoms associated with other organ symptoms. Not surprisingly, patients with medical illness and comorbid depression have 50% higher medical costs than patients with medical illness alone (Katon, 2003). Comorbid patients are more functionally impaired and have more lost workdays, poorer quality of life, and higher rates of medical utilization (Simon, 2003). Disease management is also complicated by higher rates of nonadherence to treatment and self-care regimens, as well as higher rates of risk behaviors (e.g., smoking, overeating, sedentary lifestyle). Response to antidepressant treatment may be less robust, as evidenced by patients with cardiovascular disease, stroke, and diabetes (Katon, 2003).

Diagnosis and Screening of Mood and Anxiety Disorders

Key Points

- Distinguishing unipolar from bipolar depression is critical for the proper management of depressed patients. The MDQ may aid practitioners in detecting bipolar disorder in primary care settings.
- The PHQ-9 is a common and easy-to-use screening tool for depression.
- No standard screening instrument for anxiety disorders has currently been accepted in general practice.

Diagnosis of Mood Disorders

Mood disorders are divided into depressive disorders, bipolar disorders, and disorders based on etiology (i.e., mood disorders caused by general medical conditions and substance-induced mood disorders). For primary care physicians, identification, treatment, and management of depressive disorders are essential. Bipolar disorders, which are typically more complex to identify and treat, are best referred to mental health professionals for ongoing treatment. Therefore, this chapter concentrates on identifying bipolar disorder and distinguishing between unipolar and bipolar depression, but does not delve into the specifics of treating bipolar patients.

The essential feature of a *major depressive episode* is a period lasting at least 2 weeks during which the patient experiences depressed mood or loss of interest or pleasure in almost all activities, a distinct change in usual self, and clinically significant distress or changes in functioning. It is accompanied by a constellation of other symptoms, such as changes in sleep, eating, energy, motivation, and concentration; difficulty making decisions; and often feelings of hopelessness, worthlessness and guilt (Box 47-1). Patients may ruminate about death, feel that life is not worth living, have thoughts about suicide, may make plans to kill themselves, or make attempts. Many patients complain of memory difficulties, become easily distracted, and describe an inability to

---

Box 47-1 Diagnostic Criteria for Major Depressive Episode

A. Five (or more) of the following symptoms have been present during the same 2-week period and represent a change from previous functioning; at least one of the symptoms is either (1) depressed mood or (2) loss of interest or pleasure.

Note: Do not include symptoms that are clearly due to a general medical condition, or mood-incongruent delusions or hallucinations.

1. Depressed mood most of the day, nearly every day, as indicated by either subjective report (e.g., feels sad or empty) or observation made by others (e.g., appears tearful). *Note:* In children and adolescents, can be irritable mood.
2. Markedly diminished interest or pleasure in all, or almost all, activities most of the day, nearly every day (as indicated by either subjective account or observation made by others).
3. Significant weight loss when not dieting or weight gain (e.g., a change of more than 5% of body weight in a month), or decrease or increase in appetite nearly every day. *Note:* In children, consider failure to make expected weight gains.
4. Insomnia or hypersomnia nearly every day.
5. Psychomotor agitation or retardation nearly every day (observable by others, not merely subjective feelings of restlessness or being slowed down).
6. Fatigue or loss of energy nearly every day.
7. Feelings of worthlessness or excessive or inappropriate guilt (which may be delusional) nearly every day (not merely self-reproach or guilt about being sick).
8. Diminished ability to think or concentrate, or indecisiveness, nearly every day (either by subjective account or as observed by others).
9. Recurrent thoughts of death (not just fear of dying), recurrent suicidal ideation without a specific plan, or a suicide attempt or a specific plan for committing suicide.

B. The symptoms do not meet criteria for a Mixed Episode.

C. The symptoms cause clinically significant distress or impairment in social, occupational, or other important areas of functioning.

D. The symptoms are not due to the direct physiological effects of a substance (e.g., a drug of abuse, a medication) or a general medical condition (e.g., hypothyroidism).

E. The symptoms are not better accounted for by Bereavement, i.e., after the loss of a loved one, the symptoms persist for longer than 2 months or are characterized by marked functional impairment, morbid preoccupation with worthlessness, suicidal ideation, psychotic symptoms, or psychomotor retardation.

From American Psychiatric Association. Diagnostic and Statistical Manual of Mental Disorders, 4th ed, text revision. Washington, DC, APA, 2000.

---

think clearly. Patients often pace, wring their hands or have an inability to sit still; conversely, they may become greatly slowed or immobilized. In some patients, irritable mood may predominate more than sadness, or they may have explosive, angry outbursts (Fava and Rosenbaum, 1999). Irritability is especially noted in depressed children and adolescents. In its most severe forms—major depression with psychotic features—patients may hear voices telling them to kill themselves or may develop delusional beliefs, such as having a serious illness despite numerous tests providing no evidence (APA, 2000).

The essential feature of *dysthymia* is a chronically depressed mood that occurs most days for at least 2 years. Patients may have a variety of other symptoms, such as feelings of inadequacy, generalized loss of interest or pleasure, social withdrawal, feelings of guilt or brooding about the past, and decreased activity, productivity, or effectiveness (Box 47-2). Neurovegetative symptoms such as insomnia or hypersomnia, poor appetite or overeating, low energy, and poor concentration may be present but are less common than in major depressive episodes. These patients may state that they have been depressed for as long as they can remember and cannot recall episodes of recovery or remission of symptoms. In addition, dysthymic patients may periodically have superimposed major depressive episodes, often called "double depression" (APA, 2000).

Bipolar disorder is a chronic mood disorder characterized by the presence of mania (bipolar I disorder) or hypomania and depression (bipolar II disorder). Manic episodes are distinct periods of abnormally and persistent moods that can be euphoric, expansive, or irritable. Although manic patients are often thought to be always euphoric, only about 20% of patients experience pure euphoria; most describe a mix of severe irritability, severe emotional lability, and volatility (Goodwin and Jamison, 2007). Manic patients often have greatly inflated self-esteem, confidence, decreased need for sleep, pressured speech, racing or crowded thoughts, distractibility, increased involvement in goal-directed activities (e.g., starting many projects but being unable to finish any), hypersexuality, and excessive involvement in pleasurable activities with a high potential for painful consequences (APA, 2000). Patients can exert great levels of physical activity, appear tireless, and may become extremely physically agitated. Approximately 60% of bipolar I patients will experience psychosis, which may involve delusions of grandeur (feeling omnipotent, having special powers or "gifts"), persecution, or hallucinations (more often auditory as opposed to visual) (Goodwin and Jamison, 2007). Despite mania being the defining characteristic of the disease, depressed moods tend to predominate, with bipolar I patients experiencing a 3:1 ratio of depression to mania over the course of the illness (Judd et al., 2003).

Primary care physicians are more likely to encounter patients with *bipolar II disorder* than bipolar I disorder. Bipolar II disorder is characterized by hypomanic and major depressive episodes, although over the course of the illness it is primarily a disease of depression, with depressive episodes predominating over hypomanic episodes by a 37:1 ratio (Judd et al., 2003). Symptoms of hypomanic episodes are similar to full manic episodes, but the severity of manic behaviors is attenuated, and the extreme functional, occupational, and social impairment evident in manic episodes is absent in hypomania. Current DSM-IV-TR criteria require that distinct elevations in mood must be present for at least 4 days, must be clearly different from the patient's usual nondepressed mood, and must be accompanied by a change in the patient's usual functioning. Because patients primarily seek help during their depressive episodes and typically do not report hypomanic episodes as abnormal, undiagnosed bipolar disorder remains a major difficulty in primary care settings (Manning et al., 1999). Moreover, bipolar disorder may be more common in primary care settings than in general populations. Of 649 patients being treated for depression in a primary care clinic, 21% screened positive for bipolar disorder (Hirschfeld et al., 2005), whereas 10% of patients screened positive for bipolar disorder in a general medical clinic, although 80% of these patients had been diagnosed with unipolar depression (Das et al., 2005).

Box 47-2 Diagnostic Criteria for Dysthymic Disorder

Depressed mood for most of the day, for more days than not, as indicated either by subjective account or observation by others, for at least 2 years.

Note: In children and adolescents, mood can be irritable and duration must be at least 1 year.

A. Presence, while depressed, of two (or more) of the following:
1. Poor appetite or overeating
2. Insomnia or hypersomnia
3. Low energy or fatigue
4. Low self-esteem
5. Poor concentration or difficulty making decisions
6. Feelings of hopelessness

B. During the 2-year period (1 year for children or adolescents) of the disturbance, the person has never been without the symptoms in Criteria A and B for more than 2 months at a time.

C. No Major Depressive Episode (see Criteria for Major Depressive Episode [Box 47-1]) has been present during the first 2 years of the disturbance (1 year for children and adolescents); i.e., the disturbance is not better accounted for by chronic Major Depressive Disorder, or Major Depressive Disorder, In Partial Remission.

Note: There may have been a previous Major Depressive Episode provided there was a full remission (no significant signs or symptoms for 2 months) before development of the Dysthymic Disorder. In addition, after the initial 2 years (1 year in children or adolescents) of Dysthymic Disorder, there may be superimposed episodes of Major Depressive Disorder, in which case both diagnoses may be given when the criteria are met for a Major Depressive Episode.

D. There has never been a Manic Episode, a Mixed Episode, or a Hypomanic Episode, and criteria have never been met for Cyclothymic Disorder.

E. The disturbance does not occur exclusively during the course of a chronic Psychotic Disorder, such as Schizophrenia or Delusional Disorder.

F. The symptoms are not due to the direct physiological effects of a substance (e.g., a drug of abuse, a medication) or a general medical condition (e.g., hypothyroidism).

G. The symptoms cause clinically significant distress or impairment in social, occupational, or other important areas of functioning.

From American Psychiatric Association. Diagnostic and Statistical Manual of Mental Disorders, 4th ed, text revision. Washington, DC, APA, 2000.

Unipolar Depression vs. Bipolar Depression

Distinguishing unipolar from bipolar depression remains a critical distinction and poses one of the greatest clinical challenges for professionals who treat mood disorders. Misdiagnosis of bipolar disorder can lead to mistreatment (typically with antidepressants alone), worsening of mood, switches into mania or mixed states (i.e., presence of both manic and depressive symptoms), rapid mood swings, worsening psychosocial impairment, greater suicide attempts, and higher mortality (Goldberg and Ernst, 2002; Goldberg and Truman, 2003; Schneck et al., 2008). Treatment of bipolar depression is rarely straightforward and often requires multiple medications and medication trials. Antidepressants do not appear to be especially helpful in the treatment of bipolar disorder, and antidepressants have not yet been shown to improve outcome compared to mood stabilizers alone (Sachs et al., 2007). Although no symptom is pathognomonic for bipolar depression, certain features of depression may suggest that a patient's depression is a manifestation of bipolar illness. Bipolar depression can present similar to unipolar depression, but some depression features may help distinguish the two (Ghaemi et al., 2004; Perlis et al., 2006) (Table 47-1). If a primary care physician makes a diagnosis of bipolar disorder, the patient is best served by referral to a mental health provider, preferably with expertise in treating mood disorders.

Screening Tools for Depression

Numerous screening measures have been specifically designed to detect depression, and many are sensitive to change over time when used repeatedly at follow-up visits. The integration of such tools into clinical practice, referred to as *measurement-based care,* may enhance care and improve clinical outcome. Measurement tools in the public domain and sensitive to change over time are most practical for primary care physicians because they are a cost-effective way to manage depressed patients over time (Trivedi et al., 2006). Self-report measures obviate the need for trained office personnel to administer tests. Depression screening measures do not diagnose depression but do provide critical information regarding symptom severity within a given period. Almost all measures have a statistically predetermined cutoff score at which depression symptoms are considered significant. When a depression screen is positive, an interview is necessary because screening will not include many confounding diagnostic variables (e.g., substance abuse, hypothyroidism, bereavement), and physician judgment is required. Screening measures do not address important clinical features of psychiatric illnesses (e.g., total duration of symptoms, degree of impairment) from other comorbid psychiatric conditions.

Patient Health Questionnaire 9

The Patient Health Questionnaire 9 (PHQ-9) is often used in primary care settings because of its ease of use, sensitivity to change over time, reliability, and validity (Kroenke et al., 2001). It uses only the nine depression items from the original self-report version of the PRIME-MD PHQ (Spitzer et al., 1999). Major depression is diagnosed if five or more of the depressive symptoms have been present at least "more than half the days" in the past 2 weeks, and if one of the symptoms is depressed mood or anhedonia. Other depressive syndromes (e.g., minor depression) are diagnosed if two, three, or four depressive symptoms have been present at least "more than half the days" in the past 2 weeks, and if one symptom is depressed mood or anhedonia. One of the nine test items ("thought that you would be better off dead or by hurting yourself in some way") counts if present at all, regardless of duration. Using cutoff scores from 9 to 15, sensitivity ranges from 68% to 95%, with specificity from 84% to 95%. Using the cutoff score of 9, sensitivity is 95% and specificity 84%.

Quick Inventory of Depressive Symptomatology— Self Report (QIDS-SR)

The 16-item Quick Inventory of Depressive Symptomatology Self Report (QIDS-SR$_{16}$) is an instrument designed to screen for depression and to follow the changes in severity of depression over time (Rush et al., 2006). The QIDS-SR$_{16}$ is a shortened version of the original 30-item Inventory of Depressive Symptomatology (IDS). The IDS includes criterion symptoms and symptoms typically associated with depression, such as anxiety and irritability, whereas QIDS assesses only the nine symptom domains used to characterize depressive episodes (sad mood, concentration, self-criticism, suicidal ideation, interest, energy/fatigue, sleep disturbance, changes in appetite/weight, presence of psychomotor retardation or retardation). The total score on QIDS ranges from 0 to 27 (0-5, no severity; 6-10, mild; 11-15, moderate; 16-20, severe; 21-27, very severe). The QIDS was effective in assisting management of depression in the STAR*D study, the largest depression trial conducted thus far in the United States (Trivedi et al., 2006).

Screening for Bipolar Disorder

Although no laboratory or imaging tests currently exist to distinguish unipolar depression from bipolar depression, screening questionnaires, as well as certain features of a

Table 47-1 Features Suggesting Bipolar Depression

Feature	Bipolar	Unipolar
Substance abuse	Very high	Moderate
Family history	Almost uniform	Sometimes
Seasonality	Common	Occasional
First episode before age 25 years	Very common	Sometimes
Postpartum illness	Very common	Sometimes
Psychotic features before age 35	Highly predictive	Uncommon
Atypical features	Common	Occasional
Rapid on/off pattern	Typical	Unusual
Recurrent major depressive episodes (>3)	Common	Unusual
Antidepressant-induced mania/hypomania	Predictive	Uncommon
Brief episodes (<3 months)	Suggestive	Unusual (duration usually >3 months)
Antidepressant tolerance	Suggestive	Uncommon
Mixed depression (presence of hypomanic features within depressive episode)	Predictive	Rare
Tension, edginess, fearfulness	More common	Less common
Somatic symptoms (muscular, respiratory, genitourinary)	Less common	More common

Modified from Kaye NS. Is your depressed patient bipolar? J Am Board Fam Pract 2005;18:271-281; and Perlis RH, Brown E, Baker RW, Nierenberg AA. Clinical features of bipolar depression versus major depressive disorder in large multicenter trials. Am J Psychiatry 2006;163:225-231.

patient's history and symptomatology, may prove helpful. The Mood Disorder Questionnaire (MDQ) is a tool that combines DSM-IV criteria and clinical experience to screen for bipolar disorder in primary care settings (Hirschfeld et al., 2000). It is a brief, 1-page self-report questionnaire with 13 yes/no items and two additional questions regarding functioning and timing of mood symptoms, and typically can be completed in 5 minutes or less. Seven or more positive responses to questions about manic symptoms, plus positive responses to the severity of impairment (moderate or severe) and coincident timing of symptoms yields a positive screen. Specificity and sensitivity of the MDQ vary widely by clinical setting, having the best combination of the two when given to patients with suspected mood symptoms (93% specificity; 58% sensitivity) but performs more poorly in general community samples (97% specificity; 28% sensitivity) (Hirschfeld et al., 2003; Hirschfeld et al., 2005). Other screening tools for bipolar disorder do not offer the ease of use and higher reliability and validity of the MDQ.

Diagnosis of Anxiety Disorders

The essential feature of *generalized anxiety disorder* is excessive anxiety and worry about a number of events or activities, occurring most days over 6 months. Patients have difficulty controlling the worry, report subjective distress, and may experience difficulties in social or occupational functioning. The intensity, duration, or frequency of the worry is out of proportion to the actual likelihood or impact of the feared event. Patients must have at least three associated physical symptoms, including restlessness, irritability, muscle tension, disturbed sleep, fatigability, and difficulty concentrating. The list of associated symptoms can be thought of as symptoms of inner tension (restlessness or edginess, irritability, muscle tension) and symptoms associated with the fatiguing effects of chronic anxiety (fatigue, concentration difficulties, sleep disturbance) (Box 47-3).

Panic attacks, a collection of distressing physical, cognitive, and emotional symptoms, may occur in a variety of anxiety disorders, such as specific phobias, social phobias, PTSD, and acute stress disorder. Panic attacks are discrete periods of intense fear in the absence of real danger, accompanied by at least 4 of 13 cognitive and physical symptoms (Box 47-4). The attacks have a sudden onset, build to a peak quickly, and are often accompanied by feelings of doom, imminent danger, and a need to escape. Symptoms of panic attacks can include somatic complaints (e.g., sweating, chills), cardiovascular symptoms (pounding heart, accelerated heart rate, chest pain), neurologic symptoms (trembling, unsteadiness, lightheadedness, paresthesias), GI symptoms (choking sensations, nausea), and pulmonary symptoms (shortness of breath). In addition, patients with panic attacks may worry they are dying, "going crazy," or have the sensation of being detached from reality.

Patients with panic disorder experience recurrent, unexpected panic attacks, followed by at least 1 month of persistent worry that they will suffer another panic attack. Panic disorder patients may begin to avoid places where a prior attack occurred or where help may not be available; such avoidance can lead to the development of agoraphobia and typically worsens their psychosocial functioning (Box 47-5).

Screening Tools for Anxiety Disorders

At present, screening tools for anxiety disorders have been developed to recognize anxiety as a broad syndrome, examining somatic symptoms (racing heart, lightheadedness) or cognitive symptoms (tendency to worry, intensity of worry). Other tools have been used to screen for single, distinct disorders, such as phobias or panic disorder. To date, no clear screening tool or symptom-severity measure has emerged for use in primary care settings, although newer instruments may be useful for primary care physicians. The Generalized Anxiety Disorder 7 (GAD-7) scale was developed and validated

---

Box 47-3 Diagnostic Criteria for Generalized Anxiety Disorder

Excessive anxiety and worry (apprehensive expectation), occurring more days than not for at least 6 months, about a number of events or activities.
A. The person finds it difficult to control the worry.
B. The anxiety and worry are associated with three (or more) of the following six symptoms:
   1. Restlessness and feeling keyed up or on edge
   2. Being easily fatigued
   3. Difficulty concentrating or mind going blank
   4. Irritability
   5. Muscle tension
   6. Sleep disturbance
C. The focus of the anxiety and worry is not confined to features of an Axis I disorder, e.g., the anxiety or worry is not about having a Panic Attack.
D. The anxiety, worry, or physical symptoms cause clinically significant distress or impairment in social, occupational, or other important areas of functioning.
E. The disturbance is not due to the direct physiological effects of a substance or a general medical condition.

From American Psychiatric Association. Diagnostic and Statistical Manual of Mental Disorders, 4th ed, text revision. Washington, DC, APA, 2000.

Box 47-4 Diagnostic Criteria for Panic Attack

A discrete period of intense fear or discomfort, in which four (or more) of the following symptoms developed abruptly and reached a peak within 10 minutes:
1. Palpitations, pounding heart, or accelerated heart rate
2. Sweating
3. Trembling or shaking
4. Sensations of shortness of breath or smothering
5. Feeling of choking
6. Chest pain or discomfort
7. Nausea or abdominal distress
8. Feeling dizzy, unsteady, lightheaded, or faint
9. Derealization (feelings of unreality) or depersonalization (being detached from oneself)
10. Fear of losing control or going crazy
11. Fear of dying
12. Paresthesias (numbness or tingling sensations)
13. Chills or hot flushes

From the American Psychiatric Association. Diagnostic and Statistical Manual of Mental Disorders, 4th ed, text revision. Washington, DC, APA, 2000.

Box 47-5 Diagnostic Criteria for Panic Disorder without Agoraphobia

A. Both (1) and (2):
  1. Recurrent and unexpected panic attacks
  2. At least one of the attacks has been followed by 1 month (or more) of one (or more) of the following:
     (a) Persistent concern having additional attacks
     (b) Worry about the implications of the attack or its consequences (e.g., losing control, having a heart attack, "going crazy")
     (c) A significant change in behavior related to the attacks
B. Absence of Agoraphobia.
C. The Panic Attacks are not due to the direct physiological effects of a substance or a general medical condition.
D. The Panic Attacks are not better accounted for by another mental disorder.

From the American Psychiatric Association: Diagnostic and Statistical Manual of Mental Disorders, 4th ed, text revision. Washington, DC, APA, 2000.

in primary care clinics and is a brief, seven-item self-report screening tool for GAD (Spitzer et al., 2006). The GAD-7 helps identify probable cases of GAD and measure symptom severity. A score of 10 or greater represents a reasonable cutoff point for identifying patients with GAD, and cutoffs of 5, 10, and 15 correlate to mild, moderate, and severe levels of anxiety. An extended version of the PHQ includes five questions for panic disorder (Spitzer et al., 1999), but its utility as a stand-alone tool is currently unclear. The Overall Anxiety Severity and Impairment Scale (OASIS) is a five-item continuous measure that can be used across anxiety disorders, with multiple anxiety disorders, and with subthreshold anxiety symptoms. OASIS can be used to measure the severity of anxiety symptoms, but it was not developed as a diagnostic tool for any specific disorder (Norman et al., 2006).

Assessment of the Depressed or Anxious Patient in Medical Settings

Key Points

- Patients with anxiety and depressive disorders often present with somatic complaints.
- Risk assessment includes identifying modifiable risk factors and developing a corresponding treatment plan.
- "Contracts for safety" have no empiric data to support their effectiveness in risk management.
- Worsening symptoms or suicidal ideation may require psychiatric hospitalization.

Diagnosing anxiety and depressive disorders may prove especially challenging in medical settings. The majority of patients suffering from such illnesses will more frequently present with somatic complaints, while only a minority will present with purely psychological symptoms and concerns (Bridges and Goldberg, 1985). Difficulties in diagnosis may be secondary to a patient's inability to articulate psychological problems, reticence to speak of emotional difficulties, the short time allowed for patient visits, or a primary care physician's relative lack of training in assessing and treating mental health disorders. Many presenting complaints may be consistent with symptoms of coexisting medical illnesses, further complicating assessment and likely requiring additional etiologic investigation. Of new patients presenting to an urban clinic, for example, only 17% presented with purely psychological symptoms. Of the remaining patients, 32% presented with pure somatization, 27% presented with symptoms for a coexisting medical illness, and 24% presented with an initial physical complaint that they were later able to relate to a psychological problem (Bridges and Goldberg, 1985). However, clinical clues in patients with physical complaints may identify a subgroup of patients who warrant further evaluation for an anxiety or depressive disorder. This includes patients who present with multiple physical symptoms (six or more), have higher ratings of symptom severity and lower ratings of overall health, and have an encounter that the physician perceives as "difficult" (Kroenke et al., 1997).

Assessment of anxious or depressed patients requires establishing specific psychiatric diagnosis(es), providing a thorough risk assessment (i.e., suicidality, homicidality, ability or inability to care for self), assessing the severity of the illness, identifying specific target symptoms to track over time, assessing factors that are likely complicating or exacerbating the illness (e.g. medical disorders, substance abuse), and gathering collateral information whenever possible from family, friends, or other providers (Box 47-6). Distinguishing bipolar from unipolar depression, as discussed previously, is one of the most important distinctions when establishing diagnosis. In addition, clinicians should look for the presence of comorbid anxiety disorders, because patients with such disorders often require lower initial antidepressant dosing and may have their anxiety symptoms paradoxically worsen as treatment is initiated unless lower doses are used (Table 47-2). Education on the medical nature of depression and anxiety may prove extremely helpful, because both patients and families often believe that psychiatric illness is evidence of "weakness" or indicative of some other personal failing. Information on prognosis and the expected treatment course may lessen pressure and expectations for rapid improvement and let the patient know when to expect medication benefit.

Physicians should assess the severity of illness and develop a list of target symptoms to track and measure over time, to better evaluate treatment response. Tracking specific symptoms particular to an individual patient's depression improves objective assessment of change. Often, patients' neurovegetative symptoms will improve before the subjective experience of their mood improving. Assessing sleep, appetite, energy level, anxiety, and concentration allows the physician to select a more appropriate antidepressant or anxiolytic by targeting specific symptoms. This may include using a sedating antidepressant such as mirtazapine for patients with insomnia or a more activating antidepressant such as bupropion for patients with lethargy or somnolence. Measurement tools that are symptom specific and sensitive to change over time (e.g., PHQ-9, QIDS-SR) may help the physician track such changes. In addition, assessing overall functionality (ability to shower, pay bills, shop, prepare meals) is equally important in establishing the degree of impairment caused by the patient's mood disorder.

Box 47-6 Initial Assessment of Anxious or Depressed Patients

1. Establish diagnosis.
2. Perform risk assessment.
   Suicide risk
   Risks to others
3. Establish severity of illness.
   Ability to care for self
   Functioning/functional impairment
4. Identify specific target symptoms.
   Neurovegetative symptoms (e.g., sleep, appetite, concentration)
   Use of measurement scales (e.g., QIDS)
5. Assess factors complicating illness.
   Alcohol or /drug use
   Comorbid or contributing medical conditions
6. Gather input from family and friends if possible.

Table 47-2 Dosing for Common Antidepressant and Antianxiety Agents

Medication	Usual Daily Starting Dose (mg)		Daily Dose Range
	Anxiety	Depression	
Selective Serotonin Reuptake Inhibitors (SSRIs)			
Citalopram	10	20	10-60
Escitalopram	5	10	5-30
Fluoxetine	10	20	20-80
Fluvoxamine	25	50	100-300
Paroxetine	10	20	20-60
Sertraline	25	50	50-200
Serotonin-Norepinephrine Reuptake Inhibitors (SNRIs)			
Desvenlafaxine	50	50	50-100
Duloxetine	30	30	30-120
Venlafaxine	37.5	75	150-300
Tricyclic Antidepressants (TCAs)			
Amitriptyline	25	50	100-300
Imipramine	25	50	100-300
Nortriptyline	10	25	50-200
Desipramine	25	50	100-300
Norepinephrine-Dopamine Reuptake Inhibitors			
Bupropion	—	150	300-450
Norepinephrine-Serotonin Modulators			
Mirtazapine	15	30	30-60

Differential Diagnosis

Many medical conditions may cause or mimic depression. Physical disorders that have been associated with depression include Addison's disease, acquired immunodeficiency syndrome (AIDS), coronary artery disease (especially in those with myocardial infarction), cancer, multiple sclerosis, Parkinson's disease, anemia, diabetes, acute infection, temporal arteritis, hypothyroidism, and especially dementias. It is imperative that the physician complete a neurologic evaluation to rule out an underlying disorder as the cause of the patient's depression. In addition, many medications may worsen depression, especially cardiovascular drugs, hormones, typical antipsychotic agents, anti-inflammatory agents, and anticonvulsants.

Anxiety disorders may be caused or exacerbated by medical conditions, medications taken for other psychiatric or medical disorders, and other substances with stimulant properties. For example, hyperthyroidism can mimic or exacerbate anxiety disorders, and therefore thyroid function should be carefully evaluated when patients present with anxiety symptoms. In addition, lifetime risk of thyroid dysfunction appears higher in patients with panic disorder or GAD (Simon et al., 2002). Physicians should also assess the patient's use of other medications, especially stimulants (whether prescribed or obtained from other sources), nicotine, illicit drugs, and caffeine.

Suicide Screening and Assessment

Identifying patients at risk for suicide is a complex and difficult task, particularly in the setting of a busy medical practice. Suicide is currently the 11th leading cause of death for all ages and accounts for approximately 32,000 deaths annually in the United States (CDC, 2009). It is the second leading cause of death in those 25 to 34 years old and the third leading cause in those 15 to 24. Older males 75 and older have the highest suicide rate, at 37.4 per 100,000. Males continue to take their lives at approximately four times the rate of females and account for almost 80% of all U.S. suicides. Women in their 40s and 50s have the highest rates of suicide among females (8 per 100,000), and women continue to make suicide attempts two to three times more often than men (Krug et al., 2002). Approximately 60% of all suicides are associated with patients with mood disorders, and approximately 50% of patients who completed suicide had contact with professional help in the month before their death (Isometsa et al., 1995).

Despite no definitive suicide assessment tool being available, risk factors have been defined that can help identify patients at risk for suicide. Suicide screening should include assessing current level of depression, severity of symptoms, feelings of hopelessness; current suicidal thoughts and behaviors (as well as past attempts), use of drugs or alcohol (which can increase levels of impulsivity and worsen dysphoria), current levels of anxiety and agitation, access to lethal means (especially firearms), presence of psychosis (command hallucinations, poor reality testing), recent acute stressors, and presence (or absence) of a psychosocial support system (APA, 2003). When possible, additional information from family or friends can be helpful in assessing statements or behaviors that may indicate a patient's intentions of committing suicide.

Physicians should be alert to those suicide risk factors that can be modified. Although numerous historical and biologic risk factors cannot be modified (history of suicide attempts, family history of suicide, male gender, history of childhood trauma), other risk factors are amenable to intervention. Mood, anxiety, and psychotic symptoms can be successfully treated with medications. Substance abuse referral may help the patient actively struggling with substance abuse or dependence, or for relapse prevention. Encouraging the patient to mobilize psychosocial resources, such as contacting family members for support, can provide a measure of safety while the patient is recovering from depression. Removing access to firearms can be especially helpful in preventing rapid access to lethal means during episodes of acute distress and high levels of impulsivity. Physicians should be aware that "contracts for safety" have not been shown to be effective in preventing suicide and may provide a false sense of patient safety (Rudd et al., 2006). Continued assessment of mood, hopelessness, and suicidal ideation is required throughout the course of treatment. Worsening symptoms, along with plans or active preparations for suicide, may require increased observation or hospitalization.

Management and Treatment of Major Depression and Anxiety Disorders

The key objective in treating depressive and anxiety disorders is remission of all symptoms. Studies in the treatment of major depression have consistently shown that lack of remission is associated with higher relapse rates, more severe subsequent depressions, shorter duration between episodes, continued impairment in work settings and social relationships, increased all-cause mortality, and increased risk of suicide (Judd et al., 2000). Initiation of treatment should include education about the expected temporal course of improvement; importance of regular eating, activity, social interaction, and sleep; medication selection; follow-up schedule; and safety management if symptoms worsen or suicidal ideation is evident (Box 47-7).

Box 47-7 Initiation of Treatment for Major Depression and Anxiety Disorders

1. Educate the patient.
   Details of illness
   Treatment course, prognosis, goal of treatment (remission of symptoms)
   Importance of general health: exercise, sleep hygiene, nutrition
   Inclusion of family when possible
   Coordination with other providers
   Resource lists for support groups, therapy referrals
2. Select medication from reasonable choices.
   Patient history of antidepressant use/response
   Family history of antidepressant response
   Typical time course to antidepressant response
3. Administer starting dose, and initiate dose titration.
   Common side effects of medications
4. Establish monitoring with measurement-based care (e.g., QIDS).
5. Schedule follow-up in 2 to 4 weeks.

Depression

Pharmacotherapy remains the mainstay treatment of depression. Treatment should be considered for the majority of depressed patients, especially those who are suicidal, functionally impaired from their depression, or experiencing a recurrent episode, or who have comorbid medical or psychiatric conditions likely to worsen unless their depression is treated (e.g., panic, GAD, chronic pain). Treatment of depression has clearly been shown to prevent relapse, shorten current episodes, decrease psychosocial impairment, decrease risk of suicide, and improve quality of life. Mild depression may be treated with symptomatic intervention alone (e.g., mild sedative for insomnia), although continuing depressive symptoms or inadequate response to purely symptomatic interventions warrants more aggressive treatment of the underlying depression. Patients with psychotic depression typically require treatment with both antidepressant and antipsychotic agents, or they may require electroconvulsive therapy (ECT). Often, psychotically depressed patients require hospitalization. Patients with psychotic depression should be referred to a psychiatrist, given the severity of illness and complexity of treatment.

Again, the aim of treatment is remission of all depressive symptoms and a return to the patient's previous baseline functioning. Pharmacotherapy combined with psychotherapy has been shown to be superior to either modality alone (de Maat et al., 2008; Thase, 1997); thus referral to a psychotherapist may be helpful, especially for patients with moderate to severe depression. Some patients may choose psychotherapy alone to treat depression; cognitive-behavioral therapy, interpersonal therapy, behavioral activation, and psychodynamic therapy may prove as effective as medication alone.

Selection of Medication

The effectiveness of antidepressants is generally comparable across classes, and therefore selection of an antidepressant depends mainly on patient preference, side effect profile, drug interactions, previous response to a specific medication, treatment overlap with other psychiatric conditions, and cost (Tables 47-3 and 47-4). Minimal data support the increased efficacy or speed of onset for any particular agent, with response rates across clinical trials generally 50% to 75% for patients receiving active treatment. Onset of improvement typically takes 3 to 6 weeks, although the STAR*D study indicates that patients may require up to 12 to 14 weeks to achieve remission of symptoms. In fact, 40% of patients in the multiyear, multisite STAR*D study who eventually achieved remission in the first level of treatment with citalopram did not show a response (i.e., 50% improvement in symptoms) until week 8 of treatment (Trivedi et al., 2006).

For most patients, initial treatment with a selective serotonin reuptake inhibitor (SSRI), serotonin-norepinephrine reuptake inhibitor (SNRI), bupropion, or mirtazapine is reasonable. Tricyclic antidepressants (TCAs) are more often used as second-line agents in the treatment of depression because of their potential toxicity in overdose, greater side effect burden (largely from anticholinergic, antihistaminic, and antiadrenergic properties), and potential cardiac complications (conduction delays). Monoamine oxidase inhibitors (MAOIs) are complex drugs to use given their potentially fatal drug and dietary interactions and probably should not be prescribed in family practice settings. Most antidepressant studies have been conducted in specialty settings, but a number of studies in primary care settings have also shown the superiority of antidepressants over placebo (Arroll et al., 2009). Thus, given the comparable speed and efficacy of antidepressants across classes and within classes, selection of an antidepressant agent may be primarily guided by side effect profile, possible secondary uses of antidepressants (e.g., treating pain or insomnia), and contraindications to particular agents (e.g., bupropion in seizure disorder patients). Table 47-2 gives the usual starting doses for treatment of major depression.

Serotonin reuptake inhibitors are safe, effective medications that can treat a variety of psychiatric conditions. All SSRIs operate by the same mechanism of action and are considered equally effective in the treatment of depression. However, failure of one SSRI does not necessarily imply failure of all SSRIs; patients may respond preferentially to one SSRI over another (Rush et al., 2006). SSRIs differ substantially by their potential to inhibit particular hepatic cytochrome P-450 metabolic pathways, by half-life, potency, and presence or absence of active metabolites. Clinicians should

check for drug interactions in patients receiving complex polypharmacy regimens, because drug-drug interactions are constantly being updated and changing. For example, fluoxetine is a potent 2D6 inhibitor that can triple TCA and phenytoin levels or increase the anticoagulation associated with warfarin. Fluoxetine also has the longest half-life of any SSRI; its active metabolite norfluoxetine has a half-life of 10 days. SSRIs have sexual side effects (decreased libido, delayed orgasm or anorgasmia) and GI side effects (nausea, diarrhea) (see Table 47-4). GI side effects likely will remit over time, but sexual effects typically do not attenuate and may require treatment with other agents, such as a phosphodiesterase inhibitor (e.g., sildenafil), or choosing an antidepressant less likely to cause sexual side effects.

Serotonin-norepinephrine reuptake inhibitors (venlafaxine, duloxetine, desvenlafaxine) are similar in efficacy to SSRIs, although a few studies have suggested a mild advantage of SNRIs over SSRIs (Thase et al., 2001). Although SNRIs by definition inhibit the reuptake of both serotonin and norepinephrine, dual-neurotransmitter reuptake inhibition does not occur with venlafaxine until doses reach approximately 150 mg daily; below this dose, it acts primarily as an SSRI. Venlafaxine is available in immediate-release and extended-release (XR) formulations, although most patients

Table 47-3 FDA Indications for Antidepressant Therapy

Medication	MDD	OCD	Panic	PTSD	GAD	Soc Anx	PMDD	Bulimia	Other/Off-Label Uses
Amitriptyline	X								Migraine prophylaxis, chronic pain
Bupropion	X								Smoking cessation
Citalopram	X								
Desvenlafaxine	X								
Desipramine	X								
Duloxetine	X				X				Diabetic peripheral neuropathic pain, fibromyalgia
Escitalopram	X				X				
Fluoxetine	X	X	X				X	X	X/Pediatric depression
Fluvoxamine		X							
Imipramine	X								Enuresis
Mirtazapine	X								
Nortriptyline	X								
Paroxetine	X	X	X		X	X	X		
Sertraline	X	X	X	X			X		Premature ejaculation
Venlafaxine	X		X		X				

FDA, U.S. Food and Drug Administration; *MDD*, major depressive disorder; *OCD*, obsessive-compulsive disorder; *PTSD*, posttraumatic stress disorder; *GAD*, generalized anxiety disorder; *Soc Anx*, social anxiety disorder; *PMDD*, .

Table 47-4 Common Side Effects of Antidepressant Medications

Class/Drug	Side Effects	Comments
Selective serotonin reuptake inhibitor (SSRI)	Gastrointestinal side effects (nausea, diarrhea, heartburn); sexual dysfunction (decreased libido, delayed orgasm): headache; insomnia/somnolence	Likely little difference between SSRIs in rates of sexual side effects. SSRIs have been used to treat premature ejaculation.
Serotonin-norepinephrine reuptake inhibitor (SNRI)	Hypertension, sweating, nausea, constipation, dizziness, sexual dysfunction	Risk of increased blood pressure escalates as dose is increased; abrupt withdrawal of venlafaxine may cause discontinuation syndrome.
Tricyclic antidepressant (TCA)	Dry mouth, constipation, blurry vision, orthostatic hypotension, weight gain, somnolence, headache, sweating, sexual dysfunction	Use with caution in patients with cardiac conduction delays.
Bupropion	Insomnia, dry mouth, tremor, headache, nausea, constipation, dizziness	Contraindicated in patients with seizure disorders or eating disorders; patients generally free of sexual side effects.
Mirtazapine	Somnolence, increased appetite, and weight gain, dry mouth	Sedation may be more pronounced at lower doses.
Trazodone	Sedation, orthostatic hypotension, priapism	Usually used as a sedative-hypnotic.
Benzodiazepines	Sedation, fatigue, ataxia, slurred speech, memory impairment, weakness	Risk of dependence or abuse, especially with shorter-acting benzodiazepines.

and clinicians favor use of the XR preparation, given its once-daily dosing and lower likelihood of provoking a withdrawal syndrome on discontinuation of the drug, more frequently observed with the immediate-release formulation. Desven-lafaxine, the active metabolite of venlafaxine, is more potent than its parent compound, but any advantages over venla-faxine are currently unclear. Unlike venlafaxine, duloxetine provides dual-neurotransmitter reuptake inhibition at any dose, although this does not appear to confer any advantage over other SNRIs in terms of efficacy or side effect profile. Duloxetine currently is indicated for treatment of chronic pain as well as depression, but this is likely a class effect of SNRIs and not unique to duloxetine. Side effects are similar to SSRIs (see Table 47-4), with the additional side effects with SNRIs likely caused by increased noradrenergic activity,

including dose-related hypertension, excessive sweating, and dry mouth (Thase, 2008a; Thase et al., 2005).

Mirtazapine is a serotonin-norepinephrine modulator that also blocks postsynaptic hydroxytryptamine (HT) receptors, including those in the 5-HT-3 (serotonin) class. Mirtazap-ine is sedating and can increase appetite and therefore may be favored when patients have insomnia or decreased appe-tite and weight loss. Because of a dose-dependent ratio of neurotransmitter blockade involving histamine receptors, mirtazapine is generally more sedating at lower doses than higher. Although currently indicated only for depression, mirtazapine is reported to have general anxiolytic effects and may be beneficial for patients with mild to moderate anxi-ety. With its 5-HT-3 blockade, mirtazapine may be helpful when patients complain of nausea or other GI symptoms or side effects from SSRIs. Mirtazapine also has fewer sexual side effects than SSRIs or SNRIs, and has been tried as an antidote to SSRI-induced sexual side effects. Common side effects from mirtazapine include weight gain and daytime somnolence (see Table 47-4).

Bupropion is pharmacologically unique among antidepres-sants and is manufactured in immediate-release, slow-release (SR), and XR formulations. Although its primary mechanism of action is unclear, the drug has weak norepinephrine and dopamine reuptake inhibition. Bupropion is an activating drug, making it better suited for patients with poor energy or who feel they cannot tolerate a sedating medication. It is also virtually free from sexual side effects and has been used with limited success as an antidote for patients with SSRI-induced sexual side effects (Clayton et al., 2004). Bupropion rarely causes weight gain and is therefore a good choice for patients who are obese or who feel they cannot tolerate weight gain. Unlike SSRIs, SNRIs and TCAs, bupropion does not treat anxiety disorders and may even worsen anxiety in patients because of its activating properties. Bupropion car-ries a black-box warning against its use in patients with a history of seizures or eating disorders; the latter group was shown to have a higher incidence of seizures in clinical trials. Given its greater propensity for seizures, bupropion dosing should not be pushed above the FDA-recommended dosing limits. Bupropion has also been approved for treatment of smoking cessation and therefore may have particular utility for depressed patients who also want to quit smoking.

Tricyclic antidepressants are effective medications for treat-ing depression and anxiety, with evidence of being more effective than SSRIs for severe depression, but TCAs confer a greater side effect burden than newer antidepressants and can be fatal in overdose. TCAs are divided into tertiary and secondary amines. Tertiary amines, such as amitriptyline and imipramine, have greater anticholinergic, antihistaminic and α-adrenergic blockade side effects than secondary amines, such as their respective metabolites nortriptyline and desip-ramine. TCAs offer an advantage over other antidepressants in that blood levels can readily be checked and dosing indi-vidualized. Reasonable evidence suggests TCAs may be more effective in severely depressed patients (Agency for Health Care Policy Research, 1999). In addition, nortriptyline has a therapeutic window, with superior antidepressant efficacy if levels are maintained at 50 to 150 ng/mL. Because of car-diac conduction side effects, however, TCAs must be used with caution in patients with conduction delays or who are taking class I antiarrhythmic agents, and electrocardiograms

(ECGs) should be checked and monitored in patients older than 50 or those with suspected cardiac disease. TCAs also may cause tachycardia and orthostatic hypotension and thus should be used with caution in patients at risk for tachyarrhythmias or falls. The greatest single disadvantage to TCAs is their potential lethality in overdose; a typical 10-day supply can be lethal, and therefore TCAs should be prescribed cautiously in patients at high risk for suicide. TCAs are also used in a variety of headache and pain syndromes and thus may be useful in patients with such comorbidities.

Trazodone is structurally distinct from SSRIs, TCAs, tetracyclics or MAOIs, but it still inhibits neuronal uptake of serotonin. Although the U.S. Food and Drug Administration (FDA) has approved it as an antidepressant, trazodone is most often used as a sedative-hypnotic. Dosing as an antidepressant is usually 300 to 450 mg, whereas sedative-hypnotic dosing is usually 50 to 150 mg. Risks and side effects of trazodone include sedation, priapism, and myocardial irritability; the latter effect includes the potential of inducing torsades de pointes.

KEY TREATMENT

All antidepressants are generally equally effective; selection is most often based on side effect profile, previous response, comorbid conditions, drug interactions, and cost (Arroll et al., 2009; Trivedi et al., 2006) (SOR: A).

SSRIs, SNRIs, mirtazapine, and bupropion are first-line treatments for depression (Rush et al., 2006) (SOR: A).

Antidepressant doses should be increased every 2 to 4 weeks until remission of depressive symptoms is achieved or side effects become intolerable (SOR: A).

Treatment of depressive episodes ranges from 6 to 9 months to years, depending on the number of prior episodes, severity of episodes, and risk of relapse (AHCPR, 1999; Geddes et al., 2003) (SOR:A).

Psychotherapy has proved effective in treating depression, either as monotherapy or combined with pharmacotherapy (de Maat et al., 2008; Thase, 1997) (SOR: A).

Initiation of Treatment

Once a patient has been initiated on an antidepressant, dosing should be optimized to treat depressive symptoms to remission while minimizing side effects (Box 47-8). Patients should be monitored for improvement in their mood and their specific array of depressive symptoms. Continued use of measurement-based care tools, such as the PHQ-9 or QIDS, can aid in the objective assessment of improvement. Patients should be followed more frequently on initiation of treatment, increasing time between appointments as the patient improves. Monitoring for side effects, particularly those that patients may be reluctant to bring up spontaneously, such as sexual side effects, can improve adherence and the therapeutic alliance. Patients should also be monitored for any worsening of mood, increased irritability, impulsivity, insomnia, sudden switches into euphoria, or suicidal ideation. Such symptoms may suggest *bipolar diathesis*, in which case discontinuing the antidepressant and changing to mood stabilizing agents may be indicated. Antidepressant doses should be increased every 2 to 4 weeks until the patient shows a response, maximum dose is reached, or side effects limit further dose changes. Antidepressant doses should

Box 47-8 Assessing Antidepressant Treatment

1. Monitor effectiveness of treatment.
2. Continue assessment of specific symptoms.
3. Assess need for further titration of medication.
4. Continue to use measurement-based care.
5. Assess any worsening of mood, increased irritability, or worsening suicidal ideation.
6. Assess adherence to medication regimen.
7. Assess for medication side effects.
8. Continue to emphasize nutrition, physical activity, and caring for self.
9. Minimize complexity of medication dosing (e.g., once daily or nightly, when possible).

Box 47-9 Discontinuation of Antidepressant Treatment

Remission of symptoms for 6-12 months.
Tapering of medications rather than abrupt cessation.
Discussion of relapse risks and early warning signs of recurrence.

continue to be pushed until remission is achieved, or the patient has undergone an adequate antidepressant trial, i.e., continuation of a therapeutic dose for at least 4 to 8 weeks (Nierenberg et al., 2000).

Continuation of Treatment

As noted, physicians are encouraged to push treatment until symptoms remit, maximum doses are achieved, or side effects become intolerable. Once symptoms remit, medications should continue for 6 to 9 months because risk of relapse is greater if patients discontinue medications prematurely (AHCPR, 1999; Geddes et al., 2003). Patients who have had multiple episodes of depression should continue pharmacotherapy because lifetime relapse rates for such patients are 50% to 85% (Eaton et al., 2008), and risk of recurrence increases by 16% with each successive episode (Solomon et al., 2000). Ongoing treatment should also be considered for patients who experienced severe functional impairment, severe suicidal ideation, or serious suicide attempts.

Discontinuation of Treatment

For patients who have achieved ongoing remission and want to discontinue their medications, withdrawal of treatment should be gradual and carefully monitored (Box 47-9). Timing of discontinuation often depends on a patient's current life stressors and the potential consequences of depressive relapse (e.g., loss of new job, stress on recently repaired relationship). Antidepressants should be gradually withdrawn to minimize potential withdrawal syndromes and allow for rapid upward titration should depressive symptoms recur. Physicians should discuss early warning signs of relapse (insomnia, early-morning awakening, loss of interest in activities) and instruct patients to contact the physician should such symptoms recur. Risk of relapse is greatest in the first few months of discontinuing antidepressants, and thus a scheduled appointment in this period is often needed to monitor for relapse. Patients who relapse after cessation of antidepressants should be restarted on their previous medication and again titrated to remission of symptoms.

Antidepressant Failure

Patients who fail antidepressants should be carefully reevaluated, with reconsideration of medication adherence, adequacy of dosing and treatment duration, diagnosis, comorbid psychiatric illnesses, increased stressors, and unaddressed medical or substance comorbidities. Initial antidepressant failure may be relatively common; only one third of patients achieved remission after 12 to 14 weeks of treatment with citalopram in the STAR*D study (Trivedi et al., 2006). If a patient fails an adequate antidepressant trial, the next strategy is (1) switching to a different antidepressant, within the same class or across classes; (2) augmenting the existing antidepressant with a secondary agent; or (3) adding a second antidepressant to the first. Choice of strategy depends on patient preference, assessment of benefit from current antidepressant, current side effects, and psychiatric and medical comorbidities.

Switching antidepressants is generally considered when the patient has had little to no response to the first agent or is having intolerable side effects. Across-class switches are most often considered as an initial strategy (e.g., SSRI to SNRI), although within-class switches may also prove useful (e.g., fluoxetine to sertraline). Across-class or intraclass switching may yield response rates of 20% to 50% (Thase, 2008b). In the STAR*D study, switching from citalopram to either bupropion SR, venlafaxine, or sertraline yielded remission rates of 18% to 25% (Rush et al., 2006). No clear guidelines exist as how best to cross-taper medications, although it is generally unwise to stop antidepressants abruptly because withdrawal syndromes may ensue. Medications with a short half-life, such as venlafaxine (immediate release) or paroxetine, have most often been associated with withdrawal syndromes. Typically, patients complain of flulike symptoms, electric-like shocks in the back of their heads, or dizziness (Taylor et al., 2006). Consideration of half-life and slow cross-tapers often yields the most tolerable switch.

Augmentation strategies involve adding a second agent with no intrinsic antidepressant properties to the existing antidepressant. These are often considered when a patient has had a partial response to an antidepressant but has not reached remission, and switching to an alternate antidepressant may risk loss of existing response. The two best studied augmentation strategies to date are adding lithium and triiodothyronine (T_3). Although many lithium augmentation studies are limited by methodologic considerations, response has been seen as quickly as 48 hours or as long as 2 to 4 weeks. Standard lithium levels of 0.5 to 1.0 mmol/L have most often been used. T_3 augmentation has yielded similar results, if often better tolerated than lithium, usually with doses of 25 to 50 μg/day. Overall remission rates in patients unable to achieve antidepressant-alone remission range from 15% to 50% (Nierenberg et al., 2006). Atypical antipsychotic drugs have also been used as augmenting agents in nonpsychotic major depression, with beneficial results. Aripiprazole currently has an indication as an augmenting agent, at 2 to 15 mg daily. To date, no other atypical antipsychotic has an FDA indication as an augmenting agent, though a meta-analysis

of atypical antipsychotics as augmenting agents found their efficacy superior to placebo, with a number needed to treat (NNT) of nine for both response and remission (Nelson and Papakostas, 2009). Buspirone has also been used as an augmenting agent, as its 5-HT-1A receptor agonism may enhance SSRI response. In the STAR*D study, 30% of patients who failed to achieve remission taking citalopram went on to remit with the addition of buspirone, up to 60 mg daily (Trivedi et al., 2006).

Combining two antidepressants to treat refractory depression is based on the theory that targeting a greater number of neurotransmitters will lead to improved antidepressant response. Common strategies include combining mirtazapine and venlafaxine, bupropion and SSRIs, or bupropion and SNRIs. Combining drugs of similar class (e.g., SSRI + SSRI or SNRI + SNRI) currently has few data to support its use. Venlafaxine combined with mirtazapine and citalopram plus bupropion SR were effective in the STAR*D study when patients failed to achieve remission on their current regimen. Adding bupropion to citalopram achieved a remission rate of approximately 30% in patients whose symptoms failed to remit after 12 weeks of citalopram therapy. The combination of venlafaxine plus mirtazapine was used in a highly treatment-refractory group (failed three previous medication trials) and achieved remission of symptoms in approximately 14% of patients (McGrath et al., 2006).

KEY TREATMENT

Patients who fail antidepressants should be carefully reevaluated for medication adherence, adequacy of dosing and therapy duration, diagnosis, comorbid psychiatric illnesses, increased stressors, and unaddressed comorbidities (Trivedi et al., 2006) (SOR: A). Common strategies used when patients fail an initial antidepressant treatment are switching antidepressants (either within class or across classes) (Rush et al., 2006; Thase, 2008b), augmenting with other agents (lithium, T_3, atypical antipsychotics) (Nierenberg et al., 2006; Trivedi et al., 2006), or combining different antidepressants (McGrath et al., 2006) (SOR: A).

Anxiety

There is significant pharmacologic overlap between the treatment of depression and anxiety disorders. Most antidepressants are also effective antianxiety agents, or anxiolytics (see Table 47-3), thus simplifying treatment strategies when patients have both disorders. In addition, significant overlap also exists between medications that effectively treat GAD and panic disorder. Treatment recommendations for both GAD and panic will be explored separately in order to highlight some of the treatment differences between the two disorders.

Generalized Anxiety Disorder

Antidepressants are generally considered first-line agents for treatment of GAD because of efficacy and safety, effectiveness in treating comorbid major depression, and absence of addictive or abuse potential, as seen with benzodiazepines. As a general rule, starting antidepressant doses for patients with GAD should be approximately half the lowest starting dose for treatment of depression; many experience a paradoxical worsening of their symptoms on antidepressant initiation if doses are high (see Table 47-2). Patients with anxiety disorders are typically more sensitive to antidepressant side effects (see Table 47-4), and thus starting at lower doses and titrating slowly will likely yield better results.

The SSRIs and SNRIs are considered first-line treatments, with numerous studies demonstrating both efficacy and effectiveness (Hoffman and Mathew, 2008). A Cochrane review of antidepressant treatment of GAD that included paroxetine, sertraline, venlafaxine, and imipramine found a very large effect size, with NNT of only five patients for one patient to receive benefit, with no clear evidence of one antidepressant superior to another (Kapczinski et al., 2003). At present, the SSRIs escitalopram and paroxetine and the SNRIs venlafaxine and duloxetine are the only antidepressants with an FDA indication for GAD (see Table 47-3). No randomized controlled trials (RCTs) have yet supported the efficacy of fluoxetine or citalopram in the treatment of GAD, although their clinical use is based on the assumption that SSRIs exert a class effect and are likely equally effective. The SNRI desvenlafaxine may be effective but currently is indicated only for major depression.

The TCAs, also effective agents for treating GAD, have been relegated to second-line treatment because of side effects (e.g., anticholinergic, sedative, orthostatic) and potential lethality in overdose. Imipramine has the strongest data to support its use in GAD (Kapczinski et al., 2003). Although used effectively in the treatment of anxiety disorders, monoamine oxidase inhibitors (MAOIs) have significant side effects (risk for hypertensive crisis, potential lethal interactions with other medications) and likely do not have a role in primary care and should be reserved for psychiatric practice. Mirtazapine has shown some efficacy in open-label trials (Gambi et al., 2005) but needs further study in RCTs to be considered a first-line agent in GAD. Bupropion has a less clear role in the treatment of anxiety disorders and may worsen rather than alleviate anxiety symptoms. However, a recent pilot study showed that bupropion XL had comparable anxiolytic efficacy with escitalopram in a 12-week, double-blind RCT and was well tolerated (Bystritsky et al., 2008). Bupropion may have a role in GAD treatment in the future but currently may be considered a second-line or third-line agent.

Benzodiazepines are also extremely effective for treatment of GAD and offer the advantage of rapid effect. Onset of action is typically within hours, versus weeks with antidepressants. All benzodiazepines are theoretically equally effective in GAD, and thus selection of individual agents often involves comparing half-lives, metabolic pathways, and the presence or absence of active metabolites (particularly in patients with liver disease), and speed of onset of action. Benzodiazepines with shorter half-life result in the inconvenience of multiple daily dosing, the risk of rebound anxiety, and the common need to use as-needed doses as a "rescue" medication when symptoms are inadequately controlled. Medications such as clonazepam, with a long half life, or alprazolam XR, with a slower and more prolonged onset of action, may be more effective than drugs with shorter half-life, such as immediate-release alprazolam or lorazepam. Scheduled dosing of a benzodiazepine provides for a more consistent medication blood level and may also be a more effective approach than as-needed dosing. The duration of therapeutic effect for benzodiazepines is determined by the rate and extent of drug distribution (lipophilicity) and not necessarily by the rate of

elimination. Benzodiazepines such as diazepam have a longer half-life than lorazepam, but because diazepam is more lipophilic, it has a faster onset of action and shorter duration of effect after a single dose (Schatzberg and Nemeroff, 2009). Drug elimination occurs in the liver through microsomal oxidation or glucuronide conjugation. Oxidation is sensitive to liver disease and certain medical conditions and medications (e.g., cimetidine), and therefore benzodiazepines metabolized through hepatic oxidation are more likely to show unpredictability than those metabolized via conjugation. Benzodiazepines such as temazepam, lorazepam, and oxazepam are cleared through hepatic conjugation and are safer and better tolerated when oxidative elimination has been altered.

Even though benzodiazepines offer the advantage of rapid onset and effectiveness, other disadvantages have relegated them to second-line agents. Benzodiazepines pose a significant risk of dependency and withdrawal, are potentially lethal in overdose if mixed with other sedating agents (especially alcohol), and are ineffective in treating comorbid depression. Benzodiazepines also can impair attention and vigilance and cause dose-dependent anterograde amnesia, with limited effect on psychic symptoms, including worry (Hoehn-Saric et al., 1988). Benzodiazepines should generally be considered second- to third-line agents as monotherapy in GAD, although they are often used as adjunctive agents when initiating antidepressant treatment, to provide immediate relief of anxiety symptoms until antidepressant effects begin. Symptom severity and patient preference should be considered when deciding whether to use an antidepressant as monotherapy or to start a benzodiazepine with an antidepressant. A subset of patients may benefit from long-term treatment with both an antidepressant and a benzodiazepine.

Nonbenzodiazepine and nonantidepressant treatment may also be effective in the treatment of GAD, especially for patients with mild to moderate symptom severity. *Buspirone*, an azapirone that exerts 5-HT-1A receptor agonism, carries an FDA indication for GAD. Buspirone appears useful in the treatment of GAD, particularly for patients who have not yet received a benzodiazepine (Chessick et al., 2006). In clinical practice, buspirone can be used as monotherapy in patients with mild to moderate symptoms, and it is often considered an alternative to benzodiazepines as an augmenting agent to antidepressants. *Hydroxyzine*, an antihistaminic agent, also carries an FDA indication for GAD and has shown efficacy in RCTs (Llorca et al., 2002). Its sedative properties and lack of efficacy in comorbid disorders have relegated hydroxyzine to a second-line agent. Interestingly, a meta-analysis of effect sizes in pharmacotherapy of GAD recently showed that hydroxyzine had a larger effect size (0.45) than SSRIs (0.36) (Hidalgo et al., 2007). At present, hydroxyzine may be considered an alternative to benzodiazepines when no comorbid illnesses are present as monotherapy. Recent studies of *pregabalin* have also shown efficacy in the treatment of GAD. In the meta-analysis cited, pregabalin was found to have the largest effect size (0.5) of all agents (SSRIs, SNRIs, benzodiazepines, azaspirones, antihistamines, complementary/alternative agents). The effect size of pregabalin was determined from two large RCTs. In addition, pregabalin was found to be effective in relapse prevention compared to placebo over a 6-month trial (Feltner et al., 2008). *Beta blockers* such as propranolol and pindolol have also been used in the treatment of GAD. Although these can block the physiologic effects of anxiety, such as sweating and increased heart rate, beta blockers appear ineffective in treating the underlying emotional component of anxiety, and little empiric evidence supports their use in GAD at present.

KEY TREATMENT

SSRIs and SNRIs are considered first-line treatments for generalized anxiety disorder, with starting dose typically half that used in depression (Hoffman and Mathew, 2008) (SOR: A).

TCAs are effective in treatment of GAD (SOR: A), but their side effect profile and potential lethality have relegated them to second-line agents (Kapczinski, et al., 2003).

Benzodiazepines offer the advantage of rapid effect and proven efficacy (Chessick et al., 2006; Schatzberg and Nemeroff, 2009) (SOR: A), but carry risk of abuse and dependence.

Other agents for treatment of GAD include hydroxyzine (Llorca et al., 2002) (SOR: A), buspirone (Chessick et al., 2006) (SOR: B), and pregabalin (Feltner et al., 2008) (SOR: B).

Maintenance treatment of GAD reduces the likelihood of relapse (Thuile et al., 2009) (SOR: B).

Panic Disorder

Similar to treatment of GAD, SSRIs, SNRIs, TCAs and benzodiazepines have all been found to be effective for the treatment of panic disorder. Effectiveness of these agents appears relatively equal, and thus selection of a particular agent is most often based on tolerability, cost, ability to treat comorbid disorders, potential for abuse and tolerance, and patient preference. First-line agents to treat panic are most often SSRIs and SNRIs. Fluoxetine, paroxetine, sertraline, and venlafaxine all have FDA indications for panic disorder (see Table 47-3), although all the SSRIs have data to support their use (Otto et al., 2001). The SNRIs duloxetine and desvenlafaxine do not currently have large-RCT evidence to support their use in panic disorder but may have efficacy based on class effect. TCAs are also as effective in treating panic as SSRIs, but are less well tolerated due to their anticholinergic and antihistaminic side effects (Bakker et al., 2002). Both imipramine and clomipramine have the most data to support their use in panic disorder (APA, 2009). Because of tolerability and toxicity in overdose, TCAs are second-line agents for panic.

Benzodiazepines offer several advantages over antidepressants in the treatment of panic, including rapid onset, as-needed dosing schedules, and relief of insomnia and somatic symptoms (Bruce et al., 2003). Similar to use in GAD, selection of a particular benzodiazepine is based on half-life, speed of onset of action, presence or absence of active metabolites, and metabolic pathways (particularly in patients with liver disease). All benzodiazepines are likely equally effective in treating panic, although in clinical practice, higher-potency benzodiazepines (e.g., alprazolam, clonazepam, lorazepam) are used more often than lower-potency drugs (e.g., oxazepam). Clonazepam and alprazolam both are FDA approved for panic disorder, and some clinicians prefer clonazepam to alprazolam because of clonazepam's longer half-life, less frequent dosing, and slower onset of action. Lorazepam and diazepam do not have an FDA indication for panic, but seem to be effective agents in RCTS and clinical practice (Mitte et al., 2005). Benzodiazepines may be considered as first-line monotherapy when no comorbid conditions exist with panic

disorder. Agents with rapid onset (alprazolam, lorazepam) may be preferred if taken on an as-needed basis or used as a rescue medication. However, shorter-acting agents can introduce problems with interdose rebound anxiety or more difficulty with adherence to multidose regimens. Agents with longer half-life, such as clonazepam and alprazolam XR, may be scheduled once or twice daily to provide more even coverage throughout the day, but do not provide immediate relief if taken on an as-needed basis.

Although benzodiazepines can bring quick relief from panic symptoms, their side effect profile and risk of dependency, abuse, and withdrawal must be considered when deciding on their use. Common side effects include sedation, fatigue, ataxia, slurred speech, memory impairment, and weakness. Geriatric patients taking benzodiazepines may be at higher risk for falls and fractures (Stone et al., 2008). Patients with a substance abuse history may need to be monitored closely for signs and symptoms of abuse; patients actively abusing substances should probably not be prescribed benzodiazepines. For many of these patients, discussing clear expectations that prescriptions will not be rewritten or refilled before a set date can limit later conflicts and improve treatment adherence.

Evidence for the use of beta blockers in panic disorder is sparse. Beta blockers have been used to reduce the somatic symptoms of panic attacks, such as palpitations, but do not seem to be effective in overall treatment of panic disorder.

KEY TREATMENT

SSRIs, SNRIs, TCAs, and benzodiazepines have all been found to be effective in the treatment of panic disorder (Otto et al., 2001) (SOR: A).

First-line agents for panic disorder are SSRIs and SNRIs, with starting doses typically half that for depression (APA, 2009) (SOR: A).

Benzodiazepines can be used as first-line agents when no comorbid psychiatric issues are present, including issues of substance abuse and dependence (Mitte et al., 2005) (SOR: A).

Maintenance treatment of panic disorder has been shown to reduce the likelihood of relapse (Thuile et al., 2009) (SOR: B).

Continuation of Treatment in Anxiety Disorders

Treatment for anxiety disorders should be continued for 6 months to a year; a more definitive time frame is not yet clear. Results from long-term RCTs of antidepressants in anxiety disorders indicate that maintenance treatment significantly reduces the risk of relapse, whatever the disorder (Thuile et al., 2009). Decisions on length of treatment are generally made on a case-by-case basis, taking into account the risk/benefit ratio of treatment versus no treatment. If the decision is to discontinue treatment, the medication should be tapered at a rate that takes into account its pharmacokinetics and whether the patient experiences withdrawal symptoms (see Box 47-9).

Other Considerations

Antidepressants and Suicidal Ideation

In 2004 the FDA added a black-box warning to all antidepressants indicating that the use of antidepressants in children, adolescents, and young adults under 25 years of age increased the risk of suicidal thinking and behavior. The warning on antidepressants was based on an analysis of 372 clinical trials involving 11 antidepressant medications, noting an increase in the number of patients who experienced an increase in suicidal ideation and behavior, although no increase in actual suicides was observed. Further analysis of the FDA data revealed a strong age-dependent relationship, such that the greatest risk was in patients younger than 25. In clinical terms, four additional patients in 1000, age 18 to 24 years, would be expected to experience suicidal ideation or behavior as a result of taking antidepressants, and an additional 14 patients in 1000, under age 18, would be expected to experience worsening. Patients older than 30 showed a reduction in suicidal ideation as a result of taking antidepressants, with a reduction of 6 patients of 1000 in adults over 65. The net effect of antidepressant use in patients age 25 to 64 seems moderately protective against suicidal ideation and more strongly protective for adults age 65 and older (Levenson and Holland, 2006). Antidepressants should be used cautiously in patients under age 25, with close monitoring for worsening of mood or thoughts of suicide, particularly in the days and weeks after the drug is initiated. For the majority of depressed patients, the beneficial effects of antidepressants greatly outweigh the risks (Libby et al., 2007).

Nontraditional Therapy

Interest in complementary and alternative medicine (CAM) for health disorders has been growing steadily in the last several decades. As a result, a greater number of alternative or complementary agents are being tested in more methodologically rigorous ways, allowing greater scientific assessment of such treatments. Survey evidence suggests that as many as 40% to 60% of patients may be taking CAM therapies, although patients often do not disclose such use to their physicians (Elkins et al., 2005). In addition, because production of alternative agents is unregulated, variability in product strength, dosing, and purity is common, which in turn likely affects the predictability of their outcomes. Given the widespread use of CAM agents and patients' apparent reluctance to spontaneously disclose such use to their providers, it is incumbent on physicians to inquire about such use.

The majority of CAM treatments have been used to treat depression, including St John's wort (Hypericum perforatum), S-adenosyl-methinionine, and omega-3 fatty acids. In a Cochrane review of St John's wort for treatment of major depression, great heterogeneity was found among the 29 analyzed trials (Linde et al., 2005). St John's wort was found to be superior to placebo and similarly effective as standard antidepressants, but findings were more favorable to St John's wort studies from German-speaking countries, where use of the extract has a long tradition. The more positive results may be caused by physician expertise with the medication, patient selection, or flawed methodologies in some research. The larger, placebo-controlled studies have yielded mixed results, although compared to antidepressants, St John's wort has generally been better tolerated (Shelton, 2009).

S-Adenosyl-L-methionine (SAM-e), a dietary supplement, has been used to treat a variety of illnesses, ranging from major depression to osteoarthritis to liver disease. Clinical trials have shown SAM-e to be superior to placebo and equivalent to TCAs in treating patients with depression, although the most robust findings have been shown with parenteral administration of the drug. Studies using the oral form have yielded more variable results. In adjunctive use with antidepressants, only one open-label study has been published to date. SAM-e has been shown to be safe and well tolerated thus far (Papakostas, 2009).

Omega-3 fatty acids have a variety of health benefits and may be helpful as augmenting agents in the treatment of major depression. The best-studied agents are eicosapentaenoic acid (EPA) and docosahexaenoic acid (DHA). Findings in depression are limited by variability in study design and small sample sizes, although the majority of evidence favors a positive effect in the treatment of mood disorders (Freeman, 2009).

At present, little robust evidence supports the efficacy of CAM agents in the treatment of anxiety disorders. Kava *(Piper methysticum)* has preliminary evidence of efficacy in GAD, but further testing is needed to determine its side effects and potential for hepatotoxicity (Sarris and Kavanagh, 2009). A meta-analysis found no statistically significant difference between kava and placebo (Hidalgo et al., 2007). Given the paucity of current evidence, caution should be used when considering kava as a therapeutic agent.

Other Treatments

Electroconvulsive Therapy

Electroconvulsive therapy (ECT) involves a brief electrical stimulation of the brain while the patient is anesthetized, inducing a seizure. ECT remains the most effective treatment for depression (UK ECT Group, 2003), although the stigma surrounding the treatment, misinformation about its practice, side effects, and cost have often made it a treatment of last resort. Although occasionally used as first-line therapy for severe depression, ECT is often used for multitreatment-refractory patients, those with psychotic depression, suicidal patients (imminent), and depressed patients with compromised oral intake. A typical course is six to 20 treatments, with patients receiving ECT three times a week during the acute phase, gradually increasing the time between treatments as improvement becomes apparent. After acute treatment, patients are often returned to antidepressant therapy, although medication efficacy after ECT does not appear to be enhanced (Kellner et al., 2006). Physicians should be aware that ECT is safe, well tolerated, humane, and effective.

Vagus Nerve Stimulation and Transcranial Magnetic Stimulation

Vagal nerve stimulation (VNS) involves the surgical implantation of a nerve stimulator for the left vagus nerve at the cervical level and has been approved for treatment of refractory depression. VNS is not an acute treatment, but has shown some long-term benefit for depressed patients (George et al., 2005). Transcranial magnetic stimulation (TMS) involves the introduction of repetitive magnetic impulses to the right prefrontal cortex in a series of treatments over several weeks. TMS is approved for the treatment of unipolar depression for patients who have failed one trial of antidepressants or for those patients who have exhibited marked intolerance to antidepressants (O'Reardon et al., 2007).

Psychotherapy

In addition to pharmacologic interventions for depression, panic disorder, and GAD, psychotherapy continues to be an effective tool used by psychiatrists and psychotherapists for treating mood and anxiety disorders. Although primary care physicians will not administer such treatments, it is important to be aware of general psychotherapeutic concepts and strategies. Several types of therapy have strong evidence supporting their efficacy in treating both depression and anxiety disorders, including cognitive-behavioral therapy, interpersonal therapy, psychodynamic psychotherapy, problem-solving therapy, and supportive therapy (Cuijpers et al., 2008). Some patients may prefer to begin treatment with medications alone, whereas others may prefer only psychotherapy or a combination. Combined pharmacologic and psychotherapeutic interventions have generally been shown to be superior to either approach alone in trials for both anxiety disorders and depression (Furukawa et al., 2007) (Pampallona et al., 2004).

Referral to Mental Health Providers

Which patients should be referred to mental health providers? Referrals may be made because of patient preference, severity of illness, or because of the complexity of comorbid illnesses. Patients who experience refractory depression or psychotic depression are best treated by specialty providers. Patients with bipolar disorder should be referred as well, especially those suffering from bipolar depressions, as they are often especially difficult to treat, usually require complex polypharmacy, and worsen with inappropriate treatment. Patients requesting or needing psychotherapy or behavioral therapy may be referred to a mental health provider.

Summary

For the majority of depressed patients, the beneficial effects of antidepressants greatly outweigh the risks. CAM treatments for depression may be beneficial for some patients, but study methodology limits their generalizability. ECT is still considered the most effective treatment for severe depression. VNS and TMS are emerging therapies for the treatment of depression.

KEY TREATMENT

Psychotherapy is an important and effective treatment strategy for both depression and anxiety. Psychotherapy combined with pharmacotherapy often yields superior results to either treatment alone (Furukawa et al., 2007; Pampallona et al., 2004) (SOR: A).

References

The complete reference list is available online at www.expertconsult.com.

Web Resources

Patient Resources

National Institute of Mental Health

www.nih.nimh.gov

Provides excellent up-to-date information on the symptoms, causes, course, and treatment of a number of illnesses. Provides numerous lists and links to resources.

Anxiety Disorders

Freedom From Fear

freedomfromfear.org

National non-profit mental health advocacy organization focused on anxiety and depressive disorders.

The Obsessive-Compulsive Foundation

www.ocdfoundation.org

Provides information and resources on obsessive-compulsive disorder and other mental health diagnoses.

Support for Patients, Family, and Friends

American Foundation for Suicide Prevention

www.afsp.org

Leading national non-profit dedicated to understanding and preventing suicide through education and research, and to reaching out to people with mood disorders and those impacted by suicide.

The Federation for Families for Children's Mental Health

www.coloradofederation.org

The mission of the Federation is to promote mental health for all children, youth and families. The website has numerous links to resources, articles, books, and support groups.

Healthy Minds

www.healthyminds.org

Site created by the American Psychiatric Association to provide education and resources on mental health issues.

National Alliance on Mental Illness

www.nami.org

Grass-roots, self-help, support, and advocacy group for people with severe mental illnesses, their family members, and friends.

Depression and Bipolar Support Alliance

www.dbsalliance.org

Provides education to patients and families about mood disorders; advocates research funding, improving access to care, fostering self-help, and decreasing public stigma of these illnesses.

Depression Is Real

www.depressionisreal.org

Provides information and resources about depression.

Madison Institute of Medicine

www.miminc.org

Provides information and resources on mood disorders, anxiety disorders, and dementias.

WebMD Depression

www.webmd.com/depression

Provides information on diagnosis and treatment of mood disorders.

48 CHAPTER

Delirium and Dementia

David A. Smith and David A. Brechtelsbauer

Dementia and delirium are organic brain syndromes characterized by global cognitive dysfunction. *Delirium* is the recognized terminology for what has also been called acute confusional state, acute brain syndrome, acute cerebral insufficiency, and toxic-metabolic encephalopathy. *Dementia* has commonly been called "senility" or the insufficiently specific "organic brain syndrome." It may be useful to conceptualize delirium as *acute* brain failure and dementia as *chronic* brain failure.

Delirium

Clinical Features

Key Points

- Delirium is characterized by an acute change from usual function and cognition.
- Level of consciousness varies, often dramatically, in patients with delirium.
- Delirium may be hyperactive, hypoactive, or mixed.
- Delirium is often overlooked or misdiagnosed.
- Delirium worsens prognosis and increases length of stay and likelihood of nursing home placement.

Delirium is an acute disorder of global cognitive function involving attention, consciousness, orientation, memory, sensory perception, executive function, and behavior. Misperceptions of any of the senses may occur, but auditory and visual disturbances manifesting as suggestible hallucinations or illusions are common. For example, the delirious patient may interpret spots on the floor tiles as bugs or the sound of the wind as whispering. Delirious patients have abnormal visual perception compared to cognitively normal and demented patients that is independent of the severity of cognitive impairment (Brown et al., 2009).

Delirium cases can be grouped into hyperactive, hypoactive, and mixed subtypes on the basis of psychomotor behavior (Meagher et al., 2008). It has been suggested that the *hypoactive* subtype is more often seen in elderly persons and with delirium caused by hypoxia, metabolic abnormality, and anticholinergic drugs, whereas the *hyperactive* subtype is more common in substance intoxication and withdrawal states. Cognitive impairment and generalized slowing of the electroencephalogram (EEG) are similar in hypoactive and hyperactive subtypes.

Delirium can occur at any age, although advanced age is an independent risk factor. Rather than considering chronologic age in assessing risk, a family physician may best consider biologic age and frailty.

Delirium is often overlooked or misdiagnosed. This lack of diagnostic clarity is concerning given that, independent of other variables, delirium worsens prognosis (Fong et al., 2009; McAvay et al., 2006), often leading to chronic decreased function and cognition. Only 15% of delirious hospitalized patients will regain their baseline function by discharge, and less than half will return to prior function at 6 months (Khan et al., 2009). Delirium increases hospital length of stay by 5 to 10 days (Siddiqi et al., 2006), as well as the likelihood of nursing home placement (Inouye et al., 1998). Finally, mortality increases by 10% to 37% in hospitalized elderly patients (McCusker et al., 2002; Siddiqi et al., 2006). Approximately 40% of patients with delirium during hospitalization who survive to discharge will die within 1 year (Inouye, 2006).

Delirium prevalence and incidence vary greatly across settings of care and populations served. From 10% to 15% of hospitalized elderly patients have delirium on admission, and another 5% to 10% develop it during their stay. More than half of long-term care residents will exhibit delirium on hospital admission. Postsurgical patients (e.g., hip fracture, cardiac surgery) and elderly patients cared for in an intensive care unit (ICU) are at particularly high risk (Khan et al., 2009).

Etiology

Key Points

- Central nervous system immaturity in children and CNS disease in elderly persons may explain the increased prevalence of delirium in these two groups.
- Children generally have a more acute onset of delirium, but a less fluctuating course, than adults.
- Delirium is thought to be caused by an acute cholinergic deficit; other neurotransmitter disturbances are also probably involved.

A stress-diathesis model has been proposed to explain the risk of delirium, depending on the severity of an insult to brain function and the vulnerability of the brain because of immaturity in children and central nervous system (CNS) disease or degenerative disorders most common in elderly persons. This helps explain the highest risk of delirium in the elderly population and more frequent occurrence in children than in young and middle-aged adults.

Although the phenomenology of delirium in adults and in elderly persons differs only in the severity of cognitive symptoms and resilience in recovery, the course and symptomatology in childhood are different. Childhood delirium is often associated with febrile illness and from CNS-toxic medications (anticholinergics) (Lenntjens et al., 2008). Delirium in a child is more likely to have a very acute onset, but a less fluctuating course with less disruption of the sleep-wake cycle, than in adults. Cognitive deficits may be less pronounced in children, whereas hallucinations, delusional thinking, and labile mood may be more pronounced. The different array of causes of delirium in children and adults might explain these differences. In both children and elderly patients with dementia, problematic behaviors caused by delirium are often falsely attributed to irritability associated with illness or oppositional behavior toward caregivers. When a child cannot be comforted by a parent, delirium should be suspected.

The remainder of this discussion focuses on delirium in the elderly patient.

Neurochemical Hypothesis

Cholinergic transmission in the CNS has a major role in cognition and attention, and an acute cholinergic deficit exists in delirium. Dopaminergic transmission is increased in delirium, and this or the imbalance between cholinergic and dopaminergic systems may be etiologic. Disturbances in other neurotransmitters are hypothesized, perhaps explaining subtypes or variations in presentations of delirium. Serotonin may be increased in delirium associated with serotonin syndrome and in hepatic encephalopathy, but decreased in delirium from other causes. Glutamate and γ-aminobutyric acid (GABA) are believed to be increased in alcohol withdrawal and hepatic encephalopathy. Melatonin may be increased or decreased in delirium, which may explain hypoactive and hyperactive subtypes. Norepinephrine may be increased in delirium associated with anoxia and in hepatic encephalopathy. Inflammation may also play a role in causing delirium, either by a direct neurotoxic effect or by causing disturbances in the neurotransmitters. Figure 48-1 depicts a theoretic explanation for the etiology of delirium.

Diagnostic Process

Key Points

- Tools for diagnosing and managing delirium include Confusion Assessment Method and Memorial Delirium Assessment Scale.
- Dementia is the strongest risk factor for development of delirium.
- Diagnostic testing needs to be informed by a thorough history and careful physical examination.

Diagnostic criteria for delirium are adapted from the American Psychiatric Association's *Diagnostic and Statistical Manual of Mental Disorders,* 4th edition, text revision (DSM IV-TR, 2000) (Box 48-1). Given the high prevalence of delirium in certain health care settings and clinical circumstances, diagnosis should not depend solely on a high index of suspicion. Formal evaluation of mental status to detect delirium or dementia should become part of routine assessment of elderly patients presenting with a change of condition. This not only fosters appropriate preventive and therapeutic interventions, but also alerts the *interdisciplinary team* (IDT) to plan care to ensure patient and staff safety, specific patient and family education, carefully considering cognition and function at discharge planning.

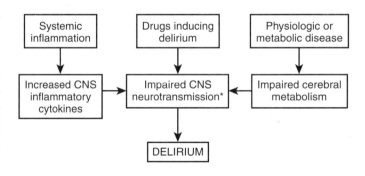

*More vulnerable in immature or already impaired brain.

Figure 48-1 Theoretic etiologic hypothesis for delirium.

Box 48-1 Diagnostic Criteria for Delirium (DSM IV-TR)

A. Disturbance of consciousness (i.e., reduced clarity of awareness of the environment) with reduced ability to focus, sustain, or shift attention.

B. A change in cognition (e.g., memory deficits, disorientation, language disturbance) or the development of a perceptual disturbance that is not better accounted for by a preexisting, established, or evolving dementia.

C. The disturbance develops over a short period (usually hours to days) and tends to fluctuate during the course of the day.

D. There is evidence from the history, physical examination, or laboratory findings that the disturbance is caused by a general medical condition, a substance intoxication, or a substance withdrawal; is the result of multiple etiologies; is caused by an etiology other than these (e.g., sensory deprivation); or cannot be determined.

Modified from American Psychiatric Association. Diagnostic and Statistical Manual of Mental Disorders, 4th ed, text revision. Washington, DC, APA, 2000.

Several standardized instruments have been developed to assess for delirium and monitor severity. The Confusion Assessment Method (CAM) is based on DSM IV-R criteria and has 94% to 100% sensitivity and 90% to 95% specificity, with good interrater reliability when used with formal cognitive testing and administered by trained interviewers (Inyoue et al., 1990). Once diagnosed, the 10-item Memorial Delirium Assessment Scale is useful to monitor severity (Breibart et al., 1997). Other scales are used in specific settings (e.g., ICU). Given the fluctuating course of delirium, it is essential to perform monitoring frequently.

History and Physical Examination

The etiology of delirium is often multifactorial. Therefore the history and physical examination must be detailed and exhaustive; stopping on discovery of one cause is inadequate. The history relevant to delirium is largely a search for risk factors. Risks may be considered as predisposing factors (vulnerability of brain) and precipitating factors (insults to brain). Dementia is the strongest risk factor for delirium (Cole, 2004); two thirds of elderly patients with delirium will also have dementia. This relationship is so strong that if delirium is diagnosed in an elderly person without known dementia, an investigation should be made once the delirium has resolved.

Severe illness, infections, sensory deprivation, medications, and substances of abuse causing either toxicity or withdrawal states can precipitate delirium. Use of medications confers risk both by number and by drug interaction. The risk of delirium is especially high in elders who have three or more medications initiated within a 24-hour period during hospitalization. Box 48-2 is a compilation of predisposing and precipitating risks for delirium, and Boxes 48-3 and 48-4 list medical illnesses and drugs, respectively, that can cause or contribute to delirium.

A comprehensive physical examination should be completed, emphasizing the neurologic exam, including objective tests of cognition (see Diagnostic Process for dementia).

An investigation for focal neurologic signs should be done. For example, *asterixis* (flapping of maximally dorsiflexed hands) is characteristic of hepatic encephalopathy, but not unique to it. Tremor may be present in withdrawal states, as are signs of autonomic dysfunction (hypertension, tachycardia, mydriasis, sweating).

Nuances of the history and physical examination are essential to hypothesizing the cause(s) of delirium and to inform decisions to order laboratory and other diagnostic studies and plan specific therapy. Broadly testing without guidance from the history and physical exam is particularly inefficient in determining the cause(s) of delirium. Neuroimaging is of extremely low yield unless done to investigate focal neurologic findings. Furthermore, history of a fall with head trauma and even the finding of a subdural hematoma on computed tomography (CT) might not fully explain a patient's delirium as caused only by acute brain injury if, for example, the fall was caused by a preexisting delirium from recent initiation of a medication.

Other investigations may be needed in specific situations. An EEG is not routinely needed but is helpful in diagnosing

---

Box 48-2 Risk Factors for Delirium

Predisposing Factors

Sensory impairment
Immobility (functional and iatrogenic)
Psychological stress
Cognitive impairment (dementia, MCI)
Lower educational status
Advanced age
Past history of delirium, CVA, falls, or neurologic disease
Multiple medical comorbidities
Male gender
Polypharmacy

Precipitating Factors

Medical conditions (see Box 48-3)
Medications (see Box 48-4)
Environmental change or stress
Pain
Profound sleep deprivation

MCI, Mild cognitive impairment; *CVA*, cerebrovascular accident (stroke).

Box 48-3 Medical Conditions that May Cause or Contribute to Delirium

Cardiovascular disease
  Arrhythmia
  Congestive heart failure
  Myocardial infarction
  Shock
  Cerebrovascular accident (stroke)
  Hypertensive encephalopathy
Central nervous system (CNS) neoplasm
Infections
  CNS infection
  Pneumonia
  Sepsis
  Urinary tract infection
Metabolic disorders
  Acidosis/alkalosis
  Anemia
  Endocrinopathies
  Fluid and electrolyte imbalance
  Hepatic failure
  Renal failure
Nutrition related
  General
  Specific deficiencies (e.g., thiamine)
Pulmonary disorders
  Hypoxia
  Hypercarbia
Sensory deprivation
  Hearing
  Vision
  "ICU psychosis"
Trauma
  Head
  Other severe injury
  Surgery

toxic encephalopathy, and it is essential in a patient with suspected nonconvulsive status epilepticus.

Prevention

Key Point

- Prevalence of delirium in high-risk settings mandates uniform implementation of unit-wide or facility-wide preventive programs.

An evaluation of risk allows caregivers to apply preventive strategies to avoid development of delirium in high-risk individuals (Box 48-5). However, given the high prevalence in hospitalized elderly patients and in long-term care patients, and the benign nature of many of the strategies for prevention, a standardized facility-wide prevention program may be more appropriate and effective. Prevention involving nonpharmacologic strategies attempts to maintain or normalize sleep patterns, stimulate physical and mental activity consistent with the elderly person's function, maintain or restore orientation to time/person/place, avoid or correct fluid and electrolyte disturbances, maximize the accuracy of sensory perceptions, and minimize the use of catheters and physical restraints.

Benzodiazepines and anticholinergic medications are best avoided when possible. Appropriate pain relief must be balanced with the risk of narcotic-induced delirium. Meperidine creates high risk from short analgesic effect but prolonged elimination of a nonanalgesic but CNS-toxic metabolite. Trials of proactive geriatrics consultation (Marcantonia et al., 2001), nurse-led IDT protocol-based interventions (Milsen et al., 2001), and preemptive low-dose haloperidol (Kalisvaart et al., 2005) have demonstrated decreases in delirium severity in elderly patients hospitalized for repair of hip fractures.

Box 48-4 Drugs that May Cause or Contribute to Delirium

Antiarrhythmics
Anticholinergics
Antidepressants
Antiemetics
Antiepileptics
Antihistamines
Antiparkinsonian agents
Antipsychotics
Antineoplastic agents
Anxiolytics
Centrally acting antihypertensive agents
Corticosteroids
Mood stabilizers
Muscle relaxants
Nonsteroidal anti-inflammatory drugs
Opioid analgesics
Sedative-hypnotics

From American Medical Directors Association. Delirium and Acute Problematic Behavior Clinical Practice Guideline. Columbia, Md, AMDA, 2008.

KEY TREATMENT

Geriatrics consultation, nurse-led interdisciplinary programs, and preemptive low-dose haloperidol decreased delirium severity (but not incidence) in randomized controlled trials (RCTs) or pre/post trials (Kalisvaart et al., 2005; Marcantonia et al., 2001; Milsen et al., 2001) (SOR: B).

Treatment

Key Points

- Nonpharmacologic management plans should be considered first when treating delirium.
- Indications for pharmacotherapy include delirium-induced behaviors that create a danger to the patient or others, or that interfere with necessary medical therapy.
- Fluctuating nature of delirium makes assessment of treatment efficacy difficult. Assessments must be objective and repeated frequently. Repeat assessment to judge drug efficacy should be consistent with time required for drug to reach steady state.

Treatment of delirium begins with maximized effort to apply strategies outlined in Box 48-5. Identifying and treating one or more potential causes of delirium are equally important (e.g., correcting fluid and electrolyte imbalance, treating an infection *and* discontinuing medications conferring risk). Many delirium-induced behaviors respond well to nonpharmacologic interventions. For example, a delirious elderly patient with repetitive vocalizations disturbing others should be managed by

---

Box 48-5 Prevention and Treatment Strategies for Delirium

1. Provide reassurance and education.
2. Optimize orientation.
    Minimize potentially ambiguous stimuli (e.g., overhead pager).
    Permit visitation (overnight family stay).
    Minimize room/facility transfers.
    Ensure consistent staff assignment.
    Provide clear instructions.
    Use frequent eye contact.
3. Optimize vision and hearing.
4. Optimize nutrition and fluid intake.
5. Optimize pain management,
6. Optimize mobility within patient's limitations,
    Minimize restraints and catheter use.
    Maximize independent function (e.g., grooming).
7. Optimize sleep hygiene.
    Ensure consistent hour of retirement.
    Use bright light during day, with dark, quiet nights.
    Prevent nocturia.
    Provide pre-retirement routine (warm milk/herb tea, relaxation techniques, back massage).
    Avoid sedative-hypnotics.
8. Provide proactive medication management.
    Avoid drugs that typically cause delirium.
    Minimize polypharmacy.

protecting others from the noise, not by sedating the delirious patient. Having a family member or sitter stay with a restless patient is better than use of physical or chemical restraints.

Pharmacologic treatment becomes necessary when patients have delirium-induced behavior that makes them a danger to self or others, or that interferes with needed medical care (e.g., maintaining bed rest after major surgery, maintaining catheter integrity). Hypoactive delirium might warrant treatment to improve oral intake of food, fluids, and medication or to avoid the medical consequences of inactivity. Additionally, some patients will require treatment for the confusion or hallucinations causing anxiety and fear. Both agitation in hyperactive delirium and lethargy in hypoactive delirium increase the risk for malnutrition and dehydration, aspiration, pressure ulcerations, and deep venous thrombosis or pulmonary embolism. The goal of pharmacologic management should be correction of neurochemical abnormalities, not simply sedation.

No medications are approved by the U.S. Food and Drug Administration (FDA) for treatment of delirium. Benzodiazepines are first-line therapy in patients with delirium induced by alcohol and sedative withdrawal. Antipsychotics are generally considered the drugs of choice in patients with most other types of delirium requiring pharmacologic management. The mode of action for antipsychotics in delirium is probably antagonism of dopamine and the resultant increase in acetylcholine. The choice of antipsychotic should be individualized based on suspected etiology, target symptoms, and patient susceptibility to adverse drug reactions (ADRs) because of age and comorbid conditions. The profile of antipsychotics regarding risk of cardiovascular events and death, QT_c prolongation, anticholinergic effects, sedation, hypotension, and resulting glucose intolerance and movement disorders must be considered when choosing a drug. Higher doses and longer duration of therapy increase the risk of ADRs, as do age, female gender, and preexisting mood disorders or dementia.

Delirious patients, particularly the elderly, often respond to fairly brief courses of low doses of antipsychotics, which decreases the chance of adverse side effects. Benzodiazepines are not recommended, but if used, low doses of short–half-life products (loratzepam, oxazepam) are preferred in elderly patients. Occasionally, methylphenidate is tried in hypoactive delirium. Delivery of medication to a delirious patient can be difficult; rapidly dissolving oral formulations are useful when cooperation with tablets or capsules is problematic. Depot injections of antipsychotics have no role in the treatment of delirium.

The fluctuating course of delirium makes evaluation of drug therapy difficult. Monitoring of mental status and behavior throughout the day using objective measures is required. The use of any of the recognized pharmacologic treatments for delirium risks further impairment of cognitive function, thereby confounding monitoring because the observer has little to differentiate an inadequate response to therapy (and need for uptitration), worsening of the delirium per se, or worsening of cognition from an adverse drug effect, compounding the original delirium.

When treating delirium, the family physician should employ nonpharmacologic strategies, medicate only when necessary, and use monotherapy. Adjust dose to age/body weight/composition and renal/hepatic function; avoid as-needed dosing; and titrate dose based on repeated objective assessments of delirium severity at intervals consistent with the time necessary for the drug to reach steady state. Treatment for 7 to 10 days after symptoms resolve is usual.

KEY TREATMENT

Benzodiazepines are indicated for the treatment of alcohol withdrawal seizures (SOR: A) but are *not recommended* for treatment of non-alcohol-related delirium (SOR: B) (Cochrane Review).

Haloperidol (<3.5 mg/day), risperidone, and olanzapine are equally effective in treating delirium, with few adverse effects (Cochrane Review) (SOR: B).

Despite plausible theoretic arguments for efficacy, no convincing evidence supports the use of cholinesterase inhibitors for delirium (Cochrane Review) (SOR: B).

Natural History of Delirium

Delirium is usually of acute onset and transient duration. Delirium often resolves a few days to a few weeks after etiologic insults are corrected. In some patients, however, delirium may persist. When chronic, delirium may result in permanent cognitive deficits, meeting the criteria for dementia (Fong et al., 2009). Hastening the progression of an existing dementia might explain this clinical observation. Delirium is persistent at hospital discharge in almost one third of patients, with almost as many still having symptoms and signs of delirium 6 months after discharge (McAvay et al., 2006; McCusker et al., 2003).

Dementia

Dementia is a syndrome characterized by multiple chronic and progressive cognitive deficits. Deficits in short-term memory and inability to learn new information are typical symptoms that first bring the patient to medical attention. The initial clinical problem is to determine if the presenting concerns are caused by dementia, and if so, to determine the type of dementia.

Clinical Features

Key Points

- Dementia is characterized by multiple areas of cognitive impairment but preserved level of alertness.
- Age-related memory loss, mild cognitive impairment, depression, delirium, and DSM Axis I psychiatric disorders should be considered in the differential diagnosis of dementia.

Dementia is caused by a heterogeneous group of brain disorders that result in global impairment of cognition. In addition to memory impairment, impairment in language (aphasia), inability to carry out motor tasks (apraxia), inability to recognize objects (agnosia), and loss of executive function are seen. Mood, personality, and behavior are often affected. Dementia is distinguished from mental retardation and developmental delay by its onset after a long period of higher, often normal cognitive function. Dementia must be differentiated from delirium, as noted earlier. Of greatest utility to the primary care physician, attention is preserved in dementia, but it is altered and labile in delirium.

Some elderly persons present with a concern about mild changes in memory (inability to recall names and slower processing of information) but have no functional deficits. This age-related memory loss is thought to be normal. Of more concern is the emerging concept of *mild cognitive impairment* (MCI). Patients with MCI have memory concerns corroborated by an informant, objective but mild memory loss, normal general cognitive function, and intact activities of daily living (ADLs). Many, but not all, patients with MCI progress to Alzheimer-type dementia. Depression in the elderly patient can masquerade as dementia. An elderly patient might present with nondysphoric depression, marked by apathy, decreased cognitive ability, nervousness, somatization, or insomnia. This condition should be recognized and treated as depression. Patients need to be carefully followed because almost half will develop dementia within 5 years (Alexopoulos et al., 1993).

Because psychotic features can occur in delirium, dementia, and depression, psychotic mental illnesses are included in the differential diagnosis of impaired cognitive status. Key features distinguishing the causes of cognitive impairment are summarized in Table 48-1.

Diagnostic Process

Key Points

- Use of clinical tools will improve the precision, efficiency, and usefulness of the clinical evaluation, as well as provide a baseline for comparison because dementia progresses over time.

- Mini-Cog is an efficient and easily interpreted tool for initial cognitive assessment.
- Demonstration of ability to perform ADLs and IADLs will provide insight into the practical problems created by dementia and allow for focused anticipatory guidance relative to patient safety and risk for exploitation.
- Initial laboratory evaluation of the dementia patient includes CBC, urinalysis, chemistry panel, TSH, B_{12}, and perhaps a syphilis serology.
- Structural imaging is appropriate, but functional imaging is still a research tool.

A casual conversation or even a medical interview is unlikely to uncover mild dementia. Patients often maintain social skills and unconsciously develop ego-protective techniques that hide cognitive deficits. Although this observation makes routine screening for cognitive dysfunction attractive, the U.S. Preventive Services Task Force, noting insufficient evidence, does not recommend *routine* screening for dementia (MCI) for any age group (USPSTF, 2003).

On the other hand, multiple guidelines strongly encourage a prompt and systematic response when family members report symptoms suggestive of cognitive decline. Use of screening tools in this context is appropriate. These tools assess cognitive and functional deficits as well as mood. Screening tools provide semiquantitative and reproducible assessments that add diagnostic certainty, document change over time, and facilitate efficient communication with other professional caregivers. The 30-item Mini–Mental State Examination (MMSE) has demonstrated utility in primary care and research settings, but is criticized as being too cumbersome for use in a busy office setting. The Mini-Cog, involving only three-word recall and clock drawing, is an attractive alternative because of its brevity, ease of scoring, and usefulness in ethnolinguistically diverse populations

Table 48-1 Comparison of Presenting Characteristics of Conditions with Altered Mental Status

Presentation	Delirium	Dementia	Depression	Psychoses[*]
Onset	Acute	Insidious	Insidious	Variable
Duration	Short to prolonged	Prolonged, progressive	Variable or recurrent	Chronic with exacerbations
Attention	Impaired, fluctuating	Normal except late stage	Normal or impaired	Normal or impaired
Consciousness	Impaired, fluctuating	Normal except late stage	Normal	Normal
Sensory perceptions	Impaired	Agnosia, misperception	Intact	Impaired
Thought content	Disorganized	Paucity of thought	Normal or ruminating	Normal or disorganized
Orientation	Impaired, fluctuating	Impaired, mostly stable	Intact	Intact
Delusional thinking	Disorganized if present	Secondary to memory loss or misperceptions	Self-depreciating if present	Systematized
Participation in exam	Distractable or unable	Tries but fails to perform	Lacks in effort	Variable
Hallucinations	Common, visual, suggestible	Uncommon, later stages, visual or global	Not in absence of psychotic features	Common, auditory (e.g., command hallucinations), visual

[*]DSM-IV-R Axis I psychotic mental illnesses.

(Borson et al., 2003). The Montreal Cognitive Assessment Test (MoCA) and the St. Louis University Mental Status Test (SLUMS) are more elaborate tools that seek to detect MCI and distinguish MCI from early dementia.

Examination and assessment of function can be accomplished by evaluating ADLs (bathing, dressing, toileting, transfers, continence, eating) and instrumental ADLs (using telephone, shopping, food preparation, housekeeping, laundry, transportation, taking medicine, money management). Functional assessment provides insight into the impact of cognitive impairment on everyday life. The Geriatric Depression Scale (GDS) offers uniform assessment for coexisting depression when MMSE score is 15 or greater. The Cornell Scale for Depression in Dementia, an observer-generated scale, provides a screen for depression in more severely impaired patients. These tests should become a familiar part of the initial evaluation and continuing care provided by the family physician.

History and Physical Examination

When obtaining the medical history, the physician should focus on the onset, trajectory, use of prescription and nonprescription drugs, history of substance abuse, vascular problems or risk factors (especially hypertension), history of head trauma, history of CNS infections or surgery, and family history of dementia. Assessment of ADLs and IADLs, whenever possible, should be demonstrated as part of the physical examination rather than rely on patient or family report. A general physical examination is appropriate to assess the status of comorbid conditions and for evidence of disease states that could be related to dementia. The cardiovascular examination is important to detect the presence of vascular disease. A careful neurologic exam, particularly to identify movement disorders and focal neurologic deficits, will impact the selection of diagnostic tests. ADL and IADL assessments often raise concerns about safety or potential for exploitation and may need to be followed up with a home visit or a referral to social services.

Laboratory and Imaging Studies

Traditionally recommended laboratory studies include a complete blood count (CBC), urinalysis, chemistry panel, thyroid-stimulating hormone (TSH) and vitamin B_{12} levels, and, if concerns are raised in the history, a syphilis serology. These studies have relatively low yield relative to defining the cause of dementia, but they can be helpful to document the severity of comorbid conditions. They also provide a convenient assessment of the patient's nutritional status. Routine use of apolipoprotein (apo) E genotyping and cerebrospinal fluid (CSF) studies are not recommended for routine use. Structural imaging with non-contrast-enhanced CT or magnetic resonance imaging (MRI) is appropriate in the early evaluation of patients with dementia. Imaging may reveal treatable conditions such as benign or malignant brain tumors or subdural hematomas or suggest normal-pressure hydrocephalus (NPH). Functional imaging remains a research tool and is not recommended in the routine dementia evaluation (Knopman et al., 2001).

Referral for formal neuropsychological testing or EEG can be useful for difficult patients. A systematic evaluation provides a basis for more precise patient and family education, aids in prognostication, and may guide therapy. It can help overcome patient and family denial and decrease "doctor shopping." Box 48-6 summarizes conditions the clinician should consider when approaching a patient with suspected dementia.

Common Types of Dementia

Clinical evaluation will establish that most patients have Alzheimer's disease (AD), Levy body disease (LBD), or vascular dementia (VaD). Autopsy study of brain tissue obtained from persons dying with dementia reveal that most patients actually have mixed dementia, with microscopic changes of AD and VaD most often reported.

Alzheimer's Disease

Key Points

- Alzheimer's disease is the most common type of dementia and the fifth leading cause of death for Americans over age 65.
- Alzheimer's disease is classified as late-onset AD (much more common) and early-onset AD (less common but stronger genetic basis).
- Age is the strongest risk factor for AD.
- Course of AD is one of slow but relentless progression.
- Life expectancy from diagnosis is 4 to 6 years, although some patients live much longer. Clinical indicators of short life expectancy include eating problems and nonremediable weight loss, repeated bouts of pneumonia, and frequent febrile episodes.
- Family medicine's commitment to continuity, a biopsychosocial approach, and recognition of the family as a unit of care allow the family physician to be particularly effective when helping caregivers.

Alzheimer's disease is the most common type of dementia. The exact cause or causes of AD are unknown, but age is the most important risk factor. Given the increasing life expectancy in the United States (and worldwide), and that

---

Box 48-6 Diagnostic Considerations for Evaluating Patient with Suspected Dementia

D—Drugs and toxins (alcohol, neuroleptics, hypnotics, anticonvulsants, analgesics, many others)

E—Environmental deprivation (poor vision and hearing, lack of assistive devices); electrolyte disorders (sodium, calcium, magnesium)

M—Metabolic and endocrine disorders (hypothyroidism, hyperammonemia); movement disorders (dementia with Lewy bodies, Parkinson's disease)

E—Emotional disorders (depression, delirium)

N—Nutritional deficiencies (vitamin B_{12}, thiamine, niacin)

T—Tumors and trauma (subdural hematoma, normal-pressure hydrocephalus, brain tumors)

I—Infections (human immunodeficiency virus, syphilis, Creutzfeldt-Jakob disease)

A—Alzheimer's disease, vascular dementia

"baby boomers" (those born between 1946 and 1966) have begun turning 65, family physicians can expect more and more patients and families seeking treatment for AD. Currently, about 5.3 million Americans have AD. Unless new discoveries facilitate prevention, delay the onset, or slow the progression of AD, it is estimated there will be 11 to 16 million persons with AD in 2050.

Most cases of AD develop in people older than 60 years. Genetics appears to have little influence in late-onset AD, although there is great research interest in the apo E E4 allele, located on chromosome 19. Patients not expressing the apo E E4 allele have the least risk for AD, heterozygous patients are at intermediate risk, and homozygous patients are at greatest risk. Apolipoprotein E is involved in lipid transport. It is a risk factor for AD, as well as LBD and VaD. The clinical relevance of this observation is unclear.

Early-onset AD patients often have changes in chromosomes 21, 14, or 1. Persons with Down syndrome (trisomy 21) often develop the symptoms and histologic findings of AD in their 40s and 50s. Other risk factors for AD include head injury with loss of consciousness and lower educational level. Various risk factors for atherosclerosis (diabetes, hypertension) have also been shown to increase the risk of AD, as well as VaD.

Histopathologic markers of AD include extracellular senile plaques (aggregations of abnormal amyloid protein), intraneuronal neurofibrillary tangles (hyperphosphorylated tau protein), and brain cell death. Neurofibrillary tangles are preferentially distributed in the medial temporal lobe, hippocampus, and amygdala, whereas senile plaques are widely scattered throughout the cerebral cortex (Clark and Karlawish, 2003). The AD patient's brain displays shrinking gyri, widening of the sulci (particularly in the frontotemporal region), and enlargement of the ventricular system in proportion to the atrophy of the cortex. Caution should be taken in using these features exclusively for the diagnosis because normal aging occurs in much the same manner, although with more diffuse atrophy and slower progression if serial studies are performed. Decreases in hippocampal volume correlate well with deteriorating clinical status (Jack et al., 2000).

Many neurotransmitters, including norepinephrine, serotonin, somatostatin, and various neuropeptides, show alterations in AD patients. The most prominent neurochemical defect appears to be a deficiency in the enzyme choline O-acetyltransferase, resulting in a deficit of acetylcholine. This is most evident in the nucleus basalis of Meynert and the hippocampus. In the absence of cholinergic stimulation from these lower centers of the brain, there is secondary atrophy in the cerebral cortex, leading to memory problems and other deficits in cognitive function. Neurochemical alterations probably contribute to the associated psychiatric symptoms of AD (depression, anxiety, agitation, psychosis). Early in the course of AD, impaired memory is the predominant finding. Changes in mood and personality can also be seen. Later, memory impairment becomes more dramatic, and word-finding difficulty (anomia) appears. These changes can be subtle, and family, co-workers, and physicians might unconsciously adapt to the person's impairment. This is helpful to the patient, but it contributes to delay in diagnosing AD. Eventually, functional performance is affected, with deterioration in skills of driving, handling finances, meal planning, and hygiene. There is further deterioration in language with disordered syntax. Executive functions, manifesting with impaired judgment, sequencing, and problem solving, become more problematic. Memory loss becomes profound, with loss of recognition of previously familiar persons or things, as illustrated in Figure 48-2.

Influenced somewhat by premorbid personality, psychiatric syndromes can develop at any point in the course of the illness. Paranoia, agitation, frustration, irritability, anxiety or restlessness, socially inappropriate behavior, delusions, and hallucinations are all common. Food preferences may change. In later stages, apraxia and probable decrease in the pleasurable, endorphin-mediated response to eating lead to a decrease in nutritional intake without suffering. Finally, near-coma deteriorates to coma. Seizures and myoclonic jerks are often observed in AD and other dementias (Scarmeas et al., 2009). Life expectancy of AD patients is generally 4 to 6 years after diagnosis (Larson et al., 2004), although some patients live for 10 years and longer. Box 48-7 summarizes diagnostic criteria for dementia and AD.

Pharmacotherapy

Early recognition of AD offers the greatest opportunity for modification of the course of the illness. Pharmacotherapy should be considered only as part of a comprehensive treatment plan that addresses comorbid medical and psychiatric conditions, behavioral management, social interventions, and support and education of caregivers. Goals of pharmacotherapy include improving memory and cognition (or at least slowing cognitive decline), alleviating behavioral disturbances, decreasing caregiver burden, and delaying need for institutionalization.

Two classes of pharmacotherapeutic agents have recognized indications for the treatment of AD, comprising four cholinesterase inhibitors and one N-methyl-D-aspartate (NMDA) receptor agonist. The first cholinesterase inhibitor developed, tacrine, has little current use because of inconvenient dosing and need for laboratory monitoring for liver toxicity. The other three, donepezil, galantamine, and rivastigmine, have shown consistent, modest beneficial effects in the domains of cognition and global assessment. Diarrhea, nausea, and vomiting, consistent with expected effects of cholinesterase inhibitors, were the most common side effects. Memantine, the NMDA receptor agonist, improves cognition and global assessment, but effect sizes were small. Other studies suggest improvement in quality of life. Common side effects include nausea, diarrhea, dizziness, and headache (Raina et al., 2008). No clinically important differences among the drugs have been demonstrated. Alternative delivery systems (rapidly dissolving tablets, liquid formulations, transdermal patches) are available.

Based on an exhaustive and comprehensive reviewed of these five FDA-approved dementia treatments, the Joint American College of Physicians/American Academy of Family Physicians Panel on dementia concluded that a decision to start therapy should be based on individual assessment, noting that all the drugs are associated with known adverse events and have shown only modest or even, in some studies, no benefit. The panel also stated treatment with memantine or a cholinesterase inhibitor is not appropriate when the goals of care no longer include slowing decline, a circumstance frequently seen when AD is advanced (Qaseem et al., 2008).

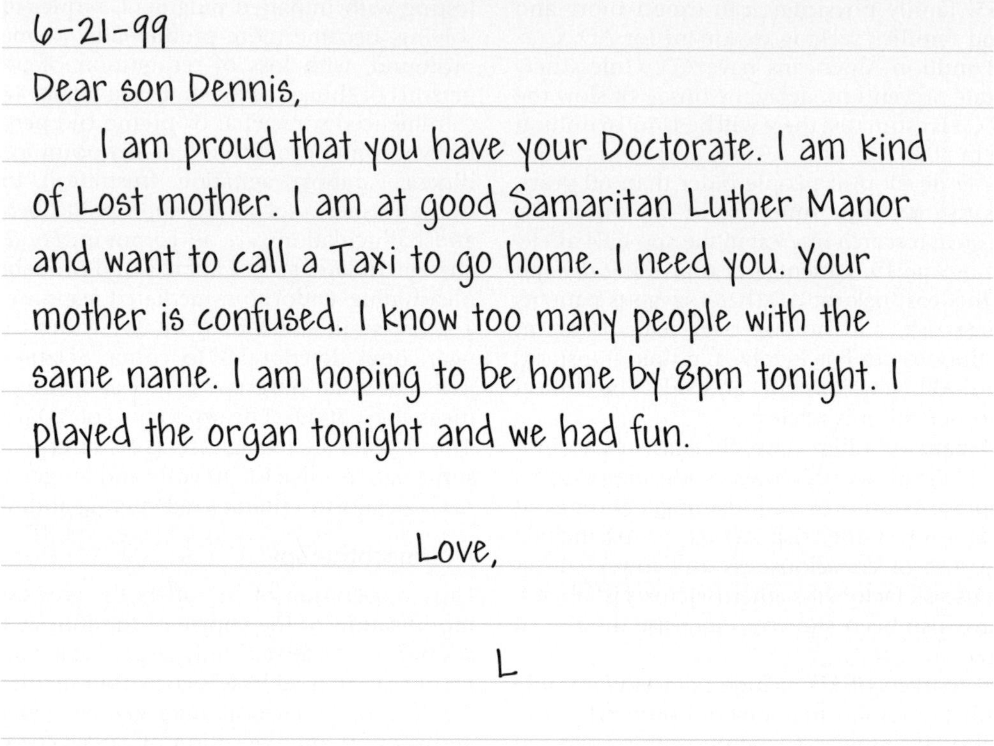

6-21-99

Dear son Dennis,

I am proud that you have your Doctorate. I am kind of Lost mother. I am at good Samaritan Luther Manor and want to call a Taxi to go home. I need you. Your mother is confused. I know too many people with the same name. I am hoping to be home by 8pm tonight. I played the organ tonight and we had fun.

Love,

L

Figure 48-2 A note, transcribed by a nursing home volunteer, from an Alzheimer's disease patient to her son.

Box 48-7 Diagnostic Criteria for Dementia and Probable Alzheimer's Disease

Dementia

Loss of memory, documented by MMSE or similar testing

and

Evidence of at least one additional impairment including:

Aphasia

Apraxia

Agnosia

Impairment of executive function

and

Resulting impairment sufficient to interfere with usual social or occupational functioning

Probable Alzheimer's Disease

Typical history, including:

Insidious onset

Gradual progression

Documented cognitive loss

Absence, documented by physical exam, laboratory testing, and neuroimaging of other diseases that could cause dementia.

Based on DSM-IV-TR and National Institute of Neurologic and Communicative Disorders and Stroke, Alzheimer's Disease and Related Disorders Association (NINCDS-ADRDA) criteria.

MMSE, Mini–Mental State Examination.

KEY TREATMENT

Three cholinesterase inhibitors and one NMDA agonist are available for the treatment of AD (Raina et al., 2008). Comprehensive literature review shows modest efficacy and predictable non-life-threatening side effects (SOR: B).

Prevention

The absence of clearly effective active treatments has created considerable interest in efforts to prevent AD and other dementias. Numerous vitamins, nutraceuticals, and pharmacologic agents have been examined for use as preventive agents for AD-related memory loss. A double-blind placebo-controlled study of vitamin E and donepezil for the treatment of MCI was unable to demonstrate a benefit from vitamin E and showed only modest and short-term benefit from donepezil (Petersen et al., 2005). No medication, nutraceutical, or vitamin has been shown to prevent AD.

Ginkgo biloba is probably the best studied of the nutraceuticals promoted for the prevention of dementia. Initially encouraging studies have not been supported by subsequent RCTs. A National Institutes of Health (NIH)–funded study involving more than 3000 volunteers age 75 and older concluded that *Ginkgo biloba* "was not effective in reducing the overall incidence rate of dementia or AD incidence in elderly individuals with normal cognition or those with MCI" (DeKosky et al., 2008; Snitz et al., 2009).

Enthusiasm for a preventive role for estrogen and nonsteroidal anti-inflammatory drugs (NSAIDs), based on epidemiologic correlations, have not been supported by follow-up studies. Neither is recommended.

A number of cohort studies suggest that educational and occupational attainment, cognitively stimulating activities such as reading, playing cards or board games, going to museums, playing musical instruments, and dancing are associated with reduced risk of developing AD. Controlled trials have not been done (and will be difficult or impossible to perform) to confirm these associations (Verghese et al., 2002; Wilson et al., 2002). Given the benign nature of the proposed interventions, it would seem prudent to encourage such activities when patients or family members raise questions about prevention.

Given the increasing awareness of the contribution of cerebrovascular pathology to disease burden of all types of dementia, aggressive management of hypertension and diabetes, as well as the management of vascular risk factors through diet, exercise, and preventive pharmacologic agents, is having the added benefit of lowering the risk of dementia (Middleton and Yaffe, 2009).

KEY TREATMENT

Cognitive, physical, and social activity; a diet rich in antioxidants and polyunsaturated fatty acids; and vascular risk factor control (particularly hypertension treatment) may have a role in the prevention of AD dementia (Middleton and Yaffe, 2009; Verghese et al., 2002; Wilson et al., 2002) (SOR: B).

Caregiver Education and Support

Family physicians are often in a particularly powerful position to address caregiver issues. In some cases the family physician is the doctor for both the dementia patient and the caregiver. Family medicine's commitment to continuity and a comprehensive biopsychosocial approach provides a useful framework for understanding and addressing the stresses that affect family members. A meta-analysis of psychosocial interventions for caregivers showed decreased levels of caregiver stress, improved knowledge, and improved patient mood, but no effect on caregiver burden. Involving both the caregiver and the patient in the intervention increased the benefit. At least four studies indicate that caregiver interventions delay nursing home admission (Brodaty et al., 2003).

Knowledge of and referral to community resources is critical to managing caregiver stress and preserving patient quality of life. Adult day care, respite care, medical and nonmedical home care, and hospice programs all play a role in the care of the AD patient and family. Particularly helpful are the Alzheimer's Association and the National Institute of Aging's Alzheimer's Disease Education and Referral (ADEAR) Center. Bibliotherapy references include *The 36-Hour Day* (Mace et al., 2006) and *Alzheimer's Disease: the Family Journey* (Caron et al., 2000).

End-of-Life Care

Alzheimer's disease is a terminal illness. It is currently the fifth leading cause of death for persons age 65 and older (Heron et al., 2009). AD progresses slowly, making it difficult to recognize when a patient goes from the advanced to terminal phase of the illness. This in turn makes it difficult

to determine when to initiate discussions with family about shifting to an exclusively palliative care approach and possible involvement of hospice. Potential clinical indicators for the shift include progressive nonremediable weight loss (White et al., 1998), eating problems, repeated episodes of pneumonia, and frequent febrile episodes (Mitchell et al., 2009). The Center for Medicare and Medicaid Services (CMS) has published guidelines to assist in the determination of terminal status in patients with dementia (Box 48-8). Once the terminal stage is recognized by the physician and acknowledged by the family and other caregivers, an appropriate end-of-life care plan can be instituted.

Lewy Body Disease

Lewy body disease (LBD) is emerging as a term to capture both dementia with Lewy bodies (DLB) and dementia associated with Parkinson's disease (PDD). This is useful because the only difference is the timing of dementia. In DLB the dementia is evident before or concurrently with the appearance of parkinsonian symptoms. In PDD, Parkinson's disease is evident for 1 year or more before dementia symptoms appear. Three core clinical features help distinguish LBD from other dementias: (1) fluctuating cognition with pronounced variations in attention and alertness, (2) recurrent visual hallucinations that are typically well formed and detailed, and (3) spontaneous features of parkinsonism (McKeith et al., 2005).

Box 48-8 Medicare Local Coverage Determination (LCD) for determining terminal state of Alzheimer's Disease (AD)*

Patients will be considered to be in the terminal stage of dementia (life expectancy of 6 months or less) if they meet the following criteria. Patients should show all the following characteristics:

1. Stage 7 or beyond according to the Functional Assessment Staging Scale (FAST)† [FAST Stage 7 represents severe AD]
2. Unable to ambulate without assistance
3. Unable to dress without assistance
4. Unable to bathe without assistance
5. Urinary and fecal incontinence, intermittent or constant
6. No consistently meaningful verbal communication: stereotypical phrases only, or the ability to speak is limited to six or fewer intelligible words

Patients should have had one of the following within the past 12 months:

1. Aspiration pneumonia
2. Pyelonephritis or other upper urinary tract infection
3. Septicemia
4. Decubitus ulcers, multiple, stage 3-4
5. Fever, recurrent after antibiotics
6. Inability to maintain sufficient fluid and calorie intake with 10% weight loss during previous 6 months or serum albumin <2.5 g/dL

From Center for Medicare and Medicaid Services (CMS). Local Medical Review Policy. www.cms.hhs.gov. Minor regional variations and modifications over time are anticipated.

*This section is specific for AD and related disorders and is not appropriate for other types of dementia, such as multi-infarct dementia.

†FAST Scale © 1984 by Barry Reisberg, MD.

In advanced stages it can be difficult to distinguish LBD and AD, both clinically and pathologically. It is important to make the diagnostic distinction, however, because use of typical antipsychotic agents in LBD can be associated with severe, even fatal, exacerbations of parkinsonism and autonomic instability. Diagnostic criteria are listed in Box 48-9.

Motor symptoms can be treated with carbidopa-levodopa, starting with low doses and proceeding cautiously. Carbidopa-levodopa itself can cause confusion, and distinguishing an adverse drug reaction from a dementia-related psychotic episode is difficult. Neurochemical changes in LBD are similar to those seen in AD, particularly the deficiency in acetylcholinesterase, suggesting that cholinesterase inhibitors would be particularly effective. Despite positive case reports, systematic review of the evidence notes that "patients with dementia with Lewy bodies who suffer from behavioral disturbances may benefit from rivastigmine, but the evidence is weak" (Wild et al., 2003).

Psychosocial interventions for LBD are similar to those used in AD. Anticipatory guidance for caregivers regarding the likelihood of waxing/waning cognition and dramatic hallucinations, as well as the need to avoid the use of typical antipsychotics, is important.

KEY TREATMENT

Cholinesterase inhibitors should be beneficial in Lewy body disease patients, but evidence supporting their efficacy is modest (Wild et al., 2003) (SOR: B).

Box 48-9 Revised Criteria for Clinical Diagnosis of Dementia with Lewy Bodies (DLB)

1. *Central features* (essential for a diagnosis of possible or probable DLB)

   Progressive cognitive decline of sufficient magnitude to interfere with usual social or occupational function

   Prominent or persistent memory impairment

   Deficits on tests of attention, executive function, and visuospatial ability

2. *Core features* (two core features are sufficient for a diagnosis of probable DLB, one for possible DLB)

   Fluctuating cognition and variations in attention and alertness

   Recurrent visual hallucinations

   Spontaneous features of parkinsonism

3. *Suggestive Features* (one core + one suggestive feature sufficient for diagnosis of probable DLB, with no core features one suggestive feature sufficient for diagnosis of possible DLB)

   Severe neuroleptic sensitivity

   REM sleep behavior disorder

4. *Supportive features* (commonly present in DLB but without proven diagnostic specificity)

   Repeated falls and syncope

   Transient, unexplained loss of consciousness

   Severe autonomic dysfunction (e.g., orthostatic hypotension, urinary incontinence)

   Systematized delusion, nonvisual hallucinations

Modified from McKeith IG, Dickson DW, Lowe J, et al. Diagnosis and management of dementia with Lewy bodies: Third Report of the DLB Consortium. Neurology 2005;65:1863-1872.

REM, Rapid eye movement.

Vascular Dementia

Vascular dementia vies with LBD as the second most common type of dementia in the United States. The rate is higher in areas with higher rates of hypertension. Conceptually, VaD refers to cases in which vascular disease produces cerebral injury severe enough to result in dementia. This fairly simple concept is made clinically challenging by the multiple types of vascular disease and the varying location and degree of the resulting cerebral injury. Cerebral damage may be hemorrhagic, hypoxic, or anoxic. The vascular disease can occur in larger arteries, medium or small arterioles, or capillaries. VaD may be the result of a sentinel infarct, multiple infarcts, Binswager's disease, or vasculitis. Hypoxic damage related to systemic episodes of hypotension can also result in VaD.

Given the variety of causes and manifestations, it is not surprising that there are no uniformly accepted criteria for the diagnosis of VaD. It may be overdiagnosed, given the high prevalence of subclinical cerebrovascular disease seen in elderly persons, or underdiagnosed, given the lack of clear criteria for diagnosis. VaD is the most common second diagnosis in mixed dementia, a finding that has clinical significance: AD + VaD or LBD + VaD = more cognitive and functional deficits than AD or LBD alone (Schneider et al., 2007).

Treatment of the resulting dementia includes off-label use of cholinesterase inhibitors and memantine, as well as treatment directed at the control of vascular risk factors. Psychosocial approaches are similar to those used with dementia in general, as described earlier. Disclosure of the diagnosis of VaD to family members creates an opportune "teachable moment" to discuss familial risk and prevention.

Less Common Causes of Dementia

The vast majority of patients seen in primary care settings will have AD, LBD, VaD, or mixed dementia. The following types are relatively rare and therefore are not discussed in detail. They should be suspected when the presentation or course of the dementia is atypical. Consultation will likely be necessary to confirm the diagnosis.

Frontotemporal Lobar Degenerations

Frontotemporal dementia (FTD), formerly called Pick's disease, is the most common of three frontotemporal lobe degenerations (FTLDs). The other two are progressive aphasia and semantic dementia. FTD often presents with disordered behavior as a result of impairment in executive function, motivation, goal setting, and sequencing of plans. Labile mood and social disinhibition are common even before cognitive testing shows an abnormality. Neuroimaging often shows frontal or temporal lobe atrophy; formal psychometric testing is useful to confirm the diagnosis. There are no specific treatments (Liscic et al., 2007).

Normal-Pressure Hydrocephalus

First described in 1965, NPH is characterized by gait disturbance (magnetic gait), urinary incontinence, and dementia. This triad does not offer help with diagnosis, because the findings are common in other dementias as well. Frequently, this is first suspected when prominent ventriculomegaly is noted on neuroimaging (Hunter-Smith et al., 2007). There is no effective pharmacotherapy, but some cases respond to ventricular shunting. Selection of patients likely to respond to shunting is difficult, and referral to a center with considerable experience is advised if surgical treatment is being considered.

Creutzfeldt-Jakob Disease

Creutzfeldt-Jakob disease (CJD) is a very rare type of dementia associated with prion infection in the brain. It is characterized by unusually rapid progression. Rapid cognitive decline suggests the diagnosis of CJD. Myoclonus, fatigue, and visual problems are associated symptoms. Precise diagnosis requires a brain biopsy, but characteristic CSF and EEG findings are helpful to increase diagnostic certainty. Iatrogenic CJD occur when prion-contaminated tissue is grafted (dura mater, cornea) or injected (human growth hormone, pituitary gonadotropins) (Prusiner, 2001).

HIV-Associated Dementia

Human immunodeficiency virus (HIV)–associated dementia (HAD) develops late in HIV infection. It is a common cause of dementia worldwide. Motor deficits are observed in addition to cognitive decline. Patients are generally younger than most other dementia patients; HAD has been diagnosed in pediatric HIV patients. The use of highly active antiretroviral therapy (HAART) has decreased the incidence of HAD, and newly diagnosed cases often respond to antiretroviral therapy (McArthur, 2004). Opportunistic CNS infections, particularly toxoplasmosis, can be a contributing factor and must be sought and treated.

Behavioral and Psychiatric Symptoms Accompanying Dementia

Key Points

- It is necessary to understand the behavior from the patient's point of view to develop a treatment plan.
- Treating distressing symptoms, such as pain or constipation, may resolve problematic behaviors.
- As the patient's dementia progresses, behaviors are likely to change.

Behavioral and psychiatric symptoms occur frequently in dementia patients. Behavioral symptoms usually increase the suffering of the patient and are very distressing for both family and professional caregivers. Common problem behaviors include wandering, repetitive movements, verbal or physical aggression, resistiveness, pestering, hoarding, inappropriate sexual behavior, and sleep disturbances.

Many patients display psychotic symptoms at some point in the course of their dementia. Simple delusions, hallucinations, and paranoia may occur because of misperceptions of the environment. True psychotic delusions and hallucinations, which are usually visual rather than auditory, may also occur. Any of these symptoms can cause considerable distress, generating requests for the physician to prescribe antipsychotic or sedating medication with the intent to suppress the problematic behavior.

The genesis of psychotic symptoms in the degenerating brain of the dementia patient probably differs from the psychotic symptoms associated with schizophrenia or other psychotic mental illness, and therefore antipsychotics are only occasionally effective. The FDA has not approved antipsychotic drugs for use in dementia patients. A clinical review concluded "pharmacological therapies are not particularly effective for the management of neuropsychiatric symptoms of dementia" (Sink et al., 2005). The safety of these agents in the frail elderly population is also a concern. In 2008 the FDA notified physicians that "both conventional and atypical antipsychotics are associated with an increased risk of mortality in elderly patients treated for dementia-related psychosis."

For all these reasons, nonpharmacologic interventions are preferred for the management of behavioral and psychiatric symptoms. This requires analysis of the problematic behavior, seeking to understand the behavior from the patient's perspective. Attention to precipitating events and consequences of the behavior can lead to a behavioral modification plan. The dementia patient's profound memory loss may be the basis for some behavioral symptoms. Repeated questioning may reflect extreme short-term memory loss. Paranoia-like verbalizations that people are stealing the patient's possessions occur when the dementia patient cannot remember where possessions are kept. Box 48-10 provides a guideline to assist the evaluation and management of behavioral problems.

Depression is typically seen in dementia patients and is often the cause of irritability, apathy, anorexia, insomnia, or other symptoms that can drive problem behaviors. Successful treatment of the depression is marked by resolution of the problematic behaviors. Unmet physical needs (e.g., pain, constipation) should also be sought as a possible underlying stimulus for problem behavior.

KEY TREATMENT

Typical and atypical antipsychotics show some benefit in dementia patients, particularly in controlling aggression and psychosis, but also carry significant risk, including increased mortality (Sink et al., 2005). (SOR: B).
If antipsychotics are used, low doses and short duration of therapy are recommended (SOR: C).

Care Settings for the Dementia Patient

Key Points

- Physicians' work will change as dementia progresses and goals of care change.
- When dementia patients are in institutional settings, the physician must consider the needs, capabilities, and risks of the institution (adult daycare program, hospital, nursing home, assisted-living center) to ensure delivery of effective care.

Office Care

Office treatment of medical issues in dementia patients is challenging. The impact of impaired decision making, inability to report adverse events, and problems with adherence can alter usual risk/benefit calculations (Brauner et al., 2000). Family members often need to be involved to help

Box 48-10 A-B-C-D Evaluation of Behavior Problems in Delirium and Dementia

A. What is (are) the *antecedent*(s) to the behavior?
B. What exactly is the *behavior*?
C. What are the *consequences* of the behavior?
D. What *disaster* might result from the behavior?

Modified from American Medical Directors Association. Delirium and Acute Problematic Behavior Clinical Practice Guideline. Columbia, Md, AMDA, 2008.

weigh the risks, burdens, and benefits of therapy, particularly therapy that does not lead directly to symptomatic improvement. Office care usually involves patients with mild to moderate disease. Goals of care typically include patient and family education and completion of formal advance directives while the patient is still able to have some input into decision-making. An RCT comparing usual care management with "medical home" care using an advanced-practice nurse–led IDT showed fewer behavioral and psychological symptoms among patients and caregivers (Callahan et al., 2006).

Hospital Care

Behavioral symptoms are often precipitated by a move from a familiar to an unfamiliar environment. Hospitals can be a particularly stressful environment for a dementia patient, as can the acute or exacerbating medical illness that creates the need for hospitalization. The physician should communicate the dementia diagnosis to the hospital staff. This knowledge can allow preemptive implementation of measures to decrease the likelihood of delirium (Inouye et al., 1999).

Patients with advanced dementia who are hospitalized with acute illnesses have a dismal prognosis. Explaining the risks and benefits of hospitalization and aggressive therapy, especially when the physician has had an ongoing relationship with the patient and family, often results in a decision to focus on aggressive symptom management without hospitalization (Morrison and Siu, 2000). A "do not hospitalize" order is often appropriate.

Nursing Home

As dementia progresses, most patients develop severe functional deficits or behavior problems that make living at home impossible, even with the most dedicated family caregivers supported by home health care workers. Nursing home admission is a traumatic experience for the patient and family even in the best of circumstances. The trauma is reduced if the admission can be anticipated and the patient and family have meaningful involvement in the decision-making process.

The physician's role in caring for the dementia patient in the nursing home includes direct patient care and IDT communication. The physician and family can help the nursing home staff learn the patient's premorbid status and personality to identify any idiosyncrasies that could be helpful when providing care (e.g., "She always calms down if she has chocolate milk"). Open and efficient communication with nursing home staff enhances patient care and promotes creative problem solving.

It is necessary to see the dementia patient in the facility for most visits because transporting the patient to the office is often burdensome for the patient and can precipitate a florid delirium. On-site visits can also facilitate communication with the nursing home staff. Professional groups have provided formal guidance for nursing home attending physicians (Besdine et al., 1996). Physician and family confidence in the care provided in the nursing home allows for quality end-of-life care without the need for hospital transfer when signs of imminent demise are evident.

References

The complete reference list is available online at www.expertconsult.com.

Web Resources

www.hospitalelderlifeprogram.org
Description and supportive information for patients, families, and professionals about delirium and a program for its management in the hospital.
www.hhs.gov/aging
Access noncommercial information on variety of aging topics; links to FDA, CDC, Administration on Aging; useful for patients and families as well as professional caregivers.
www.amda.com
Professional organization for nursing home medical directors, attending physicians, and other members of the interdisciplinary team; source of clinical and practice management information for care of patients in long-term care settings.

www.alz.org
Advocacy organization for patients and families dealing with Alzheimer's disease and other dementias; useful patient and caregiver education materials; also offers information for physicians and other professionals.
www.lbda.org
Advocacy organization for patients and families dealing with Lewy body dementia; useful patient and caregiver education materials; also offers information for physicians and other professionals.

CHAPTER 49

Alcohol Use Disorders

Kevin Sherin and Stacy Seikel

Chapter contents

Overview

Key Points

- Annual alcoholism-identified health costs are $246 billion.
- Alcoholic persons are heavy users of health care.
- Primary care screening is inadequate for alcoholic patients.

Alcoholism is a chronic and pervasive medical disorder that adds enormous cost to the U.S. health care system. Alcohol abuse and dependency are among the top-three preventable causes of death. The Centers for Disease Control and Prevention (CDC, 2004) estimates that for every alcohol-attributable death, 30 years of potential life is lost, accounting for 2.3 million years of potential life lost (YPLL) and 75,000 preventable deaths per year from identified cases. The total economic costs attributed to alcohol use disorders are $246 billion, of which $218 billion is related to alcohol-related motor vehicle crashes (MVCs), violence, and premature death (Harwood et al., 1998).

Alcoholic patients use health care resources disproportionately compared with other populations. Relative to the general population, alcoholics are heavy users of emergency department (ED) services, trauma-related services, acute hospitalization, diagnostic procedures, transfusions, and psychiatric services (Whiteman et al., 2000).

Estimates of the extent of alcohol involvement in trauma include 39% of MVC fatalities (National Highway Traffic Safety Administration, 2004), 47% of homicides, 29% of suicides (Smith et al., 1999), 20% to 40% for fatal recreational injuries (Mayhew et al., 1986), and 10% to 25% for home injuries (CDC 1983; Fell and Nash, 1989). Alcohol is involved in a substantial percentage of injuries caused by falls, drowning, and burns (Howland and Hingson, 1988). More than 5% of all hospital discharges other than childbirth include at least one alcohol-related diagnosis (Chen et al., 2005).

Cirrhosis of the liver continues to be largely attributable to alcohol abuse, with estimates of 60% to 90% of cirrhosis deaths (Johannes et al., 1987). Comorbidity with hepatitis C is frequently a factor in many of these alcoholic cirrhosis-related deaths. Hospitalizations for acute pancreatitis are frequently associated with alcohol dependency. Psychiatric comorbidity is common in the alcoholic population, especially depression and suicide. These sequelae have major implications for managed care organizations and federal and local payers alike. However, screening for alcoholism in primary care and emergency settings is not universal. The recent prospective data from the National Epidemiologic Survey on Alcohol and Related Conditions (NESARC) have provided annual incidence rates for DMS-IV alcohol abuse at 1.0 per 100 person years and alcohol dependence at 1.7 per 100 person years; data also indicate that the greatest risk for alcohol use disorders occurs during young adulthood (Grant et al., 2008).

Prevalence

Key Points

- Alcohol abuse is more common than diabetes mellitus.
- Heavy alcohol use is more common in men.
- More screening and brief interventions are needed in primary care settings, which results in decreased drinking.
- Screening in hospitals, EDs, and trauma settings can be valuable, but brief interventions in these settings have produced inconclusive results.

In the United States, an estimated 140 million persons use alcohol, making it the most popular psychoactive substance (Baldwin et al., 1993). A reanalysis of the 1994 national comorbidity study found that 8% to 10% of the U.S. population reported lifetime alcohol abuse or dependence (Narrow et al., 2002). About 61% of the U.S. population drinks alcohol (CDC, 2003). The number of U.S. adults who abuse alcohol or are alcohol dependent rose from 3.8 million (7.41%) in 1991–1992 to 17.6 million (8.46%) in 2001–2002, according to NESARC, a study directed by the National Institute on Alcohol Abuse and Alcoholism (NIAAA, 2003). Heavy use is found more frequently in men (10.3%) than women (2.5%). Ethnic variation is minimal in whites (6.4%), Hispanics (7.3%), and African Americans (4.8%) (OAS, 1995). The prevalence of binge drinking, that is, drinking five or more drinks at least once in the preceding month, is 14.2% (Winick, 1996).

The prevalence of alcohol use disorders (abuse and dependence) is almost 15% in the population who consumes alcohol. Compared with other chronic medical conditions in family medicine, alcohol use disorders appear to be of significant importance for early recognition and intervention. Hypertension is estimated to affect at least 50 million Americans, and diabetes mellitus (DM) type 2 affects more than 2% of the U.S. population, or 5.4 million adults. Alcohol use disorders rank almost as high as hypertension and much higher than DM in terms of prevalence. The key for the family physician is to increase the screening, diagnosis, and treatment of alcohol abuse in the clinical setting to the level of importance attached to hypertension or DM. Screening in hospitals, EDs, and trauma care settings can add value (ACS, 2008; Gentillelo et al., 1999; Smothers et al., 2004). However, brief interventions for alcohol use in patients with acute injuries in the ED and in hospital admissions have been inconclusive (Dappen et al., 2007; Emmen et al., 2004). A meta-analysis of *screening and brief intervention* (SBI) was found effective in reducing alcohol consumption at 6 and 12 months among non-treatment-seeking primary care patients, regardless of gender (Fleming, 2002). Some evidence suggests that SBI for prevention is also effective in pregnancy care settings (Floyd, 2007).

Causative Factors; Diagnosis and Classification

See the discussion online at www.expertconsult.com.

Screening and Assessment

Key Points

- Apply CAGE screening to all patients older than 18.
- Be aware of "negative" drinking history.
- Closely follow up positive responses.
- The AUDIT-C is a standard for quantifying alcohol use disorders in medical settings.

There is good evidence to support screening for alcohol dependency and alcohol use disorders when using standard screening tools in practice. For the family physician, the diagnosis of alcoholism often depends on clues from the history and physical examination (Box 49-1). Possible clues may include a history of driving under the influence (DUI) or an MVC; history of repetitive trauma; new-onset hypertension, gastritis, or pancreatitis; other, otherwise unexplained liver disease (AST > ALT); presence of depression; recent loss of employment or separation from family; unexplained tremor; upper gastrointestinal (GI) bleeding; recent falls or accidents; and a history of family or marital violence.

The four CAGE questions (cut down, annoyed, guilty, eye opener) are adequate for screening purposes (Box 49-2), derived from the longer Michigan Alcoholism Screening Test (MAST) questions (see **eTable 49-1** online) (Hays and Spickard, 1987; Powers and Spikard, 1984). Two positive responses are considered a positive screen and indicate that further assessment is warranted. An important point is that family physicians should not assume that someone does not have an alcohol use disorder when that person answers negatively to questions about drinking. If such patients do not use alcohol at all, it may indicate that they had to quit because they had problems with alcohol. Given the prevalence of alcohol use disorders, it is recommended that the CAGE questions be applied to all patients older than 18 years. Another brief set of screening questions is the TWEAK questionnaire: tolerance, worries, eye openers, amnesia, and cut down (Box 49-3).

Longer screening questionnaires include the MAST and the Alcohol Use Disorders Test (AUDIT: see **eTable 49-2** online) (Saunders et al., 1993). Both are considered higher in predictive value but more difficult to administer. Age-specific and population-specific survey tools are also available, including the Geriatric Alcoholism Screen and an adolescent alcoholism inventory. The 10-item Core questionnaire includes three questions on alcohol consumption (the AUDIT-C) and seven on the impact of alcohol use. The AUDIT has been shown to have good sensitivity and specificity in

---

Box 49-1 Screening Clues for Alcoholism

"Driving under the influence" (DUI) arrest
Domestic violence
Unexplained trauma
Family stress
New hypertension
Gastritis
Pancreatitis
Tremor

Box 49-2 Brief Screening Questions for Alcohol Use

CAGE*

1. Have you ever felt you should *cut down,* on your drinking?
2. Have people *annoyed* you by criticizing your drinking?
3. Have you ever felt bad or *guilty* about your drinking?
4. Have you ever had a drink first thing in the morning to steady your nerves or to get rid of a hangover (*eye opener*)?

  Scoring: Item responses on the CAGE are scored 0 for "no" and 1 for "yes" answers, with a higher score an indication of alcohol problems. A total score of 2 or greater is considered clinically significant.

  The normal cutoff for the CAGE is two positive answers; however, the Consensus Panel recommends that the primary care clinicians lower the threshold to one positive answer to cast a wider net and identify more patients who may have substance abuse disorders. A number of other screening tools are available.

CAGE Questions Adapted to Include Drugs (CAGE-AID)†

1. Have you ever felt you ought to cut down on your drinking or drug use?
2. Have people annoyed you by criticizing your drinking or drug use?
3. Have you felt bad or guilty about your drinking or drug use?
4. Have you ever had a drink or used drugs first thing in the morning to steady your nerves or to get rid of a hangover (eye-opener)?

*Ewing JA. Detecting alcoholism: the CAGE questionnaire. JAMA 1984;252:1905-1907.

†Brown RL, Rounds LA. Conjoint screening questionnaires for alcohol and drug abuse. Wis Med J 1995;94:135-140.

Box 49-3 TWEAK Screening For Alcohol Use

TWEAK is a five-item scale developed originally to screen for risk drinking during pregnancy.

Points

(1-2) *Tolerance:* How many drinks can you hold? *or* How many drinks do you need to feel high?

(1-2) *Worried:* Have close friends or relatives worried or complained about your drinking in the past year?

(1) *Eye-openers:* Do you sometimes take a drink in the morning when you first get up?

(1) *Amnesia* (blackouts): Has a friend or family member ever told you about things you said or did while you were drinking that you could not remember?

(1) *Cut down:* Do you sometimes feel the need to cut down on your drinking?

Administering and Scoring

Before administering TWEAK, drinkers are identified by a positive response to the question, "Do you consume, or have you ever consumed, beer, wine, wine coolers, or drinks containing liquor (i.e., whiskey, rum, or vodka)?"

To score the test, a 7-point scale is used.

The "tolerance-hold" question scores 2 points if the respondent is able to hold six or more drinks.

The "tolerance-high" question scores 2 points if three or more drinks are needed to feel high.

A total score of 2 or more indicates that obstetric patients are likely to be risk drinkers. However, preliminary studies suggest that cutoff points of 3 or 4 are better than 2 for identifying harmful drinking or alcoholism.

---

medical and general populations and has recently been useful for screening patients with major psychiatric disorders and as an assessment instrument for patients seeking treatment for alcohol use disorders (Cassidy et al., 2008; Donovan et al., 2006). The AUDIT-C provides an efficient standardized method for assessing the quantity and frequency of alcohol use and accounts for much of the test's discriminative power in medical populations (Rodriguez-Marros and Santamarina, 2007).

Biologic Markers

Key Points

- The MCV is higher than 100 fL.
- The AST level is higher than the ALT level.
- There is a positive response to CDT level.
- Five drinks daily for 2 weeks elevates GGT in most people.
- Using GGT and CDT in combination increases sensitivity over either marker alone by 20% without compromising specificity.

Diagnostic clues from the laboratory include a complete blood count (CBC) with an elevated mean cell volume, elevated γ-glutamyltransferase (GGT), aspartate transaminase (AST) level higher than alanine transaminase (ALT), unexplained leukopenia or thrombocytopenia, and positive response to the *carbohydrate-deficient transferrin* (CDT) level (Borg et al., 1992). It is estimated that 5 drinks/day for two weeks will yield an elevated GGT in most people (USDHHS, SAMSHA, 2006). Using CDT and GGT together increases

sensitivity by 20% of either marker alone without compromising specificity (Hitela et al., 2006). Dose-response relationships are not well established, making it difficult to use these tests as a direct quantifier for alcohol consumption (Allen et al., 2004).

Interview Questions

Guidelines for interviewing adolescents about alcohol have been reviewed (Speraw and Rogers, 1998). An atmosphere of trust and privacy must be conveyed (parents should be excluded). The questioning should be gradually moved from nonthreatening areas about general lifestyle to more specific questions about medications to questions about alcohol use. Standard interview questions for alcohol abuse include quantity of consumption; frequency of consumption; preference of alcoholic beverages; age at onset of drinking; attempts to cut down or quit; time of most recent drink; adverse sequelae related to drinking (or stopping drinking); and pattern of drinking (continuous, daily drinking, binge pattern). Quantity questions can classify binge drinking as never, less than one, one to three, three to five, and more than five per month. Vague or evasive answers, as well as rationalizations, should be "red flags." Patients can also be asked how much alcohol they purchase and how often. It is important to elicit specific, concrete information and not become derailed by certain responses.

A family history of alcohol problems must be detailed because it is a major predictive variable. When a clinician receives the answer that the patient does not drink at all, the line of questioning should still be pursued to determine whether cessation was problem based. Once it has been established that the person has a history of binge drinking or continuous daily drinking, follow-up questions are in order. These questions may include role impairment, family concerns, amnesia, self-concern, and hangovers to determine the patient's sentiments about alcohol consumption.

Detailed Assessment

Once it has been established that the patient has problems with alcohol, more detailed assessment is in order. The history should then be focused on the known harmful consequences of alcohol abuse and dependency as related to the patient's history. (For a list of complications, see Woodard, 2009). Major disorders include Wernicke's encephalopathy, withdrawal seizures, cerebellar disease, peripheral neuropathy, cardiomyopathy, cirrhosis, pancreatitis, gastritis, bone marrow suppression, and aseptic necrosis of the hip. A careful history should include an assessment of tolerance and withdrawal symptoms, including shakes, hallucinosis, seizures, and delirium tremens (DTs). The time of the last drink and quantification of daily drinking are prerequisites. A history of stage 2 to 4 withdrawal with or without a history of serious medical complications is in itself justification for acute care hospitalization. Alcohol withdrawal often includes anxiety, nausea, vomiting, diarrhea, tremors, and elevated pulse and blood pressure (BP). A history of blackout or amnesic episodes while drinking must also be elicited. A history of family, social, legal, and occupational complications should be obtained as part of the diagnosis of alcoholism.

A psychiatric evaluation is key in the assessment for alcohol abuse. Screening tools such as the Beck Depression Inventory can help identify underlying depression. Assessment of suicidal ideation must be documented, because alcoholics are at much greater risk for suicide-related deaths. The Mini–Mental Status Examination (MMSE) can be useful for assessing possible dementia or delirium and pointing to the need for more extensive neuropsychiatric testing (see Chapter 48). Cognitive damage may be a factor in denial, a trait that characterizes many patients with known alcohol dependency. A sexual history should be included, with attention to multiple partners and human immunodeficiency virus (HIV) risk assessment. A history of comorbid polysubstance abuse and intravenous (IV) drug use should also be sought. Cough hemoptysis, night sweats, fever, and weight loss suggest the need to investigate for tuberculosis.

Physical Assessment

The physical examination should pay close attention to vital signs. Elevated BP, pulse, or respiration can be a clue to the severity of alcohol withdrawal. The smell of ethanol on the breath will point to acute intoxication; the comorbid "dry mouth" may then be a local effect and not related to dehydration. Skin changes can be seen in alcoholics and may include rhinophyma, red swollen facies, and porphyria cutanea tarda. A thorough neurologic examination is in order, including cranial nerves, extraocular movements, gait, and cerebellar signs, as well as a sensory assessment of the lower extremities. Ataxia and nystagmus can be clues to possible intoxication or Wernicke's encephalopathy. Percussion and palpation

of the liver are important in alcoholism. Examination of the extremities can include visualization of Dupuytren's contractures and palmar erythema. An irregular heart rhythm suggests atrial fibrillation, or "holiday heart."

In women, diagnosis of pregnancy should also be excluded (see Alcohol Use Disorder in Women). Alcoholism in pregnancy has severe perinatal effects. Cardiovascular, liver, GI, neurologic, and other sequelae of alcohol and other drugs of abuse have been reviewed (Gordis, 2003). Alcohol abuse is frequently associated with hypertension.

KEY TREATMENT

Evidence on the effectiveness of counseling to reduce alcohol consumption during pregnancy is limited; however, studies in the general adult population show that behavioral counseling interventions are effective among women of childbearing age. The benefits of behavioral counseling interventions to reduce alcohol misuse by adults outweigh any potential harm (USPSTF, USDHHS, 2006) (SOR: B).

Management

Alcohol Intoxication

Key Points

- Naive alcohol users are impaired at lower levels.
- Always give thiamine to alcoholic patients.
- Urine toxicology is frequently helpful for concomitant drug use.

Alcohol intoxication is frequently seen as a component of trauma, domestic violence, or suicide attempts (McGinnis and Foege, 1993). The degree of intoxication is determined by the amount of alcohol ingested, the duration of the ingestion, and the patient's tolerance, if any, for the alcohol. Subtle effects occur at levels of 20 mg/dL and include mild euphoria, mild impairment of coordination, and mood alterations. At 80 to 100 mg/dL, delayed reaction times and slurred speech may be noted. This 80-mg/dL level is generally accepted as an unsafe level for motor vehicle operation. Between 100 and 200 mg/dL, ataxia, grossly slurred speech, and incoordination occur. As the level climbs to 300 mg/dL, the ataxia becomes more marked, and drowsiness, lethargy, and vomiting may occur. In naive drinkers, levels above 400 mg/dL are associated with coma, respiratory depression, hypothermia, and death from central nervous system (CNS) depression, loss of airway integrity, or pulmonary aspiration. Chronic alcoholics will have different tolerance responses than those just listed and may be in severe withdrawal at substantial levels.

Alcohol-induced coma can be managed by protecting the airway and performing basic resuscitation, if necessary. The patient should be placed in a warm protective environment, with careful monitoring of vital signs. Gastric emptying is rarely helpful because of the rapid absorption of alcohol, but it may be considered if the ingestion has occurred within 60 minutes. Alcohol is eliminated mostly by hepatic metabolism, which follows zero-order kinetics. The rate does not change with changes in the alcohol blood level. Fructose can enhance elimination but is not typically used. In extreme cases, hemodialysis may be effective in reducing the level quickly. Activated charcoal does not efficiently absorb ethanol but may be given if other toxins have been ingested (Mayo-Smith, 2009).

Thiamine and glucose should always be administered, because chronic alcoholism is associated with hypoglycemia and thiamine deficient states such as Wernicke's encephalopathy (mental confusion, cranial nerve palsies, ataxia). Thiamine should be given immediately before or with glucose to prevent hypoglycemia because glucose is metabolized with the enzyme thiamine pyrophosphorylase. The physician should look for additional drug use in all patients because the effects of other drugs may be obscured by the obvious alcohol intoxication (Mayo-Smith, 2009). A urine toxicology screen may be positive for concomitant intoxicants.

Overview of Alcoholism Treatment

Alcoholics who are actively drinking are among the highest cost users of medical services in the United States. Several studies have documented that alcohol treatment has beneficial effects on health care expenditures, primarily as a result of decreased health care use by alcoholics and their families. A Harvard Study compared 587 lifesaving interventions and ranked all substance abuse interventions, including treatment of alcoholism, in the top 10% (Tengs et al., 1995).

Physicians interface with the medical or behavioral effects of alcoholism when patients deteriorate to the point of trauma, end-organ damage, or behavioral impairment. As with other chronic disorders, alcoholism is slow but progressive. As the disease progresses, the ability to control drinking diminishes, which distinguishes an alcoholic from a nonalcoholic. Many physicians view detoxification as the treatment of this disorder, which is similar to giving diabetics one injection of insulin to control their diabetes. It treats the immediate problem but does little to address the chronic disorder in 1 week or 1 month. Although the goal for an alcoholic is complete abstinence from alcohol, the norm is alcohol consumption in increasing amounts. The family physician can view intermittent periods of abstinence or reductions in alcohol consumption as progress in treatment of the disease and encourage further efforts. Relapse must be evaluated carefully, and keys to change can open the door to further reductions or ongoing abstinence.

The American Society of Addiction Medicine (ASAM) has developed patient placement criteria (PPC) to better guide treatment of alcoholism.(Mee-Lee et al., 2001). The PPC can help to assign the appropriate level of care for detoxification and subsequent rehabilitation of those with alcohol use disorders. The ASAM criteria reflect a consensus of expert opinion for adolescents and adults in treatment. Levels of care are differentiated by three criteria: (1) degree of direct medical management provided; (2) degree of structure, safety, and security provided; and (3) degree of treatment intensity provided. The current criteria are under revision since 2007. Special populations who need consideration include pregnant and nursing women; adolescents; older adults; HIV-positive patients; patients with neurologic, cardiovascular, hepatic, or renal disorders; patients with psychiatric comorbidities; and persons in criminal justice settings (Wright et al., 2009).

Detoxification

The *alcohol withdrawal syndrome* is a somewhat predicable series of events that have a temporal relationship to the use, decrease in intake, or cessation of alcohol consumption. Alcohol withdrawal may occur in a patient who has a reduction in alcohol intake from a previously significant level or an absolute absence of alcohol. The pharmacology of alcohol and its subsequent metabolism is well known and follows zero-order kinetics, primarily through the liver and cytochrome pathways (Mayo-Smith, 2009).

Patients with mild to moderate alcohol withdrawal symptoms and no serious psychiatric or medical comorbidities can be safely treated in the outpatient setting (Asplund et al., 2004). The severity of these symptoms varies greatly among individuals, but in a majority, they are mild and transient, passing within 1 or 2 days (Driessen et al., 2005; Mayo-Smith, 2009). Westerling and colleagues (2006) developed a scale to predict severity of alcohol withdrawal.

The signs and symptoms of alcohol withdrawal vary individually but tend to be repetitive in the same person. Most alcoholics who withdraw from alcohol experience minimal symptoms, such as sleep disturbance or anxiety. A small number may have tremulousness, agitation, diaphoresis, and cognitive impairment. The tremors or shakes typically begin 12 to 14 hours after a period of heavy drinking and are usually noted in the early morning. Tremulousness may be accompanied by *alcoholic hallucinosis*, a misperception of objects in the patient's sensory arena. Other symptoms of withdrawal include nausea, vomiting, poor oral intake, sweats, and anxiety. Seizures during alcohol withdrawal tend to occur as one isolated seizure or a brief cluster of seizures. Seizures are frequently preceded by tremors and tend to recur in a similar pattern in the same patient. Seizures may be the initial manifestation of alcohol withdrawal. Seizure activity is most common 24 to 48 hours after alcohol cessation, although seizures can occur as early as 24 hours or as late as 2 weeks after cessation of alcohol (Victor, 1983) (Box 49-4). Seizures may occur even later with concomitant benzodiazepine abuse. Withdrawal seizures are typically generalized, grand mal, and self-limited. Rarely, seizures may progress to status epilepticus (<3%). Physical signs include an elevated pulse and BP along with signs of autonomic hyperactivity. Researchers have noted increased levels of catecholamine in the locus ceruleus (brainstem) and abnormalities in the neuroinhibitory hormone γ-aminobutyric acid (Mayo-Smith, 2006).

The revised Clinical Institute Withdrawal Assessment for Alcohol scale, revised (CIWA-Ar) is a validated 10-item assessment tool used to quantify the severity of alcohol withdrawal syndrome and to monitor and medicate patients going through withdrawal (Bayard et al., 2004) (Table 49-1). Patients with moderate withdrawal should receive pharmacotherapy

---

Box 49-4 Alcohol Withdrawal Seizures

Peak seizure risk is 24 to 48 hours after cessation; may occur up to 2 weeks later.

Seizures are brief or occur in a "flurry."

Dilantin is ineffective.

Use caution with medications that lower seizure threshold (e.g., tricyclics, phenothiazines).

to treat their symptoms and reduce the risk of seizures and DTs during outpatient detoxification. Benzodiazepines are the treatment of choice for alcohol withdrawal, according to U.S. and Scottish guidelines (SIGN, 2003). In healthy people with mild to moderate alcohol withdrawal, carbamazepine has many advantages, making it a first-line treatment for properly selected patients (Asplund et al., 2004).

Major alcohol withdrawal, also known as *delirium tremens,* occurs in less than 5% of alcoholics in withdrawal. Delirium tremens is usually preceded by minor withdrawal symptoms, although they may appear frankly in a patient with minimal symptomatology. The delirium often begins 3 to 4 days after the last drink and is characterized by a marked change in sensorium with agitation, frank hallucinations,

Table 49-1 Clinical Institute Withdrawal Assessment of Alcohol Scale, Revised (CIWA-Ar)*

Patient:_____ Date:_____ Time:_____ (24 hour clock, midnight = 00:00)

Pulse or heart rate, taken for 1 minute:_____ Blood pressure:_____

Nausea and Vomiting	**Tactile Disturbances**
Ask, "Do you feel sick to your stomach? Have you vomited?" Observation.	Ask, "Have you any itching, pins and needles sensations, any burning, any numbness, or do you feel bugs crawling on or under your skin?" Observation.
0 No nausea and no vomiting	**0** None
1 Mild nausea with no vomiting	**1** Very mild itching, pins and needles, burning, or numbness
2	**2** Mild itching, pins and needles, burning, or numbness
3	**3** Moderate itching, pins and needles, burning, or numbness
4 Intermittent nausea with dry heaves	**4** Moderately severe hallucinations
5	**5** Severe hallucinations
6	**6** Extremely severe hallucinations
7 Constant nausea, frequent dry heaves, and vomiting	**7** Continuous hallucinations

Tremor	**Auditory Disturbances**
Arms extended and fingers spread apart. Observation.	Ask, "Are you more aware of sounds around you? Are they harsh? Do they frighten you? Are you hearing anything that is disturbing to you? Are you hearing things you know are not there?" Observation.
0 No tremor	**0** Not present
1 Not visible, but can be felt fingertip to fingertip	**1** Very mild harshness or ability to frighten
2	**2** Mild harshness or ability to frighten
3	**3** Moderate harshness or ability to frighten
4 Moderate, with patient's arms extended	**4** Moderately severe hallucinations
5	**5** Severe hallucinations
6	**6** Extremely severe hallucinations
7 Severe, even with arms not extended	**7** Continuous hallucinations

Paroxysmal Sweats	**Visual Disturbances**
Observation.	Ask, "Does the light appear to be too bright? Is its color different? Does it hurt your eyes? Are you seeing anything that is disturbing to you? Are you seeing things you know are not there?" Observation.
0 No sweat visible	**0** Not present
1 Barely perceptible sweating, palms moist	**1** Very mild sensitivity
2	**2** Mild sensitivity
3	**3** Moderate sensitivity
4 Beads of sweat obvious on forehead	**4** Moderately severe hallucinations
5	**5** Severe hallucinations
6	**6** Extremely severe hallucinations
7 Drenching sweats	**7** Continuous hallucinations

Anxiety	**Headache, Fullness in Head**
Ask, "Do you feel nervous?" Observation.	Ask, "Does your head feel different? Does it feel like there is a band around your head?" Do not rate for dizziness or lightheadedness. Otherwise, rate severity.
0 No anxiety, at ease	**0** Not present
1 Mild anxious	**1** Very mild
2	**2** Mild
3	**3** Moderate
4 Moderately anxious, or guarded, so anxiety is inferred	**4** Moderately severe
5	**5** Severe
6	**6** Very severe
7 Equivalent to acute panic states, as seen in severe delirium or acute schizophrenic reactions	**7** Extremely severe

Continued

Table 49-1 Clinical Institute Withdrawal Assessment of Alcohol Scale, Revised (CIWA-Ar)—cont'd

Agitation	Orientation and Clouding of Sensorium
Observation.	Ask, "What day is this? Where are you? Who am I?"
0 Normal activity	**0** Oriented and can do serial additions
1 Somewhat more than normal activity	**1** Cannot do serial additions or is uncertain about date
2	**2** Disoriented for date by no more than 2 calendar days
3	**3** Disoriented for date by more than 2 calendar days
4 Moderately fidgety and restless	**4** Disoriented for place or person
5	
6	
7 Paces back and forth during most of the interview, or constantly thrashes about	

Total CIWA-Ar Score _____

Rater's Initials _____

From Sullivan JT, Sykora K, Schneiderman J, et al. Assessment of alcohol withdrawal: the revised Clinical Institute Withdrawal Assessment for Alcohol scale (CIWA-Ar). Br J Addict 1989;84:1353-1357.

*The CIWA-Ar is not copyrighted and may be reproduced freely. This assessment for monitoring withdrawal symptoms requires approximately 5 minutes to administer. The maximum score is 67 (see instrument). Patients scoring less than 10 do not usually need additional medication for withdrawal.

Box 49-5 Delirium Tremens (DTs)

Usually preceded by tremor or seizures.

Usually begin 3 to 4 days after alcohol cessation.

Delirium with severe disorientation

Autonomic hyperactivity

Disturbed sleep

Worsened by concomitant disorders (e.g., pancreatitis, pneumonia, GI bleed)

---

and severe disorientation (Box 49-5). Severe and potentially life-threatening autonomic hyperactivity leads to tachycardia, hypertension, and diaphoresis, frequently with low-grade fever. The severe disorientation may lead to self-injury or harm. Typically, the patient's actions may be appropriate to the context of the state of disorientation and hallucinosis. The patient's sleep activity is usually disturbed, along with excessive motor activity. Risk factors for DTs are a high blood alcohol level at the initial evaluation, an alcohol withdrawal seizure early in the withdrawal syndrome, and a previous history of delirium (Victor, 1983). Concomitant infections or additional medical disorders may also predispose to severe alcohol withdrawal. Fever over 101° F (38.3° C) should be evaluated further. Before the treatment of alcohol withdrawal, a complete physical examination should be performed to assess the patient, including analysis for GI blood loss.

KEY TREATMENT

Physicians should always use thiamine supplementation (Mayo-Smith, 2009 (SOR: A).

Giving benzodiazepines is the treatment of choice of alcohol withdrawal and is supported by the latest systematic reviews (Ntais et al., 2005) (SOR: A).

Carbamazepine is first-line treatment for properly selected patients (Asplund et al, 2004) (SOR: C).

Phenytoin (Dilantin) is ineffective in withdrawal seizures.

Withdrawal Treatment

Treatment of alcohol withdrawal consists of supportive and pharmacologic interventions. Supportive interventions include fostering the patient's desire for abstinence during the withdrawal process. A calm, quiet environment, reassuring and reorienting the patient if confused, decreases the risk of injury or relapse.

The preferred CNS agents for detoxification are the benzodiazepines, according to U.S. and Scottish guidelines (Asplund et al., 2004; SIGN, 2003) and Cochrane review (Ntais et al., 2005). They provide the best side effect profile and have a better risk/benefit profile than other agents. Benzodiazepines are not likely to be fatal in overdose unless mixed with another central depressant (check the urine toxicology screen). Chlordiazepoxide and diazepam are both effective agents. If liver disease is present, or to treat withdrawal in an older patient, oxazepam or lorazepam may be a safer choice because of shorter half-life. Additionally, beta blockers such as atenolol, 50 to 100 mg/day, may decrease tremulousness and sympathomimetic symptoms if there are no contraindications (Table 49-2). A scheduled regimen of chlordiazepoxide, 100 to 300 mg on day 1, followed by daily 50% dose reductions for 3 to 5 days, rather than "as needed" or on a symptom schedule, provides for a smooth withdrawal. Doses must be held for oversedation or somnolence. Monitoring for oversedation is necessary before each dosing (Sullivan et al., 1989). Aggressive regimens support patient comfort, help maintain compliance, and reduce the risk of seizures and major withdrawal. Outpatient detoxification can be performed; without supervision, however, some risk is present (e.g., seizures, self-injury, overdose), and relapse is likely if further alcohol is available.

Anticonvulsants such as phenytoin have not been demonstrated to reduce withdrawal seizures better than benzodiazepines. Anticonvulsants used for detoxification with a history of seizures received a level B of evidence in the Scottish guidelines (SIGN, 2003). Carbamazepine is superior to other anticonvulsants and results in less psychiatric distress, a faster return to work, less rebound symptoms, and reduced

Table 49-2 Alcohol Withdrawal: Stages and Treatment Summary

Stage	Intervention	Pharmacology
I. Mild	Be supportive. Contact Alcoholics Anonymous. Provide close follow-up.	Thiamine, 100 mg daily Chlordiazepoxide, 25 mg three times daily if necessary, 3 days only
II. Moderate	Allow brief inpatient visit. Make observations. Check laboratory test results (e.g., magnesium, phosphate, electrolyte, glucose levels).	As above, *plus* chlordiazepoxide, 100-300 mg/day, 3 days only Atenolol, 50-100 mg/day, 3 days only
III. Severe	Hospitalize in ICU. Delirium tremens, intermediate care. Laboratory tests as above. Monitor fluid status. May need restraint. Monitor for infection. Prevent self-harm.	As above, *plus* chlordiazepoxide, 100 mg hourly until asleep or subdued, then taper. Antipsychotics: haloperidol, 2-10 mg/day Lorazepam, 1-2 mg intravenously if unable to take orally

Box 49-6 Components of Effective Brief Intervention

Feedback of physician's assessment
Emphasis on patient *responsibility*
Clear, direct *advice to change*
Nonconfrontational physician approach
Menu of options provided

From Bien TH, Miller WR, Tonigan JS. Brief interventions for alcohol problems: a review. Addiction 1993;8:315-335.

posttreatment drinking (Malcolm et al., 2001). Anticonvulsants are not generally indicated unless a concomitant seizure disorder is present.

Antipsychotic medications such as risperidone, olanzapine, and haloperidol have benefits in patients with hallucinosis and DTs but may reduce the seizure threshold (SIGN, 2003). Ear acupuncture has not shown efficacy in alcohol withdrawal in clinical trials. However, massage therapy has reduced withdrawal scores (Kunz et al., 2007; Reader et al., 2005).

Interventions in Alcohol Disease

Interventions by family physicians have the goal of changing the natural course or outcome of the alcoholic disease process. A family physician typically performs many interventions on patients with chronic disorders over time. Interventions generally follow an assessment and consist of advice about how to manage the disorder, may include a pharmacologic agent, and usually require some type of follow-up or ongoing monitoring.

Brief Interventions

Brief interventions can be very successful in primary care (SIGN, 2003) (Box 49-6). The father of the concept of *stages of change*, Prochaska (2009) reviews motivation to change in alcohol addiction. Family physicians can apply motivational interviewing in helping patients to move to the next level in stages of change. Part of any substance abuse intervention is the physician's assessment of the patient's readiness to change. First described by Prochaska and DiClimente (1983) while studying smokers, assessing the state of change assists the family physician in targeting the interventional approach to the patient. Change consists of the following six states:

1. *Precontemplation.* The physician can plant the seed of how alcohol is harming the patient (think of creative ways to list reasons) physically or emotionally. Written

information is helpful, and support to the family and others involved must be offered. Further biologic or historical data should be collected, with follow-up at reasonable intervals and availability to help the patient when ready. A nonjudgmental approach is best.

2. *Contemplation.* The patient is aware that harm is occurring but is not yet ready for action. The physician tries to motivate patent to the action phase by listing more reasons for urgency, such as bleeding, ulcers, pancreatitis, and family violence. The physician offers referral advice if the patient is interested, collects more data, performs follow-up at a short interval, and is ready to help the patient when ready to start.

3. *Preparation.* The physician assists the patient in preparing for reduction or cessation of use.

4. *Action.* The patient is ready for referral, has "hit bottom," or is otherwise ready for change. The physician arranges inpatient or outpatient detoxification and involvement in a treatment program and completes a history and physical examination, with laboratory studies as appropriate.

5. *Maintenance.* The physician performs follow-up on the patient; reviews participation in the self-help program and use of the 12 steps as well as the frequency of Alcoholics Anonymous (AA) attendance; monitors target organ issues; performs mental status and depression screening; counsels regarding relapse prevention; monitors laboratory values (e.g., GGT, CDT); prescribes vitamins, naltrexone, acamprosate, antidepressants, or disulfiram (Antabuse) as needed; monitors urine ethylglucuronide (ETG) to determine alcohol use in the previous 72 hours; monitors and schedules; and performs follow-up regularly, as with any chronic disease.

6. *Relapse.* The physician anticipates relapse with any addictive disorder, is ready to help the patient again with entry into a recovery program, and offers nonjudgmental support.

Brief interventions can be carried out in the context of a routine office visit (Edwards and Rollnick, 1997; Fleming et al., 1999). Interventions can follow assessment of the patient. When the physician sees sufficient evidence to conclude or strongly suspect that an alcohol use disorder is present, the brief intervention can be targeted to the patient's stage of change. An encounter with a precontemplative patient would include presentation of the physician's analysis of the problem in a supportive and nonconfrontational manner, with the goal of moving the patient to another state of change. For example:

Mr. Smith, your recent accident, alcohol use pattern, liver enlargement on physical examination, and abnormal laboratory test results lead me to conclude that your use of alcohol is a problem. As your family physician, I am concerned about your ongoing health risks. What can we do to deal with this problem?

Alternatively, a patient who is in the contemplation phase of change would be asked a different set of questions, such as:

Mr. Smith, I am glad that you are able to realize the impact that your alcohol drinking is having on your health, but we need to move forward and discuss treatment options.

An effective brief intervention should include *feedback* summarizing the physician's assessment; patient responsibility should also be emphasized, followed by clear, direct advice to change given in a nonconfrontational manner. The patient is given a menu of options from which to choose (Bien et al., 1993). Authoritative approaches are generally less effective than an empathetic approach. This type of approach will take practice and refinement for busy family physicians but can be integrated into the office practice without substantial time or expense. These techniques are more generally known as *motivational interviewing*. Motivational interviewing is effective in helping family physicians to engage patients in a variety of behavioral changes, including alcohol or tobacco abuse. Motivational interviewing has been a successful technique when used with alcohol brief interventions (Vasilaki et al., 2006).

Classic Intervention

When a brief intervention is not effective, or if the circumstances demand more expeditious change, a classic intervention can be planned. The interventional goal is to break through the alcoholic denial system by providing an overwhelming amount of evidence and feedback to the alcoholic patient. Classic interventions need to be carefully orchestrated by professionals trained in chemical dependency treatment. Unless actively involved in alcoholism treatment, most family physicians will consult one of their referral treatment programs for assistance in developing a classic intervention. The family physician may be an appropriate member of the intervention group.

Treatment of Alcoholism

Key Points

- Try the least restrictive treatment first for the alcoholic patient.
- Long-term treatment is favored for alcoholism.
- The presence of other disorders increases acuity needs in the alcoholic.

The treatment options for alcoholism are extensive (Fuller et al., 2003; Kranzler et al., 2009). The medications most widely studied for alcohol use disorders are disulfiram, naltrexone, and acamprosate. Results from the COMBINE study and trials of depot naltrexone formulations and oral topiramate have provided important new information on the use of these medications in alcohol rehabilitation.

A family physician is faced with several decisions when evaluating a patient for treatment of alcoholism after successful detoxification, or if medically supervised detoxification is not needed. Should the patient go through a hospital or a nonhospital (residential) inpatient program, a day treatment program, or any outpatient program? Should the patient receive counseling, attend AA, or be involved in a cognitive program? Inpatient programs offer isolation from the drinking environment, intensive treatment, family involvement, in-depth assessment, and convenience for further medical or psychiatric assessment. However, they carry significant expense, typically occur after detoxification, remove the patient from the real-world environment, and have not been consistently shown to improve long-term outcomes. Patients who are suicidal or who have serious concomitant mental disorders that may impair recovery, as well as those unable to maintain abstinence in a less restrictive environment, should be considered for these facilities. Advantages of day treatment and outpatient treatment include reduced expense, ability to maintain work in some cases, and usually a longer period of treatment in a less restrictive environment. In general, as long as it is safe to try outpatient treatment initially, it is the least restrictive and most cost-effective method.

Access to relapse prevention treatments of established efficacy should be facilitated for alcohol-dependent patients. These therapies include outpatient programs, residential and "halfway house" milieu therapies, and partial hospitalization programs (SIGN, 2003).

Alcohol Dependency and Psychiatric Comorbidities: Dual Diagnosis

Dual diagnosis is defined as alcohol dependency with one or more other psychiatric comorbidities. Frequently, alcoholics abuse other substances, such as crack cocaine, nicotine, and even opiates (Tallia et al., 2005). Comorbidity estimates among alcoholics, gender preferences for addictive substances, and patterns of progression vary widely (Crum, 2009). Assessment of long-term outcomes highlights the impact of comorbidities on level of functioning, educational achievement, occupation, and social relationships (Crawford et al., 2008).

Patients with alcohol problems and anxiety or depression should have their alcohol problem treated first. If depressive symptoms persist for more than 2 weeks after treatment for alcohol dependence, the physician should consider use of a selective serotonin reuptake inhibitor (SSRI) or tricyclic antidepressant (TCA), or referral for supportive psychotherapy and cognitive-behavioral therapy (CBT), along with relapse prevention (SIGN, 2003). CBT has been shown to be efficacious (Longabaugh and Morgenstern, 1999; Project MATCH, 1997).

Patients with psychotic disorder and alcohol dependence should be encouraged to address their alcohol use and may benefit from motivational, CBT, family, and nonconfrontational approaches. Structured settings may offer some advantage for patients with psychotic comorbidities. Another challenge with treating alcoholics with comorbid conditions is *impulse control disorders* (ICDs). Also known as "behavioral addictions," ICDs include pathologic gambling (PG) and many other conditions (Yip and Potenza, 2009). Of interest in the treatment of alcoholics is evidence that patients with

PG can benefit from treatment with naltrexone (Kim et al., 2001).

Drug Treatment Specific to Alcohol Dependency and Recovery

Key Points

- Disulfiram can be regarded as an aversive agent.
- Naltrexone produces a surmountable opiate blockage and diminishes the reinforcing effect of alcohol.
- Depot naltrexone has greater efficacy than oral naltrexone in alcohol use disorders.
- Acamprosate reduces the urge to drink in some patients.

Treatment of alcohol abuse and dependency with medications has long been a challenging and controversial topic. Drug treatment of alcohol abuse can be divided into drugs used for detoxification (see earlier discussion) and those used to reduce or eliminate alcohol consumption after detoxification and for relapse prevention. Pharmacologic interventions for alcoholism have been reviewed (Fuller et al., 2003). The U.S. Food and Drug Administration (FDA) now approves three drugs for alcohol treatment to reduce or eliminate consumption: disulfiram (Antabuse), acamprosate (Campral), and naltrexone (ReVia) as well as long-acting naltrexone (Vivitrol).

Disulfiram

Disulfiram has been available for the treatment of alcohol dependency since the late 1940s. Given as a single daily dose, disulfiram inhibits aldehyde dehydrogenase, the second alcohol degradation enzyme. This inhibition causes acetaldehyde to increase 5 to 10 times the usual level found after alcohol consumption. Symptoms that occur in patients acquiring alcohol from any source include flushing, palpitations, respiratory difficulty, nausea, vomiting, weakness, and general uneasiness. If alcohol consumption continues or a large volume is ingested, hypotension, syncope, loss of consciousness, and death may follow. Minor reactions may occur with inadvertent exposure from nonbeverage alcohol sources such as colognes, over-the-counter (OTC) medications, or foods with uncooked alcohol. Also used in attempted and completed suicides, disulfiram can be thought of as an "incomplete poison" that will become a "complete poison" if alcohol is added.

Disulfiram works on the patient's understanding and expectation of an adverse experience if alcohol is consumed. It can be given in dosages of 125 to 500 mg daily and can be safely started 24 to 48 hours after alcohol cessation. Avoidance or extreme caution should be used in patients with known or suspected coronary artery disease, those at risk for suicide or with serious mental illness, or those unable or unlikely to comply with a complete treatment plan that includes additional forms of treatment. Disulfiram should not be used as the only treatment for alcohol abuse; it is better considered as an adjunct for carefully selected patients. An often-quoted blinded placebo-controlled study of Veterans Administration patients found that doses of 250 mg, 1 mg, and no disulfiram produced no significant differences in total abstinence (Fuller et al., 1986). Higher doses were associated with fewer drinking days than in other groups. Adverse reactions include peripheral neuropathy, optic neuritis, drowsiness, fatigue, metallic aftertaste, and infrequent hepatotoxicity, probably resulting from hypersensitivity. Evaluation of liver enzyme levels before therapy and periodically is recommended.

Supervised treatment or directly observed therapy (DOT) with oral disulfiram may be used to prevent relapse. However, patients must be informed that this treatment requires complete abstinence, and they should clearly understand the risks of disulfiram therapy.

Naltrexone

The euphoric effect of alcohol is mediated through the endogenous opioid system, with activation of the prefrontal cortex (Tuhonen et al., 1994). Naltrexone, an opioid antagonist, has documented beneficial effect in reducing relapse and craving in alcoholic patients (O'Malley et al., 1992; Swift et al., 1994; Volpicelli et al., 1992). Alcoholics taking naltrexone report a less pleasurable effect or high from alcohol consumption and do not escalate their drinking as rapidly as control groups (Volpicelli et al., 1995). A decreased craving for alcohol has not been universally reported. Naltrexone is given as a daily 50-mg tablet or a monthly 300-mg injection. This dosage provides a surmountable opioid blockage that will render other opioids ineffective unless given in greatly increased doses. Naltrexone is not an aversive agent. Many alcoholic patients report a less-than-expected pleasurable experience with alcohol consumption, whereas others report some mild aversive symptoms.

Naltrexone undergoes first-pass hepatic metabolism and is hepatotoxic in excessive doses. It should not be given to patients currently addicted to opiates because it will precipitate acute opiate withdrawal (Croop et al., 1997). The most common side effects at the usual dosage include nausea, headache, dizziness, anxiety, and somnolence. Good candidates for naltrexone are those likely to be compliant with therapy, those concomitantly addicted to opiates who have been detoxified and have not received opiate replacement therapy, and those with heavy alcohol cravings at entry to therapy (Volpicelli et al., 1997). Naltrexone should *not* be used as a single treatment agent but rather in conjunction with other behavioral or motivational treatment modalities. Questions remain about the duration of treatment with naltrexone in alcohol use disorders. Generally, prolonged abstinence rates improve after 12 months of continuous abstinence.

Poor compliance with oral naltrexone reduces its potential benefits (Volpicelli et al., 1997). In a pilot study, alcohol-dependent patients treated with subcutaneous depot formulation of naltrexone had detectable plasma concentrations of the medication for more than 3 days after injection and had reduced frequency of heavy drinking compared with the placebo group (Kanzler et al., 1998). A randomized clinical trial with depot naltrexone did not demonstrate reduced incidence of heavy drinking, although it did demonstrate significantly delayed onset of drinking, increased number of abstinent days, and increased abstinence (Kanzler et al.,

2004). The FDA approved long-acting naltrexone (Vivitrol), 380 mg each month intramuscularly (IM) in the buttock, for alcohol dependency in 2006. Patients should be abstinent when they are started on naltrexone.

An alternative opioid antagonist with some success in patients with alcohol dependency, but not as well studied, is nalmefene (Kanzler et al., 2009).

According to the Agency for Health Care Policy and Research, there is good (level B) evidence to support the use of naltrexone to reduce craving and relapse (AHCPR, 1999).

Acamprosate

Acamprosate is one of the newest drugs to be added to the formulary for the treatment of alcohol dependency. The FDA has approved acamprosate for maintenance of abstinence from alcohol in patients with alcohol dependence who are abstinent at treatment initiation. This provision includes that patients also participate in a comprehensive alcohol treatment program. Acamprosate is reasonably well tolerated and without serious adverse effects (AHCPR, 1999). European trials of acamprosate showed efficacy in alcohol dependence; acamprosate enhanced abstinence and reduced drinking days in alcohol-dependent subjects.

Acamprosate is recommended in newly detoxified dependent patients as an adjunct to psychosocial interventions. Acamprosate is approved for use in alcohol-dependent and alcohol-abusing patients. Its mechanism of action is not well known, although there is fair evidence of its benefit. Acamprosate is an analog of homotaurine, a GABA-ergic agonist. The GABA-ergic system appears to affect the action of alcohol-induced behavior. Acamprosate also appears to have effects on glutamate and NMDA receptors. Chronic alcohol exposure is thought to alter the normal balance between neuronal excitation and inhibition, and acamprosate may help restore some of this balance. Several controlled clinical trials have demonstrated the effectiveness of acamprosate as an adjunct to psychosocial therapy for alcoholics who have undergone inpatient detoxification. In these studies, acamprosate was demonstrated to be superior to placebo. Acamprosate does not appear to be effective in the treatment of polysubstance abuse (Bouza et al., 2004; Mann et al., 2004). Evaluation of renal function for those at risk, including elderly patients, is indicated before initiating treatment with acamprosate.

Two U.S. multicenter trials, including the Combining Medications and Behavioral Intervention for Alcoholism (COMBINE) study, failed to show an advantage of acamprosate over placebo on an "intent to treat" basis (Anton et al., 2006; Mason et al., 2006). Discrepancies may be caused by differences in European studies, which included heavier drinkers with longer periods of abstinence before induction in trials (Kanzler et al., 2009).

Summary

Pharmacotherapy for alcohol use disorders with strength of recommendation (SOR) is as follows:
Naltrexone (A, 1)
Long-acting naltrexone (Vivitrol) (A, 1)
Acamprosate (A, 1)
Disulfiram (B, 2)

Other Medications Used in Alcohol Treatment

Anticonvulsants (Topiramate)

Anticonvulsants likely exert beneficial effects on γ-aminobutyric acid (GABA) receptors. Placebo-controlled studies included carbamazepine (Mueller et al., 1997), divalproex (Brady et al., 2002), and topiramate (Johnson et al., 2003), with a multicenter study confirming the efficacy of topiramate and anticonvulsants for treatment of alcohol use disorders (Johnson et al., 2007). Topiramate was shown to decrease (1) drinks/day, (2) drinks/drinking day, (3) drinking days, (4) heavy-drinking days, and (5) GGT levels (Johnson et al., 2007). Side effects of anticonvulsants include numbness and tingling, metabolic acidosis, fatigue, dizziness, loss of appetite, nausea, diarrhea, weight loss, and difficulty concentrating, with memory, and in word finding. Suicidal thoughts or actions are infrequently reported, as are renal calculi and acute secondary glaucoma (Kranzler et al., 2009).

Baclofen

A GABA-B receptor agonist, baclofen has long been used as an antispasmodic. Only more recently has baclofen been investigated as a treatment for alcohol dependency. In a modest controlled trial of 1 month, baclofen was efficacious in achievement of total abstinent days compared with placebo (Addolorato et al., 2002). A follow-up study demonstrated efficacy in 84 patients with cirrhosis of the liver in maintaining abstinence (71% baclofen vs. 29% placebo) (Addolorato et al., 2007). There is potential for abuse of baclofen and withdrawal reactions, including delirium, which underscores the need for further research (Kanzler et al., 2009).

Serotonergic Agents

Most episodes of postwithdrawal depression will remit without specific treatment if abstinence from alcohol is maintained for days or weeks (Brown et al., 1988; Schukit, 1983). Whereas patients with comorbid depression often require pharmacotherapy, and although the SSRIs have a low side effect profile, they can exacerbate the tremor, anxiety, and insomnia in early-recovering alcoholics. Recovering alcoholics with comorbid depression may actually do better with TCAs (Nunes and Levin, 2004).

Special Populations

Alcohol Use Disorder in Women

Women have lower rates of alcohol abuse and dependency than their male counterparts, 1.5% overall and 1.5% in older adult women (Mouton and Espino, 1999) (Box 49-7). Women generally enter treatment later than men and have more psychiatric symptoms. Women seem to develop many pathologic effects of alcohol more rapidly than men (Blume and Zilberman, 2005), including fatty liver, hypertension, anemia, malnutrition, GI hemorrhage, and peptic ulcer requiring surgery (Zweben, 2009). For women, five to seven drinks daily is sufficient to cause significant disease progression.

Box 49-7 Women Alcoholics

Lower rates of abuse than men.

More hidden drinking than men.

TWEAK screening better than CAGE.

Less alcohol consumption than men may cause significant disease progression.

Treatment in all-women program is preferred.

Nonmedical use of prescription drugs in general and opioids in particular has been identified as a significant problem since the late 1990s. Women also have higher associated rates with first use of illicit drugs after age 24, serious mental illness, and cigarette smoking (Tetrault et al., 2008). Comorbid conditions for women include drug addiction, sexual abuse, intimate partner violence, borderline personality disorder, eating disorders, mood disorders and anxiety disorders, and HIV infection. Women who drink alcohol may be more sensitive to the behavioral effects of concomitant cocaine use (Zweben, 2009).

Family physicians generally detect alcohol use disorders in women later than in male alcoholics. Screening tests (e.g., CAGE) have less sensitivity in women and need to be interpreted differently, usually with lower cutoff points. This difference may result from the lower volume of alcohol consumed and the social stigmatization of these women (Bradley et al., 1998). Screening tests such as the TWEAK have performed better than the CAGE in women. It is important for physicians to educate women about their greater risk, even highly educated patients (Green et al., 2007). Incarcerated women often begin using drugs and alcohol at very young ages and frequently require significant educational and job-training support to make successful transitions to recovery (Zweben, 2009). Women may have better treatment outcomes if referred to all-women programs or programs specializing in women's addictions (Hodgkins et al., 1997).

Alcohol Abuse and Pregnancy

The Institute of Medicine recognizes alcohol-related birth defects (ARBDs) and alcohol-related neurodevelopmental disorder (ARND) in addition to fetal alcohol syndrome (FAS) as potential effects of alcohol use in pregnancy and the periconception period (Warren and Foudin 2001; Muchowski and Paladine, 2004). A diagnosis of FAS requires characteristic facial anomalies, growth retardation, and neurodevelopmental abnormalities. In *partial* FAS, affected children have some of these characteristics, with no other explanation. ARBD includes a confirmed history of maternal alcohol use plus one or more congenital defects, most often cardiac, renal, vision, hearing, or skeletal. ARNDs require a confirmed history of maternal alcohol use and the neurodevelopment abnormalities or cognitive-behavioral abnormalities found in partial FAS.

The prevalence of FAS in the U.S. population is estimated at 0.5 to 2 per 1000 births, with up to 10 in 1000 newborns having some effect from alcohol exposure. The rate of FAS is more than 20 times higher in the United States compared with other countries, including European countries, partially because of differences in diagnosis (Muchowski

and Paladine, 2004). Whether a safe threshold of alcohol consumption exists before or during pregnancy is controversial. Many U.S. authorities recommend against any alcohol intake before or during pregnancy. The effects of alcohol on a fetus depend on the amount of alcohol consumed at one time, timing of alcohol consumption in gestation, and duration of alcohol use in pregnancy. This is complicated by studies using various definitions of "light" and "heavy" alcohol use, with categories that often overlap among different studies. *Binge drinking*, defined as more than five drinks in a single day, even when episodic, is more dangerous to fetal brain development than non–binge drinking (Muchowski and Paladine, 2004).

Less severe problems can occur, although a high level of alcohol use in pregnancy is associated with more severely affected offspring. A 1984 study of 31,000 pregnancies showed a higher risk of growth retardation if a mother had even one drink a day. A 2001 study of more than 600 urban African American children showed continued behavioral effects of alcohol at age 6 to 7 years with low levels (one drink daily) of maternal alcohol consumption (Muchowski and Paladine, 2004).

Some intervention attempts show promise. A review of trials in which physicians briefly counseled nonpregnant women who were problem drinkers found no consistent decrease in drinking. Trials of personalized advice to pregnant women have also been found to be no more effective than written information alone. A written self-help manual, however, did improve cessation rates in women at a prenatal clinic. The CDC sponsored a pilot project to encourage alcohol cessation and effective contraception in women at risk for alcohol-exposed pregnancy (Muchowski and Paladine, 2004). Although not a controlled trial, this more extensive intervention showed promise. Of the 143 women enrolled, 68.5% had stopped their alcohol consumption or were using effective contraception by the 6-month follow-up. Women should not be discouraged from breastfeeding, if they are not using illicit drugs and do not have specific contraindications such as HIV infection (McCarthy and Posey, 2000).

Applying the Evidence

Written information about the risks of alcohol use in pregnancy should be provided to pregnant women who consume alcohol (Floyd et al., 1999; Muchowski and Paladine, 2004). Data are insufficient to recommend physician counseling for alcohol cessation before or during pregnancy. More comprehensive interventions may be more effective but have yet to be fully studied. No studies have evaluated neonatal outcomes with women counseled on alcohol cessation in the periconception period.

Emergency Contraception

The importance of making information and resources available for emergency contraception deserves more attention for women with addictions. Emergency contraception techniques are widely available and as OTC medications in some states. However, these are underused by women at risk for unintended pregnancy. An emergency hotline is available nationally for emergency contraception access for women: 1-888-NOT-2-LATE (1-888-668-2528) (http://not-2-late.com accessed 8-31-06).

Adolescents

Family physicians should develop expertise for recognizing alcohol abuse in adolescents. According to the American Academy of Family Physicians Graham Center, 38% of ambulatory adolescent health visits in the United States are made to family physicians (AAFP, 2001). Specific screening tools are available for adolescents (Comerci, 2002). Alcohol abuse in the family system can create several levels of dysfunction, including the abuse of alcohol or other drugs by adolescents. Approximately 3% of adolescents are addicted to alcohol or other drugs (NIAAA, 1997). Drinking is frequently a family matter, with 82% of drinking families raising children who drink, and 72% of families who abstain raising children to abstain (Johnson and Leff, 1999). Environmental, physiologic, and genetic factors combine to place certain adolescents at risk.

Detection of use or abuse requires reliable information from the adolescent. An atmosphere of trust must be established, and more than one visit is often necessary. Urine drug screening can be effective but is controversial. The American Academy of Pediatrics recommends involuntary testing only in limited emergency circumstances, such as altered mental status, inability to give consent (seizures, coma), acute medical problems putting the adolescent at serious risk, a preadolescent or very young adolescent, and court-ordered monitoring (AAP, 1998; Comerci, 2002). Family physician interventions for adolescents abusing alcohol or other substance must be tailored to the adolescent's specific needs. Appropriate treatment programs should have strong family involvement, total abstinence goals, and professionals experienced in adolescent care.

College student drinking is a major concern on U.S. campuses. An estimated 1700 unintentional college student deaths per year involve alcohol (Hingson et al., 2005). The NIAAA Task Force on College Drinking categorized college student drinking consequences as damage to self, others, or the institution, as well as the overlapping categories of drinking and driving, high-risk sexual behavior, and physical and sexual aggression (NIAAA, 2002). College prevention strategies include cognitive-behavioral skills–based interventions, brief motivation interventions, feedback-only interventions, and environmental interventions. Underage drinking statutes, including penalties for servers, and comprehensive campus-community approaches that involve students, all campus stakeholders, and community leaders have proved beneficial (Larimer et al., 2009).

Treatment of Older Adults

Alcohol use disorders and prescription drug abuse are prevalent in older adults (Blow et al., 2002). Specific "geriatric alcohol use disorder" screening tests can be used by family physicians, including the SMAST-G, MAST-G, AUDIT, and CAGE (see earlier discussion) (Blow et al., 2009). Older adults are often categorized as "binge drinkers." The National Institute on Alcohol Abuse and Alcoholism (NIAAA) and the Centers for Substance Abuse Treatment (CSAT) have published alcohol use guidelines for older adults (Blume, 2009). Often, comorbid affective disorders are present in older adults. Premorbid alcohol use disorders predict a more severe course of affective disorders (Cook et al., 1991).

Concomitant alcohol use disorders and depression increase late-life suicide risk, as does at-risk and problem drinking among elderly persons (Blow et al., 2004). Older persons with alcohol use disorders may respond well to brief interventions and increased socialization. The GOAl study and Health Profile Project found brief interventions in older adults to be efficacious (Blow and Barry, 2000; Blow et al., 2009; Blume, 2009).

Physician with Alcohol Use Disorders

The prevalence of alcohol use disorders among physicians is comparable to the national lifetime prevalence of 13.5% (Reiger et al., 1990). Family physicians, along with anesthesiologists, were overrepresented in a study of 1000 physicians with substance use disorders (Talbott et al., 1987).

Male physicians outnumber female physicians in studies of substance use disorders. Risk factors used in other patient groups apply to physicians as well (see online discussion of causative factors). The pattern of physician abuse differs from that in the general population by the increased use of alcohol, benzodiazepines, and prescription opiates (Hughes et al., 1992). Much of the prescription drug use is self-prescribed. Impairment is generally noted first in the alcohol-abusing physician's family and social life. Marital discord, relationship problems, and heavy drinking at social events can progress to work dysfunction and impairment (Talbott et al., 1987). The physician's thinking initially becomes impaired in spatial and constructive skills, along with negative effects on memory. Verbal skills are maintained, although cognition is affected as drinking continues. An alcoholic physician will frequently turn to benzodiazepines for relief of anxiety or stress symptoms. Further impairment leads to avoidance of responsibility, such as not returning pages while on duty, showing up late, or arriving for patient care responsibilities with alcohol on the breath.

Several studies have shown that alcohol use and abuse patterns are established early in the physician's career (Birch et al., 1998; Clark et al., 1987). In 2001, The Joint Commission (formerly Joint Commission on the Accreditation of Healthcare Organizations) pressured hospital organizations to address the wellness of their medical staff (Joint Commission, 2008). State medical societies and licensing bodies have been active in establishing physician health programs and guidelines, to assist the physician in returning to a productive career (Federation of State Physician Health Programs, 2005). Treatment outcomes for physicians in these structured programs are excellent, with sustained recovery rates of 70% to 80% or better (Paris and Cannavan, 1999). A cohort study of 100 physicians with alcohol use disorders found similar trends and an average sustained abstinence of 17.6 years (Lloyd, 2002).

As with the treatment of any chronic illness, early identification and intervention improve recovery rates of physicians with alcohol use disorders. Posttreatment behavioral and biologic (urine) monitoring, as well as attendance at physician support groups and AA meetings, are important in the recovery process (Galanter et al., 1990). The AAFP (1998) recognizes physician treatment and recovery from alcoholism or other forms of substance abuse and supports physicians who successfully complete treatment programs acceptable to the physician health program of the individual state.

Prevention

Primary prevention is the education of at-risk populations to avoid problems. Family physicians have the power to identify families with alcoholism and provide education to the children and adolescents who are at risk. Primary prevention includes the community; a Chinese proverb says the physician who also cares for the community is the "best physician." Family physicians can offer universal screening for alcoholism and alcohol abuse; this is an example of the secondary level of prevention in their practice. The evidence for effectiveness of "designated driver" and school-based drinking and driving prevention programs has been insufficient (Ditter et al., 2005; Elder et al., 2005). School prevention programs noted as effective include the Michigan Model for Comprehensive School Health Education (Shope et al., 1996).

Public Policy Recommendations

Family physicians can affect public policy advocacy on issues of alcohol abuse through professional organizations such as the AAFP and state academies. The CDC (2004) recommends that states and local jurisdictions consider adoption of effective strategies aimed at reducing excessive drinking. Family physicians can advocate policies that include (but are not limited to) increasing alcohol excise taxes, reducing DUI limits to the 0.04 blood alcohol level, toughening DUI penalties, restricting advertising along highways or in ethnic minority communities, zoning restrictions on placement of points of sale, and increasing opportunities for screening in various settings (e.g., courts, jails, EDs).

Public policy interventions can be categorized as (1) measures to reduce the availability of alcohol, such as control of hours and days of sales, outlet-density restrictions, monopoly regulatory systems, and minimum-age drinking laws, or as (2) penalties, such as increased DUI enforcement, server-liability laws, and altering the server environment through training. "Ecologic research" on environmental changes and prevention of alcohol abuse includes the Communities Mobilizing for Change on Alcohol Project, the Community Trials Project, and the Sacramento Neighborhood Alcohol Prevention Project (Treno et al., 2009). This emerging body of evidence should help communities in the future as they strive to create environments that reduce the frequency of alcohol use disorders.

KEY TREATMENT

Screening in primary care settings can accurately identify patients whose levels or patterns of alcohol consumption do not meet criteria for alcohol dependence, but place them at risk for increased morbidity and mortality. Brief behavioral counseling interventions with follow-up produce small to moderate reductions in alcohol consumption that are sustained over 6 to 12 months or longer (USPSTF, USPHS, 2000) (SOR: B).

References

The complete reference list is available online at www.expertconsult.com.

Web Resources

www.niaaa.nih.gov –
    National Institute for Alcoholism and Alcohol Abuse is a clearinghouse for information on alcohol use disorders and treatment resources and is part of the National Institutes of Health (NIH).
www.nida.nih.gov
    National Institute on Drug Abuse is a clearinghouse for substance used disorders and offers benefits for dually dependent and dual-use disorder populations and is part of NIH.

www.samhsa.gov
    Substance Abuse and Mental Health Services Administration has resources for mental health and substance abuse disorders.
www.csat.samhsa.gov
    Centers for Substance Abuse Treatment is part of SAMHSA and offers resources for Treatment Guidelines of practical use to clinicians, and treatment improvement protocols.
www.AA.org
    Alcoholics Anonymous.

CHAPTER 50

Nicotine Addiction

Robert E. Rakel and Thomas Houston

Chapter contents

Overview

Key Points

- Tobacco use is the leading cause of death in the United States.
- Toxins from cigarette smoke cause disease in most organs of the body.
- Smokers die an average of 13 or 14 years earlier than nonsmokers, and 50% of continuing smokers will die of a tobacco-related disease.
- Smoking is responsible for 40% of all deaths from cancer and 21% of deaths from cardiovascular disease.
- Almost 10% of deaths attributable to smoking occur in nonsmokers exposed to secondhand smoke.

The power of nicotine addiction became clear when I saw malnourished and hungry people trading food rations for cigarettes.

William Foege (1989), commenting on refugee camps during the Nigerian Civil War

Tobacco smoking leads to a dependence on nicotine that is indistinguishable from other forms of drug dependence. The revised fourth edition of the *Diagnostic and Statistical Manual of Mental Disorders* (DSM-IV-TR) of the American Psychiatric Association (APA, 2000) classifies tobacco dependence as an *addiction*. In such a dependency, the drug is needed to maintain an optimal state of well-being. *Nicotine*, the addictive constituent of tobacco, meets these criteria because a typical withdrawal syndrome occurs after smoking cessation, tolerance to its use develops, and most importantly, use persists

after developing symptoms attributable to the substance and in the face of its known harm. Some believe that nicotine is more addicting than cocaine or alcohol (Krasnegor, 1979; Lee and D'Alonzo, 1993; Kandel et al., 1997). However, a substantial fraction of daily smokers, perhaps as many as half, do not meet the DSM-IV criteria for nicotine dependence (Hughes et al., 2006; Donny and Dierker, 2007).

Nicotine acts on specific α4β2 nicotinic acetylcholine receptors in the mesocorticolimbic system, through neural pathways that are now seen as a common pathway for addictive drugs. Nicotine modulates the release of dopamine in the brain's reward centers in the ventral tegmental area and the nucleus accumbens, decreasing the normal rate of degradation of dopamine as well. High concentrations of nicotine are delivered to the central nervous system (CNS) within seconds of a puff during smoking, with complete saturation of nicotinic receptors with as few as three cigarettes, and lasting as long as 3 hours (Brody, 2006).

It may take only one cigarette to hook an adolescent. About one fourth of young people experience a *first-inhalation relaxation experience* (FIRE) with their first cigarette, a large percentage of whom become addicted (DiFranza et al., 2007).

For tobacco-dependent persons, craving results when nicotine occupancy on receptors declines over time (e.g., during sleep at night). Relief from craving requires that the smoker replenish the nicotine within the receptor as completely as possible, which is why the first cigarette of the morning is often the most "satisfying" to addicted smokers. Since the cigarette is the most efficient rapid-delivery device for nicotine and the concurrent relief of craving, physicians and patients need to understand that medicinal nicotine replacement products are quite inefficient, by comparison, delivering lower concentrations of nicotine and incompletely resolving cravings.

The sheer number of nicotine doses is also highly reinforcing. A typical one-pack-daily smoker receives about 100,000 reinforcing hits a year, much more than with cocaine or heroin (Brunton, 1999).

Tobacco contributes to about 443,000 deaths annually in the United States and has rightly been dubbed the "leading cause of death in the United States" (McGinnis and Foege, 1993; Mokdad et al., 2004). One third of these smoking-related deaths are from cardiovascular disease and cerebrovascular accident (CVA, stroke), 29% from lung cancer, 20% from chronic respiratory disease, and at least 8% from cancers other than lung (Fig. 50-1). Just over 10% of deaths attributable to smoking occur in nonsmokers exposed to secondhand smoke, most from cardiovascular causes (CDC, 2008). Each year, smoking is responsible for 18% of the total deaths in the United States—seven times more Americans than were killed in the Vietnam War. Smoking has killed more Americans during the 20th century than were killed in battle or died of war-related diseases in all U.S. wars ever fought (Pollin and Ravenholt, 1984). Furthermore, cigarettes kill more Americans than alcohol, car accidents, suicide, AIDS, homicide, and illegal drugs combined (ACS, 2005).

As shown by the grim, disease-specific facts, most smokers do not understand the implications for longevity involved in continued tobacco use. On the average, male smokers in the United States die 13.2 years earlier and females 14.5 years earlier than nonsmokers (Manson et al., 2000). Half of all continuing adult smokers will die of a cigarette-related illness (Doll et al., 2004). This relative lack of knowledge about tobacco harm may be in part because of the lack of publicity given to celebrities who die from smoking-related diseases (see **eTable 50-1**), although the death of news anchor Peter Jennings from lung cancer in 2005 received considerable attention and spurred increased interest in cessation.

The Centers for Disease Control and Prevention (CDC; 2009) estimated that in 2007, 19.8% of American adults smoked cigarettes (21.3% of men and 18.4% of women). Smoking prevalence is lowest among Asians (9.6%) and Hispanics (13.3%) and highest among American Indians and Alaska Natives (36.4%). Smoking prevalence is also higher among adults living below the poverty level (28.8%). Higher educational status confers additional protection against smoking, with persons holding a graduate degree smoking the least (6.2%). Thus, cigarette-related disease is increasingly becoming a set of afflictions suffered by the poor and undereducated, persons who understand the least about their risks and who have the poorest access to medical care resources (CDC, 2008).

In 2008, about one in five (20.4%) high school seniors smoked, the lowest level since monitoring started in the 1970s. Boys smoke more than girls in high school, (21.3% vs. 18.7%), and many more boys use smokeless tobacco (13.6% vs. 2.2%). The tobacco industry spends more than $12 billion annually on marketing (>$42 million/day) (Campaign for Tobacco-Free Kids, 2008).

Although few people start smoking as adults, each day 4000 children and adolescents try smoking for the first time, and 3000 of them become regular users of tobacco. Half of high school seniors who smoke started by age 14. Most smokers start smoking before 18, and only 5% start after age 20. Each year, 70% of those who smoke say that they would like to stop, and about 50% attempt to quit, but less than 5% succeed (Fiore et al., 2008). The likelihood of success in smoking cessation increases with the number of attempts, and those with a college education are twice as likely to succeed as less educated smokers. Family physicians must view tobacco addiction as a chronic disease that requires frequent intervention.

Health Risks Associated with Smoking

Toxins from cigarette smoke go everywhere the blood goes and cause disease in almost every organ of the body.

Cancer

Key Points

- A dose-response relationship exists between the number of cigarettes smoked and the risk of cancer. Those smoking more than one pack a day have 20 times the risk of nonsmokers.
- Smoking formerly labeled "low-tar" and "low-nicotine" cigarettes provides no benefit over smoking regular cigarettes.
- Less than half of all smoking deaths are from cancer; the rest are from heart disease, chronic lung disease, and stroke.
- Tobacco use increases the risk of cancer in most organs.

About 30% of all cancer deaths are attributable to cigarette smoking, with the evidence increasingly stronger. Box 50-1 lists diseases, including many cancers, for which the

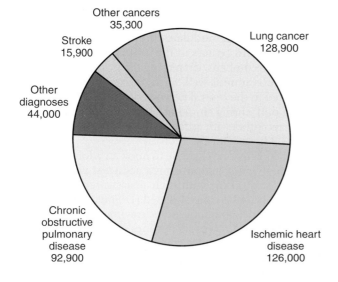

ABOUT 443,000 U.S. DEATHS ATTRIBUTABLE EACH YEAR TO CIGARETTE SMOKING*

Other cancers 35,300
Stroke 15,900
Lung cancer 128,900
Other diagnoses 44,000
Chronic obstructive pulmonary disease 92,900
Ischemic heart disease 126,000

* Average annual number of deaths, 2000—2004.

Figure 50-1 Deaths attributable each year to smoking. *(From CDC Office on Smoking and Health.* http://www.cdc.gov/tobacco/data_statistics/tables/index.htm.)

Box 50-1 Evidence-Based Relationship between Smoking and Disease

The evidence is sufficient to infer a causal relationship between smoking and:

Cancer of the bladder, cervix, esophagus, kidney, larynx, lung, oral cavity, pharynx, pancreas, stomach

Acute myeloid leukemia

Abdominal aortic aneurysm

Subclinical atherosclerosis

Stroke (cerebrovascular accident)

Coronary heart disease

Chronic obstructive pulmonary disease (COPD)

Acute respiratory infections, including pneumonia

Reduced lung function in infants

Impaired lung growth during childhood and adolescence

Respiratory symptoms in children and adolescents, including cough, phlegm, wheezing, and dyspnea

Asthma-related symptoms (e.g., wheezing) in childhood and adolescence

Premature onset of age-related decline in lung function

All respiratory symptoms among adults, including coughing, phlegm, wheezing, and dyspnea

Poor asthma control

Sudden infant death syndrome (SIDS)

Reduced fertility in women

Fetal growth restriction and low birth weight

Premature rupture of membranes, placenta previa, and placental abruption

Preterm delivery and shortened gestation

Cataracts

Increased absenteeism from work

Adverse surgical outcomes related to wound healing and respiratory complications

Hip fractures

Low bone density in postmenopausal women

Peptic ulcer disease

The evidence is suggestive of a causal relationship between smoking and:

Colorectal cancer

Liver cancer

Increased prostate cancer mortality

Acute respiratory infections in persons with COPD

Increased lower respiratory tract illnesses during infancy

Impaired lung function in childhood and adulthood (with maternal smoking)

Poorer prognosis for children and adolescents with asthma

Increased nonspecific bronchial hyperresponsiveness

Ectopic pregnancy

Spontaneous abortion

Cleft palate

Low bone density in older men

Dental caries

Erectile dysfunction

Macular degeneration

Graves' disease

From US Surgeon General. The Health Consequences of Smoking: a Report of the Surgeon General, 2004. Rockville, Md, US Department of Health and Human Services, Public Health Service, Office of the Surgeon General, 2004.

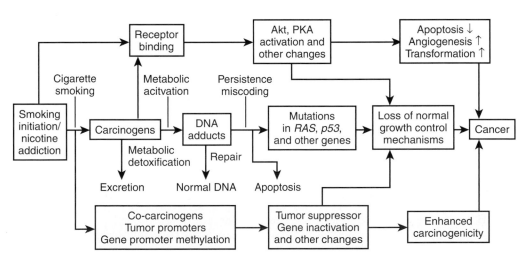

Figure 50-2 Mechanisms that contribute to tobacco-caused cancer. *(From American Chemical Society, for Stephen S. Hecht. Progress and Challenges in Selected Areas of Tobacco Carcinogenesis.)*

evidence is sufficient to *infer* a causal relationship, as well as those for which the evidence is sufficient only to *suggest* a causal relationship. Reviewing tobacco's role in carcinogenesis, Hecht (2008) discusses several mechanisms that contribute to cancer, including metabolic changes in DNA and formation of DNA-carcinogen adducts, leading to mutation; inhibition of genes such as *p53*, a tumor suppressor; and mutations in the *K-RAS* oncogene (Fig. 50-2).

Lung

A clear dose-response relationship exists between lung cancer risk and daily cigarette consumption. From 1950 to 1990, the U.S. mortality rate for lung cancer increased fourfold for men and sevenfold for women. Although the mortality rates in men have been declining since 1990, lung cancer is still the principal cause of cancer death for both genders.

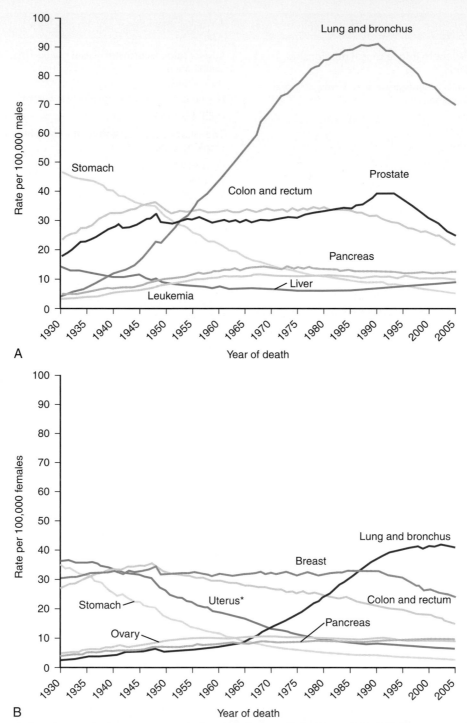

Figure 50-3 A, Annual age-adjusted cancer death rates among males for selected cancers, United States, 1930–2005 (rates are age-adjusted to the 2000 U.S. population). Because of changes in *International Classification of Disease* (ICD) coding, numerator information has changed over time. Rates for cancers of the lung and bronchus, colon and rectum, and liver are affected by these changes. **B,** Annual age-adjusted cancer death rates among females for selected cancers, United States, 1930–2005 (rates are age-adjusted to the 2000 U.S. standard population). *Uterus includes uterine cervix and uterine corpus. Because of changes in ICD coding, numerator information has changed over time. Rates for cancers of the uterus, ovary, lung and bronchus, and colon and rectum are affected by these changes. (**A** *from US mortality data, 1960 to 2005, US Mortality 1930–1959. National Cancer Institute, CDC, 2008. CA Cancer J Clin 59:233, 2009;* **B** *from US mortality data, 1960 to 2005, US Mortality 1930–1959, National Center for Health Statistics, CDC, 2008. CA Cancer J Clin 59:234, 2009.)*

In 1988, lung cancer passed breast cancer as the leading cause of death from cancer in women (Fig. 50-3). Although the lung cancer death rate has leveled off in U.S. women, in some states it is still increasing (Fig. 50-4).

Unfortunately, early detection does not improve the survival rate for lung cancer. The 5-year survival rate is only 15% and has improved only slightly since the early 1960s (ACS, 2005). Almost 60% of lung cancer patients die within a year and 85% within 5 years. By the time the diagnosis is made, three of four patients already have metastases. However, the risk of death from lung cancer is substantially reduced when smoking is discontinued. Reducing smoking from an average

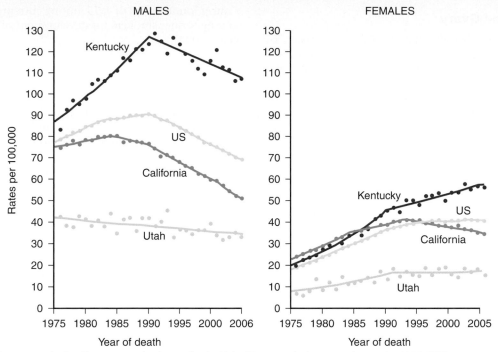

MALES   FEMALES

Figure 50-4 Trends in age-standardized lung cancer death rates for the United States and select states by gender, 1975–2005. *(From Cokkinides V et al. CA Cancer J Clin 59:357, 2009.)*

of 20 cigarettes a day to less than 10 per day reduces the lung cancer risk by 25% (Godtfredsen et al., 2005). A diminished risk for lung cancer is experienced in former smokers after 5 years of cessation; however, the risk remains higher than that of nonsmokers for as long as 15 to 20 years (US Surgeon General, 2004).

Although the amount of tar in cigarettes has declined in recent years, the risk of lung cancer has not changed. Smoking formerly labeled "low-tar" and "low-nicotine" cigarettes provides no benefit over smoking regular cigarettes, and the uptake of carcinogens is no different in "regular," "light," and "ultralight" smokers (Hecht et al., 2005), as previously marketed. However, surveys show that most people believed "light" cigarettes to be less dangerous than regular cigarettes and regular cigarettes much more likely to cause illness. The recent federal legislation banning the use of words such as "light" from tobacco advertising is beginning to dispel this myth.

Increasing data regarding the genetic predisposition to lung cancer are emerging (see Smoker's Genetics). Family aggregation related to lung cancer is likely multifactorial, including exposure to secondhand smoke, major genetic factors (e.g., chromosome 6p locus, *CYP1A1* gene), other genes that modify risk of lung cancer, and genes that may enhance nicotine addiction or modify nicotine metabolism (D'Amico, 2008; US Surgeon General, 2004).

Larynx

The risk for laryngeal cancer is 20 to 30 times greater in smokers. About 70% of oral and 85% of laryngeal cancer deaths are directly attributable to smoking. The risks of cancer of the oral cavity, pharynx, and larynx drop sharply during the first 10 years after smoking cessation. There appears to be a synergistic, multiplicative effect between smoking and drinking,

such that the risk for development of cancer of the larynx is as much as 75% higher in people who use tobacco and alcohol versus those exposed to either substance alone (US Surgeon General, 1990, 2004).

Esophagus

Cigarette smoking is a casual factor in both squamous cell carcinoma and adenocarcinoma of the esophagus. Heavy smokers (more than one pack per day) have 10 times the mortality from esophageal cancer as do nonsmokers.

Head and Neck

Cancers of the head and neck account for about 5% of all cancers diagnosed and 3% of cancer mortality each year. Tobacco use, whether smoking or chewing, is a key causal factor, with excess risks ranging from 5 to 25 times that of persons not using tobacco. Smoking accounts for 45% to 75% of all head and neck cancers (Freedman et al., 2007). The risks are dose dependent, and concurrent alcohol use multiplies the risks of developing head and neck cancer.

Pancreas

An equally dismal picture occurs with cancer of the pancreas, for which the 5-year survival rate is only 2%. Because of the nonspecific nature of the initial symptoms and the difficulty in making a diagnosis, the mean survival time after diagnosis of pancreatic cancer is less than 6 months. Smokers have two to three times the risk of pancreatic cancer as nonsmokers, and the risk is proportional to the amount smoked. Increased risk persists at least 10 years after quitting. More than one fourth of pancreatic cancer cases (27%) are attributable to cigarette smoking (Silverman et al., 1994; US Surgeon General, 2004).

Cervix Uteri and Ovary

Women who smoke cigarettes have four times the risk of cervical cancer as nonsmokers. Even women who smoke only 100 cigarettes during their lifetime more than double their risk of cervical cancer. The risk from smoking is greater in women younger than 30 than in those older than 30 (Slattery et al., 1989). Constituents from cigarette smoke, including mutagens and the carcinogen 4-(methylnitrosamino)-1-(3-pyridyl)-1-butanone (NNK), have been detected in the cervical mucus of smokers at levels 40 to 50 times those in serum. Smoking is a risk factor for cervical intraepithelial neoplasia (CIN) and cervical cancer among women who test positive as well as negative for human papillomavirus (HPV). The relative risks for CIN and cervical cancer are two to four times greater for current and former smokers compared with never-smokers (US Surgeon General, 2004). Although the risk of some types of ovarian cancer has been shown to be as much as three times greater in women who smoke cigarettes (Qian et al., 1989; Tworoger et al., 2008), the evidence is inadequate to confer a causal relationship (US Surgeon General, 2004).

Bladder and Kidney

Forty percent of bladder cancers are smoking-related, and higher rates of kidney cancers are also noted in smokers. Smokers have two to four times the risk of bladder cancer as those who never smoked. The risk for kidney cancer is strongly dose dependent. Even one to nine cigarettes per day creates a 60% excess risk of renal cell cancer in men, and the risk doubles for men smoking more than a pack a day. Overall, the relative risk (RR) for women smokers is about 1.38, and for men 1.54 (Hunt et al., 2005). Smoking accounts for most cancers of the renal pelvis and ureter in the United States (McLaughlin et al., 1996; US Surgeon General, 2004). The kidneys and bladder are the final common pathway for the concentration of toxic products of tobacco smoke and provide the longest direct exposure to carcinogens and radioactive substances, such as polonium 210, in tobacco smoke (Winters and DiFranza, 1982).

Colon and Rectum

A strong relationship has been noted between smoking and colorectal cancer, but the induction period is about 35 years. This lengthy induction would explain why it is just beginning to show up in women and indicates that efforts to prevent smoking among young people should be intensified (Giovannucci et al., 1994). The increased risk is about 20% higher for current smokers, and appears to be stronger for rectal cancer. Although the evidence is suggestive but not conclusive, a causal relationship would mean that about 12% of the colorectal cancer burden would be attributable to smoking (Tsoi et al., 2009; US Surgeon General, 2004).

Liver

Although the 2004 Surgeon General's Report concludes that the relationship between smoking and liver cancer is suggestive but not causal, a meta-analysis from the World Health Organization (WHO) International Agency for Research on Cancer found an RR of 1.55 among current smokers and 1.2 among former smokers for development of liver cancer (Lee et al., 2009).

Leukemia

Overall, smoking cigarettes increases a person's risk for leukemia by 30%. Mortality from leukemia is increased 50% in cigarette smokers (RR, 1.53), and the response is dose related. The risk is greatest for myeloid leukemia. The potent carcinogen *benzene*, a constituent of cigarette smoke, seems to be the major toxin responsible for leukemia among smokers. Approximately 14% of all cases of leukemia in the United States may be caused by cigarette smoking (Brownson et al., 1993).

Second Primary/Recurrent Cancers

Continued smoking interferes with both radiotherapy and chemotherapy used for cancer treatment. An increase in second primary tumors among continuing smokers is seen in lung (Lin et al., 2005) and head and neck cancer (Chuang et al., 2008). The emergence of contralateral breast cancer has also been linked to continued smoking among women (Li et al., 2009).

Chronic Obstructive Pulmonary Disease (COPD)

Key Points

- COPD is the leading cause of disability in the United States, and cigarette smoking is its main cause.
- The risk of COPD is directly proportional to the number of cigarettes smoked, but lung function improves with cessation of smoking, even after age 60.

Cigarette smoking is the main cause of COPD, which includes emphysema and chronic bronchitis. COPD is the fourth leading cause of death and the leading cause of disability in the United States. Women smokers are 13 times more likely to die from COPD, and male smokers have about a 12-fold increased risk (US Surgeon General, 2004). During their lifetime, smokers have about a 40% chance of developing chronic bronchitis. There may also be important racial differences, with African Americans, particularly females, having a higher risk than white smokers (Dransfield et al., 2006; Pelkonen, 2008). COPD among women is rising more quickly than among men, and since 2000, more women than men have died each year from COPD (CDC, 2008).

Changes in bronchi and the lung parenchyma are proportional to duration and intensity of smoking. Cigarette smoke inhibits ciliary activity of the bronchial epithelium and phagocytic activity of macrophages in the alveoli, resulting in decreased clearance of foreign material and bacteria from the lung, which leads to increased infection and tissue destruction. Smoking also releases inflammatory mediators, including oxidases and proteases, and inhibits pulmonary repair mechanisms. Even after age 60, smokers who quit have better pulmonary function than those who continue smoking. Lung function is inversely related to the number of cigarettes smoked over a lifetime. The rate of decline in pulmonary function is arrested by smoking cessation, the earlier the better.

Cardiovascular Disease

Key Points

- The risk of myocardial infarction is proportional to the number of cigarettes smoked.
- More than half of deaths from coronary artery disease are sudden, but the risk of sudden death is reduced immediately on cessation of smoking.
- Filter cigarettes and those with "low tar" or "low nicotine" do not reduce the risk of myocardial infarction.

Coronary Heart Disease

Heart disease is the leading cause of death in the United States, and tobacco use is a major risk factor. Up to 30% of all deaths from heart disease are caused by smoking, with a strong dose-dependent relationship. In general, smokers have two to four times the risk of coronary heart disease as nonsmokers. For women smokers, the risk may be even higher. Women who smoke only one to five cigarettes a day have 2.5 times the risk of developing coronary heart disease as nonsmokers, rising to 75 times the risk in those who smoke 40 or more cigarettes a day. Three fourths of myocardial infarctions in women younger than 50 have been attributed to smoking (Dunn et al., 1999; Slone et al., 1978). Women who smoke and use oral contraceptives (OCs) have up to 10 times greater risk of heart attack than women who do neither, depending on which generation of OC is used.

Smoking acutely raises systolic blood pressure, heart rate, and cardiac output and causes vasoconstriction. It increases inflammation, promotes thrombosis and platelet aggregation, increases atherogenesis and plaque destabilization, and promotes oxidation of low-density lipoproteins (LDLs). Both active and secondhand smoke exposure cause endothelial dysfunction, a key element in early atherogenesis. Increased levels of C-reactive protein (CRP) are found in smokers, and the low-grade inflammatory response associated with smoking also results in increased leukocyte counts. Increased blood viscosity and lower oxygen-carrying capacity from carbon monoxide (CO) in cigarette smoke further decrease the coronary reserve. CO has an affinity for hemoglobin (forming carboxyhemoglobin) that is 245 times stronger than that of oxygen. Thus, CO reduces oxygen delivery to the myocardium and has a decidedly negative inotropic effect. Carboxyhemoglobin also lowers the threshold for ventricular fibrillation and could help explain the higher incidence of sudden death in those who smoke.

More than half of all deaths from coronary heart disease are sudden deaths caused by cardiac arrhythmia. Nicotine is arrhythmogenic, because it increases serum catecholamine concentration. Those who quit smoking reduce their risk of sudden death immediately; the decline is not time dependent (Goldenberg et al., 2003).

The risk of myocardial infarction (MI) is proportional to the number of cigarettes smoked, but as few as one to four cigarettes a day raises the risk of dying from ischemic heart disease by 2.7 times in men and 2.9 times in women (Bjartveit and Tverdal, 2005). The risk of MI increases progressively to as much as 20-fold in persons smoking 35 or more cigarettes per day. Persons who smoke cigarettes containing "low" amounts of nicotine have the same degree of MI risk as those who smoke cigarettes containing larger amounts. Smokers of these "low-dose" cigarettes still have three times the MI risk as nonsmokers (Kaufman et al., 1983). Within a few years of stopping, the risk of MI decreases to a level similar to that in men who have never smoked, even in heavy smokers who have a positive family history of coronary heart disease (Rosenberg et al., 1985). The risk of coronary heart disease is reduced by about half after the first year of cessation, falling to that of never-smokers after 15 years of abstinence (US Surgeon General, 1990). Those who have coronary heart disease and stop smoking have a reduction of about 36% in both all-cause mortality and nonfatal MI (Crichley and Capewell, 2004). Women who follow lifestyle guidelines involving diet, exercise, and not smoking have a very low risk of coronary heart disease (Stampfer et al., 2000).

"Silent" ischemia probably accounts for most cardiac ischemic events. Patients with coronary heart disease who smoke have three times as many episodes of silent ischemia as nonsmokers, and the duration of each is 12 times longer (Barry et al., 1989). Frequent episodes of myocardial ischemia, even though asymptomatic, must damage the heart. Because smoking also increases platelet adhesiveness, increases levels of triglycerides and LDL cholesterol, and lowers high-density lipoprotein cholesterol, a higher incidence of MI would be expected (Chelland et al., 2008).

Benefits from stopping smoking can be demonstrated at all ages. No decrease in benefit is seen with age, so it is still worthwhile for someone older than 65 to break the addiction (Hermanson et al., 1988; LaCroix et al., 1991). This benefit can be demonstrated in the cerebral as well as the coronary circulation. Older adults who stop smoking have significantly higher cerebral perfusion levels than those who continue to smoke. Even those who have smoked for 30 to 40 years have improved cerebral circulation within a relatively short time after stopping smoking (Rogers et al., 1985).

Stroke (Cerebrovascular Accident)

Key Points

- Risk of stroke is six times greater in smokers (>1 pack/day).
- Smokers who are also hypertensive have a 20 times greater stroke risk.
- Risk of CVA declines rapidly after smoking cessation, and at 5 years is the same as for a nonsmoker.

Stroke (CVA) is the third most common cause of death in the United States. Although hypertension is the greatest risk factor for stroke, cigarette smoking is also significant. The incidence of stroke in smokers is two to four times higher than in nonsmokers. Among those screened in the Multiple Risk Factor Intervention Trial (MRFIT), smokers had twice the risk of a nonhemorrhagic stroke, and smoking was strongly associated with all forms of stroke (Neaton et al., 1993).

The risk of stroke increases in proportion to the amount of smoking. Those who smoke more than 40 cigarettes/day have twice the stroke risk of those who smoke less than 10 cigarettes/day. Compared with women who have never smoked, the risk of stroke increases 2.2-fold in women smoking 1 to 14 cigarettes/day and 3.7-fold in women smoking 25 or more cigarettes/day (Colditz et al., 1988). Noting a clear dose-response relationship, Bonita and associates (1986) found a threefold increase in the risk of stroke in smokers versus nonsmokers (see **eFig. 50-1** online). The risk is 5.6 times higher in persons smoking more than one pack daily. Cigarette smokers who are also hypertensive have a 20-fold increased risk of stroke (US Surgeon General, 2004).

Sclerosis of the carotid arteries is directly proportional to the amount of smoke exposure. Smoking increases the risk of ischemic heart disease and cerebrovascular disease regardless of the level of serum cholesterol. Low cholesterol level did not protect against smoking-related arteriosclerotic cardiovascular disease in patients in South Korea, where the prevalence of smoking is among the highest in the world (72% of men) (Jee et al., 1999). Smoking may increase the likelihood of thrombosis by increasing serum fibrinogen, enhancing platelet aggregation, and increasing blood viscosity.

The risk of stroke declines rapidly after cessation of smoking. After 5 years, risk of CVA is at the level of nonsmokers, which emphasizes that "it is never too late to quit," no matter how long the patient has been smoking.

Subarachnoid Hemorrhage

A recent systematic review of the risk factors for subarachnoid hemorrhage (SAH) shows that smoking doubles the risk for SAH (Feigin et al., 2005). About one third of all SAH was found to be attributable to smoking in a smaller case-control study, and, although the risk dropped within a few years after quitting, it may remain increased for up to 15 years in the heaviest women smokers (Anderson et al., 2004).

Older studies involving high-dose estrogen OCs showed a significant interaction with smoking, increasing the risk for stroke and SAH among women who both smoked and used OCs. Studies of women who use second and third-generation OCs find no increased risk of stroke, even among smokers (Yang et al., 2009). However, the American College of Obstetricians and Gynecologists states that "practitioners should prescribe combination hormonal contraceptives with caution, if at all, to women older than 35 years who smoke" (ACOG, 2006).

Peripheral Vascular Disease

Smoking is strongly associated with other forms of cardiovascular disease, including abdominal aortic aneurysm (AAA) and peripheral vascular disease in both men and women. Smoking causes as much as half of all peripheral artery disease, and significantly increases the failure rates after lower-limb bypass surgery. The risk of AAA rises in proportion to duration and intensity of smoking and is up to sevenfold greater at 20 pack-years (US Surgeon General, 2004). The U.S. Preventive Services Task Force (USPSTF) has recommended one-time screening for AAA by ultrasonography in men age 65 to 75 who have ever smoked. Consideration should also be given for screening women over age 65 with a history of smoking (Derubertis et al., 2007), because about 40% of the annual deaths from AAA occur among women, in whom the disease is more deadly than men. Smoking is also an independent risk factor for erectile dysfunction, an additional fact that may help motivate men to stop smoking.

Other Diseases and Conditions

Alzheimer's Disease

Studies show conflicting evidence linking smoking with Alzheimer's dementia and other causes of cognitive decline. However, a meta-analysis found that compared with never-smokers, current smokers had RRs of 1.79 for Alzheimer's disease (AD) and 1.78 for vascular dementia. Smokers in this study also had greater yearly declines in Mini–Mental State Examination (Anstev et al., 2007). Another systematic review and meta-analysis also found significant risk for AD among smokers (RR, 1.59) but less risk for developing vascular dementia (1.35) and cognitive decline (1.20) compared with never-smokers (Peters et al., 2008).

Graves' Disease

Smoking appears to be one of the many factors causing Graves' disease, particularly among women, and includes a higher risk of Graves' ophthalmopathy as well (Vestergaard, 2002).

Diabetes Mellitus

Diabetes is a rapidly growing worldwide pandemic, and cigarette smoking is responsible for about 10% of the incidence of type 2 diabetes. A dose-response relationship exists, with the risk increasing in direct proportion to the number of cigarettes smoked. People who smoke more than one pack a day have about double the risk for diabetes as nonsmokers, and the risk is still 1.5 times greater for those who smoke only 1 to 14 cigarettes a day (Manson et al., 2000; Willi et al., 2007). Smoking increases the risk for development of the metabolic syndrome and its attendant cardiovascular consequences (Chiolero et al., 2008).

Patients with diabetes who smoke are at increased risk for both micro- and macrovascular complications. Cigarette smoking increases the risk for diabetic nephropathy, retinopathy, and neuropathy. This association is strongest in patients requiring insulin for control. Smoking cessation is essential for preventing diabetic complications.

Depression

Smokers are more likely to experience major depression than nonsmokers, and the incidence increases steadily with the number of cigarettes smoked. This increased risk may result from genes that predispose to both conditions (Kendler et al., 1993). Smoking may predispose to depression and, conversely, may be an antecedent to smoking, in the adolescent population (Brook et al., 2004; Goodman and Capitman, 2000).

Wrinkles

We are not very effective in getting the message about tobacco's hazards across to adolescents. By talking about disease, we may not be speaking their language. The fact that smoking causes wrinkles, bad breath, and yellow teeth may be a more effective message than evidence that smoking kills. Premature wrinkling (crow's feet) increases with the number of cigarettes smoked; heavy smokers are five times more likely to have wrinkles than nonsmokers (Kadunce et al., 1991).

Macular Degeneration and Cataract

Macular degeneration is the leading cause of blindness after age 65, and nothing prevents or delays its progression. Smoking 20 or more cigarettes a day increases the risk of macular degeneration two- to threefold. As with other smoking-related disorders, macular degeneration also appears to be dose related, with the incidence increasing with the number of pack-years (Christen et al., 1996; Thornton et al., 2005). Smoking is also a cause of nuclear cataract, with smokers having two to three times the risk of never-smokers.

The Myth of Filtered Cigarettes

There is a mistaken popular belief that filtered brands of cigarettes, which now account for more than 97% of those sold in the United States, are safer than nonfiltered cigarettes and that formerly labeled "light" cigarettes convey a degree of health protection. "Low-tar" and "low-nicotine" filtered cigarettes are now the most commonly purchased products. Because the addiction is to nicotine, people who smoke low-nicotine cigarettes undergo "compensatory smoking," in which they inhale more frequently and more deeply to maintain their blood nicotine levels. As a result, tar intake increases, so the cigarette changes from the low-tar to the high-tar category. Smokers who take 14 puffs per cigarette inhale 58% more tar than those taking the standard 8.7 puffs per cigarette. Most manufacturers create tiny perforations in the filter to dilute the smoke with air, thus creating their "light" and "ultralight" cigarettes. Many smokers, however, block the holes with their lips or their fingers to obtain undiluted smoke with a higher concentration of nicotine (Kozlowski et al., 1980).

Cigarettes with reduced yields of nicotine and CO are not safer. The fourfold increased risk of MI does not vary according to the nicotine content. The degree of risk is proportional to the number of cigarettes smoked (Palmer et al., 1989). Similar myths about "natural" and "organic" cigarettes should be dispelled, since there is absolutely no evidence that these tobacco products confer any health protection compared with other brands.

Cigars

Key Points

- Cigars are not a safe alternative to cigarettes, causing both cancer and heart disease.
- Cigar-related health risks are related to number smoked and depth of inhalation.
- Risk of tobacco-related disease is increased when smoking is combined with alcohol consumption.

In 2004 the CDC estimated that about 9.4% of men, 1.9% of women, and 14.8% of students grades 8 to 12 were current cigar smokers. The mortality patterns from cigar smoking relate in part to the degree of inhalation by the smoker. Primary cigar smokers, or those who have never or rarely smoked cigarettes, inhale much less than secondary cigar smokers—those who have switched from or are concurrent cigarette smokers. The main reason for the difference is the pH of the smoke, which in cigars is higher than in cigarettes, allowing nicotine to be absorbed across the oral mucosa. Secondary cigar smokers, however, have learned to inhale smoke, and increase their risk of cancer and heart disease.

Cigar smokers have a risk of oral and pharyngeal cancer that is similar to cigarette smokers; their risk of esophageal cancer is several times that of never-smokers. As with cigarette smoking, the use of alcohol multiplies the risk of these cancers, accounting for about 75% of cases in developed nations (Pelucci et al., 2008).

Lung cancer risk varies with depth of inhalation and number of cigars per day. Primary cigar smokers with no or slight inhalation have about a 1.8 mortality ratio of lung cancer; moderate-deep inhalers increase this to 4.9, with an overall mortality ratio of 2.11 compared with nonsmokers. Secondary cigar smokers have a mortality ratio of 5.4; moderate-deep inhalers in this group increase the risk to 9.77. Combined cigarette-cigar smokers have an overall lung cancer mortality ratio of 11.20 (NCI, 1998).

Cigar smokers are also at higher risk for both COPD (RR, 1.45) and coronary artery disease (RR, 1.27) compared with nonsmokers (Iribarren et al., 1999). As with the cancer risk, the level of inhalation increases risk; for example, secondary cigar smokers with moderate-deep inhalation patterns have a fivefold increased risk for COPD (NCI, 1998).

Electronic Cigarettes

Electronic cigarettes (e-cigarettes), first developed in China in 2003, consist of a metal tube resembling a normal cigarette, a battery, an atomizer, and a replaceable cartridge containing liquid nicotine, propylene glycol, and flavoring. Examples of flavorings are chocolate, cherry, and bubblegum, all of which can be enticing to children. When a user puffs on the e-cigarette, an indicator light at the tip glows and the heating element vaporizes the solution from the cartridge containing nicotine and other substances. A mist is produced that is similar to cigarette smoke and contains the propylene glycol, a known pulmonary irritant used in antifreeze.

To date there are no published clinical trials and there is no quality control to limit the amounts of chemicals in e-cigarettes, including known carcinogens. The sale of electronic cigarettes containing nicotine is illegal in Australia. In the United States the American Cancer Society (ACS) and other professional organizations have called for e-cigarettes to be illegal. The U.S. Food and Drug Administration (FDA) has not approved these devices and has halted shipments of them from entering the country, but Internet sales are growing.

In 2009 the U.S. Congress granted the FDA the power to regulate tobacco products, including the authority to stop e-cigarettes from entering the country. Electronic cigarettes, even though smokeless, may contain known carcinogens and toxic chemicals. There is considerable debate as to whether these products might deliver nicotine with minimal additional harm to the smoker, becoming a "harm reduction" instrument that enables smokers to continue their nicotine dependence and reduce risk or enhance quit attempts. On the other hand, these products have little quality control; nicotine delivery is inconsistent; FDA-type testing has not yet been done; and long-term risks are not known.

Smokeless Tobacco

Key Points

- Snuff users have a 50-fold increased risk of cancer of the cheek and gum.
- The carcinogens in smokeless tobacco have a greater concentration than in cigarette tobacco; the level of nitrosamines is more than 10,000 times that allowed in bacon and beer.

Smokeless tobacco comes in two types: *snuff,* which is dry or moist, and *chewing* (spitting) tobacco, which comes as a loose leaf, plug, or twist. Smokeless tobacco contains many of the same carcinogens as cigarette tobacco, but some are present in much greater concentrations. *Nitrosamines,* which are powerful chemical carcinogens, are present at levels up to 14,000 times higher than the federal government allows in bacon and beer (Connolly et al., 1986).

A variation on smokeless tobacco is called *snus,* which contains powdered, flavored tobacco in small satchets placed under the lip, releasing nicotine through the buccal mucosa. Because of differences in manufacturing, snus has comparatively small levels of the carcinogenic compounds found in traditional smokeless products. No spitting is required. Snus marketing campaigns emphasize its use when smoking is not allowed, and most U.S. snus users also smoke cigarettes. In Sweden, snus use has eclipsed smoking, and many smokers have used snus to quit smoking but have continued using snus, and many appear to be dependent. Again, in the United States, this has sparked a fierce debate about the use of snus and similar products as agents for "harm reduction," and whether smokers should be advised to switch as a means of smoking cessation, since exclusive smokeless tobacco use avoids many of the dangers of combustible tobacco.

Treatment of smokeless tobacco use is difficult, because none of the standard medications used for smoking cessation has shown effectiveness for smokeless tobacco users, although behavioral counseling has a modest effect (Fiore et al., 2008). The nicotine patch and lozenge have been suggested, and clinical trials of combination therapy are ongoing. Behavioral interventions such as mailings, oral or dental screenings, group discussions, workplace interventions, and telephone support showed the best evidence for smokeless tobacco cessation (SOR: B). There was no benefit from the use of bupropion SR or nicotine patches or gum (Cayley, 2009; SOR: A).

Use of smokeless tobacco increases the frequency of oropharyngeal cancer and causes gum recession and tooth loss. Overall, the RR for oral cancer among snuff users is 2.6; for esophageal and pancreatic cancer, 1.6 (Boffetta et al., 2008). Leukoplakia is found in 18% to 64% of users (Connolly et al., 1986). Snus has been associated with a higher risk of oropharyngeal cancer in some studies (Roosar et al., 2008), but not others (Luo et al., 2007), and also has a small risk of pancreatic cancer. A systematic review and meta-analysis of the risk for myocardial infarction and stroke among current smokeless tobacco users found small increases in relative risk for these conditions (Boffetta and Straif, 2009).

Although educational programs have been launched by the National Cancer Institute and Major League Baseball, smokeless tobacco use has trended upward in adolescents. College athletes often believe that male peers, coaches, and professional athletes are indifferent to the use of spitting tobacco (Hilton et al., 1994). An estimated 8.6% of high school students are current smokeless tobacco users. Smokeless tobacco is more common among high school boys (14%) than girls (2.2%). As with college students, many high school spit tobacco users participate in organized sports. Enlisting the support of coaches to help with tobacco use prevention is an untapped resource that should be explored.

Involuntary (Passive) Smoking

Key Points

- Secondhand smoke contains 4000 different chemicals, of which more than 60 are carcinogenic.
- About one third of lung cancers occur in nonsmokers who live with a smoker or work in a smoky environment.
- Passive smoking is the third leading preventable cause of death, after alcohol and smoking itself.
- Passive smoking increases the risk of SIDS in infants and otitis media, cancer, and respiratory disease in older children, in direct proportion to smoke exposure.

Secondhand smoke, also called *environmental tobacco smoke* (ETS), is the combination of smoke emitted from the burning end of a cigarette, cigar, or pipe and the smoke exhaled by a smoker. Two thirds of the smoke from a burning cigarette never reaches a smoker's lungs, but instead goes directly into the air. *Sidestream smoke* is emitted into the air from a smoldering cigarette or cigar between puffs, and *mainstream smoke* is what the smoker inhales directly—the exhaled smoke also contributes to ETS. Although diluted by air before being inhaled, sidestream smoke contains greater concentrations of toxic substances than mainstream smoke because of a lower combustion temperature and lack of filtration through the cigarette.

The 2006 Report of the Surgeon General, *The Health Consequences of Involuntary Exposure to Tobacco Smoke* (USHHS, 2006), concludes the following:
1. Secondhand smoke causes premature death and disease in children and adults who do not smoke.
2. Children exposed to secondhand smoke are at increased risk for sudden infant death syndrome (SIDS), acute respiratory infections, ear problems, and more severe asthma. Smoking by parents causes respiratory symptoms and slows lung growth in their children.
3. Exposure of adults to secondhand smoke has immediate adverse effects on the cardiovascular system and causes coronary heart disease and lung cancer.
4. The scientific evidence indicates that there is no risk-free level of exposure to secondhand smoke.
5. Eliminating smoking in indoor spaces fully protects nonsmokers from exposure to secondhand smoke. Separating smokers from nonsmokers, cleaning the air, and ventilating buildings cannot eliminate exposures of nonsmokers to secondhand smoke.

Tobacco smoke contains more than 4000 different chemicals, at least 60 of which are known carcinogens (National Toxicology Program, 2005). The U.S. Environmental Protection Agency, (EPA) the National Toxicology Program, the U.S. Surgeon General, and the International Agency for Research on Cancer have determined that environmental tobacco smoke is a class A (known) human carcinogen, in the same class as asbestos, mustard gas, arsenic, and benzene. In addition to the 3000 lung cancer deaths a year in nonsmokers, almost 40,000 heart disease deaths each year are linked to secondhand smoke. Secondhand smoke exposure also causes chronic otitis media, cough, and lower respiratory illnesses in children, such as asthma, bronchitis, and pneumonia. It is estimated that tobacco smoke in the home and workplace could be responsible for the deaths of about 50,000 nonsmokers annually in the United States, making passive smoking the third leading preventable cause of death, after those from direct smoking and alcohol (Air Resources Board, 2005).

In a classic study, Hirayama (1981) was among the first scientists to demonstrate an increased risk of lung cancer in nonsmoking housewives exposed to the secondhand cigarette smoke of their husbands (see eFig. 50-2 online). Since then, many studies have shown an association between being married to a smoker and having an increased risk of lung cancer. Overall risk of lung cancer increases 20% to 30% in nonsmokers exposed to ETS in the home; combined home and work exposure further increases the risk (USDHHS [Report of the Surgeon General], 2006).

A report from the California EPA's Air Resources Board is another well-researched review of the health effects of passive smoking. Their meta-analyses of the breast cancer risk indicate that the RR for breast cancer, particularly among premenopausal women, is between 1.68 and 2.20 (Air Resources Board, 2005; Miller et al., 2006). A 2009 Canadian task force report found a causal link between passive smoke exposure and breast cancer, especially in younger, premenopausal women, and a causal relationship between active smoking and breast cancer at all ages (Johnson et al., 2011).

It is estimated that the risk of MI is up to 70% greater for a woman whose husband smokes (Wells, 1994). Relative risk estimates from meta-analysis indicate a 25% to 30% increase in the risk for coronary heart disease in exposed nonsmokers; as with lung cancer, multiple sites of exposure increase the risk (USDHHS [Report of the Surgeon General], 2006). The cardiovascular effects of even brief exposure to secondhand smoke are often nearly as great as those of direct smoking, with platelet aggregation and arterial endothelial damage occurring within 30 minutes of exposure; furthermore, secondhand smoke induces oxidative stress and promotes vascular inflammation (Barnoya and Glantz, 2005). Exposure to secondhand smoke is associated with increased levels of inflammatory markers related to the development of atherosclerosis. People exposed have higher white blood cell counts and elevated CRP levels, oxidized LDL cholesterol, homocysteine, and fibrinogen. Even occasional exposure results in elevated levels. These increases are similar to those seen in active smokers.

Reports show that the health benefits of banning smoking in public places and the workplace include a reduction in heart attacks. Examination of community MI rates after implementation of strong smoke-free legislation found a pooled random-effects estimate of the rate of acute MI hospitalization 12 months later to be 0.83 (95% CI, 0.80-0.87), with growth of this benefit expected over time (Lightwood and Glantz, 2009). With similar findings, systematic review and meta-analysis of 10 locations with smoke-free legislation concluded that the acute MI risk decreased by 17% overall,

with the greatest effect in younger individuals and nonsmokers (Meyers et al., 2009).

Secondhand Smoke: Effects on Children

Over 50% of children younger than 5 years of age live in homes with at least one adult smoker. Children of smoking parents have more bronchitis and pneumonia during their first year of life and more otitis media when older. They have increased incidence of cough, bronchitis, and pneumonia proportional to the number of cigarettes smoked by the parents, particularly the mother. In fact, children of parents who smoke at least a half-pack a day have almost twice the risk of hospitalization for a respiratory illness. Secondhand smoke causes new-onset asthma in exposed children, and young persons with asthma have more asthma episodes (Charlton, 1994; Rantakallio, 1978; USHHS [Report of the Surgeon General], 2006).

Passive smoking also increases the risk of sudden infant death syndrome. Infants exposed to secondhand smoke have twice the risk of SIDS, and infants whose mothers smoke before and after birth are three to four times more likely to die from SIDS (US Surgeon General, 2004, 2006).

Small children are victimized more by passive smoking than adults. Because of their more rapid breathing, children inhale larger amounts of harmful substances. Children exposed to their parents' cigarette smoke have six times the average number of respiratory infections. They also have deficits in growth and in intellectual and emotional development, as well as more behavior disorders, such as hyperactivity.

Physicians and health care providers who care for children should advise parents to quit smoking to limit their children's exposure to secondhand smoke, and advocate for smoke-free indoor air both at home and in cars when children are passengers, since these two locations account for the majority of childhood exposure to secondhand smoke.

Thirdhand Smoke

Thirdhand smoke occurs when cigarette smoke reacts with nitrous acid on surfaces to form *tobacco-specific nitrosamines* (TSNAs). Nitrous acid is a common indoor pollutant and, when combined with cigarette smoke, forms a carcinogen that becomes more potent over time. Thus, nicotine is converted to a dangerous carcinogen after it is absorbed on indoor surfaces in automobiles and furniture. This can be especially hazardous to infants and children who live close to the floor because the TSNAs are especially concentrated in dust and carpeting. Smokers believed that smoking only when others were not present (e.g., in car or home) created no risk to the nonsmoker who arrives later. In fact, the smoke clings to upholstery, cotton, and carpeting and actually builds up over time, exposing the nonsmoker to potent carcinogens. This thirdhand smoke can be especially dangerous because TSNAs cannot be simply inactivated by dry cleaning or washing with soap and water. Most soaps are alkaline and cleansers that dissolve nicotine must be acidic. Thus, it is almost impossible to remove TSNAs from carpeting, which will continuously uptake nicotine. Even washing smooth stone and metal with an alkaline soap will not remove nicotine residue (Dreyfuss, 2010; Sleiman et al., 2010).

Pregnancy

See the discussion online at www.expertconsult.com.

Key Points

- The more a pregnant woman smokes, the greater the risk of premature delivery and low-birth-weight infants, unless she stops smoking by the fourth month of gestation.
- Smoking during pregnancy increases the risk of congenital abnormalities, mental retardation, learning problems, and attention-deficit/hyperactivity disorder (ADHD).
- The risk is increased for spontaneous abortion, placenta previa, and premature rupture of membranes.
- Reduced fertility is proportional to the number of cigarettes smoked.

KEY TREATMENT

Because of the serious risks of smoking to the pregnant smoker and the fetus, whenever possible pregnant smokers should be offered person-to-person psychosocial interventions that exceed minimal advice to quit (Fiore et al., 2008) (SOR: A).

Although abstinence early in pregnancy will produce the greatest benefits to the fetus and expectant mother, quitting at any point in pregnancy can yield benefits. Therefore, physicians should offer effective tobacco-dependence interventions to pregnant smokers at the first prenatal visit and throughout pregnancy (Fiore et al., 2008) (SOR: B).

Smoking and Mental Health

Mental illness and substance abuse puts patients at particular risk for dying of tobacco-related illness because they are more likely to smoke, and smoke more heavily, than others in the population. Patients with psychiatric illness consume up to 70% of the cigarettes smoked in the United States, with two to four times the general prevalence of smoking (Grant et al., 2004; Kalman et al., 2005). Among mentally ill and substance-abusing patients, as many as 200,000 die each year from tobacco-related causes—almost half the total U.S. tobacco-related mortality (Williams et al., 2004). Individuals in this special population of smokers do express strong interest in quitting smoking, however. Counseling and pharmacology that is useful with other smokers is effective in mentally ill and substance-abusing patients who smoke (Ranney et al., 2006), and just as with other smokers, this part of their health care must not be neglected.

Social and Legal Action

See online text for discussion.

Smoking Cessation

Key Points

- Patients who smoke should receive advice and encouragement to stop at every visit.
- Take advantage of the teachable moment, when a patient who smokes is being treated for any medical condition.
- Multiple strategies and persistence are usually needed for successful cessation because tobacco dependence is a chronic disease.
- Brief counseling, usually lasting less than 3 minutes, is an effective way to begin intervention.

Family physicians are in a unique position to assist their patients in smoking cessation. Because 7 of every 10 smokers visit their physician at least once a year, this is a golden opportunity that should not be missed. Among smokers, 70% want to quit and about 40% make an attempt each year, but less than 5% succeed. Even brief physician advice can double the quit rate (Fiore et al., 2008). Of those who try to quit on their own and do not use recommended cessation methods, most relapse within 8 days (CDC, 2008).

A survey by the Association of American Medical Colleges (AAMC, 2007) about physician behavior related to smoking cessation is summarized as follows:

> *Most physicians consistently ask patients who smoke about their smoking status and advise them to stop (86%), but only 13% say they usually refer smokers to others for appropriate treatment and only 17% say they usually arrange for follow-up visits to address smoking. Only 31% "usually" advised use of nicotine replacement therapy, and 25% "usually" prescribed other medication for cessation. Only 7% regularly referred patients to a quit line.*

Physicians regard current smoking cessation tools as inadequate, citing the following:
- Insufficient services, resources, and organizational support
- Interventions that have only limited effectiveness
- Limited education and training for physicians on addressing tobacco use and cessation interventions

The five factors cited most often by physicians as significant barriers to successful interventions are lack of patient motivation (63%), limited coverage for interventions (54%), limited reimbursement for a physician's time (52%), time with patients is limited (41%), and too few available cessation programs (39%).

Patients should be asked about tobacco use at every visit because repeated screening increases rates of clinical intervention. Tobacco users should be advised to quit at every visit (SOR A), because there is a dose-response relationship between the number of contacts and abstinence. Tobacco use screening coupled with brief advice is one of the top-three clinical prevention measures and is cost-effective as well (Maciosek et al., 2006). Tobacco-cessation treatment may include a variety of components: counseling for behavior change in both individual and group settings, such as motivational interviewing and problem solving/skills training; use of evidence-based pharmacotherapy; and proactive telephone quit line counseling (Fiore et al., 2008; USPSTF, 2009). Patients should receive at least minimal advice and encouragement at every visit based on the five "As" approach (Box 50-2). The American Academy of Family Physicians (2005) has a campaign to encourage its members to engage themselves in smoking cessation interventions. Using two As, "Ask and Act," the AAFP program emphasizes brief counseling and effective follow-up.

Box 50-2 Five As for Tobacco Users Willing to Quit

Ask about tobacco use at every visit.
Advise to quit through clear personalized messages.
Assess willingness to quit.
Assist efforts to quit.
Arrange follow-up and support.

As part of taking the history from a patient who smokes, clinicians should ask the following three questions to assess the patient's degree of nicotine addiction:

1. How much do you smoke? (How many cigarettes or cans of "dip" per day, for how many years?)
2. When do you smoke the first cigarette of the day?
3. How long is the period between cigarettes before craving another smoke?

Patients who smoke more than 20 cigarettes a day, who light their first cigarette within 30 minutes of waking, and who have cravings within 1 hour of the most recent cigarette are likely to have significant physiologic addiction to nicotine. Smoking fewer than 10 cigarettes a day suggests less addictive behavior, and a few patients report that they smoke only during social situations and only 5 to 10 cigarettes a week. Determining the patient's pattern of smoking will provide clues into the level of addiction.

Office spirometry to obtain a forced expiratory volume in 1 second (FEV_1) can also be useful in motivating smokers to quit. Comparing the smoker's "lung age" to the age of a healthy individual who has the same FEV_1, then showing the smoker a graphic display (Fig. 50-5, *A*), more than doubled the rate of quitting smoking after 12 months (13.6% vs. 6.4%) (Parkes et al., 2008). For example, a 52-year-old smoker with a 20-pack-year history (1 pack/day for 20 years) may have the lung age of a 75-year-old. Probable age at disability and death if the person continues smoking or stops smoking can be shown (Fig. 50-5, *B*). Such a visual presentation is often effective in achieving cessation even if smokers have a normal lung age because they may think it is not too late for them to quit.

Stages of Change

Patients who begin any major behavioral or lifestyle change go through successive stages in the process, as follows:

Precontemplation: Patient is not interested in quitting smoking in the near future (within 6 months).
Contemplation: Patient is thinking about quitting within the next few months, but has taken no action.
Preparation: Patient is planning to quit in the next 30 days.
Action: Patient is in the process of quitting, or has quit during the last 6 months.
Maintenance: Patient has abstained for more than 3 months.

Family physicians should emphasize progression through the process of change to facilitate the patient's efforts to stop smoking. When a patient reaches the preparation stage, the physician can play a major role in motivating the patient, including counseling and routine use of pharmacotherapy. However, recent research indicates that many smokers do not go through sequential stages and are often successful in quitting during spontaneous, unplanned attempts, perhaps sparked by an illness or by policy changes such as price increases or clean indoor air laws. Physicians' continued

support and encouragement may help increase the frequency and success of these efforts (Ferguson et al., 2009).

Helping to Change Behavior

In addition to the support for smoking cessation activity described by the U.S. Public Health Service (Fiore et al., 2008), *motivational interviewing* is a patient-focused approach to discussing patients' ambivalence about changing their tobacco use behavior. Motivational interviewing uses empathy and a nonjudgmental style to open a dialogue that can show the importance of change and build a patient's self-motivation. Patients can build on prior success (even brief) and become more active partners in the path to abstinence (Mallin, 2002; Miller and Rollnick, 2002). A clear relationship exists between the intensity of counseling and its effectiveness. Although even brief counseling (≤3 minutes) doubles the spontaneous quit rate, intensive therapy can be more effective and should be used whenever possible (Fiore et al., 2008).

Both physicians and their patients who smoke should think of nicotine dependence as a chronic disease, usually characterized by many episodes of remission and relapse. A number of strategies are often needed, and expectations must be realistic, because smokers usually do not succeed on their first or even second attempt. Clearly, however, the chances of success increase with each attempt, and relapse should not be considered a sign of failure.

Intensive counseling is associated with a 22% smoking-cessation success rate and even minimal counseling (<3 minutes) has a 13% quit rate (Schroeder, 2005). Physicians should take advantage of the teachable moment, such as when a smoker is being seen for a respiratory or cardiovascular problem, an asthma attack in a smoke-exposed child, or the smoking-related death of a loved one (Miller and Wood, 2003). One of the most productive times for cessation advice to be received and effective is during prenatal care or after a nonfatal cardiac event. When intensive counseling and follow-up are provided to patients recovering from coronary bypass graft surgery or a heart attack, more than 60% stop smoking and stay off cigarettes, almost twice the rate of those who receive less definitive advice (Smith and Burgess, 2009; SOR A). A Cochrane review of cessation interventions among hospitalized patients shows that intensive interventions that begin in the hospital and have at least one supportive contact after discharge increase the odds of successful tobacco abstinence (Rigotti et al., 2007).

Pharmacotherapy

The updated clinical practice guideline, Treating Tobacco Use and Dependence (Fiore et al., 2008), discusses the use of the different forms of nicotine replacement therapy

---

KEY TREATMENT

Tobacco users attempting to quit should be prescribed one or more effective first-line pharmacotherapies for tobacco use cessation, including five nicotine replacement therapies (NRTs) (transdermal patch, gum, nasal spray, lozenges, or vapor inhaler) and nonnicotine replacement (bupropion sustained release [SR], or varenicline) (Eisenberg et al., 2008; Fiore et al., 2008) (SOR: A). Brief counseling (≤3 minutes) doubles the spontaneous quit rate; intensive therapy can be even more effective and should be used whenever possible (Fiore et al., 2008) (SOR: A).

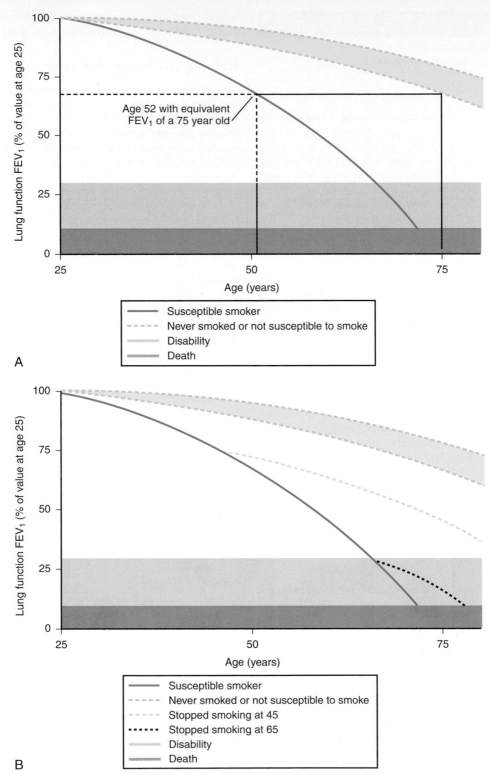

Figure 50-5 A, Explaining lung age to participants. **B,** Graph of lung function against age showing how smoking accelerates age-related decline in lung function. *(From Parkes G et al. BMJ 336:598-600, 2008, Figs. 1 and 2.)*

and the other two FDA-approved prescription medications used for tobacco cessation, bupropion and varenicline (Box 50-3). Effective second-line agents include clonidine, delivered transdermally or orally, and nortriptyline (Fiore et al., 2008), but neither is FDA approved for this indication. All these medications in randomized clinical trials have two to four times the odds ratio for success compared with placebo for smoking cessation. Medication and treatments to avoid include antidepressants such as SSRIs, benzodiazepines, mecamylamine, hypnosis, acupuncture, laser therapy, and beta-adrenergic blocking agents, none of which has been found to have a beneficial effect (Fiore et al., 2008).

Box 50-3 Clinical Guidelines for Nicotine Withdrawal

Nicotine Patch

Patches should be applied as soon as patients waken on their quit day.

At the start of each day, the patient should place a new patch on a relatively hairless location between the neck and waist.

There should be no activity restrictions while using the patch.

Treatment for 8 weeks or less is as effective as longer treatment periods.

New research indicates that starting the patch 2 weeks before quit day increases success.

Dosage

Nicoderm, Habitrol: 21 mg/24 hr for 4 wk, then 14 mg/24 hr for 2 wk, then 7 mg/24 hr for 2 wk

Nicotrol: 15 mg/16 hr for 4 wk, then 10 mg/16 hr for 2 wk, then 5 mg/16 hr for 2 wk.

ProStep: 22 mg/24 hr for 4 wk, then 11 mg/24 hr for 4 wk

Nicotine Gum

Gum should be chewed slowly until a peppery taste emerges, then parked between the check and gum to facilitate nicotine absorption through the oral mucosa. The gum should be slowly and intermittently chewed and parked for about 30 minutes.

Acidic beverages (e.g., coffee, juices, soft drinks) interfere with the buccal absorption of nicotine, so eating and drinking anything except water should be avoided for 5 minutes before and during chewing.

Instructing patients to chew the gum on a fixed schedule may be more beneficial than ad lib use. Patients often do not use enough gum to obtain the maximum benefit.

Dosage

Nicorette: Available as 2 mg and 4 mg per piece. Smokers of more than one pack a day, those who smoke within 30 minutes of awakening, and those with a history of severe withdrawal symptoms should use 4 mg; light smokers should use 2 mg.

Chew one piece every 1-2 hr (at least 9/day) for 6 wk, then one piece every 2-4 for 3 wk, then one piece every 4-8 hr for 3 wk, then discontinue.

For the 2-mg dose, do not exceed 30 pieces/day; for the 4-mg dose, 20 pieces/day.

Nicotine Lozenge

Each lozenge is one 2-mg or 4-mg dose and should be dissolved in the mouth when the urge to smoke starts; lasts 20-30 minutes.

Use 9-20/day for up to 12 weeks.

No eating or drinking during use or 15 minutes before use.

Side effects include sore teeth or gums, indigestion, throat irritation, and other symptoms similar to those with the nicotine gum.

Dosage

Commit lozenge: 2 mg and 4 mg per piece. Smokers of more than one pack a day who smoke within 30 minutes of waking, and those with prior history of severe withdrawal, should use the 4-mg form. Light smokers should start with the 2-mg strength. Do not swallow, bite, or chew the lozenge.

Nicotine Inhaler

Local irritation in the mouth and throat occurs in 40% of patients. Coughing and rhinitis are also common. The severity and frequency of these symptoms decline with continued use.

In cold weather, the inhaler and cartridges should be kept in an inside pocket or warm area, because nicotine delivery declines significantly at temperatures below 40° F (4.4° C).

Dosage

Nicotrol Inhaler: 10 mg/cartridge (4 mg delivered and 2 mg absorbed). Each cartridge lasts about 20 minutes with frequent puffing and is equivalent to about two cigarettes. Use 6 to 16 cartridges/day for the first 12 wk, then reduce gradually over 12 wk.

Nicotine Nasal Spray

Moderate nasal irritation for first 3 weeks or longer. Nasal congestion and transient changes in sense of smell and taste may also occur.

Should not be used in patients with severe reactive airways disease.

Do not sniff, swallow, or inhale through nose while administering doses.

Deliver with head tilted slightly back.

Dosage

Nicotrol NS: One spray (0.5 mg) to each nostril (1.0 mg total). Use 1-2 doses/hr and 8 to 40 doses/day (maximum, 5 doses/hr). Each bottle contains 100 doses. Usual maximum, 12 weeks.

Bupropion SR

Contraindicated in patients with a history of significant head trauma, seizure disorder, or eating disorder, and in those who have used a monoamine oxidase inhibitor (MAOI) in the past 14 days.

Side effects are insomnia and dry mouth. If insomnia is present, take the evening dose in the afternoon, but at least 8 hours after the first dose.

Dosage

150-mg tablets; one every morning for 3 days and then twice daily. Start 2 weeks before the target quit date and continue for 12 weeks.

Side effects are nausea (30% of patients), abnormal dreams, insomnia, headache, taste aversion, and flatulence.

Varenicline

Start 1 week before quit date.

Side effects are nausea (30% of patients), abnormal dreams, insomnia, headache, taste aversion, and flatulence. FDA warning addresses behavior changes and suicidal ideation.

Dosage

Chantix: 0.5 mg (white tablet) once daily for 3 days, then twice daily for 4 days, then 1.0 mg (blue tablet) twice daily, for total of 12 weeks.

Comments

Some patients may prefer the nasal spray or inhaler, because the more rapid delivery of nicotine better simulates smoking.

Others may prefer bupropion because it is nonnicotine therapy.

Bupropion should be considered especially in those with a history of depression.

Modified from US Department of Health and Human Services. Treating Tobacco Use and Dependence: Clinical Practice Update. Rockville, Md, Agency for Health Care Policy and Research, Public Health Service, 2008.

Nicotine Patch

The nicotine patch is a mainstay of treatment, often combined with other forms of replacement or psychotropic medication and counseling. The main advantages of the patch are consistent delivery, easy use, and concealment. The major disadvantage is insomnia, which can be avoided by not wearing the patch at night.

In a study by Cornish and Gariti (2002), by the second day of patch use, nicotine levels are about half or greater than those achieved by smoking. Quit rates at 4 to 8 weeks (depending on the study) are about double the rate of success for placebo—that is, up to 70% for the nicotine patch versus up to 40% for placebo. After 1 year, the abstinence rates are about 25% for the gum and patch compared with 12% for placebo. The combination of a short-acting form of NRT (gum, lozenge, nasal spray) added to the patch increases the odds of success, because it helps control cravings and gives the smoker the ability to titrate the dose. Recent evidence also indicates that smokers who begin the patch 2 weeks before the quit date may double the rate of abstinence (Rose et al., 2009).

Nicotine Gum

To obtain maximal results, the gum must be chewed slowly and then parked between cheek and gum to allow for buccal absorption. Although 2-mg and 4-mg strengths are available, the 4-mg strength is recommended for patients who smoke more than one pack a day. Absorption is decreased if the mouth is acidic, so the patient should avoid beverages such as coffee, tea, soda, and fruit juice. Abstinence rates at 4 to 6 weeks are 73% for nicotine gum compared with 49% for placebo gum. The duration of treatment, as with other NRT, should be at least 6 weeks, although a Cochrane review did not find evidence of enhanced success for the patch beyond 8 weeks (Stead et al., 2007).

Nicotine Inhaler and Nasal Spray

The nicotine inhaler resembles a cigarette and mimics the act of smoking, thus permitting perpetuation of a behavioral ritual, but the nicotine is absorbed through the buccal mucosa rather than the lungs. Its efficacy is similar to that of the patch. The nicotine nasal spray is more rapidly absorbed than the other forms of NRT and should be a first-line treatment for heavier smokers. As monotherapy, the nasal spray has a higher odds ratio for success than the other NRT used alone (Fiore et al., 2008).

Nicotine Lozenges

Nicotine lozenges deliver slightly more available nicotine than nicotine gum, are easier to use, and have fewer gastric side effects. The lozenge comes in several flavors and should be sucked like candy, slowly, until the flavor becomes intense. It is then held between the cheek and gums, like nicotine gum, and sucked again after the flavor has diminished. It should not be chewed or swallowed. The 4-mg strength lozenge should be used for those whose first cigarette is within 30 minutes of waking, with the 2-mg strength used for lighter smokers. Smokers should use seven or eight lozenges or more per day, up to 20.

Bupropion

Bupropion is a monocyclic antidepressant, thought to inhibit the reuptake of both dopamine and norepinephrine. It may exert multiple mechanisms, producing craving relief from dopaminergic activity, and antagonism of nicotinic acetylcholine receptors. The U.S. Public Health Service (PHS) guidelines and other analyses show that bupropion doubles long-term abstinence compared with placebo (Eisenberg et al., 2008; Fiore et al., 2008). Dosing begins 1 week before the quit date: 150 mg for 3 days, then 150 mg twice daily for the remainder of the week until quit day, and long-term maintenance at that dose. Bupropion may also be effective in relapse prevention, although a recent Cochrane review questions that conclusion (Hajek et al., 2008). Bupropion carries a small risk of seizures, as with other antidepressants, and is contraindicated in patients with a significant history of head trauma, eating disorders, or seizure disorders. Bupropion is effective in delaying weight gain associated with smoking cessation. The FDA has issued a black-box warning for both bupropion and varenicline, highlighting the risk of serious mental health events, including changes in behavior, depressed mood, hostility, agitation, suicidal thoughts, and attempted suicide.

Combination Therapy

Just as long-acting and short-acting NRT can be combined to augment cessation success, bupropion can be used with the patch or other forms of NRT. Combination therapy appears to be a promising approach. A 9-week study combining bupropion SR with transdermal nicotine found much greater efficacy than with either medication alone (Jorenby et al., 1999), and subsequent review in the PHS guidelines confirms the utility of combination therapy (Fiore et al., 2008). One might think of bupropion or the patch as the "controller" medication and the short-acting NRT as the "rescue" drug, much as dual therapy is used in asthma control. A recent trial of "triple therapy" using the patch, bupropion, and the nicotine vapor inhaler for up to 6 months showed a 2.57 odds ratio for abstinence compared with patch alone (Steinberg et al., 2009).

Clinicians at the Mayo Clinic Nicotine Dependence Center have routinely used combination therapy and base initial NRT patch dosing on venous cotinine levels. If that is not available, the intensity of smoking or spit tobacco use can be a useful guide (Table 50-1) (Dale et al., 2000).

Table 50-1 Recommended Dosages for Nicotine Replacement Therapy

Cigarettes (per day)	Nicotine Patch Dose (mg/day)
Less than 10	7-14
10-20	14-22
21-40	22-44
More than 40	44+

Varenicline

Varenicline is a partial agonist/antagonist that is selectively bound to the α4β2 nicotinic receptors, thus blocking nicotine from these brain cells, as well as stimulating them to release dopamine at lower levels than does nicotine itself. This leads to reduced cravings and fewer symptoms of nicotine withdrawal. A Cochrane review of its effectiveness concludes that it increases the odds of successful cessation two to three times more than attempts not using pharmacotherapy, with a pooled RR at 1 year compared to bupropion of 1.52 (Cahill et al., 2008). Varenicline is titrated over 1 week, mainly to help overcome its major side effect of nausea, ameliorated by taking varenicline with meals. Begin with 0.5 mg daily for 3 days, then 0.5 mg twice daily, then 1 mg twice daily on day 8, which is quit day for the patient. Treatment should continue for at least 12 weeks; an additional 12 weeks may be useful in patients who are insecure in their attempts and are at high risk for relapse. The longer dosing schedule was shown to increase success in clinical trials.

Concern has been raised about varenicline and its potential to cause behavior changes and suicidal thoughts. In July 2009 the FDA issued a black-box warning for both varenicline and bupropion saying that patients taking either of these drugs should be observed for symptoms of behavior change, including hostility, aggression, depressed mood, and suicidal ideation or attempts. Patients should stop taking varenicline and contact their physician if these or other unusual neuropsychiatric symptoms occur. In addition, patients should take precautions when driving or operating machinery until they know whether varenicline might adversely affect them. Pilots, air traffic controllers, and persons with commercial motor vehicle licenses cannot use varenicline, according to federal rules issued in 2008. A cohort study of more than 80,000 persons using different medications for smoking cessation, however, found no clear evidence that varenicline caused suicide or depression (Gunnell et al., 2009).

Early evidence shows that using varenicline in combination with the nicotine patch and with bupropion appears to be safe and well tolerated; however, more investigation is needed before these combinations become a mainstay of smoking-cessation therapy (Ebbert et al., 2009a, 2009b).

Second-Line Medications

Clonidine and nortriptyline are listed in the PHS guidelines as second-line drugs, and both have been shown to have significant effects on cessation compared with placebo (Fiore et al., 2008). Nortriptyline is generally titrated up to 75 to 100 mg/day and used for 8 to 12 weeks. It has the advantage of being quite inexpensive, but drug levels may be needed to avoid toxicity. Clonidine patches, 0.2 mg/day, are recommended for up to 10 weeks and should be started 1 week before the quit date. Clonidine's side effects of drowsiness may limit its usefulness in many patients. Neither is FDA approved for smoking cessation.

Quit Lines

One of the least used methods, yet one of the most effective, is telephone quit lines. Surveys have shown that 70% to 85% of smokers prefer to use a quit line to seeing a clinician, perhaps because of the convenience, anonymity, and ability to obtain counseling in their native language. The toll-free number, 1-800-QUITNOW (1-800-784-8669), is a single access point to the National Network of Tobacco Cessation Quit Lines. Callers are automatically routed to a state-run quit line, if one exists in their area. If there is no state-run line, callers are routed to the National Cancer Institute (NCI) quit line, where they may receive cessation services and other information. Quit lines are available in almost every state (Schroeder, 2005). There is also a California Smoker's Helpline at 1-800-662-8887, which links people nationwide to counselors who will give one-to-one support. Quit lines are even more effective when combined with NRT (Bush et al., 2008)

Relapse Prevention

Perhaps the most poorly understood element in smoking cessation is preventing relapse. Follow-up and ongoing contact with patients is essential, especially in the first few weeks of a cessation attempt. The first 2 weeks are the most crucial period, when smoking even one cigarette is a strong predictor of a return to regular smoking within 1 year. A return visit, proactive telephone call, or regular sessions with a quit line counselor in the early stages of cessation should be integrated into the patient's treatment. To be truly successful, family physicians should integrate tobacco-dependence treatment into their practice (Solberg, 2000). The Cochrane review on relapse prevention found that while no definitive evidence yet exists for specific interventions to sustain abstinence, efforts to help smokers identify and deal with "tempting situations" show promise (Hajek et al., 2008). However, an excellent series of materials for patients is available from the National Cancer Institute website and may be very useful in helping patients with discussions of relapse issues ("Forever Free" at www.smokefree.gov/resources.aspx).

Current Developments

Smoker's Genetics

Genetic testing may be able to indicate persons most susceptible to becoming addicted to nicotine. Addictive individuals who have a particular gene and are trying to quit may be more responsive to nicotine patches than nonnicotine measures such as bupropion (Zyban). Multiple genes are involved, however, and considerable research will be needed to create practical applications for these discoveries.

Much work is currently underway regarding genes and gene mutations that predispose cigarette smokers to lung cancer. *Gene methylation* is a chemical modification that may be a marker for the early detection of lung cancer. The gene *GPC5* has an important tumor suppressor–like function that, if insufficient, can promote lung cancer development. A variant of this gene has been found in one third of nonsmokers who develop lung cancer (Yang, 2010).

Diet

Diet may protect against gene changes in smokers. Some vitamins and green leafy vegetables serve as protective factors against lung cancer, as for colorectal cancer. Increased variety in fruit and vegetable intake may confer some protection against lung cancer among smokers (Buchner et al., 2010).

References

The complete reference list is available online at www.expertconsult.com.

Web Resources

www.askandact.org
American Association of Family Physicians website for tobacco control and cessation issues.

www.cdc.gov/tobacco
Centers for Disease Control and Prevention Office on Smoking and Health site; contains withdrawal data, U.S. Surgeon General reports, MMWR articles on tobacco.

www.cancer.gov
National Cancer Institute (NCI) site, with research data, the Smoking and Tobacco Control Monograph series, prevention and cessation information.

www.epa.gov/smokefree
Advice on how to protect children from secondhand smoke and other tobacco-related materials.

www.lungusa.org
American Lung Association offers printed quit materials, some in Spanish. Also offers the tobacco cessation program "Freedom from Smoking Online" at www.ffsonline.org.

www.cochrane.org/reviews/
Cochrane Collaboration; evidence-based systematic reviews of the medical literature, with dozens of topics related to smoking and tobacco.

www.thecommunityguide.org/index.html
The Guide to Community Preventive Services.

www.ahrq.gov/clinic/uspstfix.htm
U.S. Preventive Services Task Force; Guide to Clinical Preventive Services.

www.nicotine-anonymous.org
Information and meeting schedules of Nicotine Anonymous in your area.

www.quitnet.com
Offers free cutting-edge tobacco-cessation services to people worldwide.

www.tobaccofreekids.org
Campaign for Tobacco-Free Kids; useful reports and data on state and national issues, advocacy oriented.

www.smokefree.gov
Evidence-based information and professional assistance to help support the immediate and long-term needs of people trying to quit smoking.

www.quittobacco.org
Smoking cessation site for the public from the Center for Health Improvement and Group Health in Seattle.

www.smokefree.net
Network for tobacco control information and discussion groups.

www.no-smoke.org
The Americans for Nonsmokers Rights site; a primary spot for information on secondhand smoke.

http://smokingcessationleadership.ucsf.edu/
University of California at San Francisco (UCSF) site, promoting health professionals to help patients with cessation; many links and resources.

www.tobacco.org
A daily news service with medical articles and stories from print and broadcast media on tobacco issues.

www.scenesmoking.org
Annual monitoring of the amount of smoking in each movie category by the Breathe California of Sacramento–Emigrant Trails, Sacramento.

www.treattobacco.net
Evidence-based tobacco control site of the Society for Research on Nicotine and Tobacco.

Drug Abuse

Alicia Kowalchuk and Brian C. Reed

Scope of the Problem

Key Points

- About 8.0 % of the U.S. population, or 20.1 million Americans, reported using illicit drugs in 2008.
- Marijuana has remained the most frequently used illicit drug in the United States.
- The prevalence of illicit drug use has been greatest in those 18 to 20 years of age.
- With the exception of hallucinogens such as "ecstasy," prevalence of drug use in teenagers age 12 to 17 has decreased since 2002.
- Illicit drug use is significantly higher among people with serious mental illness.

According to the 2008 Substance Abuse and Mental Health Services Administration (SAMHSA) National Survey on Drug Use and Health, an estimated 20.1 million Americans age 12 or older were current users of illicit drugs or reported having used an illicit substance 1 month before the survey. This represented 8.0% of the U.S. population. This rate has remained essentially stable since 2002. With an estimated 15.2 million current users, marijuana was the most frequently used illicit drug. Among people who used illicit drugs, marijuana was used by an estimated 75.7% of current illicit

drug users. Following marijuana were nonmedical use of prescription psychotherapeutic drugs (6.2 million), cocaine (1.9 million), hallucinogens (1.1 million), and methamphetamine (314,000).

The age group with the greatest prevalence of illicit substance abuse was individuals age 18 to 20, at 21.5%. Rates of illicit drug use among youths age 12 to 17 decreased from 11.6% in 2002 to 9.3% in 2008. The rate of substance abuse or dependence for males age 12 and older was almost twice as high as that for females (11.5% vs. 6.4%). However, males and females had similar rates of nonmedical use of psychotherapeutic drugs, pain relievers, stimulants, and sedatives.

The prevalence of illicit drug use varies by race and ethnicity. Illicit substance use was highest among people reporting two or more races, at 14.1%. An estimated 10.1% of blacks, 9.5% of American Indians or Alaska Natives, 8.2% of whites, 7.3% of Native Hawaiians or other Pacific Islanders, 6.3% of Hispanics, and 3.6% of Asians were current illicit drug users in 2008. Illicit drug use also varies by education level. Among adults age 18 or older, the prevalence of current illicit drug use was 9.4% of adults with some college education, 8.1% of adults who did not complete high school, 8.6% of high school graduates, and 5.7% of college graduates. In 2008 an estimated 8000 people used an illicit substance for the first time each day. Most initiates were female and younger than 18. Between 2003 and 2008, the number of daily new

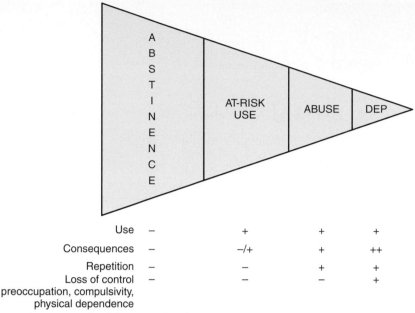

Use	−	+	+	+
Consequences	−	−/+	+	++
Repetition	−	−	+	+
Loss of control	−	−	−	+
preoccupation, compulsivity, physical dependence				

Figure 51-1 Continuum of drug use in patients with substance use disorders. *(Modified from Association for Medical Education and Research in Substance Abuse.)*

users of cocaine, psychotherapeutic drugs and inhalants had decreased. During the same 5-year interval, the number of people initiating use of hallucinogens, ecstasy, and LSD had increased significantly. Approximately, 19.6% of unemployed individuals age 18 and older were current illicit drug users. This was significantly higher than the prevalence of current drug use among individuals employed full time (8.0%) and part time (10.1%).

The prevalence of substance of abuse was also significantly higher among individuals with serious mental illness. Use of illicit drugs in the past year among adults age 18 or older with serious mental illness was 30.3%, whereas use among same-age adults without serious mental illness was 12.9%.

Terminology

The term "substance use disorder" (SUD) implies a continuum of use: from abstinence to at-risk use to abuse and dependence (Fig. 51-1). The majority of the general population, as well as family medicine patients, are "abstainers." The majority of users of illicit substances do not meet criteria for the diagnosis of abuse and dependency. This model of substance use is important for family medicine physicians to keep in mind as they talk with their patients about substance use issues. It highlights the key role played by screening for substance use and early intervention at the at-risk use level, before specialized treatment services are more likely needed. For illicit substances, unlike alcohol, no amount of use can be considered safe or healthy, in part because any use is illegal.

Box 51-1 lists the DSM IV diagnostic criteria for substance abuse and dependence. Of note, physical dependence alone does not make a diagnosis of substance abuse or dependence, nor does lack of physical dependence exclude the diagnoses.

Table 51-1 shows some common drug street names. Comprehensive lists can be found on the Office of National Drug Control Policy website, www.whitehousedrugpolicy.gov. Street names vary by region and user group. The most useful

---

Box 51-1 Diagnostic Criteria for Substance Abuse and Dependence (DSM IV)*

A maladaptive pattern of substance use leading to clinically significant impairment or distress, as manifested by:

Abuse

One or more of the following, occurring in a 12-month period, and these symptoms have never met the criteria for Substance Dependence:

Recurrent substance use resulting in a failure to fulfill major role obligations at work, school, or home

Recurrent substance use in situations in which it is physically hazardous

Recurrent substance-related legal problems

Continued substance use despite having persistent or recurrent social or interpersonal problems caused or exacerbated by the effects of the substance

Dependence

Three or more of the following, occurring in the same 12-month period:

Tolerance, as defined by either of the following: a need for markedly increased amounts of the substance to achieve intoxication or desired effect *or* markedly diminished effect with continued use of the same amount of substance

Withdrawal, as manifested by either of the following: the characteristic withdrawal syndrome for the substance *or* the same (or a closely related) substance is taken to relieve or avoid withdrawal symptoms

The substance is often taken in larger amounts or longer than intended.

There is a persistent desire or unsuccessful efforts to cut down or control substance use.

A great deal of time is spent in activities to obtain the substance, use the substance, or recover from its effects.

Important social, occupational, or recreational activities are given up or reduced because of substance use.

The substance use is continued despite knowledge of having a persistent or recurrent physical or psychological problem that is likely to have been caused or exacerbated by the substance.

*American Psychiatric Association. Diagnostic and Statistical Manual of Mental Disorders, 4th ed, text revision. Washington, DC, APA, 2000.

Table 51-1 Common Drug Street Names

		Street Names (NIDA website)	Substance
		Candy, downers, sleeping pills, sticks, handlebars	Benzodiazepines
		Blow, bump, C, candy, coke, crack, flake, rock, snow	Cocaine
		Captain Cody, school boy, pancakes and syrup	Codeine
		Robotripping, Robo, Triple C	Dextromethorphan
		Roofies, rope, rophies, forget-me pill, Mexican Valium	Flunitrazepam (Rohypnol)
		Liquid ecstasy, Georgia home boy, grievous bodily harm	GHB
		Brown sugar, dope, H, horse, junk, skag, skunk, smack	Heroin
		K, special K, vitamin K, cat Valiums	Ketamine
		Acid, blotter, boomers, cubes, microdot	LSD
		Blunt, dope, ganja, grass, herb, joints, pot, reefer, weed	Marijuana
		Adam, clarity, ecstasy, Eve, lover's speed, peace, X	MDMA
		Chalk, rank, crystal, fire, glass, go fast, ice, meth, speed	Methamphetamine
		Skippy, vitamin R, the smart drug, R-ball	Methylphenidate
		Oxy, OC, killer, vike	Oxycodone (Oxycontin), hydrocodone (Vicodin)
		Angel dust, boat, hog, love boat, peace pill	PCP

NIDA, National Institute on Drug Abuse; *GHB*, γ-hydroxybutyrate; *LSD*, lysergic acid diethylamide; *MDMA*, methylenedioxymethamphetamine; *PCP*, phencyclidine.

information is obtained on the local level, simply by asking patients what they call the drug they are using.

Screening

Screening, brief intervention, and referral to treatment (SBIRT) for alcohol use disorders in primary care has been well studied and is recommended for incorporation into routine primary care by the U.S. Preventive Services Task Force (USPSTF, SOR B). However, SBIRT in primary care for drug use has been less studied to date, and USPSTF states that there is currently insufficient evidence to recommend for or against routine screening for drug use in primary care.

With the recent increase in prescription drug misuse and abuse, interest in drug-use SBIRT incorporation into primary care has broadened and is being studied for efficacy (Insight Project, 2009). Limitations on drug-use SBIRT in primary

Table 51-2 CRAFFT Screening Tool for Adolescents

CRAFFT	Question
Car	Have you ever ridden in a **car** by someone (including yourself) who was "high" or had been using alcohol or drugs?
Relax	Do you ever use alcohol or drugs to **relax,** feel better about yourself, or fit in?
Alone	Do you ever use alcohol or drugs while you are by yourself, or **alone**?
Forget	Do you ever **forget** things you did while using alcohol or drugs?
Friends	Do family members or **friends** ever tell you that you should cut down on your drinking or drug use?
Trouble	Have you ever gotten into **trouble** while you were using alcohol or drugs?

Scoring:
A "no" response = 0 points; a "yes" response = 1 point.
0-1 point = negative screen.
2-6 points = positive screen; consider a safety contract for "yes" response to "car" question regardless of total score.

Table 51-3 CAGE-AID Screening Tool for Adults

CAGE	Question
Cut down	Have you felt you ought to **cut down** on your drinking or drug use?
Annoyed	Have people **annoyed** you by criticizing your drinking or drug use?
Guilty	Have you felt bad or **guilty** about your drinking or drug use?
Eye opener	Have you ever had a drink or used drugs first thing in the morning to steady your nerves or to get rid of a hangover **(eye opener)**?

Scoring:
A "no" response = 0 points; a "yes" response = 1 point.
0-1 point = negative screen.
2-4 points = positive screen.

Box 51-2 FRAMES intervention technique

Feedback about personal risk
Responsibility of the patient for change
Advice to change
Menu of strategies
Empathy: express empathy.
Self-efficacy: elicit and support patient's self-efficacy for change.

Box 51-3 Five "A's" Intervention Technique

Assess the risk of the behavior for the patient.
Advise the patient on their risk and how to modify.
Agree: come to an agreement with patient on treatment.
Assist the patient with the treatment plan.
Arrange follow-up or referral to treatment.

care include lower prevalence of drug use in primary care patients compared with alcohol use as well as concerns about the practicality of use and positive predictive value (PPV) of available screening instruments in the primary care setting. The American Academy of Pediatrics (AAP), the Bright Future Initiative, and American Medical Association (AMA) Guidelines for Adolescent Preventative Services (GAPS) all recommend at least annual screening of adolescents for drug use. The American College of Obstetricians and Gynecologists (ACOG) advocates regular, periodic screening for all patients, regardless of pregnancy status, although no specific screening instrument is recommended and, to date, no screening instrument has been validated for pregnant women (Lanier and Ko, 2008). Common validated screening instruments for drug use are briefly discussed below.

The CRAFFT is the only screening instrument validated for adolescents and has shown an 83% PPV (Table 51-2). It screens for alcohol as well as drug use (Knight et al., 2002).

The ASSIST, CAGE-AID, and DAST have been validated in nonpregnant adults. PPVs for the Alcohol, Smoking and Substance Involvement Screening Test (ASSIST) are not currently available (Newcombe et al., 2005). It screens for tobacco and alcohol in addition to drugs. The ASSIST is available at no cost from the World Health Organization (WHO).

The CAGE-Adjusted to Include Drugs (CAGE-AID) has shown 12% to 78% PPV, with PPV increasing with increasing prevalence of drug use in the study population (Brown and Rounds, 1995). It screens for both alcohol and drug use (Table 51-3).

The Drug Abuse Screening Test (DAST) has similarly shown a wide PPV range of 23% to 75% and is also in the public domain. It screens for drug use only (Staley and El-Guebaly, 1990).

The ASSIST and DAST are more lengthy screens than the CAGE-AID and CRAFFT and consequently have not been reproduced here. The SAMHSA SBIRT initiative recommends both the ASSIST and the DAST for drug screening. (Lanier and Ko, 2008). SBIRT models vary but typically involve a brief screen of several questions regarding tobacco, alcohol, and/or drug use, conducted by frontline staff. Recently a single-question screen for drug use has been validated for primary care: "How many times in the past year have you used an illegal drug or used a prescription medication for nonmedical reasons?" An answer of one or more is a positive screening response (Smith et al., 2010). With sensitivity of 100% and specificity of 73.5%, this single-question screen is comparable to the four-question CAGE-AID.

Patients screening positive receive more in-depth screening with a self-administered or provider-administered screening instrument, such as the DAST or ASSIST, which both allow for stratification of each patient along the SUD continuum. The physician then scores the formal screen and reviews the results with the patient. Patients screening negative are given brief feedback about the results of their screen, and their healthy choices regarding substance use are reinforced by the physician. Patients screening positive for at-risk use, but who do not meet criteria for abuse or dependence, receive a brief intervention, often using the FRAMES model (Box 51-2) or the "Five A's" model (Box 51-3). Both are useful for patients receptive to change. Motivational interviewing techniques may be more useful than the FRAMES or Five A's techniques for patients who are more ambivalent about change (Searight, 2009).

Patients screening positive and meeting criteria for abuse or dependence are offered referral to onsite or, more typically, community drug treatment programs. Referral to treatment can be time-consuming and therefore is often done by ancillary staff with knowledge of local treatment resources, or by referring the patient to a community-based agency that provides treatment-matching services.

Laboratory Testing

Key Points

- Any drug testing method involves several important considerations:
- Samples can be adulterated to mask true results: creatinine, pH, specific gravity, and temperature are often used to detect urine sample adulteration.
- A single test result is a marker of use at one point in time and does not itself make a diagnosis of abuse or dependence; laboratory detection of drug use is one tool that may be used during screening, diagnosis, treatment, and relapse prevention of substance use disorders.
- Rates of false positives and false negatives depend on the drug ingested, quantity ingested, duration of use, and specific laboratory cutoffs used; it is important to know the cutoff values of the laboratory used and to obtain a comprehensive history of drug ingestion quantity and frequency over time.

Laboratory testing is frequently used in SUD screening, treatment, and monitoring for relapse. The most common testing method is the *urine drug test.* Other options include blood, sweat, hair, and oral fluid testing. Table 51-4 lists the advantages and disadvantages of each method (Ries et al., 2009).

Table 51-5 details typical detection times and causes of false-positive results for drugs that can be detected by readily available urine drug testing. Most urine drug tests use immunoassays because these are inexpensive, fast, and easily automated. Gas chromatography with mass spectroscopy (GC/MS) is typically reserved for confirmation of a positive result. Methadone is not a part of most urine drug screen panels and does not show as a positive opiate test. Separate testing for methadone is available. Separate testing is also needed for most "club drugs," including 3,4-methylenedioxymethamphetamine (MDMA), ketamine, and γ-hydroxybutyrate (GHB). Benzodiazepines have a wide range of potencies, half-lives, and metabolites, which makes urine drug screen results less reliable (Ries et al., 2009).

Table 51-4 Drug-Testing Methods: Advantages and Disadvantages

Test	Advantages	Disadvantages
Blood	Difficult to adulterate; detects very recent ingestion	Invasive; drugs clear blood more quickly after ingestion than urine
Hair	Noninvasive; difficult to adulterate; detects patterns of use over time; frequently used in forensics and research	Not useful for recent ingestion; more difficult to process than other methods
Oral fluids	Noninvasive; direct observation easy and makes adulteration more difficult; detects recent ingestion; rapid results	Unintentional contamination from recently ingested substances; drugs clear quickly after ingestion (see Urine)
Sweat	Noninvasive; uses patch for collection; monitor for use over extended period	Quantification of drug levels difficult
Urine	Noninvasive; rapid results; relatively inexpensive vs. other methods	Easy to adulterate sample, even when observed collection method used

Table 51-5 Urine Drug Testing: Detection Times and Drugs Causing False Positives

Drug	Detection Time	False-Positive Result
Amphetamines, methamphetamine	1-3 days	Bupropion, chloroquine, chlorpromazine, ephedrine, labetalol, phenylpropanolamine, propranolol, pseudoephedrine, ranitidine, selegiline, trazodone, tyramine, Vick's inhaler
Barbiturates	Short acting: 1-4 days Long acting: several wks	Phenytoin
Benzodiazepines	Highly variable	Oxaprozin, sertraline
Cocaine	3 days	None
LSD	2-5 days	Amitriptyline, chlorpromazine, doxepin, fluoxetine, haloperidol, metoclopramide, risperidone, sertraline, thioridazine, verapamil
Marijuana (THC)	Single joint: 2 days Heavy use: 27 days	Efavirenz, pantoprazole, quinaprine
Methadone	2-3 days	Quetiapine
Opiates	1-2 days	Gatifloxacin, levofloxacin, ofloxacin, papaverine, rifampicin, poppy seeds
Phencyclidine	7 days	Dextromethorphan, diphenylhydramine, thioridazine, venlafaxine
Propoxyphene	6 hours to 2 days	Cyclobenzaprine, diphenylhydramine, doxylamine, imipramine, methadone

Pharmacology

Cocaine

Cocaine is a powerful and highly addictive stimulant derived from the leaf extract of the *Erythroxylon coca* bush. In 2008, there were an estimated 1.9 million current users of cocaine, or 0.7 % of the U.S. population. Cocaine use is highest among individuals 18 to 25 years of age.

Cocaine causes a brief, intense feeling of euphoria by blocking the reuptake of dopamine, a neurotransmitter that is associated with pleasure and movement. This blockage accordingly increases the level of dopamine in the central nervous system (CNS). The more rapidly cocaine is absorbed into the bloodstream and delivered to the CNS, the more intense the "high" experienced by the user. Cocaine can be inhaled, injected, or smoked. Injecting or smoking cocaine produces an intense, 5- or 10-minute high that is much stronger than the sensation produced by snorting powder cocaine. The euphoria induced by snorting powder cocaine typically lasts 15 to 30 minutes but is slower in onset than injecting or smoking cocaine. Small amounts of cocaine give users feelings of euphoria, increased mental alertness, and energy.

Symptoms of cocaine intoxication include euphoria, agitation, impaired judgment, bizarre behavior, paranoia, tachycardia, elevated blood pressure, dilated pupils, and diaphoresis. Increased doses of cocaine cause some cocaine users to experience auditory hallucinations, tactile hallucinations, delusions, and aggressive behavior. Sudden cardiac arrest, seizures, and respiratory arrest are examples of fatal complications from cocaine overdose. Tolerance to cocaine causes addicts to binge on cocaine or take more cocaine at increasingly frequent intervals. Withdrawal from cocaine begins with a "crash" or excessive sleep. After 1 to 2 days, the user may feel anxious, irritated, fatigued, and depressed from the absence of cocaine and decreased dopamine levels, which can also cause intense cravings, depression, and suicidal ideation.

Although cocaine has legitimate medical uses, such as local anesthesia in eye, ear, and throat surgery, nonmedical use and importation were banned by the Harrison Act in December 1914.

Marijuana

Derived from a mix of flowers, stems, seeds, and leaves of the plant *Cannabis sativa*, marijuana is the most commonly abused illicit drug in the United States. In 2008, approximately 15.2 million people over 12 years of age were current users of marijuana. Nerve cells in the brain have receptors for THC (delta-9-tetrahydrocannabinol), the main active chemical in marijuana. Once the drug enters the brain, THC causes the release of dopamine and produces feelings of euphoria. Smoking marijuana can produce a high that lasts 1 to 3 hours. Ingesting marijuana that has been mixed with food or brewed with tea can cause a longer high that lasts up to 4 hours. While high on marijuana, users may experience pleasant feelings, a feeling that time passes more slowly, and perceptions of heightened sensation with color and sound stimuli. Marijuana users may also have sudden hunger, thirst, and feelings of paranoia and anxiety. As the euphoria passes, marijuana users may feel depressed or sleepy. Long-term marijuana use can cause damage to short-term memory by altering the manner in which information is processed in the hippocampus. Marijuana can also cause respiratory problems such as chronic cough, recurrent lung infections, and lung cancer.

Methamphetamine

Methamphetamine is a highly addictive stimulant that can cause increased alertness and increased physical activity with small doses by causing the release of high levels of the neurotransmitter dopamine in the brain. Abusers of methamphetamine experience a brief "rush" by smoking or injecting methamphetamine. Oral ingestion or snorting methamphetamine can produce a high that can last approximately half a day. Due to tolerance, chronic users of methamphetamine may take higher doses of the drug or binge for several days. Long-term use of methamphetamine can cause functional and molecular changes to the brain. Chronic methamphetamine users may exhibit anxiety, violent behavior, and symptoms of psychosis, such as hallucinations, paranoia, and delusions. Fortunately, the use of methamphetamine in the United States has been decreasing. In 2008, there were approximately 314,000 users of methamphetamine, or half the number of users as in 2006.

Hallucinogens

Hallucinogens alter mood and perception. Commonly abused hallucinogens include LSD, PCP, MDMA, and hallucinogenic mushrooms. In 2008, there were 1.1 million current users of hallucinogens in the United States; use increased among youths 12 to 17 years old. *Lysergic acid diethylamide* (LSD) is sold as tablets, capsules, or liquids. It is often added to absorbent paper and dosed in small, decorated squares. Users of LSD experience unpredictable sensations of sound, color, hallucinations, and delusions. Long-term consequences of LSD usage include flashbacks, depression, and long-lasting psychosis. Users of *phencyclidine* (PCP) may smoke, ingest, inject, or snort it to experience hallucinations. PCP use may cause violent behavior, anxiety, and paranoia.

"Club Drugs"

Ketamine, MDMA, GHB, and flunitrazepam (Rohypnol) are substances used in nightclubs, "raves," and dance parties to enhance feelings of intimacy and sensory stimulation. "Ecstasy," or MDMA, produces distorted perceptions of time, enhanced enjoyment of tactile sensations, and feelings of increased energy by increasing the release of serotonin, dopamine, and norepinephrine. The sympathetic overload caused by MDMA can produce hypertension, tachycardia, tremor, diaphoresis, and arrhythmias. MDMA intoxication is also associated with a potentially fatal serotonin syndrome that causes hyperthermia, autonomic instability, and myoclonus. Users of MDMA will typically experience severe depression 2 days after its ingestion.

Ketamine is a dissociative anesthetic derived from PCP. Usually stolen from veterinarians and physician offices, illicit supplies of ketamine are dried in powder form and smoked in nightclubs with tobacco and marijuana or inhaled. "Special K" can produce sensations of floating outside one's body, visual hallucinations, and dreamlike states that last for 30 to 45 minutes after ingestion.

Gamma-hydroxybutyrate (GHB) can cause euphoria at lower doses and drowsiness, dizziness, visual disturbances, hypotonia, and amnesia at higher doses. Overdoses of GHB can cause seizures, severe respiratory depression, coma, and death. Because of its sedative and amnesic effect, GHB has been used as a "date rape" drug.

Flunitrazepam (Rohypnol) is a powerful benzodiazepine with 10 times the strength of diazepam that is capable of reducing anxiety, muscle tension, and inhibition. Higher doses of flunitrazepam can produce lack of muscle control, loss of consciousness, and anterograde amnesia. As with GHB, flunitrazepam has been used as a "date rape" drug (Gahlinger, 2004).

Benzodiazepines

Benzodiazepines are a family of depressants used therapeutically to produce sedation, relieve anxiety, induce sleep, control seizures, and alleviate muscle spasms. Abusers of benzodiazepines experience reduced inhibition and impaired judgment. Users of cocaine and amphetamines may take benzodiazepines to counter the stimulant effects. Concurrent use of benzodiazepines with alcohol and other depressants can be life threatening. Abrupt cessation of benzodiazepine use can cause seizures and a withdrawal syndrome similar to delirium tremens.

Opiates (Nonmedical Use of Prescription Drugs)

Hydrocodone (Vicodin) is the most frequently prescribed opioid in the United States. Oxycodone (Oxycontin) and hydrocodone are prescribed in the treatment of acute and chronic pain. Abusers of hydrocodone and oxycodone experience euphoria, relaxation, and sedation. Long-term use can result in tolerance. Abusers may overdose as they take increasing doses of the medication while pursuing euphoric sensations that they previously experienced. Overdoses may result in severe respiratory depression, hypotension, coma, and death. Recently, methadone, primarily diverted from prescriptions for chronic pain and not methadone maintenance treatment, has been linked to increased opiate overdoses as well. Its relatively long onset of action and long half-life make methadone-naive individuals more prone to overdose as they seek a stronger high with escalating doses, which accumulate, causing overdose.

Heroin

Heroin, or diacetylmorphine, is a synthetic opiate, first created by Bayer in the late 1800s and marketed for pain relief and treatment of morphine addicts. It has a high abuse potential because of its rapid onset of action and short half-life. Heroin is therefore a Schedule I substance (i.e., not available for therapeutic use in the United States). Heroin can be injected intravenously (IV), subcutaneously (SC, "skin popping"), or snorted intranasally, as well as smoked in freebase form. Use of the intranasal route has greatly increased, along with the purity of street heroin and

awareness of human immunodeficiency virus (HIV) infection risk associated with injecting. Heroin itself is an inactive prodrug with two active metabolites, one of which is morphine, and both of which are active at the mu opioid receptor. After intravenous (IV) injection, users describe an intense rush within 1 to 2 minutes, followed by a period of euphoric sedation lasting about 1 hour. In dependent users, withdrawal symptoms can begin within 4 to 6 hours (Ries et al., 2009).

Intoxication and Withdrawal

Signs and symptoms of intoxication and withdrawal and treatments are based on drug class. Generally, withdrawal symptoms are characterized by the opposite of intoxication, with their intensity inversely proportional to the duration of action of the drug and proportional to chronicity of use. Symptom onset is proportional to the half-life of the drug.

Treatment of intoxication for most substances is supportive and symptomatic and typically occurs in inpatient settings. Receptor antagonists are available for both opiate and benzodiazepine intoxication, with use reserved primarily for the overdose state. Treatment of withdrawal usually follows one of two principles: substituting a longer-acting less reinforcing equivalent, then tapering, or symptom control. Withdrawal treatment may occur in the inpatient or outpatient setting depending on the severity of the withdrawal anticipated, the underlying mental and physical health issues of the patient, and level of support available to the patient in the outpatient setting.

Opiates

Intoxication with opiates causes miotic pupils, euphoria, altered level of consciousness, constipation, and respiratory depression. Treatment of opiate overdose involves providing respiratory support and administering naloxone, a pure opiate antagonist. Naloxone is typically administered IV but may also be administered SC, intramuscularly (IM), via endotracheal tube, or intranasally until IV access is established (Barton et al., 2005). The initial dose is typically 0.4 to 0.8 mg, with a 2-minute onset of action when given IV. Doses are repeated and escalated as needed to reverse the overdose. After reversal, patients need to be monitored for 1 to 3 hours for repeated dosing, and sometimes longer if longer-acting opiates such as methadone have been used in the overdose. Naloxone treatment can initiate a rapid and intense withdrawal syndrome (Ries et al., 2009).

Opiate withdrawal is rarely fatal but is extremely uncomfortable and typically is accompanied by strong cravings. Withdrawal signs and symptoms include vomiting, diarrhea, body aches, rhinorrhea, thermoderegulation, insomnia, anxiety, dysphoria, gooseflesh, yawning, and pupil dilation. Treatment can be symptomatic, as with the alpha-2-adrenergic agonist clonidine, or can involve receptor agonist or antagonist activity. Methadone can be used with short- or long-taper protocols. Buprenorphine, a partial opiate agonist can similarly be used. The antagonist, naltrexone in combination with clonidine has been used effectively in both inpatient and outpatient settings (Ries et al., 2009).

Sedative-Hypnotics (including Benzodiazepines)

Intoxication with the sedative-hypnotic drug class causes slurred speech, ataxia, respiratory depression, stupor, coma, and death (mostly with mixed overdose). Treatment of overdose involves providing respiratory support and gastrointestinal (GI) tract evacuation. Activated charcoal is particularly helpful for barbiturate overdose, as is urine alkalization for phenobarbital overdose. Flumazenil, a benzodiazepine receptor antagonist, can be used in benzodiazepine overdose, but with caution because it can dramatically increase the risk of seizures and cardiac arrhythmias, especially in mixed overdoses and in patients physiologically dependent on benzodiazepines (Ries et al., 2009).

Withdrawal signs and symptoms from sedative-hypnotics include tachycardia, hypertension, fever, agitation, anxiety, hallucinations, insomnia, irritability, nightmares, sensory disturbances, tremor, tinnitus, anorexia, diarrhea, nausea, seizures, delirium, and death. Most sedative-hypnotic withdrawal is managed by either simple, slow, fixed-dose taper or substitution and taper. A *simple taper* involves decreasing the dose by no more than 10% every 1 to 2 weeks until the starting dose has been 75% decreased, then by 5% every 2 to 4 weeks for the last 25% until the taper is completed. *Substitution and taper* involves substituting a long-acting benzodiazepine (e.g., clonazepam) or phenobarbital for a shorter-acting drug and tapering as above. Conversion tables are available to calculate an approximate equivalent dose, and the dose is titrated over several days to a week, to achieve good relief of withdrawal symptoms before tapering is begun of the substitute, as with the simple taper method. Other adjunctive medications that have shown positive effects include carbamazepine, sodium valproate, propranolol, and trazodone. Because many patients dependent on benzodiazepines in particular have underlying anxiety and other psychiatric comorbidities, and because withdrawal protocols are typically prolonged, anticipation and treatment of reemergence of these symptoms must be anticipated, or relapse is more likely (Ries et al., 2009).

Other Drugs

Table 51-6 lists the signs and symptoms of intoxication and withdrawal of other drugs. There are no specific antidotes or reversal agents for the remaining drug classes. Care of the overdose patient is largely supportive and aimed at treating the medical effects of the particular overdose, such as treatment of myocardial ischemia resulting from cocaine overdose. Currently, no FDA-approved medications are available for stimulant (including cocaine and methamphetamine), marijuana, hallucinogen (e.g., LSD, PCP), or club drug (e.g., MDMA) withdrawal. Behavioral therapies are the mainstay of treatment.

KEY TREATMENT

Naloxone at 0.4 to 0.8 mg initial dose and repeated as needed is effective for opiate-intoxicated patients with inadequate spontaneous ventilation (Ries et al., 2009) (SOR: A).

Sedative-hypnotic withdrawal is managed by simple taper or substitution to phenobarbital or longer-acting benzodiazepine and taper. (SOR: C).

Medical Management (beyond Withdrawal)

Medical management of SUD after the acute withdrawal period for opiate dependence has a relatively long history, with various opioids being tried as maintenance therapies from the late 1800s until passage of the Harrison Act of 1914, which effectively outlawed prescribing opiates for treating addiction for nearly half a century. Currently, three pharmologic interventions predominate: methadone, buprenorphine, and naltrexone. Of these three therapies, methadone is the most studied and the standard of care for patients with chronic relapsing opiate dependence. However, methadone

Table 51-6 Signs and Symptoms of Intoxication and Withdrawal

Drug	Intoxication	Withdrawal
Stimulants, including cocaine	Pupil dilation, headache, hyperventilation, dyspnea, cough, chest pain, wheezing, hemoptysis, bronchospasm, pulmonary edema, psychosis, tremor, hyperreflexia, tics, myoclonus, seizures, cerebral hemorrhage or infarct, cerebral edema, nausea, vomiting, bowel infarction or perforation, diuresis, myoglobinuria, acute renal failure, fever, malignant hyperthermia, rhabdomyolysis	Depression, anxiety, fatigue, anhedonia, increased appetite, hypersomnolence, increased dreaming, increased drug craving
Marijuana	Pupil constriction, conjunctival injection, headache, tachypnea, tachycardia, orthostatic hypotension, tremor, ataxia, increased appetite, urinary retention	Irritability, insomnia, anxiety, depression, restlessness, anorexia, vivid dreams, chills, nausea, diaphoresis
PCP	Horizontal nystagmus, increased tear and saliva production, lost corneal reflex, eyes open coma, pupil dilation, absent laryngeal/pharyngeal reflexes, diaphoresis, flushing, apnea, pulmonary edema, tachypnea, tachycardia, hypertension, high output cardiac failure, stupor, hyperreflexia, nausea, vomiting, acute renal failure, malignant hyperthermia, rhabdomyolysis	Depression, anxiety, irritability, hypersomnolence, diaphoresis, tremor, dysphoria, craving
MDMA	Bruxism, headache, dye mouth, diaphoresis, flushing, tachycardia, hypertension, tremor, increased muscle tone, nausea, anorexia, acute renal failure, malignant hyperthermia, rhabdomyolysis	Depression, anxiety, fatigue, difficulty concentrating, muscle pain
LSD	Pupil dilation, piloerection, diaphoresis, hypertension, tachycardia, hyperreflexia, tremors, seizures, nausea, vomiting, urinary retention, thermodysregulation	Fatigue, irritability, anhedonia

is also the most stigmatized and has many regulatory barriers to access.

Naltrexone works as a competitive opiate receptor antagonist to block the affects of opiate agonists. It has been shown to be most useful in patients with a strong external motivator for treatment adherence, such as professionals with ongoing licensing board monitoring. In more generalized patient populations, retention in treatment with naltrexone is only 20% to 30% at 6 months. The usual dose of naltrexone is 50 mg daily or 350 mg weekly divided into three doses (100, 100, 150 mg). A reduced starting dose of 25 mg on day 1 is used to minimize GI side effects such as nausea and vomiting, which occur in 10% of patients. Liver enzymes are monitored because liver toxicity is a rare but more serious side effect, shown to resolve after stopping naltrexone (Reis et al., 2009). A monthly depot injectable form of naltrexone was approved by the U.S. Food and Drug Administration (FDA) for treating opiate-dependent patients in 2010. Studies of longer-acting naltrexone implants are ongoing for FDA approval.

Methadone is a long-acting opiate receptor agonist with strong affinity for its receptor and can be dosed once daily for most opiate-dependent patients. Currently, methadone may be used for treating opiate dependence in hospitalized patients (i.e., for withdrawal) or in licensed methadone treatment facilities. Take-home doses are regulated and depend on length of time in treatment and treatment response, including good attendance, adherence to program rules, lack of diverting behaviors, and abstinence, as verified by drug test results. Generally one take-home dose a week is allowed from the outset (many programs are closed on Sundays). Progression to increased take-home doses is determined by state and federal regulations, with the more restrictive statute taking precedent. For family physicians with patients in methadone maintenance, knowing a patient's take-home schedule can provide insight into how well they are doing in treatment. Recent increases in overdose deaths involving methadone have been explored and are more likely caused by an increase in misuse or diversion of methadone prescribed to treat chronic pain, and less likely from an increase in opiate agonist treatment facility diversion (CSAT, 2004).

Buprenorphine is a partial opiate agonist that causes a 50% activation of the opiate receptors. This is typically enough to alleviate withdrawal symptoms and prolonged abstinence symptoms, but not enough to induce euphoria for patients with opiate dependence. It binds more tightly than any of the opiate agonists and has a long half-life, making it a good candidate for blockade therapy. Buprenorphine is given as a sublingual tablet or film, most often compounded with naloxone (Suboxone), to discourage intravenous use, since the naloxone, a potent opiate antagonist, has little effect unless injected. Buprenorphine comes in 2-mg and 8-mg strengths. Unlike methadone, the Drug Abuse Treatment Act of 2000 allows physicians to prescribe buprenorphine outside a methadone treatment facility, with the goal of bringing the treatment of opiate dependence into primary care, greatly expanding treatment availability. To prescribe buprenorphine for opiate dependence, a physician needs to take an 8-hour course, now available online, and submit their application for an additional "X" number from the U.S Drug Enforcement Administration (DEA). Physicians also need to have a way to refer or provide behavioral health-based addiction treatment for their patients. The number of patients is proscribed by

statute to 30 the first year and up to 100 patients at any given time past the first year if an additional waiver is submitted. Typical doses of buprenorphine range from 8 to 16 mg daily.

Many pharmacologic interventions have been studied for stimulant dependence, but to date, none has been FDA approved. Several anticonvulsants, baclofen, disulfiram, and antidepressants have shown promise in select patient populations, have shown little effect, or are still in clinical trials. Research in treating stimulant dependence also includes maintenance therapy, with sustained-released preparations of slow-onset stimulants such as modafinil (Ries et al., 2009). Vaccine therapy also currently being studied, involves stimulating the patient's immune system to produce antibodies; for example, when bound to cocaine, antibodies prevent the drug from crossing the blood-brain barrier (Martell et al., 2009).

There is even less evidence for use of medications in the long-term management of other substances of abuse, such as hallucinogens, marijuana, and club drugs. Currently, behavioral therapies are the mainstay of treatment (Ries et al., 2009).

KEY TREATMENT

Methadone maintenance is the most studied and effective medical treatment for opiate dependence (National Consensus, 1998) (SOR: A).

Buprenorphine maintenance therapy, an alternative to methadone for treating opiate dependence, can be prescribed by appropriately trained and certified primary care physicians, but is somewhat less effective than methadone prescribed at adequate doses (Mattick et al., 2008) (SOR: A).

Oral naltrexone is typically reserved for use in patients with strong external motivators for treatment adherence, such as licensed professionals, because treatment retention is otherwise poor, and relapse is common (Minozzi et al., 2006) (SOR: B).

Behavioral Therapies for Substance Use Disorders

Behavioral therapies are a mainstay of SUD treatment. Common modalities include cognitive-behavioral therapy, contingency management, motivational enhancement therapy (MET), "therapeutic communities," and 12-step facilitation. Except for MET, these have not been adapted for use by family medicine physicians in routine office practice, but are usually available as community-based referrals.

Cognitive-Behavioral Therapy

Cognitive-behavioral therapy (CBT) is based on the assumption that the learning processes used by patients to initiate and continue their drug use behaviors can also be used to reduce or stop their drug use. CBT has been extensively studied, especially with cocaine users, and has shown good results. CBT is primarily used in the outpatient setting, usually with weekly individual sessions over several months. Sessions focus on patients learning to recognize the situations in which they are most likely to use drugs, learning to avoid those situations, and learning to cope with their problems without resorting to drug use. These lessons are accomplished through functional analysis and skills training. In functional analysis, each episode of drug use is analyzed in terms of what the patient was feeling, thinking, or doing before and after the use. This helps identify high-risk situations or coping issues. Skills training involves working on ways to avoid these situations and learn new (or reconnect with past) coping mechanisms for handling high-risk situations and other life stressors without using drugs (Carroll, 1998).

Contingency Management

Contingency management (CM) is based on operant conditioning and involves a structured and consistently administered system of consequences that are used to reinforce behaviors consistent with treatment goals. Basic principles include close temporal proximity of consequence to targeted behavior, performance of targeted behavior easy to verify and verified often, positive consequence given and escalated for continuous positive behavior change, and positive consequence removed when targeted behavior not performed. CM has been shown to be more effective when a single targeted behavior is addressed at a time and when resumption of continuous positive change is reinforced after a brief slip. Barriers include funding sources to cover the cost of rewards and determining appropriate length of treatment for this method. Advantages of CM include the breadth of behavioral changes that can be targeted and its demonstrated success in patients with severe and complex substance use disorders (Petry et al., 2001).

Motivational Enhancement Therapy

Motivational enhancement therapy (MET) engages patients in increasing their internal motivations for making healthy changes in their drug use, building on a patient's strengths and resources in making prior behavioral changes. Goals are set by the patient, although the counselor may advise specific goals when appropriate. This approach is nonconfrontational. The counselor seeks to have the patient talk about the pros and cons of the substance use, reflecting and summarizing as an active listener in a way that highlights discrepancies between the patient's life goals or beliefs and current drug use behaviors. These discrepancies are then used to increase the patient's internal desire for change or discomfort with the status quo. A patient's stage of readiness to change, whether precontemplative, contemplative, preparation, action, maintenance, or relapse, is also determined at each session. In addition, a patient's self-efficacy for change is assessed, and the patient is guided to talk about prior successful behavioral changes, and any optimism for change is reflected and highlighted (Prochaska et al., 1992). MET has been used in both inpatient and outpatient settings, from one session (brief intervention) to several months of weekly sessions.

Therapeutic Communities

Therapeutic communities (TCs) are traditionally residential facilities in which the community structure and function are agents of change, and 12-step–based self-help programs guide individual recovery. Average lengths of stay are about 12 months (6-24 months). Community members progress through varying roles and responsibilities in their recovery and collectively ensure day-to-day functioning of the community. Days are highly structured and involve group and individual sessions, as well as time for community and personal chores and self-development, such as exercise, vocational time, and educational time. TCs have been successfully adapted to serve special needs populations, such as adolescents, patients with concomitant mental health disorders, patients with HIV infection, and women with children. Successful completion of a TC program has been shown to lead to a significant decrease in SUD behaviors. Day treatment or nonresidential TCs are also available and may be more cost-effective for patients with less severe social problems to address (NIDA, 2002).

Twelve-Step Facilitation

Twelve-step facilitation (TSF) is a modality that seeks to increase the SUD patient's attendance and active involvement in 12-step self-help groups such as Cocaine Anonymous (CA) and Narcotics Anonymous (NA). TSF is used in residential treatment programs as well as outpatient settings. Sessions are highly structured, often workbook guided, and cast the counselor in the role of facilitator of change, with patient involvement the true agent of change. The underlying 12-step principles are the same: the patient's lack of control must be accepted, willpower is insufficient to stop use, and abstinence is desired. Research has shown that the more 12-step self-help group involvement, both in terms of number of meetings attended and, more robustly, the degree of active participation, the greater the success of achieving abstinence and recovery (McIntosh, 2009).

Formal TSF counseling is outside the scope of most family medicine practices. However, physicians making a 12-step self-help group referral can increase the likelihood the patient will engage by (1) contracting with the patient to attend a certain number of meetings weekly, (2) having the patient call the local CA or NA hotline during the visit to set up his or her first meeting, and (3) encouraging attendance at several different meetings to ensure a "good fit." Checking in with patients previously referred or in long-term recovery on meeting attendance and 12-step involvement, such as sponsorship and step work, is supportive of recovery and easily integrated into the primary care visit.

> **KEY TREATMENT**
>
> Cognitive-behavioral therapy and contingency management decrease cocaine use and increase treatment retention (Knapp et al., 2007) (SOR: B).
> Twelve-step involvement positively correlates with achieving abstinence and recovery (McIntosh, 2009) (SOR: C).

Primary Care of SUD Patients

The primary care of SUD patients must take into account the systemic effects of the drug(s) ingested, route of administration, methods of drug procurement, illicit drug–prescription drug interactions, and typically, higher rates of nonadherence to follow-up and prescribed regimens (Ries et al., 2009). Infectious diseases (e.g., HIV, hepatitis B and C, tuberculosis) and sexually transmitted infections (e.g., gonorrhea, chlamydia, herpes, syphilis, human papillomavirus) are more common in SUD patients than in the general population, and patients should be screened routinely. Other infections common in IV drug users include skin abscesses, cellulitis, infectious endocarditis, and pneumonia.

Cocaine and other stimulants can cause myocardial infarction and stroke, raise blood pressure, and make essential hypertension resistant to treatment. Crack cocaine use, inhaled methamphetamines, and marijuana can lead to lung injury, chronic obstructive pulmonary disease, fibrosis, and pulmonary hypertension. Seizures can stem from stimulant use, benzodiazepine withdrawal, "ecstasy" and other "club drug" intoxication (Ries et al., 2009).

Treatment for asthma, hypertension, chronic pain, and diabetes is complicated by the concomitant SUD. Patient adherence to treatment regimens is often compromised by the SUD, with "getting high" and minimizing withdrawal symptoms becoming the focus of their activities. Regular and nutritious meals may be difficult to access or may not be a priority for SUD patients, along with hygienic activities. Sleep disorders are common and can exacerbate health problems and their management. SUD patients' ability to store their medications safely and securely can be compromised by homelessness, diversion, and unsafe living environment.

Ongoing SUDs can mask symptoms, leading to late presentation of diseases such as cancer. This masking often is compounded by lack of access or utilization of primary care and preventive services by SUD patients.

Special Populations

Adolescents

In 2008, approximately 9.3% of youths age 12 to 17 were current users of illicit drugs. This continued a trend of decreased illicit substance use among adolescents. Compared with 2002 data, the prevalence of illicit drug use had decreased for several drugs, including marijuana (8.2% to 6.7%), nonmedical use of prescription drugs (4.0% to 2.9%), cocaine (0.6% to 0.4%), and methamphetamine (0.3% to 0.1%). The use of hallucinogens such as ecstasy, LSD, and PCP had slightly increased (0.7 % to 1.0 %). Concern about performance-enhancing agents and steroid use among high school and junior high school students has led to surveillance of steroid use among teenagers since 1989. Compared to previous years, overall use of anabolic steroids had decreased. Although predominantly found among young males, the proportion of anabolic steroid use attributable to young females had increased. Among teenagers, African Americans had significantly lower rates of illicit drugs compared to Caucasians. Hispanics in the 12th grade reported the highest rates of some use of crack, heroin, and crystal methamphetamine.

Most youths reported that drugs are readily available. For example, approximately 49% of teenagers 12 to 17 years old reported that it would be "fairly easy" to obtain marijuana, 22.1% reported they could obtain cocaine, and 13.8%

reported that they could obtain LSD. In 2008, 13.7 % of adolescents reported that they had been approached by someone selling drugs within the past month.

Because peer pressure is a significant factor for adolescents, their perceptions of risk associated with substance abuse and peer disapproval have also been surveyed. A majority of teenagers have strongly disapproved or somewhat disapproved of illicit drug use by their peers. However, the perceived risk of using marijuana, cocaine, hallucinogens, and other drugs has been lower in recent years. Teenagers may possess less knowledge about adverse drug effects than their predecessors and may display some "generational forgetting" (Johnston et al., 2009).

Racial and Ethnic Minorities

In 2008 the rate of current illicit drug use varied significantly among people of seven different major racial categories. Current drug use was highest among people who reported having two or more races (14.1%). An estimated 10.1% of blacks, 9.5% of American Indians or Alaska Natives, 8.2% of whites, 7.3% of Native Hawaiians or other Pacific Islanders, 6.3% of Hispanics, and 3.6% of Asians were current illicit drug users in 2008.

Pregnant Women

Approximately 5.1% of pregnant women age 15 to 44 were current users of illicit substances in 2008. Compared with nonpregnant women, the rate of drug use is significantly lower for all age groups, with the exception of adolescent women 15 to 17 years old. The rate of illicit substance use was higher among pregnant adolescents age 15 to 17 compared to same-age nonpregnant adolescents (21.6% vs. 12.9%). Use of cocaine, heroin, methamphetamine, marijuana, MDMA, inhalants, and nicotine during pregnancy has been associated with adverse outcomes such as intrauterine growth retardation, delayed cognitive development, and difficulty with attention and learning. Effects vary by substance ingested, quantity and frequency of ingested drug or drugs, and stage of fetal development when ingestion occurs. Currently, methadone maintenance is the treatment of choice for opiate dependency during pregnancy, although buprenorphine has been used when methadone is not available. Newborns are monitored for signs of withdrawal and treated if symptoms are noted.

Mental Health and Substance Abuse

The prevalence of illicit substance abuse or dependence among patients with serious mental illness was 25.2%, or an estimated 2.5 million people, in 2008. Similarly, adults age 18 and older with an episode of major depression within the last year had higher rates of illicit drug use than adults without a major depressive episode (27.2% vs. 13.0%). Having a major depressive episode within the past year was also associated with higher prevalence of dependence on illicit drugs.

References

The complete reference list is available online at www.expertconsult.com.

Web Resources

https://nsduhweb.rti.org/
National Survey on Drug Use and Health website has current and extensive database.

www.nida.nih.gov/
National Institute on Drug Abuse website has valuable resources for physicians and families.

www.jointogether.org/
Addiction medicine news and advocacy/research.

www.asam.org/
American Society of Addiction Medicine website with link to online buprenorphine training.

http://dasis3.samhsa.gov/
Substance Abuse and Mental Health Services Administration treatment locator resource.

www.cdaweb.org/
12-Step–based self-help organization.

http://nar-anon.org/Nar-Anon/Nar-Anon_Home.html
12-Step–based resource for families.

www.bu.edu/aodhealth/index.html
Boston University website offering periodic summaries of the latest SUD research findings.

Index

Page numbers followed by f indicate figures; b, boxes; t, tables.